Oh's
INTENSIVE CARE
MANUAL

Commissioning Editor: *Paul Fam*
Project Development Manager: *Shuet-Kei Cheung*
Project Manager: *Jess Thompson*
Illustration Manager: *Mick Ruddy*
Designer: *Andy Chapman*
Illustratons: *Marion Tasker*

Oh's
INTENSIVE CARE MANUAL

FIFTH EDITION

Edited by

Professor Andrew D Bersten MB BS MD FANZCA FJFICM
Department of Critical Care Medicine, Flinders Medical Centre and School of Medicine,
Flinders University, Adelaide, Australia

Dr Neil Soni MB ChB FANZCA FRCA MD FJFICM
Consultant in Intensive Care and Anaesthesia; Director and Lead Clinician, Intensive Care
Unit, Magill Department of Anaesthesia, Intensive Care and Pain Management
Hon. Senior Lecturer; Imperial College Medical School, Chelsea and Westminster Hospital,
London, United Kingdom

Consulting editor

Professor Teik E Oh MB BS MD FRCP FRCPE FRACP FRCA FANZCA
Hon FAC RCSI FJFICM FHKAM
Professor of Anaesthesia, Department of Anaesthesia and Pain Medicine, Royal Perth
Hospital, Australia

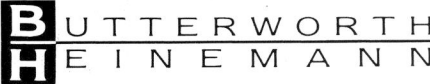

Edinburgh • London • New York • Oxford • Philadelphia • St Louis • Sydney • Toronto • 2003

BUTTERWORTH-HEINEMANN
An imprint of Elsevier Limited

© First published 1979
© Reprinted 1981
© Second edition 1985
© Reprinted 1986, 1988
© Third edition 1990
© Reprinted 1991
© Fourth edition 1997
© Reprinted 1998
© Fifth edition 2003

ISBN 0 7506 5184 9

British Library Cataloguing in Publication Data
A catalogue record for this book is available from the British Library

Library of Congress Cataloging in Publication Data
A catalog record for this book is available from the Library of Congress

Notice
Medical knowledge is constantly changing. Standard safety precautions must be followed, but as new research and clinical experience broaden our knowledge, changes in treatment and drug therapy may become necessary or appropriate. Readers are advised to check the most current product information provided by the manufacturer of each drug to be admin-istered to verify the recommended dose, the method and duration of administration, and contraindications. It is the responsibility of the practitioner, relying on experience and knowledge of the patient, to determine dosages and the best treatment for each individual patient. Neither the Publisher nor the editors assumes any liability for any injury and/or damage to persons or property arising from this publication.
The Publisher

Printed in China

The
publisher's
policy is to use
**paper manufactured
from sustainable forests**

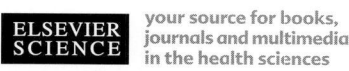

your source for books,
journals and multimedia
in the health sciences
www.elsevierhealth.com

Contents

Contributors

Rinaldo Bellomo MB BS MD
FRACP FJFICM FCCP
Director of Intensive Care Research
Dept of Intensive Care
Austin Repatriation Medical Centre
Victoria
Australia

Andrew D Bersten MB BS MD
FANZCA FJFICM
Dept of Critical Care Medicine
Flinders Medical Centre and School of
Medicine
Flinders University
Adelaide
Australia

David Bihari FRCP FRACP FJFICM
Senior Staff Specialist
Dept of Critical Care Medicine
Prince of Wales Hospital
Randwick
NSW
Australia

Stephen J Brett MD, FRCA
Consultant in Intensive Care Medicine
Dept of Anaesthesia & Intensive Care
Hammersmith Hospital
London
UK

Geoffrey M Clarke AM MBBS DA
FFARCS FANZCA FJFICM
Head of Intensive Care Unit
Intensive Care Unit
Royal Perth Hospital
Perth WA
Australia

Frances Colreavy MBBch FFARCSI
FJFICM
Mayo Clinic
Rochester
Minnesota
USA

David J Cooper BMBS MD FRACP
FANZCA FJFICM
Associate professor
Head Trauma ICU
Dept Intensive Care
Alfred Hospital
Prahran
Victoria
Australia

Simon Cottam MB ChB FRCA
Consultant in Anaesthetics and Intensive
Care
Department of Anaesthetics
Kings College Hospital
London
UK

Lester A H Critchley MD
FFARCSI FHKAM
Associate Professor in Anaesthesia and
Intensive Care
Dept Anaesthesia and ICU
Chinese Univesity of Hong Kong
Prince of Wales Hospital
Shatin
Hong Kong

Andrew R Davies MBBS FRACP
FJFICM
Intensive Care Physician
ICU
The Alfred Hospital
Melbourne
Victoria
Australia

Karl Donovan MB FRACP FRCPI
FJFICM
Specialist Intensive Care
Intensive Care Unit
Royal Perth Hospital
Perth
WA
Australia

Graeme Duke MBBS FJFICM
FANZCA
Critical Care Director
Critical Care Dept
The Northern Hospital
Epping
Australia

Alan W Duncan MBBS FRCA
FANZCA FFICANZCA FJFICM
Director
Paediatric Intensive Care
Princess Margaret Hospital for Children
Perth
WA
Australia

Cyrus Edibam MBBS FANZCA
FJFICM
Staff Specialist
Department of Intensive Care
Royal Perth Hospital
Perth
WA
Australia

Evan Everest BSc MB ChB FRACP
Senior Consultant Critical Care Unit
Flinders Medical Centre
South Australia
Australia

Malcolm M Fisher MBChB
FANZCA FRCA FJFICM MD
Clinical Professor
University of Sydney
Intensive Therapy Unit
Royal North Shore Hospital
NSW
Australia

David Fraenkel BM, BS, FRACP
Senior Staff Intensivist
Dept of Intensive Care Medicine
Royal Brisbane Hospital
Herston
Queensland
Australia

Martyn A H French MB CRB MD
FRCPath FRCP FRACP
Consultant Clinical Immunologist and
Clinical Associate Professor in Pathology
Dept of Clinical Immunology
Royal Perth Hospital
Perth
Australia

Tony Gin MB ChB BSc DipHSM
FRCA FANZCA MD
Professor & Chairman
Dept of Anaesthesia & Intensive Care
Chinese University of Hong Kong
Shatin
NT
Hong Kong

C D Gomersall MB BS MRCP(UK)
FRCA FFICANZAC EDIC
Assistant Professor
Dept of Anaesthesia & Intensive Care
The Chinese University of Hong Kong
Shatin
Hong Kong

Munita Grover BSc(Hons) MBBS
FRCA
Anaesthetic Research Fellow
Chelsea & Westminster Hospital
Fulham Road
London
UK

Geoff Gutteridge MB BS FANZCA
FJFICM
Director of Intensive Care
Austin Repatriation Medical Centre
Studley Rd
Heidelberg
Australia

Felicity Hawker MBBS FJFICM
Director Intensive Care Unit
Intensive Care Unit
Cabrini Hospital
Malvern
Victoria
Australia

Michelle Hayes MD FRCA
Consultant in Anaesthesia and Intensive
Care
Chelsea and Westminster Hospital
London
UK

Robert D Henning FRCA FJFICM
DCH
Staff Specialist
Intensive Care Unit
Royal Childrens Hospital
Parkville
Victoria
Australia

Bernard E F Hockings MB BS MD
FRACP
Cardiologist and Clinical Associate
Professor of Medicine
University of Western Australia
Perth
Australia

Andrew Holt MBBS FFARACS
Critical Care Specialist
Dept Critical Care Medicine
Flinders Medical Centre
Bedford Park
South Australia

Gillian C Hood MB ChB FRACP (Int
Care) FJFICM
Specialist Intensive
Dept Critical Care Medicine
Auckland Hospital
Auckland
New Zealand

Anwar Hussein DPhil FRCA
St Helier Hospital
Carshalton
Surrey
UK

James P Isbister MB BS BSc(Med)
FRACP FRCPA
Clinical Professor of Medicine
Royal North Shore Hospital
St Leonards
NSW
Australia

Mandy Oade Jones Ph.D MSc
GRAD DIP DHYS MCSP
Research fellow
Sleep Ventilation Unit
Royal Brompton and Harefield NHS
Trust
Sydney Street
London
UK

Gavin Joynt MB BCH FFA(SA) FHKA
FHKCA (IC) FJFICM FCCP
Associate Professor
Dept of Anaesthesia & Intensive Care
Price of Wales Hospital
Shatin
Hong Kong

James A Judson MB ChB FFARACS
FANZCA FFICANZCA FJFICM
Specialist Intensivist
Dept of Critical Care Medicine
Auckland Hospital
Auckland
New Zealand

Richard T Keays MB BS MD FRCP
FRCA
Consultant Anaesthesia and Intensive
Care
Chelsea & Westminster Hospital
London
UK

Angus Kennedy MB BS MRCP MD
Consultant Neurologist
Chelsea and Westminster Hospital
London
UK

Geoffrey J Knight MB BS FRACP
FJFICM
Paediatric Intensive Care Physician
Paediatric Intensive Care Unit
Princess Margaret Hospital for Children
Perth WA
Australia

Richard Priestley Lee MBBS
FNAZCA FJFICM
Senior Specialist
ICU
Royal North Shore Hospital
St Leonards
NSW
Australia

Richard Leonard
Department of Anaesthesia
St Mary's Hospital
London
UK

John Leong OBE FRCS FRCS(Edin)
FRACS JP
Department of Orthopaedic Surgery
The University of Hong Kong
Pokfulam
Hong Kong

Jeffrey Lipman MBBch DA FCA FFA
(Crit care) FFICANZCA
Director Intensive Care
Dept of Intensive Care Medicine
Royal Brisbane Hospital
Herston
Queensland
Australia

David Mackie MD
Specialist Anaesthesiologist/Intensivist
Red Cross Hospital
Vondellaan 13
Beverwijk
The Netherlands

Neil T Matthews
Medical Head of Unit
Paediatric Intensive Care Unit
Women's and Children's Hospital
South Australia

Colin J McArthur
Clinical Director
Dept of Critical Care Medicine
Auckland Hospital
Auckland
New Zealand

Justin McKinlay
Intensive Care Unit
Prince of Wales Hospital
Randwick
NSW
Australia

Angela McLuckie FRCA, FJFICM
Consultant Intensivist
Dept of Intensive Care
Guys and St Thomas Hospital Trust
London
UK

Cliff Morgan BM FRCA
Consultant in Critical Care and
Anaesthesia
Department of Anaesthesia
Royal Brompton Hospital
London
UK

Thomas John Morgan MBBS,
FJFICM
Deputy Director
Adult Intensive Care
Mater Misericordiae Health Services
Raymond Terrace
South Brisbane
Queensland
Australia

Peter Thomas Morley MBBS
FANZCA FJFICM FRACP
Senior Specialist
Dept Intensive Care
Royal Melbourne Hospital
Victoria
Australia

Blair Munford
NRMA Careflight
Westmead
NSW
Australia

John A Myburgh MBBCh DA(SA)
FANZCA FJFICM
Director of Research and Education
Intensive Care Unit
St George Hospital
Sydney
NSW
Australia

Michael Mythen MD FRCA
Portex Professor of Anaesthesia and
Critical Care
The Portex Unit
Institute of Child Heath
London
UK

Matthew T Naughton MBBS MD
FRACP
Associate Professor of Medicine
Department of Respiratory Medicine
Alfred Hospital
Melbourne
Victoria
Australia

W D Ngan Kee BHB MBChB MD
FANZCA FHKLA FHKAM
Associate Professor
Dept of Anaesthesia & Intensive Care
Chinese University of Hong Kong
Prince of Wales Hospital
Shatin
Hong Kong

Teik E Oh MB BS MD FRCP FRCPE
FRACP FRCA FANZCA Hon FAC RCSI
FJFICM FHKAM
Professor of Anaesthesia Research
Dept of Anaesthesia and Pain Medicine
Royal Perth Hospital
Australia

Helen Opdam MBBS FRACP
FJFICM
Staff Specialist
Dept Intensive Care
Austin & Repatriation Medical Centre
Intensive Care Unit
Heidelberg
Victoria
Australia

Simon P G Padley FRCP FRCR
Consultant Radiologist and Honorary
Senior Lecturer
Dept of Radiology
Chelsea & Westminster Hospital
London

Mark Palazzo MB FRCA FRCP MD
Director of Critical Care
Charing Cross Hospital
Fulham Palace Rd
London
UK

Michael E Pelly MSc MBBS FRCP
MRCP DIM HRCP
Consultant Physician
Chelsea & Westminster Hospital
London
UK

Didier Pittet MD MS
Professor of Medicine
Infection Control Programme
Dept of Internal Medicine
Geneva University Hospitals
Switzerland

Brad Power MBBS FRACP FJFICM
Intensive Care Specialist
Dept of Intensive Care
Sir Charles Gairdner Hospital
Perth
Australia

R Raper MB BS BA MD FRACP
FJFICM
Intensive Care Specialist
Intensive Therapy Unit
Royal North Shore Hospital
St Leonards
Australia

Bernard Riley MBE BSc MBBS
FRCA
Consultant in Adult Critical Care
Queen's Medical Centre
University Hospital
Nottingham
UK

Janice Risley BSc MSc
Senior Physiotherapist
West Dorset General Hospitals
Dorset County Hospitals
Physiotherapy Department
Dorchester
Dorset
UK

John E Sanderson MD FRCP
FACC
Professor of Medicine & Therapeutics
Head, Division of Cardiology
Dept of Medicine and Therapeutics
The Chinese University of Hong Kong
Prince of Wales Hospital
Shatin
Hong Kong

Hugo Sax MD
Attending Physician
Infection Control Programme
Dept of Internal Medicine
Geneva University Hospitals
Switzerland

Frank Shann MBBS MD FRACP
FJFICM
Professor of Critical Care Medicine
Intensive Care Unit
Royal Children's Hospital
Parkville
VIC
Australia

Timothy G Short MB ChB MD
FANZCA
Specialist Anaesthetist
Auckland Hospital
Department of Anaesthesia
Auckland
New Zealand

Ramachandran Sivakumar MD
MRCP
Specialist Registrar
Chelsea and Westminster Hospital
London
UK

Elizabeth Sizer MBBS FRCA
Senior Trainee in Intensive Care of
Anaesthetics
Institute of Liver Studies
Kings College Hospital
London
UK

George Skowronski MBBS(Hons)
FRCP FRACP FJFICM
Associate Professor Critical Care
University of New South Wales
St George Hospital
Kogarah
NSW
Australia

Anthony J Slater BMed SCMB BS
FRACP FJFICM
Senior Staff Specialist
Dept of Paediatric Critical Care
Medicine
North Adelaide
South Australia

Neil Soni MB ChB FRCA FANZCA
MD FJFICM
Consultant in Anaesthesia and Intensive
Care
Chelsea and Westminster Hospital
London
UK

Stephen J Streat BSc MB ChB
FRACP
Specialist Intensivist
Department of Critical Care Medicine
Auckland Hospital
Auckland
New Zealand

Joseph J Y Sung MD PhD FRCP
FRCPE FRACP FACP
Professor of Medicine
Dept of Medicine and Therapeutics
Prince of Wales Hospital
Shatin
Hong Kong

Ian K S Tan MBBS MRCP(UK)
FANZCA FJFICM HKCA HKCA(IC)
Director
Intensive Care Unit
Pamela Youde Eastern Hospital
Hong Kong

Christopher Theaker RGN
Clinical Research Fellow
Intensive Care
Chelsea and Westminster Hospital
London
UK

James Tibballs MD BS B.Med.Sc
(Hons) MEd MBA FANZCA FJFICM
FACTM
Associate Professor
Intensive Care Unit
Royal Children's Hospital
Parkville
Melbourne
Australia

David Treacher MB BS BA FRCP
Consultant Physician in Intensive Care
Medicine
Dept of Intensive Care
St Thomas' Hospital
London

David V Tuxen MBBS MD FRACP
Dip DHM FJFICM
Director of Intensive Care and
Hyperbaric Medicine
Intensive Care Unit
Alfred Hospital
Melbourne
Victoria
Australia

Peter V van Heerden MBBCh
MMed(Anaes) PhD DA(SA) FFARCSI
FJFICM FANZCA
Director of Intensive Care
Sir Charles Gairdner Hospital
Perth
WA
Australia

Alnis E Vedig
Head of Department of Critical Care
Medicine
Flinders Medical Centre
South Australia
Australia

Bala Venkatesh MBBS
MD(Gen. Med) FFARCSI FRCA EDICM
MD(UK) FJFICM
Associate Professor
Dept of Intensive Care
Royal Brisbane Hospital
Herston
Queensland
Australia

Carl S Waldmann MA MB BChir
FRCA EDICM
Director
Intensive Care & Consultant
Anaesthetist
ICU
Reading
UK

John R Welch BSc (Hons), MSc,
RGN, ENB 100
Consultant Nurse, Critical Care
Dept Anaesthesia
Kingaton hospital
Kingston uopn Thames
Surrey
UK

Julia Wendon MBChB FRCP
Senior Lecturer &. Consultant in
Intensive Care
Institute of Liver Studies
Kings College Hospital
London
UK

Steve Wesselingh
Director
Infectious Diseases Unit
The Alfred Hospital
Prahan
Victoria
Australia

Lindsay I G Worthley MB BS
FRACP
Critical Care Consultant
Dept of Critical Care Medicine
Flinders Medical Centre
Bedford Park
Australia

Duncan L A Wyncoll MBBS FRCA
EDIC DICM
Consultant Intensivist
East Wing Intensive Care
St Thomas' Hospital
London
UK

Steve Yentis BSc MBBS MD FRCA
Consultant Anaesthetist and Honorary
Senior Lecturer
Magill Dept of Anaesthesia, Intensive
Care & Pain Management
Chelsea and Westminster Hospital
London
UK

Foreword

The first edition of "The Manual" was conceived at the end of the 1970's from a collection of handouts for junior doctors and nurses working in the ICU. The resultant popularity of, and demand for, these notes hospital-wide indicated a need to compile a manual to manage seriously ill patients. The manual had to be concise, practical, and above all, easy to read. It had to provide more detail than a synopsis, but be unburdened as a reference tome, so that key information could be readily accessed. This "Intensive Care Manual" was launched in 1979/1980 and its immediate success guaranteed a second edition.

Today, the contents of the first edition seem basic, simplistic, and even primitive. Intensive Care Medicine was in its infancy then, and all of us involved in caring for ICU patients were on a steep learning curve. Progress since has been awesome, with new technology, devices, therapeutic agents, research, education and training, and quality improvement programs firmly establishing the specialty in modern medicine. All these were mirrored in subsequent second, third, and fourth editions of the Manual. This fifth edition reflects contemporary intensive care practice and shows how far we have come. New chapters and new facts in this edition report new knowledge and ongoing developments, all good signs of the health of the specialty. The girth of the Manual has certainly grown, but it was never intended to fit into a white coat pocket. However, its objectives and readership remain unchanged as a bedside book for doctors, nurses, and health professionals to start managing seriously ill patients. In-depth information can be sought later from reference tomes and journal articles. The fifth edition also marks my handing over the editorial reigns to Andrew Bersten and Neil Soni, whose outstanding efforts will ensure that many more editions will follow. Once again, I am indebted to my wife Lala, my children Kazia and Stefan for their support, and I thank Butterworth-Heinemann.

T E Oh
Perth, Western Australia
2003

Preface to fourth edition

This 4th edition follows the successful format of the previous three – rapid access to lucid information on the practical management of diseases and problems in an Intensive Care Unit as well as on subjects relevant to critical care medicine. Each chapter has again been planned to be self-contained, with cross-referencing between chapters. The manual is produced as a comprehensive handbook. It is not intended to be a reference tome, although topics are covered fairly extensively and sufficiently for most clinical situations.

New material in this edition present recent advances and additional chapters. The new chapters contribute to critical care aspects of nursing, infections, oxygenation and organ transplantation, and to paediatric intensive care. Some chapters have been assigned to different sections, and there are new sections on environmental injuries, pharmacological considerations, and transplantation.

The speciality of critical care medicine is now mature, with societies, qualifications, specialist recognition, and career infrastructures founded and implemented in many countries. Critical personnel, other health professionals, and students have found past editions of the book useful. I am confident that they will find this edition likewise.

T E Oh
Hong Kong, March 1996

Preface to fifth edition

This fifth edition is based on the successful format of the previous four editions. The express intention is to provide rapid access to lucid and easily read information that will assist in the practical management of diseases and problems in an intensive care unit.

'If it isn't broken, don't fix it' is the policy of the two new editors but at the same time there is recognition that new authors bring new ideas. Consequently, some chapters have been updated while others have been newly written. While not intended to be a reference tome the referencing is contemporary, relevant and will guide the reader towards more detailed literature. Originally a handbook, the exponential growth of this speciality and associated literature has mandated an increase in the size of the text. Nevertheless, we have maintained the ethos of a practical manual.

There is a lot of new material in this edition. From the seemingly complete reworking of the classification of both coronary artery disease and mechanical ventilation along with a panoply of new management, through information technology and into the increasingly relevant areas of blast injury and biological warfare. In individual chapters, emphasis has been placed on addressing relevant changes since the last edition, whether it be diagnosis or management.

Finding the balance between a comprehensive manual and a complete reference tome in arguably the most rapidly evolving medical speciality, with two editors at different ends of the world, functioning at different times of day has been an interesting task. E-mail and the internet has made an impact in facilitating our endeavours most but not all of the time. There are clear parallels between the influence of this new technology in editing a book and in the clinical environment. The power it provides in terms of accessibility at a speed and of a magnitude that is extraordinary is partially offset by the potential for both loss of focus and misinterpretation. A vast array of raw unfiltered information is easily accessible to everyone but both computers and people may download similar information in very different formats. The expectations of patients, their relatives, and clinicians from all disciplines has been changed. Everyone has access to the latest facts and figures. Paradoxically, the availability of a plethora of 'latest' facts increases the value of a practical manual full of weighed and measured information, and this should be of benefit to all members of the multi-disciplinary team that represents intensive care practice. We want this new edition to be as useful to critical care personnel across the board as its predecessors and we are confident it will match those expectations.

A D Bersten and N Soni
2003

Acknowledgements

Neither of us was under any illusions when the opportunity to edit this Manual was presented. It was always going to be hard work, frustrating at times, and the reward - to try and match the high standards and utility set by the previous four editions. We hope this has been achieved.

Our sincere thanks to Professor Teik Oh for this wonderful opportunity, and for his help and guiding hand. Without the great efforts of many individuals, authors and publishers the fifth edition would not have been completed. We also thank our wives and children (Libby, Eleanor, David and Ben; Allison, Kate and Ben) and our colleagues for their unfailing and generous support.

A D Bersten and N Soni
2003

Part One

Organisation Aspects

Design and organization of intensive care units

T E Oh

An Intensive Care Unit (ICU) is a specially staffed and equipped hospital ward dedicated to the management of patients with life-threatening illnesses, injuries or complications. It has been suggested that the ICU developed from the postoperative recovery room or the poliomyelitis epidemic in the early 1950s, when the use of long-term artificial ventilation resulted in reduced mortality. However, modern intensive care or critical care medicine is not limited to postoperative care or mechanical ventilation. It is a specialty which evolved from the experience of respiratory and cardiac care, physiological organ support, and Coronary Care Units (CCUs), which were established in the early 1960s.[1] Benefits derived from the centralizing of special equipment, staff and facilities to treat critically ill patients and to avert complications or reduce their severity became recognized. The 1970s saw a heightened interest in intensive care, with research into the pathophysiological processes, treatment regimens, and outcomes of the critically ill, and the founding of specialty journals, training programmes and qualifications dedicated to intensive care.[2–4] Intensive care today is a separate specialty,[5] and while some period of training in an ICU is valuable to all specialties, it can no longer be regarded as 'part of' anaesthesia, medicine, general surgery, or any acute discipline.

ECONOMICS OF INTENSIVE CARE[6]

Utilization of ICUs increased markedly in developed countries in the 1970s and early 1980s (e.g. annual increases of 8% in USA and 4.8% in Canada).[6] This inevitably necessitates economic considerations. There are *fixed costs* in any ICU, which are irrelevant to the workload and patient outcome. Salaries make up the bulk of fixed costs (up to 80%). *Variable costs* depend on patient admissions and the services rendered (e.g. investigations, monitoring and procedures). In both fixed and variable costs, there are components that are related to patient care (*direct costs*) and those that are not, for example, 'hotel' or administration expenditures (*indirect costs*).

Provision of intensive care services relates to *supply* and *demand*. Supply of resources to ICUs comes from government funds, private fees and insurance payments. Rising costs have resulted in restrictions on supply through reduced hospital budgets ('implicit rationing') and payments for services ('explicit rationing'). Some countries have adopted a prospective payment system based on diagnosis-related groups (DRGs) which was introduced in USA in 1983. However, DRG reimbursements for certain ICU patients fall short of actual costs. Demand for ICU services is related to demography, economy and technology, but can also be doctor generated (see *Operational policies* below). An ICU bed costs three times more per day than for an acute ward bed,[7] and the ICU uses 8% of the total hospital budget (14–20% in USA).[7] Total ICU costs per patient of US$22 000 in the USA (1978),[8] and Aus$1375 in Australia (1986),[9] have been reported. In the UK, costs are frequently quoted as between £1500 and £2000 per day (2002).

ROLE OF THE ICU

The definition and delineation of roles of hospitals in a region or area are necessary to rationalize services and optimize the use of resources. Each ICU should similarly have its role in the region defined, which should support the defined duties of its hospital. In general, small hospitals require ICUs that provide basic intensive care. An ICU that uses complex management and requires investigative backup should be located in a large tertiary referral hospital of the region. Three levels of adult ICUs can be classified as follows.[10]

1 **Level I Adult ICU – Small District Hospital.** A Level I adult ICU has a role in small district hospitals. It may also be called a 'high dependency unit' (HDU), but the role and functions of an HDU are separate from those of an ICU (see below). A Level I

adult ICU provides resuscitation and short-term cardiorespiratory support of critically ill patients, and monitors and prevents complications in 'at-risk' medical and surgical patients. It is capable of providing mechanical ventilatory support and simple invasive cardiovascular monitoring for a limited period. The medical director is an intensive care specialist.

2 **Level II Adult ICU – General Hospital.** A Level II adult ICU is located in larger general hospitals. It provides a high standard of general intensive care, including multisystem life-support, in accordance with the role of its hospital (e.g. regional centre for acute medicine, general surgery, trauma, etc). It has a resident doctor and access to physiotherapy, pathology and radiological facilities at all times, but may not have all forms of complex therapy and investigations (e.g. radiological angioplasty and MRI scans). A Level II adult ICU's medical director and at least one other consultant are intensive care specialists. Patients admitted are referred to the attending intensive care specialists for management.

3 **Level III Adult ICU – Tertiary Hospital.** A Level III adult ICU is located in a major tertiary referral hospital. It should provide all aspects of intensive care required by its referral role for indefinite periods. The unit is staffed by specialist intensivists with trainees, critical care nurses, allied health professionals, and clerical and scientific staff. Support of complex investigations and imaging, and by specialists of all disciplines required by the referral role of the hospital, is available at all times. All patients admitted to the unit must be referred to the attending intensive care specialist for management.

HIGH DEPENDENCY UNIT[11]

An HDU is a specially staffed and equipped section of an intensive care complex that provides a level of care intermediate between intensive care and general ward care. It provides for immediate resuscitation and management of unstable patients and short-term management of emergencies. Patients in an HDU typically have single-organ failure and are at risk of developing complications. The HDU may admit patients directly from the wards, operating suite or emergency areas. Those whose conditions deteriorate will be transferred to the ICU. The HDU may also admit stable patients from the ICU as a step-down prior to transfer to the wards. An HDU may be located within an ICU complex or in a separate ward adjacent or nearby to it, and is usually staffed by the ICU personnel.

PAEDIATRIC ICU

A paediatric ICU (PICU) is a separate area in the hospital capable of providing complex, multisystem life-support for indefinite periods to infants and children less than 16 years of age. It must be a tertiary referral centre for children needing intensive care, and have extensive backup laboratory and clinical services to support this tertiary role. Consultants in a PICU are paediatric intensive care specialists with expertise different from their adult intensive care colleagues. All patients admitted to the PICU are referred to the attending PICU specialists for management.

TYPE, SIZE AND SITE OF AN ICU[6,10–14]

Health planning policies may rationalize services by hospitals within a geographical region, so as not to unnecessarily duplicate expensive services. Hence, within each classification, an ICU may not be able to provide intensive care for all subspecialties, or may need to be more orientated towards a particular area of expertise (e.g. neurosurgery, cardiac surgery, burns or trauma). Also, an institution may organize its intensive care beds into multiple units, under separate management by single discipline specialists, for example, Medical ICU, Surgical ICU, Burns ICU, etc. While this may be appropriate in certain hospitals, Australasian experience has favoured the development of general multidisciplinary ICUs. Thus, with the exception of dialysis units, CCUs and neonatal ICUs, critically ill patients are admitted to the hospital's multidisciplinary ICU, and are managed by specialist intensivists or paediatric intensivists in paediatric hospitals.

There are good economic and operational arguments for a multidisciplinary ICU as against separate, single discipline ICUs.[6] Duplication of some equipment and services are avoided. Critically ill patients develop the same pathophysiological processes no matter whether they are classified as medical or surgical, and they require the same approaches to support vital organs. Problems of critically ill patients are not confined to their primary disease. Single discipline doctors lack the experience and expertise to deal with the complexities of multiorgan failure.

The number of ICU beds in a hospital usually ranges from 1 to 4 per 100 total hospital beds.[6,7,15] This would depend on the role and type of ICU. Multidisciplinary ICUs would require more beds than single specialty ICUs, especially if high dependency beds were not available elsewhere in the hospital. ICUs with less than 4 beds are considered not to be cost-effective, whereas those with over 20 non-high dependency beds may be difficult to manage.

The ICU should be sited in close proximity to relevant acute areas, that is, operating rooms, emergency department, CCU, labour ward, acute wards, and to investigational departments (e.g. radiology and organ imaging and pathology laboratories). Critically ill patients are at risk when they are moved (see Ch. 3 *Transport of the critically ill*). There should be sufficient numbers of lifts, and these, with doors and corridors, should be spacious enough to allow easy passage of beds and equipment – vital points often ignored by 'planning experts'.

DESIGN OF AN ICU[12,14]

There should be a single entry and exit point, attended by the unit receptionist. Through traffic of goods or people to other hospital areas must never be allowed. An ICU should have areas and rooms for public reception, patient management and support services (Table 1.1).

PATIENT AREAS

Each patient bed area in an adult ICU requires a minimum floor space of 20 m² (215 ft²), with single rooms being larger, to accommodate patient, staff and

Table 1.1 Physical design of a major ICU

Reception area
Reception foyer
Waiting room for visitors (with telephones and beverage facilities)
Distressed ('crying')/interview room
Overnight relatives' room

Patient areas
Open multi-bed ward(s)
Single bed isolation rooms
Central nurse station (including drugs storage)
Specialized rooms/beds if necessary, for:
  procedures/minor surgery (e.g. tracheostomy)
  haemodialysis
  burns
  use of bypass or intra-aortic balloon pump machines

Storage and utility areas
Monitoring and electrical equipment
Respiratory therapy equipment
Disposables and central sterilizing supplies
Linen
Stationery
Fluids, vascular catheters and infusion sets
Non-sterile hardware (e.g. drip stands and bed rails)
Clean utility
Dirty utility
Equipment sterilization

Technical areas
Laboratory
Workshop for repairs, maintenance, and development

Staff areas
Lounge/rest room (with facilities for meals)
Changing rooms
Toilets and showers
Offices
Doctors' on-call rooms
Seminar/conference room

Other support areas
Cleaners' room
Plant room/alcove

equipment without overcrowding. The ratio of single-room beds to open-ward beds would depend on the role and type of the ICU, but 1:6 is recommended for multi-disciplinary ICUs. Single rooms are essential for isolation cases and (less importantly) privacy for conscious long-stay patients. Positive/negative pressure air conditioning for single isolation rooms is expensive and of unproven value. Sufficient numbers of non-splash hand wash basins, one for every two ward beds, should be built close to the beds. Each single room must have its wash basin.

Bedside service outlets should conform to local standards and requirements (including electrical safety and emergency supply, such as to the Australian Standard, Cardiac Protected Status AS3003).

Utilities per bed space as recommended for a Level III ICU are:

- 3 oxygen
- 2 air
- 3 suction
- 16 power outlets
- a bedside light.

Adequate and appropriate lighting for clinical observation must be available. How the services are supplied (e.g. from floor column, wall mounted, or bed pendent) depends on individual preferences, as each design has its pros and cons. There should be room to place or attach additional portable monitoring equipment and, as much as possible, equipment should be kept off the floor. Space for charts, syringes, sampling tubes, pillows, suction catheters, and patient personal belongings are best arranged in bed dividers. Lead lining these dividers will help minimize X-ray radiation risks to staff and patients.

All central staff and patient areas must have large clear windows. Lack of natural light and windowless ICUs give rise to patient disorientation and increased stress to all. Since critical care nursing is at the bedside, manning of a central nurse station is less important than in a CCU. Nevertheless, the central station and other work areas should have adequate space for staff to work in comfort and be sited to allow all patients to be seen. This central station usually houses a central monitor, drugs cupboard, drugs/specimens refrigerator, telephones, laboratories-linked computer, and patient records. At least one multi-display X-ray viewer is needed in each multi-bed ward. Proper facilities for haemodialysis, such as filtered water, should be incorporated.

STORAGE AND SUPPORTING SERVICES AREAS

Most ICUs lack storage space. Storage areas should total a floor space of about 25–30% of all the patient and central station areas. Frequently used items (e.g. i.v. fluids and giving sets, sheets, dressing trays, etc.) should be located closer to patients than infrequently used or non-patient items (e.g. more sophisticated monitoring devices).

Floor areas for supporting services (Table 1.1) should make up about 20–25% of the patient and central station areas. Utility rooms must be clean and separate, each with its own access. Disposal of soiled linen and waste must be catered for, including contaminated items from infectious patients, using one-way traffic schemes. Facilities for estimating blood gases, electrolytes, haemoglobin, haematocrit, and osmolality, with a microscope being available, are usually sufficient for the unit's laboratory. Larger ICUs may require a satellite pharmacy within the unit. A good communication network of 'phones/intercoms is vital to locate and inform staff quickly. A special paging code, such as '1111', will enable instant summoning of ICU staff in emergencies. Adequate arrangements for offices, doctor-on-call rooms, staff lounge (with food/drinks facilities), wash rooms, education (seminar room), and a waiting room (see below) complete the unit.

EQUIPMENT

The quantity and level of equipment will depend on the role and type of ICU. Level I and II units will obviously require less than a Level III unit (Table 1.2). For example, a 2-channel bedside monitor should suffice for a small district hospital ICU, whereas a major teaching hospital ICU should be equipped with monitors able to display at least 4 physiological signals. (Monitoring devices and ventilators are discussed in Ch. 28 *Respiratory Monitoring*, and Ch. 10 *Haemodynamic Monitoring*). Equipment should be chosen by experienced intensivists, as often expensive but inappropriate or unsuitable equipment are bought by inept or less knowledgeable people.

STAFFING[2,14,16]

The level of staffing also depends on the type of hospital. A large hospital ICU requires a large team of people (Table 1.3).

MEDICAL STAFF

Career intensivists are the best senior medical staff to be appointed to the ICU.[2,4] The ICU director is one such specialist intensivist. Sufficient specialist staff with experience in intensive care are necessary to provide for administration, teaching, research, reasonable working hours, and leave of all types. In an ICU of Level II or III there must be at least one specialist exclusively rostered to the unit at all times. Specialists should have a significant or full-time commitment to the ICU ahead of clinical commitments elsewhere.

Table 1.2 Equipment in a major ICU

Monitoring
Bedside and central monitors
12-lead ECG (paper) recorder
Intravascular and intracranial pressure monitoring devices
Cardiac output computer
Pulse oximeters
Pulmonary function monitoring devices
Expired CO_2 analysers
Cerebral function/EEG monitor
Patient/bed weighers
Temperature monitors
Enzymatic blood glucose meters

Radiology
X-ray viewers
Portable X-ray machine
Image intensifier

Respiratory therapy
Ventilators, bedside and portable (including monitors and alarms for oxygen and gas supply failure, circuit disconnection, oxygen concentration, and ventilating volumes and pressures)
Humidifiers (including monitoring inspired temperature)
Oxygen therapy devices and airway circuits
Tracheal intubation trolley (airway control equipment)
Airway devices
Manual self-inflating resuscitators and other manual ventilating systems
Fibreoptic bronchoscope
Suction apparatus
Chest drainage apparatus
Anaesthesia machine

Cardiovascular therapy
Cardiopulmonary resuscitation trolleys
Defibrillators
Cardiac pacing facilities
Intra-aortic balloon pump
Infusion pumps and syringes and vascular access equipment

Support therapy
Temperature control equipment (e.g. heating/cooling blankets)
Patient transport equipment

Dialytic therapy
Haemodialysis machine (including monitors of air embolism)
Peritoneal dialysis equipment
Continuous haemofiltration sets (including monitors of air embolism)

Laboratory
Blood gas analyser
Selective ion (electrolyte) electrode analysers
Osmometer
Haematocrit centrifuge
Thromboelastograph
Microscope

Table 1.3 Staff of a major ICU

Medical
Director
Staff specialist intensivists
Junior doctors

Nurses
Nurse managers
Nurse specialists
Nurse educators
Critical care nurse trainees

Allied health
Physiotherapists
Pharmacist
Dietician
Social worker
Respiratory therapists

Technicians

Secretarial
Secretary
Ward clerk

Radiographers

Support staff
Orderlies
Cleaners

There should be a full-time junior medical staff with an appropriate level of experience available 24 hours rostered exclusively to Level II and III units at all times. Junior medical staff in the ICU may be intensive care trainees, but should ideally also include trainees of other acute disciplines (e.g. anaesthesia, medicine, and surgery). It is imperative that junior doctors are adequately supervised, with specialists being ready available.

NURSING STAFF

The level of nursing staffing will also depend on the type of ICU. Major ICUs should have a majority of their nurses experienced in critical care nursing. Courses or training programmes in critical care are valuable if creditable. The actual total numbers of nurses for an ICU must take into account night shifts, and annual, sick, or study leave. Critically ill patients on mechanical ventilation require 1:1 nursing. Level III units should be capable of providing nursing care to greater than 1:1 ratio for the most critically ill patients, whereas one nurse is often required for 2–3 stable patients (e.g. those for postoperative monitoring). Practical staff numbers can be derived from work statistics, types of patients[14] and leave allowances (see Ch. 5 *Critical care nursing*). As a rule of thumb, long-term 24-hour cover of a single bed requires a staff complement of 6 nurses.

ALLIED HEALTH

Major ICUs should have 24-hour access to physiotherapists and radiological services. Access to other therapists, dieticians, and social workers should also be available. A dedicated ward clinical pharmacist is invaluable. Respiratory therapists are allied health personnel trained in, and responsible for, the equipment and clinical aspects of respiratory therapy, a concept well established in North America, but not Britain, Europe, and Australasia. Technicians and scientists, either as a member of the ICU staff, or seconded from biophysics departments, are necessary to service, repair, and develop equipment.

OTHER STAFF

Provision should be made for adequate secretarial support. Transport and 'lifting' orderly teams will reduce physical stress and possible injuries to nurses and doctors. If no mechanical system is available to transport specimens to the laboratories (e.g. air pressurized chutes), sufficient and reliable couriers must be provided to do this day and night. Contact is made with the local interpreters, chaplains, priests, or officials of all religions, when there is need for their services. Their role in counselling and consoling distressed relatives is invaluable (see below).

OPERATIONAL POLICIES[6,13,14]

Clear-cut administrative policies are vital to the functioning of an ICU. An *open* ICU has unlimited access to multiple doctors who are free to admit and manage their patients. A *closed* ICU has admission, discharge, and referral policies under the control of intensivists. Improved cost–benefits are likely with a closed ICU, and patient outcome may be better, especially if the intensivists have full clinical responsibilities.[17–19] Some ICUs, particularly in countries that do not offer qualifications or training programmes in intensive care, adopt a 'management-in-consultation' policy. A team (usually anaesthetists) looks after the day-to-day and emergency aspects, but 'co-manages' the patients with the referring specialists. Although laudably democratic, lines of responsibility at times are unclear, and acquisition of knowledge or experience may not be optimal.

ICUs today, especially Levels II and III, should be *closed* under the charge of a medical specialist director. All patients admitted to the ICU are referred to the director and his/her specialist staff for management.

There must be clearly defined policies for admission, discharge, management, and referral of patients. Lines of responsibilities must be delineated for all staff members, and their job descriptions defined. The director must have final, overall authority of all staff and their actions, although in other respects each group may be responsible to their respective hospital heads, for example director of nursing.

Policies for the care of patients should be formulated and standardized. They should be unambiguous, periodically reviewed, and familiarized by all staff. Certain policies are universally applicable, for example, antibiotic policies and compulsory hand-washing before and after examining patients. Others depend more on local situations and personal beliefs, for example, donning gowns and over-shoes before entering the ICU, a ritual not proven to reduce cross infection.

OUTREACH INTENSIVE CARE SERVICES

Ward care of seriously ill patients, as expected, cannot compare with that in an ICU. None the less, care of seriously ill patients in the wards may be suboptimal, especially before they are admitted into the ICU.[20] Early identification of at-risk patients[21,22] or treatment by a medical emergency team or an 'at-risk team' before ICU admission may decrease mortality.[23–25] This is a team of mobile ICU staff that responds to enquiries and consultations from the wards regarding their seriously ill patients, and responds by providing resuscitation and rapid admission to the ICU. This outreach ICU care overcomes late referrals to the ICU and provides intensive care services hospital-wide, rather than just within the ICU.

QUALITY ASSURANCE, CONTINUING EDUCATION AND RESEARCH

An ICU should have formal audit, peer review and quality assurance (QA) processes. The measurement and improvement of quality of care is very much applicable to intensive care. QA programmes in the ICU can be considered under three headings.

1 *Structure.* Documentation must be available to show that the ICU functions according to its operational guidelines, and conforms to policies of training and specialist bodies (e.g. staffing establishment and levels of supervision). Data on clinical workload and case mix should be collected.
2 *Clinical process.* Audits of clinical performance are conducted as peer review meetings, clinical–pathological conferences, and critical incident reporting. A critical incident is an event that has led or would have led to patient morbidity or mortality.[26] Analysis of reports will alter practice to improve care.
3 *Outcome.* Quality of care in terms of outcome is difficult to measure. Mortality rates are not useful. The Acute Physiology and Chronic Health Evaluation II (APACHE II) scoring system for illness severity (see Ch. 2 *Assessment of severity and outcome of critical illness*) can be used across countries.[27,28] Its multivariate analysis model has been used to compare performance in terms of actual vs predicted death rates. Data on quality of life of survivors are difficult to collect and assess.

ICUs should also have on-going academic programmes. Apart from clinical reviews (above), meetings to review journals and new developments should be held regularly. Teaching programmes must be instituted for trainees, nurses and other health care workers who must be encouraged to develop their quality assurance programmes. Research programmes have to be pursued. Potential research areas are numerous, including those on basic sciences, drugs, therapies, equipment, and multi-centre trials.

CONSIDERATION OF RELATIVES[29]

Apart from a waiting room, ICUs of Level II and III should have a separate room to interview and comfort distressed relatives. Facilities for overnight accommodation should be considered. ICU care includes sensitive handling of patient relatives. Family members undergo feelings of fear, anxiety, disbelief, incomprehension, denial, anger, guilt, and 'why me?'. The ICU environment can be hostile and frightening. Antagonism and frustration can build up through concern for their critically ill family members, compounded by an inhospitable physical environment and failure by staff to provide explanations. Attention must be paid to the following considerations in handling relatives.

EFFECTIVE COMMUNICATION

One senior doctor should be identified as the ICU representative to liaise with a particular family. He/she should identify, by consensus, a spokesman for the family to whom information is normally conveyed. An ICU nurse, preferably the one caring for the patient, is a valuable member in discussions with the family. Relatives feel less daunted in the presence of a nurse, who helps in explanations and consoling distressed members. Children should not be excluded in discussions.

In each interview, the intensivist must ascertain what the family already knows or has been told. Any misinformation or misconceptions must be rectified. When providing explanations, simple, clear, consistent terms must be used. Stressed relatives 'shut out' bad news and can misunderstand or misinterpret what was said. Honesty is best; and if death is probable or imminent, say so accordingly. Failure to inform about grave prognoses and changes in condition give an impression of staff being uncaring and incompetent. The intensivist should show empathy and avoid clichés, false sympathy, and being patronizing. One should listen, encourage questions, and expect a spectrum of emotions from any family member. Worried, grieving relatives can be abusive as well as tearful. They should be enabled to cry and accept reality. Assurances that treatment for relief of pain and suffering are being given to their loved one must be made. Culture permitting, touch (e.g. holding hands of distressed members) should be appropriately applied. Request for organ donation must be made by an experienced specialist, and at an appropriate time, usually after confirmation of brain death. The time, date, and discussion of each interview should be recorded.

PHYSICAL ENVIRONMENT

Interviews should be conducted in a private, suitably furnished, dedicated room. Tissues, tea/coffee, and a telephone must be available, and relatives should have access to toilets and a cafeteria. An availability of hospital short-term accommodation for those who live far away is helpful. Visiting hours must be liberal, if not round the clock. Entry of children into the ICU would be at the discretion of the family and staff. If relatives have to wait for a prolonged period while the patient is undergoing treatment, a staff member should explain the delay.

OTHER SUPPORTIVE MEASURES

Contact with a social worker, counsellor, priest or religious minister should be arranged if appropriate. Sedatives may need to be prescribed for some family members. Follow-up counselling may be required. Emotional support for staff may be necessary and is also important. If death occurs, the family should be allowed privacy to mourn, and to view, touch and hold the deceased. Whether children should view the patient after death is best decided by the family.

REFERENCES

1 Editorial. Twenty five years of coronary care. *Lancet* 1988; ii: 830–1.
2 The Duties of an Intensive Care Specialist in Hospitals Accredited for Intensive Care Training. Policy Document IC-2, 2000, Faculty of Intensive Care, Australian and New Zealand College of Anaesthetists, Melbourne.
3 NIH. Consensus Development Conference on Critical Care Medicine. *Crit Care Med* 1983; **11**: 466–9.
4 Guidelines for Intensive Care Units Seeking Faculty Accreditation for Training in Intensive Care. Policy Document IC-3, 2000, Faculty of Intensive Care, Australian and New Zealand College of Anaesthetists, Melbourne.
5 Dudley HAF. Intensive Care: a specialty or a branch of anaesthetics? *BMJ* 1987; **294**: 459–60.
6 Oh TE. The development, utilization, and cost implications of Intensive Care medicine – strategies for the future. In: Tinker J, Browne D, Sibbald W (eds). *Critical Care – Standards, Audit and Ethics.* London: Edward Arnold; 1999: 11–20.
7 Jacobs P, Noseworthy TW. National estimates of intensive care utilization and costs: Canada and the United States. *Crit Care Med* 1991; **18**: 1282–6.
8 Cullen DJ, Keene R, Waternoux C, *et al.* Results, changes, and benefits of intensive care for critically ill patients: update 1983. *Crit Care Med* 1984; **12**: 102–6.
9 Slatyer MA, James OF, Moore PG, Leeder SR. Costs, severity of illness and outcome in intensive care. *Anaesth Intensive Care* 1986; 14: 381–9.
10 Minimum Standards for Intensive Care Units. Policy Document IC-1, 1997, Faculty of Intensive Care, Australian and New Zealand College of Anaesthetists, Melbourne.
11 Minimum Standards for High Dependency Units Seeking Accreditation for Training in Intensive Care. Policy Document IC-13, 2000, Faculty of Intensive Care, Australian and New Zealand College of Anaesthetists, Melbourne.
12 Recommendations for critical care unit design. Task Force on Guidelines, Society of Critical Care Medicine. *Crit Care Med* 1988; **16**: 796–806.
13 Recommendations for intensive care unit admission and discharge criteria. Task Force on Guidelines, Society of Critical Care Medicine. *Crit Care Med* 1988; **16**: 807–8.
14 *Standards for Intensive Care Units.* Intensive Care Society (UK); 1983.
15 Miranda DR, Langrehr D (eds). *The ICU: a Cost–Benefit Analysis.* International Congress Series 709. Amsterdam: Excerpta Medica; 1986.
16 Recommendations for services and personnel for delivery of care in a critical care setting. Task Force on Guidelines, Society of Critical Care Medicine. *Crit Care Med* 1988; **16**: 809–11.
17 Knaus WA, Draper EA, Wagner DP, Zimmerman JE. An evaluation of outcome from intensive care in major medical centers. *Ann Intern Med* 1986; **104**: 410–18.
18 Brown JJ, Sullivan G. Effect on ICU mortality of a full-time critical care specialist. *Chest* 1989; **96**: 127–9.
19 Groeger JS, Strosberg MA, Halpern NA, *et al.* Descriptive analysis of critical care units in the United States. *Crit Care Med* 1992; **20**: 846–63.
20 McQuillan P, Pilkington S, Allan A, *et al.* Confidential enquiry into quality of care before admission to intensive care. *BMJ* 1998; **316**: 1853–8.
21 Goldhill DR, Sumner A. Outcome of intensive care patients in a group of British intensive care units. *Crit Care Med* 1998; **26**: 1337–45.
22 Goldhill DR, White SA, Sumner A. Physiological values and procedures in the 24 hours before ICU admission in the ward. *Anaesthesia* 1999; **54**: 529–34.
23 Goldhill DR, Withington LM, Mulcahy AJ, Tarling MM. The patient-at-risk team: identifying and managing seriously ill ward patients. *Anaesthesia* 1999; **54**: 853–60.
24 Mercer M, Fletcher SJ, Bishop GFI. Suboptimal ward care of critically ill patients. Medical emergency teams improve care. *BMJ* 1999; **318**: 54–5.
25 Bristow PJ, Hillman KM, Chey T, *et al.* Rates of in-hospital arrests, deaths and intensive care admissions;

the effect of a medical emergency team. *Med J Aust* 2000; **173**: 236–40.

26 Short TG, O'Reagan A, Lew J, Oh TE. Critical incident reporting in an anaesthetic department quality assurance programme. *Anaesthesia* 1993; **48**: 3–7.

27 Zimmerman JE, Knaus WA, Judson JA, *et al.* Patient selection for intensive care: a comparison of New Zealand and United States hospitals. *Crit Care Med* 1988; **16**: 318–26.

28 Oh TE, Hutchinson RC, Short S, *et al.* Verification and use of the acute physiology and chronic health evaluation scoring system in a Hong Kong intensive care unit. *Crit Care Med* 1993; **21**: 698–705.

29 McLauchlan CAJ. ABC of trauma. Handling distressed relatives and breaking bad news. *BMJ* 1990; **301**: 1145–9.

2

Assessment of severity and outcome of critical illness

M Palazzo

Clinical assessment of severity of illness is an essential component of medical practice. It primarily determines whether there is a need for therapeutic intervention, its degree of urgency and may also indicate likely prognosis when other factors are considered. It is a logical step to consider whether patterns of physiological disturbance can be linked to outcome. Perhaps the earliest reference to grading illness was in an Egyptian papyrus which classified head injury by severity.[1] Modern examples such as the Ranson score for acute pancreatitis, the Child–Pugh classification of cirrhosis and the Glasgow Coma Scale for head injury, popularized the use of systems of patient descriptors which associate physiological disturbance with outcome. The earliest attempt to quantify severity of illness in a general critically ill population was by Cullen[2] who devised a therapeutic intervention score. This was followed in 1981 with the introduction of the Acute Physiology, Age and Chronic Health Evaluation (APACHE) scoring system by Knaus.[3] Subsequently, numerous systems have been designed and tested in populations across the world.

The potential advantages of quantifying critical illness include providing;

- a common language for discussion
- comparators for clinical trials
- estimates of prognosis

More controversial is the potential use of scoring systems for resource management and decision pathways in individual patients. The desire for this is hardly surprising as it has been estimated that non-survivors cost twice as much as survivors.[4]

However these systems do have a potentially important role in medical care process evaluation.

PRINCIPLES OF QUALIFYING SEVERITY OF CRITICAL ILLNESS

Severity of illness is:

- Readily associated with the degree of physiological disturbance
- Put into context with respect to outcome when related to a primary pathological process, and a patient's physiological reserve

These factors should be represented if quantification of illness is to be related to outcome.

PHYSIOLOGICAL DISTURBANCE

An insult may be initially followed by little physiological disturbance due to homeostatic and compensatory mechanisms. Changes follow when there is decompensation or if the initial insult is overwhelming. The relationship between insult and physiological response is confounded by:

- non linearity
- natural variability between patients
- variable physiological reserve

Additional considerations include:

- Whether a severity of illness should score include an element which reflects the size of the insult or simply rely on the physiological response to such an insult or both?
- Whether physiological disturbance can be represented on a linear scale (consider liver and kidney disturbance which only manifest biochemical abnormality when a significant proportion of their mass is malfunctioning)?

- Determining the relative impact of different organ disturbances when quantifying overall severity of illness?

In addition, the degree of physiological disturbance will vary depending on the moment it is assessed in the course of the illness, and this will be profoundly affected by the supportive interventions that have preceded assessment. Many systems have arbitrarily estimated severity of illness on or near admission to an intensive care unit.

PATHOLOGICAL PROCESS

The potential reversibility of a pathological process, whether spontaneous or through specific treatment, largely influences outcome and by implication qualifies and quantifies the severity of illness. For example, similar degrees of respiratory decompensation in an asthmatic and a patient with haematological malignancy indicate quite different severities of illness.

Some critical care scoring systems have included diagnostic categories to better define the relationship between physiological disturbance and outcome.

PHYSIOLOGICAL RESERVE

Physiological reserve is a surrogate term which broadly combines the effects of age and premorbid health status. Age may be associated with diminishing physiological capacity but not in a predictable fashion.

- Age alone is not a very strong influence on outcome
- Chronological or biological. The latter is a vague term usually used to imply physiological reserve below that expected for a patient of that age or that a patient appears to be physiologically older. Biological age is often related to acquired dysfunction from factors such as heavy smoking, alcohol consumption, generalized peripheral vascular disease or diabetes which prematurely reduce renal, respiratory and cardiovascular capacity

Chronic health states, such as immunosuppression, cirrhosis, cancer and haematological malignancies, all result in significant diminution of physiological reserve and may have an overwhelming influence on outcome. They are universally included in assessments of critical illness, severity.

OUTCOME: ITS MEASUREMENT AND RELATIONSHIP TO SEVERITY OF ILLNESS

Physiological disturbance, pathological process and physiological reserve can be related to outcome by statistical methods. Common outcome measures are ICU mortality, mortality at 28 or 30 days or hospital mortality. These particular measures depend heavily on the acute physiological disturbance. Patient morbidity might be at least as important an endpoint as mortality, since many patients survive with serious functional impairment.[5,6] For socio-economic reasons, there would be a strong argument to consider 1 year survival, or time to return to normal function or work as endpoints.[4,5,7] These measures have been more closely related to chronic health status. Consequently, the weighting given to the acute or chronic aspects of severity of illness scores should take account of the preferred principle outcome measure.

Hospital mortality is the most common outcome measure because it is frequent enough to act as a discriminator and is easy to define and document.

SCORING SYSTEM DESIGN

CHOICE OF INDEPENDENT VARIABLES AND TIMING

Independent variables from large patient cohorts provide the basis for scoring system models. Acute physiological diagnostic details, premorbid conditions, age and emergency status have been variably included. The original APACHE and Simplified Acute Physiology Score (SAPS) systems, chose variables based on expert opinion which were given arbitrarily determined weightings.[8,9] The later SAPS II, APACHE III and the Mortality Probability Model (MPM) systems used logistic regression to determine the variables and their weightings with respect to the primary outcome, hospital mortality.[10]

To simplify scoring the worst physiological data during the first 24 h of intensive care management were used. Other systems used trends these included, the Sickness Score, Organ Systems Failure score, Organ Failure score, and MPM, in an attempt to provide better models.[11-14]

THE INFLUENCE OF TREATMENT ON SCORES

Many patients have received treatment prior to admission to ICU which will influence the score. This introduces lead-time bias (i.e. in the time taken for the patient to arrive in ICU, therapy has reduced the physiological perturbations). This particularly affects APACHE and SAPS. MPM II, less based on acute physiology and more on pathological processes such as cardiac arrest, coma and co-morbidity, is theoretically less susceptible to lead time changes.

SCORING METHODOLOGY AND VALIDATION

A database is built up from a large critical care population and an equation derived from this developmental dataset. Special statistical techniques such as 'jack-knifing' or 'boot-strapping' allow the original developmental set to be also used for validation. However, the more recent Scoring systems have divided the patient cohort into separate developmental and validation data sets. All the major models have been based on logistic regression methodology in which a dichotomous outcome, survival or death is related to the weighted variables.

- Derived equations are sensitive to changes in validation case mix[16]
- Derived equations provide a probability model for groups of patients and not individuals

In a perfect model:

- Overall predicted and observed outcomes should be the same – a measure of calibration
- No misclassification of patients with respect to death or survival – a measure of discrimination

It is possible to assess the model for its ability to discriminate survivors from non-survivors (see Appendix). The discriminating power of a model can be determined by defining a series of threshold risks of death and using the model to predict survivors and non survivors at these thresholds or cut-off points. For example, the APACHE II system misclassification rate was 14.4, 15.2, 16.7 and 18.5% at 50, 70, 80 and 90% predicted risk of death cut-off points indicating that the model worked best at a cut-off point of 50% risk of death.

A conventional approach to displaying this is to plot sensitivity on the y-axis indicating true positive predictions against false positive predictions (1 – specificity) on the x-axis over several cut-off points, a receiver operator characteristic curve (ROC) (Fig. 2.1).

A perfect model would show no false positives and would therefore follow the y-axis. The area under the curve (AUC) under such conditions would be 1. A non discriminating graph would be indicated by a line at 45 degrees through the origin and would have AUC of 0.5. A graph with AUC greater than 0.8 is considered good.

Good calibration is observed when a model predicts a similar percentage mortality of a group of patients as that observed (Hosmer–Lemeshow goodness of fit C statistic compares the model to the patient group).[17]

COMMONLY USED SCORING SYSTEMS

GLASGOW COMA SCALE (GCS)

Ths was introduced in 1974 to quantify level of consciousness after the first 6 h of head injury. It individually scores best eye opening, verbal and motor responsiveness, providing an overall scale between 3 (profound coma) to 15 (normal alert state). Its major strengths are that it has proved to be consistent between expert and non-expert observers and has been adopted worldwide.[18–20] This consistency has allowed head injury management protocols to be based on the initial scale at presentation, decision making based on trends and, when combined with age, it provides some assessment of prognosis.

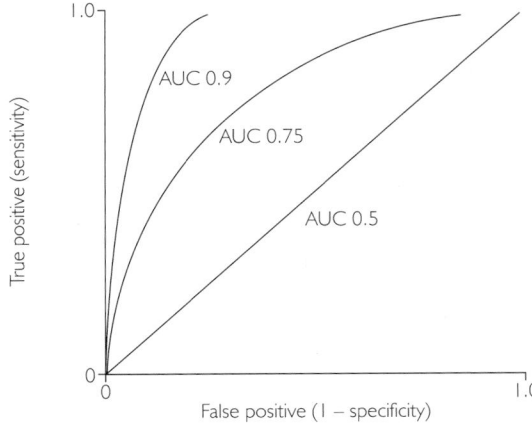

Fig. 2.1   A receiver operator curve (ROC) plots true positives against false positive rates for a series of cut-off points for risk of death. For example, a risk of death cut-off point of 10% would predict all patients with a risk greater than 10% to die and all those below to survive. This would be compared with the observed rates in those patients. The prediction would be expected to be frequently wrong and would reflect itself in the calculation of true positive and false positive rates. These calculations would represent one point on the ROC curve. The exercise is repeated at different cut-off points such as 15, 20, 25, 30, etc., from which a curve can be constructed. The resulting area under the curve reflects the ability of the model to predict survival correctly. This is a measure of discriminatory power. The best models have values greater than 0.85

Table 2.1   Ability of scores to discriminate correctly between survivors and non survivors when tested on similar case mixes. A value of 1 represents perfect prediction

Score	Area under ROC curve
APACHE II	0.85
APACHE III	0.9
SAPS II	0.86
MPM II$_0$	0.82
MPMII$_{24}$	0.84

It has been included in a number of general scoring systems. The standard form of GCS is inapplicable to infants and children below the age of 5 years and has been modified to recognise that the expected normal verbal and motor responses must be related to the patient's age.[21]

THERAPEUTIC INTERVENTION SCORING SYSTEM (TISS)

This was introduced in 1974 with the aims of estimating severity of illness, the burden work for ICU staff and nursing resource allocation.[2] It requires the daily collection of 76 listed items, primarily interventions or treatments, although a cut down version has been suggested, TISS 28.[22,23]

- Good indicator of nursing and medical work
- Poor measure of severity of illness
- Successfully used as a method of accountancy through allocation of average costs per point

ACUTE PHYSIOLOGY AGE AND CHRONIC HEALTH EVALUATION (APACHE)

In 1981, Knaus *et al.* described APACHE, a physiologically based classification system for measuring severity of illness in groups of critically ill patients. They suggested it could be used to control for case mix, compare outcomes, evaluate new therapies, and study the utilization of ICUs.[3] APACHE II, a simplified version, was introduced in 1985 and, although superseded by APACHE III in 1991,[9,24] it has remained the most widely studied and extensively used severity of illness scoring system.

APACHE II was developed and validated on 5030 non-coronary artery bypass patients admitted to intensive care units.

It is the sum of three components:

- an acute physiology score (APS)
- a chronic health score based on defined premorbid states
- a score based on the patient's age

The 12 variables of the APS and their relative weights were decided by expert opinion. These are collected in the first 24 h after admission to intensive care and should represent the worst physiological values (see Appendices). The APACHE II score can be included in a logistic regression equation with a coefficient for one of 50 precipitating diagnostic categories and a factor for emergency surgery to provide a risk of death probability.

APACHE II is able to predict hospital mortality in a wide variety of hospital patient cohorts but has been less useful with narrow diagnostic groups such as AIDS and trauma which bear little relationship to the case mix of the original database.[25,26] A recent report[27] demonstrated that APACHE II is better calibrated than SAPS and MPM I but was not as discriminating nor as well calibrated as APACHE III when applied to a 14 745 mixed patient cohort from European and American intensive care units. The fall off in calibration of APACHE II relate to the older more complex case mix that now tends to populate most ICUs.

Standardized mortality ratio (SMR) is the comparison of predicted with observed mortality rates. This was used as surrogate evidence for good quality of care and a value of 1 is considered normal but:

- standard deviations have not been defined

- SMR should be considered in the context of case mix[28–30]

Bion and Chang separately were the first to explore the possibility of using APACHE II in a dynamic scoring system. The former used a modified APACHE II in the Sickness Score System in which the day 1 score was compared with day 4 and risk of mortality was predicted.[11] Chang on the other hand used the product of daily APACHE II scores with a modified Organ Failure Score and calculated thresholds above which individual patient mortality was predicted.[12]

APACHE III

This upgrade of APACHE II based on a larger reference database was designed to:

- improve prognostic estimates by re-evaluating the selection and weighting of physiological variables
- examine how outcome is related to patient selection for ICU admission and its timing
- clarify the distinction between using the APACHE scoring system to stratify by risk of mortality within particular patient groups and using it to make individual estimates of mortality

In the new system:

- Three-fold larger database (17 440 patients) from 40 hospitals equally divided between developmental and validation groups
- Exclusions included admission for less than 4 h, age less than 16 years, burn injuries or admitted with chest pain
- Coronary artery bypass patients were a separate group
- Seventeen physiological variables and their weights were chosen through statistical analysis; diagnostic categories increased from 50 to 78
- Revised version of the GCS
- Only those co-morbidities which seem to affect the patient's immune status were included

The coefficients for the regression equations are not in the public domain, this has made independent assessment of the predictive aspect of the scoring system a little more difficult. APACHE III represents an advance over APACHE II with improved discriminatory power (ROC 0.9 vs 0.85), and better calibration.[24,27]

SIMPLIFIED ACUTE PHYSIOLOGY SCORE (SAPS)

The Simplified Acute Physiology Score (SAPS) was based on data derived from Europe.[8] The 14 physiological variables were chosen through expert opinion and the points ascribed to these variables and their deviation from normal were arbitrary. Initially, the score was not related to an equation for predicting probability of death, although later this was possible. Unlike APACHE II this system did not include a diagnostic category nor chronic health status as part of the severity of illness estimate.

In 1993, SAPS II, based on European and North American patients was introduced.[15] The database contained 13 152 patients divided 65% and 35% between developmental and validation samples. Patients under 18 years, burns patients, coronary care and post cardiac surgery patients were all excluded.

The weightings given to physiological derangements were derived from logistic regression analysis. It included 12 physiological variables and specific chronic health conditions such as the presence of AIDS, haematological malignancies, cirrhosis and metastasis. Similar to SAPS, there was no requirement for inclusion of diagnostic groups to calculate probability of hospital mortality. The probability for hospital death can be readily calculated from a logistic regression equation based on acute physiology scores and chronic health weightings. In the validation sample, the area under the ROC curve was 0.86. Equivalent in calibration and discrimination to APACHE III and MPM II. It is the most commonly used scoring system in Europe.

MORTALITY PREDICTION MODELS (MPM I–II)

This was introduced in 1985 to provide an evidence based approach to constructing a scoring system.[31,32] The data was derived from a single institution and included observations at the time of admission to ICU and within the first 24 h. MPM I_0 was based on the absence or presence of some physiological and diagnostic features at the time of admission while a further prediction model MPM I_{24} was based on variables reflecting the effects of treatment at the end of the first ICU day. Unlike APACHE and SAPS systems, it does not calculate a score but computes the hospital risk of death from the presence or absence of factors in a logistic regression equation.

MPM II is based on the same data set as SAPS II.[10,14] The system is a series of four models which provide an outcome prediction estimate for ICU patients at admission and at 24, 48 and 72 h. In common with APACHE and SAPS systems, the models excluded burns, coronary care and cardiac surgery patients. The models were derived by using logistic regression techniques to choose and weight the variables with an additional criteria that variables had to be 'clinically plausible'.

MPM II_0 and MPM II_{24} have similar discriminatory power to SAPS II, with ROC curve AUC of 0.82 and 0.84 respectively. MPM II_0 remains the only method validated for use at the time of ICU admission.

In a comparison between MPM II, SAPS II and APACHE III and the earlier versions of these systems, all the newer systems performed better than their respective older versions; however, no system stood out as being superior to the others.[27]

ORGAN FAILURE SCORES

It is possible to relate the number of failed organs and their duration to probability of mortality. The organ system failures (OSF) were defined for five organs in an all or nothing manner and the number of failures summed.[13] The outstanding observations were that:

- Single OSF lasting 1 day produced a hospital mortality rate of 30%
- Two OSFs for 1 day (medical and surgical) increased rates to 60%
- Three or more OSFs lasting 3 days produced a mortality rate of 90%
- Advanced chronologic age increased both the probability of developing OSF and the probability of death once OSF occurred

Scores to take account of grades of dysfunction and supportive therapy have been proposed including the multiple organ dysfunction score (MODS), which was based on specific descriptors in six organ systems (respiratory, renal, neurological, haematological, cardiovascular and hepatic). Progressive organ dysfunction was measured on a scale of 0 to 4; the intervals were statistically determined for each organ based on associated mortality. The summed score (maximum 24) on the first day score was correlated with mortality in a graduated fashion.[33]

ICU mortality was approximately:

- 25% at 9–12 points
- 50% at 13–16 points
- 75% at 17–20 points
- 100% at levels of >20 points

Good discrimination with areas under the ROC curve of 0.936 in the development set and 0.928 in the validation set were obtained.

SEPSIS RELATED ORGAN FAILURE ASSESSMENT (SOFA)

Originally associated with sepsis, it takes into account six organs (brain, cardiovascular, coagulation, renal, hepatic, respiratory) and scores organ function from zero (normal) to 4 (extremely abnormal). Experts defined the parameter intervals[34,35] intended to provide the simplest daily description of organ dysfunction for use in clinical trials. It has the merit of including supportive therapy and although increasing score can be shown to be associated with increasing mortality it was not designed for estimation of outcome probability. The SOFA score has subsequently been renamed 'sequential organ failure assessment'. This simple method has become a popular method by which to track and describe patient changes in morbidity.

LODS is an organ failure score that could be used for hospital outcome prediction.[36] Based on the patient cohort used to derive the SAPS II and MPM II systems, logistic regression was used on first day data to propose an organ failure score. The LOD system identified from 1–3 levels of organ dysfunction for six organ systems and between 1 and 5 LOD points were assigned to the levels of severity. The resulting LOD scores ranged from 0 to 22 points. Calibration and discrimination were good. It demonstrated that neurological, cardiovascular, and renal dysfunction carried the most weight for predictive purposes followed by pulmonary and haematologic dysfunction with hepatic dysfunction carrying the least weight. Unlike SOFA, the system takes into account the relative severity between organs and the degree of severity within an organ system by attributing different weights.

SCORES FOR INJURY AND TRAUMA

This is a relatively homogenous group for assessment of severity of illness. There are two principal methods:

1 Injury severity score (ISS) scores the extent of anatomical injury.[37] It is based on the Abbreviated Injury Scale (AIS) which assigns a code and a value from 1 (minor) to 6 (unsurvivable) to six body regions, and incorporates a modification for blunt and penetrating injury.[38] ISS is calculated from the sum of the squares of the highest AIS score in each of the three most severely injured body regions (the square of values transformation results in a relatively linear relationship with mortality and other measures of severity). The highest score is 5 (6 is fatal) in each body region and, consequently, the highest ISS is 75. Major trauma is defined as an ISS greater than 16 and this is associated with a greater than 10% risk of mortality. The ISS is a purely anatomical system that ignores physiological derangements or chronic health status.

2 Trauma Score is a physiologically based triage tool for use in the field, based on systolic blood pressure, capillary refill, respiratory rate, chest expansion and GCS. It can be used with anatomical and age data.[39]

The Revised Trauma Score (RTS)[40,41] is based on disturbances in three variables

- GCS
- Systolic blood pressure
- Respiratory rate

Each score is coded between 1 and 4. The physiological disturbances were further modified by use of a coefficient to indicate a relative weighting.

The ISS and RTS individually had flaws as indicators of outcome, but they were successfully combined by Boyd to provide the Trauma Injury Severity Score (TRISS) methodology for outcome prediction. TRISS also included the presence of penetrating injury and age in its methodology.[37,40,42,43]

It uses coefficients derived from the data of 30 000 injured patients, from which it calculates an estimated probability of survival for individual trauma victims. It also provides a comparative measure of quality of care by trauma centers, using expected and observed outcomes.

A Severity Characterization of Trauma (ASCOT) was introduced to rectify perceived problems with TRISS.[44] There are more details on injuries in the same body region, more age subdivisions and the use of emergency room acute physiology details rather than field values. ASCOT predicts survival better than TRISS particularly for blunt injury. Reluctance to use ASCOT derives from increased complexity for only a modest gain in predictive value.[45,46]

APPLICATION OF SCORING SYSTEMS

The introduction of scoring systems has brought some standardization and a new language that allows clinicians to relatively accurately describe their case mix. Such descriptions have led to numerous potential uses including:

- stratification of patients for clinical trials
- comparison of predicted and observed outcomes
- relating resource usage to severity of illness at presentation

Decision making based on the predictions of scoring systems is widely considered an inappropriate use because such systems are intrinsically flawed for use for individual patients. The logistic regression equations provide a probability for a dichotomous event, such as death or survival and not certainty, and therefore they have no potential use as a guide to further treatment or limitation orders for an individual. When APACHE II was tested against an identical case mix to that from which it was derived and used as a predictor of outcome for individuals, at best it had a misclassification rate of 15%.[9] The performance of these systems may be worse with different case mixes.[28–30]

Attempts to reduce misclassification for this have included recalibrating the APACHE II system[47] and the use of neural networks. Neural networks use ongoing patient data input to continually modify predictor equations. This approach theoretically gets closer and closer to predicting outcome for a specific case mix but never reaches certainty.

While it is important for humanitarian and economic reasons to recognize the hopelessly ill patient as early as possible, it is likely that patient management decisions will remain based on clinical judgement for the foreseeable future.

Although there are good reasons for not using severity score predictions to guide management, they can be used as a benchmark method and for stratifying comparable patient groups for clinical studies. This stratification is best based on estimates of risk of death.

Benchmark comparison of risk of death and outcome between intensive care units should be based on, some fundamental assumptions if ICU comparisons are to be robust :

- All pre ICU care is identical between hospitals and has no differential impact on ICU or hospital outcome
- Patients in the different hospitals are drawn from the same population (case mix)
- The samples are large enough to obey the mathematical principles of logistic regression calculations
- Data acquisition is both flawless with respect to the rules of the scoring system and consistent between units

Since these assumptions can rarely be made, comparisons between units can be misleading. SMR may be misleading for between hospital comparisons as a measure of ICU performance, but it remains a useful tool for within ICU comparisons where it is assumed many of the confounding factors are the same. In such circumstances, changes in ICU process or improvements prior to ICU admission while case mix remains the same may reveal themselves through improvements in SMR.

It is in such a context that scoring systems can contribute to patient management. A simple example is the reduction in secondary brain injury by use of GCS cutoff values for elective intubation and ventilation before transfer from the scene of injury.

Key points for clinical practice are indicated in Table 2.2.

Table 2.2   Key points for clinical practice

- Although hospital mortality is the end-point used in the three main scoring systems, morbidity is at least as useful but more difficult to measure
- Physiological variables reflect illness severity, but prone to bias from the effect of immediate pre critical care management and errors in data collection
- The receiver operator characteristic curve quantifies a model's ability to discriminate between survivors and nonsurvivors. Most have misclassification errors of 10–15%. Calibration estimated by goodness of fit tests indicates the suitability of the model for a particular case mix
- Standardized Mortality Ratios (SMR) reflect the whole process of care from hospital admission to discharge; critical care is a part of that process.
- Standardized mortality ratios are useful for measuring within critical care unit efficacy of care but should be used cautiously for between unit comparison where case mix may be different.
- Mortality risk estimates are useful for establishing comparability of patient groups in clinical trials
- At present, scoring systems are not sufficiently accurate to make outcome predictions for individual patients

REFERENCES

1 Breasted J. *The Edwin Smith Papyrus*. Chicago: University of Chicago; 1930.
2 Cullen DJ, Civetta JM, Briggs BA, Ferrara LC. Therapeutic intervention scoring system: a method for quantitative comparison of patient care. *Crit Care Med* 1974; **2**: 57–60.
3 Knaus WA, Zimmerman JE, Wagner DP, *et al.* APACHE-acute physiology and chronic health evaluation: a physiologically based classification system. *Crit Care Med* 1981; **9**: 591–7.
4 Sage W, Rosenthal M, Silverman J. Is intensive care worth it? An assessment of input and outcome for the critically ill. *Crit Care Med* 1986; **14**: 777–82.
5 Connors AF, Dawson NV, Thomas C *et al.* Outcomes following acute exacerbation of severe chronic obstructive lung disease. The SUPPORT investigators (Study to Understand Prognoses and Preferences for Outcomes and Risks of Treatments). *Am J Respir Crit Care Med* 1996; **154**: 959–67.
6 Hamel MB, Goldman L, Teno J, *et al.* Identification of comatose patients at high risk for death or severe disability. SUPPORT Investigators. (Study to Understand Prognoses and Preferences for Outcomes and Risks of Treatments). *JAMA* 1995; **273**: 1842–8.
7 Ridley S, Plenderleith L. Survival after intensive care. Comparison with a matched normal population as an indicator of effectiveness. *Anaesthesia* 1994; **49**: 933–5.
8 Le Gall JR, Loirat P, Alperovitch A, *et al.* A simplified acute physiology score for ICU patients. *Crit Care Med* 1984; **12**: 975–7.
9 Knaus WA, Draper EA, Wagner DP, Zimmerman JE. APACHE II: a severity of disease classification system. *Crit Care Med* 1985; **13**: 818–29.
10 Lemeshow S, Teres D, Klar J, *et al.* Mortality Probability Models (MPM II) based on an international cohort of intensive care unit patients. *JAMA* 1993; **270**: 2478–86.
11 Bion JF, Aitchison TC, Edlin SA, Ledingham IM. Sickness scoring and response to treatment as predictors of outcome from critical illness. *Intensive Care Med* 1988; **14**: 167–72.
12 Chang RW, Jacobs S, Lee B. Predicting outcome among intensive care unit patients using computerised trend analysis of daily Apache II scores corrected for organ system failure. *Intensive Care Med* 1988; **14**: 558–66.
13 Knaus WA, Draper EA, Wagner DP, Zimmerman JE. Prognosis in acute organ-system failure. *Ann Surg* 1985; **202**: 685–93.
14 Lemeshow S, Klar J, Teres D, *et al.* Mortality probability models for patients in the intensive care unit for 48 or 72 hours: a prospective, multicenter study. *Crit Care Med* 1994; **22**: 1351–8.
15 Le Gall JR, Lemeshow S, Saulnier F. A new Simplified Acute Physiology Score (SAPS II) based on a European/North American multicenter study. *JAMA* 1993; **270**: 2957–63.
16 Bastos PG, Sun X, Wagner DP, *et al.* Application of the APACHE III prognostic system in Brazilian

intensive care units: a prospective multicenter study. *Intensive Care Med* 1996; **22**: 564–70.

17 Lemeshow S, Hosmer DW Jr. A review of goodness of fit statistics for use in the development of logistic regression models. *Am J Epidemiol* 1982; **115**: 92–106.

18 Teasdale G, Jennett B. Assessment of coma and impaired consciousness. A practical scale. *Lancet* 1974; **2**: 81–4.

19 Teasdale G, Jennett B. Assessment and prognosis of coma after head injury. *Acta Neurochir (Wien)* 1976; **34**: 45–55.

20 Teasdale G, Knill Jones R, van der Sande J. Observer variability in assessing impaired consciousness and coma. *J Neurol Neurosurg Psychiatry* 1978; **41**: 603–10.

21 Reilly PL, Simpson DA, Sprod R, Thomas L. Assessing the conscious level in infants and young children: a paediatric version of the Glasgow Coma Scale. *Childs Nerv Syst* 1988; **4**: 30–3.

22 Keene A, Cullen D. Therapeutic Intervention Scoring System: update 1983. *Crit Care Med* 1983; **11**: 1–3.

23 Miranda DR, de Rijk A, Schaufeli W. Simplified Therapeutic Intervention Scoring System: the TISS-28 items – results from a multicenter study. *Crit Care Med* 1996; **24**: 64–73.

24 Knaus WA, Wagner DP, Draper EA, *et al*. The APACHE III prognostic system. Risk prediction of hospital mortality for critically ill hospitalized adults. *Chest* 1991; **100**: 1619–36.

25 Chu DY. Predicting survival in AIDS patients with respiratory failure. Application of the APACHE II scoring system. *Crit Care Clin* 1993; **9**: 89–105.

26 Vassar MJ, Holcroft JW. The case against using the APACHE system to predict intensive care unit outcome in trauma patients. *Crit Care Clin* 1994; **10**: 117–26.

27 Castella X, Artigas A, Bion J, Kari A. A comparison of severity of illness scoring systems for intensive care unit patients: results of a multicenter, multinational study. The European/North American Severity Study Group. *Crit Care Med* 1995; **23**: 1327–35.

28 Metnitz PG, Lang T, Vesely H, *et al*. Ratios of observed to expected mortality are affected by differences in case mix and quality of care. *Intensive Care Med* 2000; **26**: 1466–72.

29 Murphy Filkins R, Teres D, Lemeshow S, Hosmer DW. Effect of changing patient mix on the performance of an intensive care unit severity-of-illness model: how to distinguish a general from a specialty intensive care unit. *Crit Care Med* 1996; **24**: 1968–73.

30 Ridley S. Severity of illness scoring systems and performance appraisal. *Anaesthesia* 1998; **53**: 1185–94.

31 Lemeshow S, Teres D, Pastides H, *et al*. A method for predicting survival and mortality of ICU patients using objectively derived weights. *Crit Care Med* 1985; **13**: 519–25.

32 Lemeshow S, Teres D, Avrunin JS, Gage RW. Refining intensive care unit outcome prediction by using chang-

ing probabilities of mortality. *Crit Care Med* 1988; **16**: 470–7.

33 Marshall JC, Cook DJ, Christou NV, *et al*. Multiple organ dysfunction score: a reliable descriptor of a complex clinical outcome. *Crit Care Med* 1995; **23**: 1638–52.

34 Vincent JL, de Mendonca A, Cantraine F, *et al*. Use of the SOFA score to assess the incidence of organ dysfunction/failure in intensive care units: results of a multicenter, prospective study. Working group on 'sepsis-related problems' of the European Society of Intensive Care Medicine. *Crit Care Med* 1998; **26**: 1793–800.

35 Vincent JL, Moreno R, Takala J, *et al*. The SOFA (Sepsis-related Organ Failure Assessment) score to describe organ dysfunction/failure. On behalf of the Working Group on Sepsis-Related Problems of the European Society of Intensive Care Medicine. *Intensive Care Med* 1996; **22**: 707–10.

36 Le Gall JR, Klar J, Lemeshow S, *et al*. The Logistic Organ Dysfunction system. A new way to assess organ dysfunction in the intensive care unit. ICU Scoring Group. *JAMA* 1996; **276**: 802–10.

37 Baker SP. The injury severity score: a method for describing patients with multiple injuries and evaluating emergency care. *J Trauma* 1974; **14**: 187–96.

38 American Association for Advancement of Automotive Medicine. *The Abbreviated Injury Scale. 1990 Revision*. Arlington Heights, IL: American Association for Advancement of Automotive Medicine; 1990

39 Champion HR, Sacco WJ, Carnazzo AJ, *et al*. Trauma score. *Crit Care Med* 1981; **9**: 672–6.

40 Champion HR, Sacco WJ, Copes WS, *et al*. A revision of the Trauma Score. *J Trauma* 1989; **29**: 623–9.

41 Champion HR, Copes WS, Sacco WJ, *et al*. The Major Trauma Outcome Study: establishing national norms for trauma care. *J Trauma* 1990; **30**: 1356–65.

42 Boyd CR, Tolson MA, Copes WS. Evaluating trauma care: the TRISS method. Trauma Score and the Injury Severity Score. *J Trauma* 1987; **27**: p. 370–8.

43 Baker S, O'Neill B. The Injury Severity Score: an update. *J Trauma* 1976; **16**: 882–5.

44 Champion HR, Copes WS, Sacco WJ, *et al*. A new characterization of injury severity. *J Trauma* 1990; **30**: 539–45.

45 Champion HR, Copes WS, Sacco WJ, *et al*. Improved predictions from a severity characterization of trauma (ASCOT) over Trauma and Injury Severity Score (TRISS): results of an independent evaluation. *J Trauma* 1996; **40**: 42–8.

46 Markle J, Cayten CG, Byrne DW, *et al*. Comparison between TRISS and ASCOT methods in controlling for injury severity. *J Trauma* 1992; **33**: 326–32.

47 Rowan KM, Kerr JH, Major E, *et al*. Intensive Care Society's Acute Physiology and Chronic Health Evaluation (APACHE II) study in Britain and Ireland: a prospective, multicenter, cohort study comparing two methods for predicting outcome for adult intensive care patients. *Crit Care Med* 1994; **22**: 1392–401.

APPENDICES

Effect of prevalence of death (casemix) on predictive valves.

Appendix 1   Calculations of sensitivity and specificity for a prediction model for mortality

	Observed deaths	Observed alive	Total
Predicted deaths	450	100	550
Predicted alive	40	410	450
Total	490	510	1000

Sensitivity; the proportion of observed deaths that are predicted correctly (i.e. true positive).
   Sensitivity = 450/(490) = 0.92
Specificity; the proportion alive that are predicted to be alive (i.e. true negative).
   Specificity = 410/(510) = 0.80
1 – specificity is proportion alive predicted to be dead (i.e. false positive).
   Positive predictive value observed deaths as % of predicted
   deaths = 450/(550) = 0.82
   Negative predictive value observed alive as % of predicted to
   live = 410/(450) = 0.91
   Misclassification rate is the proportion of patients wrongly predicted
   (100 + 40)/1000 = 14%
   Correct classification rate is the proportion of patients correctly
   predicted = 450 + 410/1000 = 86%
   False positive rate = 100% – positive predictive value = 18%
   False negative value = 100% – negative predictive value = 9%
   Prevalence of death 490/1000 = 49%

Appendix 2   The effect of a 50% reduction of prevalence of death on sensitivity and specificity

	Observed deaths	Observed alive	Total
Predicted deaths	225	148	373
Predicted alive	20	607	627
Total	245	755	1000

Sensitivity = 225/(245) = 0.92
Specificity = 607/(755) = 0.80
Positive predictive value = 225/(373) = 0.60
Negative predictive value = 607/(627) = 0.97
Misclassification rate (148 + 20)/1000 = 16.8%
Correct classification rate = 225 + 607/1000 = 83.2%
False positive rate = 40%
False negative value = 3%

Appendix 3   Summary of effect of prevalence of death in an ICU population on predictive values

Prevalence of death	49%	24.5%
Sensitivity	0.92	0.92
Specificity	0.80	0.82
Positive predictive value	0.82	0.60
Negative predictive value	0.91	0.97
False positive rate	18	40
False negative rate	9	3
Correct classification	86	83.2
Misclassification rate	14	16.8

3.

Transport of the critically ill

E Everest and B Munford

All intensive care units (ICUs) are required to move critically ill patients for investigations or procedures that cannot be performed in the ICU. These patients have reduced or absent physiological reserves and even short trips can result in significant adverse events.[1,2] These events can be reduced by the use of trained personnel.[3,4]

In addition, ICU personnel are frequently involved in the stabilization and transfer of critically ill patients into an ICU,[5] while some units may be involved in the transport of patients from the site of a pre-hospital incident, or between hospitals.[6,7] The inter-hospital transfer could be due to the increasing sophistication of critical care facilities in tertiary hospitals compared with district or rural hospitals, different subspecialty capabilities, local bed shortages[3] or, in certain health systems, for insurance or financial reasons. In some cases, the complexity of these inter-hospital transfers can be further complicated by the need for rapid transport, or the distances involved. All patient movement is associated with an increase in mortality or morbidity, but with an integrated approach using high level clinical personnel who have the correct equipment and undertake sufficient planning, adverse events can be reduced.[3,4,6–8] Regular ambulances or untrained hospital staff should not be expected to manage ICU patients. Compared with specialist transport teams, standard ambulances with junior doctor escorts are associated with more cases of hypotension, acidosis and death.[9]

The hospital of the future has been described as the critical care hub of a dispersed network of facilities linked by information systems and critical care transport services.[10] Critical Care transport should be part of a regional intensive care network and adhere to promulgated minimum standards for transport of the critically ill.[11,12]

INTER-HOSPITAL TRANSPORT

The general principles of patient transport regarding equipment, patient monitoring and checking after movement are identical, whether intra-hospital or inter-hospital. In inter-hospital transport the same problems are encountered but compounded by distance and the vehicular environment.

Patients are moved from the ICU for generally two reasons: (i) diagnostic imaging that cannot be performed in the ICU, and (ii) for procedures, traditionally the operating theatre, but increasingly for radiologically guided procedures including vascular embolization, angioplasty, percutaneous drainage and stent insertion.

Moving an ICU patient is a high-risk procedure but with sufficient planning and preparation there should be little or no compromise to his or her condition. Unfortunately, this is not always achieved, as there are often a number of distractions that will divert staff from monitoring the patient, or disconnection of infusions or ventilation. In up to 70% of ICU patient transports, adverse events occur, of which:

- one-third are equipment related[13]
- acute deterioration of PaO_2/FIO_2 ratio is common
- ventilator associated pneumonia is significantly increased.[14,15]

However management is changed in 40–50% of patients, thus justifying the risk. Sufficient notification will allow the assembly of equipment, monitoring and sufficient staff who are trained and familiar with the equipment and the patient. The more complex the patient, the more capable the team required. In unstable patients the minimum team should consist of a suitably trained doctor (e.g. one capable of re-intubating a ventilated patient and able to manage any changes occurring in the patient's condition), the patient's nurse and two assistants to move the bed and help to lift the patient. For more stable, less complicated patients the patient's nurse and assistants may be sufficient.

CT SCANNING

The most common diagnostic investigations necessitating transport is computerized tomography (CT). On most occasions very little planning and preparation is required for what is almost a routine procedure. The exceptions are patients with head injuries and the administration of nasogastric contrast and the increased aspiration risk in patients with decreased gastric motility. Repeated CT scanning of head injury patients is common.

In those patients with decreased cerebral compliance, movement and changes in body position or Pa_{CO_2} can result in marked changes in intracranial pressure (ICP). Prior to transport, Et_{CO_2} should be measured on the transport monitor while the patient remains connected to the ICU ventilator. ICP changes caused by ventilator induced variations in Pa_{CO_2} when switching to the transport ventilator can be reduced by adjusting the minute volume to maintain a stable Et_{CO_2} Adequate sedation will also decrease movement induced rises in ICP. Ideally, the ICP should be measured on the transport monitor but this is often not possible. Whether a staff member remains in the scanner room or views the patient and monitor from outside depends on patient stability. Radiation exposure, is small and is not considered a risk, and depends on where personnel stand in relation to the scanner's 'doughnut', from where the radiation is emitted.

MRI SCANNING

The hazards to a patient in MRI are greater due to limitations in the proximity of infusion pumps, ventilators and monitors to the magnet, and at times on catheters and pacemakers inserted in the patient. The need for the MRI needs to be balanced with the information likely to be gained. The three main problems with transport equipment are:

- metal objects becoming projectiles when in close proximity to the magnet
- equipment interfering with the MRI
- the MRI causing failures in transport equipment.

MRI units vary in policy, from prohibiting any equipment in the room to having minimal equipment that is placed as far away from the magnet as possible. The ability of ventilators and infusion pumps to function in the MRI scan room must have been tested prior to any patient being scanned, as some modern transport ventilators have failed in the MRI. Ideally, the equipment should be left outside the room with extensions added to the infusion and ventilator tubing, but this increases the risk of disconnection. There is one reported case of the external part of a pulmonary artery catheter burning through during an MRI scan,[16] probably caused by the development of RF eddy currents. Thermodilution pulmonary artery catheters are probably safe, but although patients with internal defibrillators and permanent pacemakers have been scanned with no consequence, deaths have been reported. Prior discussion with individual MRI units on how ICU patients can be scanned is required.

INTER-HOSPITAL TRANSPORT

ORGANIZATIONAL ASPECTS

Provision of critical care transport services needs to be a part of regional ICU services. The staffing of critical care

transport teams will depend on the workload, with around 300 per year, being the threshold for a specific transport roster, depending on transport duration and regulations affecting duty times. Other factors include regional demographics, resources and geography. A team from within that unit, or from another ICU, or an emergency department, or a stand-alone transport service may provide transport of patients to a particular ICU. The merits of each system have been summarized recently.[17] Whatever arrangement is chosen, staff should not be conscripts but selected from those interested in critical care transport, and should be appropriately trained. Use of junior inexperienced staff is associated with increases in preventable mortality and morbidity.[18,19] Rostering of teams needs to be appropriate for the workload and take into account the potential for significant overtime hours when urgent requests occur near shift changeovers. If personnel are also allocated to other clinical duties, they need to be readily relieved when required. Equipment should be prechecked and the team should have a practised routine to enable prompt departure

A co-ordination centre should be used in systems involving multiple requests and transport teams.

PERSONNEL

The aim of the transport team is to at least maintain but preferably enhance the level of care. This requires transport teams to have diagnostic and procedural skills to provide the full complement of care for the full range of patients transported. Ideally, the personnel caring for the patient in transit should be equivalent to the 'front line' clinical team at the destination, implying a physician based team, although transport of well-stabilized patients by non-physician teams has been reported.[20]

The transport team should be a minimum of two people. For multiple patients a formula of $n+1$ personnel for n critical patients has been suggested.[21] Multidisciplinary teams of physicians, nurse and/or ambulance officers offer advantages of a wider range of skills and training than a team from any single profession. In certain circumstances, other specialized staff may need to be taken, for example a surgeon or obstetrician.[6] It is preferable and safer to add a specialist to the standard team because of the latter's familiarity with the practicalities of the transport environment. Other desirable attributes in staff include: good teamwork and communication skills; adaptability; reasonable body habitus and physical condition; and no significant visual or auditory impairment or susceptibility to motion sickness. Travel sickness medications such as hyoscine (scopolamine) are of limited value, needing to be taken up to 4 hours pre-transport and may cause significant side-effects.[22]

Training should encompass:

- principles and practicalities of clinical care in transport
- vehicle familiarization

- relevant communication, safety and emergency procedures.

Staff should have:

- appropriate personal protective equipment
- lightweight fireproof overalls or other clothing
- uniforms for pre-hospital responses, which should be of high visibility and bear identification.

PATIENT SELECTION

The best utilization of a critical care transport system is when it is activated for appropriate patients, which will depend on the levels of care available within the ambulance services. The need for critical care transport may be identified by:

- a diagnosis with the potential to deteriorate
- the requirement for physiological monitoring and acute interventions
- the continuation of treatment already instituted during transport.

Both receiving hospitals and ambulance services need to be alert to possible cases where critical care transport is indicated, but not identified by the referring team. A mechanism that is highly sensitive and specific at identifying patients unsuitable for standard ambulance transport is required. Triage mechanisms and tables to aid in patient selection have been described.[23,24]

COMMUNICATIONS

A systematic approach is necessary to ensure a smooth response when the need for transport of a critically ill patient is identified. A single toll-free telephone number with conference call capability is the ideal. Facsimile and teleradiology capabilities may also be of value. The one call for assistance should result in the provision of clinical advice if required, the dispatch of a transport team, and finding a bed in an appropriate hospital. Concise, simple clinical advice appropriate for the capabilities of the referring hospital by either the receiving hospital or the transport service is paramount. No matter how fast the transport team's response, without some interim care the patient with major airway, breathing or circulatory compromise will not survive.[6,7] Ongoing advice including stabilization and preparation of the patient for transport may be required prior to the arrival of the transport team. The provision to referring hospitals of a checklist for patient management and preparation for transport may assist.

The transport team should communicate with the receiving hospital, especially where changes in the patient's condition change the time of arrival, post-transport management or destination within the hospital or to another centre. Cellular telephones have revolutionized communication in transit, but their use may not be possible in all circumstances. Radio communication between ground and air ambulances and relevant hospitals is a preferred backup.

EQUIPMENT

GENERAL CONSIDERATIONS

Minimum standards for supplies, equipment and monitoring for critical care transport have been developed.[10,17] Equipment selection is a compromise between providing for every conceivable scenario and being mobile. The aim should be to have a core set of equipment plus optional items for specific scenarios plus some backup redundancy for vital supplies and equipment such as oxygen, airway devices, and basic circulatory monitoring. A suggested equipment schedule is appended in Table 3.1. Meticulous checking of equipment after each use and on a regular basis is essential.

Transport monitors, infusion pumps and ventilators must work outside the transport vehicle. This requires equipment to be battery powered and readily portable. Although newer monitors and other devices have rechargeable batteries with improved endurance, problems can still occur. The equipment checking process includes different charging regimes. Nickel cadmium (NiCad) batteries need to be fully discharged before recharging to decrease memory effect, which reduces endurance, whereas sealed lead–acid or lithium batteries perform best when continually charged between uses.[25]

Internal batteries should not be relied upon unless transport duration is less than half the estimated battery life. For longer trips, a supplementary power source from either an external battery pack or the transport vehicle should be available to reduce battery use or even charge the batteries. An external supply combined with a wiring harness to run and recharge internal batteries on all devices is preferable. Spare batteries are not ideal, as many devices are not amenable to rapid 'on the job' battery swaps without interruption of monitoring and therapy.

Portability can be addressed in two ways. Equipment can be vehicle mounted but readily detachable to accompany the patient, either as individual devices or more conveniently as a modular unit.[26] Alternatively, a mobile intensive care module can be incorporated into the stretcher; either in the base[27] or as a 'stretcher bridge' straddling the patient.[28] Such designs are now widely used and allow the patient and equipment to be assembled into one unit at the referral point; this reduces loading and unloading time, ventilator and other device disconnections, and the risk of leaving equipment behind. Minor disadvantages include the increase in weight (25–30 kg), with corresponding reduction in maximum patient weight; and slight top heaviness of the stretcher/patient combination.

MONITORING

Clinical observation by experienced personnel remains the mainstay of monitoring,[10] but some clinical assessments such as auscultation are impossible during transit. Hence monitoring by appropriate equipment should be at the same or higher level than what the patient receives in the stationary setting. Referring institutions should

Table 3.1 Suggested equipment schedule for inter-hospital critical care transport

RESPIRATORY EQUIPMENT

Intubation kit:
  Endotracheal tubes & connectors – adult & paediatric sizes
  Introducers, bougies, Magill forceps
  Laryngoscopes, blades, spare globes & batteries
  Ancillaries: cuff syringe & manometer, clip forceps,
  'gooseneck' tubing, HME/filter(s), securing ties, lubricant
Alternative airways:
  Simple: Guedel & nasopharyngeal
  Supraglottic: laryngeal masks &/or Combitube
  Infraglottic: cricothyrotomy kit & tubes
Oxygen masks (including high FiO_2 type), tubing, nebulizers
Suction equipment:
  Main suction system – usually vehicle mounted
  Spare (portable) suction – hand, O_2, or battery powered
  Suction tubing, handles, catheters & spare reservoir

Self-inflating hand ventilator, with masks & PEEP valve
Portable ventilator with disconnect & overpressure alarms
Ventilator circuit & spares
Spirometer & cuff manometer
Capnometer/capnograph.
Pleural drainage equipment:
  Intercostal catheters & cannulae
  Surgical insertion kit & sutures (see below)
  Heimlich type valves & drainage bags
Main oxygen system (usually vehicle mounted) of adequate
  capacity with flowmeters and standard wall outlets
Portable/reserve oxygen system with flowmeter & std outlet

CIRCULATORY EQUIPMENT

Defibrillator/monitor/external pacemaker, with leads, electrodes
  & pads
i.v. fluid administration equipment:
  Range of fluids: isotonic crystalloid, dextrose, colloids
  High flow & metered flow giving sets
  i.v. cannulae in range of sizes: peripheral & central/long lines
  i.v. extension sets, 3 way taps & needle free injection system
  Syringes, needles & drawing up cannulae
  Skin preparation wipes, i.v. dressings & bandaids
  Pressure infusion bags (for arterial line also)

Blood pressure monitoring equipment:
  Arterial cannulae with arterial tubing & transducers
  Invasive & non-invasive (automated) BP pressure monitors
  Aneroid (non-mercury) sphygmomanometer & range of
    cuffs (preferably compatible with NIBP also)
Pulse oximeter, with finger & multi-site probes
Syringe/infusion pumps (minimum 2) & appropriate tubing

MISCELLANOUS EQUIPMENT

Urinary catheters & drainage/measurement bag
Gastric tubes & drainage bag
Minor surgical kit (for ICC, CV lines, cricothyrotomy, etc):
  Sterile instruments: scalpels, scissors, forceps, needle holders
  Suture material & needles
  Antiseptics, skin preparation packs & dressings
  Sterile gloves (various sizes); drapes +/− gowns
Cervical collars, spinal immobilization kit, splints
Pneumatic anti-shock garment (MAST suit)

Thermometer (non-mercury) &/or temperature probe/monitor
Reflective (space) blanket & thermal insulation drapes
Bandages, tapes, heavy duty scissors (shears)
Gloves and eye protection
Sharps & contaminated waste receptacles
Pen & folder for paperwork
Torch +/− head light.
Drug/additive labels & marker pen
Nasal decongestant (for barotitis prophylaxis)

PHARMACOLOGICAL AGENTS

CNS drugs:
  Narcotics +/− non narcotic analgesics
  Anxiolytics/sedatives
  Major tranquillizers
  Anticonvulsants
  i.v. Hypnotics/anaesthetic agents
  Antiemetics
  Local anaesthetics
Cardiovascular drugs:
  Antiarrhythmics
  Anticholinergics
  Inotropes/vasoconstrictors
  Nitrates
  α & β blockers; other hypotensives
Electrolytes & renal agents:
  Sodium bicarbonate
  Calcium (chloride)
  Magnesium

  Potassium
  Loop diuretics
  Osmotic diuretics
Endocrine & metabolic agents:
  Glucose (concentrate) +/− glucagon
  Insulin
  Steroids
Other agents:
  Neuromuscular blockers: depolarizing & non-depolarizing
  Anticholinesterases (neuromuscular block reversal)
  Narcotic & benzodiazepine antagonists.
  Bronchodilators
  Antihistamines
  H_2 blockers/proton pump inhibitors
  Anticoagulants
  Thrombolytics
  Vitamin K

Table 3.1 *(cont'd)*

PHARMACOLOGICAL AGENTS *(cont'd)*	
Antibiotics	Tocolytics
Oxytocics	Diluents (saline & sterile water)

ADDITIONAL/OPTIONAL EQUIPMENT	
Transvenous temporary pacing kit & pacemaker	Additional paediatric equipment (depending on capability of basic kit)
Blood (usually O negative) &/or blood products	Antivenene (polyvalent or specific)
Additonal infusion pumps & associated i.v. sets	Specific drugs or antagonists
Obstetrics kit	

Intercostal catheter (ICC), Central venous (CV), Heat moisture exchanger (HME). For other abbreviations, see text.

not allow patients to be transported by teams with inferior monitoring capability. Compact transport monitors offering ECG, SpO_2, non-invasive and multi-channel invasive pressures, capnography and temperature monitoring have largely superseded older techniques, such as systolic pressure estimation by palpation and mean arterial pressure monitoring via an aneroid interface and gauge. These older techniques can still be used for backup, as can defibrillators for ECG, while small hand-held pulse oximeters and $EtCO_2$ detector are also available. Non-invasive blood pressure and pulse oximetry devices are susceptible to artefact[29,30] and the use of invasive arterial monitoring or shielding pulse oximetry probes may be required. Mercury-containing devices are unsuitable especially in aircraft. For longer transports, or patients with major biochemical or respiratory disturbances, compact biochemical and blood gas analysers may be valuable.[31]

VENTILATION AND RESPIRATORY SUPPORT

A mechanical ventilator should be used on all ventilated patients during transport. Manual ventilation occupies one team member fully and cannot reliably deliver constant tidal volumes and stable $EtCO_2$.[32] Transport ventilators are a compromise between portability and features.

Table 3.2 Features of an ideal transport ventilator[a]

- Small, light, robust, and cheap.
- Not dependent on external power source.
- Easy to use and clean, with foolproof assembly.
- Economical on gas consumption.
- Suitable for patients from neonates to large adults.
- FiO_2 continuously variable from ambient air to 100% oxygen.
- Able to deliver PEEP, CPAP, SIMV & pressure support.
- Variable I:E ratios
- Flow or pressure generator modes
- Integrated monitoring & alarm functions with audio & visual signals
- Altitude compensated

[a] For abbreviations, see text.

The characteristics of an ideal transport ventilator are outlined in Table 3.2. No currently available transport ventilator meets all of these, and different models are optimized for different scenarios, so selection of a transport ventilator should take into account likely clinical and operational requirements. Backup manual ventilation equipment must be available. In some cases of severe respiratory disease, a standard ICU ventilator may be needed. This may require medical air and AC power although newer hybrid ICU/transport ventilators can provide enhanced ventilation capability without supply of these.[33] Similar requirements will apply to transport of patients on extracorporeal membrane oxygenation.

The provision of continuous positive airways pressure (CPAP) in transport remains problematic. 'Clapper board' type systems are economical on gas consumption, but being gravity driven perform poorly during movement. Conventional CPAP systems have extremely high gas consumption, rendering them impractical except for short road transports. Electronically triggered CPAP is a feature of some newer transport ventilators; however, though they have been successfully used on occasions, poor performance with mask CPAP has been reported,[34] and some patients may need to be converted to SIMV or intermittent positive pressure ventilation (IPPV) for transport.

Maintenance of humidification of inspired gases is important during transport. In most cases, heat and moisture exchangers should provide adequate protection for intubated patients.[35] In special circumstances, for example, in neonates and cystic fibrosis patients, it may be necessary to use active humidification.

A suction system and preferably a reserve are needed during all phases of transport. These may be venturi systems, electrical powered pumps or manual aspirators. Oxygen venturi systems are lighter than electrical systems and outperform manual aspirators, but have high oxygen consumption, >40 l/min.[36]

INFUSIONS

Critically ill patients often have multiple drug infusions which need to be continued during transport.

A reduction in pumps may be obtained by combining sedation infusions or by suspending some infusions for transport and giving them as intermittent boluses.

During the referral process it is important to ascertain the number of infusions running to ensure sufficient pumps are taken. Modern lightweight syringe drivers are preferable for most infusions but a volumetric pump is superior if an infusion of large volumes of fluid is required. Older 'drop counting' type infusion pumps are susceptible to disruption by movement and ambient pressure change and should not be used. Infusion pressure bags should also be available to maintain i.v. flow rates, as only minimal elevation of fluid bags is possible in most transport vehicles.

MISCELLANEOUS EQUIPMENT

Transcutaneous pacing is adequate in an emergency, or during very short transports, but in other circumstances elective trans-venous pacing should be instituted. Equipment to institute or maintain other specialized therapy en route should be carried if required. In some cases situations such as with an intra-aortic balloon pump, the equipment may be bulky and can influence the selection of the transport vehicle.[37]

Heimlich or similar one-way flap valves for pleural drainage are essential, as underwater seal drainage systems are not suitable for transport, owing to the likelihood of tipping and/or syphoning. Equipment to maintain nasogastric, urinary, and wound drainage is also required.

MODE OF TRANSPORT

Three types of transport vehicles are commonly employed: road, aeroplane (fixed wing), and helicopter (rotary wing). Basic requirements for critical care transport vehicles are listed in Table 3.3. Ideally, dedicated vehicles for all transport modes should be used, but the workload may not justify this and often vehicles that can be readily converted for mobile ICU use are seconded as required. The mode of transport depends on distances involved between referring and receiving hospitals and transport team locations; also the urgency of the case, which is often influenced by the clinical capability of the referring centre. Guidelines for vehicle utilization should be developed but should have some flexibility for special circumstances e.g. workload, traffic congestion, weather. Features and limitations of different modes of transport are summarized in Table 3.4.

ROAD TRANSPORT

The ground ambulance remains the most commonly used critical care vehicle. With patients for whom time is not critical and level of care in transit is more important than speed, road transport over considerable distances is feasible and may be safer in some patient groups.[38]

Table 3.3 Essential features of transport vehicles

- Readily available
- Adequate operational safety
- Capable of carrying (at least one) stretcher and mobile intensive care equipment set
- Safe seating for full medical team, including at head and side of patient
- Adequate space and patient access for observation & procedures
- Equipped with adequate supply of oxygen/other gases for duration of transport
- Fitted with medical power supply of appropriate voltage and current capacity
- Appropriate speed (coupled with) comfortable ride, without undue exposure to accelerations in any axis
- Acceptable noise and vibration levels
- Adequate cabin lighting, ventilation and climate control.
- Fitted with overhead i.v. hooks, and sharps/biohazard waste receptacles
- Straightforward embarkation & disembarkation of patient and team
- Fitted with appropriate radios and mobile telephone

FIXED WING TRANSPORT

Conventional aircraft are the most suitable for long-range transport. Their faster speed is offset by the secondary ambulance transport at both ends. Advantages over helicopters include pressurized cabins (in most models), decreased cabin noise compared with helicopters and the ability to fly in icing conditions.

ROTARY WING TRANSPORT

Helicopters remain the most controversial, high profile and expensive vehicles which require significant internal adaptations by clinical teams to enable them to perform patient care. Smaller helicopters are relatively or totally unsuitable as air ambulances. Appropriate helicopters are versatile vehicles, with the ability to perform transport both inside and beyond their 50–300 km optimum range 'doughnut'. Maximum value is obtained with a high workload, ensuring efficient clinical team utilization and between hospitals with on-site helipads to avoid secondary transport.

SAFETY AND TRAINING

Transport by any mode involves risk to staff and patients, and also imposes limitations on the delivery of care. In the aeromedical environment unfamiliar personnel perform clinical tasks poorly,[39] so teams must be appropriately trained and equipped to function effectively and safely in each mode of transport. They need to be familiar with use of the various transport vehicles' oxygen, suction, medical power, communications systems, and other equipment and stores. A senior member of their own professional group should train and accompany new personnel for several missions. Other specialist staff added to a team should receive a thorough safety brief

Table 3.4   Properties of transport vehicles

	Road	Helicopter	Fixed wing
Launch time	3–5 min	5–10 min (more if IFR)	30–60 min
Speed	10–120 km/h dependent on roads & traffic	120–150 knots (220–290 km/h), straight line	140–180 knots (piston) 230–270 knots (turboprop) 375–460 knots (jet)
Secondary transport	Not applicable	Sometimes	Inevitable
Effective range	0–100 km (longer if required)	50–300 km (longer or shorter in special cases)	200–2000 km
Noise	Low, except at high speed	Moderate to high (headsets required)	Low to moderate (cruise). Higher on takeoff/landing
Vibrations	Variable with speed & road surface	Moderate in most phases (varies with rotor type)	Low in cruise, moderate or high on takeoff/landing
Accelerations	Variable and sometimes unpredictable in all axes	Minimal & usually vertical only	Significant (fore/aft) on takeoff & landing
Special features	Base vehicles readily available	Versatility; point to point capability	Cabin pressurization & all weather capability (most)
Acquisition cost	Lowest	High (US$1–4.5 million new) depending on capabilities	Moderate (piston) to very high (jet)
Operating costs (per km)	Intermediate	Intermediate to high	Low to intermediate

and work under the direction of regular transport team members. Aeromedical crew training should encompass safety equipment, crash response, emergency egress and survival. Safety should be a foremost consideration in any transport. Activities that compromise road and air safety such as hazardous driving or flying below safe minima are not acceptable, and clinical teams must avoid attempting to coerce drivers or pilots to take risks. This has been recognized as a contributor to air ambulance accidents.[40]

ALTITUDE AND TRANSPORT PHYSIOLOGY

All transport modes result in increased noise, vibration, turbulence and accelerations in various or all axes (see Table 3.4). Personnel need to be aware of altitude-related complications that can occur with air transport. Increasing altitude results in decreasing oxygen partial pressure in accordance with Dalton's Law; while gas volumes increase or where volume change is restricted relative increases in pressure occur in accordance with Boyle's Law (see Table 3.5). Good introductory[41,42] and more detailed[43,44] aviation physiology texts are available.

OXYGENATION AND HYPOXIA

Critical patients who are already dependent on an increased FIO_2 will be compromised by reduction in atmospheric pressure. Further oxygen supplementation will be required to maintain arterial PaO_2. Only in special or unexpected circumstances, for example, alpine helicopter

operations or cabin decompression, would hypoxia be expected to affect the medical crew; however, they should be aware of the risk and alert to symptoms. The manifestations of hypoxia are well described elsewhere.[37–40]

GAS EXPANSION

Expansion of trapped gases can manifest in (a) physiological air spaces, (b) pathological air spaces, and (c) air-containing equipment.

The first category includes the middle ear, nasal sinuses, and the gastrointestinal tract. These manifestations can affect crew as well as patients; consequently staff with upper respiratory tract infections or gastrointestinal disturbances should not fly.

The second category includes pneumothoraces, emphysematous lung cysts or bullae, intraocular or intracranial air from open injuries, bowel obstruction or rupture, and gas emboli. Such patients should be transported at the lowest possible cabin or ambient altitude, with close monitoring and extreme care, especially on the ascent phase. The effect of trapped gas expansion can be reduced with denitrogenation by breathing 100% O_2 before and during flight.

Air-containing equipment includes: endotracheal and tracheostomy tube cuffs; Sengstaken–Blakemore tubes; pulmonary artery catheter balloons; air splints, pneumatic antishock garments (MAST suit) and pleural, gastric and some wound drainage bags. Endotracheal cuff pressures need to be adjusted during flight, or filled

Table 3.5 Changes with altitude

Altitude (feet)	Pressure (mmHg)	Alveolar Po_2		Gas space expansion	Std Temp (°Celcius)	Notes
		(on air)	(100% O_2)			
Sea Level	760	103	663	–	15	15°C is 'reference' average temp – actual obviously varies.
1000	733	98	636	+3.6%	13	Minimum altitude above ground level for helicopter transports
2000	706	94	609	+8%	11	Likely altitude for most (VFR) helicopter flights over sea level terrain
3000	681	89	584	+12%	9	Likely range of cabin altitude for standard flights in most turboprop air ambulance craft (e.g. Raytheon–Beech King Air series)
4000	656	85	559	+16%	7	
7000	586	73	489	+29%	1	Standard cabin altitude for airliners & most jet air ambulances (e.g. Lear 35)
10 000	523	61	426	+45%	−5	Likely ceiling of helicopter operations & hypoxic threshold in normal individuals
15 000	429	45	332	+77	−14.5	Threshold for hypoxic decompensation in non acclimatized individuals
20 000	349	34	252	+117	−24.5	Likely upper range of cruise altitude for turboprop aircraft. Decompression at these altitudes causes rapid loss of consciousness & death without O_2
25 000	282	30	185	+170	−34	
40 000	141	<10	61	+439	−56	Cruise ceiling for airliners & jets. Limit for survivable decompression, even with 100% O_2 for flight crew

with water. Increases in tidal volume in pneumatically controlled ventilators can occur with altitude, necessitating setting changes.[45]

CABIN PRESSURIZATION

Most fixed wing air ambulances have pressurized cabins, which decreases hypoxia and gas expansion. The pressurization creates a cabin pressure equivalent to flying at a lower altitude, hence the term 'cabin altitude'. The maximum pressure differential that can be generated depends on the aircraft model. Most turboprop air ambulances can provide around 350 mmHg (46.7 kPa) differential, or cabin altitude of 1000 m (3000 ft) while flying at 6500 m (20 000 ft). Once maximum differential has been achieved lower cabin altitude can only be provided by lower flight, which may be relatively or absolutely contraindicated – for example, a slower more turbulent flight or beneath lowest safe altitude, respectively. The medical team should not request a lower cabin altitude than what is required, with the final decision resting with the pilot. Failure of cabin pressurization is rare, but if sudden can have dramatic consequences, and teams should be aware of procedures to follow.

OTHER CONSIDERATIONS

Temperature falls by 2°C for every 300 m (1000 ft) altitude increase. Water partial pressure also falls and is not corrected by cabin pressurization. Respiratory and other exposed mucosa can become dehydrated and could eventually lead to systemic hypovolaemia. All intubated patients should have at least passive humidification. On prolonged journeys, staff may also be affected. Staff rostered for air transport should refrain from compressed gas diving for at least 24 hours prior to the shift.[46]

PATIENT PREPARATION FOR TRANSPORT

The preparation phase for transport will depend on the patient's diagnosis and condition. If possible, the patient should be stable; and efforts, which may include surgery, should be undertaken to obtain stability. The exception would be a patient requiring time-critical intervention at the receiving hospital. These transports are riskier, but are likely to be less futile than attempting to stabilize an inevitably deteriorating patient. All patients prior to any transport must have a secure airway, either self-maintained or intubated and ventilated, and intravenous access. Any external bleeding should be controlled.

Table 3.6 Suggested pre-departure checklists

A. BEFORE LEAVING HOSPITAL

Patient identity & next of kin	Recorded
Consent for transport	Obtained & documented
Paperwork & X-rays	Collected
Drugs for transport	Present & sufficient
Emergency drugs/equipment	Available
Medical equipment	Collected & repacked
Monitors, ventilator & infusions	Connected & on
Tubes, lines, drains & catheters	Secured
Altitude request (if applicable)	Passed to pilot
Receiving unit	Contacted & updated

B. IN VEHICLE & PRE-DEPARTURE

Stretcher & patient restraints	Secured & checked
Oxygen supply	On & sufficient
Monitors, ventilator & infusions	Working & secure
Emergency drugs/equipment	Stowed & accessible
Other medical packs	Stowed
i.v. fluids	Hung & running
i.v. injection port	Accessible
Medical power	On & connected
Communications	Checked as applicable
Seatbelts	On & checked
Staff/patient headsets	On/checked (if applicable)

Urgent investigations (e.g. X-rays, arterial blood gases) should be obtained where indicated, and possible in the time available. The patient should be secured on the stretcher and connected to ventilators and monitoring commensurate to the degree of stability and time constraints. Infusions should be rationalized and sedation may need to be increased during the trip.

Intercostal drains, if present or placed, should be connected to Heimlich type valves. If parenteral nutrition is discontinued, an appropriate dextrose infusion should be substituted, with interval blood glucose estimation.

Appropriate documentation including a referral letter, results of investigations and hospital and ambulance observations needs to accompany the patient. The team should ensure that any relevant legal requirements have been complied with and, where possible, consent for transport obtained.[47] The final step prior to transport should be a series of checks as listed in Table 3.6.

PATIENT CARE DURING TRANSPORT

If the patient is adequately prepared this phase should be uneventful. Special vigilance should be employed in the initial stages of movement, as this is the most likely time for either physiological decompensation, or technical problems such as disconnections to occur. Once in the transport vehicle, a further set of checks is advisable (see Table 3.6). Therapy, monitoring and documentation should continue during transport. Transported patients are vulnerable to hypothermia, especially if intubated and/or paralysed and/or receiving multiple infusions.[2,48] Active heating in-transit may be possible using the vehicle heating, while passive heat conservation should be practised during loading and unloading. Transport crews should be restrained during transport. If a critical event occurs necessitating the crew leaving their seats, the driver or pilot should be informed.

Death in transport should be a rare occurrence.[6,7] If it does occur, distance and the expectations and location of relatives should be taken into account in making the decision whether or not to continue transport to the destination. Carriage of relatives remains a controversial issue. For conscious patients, especially children, the presence of family members may have a beneficial effect. For unconscious patients it is less clear and needs to be balanced against space constraints in the mobile ICU vehicle, and the potential reaction of relatives in case of a critical event. Transport services should have policies in place both for carriage of relatives and for death in transit.

QUALITY ASSURANCE IN EDUCATION AND RESEARCH

Critical care transport is a recent development where accepted standards and guidelines are still evolving.[49] This means there is still considerable likelihood of problems, errors and critical incidents; with corresponding scope for research and quality improvement. This requires good clinical and operational data collection and patient outcomes. The process should be sensitive to the existence of system errors as well as individual patient, equipment or staff incidents. Preliminary results from the use of a critical incident monitoring system have been reported.[13] Users of the service must be informed of recommendations and system changes resulting from this process. Innovation and research by staff involved in this area should be encouraged.

SPECIAL TRANSPORT SITUATIONS

PERINATAL TRANSPORT

This encompasses both *in utero* and extrauterine transport of the neonate. Specialized neonatal teams normally perform neonatal transport.[50] Alternatively, part or all of the regular transport team may accompany specialist neonatal personnel. Neonatal transport stretchers are bulky and heavy, and require a vehicular power output of up to 250 W for the incubator and active humidifier as well as monitors, ventilator and infusion pumps. They also require a supply of medical air to allow precise regulation of FIO_2.[51] Transport of the pregnant patient carries the risk of precipitating labour, and in rare cases, delivery in transit.[52] This is suboptimal, especially where the baby is premature or otherwise at risk. Where labour cannot be suppressed, consideration should be given to delivery at the referring hospital, with subsequent neonatal and maternal transport.

TRANSPORT OF DIVING INJURY PATIENTS

Patients with decompression sickness or arterial gas embolus require expeditious transport to a recompression facility. This must be balanced against the risk of even small decreases in ambient pressure; even a 100 m (300 ft) increase in altitude can exacerbate pathogenesis.[42] Divers with other problems such as marine animal envenomation, or other medical conditions will still have increased total body nitrogen stores and can be at risk of developing evolved gas disorders during air transport. The use of transportable hyperbaric chambers has been reported[53] but their use severely compromises speed of response, and therapy possible in transit. Transport at or very near sea level cabin pressure on 100% oxygen is the usual procedure.

INTERNATIONAL AND LONG DISTANCE TRANSPORTS

International transport of critically ill patients is becoming increasingly common. There are often complex medical, social and economic factors to return a patient to their own medical system. These must be balanced against the immigration, visa, and logistic requirements, and medical problems of ultra-long distance transport.[54] A physician based team is less likely to have problems relating to drug carriage and status compared with a paramedical team. Logistic problems include carriage of sufficient supplies, and clinical staff to work shifts for prolonged transports. Pressure may be exerted to utilize cheaper regular passenger transport services instead of much more expensive air ambulances. Most international airlines will accept a stable seated patient; but there is considerable variation among airlines willing to carry stretcher patients and associated equipment. Such transports require considerable planning to arrange stretcher fitment and sufficient supplies of oxygen and electric power. A separate oxygen system for critical care transports is required as the aircraft's emergency oxygen system is not permitted for patient care and the oxygen systems for inflight use by passengers with medical conditions can only deliver up to 4 l/min.[50] Airline engineering clearance of medical equipment is often required. Aircraft power needs to be negotiated or sufficient batteries carried. An air ambulance may be indicated for cases that are urgent, infective or require low cabin altitude; whereas stable post myocardial patients can be safely transported in commercial aircraft with appropriate escorts.[55]

CRITICAL CARE SCENE RESPONSES

Critical care teams offer a wide range of measures to complement standard pre-hospital providers, especially for major trauma; including: sedative/relaxant assisted intubation; cricothyrotomy; tube thoracostomy; intravenous cutdown or central line insertion; and blood administration; as well as triage to an appropriate hospital.[56] These teams are useful only for trapped patients in the urban setting,[57] but combined with helicopter transport can improve outcomes in rural patients with blunt trauma.[56,58,59] In these situations the team should include an experienced pre-hospital provider. With appropriate activation the team may reach the patient at the scene or supplement management at the local hospital.

Critical care teams may also be of value in disaster situations.[60] Disaster medicine involves a change in emphasis to performing a small number of basic life-saving procedures on a large number of patients. Personnel with transport/pre-hospital experience are likely to be better trained and equipped to work at disaster scenes than traditional hospital disaster teams.[61] The order of priority remains the same as traditional critical care transport: triage, treatment, and then transport.

REFERENCES

1 Braman S, Dunn S, Amico CA, Millman RP. Complications of intrahospital transport in critically ill patients. *Ann Intern Med* 1987; **107**: 469–73.
2 Ridley S, Carter R. The effects of secondary transport on critically ill patients. *Anaesthesia* 1989; **44**: 822–7.
3 Duke GJ, Green JV. Outcome of critically ill patients undergoing interhospital transfer. *Med J Aust* 2001; **174**: 122–5
4 Edge WE, Kantar RK, Weigle CG, Walsh RF. Reduction of morbidity in interhospital transport by specialised paediatric staff. *Crit Care Med* 1994; **22**(1): 186–91.
5 Hourihan F, Bishop G, Hillman KM, *et al.* The Medical Emergency Team: a new strategy to identify and intervene in high risk patients. *Clin Int Care* 1995; **6**: 269–72.
6 Gilligan JE, Griggs WM, Jelly MT, *et al.* Mobile intensive care services in rural South Australia. *Med J Aust* 1999; **171**: 617–20.
7 Havill JH, Hyde PR, Forrest C. Transport of the critically ill: example of an integrated model. *NZ Med J* 1995; **108**: 378–380.
8 Flabouris A. Patient referral and transportation to a regional tertiary ICU: patient demographics, severity of illness and outcome comparison with non-transported patients. *Anaesth Intensive Care* 1999; **27**: 385–90.
9 Bellingan G, Olivier T, Batson S, Webb A. Comparison of a specialist retrieval team with current United Kingdom practice for the transport of critically ill patients. *Intensive Care Med* 2000; **26**: 740–4.
10 Goldsmith JC. The US health care system in the year 2000. *JAMA* 1986; **256**: 3371–5.
11 Faculty of Intensive Care, Australian and New Zealand College of Anaesthetists, and Australasian College of Emergency Medicine. Minimum Standards for Transport of the Critically Ill. Policy Document IC-10, 1996.
12 Commission on Accreditation of Medical Transport Systems. Accreditation Standards. Anderson, SC: CAMTS; 1997.

13 Waydhas C. Intrahospital transport of critically ill patients. *Crit Care* 1999; **3**: R83–9.

14 Predictors of respiratory function deterioration after transfer of critically ill patients. *Intensive Care Med* 1998; **24**: 1157–62.

15 Kollef MH, Von Harz B, Prentice D, *et al.* Patient transport from intensive care increases the risk of developing ventilator-associated pneumonia. *Chest* 1997; **112**: 765–73

16 ECRI. A new MRI complication. Health Devices Alert 1988. ECRI

17 Flabouris A, Seppelt I. Optimal Interhospital Transport Systems for the Critically Ill. In: Vincent JL (ed.) 2001 *Yearbook of Intensive Care and Emergency Medicine*. Berlin, Heidelberg: Springer-Verlag; 2001: pp. 647–60.

18 Deane SA, Gaudry PL, Woods WPD, *et al.* Interhospital transfer in the management of acute trauma. *Aust NZ J Surg* 1990; **60**: 441–6.

19 Gentleman D, Jennett B. Hazards of interhospital transfer of comatose head injured patients. *Lancet* 1981; **2**: 853–5.

20 Beyer AJ IIIrd, Land G, Zaritsky A. Non-physician transport of intubated paediatric patients: a system evaluation. *Crit Care Med* 1992; **20**: 961–6.

21 International Society of Aeromedical Services Australasian chapter. Aeromedical Standards. Arncliffe, Sydney: ISAS Australasia; 1993.

22 Benson AJ. Motion Sickness. In: Ernsting J, King PF (ed.) *Aviation Medicine*. Oxford: Butterworth-Heinemann; 1988: pp. 318–38.

23 Lee A, Lum ME, Beehan SJ, Hillman KM. Inter-hospital transfers: decision making analysis in critical care areas. *Crit Care Med* 1996; **24**: 618–23.

24 New South Wales Health Department/Ambulance Service. Guidelines for Retrieval of the Critically Ill. Sydney: NSW Health Dept; 1995.

25 Gates Energy Products Technical Marketing Staff. *Rechargeable Batteries Applications Handbook*. Stoneham, MA: Butterworth-Heinemann; 1992.

26 Noy-Man Y, Papa MZ, Margaliot SZ. Portable air mobile life support unit. *Aviat Space Environ Med* 1985; **56**: 598–600.

27 Grant-Thompson JC. The Mobile Intensive-care Rescue Facility (MIRF): a close look at the intensive care aeromedical evacuation capability. *US Army Med Dept J* 1997; Sept–Oct: 23–6.

28 Wishaw KJ, Munford BJ, Roby HP. The Care Flight stretcher bridge: a compact mobile intensive care module. *Anaesth Intensive Care* 1990; **18**: 234–8.

29 Rutten AJ, Isley AH, Skowronski GA, Runciman WB. A comparative study of mean arterial blood pressure using automatic oscillometers, arterial cannulation, and auscultation. *Anaesth Intensive Care* 1986; **14**: 58–65.

30 Lawless ST. Crying wolf: false alarms in a paediatric intensive care unit. *Crit Care Med* 1994; **22**: 981–5.

31 Hankins DG, Herr DM, Santrach PJ, *et al.* Utilisation of a portable clinical analyser in air rescue. In: ADAC/International Society of Aeromedical Services AIRMED 96 Congress Report. Munich: Wolfsfellner Medizin Verlag; 1997: pp. 109–11.

32 Erler CJ, Rutherford WF, Rodman G, *et al.* Inadequate respiratory support in head injury patients. *Air Med J* 1993; **12**: 223–6.

33 Wong LS, McGuire NM. Laboratory assessment of the Bird T–Bird VS ventilator performance using a model lung. *Br J Anaesth* 2000; **84**: 811–17.

34 Porges KJ, Kelly SL. A comparison of the imposed work of breathing in continuous positive pressure ventilation mode between three different ventilators. *Emerg Med* 1999; **1**: 111–17.

35 Hedley RM, Allt-Graham J. Heat and moisture exchangers and breathing filters; a review. *Br J Anaesth* 1994; **73**: 227–36.

36 Russell WJ. Venturi suction. In: *Equipment for Anaesthesia and Intensive Care*. Adelaide, SA: WJ Russell; 1997: pp. 27–9.

37 Mertlich G, Quaal SJ. Air transport of the patient requiring intra-aortic balloon pumping. *Crit Care Nursing Clin N Am* 1989; **1**: 443–58.

38 Schneider NS, Borok Z, Heller M, *et al.* Critical cardiac transport: air versus ground. *Am J Emerg Med* 1988; **6**: 449–52.

39 Harris BH. Performance of aeromedical crew members: training or experience? *Am J Emerg Med* 1986; **4**: 409–13.

40 National Transportation Safety Board (US) Safety Study: Commercial Emergency Medical Services Helicopter Operations. SS/88/01. USA: NTSB; 1988.

41 Blumen IJ. Altitude and flight physiology: a reference for air medical physicians. In: Blumen IJ, Rodenberg H (eds) *Air Medical Physician Handbook*. Salt Lake City, UT: AMPA/Chicago University Press; 1994: pp. 000–000.

42 Rodenberg H. The physiological effects of altitude. In: Martin TE (ed) *Aeromedical Transportation: a Clinical Guide*. Aldershot, UK and Brookfield, Vt: Avebury Aviation; 1996: pp.000–000.

43 De Hart RL (ed.) *Fundamentals of Aerospace Medicine*. Philadelphia: Lea & Febiger; 1985.

44 Ernsting J, King PF (eds) *Aviation Medicine*. Oxford: Butterworth-Heinemann; 1988.

45 Thomas G, Brimacombe J. Function of the Drager Oxylog ventilator at high altitude. *Anaesth Intensive Care* 1994; **22**: 276–80.

46 Edmonds C, Lowry C, Pennefather J. (eds) *Diving and Subaquatic Medicine*, 3rd edn. Oxford, UK: Butterworth-Heinemann; 1992: 000–000.

47 Dunn JD. Legal aspects of transfers. *Problems Crit Care* 1990; **4**: 447–8.

48 Fiege A, Rutherford WF, Nelson DR. Factors influencing patient thermoregulation in flight. *Air Med J* 1996; **15**: 18–23.

49 Gabram SGA, Benson N. Quality Improvement: An Introductory Guide for Air Medical Physicians. In: Blumen IJ, Rodenberg H (eds) *Air Medical Physician Handbook*. Salt Lake City, UT: AMPA/Chicago University Press; 1994.

50 American Academy of Pediatrics Task Force on Interhospital Transport. Guidelines for Air and Ground Transport of Neonatal and Pediatric Patients. Elk Grove, IL: American Academy of Pediatrics; 1993.

51 James AG. Neonatal resuscitation, stabilisation and emergency neonatal transportation. *Intensive Care World* 1995; **11**: 53–7.

52 Low RB, Martin D, Brown C. Emergency Air Transport of Pregnant Patients: The National Experience. *Am J Emerg Med* 1988; **6**: 41–8.

53 Gilligan JE, Gorman DF, Millar I. Use of an airborne recompression chamber for transfer under pressure to a major hyperbaric facility. In: Shields TG (ed.) Proceedings of the XIV Meeting of the European Undersea Biomedical Society. Aberdeen, UK: European Undersea Biomedical Society; 1988.

54 Roby HP, Bentley L, Munford BJ. Considerations in international air medical transport. In: Blumen IJ, Rodenberg H (eds) *Air Medical Physician Handbook.* Salt Lake City, UT: AMPA/Chicago University Press; 1994.

55 Essebag V, Lutchmedial S, Churchill-Smith M. Safety of long distance aeromedical transport of the cardiac patient: a retrospective study. *Aviat Space Environ Med* 2001; **72**: 182–7.

56 Garner A, Rashford S, Lee A, Bartolacci R. Addition of physicians to paramedic helicopter services decreases blunt trauma mortality. *Aust NZ J Surg* 1999; **69**: 697–700.

57 Hanrahan BJ, Munford BJ. Air medical scene response to the entrapped trauma patient. In: *AIRMED 96.* ADAC/International Society of Aeromedical Services Congress Report. Munich: Wolfsfellner Medizin Verlag; 1997: pp. 375–80.

58 Baxt WG, Moody P. The impact of a physician as part of the aeromedical prehospital team in patients with blunt trauma. *JAMA* 1987; **257**: 3246–50.

59 Schmidt U, Scott BF, Nerlich ML, *et al.* On-scene helicopter transport of patients with multiple injuries – comparison of a German and American system. *J Trauma* 1992; **33**: 548–55.

60 Nocera A, Dalton AM. Disaster alert! The role of physician staffed helicopter emergency medical services. *Med J Aust* 1994; **161**: 689–92.

61 Garner A, Nocera A. Should New South Wales hospital disaster teams be sent to major incident sites? *Aust NZ J Surg* 1999; **69**: 702–7.

4.

Physiotherapy in intensive care

J G Risley and M O Jones

Historically, physiotherapy in the ICU was confined to the treatment of respiratory problems performed routinely on all patients. Evidence based practice has demonstrated that there is no longer a place for routine physiotherapy treatment in the ICU. Physiotherapeutic intervention is based on clinical reasoning following the identification of problems amenable to physiotherapy, which are elucidated from a thorough systematic assessment.

There is still some debate about the precise role of the physiotherapist within ICU, which may vary,[1] but the main features include:

- optimization of ventilation/cardiopulmonary function
- assistance in the weaning process, utilizing ventilatory support and oxygen therapy
- advice on positioning to optimize ventilation/perfusion matching and oxygenation
- advice on positioning to protect joints, and to minimize potential muscle and soft tissue shortening/injury and nerve damage
- optimization of body position to effect muscle tone in the brain injured patient
- instigation of an early rehabilitation/mobilization programme to assist in preventing the consequences of enforced immobility and optimize voluntary movement to promote functional independence and improve exercise tolerance
- assessment/treatment/advice on presenting musculoskeletal pathology
- enlisting as appropriate other specialist physiotherapists to optimize patient care (e.g. orthopaedic/neurological/HIV)
- involvement as required carers/partners/family/other professions allied to medicine
- liaison with medical and nursing staff on the continuation and monitoring of ongoing physiotherapy devised careplans.

PHYSIOTHERAPEUTIC TECHNIQUES

TREATMENT MODALITIES TO OPTIMIZE CARDIOPULMONARY FUNCTION

Physiotherapy treatment modalities may differ depending on the presence of an endotracheal tube. Each intervention is rarely used in isolation, but as part of an effective treatment plan. Some physiotherapeutic techniques may have short-lived beneficial effects on pulmonary function, and some have no clear evidence to validate their effectiveness (Table 4.1).

MANUAL HYPERINFLATION (MHI)

In this technique, a Waters-type bag is used to deliver a volume of gas greater than tidal volume (V_T) via an endotracheal or tracheostomy tube. MHI delivery

Table 4.1 Treatment modalities to optimize cardiopulmonary function

Invasively ventilated patients	Non-invasive/self-ventilating patients
Manual hyperinflation (MHI)	Active Cycle of Breathing Technique (ACBT)
Suction	
Manual techniques	Manual techniques
Positioning	Positioning
Mobilization/rehabilitation	Intermittent Positive Pressure Breathing (IPPB)
	Continuous Positive Airways Pressure (CPAP)
	Bi-level non-invasive ventilation
	Nasopharyngeal/oral suction
	PEP mask, flutter valve, cornet
	Autogenic drainage
	Mobilization/rehabilitation

Table 4.2 Potential advantages and complications of MHI

Potential advantages
Reversal of acute lobar atelectasis[2]
Alveolar recruitment via channels of collateral ventilation
Improvement in arterial oxygen saturation[3] and gaseous exchange
Mobilization of secretions and contents of aspiration
Improved static lung compliance[3,4]
Effectiveness may be increased when combined with appropriate positioning and manual techniques[5,6]

Potential complications
Absolute contraindications include undrained pneumothorax and unexplained haemoptysis
Cardiovascular and haemodynamic instability[7]
Loss of positive and expiratory pressure (PEEP), inducing hypoxia and potential lung damage. This can be minimized by incorporating a PEEP valve into the circuit of a 'PEEP dependent' patient
Risk of volutrauma, barotrauma and pneumothorax[8], which can be reduced by including a manometer in the circuit[9]
Risk of increased intracranial pressure (ICP)
Increased patient stress and anxiety

techniques vary according to the underlying pathology and desired outcome. For example, a slow inspiration/quick release may mobilize secretions by increasing the expiratory flow rate and/or stimulating a cough, whereas a slow inspiration with/without an inspiratory hold may assist the reversal of atelectasis. In an emergency situation, an Ambu-bag and facemask can be used to perform MHI in the self-ventilating patient. However, an alternative technique such as intermittent positive pressure breathing (IPPB), should be considered when an aug-mented V_T is required during a therapeutic intervention (Table 4.2).

SUCTION

Suction is used to clear secretions from central airways when a cough reflex is impaired or absent. A suction catheter is passed via an endotracheal or tracheostomy tube, or via a nasal/oral airway to the carina which may stimulate a cough in a non-paralysed patient. The catheter is pulled back 1 cm before suction is applied on withdrawal. The suction catheter diameter should not be greater than 50% of the diameter of the airway through which it is inserted, as large negative pressure can be generated intrathoracically without air entrainment (Table 4.3).

MANUAL TECHNIQUES
Chest shaking and vibrations

Shaking and vibrations are oscillatory movements of large and small amplitude performed during expiration, which are thought to increase expiratory flow rate, aiding mucociliary clearance. These techniques are believed to be more effective when performed at high lung volumes.

Chest wall compression

Compression of the chest wall can be used to augment an expiratory manoeuvre such as a 'huff' (see section below on ACBT) or a cough by providing tactile stimulation, or wound support.

Chest clapping/percussion

Chest clapping is a rhythmical percussion applied over specific areas of the chest, which may stimulate a cough reflex by mobilizing secretions. It should be considered for patients who have copious sputum production.[11]

Neurophysiological facilitation (NPF) of respiration

NPF of respiration is a set of techniques designed for the treatment of the neurologically impaired adult. Manual externally applied stimuli to the thorax, abdomen and mouth can be used to stimulate increased V_T, a cough reflex, augmented contraction of the abdominal muscles, or an increased conscious level (Table 4.4).

POSITIONING

Positioning can be utilized to achieve several different goals: drainage of secretions (using gravity assisted positioning), a reduced work of breathing/breathlessness or to maximize ventilation/perfusion ($\dot{V}/\dot{Q}$) ratio.

Gravity assisted positioning (GAP)

GAP facilitates the removal of excess bronchial secretions by positioning a specific bronchopulmonary segment perpendicular to gravity. An individual position exists for each segment, based on the anatomy of the bronchial tree.[11] (Table 4.5).

Table 4.3 Potential advantages and complications of suction

Potential advantages
Stimulation of a cough when reflex is impaired by mechanical stimulation of the larynx, trachea or large bronchi[10]
Removal of secretions from central airways when cough is ineffective or absent

Potential complications
Tracheal suction is an invasive procedure and should only be undertaken when there is a clear indication to do so
Absolute contraindications to suctioning are unexplained haemoptysis, severe coagulopathies, severe bronchospasm, laryngeal stridor, base of skull fracture and a compromised cardiovascular system
Hypoxaemia can be induced secondary to suctioning. This can be limited by pre- and post-oxygenation
Cardiac arrhythmias may be more common in the presence of hypoxia
Tracheal stimulation may produce increased sympathetic nervous system activity or a vasovagal reflex producing cardiac arrhythmias and hypotension

Table 4.4 Potential advantages and complications of chest shaking and vibrations, compression, chest clapping and NPF

Potential advantages
Stimulation of a cough reflex facilitates movement of secretions
Improved arterial blood gases (ABGs) when clapping, shaking and vibrations are combined with ACBT[12]
Slow one-handed clapping may reduce intracranial pressure in head injured patients
NPF may improve ventilation and sputum clearance in self-ventilating neurologically impaired adults[13]
Effectiveness may be increased when used in conjunction with gravity assisted positioning and ACBT

Potential complications
Arterial oxygen de-saturation[3] and cardiac arrhythmias
Bronchospasm in patients with reactive airways[14]
Reduced pulmonary compliance
Patient discomfort

Work of breathing/breathlessness

A reduction in the work of breathing/breathlessness can be achieved by putting a patient in a position that optimizes the length–tension relationship of the diaphragm, promotes relaxation of the shoulder girdle and upper chest, and facilitates the use of breathing control Adequately supported high side lying using pillows is a useful position to promote relaxation of the breathless patient. In addition, it can discourage the overuse of accessory muscles of respiration, which may reduce energy expenditure. Some patients prefer forward lean sitting with their arms placed in front of them on a high table. In this position the length–tension relationship of the diaphragm is optimized secondary to forward displacement of the abdominal contents (Table 4.6).

Ventilation/perfusion

Appropriate positioning of a patient can maximize $\dot{V}/\dot{Q}$. In self-ventilating adults, $\dot{V}/\dot{Q}$ matching increases from non-dependent to dependent areas of lung.[16] However, in adults receiving positive pressure ventilation, lung mechanics are altered, producing $\dot{V}/\dot{Q}$ inequality. In this situation, non-dependent areas of lung are preferentially

Table 4.5 Potential advantages and complications of GAP

Potential advantages
Maximizes removal of excess bronchial secretions when combined with ACBT
Allows accurate treatment of specific bronchopulmonary segments
Self-treatment can be included in a home programme

Potential complication
Positions need modification when used in the presence of cardiovascular/neurological instability, haemoptysis or gastric reflux

Table 4.6 Potential advantages and complications of positioning to affect work of breathing/breathlessness

Potential advantages
Decreases the work of breathing by reducing the use of accessory muscles of respiration, improving lung volumes and decreasing airway resistance
Improved ABGs
Potential complication
Positions may need modification in the presence of other existing pathology

Table 4.7 Potential advantages and complications of positioning to affect ventilation/perfusion

Potential advantages
Improved ABGs
Reduction in oxygen therapy
Drainage of pulmonary secretions can occur simultaneously

Potential complications
An optimal position may not be possible in the presence of cardiovascular/neurological instability or multiple pathology
Constant adjustment to maintain optimal positioning may be required

ventilated while dependent regions are optimally perfused (Table 4.7).

ACTIVE CYCLE OF BREATHING TECHNIQUE (ACBT)
The ACBT is a cycle of specific breathing exercises adapted for each patient according to existing underlying pathology. It consists of:

- breathing control (normal tidal breathing using the lower chest minimizing the use of accessory muscles of respiration)
- thoracic expansion, emphasizing inspiration (with/without an inspiratory hold)
- forced expiration, emphasizing expiration with an open glottis ('huff') and combined with breathing control.

Although mainly used in the self-ventilating patient, alert, co-operative, ventilated patients can be taught the technique (Table 4.8).

INTERMITTENT POSITIVE PRESSURE BREATHING (IPPB)
IPPB is a patient-triggered, pressure cycled mechanical device, mainly used in self-ventilating patients to mobilize bronchial secretions and re-expand lung tissue by augmenting V_T. Positive airway pressure is maintained throughout inspiration, whereas expiration is passive. IPPB requires constant adjustment of pressure and flow rates and careful patient monitoring to maintain effectiveness and co-operation. Effectiveness is increased when

Table 4.8 Potential advantages and complications of ACBT

Potential advantages
Mobilizes and clears excess bronchial secretions[14,17]
Improves lung function[18]
Minimizes the work of breathing
Individual components of the cycle can be utilized/emphasized to target specific problems
Can be used in combination with other manual techniques, GAP, V/Q matching, positioning to reduce breathlessness, and during activities such as walking
Self-treatment can be included in a home programme

Potential complications
Without adequate periods of breathing control, bronchospasm and de-saturation can occur.
Poor technique can lead to ineffective treatment and unnecessary energy expenditure

Table 4.10 Potential advantages and complications of IPPB, CPAP and bi-level non-invasive ventilation

Potential advantages
Improves lung volumes
Improves gaseous exchange
Decreases the work of breathing
IPPB and bi-level non-invasive ventilation can mobilize excess bronchial secretions by improving V_T
IPPB and bi-level non-invasive ventilation can improve lung and chest wall compliance
CPAP reduces left ventricular afterload by reducing the transmural pressure gradient
Patients can be mobilized while on CPAP and some modes of bi-level non-invasive ventilation. Alteration of ventilator settings might be indicated to maximize patient potential/exercise tolerance during treatment
Settings can be adjusted to augment physiotherapy intervention e.g. increased IPAP to assist removal of secretions

Potential complications
Absolute contraindications include severe bronchospasm, undrained pneumothorax, pneumomediastinum, unexplained haemoptysis and facial fractures. Use with care in pre-existing bullous lung disease.
Haemodynamic/neurological instability
Risk of decreased urine output with CPAP and bi-level non-invasive ventilation
Risk of carbon dioxide retention with CPAP
Risk of aspiration

used in conjunction with positioning, ACBT and manual techniques.

CONTINUOUS POSITIVE AIRWAYS PRESSURE (CPAP)

CPAP maintains a positive airway pressure throughout inspiration and expiration. It is used in both intubated and self-ventilating patients to reverse atelectasis by recruiting lung units and increasing/normalizing functional residual capacity (FRC). Effectiveness is increased when used in conjunction with appropriate positioning.

BI-LEVEL NON-INVASIVE VENTILATION

Bi-level non-invasive ventilation is used in both ventilated and self-ventilating patients. Separate levels of positive pressure are delivered to the patient, one on inspiration (IPAP) and another on expiration (EPAP). Bi-level non-invasive ventilators function in one of four modes: CPAP, spontaneous assisted ventilation, spontaneous/timed (assist/control) ventilation, and controlled ventilation. Effectiveness is increased when used in conjunction with positioning for optimum $\dot{V}/\dot{Q}$ (Tables 4.9 and 4.10).

TREATMENT ADJUNCTS AND TECHNIQUES

PEP mask, flutter, cornet and autogenic drainage are specialized mucociliary clearance devices/techniques used by some patients with chronic lung disease. These devices/techniques are rarely introduced in the ICU setting.

TREATMENT MODALITIES TO OPTIMIZE FUNCTIONAL ABILITY

MOBILIZATION/REHABILITATION

A rehabilitation programme aims to overcome the well-documented affects of immobility, encourage normal movement and optimize functional independence. It includes:

- positioning for the prevention of pressure sores, soft tissue shortening, joint contractures, to minimize nerve damage, and to normalize tone in the brain injured patient
- passive/active-assisted/active movements to assess for changes in joint range, muscle power, muscle tone and muscle/soft tissue/tendon length
- specific treatment modalities to help reverse identified musculoskeletal problems (e.g. splinting, positioning,

Table 4.9 Site and action of IPPB, CPAP and bi-level non-invasive ventilation

	IPPB	CPAP	Bi-level non-invasive ventilation
Lung volume affected	↑ V_T	↑ FRC	↑ V_T and FRC
Action	Assists removal of excess bronchial secretions	Reverses atelectasis	Ventilatory support

passive joint mobilizations, muscle lengthening and soft tissue mobilization techniques, active-assisted or active exercises)

● specific exercises as part of a strengthening/stability-based programme
● functional activities linked to activities of daily living;
● postural advice/education
● gait re-education.

Treatment can be divided into two stages:

Stage I starts from the initial assessment and treatment, and includes a full neurological and musculoskeletal assessment. Aims of treatment are to maintain muscle and joint range and encourage active movements. Splinting, passive/active-assisted movements and/or passive joint mobilizations may be indicated.

Stage II starts when the patient is stable but may still be requiring respiratory support – this will not affect the aims of rehabilitation (Figs 4.1 and 4.2).

Potential advantages

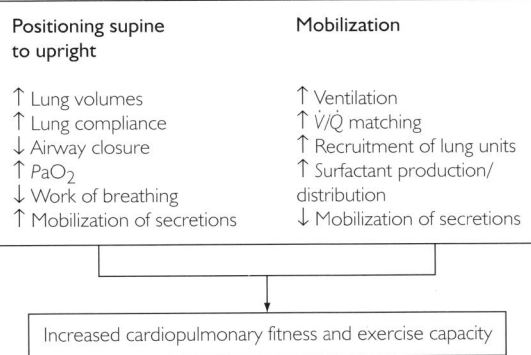

Positioning supine to upright	Mobilization
↑ Lung volumes	↑ Ventilation
↑ Lung compliance	↑ $\dot{V}/\dot{Q}$ matching
↓ Airway closure	↑ Recruitment of lung units
↑ PaO_2	↑ Surfactant production/distribution
↓ Work of breathing	↓ Mobilization of secretions
↑ Mobilization of secretions	

Increased cardiopulmonary fitness and exercise capacity

Potential complications

Cardiovascular/neurological/haematological instability
Increased oxygen/ventilatory requirement

Fig. 4.2   Potential advantages and complications of mobilization. (Adapted from Dean.[19])

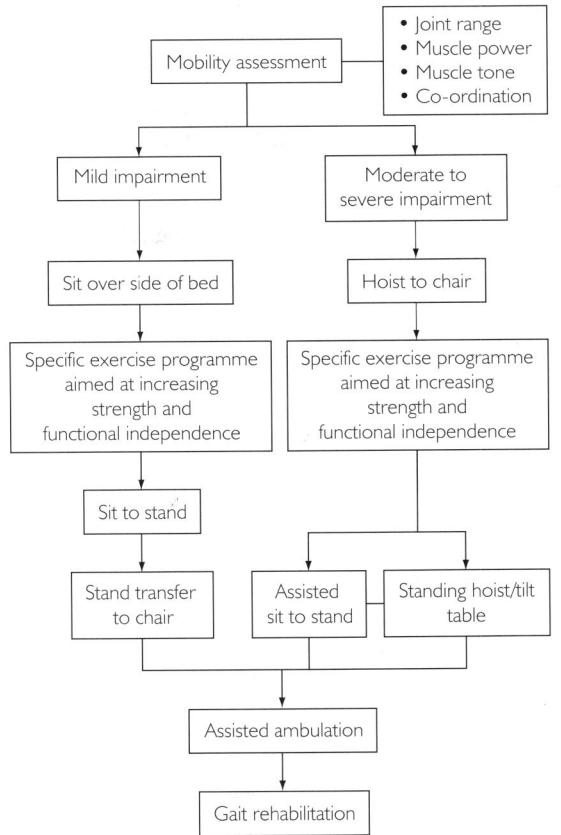

Fig. 4.1   Example of a mobility/rehabilitation treatment progression plan for the mildly impaired and moderate-to-severely impaired patient at Stage II (see text).

PHYSIOTHERAPY TREATMENT FOR SPECIFIC PATIENT GROUPS

ACUTE RESPIRATORY DISTRESS SYNDROME (ARDS)

Disruption of the alveolar–capillary membrane secondary to a variety of causal factors, produces three distinct clinical features: hypoxaemia, reduced respiratory compliance and diffuse radiographical infiltrates. In the acute phase these problems are not amenable to physiotherapeutic intervention. As ARDS progresses, fibrosis is the main clinical feature. During this time respiratory physiotherapy treatment may help to reverse atelectasis and assist in the removal of bronchial secretions.

TREATMENT MODALITIES TO OPTIMIZE CARDIOPULMONARY FUNCTION

Treatment modalities previously discussed require modification when used with this patient group.

ACUTE PHASE:

● Patients should only be disconnected from the ventilator when it is absolutely essential. This is in order to maintain 'lung recruitment' ventilatory strategies (positive end-expiratory pressure [PEEP]/inverse ratio ventilation or continuous inhaled vasodilator therapy [nitric oxide, prostacyclin]).
● A change of position from supine to prone and/or prone to supine may be required to re-distribute dependent atelectasis and maximize $\dot{V}/\dot{Q}$ matching.

- If suction is required in the presence of infected bronchial secretions, a closed-circuit system should be used.

FIBROTIC/RECOVERY PHASE:

If physiotherapy treatment is indicated in a patient who remains 'PEEP dependent' for adequate oxygenation, a PEEP valve should be incorporated in the MHI circuit. However, MHI will be ineffective in some patients who have multiple chest drains secondary to pneumothoraces with significant air leaks.

TREATMENT MODALITIES TO OPTIMIZE FUNCTIONAL ABILITY

Treatment modalities previously discussed can be used to optimize functional ability in this patient group. However, some modifications may be indicated:

- passive mobilization of the thoracic spine and ribs to help reduce joint stiffness secondary to reduced chest wall compliance
- commencement of a rehabilitation programme once the patient is medically stable.

THE ACUTE NEUROLOGICAL PATIENT

As all patient interventions may potentially lead to an increase in intracranial pressure (ICP), a clinically significant respiratory problem must be identified through a thorough systematic assessment before undertaking any treatment.

TREATMENT MODALITIES TO OPTIMIZE CARDIOPULMONARY FUNCTION

Treatment modalities previously discussed may be used with this patient group. However, some modifications may be indicated:

Position the patient at 15–30 degrees, head up with the head and neck in midline to facilitate venous return and limit ICP increases.

Undertake appropriate re-positioning and close assessment of the patient's response prior to any further intervention.

Where appropriate, a bolus of sedation may prevent neurological instability during treatment.

Oxygenate before and after suctioning.

Give suction for a maximum of 10 seconds to decrease risk of hypoxia.

Hyperventilation performed between MHI breaths may help decrease ICP.

Continued assessment during treatment (e.g. pupil reaction) can prevent detrimental effects of treatment intervention and neurological instability.

Continued monitoring during treatment of cardiovascular parameters can ensure adequate mean arterial pressure and cerebral perfusion pressure.

TREATMENT MODALITIES TO OPTIMIZE FUNCTIONAL ABILITY

Specific modifications/considerations to previously discussed treatment modalities are usually indicated in this patient group:

- Appropriate positioning with pillows/rolls will assist in maintaining extensibility of the nervous system, challenge the recovering central nervous system and encourage normal movement.
- Passive/active movements, together with positioning, will promote meaningful sensory input and assist in preventing contractures.
- Splinting to prevent contractures by maintaining joint and muscle range may be indicated, particularly in the presence of changes in muscle tone.
- Sitting patients up and standing patients may have a beneficial effect on ICP pressures.
- Joint therapy sessions with other MDT members, for example, swallow/communication assessments and treatment with speech and language therapists.

THE SPINAL INJURED PATIENT

The level of injury and stability will dictate patient presentation and consequent treatment. Higher level lesions can affect respiratory muscles and alter rib cage mechanics, leading to a decrease in FRC, V_T, chest wall compliance and $\dot{V}/\dot{Q}$ imbalance.

Treatment is aimed at:

- maintaining respiratory and neurological status
- preventing contractures
- commencing an early rehabilitation programme.

Unopposed muscle groups can potentially lead to contractures developing, therefore early management is essential. Treatment modalities already discussed may be considered for use with this patient group; however, some modifications may be indicated.

SPECIFIC TREATMENT MODIFICATIONS

These include:

- assisted coughing
- 24-hour positioning regime
- bi-lateral treatment interventions
- passive/active-assisted/active movements/exercises relevant to the level of injury
- splinting
- early rehabilitation, maximizing functional ability.

Potential complications are:

- autonomic dysreflexia
- hetertrophic ossification
- muscle tear/damage
- joint pain.

Table 4.11 Psychological, cardiopulmonary and functional problems often encountered in patients after discharge from the ICU

Psychological	Cardiopulmonary	Functional
Depression	Compromised cardiopulmonary system	Back pain
Fear	Difficulty clearing retained secretions	Shoulder pain
Anxiety	(trache tube, mini-trach *in situ*)	Muscle atrophy/decreased strength
Confusion	Decreased lung volumes	Inability to carry out activities of daily living
Disorientation	Oxygen dependency	independently
Flashbacks		Limited mobility
Lack of motivation		Poor exercise tolerance
Functional dependence		Poor gait pattern

Over-vigorous passive movements and poor positioning can cause the last three complications.

PROBLEMS AFTER PATIENT DISCHARGE FROM THE ICU

A prolonged stay in the ICU can be debilitating mentally and physically and can affect recovery after discharge (Table 4.11). In order to optimize a fast and effective recovery, a patient's careplan should be multidisciplinary.

SUMMARY

The physiotherapist has an important and varied role within the ICU or high dependency unit setting, working as part of the multidisciplinary team to optimize cardiopulmonary function and functional ability. The physiotherapist is often uniquely placed to follow and treat a patient from the acute stages at ICU admission, through the rehabilitation process to his or her subsequent discharge from hospital and, if necessary, treatment can be continued in the outpatient setting.

There is no longer a place for routine physiotherapy treatment. Regular systematic assessment will identify physiotherapy amenable problems that contribute to a multidisciplinary careplan. Implementation of any physiotherapy treatment should always utilize continuous analytical re-assessment.

ACKNOWLEDGEMENT

The authors wish to acknowledge the assistance of Jane Milligan for her contribution.

REFERENCES

1 Norrenberg M, Vincent JL. A profile of European intensive care unit physiotherapists. European Society of Intensive Care Medicine. *Intensive Care Med* 2000; **26**(7): 988–94.

2 Marini J, Pierson D, Hudson L. Acute lobar atelectasis; a prospective comparison of fiberoptic bronchoscopy and respiratory therapy. *American Review of Respiratory Disease* 1979; **119**: 971–7.

3 Jones AYM, Hutchinson RC, Oh TE. Effects of bagging and percussion on total static compliance of the respiratory system. *Physiotherapy* 1992; **78**(9): 661–5.

4 Hodgson C, Denehy L, Ntoumenopoulos G, *et al*. An investigation of the early effects of manual lung hyperinflation in critically ill patients. *Anaesth Intensive Care* 2000; Jun 28(3): 255–261.

5 Stiller K, Geake T, Taylor J, *et al*. Acute lobar atelectasis. A comparison of two chest physiotherapy regimens. *Chest* 1990; **98**(6): 1336–40.

6 Denehy L. The use of manual hyperinflation in airway clearance. *Eur Respir J* 1999; **14**(4): 958–65.

7 Singer M, Vermaat J, Hall G, *et al*. Hemodynamic effects of manual hyperinflation in critically ill mechanically ventilated patients. *Chest* 1994; **106**(4): 1182–7.

8 Clarke RCN, Kelly BE, Convery PN, Fee JPH. Ventilatory characteristics in mechanically ventilated patients during manual hyperventilation for chest physiotherapy. *Anaesthesia* 1999; **54**: 936–40.

9 King D, Morrell A. A survey on manual hyperinflation as a physiotherapy technique in intensive care units. *Physiotherapy* 1992 **78**(10): 747–50.

10 Widdicombe JG. Mechanism of cough and its regulation. *Eur J Respirat Dis* 1980; **61**(Supp110): 11–15.

11 Gallon A. The use of percussion. *Physiotherapy* 1992; **78**(2): 85–9.

12 Pryor JA, Webber BA, Hodson ME. Effect of chest physiotherapy on oxygen saturation in patients with cystic fibrosis. *Thorax* 1990; **45**: 77.

13 Bethune D. Neurophysiological facilitation of respiration in the unconscious adult patient. *Physiotherapy Canada* 1975; **27**(5): 241–5.

14 Webber BA, Pryor JA. Physiotherapy techniques. In: Pryor JA, Webber BA (ed.) *Physiotherapy for Respiratory and Cardiac Problems*, 2nd edn. Ch. 8. Edinburgh: Churchill Livingstone; 1998: pp. 137–209.

15 Thoracic Society. The nomenclature of bronchopulmonary anatomy. *Thorax* 1950; **5**: 222–8.

16 West JB. Ventilation–perfusion relationships. In: *Respiratory Physiology*, 5th edn. Baltimore: Williams & Wilkins, 1995: pp. 51–69.

17 Pryor JA, Webber BA, Hodson ME, Batten JC. Evaluation of the forced expiration technique as an adjunct to postural drainage in treatment of cystic fibrosis. *BMJ* 1979; **2**: 417–18.

18 Webber BA, Hofmeyr JL, Morgan MDL, Hodson ME. Effects of postural drainage, incorporating forced expiratory technique on pulmonary function in cystic fibrosis. *Br J Dis Chest* 1986; **80**: 353–9.

19 Dean E. The effects of positioning and mobilization on oxygen transport. In: Pryor JA, Webber BA (eds) *Physiotherapy for Respiratory and Cardiac Problems*, 2nd edn, Ch. 7. Edinburgh: Churchill Livingstone; pp. 125.

5.

Critical care nursing
J R Welch and C Theaker

The recent UK modernization plan for critical care (CC) openly acknowledged the contribution of nursing to the specialty.[1] This analysis asserts that all critically ill patients in the ICU *and* elsewhere in the hospital should receive 'skilled critical care nursing', but noted that many designated CC units are short staffed, even before provision is made for patients in other areas.[1] Despite wide variation in staffing levels and salaries across the world, nursing staff generally comprise the biggest single expense for CC. The value and development of CC nursing is under growing scrutiny and there is a need to consider key priorities for CC nurses in the future. These priorities include:

- attention to service delivery and organization
- clinical effectiveness, research and development
- education, training, and workforce development
- human resource issues and career pathways
- leadership development at all levels of the nursing team.[2]

THE NATURE AND FUNCTION OF CRITICAL CARE NURSING

CC nursing is influenced both by the fundamental nature of nursing and the specific characteristics of the field. Basic concerns for all nurses are said to take in:

- the concept of holism
- a proper appreciation of the whole range of influences on all areas of life
- the pursuit of health rather than treatment of illness.[3]

Such thinking is claimed to differentiate nursing from medicine and other healthcare disciplines founded on mechanical, reductionist principles. There is inevitably a degree of fixation on technology in CC, sometimes at the expense of holism. A former ICU patient described the experience as 'rooted in the minute analysis of charts and the balancing of chemicals, not so much in the warmth of human contact'.[4]

Nurses act as a round-the-clock constant for CC patients and their families, often functioning as the 'glue' that holds together and maintains the different components of the service by ensuring safety, providing continuity, and co-ordinating patient care and therapies.

CC nurses provide:

- continuous, close monitoring of patients and the attached apparatus
- dynamic analysis and synthesis of complex data
- anticipation of complications
- decision-making, execution and evaluation of interventions to minimize adverse effects
- enhancement of the speed and quality of recovery
- support of the dying patient.[5]

Such activities must be performed with awareness of the essential human elements of care, as shown by a study of CC expertise that revealed the value of 'presencing': connecting with patients both psychologically and physically.[6] Fundamental care (e.g. personal cleansing, protection of tissue integrity, prevention of infection) is generally undertaken or supervised by nurses. Other key needs (e.g. chest physiotherapy, mobilization, delivery of nutrition) are managed by different specialists in some systems, but it is nurses who integrate these treatments into the complete package of care.

There is no body of evidence comprising large-scale studies to demonstrate the undeniable advantages of particular systems of CC nursing, or a main effect of CC nursing that is entirely distinct from other variables that influence patient outcomes. The interdependence of different CC personnel was seen in a multicentre investigation where interaction and communication between members of the CC team were more significant correlates of patient mortality than the therapies used or the status of the institution.[7] None the less, a 4-year retrospective study has shown a significant relationship between varying levels of nursing workload and deaths in ICU, suggesting that insufficient staffing and deficiencies in care can have a direct effect on mortality.[8]

It should be apparent from the above that CC nursing is a highly complex field. It is vital therefore to structure the patient review in order to clarify and prioritize patient needs, and to make sure that the whole range of patient function – and dysfunction – is addressed.

In acute situations, the novice may find that assessment in turn of the fundamental A-B-C-D-E aspects of physiology is a useful method; thus:

- airway – establishment and maintenance of airway patency; usually with the use of artificial devices, removal of pulmonary secretions, etc.
- breathing – adequacy of oxygenation and ventilation
- circulation – perfusion of brain, heart, lungs, kidneys, gut and other organs; control of bleeding, haematology, etc.
- disability – consciousness and the factors that affect it; systemic and localized neurology
- exposure – hands-on examination; and everything else (!); electrolytes and biochemistry, renal function; wounds, etc.

Appropriate treatment strategies can also be prioritized using this schema, which has the additional benefit that it will be familiar to nursing and medical colleagues trained in various of the medical emergency algorithms.

Further detail may then be gained from review of:

- fluid balance, fluid administration, urine output
- gastrointestinal tract function – nutritional needs and elimination
- history and holistic overview of the person
- infection and microbiology
- lines – utility and risks
- medications
- psychology – pain and comfort, rest and sleep
- relatives – communication of plan and prognosis in short term, medium term and longer term.[9]

There are more sophisticated models that can be used to frame a wider impression of the patient; and also to reflect a particular philosophy or approach to CC nursing. For example, the Roy model[10] expresses a view of nursing as a vehicle for enabling adaptive adjustments to any dysfunction. The model prompts analysis of both immediate and other contributing influences in a systematic consideration of oxygenation, nutrition, elimination, activity and rest, protective mechanisms, sensory function, fluid, electrolyte and acid–base balance, neurological and endocrine function; as well as the patient's self-concept, role-mastery, and psycho-social interdependence.[10] Such an approach can be commended for its breadth of vision, but may appear too complex for the novice. Coherent articulation of patient problems may be aided by use of validated 'nursing diagnoses', as developed in North America. This system provides definitions and recommended nursing responses for many problems, and helps specify appropriate outcome measures.

What is most important is that the system used promotes unambiguous definition of patient problems and a clear statement of specific, measurable therapeutic goals.

EVOLVING ROLES OF CRITICAL CARE NURSES

CC nurses' range of practice has evolved rapidly with progress in technology and also with changes to the working of their professional colleagues.[11] The benefits of developing specific expertise in some therapies and technical tasks must be balanced against maintenance of nursing roles involving essential patient care.[12] There remains a large variation in the array of tasks undertaken by CC nurses, with drug prescriptions and invasive procedures still mainly done by doctors. At present, the law in Britain and most other countries does not support nurse prescribing in CC, but there is increasing interest in developing independent nurse prescribing in acute care,[13] which may eventually extend into CC areas.

CC nurses have a larger and developing role in decision-making regarding the ongoing fine-tuning, trouble-shooting and titration of such key treatments as ventilation, fluid and inotrope administration, and renal replacement therapy. The use of less invasive techniques (e.g. trans-oesophageal Doppler ultrasonography for cardiac output estimation) means that it is possible for nurses to institute relatively sophisticated monitoring and administer appropriate therapies for restoration of homeostasis. Indeed, there is evidence that CC nurses can achieve good outcomes in some of these areas, especially with the use of clinical guidelines and protocols; for example, by reducing the time to wean respiratory support.[14] This indicates that further development of protocols, guidelines, care pathways and the like can be used to enhance the nursing contribution to CC.

NEW NURSING ROLES IN CRITICAL CARE

Medical and nursing staffing in the ICU is an ongoing problem in many countries and has led to various initiatives to facilitate delivery of both fundamental and more sophisticated modes of care.[15] New nursing roles in CC include those that essentially substitute for medical roles, as well as those that retain a nursing focus and aim to fill gaps in health care with nursing practice rather than medical care.[16] For example, the UK has designated a relatively small number of generally well-rewarded nurse consultant posts in all areas of health care, partly in order to try to retain experts in practice settings. At present, the largest proportion of nurse consultants are employed in CC, particularly CC outreach (see below). These are advanced practitioners focusing primarily on clinical practice, who are also required to demonstrate professional leadership and consultancy, development of appropriate education and training, macro-level practice and service development, research and evaluation.[17]

Other sorts of non-nursing staff are increasingly being used to deliver what has been seen as 'basic' nursing care (e.g. oral and ocular care, recording of vital signs), in order to support trained nurses and enable them to concentrate on more advanced activities.[18] Nursing shortages may make such developments inevitable in some areas, but it is imperative that nurses continue to ensure best outcomes for patients with proper arrangements for training, support, and working systems.

CRITICAL CARE NURSING BEYOND THE ICU: CRITICAL CARE OUTREACH

It is evident that acutely ill patients who are not accommodated in CC facilities can benefit from CC nursing skills for some period of their hospital stay. Analysis of acute admissions to ICU from general wards found that most suffered substandard care before transfer to ICU. Cited as particular problems were:

- failure to recognize the urgency of the situation
- lack of knowledge and
- organizational issues, leading to a subsequent hospital mortality of 56%.[19]

Another review of deaths in a medium-sized hospital with very low mortality overall suggested that there were still two unexpected, potentially avoidable deaths a month in general wards, due to, basic, recorded, but untreated problems such as hypotension, hypokalaemia, hypoxia and hypoglycaemia over some hours or days.[20] In the main, it is nurses who record these signs, so this work suggests either poor understanding of the seriousness of such indicators, or a failure to communicate effectively with medical staff, or difficulty in ensuring that appropriate treatment is prescribed and administered.

These issues and considerations of equity of care have fuelled demands for CC outreach services to facilitate care of at-risk and deteriorating patients on general wards: before, after, or sometimes instead of admission to a designated CC facility.[11] The intention is to reduce the numbers and severity of illness of CC admissions by predicting and intervening promptly early in the course of critical illness. Similarly, patient discharges from CC at problematic times or when the patient is not completely ready are associated with worse outcomes[21] that might be improved by an outreach service. Such teams could also support patients during longer term recovery, and obtain feedback for use in future care. Perhaps more important is that outreach is about sharing CC skills with staff in other areas.[1]

Several Australian hospitals have for some time used an outreach approach, usually with an acute care team responding to referrals made on the basis of deranged physiology[22]: one recent medical study showed a halving of unexpected cardiac arrests, reducing the mortality by

2 per 1000 hospital admissions.[23] Such services can be staffed by CC nurses, who appraise acute hospital admissions, patients discharged from CC areas after major surgery, patients displaying abnormal vital signs, etc., in order to identify those at particular risk and in need of close attention. Outreach aims to support ward staff in the management of these patients where possible, or to facilitate transfer to CC when appropriate. Potential problems include:

- loss of CC staff to such systems
- ensuring that team-members have the necessary skills
- restrictions faced by nurses in terms of prescribing and administering treatments in these areas.

PATIENT FOLLOW-UP

Recovery from critical illness can be a slow and painful process with many patients debilitated for long periods. Two-thirds of survivors experience significant problems with various aspects of physical health, work issues, or mental health; while 13% are severely limited in everyday life, experience post traumatic stress, etc.[11] There is encouraging evidence that relatively inexpensive and easy-to-administer nurse-led rehabilitation schemes can significantly improve recovery. One trial tested an essentially self-help rehabilitation package for survivors of CC.[24] The package consisted of a manual with general advice (about drugs, psychological issues, relationships, nutrition, etc.); detailed information about exercise routines; and week-by-week programmes involving self-assessment of physical function, exercise regimens and stress management techniques. Use of the manual gave measurably better physicality at 2 and 6 months, and some benefit in reducing depression in the first weeks of the recovery period.[24]

NURSE EDUCATION

In many countries, CC nurses have benefited more than some of their colleagues from long-standing specialist educational programmes available through diverse institutions. Analysis reveals considerable inconsistency in the content, demands, and quality of different versions of such training. Nurses clearly desire to attain formal academic credentials. There is an important role for study of relevant philosophy, nursing theory, research methods, etc. but there is also a renewed appreciation of the importance of learning that focuses on clinical practice issues and problem-solving that can benefit patients.[25] It is recognized that there needs to be more widespread deployment of CC nursing skills: the British CC modernization plan requires 'competence based high dependency care training' by 2004 for all general ward staff.[1] These imperatives drive a need to produce unambiguous statements about the standards necessary for proper nursing assessment and nursing management of CC patients.

Summarized examples of competencies for CC nurses might include the following.[26]

1 Safe, effective and appropriate nursing management of patient requiring invasive ventilation, using:
   * a range of suitable ventilatory modes
   * pulmonary recruitment manoeuvres (e.g. prone positioning)
   * strategies for weaning
   * consideration of patient comfort (sedation, etc).
2 Safe, effective and appropriate nursing management of patient suffering from cardiovascular instability, including:
   * acute coronary syndromes
   * cardiac dysrhythmias
   * haemodynamic instability secondary to other factors
   * circulatory failure
   * peri-arrest situations
   * cardiopulmonary arrest.
3 Safe and effective management of pre-renal failure, intrinsic renal failure and post-renal failure, with appropriate nursing care, including:
   * fluid and drug therapies
   * urinary drainage devices
   * renal replacement techniques (in appropriate setting).

These statements outline the types of competencies that might be required by CC nurses, and can be used to structure in-depth descriptions of the skills, applied knowledge and attitudes needed to achieve appropriate patient outcomes. Clear detailing of specific skills is essential, but there also needs to be consideration of how individual actions are integrated into holistic care, and the degree of independent clinical judgement displayed in practice by the CC nurse. Appraisal of performance requires suitable assessors to observe and question the nurse in practice rather than examination of written work; but this places great demands on hard-pressed clinical areas. It may be that increasingly sophisticated simulators can be used to test performance away from the practice setting.

Various frameworks to identify different levels of performance have been developed, for example, based on Benner's hierarchy (see Table 5.1).[6] These can be used to mark progression to particular standards in core skills.

CRITICAL CARE NURSING RESEARCH

One hundred and forty years ago, Florence Nightingale emphasized the importance of rigorous audit and evaluation with the purpose of improving patient outcomes.

Table 5.1   Assessment of performance in CC nurses. (After Benner 1984)[6]

Rating	Definition	Observed behaviour	Prompts
Novice	Limited skill and/or knowledge, inconsistent practice, variable interpersonal skill. Limited understanding of wider context, inflexible rule governed behaviour	Lacks co-ordination and confidence. Potential for omissions or inaccuracies. Unable to demonstrate accurate and safe performance despite repeated attempts.	Requires frequent directive prompts, supervision and advice.
Advanced beginner	Some skill and knowledge, generally consistent practice and interpersonal skill; variable ethical thought. Some appreciation of situational influences	Co-ordinated and confident in fundamental tasks. Easily distracted or unable to integrate other aspects of patient care.	Requires occasional directive prompts and some supervision.
Competent	Consistent safe, accurate and effective practice, interpersonal skill and ethical thought. Conscious and deliberate planning with consideration of immediate context	Skilful, confident and co-ordinated patient focused practice, with evident integration of other aspects of care. Prioritization of workload.	Self-directing without supervision.
Proficient	Consistent safe, accurate and effective practice, higher level of interpersonal skill and ethical reasoning. Conscious and deliberate planning with consideration of longer-term goals. Adapts care in response to changing situations	Skilled and accomplished practice, proactive and flexible approach to care. Problem solving and decision making through reflection. Role model.	Capable of supporting and demonstrating skills to others.

Nightingale described length of stay and complications after surgery at different hospitals, highlighting the association between the clinical environment and survival. In the 21st century, it is essential that CC nurses engage with research in order to justify and advance their methods with a theoretical base that supports best nursing practice. Many aspects of CC warrant examination.

Critical Care:

- treats comparatively small numbers of patients – at a high cost
- has great physical and psychological impact
- frequently uses somewhat untested therapies
- results are often poor or questionable
- outcomes are subject to a multitude of treatment methods, patient variables, and human factors
- is delivered by sundry means of planning, resourcing, and organizing the service.

The many variables evident in such an environment mean that a whole range of quantitative and qualitative investigative procedures may be required to obtain a comprehensive understanding of the issues. The approach chosen depends on the objectives of the researcher, the nature of the research question and the resources available. What then are the procedures that yield good quality research that can be used to develop practice? Research studies are essentially based on the creation of a specific question or hypothesis, then an investigation, and findings developed to a conclusion. Thus:

- successful research requires that the overall objectives and the specific research questions are clearly understood and articulated
- new researchers should consult an experienced researcher at the outset
- ethics committee approval is almost always needed.

The research process can be followed through seven stages:

Stage 1. Identify and develop the topic that needs to be examined. Research in clinical settings is most valued when it is seen to have a real relevance to practice, and therefore the researcher may gain most support for investigation of high risk and high cost processes. However, many everyday, fundamental methods and treatments warrant examination too, particularly when there are significant variations in practice. The researcher should then determine how the topic of interest might be described in a measurable way, and formulate the topic as a question – with some consideration about how answers may be obtained.

Stage 2. Gather relevant background information. This can be done in various ways, with the hospital library usually a good starting point. It is usually important to collect information that enables an understanding of the issues under investigation, and helps justify that investigation. Indexes for journals and books are found in print and computer-based formats, with data-bases and texts also increasingly available through the Internet:

- PubMed is a service that includes the MEDLINE (Medical Literature, Analysis, and Retrieval System Online) biomedical database and links to other practical websites. It can be accessed via the US National Library of Medicine site: http://www.nlm.nih.gov/
- CINAHL is the Cumulative Index to Nursing and Allied Health: http://www.cinahl.com
- The Cochrane collaboration contains systematic reviews of healthcare interventions: http://www.cochrane.org/

Some training in the use of such systems is highly recommended in order that the literature search is performed most effectively and efficiently.

Evaluate the information: different types of research designs carry with them particular weight. For example, results obtained from randomized controlled trials are considered to be evidence of the highest grade, while observational studies are deemed to be less useful.[27] This scheme is not always applicable and may be seen to devalue some sorts of useful work; but it does emphasize the need to critically examine the credibility of research.

Stage 3. Design a method that will:

- provide data that will answer the question
- be adequate to answer the question (the numbers required will require statistical input to determine the power of the study, i.e. the numbers needed to demonstrate a difference)
- be feasible to do in practice
- be ethical.

Stage 4. Collect the data. This is usually relatively simple provided that the data points to be collected are clearly established at the planning stage of the study. A common pitfall is to collect vast amounts of unnecessary data and lose the focus of the original research question. Collect the data in a manageable format. This may require a database.

Stage 5. Organize and present your information. By this stage of the research process, a large amount of material may have been gathered from primary and secondary sources. It is important:

- to employ a system of categorization and analysis that meets the objectives of the investigation
- that the analysis should address the original question
- that appropriate statistical methods should be used, for which special expertise or advice might be needed
- conclusions should be derived from the analysis, with no extrapolation.

Stage 6. Present and explain the data. This can take many forms, but it is always necessary to set out the question asked, to describe the research method, illustrate the results and their analysis, and finally present the key findings and conclusions. This must be in a succinct and constructive manner and any shortcomings or problems with the study should be discussed. The goal is that the reader can understand the methodology and interpret the results, while acknowledging any limitations of the study.

Stage 7. Evaluate the project. This final phase is reflective. Conducting research is a process that can always be improved in later work. Constructive feedback from colleagues is the most effective way of determining the value of a study. The researcher should review what has been learnt from the process as well as from the results of the study, and consider how the work might be further developed in the future.

REVIEWING RESEARCH STUDIES

The methods used to appraise research depend partly on the type of work under review. The questions outlined below may be used to guide a critique.

- Scientific content: Is there a specific hypothesis and a specific question? Is the background well researched and the rationale for the study clearly established?
- Originality: Is it a new idea? It does not need to be new, and may be re-examining an old problem differently or better.
- Methodology and study design: Are the methods appropriate and are they likely to produce an answer to the question?
- Is the research method described in a way that can be readily understood – or replicated?
- Are the relevant results shown? Are other important data such as the demographics of the population shown?
- Is the analysis appropriate and is the power of the study adequate? (This is usually determined by the numbers involved and the size of the difference being examined.)
- Interpretation and discussion: Are the conclusions and comments reasonable in the light of the results? Do the conclusions lead from the analysis shown?
- Are any references to the literature reasonably comprehensive and appropriate?
- What can be taken from the study, that is, what value does the study have in terms of supporting or developing clinical practice?
- What is the overall impression of the work? Are the sources credible? Is the presentation clear and informative?
- If evaluating a paper – has the work undergone proper peer review?

CRITICAL CARE NURSING MANAGEMENT

The responsibilities, role, and challenges of the CC nurse manager vary across different national systems and individual hospitals, but it is evident that the nurse manager role is crucial to the performance of the department. The most fundamental concern for the CC manager is probably the problem of attracting and retaining a flexible, developing, and effective nursing team that works well with other CC healthcare professionals to meet fast-changing patient needs – within a limited budget. The manager is typically responsible for:

- the cohesive and co-ordinated operational management of the area
- the quality of nursing care
- management of nursing pay and non-pay budget
- personnel management.

Such functions take place in the context of dynamic political, social, and economic forces which are specific to the organizational objectives and resources of the hospital. The nurse manager needs to be aware and considerate of these factors both within and without the unit in order to provide both the practical means of delivering patient care and a healthy environment for nurses' development. Within a coherent unit the nurse manager ensures that this rationale or strategy is communicated to the staff, so that there is a shared understanding of exactly what needs to be done in practice, and where each team-member fits into the plan. Externally, the manager represents the CC service and ensures that other disciplines and the organization are informed about CC issues.

Teams perform most effectively when individuals believe that they are working toward some common and worthwhile goals. A key role of the manager is to provide such coherence not just within the unit but also by integrating the views of all users of the service including patients and their families into the departmental plan. The principles of shared governance can be usefully applied in this perspective, whereby staff collectively review and learn from existing practices in order to develop and improve patient care within the unit. This has to be in the context of:

- the strategic agendas of the unit and the hospital
- the development of the service
- financial issues, budgets and budgetary restraints
- appreciation of day-to-day working issues.

Not surprisingly, the complexity and range of requirements may be too much for one person in some cases, so that different individuals are employed to take responsibility for particular aspects of management.

STRESS MANAGEMENT AND MOTIVATION

The ICU can be extremely stressful, demanding considerable cognitive, affective and psychomotor effort. Supervisory arrangements and feedback mechanisms should be in place that alleviate such demands, and enable prompt recognition of staff that are having difficulties at work. Regular individual performance reviews and formulation of development plans provide positive assurance, encouragement and can identify an individuals personal requirements, such as educational needs. It also provides an opportunity to identify poor practice which can then be rectified in a constructive manner.

Occupational psychology suggests that providing staff at all levels with opportunities to feel that they can influence and perhaps change the working environment tends to decrease stress and increase motivation. An example might be giving choice regarding rostering, so that a nurse may deliberately choose to work with particular patients on an ongoing basis to promote continuity and co-ordination of care. This can also have real benefits for patients and their families.

Developing nurses' critical thinking and decision-making skills is important for most effective working so that the nurse manager should provide a system that faciliates such training, while safeguarding the patients.

Flexibility to work in different ways at different times, so that the overall demands of the department can be met, is increasingly important. It is the manager's job to balance and meet the needs of staff, patients and the organization.

FURTHER READING

Wedderburn Tate C (1999) *Leadership in Nursing*, Edinburgh, Churchill Livingston.

REFERENCES

1 Department of Health. *Comprehensive Critical Care: a Review of Adult Critical Care Services.* London: Department of Health; 2000. [http://www.doh. gov.uk/pdfs/criticalcare.pdf]

2 Department of Health. *The Nursing Contribution to the Provision of Comprehensive Critical Care for Adults: a Strategic Programme of Action.* London: Department of Health; 2001. [http://www.doh.gov.uk/cno/critical-carenurs.pdf]

3 Chinn P, Kramer M. *Theory and Nursing: Integrated Knowledge Development.* St Louis, MO: Mosby; 1999.

4 Watt B. *Patient: the True Story of a Rare Illness.* London: Penguin; 1996.

5 Royal College of Nursing Critical Care Forum. Guidelines for nurse staffing in intensive care: a consultation document [3rd draft, July 2001] *Intensive Crit Care Nursing* 2001; **17**(5): 254–62.

6 Benner P. *From Novice to Expert: Excellence and Power in Clinical Nursing Practice.* Menlo Park: Addison-Wesley; 1984.

7 Knaus W, Draper E, Wagner D, Zimmerman J. An evaluation of outcome from intensive care in major medical centers *Ann Int Med* 1986; **104**(3): 410–18.

8 Tarnow-Mordi W, Hau C, Warden A, Shearer A. Hospital mortality in relation to staff workload: a 4-year study in an adult intensive care unit. *Lancet* 2000; **356**(9225): 185–9.

9 Hillman K, Bishop G, Flabouris A. Patient examination in the intensive care unit. *Yearbook of Intensive Care and Emergency Medicine* 2002. Berlin: Springer-Verlag; 2002.

10 Roy C, Andrews H. *The Roy Adaptation Model.* Englewood Cliffs, NJ: Prentice-Hall; 1999.

11 Audit Commission. *Critical to Success: the Place of Efficient and Effective Critical Care Services within the Acute Hospital.* London: Audit Commission; 1999. [http://www.audit-commission.gov.uk/publications/pdf/nrccare.pdf]

12 Mullally S. Improving the quality of clinical practice. *Nursing Ethics* 2000; **7**(6) 531–2.

13 Department of Health. *Extending Independent Nurse Prescribing within the NHS in England. A Guide for Implementation.* London: Department of Health; 2002. [http://www.doh. gov.uk/nurseprescribing/implementationguide.pdf]

14 Kollef M, Shiparo S, Silver P, *et al.* A randomized, controlled trial of protocol directed versus physician directed weaning from mechanical ventilation *Crit Care Med* 1997; **25**(4): 567–74.

15 Scholes J, Furlong S, Vaughan B. New roles in practice: charting three typologies of role innovation. *Nursing Crit Care* 1999; **4**(6): 268–75.

16 Smith M. The core of advanced practice nursing. *Nursing Sci Q* 1995; **8**(1): 2–3.

17 NHS Executive. Health Service Circular 1999/217. *Nurse, Midwife and Health Visitor Consultants.* Leeds: NHS Executive; 1999. [http://www.nursingleadership.co.uk/pubs/HSC%201999%20217.pdf]

18 Hind M, Jackson D, Andrews C, *et al.* Health care support workers in the critical care setting. *Nursing Crit Care* 2000; **5**(1): 31–9.

19 McQuillan P, Pilkington S, Allan A, *et al.* Confidential inquiry into quality of care before admission to intensive care. *BMJ* 1998; **316**(7148): 1853–8.

20 McGloin H, Adam S, Singer M. Unexpected deaths and referrals to intensive care of patients on general wards. Are some cases potentially avoidable? *J Roy Col Physicians Lond* 1999; **33**(3): 255–9.

21 Daly K, Beale R, Chang R. Reduction in mortality after inappropriate early discharge from intensive care unit: logistic regression triage model. *BMJ* 2001; **322**(7297): 1274–8.

22 Lee A, Bishop G, Hillman K, Daffurn K. The medical emergency team. *Anaesth Intensive Care* 1995; **23**(2): 183–6.

23 Buist M, Moore G, Bernard S, *et al.* Effects of a medical emergency team on reduction of incidence of and mortality from unexpected cardiac arrests in hospital: preliminary study. *BMJ* 2002; **324**(7334): 387–90.

24 Griffiths R, Jones C. *Intensive Care Aftercare.* Oxford: Butterworth-Heinemann; 2002.

25 Wigens L, Westwood S. Issues surrounding educational preparation for intensive care nursing in the 21st century. *Intensive Crit Care Nursing* 2000; **16**(4): 221–7.

26 SW London Critical Care Nursing Curriculum Planning Group. *Critical Care Competencies.* London: Kingston University & St. George's Hospital Medical School Faculty of Healthcare Sciences; 2002.

27 Concato J, Shah N, Horwitz R. Randomized, controlled trials, observational studies, and the hierarchy of research designs. *New Engl J Med* 2000; **342**(25) 1887–92.

6.

Ethics in intensive care
T E Oh

DEFINITION

Ethics is a science of moral behaviour that analyses the theories of moral thinking to examine rights and wrongs. Medical ethics is the application of ethics and moral theories to the practice of medicine, and such ethical obligations govern the practice of intensive care. Consideration of medical ethics is highly important, because of medical advances, high health care costs, restrictive governments, and a more knowledgeable and demanding public. Medical ethics generally refer to decisions concerning patient care, but ethical and moral obligations also apply to conduct and behaviour ('professionalism') and the business side of managing a practice.

ETHICAL PRINCIPLES

The intensivist may encounter ethical dilemmas in following his/her goal to maintain the highest standards of practice, teaching and research; the principal driving force of intensive care must be the welfare of the patient. This goal may at times be in conflict with personal beliefs, workload pressure, behaviour, expediency, financial interest, and indeed some ethical principles themselves (see below). In nearly all cases, the intensivist has to make a decision. Ethical principles, which are general guides that provide a framework for reasoning and analysis, can then be considered. Each clinical ethical dilemma is considered in the context of these principles, which are:

1 *Autonomy* or the respect for patients to determine their medical treatment (as against *paternalism* whereby 'the doctor knows best').
2 *Beneficence* or the principle of 'doing good' to our patients – an obligation to do our best to cure, to alleviate pain and suffering, to save lives and, most importantly, to act in the best interests of our patients.
3 *Non-maleficence* or the duty not to do any harm to patients or members of the healthcare team.

4 *Fidelity* or faithfulness to our duties and obligations, a principle underlying confidentiality, telling the truth, keeping up with medical knowledge (i.e. continuing professional development), and not to neglect patient care.
5 *Social justice* or the right of all patients to be fairly treated and entitled to medical care according to medical need.
6 *Utility* or the principle of doing most good for the most number of people, that is, achieving maximum benefits for society without wasting health resources.

Medical ethics are intertwined with legal requirements. Laws relating to medical ethical issues vary between countries, and indeed, even between regions, states, and provinces of a country. Every intensivist must be aware of universal ethical requirements imposed by professional bodies and laws that apply locally. Local laws may take precedence over some practice principles and guidelines. Seeking legal opinion is often advisable. In intensive care, important ethical and legal issues include consent, confidentiality, and end-of-life decisions.

CONSENT

The patient's consent to treatment underpins the relationship between physician and patient. Consent is both a legal and moral requirement in delivering medical care. Some principles of consent can be established.[1,2]

PRINCIPLES

- The patient's consent must be obtained on every occasion the intensivist wishes to initiate treatment, except in emergencies. Minor procedures may be excluded if considered part of basic supportive care.
- In an emergency when the patient is unable to give consent, treatment may be provided that is immediately necessary to save life or avoid significant deterioration of condition.

- In seeking consent, the intensivist must provide adequate information about the intervention, including benefits and risks.
- Patient consent must be voluntary and free from pressure.
- Consent forms are evidence of the consent process, but consent itself need not be in writing, unless specifically required by a local authority. None the less, consent given should be recorded each time in the patient's notes.
- Competent patients are entitled to refuse consent to treatment even when doing so may result in death.
- Intensivists may treat an incompetent patient without consent in some jurisdictions, if it is necessary and in the patient's best interests. Other jurisdictions allow a proxy or surrogate to give consent on behalf of an incompetent adult patient, but the surrogate cannot demand treatment which is judged to be against the patient's interests. Surrogates in order of priority are partners, adult offsprings, parents, and the nearest living relative.
- An enduring power of attorney can make decisions on an individual's financial affairs but normally has no legal right to consent treatment.
- Depending on the jurisdiction, competent minors may or may not have rights to consent to, or refuse, treatment. The legal age that defines a minor varies. Otherwise, and for incompetent minors, consent may be given by parents or a person or local authority with parental responsibility. Parental involvement should be encouraged, but a competent minor's request for confidentiality should be respected.
- Consent is required to involve a patient in research, using proper research consent forms and protocols.
- Consent is required for teaching purposes, such as video recording and photographing patients and teaching of practical procedures.
- Testing for HIV/AIDS, hepatitis B and C, and other conditions in many jurisdictions requires consent, even if the patient is unconscious or if a staff member has suffered a needlestick injury.

ADVANCE STATEMENT[3]

An advance statement is a written document, a witnessed oral statement, or a recorded discussion, made by a competent patient regarding his/her choices of treatment when incapacitated. This may reflect the patient's preferences or give clear instructions refusing medical procedures. The latter is sometimes called an advance directive. As these 'living wills' are made in advance without knowing the nature of one's future incapacitation (or indeed that it will occur), they can lack precision. For example, an advance directive to refuse 'life support' could prevent effective management of diabetic or anaphylactic shock, both treatable conditions with

potentially excellent outcomes. Also, in the ICU, medical treatment decisions are seldom made once and for all, as the critically ill patient's condition may continually change. None the less, the intensivist should observe guidelines below.

- ICU staff may be legally liable if they disregard an advance directive refusing treatment that it is applicable to the clinical situation, except in cases where refusal harms others (e.g. spread of infection) or conflicts with local legislation.
- Advance statements of preferences and general beliefs that do not refuse treatment may have no legal binding but should be respected. Demands for continuation of futile treatment or treatment that does not serve the patient's best interests, usually have no legal force.
- Minors do not have the same rights at law as adults.
- An advance statement or directive is superseded by a clear and competent contemporaneous decision by the patient concerned.
- Relatives or surrogates cannot overrule an advance directive.

CONFIDENTIALITY[4]

ICU staff have a moral and legal duty to observe patient confidentiality. Important principles of confidentiality applicable in intensive care are:

- ICU staff can record only patient information that is necessary for patient care. Consent is required to use information for research, quality assurance, or other stated purposes, unless anonymity is applied.
- Patient consent is needed for disclosure of information to third parties. Consent for disclosure to other health care providers can be obtained when consent is sought for medical care in (1) above.
- Patient information may only be used or disclosed for the purposes that it was collected, unless the patient's consent is obtained.
- For incompetent adult patients and minors, consent may be given by an authorized third party.
- Anonymous information should be used whenever possible.
- Patient information must be accurate, up-to-date and safeguarded against unauthorized access or misuse.

END-OF-LIFE DECISIONS[5]

End-of-life decisions in the ICU can be considered under withdrawal or withholding of treatment and euthanasia. These issues are highly controversial and fraught with ethical, moral and legal dilemmas. The law is sometimes unclear. Groups with unbending convictions (e.g. 'right-to-life' and 'voluntary euthanasia' believers), public misconceptions, different interpretations of terminology and irresponsible public media add to difficulties.

WITHDRAWAL OR WITHHOLDING THERAPY[6–10]

The withdrawal or withholding of treatment which sustains or prolongs life has been called, unfortunately, 'passive euthanasia', a term which is misleading. Allowing a patient to die by withdrawing failed treatment or forgoing treatment that offers no net benefit, when death is inevitable, is not euthanasia, as the intentions are different. The situation in intensive care differs from that outside the ICU. Withdrawing and withholding therapy when death is not imminent, but because it is intolerably burdensome or because the patient is in a state of worthless existence (e.g. persistent vegetative state), are not considerations in the ICU. Discussions of withdrawing or withholding therapy are not relevant to patients declared brain dead. These patients are legally dead and any continuing treatment is pointless.

Withdrawing or withholding therapy accords with ethical principles above. It puts the welfare of the patient foremost, avoids harm from continuing treatment, and applies equity in use of ICU resources. The law is unclear in some circumstances, but intensivists differentiate withdrawing therapy from physician-assisted suicide (see below). Withdrawing life support is widely practised in North America and Australasia.[6–8,11–13] Indeed, withdrawing or withholding life support is the most common cause of death in US ICUs.[11]

Important considerations in withdrawal or withholding therapy are as follows.

- The intensivist has to decide whether the treatment can be justified, weighing up prognosis, benefits and burdens. Caring for the patient and family should take precedence over an all-out preservation of life *per se*.
- A patient's wish and a valid advance directive to refuse some or all treatment must be followed (principle of autonomy). However, but there is no right to inappropriate treatment such as continuing futile treatment.
- The public, local laws and some clinicians[14] may differentiate between withdrawing therapy and withholding therapy, but there is no moral difference.
- Relatives of an incompetent patient, ICU staff, and other involved specialists are to be consulted. The patient's dignity, comfort, rights, cultural and religious beliefs, and known wishes must be protected and respected. Effective communication between the ICU team and the patient's family must be maintained. Discussions should be recorded.
- A management plan to withdraw and withhold therapy should be formulated. There are no moral differences between categories of withdrawal. Removal of the endotracheal tube as the first step has been

reported,[15] and may be a common practice. However, it may be less distressing for the patient, family and staff, if the process is sequential rather than a single step. Plans to withdraw life support vary among intensivists.[7,16,17] A common first step is to discontinue dialytic therapy, inotropic drugs, bedside monitoring, laboratory tests, and antibiotics. Discontinuation of nutrition and mechanical ventilation then follows some hours or even days later, with the endotracheal tube left *in situ*. Administration of muscle relaxants has been reported[18] but is illogical and unnecessary. Morphine and sedatives must be given liberally, even it they hasten death (see below). A plan appropriate to each patient should be applied. Use of slang and colloquial terms such as 'terminal weaning' is best avoided as they mean different things to different people.

EUTHANASIA

Euthanasia can be defined as '*a direct act to terminate life with primary intent*' and can be viewed as three types:

1. 'Voluntary euthanasia', or intentional killing of those who have expressed a competent, freely made wish to be killed
2. Physician-assisted suicide and
3. 'Non-voluntary euthanasia', or homicide by agreement of all parties except the patient.

There is enormous debate on euthanasia. The public and the media generally refer to voluntary euthanasia, but are often confused with terms and concepts. Requests for euthanasia in the ICU are rare. Advocates of euthanasia argue that it is morally justified in certain cases, as the ultimate outcome is 'best' for the patient, and that there is no moral difference between letting die on request and killing on request. However, if society allows euthanasia, it cannot guarantee safeguards against non-voluntary euthanasia (either accidental or intentional) in vulnerable patients such as the elderly and those with chronic debilitating diseases. Patients' trust in their physicians may be irreparably harmed. In most jurisdictions, all types of euthanasia are illegal, and at present they have no place in intensive care. It must be emphasized again that withdrawal or withholding therapy is not euthanasia, as a direct act is absent and the primary intent is not to kill. Also, death in terminally ill patients, hastened by respiratory depression from liberal doses of opioids, is not euthanasia. The intention in administrating the opioids is to relief pain and discomfort at the end of life, and not to kill ('double effect' doctrine).[19]

RESOLVING ETHICAL CONFLICTS

Making medical ethical decisions is not simple and cannot always be derived from set protocols. The following guidelines may be useful.

- The intensivist can start with his/her own personal beliefs and values, but in multicultural societies such as Australia and the USA, concepts of life will be diverse.
- It may be helpful to refer to relevant State and Federal laws and the regulations and guidelines of professional bodies, such as the Australian & New Zealand College of Anaesthetists and the Faculty of Intensive Care's *Statement Relating to the Relief of Pain and Suffering and End of Life Decisions*.[20] However, many ethical issues in medical practice are not covered by laws, regulations, or guidelines, and the law may contradict ethical principles.
- The intensivist may turn to case-based ethical reasoning, whereby the ethical issue is considered in terms of other cases previously decided by consensus. The analysis covers the areas of medical indications, patient preferences, quality of life, and contextual features (external socio-economic factors) in the background of ethical principles and applicable laws. However, case reviews can be subjective and a consensus, which is a majority view, may be unfair to minorities or the weak and defenseless.
- The intensivist may require the advice and guidance of close colleagues, institutional ethics committees, or professional bodies. He/she may even need to turn to a court of law for ruling. The International Code of Medical Ethics, which is a modern-day Hippocratic oath, is given below for reference (Table 6.1).
- Consultation with patients' families and ICU staff is good practice.

Table 6.1 International Code of Medical Ethics[21]

- I solemnly pledge myself to consecrate my life to the service of humanity
- I will give to my teachers the respect and gratitude which is their due
- I will practise my profession with conscience and dignity
- The health of my patient will be my first consideration
- I will respect the secrets which are confided in me, even after the patient has died
- I will maintain by all means in my power, the honour and the noble traditions of the medical profession
- My colleagues will be my sisters and brothers
- I will not permit consideration of age, disease or disability, creed, ethnic origin, gender, nationality, political affiliation, race, sexual orientation, or social standing to intervene between my duty and my patient
- I will maintain the utmost respect for human life from its beginning even under threat and I will not use my medical knowledge contrary to the laws of humanity
- I make these promises solemnly, freely and upon my honour

REFERENCES

1 Consent. Report of the Working Party 2001. London: British Medical Association; 2001.

2 Coulter A, Entwistle V, Gilbert D. Sharing decisions with patients: is the information good enough? *BMJ* 1999: 318; 318–22.

3 Advance Statements about Medical Treatment. Report of the Working Party 1995. London: British Medical Association; 1995.

4 Confidentiality and Disclosure of Health Information. Report of the Working Party 1999. London: British Medical Association; 1999.

5 Sprung CL. End-of-life decisions in critical care medicine – where are we headed? *Crit Care Med* 1998; **28**: 200–2.

6 Brody HML, Campbell ML, Faber-Langendoen K, Ogle KS. Withdrawing intensive life-sustaining treatment – recommendations for compassionate clinical management. *N Engl J Med* 1997; **336**: 652–7.

7 Faber-Langendoen K, Lanken P. Dying patients in the intensive care unit: foregoing treatment, maintaining care. *Ann Intern Med* 2000; **133**: 886–93.

8 Fisher MM, Raper RF. Withdrawing and withholding treatment in intensive care. *Med J Aust* 1990; **153**: 217–29.

9 Winter B, Cohen S. ABC of intensive care. Withdrawal of treatment. *BMJ* 1999; **319**: 306–8.

10 American Thoracic Society. Withholding and withdrawing life-sustaining therapy. *Ann Intern Med* 1991; **115**: 478–85.

11 Prendergast TJ, Claessens MT, Luce JM. A national survey of end-of-life care for critically ill patients. *Am J Respir Crit Care Med* 1998; **158**: 1163–7.

12 Keenan SP, Busche KD, Chen L, *et al.* A retrospective review of a large cohort of patients undergoing the process of withholding or withdrawal of life support. *Crit Care Med* 1997; **25**: 1324–31.

13 Eschun GM, Jacobson E, Roberts D, Sneiderman B. Ethical and practical considerations of withdrawal of treatment in the intensive care unit. *Can J Anaesth* 1999; **45**: 405–8.

14 Keenan SP, Busche KD, Chen L, *et al.* Withdrawal and withholding of life support in the intensive care unit: a comparison of teaching and community hospitals. *Crit Care Med* 1998; **26**: 245–51.

15 Mayer SA, Kossoff SB. Withdrawal of life support in the neurological intensive care unit. *Neurology* 1999; **52**: 1602–9.

16 Asch DA, Faber-Langendoen K, Shea JA, Christakis NA. The sequence of withdrawing life-sustaining treatment from patients. *Am J Med* 1999; **107**: 153–6.

17 Vincent J-L. Forgoing life support in Western European intensive care units: the results of an ethical questionnaire. *Crit Care Med* 1999; **27**: 1626–33.

18 Truog RD, Burns JP, Mitchell C *et al.* Pharmacologic paralysis and withdrawal of mechanical ventilation at the end of life. *N Engl J Med* 2000; **342**: 508–11.

19 Luce JL, Alpers A. End-of-life care: what do the American courts say? *Crit Care Med* 2001; Feb Suppl **29**(2): N40–N45.

20 Statement Relating to the Relief of Pain and Suffering and End of Life Decisions. Professional document PS38 1999. Melbourne: Australian & New Zealand College of Anaesthetists; 1999.

21 International Code of Medical Ethics. Declaration of Geneva: World Medical Association; 1994.

7.

Common problems after ICU

C S Waldmann

Until recently, an intensive care unit (ICU) stay was deemed successful if a patient survived to go to the ward. No consideration was taken of the patient dying on the ward or soon after leaving hospital or indeed if the patient went home with an appalling quality of life.

Mortality figures for patients leaving our own ICU recently are shown in Fig. 7.1.

A Kings Fund report[1] in 1989 concluded that it was necessary to look at the morbidity following critical illness as well as mortality: 'There is more to life than measuring death'.

Recent publications such as that of the Audit Commission (Critical to Success)[2] and that of the National Expert Group[3] (Comprehensive Critical Care) have supported the development of follow-up for patients following a stay in intensive care.

We have been following-up patients after critical illness for 8 years. The service 'Intensive After Care After Intensive Care' until recently fell between too many

stools. Following multiorgan dysfunction, it is difficult to categorize a patient to an individual speciality such as Cardiac, Respiratory or the Stroke Rehabilitation Teams.

SETTING UP A FOLLOW-UP SERVICE

Funding what is essentially a new service may pose local problems in different health services. Our service was initially funded by local then regional Audit Committees.

The service is staffed by a follow-up sister helped by a staff nurse 1 day per week and an ICU consultant for the clinics held as a formal outpatient clinic twice monthly.

Patients who were in ICU more than 4 days are followed up at 2 months, 6 months and 1 year after discharge and, occasionally, we will see referrals from other hospitals. It is important to identify clerical and IT support, to achieve good collaboration with other hospital departments and GPs to ensure patients do not make unnecessary journeys to the hospital and ensure that transport is organized where necessary. Very often, patients will voluntarily come from long distances if they had initially been admitted from other geographical locations, 'Out of Area Transfers'.

The logistics of running the service include prospectively arranging specific tests that may be required for the visit, such as pulmonary function tests, swabs for MRSA, blood/urine for creatinine clearance. There may be special tests such as magnetic resonance imaging (MRI)[4] for patients who had a tracheostomy in ICU.

The costs last year were estimated at £30 000 which in the context of the bigger picture (£3.1 million budget for our ICU) is a small price to pay (Fig. 7.2).

SPECIFIC PROBLEMS POST ICU

The range of problems seen after intensive care is vast and ranges from nightmares and sleep disturbance through to ill-fitting clothes. Many of the problems are very specific

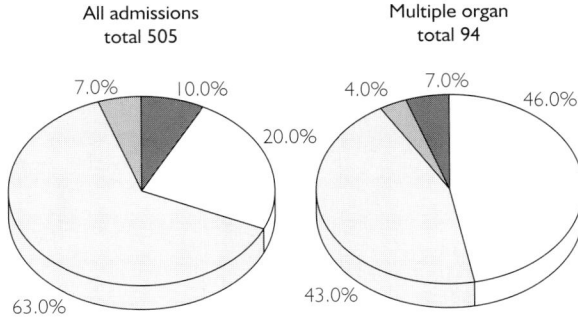

All admissions total 505 — 7.0%, 10.0%, 20.0%, 63.0%

Multiple organ total 94 — 4.0%, 7.0%, 46.0%, 43.0%

Mortality in ICU
Mortality in hospital after discharge from ICU
Mortality within 1 year after discharge from ICU
Survivors 1 year after discharge

Fig. 7.1 Mortality rates for leaving ICU

Follow-up clinic	
Nursing	£18 000
Medical	£6 000
Administration	£4 000
Laboratory tests and X-rays	£2 000
Total	£30 000

Fig. 7.2   Costs of running a service

Table 7.1   Quality of Life tool examples

Objective	QALY	Quality of Life tool[5]
Subjective	HAD	Hospital Anxiety and Depression[6]
	PQOL	Perceived Quality of Life[7]
	EuroQol	'European' tool[8]
	SF 36	36 item short-form survey[9]

to the individual but there are also recurrent themes. Flashbacks are common as are taste loss, poor appetite, nail and hair disorders and sexual dysfunction.

There are several Quality of Life tools used in follow-up studies (Table 7.1). Objective measurements may be inappropriate because they look at aspects such as return to work; often, patients in their fifties may not return to work after a traumatic episode including ICU and subjective measures would be more applicable, such as perceived quality of life (PQOL).

TRACHEOSTOMY

Since percutaneous techniques performed by intensivists started to replace surgical tracheostomy in 1991, we have seen an increasing number of patients tracheostomized earlier in their ICU stay.

The long-term sequelae have been assessed by lung function tests, nasendoscopy and MRI screening (Fig. 7.3). There are minor cosmetic problems, such as tethering (Fig. 7.4). Tethering is easily dealt with in ENT outpatients under local anaesthetic.

More difficult to manage is tracheal stenosis, defined as a 15% reduction in tracheal diameter. However, there have been only two cases to date out of over 100 patients with tracheostomy. These were seen in the first series of 30 cases.[4]

MOBILITY

Even in the absence of trauma, patients can expect to need 9 months to 1 year to regain full mobility. This is usually due to a mixture of joint pain, stiffness and muscle weakness. In a recent study,[10] the duration of ICU stay was associated with mobility problems probably associated with loss of muscle mass. Often patients, if

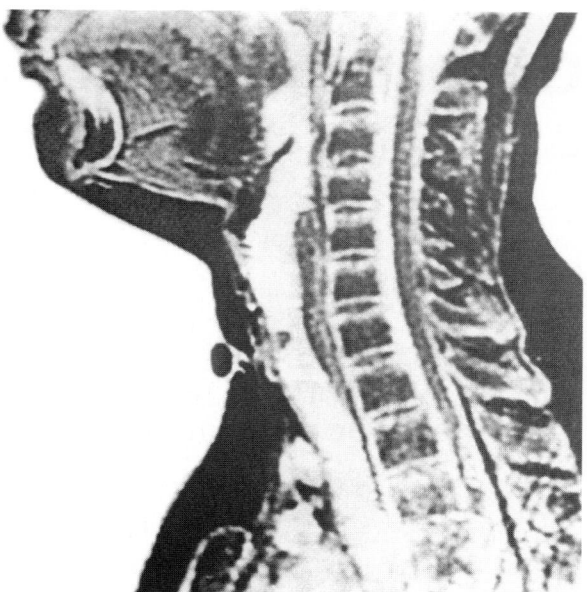

Fig. 7.3   Assessment of long-term sequelae

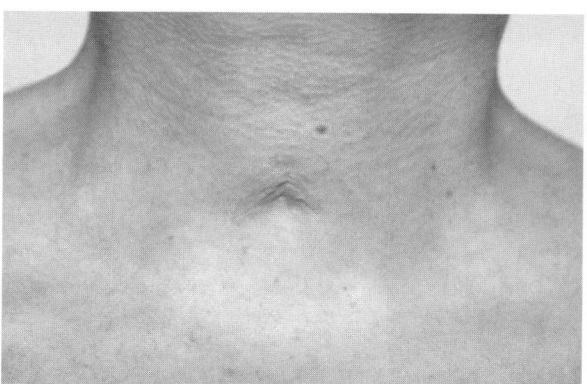

Fig. 7.4   Tethering

questioned, will report climbing stairs on all fours and descending on their bottoms (Fig. 7.5).

Critical illness polyneuropathy (CIP)[11] may be responsible for prolonged weaning times from ventilatory support and may delay rehabilitation. Muscle wasting can present as a severe localized problem.

The part played by muscle relaxants in the development of CIP has been previously emphasized[12] but recently has been shown to be statistically insignificant in terms of delayed weaning of intermittent positive-pressure ventilation and duration of stay in ICU.[13]

Until now, there have been no specific rehabilitation programmes for patients recovering from critical illness, whereas rehabilitation programmes for heart attack,

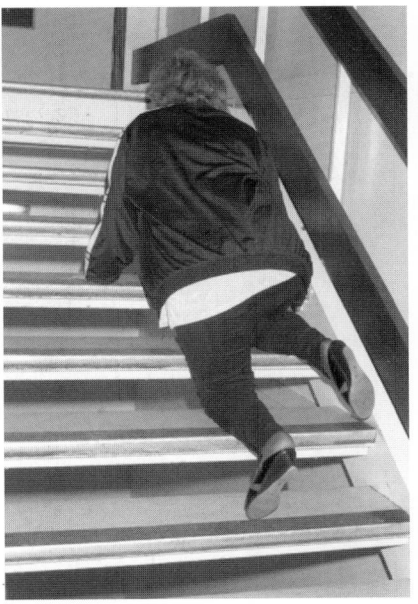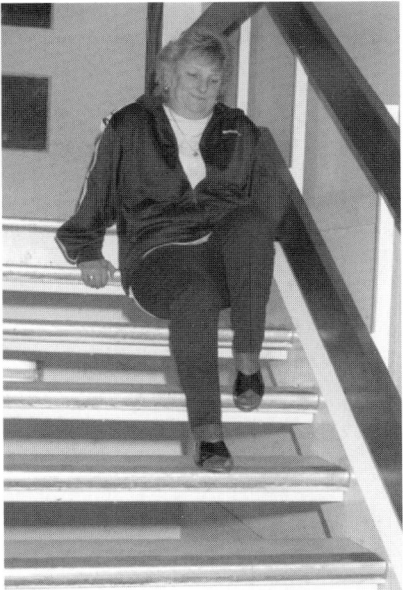

Fig. 7.5   Climbing and descending stairs

stroke and respiratory disease are well established. A recent three centre study has shown that a self-help, guided rehabilitation exercise programme will speed up physical recovery after intensive care.[14]

It is important for a member of the team to spend time with patients at their homes to assess their special needs and liaise with the GPs, district nurses, community physiotherapists and occupational therapists.

SKIN

Patients complain of a variety of non-specific disorders including hair loss or nail ridging. Severe pruritis used to be common and not amenable to treatment and traced back to the use of starch solutions in ICU. This was confirmed by a study published in 2000,[15] which looked at 85 cardiac surgical patients. Pruritis was absent in the 26 patients who did not receive starch, but there was a 22% incidence in the 59 patients who did receive starch.

Colonization with methicillin-resistant *Staphylococcus aureus* (MRSA) presents problems. It often takes 9 months for patients to lose their MRSA status (Fig. 7.6). It is common to find patients being treated as 'lepers' by their own family.

SEXUAL DYSFUNCTION

Any patient who estimates their sex-life activity to be less active than before ICU admission is deemed to have sexual dysfunction.

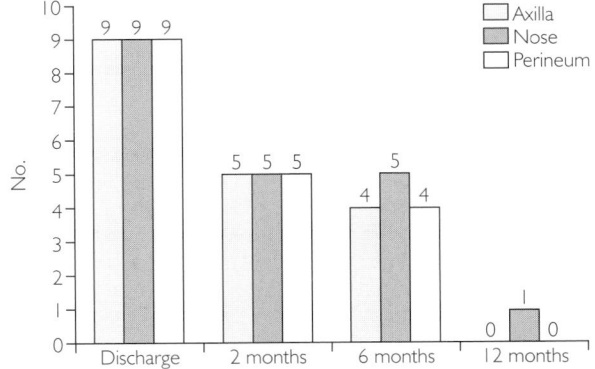

Fig. 7.6   Colonization with MRSA

In a recent study,[16] there was a 39% incidence of sexual dysfunction in a group of 57 patients. In four patients, sex-life had improved. Sexual dysfunction improves with time, about 26% at 2 months post ICU down to 16% at 1 year.[17] Sexual dysfunction is thought to be a psychological problem but interestingly, following severe burns, it has been reported that there is no correlation between the incidence of post-traumatic stress syndrome and sexual dysfunction.[18] Nevertheless, withdrawing sexual intimacy because of fear of failure can damage relationships. Often sexual dysfunction may go untreated because people are too embarrassed to mention the problem when they have recovered from a life-threatening illness.

Sexual dysfunction can effect women as well as men. In the latter, it usually manifests itself as impotence or inability to maintain an erection sufficient for satisfactory sexual activity. There are now UK management guidelines for erectile dysfunction.[19]

In investigating sexual dysfunction, it is important to eliminate causes such as use of drugs e.g., L-Dopa and H_2-blockers and certain types of surgery (aortic aneurysm) or trauma/radiotherapy to the pelvic region. The patients may be diabetic.

Treatments available include intracavernous or trans-ureteral alprostadil or oral Viagra. Patients with cardio-vascular dysfunction have to be carefully assessed before being given Viagra. Non-pharmacological therapies include the use of vacuum devices and inflatable penile prostheses.

In females, sexual dysfunction may occur due to surgery or trauma to the pelvis. More commonly, there is a reduction in desire. Various lubricating gels can be used. As yet, the role of Viagra for women has to be determined.

OTHER PHYSICAL PROBLEMS

A variety of other problems have been seen during follow-up:

- In patients who have been profoundly hypotensive, visual problems may occur. Occasionally ischaemic changes may be seen on fundoscopy (Fig. 7.7a), which may be amenable to laser therapy (Fig. 7.7b).
- Severe scarring where the tape fixing in the endotracheal tube is too tight. This scarring can be the whole thickness of the cheek.
- It is not uncommon to discover patients on medication started in ICU as a temporary measure that have not been discontinued (e.g. Amiodarone started for sepsis-related arrhythmias).

PSYCHOLOGICAL PROBLEMS

Most patients admitted to ICU have no warning of their admission (emergency admission) and these are the patients very much at risk of psychological sequelae post ICU.

The majority of patients do not have a structured memory of their ICU stay. Those that do may have upsetting memories which may be relatively innocuous, such as being thirsty and hearing a can of coke being opened, or of a far more profound nature.

The story of 'torture' experiences is not unusual when you talk to an ex-ICU patient. The psychological impact of the experience may be formidable and may be resented by the patient. The memory of hearing that a patient is about to be 'bagged' was interpreted as being put into a body bag rather than a physiotherapy manoeuvre and the

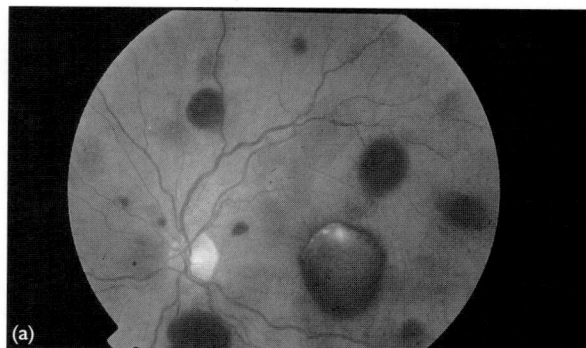
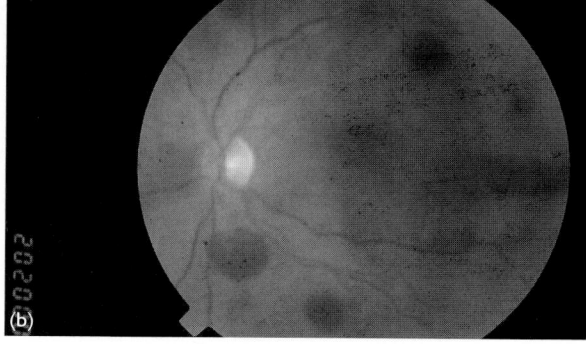

Fig. 7.7 Ischaemic changes in fundoscopy

use of a tape-measure was interpreted as being measured for a coffin and not as part of the cardiac output measurements. Previous studies demonstrate a high incidence of anxiety, depression and post-traumatic stress.[20] It is common for patients to have memories of being trapped, of being unable to move easily, of being unable to see what is happening and of feeling intensely vulnerable. The anxiety of impending death is also reported.

Below is a typical nightmare of one of our patients:

'I was in a tunnel knee-deep in mud. It was pitch black, but I could see light at the end. I felt a cold chill on my neck as if someone was breathing down my neck. I thought it was the grim-reaper, I knew I had to get to the light.'

There may be several reasons for these experiences (Table 7.2).

There is a common belief that, when on ICU, it is better that a patient does not remember anything. However, it is increasingly realized that false memories or delusions during an ICU stay can have a significant impact on psychological recovery after ICU[21] and factual memories of ICU may reduce anxiety.[22]

It now seems likely that delusional memories of ICU and nightmares are associated with post-traumatic stress disorder (PTSD).

Table 7.2 Psychological problems

Illness
Sedation technique
Withdrawal
No communication aids
Lack of clear night/day
Continuous noise of alarms
Sleep disturbance – lack of REM sleep

PTSD is a normal reaction to severe stress and is similar to a grief reaction to bereavement. It occurs in about 1% of the population and increases to 10% in victims of road traffic accidents and 65% in prisoners of war. About 15% of patients have the typical disorder post ICU. In those with adult respiratory distress syndrome, the incidence increases to 27.5%.

PTSD is the development of characteristic symptoms after being subjected to a traumatic event. PTSD can be triggered by any memory or mention of something to do with the traumatic event and is characterized by intrusive recollections, avoidance behaviour and hyper-arousal symptoms.[23]

Chronic fatigue syndrome (CFS), previously known as ME, is thought to describe the condition of many patients post-ICU who have had a period of prolonged inactivity. CFS is diagnosed by the presence of fatigue at 6 months post ICU with impairment of daily living, social and leisure pursuits and with no medically significant cause of the fatigue. There is no doubt that a graded exercise programme is of benefit to aid physical recovery in such ICU patients.[14] Drugs such as fluoxetime (Prozac) do not seem to benefit such patients, even though there is a great temptation to use antidepressants in these patients.[24]

Various strategies to deal with the psychological sequelae of ICU stay have been tried.

DURING ICU STAY

● There is no doubt that continuous i.v. sedation has been identified as an independent predictor of a longer duration of mechanical ventilation, ICU stay and total hospital stay.[25] Kreiss *et al.*[26] demonstrated that, in 128 adults, ICU stay was reduced from an average of 7.3 to 4.9 days by the daily interruption of the sedative regime. This regime may have had an impact by reducing PTSD as the patients are more likely to have some recollection of their ICU stay, thus helping them to understand the reasons for the need for their prolonged rehabilitation period. Concerns have been raised as to the type of sedative agent used in ICU. It is well know that Etomidate may cause an excess in mortality in trauma patients in ICU[27] and propofol may do the same in head-injured

patients at doses greater than 5 mg/kg per h.[28] The decision to increasingly use benzodiazepines such as midazolam may be associated with dependency. In a study in Manchester, 21 out of 148 ICU patients were discharged home on oral benzodiazepine, of which 10 were still taking them at 6 months post discharge having not been on them pre-ICU.[29] More recently, lorazepam has been promoted as the benzodiazepine of choice for sedation in ICU[30] and is preferred by a task force in the USA for adult patients in ICU.[31]

● Encouraging the use of communication aids, involving speech therapists particularly in patients with tracheostomies[32] and training more nurses to lip-read can be invaluable.

● When building or modifying ICUs, remember that windows and 24-hour clocks visible to patients may help re-establish circadian rhythms and the use of curtains to ensure patient dignity should not be forgotten. There has been some interest in appropriate colours that should be used in ICU décor with avoidance of colours that cause alarm in the animal kingdom such as red, yellow and black.

● Use of aromatherapy and massage whilst patients receive their ICU does seem to reduce stress levels and encourage contact between the patient and relatives, reducing the feeling of isolation.[33]

POST ICU DISCHARGE

Visiting patients on the ward post ICU discharge and giving them an information booklet helps to prepare them better for the long rehabilitation process ahead.

As well as three ICU Follow-Up Clinic appointments in the year after their discharge, patients with PTSD are encouraged to visit the ICU and, with the help of a diary, reconstruct the lost period of time in the patient's life. We are considering the use of photos of patients whilst they are on ICU to help them understand how ill they actually were.

CONCLUSION

It is important to assess patient satisfaction or dissatisfaction with their follow-up. This may be audited by questionnaire during their third visit to the Follow-Up Clinic at 1 year post-ICU discharge.[34]

The response rate was 87 out of 88 patients and all but one of the 87 patients found benefit from the Clinic specifically because questions could be answered (often their GP could not help); 28% benefited from referral to other specialists and 26% from PTSD counselling. About 25% felt they benefited from returning to the ICU and having a diary written for them. Nearly half (48%) felt they were helping the staff of the ICU.

The comments were very useful e.g.:

- 'You helped me fill in the time lost whilst under sedation'
- 'It was frightening leaving ICU to go back to the ward. My wife slept next to me in the ward on a mattress on the floor'

There is no end to the surprises and unexpected problems that arise in patients after intensive care. It is not unusual to see patients who were initially deemed inappropriate for surgery and ICU, who have done well and who on questioning have an excellent quality of life. It is only by the ICU specialists undertaking to follow-up patients that we can assess the appropriateness of our decision making and treatments.

REFERENCES

1 Kings Fund. Intensive Care in the United Kingdom; a report from the Kings Fund Panel. *Anaesthesia* 1989; **44**: 428–30.
2 Critical to Success. *The Place of Efficient and Effective Critical Care Services within the Acute Hospital.* London: Audit Commission; October 1999.
3 Comprehensive Critical Care. A Review of Adult Critical Care Services. Department of Health Publication 2000 (www.doh.gov.uk/nhsexec/comparitcare.htm).
4 Bernau F, Waldmann CS, Meanock C, Thomas J. Long-term follow-up of percutaneous tracheostomy using flow-loop and MRI scanning. *Intensive Care Med* 1996; **22**: S295.
5 Harris J. Qualyfying the value of life. *J Med Ethics* 1987; **13**: 117–73.
6 Zigmond AS, Snaith RP. The hospital anxiety and depression scale. *Acta Psychiatry Scand* 1983; **67**: 361–70.
7 Patrick DL, Davis M, Southerland LI, Hong G. Quality of life following intensive care. *J Gen Int Med* 1988; **3**: 218–23.
8 Williams A. The Euro Qol – a new facility for the measurement of health related quality of life. *Health Policy II* 1990; **16**: 199–208.
9 Ware JE, Sherbourne CD. The MOS 36-item short-form health survey (SF-36): I. Conceptual framework and item selection. *Med Care* 1992; **30**: 473–81.
10 Jones C, Griffiths RD. Identifying post intensive care patients who may need physical rehabilitation. *Clin Intens Care* 2000; **11**: 35–8.
11 Leijten FSS, de Weerd AW. Critical illness polyneuropathy. A review of literature, definition and pathophysiology. *Clin Neurol Neurosurg* 1994; **96**: 10–19.
12 Barohn RJ, Jackson CE, Rogers SJ, *et al.* Prolonged paralysis due to non-depolarising neuromuscular blocking agents and corticosteroids. *Muscle Nerve* 1994; **17**: 647–54.
13 Zifko UA, Zipko HT, Bolton CF. Clinical and electrophysiological finding in critical illness polyneuropathy. *J Neurol Sci* 1998; **159**: 186–93.
14 Jones C, Skirrow P, Griffith RD. Rehabilitation after critical illness, a randomised controlled trial. *BJA* 2001; **87**: 330.
15 Morgan PW, Berridge JC. Giving long-persistent starch as volume replacement can cause pruritis after cardiac surgery. *BJA* 2000; **85**: 676–99.
16 Quinlan J, Gager M, Fawcett D, Waldmann CS. Sexual dysfunction after intensive care. *BJA* 2001; **87**: 348.
17 Quinlan J, Waldmann CS, Fawcett D. Sexual dysfunction after intensive care. *BJA* 1998; **81**: 809–810.
18 De Rios MD, Norac A, Achauer BH. Sexual dysfunction and the patient with burns. *Burn Care Rehabilit* 1997; **18**: 37–42.
19 Ralph D, McNicholas T. UK Management Guidelines for Erectile Dysfunction. *BMJ* 2000; **321**: 499–503.
20 Koshy G, Wilkinson A, Harmsworth A, Waldmann CS. Intensive care unit follow-up program at a district general hospital. *Intensive Care Med* 1997; **23**: S160.
21 Griffiths RD, Jones C, McMillan I. Where is the harm in not knowing? Care after intensive care. *Clin Intens Care* 1996; **7**: 144–45.
22 Jones C, Griffiths RD, Humphries G. Factual memories of intensive care may reduce anxiety post-ICU. *BJA* 2000; **82**: 793.
23 Horowitz M J. Stress response syndromes – a review of post-traumatic stress and adjustment disorders. In: Wilson JP, Raphael B (eds). *International Handbook of Traumatic Stress Syndromes.* New York: Plenum Press; 1993: pp. 49–60.
24 Jones C, Skirrow P, Griffiths RD, *et al.* The characteristics of patients given antidepressants while recovering from critical illness. *BJA* 2000; **84**: 666.
25 Kollef MH, Levy NT, Ahrens TS, *et al.* The use of continuous IV sedation is associated with prolongation of mechanical ventilation. *Chest* 1998; **114**: 541–8.
26 Kreiss JP, Pohlman AS, O'Connor MF, Hall JB. Daily interruption of sedative infusions in critically ill patients undergoing mechanical ventilation. *N Engl J Med* 2000; **342**: 1471–7.
27 Ledingham IM, Watt I. Influence of sedation in multiple trauma patients. *Lancet* 1983; editorial: 1270.
28 Cremer OL, Moons GM, Bouman EAC, *et al.* Long-term propofol infusion and cardiac failure in adult head-injured patients. *Lancet* 2001; **357**: 117–118.
29 Conway DH, Eddleston J, Turner S. Prevalence of oral sedation dependency following intensive care. *Intensive Care Med* 1999; **25** (suppl. 1): S169.
30 Meagher DJ. Delirium: optimising management. *BMJ* 2001; **322**: 144–9.
31 Shapiro BA, Warren J, Egol AB, *et al.* Practice parameters for intravenous analgesia and sedation in the Intensive Care Unit: an executive summary. *Crit Care Med* 1995; **23**: 1596–600.

32 Etchels MC (Personal Communication) ICU Talk (www.computing.dundee.ac.uk/projects/icutalk).

33 Waldmann CS, Tseng P, Meulman P, Whittet H. Aromatherapy in the intensive care unit. *Care Crit Ill* 1993; **9**: 170–4.

34 Hames KC, Gager M, Waldmann CS. Patient satisfaction with specialist ICU follow-up. *BJA* 2001; **87**: 372.

8

Clinical information systems

D Fraenkel

Clinical record keeping necessitates an integrated system to manage the information, including its acquisition during clinical care, and archiving and availability for future clinical, business, and research uses.

The term 'clinical information system' (CIS) usually refers to a computerized system for managing the clinical record, often within geographically or specialty defined areas of a hospital, such as intensive care, emergency medicine, operating theatres or cardiology. The electronic medical record (EMR) and the electronic healthcare record (EHCR) refer respectively to hospital and community wide electronic systems for storing and accessing patient records.

CIS for intensive care units (ICUs) have been developed and evaluated since the late 1980s; however, their implementation was sparing and erratic through the 1990s.[1-7]

The reasons for this slow uptake include:

- Financial cost
- Rapidly changing nature of the technology
- Lack of computer literacy amongst clinicians
- Limited ability of CIS to meet the standards and requirements of their clinical users[1,3,5,7-8]

More recently developed systems seem to be approaching the required functionality and CIS implementations are increasing, but the financial and human resources required to implement CIS are significant. This includes a substantial change in practice and infrastructure, similar in scope to the redevelopment of ICU facilities themselves.

FUNCTIONS AND ADVANTAGES OF CIS

CIS seek to deliver several key benefits (Table 8.1).[1,7,9] These include the automation of repetitive manual tasks, improved accuracy through reductions in human error, attributable records simultaneously available from multiple points of care, and integration with other bedside equipment and information systems. The built in error checking and knowledge-based systems should also provide a safer and higher quality clinical process. The

Table 8.1 CIS benefits

1. Recording of bedside observations
   - (a) automation of physiological data collection
   - (b) reduction in transcription and arithmetic errors
   - (c) downloading from bedside therapeutic devices (e.g. pumps, ventilators)
2. Clinical documentation
   - (a) legible and attributable clinical record
   - (b) structures and cues encourage comprehensive documentation
   - (c) electronic record of drug prescription and administration
   - (d) attributable record simultaneously available from multiple points of care
3. Access to additional clinical information at the bedside
   - (a) pathology results
   - (b) digitized medical imaging and reports
   - (c) digital clinical photographs
   - (d) other hospital systems (e.g. ADT, CIS)
4. Bedside decision support systems
   - (a) passive
     - (i) improved and accessible clinical record
     - (ii) online clinical policies and procedures
     - (iii) online knowledge bases
     - (iv) online literature searches
   - (b) active
     - (i) investigative and therapeutic management algorithms
     - (ii) clinical pathways
     - (iii) drug allergy and interaction alerts
     - (iv) drug dosing and monitoring support
     - (v) antibiotic selection and prescribing
     - (vi) ventilation and haemodynamic management systems
5. Medicolegal archiving
   - (a) audit trail for all changes during episode of care
   - (b) no ability to change once archived
   - (c) secure long term storage and ensured availability
6. Clinical databases
   - (a) long term accessible storage of relevant clinical data
   - (b) industry standard database format
   - (c) efficient and flexible query and reporting solutions
   - (d) scheduled and ad-hoc reports
   - (e) clinical, research and management requirements

CIS electronically captures the data and makes it potentially available to a multitude of systems. This obviates the need for repetitive manual data entry or transcription, while making the data accessible for a range of purposes which may include clinical, business and research reporting.

The ICU is already a technology rich environment, where bedside devices process and provide data elements in electronic format. Similarly, many clinical measurements are available on monitors, ventilators and pumps. Traditionally, these electronically derived values are transcribed onto observation charts and paper-based clinical records, as are repetitive clinical observations and arithmetic calculations which are often performed manually or with the aid of a calculator. The voluminous observation charts present a challenge for both storage and access, and transcription errors and arithmetic errors are prolific in these paper systems.

The CIS automates the process of electronic data collection from monitors, ventilators, infusion pumps, dialysis/filtration equipment, cardiac assist devices and other bedside devices and provides a real time spreadsheet with arithmetic accuracy.[10] Incorporation of clinical documentation and progress notes provides a legible and attributable record of events.

The patient record can then be accessed from geographically distant workstations in the ICU, the hospital, and even from other more remote sites. As long as the system is running, the record is easy to locate and always available.

A major contribution of CIS to clinical safety and quality is through the provision of an electronic prescribing and administration record for drugs and fluids. Errors in prescription and administration are a leading cause of adverse events with associated morbidity.[11-13] CIS provides both legibility and varying levels of decision support. These can range from defining usual dosages and administration routes to preventing prescribing in cases of known allergy or likely drug interaction. Despite evidence that such prescribing systems reduce pharmaceutical adverse events, the expense and often limited levels of decision support have impeded widespread implementation.[14]

ARCHITECTURE AND COMPONENTS OF CIS

BASIC CIS ARCHITECTURE

All CIS share certain basic components consisting of workstations, a network and central servers[9] (Fig. 8.1). The user interface is presented at the workstation which is usually at each bedside but may also be in nearby central and administrative areas, such as the nurses' station, or more distant in the offices of clinical or administrative staff. Workstations most commonly consist of standard personal computer (PC) hardware, often only requiring some additional RAM, video-cards or network cards. They may be placed at any convenient location.

Wireless systems are desirable but are not currently widely available and present technical challenges related to the speed and reliability of data transfer in an electromagnetically 'hostile' environment. Most CIS allow other

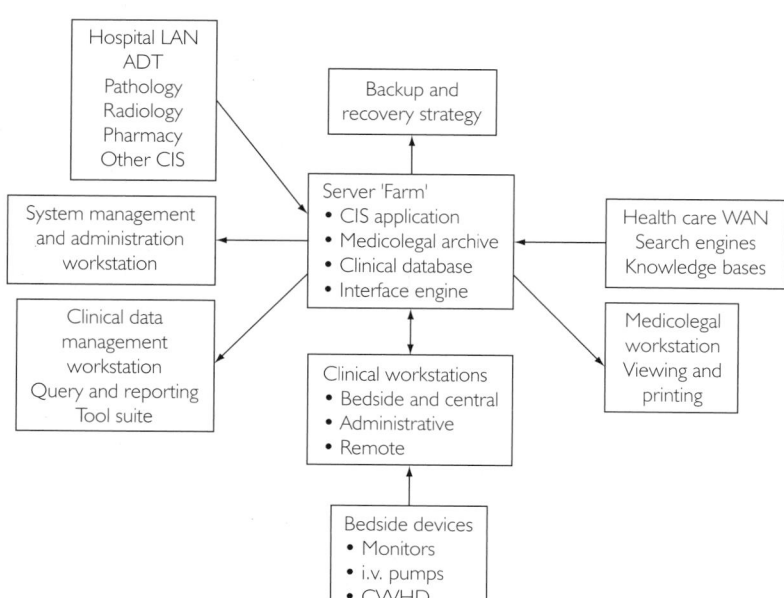

Fig. 8.1 CIS architecture. LAN, Local area network; WAN, wide area network; ADT, admission/discharge/transfer; CVVHD, continuous venovenous haemodialysis

applications, such as word processing or e-mail, to be run on the same PC, but this is potentially a rich source of system conflicts and requires careful administration.

Workstations are linked to each other and a centralized set of servers through a network of communication cables. Hubs, switches and routers control network traffic. A dedicated network, either actual or virtual, enhances system performance but it is important to ensure built in redundancy in network loops and power sources to minimize potential interruptions from physical disruption or component failure.

The configuration of computer servers varies widely but it is common to have 'paired' or 'mirrored' servers, which duplicate their partner's function. This provides protection from hardware failure, minimizing system down time, and provides some degree of data protection. Servers have a finite capacity to process data from multiple workstations and other peripheral connections, and so larger systems may require multiple server pairs.

CIS usually requires a separate workstation or server to manage the interfaces with other systems. These include hospital demographics (ADT systems for admission/ discharge/transfer), pathology laboratory, pharmacy, radiology and hospital finance.[1,9] Interfacing requires a software platform known as an 'interface engine'. Additional software identifies the relevant data and directs and processes it to the correct field in the appropriate format. Due to the huge variety of current and legacy systems, this process almost always requires custom written code and programming, representing one of the major risks and expenses of systems integration.[15]

Bedside monitoring systems usually include a central station or server that can be linked with the CIS servers to transfer their downloaded information back to the bedside. Transferring data from other bedside devices is usually achieved by a cable connection from the device to a bedside concentrator in the patient bay. The connection requires an electronic decoder, specific to the manufacturer and model of the device. The concentrator must then communicate with the central servers via a subsidiary server that provides the software translator to complete the interface. A selection of established interfaces to commonly utilized equipment exist but often additional customized interfaces must be written.

MEDICOLEGAL STORAGE

Electronic data capture does not necessarily result in long term electronic data storage. Many CIS sites continue to require the printing out of all reports from the patient episode to store in the paper-based hospital medical record.[1,8,9] Modern servers have extensive storage capacity but this can be rapidly consumed by the equally enormous amount of data being collected from every patient. Some server pairs can only hold 2–3 months of data before data begins to be purged or overwritten. An additional storage system such as extra hard disk arrays, more efficient database formats, CD-ROM jukeboxes, or digital tapes may be needed. When the choice of storage solution is made, it is equally important to be aware that the format of data storage is determined by the anticipated use of the data.

Data archiving for medicolegal purposes requires that the clinical information be readily accessible and preferably presented in exactly the same format as it was recorded and reviewed by the clinicians during the episode of patient care. Any changes to the clinical record during the patient episode must be clearly displayed and attributable – this is known as an audit trail or change history. An audit trail is a standard feature of most CIS and actually offers improved accountability over paper-based systems. It may be desirable to make it impossible to alter the record after the patient episode, which requires specialized storage formats or strict access restrictions to the data archive.

One solution to medicolegal archiving is to utilize electronic document management solutions (EDMS) which function much as computerized microfiche. Complete and timely storage of all CIS reports also requires a file registry on the CIS server and a rigorous file transfer system, together with a means of indexing, retrieving and reviewing the reports on the archival server. An alternative solution is to acquire enough memory in the CIS application server, or its subsidiary servers, to allow the storage of CIS data in its original format for a decade or so. As well as requiring more secure and restricted user access, this system requires guaranteed retrospective compatibility of any software revisions of the CIS application software.

Once the record is stored, by whatever method, it must be protected from accidental loss. This usually requires a carefully engineered and documented management plan with regular scheduled backups, off-site storage of duplicates, and robust recovery strategies. When these requirements are fulfilled, the electronic medicolegal archive can readily exceed the performance of a paper-based record through its assured availability and authenticity.

CLINICAL DATABASE STORAGE

A major objective of CIS is to provide a comprehensive clinical database which will accumulate data in real time that can be stored and queried for a wide range of reports for a variety of purposes.[1,6,8,9,16] The relevant data needs to be held in an accessible and readily searchable database that will allow a variety of sophisticated reports to be prepared on both a scheduled and *ad hoc* basis. These requirements are quite different from those of medicolegal storage and usually require a separate form of data storage commonly known as a clinical database or clinical data management solution.

It may be desirable to adopt a significantly different database structure from the core CIS database that is after used for only temporary storage. The CIS database table structure may have been designed with prospective user configurability in mind, rather than allowing easy location of data fields in a structure designed for rapidly processing queries. The design of the clinical database is a compromise between saving effectively the large amount of data collected while maintaining speed and ease of use in running queries. Even when the vendor has utilized an industry standard database application, such as Oracle™ or Sybase™, in the core CIS application, designing and running queries may still present a challenging specialist task because of the complexity of the table structure or the huge amount of aggregated data.

The clinical data management solutions currently offered are quite diverse. One solution simply provides an industry standard data transfer protocol (e.g. 'ODBC driver'). The local circumstances of each hospital then dictate a customized design for local use. Alternatively, an industry standard query tool is used to generate reports from the core CIS database, but the number of queries that can be designed and preconfigured in this fashion is relatively limited, particularly as the user configurations of the CIS vary widely. There is inevitably a compromise between standardization and flexibility. Data fields must be defined in the user configuration of the CIS, and then located in the table structure, to allow standard queries to be performed. Some CIS solutions offer a subsidiary database containing selected clinical data with a wider range of reports preconfigured into the query tool.

EVALUATION AND IMPLEMENTATION OF CIS

Clinicians frequently underestimate the financial, human resource, and opportunity costs of CIS purchase and implementation.[7,17] The process should be viewed as a major project requiring advanced planning and management skills[18,19] (Table 8.2). The project team must be multidisciplinary and consult widely or else a suboptimal result is guaranteed.[7,20] The CIS will impact on medical, nursing, allied health, managerial and technical staff within the ICU, together with those from other clinical disciplines. Involvement of hospital information management and medical records staff is strongly recommended. Extensive documentation and continued scheduled reviews are required throughout the process.

Business case development to secure funding is difficult. Many of the benefits of CIS are improvements in quality rather than outright financial savings.[21] The most basic system can be expected to cost in the order of AUD $25 000 per bed, while more advanced systems may be two to three times that cost. Annual recurrent costs are significant and usually exceed 20% of the capital cost of the system.

Table 8.2 CIS implementation

1 Professional project management
  (a) structured multidisciplinary team
    (i) sponsor, director, manager, representatives
    (ii) medical, nursing, allied health, managerial
  (b) comprehensive documentation
  (c) consultative approach
    (i) medical records department
    (ii) IT/IM department
    (iii) hospital and business managers
2 Project framework
  (a) needs analysis
  (b) definition of scope
  (c) management of expectations and scope creep
3 Tender evaluation (Table 8.3)
4 Implementation process
  (a) implementation plan and schedule
  (b) training
  (c) installation
  (d) schedule of payments
  (e) quality monitoring of process
5 Post-implementation review
  (a) actual outcomes cf plan
  (b) unresolved issues
  (c) process improvement
6 System management plan
  (a) identification of system components
  (b) departmental and individual roles and responsibilities
  (c) identification of vendor responsibilities
  (d) backup schedules and recovery plans
7 Support contracts
  (a) scope and level of support
  (b) pricing
8 Future issues
  (a) ongoing management of 'special projects'
  (b) continued development and innovation
  (c) system upgrades
  (d) scheduled hardware replacement
  (e) system obsolescence and replacement

The CIS industry is subject to the same vagaries as other parts of the information technology industry. These include:

- rapid product development
- high turnover of personnel
- frequent inability to deliver on promised functionality and time lines[2,3,7,22]

CIS selection is best conducted as a formal tender process, and the evaluation of submissions is a complex task[20] (Table 8.3). Availability and expense of on-site support during and following implementation is also a critical factor.[15,22]

Implementation planning should be detailed and requires a full time project officer on site.[17,23] A standard implementation needs 4–6 months prior to the 'go live' date with hospital wide consultation, issue management

Table 8.3 CIS evaluation

1 Vendor characteristics
  (a) monitoring cf. software expertise
  (b) niche specialty products cf. healthcare wide
  (c) development base by specialty and geography
2 Preliminary evaluation
  (a) evaluate tender documents
  (b) product demonstration
  (c) prepared and impromptu scenario testing of product
  (d) ensure all required components identified e.g. database, interfaces, etc.
  (e) comparative levels of best fit for needs and specifications
3 Site visits to installed customer base
  (a) reference sites and 'sites like us'
  (b) demonstrations with vendor
  (c) candid visits without vendor
  (d) observe functionality
  (e) examine interfaces
  (f) explore support issues
4 Interfaces
  (a) identify requirements
  (b) assess vendor capabilities
  (c) inspect working interfaces
  (d) customization scope and cost
5 Technical issues
  (a) industry standard hardware and software
  (b) local acceptability
  (c) integration with existing systems
  (d) upgrade paths
  (e) network specifications
  (f) network costs and management
6 Support issues
  (a) location and availability
  (b) product support specialists
  (c) technical engineers
  (d) level of risk sharing
  (e) whole of life costing

and carefully scheduled staff training. It is desirable to have as many as possible of the interfaces and bedside devices linked to the CIS at the implementation date. This will maximize perceived benefits early and thereby encourage acceptance of the system. It should be implemented through the whole ICU as partial implementations are rarely successful.

Post-implementation review is essential to progress outstanding issues, which are usually prolific, and help establish the arrangements for the support and continued development of the system. A system management plan identifies the responsibility centres for management of the CIS components and clarifies requirements and expectations. A permanent on-site system management position is required for system maintenance, progressing outstanding issues, and managing future upgrades and developments.

BENEFITS OF CIS: THE STATE OF THE ART

Basic CIS requirements are fulfilled by the majority of systems currently available.

- Charting, including tabulation of bedside observations and measurements such as fluid balance. The flow sheets are usually more than adequately flexible and configurable to meet local requirements
- Bedside device interfaces. New devices may not have the necessary decoders and software. The expense of developing new interfaces can be considerable when calculated on a per bed basis
- Clinical progress notes. Adequate but the free text may not be 'searchable', and structured text only marginally better.
- Keyboard skills are increasingly widespread but may still be an issue with some clinicians
- Drug and fluid prescription and administration is good but not always incorporated in some systems, necessitating a separate system

Given these basic achievements there is an expectation that CIS will demonstrably reduce *staff workloads* and will provide savings in expenditure on salaries.

There is little literature to support this and this is generally found not to be the case.[10,24] Some aspects of documentation may in fact take longer, as they are being conducted more thoroughly than previously and the quality and consistency of documentation has been demonstrated to increase.[10,21,25]

CIS will provide improved access to a legible, attributable and more complete record of care with subsequent important *quality improvements*. There is some evidence to support this. Reductions in adverse events related to drug administration[14,21] and ventilator orders[21] have been described.

System interfaces remain a difficult area. There is a plethora of new and legacy ADT, hospital and pathology systems throughout most hospitals. Hospital IT standards such as HL7 are really in their infancy and do not guarantee system compatibility.

The consequence is that almost every implementation will require a significant degree of customized interfacing. This results in both expense and difficulty.

Decision support has been generally disappointing.[1,5] Drug allergies and interactions should be routinely flagged and prescription impeded but this has not happened yet. Systems integrating information, such as baseline renal function, recent urine output, last measured creatinine and required dose of aminoglycoside, are not generally available.[6] Decision support systems to recommend antimicrobial prescribing, ventilatory therapy or haemodynamic measurement have been developed in dedicated centres of excellence, but are also not generally available nor necessarily able to be migrated successfully across boundaries of international practice.[26,27]

An improved record of previous and ongoing care does offer a primitive level of improved decision support. Access to knowledge based systems through CIS and hospital intranets, as well as resources such as pharmacopoeia, literature search engines, and online texts and journals, are widely available. It is intuitive that these resources would improve the quality of clinical outcomes; but there is little evidence to support this.[18]

Comprehensive electronic storage of the CIS patient records has also been difficult to achieve and many otherwise sophisticated systems have their records archived to paper. This problem is perpetuated by various jurisdictions' reluctance to accept electronic storage for medicolegal purposes although there is now increased acceptance of electronic security and longevity. Archiving in a report format utilizing an EDMS is currently the preferred option.

Clinical databases remain a problem.[1,5,8,9] While many products are purported to include data management and query solutions, those that are available 'off the shelf' are quite rudimentary. In addition, they are not consistent with the level of sophistication seen in financial and business systems. This can be achieved but requires additional expenditure and a major commitment from the clinical staff.

Part of the problem is the need for clinicians to prospectively define what is expected of the system. This requires exhaustive definition of the questions that the system should be able to answer and therefore also specification of the detailed nature of the data and queries that will be required.[7,19]

Accurate analysis of diagnoses and procedures requires that key information is entered correctly and consistently and that reliable and high quality data capture is achieved.[5,16] Data entry should be 'once-only', simple, and robust, and should be easily performed as the clinical scenario unfolds. There is very limited agreement and standardization between clinicians with respect to mandatory data fields, diagnostic criteria and classifications. Standardized reports are therefore difficult to develop in different clinical environments, let alone states or countries. Current installations with significant database and querying capabilities have all required additional expertise and a variety of subsidiary data extraction, management, query and reporting solutions.[4,6,16] Acceptance of a mandatory set of fields and a minimum obligatory standard configuration would facilitate solution design.

FUTURE DEVELOPMENTS

CIS is a potentially powerful agent for organizational and work process change. To realize this potential, it needs to achieve the current expectations of clinicians and managers, which have been shaped by the capabilities of IT in other areas.

As hospital and healthcare systems develop, it becomes critical for CIS in specialty areas to be able to integrate, obtain and share information with other systems.

The ability to provide full electronic documentation and data capture has already gone some way to delivering the quality improvements expected by clinicians and managers. CIS archiving, databases and reporting still have some way to go. They remain the most potentially rewarding benefits of CIS implementation. Improvements in software applications, disciplined approaches by clinicians, and more sophisticated systems management will offer better outcomes in the future.

REFERENCES

1 Metnitz PGH, Lenz K. Patient data management systems in intensive care – the situation in Europe. *Intensive Care Med* 1995; **21**: 703–15.

2 Petty GK. Shopping for a clinical information system (CIS): tips from an expert. *J Emerg Nursing* 1994; **20**: 564–66.

3 Anonymous. Buyer beware when purchasing clinical information systems. *Health Manag Technol* 1996; **17**: 20–4.

4 Shabot MM. The HP CareVue clinical information system. *Int J Clin Monitor Comput* 1997; **14**: 177–84.

5 de Keizer NF, Stoutenbeck CP, Hanneman LAJBW, de Jonge E. An evaluation of patient data management systems in Dutch intensive care. *Intensive Care Med* 1997; **24**: 167–71.

6 Teich JM, Glaser JP, Beckley RF, *et al*. The Brigham integrated computing system (BICS): advanced clinical sytems in an academic hospital environment. *Int J Med Inform* 1999; **54**: 197–208.

7 Snyder-Halpern R, Wagner MC. Planning for implementation of a vendor-based clinical information system: case study. *Comput Nursing* 2000; **18**: 9–12.

8 Urschitz M, Lorenz S, Unterasinger L, *et al*. Three years experience with a patient data management system at a neonatal intensive care unit. *J Clin Monitor Comput* 1998; **14**: 119–25.

9 Fraenkel DJ. Clinical information systems in intensive care. *Crit Care Resuscit* 1999; **1**: 173–9.

10 Hammond J, Johnson HM, Varas R, Ward CG. A qualitative comparison of paper flowsheets vs a computer-based clinical information system. *Chest* 1991; **99**: 155–7.

11 Leape LL, Brennan TA, Laird NM, *et al*. The nature of adverse events in hospitalised patients: results of the Harvard Medical Practice Study II. *N Engl J Med* 1991; **324**: 377–84.

12 Wilson RM, Runciman WB, Gibberd RW, *et al*. The quality in Australian health care study. *Med J Aust* 1995; **163**: 458–71.

13 Bates DW, Cullen DJ, Laird N, *et al*. Incidence of adverse drug events and potential adverse drug events: Implications for prevention. *JAMA* 1995; **274**: 29–34.

14 Bates DW, Teich JM, Lee J, *et al*. The impact of computerised physician order entry on medication error prevention. *J Am Med Inform Assoc* 1999; **6**: 313–21.

15 Bradley V. Preparing a cost estimate for a clinical information system. *J Emerg Nursing* 1998; **24**: 577–80.

16 Metnitz PGH, Laback P, Popow C, *et al*. Computer assisted data analysis in intensive care: the ICDEV project – development of a scientific database system for intensive care. *Int J Clin Monitor Comput* 1995; **12**: 147–59.

17 Staggers N. Notes from a clinical information system manager: a solid vision makes all the difference. *Computers Nursing* 1997; **15**: 232–5.

18 Aarts J, Peel V. Using a descriptive model of change when implementing large scale clinical information systems to identify priorities for further research. *Int J Med Inform* 1999; **56**: 43–50.

19 Goldberger D, Kremsdorf R. Clinical information systems – developing a systematic planning process. *J Ambul Care Manage* 2001; 24: 67–83.

20 Staggers Ny, Repko KB. Strategies for successful clinical information system selection. *Comput Nursing* 1996; **14**: 146–155.

21 Fraenkel JJ, Cowie M, Daley P. Quality benefits of an intensive care clinical information system. *Crit Care Med* 2003; in press.

22 Snyder-Halpern R, Wagner MC. Evaluating return-on-investment for a hospital clinical information system. *Comput Nursing* 2000; **18**: 213–219.

23 Staggers N. Notes from a clinical information system project manager: requisite survival skills. *Comput Nursing* 1998; **16**: 244–6.

24 Peirpoint GL, Thilgen D. Effect of computerised charting on nursing activity in intensive care. *Crit Care Med* 1996; **23**: 1067–73.

25 Nahm R, Poston I. Measurement of the effects of an integrated, point-of-care computer system on quality of nursing documentation and patient satisfaction. *Comput Nursing* 2000; **18**: 220–9.

26 Sittig DF, Pace NL, Gardner RM *et al*. Implementation of a computerised patient advice system using the HELP clinical information system. *Comput Biomed Res* 1989; **22**: 474–87.

27 Evans RS, Pestotnik SL, Classen DC, *et al*. A computer-assisted management program for antibiotics and other antiinfective agents. *N Engl J Med* 1998; **338**: 232–8.

Part Two

Shock

9

Shock: An overview

A McLuckie

Shock is a clinical state, with characteristic symptoms and signs, that occurs when an imbalance between oxygen supply and demand leads to the development of tissue hypoxia. Although changes in systemic perfusion are always present in shock, oxygen delivery to the tissues is not invariably reduced, and indeed may be increased in shock due to severe sepsis.[1]

CLASSIFICATION

Traditionally, shock is classified according to its aetiology, the main subdivisions being cardiogenic, hypovolaemic and septic, with neurogenic and anaphylactic shock occurring less frequently.

Most often, cardiogenic shock is the result of myocardial disease (infarction, ischaemic ventriculo-septal defect, myocarditis). However, valvular abnormalities, such as mitral regurgitation due to papillary muscle rupture, and mechanical problems (pulmonary embolus and cardiac tamponade) may also be implicated. The term obstructive shock can be used to distinguish shock due to a PE or cardiac tamponade from that due to primary myocardial pathology.

Hypovolaemic shock is commonly the result of uncontrolled haemorrhage, but may be due to excessive fluid loss from the gastrointestinal and urinary tracts, and even the skin in severe burns.

Any type of infection, bacterial, fungal or viral can be complicated by the development of shock. The clinical findings, perhaps with the exception of the cutaneous manifestations of meningococcal disease, are not specific to the type of organism involved, and it is not generally possible to determine the nature of the infecting organism from clinical examination alone.[2]

In practice, there is often considerable overlap between the different types of shock and it is not unusual, for example, to find both hypovolaemia and myocardial dysfunction in patients with predominately septic shock. Even in cardiogenic shock, some improvement in cardiac function may be achieved with a careful volume challenge if the patient has been over-aggressively diuresed.

PATHOPHYSIOLOGY

Oxygen delivery to the tissues (DO_2) is reduced in both hypovolaemic and cardiogenic shock. Several factors contribute to this, including low cardiac output, anaemia and hypoxaemia. In hypovolaemic shock, the diminished cardiac output is secondary to a reduction in myocardial preload, while in cardiogenic shock impaired contractility predominates.

During the initial stages of hypovolaemic and cardiogenic shock, as DO2 begins to fall, the tissues are able to maintain their oxygen uptake (VO_2) at a normal level (14 ml/kg per min), by extracting more oxygen from each unit of blood (supply-independent VO_2). However, once DO_2 falls below a critical value of 8–10 ml/kg per min, this compensatory mechanism is insufficient and oxygen uptake begins to decline (supply-dependent VO_2). This phase is associated with the accumulation of an 'oxygen debt', and its severity may be gauged by the degree to which blood lactate is elevated (Figure 9.1).

In septic shock, microbial components or their toxins are recognized by soluble cell-bound receptors, such as CD14 and toll-like receptors. This stimulates the release of pro-inflammatory (TNFα, IL-1, Il-6) and

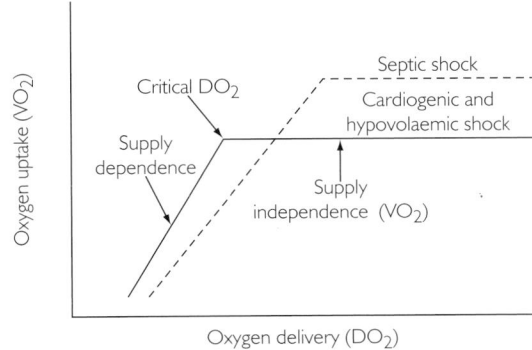

Fig. 9.1 Relationship between VO_2 and DO_2 in cardiogenic, hypovolaemic and septic shock.

anti-inflammatory (Il-10, IL-1ra, TNF receptors) cytokines, generation of complement, activation of coagulation and platelet aggregation. There is also increased synthesis of arachidonic acid metabolites, reactive oxygen species and nitric oxide.[3] The combined effect of these changes is to produce vasodilatation, increased cardiac output despite impaired contractility, and reduced intravascular volume secondary to increased capilliary permeability.

DO_2 in septic shock is supra-normal, mainly as a result of the elevated cardiac output. VO_2 is also raised, due to an increase in tissue metabolic activity. At levels of DO_2 above the normal critical threshold, although VO_2 is increased, it appears to be inadequate and a lactic acidosis develops. Supply-dependency is thus observed over a wider range of DO2 values than usual. This may be explained by abnormalities in perfusion at a microcirculatory level, resulting in locally reduced DO2 despite a supra-normal global value. Alternatively, sepsis induced mitochondrial dysfunction may prevent oxygen utilization at a cellular level.

In all forms of shock, anaerobic cellular metabolism leads to depletion of adenosine triphosphate and failure of the cell membrane sodium-potassium pump. Cell swelling occurs due to the influx of sodium and water. Anaerobic metabolism also leads to a worsening lactic acidosis. Mitochondrial calcium loss further impairs the efficiency of oxidation and phosphorylation, and may interfere with other organ specific functions such as myocardial contractility. If untreated, or sub-optimally treated, shock will eventually progress via multiple organ dysfunction to frank failure.

CLINICAL PRESENTATION

The clinical picture observed with the different types of shock can be divided into two categories, depending upon whether cardiac index (CI) is reduced (hypodynamic shock) or increased (hyperdynamic shock).

Hypovolaemic and cardiogenic shock are both usually associated with a low cardiac index, however blood pressure may be normal due to compensatory sympathetic and neuro-hormonal responses. Classically, the patient is confused, pale, tachycardic, tachypnoeic, poorly perfused and oliguric. The combination of extreme respiratory difficulty and inspiratory crepitations on auscultation of the chest should alert the physician to the possibility of pulmonary oedema due to left ventricular failure, which occurs frequently in cardiogenic shock. Clinically, estimation of central venous pressure may help to differentiate between hypovolaemic and cardiogenic shock, since it is invariably low in the former and often raised in the latter.

Septic shock in contrast is usually hyperdynamic, unless the patient is also significantly hypovolaemic. By definition, the patient must have a proven source of infection, be hypotensive (or requiring vasopressors to maintain a systolic blood pressure of 90 mmHg), exhibit two or more signs of systemic inflammation (tachycardia, tachypnoea, hypo/hyperthermia, leukocytosis/leukopaenia), and have dysfunction of at least one end organ.[4] As with other forms of shock, the patient is often confused, tachycardic, tachypnoeic and oliguric. However, in contrast to hypovolaemic and cardiogenic shock, peripheral pulses are bounding and the extremities are warm to touch. In meningococcal septecaemia a characteristic purpuric rash may be visible.

INVESTIGATIONS

LABORATORY, RADIOLOGICAL AND NON-INVASIVE CARDIAC INVESTIGATIONS

Investigations should be tailored to the history and clinical findings. In most cases, a few simple blood tests (FBC, clotting, electrolytes, urea and creatinine, arterial blood gas, lactate, troponin and blood cultures), in conjunction with an ECG and chest X-ray will be sufficient to confirm the nature of the shock.

In cardiogenic shock, echocardiography is invaluable, since it provides an objective measure of ventricular function, can identify and quantify abnormalities of regional wall motion and valvular function, and exclude cardiac tamponade or pulmonary embolus. Where the history and preliminary findings raise the suspicion of pulmonary embolus, alternative confirmatory tests include spiral CT, which is readily available in most hospitals, and pulmonary angiography.[5]

Hypovolaemic shock, due to concealed haemorrhage, may require further invasive and radiological investigations such as diagnostic peritoneal lavage, abdominal ultrasound, or CT scanning. When hypovolaemia is due to excessive gastrointestinal or renal losses, electrolyte disturbances can be severe, and urea and creatinine are often markedly elevated. Haemo-concentration may also be noted. Further investigations will depend upon the likely pathology, but may include supine and erect abdominal X-rays in bowel obstruction, abdominal ultrasound in acute cholecystitis and serum amylase and abdominal CT scan in pancreatitis.

Septic shock can lead to a rise or fall in the WCC, the latter being associated with a particularly poor prognosis. Blood and other relevant cultures should be taken prior to initiating antibiotic therapy wherever possible, and in certain cases measurement of C-reactive protein and procalcitonin may be of value.[6,7] Disseminated intravascular coagulation (DIC), diagnosed by the combination of prolonged clotting, thrombocytopaenia and reduced fibrinogen is often present. When measured, antithrombin III, protein C and protein S levels are commonly low.

Blood lactate may be elevated in all forms of shock, and usually indicates the presence of tissue hypoxia. The degree to which it is elevated corresponds to the severity of the shock, and it is frequently used as a guide to the effectiveness of therapeutic interventions.[8] Furthermore, lactate, base excess, or a combination of the two can be used to predict outcome in patients admitted to the ICU.[9]

INVASIVE HAEMODYNAMIC MEASUREMENTS

While the therapeutic efficacy of the pulmonary artery catheter (PAC) remains controversial,[10] the measurements obtained from it are undoubtedly extremely useful in differentiating between the three major types of shock (Table 9.1).

Pulmonary artery catheterization is rarely required to aid in the diagnosis of uncomplicated hypovolaemic shock. The clinical picture and presence of a low central venous pressure are usually sufficient. However, the additional information obtained from a PAC may be invaluable in differentiating cardiogenic shock due to acute myocardial infarction (PAoP elevated, CVP normal or elevated, PAP normal), from pulmonary embolus (PAoP normal, CVP and PAP elevated) and cardiac tamponade (PAoP and CVP identical and elevated).

It may also be helpful in cases of septic shock that are not clinically hyperdynamic, particularly in relation to optimizing fluid, inotrope and vasopressor therapy.

PRINCIPLES OF MANAGEMENT

Management may be considered in terms of general measures that are applicable to all shocked patients, and specific measures that are appropriate in shock of a particular aetiology. Irrespective of the type of the shock, it should be treated as a medical emergency. Resuscitation and investigation must therefore proceed in parallel and not in series.

GENERAL MEASURES

OXYGEN THERAPY AND MECHANICAL VENTILATION

All shocked patients should be given high flow oxygen via a facemask, with the aim of improving arterial oxygen saturation and DO_2 to the tissues. Tachypnoea is common, and

work of breathing is greatly increased, particularly in those cases with either cardiogenic or non-cardiogenic pulmonary oedema. Mechanical ventilation has much to commend it in this situation, since it will reduce VO_2 by the respiratory muscles at a time when their oxygen supply is compromised. Intubation at an early stage will also facilitate the insertion of invasive haemodynamic monitoring devices, that are invariably required to monitor and deliver fluid and inotrope therapy, but may be difficult to insert safely in a confused, agitated patient.

FLUID THERAPY

Optimizing cardiac pre-load, and restoring circulating volume are fundamental aspects of correcting tissue hypoxia in patients with shock. In cases of hypovolaemic and septic shock several litres of fluid are usually needed to achieve this, but occasionally even some patients with cardiogenic shock may benefit from judicious volume loading in conjunction with monitoring of PAoP and cardiac index (CI). In patients with severe sepsis, aggressive volume replacement within 6hrs of presentation in conjunction with targeting a central venous oxygen saturation >70% ($SvO_2 > 70$) and haemoglobin level >10 g/dl can reduce hospital mortality by up to 16%.[11]

In uncomplicated hypovolaemic shock CVP is often used as a surrogate for myocardial preload, however in patients with ischaemic heart disease PaoP is usually preferred. Intrathoracic blood volume, an alternative measure of cardiac preload, offers theoretical advantages over the use of CVP and PAoP, particularly in mechanically ventilated patients. This measurement can be made using either a double (COLD) or single (PiCCO) indicator dilution system.[12,13]

Logically, the fluid used to correct any deficit should reflect the type of fluid lost, and most patients with haemorrhagic shock will require blood transfusion. In intensive care patients without acute coronary syndromes, it appears safe to aim for a haemoglobin level of 7–9 g/dl, indeed it is associated with a lower mortality than a level of 10–12 g/dl.[14] At present, the use of blood substitutes such as diasprin cross linked haemoglobin (DCLHb) is not recommended in haemorrhagic shock, since they result in a significantly higher death rate.[15]

Given that blood is usually supplied in the form of red cell concentrates, the clinician must decide whether to combine it with crystalloid, human albumin or a synthetic colloid in order to restore circulating volume. The

Table 9.1 Values obtained from the pulmonary artery catheter in the three major types of shock.

	Septic shock	Cardiogenic shock	Hypovolaemic shock
Cardiac index	↑	↓	↓
Pulmonary artery occlusion pressure (PAoP)	N or ↓	↑	↓
Central venous pressure (CVP)	N or ↓	N or ↑	↓
Systemic vascular resistance (SVR)	↓	↑	↑
Oxygen delivery (DO_2)	↑	↓	↓

N, normal.

same dilemma, over whether to use crystalloid or colloid during resuscitation, also arises in patients with septic shock. One property in favour of colloids is that they restore circulating volume more efficiently than crystalloids, since approximately three times as much crystalloid must be infused to achieve the same haemodynamic end-point. In recent times, with this in mind, it has become popular to begin resuscitation with a colloid to restore intra-vascular volume, and to continue with crystalloid to correct interstitial and intracellular losses. There is no compelling evidence however, to suggest that patients who are resuscitated with crystalloids alone have worse outcomes, and crystalloids are undoubtedly much cheaper to use.

In addition, several papers have raised concerns regarding the safety of colloids. A systematic review of randomized studies that compared the use of crystalloids vs colloids in the resuscitation of crtically ill patients, concluded that the use of colloid was associated with a 4% increase in mortality.[16] The use of human albumin specifically in this situation has been questioned, with a systematic review of its use in the treatment of patients with hypovolaemia, hypo-albuminaemia and burns suggesting that it increased the risk of death by 6%.[17] Doubts have also been raised about the synthetic colloid hydroxyethylstarch (MMW-HES 200 kDa, 0.6–0.66 substitution), with a randomized controlled study comparing it to 3% gelatin in patients with sepsis and septic shock demonstrating a higher incidence of renal failure in the HES group.[18] The use of high molecular weight hydroxyethylstarch (HMW-HES 450 kDa, 0.5 substitution) has also been associated with abnormal clotting and increased bleeding.[19]

A number of recent publications have focused on the use of hypertonic crystalloids, such as 7.5% NaCl alone or in conjunction with dextran 70, for initial resuscitation. While most of the large studies have failed to show a clear survival benefit in the general trauma population, hypertonic solutions may be useful in certain subgroups such as those with severe head injuries, in whom the administration of large volumes of isotonic crystalloid may worsen cerebral oedema.[20,21] Most studies also show that the use of hypertonic solutions is associated with a reduction in fluid and blood transfusion requirements.[22]

INOTROPIC SUPPORT

Inotropic support is rarely required in hypovolaemic shock, except when it is severe and surgical control of bleeding is delayed. In most instances, fluid replacement alone is sufficient to restore cardiac output and blood pressure. While fluid therapy is also important in patients with septic shock, it is rarely helpful in those with cardiogenic shock, and in both septic and cardiogenic shock vasoactive drugs are often required to improve tissue perfusion and reverse tissue hypoxia.

In cardiogenic shock, cardiac output and blood pressure are characteristically low and systemic vascular resistance increased. Ideally an inodilator, for example dobutamine or milrinone should be selected, provided that blood pressure is not unduly compromised. When hypotension is a prominent feature, the use of an inoconstrictor, for example adrenaline or dopamine, or a vasopressor inotrope in combination with an inodilator, for example noradrenaline and dobutamine, is often preferred. A number of adverse side-effects are to be expected with adrenaline, including hyperglycaemia, hypokalaemia and hyperlactataemia.[23,24] Consequently, use of adrenaline should be taken into account when interpreting blood lactate measurements.

Septic shock classically results in a high cardiac output and low blood pressure due to excessive peripheral vasodilatation. This so called 'peripheral circulatory failure' is mediated via increased production of nitric oxide due to stimulation of inducible nitric oxide synthase in vascular smooth muscle and endothelium. Once cardiac preload is optimized, use of a vasopressor inotrope, for example noradrenaline, is recommended. If cardiac output is reduced, it is often helpful to combine noradrenaline with dobutamine. Theoretically, the inoconstrictor dopamine could also be used in this situation, if it were not for a number of problematic side effects. These include adverse effects on pituitary function (reduced prolactin, GH and TRH), T-cell function, gut mucosal perfusion and renal medullary VO_2.[25,26]

DIURETICS

The use of 'low-dose' or 'renal-dose' dopamine, to prevent renal failure in shocked patients, does not reduce the number of patients who subsequently require renal replacement therapy, and given the concern about possible adverse effects of dopamine should be abandoned.[27,28] If a natriuresis is desired, this can usually be achieved with frusemide, given by intermittent bolus (10–80 mg) or continuous infusion (3–10 mg/h). Care should be taken to ensure that the patient is adequately volume resuscitated before a diuretic is given, so that hypovolaemia is not exacerbated by an inappropriate diuresis.

SPECIFIC MEASURES

HYPOVOLAEMIC SHOCK

Surgical, radiological or endoscopic intervention may be required in haemorrhagic shock, and should be undertaken in a timely fashion. In most situations fluid resuscitation precedes definitive intervention, but in some trauma patients outcome may be improved if fluid resuscitation is delayed until bleeding is controlled.[29] Hypovolaemic shock due to other intrabdominal pathologies, for example perforation/obstruction, may also warrant surgery. In these cases, measures taken to improve the condition of the patient preoperatively, such as correcting hypovolaemia, hypoxia and anaemia, and increasing DO_2 can reduce perioperative mortality substantially.[30,31]

SEPTIC SHOCK
Source Control

Infected fluid collections should be drained, either radiologically or surgically. Surgical intervention may also be required for other sources of sepsis, for example bowel perforation.

Antibiotics

It is vital to select an appropriate antibiotic(s) and to ensure that the dosing regimen is optimal. This latter task is often the more difficult, especially when re-dosing depends upon monitoring of drug levels. Any delay in obtaining a level can expose the patient to a significant period of sub-optimal antibiotic therapy. In order to reduce this problem, antibiotics whose efficacy does not depend upon peak levels, for example vancomycin, may be given by continuous infusion (0.5–2 g/d, depending on renal function) with a random level taken once daily.[32] In the absence of culture results, initial antibiotic therapy is designed to cover a broad range of likely pathogens. However, once culture results are available, antibiotic cover should be narrowed and directed at the identified organism(s).

Steroids

Large doses of steroid, for example 30–120 mg/kg of methylprednisolone given within 24 h of the onset of septic shock, result in haemodynamic improvement but not increased survival. This finding may be explained by the increased incidence of secondary infection associated with their use.[33,34] Smaller doses of steroid (100 mg hydrocortisone 8 hrly), given 24–72 h after the onset of shock in those patients who still require significant doses of vasopressor and exhibit a sub-normal rise in their serum cortisol in response to ACTH (Short Synacthen Test), improves both haemodynamic state and outcome.

L-NMMA

The results of Phase 1 and 2 trials of N-methyl-L-arginine (L-NMMA), a non-selective nitric oxide synthase inhibitor, in septic shock appeared promising. When infused at a maximum rate of 20 mg/kg per h for 8 h, there was a 60–80% reduction in the amount of noradrenaline required to maintain a mean arterial pressure of 70 mmHg or greater.[36] Unfortunately, the subsequent Phase 3 study demonstrated an increased mortality in the L-NMMA group. This was largely due to L-NMMA-induced increases in both systemic and pulmonary vascular resistances that resulted in cardiac failure.[37] Further investigations in this area are likely to focus on the development of a selective inducible NO synthase inhibitor.

Vasopressin

In cases of septic shock with refractory hypotension, despite high doses of catecholamines, the addition of an intravenous infusion of vasopressin (0.04 U/min) can increase blood pressure, systemic vascular resistance and urine output.[38] Vasopressin secretion from the posterior pituitary is an important homeostatic mechanism for restoring blood pressure in various forms of shock. In septic shock vasopressin levels may be abnormally low, due to either impaired secretion or depletion. To date, use of vasopressin in refractory shock has only been reported in small numbers of patients, and its routine use in this situation cannot be recommended until further safety data relating to cardiac function and tissue ischaemia are available.

Activated Protein C

Activated protein C (APC) is an endogenous protein capeable of promoting fibrinolysis and inhibiting thrombosis and inflammation. In sepsis, the conversion of protein C from an inactive to active from, which is stimulated by thrombin bound to throbomodulin, is impaired due to downregulation of thrombomodulin by inflammatory cytokines. In patients with severe sepsis, infusing APC (24 mcg/kg per h) for up to 96 h reduces absolute risk of death by 6%. Administering it in this fashion, does however result in an increased risk of serious bleeding, and its effect on mortality has not been studied in patients who are at increased risk of bleeding, including those who have had recent surgery or trauma.[39]

High Volume Haemofiltration

Haemofiltration is frequently used to manage severe metabolic acidosis, as well as renal failure itself, in patients with septic shock. Numerous studies have demonstrated that haemodynamic status often improves following commencement of haemofiltration, and it is postulated that this is due to cytokine removal in the ultrafiltrate and by adsorption onto the filter.[40,41] In patients with sepsis, there is some evidence to suggest that using a higher dose of haemofiltration (45 ml/kg/hr) may improve outcome.[42] However, a rigorous, randomized, controlled study of high volume haemofiltration in septic patients has not been undertaken to date.

CARDIOGENIC SHOCK
Thrombolysis/Angiography/PTCA/CABG

Cardiogenic shock complicating acute myocardial infarction carries a high mortality, which is not reduced to any significant extent by thrombolytic therapy (55% at 30 d).[43] In these cases, where facilities are available, angiography should be undertaken without delay, and angioplasty or CABG performed if appropriate.

IABP

The intra-aortic balloon pump provides a useful bridge to surgery in cases of cardiogenic shock due to papillary muscle rupture and ischaemic ventricular septal defect. Its use as a supportive therapy, in conjunction with other aggressive invasive treatments, in the wider population of patients with acute myocardial infarction is also associated with a reduction in 1 year mortality.[44]

OUTCOME

Outcome in shock depends upon a multitude of factors, including aetiology, severity of illness at presentation, response to therapy and co-morbidity. In general terms, the mortality associated with hypovolaemic shock is considerably lower than that for either cardiogenic or septic shock, provided that the source of bleeding can be controlled. Even in good centres, where patients receive aggressive therapy, mortality from septic shock is approximately 30–50%, and often higher for cardiogenic shock.[45]

REFERENCES

1 Vincent JL, Van der Linden P. Septic shock: Particular type of acute circulatory failure. *Crit Care Med* 1990; **18**: S70–4.

2 Wiles JB, Cerra FB, Siegel JH, Border JR. The systemic septic response: does the organism matter? *Crit Care Med* 1980; **8**: 55–60.

3 Vincent JL, De Backer D. Pathophysiology of septic shock. *Advances in Sepsis* 2001; **1**: 87–92.

4 Members of the American College of Chest Physicians/Society of Critical Care Medicine Consensus Conference Committee. ACCP/SCCM Consensus Conference: Definitions for sepsis and organ failure and guidelines for the use of innovative therapies in sepsis. *Crit Care Med* 1992; **20**: 864–74.

5 Pruszczyk P, Torbicki A, Pacho R, *et al*. Non-invasive diagnosis of suspected severe pulmonary embolism: Transoesophageal echocardiography vs spiral CT. *Chest* 1997; **112**: 722–28.

6 Povoa P, Almeida E, Moreira P, *et al*. C-reactive protein as an indicator of sepsis. Intensive Care Med 1998; **24**: 1052–6.

7 Assicot M, Gendrel D, Carsin H, *et al*. High serum procalcitonin concentrations in patients with sepsis and infection. *Lancet* 1993; **341**: 515–8.

8 Bakker J. Lactate: May I have your votes please? *Intensive Care Med* 2001; **27**: 6–11.

9 Smith I, Kumar P, Molloy S, *et al*. Base excess and lactate as prognostic indicators for patients admitted to intensive care. *Intensive Care Med* 2001; **27**: 74–83.

10 Connors AF, Speroff T, Dawson NV, *et al*. The effectiveness of right heart catheterisation in the initial care of critically ill patients. *JAMA* 1996; **276**: 889–97.

11 Rivers E, Nguyen B, Havstad S. Early goal-directed therapy in the treatment of severe sepsis and septic shock. *N Engl J Med* 2001; **345**: 1368–77.

12 Lichtwarck-Aschoff M, Zeravik J, Pfeiffer UJ. Intrathoracic blood volume accurately reflects circulatory volume status in critically ill patients with mechanical ventilation. *Intensive Care Med* 1992; **18**: 142–7.

13 Sakka SG, Ruhl CC, Pfeiffer UJ, *et al*. Assessment of cardiac preload and extravascular lung water by single transpulmonary thermodilution. *Intensive Care Med* 2000; **26**: 180–7.

14 Hebert PC, Wells G, Blajchman MA, *et al*. A multicentre, randomized, controlled clinical trial of transfusion requirements in critical care. *N Engl J Med* 1999; **340**: 409–17.

15 Sloan EP, Koenigsbers M, Gens D, *et al*. Diaspirin cross-linked haemoglobin (DCLHb) in the treatment of severe traumatic haemorrhagic shock. A randomised controlled efficacy trial. *JAMA* 1999; **282**: 1857–64.

16 Schierhout G, Roberts I. Fluid resuscitation with colloid or crystalloid solutions in critically ill patients: a systematic review of randomised trails. *BMJ* 1998; **316**: 961–4.

17 Cochrane Injuries Group Albumin Reviewers. Human albumin administration in critically ill patients: systematic review of randomised controlled trials. *BMJ* 1998; **317**: 235–40.

18 Schortgen F, Lacherade J-C, Bruneel F, *et al*. Effects of hydroxyethylstarch and gelatin on renal function in severe sepsis: a multicentre randomised study. *Lancet* 2001; **357**: 911–16.

19 Boldt J, Knothe C, Zickmann B, *et al*. Influence of different intravascular volume therapies on platelet function in patients undergoing cardiopulmonary bypass. *Anaesth Analg* 1993; **76**: 1185–90.

20 Vassar MJ, Perry CA, Gannaway WL, Holcroft JW. 7.5% sodium chloride/dextran for resuscitation of trauma patients undergoing helicopter transport. *Arch Surg* 1991; **126**: 1065–72.

21 Vassar MJ, Fischer R, O'Brien P, *et al*. A multicentre trial for resuscitation of injured patients with 7.5% sodium chloride. The effect of added dextran 70. The multicentre group for the study of hypertonic saline in trauma patients. *Arch Surg* 1993; **128**: 1003–11.

22 Younes RN, Aun F, Accioly CQ, *et al*. Hypertonic solutions in the treatment of hypovolaemic shock: a prospective randomised study in patients admitted to the emergency room. *Surgery* 1992; **111**: 380–5.

23 Day NPJ, Phu NH, Bethel DP, *et al*. The effects of dopamine and adrenaline infusions on acid-base balance and systemic haemodynamics in severe infection. *Lancet* 1996; **348**: 219–23.

24 Totaro RJ, Raper RF. Epinephrine-induced lactic acidosis following cardiopulmonary bypass. *Crit Care Med* 1997; **25**: 1693–9.

25 Van den Berge G, De Zegher F. Anterior pituitary function during critical illness and dopamine treatment. *Crit Care Med* 1996; **24**: 1580–90.

26 Pawlik W, Mailman D, Shanbour L, *et al*. Dopamine effects on the intestinal circulation. *Am Heart J* 1976; **75**: 325–31.

27 ANZICS clinical trials group. Low-dose dopamine in patients with early renal dysfunction: a placebo-controlled randomised trial. *Lancet* 2000; **356**: 2139–43.

28 Kellum JA, Decker JM. Use of dopamine in acute renal failure. *Crit Care Med* 2001; **29**: 1526–31.

29 Bickell WH, Wall MJ, Pepe PE, *et al*. Immediate versus delayed fluid resuscitation for hypotensive patients with penetrating truncal injuries. *N Engl J Med* 1994; **331**: 1105–09.

30 Shoemaker WC, Appel PL, Kram HB, *et al*. Prospective trail of supranormal values of survivors as therapeutic goals in high-risk surgical patients. *Chest* 1988; **94**: 1176–86.

31 Boyd O, Grounds RM, Bennett ED. A randomised clinical trial of the effect of deliberate perioperative increase of oxygen delivery on mortality in high-risk surgical patients. *JAMA* 1993; **270**: 2699–2707.

32 James JK, Palmer SM, Levine DP, *et al*. Comparison of conventional dosing versus continuous-infusion vancomycin therapy for patients with suspected or documented gram-positive infections. *Antimicrob Agents Chemother* 1996; **40**: 696–700.

33 Sprung CL, Caralis PV, Marcial EH, *et al*. The effects of high-dose corticosteroids in patients with septic shock. A prospective, controlled study. *N Engl J Med* 1984; **311**: 1137–43.

34 Bone RC, Fisher CJ, Clemmer TP, *et al*. A controlled clinical trial of high-dose methylprednisolone in the treatment of severe sepsis and septic shock. *N Engl J Med* 1987; **317**: 653–8.

35 Annane D, Sebille V, Charpentier C *et al*. (2002). Effect of treatment with low doses of hydrocartisone and fludrocortisone on mortality in patients with septic shock. *JAMA* **288**: 862–871.

36 Grover R, Zaccardelli D, Colice G, *et al*. An open-label dose escalation study of the nitric oxide synthase inhibitor, N-methy-L-arginine hydrochloride (546C88), in patients with septic shock. *Crit Care Med* 1999; **27**: 913–22.

37 Grover R, Lopez A, Lorente J, *et al*. Multicentre, randomised, placebo-controlled, double blind study of nitric oxide synthase inhibitor 546C88: Effect on survival in patients with septic shock. *Crit Care Med* 1999; **27(Suppl. 1)**: A33.

38 Tsuneyoshi I, Yamada H, Kakihana Y, *et al*. Haemodynamic and metabolic effects of low-dose vasopressin infusions in vasodilatory septic shock. *Crit Care Med* 2001; **29**: 487–93.

39 Bernard GR, Vincent JL, Laterre P-F, *et al*. Efficacy and safety of recombinant human activated protein C for severe sepsis. *N Engl J Med* 2001; **344**: 699–709.

40 Heering P, Morgera S, Schmitz FJ, *et al*. Cytokine removal and cardiovascular haemodynamics in septic patients with continuous venovenous haemofiltration. *Intensive Care Med* 1997; **23**: 288–96.

41 Honore PM, Jamez J, Wauthier M, *et al*. Prospective evaluation of short-term, high-volume isovolaemic haemofiltration on the haemodynamic course and outcome in patients with intractable circulatory failure resulting from septic shock. *Crit Care Med* 2000; **28**: 3581–7.

42 Ronco C, Bellomo R, Homel P, *et al*. Effects of different doses in continuous veno-venous haemofiltration on outcomes of acute renal failure: a prospective randomised trial. *Lancet* 2000; **355**: 26–30.

43 Holmes DR, Bates ER, Kleinman NS, *et al*. Contemporary reperfusion therapy for cardiogenic shock: the GUSTO-I trial experience. *J Am Coll Cardiol* 1995; **26**: 668–74.

44 Holmes DR, Califf RM, Van de Werf F, *et al*. Difference in countries' use of resources and clinical outcome for patients with cardiogenic shock after myocardial infarction: results from the GUSTO trial. *Lancet* 1997; **349**: 75–8.

45 Brun-Buisson C, Doyon F, Carlet J, *et al*. Incidence, risk factors, and outcome of severe sepsis and septic shock in adults. *JAMA* 1995; **274**: 968–74.

10

Haemodynamic monitoring

T J Morgan

The arterial system is pressurized by the pumping action of the heart, the elastance of the vascular tree and vasomotor tone. The cerebral and coronary circulations in particular require continuously maintained perfusion pressures, and haemodynamic servo-loops defend arterial pressure as a priority. When mean arterial pressure (MAP) is threatened, autoregulation in most other tissues is variably over-ridden by the effects of the neurohumoral response. Haemodynamic disturbances cause changes in organ function, such as altered cerebration and oliguria (<0.5 ml/kg per h), and regular clinical evaluation is of itself an important component of haemodynamic monitoring.

As circulatory compromise escalates, particularly if there is accompanying tissue dysoxia, it is usually necessary to increase the number, complexity and invasiveness of monitoring sites and the frequency of data sampling. Monitoring should remain as low risk as possible, yet be sufficient to provide early warning of circulatory dysfunction, determine appropriate interventions (usually manipulation of fluids and/or vasoactive drugs) and track responses to therapy.

Haemodynamic data are analysed in the context of a circulatory model. This normally consists of a non-pulsatile pump and a hydraulic circuit with discrete sites of flow resistance, and incorporates the Frank-Starling mechanism with its concepts of preload, contractility and afterload. However, precise *in vivo* quantification of these parameters is difficult, either clinically or in the laboratory. The model itself is simplistic, and does not allow for the pulsatile interaction of the cardiac pump with the elastance of the arterial tree. Even more complex models based on electrical circuits are insufficient to quantify afterload and contractility precisely.

At the bedside the clinician must work with inexact surrogates for all three parameters (Table 10.1), derived from measurements of arterial blood pressure (systemic or pulmonary), cardiac output, volume or pressure indices of cardiac filling and various markers of tissue wellbeing. In this chapter, we focus on all these measurements except for those of tissue wellbeing, which are discussed in a separate chapter.

ARTERIAL BLOOD PRESSURE

The systemic pulse wave moves out from the aortic valve at 6–10 m/s. During its passage into the peripheral vasculature there is a progressive increase in systolic and reduction in diastolic pressures, as standing and reflected waves become incorporated into the waveform. Consequently, systemic arterial pressure measurements vary according to the site of measurement. MAP is arguably a more relevant index to monitor than either systolic or diastolic pressures for three reasons:

- MAP is least dependent on measurement site or technique (invasive versus non-invasive).
- MAP is least altered by measurement damping.
- MAP determines tissue blood flow via autoregulation (apart from the left ventricle, which autoregulates from diastolic pressure).

NON-INVASIVE ARTERIAL BLOOD PRESSURE MEASUREMENT (NIBP)

In most intensive care units, the standard NIBP instruments are automated intermittent oscillometric devices. Finger photoplethysmography and arterial tonometry can monitor both arterial pressure and waveforms continuously, but there are concerns regarding their accuracy. To make an oscillometric blood pressure measurement, a pneumatic cuff is inflated around a proximal limb until all oscillations in cuff pressure are extinguished. The occluding pressure is then lowered stepwise, so that oscillations reappear over a discrete interval. Proprietary algorithms compute mean, systolic and diastolic pressures from the alterations in oscillatory amplitude during deflation.

Oscillometry overestimates low pressures and underestimates high pressures, but for the normotensive range the 95% confidence limits are ± 15 mmHg (2 kPa). Dysrhythmias increase the likelihood of error. Cuff width should be 40% of the mid-circumference of the limb. Narrower cuffs overestimate and wider cuffs underestimate blood pressures.

Table 10.1 Bedside indices of preload, contractility and afterload

Monitoring device	Preload	Contractility	Afterload
Clinical	Skin turgor Urine output JVP Response of blood pressure, skin perfusion and urine output to fluid challenge	Urine output JVP Skin perfusion Ability to respond to a fluid challenge	Skin perfusion Core-peripheral temperature gradient
Direct intra-arterial pressure	Response to fluid challenge. Systolic pressure variation and Δdown component.	Pre-ejection period (with Q wave from ECG)	
Central venous line	CVP + response to fluid challenge		
PA catheter	PAoP, RAP	LVSWI, RVSWI	SVRI, PVRI
Volumetric PA catheter (additional information)	RVEDVI	RVEF	
Transpulmonary thermodilution	Intrathoracic blood volume. Global end-diastolic volume		
Pulse contour continuous cardiac output	Stroke volume variation		
Echocardiography	Ventricular end-diastolic areas	Ejection fraction. Regional wall motion abnormalities.	
Oesophageal Doppler	Flow time (left ventricular ejection time)	Peak flow-velocity	Peak flow-velocity. Flow time.

PAoP, pulmonary artery occlusion pressure; RAP, right atrial pressure; LVSWI, left ventricular stroke work index, RVSWI, right ventricular stroke work index; SVRI, systemic vascular resistance index; PVRI, pulmonary vascular resistance index.

Complications are unusual. Repeated cuff inflations can cause skin ulceration, oedema and bruising, more so when the conscious state is obtunded by illness and sedation. Ulnar nerve injury is also possible, especially with low cuff placement.

INVASIVE BLOOD PRESSURE MEASUREMENT: SYSTEM REQUIREMENTS

A cannula inserted into the relevant blood vessel is connected via fluid-filled non-compliant tubing <1 m in length to a linearly responsive pressure transducer.[1] The system is zeroed with reference to the phlebostatic axis. This is normally the mid-axillary line at the fourth intercostal space. Ideally, the natural resonant frequency of the system should exceed 30 Hz for heart rates up to 180 beats/min, and 20 Hz for heart rates up to 120 beats/min. Damping should be adjusted (Table 10.2) without causing unacceptable reductions in the resonant frequency.

Modern disposable transducers are pre-calibrated using electrical signals, and in normal clinical practice are not calibrated further against known pressures.

DIRECT INTRA-VASCULAR PRESSURE MEASUREMENT

Vascular cannulation allows real-time blood pressure measurement, beat to beat waveform display and regular sampling of blood for laboratory analysis.

RADIAL ARTERY CANNULATION

This is the most common site. Nothing larger than a 20-gauge cannula is advisable, and either a modified

Table 10.2 Assessment of the resonant frequency and damping coefficient of arterial pressure monitoring systems

Make a paper record of transducer output
Snap the valve of the continuous flush system. This produces a square wave on the output trace.
Repeat the process at least twice.
Resonant frequency is the distance between successive peaks divided by the paper speed in millimetres per second.
Damping is satisfactory if each snap test has two to three oscillation waves, with each wave one third or less the size of the preceding wave.

Seldinger technique or direct cannulation can be used. Unfractionated sodium heparin 3 U/ml in 0.9% saline is infused at 3 ml/h, with a snap flush rate of 30–60 ml/h. If heparin-induced thrombosis thrombocytopenia syndrome is suspected, the heparin should be omitted. Necrosis requiring amputation occurs in less than 1 in 2000 cases,[2] despite the fact that partial or complete arterial occlusion is detectable in over 25% of patients following decannulation.[3] Longer cannulas reduce the thrombosis rate.[4] The modified Allen's test is of no value, since it requires patient cooperation and even when correctly performed it does not predict subsequent distal ischaemia.[3] In view of the low rate of serious distal ischaemia, evaluation of the ulnar collateral circulation by Doppler ultrasound is rarely performed.

OTHER SITES

The axillary, brachial, femoral, posterior tibial and dorsalis pedis arteries can all be used without apparently raising the complication profile (Table 10.3). In severe circulatory compromise, gaining peripheral arterial access may be difficult and time consuming. Rapid femoral cannulation by the Seldinger percutaneous technique usually remains feasible, with the added advantage that femoral arterial monitoring reflects aortic pressure more accurately in low output states.

COMPLICATIONS

Complications of arterial cannulation (Table 10.3) must be weighed against those of repeated arterial puncture. Cannulas should be removed or resited between day 5–7, or earlier if a complication is suspected. In particular distal perfusion should be checked at least 8-hourly, and the cannula removed if there is persistent distal blanching, coolness with sluggish capillary refill, loss of distal pulses, or evidence of raised muscle compartment pressures.

Table 10.3 Complications of invasive arterial pressure measurement

Haematoma (including retroperitoneal bleeding from femoral lines)
Distal ischaemia (risk factors include shock, sepsis, embolus of air or clot, hyperlipoproteinaemia, vasculitis, female sex, prothrombotic states, accidental intra-arterial injection of drugs)
Infection
Retrograde embolisation (e.g. cerebral embolus from retrograde flow of air or clot during flush – radial, brachial or axillary lines)
Pseudoaneurysm
Arteriovenous fistula
Compartment syndrome
Damage to neighbouring structures, e.g. median nerve, bowel (femoral approach)
Exsanguination from accidental disconnection

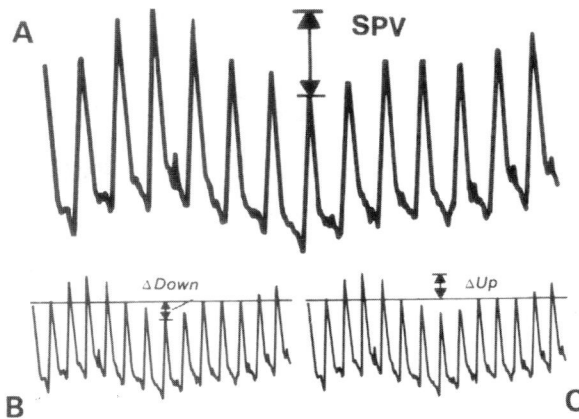

Fig. 10.1 Systolic pressure variation (SPV) during one ventilatory cycle. The horizontal line is end-expiratory systolic pressure. (Reproduced with permission from Perel A, Segal E, Pizov R. Assessment of cardiovascular function by pressure waveform analysis. In: Vincent J-L (ed.) *Update in Intensive Care and Emergency Medicine.* Berlin: Springer-Verlag; 1989: 542.)

FURTHER INFORMATION FROM THE ARTERIAL WAVEFORM

Measurement systems used in intensive care do not precisely quantify the rate of arterial pressure rise and fall. Nevertheless, the wide pulse pressure of aortic regurgitation and the slowed upstroke of severe aortic stenosis may be detected. Pulsus paradoxus can readily be quantified in the spontaneously breathing patient. Systolic time intervals can provide an indication of ventricular contractility.

SYSTOLIC PRESSURE VARIATION

During mechanical ventilation, a positive pressure breath causes first a rise and then a fall in systolic pressure (Figure 10.1). This is the opposite of what happens in normal breathing. The difference between the maximum and minimum systolic pressures generated by a single positive pressure breath has been termed the systolic pressure variation. Systolic pressure variation of >10 mmHg suggests reduced left ventricular preload, particularly when there is a fall below the systolic baseline of >5 mmHg (the 'Δdown' component).[5] These indices are at least as sensitive to reductions in left ventricular preload as alterations in PAoP and CVP,[6,7] although specificity is reduced by large tidal volumes or reduced chest wall compliance.

STROKE VOLUME

Stroke volume estimations from the arterial pulse contour form the basis of newer continuous cardiac output measurement techniques and are dealt with below.

CENTRAL VENOUS PRESSURE

Central venous pressure (CVP) is normally monitored by placing a catheter in the superior vena cava via the subclavian, internal jugular or external jugular veins.[8] The median cubital and basilic veins are used less commonly. Access to the subclavian vein is usually via the infraclavicular approach, but the supraclavicular approach is safe and reliable in experienced hands. The right tracheobronchial angle and carina are common radiological markers of insertion depth. Below this level, a catheter tip eroding through the superior vena cava can enter the pericardial sac causing cardiac tamponade. However, although tamponade is rapidly fatal and rarely diagnosed antemortem, it is rare. In addition, traditional higher catheter tip positioning may increase the likelihood of superior vena caval erosion and thrombosis, particularly with left-sided catheter placement. Some practitioners therefore place the catheter tip lower in the superior vena cava or even in the upper right atrium, ensuring that the catheter is parallel to the long axis of the vein so that the tip does not abut the vein or heart wall end-on.[9]

Femoral venous catheterization with radiological positioning of the tip close to the right atrium produces pressure measurements in good agreement with the subclavian CVP.[10] However, a 26% incidence of catheter-related femoral deep venous thrombosis has been reported.[11] Complications associated with CVP monitoring are listed in Table 10.4.

Although fluid manometry is sufficient to measure the CVP, the frequency response is low and waveform analysis impossible (Table 10.5). Therefore, an electrical transducer system is normally used.

USING THE CENTRAL VENOUS PRESSURE

The normal CVP in the spontaneously breathing supine patient is 0–5 mmHg, while 10 mmHg is generally accepted as the upper limit during mechanical ventilation.

Table 10.4   Complications associated with CVP monitoring

Early
Pneumothorax / haemothorax / chylothorax / hydrothorax
Arterial puncture
Injury to subclavian artery, aorta or pulmonary artery
Dysrhythmias, right bundle branch block
Nerve injury (e.g. phrenic, recurrent laryngeal, Horner's syndrome)
Air embolism
Tracheal injury

Late
Catheter-related sepsis
Disconnection (bleeding or air embolism)
Superior vena caval erosion (hydrothrax, cardiac tamponade)
Arteriovenous fistula
Thrombosis (superior vena cava, subclavian vein)

In health there is a good correlation between CVP and pulmonary artery occlusion pressures (PAoP), but this is lost in many types of critical illness such as pulmonary hypertension, pulmonary embolism, right ventricular infarction, left ventricular hypertrophy and myocardial ischaemia. Even as a specific measure of right ventricular preload, the CVP has significant deficiencies. This is because the relationship between CVP and right ventricular end-diastolic volume is altered by changes in right ventricular diastolic compliance and juxta-cardiac pressures.

At best, the CVP can be used as a guide to right ventricular preload, with a greater emphasis on dynamic changes rather than absolute values. For example, after a fluid load, continued hypotension with a CVP rise of <3 mmHg indicates the need for more volume, whereas a sustained CVP rise of >7 mmHg is less supportive (but not exclusive) of this need. Conversely, severe hypotension with a low or normal CVP is unlikely to be due to acute pulmonary embolism, cardiac tamponade or tension pneumothorax.

Table 10.5   Analysis of CVP waveform

Condition	Pressure changes	Waveform changes
Tricuspid regurgitation	Increased RA pressure	Prominent *v* wave, *x* descent obliterated, *y* descent steep
Right ventricular infarction	RA and RV pressure elevated. RAP does not fall and may rise in inspiration	Prominent *x* and *y* descents
Constrictive pericarditis	RA, RV diastolic, PA diastolic and occlusion pressures elevated and equalized. RAP may rise in inspiration	Prominent *x* and *y* descents
Pericardial tamponade	RA, RV diastolic, PA diastolic and occlusion pressures elevated and equalized. RAP usually falls in inspiration	*y* descent damped or absent

RA, right atrial; RV, right ventricular; RAP, right atrial pressure; PA, pulmonary artery.

PULMONARY ARTERY CATHETER[12]

Bedside flow-directed right heart catheterization has become part of the culture of intensive care, especially in the United States. Acceptance in Europe has also been impressive. In 1995, a snapshot revealed that 12.8% of European intensive care patients had pulmonary artery (PA) catheters *in situ*.[13] Information gained from bedside PA catheterizaton can generate insights into cardio-pulmonary pathophysiology (Tables 10.1, 10.6, 10.11). Measurements prompt changes in therapy in over 50% of cases,[14] and have proven difficult to predict prior to catheter insertion.[15] However, there is debate over whether this translates into a beneficial effect on outcome.[16,17]

In 1996, a prospective non-randomized cohort study of PA catheterization in American teaching hospitals appeared to show that, in any of nine major disease categories, PA catheterization in the first 24 h increased 30-d mortality (odds ratio 1.24, 95% CI 1.03–1.49), mean length of stay and mean cost per hospital stay.[18] A simultaneous editorial called for a moratorium on PA catheter use, and for a prospective multi-centre trial.[19] Subsequent debate included criticism from Europe that the study data were generated mainly in 'open' units, where staff may lack proper training in PA catheter use and interpretation, and where medico-legal considerations and financial rewards may stimulate inappropriate catheter insertions.[20] In a more recent British single-centre retrospective study of over 400 patients, PA catheterization appeared not to influence mortality.[21] At the time of writing the catheters are still used by many clinicians, and there are presently at least two randomized, controlled trials into the utility of PA catheterization under way.

MONITORING INDICATIONS

PA catheter insertion may be required to:

- Characterize a haemodynamic perturbation (e.g. distributive, cardiogenic, obstructive and hypovolaemic shock or combinations)
- Differentiate cardiogenic from non-cardiogenic pulmonary oedema.
- Guide use of, vasoactive drugs, fluids (including renal replacement therapy) and diuretics, especially when haemodynamic disturbances are coupled with increased lung water, RV or LV dysfunction, pulmonary hypertension and organ dysfunction.

In practice, PA catheterization is often confined to those patients where a satisfactory haemodynamic response has not been achieved despite establishing a working diagnosis and the administration of appropriate fluid and/or vasoactive drug therapy.

Table 10.6 Pressures measured by a pulmonary artery catheter

Site	mmHg	(kPa)
Right atrium mean	–1–7	(0.13–0.93)
Right ventricle: systolic	15–25	(2.0–3.3)
Right ventricle: diastolic	0–8	(0–1.1)
Pulmonary artery: systolic	15–25	(2.0–3.3)
Pulmonary artery: diastolic	8–15	(1.1–2.0)
Pulmonary artery: mean	10–20	(1.3–2.6)
Pulmonary artery occlusion pressure	6–15	(0.8–2.0)

CATHETER INSERTION

A 7.5–9 F, 15 cm introducer sheath is first inserted by the Seldinger technique.[22] The subclavian and internal jugular veins are most commonly used. Access is feasible with the 110 cm catheter via the median cubital, basilic and femoral veins. The external jugular veins can also be used, although difficulty may be encountered passing the introducer both into the vein and then subsequently below the clavicle into the subclavian vein.

Balloon volume is 1.5 ml. The balloon should be inflated with air before passage through the heart, to assist flow guidance and protect against myocardial injury and dysrhythmias. Inflation should not be forced, and should not alter the waveform prior to wedging. The right atrium is reached at 15–20 cm from the internal jugular vein, 10–15 cm from the subclavian vein, 30–40 cm from the femoral vein, and 40 and 50 cm respectively from the right and left basilic veins. The right ventricle and pulmonary artery are then entered at additional 10 cm intervals, with a further 10 cm to pulmonary artery occlusion.[23] Looping is likely and knotting can occur if continued insertion is attempted without passing these landmarks.

Measurements of PAoP should be performed by slow injection of air into the balloon while watching the pulmonary artery waveform. Over-wedging can lead to falsely high occlusion pressures or pulmonary arterial rupture, and less than 1.5 ml air may be required. Deflation after PAoP measurement should re-establish the normal pulmonary arterial waveform. If not, distal migration has occurred and the catheter should be withdrawn until the waveform is re-established.

Waveforms seen as the catheter floats to the wedged position are shown in Figure 10.2.

PULMONARY ARTERY CATHETER: MEASURED VARIABLES

Normal pressures are given in Table 10.6.

PULMONARY ARTERY OCCLUSION PRESSURE

Pulmonary artery occlusion pressure (PAoP) should be measured during end-expiration and ideally in end-diastole, using the ECG p-wave as a marker. PAoP has been termed the back-pressure to pulmonary blood flow,[24] and is also a key determinant of pulmonary capillary pressure (see below) and hence extravascular lung water. When the catheter wedges in a branch of the pulmonary artery it creates a static column of blood which equilibrates with downstream pressure at the site where it rejoins the flowing pulmonary venous system (the j point). Here the blood is very near the left atrium. PAoP therefore closely approximates left atrial pressure (LAP), which approximates left ventricular end-diastolic pressure (LVEDP). However, there are times when PAoP is a poor reflection of LVEDP (Table 10.7).

Zone 3 or not?

The catheter tip usually floats to a level at or below the left atrium. The tip should then be in West's zone 3, so that alveolar pressure < pulmonary venous pressure, where pulmonary venous pressure = LAP + distance of catheter tip below the left atrium. When there is reduced lung compliance as in ARDS, high PEEP does not usually cause loss of zone 3 positioning. Factors which do increase the likelihood of wedging in zones 1 and 2 include high intrathoracic pressures when there is normal or increased lung compliance (eg obstructive airways disease and high intrinsic PEEP), and low cardiac output states. Here, rotating the relevant lung down maximizes the likelihood of zone 3 positioning.

At the bedside, tests which suggest appropriate zone 3 catheter tip positioning include:

Table 10.7 Conditions where PAoP may misrepresent LVEDP

Catheter tip outside West's zone 3 (i.e. Alveolar pressure > pulmonary venous pressure)
Pulmonary venous obstruction
   Atrial myxoma
   Pulmonary fibrosis
   Vasculitis
Valvular heart disease
   Mitral stenosis (PAoP > LVEDP)
   Mitral regurgitation (PAoP > LVEDP)
   Aortic regurgitation (PAoP < LVEDP)
Markedly reduced pulmonary vascular bed
   Pneumonectomy
   Massive pulmonary embolism
LV dysfunction (PAoP < LVEDP)

- Respiratory swings in PAoP during positive pressure ventilation which do not exceed respiratory swings in pulmonary artery diastolic pressure[24]
- PAoP < pulmonary artery diastolic pressure
- PAoP alters by <50% of PEEP alterations
- PAoP increases by <50% of change in alveolar pressure
- Distally aspirated blood in the wedge position is 'arterialized' compared with mixed venous blood (unless the catheter wedges in an area of low ventilation/perfusion).

If the phasic waveform also has a and v waves (consistent with an atrial pressure waveform), PAoP should be a reliable representation of LAP.[23] However, it must be remembered that the best representation of left ventricular preload is not LAP or LVEDP but left ventricular end-diastolic volume (LVEDV). Unfortunately LVEDP

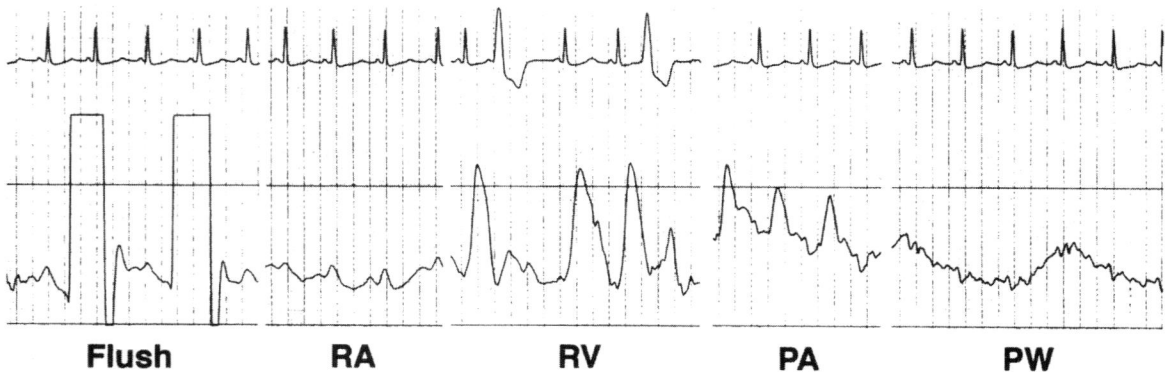

Flush   **RA**   **RV**   **PA**   **PW**

Fig. 10.2 Pressure tracings and ECG trace obtained on insertion of a pulmonary artery catheter. The snap flush test confirms an appropriate frequency response and degree of damping. RA, right atrial trace; RV, right ventricular trace. (Note simultaneous premature ventricular contractions during RV passage of the catheter.) PA, pulmonary artery trace; (note dichrotic notch and elevated diastolic pressure). PW, wedge trace (note respiratory variation). (Reproduced with permission from Leatherman JW, Marini JJ Pulmonary artery catheterization: Interpretation of pressure recordings. In: Tobin MJ (ed.) *Principles and Practice of Intensive Care Monitoring*. New York: McGraw Hill; 1998: 822.)

Table 10.8 Factors confounding a direct relationship between LVEDP and LVEDV

The normal curvilinear LVEDV/LVEDP compliance curve
Increased juxta-cardiac pressures (reducing ventricular transmural pressure)
    Extrinsic PEEP
    Intrinsic PEEP
    Active expiration
    Cardiac tamponade
    Pneumothorax
Reduced diastolic ventricular compliance
Myocardial ischaemia
Sympathetic stimulation – tachycardia
LV preload and afterload
Diastolic ventricular interaction (pericardial constraint, interventricular septal deviation)
Sepsis
Ageing
    Left ventricular hypertrophy
    Cardioplegia, e.g. post coronary artery bypass
    Inotropic drugs
    Cardiomyopathy – hypertrophic cardiomyopathy, cardiac infiltrations
Increased ventricular compliance
    Dilated cardiomyopathy

and thus PAoP are poor surrogates for LVEDV in many situations (see Table 10.8).

Effect of Raised Airway Pressures

Increased juxta-cardiac pressures reduce cardiac transmural pressures and thus preload and afterload. However, without oesophageal manometry it is difficult to predict how much PEEP is transmitted to juxta-cardiac pressures. In the absence of severe airway obstruction the nadir PAoP during transient disconnection from the ventilator eliminates the contribution of PEEP,[25] but this practice alters preload and afterload and may cause lung de-recruitment. As a rule of thumb, when lung and chest wall compliances are normal, about half of the total PEEP (extrinsic plus intrinsic) is transmitted. When chest wall compliance is reduced, more total PEEP is transmitted, and when lung compliance is reduced, less is transmitted. In acute lung injury, transmission of PEEP to intra-thoracic pressure varies from 24%–37%.[26]

Waveform Analysis

As with CVP, analysis of the PAoP waveform may give some indication of cardiac pathology. Constrictive pericarditis and pericardial tamponade show the same abnormalities (but less clearly) as in the CVP trace. Mitral regurgitation may cause a large *v* wave, which may be confused with the PA waveform. The two can be distinguished by examining the timing of the waves relative to the T wave of the ECG. The peak of the PA systolic wave occurs before and the *v* wave occurs after the T wave.

Large *v* waves may also be associated with mitral stenosis, congestive heart failure or ventricular septal defect.

PULMONARY CAPILLARY HYDROSTATIC PRESSURE

Pulmonary capillary hydrostatic pressure (PCP)[27,28] is an important determinant of extravascular lung water and thus pulmonary oedema. Because of post-capillary resistance, PCP must always exceed PAoP. The simplified Gaar equation, determined from isolated isogravimetric dog lung experiments, is as follows:

$$PCP = PAoP + 0.4 \times (Pulmonary\ MAP - PAoP)$$

The value of 0.4 represents the post-capillary contribution to the total pulmonary vascular resistance. PCP thus normally exceeds PAoP by only a few mmHg. However, with increased pulmonary vascular resistance PAoP may greatly under-estimate PCP, depending on the pre:post-capillary resistance ratio. If most of the increased resistance is pre-capillary (so that the ratio is low), PCP may still be quite close to PAoP. However, if the ratio is high, a low PAoP conceals a significant hydrostatic component to increases in lung water. Factors increasing the ratio include histamine release, inflammatory mediators and pulmonary veno-occlusive disease.

Measurement of Pulmonary Capillary Hydrostatic Pressure

PCP can be measured by methods of varying complexity.[27] The simplest involves finding the inflection point by inspection of the bi-exponential decay trace of the PA pressure waveform during a wedge manoeuvre (Figure 10.3). The inflection point marks the transition from the fast decay phase (rapid equilibration of pre-capillary, capillary and post-capillary pressures) to the slow phase (drainage of blood from capillaries through post-capillary resistance). Even this task is not simple. Correct performance

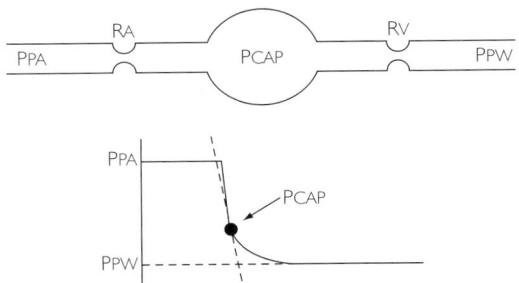

Fig. 10.3 A bedside method of determining pulmonary capillary pressure (see text). PPA, pulmonary artery pressure; R_A, pre-capillary resistance; PCAP, pulmonary capillary pressure; R_V, post-capillary resistance; PPW, pulmonary capillary wedge pressure. (Reproduced with permission from Leatherman JW, Marini JJ. Pulmonary artery catheterization: Interpretation of pressure recordings. In: Tobin MJ (ed.) *Principles and Practice of Intensive Care Monitoring.* New York: McGraw Hill; 1998: 824.)

requires the absence of respiratory movement (neuromuscular paralysis or at least very heavy sedation), a dedicated physiologic pressure recorder, and the averaging of several consecutive tracings.[27] The inflection point can still be quite difficult to identify.

PULMONARY ARTERIAL DIASTOLIC PRESSURE (PADP): SUBSTITUTE FOR PAoP?

The normal PADP–PAoP gradient is <5 mmHg, so that PADP may normally be used as a close approximation for PAoP. However tachycardia (>120/min) and conditions which increase pulmonary vascular resistance (such as ARDS, chronic obstructive pulmonary disease and pulmonary embolism) variably increase this gradient, invalidating direct substitution of PADP for PAoP. An increased gradient tends to be stable over hours, so that once it is ascertained PADP can be used to track PAoP with reasonable accuracy in the short term without repeated wedge manoeuvres.

COLD THERMODILUTION CARDIAC OUTPUT

A bolus injection into the right atrium of cold injectate (usually 5% dextrose) transiently decreases blood temperature in the pulmonary artery (monitored by a thermistor proximal to the balloon). The mean decrease in temperature (calculated by integrating temperature over time) is inversely proportional to the cardiac output, which can be determined by a modification of the Stewart–Hamilton equation:

$$Q = \frac{V \times (Tb - Ti)K1 \times K2}{Tb(t)dt}$$

Q = cardiac output; V = volume injected; Tb = blood temperature; Ti = injectate temperature; $K1$ and $K2$ = corrections for specific heat and density of injectate and for blood and dead space volumes; $Tb(t)dt$ = change in blood temperature as a function of time.

This is an indicator dilution method, using temperature change instead of indocyanine green dye, radio-isotopes, or chemicals such as sodium thiocyanate and hypertonic saline. Advantages are:

- The indicator is non-toxic.
- It does not recirculate. Repeat measurements are limited only by volume constraints and the time to regain temperature stability between injections.
- The method shows good agreement with the Fick and indocyanine green methods. However, there is considerable variability. A clinically significant change in cardiac output cannot be diagnosed with certainty unless there is a difference of at least 15% between the mean of three cardiac output determinations and the previous mean.

Too much or too little injectate will respectively underestimate and over-estimate cardiac output. Cold injectate

Table 10.9 Causes of inaccurate cold thermodilution cardiac output measurements

Catheter malposition
Wedge position
Thermistor impinging on vessel wall
Abnormal respiratory pattern
Intracardiac shunts
Tricuspid regurgitation (moderate to severe tricuspid regurgitation with caval backward flow has ben reported in 50% of mechanically ventilated patients)[30]
Cardiac dysrhythmias
Incorrect recording of injectate temperature (minimized by siting thermistor on injection port)
Rapid intravenous infusions, especially if administered via the introducer sheath
Injectate port close to or within introducer sheath
Abnormal haematocrit values (affecting $K2$ value)
Extremes of cardiac output (room temperature injectate)
Poor technique
Slow injection (>4 s)
Incorrect injectate volume

(preferably 0–4°C, but up to 12°C is usually accepted) improves the signal to noise ratio, but causes brief bradycardia, reducing cardiac output while it is being measured. Room temperature injectate introduces a small decrement in bias and precision, but has acceptable accuracy. However, the accuracy using room temperature injectate is further degraded at extremes of cardiac index, high ambient temperatures (and thus injectate temperature) or in patient hypothermia.[29]

Respiration causes fluctuations in cardiac output and PA temperature, so that measurements should ideally be made in expiration. This is difficult, and in practice an average of three evenly spaced measurements is taken. Causes of inaccurate measurements are listed in Table 10.9.[30]

WARM THERMODILUTION CARDIAC OUTPUT

This method[31] uses the same principles as cold thermodilution, but allows semi-continuous measurement. A thermal filament wrapped around the right ventricular segment of the catheter transmits low power pulses of heat. 'On–off' heat pulses in pseudo-random binary code are delivered in cycles, with a 50% total 'on' time per repetition. The downstream thermistor detects the heat pulses, which are then cross-correlated with the input sequence and power. Pulse randomization allows stochastic or spread spectral signal processing,[32] optimizing the signal to noise ratio and minimizing the amount of heat required.

Because no bolus injections are required, infection risks to both patients and health-care workers are reduced. The method shows good experimental agreement with the Fick and bolus thermodilution methods, with bias and precision (SD of bias) in the ranges of

−0.08 to +0.35 l/min and 0.5 to 1.2 l/min, respectively. Comparisons with the cold thermodilution method are hampered by the inability to make simultaneous measurements. Precision is probably closer to that of room temperature injectate, with a similar reduction of accuracy at high cardiac outputs (e.g. >10 l/min).

The main advantage is the semi-continuous cardiac output signal. However, because the measured cardiac output represents an average over the preceding 3–6 min, updated at 30-s intervals, more than 10 min must elapse before the full magnitude of any acute haemodynamic change is revealed. This interval can now be reduced to 3 min using a non-stochastic algorithm and shorter averaging times, without unacceptable loss of accuracy.[33]

Drawbacks of the technique are:

- Inaccuracy during thermal disequilibrium, such as rewarming post cardiac bypass and rapid infusions of cool fluids.
- Delay in detecting sudden changes in cardiac output.
- Magnetic resonance imaging is contra-indicated (it can melt the thermal filament).
- Electro-cautery can interfere with measurements.

DERIVED VARIABLES

A number of variables can be derived from the measurements obtained with a standard PA catheter (Table 10.11).

THE VOLUMETRIC PULMONARY ARTERIAL CATHETER

This is a standard PA catheter,[34,35] which has been altered to measure right ventricular ejection fraction (RVEF) and right ventricular end-diastolic volume index (RVEDVI). Modifications include a fast response thermistor, an ECG connection to time the R–R interval, and a multi-holed proximal lumen to maximize right atrial thermal equilibration. The principle is that following a cold bolus injection, thermal recovery in the right ventricle and pulmonary artery is pulsatile, with diastolic plateaus. Each temperature increment represents diastolic mixing of inflowing right atrial blood at core temperature with cooler right ventricular end-systolic blood. From the thermal recovery data an algorithm calculates the mean residual fraction (MRF), after corrections for the caloric inertia of the catheter body. RVEF is then 1−MRF. The method shows reasonable agreement with other RVEF methods (radionuclide techniques, echocardiography, ventriculography, magnetic resonance imaging), with a tendency to under-estimation. RVEDVI can be calculated from RVEF, since stroke index (CI/HR) is known.

RVEF is an unreliable measure of right ventricular contractility, since it is dependent on right ventricular afterload. However, RVEDVI is a volumetric index of right ventricular preload. Its interpretation is thus independent of right ventricular compliance and changes in juxta-cardiac pressures, unlike CVP. RVEDVI based predictions of CI responses to fluid challenges are superior to those made from CVP or PAoP, particularly when juxta-cardiac pressures are abnormal. If RVEDVI < 140 ml/m^2, cardiac index is said to be 'preload recruitable'.[36] RVEDVI may also improve interpretation of haemodynamic status in situations where right ventricular performance plays a crucial role, such as severe pulmonary hypertension.

However, there are many limitations to the clinical utility of this device:

- The injection port must be positioned in the right atrium as close as possible to the tricuspid valve to minimize inaccuracy.
- There is a theoretical potential for mathematical coupling in the relationship between RVEDVI and cardiac output.
- Tricuspid regurgitation invalidates RVEF and RVEDVI estimations. This is unfortunate, since moderate to severe tricuspid regurgitation and backward caval blood flow have been reported in 50% of patients subjected to mechanical ventilation.[30] Tricuspid incompetence is also common in severe right ventricular dysfunction, the very time when accurate RVEDVI determinations are most desirable.
- R–R interval sensing must be accurate. Tachycardia (>150 beats/min), atrial fibrillation and frequent ectopy can cause marked inaccuracy.
- RVEDVI is not a measure of left ventricular preload.
- Additional information on RVEDVI rarely changes treatment.

COMPLICATIONS OF PULMONARY ARTERIAL CATHETERS

These are listed in Table 10.10. A catheter may not actually be knotted, despite a chest X-ray appearance to suggest this. If knotting is suspected, other catheters should be removed in reverse order to which they were inserted, and the chest X-ray repeated. If a true knot exists, an attempt is made to pull the knot into the introducer sheath, whereupon the sheath and catheter are removed. If a sheath was not used, the catheter is pulled as far back as possible, and a cut-down to vein under local anaesthesia is undertaken. When these attempts are unsuccessful (5% of occasions), exploration by a vascular surgeon is indicated.

TRANSPULMONARY INDICATOR DILUTION

With this technique,[37] thermal and other indicators injected into a central vein are detected in a major artery. Because the indicators pass through all chambers of the heart as well as the entire pulmonary circulation, infor-

Table 10.10 Complications associated with PA Catheters. Complications of central venous catheterization (see Table 10.4)

Complications of catheter insertion
Dysrhythmias
Knotting/kinking
Valve damage
Perforation of pulmonary artery
Right bundle branch block
Complete heart block

Complications post insertion
Thrombosis
PA rupture (0.2%)
Sepsis
Endocarditis
Pulmonary infarction
Dysrhythmias (37%)
Air embolus (due to repeated attempts to fill ruptured balloon)

Risk factors for major morbidity (in particular PA rupture)
Pulmonary hypertension
Anticoagulation
In situ duration >3 days

mation additional to cardiac output can be gained. In particular, central blood volumes and indices of extravascular lung water can be measured (Figure 10.4).

TRANSPULMONARY THERMODILUTION

A fibre-optic thermistor is positioned in the femoral artery at the tip of a modified 4F arterial catheter. Cardiac output is measured by administering a central venous bolus of cold injectate, constructing an arterial thermodilution curve and applying the Stewart–Hamilton equation. The axillary artery can also be used, but placing the sensor in more peripheral arteries such as the radial causes over-

estimation of cardiac output. Curves are longer and flatter than PA catheter curves due to thermal equilibration with intrathoracic blood and extravascular lung water, but are unaffected by the respiratory phase of injection. Measurements are in good agreement with pulmonary thermodilution and direct Fick methods. There is a positive bias of about 5%, perhaps because of indicator loss, or because transpulmonary measurements are less affected by the transient bradycardia induced by cold thermodilution.

USE OF A SECOND INDICATOR

Combining thermal dilution with simultaneous dye dilution is the basis of the double indicator technique. Indocyanine green is used because it is non-toxic and highly albumin bound, remaining confined to the intravascular space on its initial circulation. Rapid response measurements can now be achieved without *ex vivo* analysis of aspirated blood, using a fibre-optic sensor at the catheter tip.

CALCULATIONS

The equilibration volumes for each indicator between injection and detection points are calculated as the product of the thermodilution cardiac output CO_{TD} and the mean transit time (MTT), where MTT is first determined from a semi-logarithmic transformation of the indicator dilution curve. Hence:

$$CO_{TD} \times MTT_{dye} = \text{intrathoracic blood volume (ITBV)}$$

$$CO_{TD} \times MTT_{thermal} = \text{intrathoracic thermal volume (ITTV)}$$

$$ITTV - ITBV = \text{extravascular lung water (EVLW)}$$

Indocyanine green concentrations after complete mixing can then be used to calculate the circulating blood

Table 10.11 Derived haemodynamic variables

Parameter	Abbreviation	Formula	Normal range	Units
Mean arterial pressure	MAP	DBP + 0.33 × (SBP − DBP)	70–105	mmHg
Mean pulmonary artery pressure	MPAP	PADP + 0.33 × (PASP − PADP)	9–16	mmHg
Mean right ventricular pressure	MRVP	CVP + 0.33 × (PASP − CVP)		mmHg
LV coronary perfusion pressure	LVCCP	DBP − PAoP		mmHg
RV coronary perfusion pressure	RVCCP	MAP − MRVP		mmHg
Cardiac index	CI	CO/BSA	2.8–4.2	l/min per m²
Stroke volume index	SVI	CI/HR	35–70	ml/beat per m²
Systemic vascular resistance index	SVRI	(MAP − CVP)/CI × 79.92	1760–2600	dyn s/cm⁵ per m²
Pulmonary vascular resistance index	PVRI	(PAP − PAoP)/CI × 79.92	44–225	dyn s/cm⁵ per m²
Left ventricular stroke work index	LVSWI	SVI × MAP × 0.0144	44–68	g m/m² per beat
Right ventricular stroke work index	RVSWI	SVI × PAP × 0.0144	4–8	g m/m² per beat
Body surface area	BSA	Weight(kg) 0.425 × Height(cm) 0.725 × 0.007184		m²

HR, heart rate; CVP, central venous pressure; PAoP, pulmonary artery occlusion pressure; SBP, systolic blood pressure; DBP, diastolic blood pressure; PADP, pulmonary artery diastolic pressure; PASP, pulmonary artery systolic pressure; MRVP, mean right ventricular pressure

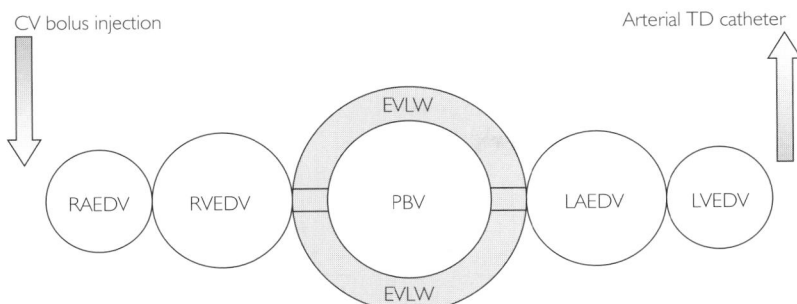

Fig. 10.4 Intravascular and extravascular equilibration volumes during transpulmonary indicator dilution. CV, central venous; EVLW, extravascular lung water; LAEDV, left atrial end-diastolic volume; LVEDV, left ventricular end-diastolic volume; PBV, pulmonary blood volume; RAEDV, right atrial end-diastolic volume; RVEDV, right ventricular end-diastolic volume. (Reproduced with permission from Hudson E, Beale R. Lung water and blood volume measurements in the critically ill. *Curr Opin Crit Care* 2000; **6**: 223.)

volume, and the subsequent concentration decay can serve as a liver function test. A device has been marketed which combines all of these features (COLD Z-021, Pulsion Medizintechnik, Munich, Germany).

INTRATHORACIC BLOOD VOLUME AS AN INDEX OF CARDIAC PRELOAD

Unlike CVP and PAoP, ITBV is a volumetric preload index. Interpretation is thus independent of alterations in juxta-cardiac pressures or myocardial compliance, and should be superior to conventional pressure indices. There is experimental and clinical evidence that this is so.

EXTRAVASCULAR LUNG WATER

EVLW is a marker of the severity of illness. Mortality is increased if EVLW is high (>14 ml/kg), and EVLW fluctuations may track lung water more closely than portable chest X-rays. Following EVLW instead of PAoP as a therapeutic endpoint may reduce positive fluid balances and ventilator and ICU days, although evidence is still limited.[38]

TRANSPULMONARY THERMODILUTION AS A SINGLE INDICATOR-EXTENDED APPLICATION

Pulmonary thermal volume (the largest thermal equilibration volume, Figure 10.4) can be determined from the cardiac output and the 'exponential downslope time' (DST) on the semi-logarithmic thermodilution curve:

$$CO_{TD} \times DST_{thermal} = \text{pulmonary thermal volume (PTV)}$$

This allows calculation of the global end-diastolic volume (GEDV), which is said to represent the volume of blood in all chambers of the heart at end-diastole. Hence:

$$ITTV - PTV = GEDV$$

Like ITBV, GEDV has a better correlation with cardiac index than CVP and PAoP. In fact ITBV can be derived as a linear function of GEDV:[39]

$$ITBV^* \text{ (ml)} = 1.25 \times GEDV - 28.4$$

Thus ITBV*, GEDV and EVLW* can be determined from transpulmonary thermodilution alone. However, thermodilution EVLW* is inaccurate in the presence of marked reductions in the pulmonary vascular bed, such as pulmonary embolism and pneumonectomy.[39]

A device is now available (PiCCO, Pulsion Medizintechnik, Munich, Germany) which employs transpulmonary thermodilution both to measure EVLW* and the preload indices ITBV* and GEDV, and to calibrate continuous cardiac output measurements by the pulse contour technique (see below). Therapeutic guidelines for this methodology have been published (Figure 10.5). The method is suitable for small children, in whom PA catheterization is not feasible. The place of devices of this type in the monitoring armamentarium is under evaluation.

LITHIUM

Lithium[40] can also serve as a transpulmonary indicator. The main advantage over thermodilution is that more peripheral arteries such as the radial can be used without loss of accuracy.

Disadvantages include:

- Corrections for packed cell volume are necessary, since lithium is distributed only in plasma.

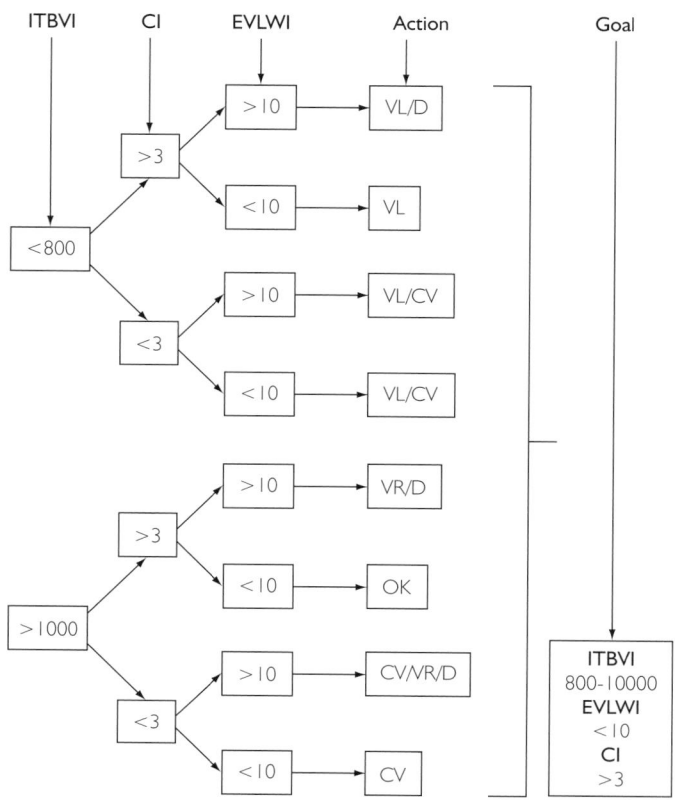

Fig. 10.5 Haemodynamic decision tree for continuous cardiac output and transpulmonary thermodilution indices. VL, volume loading; D, diuretic; VR, volume restriction; CV, cardiovascular drugs; ITBVI, intrathoracic blood volume index; EVLWI, extravascular lung water index; CI, cardiac index. (Adapted with permission from Della Rocca, Costa MG, Pietropaoli P. Clinical applications of the transpulmonary thermodilution technique. In: Gullo A (ed.) *Proceedings of the 15th Postgraduate Course in Critical Care Medicine. APICE.* Milan: Springer-Verlag; 2000: 103.)

- Blood is toxic following assay in the lithium sensitive electrode and must be discarded, introducing an infection risk and making the technique less suitable for small children.
- The method is inaccurate in patients receiving oral lithium medication.
- Electrode drift is a problem in patients receiving muscle relaxants.

CONTINUOUS CARDIAC OUTPUT

PULSE CONTOUR ANALYSIS

Modern pulse contour analysis[41] is based on the method of Wesseling, which uses a three-element model of aortic impedence, incorporating arterial compliance and systemic vascular resistance. Stroke volume is derived by analysis of the systolic area (area above diastolic pressure) of the arterial waveform, with corrections for age and

heart rate. Calibration against a simultaneous method such as thermodilution allows pulse contour analysis to be used on peripheral arterial waveforms, even non-invasive finger blood pressure waveforms. Cardiac output is computed as $HR_{mean} \times SV_{mean}$ over the preceding 30 s.

DISADVANTAGES

- Another method such as thermodilution is required for calibration.
- Recalibration is advisable every few hours to allow for changes in systemic vascular resistance. This is especially important if there is haemodynamic instability and during the administration of vasoactive drugs.
- Alterations in abdominal pressure or changes in body position, particularly in the obese, can alter aortic compliance, necessitating recalibration.
- Aortic aneurysms and significant aortic regurgitation are difficult to model and invalidate the technique.

Comparisons with PA catheter cardiac output measurements have shown good agreement, with mean bias values ≥ 0.1 L/min and precision (SD of bias) of the order of 0.6 l/min.

Another pulse contour algorithm based on frequency analysis studies of the arterial system has been developed.[42] The limits of agreement with thermodilution cardiac output (after initial calibration against this method) are −26% to +21%. The main advantage appears to be a reduced sensitivity to alterations in systemic vascular resistance.

OESOPHAGEAL DOPPLER

In the past, stroke volume and cardiac output have been measured with varying success by placing Doppler probes externally at the cardiac apex and suprasternal notch, as well as internally within the trachea and in the pulmonary artery.[43,35] Currently, oesophageal placement via the oral or nasal route seems to provide the best combination of stability and non-invasiveness.

OPERATING PRINCIPLES

There are two types of Doppler devices, continuous and pulsed wave. Oesophageal Doppler is of the continuous wave variety, emitting about 5 MHz. A piezo-electric crystal transmits the ultrasound beam while another measures the frequency of reflected waves. Flow velocity (V) of aortic red cells can be determined from the Doppler shift in the frequency of reflected waves:

$$V = (2F \times \cos\theta)^{-1} \times C\Delta F$$

where C is the speed of ultrasound in tissue, ΔF is the frequency shift, F is the emitted ultrasound frequency, and θ is the angle of incidence. The probe is positioned in the oesophagus about 30–40 cm from the teeth, where the aorta runs parallel to the oesophagus and the systolic cross-sectional area varies least. Stroke volume is calculated as the product of the mean systolic red cell velocity and the aortic cross-sectional area, assuming the descending aorta carries 70% of cardiac output. The aortic cross-sectional area is either determined from nomograms of age, weight and height, or calculated from a measured diameter. Calibration against other cardiac output methods is also possible.

ADDITIONAL INFORMATION OBTAINABLE FROM OESOPHAGEAL DOPPLER

Analysis of the velocity/time waveform provides information on:

1 Preload (flow time corrected for heart rate FTc)
2 Contractility (peak velocity)
3 Afterload (both FTc and peak velocity) (see Figure 10.6).

Early validation studies showed generally good agreement with thermodilution cardiac output. However, it is now known that agreement is poor when upper/lower body blood flow distributions are altered, or when estimates of aortic cross-sectional area are inaccurate. For example, a study of preeclamptic patients revealed consistent under-estimation of cardiac output by 40%.[44] In another study, lumbar epidural anaesthesia converted a negative bias and narrow limits of agreement with thermodilution prior to anaesthesia (bias −0.89 l/min, limits of agreement −2.67 l/min to +0.88 l/min) to a positive bias with wide limits of agreement (0.55 l/min, −3.21 l/min to +4.30 l/min).[45]

However, oesophageal Doppler has successfully guided peri-operative volume expansion in elective cardiac surgery and proximal femoral fracture repair, with reductions in both hospital stay and complication rates.[46,47] Being a volumetric index, FTc provides information on ventricular preload which should be more reliable on trend analysis than PAoP or CVP, especially in conditions such as mitral stenosis or where juxta-cardiac pressures are elevated.

ADVANTAGES

- Only a short period of training is required. Nurses at the bedside can follow volume challenge protocols guided by Doppler indices.
- The probes (6 mm diameter) are minimally invasive, and can be inserted nasally or orally. Oral insertion is usually reserved for intubated patients receiving sedation.
- Contraindications are few. They include pharyngo-oesophageal pathology, aortic balloon counterpulsation and severe aortic coarctation.[43]
- Insertion is simple, allowing reduced time to data acquisition and treatment.
- Probes are relatively stable once placed. If displaced they can be repositioned quickly, and can be left in place for days in a sedated, ventilated patient.

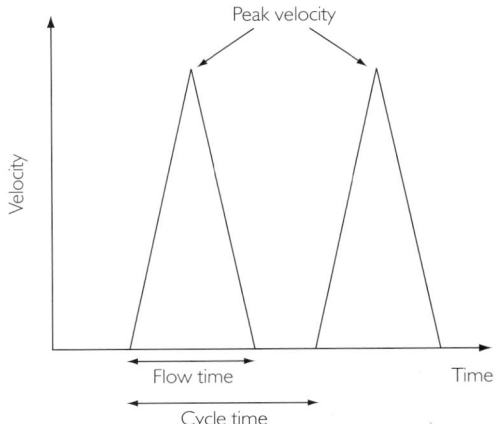

Fig. 10.6 Schematic oesophageal Doppler waveform, showing indices of preload, contractility and afterload (see text).

DISADVANTAGES

- Assumptions that descending aortic flow is 70% of total cardiac output and that nomograms accurately determine aortic cross-section can be incorrect. This limits usefulness when there is aortic pathology or compression, or abnormal upper/lower body blood flow distributions.
- In children aortic cross-section fluctuates in systole, making the assumption of a fixed systolic aortic cross-section unreliable.
- Finding and maintaining optimal probe positioning is important for consistency in trend measurements.

Other methods of determining continuous or semi-continuous cardiac output include those dependent on the Fick principle, and impedence and inductance cardiography.

THE FICK PRINCIPLE

The Fick[31] equation can be expressed as:

$$CO = VO_2/(CaO_2 - CvO_2)$$

where VO_2 is whole body oxygen consumption, and CaO_2 and CvO_2 are the oxygen contents of arterial and mixed venous blood respectively. By measuring VO_2 by indirect calorimetry under steady state conditions, plus CvO_2 (PA catheter) and CaO_2, it is possible to derive cardiac output. This method has traditionally been considered the 'gold standard', but in most ICU patients the stringent preconditions for accuracy are not met. Further error is introduced by the elevated oxygen consumption of inflamed lungs. Use is therefore mainly confined to cardiac laboratories

Various modifications can generate continuous or semi-continuous cardiac output measurements. Apart from the partial CO_2 rebreathing method, all require a PA catheter and reflectance oximetry of mixed venous blood, thus offering little or no advantage over the conventional warm thermodilution semi-continuous method.

PARTIAL CO₂ REBREATHING METHOD

With this method,[31] cardiac output can be measured every 3 min. A segment of dead space (150 ml) is introduced into the breathing circuit of an intubated, ventilated patient for 30–50 s. It is assumed that although pulmonary end-capillary, arterial and end-tidal PCO_2 rise promptly, mixed venous PCO_2 does not change during this brief period of rebreathing. Cardiac output is determined from a modification of the differential Fick equation:

$$CO = \Delta CO_2 \text{ elimination}/(S \times \Delta \text{ end-tidal } PCO_2)$$

where S is the slope of the blood CO_2 dissociation curve. Partial CO_2 rebreathing really measures non-shunted pulmonary capillary blood flow rather than total cardiac output.[48] Therefore a correction for venous admixture is

added based on FiO_2 and SaO_2 (measured by pulse oximetry).

The method appears to have reasonable accuracy post cardiac surgery and in acute lung injury.[48]

Problems with the Partial CO₂ Re-breathing Method

- Unsuitable for non-intubated patients (who have variable tidal volumes and leakage around face-masks).
- $P E' CO_2$ may not accurately reflect change in pulmonary end-capillary and arterial PCO_2, especially in chronic lung disease.
- CO_2 elimination may not reach steady state in the time available (especially in chronic lung disease).
- The value of S varies with haemoglobin concentration and PCO_2.
- Venous admixture cannot be calculated reliably from FiO_2 and SaO_2 when there is significant V/Q scatter (e.g. chronic lung disease).
- Overall lack of validation in chronic lung disease.

IMPEDANCE THORACOCARDIOGRAPHY

A constant, low amplitude high-frequency alternating current is passed through the thorax. The ECG is recorded simultaneously. Current is kept constant and fluctuations in electrical impedance are measured. By modeling the thorax as a conductor in the shape of a cylinder or truncated cone, stroke volume can be determined from the variation of impedance through the cardiac cycle. Respiratory artefact is eliminated by averaging values over several cardiac cycles using the R–R interval as a synchronizing signal. The addition of phonocardiography allows calculation of ventricular ejection times.[49]

Inaccuracies arise from many sources. They include motion artefact, electrical interference, tachycardia, dysrhythmias, conduction defects, variations in functional residual capacity, chest deformities, pneumonectomy, pleural and pericardial effusions, pulmonary oedema, chest tubes, pregnancy, metal prostheses, valvular regurgitation and intracardiac shunts. Despite this impressive list, the method has shown good agreement with the thermodilution technique in a cross section of acute medical and surgical patients, with calculated bias and precision of –0.124 l/min and 0.75 l/min, respectively. Measuring whole body, rather than truncal impedance by placing electrodes on wrists and ankles also appears successful.

INDUCTANCE CARDIOGRAPHY

Left ventricular volume curves are generated by an inductive plethysmographic transducer transversely encircling the chest near the xiphoid process.[50] Calibration against an independent technique such as thermodilution is necessary. With this technique, it is also possible to monitor trends in indices of left ventricular filling, such as the E/A ratio and the isovolaemic relaxation time. These can otherwise only be derived intermittently by Doppler echocardiography.

REFERENCES

1 Gardner R, Hollingsworth K. Optimizing the electrocardiogram and blood pressure monitoring. *Crit Care Med* 1986; **14**: 651–8.

2 Schlichtig RI. Arterial catheterization: complications. In: Tobin MJ (ed.) *Principles and Practice of Intensive Care Monitoring*. New York: McGraw Hill; 1998: pp. 751–6.

3 Slogoff S, Keats AS, Arlund C. On the safety of radial artery cannulation. *Anesthesiology* 1983; **59**: 42–7.

4 Dahl MR, Smead WL, McSweeney TD. Radial artery cannulation: a comparison of 15.2- and 4.45- cm catheters. *J Clin Monit* 1992; **8**: 193–7.

5 Coriat P, Vrillon M, Perel A, *et al*. A comparison of systolic blood pressure variations and echocardiographic estimates of end-diastolic left ventricular size in patients after aortic surgery. *Anesth Analg* 1994; **78**: 46–53.

6 Ornstein E, Eidelman LA, Drenger B, Elami A, Pizov R. Systolic pressure variation predicts the response to acute blood loss. *J Clin Anesth* 1998; **10**: 137–140.

7 Tavernier B, Makhotine O, Lebuffe G, Dupont J, Scherpereel P. Systolic pressure variation as a guide to fluid therapy in patients with sepsis-induced hypotension. *Anesthesiology* 1998; **89**: 1313–21.

8 Venus B, Satish P. Vascular cannulation. In: Civetta JM, Taylor RW, Kirby RR (eds) *Critical Care*. Philadelphia: Lippincott-Raven; 1997: pp. 521–44.

9 Fletcher SJ, Bodenham AR. Safe placement of central venous catheters: where should the tip of the catheter lie? *Br J Anaesth* 2000; **85**: 188–91.

10 Joynt GM, Gomersall CD, Buckley TA, Oh TE, Young RJ, Freebairn RC. Comparison of intrathoracic and intra-abdominal measurements of central venous pressure. *Lancet* 1996; **347**: 1155–7.

11 Mian NZ, Bayly R, Schreck DM, Besserman EB, Richmond D. Incidence of deep venous thrombosis associated with femoral venous catheterization. *Acad Emerg Med* 1997; 12: 1118–21.

12 Gomez CMH, Palazzo MGA. Pulmonary artery catheterization in anaesthesia and intensive care. *Br J Anaesth* 1998; 81: 945–56.

13 Vincent JL, Bihari D, Suter PM, *et al*. The prevalence of nosocomial infection in intensive care units in Europe – the results of the European Prevalence of Infection in Intensive Care (EPIC) study. *JAMA* 1995; **274**: 639–44.

14 Mimoz O, Rauss A, Rekik N, Brun-Buisson C, Lemaire F, Brochard L. Pulmonary artery catheterization in critically ill patients: a prospective analysis of outcome changes associated with catheter-prompted changes in therapy. *Crit Care Med* 1994; **22**: 573–79.

15 Steingrub JS, Celoria G, Vickers-Lahti M, Teres D, Bria W. Therapeutic impact of pulmonary artery catheterization in a medical/surgical ICU. *Chest* 1992; **99**: 1451–5.

16 Del Guercio LRM. Does pulmonary artery catheter use change outcome? Yes. *Crit Care Clin* 1996; 12: 553–7.

17 Leibowitz AB. Do pulmonary artery catheters improve outcome? No. *Crit Care Clin* 1996; 12: 559–68.

18 Connors AE, Speroff T, Dawson NV, *et al*. The effectiveness of right heart catheterisation in the initial care of critically ill patients. SUPPORT investigators *JAMA* 1996; **276**: 889–97.

19 Dalen JE, Bone RC. Is it time to pull the pulmonary artery catheter? *JAMA* 1996; **276**: 916–8.

20 Vincent J-L, Dhainaut J-F, Perret C, Suter P. Is the pulmonary artery catheter misused? A European view. *Crit Care Med* 1998; **26**: 1283–7.

21 Murdoch SD, Cohen AT, Bellamy MC. Pulmonary artery catheterization and mortality in critically ill patients. *Br J Anaesth* 2000; **85**: 611–5.

22 Preas II HL, Suffredini AF. Pulmonary artery catheterization: insertion and quality control. In: Tobin MJ (ed.) *Principles and Practice of Intensive Care Monitoring*. New York: McGraw Hill; 1998: pp. 773–95.

23 Worthley LIG. Vascular cannulation and haemodynamic pressure. In: Worthley LIG (ed.) *Synopsis of Intensive Care Medicine*. Edinburgh: Churchill Livingstone; 1994: pp. 83–95.

24 Pinsky MR. Hemodynamic profile interpretration. In: Tobin MJ (ed.) *Principles and Practice of Intensive Care Monitoring*. New York: McGraw Hill; 1998: pp. 871–88.

25 Pinsky M, Vincent J-L, De Smet JM. Estimating left ventricular filling pressure during positive end-expiratory pressure in humans. *Am Rev Resp Dis* 1991; **143**: 25–31.

26 Jardin F, Genevray B, Brun-Ney D, Bourdaris JP. Influence of lung and chest wall compliances on transmission of airway pressures to the pleural space in critically ill patients. *Chest* 1985; **88**: 653–8.

27 Cope DK, Grimbert F, Downey JM, Taylor AE. Pulmonary capillary pressure: a review. *Crit Care Med* 1992; **20**: 1043–56.

28 Levy MM. Pulmonary capillary pressure. *Crit Care Clin* 1996; **12**: 819–39.

29 Magder S. Cardiac output. In: Tobin MJ (ed.) *Principles and Practice of Intensive Care Monitoring*. New York: McGraw Hill; 1998: pp. 797–810.

30 Jullien T, Valtier B, Hongnat JM, Dubourg O, Bourdarias JP, Jardin F. Incidence of tricuspid regurgitation and vena caval backward flow in mechanically ventilated patients. A color Doppler and contrast echocardiographic study. *Chest* 1995; **107**: 488–93.

31 Kees Mahutte C. Continuous cardiac output monitoring via thermal, Fick, Doppler, and pulse contour methods. In: Tobin MJ (ed.) *Principles and Practice of Intensive Care Monitoring*. New York: McGraw Hill; 1998: pp. 901–13.

32 Yelderman M. Continuous measurement of cardiac output with the use of stochastic system identification techniques. *L Clin Monit* 1990; **6**: 322–32.

33 Zollner C, Polasek J, Kilger E, *et al.* Evaluation of a new continuous thermodilution cardiac output monitor in cardiac surgical patients: a prospective criterion standard study. *Crit Care Med* 1999; **27**: 293–8.

34 Cariou A, Laurent I, Dhainaut J-FA. Pulmonary artery catheterization: modified catheters. In: Tobin MJ (ed.) *Principles and Practice of Intensive Care Monitoring.* New York: McGraw Hill; 1998: pp. 811–9.

35 Marik PE. Pulmonary artery catheterization and esophageal Doppler monitoring in the ICU. *Chest* 1999; **116**: 1085–91.

36 Diebel LN, Wilson RF, Tagett MG, Kline RA. End-diastolic volume: A better indicator of preload in the critically ill. *Arch Surg* 1992; **127**: 817–21.

37 Hudson E, Beale R. Lung water and blood volume measurements in the critically ill. *Curr Opin Crit Care* 2000; **6**: 222–6.

38 Mitchell JP, Schuller D, Calandrino FS, Schuster DP. Improved outcome based on fluid management in critically ill patients requiring pulmonary artery catheterization. *Am Rev Respir Dis* 1992; **145**: 990–8.

39 Sakka SG, Reinhart K, Meier-Hellman A. Comparison of pulmonary arterial and arterial thermodilution cardiac output in critically ill patients. *Intensive Care Med* 1999; **25**: 843–6.

40 Linton RA, Band DM, Haire KM. A new method of measuring cardiac output in man using lithium dilution. *Br J Anaesth* 1993; **71**: 262–266.

41 Van Lieshout JJ, Wesseling KH. Continuous cardiac output by pulse contour analysis? *Br J Anaesth* 2001; **86**: 467–9.

42 Linton NWF, Linton RAF. Estimation of changes in cardiac output from the arterial blood pressure waveform in the upper limb. *Br J Anaesth* 2001; **86**: 486–96.

43 Venn R, Rhodes A, Bennett ED. The esophageal Doppler. In: Vincent J-L (ed.) *1999 Yearbook of Intensive Care and Emergency Medicine.* Berlin: Springer-Verlag; 1999: pp. 482–93.

44 Penny JA, Anthony J, Shennan AH, De Swiet M, Singer M. A comparison of hemodynamic data derived by pulmonary artery flotation catheter and the esophageal Doppler monitor in preeclampsia. *Am J Obstet Gynecol* 2000; **183**: 658–61.

45 Leather HA, Wouters PF. Oesophageal Doppler monitoring overestimates cardiac output during lumbar epidural anaesthesia. *Br J Anaesth* 2001; **86**: 794–7.

46 Mythen MG, Webb AR. Perioperative plasma volume expansion reduces the incidence of gut mucosal hypoperfusion during cardiac surgery. *Arch Surg* 1995; **130**: 423–9.

47 Sinclair S, James S, Singer M. Intraoperative intravascular volume optimisation and length of hospital stay after repair of proximal femoral fracture. *BMJ* 1997; **315**: 909–12.

48 de Abreu, MG, Quintel M, Ragaller M, Albrecht DM. Partial carbon dioxide rebreathing: a reliable technique for noninvasive measurement of nonshunted pulmonary capillary blood flow. *Crit Care Med* 1997; **25**: 675–83.

49 Bloch KE. Impedance and inductance monitoring of cardiac output. In: Tobin MJ (ed.) *Principles and Practice of Intensive Care Monitoring.* New York: McGraw Hill; 1998: pp. 915–30.

50 Bloch KE, Jugoon S, Sackner MA. Inductance cardiography (thoracocardiography): a novel, noninvasive technique for monitoring left ventricular filling. *J Crit Care* 1999; 14: 177–85.

Monitoring oxygenation

T J Morgan and B Venkatesh

THE ROLES OF OXYGEN IN AEROBIC ORGANISMS

The roles of oxygen in metabolic processes should be kept in mind when considering how and why oxygenation is monitored in critical illness.

- Electron transfer oxidase systems – in particular mitochondrial cytochrome oxidase Complex IV.[1] The generation of adenosine triphosphate (ATP) by oxidative phosphorylation accounts for approximately 90% of oxygen consumption. Here oxygen is the terminal electron acceptor for the electron transport chain, combining with two protons to produce water.
- Oxygen transferase systems, in which oxygen is incorporated into substrates. Examples are the production of prostanoids, catecholamines and some neurotransmitters.
- Mixed function oxidase systems. These are degradation and detoxification reactions requiring oxygen and a co-substrate (e.g. NADPH). The cytochrome P-450 hydroxylases are an example.

DYSOXIA

As originally defined[2] there are three subtypes:

- 'Hypoxic' dysoxia, defined as oxygen delivery inadequate for oxygen demand. As oxygen delivery is reduced, the oxygen transferase and mixed function oxidase systems succumb first. Below a critical mitochondrial PO_2 (0.1–1 mmHg), oxidative phosphorylation also ceases. Stopgap energy production is maintained by anaerobic glycolysis, but without oxygen there is progressive ATP depletion, lactic acidosis and eventual cell death by apoptosis and necrosis. On reoxygenation, injury from massive release of reactive oxygen species may overshadow the original hypoxic insult.
- 'Normoxic' dysoxia, defined as abnormal cellular oxygen utilization despite adequate oxygen delivery.

For example cyanide blocks the normal reduction of oxygen by binding to cytochrome oxidase.
- 'Hyperoxic' dysoxia, defined as abnormal cell function due to the high oxygen tensions (oxygen toxicity).[3]

Nowadays the term 'dysoxia' usually refers to 'hypoxic' dysoxia.

THE OXYGEN CASCADE

In unicellular organisms, oxygen reaches the mitochondria across a short diffusion path with a steep partial pressure gradient. In multi-cellular animals the diffusion path is lengthened, but the gradient is broken up into a series of smaller partial pressure reductions. This is the oxygen cascade. As a result, oxygen normally arrives at the intracellular organelles of all tissues at tensions still above the anaerobic threshold.

Important steps in the oxygen cascade include:

- inspired gas
- alveolar gas
- arterial blood
- microcirculation
- interstitium
- mitochondria and other intracellular organelles.

Threats to tissue oxygenation can arise at any of these points, causing downstream oxygen deprivation of mitochondria and other intracellular organelles. In this chapter we will consider how oxygenation can be monitored at strategic points along the cascade.

INSPIRED GAS

Monitoring the fraction of inspired oxygen (FiO_2) is necessary to prevent hypoxaemia, while minimizing the adverse effects of excess oxygen. The inspired oxygen tension (PiO_2) of humidified gas is determined by the FiO_2, the barometric pressure (BP) and the saturated vapour pressure of water (47 mmHg).

$$PiO_2 = FiO_2 \times (BP - 47) \qquad (1)$$

Gas supply pressures are monitored continuously. Ventilators incorporate input pressure alarms and oxygen analysers (usually fuel cells) within the inspiratory module to identify oxygen source failure. Additional direct measurement of circuit oxygen concentration can be performed.

TRANSFER OF INSPIRED GAS TO ALVEOLI

Communication between oxygen delivery system and pulmonary alveoli is open if:

- There are no signs of upper airway obstruction.
- Expired tidal and minute volumes and airway pressures for the ventilated patient are within correctly set alarm limits.
- There is an appropriate waveform on an end-tidal CO_2 monitor.

ALVEOLAR GAS

Alveolar PO_2 in individual lung units ranges from approximately 80 mmHg to 130 mmHg in healthy young subjects breathing air. In a critically ill patient with severe ventilation/perfusion ($\dot{V}/\dot{Q}$) mismatch receiving 100% oxygen, alveolar PO_2 can range from <40 mmHg to >600 mmHg. Consequently, end-tidal PO_2 monitoring is of no value.

THE IDEAL ALVEOLUS

A parameter used in more than one index of pulmonary oxygen transfer is the alveolar PO_2 in an imaginary ideal lung unit (PAO_2). PAO_2 is derived from the alveolar gas equation:

$$PAO_2 = PiO_2 - (1-FiO_2 \times (1-R)) \times PaCO_2/R \qquad (2)$$

where R is the respiratory exchange ratio, either measured by indirect calorimetry or assumed to be 0.8. PiO_2 is calculated as in Equation (1). $PaCO_2$ is arterial PCO_2.

Most clinicians use the following approximation:

$$PAO_2 = PiO_2 - PaCO_2/0.8$$

TRANSFER FROM ALVEOLI TO ARTERIAL BLOOD (PULMONARY OXYGEN TRANSFER)

The best measure of pulmonary gas transfer is by the multiple inert gas elimination technique,[4,5] although this is not normally available at the bedside. The method has identified $\dot{V}/\dot{Q}$ mismatch and intrapulmonary shunt as the two main causes of reduced pulmonary oxygen transfer in critical illness. Intrapulmonary shunt predominates in the acute respiratory distress syndrome (ARDS), in lobar pneumonia and after cardio-pulmonary bypass, whereas $\dot{V}/\dot{Q}$ mismatch is more prominent in chronic lung disease.

BEDSIDE INDICES OF PULMONARY OXYGEN TRANSFER

These are either tension-based or content-based.

TENSION-BASED INDICES
A-a Gradient

The A-a gradient is part of the APACHE II score.[6] It is calculated as $PAO_2 - PaO_2$, where PAO_2 has been determined from the alveolar gas equation (Eqn. 2).

Hypoxaemia with a normal A-a gradient occurs under two conditions:

- Alveolar hypoventilation (elevated $PACO_2$).
- Low FiO_2 ($FiO_2 <0.21$ or altitude).

Hypoxaemia with a raised A-a gradient can be due to:

- diffusion defect (rare)
- $\dot{V}/\dot{Q}$ mismatch
- shunt (intrapulmonary or cardiac)
- increased arterio-venous oxygen extraction (CaO_2-CvO_2).

Drawbacks of the A-a gradient include:

- It is both FiO_2 and age dependent. The normal value breathing air ranges from 7 mmHg in young adults to 14 mmHg in the elderly. On 100% oxygen, these values become 31 mmHg and 56 mmHg, respectively.
- For lungs with an unchanging intrapulmonary shunt the A-a gradient alters markedly with FiO_2 (Figure 11.1)
- In constant $\dot{V}/\dot{Q}$ mismatch the relationship between the A-a gradient and FiO_2 is even more complex (Figure 11.2)

PaO₂/FiO₂ Ratio

The PaO_2/FiO_2 ratio forms part of the definition of acute lung injury and ARDS.[7] It is also an input variable in the SAPS 2[8] and lung injury scoring systems.[9] At sea-level, the normal value is ≥500 mmHg. Its main advantage is simplicity. Unlike the A-a gradient, the PaO_2/FiO_2 ratio cannot distinguish hypoxaemia due to alveolar hypoventilation from other causes. In conditions, such as ARDS, where the predominant defect is intrapulmonary shunt, the PaO_2/FiO_2 ratio is unreliable unless estimated when FiO_2 >0.5, PaO_2 <100 mmHg and CaO_2-CvO_2 is constant.[10]

Further disadvantages are that it alters markedly *in exactly the same lungs* when:

- at altitude
- there are fluctuations in CaO_2-CvO_2, particularly at low oxygen extraction when FiO_2 is also varying.[11] This is common in sepsis.

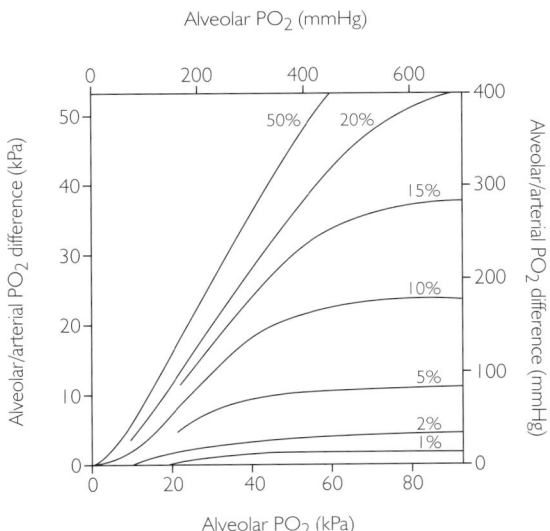

Fig. 11.1   Effect of varying FiO_2 (via alveolar PO_2) on A-a gradient with different degrees of intrapulmonary shunt. (Reproduced with permission from Nunn JF. Oxygen. In: Nunn JF (ed.) *Applied Respiratory Physiology*, 4th edn. Oxford: Butterworth-Heinemann; 1993: p. 264)

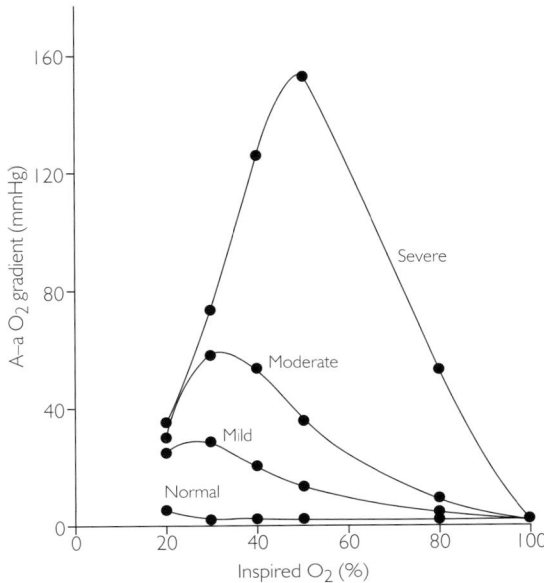

Fig. 11.2   Effect of varying FiO_2 on A-a gradient with mild, moderate and severe $\dot{V}/\dot{Q}$ mismatch. No allowance has been made for absorption atelectasis or alterations in hypoxic pulmonary vasoconstriction. (Figures 11.2 and 11.3 reproduced with permission from D'Alonzo GE, Dantzker DR. Respiratory failure, mechanisms of abnormal gas exchange, and oxygen delivery. *Med Clin North Am* 1983; **67**: 557–71.)

- FiO_2 is varied in lungs in which $\dot{V}/\dot{Q}$ mismatch is the predominant lesion. For this reason the PaO_2/FiO_2 ratio is particularly unreliable in chronic obstructive pulmonary disease.

There are other tension-based indices, such as the respiratory index (A-a gradient/PaO_2) and the arterial–alveolar oxygen tension ratio (PaO_2/PAO_2). They provide no particular advantages and are not in common use.

CONTENT-BASED INDICES
Venous Admixture ($\dot{Q}s/\dot{Q}t$)

Venous admixture is a calculation derived from a three-compartment model of the lung, the compartments consisting of:

- Alveoli with perfectly matched perfusion and ventilation ($\dot{V}/\dot{Q} = 1$, ideal compartment)
- Perfused but unventilated alveoli ($\dot{V}/\dot{Q} = 0$, venous admixture or shunt compartment)
- Ventilated but unperfused alveoli. ($\dot{V}/\dot{Q} = \infty$, alveolar dead space compartment).

Venous admixture is the proportion of mixed venous blood flowing through the theoretical shunt ($\dot{V}/\dot{Q} = 0$) compartment. It is determined according to the formula:

$$\frac{\dot{Q}_S}{\dot{Q}_T} = \frac{Cc'O_2 - CaO_2}{Cc'O_2 - CvO_2} \qquad (3)$$

$Cc'O_2$, CaO_2 and CvO_2 represent the oxygen contents of pulmonary end-capillary, arterial and mixed venous blood respectively. CaO_2 and CvO_2 are calculated from arterial and mixed venous blood gas analysis and CO-oximetry (see Table 11.4). $Cc'O_2$ is derived differently, since pulmonary end-capillary blood cannot be sampled. PcO_2 is therefore assumed to equal PAO_2 as derived from the alveolar gas equation (Eqn. 2). ScO_2 (normally close to 1) can then be computed from an algorithm for the HbO_2 dissociation curve.[12]

Advantages of venous admixture:

- Unaffected by barometric pressure
- Unaffected by alveolar hypoventilation
- Provided intrapulmonary shunt is the dominant pathology, it is stable across the entire FiO_2 range despite variations in CaO_2–CvO_2.

Disadvantages:

- Sampling mixed venous blood necessitates insertion of a PA catheter
- It is highly variable with FiO_2 in $\dot{V}/\dot{Q}$ mismatch. In $\dot{V}/\dot{Q}$ mismatch without shunt, venous admixture virtually disappears at $FiO_2 > 0.5$ (Figure 11.3).

When determined at $FiO_2 = 1$, venous admixture is an accurate measure of true shunt. However, at high FiO_2 true shunt is increased by absorption atelectasis, particularly if there are large numbers of low $\dot{V}/\dot{Q}$ lung units.

VQI: The Dual Oximetry Method[13]

By assuming $ScO_2 = 1$, the equation for venous admixture can be simplified. $\dot{Q}s/\dot{Q}t$ calculated in this way is termed 'VQI'. Unless SaO_2 is very close to 1, VQI is a linear function of $\dot{Q}s/\dot{Q}t$. The advantage is that VQI can be monitored continuously, by combining pulse oximetry with mixed venous oximetry and providing regular inputs of haemoglobin concentration and FiO_2.

Others have simplified the venous admixture equation still further by ignoring the dissolved oxygen components:[14]

$$VQI \text{ (simplified)} = (1-SaO_2)/(1-SvO_2)$$

This is less successful since dissolved oxygen is an important determinant of $\dot{Q}s/\dot{Q}t$ at higher FiO_2.

Estimated Shunt Fraction

If a fixed CaO_2-CvO_2 can be assigned, no PA catheter is necessary. However, in critical illness measured CaO_2-CvO_2 can range from 1.3 ml/dl to 7.4 ml/dl.[15]

As a result, estimated shunt fractions are not only inaccurate, but can incorrectly track directions of change.

DIFFERENCE BETWEEN END-CAPILLARY AND ARTERIAL OXYGEN CONTENT (CCO_2–CAO_2)

This content-based index provides no particular advantages.

ARTERIAL BLOOD

Indices of arterial oxygenation are PaO_2 and SaO_2. They are linked by the HbO_2 dissociation curve (Figure 11.4).

Clinically significant hypoxaemia is defined as PaO_2 <60 mmHg or SaO_2 <0.9. These values lie near the descending portion of the HbO_2 dissociation curve (assuming normal haemoglobin-oxygen affinity), so that a further drop in PaO_2 leads to a marked fall in SaO_2 and thus CaO_2.

BLOOD GAS ANALYSIS AND CO-OXIMETRY

Arterial blood is collected in a purpose-designed syringe, containing lyophilized heparin to a final concentration of 20–50 U/ml. Measurements are made by a Clark electrode (PaO_2) and by CO-oximetry (SaO_2). The Clark electrode works on polarographic principles, and CO-oximeters compute the concentrations of each of the four main haemoglobin species (HbO_2, Hb, COHb, MetHb) from light absorbances of haemolysed blood

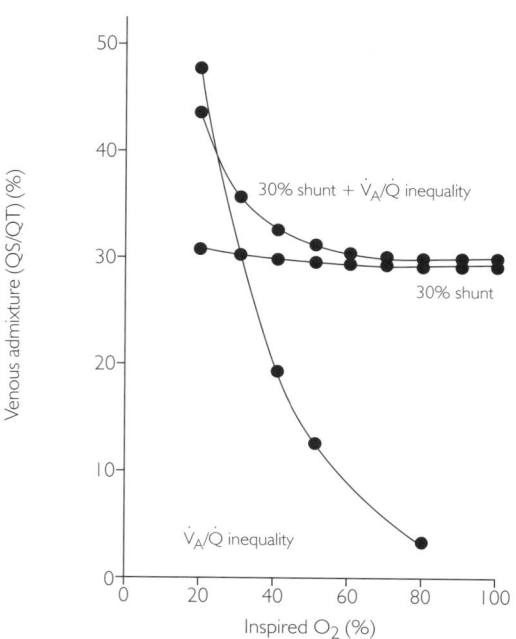

Fig. 11.3 Effect of varying FiO_2 on venous admixture in various combinations of $\dot{V}/\dot{Q}$ mismatch and shunt. No allowance has been made for absorption atelectasis or alterations in hypoxic pulmonary vasoconstriction.

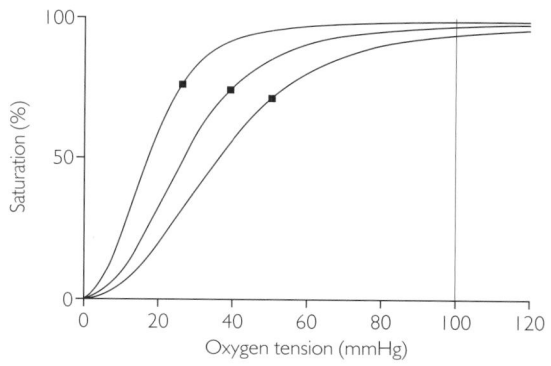

Fig. 11.4 Three HbO_2 dissociation curves: Normal (P50 = 26.7 mmHg), left-shifted (P50 = 17 mmHg) and right-shifted (P50 = 36 mmHg). The vertical line represents the normal oxygen loading tension (PO_2 = 100 mmHg). The filled squares represent an oxygen extraction of 5 ml/dl blood, assuming a haemoglobin concentration of 150 g/l. (Reproduced with permission from Morgan TJ. The HbO_2 dissociation curve in critical illness. *Critical Care and Resuscitation* 1999; 1:93–100.)

over six or seven wavelengths. SaO_2 is functional saturation, determined from concentrations of HbO_2 and Hb (see Table 11.4). Interference to CO-oximetry arises from substances with competing absorbance spectra, such as bilirubin, HbF, lipid emulsions and intravenous dyes. Newer multi-wavelength techniques reduce or eliminate this interference.

SaO_2 should always be measured rather than calculated. Calculating SaO_2 from PaO_2 is unreliable,[16] even after factoring in shifts in haemoglobin-oxygen affinity due to acid-base disturbances. The problem is that normal 2,3-diphosphoglycerate concentrations must be assumed. In critical illness, this is often incorrect.[17]

For errors, see Table 11.1.[18]

TEMPERATURE CORRECTION

All measurements are made at 37°C. Temperature-corrected values can be calculated if the core temperature of the patient is entered into the device software. Evidence for and against using temperature-corrected values is confusing and inconclusive. Most clinicians interpret blood gas data at 37°C, except when evaluating the A-a gradient.

CONTINUOUS INTRA-ARTERIAL BLOOD GAS MONITORING

Multiparameter fibre-optic sensors can be placed in the arterial stream for continuous blood gas monitoring.[19] Fibre-optic sensors are called 'optodes', and those measuring PO_2 normally operate by fluorescence quenching. They require calibration with precision gases or solutions before use. Typical sensors (Paratrend 7, Diametrics Medical, Bucks, UK) are 0.5 mm diameter, and can be inserted through 20-G arterial cannulae. Accuracy on *in vitro* and animal testing is good. The 90% *in vitro* response time to a change in PO_2 is 78 s. PO_2 drift *in vivo* is 0.03 mmHg/h. Recalibration *in vivo* can be performed against conventional blood gas analysis. See Table 11.2 for advantages and disadvantages of continuous intra-arterial PaO_2 monitoring.

PULSE OXIMETRY

Pulse oximetry[20,21] determines SpO_2 from the absorbance of light at wavelengths 660 nm (red) and 940 nm (infra-red) passed through tissue capillary beds such as fingers, earlobes and the nasal septum. Two light emitting diodes cycle on and off at multiples of the mains frequency. A third interval is inserted to allow quantification of background ambient light. A single photo-diode detects the transmitted light. The emergent signal is pulsatile due to arterial volume fluctuations. Subtraction of the background signal (tissue, capillary blood and venous blood) isolates the arterial component.

For both wavelengths, absorbance (A) is determined as follows:

$$A = \log_{10}(I_0/I)$$

I_0 = incident light intensity, and I = emergent light intensity. For a given chromophore, A is proportional to its concentration (Beer's law) and to the path length (Lambert's law). From the pulsatile (AC) and background (DC) absorbance signals at both wavelengths, a ratio (R) is derived:

$$R = (AC_{660}/DC_{660})/(AC_{940}/DC_{940})$$

Table 11.1 Pre-analytic and analytic errors in PO_2 measurement

Pre-analytic	Analytic
Exposure to air bubbles, with oxygen diffusing in or out according to the tension gradient. Contamination with line flush solution, prevented if the discard volume is 2–3 times the internal volume of cannula and tubing. Extreme leukocytosis causing pseudohypoxaemia by excessive *in vitro* oxygen consumption. Iced storage in polypropylene syringes (rather than glass) causing artefactual PaO_2 elevations. Cold increases plasma oxygen solubility, and the semi-permeability of the plastic allows oxygen ingress.[18]	Inter-analyser variability is significant, with 7–8% measurement variation on the same sample. Inadequate blood heparinization, allowing protein deposition on the electrodes. Significant non-linearity of the Clark electrode when PO_2 >150 mmHg. Maintenance of electrode temperature within narrow limits (37 ± 0.1°C) is critical. PO_2 changes by 7% for every degree Celsius temperature change.
	Interference by nitrous oxide and halothane is minimal, provided the polarizing voltage of the electrode does not exceed 600 mV. Quality control materials such as aqueous, perfluorocarbon and bovine haemoglobin solutions are used for convenience, but tonometry is the primary reference method. Arterial blood gas tensions fluctuate constantly even in stable patients. Intermittent blood gas analysis provides only a snapshot of a continuously changing variable.

Table 11.2 Advantages and disadvantages of continuous intra-arterial PaO_2 monitoring

Advantages	Disadvantages
Eliminates pre-analytic errors of intermittent blood gas analysis. More sensitive than pulse oximetry to changes in arterial oxygenation when PaO_2 >70 mmHg (the flat part of the HbO_2 dissociation curve). Free from the sources of error of pulse oximetry (see Table 11.3). Near real time PaO_2 allows prompt tracking of responses to changed ventilator settings. Reduced exposure of personnel to potentially infected blood. Reduced blood loss for diagnostic purposes.	The 'wall' effect – a sudden decrease in measured PaO_2 due to contact with the arterial wall, with averaging of arterial and wall oxygen tensions. The problem is reduced in larger arteries such as the femoral artery. The 'flush' effect. Unless the sensor is inserted a sufficient distance beyond the cannula tip, measured PaO_2 can be altered by contamination with the continuous flush solution. Damping of the arterial wave-form. Large footprint of the free-standing monitor.

SpO_2 is then computed from this R value, using software 'look-up' tables. The tables record empirically-derived relationships between R and either SaO_2 or $FHbO_2$ measured in the arterial blood of volunteers breathing hypoxic gas mixtures.

SpO_2 is usually displayed as a percentage. Only two wavelengths are used, so that it is assumed that the only haemoglobin species in the light path are HbO_2 and Hb. This is always incorrect, but with normal dyshaemoglobin concentrations, the error is trivial. Some manufacturers calibrate R against $FHbO_2$ (fractional saturation) rather than SaO_2 (functional saturation). There is debate over which calibration is correct, based on which parameter is thought to have the most clinical relevance. Again, because volunteers generating the data have normal dyshaemoglobin concentrations, differences between the two calibrations are small.

SPEED OF RESPONSE
SpO_2 is averaged over 3–6 s, and updated every 0.5–1 s. With forehead probes, a sudden reduction in FiO_2 produces a response within 10–15 s, whereas with finger probes and peripheral vasoconstriction the delay can exceed 1 m.

ACCURACY
In the 90–97% saturation range, SpO_2 has a mean absolute bias of <1%, and a precision (SD of bias) of <3%. At SaO_2 <80%, there is significant imprecision and a tendency towards negative bias.[22] This is because very low SaO_2 values are unsafe in volunteers, necessitating extrapolation from SpO_2/R relationships at higher saturations.

ERROR
Causes of error are set out in Table 11.3. A falsely high SpO_2 is of greatest concern. Unlike CO-oximetry, pulse oximetry is not subject to interference from bilirubin, lipid emulsions and HbF.

Dyshaemoglobins and Pulse Oximetry
Pulse oximeters cannot distinguish COHb from HbO_2. When [COHb] is elevated this creates a tendency for

Table 11.3 Causes of error in SpO_2 readings

Factor	Comment
COHb	Measured as HbO_2 – SpO_2 may be falsely high – see text
MetHb	Absorbs both wavelengths – see text
Low saturations	Progressive inaccuracy below 80%, usually falsely low SpO_2
Prominent venous signal	Dependent limb, tricuspid regurgitation (venous pulsations) – falsely low SpO_2
Non-pulsatile flow	Cardiopulmonary bypass – poor signal
Vasoconstriction, limb ischaemia, shock states	Low pulsatile signal
Motion artefact	Tremor, voluntary movement – falsely low SpO_2
Ambient light	Strong sunlight, fluorescent light, flickering light – falsely low SpO_2
Anaemia	Effect unclear
Dyes	Methylene blue, indocyanine green – falsely low SpO_2
Black skin pigmentation	Variable precision and bias. May require separate calibration
Nail polish	Especially blue. Falsely low SpO_2
Optical shunting	Due to inadequate probe contact – falsely low SpO_2
Radio-frequency interference	Has been reported with MRI scanners – falsely high SpO_2

SpO_2 to over-estimate SaO_2 and particularly $FHbO_2$. SpO_2 can thus provide false reassurance when hypoxaemia is combined with very high [COHb] (for example after a burn with a severe inhalational injury), particularly if SpO_2 is taken as a measure of fractional rather than functional saturation.

MetHb has more complex effects, since it absorbs both wavelengths. Over-estimation of $FHbO_2$ by SpO_2 is the rule. At normal saturations, increased [MetHb] causes under-estimation of SaO_2, but over-estimation at very low oxygen tensions is possible. At high [MetHb] ($\geq 35\%$), the R value becomes unity, which translates to $SpO_2 = 85\%$.

IMPORTANCE OF PULSE OXIMETRY

Pulse oximeters generate accurate real-time information without calibration, within moments of sensor placement. Their use is mandatory in high acuity areas such as operating and recovery rooms, intensive care units, and in patient transport. On the down side, pulse oximeters are the most common source of false alarms in intensive care. They are also insensitive to changes in arterial oxygenation at higher PaO_2 values ($>70–100$ mmHg). Of note, studies on nearly 21 000 perioperative patients have not shown a clear reduction in post-operative morbidity or mortality.[23] It is difficult to demonstrate improved outcome from any monitoring technique.

MONITORING HAEMOGLOBIN-OXYGEN AFFINITY

Haemoglobin-oxygen affinity[24] is the relationship between the oxygen tension of blood and its oxygen content, described by the sigmoid shaped HbO_2 dissociation curve (Figure 11.4). The P50 is the oxygen tension at $SO_2 = 0.5$. The normal value in man is 26.7 mmHg. Factors increasing the P50 include acidaemia (the Bohr effect), hypercapnia, high levels of erythrocytic 2,3-DPG, and fever, whereas P50 is decreased by alkalaemia, hypocapnia, low 2,3-DPG levels and hypothermia.

In the intensive care unit, it is possible to calculate reasonably accurate P50 values from one single-point measurement of blood gases and SO_2. The Oxygen Status Algorithm[12] remains accurate for clinical purposes up to $SaO_2 = 0.97$. Using simple modeling it can be shown that an increased *in vivo* P50 is of theoretical benefit at all points along the oxygen cascade downstream of PAO_2 (Figure 11.4).

OXYGEN DYNAMICS

Common indices of oxygen dynamics[25] are set out in Table 11.4.

DO$_2$/VO$_2$ RELATIONSHIPS

Late in the twentieth century, it became apparent that there was an association between hyperdynamic oxygen flow patterns and survival after high-risk non-cardiac surgery.[26] This led to the hypothesis that an induced peri-operative state of supra-normal oxygen delivery/consumption is protective. Typical therapeutic goals were CI >4.5 l/min per m², $DO_2I >600$ ml/min per m², $VO_2I >170$ ml/min per m².[27]

A related concept was that of pathologic supply dependency of oxygen consumption. In normal tissues, oxygen consumption is independent of supply until the critical

Table 11.4 Oxygen dynamics: measured and derived indices

Parameter	Abbreviation	Formula	Normal range	Units
Functional haemoglobin concentration	[Hb$_{funct}$]	[HbO$_2$] + [Hb]	12.0–18.0	g/dl
Arterial oxygen tension	PaO$_2$	Measured	95 ± 5	mmHg
Mixed venous oxygen tension	PvO$_2$	Measured	40 ± 5	mmHg
Functional saturation	SO$_2$	[HbO$_2$]/([HbO$_2$] + [Hb])		
Fractional saturation	FHbO$_2$	[HbO$_2$]/([HbO$_2$] + [Hb] + [COHb] + [MetHb])		
Arterial functional saturation	SaO$_2$		0.97 ± 0.02	
Mixed venous functional saturation	SvO$_2$		0.75 ± 0.05	
Blood oxygen content	CO$_2$	1.39 × [Hb$_{funct}$] × SO$_2$ + 0.0031 × PO$_2$		ml/dl
Arterial oxygen content	CaO$_2$		16–22	ml/dl
Mixed venous oxygen content	CvO$_2$		12–17	ml/dl
Cardiac index	CI	CO/BSA	2.5–4.2	l/min per m²
Oxygen delivery index	DO$_2$I	CI × CaO$_2$ × 10	460–650	ml/min per m²
Oxygen consumption index	VO$_2$I	CI × (CaO$_2$ – CvO$_2$) × 10	96–170	ml/min per m²
Oxygen extraction ratio	O$_2$ER	(CaO$_2$ – CvO$_2$)/CaO$_2$ or VO$_2$/DO$_2$	0.23–0.32	

HbO$_2$, oxyhaemoglobin; Hb, reduced haemoglobin; COHb, carboxyhaemoglobin.

DO_2I, when oxygen delivery falls below the anaerobic threshold.[28] However, supply dependency at flows well above the normal critical DO_2I has been reported during major surgery,[29] in sepsis,[30] in ARDS,[31] and in other conditions such as cancer or liver disease (Figure 11.5). It was felt that covert dysoxia might be operating in these individuals.[32] This provided the impetus to extend the concept of supra-normal goal-directed therapy from high-risk surgery to the broader range of critical illness.[33]

However, certain studies may have created a false impression of pathological DO_2/VO_2 dependency, for the following reasons:

● The reverse Fick measurement of VO_2I promotes mathematical coupling of VO_2I and DO_2I (CI and CaO_2 are common to both calculations, Table 11.4).[34]
● Spontaneous variability in VO_2I stimulates changes in DO_2I more often than the other way round.
● Vasoactive agents themselves increase VO_2I (the calorigenic effect).[35]

A number of subsequent trials of goal-directed therapy showed no survival benefit,[36] and many practitioners have abandoned goal-directed therapy in the broader categories of critical illness such as sepsis.

However, there is still some evidence that goal-directed therapy can improve outcome in specific groups of patients.[37] Benefit has been demonstrated if the therapy is commenced before a planned insult such as high-risk surgery,[38–40] or in the early hypodynamic phase of severe sepsis and septic shock.[41] Much of this benefit may be due to the effects of aggressive fluid loading.

MEASURING DO_2I AND VO_2I

Although DO_2I determinations require accurate measurements of CI and CaO_2, a PA catheter is not essential.

Normal ranges can be quoted (Table 11.4), but oxygen demand in critical illness is so variable that isolated DO_2I measurements are difficult to interpret.[42]

The two methods of measuring VO_2I are:

● The reverse Fick method (Table 11.4)
● Indirect calorimetry

The reverse Fick method requires a PA catheter, and has large random errors, ranging from 17% over-estimation to 13% under-estimation. Changes in VO_2I cannot be detected reliably unless they exceed 20%. The error is increased by lung inflammation, when up to 20% of VO_2I can arise from the lungs alone.

In indirect calorimetry, VO_2I is determined from the volumes and oxygen concentrations of inspired and expired gas. This method has better accuracy. However, high FiO_2 settings introduce error. Newer devices retain their accuracy up to $FiO_2 = 0.8$.

MIXED VENOUS BLOOD

Mixed venous blood must be sampled by gentle aspiration of blood from the distal port of an unwedged PA catheter. This ensures complete admixture of blood from superior and inferior venae cavae and coronary sinus. Mixed venous O_2 and CO_2 tensions and content are flow-weighted averages of the venous effluents from a wide variety of tissues. The integrating process can conceal significant pockets of dysoxia.

MIXED VENOUS PO_2 (PVO_2)

Venous gas tensions reflect post-capillary and tissue gas tensions. At a PvO_2 of 26 mmHg, the average intracellular PO_2 has fallen from 11 mmHg to 0.8 mmHg.[43] A PvO_2 below this value is thus highly suggestive of tissue dysoxia. However, a normal or high PvO_2 can also

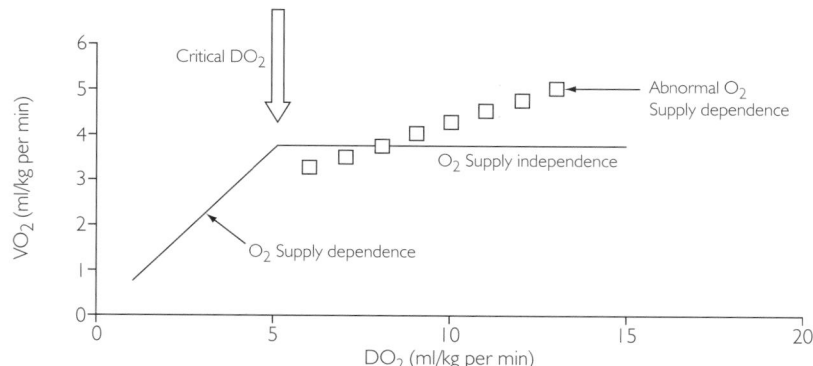

Fig. 11.5 The relationship between oxygen delivery (DO_2) and oxygen consumption (VO_2) in health (solid line) and with abnormal oxygen supply dependence (interrupted squares). VO_2 normally remains independent of DO_2 until a critical DO_2 and oxygen extraction ratio is reached. From then on there is VO_2/DO_2 dependence. Pathological VO_2/DO_2 dependence occurs at values of DO_2 above the normal critical DO_2 (see text).

co-exist with tissue dysoxia, especially in high flow states such as sepsis.

MIXED VENOUS OXYGEN SATURATION

SvO_2 is measured either intermittently by CO-oximetry on mixed venous samples or continuously by fibre-optic reflectance oximetry using a modified PA catheter.[44] SvO_2 measurements have a number of uses:

- To calculate CvO_2 (see Table 11.4). CvO_2 can then be used to determine $\dot{Q}s/\dot{Q}t$ and VQI, VO_2I by the reverse Fick method, the oxygen extraction ratio (Table 11.4), and cardiac output by the Fick method.
- As an indirect index of tissue dysoxia, acting as a surrogate for PvO_2. SvO_2 values between 0.7 and 0.8 represent a desirable balance between global oxygen supply and demand (Table 11.4). A value of 0.5 corresponds to the theoretical critical PvO_2 of 26 mmHg.[43] SvO_2 values exceeding 0.8 are generally seen in high flow states such as sepsis, hyperthyroidism and severe liver disease.

SvO_2 as a therapeutic target has shown promise,[45,46] but failed to improve survival in a large multi-centre trial.[47]

VENO-ARTERIAL PCO$_2$ GRADIENT

ΔPCO_2 (normally about 6 mmHg) is markedly increased during cardiac arrest and in experimental low output states, but has been disappointing as a global index of tissue dysoxia, lacking both sensitivity and specificity.[48] A sudden increase in the respiratory quotient (VCO_2/VO_2) is a more reliable marker of the onset of anaerobic metabolism.[49]

REGIONAL OXYGENATION INDICES

REGIONAL PCO$_2$

As tissue blood flow is lowered, the initial increase in regional PCO_2 is due to reduced clearance of aerobically generated CO_2 (flow stagnation).[50] With the onset of anaerobic metabolism, aerobic CO_2 production ceases, and continuing CO_2 generation is by proton titration of tissue and capillary HCO_3^-.

GASTRIC TONOMETRY

The gastric tonometer[51–53] is a sterile, disposable, polyvinyl chloride nasogastric tube with a silicone balloon 11.4 cm from the distal end. Gastric luminal PCO_2 is measured in a fluid equilibration medium placed in the silicone balloon.

During splanchnic hypoperfusion, intramucosal PCO_2 increases and intramucosal pH is reduced. CO_2 diffuses into the gut lumen, through the silicone membrane into the equilibration medium. Originally this medium was saline, which was aspirated after a minimum of 30 min to measure PCO_2 in a blood gas analyser. A time-based correction factor converted the measured PCO_2 to a steady state value ($PCO_{2(ss)}$), assumed to equal intramucosal PCO_2. The intramucosal pH (pHi) was then calculated from the Henderson-Hasselbalch equation, using arterial $[HCO_3^-]$ as a surrogate for mucosal $[HCO_3^-]$. Intramucosal acidosis was defined as pHi <7.3, and taken to indicate inadequate splanchnic perfusion.

Despite more than 15 years of accumulated data linking low pHi with bleeding from stress ulceration, weaning failure, post-traumatic ARDS trauma, morbidity after liver transplantation, major complications post elective cardiac surgery, and multiple organ dysfunction syndrome and death, gastric tonometry is yet to find wholesale acceptance.[54] Changing the monitoring endpoint from pHi to the mucosal–arterial CO_2 gap[55–57] has removed a fundamental flaw – the use of arterial $[HCO_3^-]$ as a surrogate for mucosal $[HCO_3^-]$. The normal CO_2 gap is about 8–10 mmHg. Automated air tonometry using infra-red absorbance reduces equilibration time and eliminates the need for correction factors.[58,59]

There are further unresolved concerns:

- Continuing uncertainty about the true dysoxic threshold.[60,61] Current recommendations are to maintain a CO_2 gap <25 mmHg.
- Regional PCO_2 is insensitive to tissue dysoxia if blood flow is preserved.[62]
- A lack of convincing evidence that titrating therapy to pHi (or to the CO_2 gap, although here data are limited) improves outcome.[63,64]

CONTINUOUS REGIONAL PCO$_2$ MEASUREMENT

Continuous measurement of regional PCO_2 using rapidly responsive fibre-optic sensors has been investigated in the small gut, oesophagus, muscle, sublingual tissue, subcutaneous tissue and the brain.[65] While preliminary data are encouraging, these techniques are yet to reach routine clinical application.

TISSUE PO$_2$

Tissue PO_2 measurements have been recorded in the brain, subcutaneous tissue, muscle and renal beds under a variety of perfusion insults mostly in animal models. There is limited clinical application at this stage.[66]

OTHER REGIONAL TECHNIQUES

Orthogonal polarization spectroscopy (OPS) allows the real-time *in vivo* imaging of microcirculatory blood flow.[67] Tissue beds visualized in intensive care have included the sublingual, rectal, oral and ileal (via stoma) microcirculations. Although presently a research investigation, OPS has potential to make the transition to a clinical monitoring tool.

Other regional techniques under investigation include optical spectroscopy,[68] laser Doppler flowmetry,[69] measurement of hepatosplanchnic blood flow,[70] and evaluation of mitochondrial redox state (cytochrome a, a_3) by near infrared spectrophotometry[71] or by ^{31}PNMR spectroscopy.

REFERENCES

1 Nathan A, Singer M. Coping with hypoxia. In: Vincent J-L (ed.) *Yearbook of Intensive Care and Emergency Medicine*. Berlin: Springer-Verlag; 1999: pp. 373–85.

2 Robin ED. Of men and mitochondria: Coping with dysoxia. *Am Rev Resp Dis* 1980; **22**: 517–31.

3 Deby-Dupont G, Deby C, Lamy M. Oxygen therapy in intensive care patients: A vital poison? In: Vincent J-L (ed.) *Yearbook of Intensive Care and Emergency Medicine*. Berlin: Springer-Verlag; 1999: pp. 417–32.

4 West JB. Ventilation-perfusion relationships. *Am Rev Resp Dis* 1977; **116**: 919–43.

5 D'Alonzo GE, Dantzker DR. Respiratory failure, mechanisms of abnormal gas exchange, and oxygen delivery. *Med Clin North Am* 1983; **67**: 557–71.

6 Knaus WA, Draper EA, Wagner DP, Zimmerman JE. APACHE II: a severity of disease classification system. *Crit Care Med* 1985; **13**: 818–29.

7 Bernard GR, Artigas A, Brigham KL, *et al.* Report of the American-European consensus conference on ARDS: definitions, mechanisms, relevant outcomes and clinical trial coordination. *Intensive Care Med* 1994; **20**: 225–32.

8 Le Gall J-R, Lemeshow S, Saulnier F. A new simplified acute physiology score (SAPS II) based on a European/North American multicentre study. *J Am Med Assoc* 1993; **270**: 2957–63.

9 Murray JF, Mathay MA, Luce JM, Flick M. An expanded definition of the adult respiratory distress syndrome. *Am Rev Resp Dis* 1988; **138**: 720–3.

10 Gowda MS, Klocke RA. Variability of indices of hypoxemia in adult respiratory distress syndrome. *Crit Care Med* 1997; **25**: 41–5.

11 Nirmalan M, Willard T, Columb MO, Nightingale P. Effect of changes in arterial-mixed venous oxygen content difference ($C(a\text{-}v)O_2$) on indices of pulmonary oxygen transfer in a model ARDS lung. *Br J Anaesth* 2001; **86**: 477–85.

12 Siggaard-Andersen O, Siggaard-Andersen M. The oxygen status algorithm: a computer program for calculating and displaying pH and blood gas data. *Scand J Clin Lab Invest* 1990; **50(Suppl 203)**: 29–45.

13 Räsänen J, Downs JB, Malec DJ *et al.* Real-time estimation of gas exchange by dual oximetry. *Intensive Care Med* 1988; **14**: 118–22.

14 Civetta JM, Nelson LD. Venous saturation monitoring and usage. In: Civetta JM, Taylor RW, Kirby RR (eds) *Critical Care*. Philadelphia: Lippincott-Raven; 1997: pp. 909–20.

15 Nirmalan M, Willard T, Khan A, Nightingale P. Changes in arterial-mixed venous oxygen content difference ($CaO_2 - CvO_2$) and the effect on shunt calculations in critically ill patients. *Br J Anaesth* 1998; **80**: 829–31.

16 Breuer H-WM, Groeben H, Breuer J, Worth H. Oxygen saturation calculation procedures: a critical analysis of six equations for the determination of oxygen saturation. *Intensive Care Med* 1989; **15**: 385–9.

17 Morgan TJ, Koch D, Morris D *et al.* Red cell 2,3-diphosphoglycerate concentrations are reduced in critical illness without net effect on *in vivo* P50. *Anaesth Intens Care* 2001; **29**: 479–83.

18 Mahoney JJ, Harvey JA, Wong RJ, Van Kessel AL. Changes in oxygen measurements when whole blood is stored in iced plastic or glass syringes. *Clin Chem* 1991; **37**: 1244–8.

19 Venkatesh B, Hendry S-P. Continuous intra-arterial blood gas monitoring. *Intensive Care Med* 1996; **22**: 818–28.

20 Jubran A. Pulse oximetry. In: Tobin MJ (ed.) *Principles and Practice of Intensive Care Monitoring*. New York: McGraw Hill; 1998: pp. 261–87.

21 Hanning CD, Alexander-Williams JM. Pulse oximetry: a practical review. *BMJ* 1995; **311**: 367–70.

22 Severinghaus JW, Naifeh KH. Accuracy of response of six pulse oximeters to profound hypoxia. *Anesthesiology* 1987; **67**: 551–8.

23 Pedersen T, Pedersen P, Moller AM. Pulse oximetry for perioperative monitoring (Cochrane Review). *Cochrane Database Syst Rev* 2001; **2**: CD002013.

24 Morgan TJ. The significance of the P50. In: Vincent J-L (ed.) *Yearbook of Intensive Care and Emergency Medicine*. Berlin Heidelberg: Springer-Verlag; 1999: pp. 433–44.

25 Chittock DR, Ronco JJ, Russell JA. Monitoring of oxygen transport and oxygen consumption. In: Tobin MJ (ed.) *Principles and Practice of Intensive Care Monitoring*. New York: McGraw Hill; 1998: pp. 317–43.

26 Shoemaker WC, Montgomery ES, Kaplan E, Elwyn DH. Physiologic patterns in surviving and nonsurviving shock patients. *Arch Surg* 1973; **106**: 630–6.

27 Shoemaker WC, Appel PL, Kram HB *et al.* Prospective trial of supranormal values of survivors as therapeutic goals in high-risk surgical patients. *Chest* 1988; **94**: 1176–86.

28 Vincent JL. The relationship between oxygen demand, oxygen uptake, and oxygen supply. *Intensive Care Med* 1990; **16**: S145–8.

29 Lugo G, Arizbe D, Dominguez G, *et al.* Relationship between oxygen consumption and delivery during anaesthesia in high-risk surgical patients. *Crit Care Med* 1993; **21**: 64–9.

30 Astiz ME, Rackow EC, Falk JL, *et al.* Oxygen delivery and consumption in patients with hyperdynamic septic shock. *Crit Care Med* 1987; **15**: 26–8.

31 Annat G, Viale JP, Percival C, *et al.* Oxygen delivery and uptake in the adult respiratory distress syndrome. *Am Rev Respir Dis* 1986; **133**: 999–1001.

32 Bihari D, Smithies M, Gimson A, Tinker J. The effects of vasodilation with prostacyclin on oxygen delivery and uptake in critically ill patients. *N Engl J Med* 1987; **317**: 397–403.

33 Dhainut FJ, Edwards JD, Grootendorst AF, *et al.* Practical aspects of oxygen transport: Conclusion and recommendations of the round table conference. *Intensive Care Med* 1990; **16**: S179–80.

34 Phang PT, Cunningham KF, Ronco JJ *et al.* Mathematical coupling explains dependence of oxygen consumption on oxygen delivery in ARDS. *Am J Respir Crit Care Med* 1994; **150**: 318–23.

35 Green CJ, Frazer RS, Underhill S *et al.* Metabolic effects of dobutamine in normal man. *Clin Sci* 1992; **82**: 77–83.

36 Gattinoni L, Brazzi L, Pelosi P. Does cardiovascular optimization reduce mortality? In: Vincent J-L (ed.) *Yearbook of Intensive Care and Emergency Medicine.* Berlin Heidelberg: Springer-Verlag; 1996: pp. 308–18.

37 Heyland DK, Cook DJ, King D *et al.* Maximizing oxygen delivery in critically ill patients: a methodologic appraisal of the evidence. *Crit Care Med* 1996; **24**: 517–24.

38 Boyd O, Grounds M, Bennett D. A randomized clinical trial of the effect of deliberate perioperative increase of oxygen delivery on mortality in high-risk surgical patients. *JAMA* 1993; **270**: 2699–707.

39 Wilson J, Woods I, Fawcett J, *et al.* Reducing the risk of major elective surgery: randomised controlled trial of preoperative optimisation of oxygen delivery. *BMJ* 1999; **318**: 1099–103.

40 Lobo SM, Salgoda PF, Castillo VGT, *et al.* Effects of maximizing oxygen delivery on morbidity and mortality in high-risk surgical patients. *Crit Care Med* 2000; **28**: 3396–404.

41 Rivers E, Nguyen B, Havstad S, *et al.* for the Early Goal-Directed Therapy Collaborative Group. Early goal-directed therapy in the treatment of severe sepsis and septic shock. *N Engl J Med* 2001; **345**: 1368–77.

42 Schlichtig R. Oxygen delivery and consumption in critical illness. In: Civetta JM, Taylor RW, Kirby RR (eds) *Critical Care.* Philadelphia: Lippincott-Raven; 1997: pp. 337–42.

43 Siggaard-Andersen O, Fogh-Andersen N, Gøthgen IH, Larsen VH. Oxygen status of arterial and mixed venous blood. *Crit Care Med* 1995; **23**: 1284–93.

44 Bowton DL, Scuderi PE. Monitoring of mixed venous oxygenation. In: Tobin MJ (ed.) *Principles and Practice of Intensive Care Monitoring.* New York: McGraw Hill; 1998: pp. 303–15.

45 Polonene P, Ruokonen E, Hippelainen M *et al.* A prospective, randomized study of goal-orientated hemodynamic therapy in cardiac surgical patients. *Anesth Analg* 2000; **90**: 1052–9.

46 Kremzar B, Spec-Marn A, Kompan L, Cerovic O. Normal values of SvO_2 as therapeutic goal in patients with multiple injuries. *Intensive Care Med* 1997; **23**: 65–70.

47 Gattinoni L, Brazzi L, Pelosi P, *et al.* for the SvO_2 Collaborative Group (1995) A trial of goal-orientated hemodynamic therapy in critically ill patients. *N Engl J Med* **333**: 1025–32.

48 Teboul JL, Michard F, Richard C. Critical analysis of venoarterial CO_2 gradient as a marker of tissue hypoxia. In: Vincent J-L (ed.) *Yearbook of Intensive Care and Emergency Medicine.* Berlin Heidelberg: Springer-Verlag; 1996: pp. 296–307.

49 Beaver WL, Wasserman K, Whipp BJ. A new method for detecting anaerobic threshold by gas exchange. *J Appl Physiol* 1986; **60**: 2020–27.

50 Vallet B, Tavernier B, Lund N. Assessment of tissue oxygenation in the critically ill. *Eur J Anaesthesiol* 2000; **17**: 221–9.

51 Kolkman JJ, Otte JA, Groeneveld ABJ. Gastrointestinal luminal PCO_2 tonometry: an update on physiology, methodology and clinical applications. *BJA* 2000; **84**: 74–86.

52 Knichwitz G, Van Aken H, Brussel T. Gastrointestinal monitoring using measurement of intramucosal PCO_2. *Anesth Analg* 1998; **87**: 134–42.

53 Lebuffe G, Robin E, Vallet B. Gastric tonometry. *Intensive Care Med* 2001; **27**: 317–19.

54 Benjamin E, Oropello JM. Does gastric tonometry work? No. *Crit Care Clin* 1996; **12**: 587–601.

55 Vincent J-L, Creteur J. Gastric mucosal pH is definitely obsolete – please tell us more about gastric mucosal PCO_2. *Crit Care Med* 1998; **26**: 1479–81.

56 Schlichtig R, Mehta N, Gayoski TJP. Tissue-arterial PCO_2 difference is a better marker of ischemia than intramural pH (pHi) or arterial pH-pHi difference. *J Crit Care* 1996; **11**: 51–6.

57 Heino A, Hartikainen J, Merasto ME, *et al.* Systemic and regional PCO_2 gradients as markers of intestinal ischemia. *Intensive Care Med* 1998; **24**: 599–604.

58 Bennet-Guerrero E, Panah MH, Bodian CA, *et al.* Automated detection of gastric luminal partial pressure of carbon dioxide during cardiovascular surgery using the Tonocap. *Anesthesiology* 2000; **92**: 38–45.

59 Venkatesh B, Morgan TJ. Blood in the gastrointestinal tract delays and blunts the PCO_2 response to transient mucosal ischemia. *Intensive Care Med* 2000; **26**: 1108–15.

60 Rozenfeld RA, Dishart MK, Tønnessen TI, Schlichtig R. Methods for detecting local intestinal ischemic anaerobic metabolic acidosis by PCO_2. *J Appl Physiol* 1996; **81**: 1834–42.

61 Miller PR, Kincaid EH, Meredith JW, Chang MC. Threshold values of intramucosal pH and mucosal-arterial CO_2 gap during shock resuscitation. *J Trauma* 1998; **45**: 868–72.

62. Vallet B, Durinck L, Chagnon JL, Neviere R. Effects of hypoxic hypoxia on veno and gut mucosal arterial PCO_2 difference in pigs. *Anesthesiology* 1996; **85**: A607.

63 Pargger H, Hampl KF, Christen P *et al.* Gastric intramucosal pH-guided therapy in patients after elective repair of infrarenal abdominal aneurysms: is it beneficial? *Intensive Care Med* 1998; **24**: 769–76.

64 Gomersall CD, Joynt GM, Freebairn RC, *et al.* Resuscitation of critically ill patients based on the results of gastric tonometry: a prospective, randomized, controlled trial. *Crit Care Med* 2000; **28**: 607–14.

65 Venkatesh B, Morgan TJ. Measuring tissue gas tensions in critical illness. In: Vincent J-L (ed.) *Yearbook of Intensive Care and Emergency Medicine*. Berlin Heidelberg: Springer-Verlag; 2001: pp. 251–68.

66 Greif R, Akca O, Horn EP *et al*. Supplemental perioperative oxygen to reduce the incidence of surgical-wound infection. Outcomes Research Group. *N Engl J Med* 2000; **342**: 161–7.

67 Mathura KR, Alic L, Ince C. Initial clinical experience with OPS imaging for observation of the human microcirculation. In: Vincent J-L (ed.) *Yearbook of Intensive Care and Emergency Medicine*. Berlin Heidelberg: Springer-Verlag; 2001: pp. 233–44.

68 Ince C, Sinaasappel M. Microcirculatory oxygenation and shunting in sepsis and shock. *Crit Care Med* 1999; **27**: 1369–77.

69 Neviere R, Chagnon JL, Vallet B, *et al*. Dobutamine improves gastrointestinal mucosal blood flow in a porcine model of endotoxic shock. *Crit Care Med* 1997; **25**: 1266–7.

70 Uusaro A, Ruokonen E, Takala J. Estimation of splanchnic blood flow by the Fick principle in man and problems in the use of indocyanine green. *Cardiovasc Res* 1995; **30**: 106–12.

71 Kruse JA. Searching for the perfect indicator of dysoxia. *Crit Care Med* 1999; **27**: 469–71.

12

Lactic acidosis

D J Cooper

Lactic acidosis is defined by convention as the combination of an increased blood lactate concentration (>5 mmol/l), and acidaemia (arterial blood pH of <7.35).[1,2] Hyperlactaemia however occurs whenever the blood lactate concentration is above the normal range (>2 mmol/l). Lactic acidosis may be masked by coincident metabolic or respiratory alkalosis. Critically ill patients with lactic acidosis usually have a high mortality and blood lactate concentrations >8 mmol/l predict fatality.[3] A recent prospective study reported 83% mortality in patients with blood lactate concentrations of >10 mmol/l.[2] In each individual patient however, prognosis is completely dependent on the underlying condition, with lactic acidosis being an indicator of shock severity, and of response to therapy. It is important to remember that in healthy athletes, severe lactic acidosis during exercise is a normal, self-limited, observation.

PATHOPHYSIOLOGY

There is a continuous cycle of lactate production and metabolism. Lactate is produced at about 0.8 mmol/kg per h, while simultaneous metabolism in liver, kidneys skeletal muscle, brain and red blood cells ensures that blood lactate concentrations are normally low (<1 mmol/l). Lactic acidosis occurs when lactate production exceeds metabolic capacity, or when metabolic capacity is decreased by organ dysfunction. The liver has a key role in lactate homeostasis and many patients who develop lactic acidosis have decreased metabolic capacity due to liver disease.[4]

Formation and metabolism of lactate in cells is catalysed by lactate dehydrogenase:

$$\text{Pyruvate} + \text{NADH} + \text{H}^+ \leftarrow \text{LDH} \rightarrow \text{Lactate} + \text{NAD}^+$$

Lactate formation is in part dependent upon pyruvate concentrations and pyruvate is sourced from glycolysis (85%) and proteolysis (15%). Glucose is derived from absorption, glycogen, and gluconeogenesis. The rate of glycolysis is controlled by three unidirectional enzymes

and the activity of one of these enzymes is increased by increasing intracellular pH. Acidosis, therefore, decreases (and alkalosis increases) glycolysis and lactate and pyruvate production. In oxygen excess, pyruvate is oxidized and lactate does not accumulate. Anaerobic metabolism, however, causes lactate accumulation and an increased lactate/pyruvate ratio. However, this ratio is a poor indicator of mitochondrial concentrations, and is not of clinical use.

In critically ill patients, lactic acidosis is often due to shock. In cardiogenic and hypovolaemic shock, hypoperfusion and tissue hypoxia increase lactic acid production while decreased hepatic perfusion decreases lactic acid metabolism. In septic shock, lactic acidosis is multi-factorial. Contributors include global hypoperfusion, microvascular disruption causing regional hypoperfusion and impaired cellular oxygen utilisation by mitochondria.

CLASSIFICATION (TYPES A AND B)

The Cohen and Woods classification of lactic acidosis[5] defines two subgroups depending on the presence (Type A) or absence (Type B) of tissue hypoxia (Table 12.1). Type A lactic acidosis, due to tissue hypoxia, is common in critically ill patients. Type B (no tissue hypoxia) is much less common. Some patients with type B lactic acidosis have increased lactate generation (some malignancies and toxins impair oxygen utilization by cells, despite adequate oxygen delivery), and others patients have decreased lactate clearance (liver disease). Patients with liver disease have greater hyperlactemia during states of increased lactate production than those with normal liver function.[4]

COMBINED ABNORMALITIES (TYPES A AND B)

In clinical practice, separation of types A and B lactic acidosis is usually not helpful, because many critically ill patients have combined abnormalities. Increased lactate

Table 12.1 Classification of lactic acidosis

	Cause
Type A	Shock
	Very severe hypoxaemia
	Very severe anaemia
	Regional hypoperfusion
	Carbon monoxide poisoning
Type B1 (underlying disease)	Sepsis
	Liver failure
	Thiamine deficiency
	Malignancy
	Phaechromocytoma
	Diabetes
Type B2 (drug or toxin)	Epinephrine
	Salbutamol
	Ethanol
	Methanol
	Paracetamol
	Nitroprusside
	Salicylates
	Ethylene (and propylene) glycol
	Biguanides
	Fructose
	Sorbitol
	Xylitol
	Cyanide
	Isoniazid
Type B3 (rare inborn errors of metabolism)	Glucose-6 phosphatase deficiency
	Fructose-1,6 diphosphatase deficiency
	Pyruvate carboxylase deficiency
	Deficiency of enzymes of oxidative phosphorylation

formation from tissue hypoxia and decreased lactate clearance often occur together. In patients with cancer, anaerobic glycolysis may be increased, while hepatic lactate metabolism is impaired by tumour replacement. Diabetic patients may present with shock, but in non-insulin dependent diabetes there may also be a defect in pyruvate oxidation, and in diabetic ketoacidosis ketones may also inhibit hepatic lactate uptake. Thiamine and biotin are essential cofactors for pyruvate dehydrogenase activity and for conversion of pyruvate to oxaloacetate. Malnutrition and inadequate parenteral nutrition have therefore been associated with lactic acidosis due to deficiencies of these cofactors. In these cases, pyruvate accumulation increases lactate production. In alcoholics, ethanol oxidation increases the conversion of pyruvate to lactate and inhibits other pathways of pyruvate metabolism. Phenformin therapy is associated with lactic acidosis for several reasons: phenformin increases glycolysis in peripheral tissues, inhibits pyruvate oxidation, increases splanchnic lactate production, and decreases hepatic lactate clearance. Phenformin was therefore used to induce lactic acidosis in older animal models until it was

recognized that phenformin is also a potent cardiac depressant. These studies reporting the effects of lactic acidosis on cardiac function were flawed. Both endogenous and infused catecholamines may cause hepatic vasoconstriction and impair hepatic lactate clearance, and epinephrine also increases hepatic glycogenolysis to lactate.[6] Importantly, acidosis also stimulates adrenal catecholamine release – which may mask other cardiac effects of acidosis.

SEPSIS

Both impaired regional microvascular blood flow and autoregulation, and mitochondrial dysfunction have been implicated in the pathogenesis of lactic acidosis during sepsis. Excess catecholamines may impair hepatic lactate extraction (by reducing regional hepatic blood flow) and increase lactate production (increased glycogenolysis). At the same time, lactate clearance is decreased because pyruvate dehydrogenase activity is reduced in both skeletal muscle and liver. Mitochondrial pyruvate oxidation is impaired.

Tissue hypoxia may not be a major mechanism for regional lactate production during sepsis, with hyperlactaemia thought to be a marker of severity of the septic hypermetabolic state.[7] Net lactate production from the hepatosplanchnic bed is uncommon in septic patients,[8] and, NMR spectroscopy suggests that hyperlactaemia may occur without tissue hypoxia.[9]

LUNG INJURY

The lung is a primary source of lactate production in patients with acute lung injury, with pulmonary release of lactate being directly related to the severity of lung injury[10,11] supporting the view that the primary contributors are the tissues with the most inflammation or injury. Recent laboratory data suggests that both metabolic and respiratory acidosis protect the lung against injury. Correction of acidosis compounded the injury.[12]

ASTHMA

Lactic acidosis often occurs in patients with acute severe asthma.[13] Fatiguing respiratory muscles have been implicated, but severe lactic acidosis also occurs in sedated, paralysed mechanically ventilated patients who have no endogenous respiratory muscle activity.[14] β-agonists including salbutamol and epinephrine cause lactic acidosis by increasing gluconeogenesis, glycogenolysis, lipolysis and cyclic-AMP activity. Clinical experience suggests that high dose β-agonists are the primary cause of lactic acidosis in patients with asthma because decreasing intravenous salbutamol infusions to less than 10 μg/min usually is associated with resolution of the acidosis. In asthma, lactic acidosis does not have specific prognostic implications.

CARDIAC SURGICAL PATIENTS

The use of epinephrine after cardiopulmonary bypass precipitates lactic acidosis in some patients.[15] This phenomenon is probably β-agonist mediated, is associated with increased whole body blood flow, and resolves after substitution of norepinephrine. Similar to asthma, lactic acidosis in this setting does not have the adverse implications of lactic acidosis associated with shock.

CLINICAL PRESENTATION

Patients present with clinical signs appropriate to their primary disorder. Their lactic acidosis is usually only evident after laboratory testing. In critically ill patients with shock, the severity of lactic acidosis can be a valuable monitor of the efficacy of resuscitation. Repeated measures of arterial blood gases and blood lactate concentrations are required. A single blood gas or lactate measurement, especially in patients with decreased lactate clearance, may be misleading. In hypovolaemic shock, resolving lactic acidosis along with the clinical signs of improving perfusion, is one of several indicators of successful resuscitation. Conversely, failure of lactic acidosis to resolve in hypovolaemic shock suggests inadequate resuscitation or another undetected or unresolved clinical problem. In patients with severe lactic acidosis[2] a blood lactate concentration of 5 mmol/l indicated a mortality approaching 80%, and survival was best in patients whose hyperlactaemia resolved. In septic shock there are many contributors to lactic acidosis, so the time course of acidosis resolution in this setting is a less reliable indicator of the adequacy of shock resuscitation.

Lactic acidosis may also occur in critically ill patients in the absence of shock. Examples include hypermetabolic states where accelerated aerobic glycolysis may contribute (trauma, burns, sepsis), conditions with increased muscle activity (seizures) and during exogenous lactate administration (lactate buffered haemofiltration fluid). In many of these patients (for example, patients with seizures) very high blood lactate concentrations have no prognostic implications because the acidosis is rapidly cleared.

CARDIAC DYSFUNCTION: ASSOCIATION, CAUSE OR RESULT OF LACTIC ACIDOSIS

Cardiac dysfunction is common in shocked patients with lactic acidosis, and it has often been assumed that thera-

pies for lactic acidosis would improve cardiac function. However, cardiac dysfunction in these patients is very likely due to other factors such as cytokines (TNF-α, interleukins), with lactic acidosis a consequence or association, rather than a cause of cardiac dysfunction.

In lactic acidosis, some clinicians advocate rapid normalization of arterial pH based on two assumptions: (i) that acidosis causes cardiac dysfunction, and (ii) that patients are better with 'normal' laboratory values.[16,17] Both of these assumptions are incorrect in most critically ill patients. While early research in isolated muscle, isolated heart preparations, animal models and clinical case reports supported the view that acidosis decreased cardiac function and decreased the haemodynamic response to catecholamines, more recent large animal studies in which preload, afterload and heart rate were carefully controlled, found only marginal effects of lactic acidosis on contractility.[1,18] Also, laboratory reports of deceased cardiac function during acidosis, studied an arterial pH much lower (pH 6.6–6.9) than that usually observed in critically ill patients.[19] Further, increasing experience with permissive hypercapnia in ARDS and asthma has supported the view that patients with respiratory acidosis have less complications and better outcomes when normal values are not targeted. The major haemodynamic effect of acute hypercapnic acidosis in ARDS and asthma was increased cardiac output and vasodilation, not cardiac depression.[20,21] Therefore, targeting normal values in lactic acidosis may not be beneficial, and may be harmful.

MANAGEMENT

GENERAL

Lactic acidosis is often an indicator of major patient pathology. The main focus is to rapidly identify and treat the cause. A clinical examination and search for occult sepsis, inadequate resuscitation, or cardiovascular failure is urgently required. After diagnosis and initial management, lactic acidosis may then be used as an ongoing monitor of disease progression or resolution. pH correction with sodium bicarbonate has the disadvantage of removing this useful clinical monitor.

TREAT THE PRIMARY DISORDER

Specific therapies and supports must be directed at each underlying cause. In hypovolaemic and cardiogenic shock, restoration of an adequate global oxygen delivery is required. Vasoconstrictors may worsen tissue perfusion and should follow adequate intra-vascular volume and appropriate cardiac supports. In septic shock, antibiotics appropriate to cover all likely sources of infection are a priority and in patients with possible ischaemic gut, surgery may be required both for diagnosis and for therapy. Post surgical gastrointestinal leaks may sometimes be difficult to diagnose, may not be detectable on CT and require early laparotomy. In status epilepsy, lactic acidosis is a result of muscle activity and rapid use of effective anticonvulsants is indicated. In diabetic keto-acidosis, insulin, appropriate fluid, and treatment of precipitants enables resolution of all metabolic abnormalities including associated lactic acidosis. Thiamine deficiency has been recently highlighted during a nationwide American shortage of multivitamins for patients receiving TPN.[22] High dose intravenous thiamine corrects both the vasodilated shock and associated lactic acidosis. In acute severe asthma, lactic acidosis is commonly a result of high dose β-agonist therapy, and dose reduction usually resolves the problem. In vasodilated patients after cardiopulmonary bypass, lactic acidosis is also related to β-agonist therapy[15] and resolves after substitution of intravenous adrenaline with noradrenaline. In these cases, lactic acidosis is not related to decreased tissue perfusion and adverse effects upon prognosis have not been noted.

HYPERVENTILATION

Hyperventilation is a normal compensatory response to metabolic acidosis in conscious patients. Therefore, in mechanically ventilated patients with lactic acidosis, most clinicians will use some hyperventilation to partially correct acidaemia. In patients with pulmonary pathology, hyperventilation may, however, be difficult or inappropriate, and in some patients hyperventilation increases intrathoracic pressure, decreases venous return, decreases cardiac output and exacerbates the cause of lactic acidosis.

BICARBONATE

Bicarbonate therapy for lactic acidosis continues to be controversial.[1,16,23] A correction of acidosis with bicarbonate might reverse depressed cardiac performance, however, there is no evidence that lactic acidosis depresses cardiac function in critically ill patients, and recent laboratory studies also report minimal depression in large animals.[18,24] Importantly, two randomized studies of bicarbonate therapy in critically ill patients with lactic acidosis and shock found no improvement in cardiac function or any other beneficial effects of pH correction.[19,25] One reason for these findings is that sodium bicarbonate has adverse effects, which outweigh potential benefits. The patient study[19] reported side-effects of acute hypercapnia and ionized hypocalcaemia. Hypercapnia may increase intracellular acidosis (CO_2 crosses cell membranes rapidly), and hypocalcaemia decreases myocardial contractility.[26] Other side-effects of bicarbonate occur because bicarbonate is a

hypertonic solution and include acute intravascular volume overload and cardiac depression. In addition, bicarbonate increases lactate production by increasing the activity of the rate limiting enzyme phosphofructokinase, shifts the haemoglobin-oxygen dissociation curve, increases oxygen affinity of haemoglobin and thereby decreases oxygen delivery to tissues. Adverse effects of bicarbonate can be reduced by using slow infusions in preference to rapid boluses, and by correcting side-effects, by increasing minute volume in ventilated patients and by correcting ionized hypocalcaemia.

Importantly however, despite decades of debate, bicarbonate has never been shown to be beneficial in any clinical trial and its use in patients with lactic acidosis is now not recommended, regardless of the degree of acidaemia.[1]

There are two subgroups of patients with lactic acidosis where bicarbonate may be considered. Patients with pulmonary hypertension and right heart failure (e.g. lung transplant recipients) may have pulmonary vasoconstriction which is exacerbated by acidosis. In these patients, although there are other useful therapies including inhaled nitric oxide, partial pH correction may improve right heart function. Second, patients with significant ischaemic heart disease and lactic acidosis may be at increased risk of major arrhythmias, because severe acidosis lowers the myocardial threshold. In both of these subgroups, bicarbonate infusions to keep the arterial pH above 7.10, could currently be justified.

ALTERNATIVE THERAPIES

CARBICARB

Carbicarb is an equimolar combination of sodium carbonate and sodium bicarbonate, which generates less carbon dioxide than bicarbonate. It may have less adverse effects. Although carbicarb more consistently increases intracellular pH, it has inconsistent effects on haemodynamics, and like bicarbonate, does not address the underlying cause of lactic acidosis. It is not in clinical usage.

DICHLOROACETATE

DCA stimulates the activity of the phosphate dehydrogenase complex, the rate-limiting enzyme that regulates entry of pyruvate into the tricarboxylic acid cycle. DCA does increase arterial pH and decrease lactate concentrations.[27] Nevertheless, a large multi-centre randomized clinical trial in patients with lactic acidosis found no haemodynamic benefit or improvement in patient outcome.[28] This study is really the best evidence currently available to support the view that correction of lactic acidosis in critically ill patients without improving the underlying primary disorder has no overall effect on patient outcome. DCA is not available commercially.

TRIS/THAM

Tris-hydroxymethyl aminomethane is a commercially available weak alkali, which is rarely used as a clinical therapy because of concerns about side-effects. These include hyperkalaemia, hypoglycaemia, extravasation-related necrosis, and neonatal hepatic necrosis.

DIALYSIS/HAEMOFILTRATION

Peritoneal dialysis has been reported to be effective at removing lactate, but bicarbonate buffered haemofiltration is completely ineffective, contributing to less than 3% of lactate clearance.[29,30] Indeed haemofiltration was so ineffective that it has been noted that lactate concentrations remain a useful clinical marker of disease progression in patients on bicarbonate buffered haemofiltration.[30]

REFERENCES

1 Forsythe SM, Schmidt, GA. Sodium bicarbonate for the treatment of lactic acidosis. *Chest* 2000; **117**: 260–7.
2 Stacpoole P, Wright E, Baumgauter T, *et al*. Natural history and course of acquired lactic acidosis in adults. *Am J Med* 1994; **97**: 47–54.
3 Broder G, Weil M. Excess lactate: an index of reversibility of shock in human patients. *Science* 1964; **143**: 1457–9.
4 Berry MN. The liver and lactic acidosis. *Proc Royal Soc Med* 1967; **60**: 1260–2.
5 Cohen RD, Woods HF. Lactic acidosis revisited. *Diabetes* 1983; **32**: 181–91.
6 Stacpoole P. Lactic acidosis. *Endo Metab Clin Nth Am* 1993; **22**: 221–45.
7 Mizock BA. The hepatosplanchnic area and hyperlactemia: a tale of two lactates. *Crit Care Med* 2001; **29**: 447–9.
8 De Backer D, Creteur J, Silva E, Vincent JL. The hepatosplanchnic area is not a common source of lactate in patients with severe sepsis. *Crit Care Med* 2001; **29**: 256–61.
9 Hotchkiss R, Karl I. Revaluation of the role of cellular hypoxia and bioenergetic failure in sepsis. *JAMA* 1992; **267**: 1503–10.
10 Kellum JA, Kramer DJ, Lee K, *et al*. Release of lactate by the lung in acute lung injury. *Chest* 1997; **111**: 1301–5.
11 De Backer D, Creteur J, Zhang H, *et al*. Lactate production by the lungs in acute lung injury. *Am J Respir Crit Care Med* 1997; **156**: 1099–104.
12 Laffey JG, Engelberts D, Kavanagh BP. Buffering hypercapnic acidosis worsens acute lung injury. *Am J Respir Crit Care Med* 2000; **161**: 141–6.
13 Mountain RD, Heffner JE, Brackett NC, *et al*. Acid base disturbances in acute asthma. *Chest* 1990; **98**: 651–5.
14 Manthous CA. Lactic acidosis in status asthmaticus. *Chest* 2001; **119**: 1599–1602.
15 Totaro RJ, Raper RF. Epinephrine-induced lactic acidosis following cardiopulmonary bypass. *Crit Care Med* 1997; **25**: 1693–9.
16 Narins R, Cohen J. Bicarbonate therapy for organic acidosis: the case for its continued use. *Ann Intern Med* 1987; **106**: 615–18.
17 Cuhaci B, Lee J, Ahmed Z. Sodium bicarbonate controversy in lactic acidosis. *Chest* 2000; **118**: 882–4.
18 Cooper DJ, Herbertson M, Werner H, Walley K. Bicarbonate does not increase left ventricular contractility during L-Lactic acidemia in pigs. *Am Rev Resp Dis* 1993; **148**: 317–22.
19 Cooper DJ, Walley K, Wiggs B, Russell J. Bicarbonate does not improve hemodynamics in critically ill patients who have lactic acidosis: a prospective controlled clinical study. *Ann Intern Med* 1990; **112**: 492–8.
20 Thorens J-B, Jolliet P, Ritz M, *et al*. Effects of permissive hypercapnia on hemodynamics, gas exchange and oxygen transport and consumption during mechanical ventilation for the acute respiratory distress syndrome. *Intensive Care Med* 1996; **22**: 182–91.
21 Cooper DJ, Cailes JB, Scheinkestel CD, Tuxen DV. Does bicarbonate improve cardiac or respiratory function during respiratory acidosis and acute severe asthma. *Am Rev Respir Dis* 1993; **147**: A614.
22 Centers for Disease Control and Prevention. Lactic acidosis traced to thiamine deficiency related to nation-wide shortage of multivitamins for total parenteral nutrition – United States. *J Am Med Assoc* 1997; **278**: 109–10.
23 Stacpoole P. Lactic acidosis: the case against bicarbonate therapy. *Ann Intern Med* 1986; **105**: 276–9.
24 Walley K, Cooper DJ, Baile E, Russell J. Bicarbonate does not improve left ventricular contractility during resuscitation from hypovolemic shock in pigs. *J Crit Care* 1992; **7**: 14–21.
25 Mathieu D, Neviere R, Billard V, *et al*. Effects of bicarbonate therapy on hemodynamics and tissue oxygenation in patients with lactic acidosis: a prospective, controlled clinical study. *Crit Care Med* 1991; **19**: 1352–6.
26 Lang RM, Fellner SK, Neumann A, *et al*. Left ventricular contractility varies directly with blood ionized calcium. *Ann Intern Med* 1988; **108**: 524–9.
27 Stacpoole P, Harman E, Curry S, *et al*. Treatment of lactic acidosis with dichloroacetate. *N Engl J Med* 1983; **309**: 390–6.
28 Stacpoole PW, Wright EC, Baumgauter TG, *et al*. A controlled clinical trial of dichloroacetate for treatment of lactic acidosis in adults. *N Engl J Med* 1992; **327**: 1564–9.
29 Levraut J, Ciebiera J-P, Jambou P, *et al*. Effect of continuous hemofiltration with dialysis on lactate clearance in critically ill patients. *Crit Care Med* 1997; **25**: 58–62.
30 Benjamin E. Continuous venovenous hemofiltration with dialysis and lactate clearance in critically ill patients. *Crit Care Med* 1997; **25**: 4–5b.

13

Multiple organ dysfunction

J McKinlay and D Bihari

Some 50 years ago (1950s), multiple organ failure did not exist as a clinical entity. Patients could not be kept alive long enough for sequential disturbances in the function of distal organs to occur. In the 1960s, acute respiratory failure with bilateral infiltrates on chest radiograph, now termed 'Acute Respiratory Distress Syndrome' (ARDS), was described following a variety of non-pulmonary insults. Finally, in 1973, the first descriptions of multiple organ failure appeared in the surgical literature – describing the course of three patients who subsequently died following surgery for ruptured aortic aneurysm.[1]

The American College of Chest Physicians/Society of Critical Care Medicine (ACCP/SCCM) consensus conference in 1992[2] proposed, 'the detection of altered organ function in the acutely ill patient constitutes a syndrome that should be termed *multiple organ dysfunction syndrome*. The terminology *dysfunction* identifies this process as a phenomenon in which organ function is not capable of maintaining homeostasis.' Since organ failure is not an 'all-or-none' phenomenon, because 'dysfunction' usually precedes and progresses to gross organ failure, the old term 'multiple organ failure' was deemed unsatisfactory. Critical illness is often associated with a downward spiral through a systemic inflammatory response (SIRS) towards frank organ failure and death.[3] The mortality from multiple organ dysfunction syndrome (MODS) is related to the numbers and duration of organ systems in failure,[4] and remains the leading cause of death in non-coronary intensive care units.[5]

The consensus committee's definition of MODS facilitates 'early detection of the disease' and thus 'allows early therapeutic intervention.' However, it should be remembered, it is only a descriptive or 'phenotypic' definition and does not provide any insight into aetiology or pathogenesis of MODS.[6]

AETIOLOGY

A wide range of physiological and pathological insults may lead to MODS (see Table 13.1).

PATHOGENESIS

RANGE OF CLINICAL RESPONSES

There are four phenotypic responses following a severe insult known to cause MODS.[7]

1 Patients showing little evidence of a systemic reaction. Their clinical course may be prolonged but overt organ dysfunction does not develop.
2 Patients who develop a mild form of SIRS and show some degree of organ dysfunction early in their illness. Organ dysfunction resolves within a few days.
3 Patients who experience a massive inflammatory response rapidly after the insult and die within a few days with refractory shock and MODS.

Table 13.1 Causes of MODS

Infectious causes	Trauma	Non-infectious inflammation	
Bacteraemia	Multiple trauma	Pancreatitis	Cancer
Viraemia	Post surgery	Vasculitides	Cytokine infusions
Fungaemia	Visceral ischaemia	HIV	Drug reactions
Rickettsial diseases	Status epilepticus	Eclampsia	Reperfusion syndromes
Mycobacteria	Head injury	Hepatic failure	Transfusion reactions
Protozoan infections	Abdominal compartment syndrome	Cardiopulmonary bypass	Aspiration syndromes
Solid organ infections		Massive transfusion	

4 Patients who display a less severe initial course but nevertheless deteriorate with evidence of one or more organ involvement. Many of these die.

Patients in the first two groups mount an inflammatory response of appropriate magnitude to the insult to which they are exposed, and in addition, this response is down-regulated appropriately leading to a net beneficial response. Meanwhile, in patients displaying either of the last two phenotypic responses, something goes wrong resulting in an inappropriate and uncontrolled response that becomes auto-destructive leading to MODS and death.

OLD THEORY OF MODS

A massive inflammatory reaction underlies both SIRS and MODS, and the similarity of inflammatory response, despite the variety of aetiologies, is suggestive of a common pathophysiology. However, earlier theories accounting for the development of MODS were based upon experiments in which endotoxin or proinflammatory mediators were injected into human volunteers or experimental animals together with studies that assayed serum levels of proinflammatory mediators in patients with SIRS or MODS. This led to a relatively simplistic paradigm for sepsis (see Figure 13.1).[8]

This model of SIRS/MODS was too simplistic and indeed too linear. Studies intermittently assaying systemic cytokine levels fail to reflect what is occurring within the microvasculature. Studies in patients using 'magic-bullets' to block cytokines and endotoxin have failed to

show any benefits in sepsis induced MODS (*vide infra*). Finally, new evidence has revealed a compensatory anti-inflammatory cascade, which is also involved in the pathogenesis of MODS.[9]

CURRENT THEORY OF MODS

Initially, following local injury or infection, proinflammatory mediators are released locally to combat foreign antigens and promote wound healing. Anti-inflammatory mediators are released concurrently to downregulate this process. Homeostasis is maintained and the patient recovers. If the pathophysiological insult is large, and local defence mechanisms are unable to contain it, then inflammatory mediators appear within the systemic circulation and recruit additional leukocytes to the site of inflammation. A whole body stress response ensues. Once again, systemic release of anti-inflammatory mediators serves to ameliorate the proinflammatory cascades and homeostasis is restored.

If, however, the systemic proinflammatory response is massive, or if the compensatory anti-inflammatory response is inadequate and so fails to achieve appropriate down-regulation, there follows a proinflammatory imbalance in the inflammatory response. At this stage patients have signs of SIRS, as well as evidence of incipient organ dysfunction. This clinical (phenotypic) response may also be seen if the anti-inflammatory response predominates, resulting in anergy and immunosuppression. Survival subsequently depends upon homeostasis being restored. If homeostasis remains disturbed then a final stage of the pathogenic process, 'immunological dissonance', occurs. At this stage, the balance between pro- and anti-inflammatory processes has been lost. Some patients experience massive inflammation, others immunosuppression and secondary infections. Clinically, patients will have signs of MODS and survival again depends upon a restoration of immunological/inflammatory homeostasis (Figure 13.2).[10]

SIGNAL TRANSDUCTION

In a minority of Gram-positive infections, 'super antigens' such as toxic shock syndrome toxin-1 or streptococcal pyrogenic exotoxin induce T cell proliferation without regard to the antigenic specificity of the T cell.[11] Up to 20% of all T cells are potentially stimulated in this way[12] with a consequent enormous release of cytokines resulting in staphylococcal or streptococcal toxic shock syndrome.

However, generally bacterial cell wall products bind macrophage CD14 receptors, and activate cellular expression of cytokines. With Gram-negative infections, the lipopolysaccharide (LPS) component of endotoxin binds lipopolysaccharide-binding protein (LBP) before interaction with CD14. Similarly, Gram-

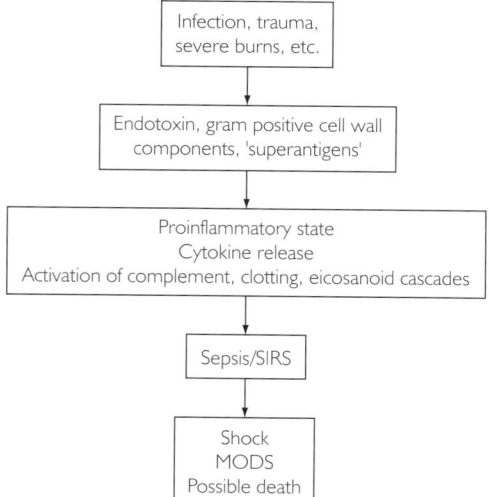

Fig. 13.1   Old 'linear' sepsis paradigm. (From Bone *et al*.,[8] with permission.)

positive cell wall components, for example peptidogly-cans, teichoic and lipoteichoic acids are presented to the CD14 receptor which then activates cell signaling.[13] In either case, the activated CD14/bacterial-product complex interacts with a member of the Toll-like receptor family (TLR) to signal gene expression of cytokines such as tumour necrosis factor α (TNF-α), and interleukin-1 (IL-1).[14] Human TLR-4 is responsible for signal mediation with LPS whilst TLR-2 mediates Gram-positive recognition.

Toll-like receptors are evolutionarily conserved receptors, which recognize whole subsets of pathogens, and represent a phylogenetically ancient defence mechanism – the innate immune system.[15] Whereas acquired immunity requires previous encounters with specific pathogens and the generation of a large repertoire of antigen receptors (antibodies), the innate immune system relies upon a number of 'pattern recognition receptors.' This furnishes multicellular organisms with a generalized defence mechanism against a broad range of organisms. Indeed,

the ligand for TLR-9 is as non-specific as bacterial DNA and TLR-2 is capable of recognizing product from *Mycobacteria*, *Treponema pallidum*, *Borrelia* species, and zymosan particle from yeast in addition to Gram-positive cell products. Toll-receptors then mediate cell signalling through the same intracellular pathways as cytokines themselves, namely the activation of the transcription factor NF-$\kappa\beta$ (Figure 13.3).

Lipopolysaccharide (LPS) released from bacterial membranes binds CD14 through an intermediary lipopolysaccharide binding protein (LBP). CD14 is anchored to the cell membrane by a glycosylphosphatidylinositol anchor. Signal transduction between the LPS-LBP/CD14 complex and intracellular pathways is via a Toll-receptor TLR-4. Nuclear factor kappa B (NF-$\kappa\beta$) is a primary transcription factor pre-existent in the cellular cytoplasm complexed with the inhibitory subunit IκBα. Activation of TLR-4 mediates proteolysis of IκBα. Free NF-$\kappa\beta$ translocates into the nucleus and binds to the promoter region of its target gene.

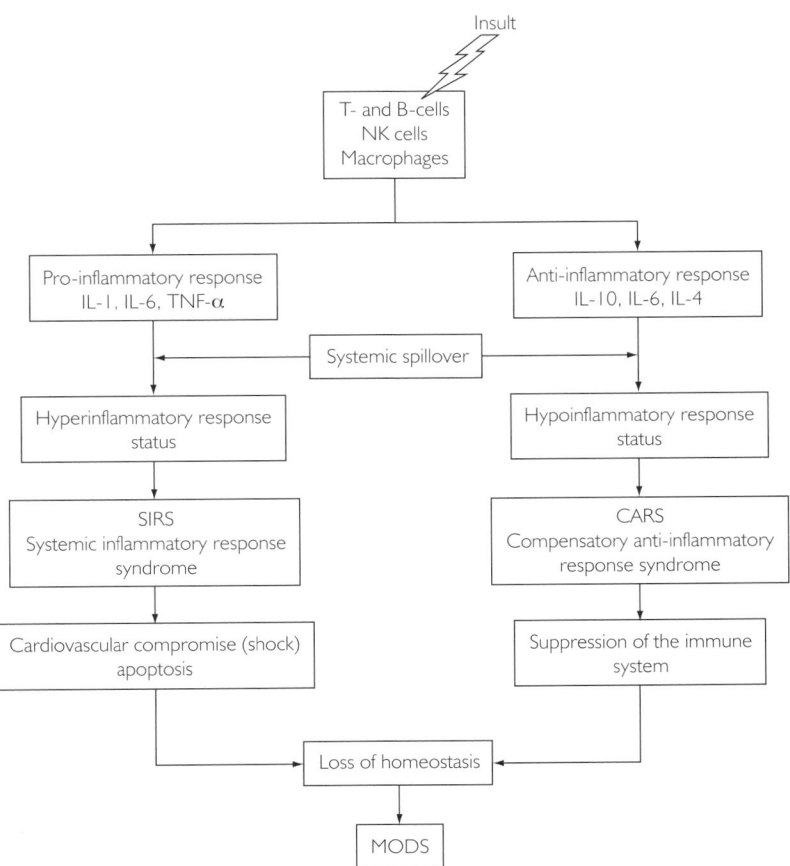

Fig. 13.2 New model of sepsis. NK cells are natural killer cells. (From Oberholzer,[10] with permission.)

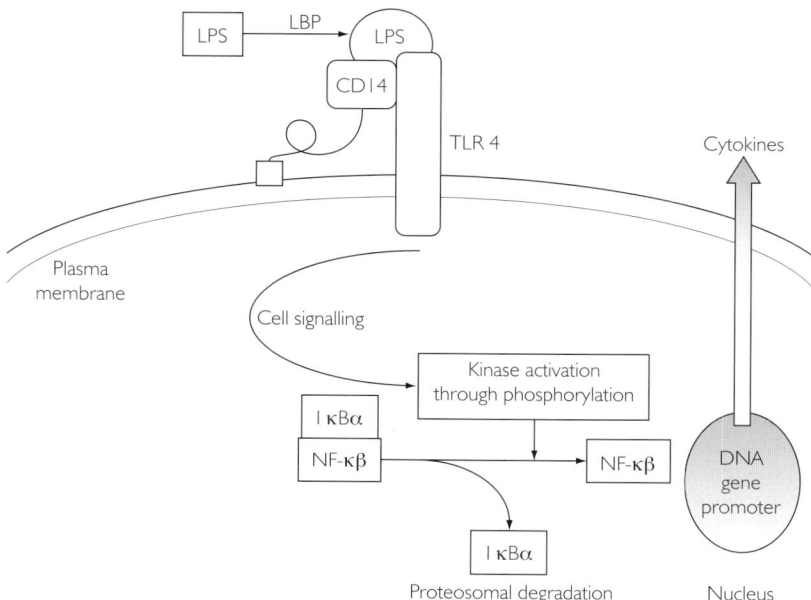

Fig. 13.3 Signal transduction in sepsis.

CYTOKINES

Cytokines are soluble, low molecular weight glycoproteins, which serve to regulate the innate and specific immune systems. Their actions are pleiotropic acting on multiple target cells in different ways depending on timing and concentration. At low concentrations they have paracrine effects whilst at higher concentrations they have endocrine effects.

Any exhaustive list of cytokines involved in sepsis will inevitably be dated and inaccurate. However, several cytokines have been implicated in the development of SIRS and MODS, including TNF-α, IL-1β, IL-8, IL-6, IL-10, whose concentrations seem to be linked to morbidity and mortality in sepsis[16] (see Table 13.2).

TNF-α and IL-1β are produced largely from mononuclear cells in response to signal transduction from pattern recognition receptors. In addition to mediating fever, they activate clotting, induce expression of adhesion molecules, potentiate the synthesis of each other and stimulate IL-6, -8, and IL-10 production. IL-6 stimulates acute phase protein production and down regulates TNF-α and IL-1β production. Control of the expression of inflammatory cytokines, from their respective genes, is controlled by intracellular transcription factors, in particular NF$\kappa\beta$, high levels of which have been associated with poor outcomes.[17]

In response to pro-inflammatory mediators, there is endogenous production of anti-inflammatory cytokines and cytokine antagonists. IL-4, IL-10, and IL-13 inhibit host leukocyte cytokine production. IL-1 receptor antagonist (IL-1 ra) and soluble TNF receptors may, at low concentrations, serve as carrier molecules but at higher concentrations are proposed to bind IL-1 and TNF thereby preventing their biological actions. Administration of IL-10 attenuates the production of TNF-α and decreases mortality whereas anti-IL-10 worsens mortality in animal models of sepsis.[18] An excess of IL-10, presumably predisposing to immunosuppression, is found in patients who die of sepsis.[19] On the other hand, low concentrations of IL-10, presumably favouring unchecked inflammation, correlate with poorer outcomes in ARDS.[20]

Apart from the instances where the initial insult is severe enough to generate an inflammatory response immediately, exceeding the in-built mechanisms of homeostasis and prompting the immediate development of SIRS/MODS, it seems that the prevailing *internal milieu* is likely to be more important than any absolute levels of one cytokine or another. This would account for observations that patients who are elderly or with underlying illnesses are known to be at increased risk for SIRS/MODS. These conditions (including advanced age) are associated with abnormal cytokine levels,[21] and it has been shown that the ability of a cell to synthesize pro- or anti-inflammatory mediators is influenced by its previous state of activation. This would explain the 'two-hit' model of pathogenesis, where an initial insult, insufficient to cause MODS nevertheless pre-primes an individual such that a secondary infection, or cytokine release from the gut or the lungs is sufficient to overwhelm homeostasis. Attempts to block one cytokine, in isolation of concurrent events, have, not surprisingly, failed to alter the outcome of SIRS/MODS.

LIPID MEDIATORS IN MODS

When the inflammatory cascade is activated, phospholipase A_2 (PLA_2) metabolizes membrane phospholipid of inflammatory cells to produce platelet-activating factor (PAF) and arachidonic acid (AA). AA is further metabolized by cyclooxygenase or 5′ lipoxygenase to produce a number of prostaglandins and leukotrienes, which like cytokines have a number of pro- and anti-inflammatory effects.

Thromboxane A_2 (TXA_2) plays a significant role in the early acute-phase organ injury, in part due to stimulation of platelet aggregation leading to microvascular thrombosis and tissue injury. TXA_2 may be responsible for abnormal pulmonary bronchoconstriction, with subsequent V̇/Q̇ mismatching, and is proposed to have myocardial depressant effects.[22] High levels of TXB_2, the stable metabolite of TXA_2, have been associated with non-survival in human sepsis.[23] Unlike TXA_2, PGE_2 and prostacyclin (PGI_2) may have some beneficial effects. While their negative effects are primarily due to vasodilatation, they may provide important counter-regulatory control through stabilizing lysosomes and hence antiproteolysis, inhibition of T- and B-cell activation and inhibition of macrophage cytokine production.[24]

PAF interacts with other cytokines, augmenting macrophage response to LPS and TNF, and enhancing monocyte production of IL-1. It also has direct inflammatory effects upon the endothelium influencing polymorphonuclear cell adhesion and endothelial cell architecture contributing to the increase in vascular permeability seen in sepsis.[22]

GENETIC INFLUENCE

If a relative excess or deficiency of mediator expression can upset inflammatory homeostasis, then it is not surprising to find a strong genetic component to fatal infectious disease. Families characterized by low TNF production have a tenfold increased risk for fatal outcome in meningococcal disease, whereas high IL-10 production increases the risk 20-fold.[25] TNF-α and IL-1ra polymorphisms are associated with greater susceptibility and worse outcomes to severe sepsis.[26] Unfortunately, genetic determinants of outcome in sepsis, and hence MODS, is likely to be more complicated than simple quantitative expression of one cytokine or another.

TISSUE INJURY

Tissue injury occurs during inflammation and is a progressive process that may culminate in organ dysfunction

Table 13.2   Partial list of pro-inflammatory and anti-inflammatory molecules involved in SIRS/MODS

Pro-inflammatory molecules	Anti-inflammatory molecules
TNF-α	IL-1 ra
IL-1β	IL-4
IL-2	IL-10
IL-6	IL-13
IL-8	Type II IL-1 receptors
IL-15	Transforming growth factor β
Neutrophil elastase	Soluble TNF-α receptors
IFN-γ	LPS binding protein
Protein kinase	Soluble CD-14
MCP-1	Prostaglandin E_2
MCP-2	Leukotriene B_4-receptor antagonism
Leukaemia inhibitory factor (D-factor)	
Thromboxane	
Platelet activating factor	
Soluble adhesion molecules	
Vasoactive neuropeptide	
Phospholipase A_2	
Tyrosine kinase	
Free radical generation	
Neopterin	
CD14	
Plasminogen activator inhibitor-1	

MCP, monocyte chemoattractant protein; IL, interleukin; LPS, lipopolysaccharide;
(From Bone[7]).

and failure. Vascular endothelial cells express adhesion molecules that divert leukocytes from the circulation into the tissues. They accumulate in response to chemokines, such as IL-8, and tissue injury occurs secondary to degranulation of leukocytes producing elastases and matrix metalloproteinases that degrade structural proteins.[18] Activated leukocytes also produce reactive oxygen species (ROS), from membrane bound NADPH oxidase that contribute to the tissue injury.

ROLE OF NITRIC OXIDE

Inducible nitric oxide synthase (iNOS), in response to inflammatory cytokines, generates excessive amounts of nitric oxide (NO). This is responsible for vasodilatation,[27] negative inotropy and depressed luistropy,[28] and, via toxic by-products of NO formed under acidic conditions, tissue nitrosylation. Myocytes from patients with sepsis have nitrosylation of intracellular proteins.[29] A prerequisite of normal organ function is that epithelial cells maintain a tight control of paracellular permeability, and nitrosylation mediated disruption of the epithelial cytoskeleton ring results in increased intestinal mucosal permeability.[30] Loss of compartmentalization has been implicated in ARDS, acute renal failure and intrahepatic cholestasis.

TISSUE HYPOXIA AND REPERFUSION INJURY

Hypoxic mediated cell death will generate an inflammatory response. In addition, hypoxia *per se* causes epithelial cells to release TNF-α and IL-8 resulting in pathological changes in epithelial permeability. IL-8 acts as a chemoattractant to neutrophils, and blocking the autocrine effect of TNF-α preserves barrier function.[31] Hypoxia also induces the release of IL-6, which is the main cytokine responsible for generating the acute-phase response.[32]

Following reperfusion of ischaemic tissues the formation of ROS follows metabolism of xanthine and hypoxanthine by xanthine oxidase, and the metabolism of arachidonic acid and the production of superoxide by activated neutrophils.[33] Additionally, there is calcium influx into cells, with calcium mediated cell damage.

APOPTOSIS

Apoptosis, or programmed cell death, is an important mechanism of cellular homeostasis in the multicellular organism. It is a genetically conserved, energy requiring mechanism that permits control of cell numbers without 'collateral' tissue injury, in contrast to the acute inflammatory response. The inflammatory response of MODS is associated with changes in the dynamics and regulation of apoptosis in comparison with the non-inflammatory state[34] (Table 13.3).

ROLE OF DISORDERED COAGULATION

Studies of the hepatic microcirculation have confirmed that microthrombi develop within 5 min of an endotoxin challenge.[35] If systemic endotoxin challenge continues, multiple fibrin clots begin to accumulate. Focal areas of hypoperfusion result, and coagulation necrosis with irreversible tissue injury ensues. Sensitive measures of coagulation activation indicate that some clotting occurs in virtually every patient in septic shock.[36]

The protein C anticoagulant pathway is a major mechanism in controlling thrombin generation. Thrombin, in turn, is proinflammatory, pro-coagulant and also regulates cellular proliferation by stimulating growth factor release.[37] Protein C deficiency in SIRS/MODS facilitates thrombin generation, and contributes to endothelial cell dysfunction (Figure 13.4).[37]

Table 13.3 Apoptosis in the pathophysiology of sepsis

Observation	Hypothesis	
Delayed neutrophil apoptosis	Beneficial	Enhanced function
		Prolonged function
	Detrimental	Prolonged elaboration of toxic metabolites
		May result in neutrophil necrosis
Increased lymphocyte apoptosis	Beneficial	Decreased autoreactive clones
		Decrease in effectors, which can perpetuate inflammation
	Detrimental	Immunosuppressive
Parenchymal apoptosis	Beneficial	Decreases burden of dying or senescent cells
		No bystander inflammation
	Detrimental	Decreases functional capacity of the organ

(From Mahidhara[34]).

IMPORTANCE OF THERAPY RELATED SIDE-EFFECTS TO TISSUE INJURY

There may be many detrimental effects arising as a consequence of the life support provided in the ICU that contribute to declining organ function (Table 13.4).[38]

CLINICAL PRESENTATION

Many of the clinical features of MODS can be explained by components of the innate immune response (Table 13.5).[39]

CARDIOVASCULAR DYSFUNCTION

Nitric oxide is responsible for the decreased systemic vascular resistance seen in MODS, and, along with TNF-α and IL-1β, the depressed myocardial function. Poor perfusion will naturally impact on other organ systems. Loss of endothelial barrier function is responsible for oedema formation and fluid redistribution. There is myocardial dilatation following fluid resuscitation and despite the high cardiac indices seen in septic patients, as many as a third have evidence of myocardial dysfunction.[40]

RESPIRATORY DYSFUNCTION

Pulmonary dysfunction is common in patients with SIRS and is manifested as tachypnoea, hypoxaemia (reduced PaO_2/FiO_2 ratio) and hypocarbia. When it is severe it may progress to acute lung injury (ALI) with ARDS complicating 60% of cases of septic shock.[41]

RENAL DYSFUNCTION

Acute renal failure in the setting of critical illness is nearly always multifactorial. In common with other tissues, the kidney is susceptible to leukocyte mediated tissue injury through the production of proteases and ROS. Hypovolaemia, low cardiac output states, nephrotoxic drugs, elevated intra-abdominal pressure and rhabdomyolysis will all contribute to renal dysfunction. The heterogeneity of blood flow within the kidney means the metabolically active medulla receives proportionately less blood flow than the filtering cortex making it extremely susceptible to ischaemic injury.[38]

GASTROINTESTINAL DYSFUNCTION

Splanchnic hypoperfusion is a common finding after trauma, sepsis and in shocked states. Gut mucosal ischaemia increases intestinal permeability with the translocation of bacteria and other mediators into the systemic circulation again contributing to any 'two-hit' component of pathogenesis.[42] There is nitrosylation of gut epithelial cell cytoskeleton and altered mucosal permeability[43] together with a close relationship between increased intestinal permeability on ICU admission and the subsequent development of MODS.[44]

Splanchnic ischaemia may manifest as stress ulcer bleeding, ileus, ischaemic hepatitis, acalculous cholecystitis, and pancreatitis.[45] Hyperglycaemia results from increased gluconeogenesis and impaired glucose clearance. Lipolysis increases plasma glycerol and free fatty acids, while ketones are low. Moreover, there is a shift in the ketone body ratio towards hydroxybuyrate indicating a reduction in hepatocyte redox potential. With progression of MODS, hypertriglyceridaemia occurs from reduced triglyceride clearance and preterminally gluconeogenesis fails, causing hypoglycaemia.[46]

NEUROLOGICAL DYSFUNCTION

Encephalopathy is very common and correlates with mortality in sepsis.[47] Heterogeneous neuropathies and myopathies may occur in the setting of MODS. In a

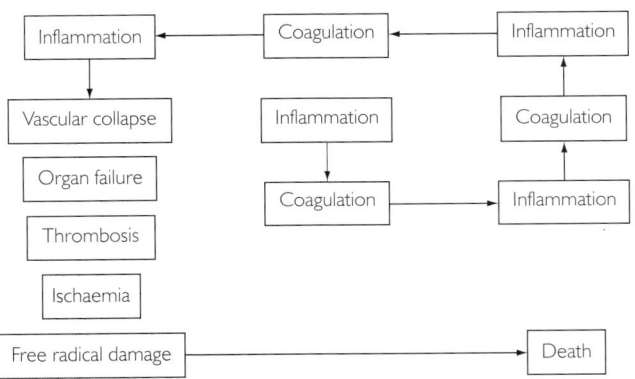

Fig. 13.4 Progression of the inflammation-coagulation auto-amplification loop. (From Esmon,[37] with permission.)

Table 13.4   Iatrogenic factors contributing to tissue injury in the pathogenesis of MODS

Medical intervention	Associated complications and tissue injury
Complications of central venous and pulmonary artery catheterization	Pneumothorax
	Arterial puncture with bleeding
	Infection
	Knotting of PA catheter
	Arrhythmias
	Pulmonary infarction, pulmonary artery rupture
	Inappropriate therapy (e.g. 'goal directed therapy')
Complications of intravenous fluid therapy	Unrecognized hypovolaemia
	Overtransfusion with crystalloid or colloid
	Excessive reductions in colloid oncotic pressure
	Massive generalized oedema
	Pulmonary oedema
Complications of inotropes and vasopressors	Arrhythmias
	Myocardial ischaemia/infarction
	Inappropriate vasoconstriction (especially dopamine and norepinephrine)
	Hyperglycaemia
	Metabolic acidosis (especially epinephrine)
	Dopamine-induced pituitary suppression
Complications of mechanical ventilation	'Volutrauma'
	Haemodynamic disturbances
	Systemic cytokine release
	Immune suppression
	Hypotension and muscle wasting related to sedatives and muscle relaxants
Complications of parenteral nutrition	Hyperglycaemia
	Hepatic steatosis and dysfunction
	Excessive CO_2 production
	Immunosuppression
	Gastrointestinal mucosa and lymphoid atrophy
Administration of toxic substances	Pulmonary oxygen toxicity
	Aminoglycosides
	High dose steroids
	NSAIDs

(From Bihari[38]).

systematic review of eight studies and 242 patients, electrophysiological abnormalities were reported in 76% of patients ventilated for more than 5 d. Two studies showed that duration of ventilation was statistically prolonged in patients with neuromuscular abnormalities, and mortality twice as high.[48]

MANAGEMENT

PREVENTION

Preventing the development of MODS must be seen as axiomatic in its management. Good surgical technique is essential; one of the earliest studies of post-surgical multiple organ failure found that surgical error contributed to the development of MODS in as many as 40% of cases.[49] Nosocomial infections, once acquired, increase the risk of death for patients 2-fold.[50] Meticulous hand washing by all staff and the use of isolation rooms, to prevent airborne spread of infectious agents, reduce cross-infection rates.[51] Modern antibacterial coatings on indwelling intravenous catheters can reduce the incidence of line-related sepsis.[52]

SOURCE CONTROL

The mainstay of the treatment of impending or established MODS is the elimination of precipitating factors along with any underlying cause or source of infection.

SURGERY

This may entail early fixation of fractures,[53] debridement of burns,[54] resection of ischaemic gut or dead tissue, and the

Table 13.5 Components of the innate immune response

Innate immune system component	Clinical feature
Neuroendocrine changes	Fever and somnolence, anorexia
	Increased adrenal secretion of catecholamine and corticosterone
	Altered growth hormone periodicity and IGF-1 production
	Altered secretion of arginine vasopressin
	Insulin resistance, increased glucagon release
Haemopoietic changes	Neutrophilia and release of immature neutrophils
	Delayed apoptosis of neutrophils
	Thrombocytosis
	Increased clearance of non-senescent RBCs
	Anaemia of chronic disease
	Increased lymphocyte apoptosis
Metabolic changes	Loss of skeletal muscle protein and lean tissue wasting
	Increased amino acid flux; increased gluconeogenesis
	Increased hepatic lipogenesis
	Increased lipolysis in adipose tissue
	Decreased lipoprotein lipase activity
	Development of cachexia
	Decreased bowel barrier function
	Trace mineral redistribution, hypoferraemia, hypozincaemia, hypercuperaemia
Hepatic changes	Albumin concentrations decline, increased albumin degradation and vascular loss
	Increased acute phase protein synthesis
	Decreased phosphoenolpyruvate carboxykinase
	Increased inducible nitric oxide synthesis
	Increased manganese superoxide dismutase
	Increased TIMP synthesis
	Increased haem oxygenase synthesis

IGF, insulin like growth factor; RBCs, red blood cells; TIMP, tissue inhibitors of metalloproteases. (Modified from Gabay and Krushner[39])

drainage of pus. Aggressive resuscitation before definitive control of bleeding may worsen survival prompting early definitive surgery.[55] Unfortunately, the source of the acute inflammatory response is not always obvious. Early surgical exploration, in spite of the current radiological techniques, should not be undervalued in the critically ill patient, particularly with a suspicious abdomen.

ANTIBIOTICS

Efforts to arrive at the correct identification of pathogens should be undertaken including blood and body fluid culture, acute and convalescent serology, and percutaneous aspiration of fluid collections. There is considerable evidence to support the view that appropriate antimicrobial therapy given early in the course of an infective illness improves outcome. Many large surveys of bacteraemia and severe pneumonia have shown that if the initial antimicrobial therapy is inappropriate, the relative risk or odds ratio for death is significantly increased.[56,57] Pre-hospital antibiotics for suspected meningococcal sepsis, compared with post-hospital administration, confer significant reductions in mortality.[58] In addition to appropriate early antibiotic administration, correct dosing is also important. The peak levels of aminoglycosides are critical in patients with Gram-

negative pneumonia, an inadequate peak (<6 mg/l for gentamicin) after the first dose being associated with a poor outcome.[59]

SUPPORTIVE CARE

Mortality due to sepsis may be declining because of improvements in supportive treatment, and prevention of complications, even in the absence of any single therapeutic advance. The prevention of skin breakdown, deep venous thrombosis[60] and the judicious use of sedation[61] may play a more important part in outcome than was once appreciated.

Details of organ specific supportive care can be found in the appropriate chapters in this manual.

INNOVATIVE THERAPIES

IMMUNE MODULATION

Based upon linear models of MODS (Figure 13.1) – activation of the innate immune system leading to progressive and inexorable inflammation – extensive investigation has been undertaken with monoclonal antibodies, and other drugs, targeted at manipulating the immune system, to see whether the harmful effects of uncontrolled inflammation could be prevented (Table 13.6).[62–74]

This 'magic bullet' approach has failed to improve mortality in MODS, largely because this linear approach is too simplistic, failing to take account of the complex network and interaction of inflammatory and compensatory anti-inflammatory cascades. Some studies that have shown trends toward marginal benefits (e.g. the 10% reduction in mortality rate seen with IL-1ra[71]) but would need 6000 to 7000 septic patients to demonstrate such a modest beneficial effect on survival. At the same time, such a small benefit makes the number of patients needed to treat (NNT = 1/actual rate reduction) to save one life very high so such agents are not cost effective.

NITRIC OXIDE INHIBITORS

A small open label study has confirmed that nitric oxide synthase inhibition, by N^G-monomethyl-L-arginine hydrochloride (L-NMMA) can restore the balance of vasomotor tone, thereby improving blood pressure. However, it is also associated with significant adverse myocardial events: decreased cardiac index, despite dobutamine infusion, increased pulmonary hypertension, and potential myocardial ischaemia.[75] Similar adverse myocardial effects of L-NMMA have resulted in the discontinuation of a large multicentre trial after interim analysis revealed an increased mortality ($P<0.005$) in the treatment group.[76] Excessive NOS inhibition has also been shown to reduce renal plasma flow and glomerular filtration rate.[77] While selective inhibitors of the inducible form of NOS might have a role in the future, there is clearly no role for indiscriminate NOS inhibition.

BLOOD PURIFICATION

Continuous high volume haemofiltration (2–6 l filtration/h) with highly permeable biocompatible membranes might remove cytokines and inflammatory mediators from the blood stream *en masse*. Unfortunately, there is little evidence that this technique significantly reduces the circulating concentrations of toxic mediators.[78] Nevertheless, while improvement in cardiovascular haemodynamics have been observed,[79] this may be related to many other factors, such as control of hyperthermia, and correction of fluid overload, metabolic acidosis and other electrolyte abnormalities.

STEROIDS

High-dose glucocorticoids (30 mg/kg methyl-prednisolone) significantly increased mortality rates in sepsis and septic shock.[80] However, after reports that corticosteroids reduce mortality rates during meningitis, *Pneumocystis carinii* pneumonia in patients with AIDS, typhoid fever, and as a late rescue therapy in ARDS,[81] new interest in steroid therapy in MODS and SIRS has emerged. Two small randomized, placebo controlled studies using adrenal replacement doses of hydrocortisone have shown more frequent reversal of shock with a trend to earlier resolution of sepsis-induced organ dysfunction.[82,83] Neither study was powered to show a significant effect upon mortality but larger studies are currently underway. The mechanisms by which physiological, and possibly beneficial, doses of corticosteroids are though to act include: (i) anti-inflammation via a decreased transcription of pro-inflammatory cytokines; (ii) treatment of relative adrenocortical deficiency; (iii) restoration of catecholamine receptor sensitivity. Such effects could be mediated through steroids known inhibition of NF-$\kappa\beta$.[83]

MANIPULATION OF THE CLOTTING CASCADE

A recent randomized, controlled trial of recombinant, activated protein C (aPC), involving 1690 patients has yielded an impressive, if somewhat surprising, result. The mortality in the treatment group was 24.7%, while in the placebo group it was 30.8%, with a reduction in the relative risk of death of 19.4% and an absolute reduction in the risk of death of 6.1% ($P=0.005$).[84] Although there was a significant increase in incidence of serious bleeding associated with aPC, the treatment effect, albeit at 28 d, was considerable.

Immune modulating therapies have failed to alter outcome in severe sepsis, and other clotting-cascade based therapies have also failed to improve survival – an antithrombin III (AT III) trial involving 2314 patients has recently failed to show beneficial effects with mortality rates of 38.7% and 38.9% in the placebo and treatment groups respectively.[85] The critical clinical question becomes: are there unique properties to the protein C anticoagulant pathway, distinct from other anticoagulants that make it central to the pathogenesis of the tissue injury associated with sepsis and MODS? The aPC trial has led many to rethink the pathogenesis of sepsis, promoting to 'centre-stage' the role played by the coagulation system. Further clinical investigation is needed to corroborate this result and elucidate more fully the role of protein C.

OUTCOME

Although many new therapies have been investigated over the last two decades and have appeared to offer some encouragement, none have been so miraculous that they have found their way into everyday practice. In the intervening period, resuscitation and supportive therapies have continued to improve, which can only be of benefit in the management of this high-risk group of patients in the ICU.

Has outcome from MOF improved? An analysis of the APACHE II and III databases suggests that patients with three or more organ systems in failure do indeed have a better outcome in the later APACHE III database.[86] Similarly, a study of 3815 patients with organ

Table 13.6 Trials of anti-sepsis therapies

Therapy	Year	No. of patients	Design	Findings	Ref.
Anti-endotoxin therapy					
Anti-endotoxin monoclonal antibody (HA-1A)	1994	600	Retrospective analysis with APACHE II predicted mortality comparisons	No significant effect on mortality from Gram −ve infections. Possible increase in mortality in non-Gram −ve infections	62
Anti-endotoxin monoclonal antibody (E5)	1995	847	RCT in Gram −ve infections	No significant effect on 28-d mortality	63
Anti-TNF therapy					
Anti-TNF monoclonal antibody (MAK 195F)	1996	122	RCT in severe sepsis/septic shock	No significant effect on overall mortality. Possible subgroup benefit for patients with raised IL-6 levels	64
Anti-TNF monoclonal antibody	1998	1879	RCT in septic shock	No significant effect on mortality. Reduction in coagulopathy	65
Soluble TNF receptor therapy					
TNF receptors p75TNFr	1996	141	RCT in septic shock	No reduction in mortality. Possible increase in mortality at higher treatment doses	66
TNF receptors p55TNFr	1997	498	RCT in severe sepsis/septic shock	No significant effect on overall mortality. Possible subgroup benefit for patients with early septic shock	67
Other therapies					
Platelet activating factor antagonist	1998	609	RCT in Gram −ve sepsis	No significant effect on 28-d mortality	68
Recombinant G-CSF	1998	61	RCT of prophylaxis in brain injury/haemorrhage	Significant reduction in bacteraemias. No effect on mortality or length of stay	69
Interferon-γ	1998	216	RCT of prophylaxis in burns patients	No significant reduction in infections or mortality	70
IL-1 receptor antagonist	1997	696	RCT in severe sepsis/septic shock	No significant effect on 28-d mortality	71
Bradykinin antagonist	1997	504	RCT in SIRS with presumed sepsis	No significant overall effect on 28-d mortality. Possible effect in Gram −ve infections	72
Ibuprofen					
Anti-prostaglandin therapy	1997	455	RCT in SIRS	No effect on survival, ARDS or shock. Dramatic benefit on survival in hypothermic subgroup with sepsis	73

G-CSF, granulocyte colony-stimulating factor; RCT, randomized controlled trial. (Adapted from Callister[74])

failure treated in 25 Australian ICUs between June and December 1994, found an improved prognosis in patients with three or more organ systems in failure compared with the APACHE II database.[87] Survival does seem to be improving in this very sick population of patients who end up at the bottom of the slippery slope, but whether MODS can be prevented by any new specific therapy remains to be seen.

REFERENCES

1 Tilney NL, Bailey GL, Morgan AP. Sequential system failure after ruptured abdominal aortic aneurysms: an unsolved problem in postoperative care. *Ann Surg* 1973; **178**: 117–22.

2 Bone RC, Balk RA, Cerra FB, *et al.* Definitions for sepsis and organ failure and guidelines for the use of innovative therapies in sepsis. The ACCP/SCCM consensus conference committee. *Chest* 1992; **101**: 1644–55.

3 Rangel-Frausto MS, Pittet D, Costigan M, *et al.* The natural history of the systemic inflammatory response syndrome (SIRS): A prospective study. *JAMA* 1995; **273**: 117–23.

4 Knaus WA, Draper EA, Wagner DP, Zimmerman JE. Prognosis in acute organ-system failure. *Ann Surg* 1985; **202**: 685–93.

5 Marshall JC, Cook DJ, Christou NV, *et al.* Multiple organ dysfunction score: a reliable descriptor of a complex clinical outcome. *Crit Care Med* 1995; **23**: 1638–52.

6 Teplick R, Rubin R. Therapy of sepsis: why have we made such little progress? *Crit Care Med* 1999; **27**: 1682–3.

7 Bone RC. Immunologic dissonance: a continuing evolution in our understanding of the systemic inflammatory response syndrome (SIRS) and the multiple organ dysfunction syndrome (MODS). *Ann Intern Med* 1996; **125**: 680–7.

8 Bone RC, Grodzin CJ, Balk RA. Sepsis: A new hypothesis for pathogenesis of the disease process. *Chest* 1997; **112**: 235–43.

9 Goldie AS, Fearon KC, Ross JA, *et al.* Natural cytokine antagonists and endogenous antiendotoxin core antibodies in sepsis syndrome. *JAMA* 1995; **274**: 172–7.

10 Oberholzer A, Oberholzer C, Moldawer LL. Cytokine signaling – regulation of the immune response in normal and critically ill states. *Crit Care Med* 2000; **28**(**Suppl**): N3–12.

11 Bernal A, Proft T, Fraser JD, Posnett DN. Superantigens in human disease. *J Clin Immunol* 1999; **19**: 149–57.

12 Li H, Llera A, Malchiodi EL, Mariuzza RA. The structural basis of T cell activation by superantigens. *Ann Rev Immunol* 1999; **17**: 435–66.

13 Schwandner R, Dziariski R, Wesche H, *et al.* Peptidoglycan- and lipoteichoic acid-induced cell activation is mediated by toll-like receptor 2. *J Biol Chem* 1999; **274**: 17406–9.

14 Le-Barillec K, Henneke P, Golenbock DT. Toll receptors: Guardians of the immune system and effectors of septic shock. *Adv in Sepsis* 2000; **1**: 23–30.

15 Glauser MP. Pathophysiologic basis of sepsis: considerations for future strategies of intervention. *Crit Care Med* 2000; **28**(**Suppl**): S4–8.

16 Pinsky MR, Vincent JL, Deviere J, *et al.* Serum cytokine levels in human septic shock. Relation to multiple-system organ failure and mortality. *Chest* 1993; **103**: 565–75.

17 Paterson RL, Galley HF, Dhillon JK, Webster NR. Increased nuclear factor kappa B activation in critically ill patients who die. *Crit Care Med* 2000; **28**: 1047–51.

18 Paterson RL, Webster NR. Sepsis and the systemic inflammatory response syndrome. *J R Coll Surg Edin* 2000; **45**: 178–82.

19 Lehmann AK, Halstensen A, Sornes S, *et al.* High levels of interleukin-10 in serum are associated with fatality in meningococcal disease. *Infect Immune* 1995; **63**: 2109–12.

20 Donnelly SC, Strieter RM, Reid PT, *et al.* The association between mortality rates and decreased concentrations of interleukin-10 and interleukin-1 receptor antagonist in the lung fluids of patients with the adult respiratory distress syndrome. *Ann Intern Med* 1996; **125**: 191–6.

21 Bone RC. Toward a theory regarding the pathogenesis of the systemic inflammatory response syndrome: what we do and do not know about cytokine regulation. *Crit Care Med* 1996; **24**: 163–72.

22 Bulger EM, Maier RV. Lipid mediators in the pathophysiology of critical illness. *Crit Care Med* 2000; **28**(Suppl): N27–36.

23 Reines HD, Halushka PV, Cook JA, *et al.* Plasma thromboxane concentrations are raised in patients dying with septic shock. *Lancet* 1982; **2**(8291): 174–5.

24 Jaffe BM, LaRosa CA, Kimura K. Prostaglandins and surgical disease: Part II. *Curr Probl Surg* 1988; **25**: 711–47.

25 Westendorp RGJ, Langermans JAM, Huizinga TWJ, *et al.* Genetic influence on cytokine production and fatal meningococcal disease. *Lancet* 1997; **349**(9046): 170–3.

26 Freeman BD, Buchman TG. Gene in a haystack: tumor necrosis factor polymorphisms and outcome in sepsis. *Crit Care Med* 2000; **28**: 3090–1.

27 Lorente JA, Landin L, De Pablo R, *et al.* L-arginine pathway in the sepsis syndrome. *Crit Care Med* 1993; **21**: 1287–95.

28 Helmut, D. Nitric oxide synthases in the failing heart: a double-edged sword? *Circulation* 1999; **99**: 2972–5.

29 Ungureanu-Longrois D, Balligand JL, Kelly RA, Smith TW. Myocardial contractile dysfunction in the systemic inflammatory response syndrome: Role of cytokine-induced nitric oxide synthase in cardiac myocytes. *J Mol Cell Cardiolog* 1995; **27**: 155–67.

30 Marik PE, Iglesias, J. Intestinal mucosal permeability: Mechanisms and implications for treatment. *Crit Care Med* 1999; **27**: 1650–1.

31 Taylor CT, Dzus AL, Colgan SP. Autocrine regulation of epithelial permeability by hypoxia: role for polarized release of tumor necrosis factor alpha. *Gastroenterology* 1998; **114**: 657–68.

32 Bertges DJ, Fink MP, Delude RL. Hypoxic signal transduction in critical illness. *Crit Care Med* 2000; 28(**Suppl**): N78–86.

33 Bonventre JV. Mechanisms of ischaemic acute renal failure. *Kidney Int* 1993; **43**: 1160–78.

34 Mahidhara R, Billiar TR. Apoptosis in sepsis. *Crit Care Med* 2000; **28** (**Suppl**): N105–113.

35 Asaka S, Shibayama Y, Nakata, K. Pathogenesis of focal and random hepatocellular necrosis in endotoxemia: microscopic observations *in vivo*. *Liver* 1996; **16**: 183–7.

36 Opal S M. Therapeutic rationale for antithrombin III in sepsis. *Crit Care Med* 2000; 28(**Suppl**):S34–37.

37 Esmon, C. The protein C pathway. *Crit Care Med* 2000; 28(**Suppl**): S44–48.

38 Breen D, Bihari, D. Acute renal failure as a part of multiple organ failure: the slippery slope of critical illness. *Kidney Int* 1998; **66**(**Suppl**): S25–33.

39 Gabay C, Krushner, I. Acute-phase proteins and other systemic responses to inflammation. *N Engl J Med* 1999; **340**: 448–54.

40 Parrillo JE, Parker MM, Natanson C, *et al*. Septic shock in humans. Advances in the understanding of pathogenesis, cardiovascular dysfunction and therapy. *Ann Internal Med* 1990; **113**: 227–42.

41 Kollef MH, Schuster DP. The acute respiratory distress syndrome. *N Engl J Med* 1995; **332**: 27–37.

42 Pastores SM, Katz DP, Kvetan, V. Splanchnic ischemia and gut mucosal injury in sepsis and multiple organ dysfunction syndrome. *Am J Gastroenterol* 1996; **91**: 1697–1710.

43 Unno N, Hodin RA, Fink MP. Acidic conditions exacerbate interferon-γ-induced intestinal epithelial hyperpermeability: role of peroxynitrous acid. *Crit Care Med* 1999; **27**: 1429–36.

44 Doig CJ, Sutherland LR, Sandham JD, *et al*. Increased intestinal permeability is associated with the development of multiple organ dysfunction syndrome in critically ill ICU patients. *Am J Resp Crit Care Med* 1998; **158**: 444–51.

45 Bersten A, Sibbald WJ. Circulatory disturbances in multiple system organ failure. *Crit Care Clin* 1989; **5**: 233–54.

46 Cerra FB. Metabolic manifestations of multiple systems organ failure. *Crit Care Clin* 1989; **5**: 119–31.

47 Bolton CF, Young GB, Zochodne DW. The neurological complications of sepsis. *Ann Neurol* 1993; **33**: 94–100.

48 De Jonghe B, Cook D, Sharshar T, *et al*. Acquired neuromuscular disorders in critically ill patients: a systematic review. *Intensive Care Med* 1998; **24**: 1242–50.

49 Eiseman B, Beart R, Norton, L. Multiple organ failure. *Surg Gynecol Obstetr* 1977; **144**: 323–26.

50 Bueno-Cavanillas A, Delgado-Rodriguez M, Lopez-Luque A, *et al*. Influence of nosocomial infection on mortality rate in an intensive care unit. *Crit Care Med* 1994; **22**: 55–60.

51 Woeltje KF, Fraser VJ. Preventing nosocomial infections in the intensive care unit – lessons learned from outcome research. *New Horizons* 1998; **6**: 84–90.

52 Maki DG, Stolz SM, Wheeler S, Mermel LA. Prevention of central venous catheter-related bloodstream infection by use of an antiseptic-impregnated catheter. *Ann Internal Med* 1997; **127**: 257–66.

53 Border JR, Bone LB. Multiple trauma: major extremity wounds; their immediate management and its consequences. *Adv Surg* 1988; **21**: 263–91.

54 Herndon DN, Barrow RE, Rutan RL, *et al*. Comparison of conservative versus early excision. Therapies in severely burned patients. *Ann Surg* 1989; **209**: 547–52.

55 Stern SA, Dronen SC, Birrer P, Wang X. Effect of blood pressure on hemorrhage volume and survival in a near-fatal hemorrhage model incorporating a vascular injury. *Ann Emerg Med* 1993; **22**: 155–63.

56 Ispahani P, Pearson NJ, Greenwood, D. An analysis of community and hospital acquired bacteraemia in a large teaching hospital in the United Kingdom. *Q J Med* 1987; **63**: 427–40.

57 Alvarez-Lerma F. Modification of empiric antibiotic treatment in patients with pneumonia acquired in the intensive care unit. The ICU Acquired Pneumonia Study Group. *Intensive Care Med* 1996; **22**: 387–94.

58 Cartwright K, Strang J, Gossain S, Begg, N. Early treatment of meningococcal disease. *BMJ* 1992; **305**: 774.

59 Moore RD, Lietman PS, Smith CR. Clinical response to aminoglycoside therapy: Importance of the ratio of peak concentration to minimal inhibitory concentration. *J Infect Dis* 1987; **155**: 393–9.

60 Saint S, Matthay MA. Risk reduction in the intensive care unit. *Am J Med* 1998; **105**: 515–23.

61 Kolleff MH, Levy NT, Ahrens TS, *et al*. The use of continuous i.v. sedation is associated with prolongation of mechanical ventilation. *Chest* 1998; **114**: 541–8.

62 The French national registry of HA-1A (Centoxin) in septic shock. A cohort study of 600 patients. The National Committee for the Evaluation of Centoxin. *Arch Intern Med* 1994; **154**: 2484–91.

63 Bone RC, Balk RA, Fein AM, *et al*. A second large controlled clinical study of E5 a monoclonal antibody to endotoxin: results of a prospective multicenter, randomized, controlled trial. The E5 Sepsis Study Group. *Crit Care Med* 1995; **23**: 994–1006.

64 Reinhart K, Wiegand-Lohnert C, Grimminger F, *et al*. Assessment of the safety and efficacy of the monoclonal anti-tumor necrosis factor antibody fragment, MAK 195F, in the patients with sepsis and septic shock: a multicenter, randomized, placebo-controlled, dose-ranging study. *Crit Care Med* 1996; **24**: 733–42.

65 Abraham E, Wunderink R, Silverman H, *et al*. Efficacy and safety of monoclonal antibody to human tumor necrosis factor alpha in patients with sepsis syndrome. A randomized, controlled, double-blind, multicenter clinical trial. TNF-alpha MAb Sepsis Study Group. *JAMA* 1995; **273**: 934–41.

66 Fisher CJ, Agosti JM, Opal SM, *et al.* Treatment of septic shock with the tumor necrosis factor receptor: Fc fusion protein. *N Engl J Med* 1996; **334**: 1697–702.

67 Abraham E, Glauser MP, Butler T, *et al.* p55 Tumor necrosis factor receptor fusion protein in the treatment of patients with severe sepsis and septic shock. A randomized controlled multicenter trial. RO 45–2081 Study Group. *JAMA* 1997; **277**: 1531–8.

68 Dhainaut JF, Tenaillon A, Le-Tulzo Y, *et al.* Platelet-activating factor receptor antagonist BN 52021 in the treatment of severe sepsis: a randomized, double-blind, placebo-controlled, multicenter clinical trial. *Crit Care Med* 1994; **22**: 1720–8.

69 Heard SO, Fink MP, Gamelli RL, *et al.* Effect of prophylactic administration of recombinant human granulocyte colony-stimulating factor (filgrastim) on the frequency of nosocomial infections in patients with acute traumatic brain injury or cerebral hemorrhage. The Filgrastim Study Group. *Crit Care Med* 1998; **26**: 748–54.

70 Wasserman D, Ioannovich JD, Hinzmann RD, *et al.* Interferon-gamma in the prevention of severe burn-related infections: a European phase III multicenter trial. The severe Burns Study Group. *Crit Care Med* 1998; **26**: 434–9.

71 Opal SM, Fisher CJ, Dhainaut JF, *et al.* Confirmatory interleukin-1 receptor antagonist trial in severe sepsis: a phase III, randomized, double-blind, placebo-controlled, multicenter trial. *Crit Care Med* 1997; **25**: 1115–24.

72 Fein AM, Bernard GR, Criner GJ, *et al.* Treatment of severe systemic inflammatory response syndrome and sepsis with a novel bradykinin antagonist, deltibant (CP-0127). Results of a randomized, double-blind, placebo-controlled trial. CP-0127 SIRS and Sepsis Study Group. *JAMA* 1997; **277**: 482–7.

73 Bernard GR, Wheeler AP, Russell, *et al.* The effects of ibuprofen on the physiology and survival of patients with sepsis. *N Engl J Med* 1997; **336**: 912–18.

74 Callister MEJ, Evans TW. Septicaemia. Haemodynamic and ventilatory support in severe sepsis. *J R Coll Physicians Lond* 2000; **34**: 522–8.

75 Grover R, Zaccardelli D, Colice G, *et al.* An open-label dose escalation study of the nitric oxide synthase inhibitor, N^G-methyl-L-arginine hydrochloride (546C88), in patients with septic shock. *Crit Care Med* 1999; **27**: 913–22.

76 Grover R, Lopez A, Lorente J, *et al.* Multi-center, randomized, placebo-controlled, double blind study of the nitric oxide synthase inhibitor 546C88: effect on survival in patients with septic shock. Abstract. *Crit Care Med* 1999; **27**(**Suppl**):A33.

77 Bech JN, Nielsen CB, Pedersen EB. Effects of systemic NO synthesis inhibition on RPF, GFR, U$_{Na}$, and vasoactive hormones in healthy humans. *Am J Physiol* 1996; **270**: F845–51.

78 Bellomo R, Tipping P, Boyce, N. Continuous veno-venous haemofiltration with dialysis removes cytokines from the circulation of septic patients. *Crit Care Med* 1993; **21**: 522–6.

79 Heering P, Morgera S, Schimtz FJ, *et al.* Cytokine removal and cardiovascular haemodynamics in septic patients with continuous venovenous haemofiltration. *Intensive Care Med* 1997; **23**: 288–96.

80 Zeni F, Freeman B, Natanson, C. Anti-inflammatory therapies to treat sepsis and septic shock: a reassessment. *Crit Care Med* 1997; **25**: 1095–1100.

81 Carlet J. From mega to more reasonable doses of corticosteroids: a decade to recreate hope. *Crit Care Med* 1999; **27**: 672–4.

82 Bollaert PE, Charpentier C, Levy B, *et al.* Reversal of late septic shock with supraphysiological doses of hydrocortisone. *Crit Care Med* 1998; **26**: 645–50.

83 Briegel J, Forst H, Haller M, *et al.* Stress doses of hydrocortisone reverse hyperdynamic septic shock: a prospective, randomized, double-blind, single centre study. *Crit Care Med* 1999; **27**: 723–32.

84 Bernard GR, Vincent JL, Laterre PF, *et al.* Efficacy and safety of recombinant human activated protein C for severe sepsis. *N Engl J Med* 2001; **344**: 699–709.

85 Warren BL, Eid A, Singer P, *et al.* High dose antithrombin III in severe sepsis. A randomized controlled trial. *JAMA* 2001; **286**: 1869–78.

86 Zimmerman JE, Knaus WA, Wagner DP, *et al.* A comparison of risks and outcomes for patients with organ system failure: 1982–1990. *Crit Care Med* 1996; **24**: 1633–41.

87 Smith SM, Churches T, McWilliam D, Herkes R. The Commonwealth Critical Care Casemix Study Group: Prognosis for multiple organ failure in Australian intensive care units (ICU). *Anaesth Int Care* 1996; **24**: 270–1.

Part Three

Acute Coronary Care

14

Acute myocardial infarction

B Power

Coronary artery disease (CAD) accounts for over 30% of all deaths in Western industrialized society with most of these deaths being due to acute myocardial infarction. Many deaths occur within the first 24–48 hours of onset of symptoms. Lowering mortality from CAD requires us to rapidly identify patients at risk and to implement evidence based treatment regimens.

Acute coronary syndrome (ACS) describes the spectrum of patients who present with chest discomfort or other symptoms caused by acute myocardial ischaemia (see Table 14.1). ACS can be further divided into unstable angina and acute myocardial infarction (AMI). Both represent medical emergencies and are one of the most frequent causes of hospital and coronary care (CCU) admission. Both are invariably caused by recent thrombus formation on pre-existing coronary artery plaque leading to impaired myocardial oxygen supply. In this sense they differ from stable angina which is usually precipitated by increased myocardial oxygen demand with background coronary artery narrowing.

Table 14.1 Classification of Acute Coronary Syndromes.

Acute Coronary Syndrome (ACS). A spectrum of acute clinical conditions characterized by a recent change in the frequency or duration of ischaemic chest pain. They range from myocardial infarction that occurs in the presence of ST segment elevation (STEMI), to myocardial infarction in the absence of ST Segment Elevation (Non-STEMI) through to unstable angina (USA).

Unstable angina (USA). Ischaemic type chest pain, which is of recent origin, is more frequent, severe, or prolonged than the patient's usual angina; is more difficult to control with drugs; or is occurring at rest or minimal exertion. Cardiac biomarkers are not elevated.

Myocardial infarction. Ischaemic symptoms with evidence of raised cardiac biomarkers. Myocardial infarction may be further categorized as
(A.) **STEMI.** Myocardial infarction with ST-segment elevation on the presenting or subsequent 12 lead ECGs
(B.) **NonSTEMI.** Myocardial infarction occurring without ST-segment elevation on presenting or subsequent 12 lead ECGs

AETIOLOGY AND RISK FACTORS

Atheroma deposits in the walls of coronary arteries provide the substrate for the development of ACS. Major risk factors for the development of coronary artery atheroma are seen in Table 14.2. Despite the strong association of these risk factors with CAD, many patients who present with myocardial infarction (MI) do not possess any of them.

Cessation of smoking, lowering plasma cholesterol (diet and medications) and adoption of a more active lifestyle can all help prevent the development of CAD. Antihypertensive therapy in hypertensive patients produces a large and early reduction in stroke mortality. The benefit upon coronary events is smaller but still significant.[1,2]

Table 14.2 Risk factors for the development of Atherosclerosis and CAD.

Modifiable	Non modifiable

By life-style
  Smoking
  Obesity
	Increasing age
	Male sex
	Family History (genetic)
	  an immediate relative
	  having CAD, male
	  <55 years, female <65.

Physical Inactivity	

By pharmacotherapy or lifestyle
  Hypertension
  Lipid Disorders
    (Elevated LDL, Low HDL,
    Elevated plasma TGs)
  Diabetes and insulin resistance
  Hyperhomocysteinaemia	

Other Factors: Increased plasma viscosity, chronic inflammation	

LDL = Low-density Lipoprotein; HDL = High-density Lipoprotein; TG = Trigylceride

Other causes of acute MI are:

- coronary artery embolus,
- aortic dissection involving coronary arteries at their origin,
- coronary artery spasm,
- vasculitis,
- cocaine or ergotamine abuse,
- blunt trauma.

PATHOPHYSIOLOGY

Formation of thrombus upon disrupted, fissured or eroded atheromatous plaque is the usual precipitant of unstable angina or MI.[3] Atherosclerotic plaque formation is probably initiated by injury to the vessel wall that may commence even as early as childhood.[4] Highly activated macrophages are attracted to the site of injury and differentiate into tissue macrophages. Macrophages incorporate bloodstream lipids into the connective tissue fibres of plaque, forming a thrombogenic soft lipid core. Plaque development is slow, but is rapidly accelerated in people with risk factors (Table 14.2).

'Vulnerable plaque' is often rich in lipid and covered by a thin fibrin cap. The cause of plaque rupture or fissuring is unknown but exposes thrombogenic lipid and collagen which are potent activators of platelets. Development of thrombus upon this eroded plaque results from:

(a) platelet adherence and activation
(b) coagulation pathway activation.

While many pathways stimulate platelet activation, the final common pathway of thrombus formation is via activation of the glycoprotein (GP) IIb/IIIa receptor, the platelet surface membrane receptor for fibrinogen. Activated GP IIb/IIIa receptors cross-link fibrinogen between activated platelets, leading to the formation of platelet thrombi. Accumulation of platelets forms '*white thrombus*' but seldom is this thrombus totally occluding. Activation of coagulation pathways by exposed lipid and fibrin as well as by the now activated platelets, leads ultimately to thrombin activation and the laying down of fibrin clot. Red cells are enmeshed in this so-called '*red thrombus*' complex which surrounds the 'white thrombus'. Sudden artery occlusion by thrombus may thus complicate even only moderate-sized plaque. (See Fig. 14.1a, b.)

The process has immediate relevance to treatment.

- Anti-platelet agents prevent platelet adherence and heaping which limits and even reverses the development of 'white thrombus'. They may target the adenosine diphosphate receptor (e.g. ticlopidine and clopidogrel) or may inhibit cyclo-oxygenases (e.g. aspirin).
- Fibrinolytic agents clear 'red thrombus'.

Current thrombolysis agents lyse fibrin and red cell thrombus, but paradoxically may increase thrombin activation. Concomitant administration of anti-thrombin agents (e.g. heparins) may limit thrombin activation.

Totally occluding thrombus causes myocardial necrosis, unless rapidly cleared or there is good collateral flow. Occlusion is often accompanied by ST-segment elevation on the electrocardiogram (ECG). If thrombus is largely 'white thrombus' with only small non-occlusive 'red thrombus', ST-segment elevation is far less likely. Non-occlusive thrombus may be asymptomatic, may cause unstable angina or may cause MI, especially if spasm or distal embolization of thrombus occurs. While non-occlusive thrombus is less likely to be associated with early or sudden death, it is a strongly associated with later re-infarction and death.

Ischaemia results in cellular disruption, loss of function, thinning and softening of the affected myocardium, and later fibrosis and ventricular remodelling.

Infarct size determines:

- left ventricular (LV) systolic function impairment;
- stroke volume decrease;
- ventricular filling pressure rise (leads to pulmonary congestion and hypotension, which may impair coronary perfusion pressures and exacerbate the myocardial ischaemia);
- LV diastolic dysfunction.

Initially, infarcted muscle is softened leading to an increase in ventricular compliance, but as fibrosis takes place compliance is decreased. With time, there is often expansion of the infarcted segment and compensatory hypertrophy of unaffected myocardial cells (i.e. ventricular remodelling). This can commence early after infarction and can affect overall ventricular function and prognosis.

CLINICAL PRESENTATION

The diagnosis of myocardial ischaemia is usually made on the basis of history and ECG.

HISTORY

Patients with myocardial ischaemia can present with chest pain or pressure, syncope, palpitations, dyspnoea or sudden death. Prodromal symptoms of unstable angina occur in the days preceding infarction in 20–60% of patients.[5]

Typically, the pain of acute MI is:

- severe, constant and restrosternal, spreading across the chest;
- lasts for more than 20 minutes;
- may radiate to the throat and jaw, down the ulnar aspect of both arms and to the interscapular area;

(a)

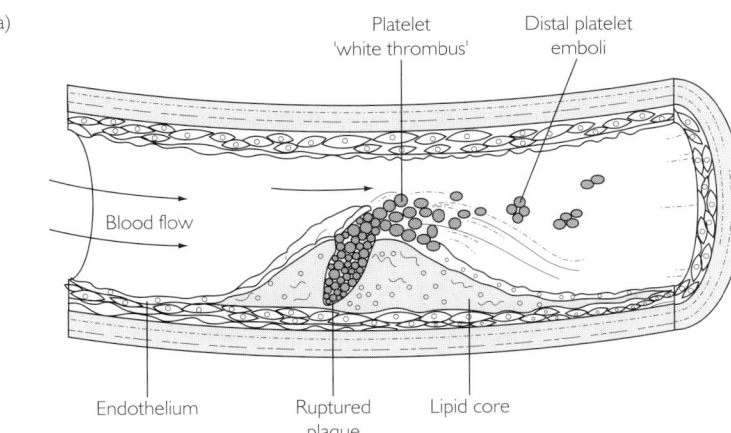

Fig. 14.1a Plaque rupture exposes thrombogenic lipid. "White thrombus" is formed by adhering activated platelets. Coronary artery narrowing, distal platelet embolization or arterial spasm can cause ischaemic myocardial pain and possible myocardial necrosis. This lesion is unstable and may lead to thrombin activation. "White thrombus" is not removed by thrombolytic therapy. **Modified from Braunwald's Atlas of Cardiology, with permission.**

(b)

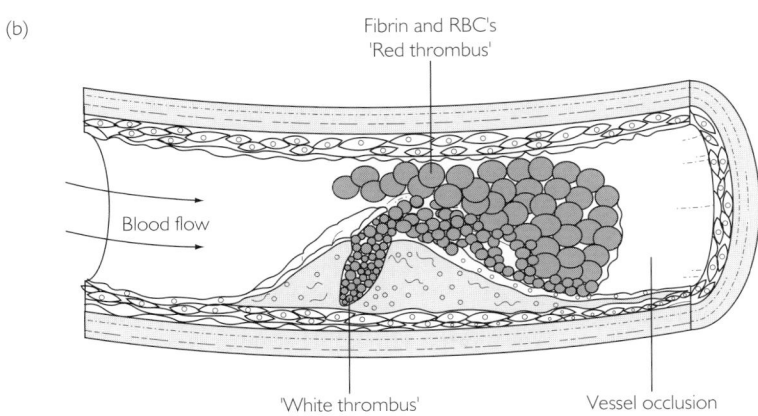

Fig. 14.1b Thrombin activation leads to a mesh of fibrin and red blood cells or "red thrombus". Arterial occlusion may occur and in arteries without adequate collateral, distal myocardial necrosis and ST segment elevation on the 12 lead ECG, result. Re-perfusion may be achieved with thrombolytic therapy or with invasive coronary procedures. **Modified from Braunwald, with permission.**

- sweating, nausea, pallor, dyspnoea and anxiety are common;

The pain of unstable angina may be similar but milder in nature. Features that may suggest it to be ischaemic are:

- waxing and waning characteristics;
- reproducibility upon minimal exertion or with emotion;
- association with autonomic symptoms.

The 'pain' may sometimes be atypical:

- epigastrium (leading to possible misdiagnosis);
- confined to the jaw, arms, wrists or interscapular region;
- burning or a 'pressure';
- sharp or stabbing in nature;
- reproduced by chest pressure.

These features do not necessarily exclude infarction.[6] Aortic dissection and pericarditis are two important differential diagnoses.

Atypical or silent presentations are common; 20–60% of non-fatal infarctions are unrecognized at onset. This presentation is more common in the elderly, diabetes, hypertension, those who smoke or take non-steroidal anti-inflammatory agents.

The assessment of clinical symptoms alone is insufficient for risk stratification and severity of pain does not usually correlate with the extent of infarction.

PHYSICAL EXAMINATION

Examination of patients with unstable angina is often unremarkable. With more severe infarction and extensive myocardial injury, signs of autonomic activation (pallor, sweating, agitation, clamminess) as well as heart failure and even shock may be apparent. Pericardial friction rubs occur frequently after MI but are usually transient.

LV failure is associated with a higher mortality. Signs include gallop rhythm, tachycardia, tachypnoe and basal crackles. A fourth heart sound is often heard, but a third heart sound usually indicates a large infarction with extensive muscle damage. A systolic murmur may be present and may be transient or persistent. These murmurs usually result from mitral regurgitation, either due to papillary muscle dysfunction or LV dilatation and have prognostic significance.

Cardiogenic shock, hypotension, oliguria and features of low cardiac output are associated with particularly poor outcome. Shock may be present without hypotension[7] and may develop many hours after onset of symptoms. Right ventricle (RV) infarction results in hypotension and marked elevation of the jugular venous pressure (also seen with major LV dysfunction usually in association with marked pulmonary venous congestion.)

Conditions with similar presentations that do not benefit from thrombolysis are:

- pericarditis (auscultate for pericardial rub);
- acute aortic regurgitation due to aortic dissection (arterial pulses are compared).

INVESTIGATIONS

The presence of MI should also be qualified by:

- size
- causation (e.g. acute, post-surgery, post-angiography)
- time from occurrence (acute, early, late).

Technological advances allow accurate detection of very small infarcts, myocardial necrosis <1.0 g[8] that would not have been detected in earlier eras.

ELECTROCARDIOGRAPHY (ECG)

Acute and complete occlusion of a coronary artery usually leads to serial ECG changes in leads subtending the area of ischaemia. (see Fig. 14.2).

- The number of leads involved broadly reflects the extent of myocardium involved.

- The height of initial ST-segment elevation is modestly correlated with the degree of ischaemia.

Identification of classical acute and early changes where ST-segment elevation is present identifies patients in whom reperfusion therapy may interrupt, prevent or minimize myocardial necrosis. These are:

- **Hyperacute** (0–20 minutes): tall peaking T waves and progressive upward curving and elevation of ST-segments.
- **Acute** (minutes to hours): persisting ST-segment elevation, gradual loss of R wave in the infarcted area. ST-segments begin to fall and there is progressive inversion of T waves
- **Early** (hours to days): loss of R wave and development of pathological Q waves in area of ischaemia. Return of ST-segments to baseline. Persistence of T wave inversion
- **Indeterminate** (days to weeks): pathological Q waves with persisting T wave inversion. ST-segments normalize (unless there is aneurysm).
- **Old** (weeks to months): persisting deep Q waves with normalized ST-segments and T waves.

Other causes of acute ST elevation and T wave changes that should not receive thrombolytic therapy are:

- normal variant,
- metabolic disturbance,
- drug toxicity, pericarditis,
- LV hypertrophy,
- LV aneurysm,
- Wolff–Parkinson–White syndrome and conduction defects.

ACS patients without or with minimal ST elevation who are not eligible for thrombolysis may still be at high risk of infarction and death. They likely have active, non-occluding thrombus. ECGs in these patients may be normal or display:

- ST-segment depression;
- ST-segment elevation (insufficient to meet thrombolysis criteria);

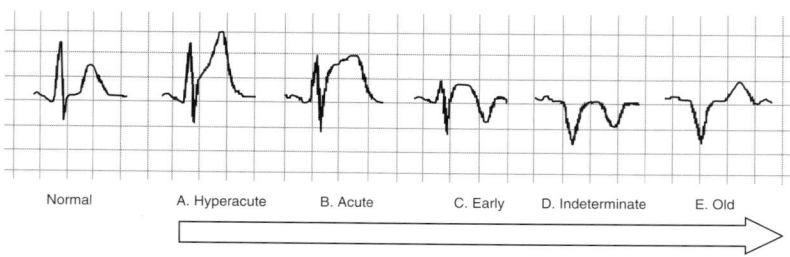

Normal   A. Hyperacute   B. Acute   C. Early   D. Indeterminate   E. Old

Fig. 14.2 Total acute coronary artery occlusion leads to serial ECG changes. Their evolution is variable and may be interrupted or altered by successful reperfusion. ST segment elevation is an early and relatively specific indicator of the need for thrombolysis in patients with ACS.

- T-wave inversion or 'normalization' of previous inverted T waves.

A normal ECG does not exclude MI. Despite the absence of ST elevation, a small percentage of patients progressively lose R-wave height and develop evidence of Q waves.

ANATOMY

There is a broad correlation between the site of infarction as suggested by the ECG and the occluded coronary artery (see Fig. 14.3). Anterior MI usually results from occlusion of the left anterior descending artery; inferior, true posterior and right ventricular (RV) infarction result from occlusion of the right coronary or circumflex arteries. The pattern of lead involvement may assist with 'localization' of the MI.[9] (See Fig. 14.4.)

- Anterior infarction – changes in leads V_2–V_4.
- Inferior infarction – leads II, III and aVF.
- Lateral infarction – leads I and aVL.
- True posterior infarction involves 'mirror' changes in leads V_1 and V_2.
- 8% of patients with MI will only display ST elevation in posterior (V_7–V_9) or in right precordial leads (V_3R–V_6R).[9]
- RV infarction is usually concurrent with inferior wall infarction and very rarely in isolation. A V_4R lead (V_4 lead in an equivalent position on the right anterior chest wall) is sensitive and specific for RV infarction.[9,10]

Other recognized sites of infarction include anteroseptal, anterolateral and infer-lateral, inferoposterior and extensive anterior (see Table 14.3).

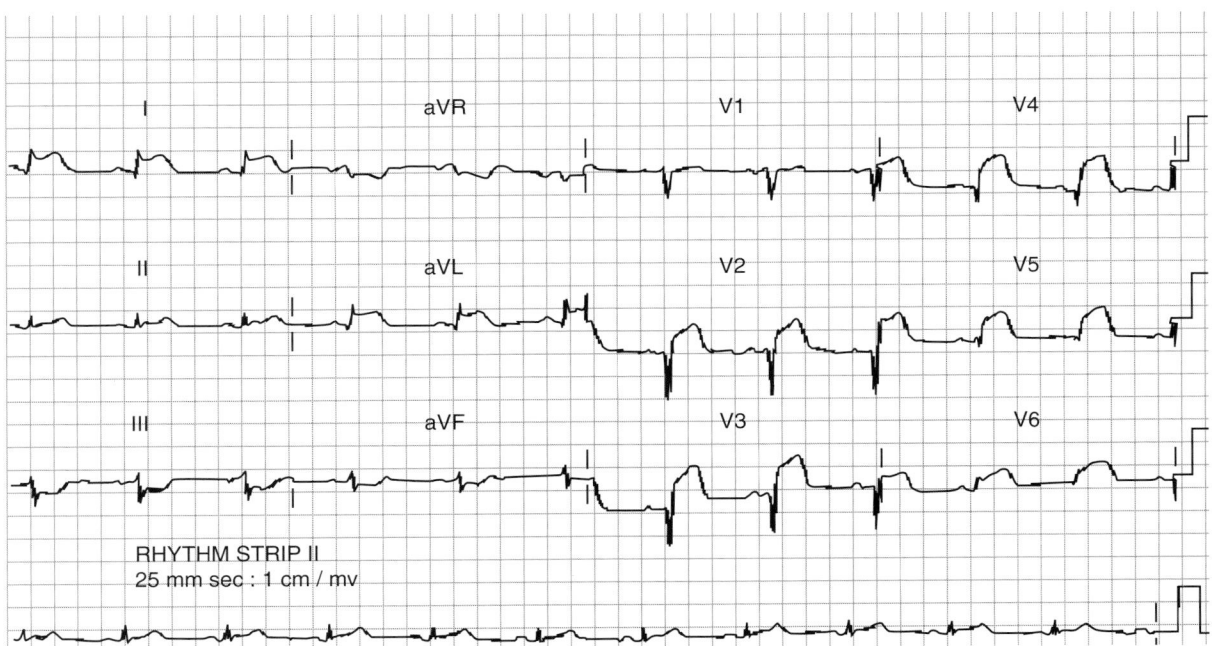

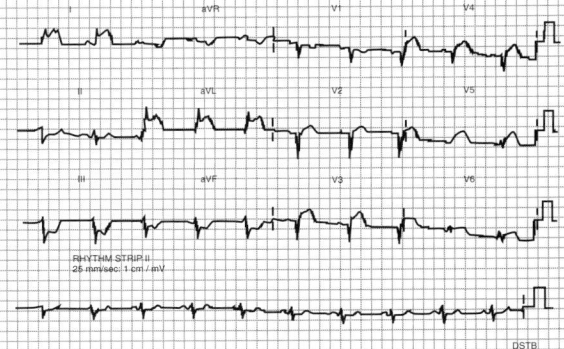

Fig. 14.3a Acute anterior myocardial Infarction with ST elevation in I, aVL, V_2 – V_6. There is ST depression in inferior leads III and aVF)

Fig. 14.3b True posterior myocardial infarction. Tall R wave in V_1. Associated acute inferior infarction with ST elevation in II, III, aVF (and ST depression in leads I, aVL and across the chest leads). The patient is in sinus rhythm with first-degree atrioventricular block and episodes of Wenckeback block.

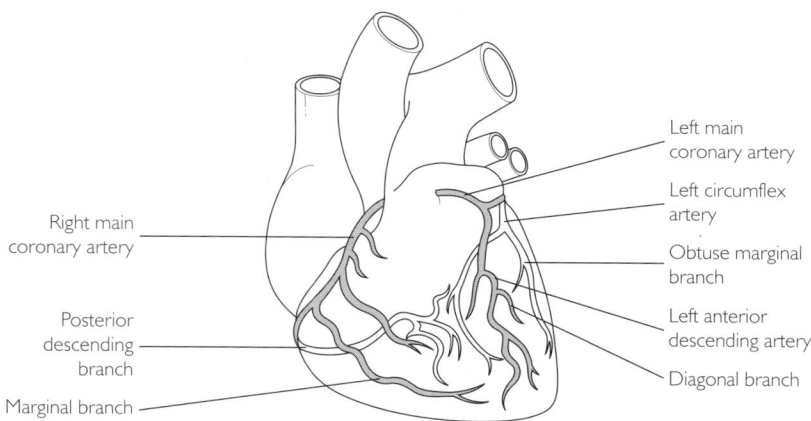

Fig. 14.4 Coronary Artery Anatomy.

Table 14.3 Anatomical patterns of myocardial injury

Location of injury	affected Leads	Infarct-related artery
Anterior/Septal	V_2, V_3, V_4	Mid LAD or Diagonal branch of LAD
Inferior	II , III, aVF	RCA or posterolateral branch of Cx
Lateral	I, aVL, V_5, V_6	Cx or LV branch of Cx
True Posterior*	V_1 and V_2	Posterolateral branch of Cx or Posterior Descending Branch of RCA
Anterolateral	I, aVL, $V_2 - V_6$	Proximal LAD
Inferolateral	II, III, aVF	
	aVL, V_5, V_6	Proximal Cx or large LV in left dominant system
Right Ventricular	V_3R, V_4R	RCA

RCA = Right Coronary Artery, LAD = Left Anterior Descending Coronary Artery, Cx = Circumflex Coronary Artery. LV = Lateral Ventricular Artery
* ST segment depression with tall R waves. T wave is inverted initially and then becomes upright.
The sensitivity, specificity and predictive value of the above in localizing infarction is least for occlusions of the RCA and Cx.

The resting ECG does not have sufficient sensitivity to identify patients with non-STEMI, and cardiac biomarkers are necessary to confirm MI.

CARDIAC BIOCHEMICAL MARKERS
(see Fig. 14.5)

Biochemical evidence of ischaemia should be considered as evidence of myocardial infarction and necrosis.[8] The typical rise and fall of cardiac markers after infarction is shown in Fig. 14.5.

TROPONINS (CTN)
Two (cTnT, cTnI) of the three isoforms of the cTn complex are exclusively expressed in cardiac myocytes (*specific*). Troponin levels allow early and sensitive detection of myocardial necrosis.

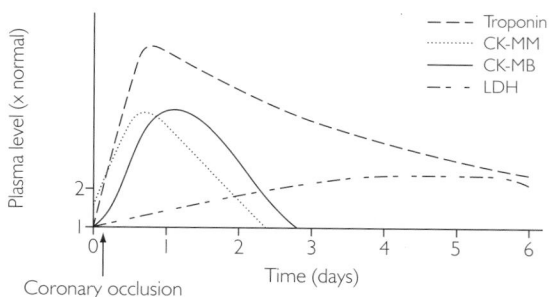

Fig. 14.5 Serum biochemical marker changes after acute myocardial infarction. The sensitivity and specificity of cardiac troponins makes them useful for the early diagnosis of MI. Their delayed fall may allow diagnosis where presentation is late. CK or CK-MB are useful if re-infarction with secondary enzyme rise is queried. Myoglobin (not shown) may prove to be a clinically useful marker.

- They are more sensitive indicators than creatine kinase (CK) and its CK-MB isomer. Up to 20–40% of patients with ACS and normal CK-MB may have elevated cTn levels, indicating 'minor' myocardial damage. Up to a third of patients previously considered to have unstable angina are now found to have evidence of myocardial necrosis.
- Their specificity is better than CK and similar to that of CK-MB. They do not differentiate the cause of the myocardial injury (e.g. ischaemia, myocarditis, trauma) and thus clinical context must always be considered.
- Their levels rise slightly earlier than CK and CK-MB.
- They are more persistent in serum (remain elevated for 7–10 days) and useful for diagnosis when presentation is late.
- They are less useful for determination of re-infarction or infarct extension – a shorter lasting biomarker such as CK or CK-MB should be measured serially.
- They are useful in risk stratification and guiding therapy. There is a continuous relationship between minimal myocardial damage characterized solely by elevation of cTn (with normal CK and CK-MB), through to extensive MI with elevated cTn and very high CK, characterized by complications such as heart failure or shock.[8]

CREATINE KINASE

- Will miss small amounts of necrosis. If negative measure cTn.
- Serial measurements of CK are useful for monitoring the course of established MI.

All biomarkers may rise following successful thrombolysis.

ECHOCARDIOGRAPHY

Echocardiography detects regional wall motion abnormalities, which can help confirm the diagnosis of MI. Regional wall motion abnormality and loss of wall thickening with contraction often precede overt ECG changes, while its absence suggests that ischaemia is not significant. It is useful for excluding differential diagnoses (e.g. aortic dissection or pericardial effusions).

Echocardiography is useful to:

- diagnose infarction, for example, where there is left bundle branch block (LBBB) or non-diagnostic ECG changes and the cause of biomarker elevation is uncertain;
- assess MI size, if thrombolysis has interfered with biomarker measurement;
- diagnose RV infarction and infarct extension;
- manage the infarction, by bedside assessment of LV function;
- diagnose specific complications, for example, mitral regurgitation, pericardial effusion and myocardial rupture, including VSD formation.

Transoesophageal echocardiography may have an increasing role in the therapy of cardiogenic shock, giving some guide to volume therapy.

Dynamic or graded intravenous dobutamine stress echocardiography (2–10 days after MI) can assess myocardial viability and distinguish non-viable myocardium from stunned myocardium.[11] Superiority to standard exercise testing has not been proven.

RADIONUCLIDE STUDIES

Radionuclide angiography, perfusion scintigraphy, infarct-avid scintigraphy and positron emission tomography can all be used to help diagnose the presence and size of MI. A technetium pyrophosphate uptake 'hotspot' scan of the myocardium can be helpful in detecting myocardial necrosis if the diagnosis is uncertain (e.g. LBBB) or if presentation is delayed many days. These scans are best-performed 24–72 hours post-infarction.

Dynamic or functional radionuclide studies (myocardial perfusion imaging studies) are also useful in post-infarction risk stratification and are able to detect 'threatened myocardium'.

STRESS TESTING

Stress testing may be useful in risk stratification and diagnosis of stable angina. After infarction, the following may be of use.

- Submaximal stress testing (to a heart rate of ≈120 bpm), pre-discharge, upon patients with an uncomplicated course.
- Maximal symptom limited stress test 3–6 weeks post-infarction

CORONARY ANGIOGRAPHY AND LEFT VENTRICULOGRAPHY.

In the appropriate clinical setting, coronary angiography will usually identify a culprit artery subtending an area of regional wall motion abnormality. These investigations are reserved for high-risk patients in whom percutaneous transluminal coronary angioplasty (PTCA) or urgent grafting is proposed to re-establish flow to the infarcted myocardium.

RISK STRATIFICATION OF CHEST PAIN AND TERMINOLOGY (See Fig. 14.6.)

In patients with ACS, early ECGs will allow stratification to those with:

(a) **ST-segment elevation (or new, presumed new, LBBB)** with persistent pain. Later development of non-resolving ST elevation should also be stratified to this group. This indicates complete occlusion of a

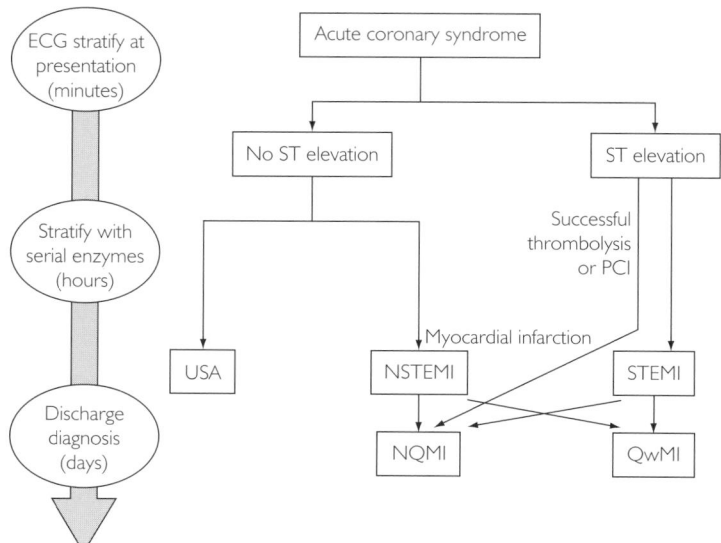

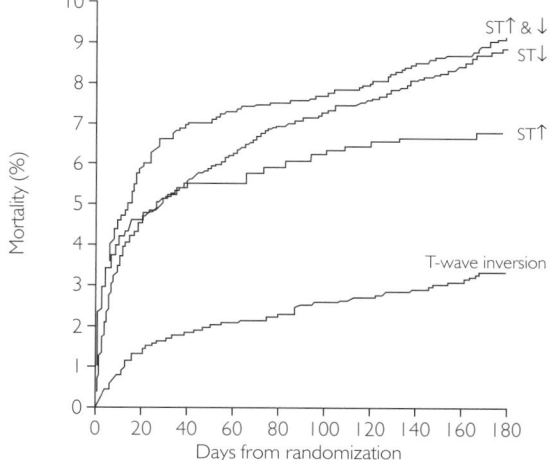

Fig. 14.6 Immediate stratification of ACS into those with and without ST segment elevation identifies patients requiring thrombolysis. Early and serial biomarker results in patients without ST segment elevation identify those with USA (normal levels) and those with NSTEMI (elevated levels). Later ECG review identifies patients who have sustained Qwave myocardial infarction (QwMI) and nonQwave myocardial infarction (NQWMI). Successful reperfusion therapy may avert of limit the extent of Q wave development.

coronary artery (>90% of patients); an indication for urgent reperfusion therapy.

(b) **No ST-segment elevation**. Patients have ischaemic chest pain but have 'non-specific' ECG changes (normal, ST depression, T-wave inversion). After later serial biomarker testing, these patients will prove to have either (i) unstable angina pectoris if biochemical markers remain normal, or (ii) non-STEMI (non-ST-segment elevation myocardial infarction) if they develop a significant rise of cTn (± elevation of CK).

Interventional strategies and treatments for both are similar and are directed at platelet inactivation and symptom control. Thrombolytic therapy is not beneficial in this group and produces worse outcomes.

Figure 14.7 displays the incidence of major coronary events over the following 6 months in patients presenting with and without ST-segment elevation. ST-segment depression has lesser early mortality but a higher mortality at 6 months and at 10 years than those presenting with ST-segment elevation.[12,13]. Features which correlate with risk are:

- Refractory angina with ischaemic ECG changes;
- Ischaemia associated with haemodynamic instability or arrhythmia;
- Recurrent ST-segment change with elevated cTn levels.

(c) **Q wave (QwMI) or non-Q wave (NqwMI) myocardial infarction**. The 10-year mortality of NqwMI (70%) is 10% higher than that of QwMI.[13] Early diagnostic classifications using both ECGs and troponins allow early risk stratification and evidence-based therapy. They recognize that unsta-

Fig. 14.7 Six-month mortality among patients with an acute coronary syndrome by presentation ECG. Although patients with ST-segment depression (ST↓) have a better early (5 day) survival than those with ST-segment elevation (ST↑), their long-term outlook is as bad, if not worse. **Reprinted with permission from Fitchett.**[14]

ble angina and MI are often clinically indistinguishable at presentation.

IMMEDIATE MANAGEMENT OF ACS

PRE-HOSPITAL CARE

About 50% of deaths from MI occur within the first hour of onset of symptoms. These deaths are usually due to ventricular fibrillation (VF). Treatment is defibrillation.

Thrombolytic therapy should be given as early as possible after hospital arrival. Meta-analysis of pre-hospital thrombolysis trials found a 17% decrease (95% CI, 2–29%) in 30-day mortality.[14a]

IMMEDIATE HOSPITAL CARE

1   Cardiac monitoring.
2   Oxygen via facemask (6–8 l/min).
3   ECG (12-lead) should be taken within 5 minutes of arrival.
4   Aspirin at 160–325 mg should be chewed and swallowed on arrival.[15]
5   Sublingual nitroglycerin (GTN) may have beneficial effects. Side-effects include hypotensive reactions and a hypotensive bradycardic response (the Bezold–Jarisch reflex).
6   Venous access is usually established.
7   Pain relief should be provided. Pain produces catecholamines which increase ischaemia. GTN, reassurance, and small incremental boluses (1–2 mg) of morphine, repeated until pain is relieved, can be given.
8   Thrombolytic therapy should be considered for all those patients with ST-segment elevation or presumed new LBBB (STEMI) who have no major contraindication (see Table 14.4.) and arrive within clinical timeframes.
9   Emergent angioplasty (or rapid transfer to a centre capable of this) should be considered for patients with:

   ● contraindication to thrombolytic therapy
   ● cardiogenic shock.
   ● high risk (e.g. previous CABG, early presentation of large anterior MI) in specialist cardiological units.

Table 14.4   Typical Indications for thrombolytic therapy in AMI

Thrombolytic therapy.
Presentation ≤ 12 hours with ACS, unrelieved by GTN and:

● ST segment elevation in 2 or more contiguous leads >0.2 mm in chest leads ($V_2 - V_6$),
   Or >0.1 mm in limb leads (I, aVL, II, III, aVF)   **OR**

● New-onset LBBB (include presumed new-onset)   **OR**

● Posterior infarction (Dominant R wave and ST depression ≥ 2 mm in $V_1 - V_2$)   **OR**

● Presentation 12–24 hours after onset of ACS with continuing pain and evidence of evolving infarction

10   β-adrenergic blockers should be commenced as soon as possible (usually after thrombolytic therapy) has been given.
11   Pulmonary oedema if present is treated with upright posture, intravenous furosemide (40 mg (frusemide) i.v.), GTN or i.v. nitrates and if severe, with CPAP.
12   Prophylactic anti-arrhythmics are *not* administered.

ACUTE MANAGEMENT OF STEMI
(See Fig. 14.8.)

REPERFUSION THERAPY

Reperfusion therapy should be considered for all patients presenting within 12 hours after the onset of STEMI.[16] Indications are given in Table 14.4. Restoration of patency reduces infarct size, preserves LV function, reduces mortality and prolongs survival.

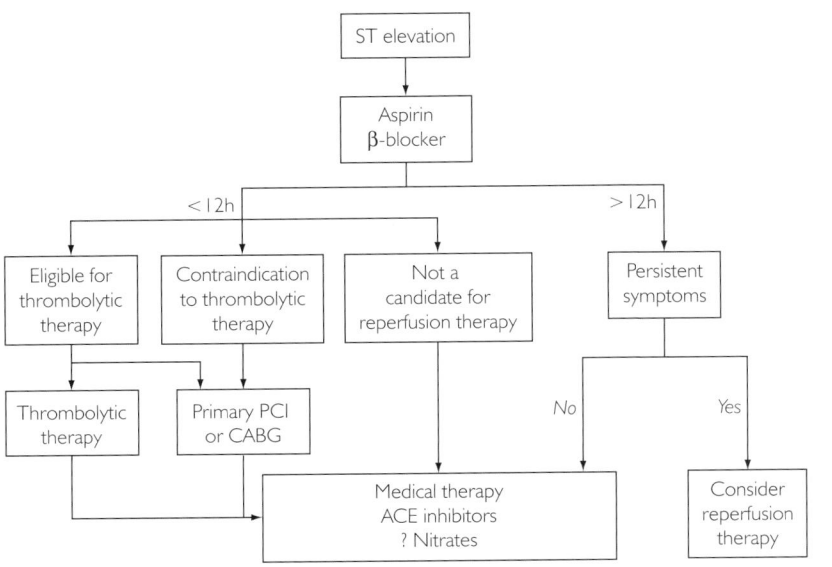

Fig. 14.8   Management of ACS with ST Segment Elevation (STEMI). Aspirin, β-blockers and a heparin (except if Streptokinase used) should be given to all patients without contraindications. Immediate reperfusion with thrombolysis (available in all centers) or with PCI (if in an expert center) should be commenced. Immediate PCI is the treatment of choice when thrombolysis is contraindicated. IV GPIIb/IIIa blockade may reduce complications during PCI. **Modified from Ryan with permission[6]**

Strategies to achieve reperfusion can include:

- fibrinolytic (thrombolytic) therapy
- percutaneous transluminal coronary interventions (PCI) e.g. angioplasty
- urgent surgery and coronary artery bypass graft.

Factors that influence treatment choice and outcome are[6,16]:

- skill and expertise of admitting hospital,
- time since onset of symptoms,
- patient age,
- comorbid illness (particularly risk of bleeding and stroke;
- previous surgery,
- haemodynamic status.

THROMBOLYSIS

A goal is 'door to needle time' of less than 30 minutes. Delay is associated with excess mortality.

Mortality. Reduction in death rate at 35 days of about 21% (reduction of approximately 20 deaths per 1000 patients treated).[6,16]

Table 14.5 Typical contraindications to thrombolytic therapy.

Absolute.

- Previous haemorrhagic stroke:
- Other stroke or cerebrovascular accident ≤ 6 months.
- Intracranial neoplasm.
- Active internal bleeding ≤ 2 weeks. (menses excluded)
- Aortic dissection, known or suspected.

Relative Contraindications. (Advisory following clinical consideration)

- Severe uncontrolled hypertension on presentation (≥ 180/110 mmHg)
- Oral anticoagulation therapy (INR > 2.5); known bleeding diathesis.
- Recent major trauma, surgery (≤ 4 weeks) including head trauma.
- Pregnancy
- Traumatic CPR
- Active peptic ulcer disease
- Previous allergic reaction to drug to be used
- Recent Streptokinase or Anistreplase (≤ 5 days). Use different agent (risk of allergy, antibodies may reduce effectiveness)
- History of prior CVA or intracerebral pathology not covered in contraindications.
- History of chronic hypertension

Specialist opinion should be sought urgently where doubt exists. Patients with contraindications may still benefit from urgent coronary angioplasty.

Effect of timing. Meta-analysis suggests that if thrombolysis could be administered within 6 hours, 30 lives per 1000 patients treated would be saved rates decreasing with delay.[6,16]

Age. Mortality reduction from 22% in patients <55 years of age; to 16% (age 65–74 years) to 4% for patients ≥75 years.[6,16] In the elderly, there is a high incidence of relative risk factors, such as stroke (Table 14.5).

THROMBOLYTIC AGENTS (FIBRINOLYTIC AGENTS)

Streptokinase (SK) and anistreplase (anisoylated plasminogen streptokinase activator complex, or APSAC) are first generation fibrinolytic drugs. They induce a 'lytic' state by generating plasmin and are considered 'non-specific' and offer:

- slightly lower efficacy
- less cerebral haemorrhage and bleeding.
- anaphylaxis and hypotension, which may complicate SK use. Hypotension is managed by temporary interruption of infusion, supine positioning and if necessary, elevation of the legs. Volume expansion and occasionally atropine may be indicated. Hydrocortisone is not required.

Second generation fibrinolytic agents (e.g. alteplase; recominant t-PA or rt-PA) are engineered from tissue plasminogen activator (tPA), a naturally occurring substance produced by vascular endothelium.

- They are more fibrin-specific than SK, act more directly at the fibrin surface and degrade less circulating fibrinogen.
- They are less antigenic.
- Weight adjusted, accelerated regimens of rt-PA produce better vessel patency rates than SK. In the GUSTO trial, r-TPA mortality (6.9%) was 14% lower than SK mortality (7.8%), saving an estimated 10 additional survivors per 1000 patients treated.[17]

Third generation fibrinolytic agents are in evolution and are bioengineered products of t-PA with longer half-lives. It is hoped that they will be more fibrin specific, produce more rapid clot lysis and be associated with less bleeding. They may be given by simple bolus injection. Reteplase (r-PA), tenecteplase and lanetoplase have been studied.

Major and minor contraindications are shown in Table 14.5.

SIDE-EFFECTS AND CHOICE OF AGENT

Benefit is confined to ACS with ST-segment elevation or new LBBB. Worsened outcomes are achieved if routinely administered to patients with unstable angina or non-STEMI.

A reasonable approach is shown in Fig. 14.9 although many cardiologists now routinely use second and third generation agents for all patients.

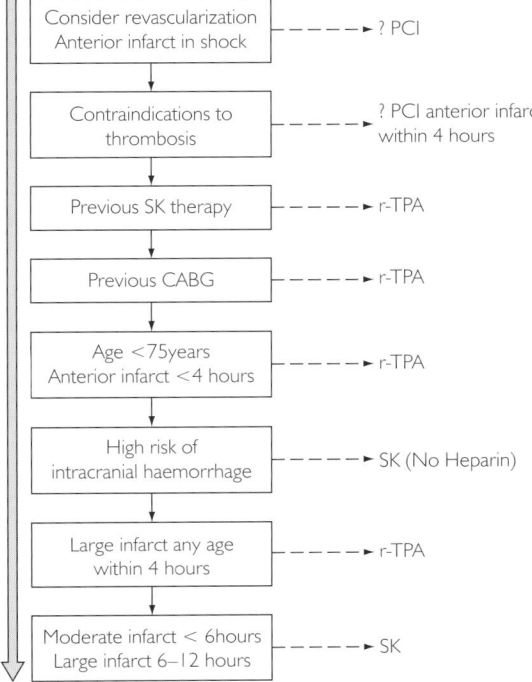

Choice of thrombolytic for ST elevation ACS

- Consider revascularization Anterior infarct in shock — — — — ► ? PCI
- Contraindications to thrombosis — — — — ► ? PCI anterior infarct within 4 hours
- Previous SK therapy — — — — ► r-TPA
- Previous CABG — — — — ► r-TPA
- Age <75years Anterior infarct <4 hours — — — — ► r-TPA
- High risk of intracranial haemorrhage — — — — ► SK (No Heparin)
- Large infarct any age within 4 hours — — — — ► r-TPA
- Moderate infarct < 6hours Large infarct 6–12 hours — — — — ► SK

Fig. 14.9 A strategy for the choice of reperfusion therapy in ST Elevation ACS. **Modified from Granger (with permission)**[49]

- 'Aggressive' thrombolysis regimens are associated with lower mortality but higher rates of cerebral haemorrhage[6,16] that are fatal in 40–60% of cases.[18]
- Severe disability occurs in ≈ 50% of non-fatal cerebral haemorrhages.[6,18]
- Of those treated with t-PA, 5 disabled stroke survivors per 1000 patients; SK with subcutaneous heparin, 3 per 1000 patients treated.[18]

SK has a lower rate of bleeding and cerebral haemorrhage[6] and so may be used in selected groups of patients such as the elderly, 'smaller' MI or thrombolysis beyond 6 hours.

Age, recent stroke and hypertension on arrival significantly increase the risk of both lethal and non-lethal stroke:

1 Patients for whom t-PA is superior to SK[17,19]:
   – anterior MI (up to 10 extra lives saved per 1000 patients treated).
   – complicated inferior MI
   – previous bypass grafting
   – SK allergy or previous SK treatment.
2 Patients for whom either t-PA or SK may be used:
   – non-anterior MI, which is uncomplicated

3 Patients in whom SK may be preferred to t-PA:
   – age >75 years
   – thrombolysis beyond 6 hours.

TREATMENT OF BLEEDING COMPLICATIONS FOLLOWING THROMBOLYSIS

Most bleeding is mild and easily controlled by simple procedures, such as pressure and volume infusion. Fibrinolytic infusions and heparin should be ceased where bleeding is severe. Surgery may be required in some cases to control bleeding vascular access sites. Therapy should be guided by repeated monitoring of coagulation studies and clinical context:

REVERSAL OF HEPARIN

(a) 1 mg protamine is usually given for every 80–100 units of heparin administered within the preceding 4 hours. Monitor activated partial thromboplastin time (APTT).

(b) 1 mg protamine neutralizes 100 IU Fragmin or 1 mg Clexane induced elevation of APTT and thrombin time, but only partially neutralizes the effect on factor Xa. The latter cannot be neutralized by increasing the dose of protamine.

- Consider cryoprecipitate 10 units (each unit contains ~200–250 mg fibrinogen and 80 units of factor VIII). Aim for fibrinogen >1.0 g/l. Repeat if necessary.
- Give 2–4 units FFP where uncontrolled and repeat as necessary.
- Correct blood loss with packed cells or fresh whole blood.
- Give platelet transfusions (aliquots of 6–12 units) where platelet defect suspected or proven.

If these are unsuccessful and bleeding is immediately life-threatening, consider:

ε-Amino-caproic acid (EACA) 5 g (or 0.1 g/kg) i.v. infused over 30–60 min. Infuse 0.5–1 g/h for 8 h or until bleeding has been controlled. Total dose in 24 h to be <30 g.

aprotonin (intravenous).

Both aprotinin and EACA are thought to increase the risk of coronary re-thrombosis. While they prevent further fibrinolysis, they do not correct they hypocoagulable state that is the immediate cause of bleeding.

PRIMARY PERCUTANEOUS TRANSLUMINAL CORONARY INTERVENTION (PCI)

Urgent coronary angioplasty offers advantages of more definitive treatment of coronary stenosis and better rates of arterial 're-opening' with lesser risk of cerebral haemorrhage.

Urgent PCI in STEMI should be considered in:

- patients with contraindications to thrombolysis
- patients with cardiogenic shock[20] within 36 hours of infarction. (see Ch. 18)
- patients presenting to cardiological centres for PTCA
- failed thrombolysis
- the elderly[21]
- diabetics – require caution with contrast use.

In centres of excellence with skilled operators and 'door to PTCA time' <90 minutes, results exceeding those of thrombolysis have been achieved.[21] Improved outcomes may reflect true advantage or better adjunctive care at such 'teaching' centres.[22] Randomized trial comparison is not yet available. Very few patients have contraindications to PCI although caution is needed in those at risk of contrast associated renal failure.

ADJUNCTIVE THERAPY USED WITH THROMBOLYSIS AND REPERFUSION
(see Fig. 14.10)

Adjunctive therapy is necessary after thrombolysis due to the following.

- About 50% of patients fail to obtain or sustain coronary artery patency.
- The underlying artery remains unstable, evidenced by:
  - angiographic re-occlusion in 30% of cases
  - recurrence of ischaemia in 20% of cases.
- Current plasminogen activators ('thrombolytics') destroy fibrin strands of 'red thrombus'. They have little effect on underlying exposed thrombin and indeed may be 'pro-thrombotic', requiring concomitant heparin (anti-thrombin) therapy.
- Anti-platelet therapy will 'pacify' underlying platelet rich 'white thrombus'

Note, however, that synergistic therapy carries the risk of increasing bleeding.

ASPIRIN
Aspirin given acutely in the ISIS-2 trial reduced mortality by 23%.[15] Streptokinase also reduced mortality (by 25%), while the combination had an additive effect and reduced mortality by 42%.[23-25] It does not appear to increase bleeding and the benefit is still present after 10 years. Aspirin should be given as soon as possible after the diagnosis of MI or ACS.

UNFRACTIONATED HEPARIN (UFH, STANDARD) AND LOW-MOLECULAR-WEIGHT HEPARIN (LMWH)

LMWHs are produced by chemical or enzymatic depolymerization of UFH. Their theoretical advantages include:

- Predictable, consistent pharmacokinetic profiles and anticoagulant response;
- Enhanced anti-Xa activity and are less affected by platelet factors;
- Weight adjusted dosing and do not require APTT monitoring;
- Convenient to administer and do not require an i.v. line, although acquisition costs are higher than for UFH

Early treatment of acute myocardial infarction

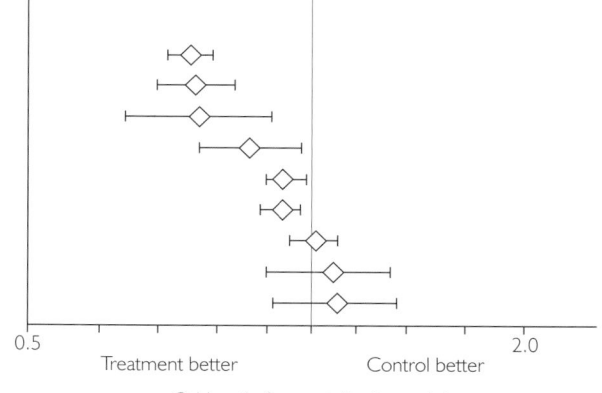

Acute intervention	Patients (n)	RCTs (n)
i.v. thrombolytics	58 600	9
Aspirin	18 773	9
Anticoagulant	4 075	7
β-blocker	28 970	29
Nitrates	81 908	22
ACE inhibitors	100 963	15
Magnesium	60 366	2
Prophylactic lignocaine	12 385	21
Calcium antagonists	6 420	16

Fig. 14.10   Effect of acute interventions upon mortality following acute myocardial infarction. Results are from meta-analyses of trials.

- Lower incidence of thrombocytopenia, skin necrosis, hypersensitivity reactions and catheter related infections.

Heparins do not lyse clot, but decrease re-thrombosis. In 'pre-thrombolysis' trials, heparin reduced mortality from 13.1 to 9.2% (20–25% relative reduction).[26] In the post-thrombolysis and aspirin era, the effect of heparins is significant but more modest.[25] Heparins administered with t-PA produce the best vessel patency rates and a small survival benefit over streptokinase.

Heparin is usually administered for 24–48 hours after alteplase, reteplase or tenecteplase. Enoxaparin (a LMWH) or UFH given in combination with t-PA have similar safety profiles and outcomes.[27] Streptokinase has a prolonged anti-thrombolytic effect and concomitant i.v. heparin increases bleeding and cerebral haemorrhage without improving survival.[6,8,25] The ASSENT III trial confirmed the efficacy and safety of enoxaparin with single bolus dose of tenecteplase,[28] a very convenient regimen.

Complications: In the GUSTO-I trial, 1.8% of patients had severe bleeding (intracranial haemorrhage, haemodynamic compromise),[17] and 11.4% of patients had moderate haemorrhage (requiring transfusion). Vigilant APTT monitoring is always required. Weight-adjusted dosing may lessen bleeding.

GLYCOPROTEIN IIB/IIIA INHIBITORS

In theory; these agents override the platelet activation caused by plasminogen activators, improving patency rates and allowing better reperfusion of small vessels beyond the occluding thrombus. They have an important role following acute interventions such as PTCA and coronary artery stenting but their role after STEMI is only evolving.

β-BLOCKERS

Given at the time of MI and continued orally, β-blockers have an early and significant effect on mortality, apparent at 7 days.[29] All patients without contraindications (pulmonary oedema, asthma, hypotension, bradycardia, advanced atrioventricular block) should be treated with β-blockers within 24 hours of the onset of symptoms.

COMPLICATIONS OF MI

ARRHYTHMIAS

Rhythm disturbance occurs in nearly all patients following acute MI and is most likely within the first few hours of onset and during reperfusion. There has been a decline in the incidence of VF from approximately 4.5% of admissions to 1% of admissions with MI. This decrease probably reflects the effect of thrombolytic therapies and better maintenance of electrolytes.

Correct hypoxia, hypovolaemia or acid–base disturbances. Maintain serum potassium levels in the normal range (4.0–5.0 mmol/l).

Maintain the serum magnesium level.

Prophylactic lignocaine tends to increased mortality and is thus reserved for the treatment of VT and VF. Prophylactic intravenous magnesium (<4 h) was of benefit in the LIMIT II study but not in the ISIS-4 trial[30] and is not recommended.

CARDIAC FAILURE

With large MI there is progressive thinning of the affected myocardium, with stretching and dilatation of the ventricle, and sometimes frank aneurysm formation. ACE inhibitors appear to limit dilatation, preserve LV function and improve prognosis. Benefits are maximal in those with poor LV function. ACE inhibitors are thus recommended for all patients with significant LV dysfunction and are usually started early following MI. Captopril has a short half-life and may be started at very small doses (3–6.25 mg t.d.s) if the systolic blood pressure is >100 mmHg (13.3 kPa). Lower starting doses may be considered (e.g. 1 mg t.d.s.) in hypotensive but otherwise stable patients. The dose is titrated upwards and a longer acting agent may be substituted prior to discharge.

RV failure secondary to RV infarction should be distinguished from RV failure secondary to LV failure and should be considered in any patient with inferior MI. These patients have a markedly elevated jugular venous pressure with little or no pulmonary congestion. Patients with RV infarction often respond to volume loading. The latter is guided by clinical response, echocardiography or by the use of a pulmonary flotation catheter, seeking to maintain an optimal LV filling pressure at around 16–18 mmHg (2.1–2.4 kPa). Diuretic therapy, afterload reduction and unrecognized hypovolaemia may aggravate hypotension and renal insufficiency in these patients.

CARDIOGENIC SHOCK

Mortality from cardiogenic shock remains very high (55–70%)[31] and is the major cause of hospital mortality from STEMI. Survival at 12 months appears improved when patients presenting with cardiogenic shock are treated with acute interventional revascularization (PCI or CABG) rather than thrombolysis and medical management.[20]

POST-INFARCTION ANGINA AND RE-INFARCTION

Post-infarction angina unresponsive to medical therapy or with significant ECG changes is an indication for aggressive anti-ischaemic therapy and early PCI. Reinfarction in the 10 days following MI occurs in up to 5–10%; can be treated with further thrombolysis or angioplasty. Where streptokinase has previously been given, t-PA is preferred because of the possible presence of antibiodies which may netralize activity or cause anaphylaxis.

CARDIAC RUPTURE

Transient mitral valve dysfunction is common after MI. More severe rupture of the papillary muscles and severe mitral regurgitation occurs in about 4% of patients.

- It can complicate even relatively small MI.
- Consider diagnosis when heart failure is disproportionate to the size of the infarction, even if a significant murmur cannot be heard.
- Surgery after medical stabilization is usually required.

Rupture of the interventricular septum occurs in about 1–2% of cases of MI, usually in large infarctions (60% of cases).

- It is often heralded by a new systolic murmur, which initially may be soft or absent and the patient may not be haemodynamically compromised.
- Diagnosis is best made by echocardiography.
- Almost always there is progressive clinical deterioration.
- Surgical repair is considered as soon as the diagnosis is made; intra-aortic balloon counter pulsation often provides a bridge to surgery.

Free wall rupture occurs in 1–3% of all hospitalized patients with MI and often occurs very early.

- Acute rupture of the LV free wall is usually catastrophic resulting in PEA.
- Subacute rupture (leaking blood is contained by pericardium forming a false aneurysm) is less common but requires urgent surgery.
- Chest pain, ST-segment change and haemodynamic deterioration may mimic re-infarction.

Thromboembolism

Embolic stroke occurs in approximately 1–3% of patients, most of these occurring following extensive anterior myocardial infarction.[32]
30–40% of anterior Q-wave MIs may be complicated by mural thrombus (echocardiography)
5–10% of these may undergo embolization, usually within the first 10 days.
Embolization is uncommon following inferior infarction.

Management

- The patient is usually put on anticoagulation therapy for 3 months for extensive anterior regional wall motion abnormality, or if mural thrombus is proven.
- The patient isusually treated with heparin, then discharged on warfarin.

- Extensive anterior wall motion abnormality is best confirmed proven by echocardiography, or instead may be presumed where CK > 1000 U/l (in the absence of thrombolysis)
- Patients with poor LV function remain at long-term risk of embolic stroke.[32]

POST-MI INJURY SYNDROME (DRESSLER'S SYNDROME) AND PERICARDITIS

Pericarditis is a common early complication of extensive anterior and inferior infarction.

- Pericardial rub may be heard in 10–15% of patients with anterior MI, less often with inferior MI.
- It occurs 24–72 hours after infarction and may mimic ischaemia
- It is best treated with high dose aspirin or NSAIDs.

Dressler's syndrome is now uncommon but is thought to be an immunopathic response to myocardial necrosis. It is characterized by fever, elevated ESR, a pericardial rub, pleuro-pericardial pain and arthralgia and may occur some weeks after MI.

ONGOING AND DISCHARGE CARE (SECONDARY PREVENTION)
(see Fig. 14 11)

A number of therapies have been studied in the long-term (secondary) treatment of MI (see Fig. 14.7.)

1 **Aspirin** at 75–160 mg daily should be continued unless there are strong contraindications.[23] In the first 2 years after MI, aspirin therapy results in an absolute decrease of approximately 36 vascular events (vascular death or non-fatal MI or stroke) for every 1000 patients treated.[24]

2 **β-blockers** significantly reduce the incidence of sudden and non-sudden cardiac death in survivors of MI.[33] Benefit is prolonged and is most marked in high-risk patients, for example, those with extensive anterior infarction.

3 **ACE inhibitors** significantly reduce mortality in high-risk patients when commenced during recovery from MI. Patients with anterior MI and Ejection Fraction <40% maintained on long term ACE inhibitor therapy, may experience a 20% relative reduction in mortality[34,35] and a significant reduction in the incidence of LVF. Benefit is still seen at 4 years post treatment.[34] Benefit is more modest in lower risk groups. Very early introduction of ACE inhibitors (within 36 hours of infarction) may also reduce mortality (7% relative reduction at 30 days).[36]

4 **Lipid lowering agents** given for elevated cholesterol concentrations after MI results in a decrease in mortality and re-infarction.

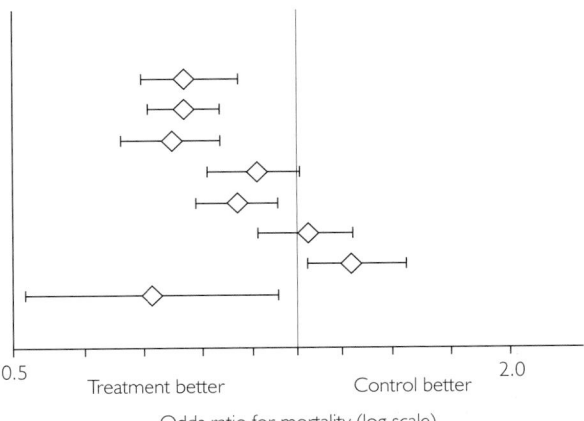

Late interventions in acute myocardial infarction

Late intervention	Patients (n)	RCTs (n)
Anticoagulant	10056	16
β-blockers	24298	26
ACE inhibitors	3966	3
Anti platelet agents	18411	10
Cholesterol reduction	10775	8
Calcium antagonists	13114	6
Class I anti-arrhythmics	6300	18
Amiodarone	1557	9

Fig. 14.11 Effect of long term therapy upon mortality following acute myocardial infarction. Results of meta-analyses of trials.[26,29,34,39] Beneficial effects of ACE inhibitors shown were achieved in patients with poor LV function. Lipid lowering therapy (not shown) also favourable decreases mortality.[47]

5 Other anti-ischaemic agents

- Nitrates may be continued where angina is refractory to ß-blockade.
- Routine use of calcium antagonists does not improve outcome.
- Agents that increase heart rate (e.g. dihydropyridines) may increase death and re-infarction.
- Agents that reduce heart rate (verapamil, diltiazem) have a neutral effect on mortality but may reduce re-infarction rates.[37]

6 Anti-arrhythmic therapy

is not routinely continued. The CAST study revealed higher mortality[38] with use of prophylactic flecainide, even though it reduced ventricular ectopy. Amiodarone in low doses (200 mg daily) may reduce mortality, but results of definitive trials are awaited and it has significant side-effects. It cannot currently be recommended as routine therapy.

7 Warfarin

is given to patients with large anterior infarction or with suspected or demonstrated thrombus. High dose regimens have been proven better than control for decreasing reinfarction, stroke and mortality after MI.[39] Moderate and high dose regimens have given outcomes comparable to but not superior to aspirin.[39]

8 Lifestyle advice

is most important and all patients should cease smoking and receive advice on exercise and diet.

MANAGEMENT OF UNSTABLE ANGINA AND NON-STEMI (See Figs 14.12 and 14.13.)

Non-ST-segment elevation ACS usually results from the development of non-occluding thrombus upon

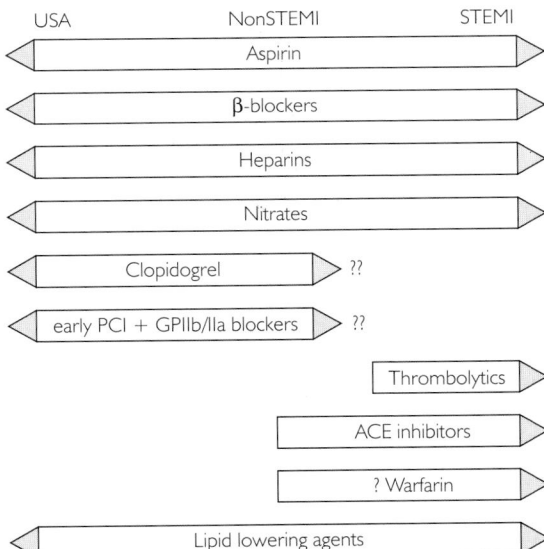

Acute coronary syndromes

Fig. 14.12 Overview of current ACS therapies. Differential benefit may occur in different groups of patients. **Modified with permission from Braunwald Atlas of Cardiology.**

unstable plaque. Superimposed vasospasm and micro-embolization may aggravate myocardial ischaemia. Therapies are directed at plaque stabilization and at reducing myocardial oxygen demand.

The immediate relief of symptoms requires anti-ischaemic therapy while prevention of complete artery

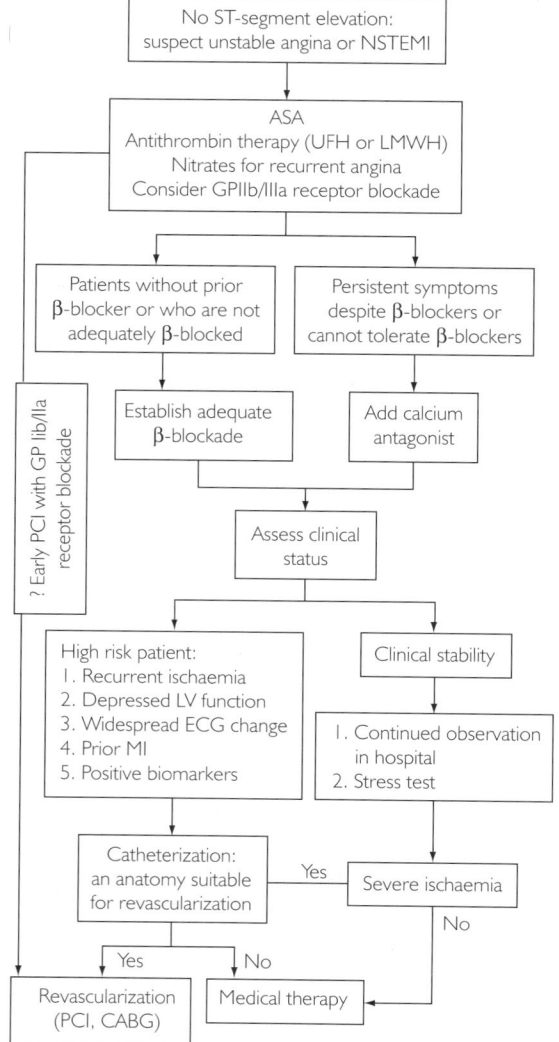

Fig. 14.13 Management ACS without ST segment Elevation. Aspirin, heparin and beta-blockers are administered to all without contraindications, nitrates being given for symptom control. Patients at intermediate or high risk may have best outcomes following early PCI with intravenous GPIIb/IIIa Receptor blockade. Patients who stabilize may be treated medically followed by stress testing to screen for inducible myocardial ischaemia. **Modified from Ryan (AHA Guidelines with permission)[6]**

occlusion requires anti-thrombotic therapy, stabilization of plaque and increasingly, acute revascularization.

ANTI-ISCHAEMIC AGENTS

1 **β-blockers** provide good symptom control. Intravenous therapy is recommended for high-risk patients (e.g. ongoing pain) without contraindications to

therapy. In these patients, metoprolol at 5 mg i.v. is commonly given incrementally every 5 min until symptoms are relieved, side effects are experienced or a dose of 15 mg is reached.

2 **Nitrates.** Sublingual nitroglycerin 300–600 μg is usually given in 2 doses, at least some minutes apart (monitoring blood pressure), to relieve ischaemic pain. Patients with ongoing pain may receive intravenous nitrates.

3 **Calcium-channel blockers** may provide symptom relief when there are problems with β-blockers and nitrates. They may have a neutral or negative effect on mortality and progression to MI.[40,41] Nifedipine without concomitant beta-blocker may increase mortality (HINT).[42] As sole agent, only those agents that reduce heart rate should be used (e.g. diltiazem or verapamil).

ANTI-THROMBOTIC THERAPY

1 **Aspirin** should be given immediately and continued long term in all ACS patients unless there is a clear contraindication.[32] It decreases death or non-fatal MI in patients with unstable angina by approximately 50%.[23,24]

2 **Ticlopidine and clopidogrel (thienopyridins)** are second-generation platelet inhibitors acting independently and, theoretically, synergistically to aspirin. Clopidogrel has a better safety profile than ticlopidine. In the CURE trial in patients with unstable angina, clopidogrel administered with aspirin produced a sustained 20% relative mortality reduction compared to aspirin alone.[43] Clopidogrel is especially useful in high-risk patients, in patients undergoing PCI and in patients with aspirin sensitivity.

3 Glycoprotein 11b/111a receptor blockers reduce the 30-day risk of non-fatal MI by 38%[44] in NSTEMI patients undergoing PCI. They have not been shown to be beneficial in the routine managament of 'medically treated' patients (GUSTO-IV-ACS).[45] There are two classes of glycoprotein IIb/IIIa inhibitors: (i) murine monoclonal, for example, abciximab; and (ii) 'small molecule' inhibitors, for example, tirofiban and eptibatide. Platelet infusion may treat significant bleeding in patients receiving abciximab, but not in those receiving more specific blockers (e.g. tirofiban, eptifibatide). Thrombocytopenia may complicate the course of some patients receiving intravenous therapy.

4 **Heparins.** Both UFH and LMWHs reduce the risk of death or MI in patients with unstable angina receiving aspirin.[46] Meta-analysis of trials comparing various LMWHs to UFH found a modest and not significant reduction of the composite of death, MI and need for urgent revascularization.[46] However, despite higher acquisition costs, their simplicity, lack of need for monitoring and acceptable safety profile perhaps favours their administration.

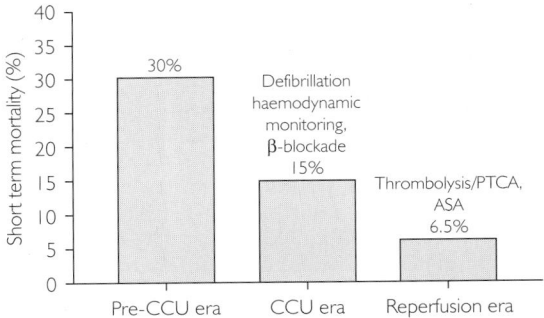

Fig. 14.14 The advent of the coronary care unit era in the early 1960s led to co-ordinated treatment of arrhythmias and of complications. Improvement in survival was continued with the introduction of thrombolysis and trial proven therapies. Better risk stratification, control of risk factors and tailored intervention will hopefully see continued improvement in outcomes. **Modified from Braunwald (with permission)**

5 **Thrombolytic agents** are generally contraindicated in the treatment of Non-ST Elevation ACS; their routine administration is associated with poorer outcome.[47]

ROLE FOR ACUTE INTERVENTIONAL THERAPY IN NON-STEMI

Early PCI now has a clinical role because of the development of better plaque stabilizing agents ('upstream therapy') with proven benefit from glycoprotein IIb/IIIa blockade[48] and LMWH. 'Emergent' PCI may offer even greater clinical benefit[48] and may well be justified in patients with high-risk featues.

OUTCOME OF MI (See Fig. 14.14.)

The in-hospital mortality from acute MI has been steadily decreasing over the past 3 decades from 15 to 30% in the 1970s to approximately 10% in 1980 and now to around 6% in the new millennium. Despite improved mortality, 60% of all deaths occur within the first hour (usually from VF), and usually before reaching a medical facility. Modern management of acute MI has undoubtedly contributed to decreased mortality, but further significant reduction in mortality must come from management strategies within the first hour of the onset of symptoms.

REFERENCES

1 Collins R, Peto R, MacMahon S, *et al*. Blood pressure, stroke, and coronary heart disease. Part 2. Short-term reductions in blood pressure: overview of randomised drug trials in their epidemiological context. *Lancet* 1990; **335**: 827–38.

2 Pocock SJ, McCormack V, Gueyffier F, *et al*. A score for predicting risk of death from cardiovascular disease in adults with raised blood pressure, based on individual patient data from randomised controlled trials. *BMJ* 2001; **323**: 75–81.

3 Davies MJ. The pathophysiology of acute coronary syndromes. *Heart* 2000; **83**: 361–6.

4 Rauch U, Osende JI, Fuster V, *et al*. Thrombus formation on atherosclerotic plaques: pathogenesis and clinical consequences. *Ann Int Med* 2001; **134**: 224–38.

5 Muller DWM, Topol EJ, Califf RM, *et al*. Relationship between antecedent angina pectoris and short-term prognosis after thrombolytic therapy for acute myocardial infarction. Thrombolysis and Angioplasty in Myocardial Infarction (TAMI) Study Group. *Am Heart J* 1990; **119**: 224–31.

6 Ryan TJ, Antman EM, Brooks NH, *et al*. 1999 update: ACC/AHA guidelines for the management of patients with acute myocardial infarction. A report of the American College of Cardiology/American Heart Association Task Force on Practice Guidelines (Committee on Management of Acute Myocardial Infarction). *J Am Col Cardiol* 1999; **34**: 890–911.

7 Menon V, Slater JN, White HD, *et al*. Acute myocardial infarction complicated by systemic hypoperfusion without hypotension: report of the SHOCK trial registry. *Am J Med* 2000; **108**: 374–80.

8 Alpert JS, Thygesen K. Myocardial infarction redefined – a consensus document of The Joint European Society of Cardiology/American College of Cardiology Committee for the redefinition of myocardial infarction. *J Am Coll Cardiol* 2000; **36**: 959–69.

9 Sgarbossa EB, Birnbaum Y, Parrillo JE. Electrocardiographic diagnosis of acute myocardial infarction: Current concepts for the clinician. *Am Heart J* 2001; **141**: 507–17.

10 Haji SA, Movahed A. Right ventricular infarction – diagnosis and treatment. *Clin Cardiol* 2000; **23**: 473–82.

11 Cheitlin MD, Alpert JS, Armstrong WF, *et al*. ACC/AHA Guidelines for the Clinical Application of Echocardiography. A report of the American College of Cardiology/American Heart Association Task Force on Practice Guidelines (Committee on Clinical Application of Echocardiography). Developed in colloboration with the American Society of Echocardiography. *Circulation* 1997; **95**: 1686–744.

12 Klootwijk P, Hamm C. Acute coronary syndromes: diagnosis. *Lancet* 1999; **353**(Suppl 2): 10–15.

13 Herlitz J, Karlson BW, Sjolin M, Lindqvist J. Ten year mortality in subsets of patients with an acute coronary syndrome. *Heart* 2001; **86**: 391–6.

14 Fitchett D, Goodman S, Langer A. New advances in the management of acute coronary syndromes: Matching treatment to risk. *CMAJ* 2001: 164: 1309–16.

14a Morrison LJ, Verbeek PR, McDonald AC, *et al*. Mortality and prehospital thrombolysis for acute myocardial infarction: a meta-analysis. *JAMA* 2000; **283**(20): 2686–92.

15 ISIS-2 (Second International Study of Infarct Survival) Collaborative Group. Randomised trial of intravenous streptokinase, oral aspirin, both, or neither among 17 187 cases of suspected acute myocardial infarction: ISIS-2. *Lancet* 1988; **2**(8607): 349–60.

16 Fibrinolytic Therapy Trialists' (FTT) Collaborative Group. Indications for fibrinolytic therapy in suspected acute myocardial infarction: collaborative overview of early mortality and major morbidity results from all randomised trials of more than 1000 patients. *Lancet* 1994; **343**: 311–22.

17 GUSTO Investigators. An international randomized trial comparing four thrombolytic strategies for acute myocardial infarction. *N Engl J Med* 1993; **329**: 673–82.

18 Gore JM, Granger CB, Simoons ML, *et al.* Stroke after thrombolysis. Mortality and functional outcomes in the GUSTO-1 trial. *Circulation* 1995; **92**: 2811–18.

19 Labinaz M, Sketch MHJr, Ellis SG, *et al.* Outcome of acute ST-segment elevation myocardial infarction in patients with prior coronary artery bypass surgery receiving thrombolytic therapy. *Am Heart J* 2001; **141**: 469–77.

20 Hochman JS, Sleeper LA, White HD, *et al.* One-year survival following early revascularization for cardiogenic shock. SHOCK Investigators.Should we emergently revascularize occluded coronaries for cardiogenic shock? *JAMA* 2001; **285**: 190–2.

21 DeGeare VS, Dangas G, Stone GW, Grines CL. Interventional procedures in acute myocardial infarction. *Am Heart J* 2001; **141**: 15–24.

22 Alter DA, Naylor CD, Austin PC, Tu JV. Long-term MI outcomes at hospitals with or without on-site revascularization. *JAMA* 2001; **285**: 2101–8.

23 Awtry EH, Loscalzo J. Aspirin. *Circulation* 2000; **101**: 1206–18.

24 Antiplatelet Trialists' Collaboration. Collaborative overview of randomised trials of antiplatelet therapy. I: Prevention of death, myocardial infarction, and stroke by prolonged antiplatelet therapy in various categories of patients. *BMJ* 1994; **308**(6921): 81–106.

25 Collins R, Peto R, Baigent C, Sleight P. Aspirin, heparin, and fibrinolytic therapy in suspected acute myocardial infarction. *N Engl J Med* 1997; **336**: 847–60.

26 Antman EM, Lau J, Kupelnick B, *et al.* A comparison of results of meta-analyses of randomized control trials and recommendations of clinical experts. Treatments for myocardial infarction. *JAMA* 1992; **268**: 240–8.

27 Ross AM, Molhoek P, Lundergan C, *et al.* Randomized comparison of Enoxaparin, a Low-Molecular-Weight Heparin, with Unfractionated Heparin adjunctive to Recombinant Tissue Plasminogen Activator thrombolysis and aspirin. *Circulation* 2001; **104**: 648–52.

28 The Assessment of the Safety and Efficacy of a New Thrombolytic Regimen (ASSENT)-3 Investigators. Efficacy and safety of tenecteplase in combination with enoxaparin, abciximab or unfractionated heparin: the ASSENT-3 randomised trial in acute myocardial infarction. *Lancet* 2001; **358**: 605–13.

29 Hennekens CH, Albert CM, Godfried SL, *et al.* Adjunctive drug therapy of acute myocardial infarction – evidence from clinical trials. *N Engl J Med* 1996; **335**: 1660–8.

30 Anonymous, ISIS-4: a randomised factorial trial assessing early oral captopril, oral mononitrate, and intravenous magnesium sulphate in 58 050 patients with suspected acute myocardial infarction. ISIS-4 (Fourth International Study of Infarct Survival) Collaborative Group. *Lancet* 1995; **345**(8951): 669–85.

31 Dauerman HL, Goldberg RJ, Malinski M, *et al.* Outcomes and early revascularization for patients ≥ 65 years of age with cardiogenic shock. *Am J Cardiol* 2001; **87**: 844–8.

32 Cairns JA, Theroux P, Lewis HDJ, *et al.* Antithrombotic agents in coronary artery disease. *Chest* 2001;**119**(1 Suppl): 228S–52S.

33 Roberts R, Rogers WJ, Mueller HS, *et al.* Immediate versus deferred beta-blockade following thrombolytic therapy in patients with acute myocardial infarction. Results of the Thrombolysis in Myocardial Infarction (TIMI) II-B Study. *Circulation.* 1991; **83**: 695–7.

34 Flather MD, Yusuf S, Kober L, *et al.* Long-term ACE-inhibitor therapy in patients with heart failure or left-ventricular dysfunction: a systematic overview of data from individual patients. ACE-Inhibitor Myocardial Infarction Collaborative Group. *Lancet* 2000; **355**: 1575–81.

35 Latini R, Tognoni G, Maggioni AP, *et al.* Clinical effects of early angiotensin-converting enzyme inhibitor treatment for acute myocardial infarction are similar in the presence and absence of aspirin: systematic overview of individual data from 96 712 randomized patients. Angiotensin-converting Enzyme Inhibitor Myocardial Infarction Collaborative Group. *J Am Coll Cardiol* 2000; **35**: 1808–12.

36 ACE Inhibitor Myocardial Infarction Collaborative Group. Indications for ACE inhibitors in the early treatment of acute myocardial infarction: systematic overview of individual data from 100 000 patients in randomized trials. *Circulation* 1998; **97**: 2202–12.

37 Held PH, Yusuf S. Effects of beta-blockers and calcium channel blockers in acute myocardial infarction. *Eur Heart J* 1993; Suppl F: 18–25.

38 Pratt CM, Moye LA. The Cardiac Arrhythmia Suppression Trial: background, interim results and implications. *Am J Cardiol* 1990; **65**: 20B–9B.

39 Anand SS, Yusuf S. Oral anticoagulant therapy in patients with coronary artery disease: a meta-analysis. *JAMA* 1999; **282**: 2058–67.

40 Held PH, Yusuf S, Furberg CD. Calcium channel blockers in acute myocardial infarction and unstable angina: an overview. *BMJ* 1989; **299**(6709): 1187–92.

41 Yusuf S, Wittes J, Friedman L. Overview of results of randomized clinical trials in heart disease. II. Unstable angina, heart failure, primary prevention with aspirin, and risk factor modification. *JAMA* 1988; **260**: 2259–63.

42 Anonymous. Early treatment of unstable angina in the coronary care unit: a randomised, double blind, placebo

controlled comparison of recurrent ischaemia in patients treated with nifedipine or metoprolol or both. Report of The Holland Interuniversity Nifedipine/Metoprolol Trial (HINT) Research Group. *Br Heart J* 1986; **56**: 400–13.

43 The Clopidogrel in Unstable Angina to Prevent Recurrent Events (CURE) Trial Investigators. Effects of Clopidogrel in addition to aspirin in patients with acute coronary syndromes without ST-Segment elevation. *N Engl J Med* 2001; **345**: 494–502.

44 Topol EJ, Moliterno DJ, Herrmann HC, *et al.* Comparison of two platelet glycoprotein IIb/IIIa inhibitors, tirofiban and abciximab, for the prevention of ischemic events with percutaneous coronary revascularization. *N Engl J Med* 2001; **344**: 1888–94.

45 Simoons ML. Effect of glycoprotein IIb/IIIa receptor blocker abciximab on outcome in patients with acute coronary syndromes without early coronary revascularisation: the GUSTO IV-ACS randomised trial. *Lancet* 2001; **357**(9272): 1915–24.

46 Eikelboom JW, Anand SS, Malmberg K, *et al.* Unfractionated heparin and low-molecular-weight heparin in acute coronary syndrome without ST elevation: a meta-analysis. *Lancet* 2000; **355**(9219): 1936–42.

47 Anonymous. Effects of tissue plasminogen activator and a comparison of early invasive and conservative strategies in unstable angina and non-Q-wave myocardial infarction. Results of the TIMI IIIB Trial. The TIMI MB Investigators. *Circulation* 1994; **89**: 1545–56.

48 Cannon CP, Weintraub WS, Demopoulos LA, *et al.* Comparison of early invasive and conservative strategies in patients with unstable coronary syndromes treated with the Glycoprotein IIb/IIIa inhibitor tirofiban. *N Engl J Med* 2001; **344**: 1879–87.

49 Granger CB. Heparin management in acute myocardial infarction (AMI). *Aust NZ J Med* 1998; **28**(4): 541–7.

15

Adult cardiopulmonary resuscitation

R P Lee and P Morley

Cardiac arrest is the cessation of clinically detectable cardiac output. It is unpredictable and rarely occurs with doctors in attendance. The initial rhythm found may be ventricular fibrillation (VF), ventricular tachycardia (VT), asystole or pulseless electrical activity (PEA, previously called electromechanical dissociation). Bystanders need to commence cardiopulmonary resuscitation (CPR) immediately if the victim is to survive. CPR incorporates basic life support (BLS), that is, making use of basic equipment (e.g. pocket mask) and advanced life support (ALS), that is, using advanced equipment, including defibrillator and drugs to treat cardiac arrest.

The 'Chain of Survival'[1] describes the events needed to achieve a good outcome: (i) early access to emergency services; (ii) early bystander CPR; (iii) early defibrillation; and (iv) early ALS.

Comprehensive, internationally-accepted guidelines for CPR[2,3] and symposia detailing the scientific basis for CPR interventions[4–8] have been published recently.

Between 40 and 120 people per 100 000 of the general population will die from cardiac arrest each year.[9]

When CPR is attempted in out-of-hospital cardiac arrest, survival-to-discharge rates vary markedly between communities: in the USA from 2% (New York, Chicago) to 18% (King County). To help under-stand these differences, the epidemiology of cardiac arrest and the effects of interventions, it is important that data are reported uniformly according to the Utstein style.[10,11]

Survival varies 12-fold in subgroups defined by age, type of arrest and place of arrest. Victims below 65 years of age who arrest in acute hospital areas have initial resuscitation rates > 50% and 1-year survival > 30%.[12] Asystole has a dismal outcome, and survival in PEA is < 5% and dependent on finding a reversible cause.

AETIOLOGY

Cardiac arrest may be due to primary cardiac disease or secondary to a systemic problem (Table 15.1). Coronary artery disease (CAD) is the cause in 80% of cases.

The typical patient is male (female : male ratio is 1.5:1), and approximately 65 years of age. In population studies, 65% of arrests occur out of hospital.

Only 20–30% of victims have a clinical acute myo-cardial infarction, but at post-mortem up to 95% will have acute coronary lesions. Spaulding[13] reported find-ings in 1762 arrests: 52% received CPR and 18% achieved initial resuscitation; 11% were admitted to hospital and 84 underwent cardiac investigation, which showed severe CAD in 60.

Table 15.1 Causes of cardiac arrest in adults

Primary cardiac
Ischaemic heart disease
Cardiomyopathy
Coronary spasm
Congenital heart disease, Brugada syndrome, prolonged QT, Wolff–Parkinson–White Syndrome
Secondary
Overdose (tricyclic antidepressant)
Shock: exsanguination (traumatic), anaphylaxis, septic
Hypoxia, hypercarbia (near drowning, narcotic O/D)
Metabolic / electrolyte disturbances
Hypothermia
Electrocution

Table 15.2 Causes of cardiac arrest in adolescents

• **Congenital heart disease**
Fallot's tetralogy
Eisenmenger complex
• **Arrhythmias**
Brugada syndrome
Congenital QT syndrome
Wolff–Parkinson–White syndrome
• **Myocarditis**
Viral

Cardiac arrest in adolescents is a rare but devastating occurrence, which may be due to congenital heart disease, congenital rhythm disturbances or myocarditis (Table 15.2) as well as non-cardiac events, such as drug overdose.

PATHOPHYSIOLOGY[14]

In a cardiac arrest of cardiac origin it is presumed that in the majority of patients myocardial ischaemia leads to ventricular irritability then ventricular tachycardia (VT) or ventricular fibrillation (VF) which, in the absence of CPR, eventually leads to asystole. Less commonly, exsanguination, pulmonary embolus or tamponade among others may lead to absence of cardiac output in the presence of a cardiac rhythm (i.e. PEA). The no-flow situation produces increasing tissue hypoxia and ischaemia with arterial hypoxia, respiratory and metabolic acidosis.

In normal brain, autoregulation maintains global cerebral blood flow at about 50 ml/100 g of brain per minute, despite variation in perfusion pressure between 50 and 150 mmHg (6.5 and 19.5 kPa). When cerebral perfusion pressure (CPP) falls below 50 mmHg (6.5 kPa), cerebral blood flow decreases. Viability of neurones is threatened by CPP below 30 mmHg (4.0 kPa) but low flow is tolerated better than no-flow. No-flow leads to loss of oxygen stores and unconsciousness within 10 seconds and an isoelectric EEG in 10–20 seconds. The concept that after 4–5 minutes of no-flow there is irreversible loss of neurones is supported by evidence of depletion of brain ATP and glucose stores. There is failure of the membrane pump, release of arachidonic acid products and cell death. During CPR and following resuscitation there may be incomplete ischaemia or reperfusion associated with release of calcium and oxygen free-radicals, which may further damage neurones. On reperfusion an initial cerebral hyperaemia is followed by persistent hypoperfusion with cytotoxic oedema.

RATIONALE FOR CPR

Immediate BLS prolongs VF and delays the progression to asystole. Rapid defibrillation/ALS has the capacity to establish the return of spontaneous circulation (ROSC).

The early pioneers implemented these principles and achieved excellent results. Kowenhoven[15] reported 70% survival for in-hospital cardiac arrest and Pantridge[16] reported 43% survival for out-of-hospital arrest associated with acute myocardial infarction. They coined the term 'hearts too good to die'.

Delay due to lack of a witness to the event or inability or refusal of the bystanders to commence CPR will lead to progressive myocardial and cerebral ischaemia/ hypoxia. For every minute of untreated VF, survival

declines by 10%.[17] If witnessed, the victim collapses and immediately loses consciousness. A convulsion may occur and a few gasping breaths may be taken. Pulselessness, apnoea and cyanosis follow.

CURRENT GUIDELINES

An algorithm approach is important to facilitate timely therapy. It provides logical stepwise assessment and treatment. Guidelines have been previously promulgated by the American Heart Association (1966, 1974, 1980, 1985, 1992), Australian Resuscitation Council,[18] British Resuscitation Council and others reflecting local opinion and habits and some scientific evidence. Recently, consensus conferences of experts from around the world have produced internationally accepted guidelines. First, the International Liaison Committee on Resuscitation[2] and more recently the American Heart Association[3] with 500 experts, 40% of whom were from outside the USA, produced guidelines based on graded available evidence:

Level I – always useful with good supporting data
Level IIa – probably useful with good supporting data
Level IIb – possibly useful with fair supporting data
Level III – probably harmful
Indeterminate – indeterminate with inconclusive supporting data

MANAGEMENT

A collapsed victim requires an immediate response, which is dependent on the environment. For example, in the monitored Coronary Care/ICU environment this may mean immediate defibrillation but, in the case of a near-drowning or drug overdose, best practice would dictate immediate care of ABC and then call for help.

BASIC LIFE SUPPORT (BLS)

- **Remove from immediate danger** – out of gas-filled room, etc.
- **Check for responsiveness** – shake and shout at the patient
- **Call for help** and resuscitation equipment (call first if VF/VT is likely)
- **Airway**
  – foreign material in the mouth is cleared and loose dentures removed
  – the airway is opened with head extension and chin lift.
- **Breathing**
  – breathing is assessed by *looking* for co-ordinated chest movement, and *listening* and *feeling* for air movement at the mouth.

– If there is no breathing, two effective slow breaths are given by mouth to mouth or mouth to mask. This is expired air resuscitation (EAR).
– To minimize gastric distension and the risk of pulmonary aspiration, a slow inspiratory time and low inflation pressure are necessary.
– If there is airway obstruction, a finger sweep of the mouth and jaw lift are performed. Back blows or abdominal thrusts are used in the awake, upright victim who may have had preceding aphonia, stridor or throat clutching, indicating foreign body airway obstruction (FBAO) or a 'café coronary'.

• **Circulation**
– Circulation is assessed by feeling for a carotid pulse at the angle of the jaw, between the trachea and the sternomastoid.
– If there is no pulse, external cardiac compression (ECC) is commenced at a rate of 100/min. The heel of one hand is placed in the midline, two finger-breadths above the xiphisternum, with the other hand on top. The sternum is depressed 4–5 cm with straight arms. 50% of the cycle is compression and 50% relaxation.
– Breathing is continued at a rate of 10–12 breaths/min and in unintubated victims the ratio of compressions to ventilation is 15:2.

ECC produces a cardiac output either by compressing the heart with competent cardiac valves against the spine (cardiac pump), or by increasing intrathoracic pressure to squeeze blood out of the heart as a valveless conduit (thoracic pump). Both mechanisms are involved at various stages. Early the valves are competent and the cardiac pump mechanism is active.[19,20]

CHEST COMPRESSION-ONLY CPR

The majority of CPR by laypersons is performed in the home on a relative. Only 15 reports of CPR-related infection have been published in scientific journals.[3] Mouth-to-mouth EAR is generally safe and effective but there is reluctance on the part of various groups, including paramedics, to perform EAR[21] for aesthetic or infectious reasons. If a rescuer is unwilling to perform mouth to mouth, chest compression-only CPR should be provided. It is significantly better than providing no CPR while awaiting the emergency team.[22,23]

ADVANCED LIFE SUPPORT (ALS)

BLS provides a cardiac output around 25% of normal and delivers an FiO$_2$ of approximately 0.10 and, although supportive, will not produce return of spontaneous circulation (ROSC) for the majority of adult patients. ALS uses equipment to help support the patient and ensure ROSC (Fig. 15.1).

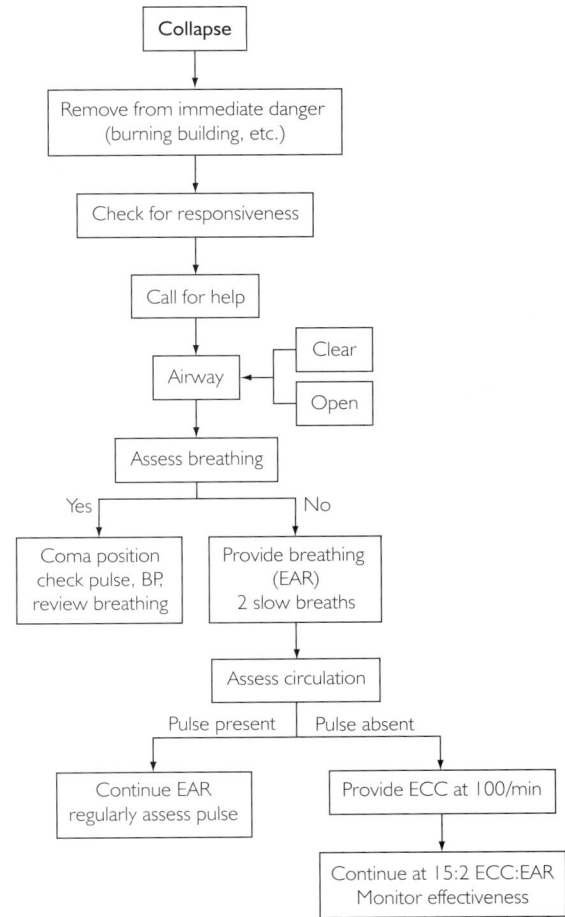

Fig. 15.1 Basic life support of the collapse victim.

Current guidelines for ALS recognize that there are two lines of therapy: (a) continued attempts at defibrillation for VF and pulseless VT; (b) attempts to improve myocardial performance and reversal of the underlying disease process for non-VF/VT (i.e. in asystole and PEA). Since the majority of patients have VF or pulseless VT due to CAD and defibrillation is the most effective therapy, defibrillation and rhythm diagnosis are the priority interventions.

COUGH CPR

Patient initiated 'cough CPR' is possible in the monitored patient who is still alert enough to generate a strong cough.

PRECORDIAL THUMP

This is recommended for witnessed VF and electrocution-associated collapse if a defibrillator is not immediately available.

DEFIBRILLATION

Direct current counter-shock produces simultaneous depolarization of the mass of myocardial cells and enables resumption of organized electrical activity. The current delivered is proportional to the energy set and inversely proportional to thoracic impedance. Impedance is increased by CAL, obesity, hirsutism and poor skin contact due to lack of pressure or dry pads.

All healthcare providers should be capable of defibrillating, and hospitals need to establish programmes for early CPR and defibrillation. Defibrillation is the priority intervention for pulseless VT/VF and the benchmarks for timing are:

- within 5 minutes of call for out-of-hospital arrest
- within 3 minutes of call for in-hospital arrest.[3]

If the rhythm is undetermined, or if there is delay in diagnosis, a blind shock should be delivered.

Technique. Paddle placement should maximize the current traversing the myocardium. Right parasternal to left axilla or anterior to posterior positioning is suggested. Gel pads should be used for skin contact.

Energy. The initial energy chosen is 200 J, the rhythm is checked, and if VF/VT persists a shock of 200 J is rapidly repeated. If VF/VT is still apparent the maximum energy is delivered (360–400 J).

Precautions. It is important to avoid:

- charging the paddles in the air
- defibrillating over ECG electrodes, nitrate patches or implanted devices such as pacemakers
- making physical contact with the patient during defibrillation.

Defibrillation failure. Causes of defibrillation failure are:

- myocardial unresponsiveness (prolonged hypoxia or ischaemia)
- failure to deliver the current (synchronization on, dead battery, broken leads)
- high thoracic impedance (obesity, etc.).

If defibrillation is unsuccessful:

1 Check paddle position and skin contact. Shave the hirsute chest.
2 Check that the shock is delivered by the presence of a myoclonic jerk
3 Check for inadvertent synchronizing or flat battery
4 Deliver two rapid shocks to reduce thoracic impedance
5 Improve myocardial metabolism
   – intubate,
   – ventilate with 100% O_2,
   – give epinephrine
   – maximize ECC

The future. Post-resuscitation myocardial depression (PRMD), manifested as histologic, metabolic and functional impairment of myocardium correlates with the total electrical energy delivered.

Implanted defibrillator technology has led to the production of low energy current based defibrillators with more efficacious, biphasic waveforms. Laboratory evidence suggests that they are more efficient, use lower energy and produce less myocardial stunning.[24,25,26] As yet there is no published clinical work to show improved outcome with the use of a particular defibrillator.[27] Early access is the most important factor at present.

Public access defibrillation (PAD)

PAD is aimed at achieving rapid defibrillation. A survival to hospital discharge rate of 59% has been recorded with PAD in witnessed arrest with an initial rhythm of VF.[28]

Placement of automatic external defibrillators (AEDs) in public locations, guided by the site-specific risk of cardiac arrest, has produced some success and may be cost effective.[29,30]

ADVANCED AIRWAY CARE

Endotracheal intubation is the gold standard technique to secure and protect the patient's airway. It also facilitates intermittent positive pressure ventilation and allows delivery of 100% oxygen. If the skills and equipment are available, it should be performed in all unconscious victims after the first three defibrillation attempts have failed. To maintain intubation skills it is important that the resuscitator performs at least 6–12 intubations per year.[3]

If intubation is not possible then lesser alternatives are[31]:

Laryngeal mask airway. This device has achieved level IIa status in AHA guidelines. It is easily inserted by infrequent users and facilitates IPPV but provides only minimal airway protection

Oesophageal tracheal combitube

Bag-valve-mask with Guedel airway. This should be a two-person technique, as maintenance of airway and seal while squeezing the bag is difficult for infrequent users.

DRUGS

Administration of drugs by central access is preferable, but peripheral access may be more readily attained. Peripheral administration should be into a fast flowing drip and followed by a 20 ml flush. Endobronchial administration requires initial airway suctioning and deep instillation of drug via a suction catheter. Epinephrine, vasopressin, lignocaine and atropine may be given by this route, but all except vasopressin are given as 2–3 times the normal dose diluted to 10 ml.

Vasopressor drugs[32,33]

Epinephrine use is supported by animal studies. Its efficacy is due to its alpha effect but there is potential for harm due to increased myocardial oxygen consumption, arrhythmias and PRMD. Epinephrine, phenylephrine and neosynephrine have equal efficacy. There are no randomized placebo-controlled trials that support its use in humans, and one negative trial. Serum epinephrine levels are also higher in non-survivors. The dose chosen is empirical and less than that used in animal studies. Eight RCTs of 1 mg versus 5 mg boluses have not shown advantage for the higher dose in terms of long-term survival. The very low survival rate in victims who failed initial defibrillation and were randomized to variable epinephrine doses supports the priority for defibrillation.

Vasopressin has achieved level IIb status as a vasoconstrictor to improve myocardial and cerebral blood flow in VF unresponsive to defibrillation. There are no data for use in asystole or PEA. It acts as a V_1 receptor agonist to produce selective peripheral vasoconstriction of skin, skeletal muscle and fat. Animal studies and one small human trial have shown improved haemodynamics and tendency to improved outcome with its use. Serum levels are higher in survivors. It is equally effective via endobronchial, intravenous and intraosseus routes. A large European trial comparing epinephrine with vasopressin is underway.

Antiarrhythmic agents[34]
Amiodarone has achieved an elevation in recommendation to first-line treatment of shock-resistant or recurrent VF based on trials suggesting improved initial resuscitation.[35] Although classified as a class III agent, it has α, β and calcium-channel blocking effects.

Bretylium has been withdrawn from recommendations because of its unavailability worldwide.

Lignocaine has not been shown to improve outcome in CPR human trials and in the laboratory is associated with an elevation in defibrillation threshold. Its level of recommendation has been reduced.

NaHCO₃
This drug should not be given routinely. It may cause hypernatraemia, hyperosmolarity and intracellular acidosis due to rapid ingress of CO_2 generated from its dissociation It is indicated in specific situations:

- sodium bicarbonate
- hyperkalaemia
- tricyclic overdose
- prolonged arrest (based on arterial blood gases)
- pre-existing severe metabolic acidosis.

Atropine
There are isolated case reports and one retrospective study suggesting increased initial resuscitation from epinephrine resistant asystole. There is no evidence of improved survival with its use.

Calcium
Its use is reserved for arrest associated hyperkalaemia, hypocalcaemia and calcium-channel blocker overdose.

Broad complex PEA may suggest that the use of calcium is indicated.

CARDIAC COMPRESSION MANOEUVRES

Active compression–decompression[36] or toilet plunger CPR, using a hand-held device with suction cup, aims to lower the intrathoracic pressure during the relaxation phase of ECC to enhance venous return. Animal studies have shown a clear improvement in survival for this use and, although most human studies are disappointing, a group of French enthusiasts has doubled survival in out-of-hospital arrest.[37]

Interposed abdominal compression in early animal studies has produced improved survival.

Open chest massage is for reserved cardiac arrest associated with cardiac surgery. Laboratory studies showed greater coronary perfusion pressure (CPP), initial resuscitation and 7-day survival but general application to CPR is limited by feasibility and major complications.

COMMENCING CPR[38,39]

Because of the time dependence of chance and quality of survival, CPR should be commenced immediately in all collapsed victims unless:

there is an active Do-Not-Resuscitate order
death is evidenced by
    – livido, rigor, putrefaction
    – decapitation
    – incineration.

CEASING CPR

CPR is terminated when resuscitation is:

(a) *Successful*. When a palpable pulse and rhythm return (i.e. ROSC), it becomes important to seek and treat the underlying cause and to maintain homeostasis (normal ventilation, normal blood pressure and normal electrolytes/fluid states, avoiding hyperglycaemia). It is important to treat hyperthermia and hypotension actively.

(b) *Inappropriate*. Resuscitation is ceased when it becomes apparent that the victim suffered from end-stage disease with no chance of functional survival (e.g. NYHA IV heart disease, disseminated terminal cancer, dependent bed-bound lifestyle, severe dementia). Age is not an independent predictor of poor outcome.

(c) *Futile*. Futility requires the definition of an acceptable chance of survival ($< 1\%$, $< 10\%$?). No scoring system, clinical criteria or time limit absolutely precludes survival in all patients.[40]

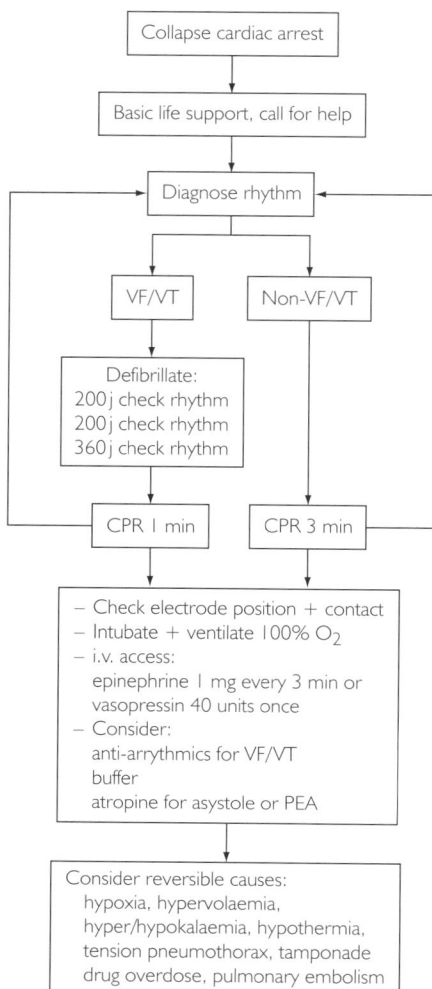

Fig. 15.2 Advanced life support.

Low survival rates have been documented if the arrest is unwitnessed, CPR is delayed or the initial rhythm is PEA or asystole, particularly if it occurs out-of-hospital.

It is recommended that CPR be ceased after 20 minutes of efficient interventions if the victim has not experienced recurrent or refractory VT or VF and is not hypothermic[41] and the arrest is not due to a drug overdose in a victim older than 45 years of age.

OBJECTIVE MEASURES OF CPR EFFICACY/EFFICIENCY

End tidal CO₂. Excretion of CO_2 is dependent on cardiac output during CPR. End tidal P_{CO_2} of <10 mmHg (1.3 kPa) precludes successful resuscitation according to human trials in PEA.[42]

Coronary perfusion pressure (CPP). CPP is best estimated by aortic diastolic (ADP) to right atrial pressure gradient. CPP threshold appears to be 15 mmHg (2.0 kPa). Unless this level is reached the likelihood of initial resuscitation is remote.[43] Early work suggested that an ADP >40 mmHg (5.2 kPa) is associated with a high initial resuscitation rate but it is not as reliable as CPP.

ECG analysis. VF amplitude has been shown to be a powerful predictor of survival after out-of-hospital cardiac arrest.[44]

POST-RESUSCITATION THERAPY

After the return of a patient-generated pulse resuscitation continues. If the patient is unable to maintain and protect the airway, intubation and ventilation are continued or established. Blood pressure is checked and maintained at pre-arrest levels or a systolic pressure at least greater than 100 mmHg (10.3 kPa) (see Ch 9 on *Shock.*) The cause of the arrest is sought and treated: full history and head-to-toe examination guide investigations such as lung scan and coronary angiography.

Electrolytes and blood sugar are normalized and hyperthermia and uncontrolled restlessness, which may lead to secondary brain injury, are rapidly treated. There is as yet no specific therapy proven for brain resuscitation after hypoxic–ischaemic injury.[14]

HYPOTHERMIA

In patients who have been successfully resuscitated after cardiac arrest due to VF, mild therapeutic hypothermia may increase the rate of a favourable neurologic outcome.[45,46]

OUTCOME

Determinants of successful resuscitation. Outcome is dependent on many factors, most importantly whether the event was witnessed, time to BLS, time to ALS and initial rhythm. The site of the event, quality of CPR, and comorbidities are also important. As reported in the literature mortality from cardiac arrest has not changed since inception in the 1960s.[9]

Under ideal circumstances (witnessed, immediate BLS, defibrillation within 3 min) 60% and 30% long term survival have been reported for in and out-of-hospital respectively.

Survival rates < 1% are reported for out-of-hospital asystole.[47,48]

Cerebral prognostication (after 'successful' resuscitation).[49–53]
Determining whether the victim will regain consciousness
and a functional existence becomes important in the hours
to days after cardiac arrest but this process is imprecise.

Motor responses less than localizing and spontaneous
eye movements neither orienting nor conjugate-roving
at 24 hours are associated with a less than 10% chance of
functional recovery. Absent pupillary light reflexes on day
3, absent motor response to pain on day 3 and bilateral
absence of early cortical somatosensory evoked potentials
(SSEP) in the first week predict death or vegetative
survival. A recording of long latency in the SSEP at
24 hours has sensitivity and specificity > 90% for predicting vegetative recovery.

REFERENCES

1 Cummins RO, Ornato JP, Thies WH, Pepe PE. Improving survival from sudden cardiac arrest. Circulation 1991; **83**(5): 1832–47.
2 The ILCOR Advisory Statements. *Resuscitation* 1997; **34**: 97–126.
3 International Guidelines 2000 for CPR and ECC. A Consensus on Science. *Circulation* 2000; **102**(Suppl), 1–165.
4 Weil MH, Tang W, Wolf Creek. Conference on cardio-pulmonary resuscitation. Addressing the scientific basis of reanimation. *Crit Care Med* 2000; **28**(Suppl): N181–232.
5 International Guidelines 2000: The story and the science. *Baillière's Clin Anaesthesiol* 2000; **14**(3).
6 Proceedings of the International Guidelines Conference for Cardiopulmonary Resuscitation and Emergency Cardiac Care. *Ann Emerg Med* 2001; **37**: S3–200.
7 Kern K, Halperin HR, Field J. New guidelines for cardiopulmonary resuscitation and emergency cardiac care. *JAMA* 2001; **285**(10): 1267–9.
8 Eisenberg MS, Mengert TJ. Primary care: cardiac resuscitation. *NEJM* 2001; **344**(17): 1304–13.
9 Becker LB. The epidemiology of sudden death in cardiac arrest. In: Paradis NA, Halperin HR, Novak RM (eds). *Cardiac Arrest. The Science and Practice of Resuscitation*. Baltimore: Williams and Wilkins; 1996: pp. 28–47.
10 Cummins RO, Chamberlain DA. Abramson NS, *et al*. Recommended guidelines for uniform reporting of data from out-of-hospital cardiac arrest: the Utstein Style. *Circulation* 1991: **84**(2): 960–75.
11 Cummins RO, Chamberlain DA, Hazinski MF, *et al*. Recommended guidelines for reviewing, reporting and conducting research on in-hospital resuscitation: the in-hospital 'Utstein Style'. *Resuscitation* 1997; **34**(2): 151–83.
12 Tunstall-Pedoe H, Bailey L, Chamberlain DA, *et al*. Survey of 3765 cardiopulmonary resuscitations in British hospitals (the BRESUS study): methods and overall results. *BMJ* 1992; May **304**: 1347–51.
13 Spaulding CM, Joly L-M, Rosenberg A, Monchi M, Weber SN, Dhainaut JFA, Carli P. Immediate coronary angiography in survivors of out of hospital cardiac arrest. *New Engl J Med* **336**(23): 1629–33.
14 Safar P. Prevention and Therapy of Postresuscitation Neurologic Dysfunction and Injury. In: Paradis NA, Halperin HR, Nowak RM (eds). *Cardiac Arrest. The Science and Practice of Resuscitation*. Baltimore: Williams and Wilkins; 1996: pp. 859–857
15 Kuowenhoven WB, Jude Jr, Knickerbocker GG. Closed chest cardiac massage. *JAMA* 1960; **173**: 1064–7.
16 Pantridge JF, Geddes JS. A mobile intensive care unit in the management of myocardial infarction. *Lancet* 1967; **2**: 271–3.
17 Pell JP, Sirel JM, Marsden AK, *et al*. Effect of reducing ambulance response times on deaths from out-of-hospital cardiac arrest: cohort study. *BMJ* 2001; **322**: 1385–8.
18 The Advanced Life Support Committee of the Australian Resuscitation Council. Adult advanced life support. *Med J Austr* 1993; **159**: 616–21.
19 Ma MHN. Transoesophageal echocardiographic assessment of mitral valve position and pulmonary venous blood flow during cardiopulmonary resuscitation in humans. *Circulation* 1995; **92**: 854–61.
20 Feneley MP, Maier GW, Gaynor JW, *et al*. Sequence of mitral valve motion and transmitral blood flow during cardiopulmonary resuscitation in dogs. *Circulation* 1987; **76**: 353–75.
21 Hew P, Brenner B, Kaufman J. Reluctance of para-medics and emergency medical technicians to perform mouth-to-mouth resuscitation. *J Emerg Med* 1997; **15**: 279–84.
22 Noc M, Tang W, Turner T, *et al*. Mechanical ventilation may not be essential for initial cardiopulmonary resuscitation. *Chest* 1995; **108**: 821–7.
23 Kern KB. Cardiopulmonary resuscitation without ventilation. *Crit Care Med* 2000; **28**(11): N186–9.
24 Walcott GP, Melnick SB, Chapman FW, *et al*. Relative efficacy of monophasic and biphasic waveforms for transthoracic defibrillation after short and long durations of ventricular fibrillation. *Circulation* 1998; **98**: 2210–5.
25 Kroll M, Brewer J. Automated external defibrillators: design considerations. *New Horiz* 1997; **5**(2): 128–144.
26 Tang W, Weil MH, Sun S. Low-energy biphasic wave-form defibrillation reduces the severity of post resuscitation myocardial dysfunction. *Crit Care Med* 2000; **28**(11) Suppl: N222–4.
27 Automated External Defibrillator Considerations. *Health Devices* 1999; **28**: 220–2.
28 Valenzuela TD, Roe DJ, Nichol G, *et al*. Outcomes of rapid defibrillation by security officers after cardiac arrest in casinos. *NEJM* 2000; **343**(17): 1206–9.
29 O'Rourke MF, Donaldson E, Geddes JS. An airline cardiac arrest program. *Circulation* 1997; **96**: 2849–53.
30 Nichol G, Mallstrom AP, Cerratou P, *et al*. Potential cost effectiveness of public access defibrillation in the United States. *Circulation* 1998; **97**: 1315–20.

31 Barnes TA, MacDonald D, Nolan J. Airway devices. *Ann Emerg Med* 2001; **37**: 5145–51.

32 Krismer AC, Wenzel V, Mays VD. Use of vasopressor drugs during cardiopulmonary resuscitation. *Baillière's Clin Anaesthesiol* 2000; **14**(3): 497–509.

33 Babbs CF, Berg RA, Kettle F. Use of pressors in the treatment of cardiac arrest. *Ann Emerg Med* 2001; **37**: 5152–62.

34 Robertson C, Summers IR. The use of antiarrhythmic agents in cardiopulmonary resuscitation. *Baillière's Clin Anaesthesiol* 2000; **14**(3): 567–75.

35 Kudenchule PJ, Cobb LA, Copass MK, *et al.* Amiodarone for resuscitation after out of hospital cardiac arrest due to ventricular fibrillation. *N Engl J Med* 1999; **341**: 871–8.

36 Kern KB, Morley PT, Babbs CF, *et al.* Use of adjunctive devices in cardiopulmonary resuscitation. *Ann Emerg Med* 2001; **37**: 568–77.

37 Plaisance P, Lurie K, Vicaut E, *et al.* Comparison of standard cardiopulmonary resuscitation and active compression decompression for out of hospital cardiac arrest. *N Eng J Med* 1999; **341**: 569–75.

38 Basket PJF. Ethics in cardiopulmonary resuscitation. *Resuscitation* 1993; **25**: 1–8.

39 Ethical issues in adult resuscitation. *Ann Emerg Med* 1993; **22**(2): 229–35.

40 Maleck WH, Piper SN, Triem J, Boldt Jl, Zittel FU. Unexpected return of spontaneous circulation after cessation of resuscitation (Lazarus phenomenon) *Resuscitation* 1998; **39**: 125–8.

41 Beat HW, Walpoth-Aslan BN, Mattle HP, *et al.* Outcome of survivors of accidental deep hypothermia and circulatory arrest treated with extracorporeal blood warming. *N Engl J Med* 1997; Nov **357**(21): 1501–5.

42 Levine RL, Wayne MA, Miller CC. End-tidal carbon dioxide and outcome of out-of-hospital cardiac arrest. *New Engl J Med* **357**(5): 301–7.

43 Paradis NA. Coronary perfusion pressure and the return of spontaneous circulation in human cardiopulmonary resuscitation. *JAMA* 1990; **263**: 1106–13.

44 Weaver WD. Amplitude of ventricular fibrillation waveform and outcome after cardiac arrest. *Ann Int Med* 1985; **102**: 53–5.

45 The Hypothermia after cardiac arrest group. Mild therapeutic hypothermia to improve the neurologic outcome after cardiac arrest. *N Engl J Med* 346(8): 549–556.

46 Bernard SA, Gray TW, Buist MD *et al.* Treatment of comatose survivors of out-of-hospital cardiac arrest with induced hypothermia. *N Engl J Med* 2002; **346**: 557–563.

47 Gray WA, Capone RJ, Most AS. Unsuccessful emergency medical resuscitation – are continued efforts in the emergency department justified? *New Engl J Med* 1991; **325**(20): 1393–8.

48 Van der Hoeven J, Waanders H, Compier E, van der Weyden PKC, Meinders AE. Prolonged resuscitation efforts for cardiac arrest patients who cannot be resuscitated at the scene: who is likely to benefit? *Ann Emerg Med* 1993; **22**(11): 1660–4.

49 Graves JR, Herlitz J, Bang A, *et al.* Survivors of out of hospital cardiac arrest: their prognosis, longevity and functional status. *Resuscitation* 1997; **35**: 117–21.

50 Zandbergen EG, De Haan RJ, *et al.* Systematic review of early prediction of poor outcome in anoxic–ischaemic coma. *Lancet* 1998; **352**: 1808–12.

51 Attia J, Cook DJ. Prognosis in anoxic and traumatic coma. *Crit Care Clin* 1998; **14**: 497–511.

52 Madl C, Kramer L, Oomanovits H, *et al.* Improved outcome prediction in unconscious cardiac arrest survivors with sensory evoked potentials compared with clinical assessment. *Crit Care Med* 2000; **28**: 721–6.

53 Levy DE, Caronna JJ, Singer BH, *et al.* Predicting outcome from hypoxic–ischaemic coma. *JAMA* 1985; **253**: 1420–6.

16

Management of cardiac arrhythmias

A Holt

CARDIAC ELECTROPHYSIOLOGY

The electrophysiological properties of cardiac cells is important in understanding cardiac arrhythmias and their management. Cardiac cells undergo cyclical depolarization and repolarization to form an action potential. The shape and duration of each action potential are determined by the activity of ion channel protein complexes on the myocyte surface.

Ion channel function can be affected by:

- Acute ischaemia
- Autonomic tone
- Myocardial scarring
- Electrolyte concentration

The spectrum of cardiac action potentials varies from 'fast response' cells; conducting and contractile myocytes (Fig. 16.1a) to 'slow response' cells of pacemaker myocytes; sino-atrial (SA) and atrioventricular (AV) nodes (Fig. 16.1b). Fast myocytes lose their characteristic action potential and behave more like slow myocytes when ischaemic. The action potential is divided into five phases:

Phase 0: In fast myocytes (Fig. 16.1a) rapid depolarization occurs due to activation of voltage dependent Na^+ channels. Activation is initiated in an all-or-none response once the threshold is reached. The Na^+ channels are inactivated as membrane potential rises to +30 mV and remain inactivated until repolarization occurs. Rapidity of depolarization determines speed of conduction. In slow myocytes depolarization does not involve Na^+ channels and the slower rate of depolarization is due to a slow inward Ca^{2+} current via L- and T-type voltage dependent Ca^{2+} channels.

Phase 1: Early rapid incomplete repolarization to approximately 0 mV occurs due to activation of transient outward current due to I_{TO1} and I_{TO2} K^+ channels. Slow myocytes do not exhibit phase 1 or 2 characteristics (Fig. 16.1b).

Phase 2: The prolonged plateau repolarization of fast myocytes is a consequence of low membrane conductance to all ions. The decreasing inward Ca^{2+} current of L- and T-type Ca^{2+} channels is initially balanced and then

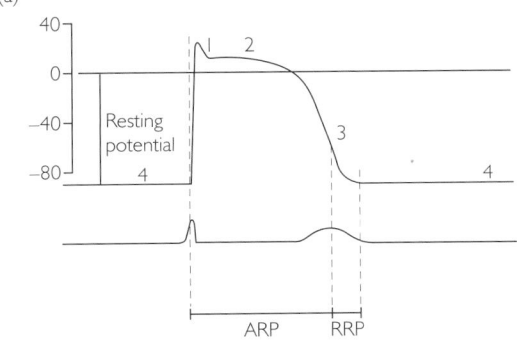

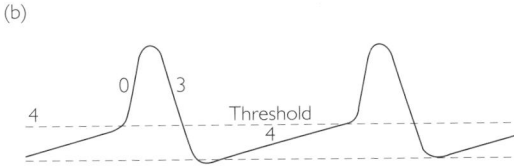

Fig. 16.1 (a) Action potential in a 'fast response', non-pacemaker myocyte: phases 0–4, resting membrane potential –80 mV, absolute refractory period (ARP) and relative refractory period (RRP). (b) Action potential in a 'slow response', pacemaker myocyte. The upward slope of phase 4, on reaching threshold potential, results in an action potential

overcome by the outward K^+ current of the delayed rectifiers or the I_k family of K^+ channels. During this phase the rise in $[Ca^{2+}]_i$ is the trigger to release sarcoplasmic reticulum stores of Ca^{2+} and initiate the contractile process.

Phase 3: Relatively rapid repolarization occurs as outward K^+ current of the delayed rectifiers increases. The I_{kr} K^+ channel, one of the I_k delayed rectifiers, is the common mechanism whereby anti-arrhythmic drugs prolong the action potential and refractoriness.

Phase 4: This is a stable electrical state in fast non-pacemaker myocytes. In slow pacemaker myocytes the resting membrane potential slowly depolarizes until the action potential threshold is reached (Fig. 16.1b). This inward or pacemaker current is due to I_f K^+ channels.

Fast-response and slow-response myocytes also have important differences in properties of refractoriness. In fast myocytes Na⁺ channels are progressively reactivated during phase 3 repolarization as the membrane potential becomes more negative. When an extra stimulus occurs during phase 3, the magnitude of the resulting inward Na⁺ current and likelihood of impulse propagation depends on the number of reactivated Na⁺ channels. Refractoriness is therefore determined by the voltage-dependent recovery of Na⁺ channels. The absolute refractory period (Fig. 16.1) is that minimum time needed for recovery of sufficient Na⁺ channels for a stimulus to result in impulse propagation. However, once propagation in fast myocytes occurs, conduction velocity is normal. In contrast, slow-response or Ca^{2+} channel-dependent myocytes exhibit time-dependent refractoriness. Even after full repolarization further time is needed before all Ca^{2+} channels are reactivated. Stimuli during this period produce reduced Ca^{2+} current and the propagation velocity of any resulting impulse is reduced. The conduction velocity independence of premature action potentials with fast-response myocytes is lost in the setting of Na⁺ channel blocking drugs or ischaemia because they behave increasing like slow-response myocytes, thereby resulting in slowed impulse conduction.

ARRHYTHMOGENIC MECHANISMS[1-3]

Many factors in isolation or combination give rise to the substrate of arrhythmogenesis (Fig. 16.2). Arrhythmia may arise from abnormalities of impulse generation or conduction. Table 16.1 demonstrates the relationship between mechanism and type of arrhythmia, and desired anti-arrhythmic effect.

ABNORMAL IMPULSE GENERATION
(Table 16.2)

Enhanced normal automaticity. Automaticity is the property of spontaneous impulse generation by cardiac fibres. This results from spontaneous depolarization during phase 4, secondary to an inward current carried by K⁺ in SA node or subsidiary pacemaker myocytes.

Abnormal automaticity: Abnormal automaticity is the mechanism by which spontaneous impulses are generated in fibres that are partially depolarized by a pathological process. This less negative resting membrane potential (RMP) is associated with inactivation of the normal ionic currents of phase 4 depolarization and the pacemaker potential results from inward Na⁺ and Ca^{2+} currents and is not readily susceptible to overdrive suppression from normal pacemaker activity. The abnormal automatic fibres, due to their less negative membrane potentials inactivate the phase 0 fast inward Na⁺ current, resulting in an impaired rate of impulse conduction (as well as contractility) which further contributes to arrhythmia. In this setting, Ca^{2+} carries the major inward current on depolarization in these fibres.

Triggered activity: Abnormal impulse generation from triggered activity originates from oscillations in the membrane potential that are initiated or triggered by a preceding action potential. There are 2 types of oscillations, early after-depolarizations (EAD) and delayed after-depolarizations (DAD). EAD occurs during phase 2 or 3 of the action potential, whereas DAD occurs after the termination of depolarization. The signal-averaged electrocardiograph (ECG) (see below) can detect after-depolarizations.

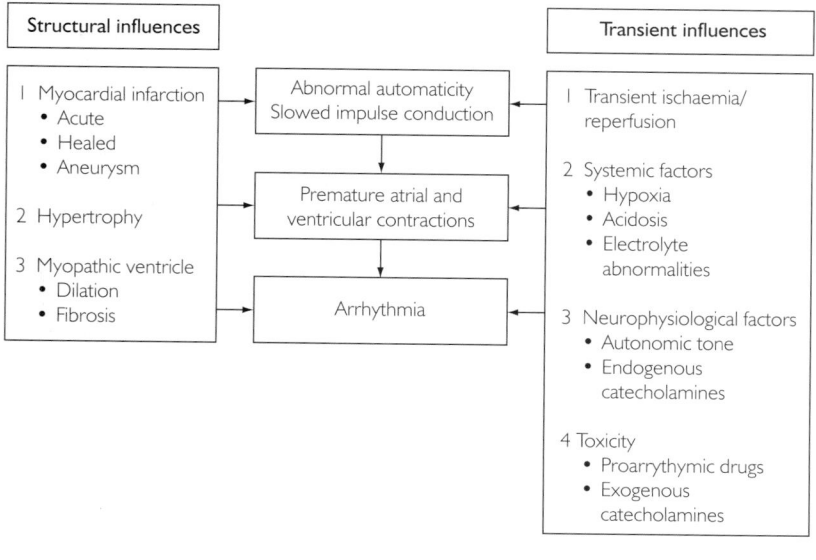

Fig. 16.2 Factors that combine to form the substrate of arrhythmogenesis

Table 16.1 Classification of mechanisms of arrhythmia and desired anti-arrhythmic drug action. Modified with permission from Task Force of the Working Group on Arrhythmia of the European Society of Cardiology[1]

Mechanism of arrhythmia	Arrhythmia	Anti-arrhythmic effect	Representative drugs
Automaticity enhanced			
Normal	Inappropriate sinus tachycardia	Decrease phase 4 depolarization	β-blocker
	Unifocal atrial tachycardia		Sodium channel blockers
Abnormal	Unifocal atrial tachycardia	Hyperpolarize or decrease phase 4 depolarization	Calcium or sodium channel blockers
	Accelerated idioventricular rhythms		M_2 agonists
	VT post myocardial infarction		
Triggered activity			
EAD	Torsade de pointes	Shorten action potential or suppress EAD	Increase heart rate with β-agonists or vagolytic agents, calcium channel blockers, β-blockers or magnesium
DAD	Digitalis-induced arrhythmias	Decrease calcium overload or suppress DAD	Calcium or sodium channel blockers, β-blockers, adenosine
	Some VT		
Re-entry: sodium channel dependent			
Long excitable gap	Afl type I	Depress conduction and excitability	Sodium channel blockers
	Circus movement tachycardia in WPW		
	Monomorphic VT		
Short excitable gap	Afl type 2	Prolong refractory period	Potassium channel blockers
	AF		
	Circus movement tachycardia in WPW		
	Polymorphic and monomorphic VT		
	Bundle branch re-entry		
	VF		
Re-entry: calcium channel dependent	AV nodal re-entrant tachycardia	Depress conduction and excitability	Calcium channel blockers
	Circus movement tachycardia in WPW		
	VT		

Table 16.2 Causes of abnormal impulse generation

Enhanced normal automaticity	Adrenergic stimulation
Abnormal automaticity	Ischaemia
Early after-depolarizations	Hypoxia
	Hypercapnia
	Catecholamines
	Class IA anti-arrhythmic drugs
	Class III anti-arrhythmic drugs
	Other drugs that prolong re-polarization
Delayed after-depolarizations	Digoxin toxicity
	Increased intracellular Na^+
	Decreased extracellular K^+
	Increased intracellular Ca^{2+}
	Intracellular Ca^{2+} overload
	Myocardial infarction
	Myocardial hypertrophy
	Reperfusion after ischaemia

(a) *EAD* appear as subthreshold humps during the plateau or depolarization phases. On reaching threshold, single or multiple action potentials can be induced. Plateau EAD are caused by an increased inward Ca^{2+} current (at this level of membrane potential fast inward Na^+ channels are inactivated) and produce slow rising and propagating action potentials. Phase 3 EAD are caused by reduction in outward K^+ currents and produce relatively rapidly rising and propagating action potentials. EAD amplitude and likelihood of triggered arrhythmia increases as driving rate decreases and action potential is prolonged. Tachyarrhythmias induced by EAD are more likely to occur on the background of a bradycardia.

(b) *DAD* are produced by Na^+–Ca^{2+} exchanger current induced oscillations in inward calcium current. These oscillations are caused by $[Ca^{2+}]_i$ overload saturating sarcoplasmic reticulum sequestration mechanisms thereby leading to Ca^{2+} induced Ca^{2+} release. DAD unlike EAD, depend on previous rapid rhythm for their initiation.

ABNORMAL IMPULSE CONDUCTION[4]

Abnormal impulse conduction may cause an arrhythmia by the phenomena of re-entry. Re-entry describes the re-excitation of an area or entire heart by a circulating impulse. While the classic 'bifurcating Purkinje fibre' model of Schmitt and Erlanger has given way to a much more complex picture, the essential electrophysiological requirements for re-entrant excitation remain. Requirements for re-entry are (Fig. 16.3):

- Conduction block in one limb of the circuit
- Slowed conduction in the other limb

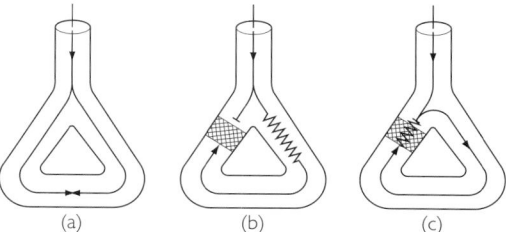

Fig. 16.3 Re-entrant excitation. (a) Normal cardiac impulse conduction results in the impulse being extinguished. (b) Conduction down one limb is blocked by segment of refractory tissue (excitable gap). (c) The impulse is conducted back up the limb and arrives at the excitable gap which has recovered from refractoriness and retrograde conduction is complete. If geometry and electrical properties are favorable the excitable gap circulates around the re-entry loop and arrhythmia is initiated

- The impulse returns back along the limb initially blocked to re-enter and re-excite the pathway proximal to the block and complete the re-entry pathway

When these properties are present, the chance of a circulating impulse producing re-entrant excitation depends on pathway geometry, the electrical properties and length of the depressed area and conduction velocity within each component. The segment of the re-entry pathway that is initially refractory and therefore blocks conduction down one limb and recovers in time to conduct the return impulse is termed the 'excitable gap'. Therefore, the generation and subsequent maintenance of a circuit depends on this excitable gap of non-refractory tissue circulating between the advancing depolarizing wave front and the re-polarizing tail. The resulting re-entrant impulse can be self-terminating causing ectopic beats or lead to atrial or ventricular tachyarrhythmias.

Re-entry may be terminated by:

- Increasing conduction velocity: the excitable gap is abolished by the wave front arriving too early and meeting refractory tissue
- Increasing refractory period: the excitable gap is lost
- Slowing conduction: a unidirectional block can be converted into a complete block

Ordered re-entry occurs along anatomical pathways which are 'macroscopic' loops (macro-re-entry) as in Wolff–Parkinson–White syndrome. Functional circuits can be created following myocardial infarction resulting in ventricular tachycardia (VT). 'Microscopic' loops (micro-re-entry), occurs at the level of single fibres where antegrade and retrograde impulse propagation occurs in parallel fibres. Random re-entry refers to the generation of a circulating impulse, not from a fixed circuit but from constantly changing electrophysiologically distinct fibres or pathways created by the circulating impulse, resulting in atrial or ventricular fibrillation.

The cellular properties that lead to impaired conduction include:

- Inactivation of the phase 0 fast Na^+ channels which reduces both the magnitude and rate of propagation of any resultant action potential
- Intercellular uncoupling increases resistance to action potential propagation and slows conduction. Intercellular coupling is reduced by ischaemia, $[Ca^{2+}]_i$ overload and acidosis

ELECTROPHYSIOLOGICAL EFFECTS OF ISCHAEMIA

Both hypoxia and acidosis are implicated in the production of a less negative RMP in ischaemia. A rise in extracellular K^+ results from impairment of the ATP-dependent K^+ inward channels. As $[K^+]_o/[K^+]_i$ is the major determinant of the RMP, ultra cellular K^+ loss results in a less negative RMP.

The consequences of this are:

- Abnormal automaticity
- Inactivation of the fast inward Na^+ channels, which slows the conduction velocity

ELECTROLYTE ABNORMALITIES AND ARRHYTHMIA[5]

POTASSIUM

Hyper and hypokalaemia both cause arrhythmia mediated by the resultant changes in RMP (Table 16.3). In ischaemia, hyperkalaemia at the local tissue level caused by a pathological extracellular shift of K^+ is the major factor contributing to ventricular re-entrant arrhythmia in this setting. In hypokalaemia, the dispersion of pacemaker activity and the effect on repolarization are similar to the electrophysiological effects of cardiac glycosides and β-adrenergic agonists, and it is not surprising that a combination of these factors is associated with an increased incidence of arrhythmia. The increased risk of death in hypertensive patients treated with thiazide diuretics (Multiple Risk Factor Intervention Trial) has been attributed to hypokalaemic (and possibly hypomagnesaemic) induced arrhythmia. Thiazide induced hypokalaemic ventricular ectopy is worsened by exercise.[6] Hypokalaemia is associated with ventricular fibrillation (VF) and VT following acute myocardial infarction. The increased incidence of VF/VT with a serum K^+ less than 3.5 mmol/l is clearly established and the probability of VT increases as the serum K^+ decreases. During acute myocardial infarction the incidence of VF/VT was 15% at 4.5 mmol/l, 38% at 3.5 mmol/l, 55% at 3.0 mmol/l and 67% at 2.5 mmol/l.[7]

MAGNESIUM

The anti-arrhythmic properties of Mg^{2+} are clearly established but a causal relationship between hypomagnesaemia and arrhythmia is largely circumstantial. Decreased extracellular Mg^{2+} by itself has little effect on the electrophysiological properties of myocytes or the ECG. Hypomagnesaemia has been implicated in the genesis of VT/VF in patients with hypertension and heart failure receiving thiazide or loop diuretics, acute alcohol intoxication or withdrawal and possibly with acute myocardial infarction. The product of K^+ and Mg^{2+} is the best predictor of arrhythmia in hypertensive patients taking thiazide diuretics.[8]

Table 16.3 Arrhythmogenic effects of potassium disturbance

	Arrhythmogenic effects	ECG changes	Arrythmia
Hyperkalaemia	Less negative RMP Inactivation of fast Na^+ channels Slowed conduction velocity	Peaked T-waves Widening of P-wave and QRS complex	Sinus node suppression AV block VF
Hypokalaemia	Prolongation of rapid repolarization Hyperpolarization of RMP Increased pacemaker activity in Purkinje and ventricular fibres	U waves ST segment and T-wave changes	Atrial and ventricular ectopy Atrial and ventricular tachyarrhythmias

AUTONOMIC NERVOUS SYSTEM AND VENTRICULAR ARRHYTHMIA[9]

The autonomic nervous system, particularly vagal tone, has a significant effect on the occurrence of post myocardial infarction VF as seen by:

- High vagal tone is associated with better outcome and less susceptibility to exercise-induced VF with new ischaemia in animal models
- Post myocardial infarction exercise training results in an increased vagal tone, which inhibits induced VF
- Implantable electrical vagal stimulation and muscarinic agents, including edrophonium, are protective
- The protection is not heart rate related as the protection remains even when atrial pacing is used to maintain the heart rate
- The administration of atropine increases the likelihood of developing VF

Vagal tone can be measured by variability in the heart rate (RR interval) or blood pressure rise induced by the pressor agent phenylephrine. Heart rate variability is considered a measure of tonic vagal activity whereas the phenylephrine method is considered a measure of magnitude of the vagal reflex in response to stimulus. A reduced vagal tone has been found post-infarction in humans, which returns to normal over a 3–6-month period. There is no relationship between vagal tone and ejection fraction and the origin of reduced vagal tone post-infarction appears to be due to afferent stimulation in response to necrotic tissue and impaired cardiac contractile geometry. This reduced vagal tone has also been shown to be predictive of mortality and inductility of arrhythmia at electrophysiological study (EPS).

PROARRHYTHMIC EFFECTS OF ANTI-ARRHYTHMIC DRUGS[10,11]

Concomitant proarrhythmia with the use of anti-arrhythmic drugs is increasingly recognized. The recognition of 'quinidine syncope' due to VF and polymorphic VT at therapeutic concentrations was also seen with disopyramide. The Cardiac Arrhythmia Suppression Trial (CAST) clearly defined the magnitude of this deleterious side effect in drugs that were previously perceived to be of benefit.[12] This placebo-controlled randomized study which involved flecainide, encainide and moricizine (a class IA drug) was terminated early because of adverse outcome in the flecainide and encainide groups (relative risk of arrhythmic death or non-fatal cardiac arrest of 3.6, 95% confidence interval 1.7 to 8.5). Proarrhythmia is reported between 5.9% and 15.8% depending on agent, clinical setting and definition of proarrhythmia, and now considered ubiquitous with all anti-arrhythmic drugs.

Proarrhythmia has been defined as an increase in frequency of ventricular ectopic beat (VEB) or aggravation of the target arrhythmia on Holter monitor or exercise test. Manifestations of proarrhythmia not only includes VEB, monomorphic and polymorphic VT and VF, but also bradyarrhythmias and atrial flutter (Afl) with 1:1 atrioventricular conduction. Most proarrhythmic events occur soon after starting the drug, but late arrhythmias are also a significant problem.

Proarrhythmia appears to be correlated with the degree of drug induced QT prolongation or the time constant of recovery of any sodium channel blockade. Agents with short time constants of sodium channel block where sodium channel blockade is more pronounced at fast heart rates (e.g. class IB, lignocaine and mexiletine) are less proarrhythmic than drugs with long time constants (e.g. class IC, flecainide and propafenone). Class III drugs and quinidine proarrhythmia correlate with degree of QT prolongation.

The mechanism of drug proarrhythmia is probably via both slowing of conduction and abnormal automaticity. Paradoxically slowing conduction, which may block a re-entry circuit, may also create the very substrate needed for re-entry, unidirectional block and an excitable gap. The existence of a re-entrant circuit requires the circulating wave front of the impulse not to catch up with the refractory tissue behind the tail. Re-entry is more likely to occur with a shorter refractory period and reduced conduction velocity (Fig. 16.4).[10]

Increasing conduction velocity is an ideal anti-arrhythmic property but there are no anti-arrhythmic drugs that accelerate conduction. The degree of conduction slowing and therefore proarrhythmic and anti-arrhythmic properties correlates with potency and time constant of recovery of sodium channel blockade. Agents with a slow constant of recovery, Class IC drugs, cause pronounced blockade of sodium channels even at slow heart rates and are most proarrhythmic.

Prolonging the refractory period is also an ideal anti-arrhythmic property, which increases the likelihood of abolishing any excitable gap by ensuring the wave front of a re-entrant circuit meets refractory tissue. The potency of class IA and III anti-arrhythmic agents is dependent on the prolongation of the refractory period. This property is also protective against proarrhythmia due to re-entry mechanism. The effect of class IB agents to shorten the refractory period will contribute to proarrhythmia in this class.

Surface mapping of the heart has been used to quantify proarrhythmic effect. The scale of potency of proarrhythmia has been found to be flecainide > propafenone > quinidine > disopyramide > procainamide > mexiletine > lignocaine > sotalol.[11] Amiodarone was not included in this study but presumably its proarrhythmia potential is similar to other class III agents and less than the class I agents.

Anti-arrhythmic drugs are effective at suppressing abnormal automaticity, with the exception of triggered automaticity due to EAD. Class IA, class III and many non-anti-arrhythmic drugs can produce proarrhythmia via EAD. These drugs not only increase the frequency of EAD, but also the likelihood of them leading to triggered

(a)

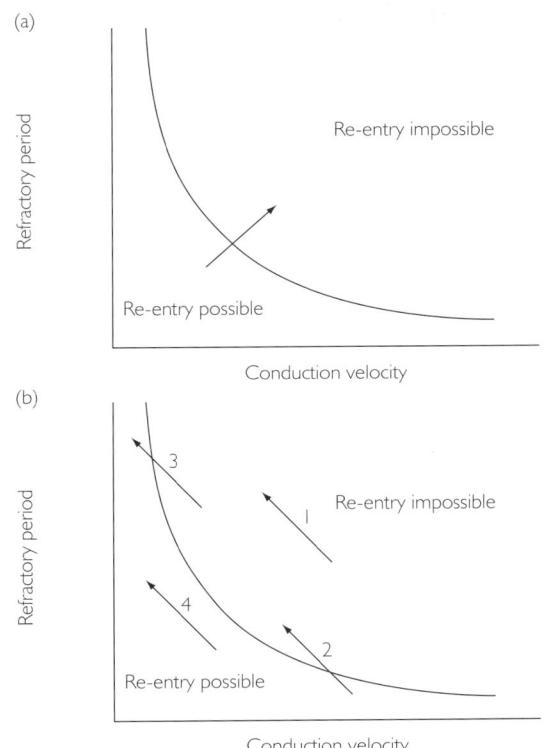

(b)

Fig. 16.4 (a) Graph of refractory period of an excitable gap versus its conduction velocity around a theoretical re-entrant circuit. When conduction velocity is high enough so that refractory period of excitable gap exceeds circuit time, re-entry is impossible. Arrow demonstrates the action of an 'ideal' anti-arrhythmic drug, which prolongs refractory period and increases conduction velocity. (b) With anti-arrhythmic drugs that increase refractory period and slow conduction, the net effect of an anti-arrhythmic drug may have no effect on proarrhythmia (arrows 1 and 4), decrease proarrhythmia (arrow 2), or increase proarrhythmia (arrow 3) depending on properties of a potential re-entrant circuit (adapted with permission[10])

tachyarrhythmias. Slowing repolarization, which leads to QT prolongation and slower heart rate, is central to this increased frequency and sensitivity to EAD. EAD manifests as prominent and bizarre T–U waves on the ECG and, if triggered activity results, VEB and ventricular tachyarrhythmias may occur. Torsade de pointes is the classical resulting arrhythmia, although less classical polymorphic VT and VF result. Risk of proarrhythmia via this mechanism correlates with the degree of QT prolongation.

All anti-arrhythmic drugs are capable of producing bradyarrhythmias via decreasing normal automaticity and slowing conduction. Digoxin can be proarrhythmic via the production of triggered activity due to DAD.

Anti-arrhythmic drug proarrhythmia is facilitated by several factors, which are frequently found in patients on anti-arrhythmic drugs or with heart disease (Table 16.4).

Table 16.4 Factors facilitating anti-arrhythmic drug proarrhythmia (adapted with permission)[10]

Toxic blood levels due to excessive dose or reduced clearance from old age, heart failure, renal disease or hepatic disease
Severe left ventricular dysfunction. Ejection fraction less than 35%
Pre-existing arrhythmia or arrhythmia substrate
Digoxin therapy
Hypokalaemia or hypomagnesaemia
Bradycardia
Combinations of anti-arrhythmic drugs and concomitant drugs with similar toxicity

MANAGEMENT OF THE PATIENT WITH A CARDIAC ARRHYTHMIA

HISTORY AND PHYSICAL EXAMINATION

A careful history is important. Specific questions should confirm or exclude palpitations, syncope, chest pain, shortness of breath, ischaemic heart disease (especially previous myocardial infarction), congestive cardiac failure, valvular heart disease, thyrotoxicosis and diuretic therapy without adequate potassium supplements. A family history is helpful for arrhythmias associated with inherited disorders (e.g. long QT syndrome and hypertrophic obstructive cardiomyopathy). The physical examination looks for underlying structural heart disease and signs to assist diagnosis, and assesses haemodynamic consequences of the arrhythmia.

VAGAL MANOEUVRES

Vagal manoeuvres may be undertaken during examination. These reflexly increase vagal tone, thereby prolonging AV node conduction and refractoriness. The effect may be:

- Transient slowing of sinus tachycardia as SA nodal discharge rate is slowed
- Termination of AV nodal re-entry (AVNRT) and AV re-entry tachycardias (AVRT)
- Unmasking (but not reversion) of atrial tachycardia, flutter (Fig. 16.5) and fibrillation

VT is not affected. Carotid sinus massage is most commonly used. Valsalva manoeuvre or iced water to the face may be useful. Eyeball pressure should be avoided as eye damage may result. Carotid sinus massage is performed with the patient supine, with head extended and turned away from the side to be massaged. After auscultation to exclude carotid bruits, the carotid bifurcation is gently palpated by placing two fingers anterior to the sternocleidomastoid muscle, just below the angle of the jaw. Massage is applied one side at a time, and never both sides simultaneously. It is

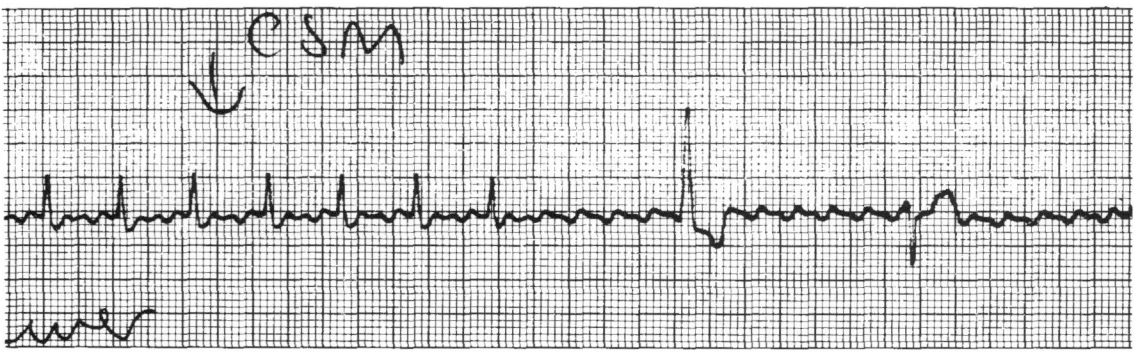

Fig. 16.5 Atrial flutter with 2 : 1 atrioventricular (AV) block. Carotid sinus massage (CSM) increases AV block and unmasks flutter waves

contraindicated in those with known or suspected cerebrovascular disease.

INVESTIGATIONS

A 12-lead ECG should be recorded with a longer rhythm strip (usually lead II or V_1). If P-waves are not visible, atrial activity may be recorded using an oesophageal electrode or pacing lead, or via a central venous catheter or the right atrial injectate port of a pulmonary artery catheter, using 20% saline and a bedside monitor.[13] Holter monitoring requires prolonged (usually 24–72 h), non-invasive, ambulatory ECG monitoring, sometimes combined with exercise testing. EPS, which involves invasive electrophysiological testing with programmed electrical stimulation, attempts to reproduce the spontaneously occurring arrhythmia.[14,15] EPS is not clearly superior to Holter monitoring in evaluating drug treatment for ventricular arrhythmias. Other investigative techniques being studied include signal-averaged ECG, heart rate variability and electrical alternans measurement.[9,16]

MANAGEMENT OF SPECIFIC ARRHYTHMIAS

Treatment has two aspects: acute termination of the arrhythmia and long-term prophylaxis. The decision whether to treat depends on the rhythm diagnosis, haemodynamic consequences, aetiology of the arrhythmia and the prognosis (e.g. risks of sudden death or long-term complications).

ECTOPIC BEATS

Premature impulses originating from the atria, AV junction or ventricles. The coupling interval (time between the ectopic and the preceding beat) is shorter than the cycle duration of the dominant rhythm.

PREMATURE VENTRICULAR ECTOPIC BEATS

Also known as ventricular premature beats and ventricular premature complexes. The ventricle is not activated normally via the rapidly conducting bundle branches, and a wide QRS complex results from slow ventricular conduction.

ECG
No preceding P-wave.

- Premature complexes occurring before the next expected QRS
- QRS is wide (>120 ms)
- T-wave of opposite polarity to the QRS (Fig. 16.6)
- VEB is not conducted retrogradely to the SA node

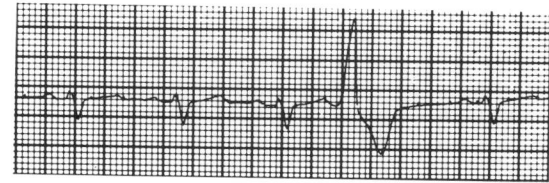

Fig. 16.6 Sinus rhythm with ventricular ectopic beat. Note complete compensatory pause

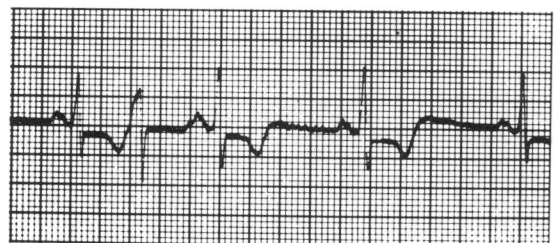

Fig. 16.7 Sinus rhythm with interpolated ventricular ectopic beat. Note absence of any compensatory pause

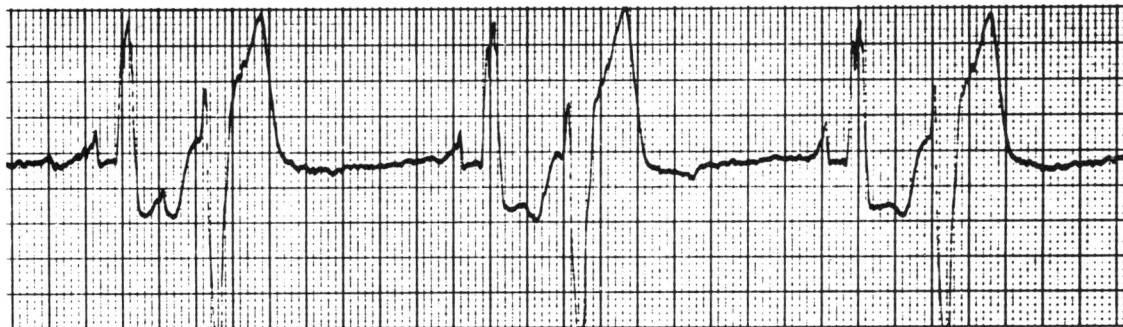

Fig. 16.8   Ventricular bigeminy

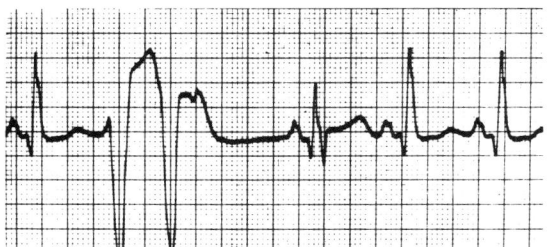

Fig. 16.9   Ventricular couplet. Note independent atrial activity continues during the couplet (see P-wave buried in T-wave after second ventricular ectopic beat)

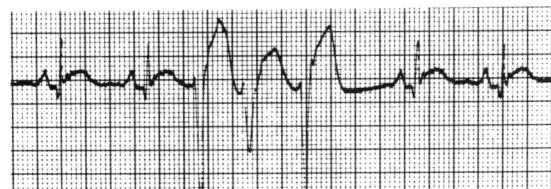

Fig. 16.10   Ventricular triplet

- SA node is therefore not reset, and there is temporary AV dissociation with a full compensatory pause; the interval between the normal QRS complexes on either side of the VEB will usually be twice that of the dominant sinus rhythm

Occasionally VEB may not produce any pause, and are said to be interpolated (Fig. 16.7). A VEB following each sinus beat is ventricular bigeminy (Fig. 16.8). Ventricular trigeminy refers to recurring sequences of a VEB followed by two sinus beats. Two VEB in succession are a couplet (Fig. 16.9), and three, a triplet (Fig. 16.10).

CLINICAL

VEB, even when frequent, complex, or in short runs of non-sustained VT, are not associated with risk of sudden death in asymptomatic healthy adults.[17] However, there is increased risk of cardiovascular death:

- Exercise induced VEB: risk of death 2.53 (95% CI 1.65–3.88)[18]
- Acute myocardial infarction (AMI), frequent and complex VEB often precede VF or sustained VT and are a marker of risk of subsequent sudden cardiac death

Apart from ischaemic heart disease, VEB may be associated with cardiomyopathy, valvular disease, myocarditis and non-cardiac precipitating factors (e.g. electrolyte and acid-base disturbances, hypoxia and drugs such as digoxin).

TREATMENT
Drug treatment of VEB is rarely indicated and may be dangerous.

- Correct potassium and magnesium
- Severely symptomatic patients with frequent complex VEB may benefit from judicious β-blockade
- The underlying cause of VEB is often more clinically relevant than the arrhythmia. Following myocardial infarction, β-adrenergic blockers, which are indicated for long-term benefit, will also likely suppress VEB
- Prophylactic lignocaine following AMI will increase total mortality and has been abandoned[19,20]
- Attempts at long-term VEB suppression with Class IC agents (flecainide and encainide), even if successful, increase mortality[12]

SUPRAVENTRICULAR TACHYCARDIAS (SVT)[21,22] (Table 16.5)

SVT are any tachycardias that require atrial or AV nodal tissue for their initiation and maintenance.

- SVT are usually conducted rapidly through the bundle branches so that QRS complexes are narrow
- All narrow complex tachycardias are SVT and wide complex tachycardias are usually ventricular

Table 16.5 Classification of supraventricular tachycardias

AV node dependent
  AV nodal re-entry tachycardia: re-entry within the AV node
  AV re-entry tachycardia: re-entry includes accessory pathway between atria and ventricles.
  Accelerated idio-nodal rhythm: increased automaticity of AV node
AV node independent
  Atrial flutter: re-entry confined to atria
  Atrial fibrillation: multiple re-entry circuits confined to atria
  Unifocal atrial tachycardia: usually due to increased automaticity
  Multifocal atrial tachycardia: increased automaticity or triggered activity
  Others: sinus node re-entry tachycardia

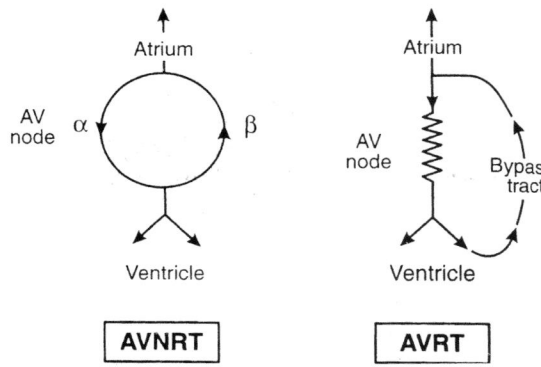

Fig. 16.11   (a) Atrioventricular (AV) nodal re-entry tachycardia (AVNRT). Re-entry circuit with both pathways within the AV node. (b) AV re-entry tachycardia (AVRT). Re-entry circuit involves the AV node and an accessory pathway external to AV node. The impulses usually pass antegrade through the AV node and retrograde up the accessory 'bypass' tract

- However, SVT may be wide complex in the setting of bundle branch block and pre-excitation

A clinically useful classification divides SVT into AV node dependent and AV node independent.

AV NODE DEPENDENT SVT
In these SVT, sometimes referred to as junctional tachycardias, the re-entry circuit or ectopic focus involves the AV node or junction. Blocking the AV node with drugs such as adenosine or vagal manoeuvres will terminate these SVT.

AV NODE INDEPENDENT SVT
In these SVT, also referred to as atrial tachycardias, the atrial tissue only is required for the initiation and maintenance of the tachycardia. Blocking the AV node will not terminate these SVT, merely slowing ventricular rate. Distinguishing between AV node dependent and independent SVTs can be difficult. Vagal manoeuvres or drugs that prolong AV nodal refractoriness (e.g. adenosine) may assist in diagnosis:

- Temporary AV block with unchanged atrial rate indicates AV node independence
- Slowing or reversion of the tachycardia diagnoses AV dependence

AV NODAL RE-ENTRY TACHYCARDIA
(Fig. 16.11a)

Re-entry tachycardia is confined to the AV node. Antegrade conduction to the ventricles usually occurs over the slow (α) pathway and retrograde conduction over the fast (β) pathway.

ECG
Regular narrow-complex tachycardia (140–220 beats/min) with abrupt onset and termination. P-waves are usually not observed as they are buried in the QRS complexes (Fig. 16.12).

CLINICAL
AVNRT is a common arrhythmia that is usually not associated with structural heart disease. The major symptom is palpitations.

TREATMENT
Vagal manoeuvres slow conduction through the AV node and may 'break' the tachycardia. If carotid sinus massage fails, adenosine is the drug of choice and nearly all AVNRTs will revert with adenosine.[23,24] Verapamil has been used in the past, but causes hypotension, which may be prolonged if cardiac function is depressed or patients are receiving β-adrenergic blockers. Sotalol, amiodarone and flecainide may also be effective but are rarely used. Rapid atrial pacing will usually terminate AVNRT but is rarely needed.

Cardioversion is occasionally necessary when drugs are ineffective or when severe haemodynamic instability is present.

PREVENTION
Troublesome recurring episodes of AVNRT can be cured by radio-frequency ablation, using a transvenous catheter to interrupt the re-entrant circuit permanently.[25]

AV RE-ENTRY TACHYCARDIA (Fig. 16.11b)

The re-entry pathway consists of the AV node and an accessory pathway, which bypasses the AV node. The accessory pathway may be evident during sinus rhythm with the ECG showing pre-excitation; short PR interval, delta wave and widening of the QRS (see Wolff–Parkinson–White (WPW) syndrome, below, under pre-excitation syndrome). However, in 25% of cases, the accessory pathway conducts only retrogradely from ventri-

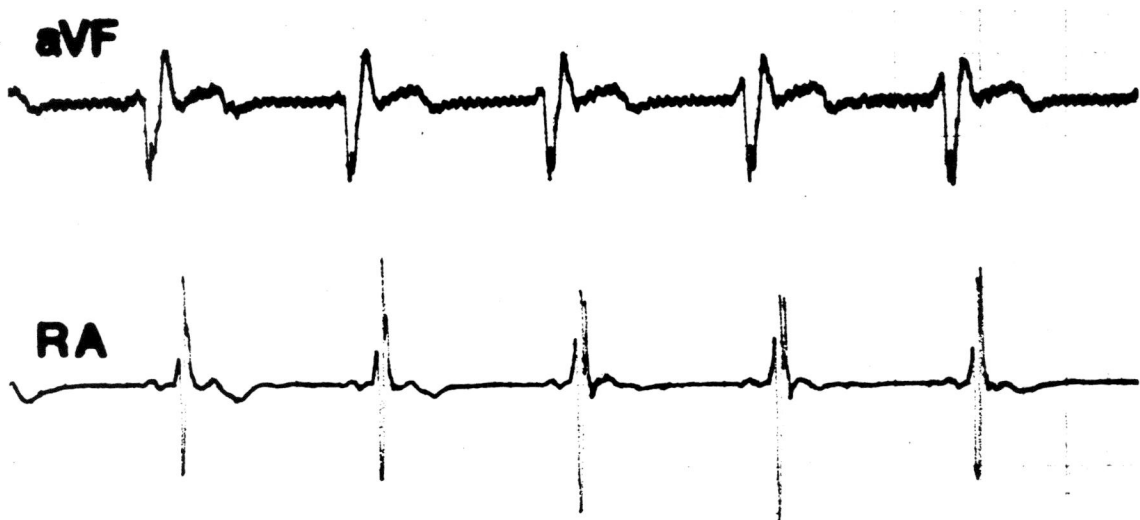

Fig. 16.12 Rhythm strip (aVF) shows narrow-complex tachycardia (paper speed 50 mm/s; rate 133 per min). There is no recognizable P-wave. Intracardiac trace from right atrium (RA) shows P-wave immediately after QRS, indicating the rhythm is AV nodal re-entry tachycardia.

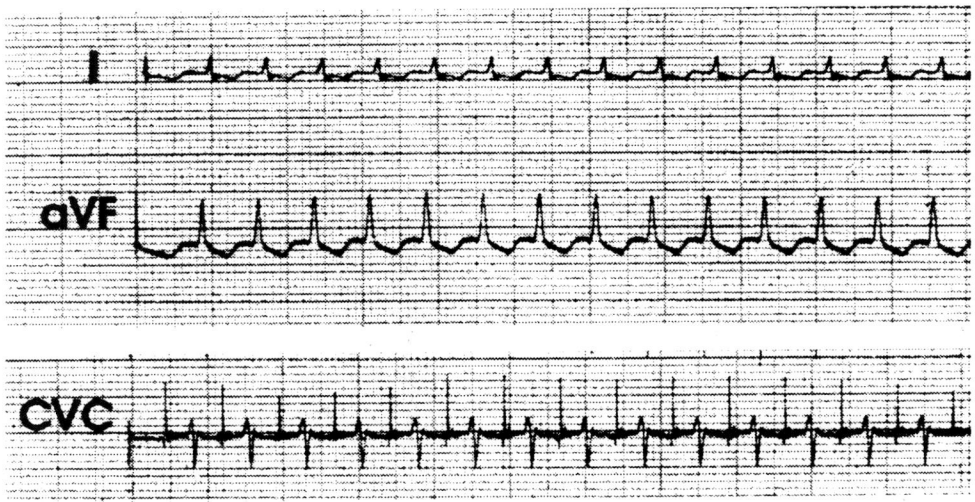

Fig. 16.13 No P-waves are evident in the surface leads (I, aVF). The trace from the central venous catheter (CVC) shows P-wave some time after the QRS, indicating the rhythm is atrioventricular re-entry tachycardia

cle to atria and the ECG pre-excitation will be concealed in sinus rhythm. Orthodromic AVRT, with antegrade nodal and retrograde accessory pathway circuit, is the most common regular SVT in patients with accessory pathway.

ECG
The ECG is similar to AVNRT. The length of the re-entry circuit is however greater, and the accessory AV pathway is some distance from the AV node. It therefore takes longer for the impulse to be conducted backwards to the atria, and so the retrograde P-wave usually occurs after the QRS, sometimes at some distance and is inverted in leads II, III and aVF (Fig. 16.13).

CLINICAL
AVRT is similar to AVNRT, although antegrade conduction over the accessory pathway may be very rapid with WPW syndrome, should AF occur.

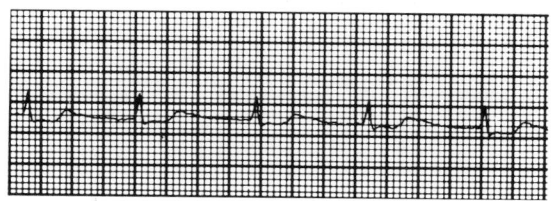

Fig. 16.14 Accelerated junctional rhythm (rate 84 per min)

TREATMENT[23,24]

Acute treatment is identical to AVNRT, but verapamil should be avoided in WPW syndrome, as it may block the AV node, facilitating very rapid conduction to the ventricles via the accessory pathway.[26]

PREVENTION

Drugs such as sotalol and flecainide may prevent recurrence of the tachycardia. Radio-frequency ablation of the accessory pathway is usually curative.[25]

ACCELERATED IDIONODAL RHYTHM

Increased automaticity of the AV junction (above the inherent discharge rate of 40–60 per min) is the usual cause of this arrhythmia. The often-used term non-paroxysmal AV junctional tachycardia is cumbersome and misleading; junctional rate is commonly 60–100 per min, not strictly a tachycardia. AV dissociation is often present, but there may be synchronization of the two pacemakers; so-called iso-rhythmic dissociation.

ECG

There are narrow complexes on the ECG at a regular rate (60–130 min) (Fig. 16.14), often with independent atrial activity. With iso-rhythmic dissociation, P-wave is either fixed relative to the QRS complex (usually just after) or oscillates to and fro across the QRS in a rhythmical manner.

CLINICAL

It may be observed in normal persons, but is often associated with structural heart disease, especially following

inferior myocardial infarction. Digoxin intoxication is another important cause.

TREATMENT

In most cases, the rhythm is transient and well tolerated, and no treatment is required. Treatment is otherwise directed towards the underlying cause.

UNIFOCAL ATRIAL TACHYCARDIA

This is sometimes called ectopic atrial tachycardia to distinguish it from the atrial tachycardias (referring collectively to unifocal atrial tachycardia, Afl and atrial fibrillation (AF)). However, it is inappropriate to call atrial tachycardia paroxysmal atrial tachycardia. Paroxysmal, by definition, indicates an abrupt onset and termination, which applies less commonly to unifocal atrial tachycardia. Vagal manoeuvres will not terminate this arrhythmia, but AV block may be induced, or increased if already present.

ECG

P-wave morphology is abnormal but monomorphic. Atrial rate is often 130–160 per min, and may occasionally exceed 200 per min. QRS complexes will usually be narrow (Fig. 16.15). AV block is common (Fig. 16.16).

CLINICAL

Digitalis intoxication is the most common cause, especially when AV block is present. Other causes include myocardial infarction, chronic lung disease and metabolic disturbances.

TREATMENT[24]

If applicable, digitalis is stopped and the toxicity treated. Otherwise digoxin may be used to control the ventricular rate. β-adrenergic blockers or amiodarone are alternatives. Rapid atrial pacing may be ineffective if the arrhythmia is due to increased automaticity, although it may increase AV block, thereby slowing ventricular rate. Synchronized direct current (DC) shock may be necessary, but is avoided if digitalis intoxication is suspected.

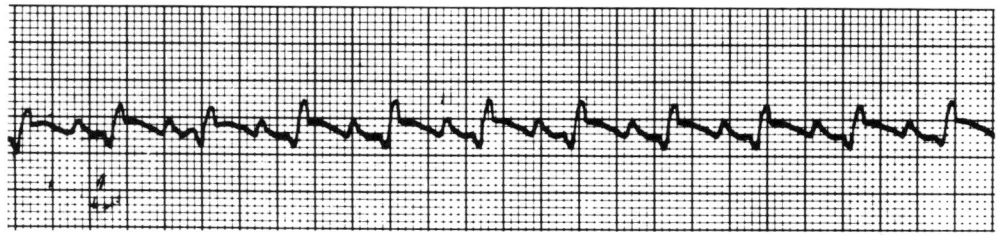

Fig. 16.15 Unifocal atrial tachycardia with 1 : 1 atrioventricular conduction (rate about 125 per min)

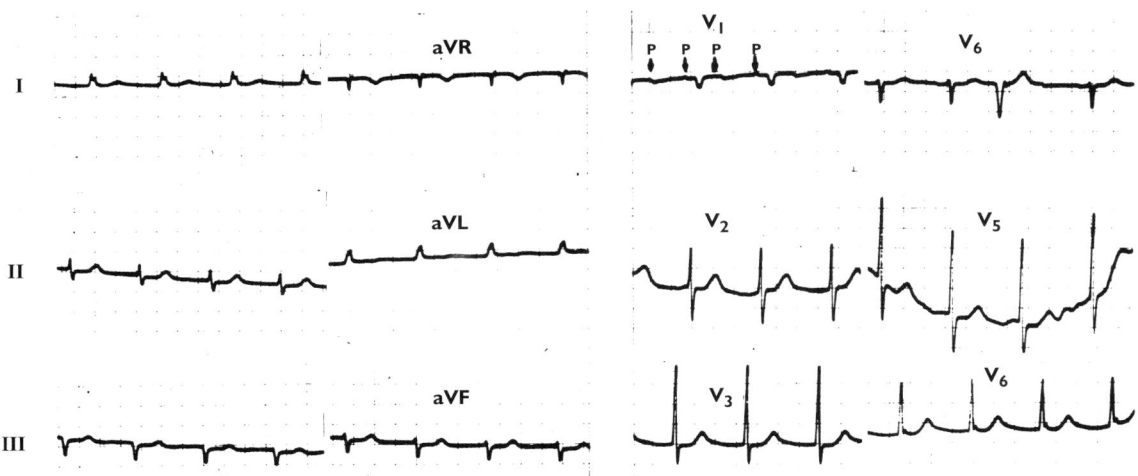

Fig. 16.16 Unifocal atrial tachycardia (atrial rate about 185 per min) with 2:1 atrioventricular block. P-waves are best seen in V_1

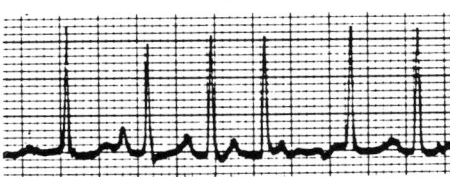

Fig. 16.17 Multifocal atrial tachycardia. Note irregular P-waves (atrial rate about 160 per min) with differing morphology. Most P-waves are conducted to the ventricles

MULTIFOCAL ATRIAL TACHYCARDIA (MAT)[27]

MAT is defined as an atrial rhythm, rate greater than 100 per min, with organized, discrete non-sinus P-waves having at least three different forms in the same ECG trace. The baseline between P-waves is iso-electric, and the PP, PR and RR intervals are irregular. This is an uncommon arrhythmia, also known as chaotic or mixed atrial tachycardia.

ECG

There are irregular atrial rates, usually 100–130 per min, with varying P-wave morphology and some degree of AV block (Fig. 16.17). Most P-waves are conducted to the ventricles, usually with narrow QRS complexes.

CLINICAL

MAT is often misdiagnosed and inappropriately treated as AF. This rhythm occurs most commonly in critically ill elderly patients with chronic lung disease and often cor pulmonale, and is associated with a very high mortality from underlying disease. Theophylline has been implicated as a precipitating cause, and rarely digoxin.

TREATMENT

Treatment should correct the underlying cause (e.g. treatment of cardio-respiratory failure, electrolyte and acid–base abnormalities and theophylline toxicity). Spontaneous reversion is common, and few patients require anti-arrhythmic therapy. Magnesium is the drug of choice for acute control.[28] β-Blockers are probably more effective than diltiazem, but because of the common association of MAT with obstructive lung disease have limited utility.[29] Digoxin and cardioversion are ineffective which highlights the need to differentiate MAT from AF. Longer-term control is best achieved with diltiazem in patients with good left ventricular function and amiodarone in those without.

ATRIAL FLUTTER[30]

Atrial rate during classical Afl is 250–350 per min, and in most cases, close to 300 per min. Afl is due to a single re-entry circuit lying within the right atrium and the wave of depolarization in most patients is anti-clockwise. If the right atrium is significantly enlarged the rate may be considerably slower. Studies in patients who had recently undergone cardiac surgery has subdivided Afl into type I and II on the basis of rate and typical responses to atrial pacing.

Type I flutter was slower, rate 240–320 beats/min, and was readily entrained with overdrive pacing. Type II flutter was faster than type I, with rates of 340–430 beats/min. Type II flutter could not be entrained or terminated by pacing. Type II is thought to arise from a circus pathway with a very short excitable gap.

ECG

Atrial flutter waves (characteristic saw-tooth appearance with no iso-electric baseline) are best seen in V_1

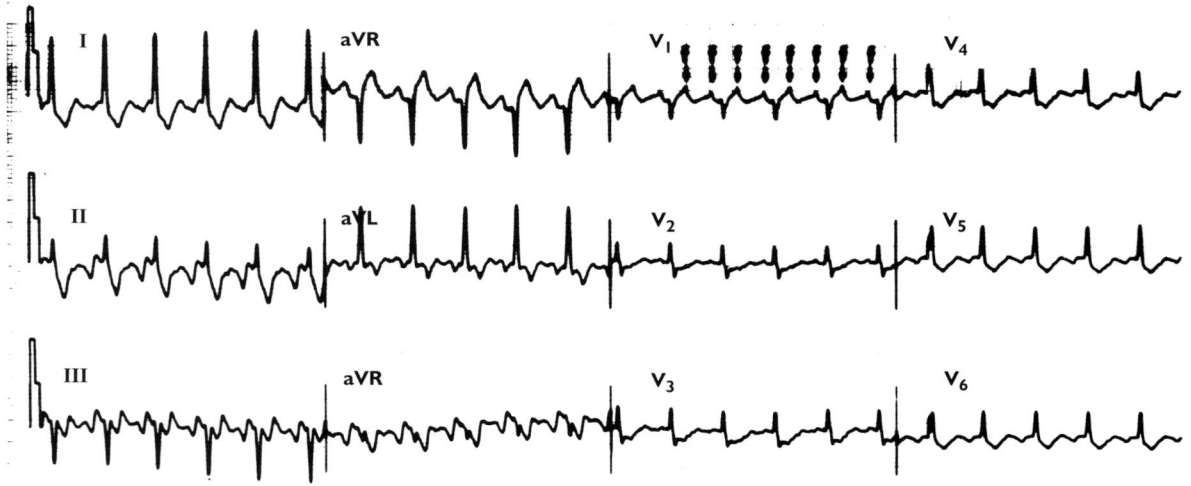

Fig. 16.18   Atrial flutter with 2 : 1 atrioventricular block. The flutter (f) waves are best seen in VI

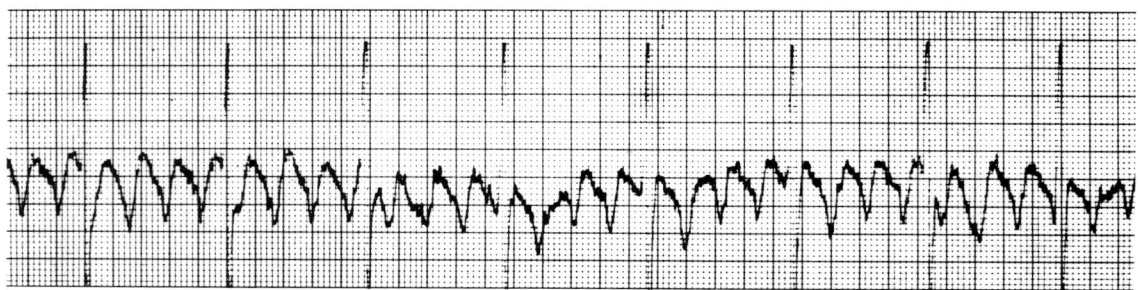

Fig. 16.19   Atrial flutter: typical flutter waves. Atrioventricular (AV) block (4 : 1) is due to drug effect on the AV node

(Fig. 16.18) or aVF, but leads II and III may also be useful. The flutter waves are usually negative in aVF. Rapid QRS waves may obscure typical flutter waves, and vagal manoeuvres may unmask them (Fig. 16.5). AV conduction block (usually 2:1) is usually present, so that alternate flutter waves are conducted to the ventricles, with a ventricular rate close to 150 beats/min. Treatment with drugs that affect AV node conduction may lead to higher degrees of AV block (Fig. 16.19) and/or variable AV block with irregular QRS duration. Rarely, Afl with 1:1 conduction occurs (Fig. 16.20). This is usually associated with sympathetic over-activity or Class I anti-arrhythmic drugs (which slow atrial discharge rate to 200 per min, thereby allowing each atrial impulse to be conducted). QRS complexes are usually narrow, as conduction through the bundle branches is normal.

CLINICAL

Afl is less common than AF. It may occur in ischaemic heart disease, cardiomyopathy, rheumatic heart disease, thyrotoxicosis, and after cardiac surgery.

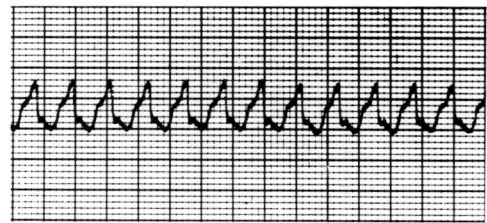

Fig. 16.20   Atrial flutter with 1 : 1 atrioventricular conduction. Heart rate approaches 300 beats per min

TREATMENT[24]

No drug will reliably terminate Afl, although ibutillide has been shown to be most likely to result in pharmacological reversion. Attempts at slowing ventricular rate by drugs that will increase degree of AV block are worthwhile in the first instance. Drugs such as digoxin, diltiazem, β-adrenergic blockers, sotalol and amiodarone may be tried, the choice depending on left ventricular function. Flecainide and procainamide may occasionally be effective at terminating Afl. However, Class IA and IC drugs may lead to 1:1 AV conduction. Class I drugs should probably be avoided unless ventricular response has been slowed with calcium channel or β-adrenergic blocking drugs.

Synchronized DC cardioversion, often with low energies (25–50 J), is a reliable treatment option. Rapid atrial pacing faster than the flutter rate will terminate classical or type I Afl in most patients.

PREVENTION

Prevention is difficult. Drugs used include sotalol and amiodarone at low doses. Class IC agents (e.g. flecainide) may be used in patients without significant structural heart disease. Increasingly recurrent or refractory Afl may be cured by radio-frequency ablation to create a linear lesion between the inferior tricuspid annulus and the eustachian ridge at the anterior margin of the inferior vena cava to interrupt the re-entry circuit.[25]

ATRIAL FIBRILLATION[31]

AF is the most common arrhythmia requiring treatment and/or hospital admission. The incidence increases with age; 5% of individuals over 70 years have this arrhythmia.

AF is common in:

- Congestive cardiac failure (40%)
- Coronary artery bypass grafting (25–50%)
- Critically ill patients (15%)

Idiopathic or lone AF (i.e. with no structural heart disease or precipitating factor) in someone aged under 60 years has an excellent prognosis, however, AF developing after cardiac surgery for instance, is associated with increased stroke, life-threatening arrhythmias and longer hospital stays.

ECG

Atrial activity is chaotic with rapid (350–600 per min) and irregular depolarizations varying in amplitude and morphology (fibrillation waves). Ventricular response is irregularly irregular (Fig. 16.21). Most atrial impulses are not conducted to the ventricles, resulting in an untreated ventricular rate of 100–180 per min (Fig. 16.22). QRS complexes will usually be narrow. When the ventricular rate is very rapid or very slow, ventricular irregularity may be missed (Fig. 16.22).

CLINICAL

AF is more common in patients with underlying heart disease (particularly those with a dilated left atrium) and abnormal atrial electrophysiology. Causes include ischaemic and valvular heart disease, hypertension, cardiac failure, thyrotoxicosis and alcohol abuse. AF may also occur after cardiac surgery and thoracotomy. AF can be chronic, or intermittent with paroxysmal attacks. Chronic AF has a poorer prognosis. AF is associated with:

- Adverse haemodynamic effects. Rapid ventricular rate and loss of atrial systole may increase pulmonary capillary wedge pressure, while stroke volume and cardiac output decline
- Systemic embolism and stroke. AF increases the risk of non-haemorrhagic stroke five-fold
- Tachycardiomyopathy. Reversible global cardiomyopathy secondary to rapid heart rate

TREATMENT[24,32,33]

The goals of treatment are ventricular rate control, anticoagulation where appropriate and conversion to sinus rhythm.

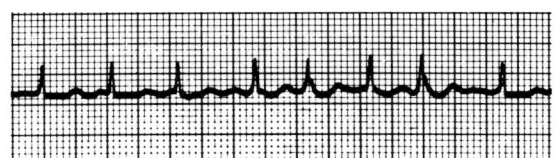

Fig. 16.21   Atrial fibrillation: wavy baseline and irregular QRS complexes

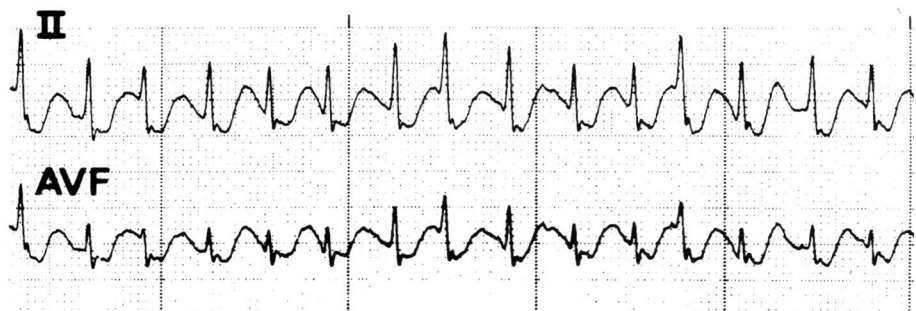

Fig. 16.22   Atrial fibrillation with rapid ventricular response. Fibrillation waves are not obvious. QRS irregularity may be missed as ventricular rate is rapid

RECENT ONSET OR PAROXYSMAL AF

VENTRICULAR RATE CONTROL

The urgency of ventricular rate control depends on the clinical situation and spontaneous reversion of AF is common. Treatment may not be necessary, and a reasonable strategy is based on clinical status:

- Haemodynamically unstable with rapid ventricular rate requires immediate synchronized DC shock to urgently control rate.
- Haemodynamically stable, symptomatic with depressed left ventricular function: semi-urgent synchronized DC shock or drug therapy, digoxin or amiodarone to control ventricular rate until spontaneous reversion occurs.
- Haemodynamically stable, symptomatic, normal left ventricular function: control of ventricular response with β-adrenergic blockers, diltiazem, digoxin, magnesium, amiodarone or sotalol.
- Haemodynamically stable, with minimal or no symptoms: no immediate treatment. Most cases will revert spontaneously within 24 h.

ANTICOAGULATION[34,35]

Once AF has been present for more than 48 h, some authors stipulate 24 h, anticoagulation is required prior to DC shock cardioversion. Anticoagulation should be continued for 3 weeks prior to DC shock cardioversion. This period can be shortened to 1 day for heparin and 5 days for warfarin if the left atrium can be demonstrated free of clot on trans-oesophageal echocardiography. Heparin dose should be titrated to an activated partial thromboplastin time 2–3 times control and warfarin to produce an international normalized ratio (INR) of 2.0–3.0. Many clinical situations dictate delay in anticoagulation, such as recent surgery or other bleeding risks, and elective DC shock cardioversion should also be delayed.

CONVERSION TO SINUS RHYTHM

Anti-arrhythmic drugs or DC shock cardioversion can be used. The likelihood of short and long term success depends on the clinical situation.

DC SHOCK CARDIOVERSION

Is indicated either before 24–48 h or after appropriated anticoagulation protocol. Combining DC shock with anti-arrhythmic drugs to promote maintenance of sinus rhythm is favored especially if risk factors for relapse exist. Cardioversion is less likely to be successful if AF has been present for over 1 year, left atrial size is greater than 45 mm, and untreated conditions are present (e.g. thyrotoxicosis, valvular heart disease and heart failure). Critically ill patients who are septic, postoperative or on drugs such as catecholamines are likely to relapse.

ANTI-ARRHYTHMIC DRUGS

The drugs used for ventricular rate control, digoxin, diltiazem and β-adrenergic blockers are unlikely to result in pharmacological cardioversion.

Anti-arrhythmic drugs that may cardiovert are unfortunately relatively ineffective and may possibly be dangerous. They are more effective at retaining sinus rhythm. About 50% will remain in sinus rhythm 1 year after cardioversion with drugs and 25% without drugs.

Quinidine is more effective than placebo, but increases mortality through proarrhythmia. Ibutilide is a new anti-arrhythmic drug with particular success at pharmacological cardioversion. Pre-treatment with ibutilide increased cardioversion from 72% for placebo to 100%. In placebo failures, crossover to ibutilide resulted in a 100% success rate with subsequent cardioversion. Ibutilide also resulted in reduction in DC shock energy required from 228 ± 93 J to 166 ± 80 J. However, ibutilide was associated with a 3% incidence of sustained polymorphous VT.[36]

Other drugs currently used to promote onset of sinus rhythm and prevent AF relapse include amiodarone, sotalol, procainamide, flecainide and propafenone. Amiodarone was found to be superior in preventing AF recurrence with a recurrence rate of 35% compared to a recurrence rate of 63% for sotalol and propafenone.[37]

The factors dictating choice are:

- degree of left ventricular depression; amiodarone having the least and flecainide the greatest
- risk of proarrhythmia; worse with flecainide and propafenone
- long term side-effect profile; amiodarone being the worst

When using amiodarone for prevention of AF recurrence there was an 18% incidence of adverse effects versus 11% for sotalol and propafenone.[37]

RADIO-FREQUENCY CATHETER ABLATION

It has been recognized, particularly in younger patients with 'lone' AF that a single arrhythmogenic focus initiates paroxysmal AF. These foci have been localized by atrial mapping, typically around the atrial orifice of pulmonary veins, and are suitable for radio-frequency ablation. Early results are promising; however, there is a risk of pulmonary vein stenosis.[25]

CHRONIC AF

While most patients undergo at least one attempt at cardioversion to sinus rhythm, many are left in chronic AF, particularly those with dilated atria, poor left ventricular function and valvular heart disease. In this setting, treatment aims at ventricular rate control and prevention of embolic stroke.

VENTRICULAR RATE CONTROL

Digoxin is often the drug of choice, particularly in patients with poor left ventricular function. It is often ineffective at controlling ventricular rate during exercise and physiological stress. Judicious addition of a small dose of a β-adrenergic blocker may improve digoxin control. Amiodarone is particularly useful in patients with poor left ventricular function. Higher dose β-adrenergic blocker, diltiazem, sotalol or flecainide can be used in patients with good left ventricular function. Rarely, His-bundle ablation with permanent cardiac pacing may be required for severe cases refractory to drug therapy.

ANTICOAGULATION

Consider for all patients. Risk of embolic stroke is increased with:

- enlarged left atrium (>45 mm)
- congestive cardiac failure
- valvular heart disease

Warfarin decreases the incidence from 8% to 3%, although intracranial haemorrhage occurs (0.3% per year). Low-dose warfarin (international normalized ratio 1.5–2.0) is less effective than an INR of 2.0–3.0 but has fewer haemorrhagic complications. Embolic stroke rate doubles as INR falls from 2.0 to 1.7, and is markedly higher at an INR of 1.3 compared to 2.0.[34] The risk of intracranial haemorrhage has to increase six-fold to justify withholding warfarin. Patients aged under 60 years with lone AF have a very low incidence of non-haemorrhagic stroke, and aspirin (e.g. 325 mg/day) is recommended. Patients over 75 years, or those with diabetes, hypertension or previous embolic episodes, have a stroke incidence of 10%, and should probably receive warfarin unless haemorrhagic risks are deemed unacceptably high.

PRE-EXCITATION SYNDROME

Pre-excitation syndromes have an additional or accessory AV pathway. The term WPW syndrome is usually applied when tachyarrhythmias are present.

ECG

During sinus rhythm, an atrial impulse will reach the ventricles via both the AV node and the accessory AV pathway. The latter conducts the atrial impulse to the ventricles before the AV node (Fig. 16.11b), resulting in ventricular pre-excitation and a short PR interval. On reaching the ventricles, the pre-excitation impulse is not conducted via the specialized conducting system. Hence, early ventricular activation will be slow (resulting in δ-wave and T-wave abnormalities) (Fig. 16.23). δ-wave polarity in a 12-lead ECG may help localize the anatomical position of the accessory pathway. Classification into type A (positive complex in V_1) and type B (negative complex V_1) is not helpful.

CLINICAL

AVRT or AF (Fig. 16.24) can occur with WPW. During AVRT, the re-entry impulse usually travels down the AV

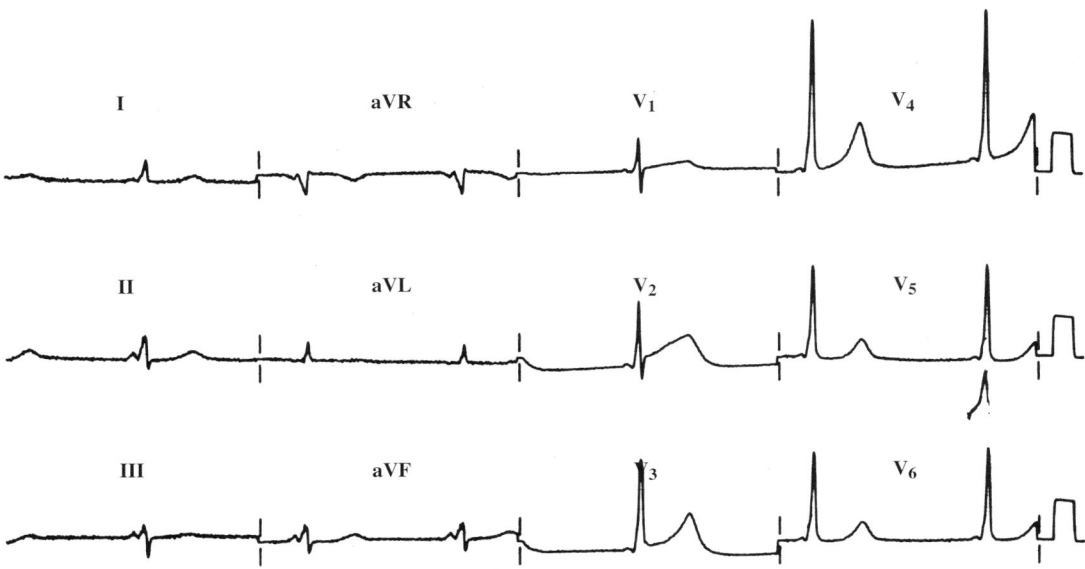

Fig. 16.23 Wolff–Parkinson–White syndrome. Note the short PR interval, wide QRS and δ wave

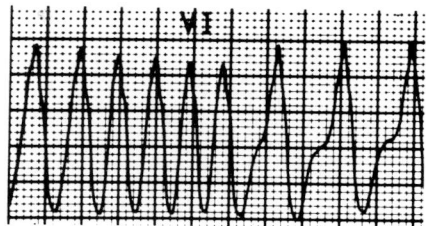

Fig. 16.24 Atrial fibrillation with Wolff–Parkinson–White syndrome. Note the irregular and wide QRS complexes

node and back up the accessory pathway; δ-waves will not be present. Occasionally, the re-entry impulse may pass in the opposite direction (down the accessory pathway and up the AV node), resulting in a wide QRS complex tachycardia. Treatment is the same as for AVRT (i.e. IV adenosine). AF is uncommon in WPW, but may be life-threatening. Most impulses are conducted via the accessory pathway, leading to wide QRS complexes (δ-waves). The ECG of WPW with AF usually shows rapid, irregular QRS complexes with variable QRS width (Fig. 16.24). Ventricular response is very rapid, leading to hypotension or cardiogenic shock. This arrhythmia may degenerate to VF.

TREATMENT[24]
Usually involves synchronized DC shock. Anti-arrhythmic drugs may be used when patients are haemodynamically stable and the ventricular rate is not excessively rapid.

- Drugs that prolong the refractory period of the accessory pathway are useful (e.g. sotalol, amiodarone, flecainide and procainamide)
- Drugs that shorten the refractory period (e.g. digoxin) are contraindicated as they may accelerate ventricular rate
- Verapamil and lignocaine may increase the ventricular rate during AF, and are also best avoided[26]
- β-Adrenergic blockers have no effect on the refractory period of the accessory pathway

Long-term management by radio-frequency ablation of the accessory pathway is effective in selected patients.[25]

VENTRICULAR TACHYCARDIA

VT is defined as three or more VEB at a rate greater than 130 per min, and may exceed 300 per min. VT lasting over 30 s is considered to be sustained. Non-sustained VT may not cause symptoms, but is associated with increased mortality in certain patients (e.g. after myocardial infarction). VT may be monomorphic (i.e. same QRS morphology) (Fig. 16.25) or polymorphic (varying QRS morphology).

MONOMORPHIC VT

This is the most common form of VT. It is commonly associated with previous myocardial infarction, and often causes symptoms (e.g. palpitations, shortness of breath, chest pain or syncope). It may result in cardiac arrest, due to the tachycardia itself or degeneration into VF. The most common mechanism is re-entry secondary to inhomogeneous activation of the myocardium and slow conduction through scar tissue from a previous myocardial infarction. AV dissociation (i.e. independent atrial and ventricular activity) (Fig. 16.26) is present in about 75% of instances, whereas retrograde ventricle to atrial conduction occurs in about 25%. AV dissociation is virtually diagnostic for VT during a wide-complex tachycardia, but ECG recognition of independent (and slower) atrial activity is difficult. VT is the most common cause of a wide-complex tachycardia (QRS >120 ms) and any such tachycardia should be considered VT until proven otherwise. Mistakes in diagnosis are common: SVT with aberrant conduction is often mistaken for VT. Inappropriate treatment based on incorrect diagnosis can have disastrous consequences.

ECG
Older criteria (e.g. QRS >140 ms and extreme electrical axis changes) are unhelpful in rhythm diagnosis.[38] New ECG criteria permit accurate diagnosis in four steps (Fig. 16.27).[39,40,41]

1 Is a RS complex present in any precordial lead? (QR, QRS, QS, monophasic R and rSR are not considered RS complexes.) If not (Fig. 16.28), the diagnosis is VT.

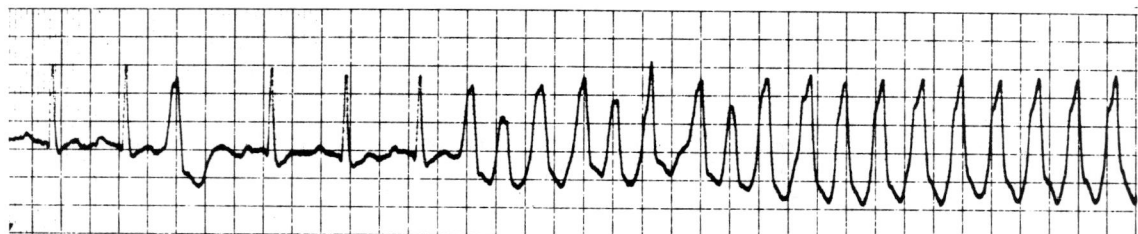

Fig. 16.25 Monomorphic ventricular tachycardia. Sinus rhythm with ventricular ectopic beats (third and seventh beats) of identical morphology are followed by ventricular tachycardia

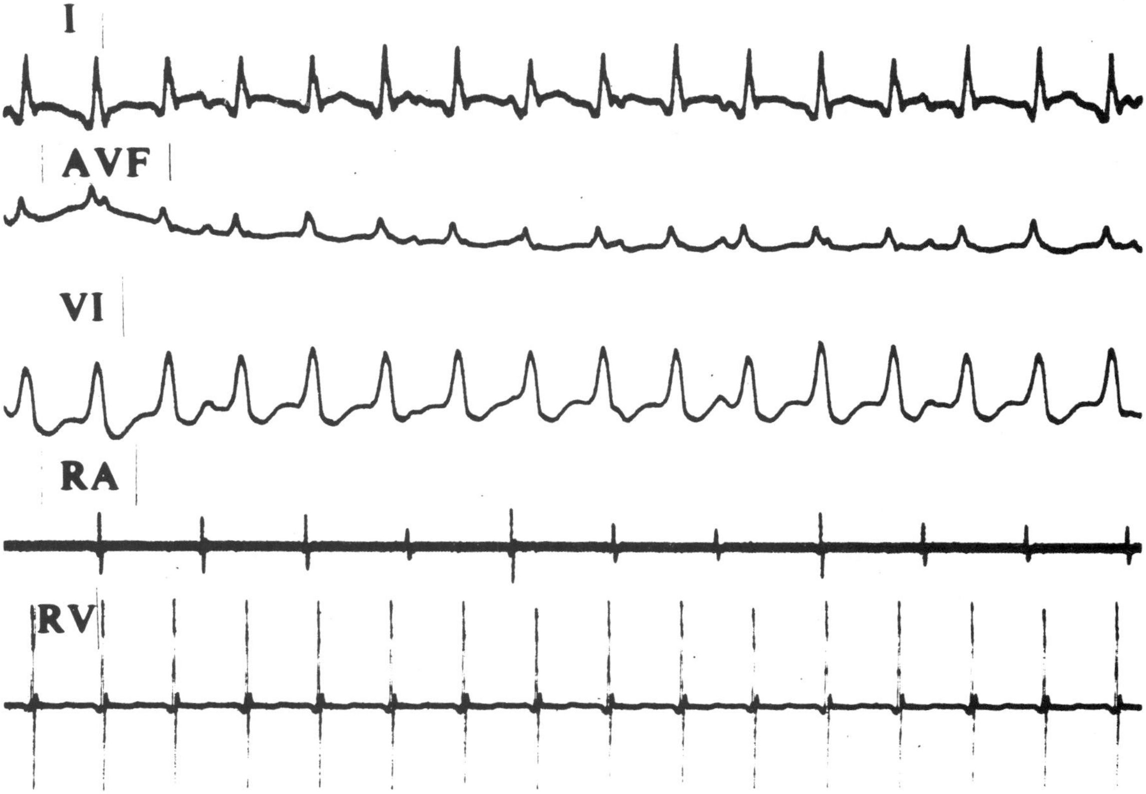

I

AVF

VI

RA

RV

Fig. 16.26 Atrioventricular ventricular (AV) dissociation in ventricular tachycardia. Leads I, aVF, and V₁ show AV dissociation with regular P-waves (rate 94 per min) unrelated to QRS complexes (135 per min). AV dissociation confirmed by intracardiac traces from pacing electrodes. Right atrial (RA) trace shows atrial activity independent of ventricular activity on the right ventricular (RV) trace

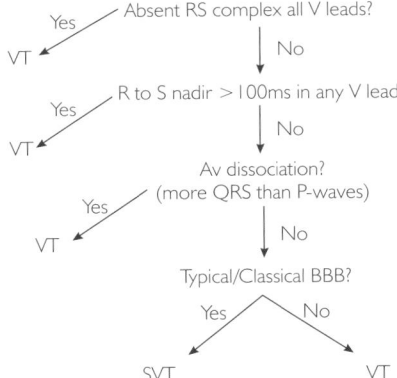

Fig. 16.27 Algorithm to diagnose a regular wide-complex tachycardia. VT, Ventricular tachycardia; AV, atrioventricular; BBB, bundle branch block; SVT, supraventricular tachycardia

2 If a RS is present, then measure the duration of the R to S nadir (lowest part of the S-wave). If this duration >100 ms in any V lead (Fig. 16.29), the rhythm is VT.

3 If RS <100 ms, then AV dissociation is searched for (more QRS complexes than P-waves (Fig. 16.26)). Indirect evidence of AV dissociation such as capture or fusion beats may be present. Capture beats occur when atrial impulses via the AV node activate the ventricle before the ventricle can be completely depolarized from the VT focus or circuit. Even a single capture or fusion beat confirms AV dissociation and VT (Fig. 16.30).

4 If AV dissociation is not present, then decide whether the wide QRS has a right or left bundle branch block (BBB) pattern. If the BBB is typical in both V₁ and V₆ leads, the rhythm is supraventricular in origin. Typical left BBB pattern requires an rS or QS nadir <70 ms in V₁ and R-wave, with no Q-wave in V₆. Typical right BBB pattern requires an rSR¹ pattern with R¹ > r in V₁ and R > S in V₆ (see the section on bundle branch block, below). If there are any atypical features, the rhythm is considered to be VT (Fig. 16.31).

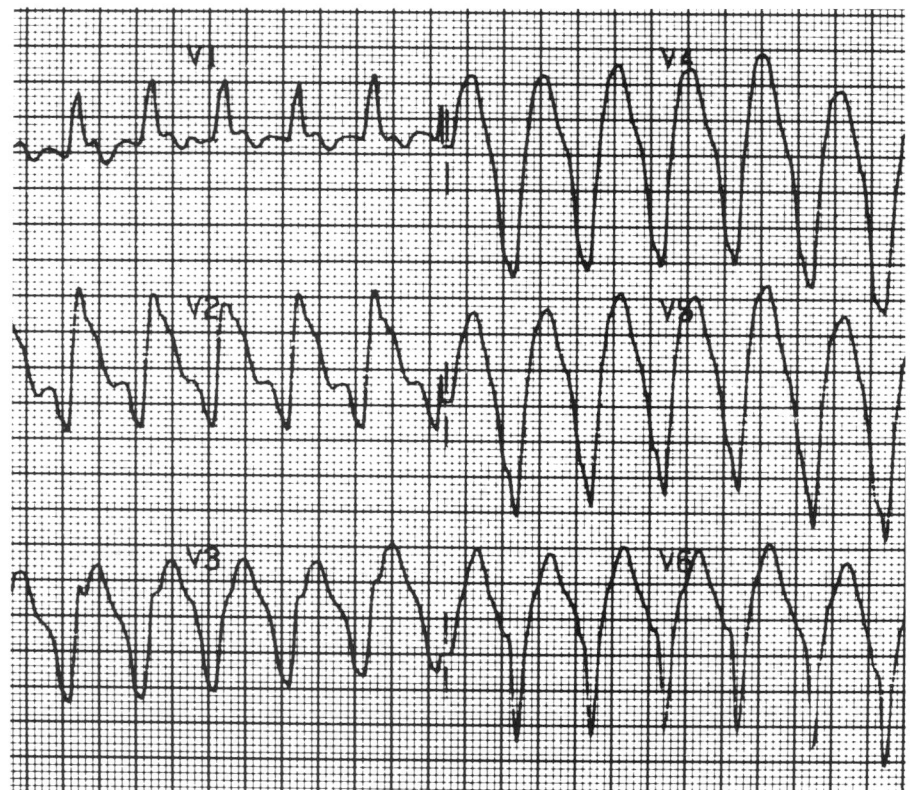

Fig. 16.28   Regular wide-complex tachycardia. No RS complex is present in any V lead. Diagnosis is ventricular tachycardia

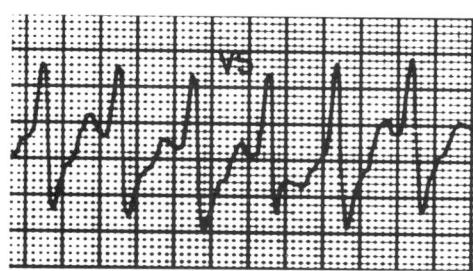

Fig. 16.29   Regular wide-complex tachycardia. RS nadir >100 ms. Diagnosis is ventricular tachycardia

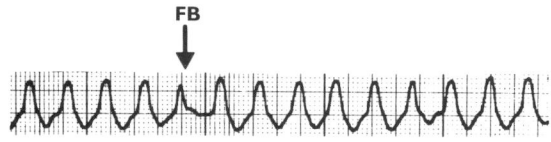

Fig. 16.30   Ventricular tachycardia. Fusion beat (FB) indicates atrioventricular dissociation

Termination of a wide-complex tachycardia by IV adenosine strongly suggests the arrhythmia as SVT. However, adenosine in this setting has the risk of destabilizing VT when blood pressure is barely compensated by vasodilatation or acceleration of accessory pathway conduction and is not recommended by International Liaison Committee on Resuscitation (ILCOR) as a diagnostic strategy in wide complex tachycardia.[25] Demonstration of AV dissociation by intracardiac ECG from a central venous catheter or a transvenous pacing lead signifies VT.

CLINICAL

The major cause of VT is significant coronary artery disease. Other causes include cardiomyopathy, myocarditis and valvular heart disease. Symptoms will depend on the ventricular rate, duration of tachycardia and underlying cardiac function. There are not necessarily any haemodynamic differences between VT and SVT with aberrant conduction but haemodynamic instability mandates management as for VT.

TREATMENT[24,42]

DC shock is indicated if a patient is haemodynamically unstable. Anti-arrhythmic drug trial is indicated in haemodynamically stable VT.

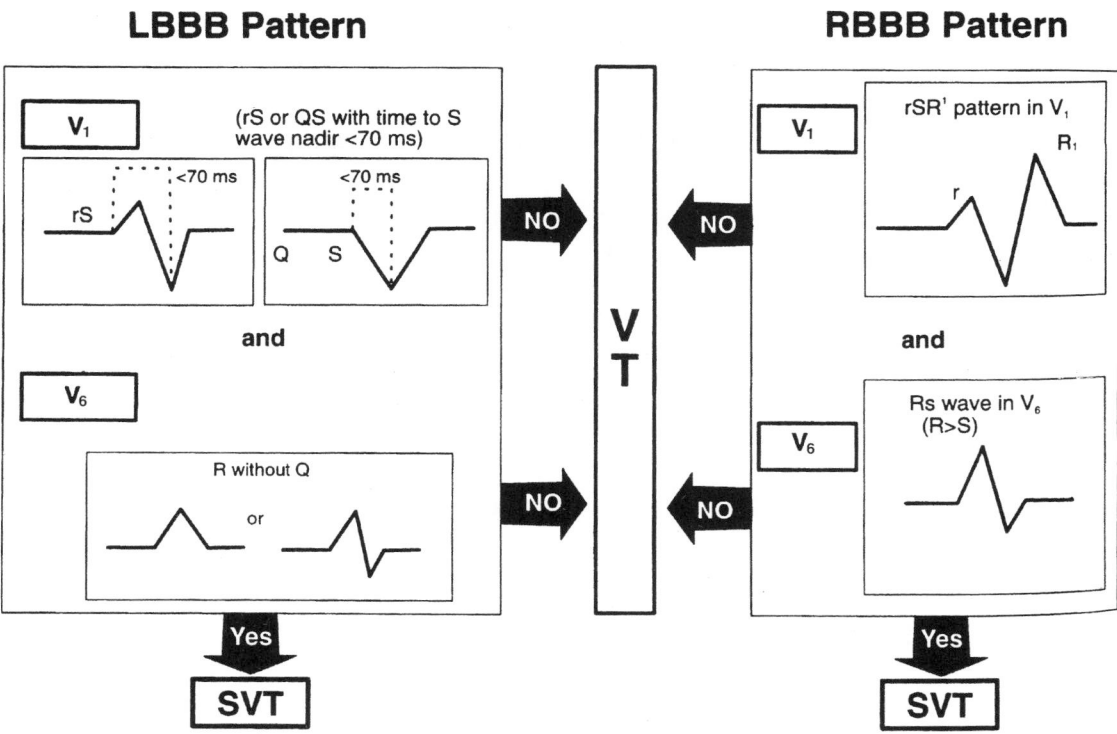

Fig. 16.31   Bundle branch block pattern with wide-complex tachycardia. If the pattern is classical (typical) in both V_1 and V_6, the diagnosis is supraventricular tachycardia. Otherwise, the rhythm is considered ventricular tachycardia. LBBB, Left bundle branch block; RBBB, right bundle branch block; SVT, supraventricular tachycardia

- Amiodarone may terminate VT; less negative inotropy action but delayed effect
- Sotalol and procainamide are more effective than lignocaine but are associated with significant myocardial depression
- Lignocaine, while traditionally indication, there are now doubts about its efficacy

If drugs are ineffective, synchronized DC shock is indicated. Rapid right ventricular pacing may also be effective.

Long-term prevention of VT and sudden death is difficult. Sotalol guided by Holter ECG or electrophysiological testing, and empirical (i.e. non-guided) amiodarone are superior to other drugs in preventing arrhythmia recurrences. Empirical β-adrenergic blockers also have a role. Implantable defibrillators can recognize and automatically terminate VT by rapid ventricular pacing or, should this fail, by internal DC cardioversion, which may be life-saving.

POLYMORPHIC VT AND TORSADE DE POINTES

This arrhythmia has QRS complexes at 200 per min or greater, which change in amplitude and axis so that they appear to twist around the baseline (Fig. 16.32). Torsade de pointe usually has prolonged QT during sinus rhythm, and U-waves are often present (see below; Long QT syndrome). However, polymorphic VT may be associated with a normal QT interval in settings such as myocardial ischaemia, infarction or post-cardiac surgery.

TREATMENT
Polymorphic VT associated with a normal QT interval during sinus rhythm (e.g. following acute myocardial infarction) should be treated in the same way as monomorphic VT. (See below treatment long QT polymarphic VT.)

ACCELERATED IDIOVENTRICULAR RHYTHM (AIVR)

This is often inappropriately called slow VT. Increased automaticity is probably the mechanism responsible for this relatively benign arrhythmia.

ECG
Wide QRS with a rate of 60–110 beats/min (Fig. 16.33). Sinus rate is often only slightly slower than the arrhythmia,

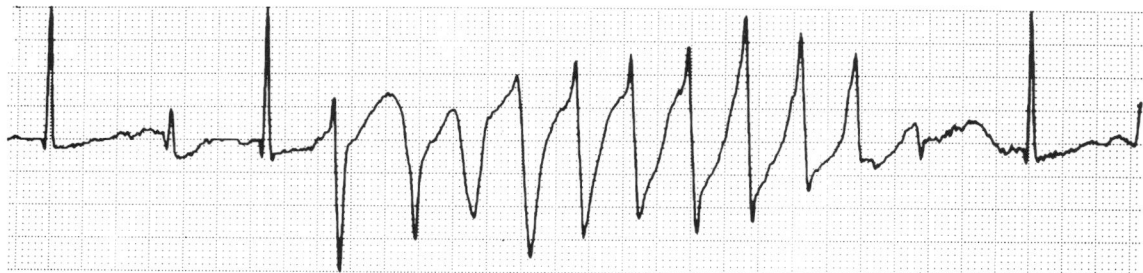

Fig. 16.32 Torsade de pointes. Note prolonged QT$_c$ interval

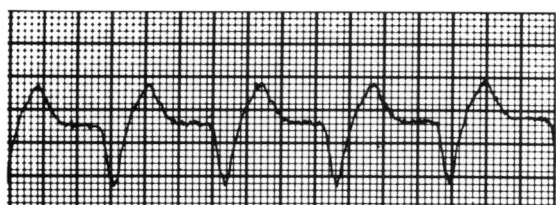

Fig. 16.33 Accelerated idioventricular rhythm (ventricular rate 88 per min)

so the dominant rhythm may be intermittent AIVR and sinus rhythm. Fusion beats are therefore common.

CLINICAL

The rhythm is commonly encountered in inferior myocardial infarction. AIVR may be misdiagnosed as VT. Occasionally, AIVR causes haemodynamic deterioration, usually due to loss of atrial systole. Increasing the atrial rate with either atropine or atrial pacing may then be necessary.

VENTRICULAR FIBRILLATION

VF always causes haemodynamic collapse, loss of consciousness and death if not immediately treated. Of patients resuscitated from VF, 20–30% have sustained an acute myocardial infarction, and 75% have coronary artery disease. VF (and VT) unassociated with acute myocardial infarction, is likely to be recurrent; 50% die within 3 years.

ECG

The ECG shows irregular waves of varying morphology and amplitude (Fig. 16.34).

CLINICAL

VF is usually associated with ischaemic heart disease, although other causes include cardiomyopathy, anti-arrhythmic drugs, severe hypoxia and non-synchronized DC cardioversion.

TREATMENT[42]

Immediate non-synchronized DC shock at 200 J, and if ineffective, repeated at 200–360 and 360 J (or biphasic equivalent). Time should not be wasted with basic life support if immediate defibrillation can be delivered.

If DC shock sequence fails basic and advanced life support aiming to maximize coronary blood flow with chest compressions and vasopressors is crucial to cardiac success. Until recently, any role of anti-arrhythmic drugs in DC shock resistant VF has been traditional rather than proven. Recommendations have varied from lignocaine, bretyllium to amiodarone. The ILCOR currently recommends consideration of a range of anti-arrhythmic drugs, including amiodarone, lignocaine, magnesium and procainamide. Recent studies indicate amiodarone as the drug of choice for DC shock resistant VF. Amiodarone (300 mg) was superior to lignocaine and, in another study, 5 mg/kg followed by 2.5 mg/kg if required was superior to lignocaine. There is an incidence of bradycardia and hypotension but no difference in adverse effect profile between lignocaine and this

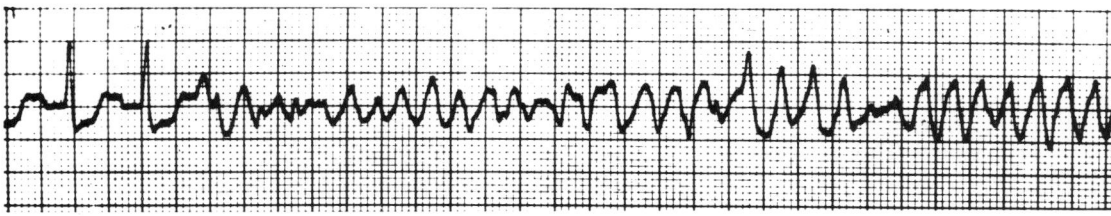

Fig. 16.34 Ventricular fibrillation

sizable amiodarone dose.[43,44] After return of circulation, appropriate anti-arrhythmic therapy is less clear but the role of lignocaine continues to disappear. Precipitating factors should be sought and treated (for long-term management issues, see the section on Sudden cardiac death).

RIGHT BUNDLE BRANCH BLOCK (RBBB)
(Fig. 16.35)

In RBBB, activation of the right ventricle is delayed.

ECG

The ECG shows wide QRS (>120 ms), rSR[1] in right ventricular leads V_1 or V_2 (often M-shaped), and a broad S-wave in left ventricular leads, especially I and V_6. Partial RBBB is identical, except the QRS duration is 110–120 ms.

CLINICAL

This is a normal variant, but may occur with massive pulmonary embolism, right ventricular hypertrophy, ischaemic heart disease and congenital heart disease (note that myocardial infarction can be diagnosed in the presence of RBBB).

LEFT BUNDLE BRANCH BLOCK (LBBB)
(Fig. 16.36)

In LBBB, the interventricular septum is activated from right to left (i.e. in the opposite direction to normal).

ECG

There is a wide QRS (>120 ms), primary and secondary R-waves (RR′, often M-shaped in left ventricular leads, especially V_6). Q-waves are never seen in left ventricular leads (V_4–V_6) (note that myocardial infarction usually cannot be diagnosed in the presence of LBBB). Partial LBBB is similar, except that the QRS duration is 110–120 ms.

CLINICAL

LBBB is often associated with heart disease such as coronary artery disease, cardiomyopathy or left ventricular hypertrophy. LBBB makes diagnosis of myocardial infarction difficult and the development of a new LBBB fulfills ECG criteria of acute infarction.

HEMIBLOCKS

The left branch of the bundle of His conducts impulses to the anterior superior left ventricle via the left anterior division, and to the posterior inferior part of the left ventricle via the posterior inferior division. Block can occur in either division.

LEFT ANTERIOR HEMIBLOCK (Fig. 16.37)
Left axis deviation (usually lead I predominantly positive, leads II and III predominantly negative) with initial R-wave in inferior leads (II, III, aVF).

LEFT POSTERIOR HEMIBLOCK
There is usually right axis deviation (lead I predominantly negative and lead III predominantly positive).

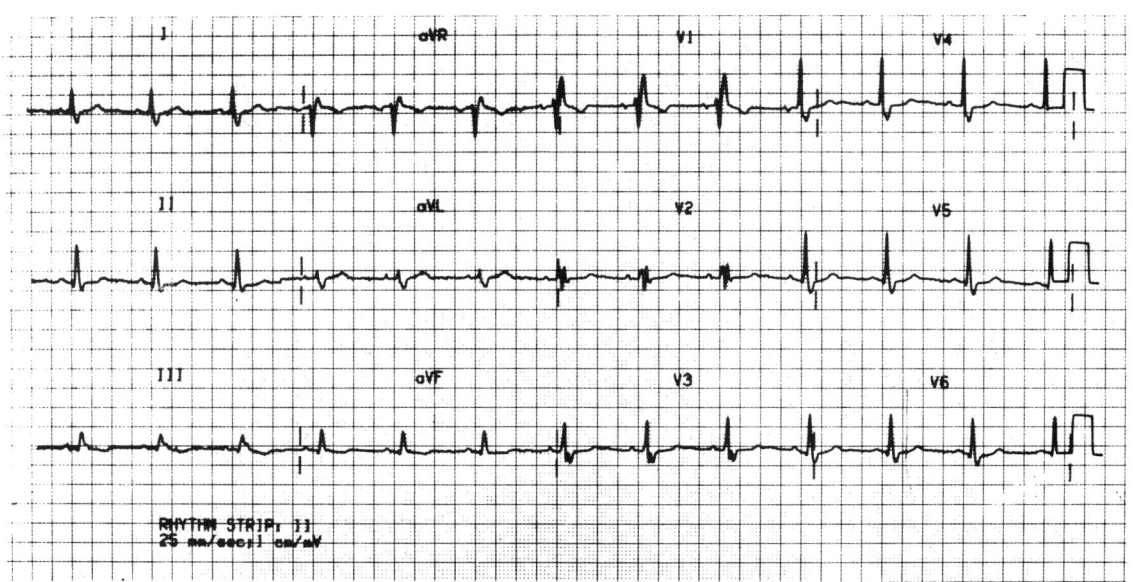

Fig. 16.35 Right bundle branch block

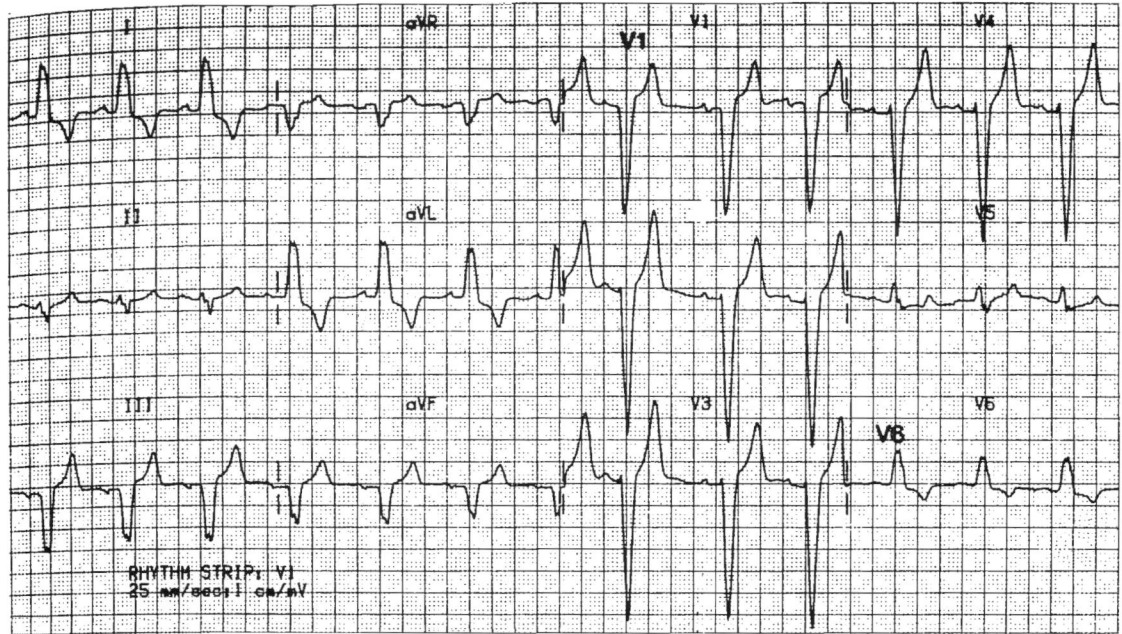

Fig. 16.36   Left bundle branch block

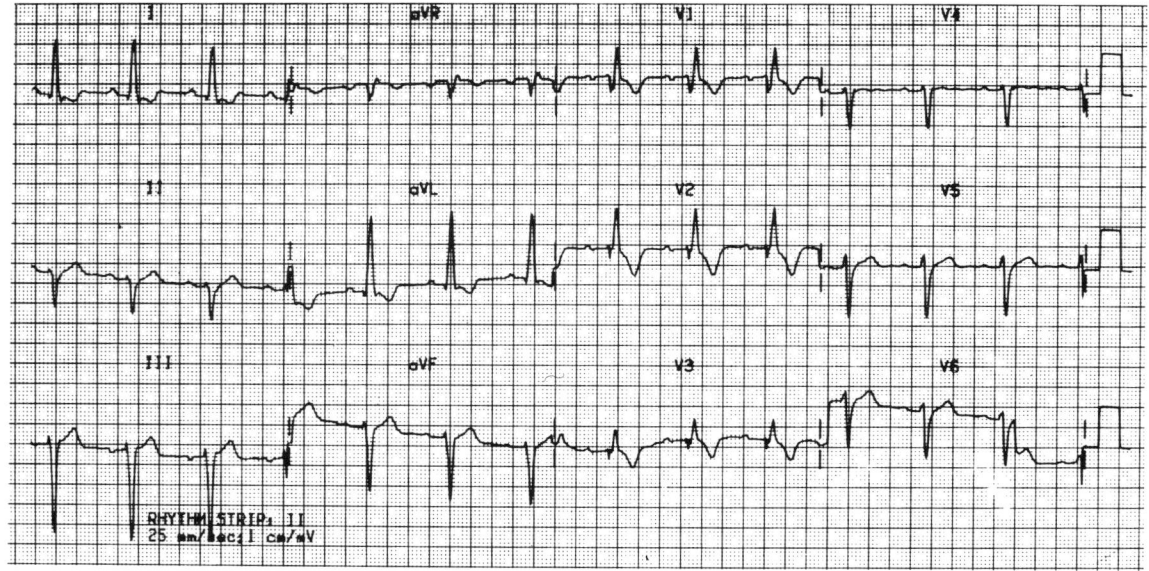

Fig. 16.37   Right bundle branch block with left anterior hemiblock. Note left axis deviation with R waves in II, III and aVF

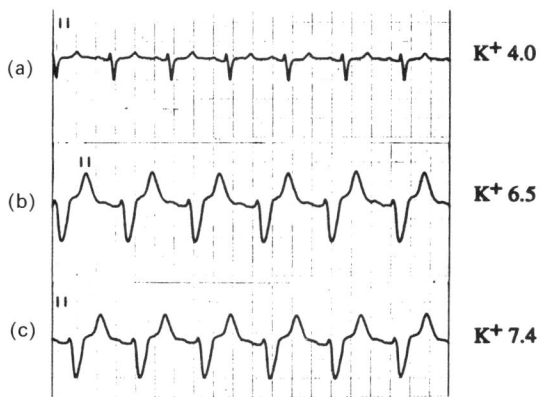

Fig. 16.38   Hyperkalaemia: ECG changes. (a) K⁺ 4.0 mmol/l, normal ECG; (b) K⁺ 6.5 mmol/l, P-waves less prominent, widening of QRS and peaked T-waves; (c) K⁺ 7.4 mmol/l, P-waves obscured, QRS complexes nearly 200 ms

Other causes of right axis deviation (e.g. right ventricular hypertrophy) need to be excluded.

CLINICAL

RBBB with either left anterior hemiblock or left posterior hemiblock indicates an extensive conduction defect and a poor prognosis (high risk of complete heart block), especially in acute myocardial infarction.

HYPERKALAEMIA

A high serum K⁺ can produce ECG changes (Fig. 16.38). Early changes consist of tall peaked T-waves with reduced P-wave amplitude. Progressive widening of the QRS may be confused with BBB. Cardiac arrest may eventually occur.

ATRIOVENTRICULAR BLOCK⁴²

AV block is a delay or failure of impulse conduction from the atria to the ventricles. AV block is classified according to whether conduction of atrial impulses is delayed (first-degree), blocked intermittently (second-degree) or blocked completely (third-degree).

FIRST-DEGREE AV BLOCK

ECG

PR interval (measured from the onset of the P-wave to the onset of the QRS) exceeds 200 ms (Fig. 16.39). Each P-wave is followed by a QRS. PR intervals may be prolonged to such a degree that the P-wave is buried in the previous T-wave or even QRS (Fig. 16.40).

CLINICAL

First-degree AV block is commonly associated with increased vagal tone, and occasionally with drugs (especially digoxin), ischaemic heart disease (particularly inferior myocardial infarction) and rheumatic fever. It usually causes no symptoms and requires no treatment. If associated with digoxin, the drug should be ceased or the dose decreased.

SECOND-DEGREE AV BLOCK

Second-degree AV block is classified into Mobitz types I and II.

MOBITZ TYPE I (WENCKEBACH)

Delay in AV conduction increases with each atrial impulse until an atrial impulse fails to conduct. This is usually a repetitive pattern.

ECG

There is progressive lengthening of the PR interval over successive cardiac cycles, culminating in a non-conducted P-wave, resulting in a missed beat (Fig. 16.41).

CLINICAL

The condition is generally benign, although it may occur with inferior infarction. Treatment is rarely necessary.

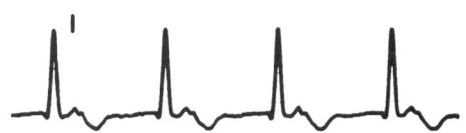

Fig. 16.40   First-degree atrioventricular block. P-wave is hidden in initial part of the T-wave

Fig. 16.39   First-degree atrioventricular block. PR interval is 320 ms

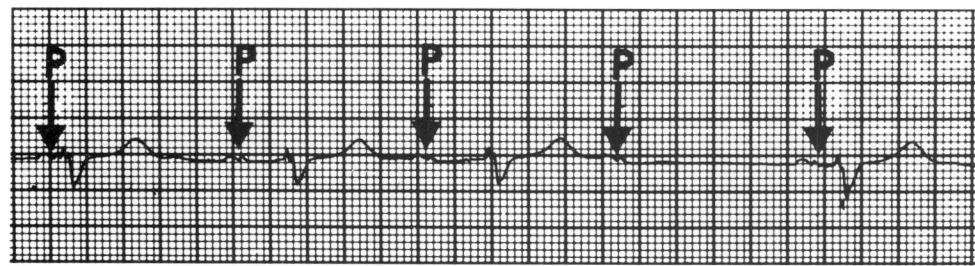

Fig. 16.41   Mobitz type I (Wenckebach) atrioventricular block. PR interval increases until a P-wave (see fourth P-wave) fails to be conducted

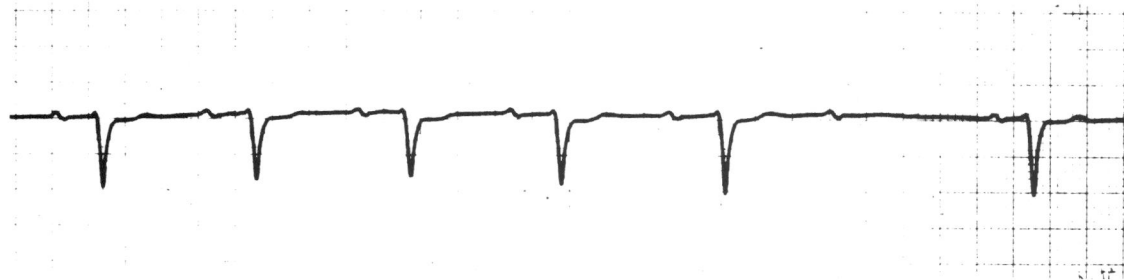

Fig. 16.42   Mobitz type II atrioventricular block. PR interval in sinus rhythm is prolonged in this example

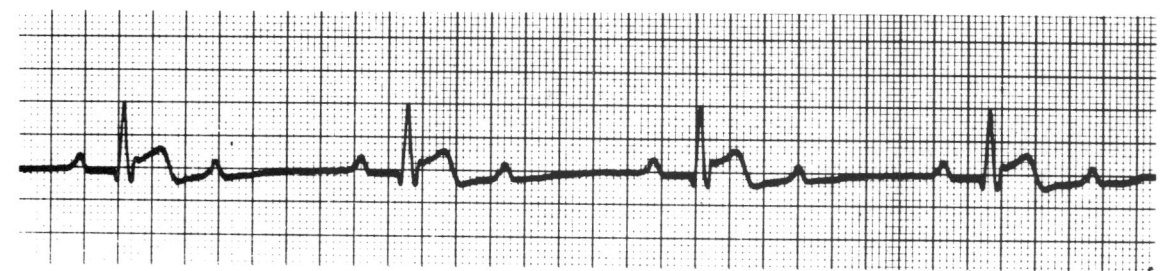

Fig. 16.43   Second-degree (2 : 1) atrioventricular block. Atrial rate is 76 per min, ventricular rate 38 per min

MOBITZ TYPE II

There is intermittent failure of conduction of atrial impulses to the ventricles without preceding increases in the PR interval. The ratio of conducted to non-conducted atrial impulses varies, e.g. every second or fourth atrial impulse may be conducted (i.e. 2 : 1 or 4 : 1 second-degree AV block).

ECG

PR interval remains constant prior to the blocked P-wave (Fig. 16.42). There is always a constant P-QRS wave ratio with the P-waves two (Fig. 16.43), three (rare) or four times more frequent than QRS waves.

CLINICAL

It is likely to be associated with structural heart disease. Slower symptomatic ventricular rates may require pacing.

The AV block may be intermittent (Fig. 16.42) or persistent (Fig. 16.43).

THIRD-DEGREE (COMPLETE) AV BLOCK

This rhythm occurs when no atrial impulses are conducted to the ventricles; atrial and ventricular contraction are dissociated. The SA node usually continues to depolarize the atria, whereas ventricular activation depends on a standby escape pacemaker located below the block. The escape pacemaker may be close to the His bundle (narrow QRS, stable pacemaker usually 40–60 per min) (Fig. 16.44), or more distal in ventricular tissue (wide QRS, relatively unstable pacemaker with a rate 20–40 per min) (Fig. 16.45). Should no ectopic escape pacemaker emerge, ventricular asystole will occur (Fig. 16.46), resulting in a Stokes-Adams

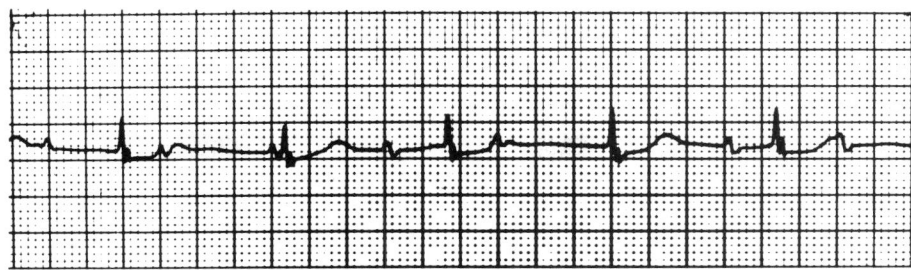

Fig. 16.44   Third-degree (complete) atrioventricular block with a junctional (narrow QRS) escape rhythm. Note independent atrial and ventricular activity (atrial rate 100 per min; ventricular rate 68 per min)

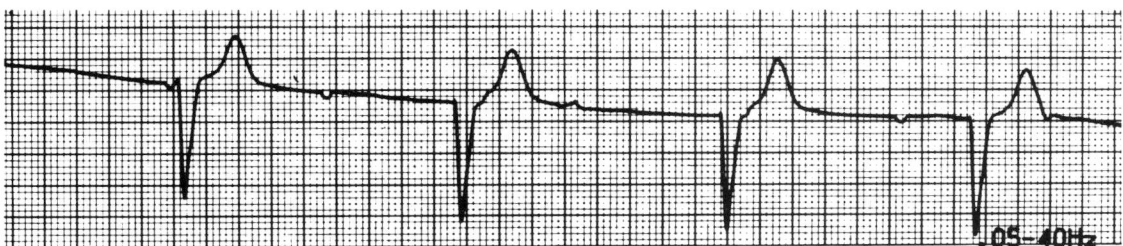

Fig. 16.45   Third-degree (complete) atrioventricular block. Atria and ventricles are dissociated. The ventricular escape pacemaker is discharging at about 38 beats per min

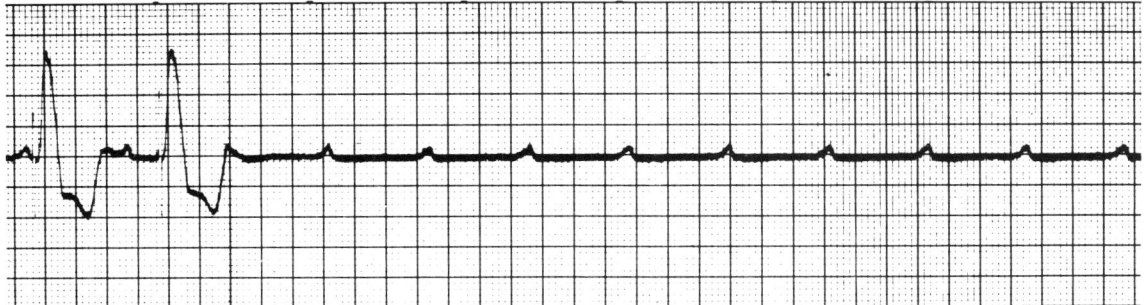

Fig. 16.46   Third-degree (complete) atrioventricular block. Failure of ventricular pacing is followed by complete heart block. Sinoatrial node discharge continues (P-waves) but no ventricular escape pacemaker emerges

attack, or death if the episode is prolonged. Torsade de pointes may also occur associated with the bradycardia.

ECG
The ECG shows normal regular P-waves completely dissociated from QRS complexes. The QRS rate is always significantly slower than the P-wave rate and may be very slow at times.

CLINICAL
Idiopathic fibrosis of the conduction system is the most common cause. Other causes include myocardial infarction, valvular heart disease, cardiac surgery and a congenital form of complete heart block. Cardiac pacing is

usually required to increase heart rate and cardiac output. Congenital forms often have a relatively fast escape ventricular rate, and patients may remain asymptomatic for many years.

SICK SINUS SYNDROME (SSS)

This consists of a number of sinus node abnormalities including inappropriate sinus bradycardia, SA blocks or sinus arrest. When sinus bradycardia or SA block occurs, junctional escape rhythms are common. There may also be abnormalities of AV conduction. Paroxysms of AF or atrial flutter may alternate with episodes of bradycardia (bradycardia–tachycardia syndrome).

CLINICAL

The bradycardias associated with SSS may result in syncope or near-syncope. SSS is often not associated with structural heart disease, but may occur with ischaemic and congenital heart disease.

TREATMENT

Cardiac pacing is usually required to control bradycardia symptoms. Atropine and low-dose isoprenaline may be useful prior to pacing, in the haemodynamically compromised patient. Bradycardia–tachycardia syndrome may require both pacing (for the bradycardia) and anti-arrhythmic drugs (for the tachycardia). Anticoagulation needs to be considered if episodes of AF occur.

CRITICALLY ILL PATIENTS AND ARRHYTHMIA[45]

In the general critically ill patient (CIP) population, excluding acute coronary syndromes and cardiac surgical patients, arrhythmia is common. The documented incidence is as high as 78%; however, the incidence of arrhythmia that requires treatment is much lower at 15–30%. SVT are by far the most common arrhythmia that require treatment. AF, Afl and unifocal atrial tachycardias are the most frequent in descending order. These SVT are rarely the cause of admission but develop early in the admission, the majority by day 2. In CIP, SVT often result in:

- adverse myocardial oxygen supply-demand balance
- compromised blood pressure, cardiac output and systemic oxygen delivery
- impaired end organ function such as oliguria and worsening gas exchange

The development of SVT in a critically ill patient is associated with a significant increase in mortality, especially in patients with sepsis and respiratory failure. Incidence of SVT is increased with:

- elderly patients
- evidence or past history of heart disease
- haemodynamic features of diastolic failure with elevated pulmonary artery occlusion pressure
- catecholamine infusion

The actual dose of the catecholamines infusion does not appear to be important and while electrolyte disturbances are common in CIP low plasma potassium and magnesium levels do not appear to be important predictors of SVT development. The incidence of SVT, particularly AF, is so high in elderly patients with heart disease on a catecholamine infusion that consideration of prophylactic strategies is worthwhile.

TREATMENT OF SVT IN CIP

Continuing arrhythmogenic and chronotropic factors make rate control difficult.

- Digoxin often results in poor rate control due to persisting endogenous and exogenous sympathomimetic tone. The inotropic and vasopressor effects of acute digitalization are beneficial. Digoxin, 10 µg/kg, has been shown to provide superior circulatory support to dopamine at 8 µg/kg per min, in septic patients.[46]
- Magnesium, irrespective of plasma levels has been shown to be effective at rate control; however, hypotension due to vasodilatation can be seen.
- Amiodarone is particularly effective and has allowed reliable acute rate control over a period of days in CIP with circulatory shock requiring catecholamines infusions.[47] It can cause hypotension if patients are rapidly loaded. In another study, magnesium was at least as effective as amiodarone in rate control and time to reversion to sinus rhythm.[48]
- Other agents such as diltiazem, sotalol and procainamide are associated with prohibitive myocardial depression and hypotension.

Urgent cardioversion is indicated in unstable patients. The likelihood of remaining in sinus rhythm in the setting of high endogenous and exogenous sympathomimetic tone is low without concomitant use of an anti-arrhythmic drug. Cardioversion is best reserved for hastening onset of sinus rhythm once a drug like amiodarone has controlled rate. Cardioversion should at least be attempted within 24–48 h of onset in the hope that embolic and anticoagulation issues are avoided.

MYOCARDIAL INFARCTION AND ARRHYTHMIA[20]

Arrhythmia is common following acute myocardial infarction (AMI). While early arrhythmia contributes significantly to mortality, treatment is largely expectant and secondary to re-establishing coronary blood flow, minimizing infarct size and treating ongoing ischaemia and heart failure. Late ventricular arrhythmia is particularly challenging, as selecting patients at risk is difficult and treatment options are limited.

MANAGEMENT OF ACUTE MYOCARDIAL INFARCTION AND ARRHYTHMIA CONTROL

Modern management of AMI, while targeted to prevent or reduce infarct size has also been very effective in reducing arrhythmia incidence and sequelae. Numerous studies have documented transient ventricular arrhythmias at the time of reperfusion resulting from thrombolysis and acute angioplasty. However, the most common arrhythmias seen in this setting are VEB, accelerated idioventricular rhythms and non-sustained VT, rather than VF or sustained VT.

Meta-analysis of thrombolytic trials has shown no increase in early VF following thrombolytic therapy in the first 24 h. The likelihood of developing VF at any time during a hospital episode is reduced following thrombolytic therapy but the risk of developing VT is increased. The mechanism of reperfusion arrhythmia is believed to be related to intracellular calcium overload and the resulting triggered activity in the form of DAD. Dipyridamole, which inhibits the cellular uptake of adenosine, has been shown to be effective in preventing and treating reperfusion ventricular arrhythmia.

Prior to the introduction of thrombolytic therapy, β-adrenergic receptor blockers significantly reduced the incidence of early VEB and VF. However, following routine use of thrombolytic therapy, the benefit of β-blockers relates to a reduction in post-infarction ischaemia and subsequent infarction.

The early work demonstrating survival benefit of magnesium was initially thought to be due to the prevention of arrhythmia.[49] However, the Leicester Intravenous Magnesium Intervention Trial (LIMIT-2) found the improved survival not to be related to a reduction in arrhythmia.[50] Subsequent studies in the thrombolytic era have failed to show any benefit at all with magnesium, although debate regarding optimal time of administration persists. Magnesium may have a role in patients in whom β-adrenergic blockers or thrombolytic therapy are contraindicated.

ELECTROLYTE CONCENTRATIONS AND ARRHYTHMIA FOLLOWING ACUTE MYOCARDIAL INFARCTION

Serum potassium following acute myocardial infarction is negatively correlated with the incidence of VEB and VT, with probability of VT falling until serum potassium exceeds 4.5 mmol/l.[7] There is no evidence that magnesium levels in this setting have any effect on ventricular arrhythmia. Nonetheless, ILCOR recommendations not only include the maintenance of serum potassium greater than 4.0 mmol/l, but also serum magnesium levels greater than 1.0 mmol/l.

BRADYARRHYTHMIAS POST ACUTE MYOCARDIAL INFARCTION

One third of patients with AMI develop sinus bradycardia because of increased vagal tone. In inferior infarcts due to occlusion of the right coronary artery, bradyarrhythmia is due to ischaemia of the SA and AV nodes. Reperfusion of the right coronary artery can also lead to sinus bradycardia and heart block that is due to accumulation of adenosine in nodal tissue. Bradycardia in this setting is resistant to atropine.

Second- or third-degree AV block occurs in approximately 20% of AMI patients. High-degree AV block occurs early when present, with 42% presenting with AV block and most, 66%, developing in the first 24 h. Similar to all post AMI arrhythmias, thrombolytic therapy has reduced the incidence down to 12%. When present, high-degree AV block is associated with an increased mortality. However, high-degree AV block is not an independent predictor, rather a marker of extensive infarction and left ventricular dysfunction.

Treatment is only indicated for sinus bradycardia associated with symptoms, hypotension or signs of poor cardiac output. Most often, first and second-degree block also do not need treatment. Mobitz type 1 second-degree block may require treatment and atropine is indicated. However, in Mobitz type 2, atropine usually has no effect on infra-nodal block and may precipitate third-degree block by increasing sinus rate and enhancing block. Atropine may improve heart rate with AV block occurring at the AV node, as demonstrated by a narrow QRS complex, by improving AV conduction or accelerating escape rhythm. Atropine is not indicated for infra-nodal third-degree block, which is diagnosed by the presence of a new wide QRS complex. When required, atropine is administered, 0.5–1.0 mg every 3 min until signs or symptoms are resolved, up to a maximum of 0.03–0.04 mg/kg. If atropine is not indicated or effective, cardiac pacing is required (Table 16.6). Transcutaneous pacing is indicated for initial management as a bridge until a transvenous temporary pacing wire can be inserted safely and with appropriate sterile technique. With the ready availability of transcutaneous pacing, intravenous catecholamines for bradyarrhythmias are to be avoided in the setting of AMI.

ATRIAL FIBRILLATION POST AMI

New onset AF occurs in 10–15% of AMI. The incidence increases with age, large infarcts, left ventricular hypertrophy and congestive cardiac failure. It is also related to atrial infarction with occlusion of the right coronary artery proximal to the sinus node branch or circumflex proximal to the left atrial circumflex branch. Later in the course of myocardial infarction, AF is related to post-infarct pericarditis.

Thrombolytic therapy has reduced the incidence of AF. In the setting of AMI, AF is usually self-limiting and requires no treatment. If rapid ventricular rates are associated with further ischaemic symptoms or haemodynamic compromise cardioversion is indicated. β-Blockers, which are indicated in the treatment of acute myocardial infarction anyway, are the initial

Table 16.6   Indications for pacing following myocardial infarction

Haemodynamically unstable bradycardia (<50 beats/min)
Mobitz type II second-degree AV block
Third-degree heart block
Bilateral bundle branch block
Left anterior fascicular block
New left bundle branch block
Bundle branch block and first-degree AV block

treatment of choice. Digoxin is not indicated in the setting of acute ischaemia as the likelihood of triggered activity associated with intracellular calcium overload is increased. AF following acute myocardial infarction is associated with an increase in mortality. Systemic emboli following acute myocardial infarction are three times more likely with AF and 50% occur in the first 24 h of onset of AF. For this reason, sustained AF is an indication for anticoagulation prior to the normal 48-h period following acute myocardial infarction.

VENTRICULAR ARRHYTHMIA POST AMI[19,51,52]

VF/VT is the leading cause of mortality following AMI. 50% of patients dying from AMI do so pre-hospital due to VF/VT. Pre-hospital mortality is being reduced by improved community education, wider application of basic life support and availability of automated external defibrillators (AED). Following admission to hospital, left ventricular failure is the most common cause of death.

The major risk period for VF is the first 4 h following onset of symptoms, with 4–18% of patients having VF in this period. Once admitted to hospital, 5% develop VF, mostly in this first 4-h period. VF in this early 4-h period is termed primary VF. VF later in the course of an AMI, usually association with left ventricular failure or cardiogenic shock, is called secondary VF.

Thrombolytic therapy has reduced VF incidence. The GISSI study found an incidence of 'primary' VF of 3.6% and 'secondary' 0.6%. The overall incidence of ventricular arrhythmia in GUSTO-1 was VF, 4.1%, VT, 3.5% and both 2.7%.

Primary VF increases in-hospital mortality and complications but not long-term mortality. Complex ventricular arrhythmias, defined as multiform VEB, couplets and non-sustained VT, occur in 35–40% of patients during hospital stay. They occur equally with Q-wave and non Q-wave infarction. Complex ventricular arrhythmia is a risk factor for subsequent VF/VT and sudden cardiac death (SCD), particularly in non Q-wave infarction. Polymorphous VT is less common after AMI and does not appear to be related to QT prolongation or electrolyte disturbances in the reported cases.

Lignocaine reduces primary VF by 33% but mortality is increased by a similar amount such that there is no net benefit and ISIS-3 reported an overall trend to increased mortality.[53] Being more selective as to which patients receive lignocaine has not been possible as only 50% of patients who develop VF have 'warning' ventricular arrhythmia. In the 'thrombolytic and β-blocker' era of treatment of AMI, the use of prophylactic lignocaine, or any other anti-arrhythmic drug, to prevent VF will have even less benefit. There is no conclusive data to support the use of lignocaine to prevent recurrent VF in those patients who have already suffered an episode of VF. Despite this, a short period of 6–24 h of lignocaine has been advocated.

Patients who survive a late or secondary episode of VF/VT following myocardial infarction require full evaluation for preventative strategies, as do survivors of SCD. All survivors of a myocardial infarction are at an increased risk for SCD but accurate prediction is not feasible. Risk factors that have been shown to be associated with increased risk of a subsequent episode of VF/VT after myocardial infarction include:

- age
- holter monitoring and demonstration of non-sustained VT, couplets and frequent VEB (i.e. >10 per min)
- impaired left ventricular function (i.e. ejection fraction less than 30–40%)
- signal-average ECG and detection of delayed after-potentials. In patients presenting with SCD after myocardial infarction, 68–87% have an abnormal signal-average ECG. However the positive predictive value is poor at 15–25%
- demonstrated inducibility of VT post-infarction is associated with increased risk of SCD. However, the positive predictive value is again poor at 20–30%.

Combinations of these risk factors have been evaluated to predict risk after infarction. The combination of delayed potentials on signal-average ECG, left ventricular ejection fraction of less than 40% and non-sustained VT on Holter monitor has been shown to be associated with up to 50% risk of SCD. Currently, there is no agreement on which patients require primary preventative strategies for VF/VT following myocardial infarction.

Using frequent VEB to identify patients at risk following myocardial infarction has been extensively used. There have been 54 randomized trials reported involving more than 20 000 patients using 11 different Class I agents.

Class I agents showed no overall benefit on all-cause mortality and Class IC agents have excess mortality despite arrhythmia suppression.[12]

Class II anti-arrhythmics, β-blockers, have an established and broadening role, with recent evidence showing significant benefit.[54]

Class III agents lack a consistent Class effect. Sotalol (SWORD) was found to increase all-cause mortality and arrhythmia deaths.[55] Amiodarone (CAMIAT) reduces all-cause mortality, in patients with frequent VEB post myocardial infarction[56] but another study (EMIAT) evaluated amiodarone in patients with ejection fraction less than 40% and found no effect on all-cause mortality but a 35% reduction in arrhythmia deaths.[57] Subsequent analysis of combined CAMIAT and EMIAT data has emphasized the importance of β-blockers. The combination of amiodarone and β-blockers in these post infarct patients was better than either drug alone.[58]

CARDIOTHORACIC SURGERY AND ARRHYTHMIA

SVT AFTER CARDIOTHORACIC SURGERY[59]

AF predominates, with AFl and unifocal atrial tachy-arrhythmia also occurring commonly after coronary artery bypass grafting, with an incidence of 11–40% and in over 50% following valvular surgery. In addition to mechanisms found in non-surgical patients, pericardial inflammation or effusion, increased catecholamine production and postoperative autonomic changes are implicated. Major risk factors include:

- previous history of AF
- increasing age
- post-operative withdrawal of β-blocker therapy

Extent of coronary artery disease, postoperative ischaemia, duration of aortic cross clamping or cardiopulmonary bypass and method of myocardial protection do not influence incidence. SVT post-cardiothoracic surgery is not a benign event with the major consequence being thromboembolic complications. Stroke occurs following coronary artery bypass grafting in 1–6% of patients and postoperative atrial tachyarrhythmias increases the incidence three-fold. Other adverse effects include:

- haemodynamic instability
- prolonged inotropic support
- need for intraaortic balloon pump
- re-operation for bleeding
- longer and more expensive critical care unit and hospital episodes

PREVENTION OF SVT[60,61]

Pre-operative β-blocker treatment should be continued post operatively. β-Blockers consistently reduces SVT across many studies with differing agents.

Amiodarone prophylaxis after elective cardiac surgery reduced postoperative AF from 53% to 25%. Diltiazem has also been shown to be effective at SVT prevention and there was associated improvement in haemodynamic variables and rates of myocardial ischaemia. Verapamil is not effective. Esmolol was found to be more effective than diltiazem.

There is no relation between SVT incidence and serum magnesium levels and there is conflicting data relating to the efficacy of prophylactic magnesium. Digoxin has no role in prevention.

TREATMENT OF SVT

Treatment is aimed at control of ventricular rate, prevention of thromboembolism and cardioversion.

Digoxin, atenolol, diltiazem or magnesium are appropriate choices to control rate.

In persisting AF, the timing of electrical cardioversion is debatable. Early electrical cardioversion, inside 24–48 h, avoids the need for anticoagulation but is associated with a significant recurrence rate as postoperative arrhythmogenic factors remain. In persistent or recurrent AF, sotalol or amiodarone, depending on myocardial function, are suitable anti-arrhythmic drugs and should be continued for 6–12 weeks following cardioversion.

Timing of safe anticoagulation following cardiac surgery is also debatable. Many advocate delaying anticoagulation till 72 h post surgery, which may be greater than 24–48 h after onset of SVT. Most cardiac surgical patients receive aspirin and low dose heparin in the early postoperative period, which is likely to reduce risk. However, it is worth noting that, in other AF settings, 325 mg of aspirin decreased thromboembolic but 75 mg did not.

VENTRICULAR ARRHYTHMIA FOLLOWING CARDIAC SURGERY

Ventricular arrhythmia requiring treatment, DC shock or drug, is common following cardiac surgery occurring in 23% of patients.[62] Arrhythmias requiring DC shock occur in the first 36 h and are associated with:

- Advanced age
- Failure to use an internal mammary artery conduit (which is likely to reflect preoperative assessment of high risk)
- SVT

The incidence was not related to previous myocardial infarction, ejection fraction of less than 50%, prolonged operative time, perioperative myocardial infarction or less number of vessels bypassed. In patients undergoing coronary artery bypass, grafting patients at high risk for sudden death, left ventricular ejection fraction less than 36% and abnormalities on signal-averaged ECG had a 6.3% incidence of sustained VT and 4.3% VF.

Episodes are common early on return from surgery with frequent or complex ectopy associated with adrenergic effects of emerging from anaesthesia and hypokalaemia. The threshold to treat these arrhythmia varies with clinicians. Potassium must be regularly checked and maintained above 4 mmol/l.

If there is accompanying emergent hypertension, in addition to the anti-arrhythmic action, the vasodilating properties of magnesium provide an ideal profile at this stage. Patients with VT/VF reverting with DC shock who are haemodynamically stable should have prophylactic anti-arrhythmic cover until adrenergic stimulation associated with awakening and weaning from mechanical ventilation is past. Lignocaine has been the agent of choice, but magnesium, amiodarone and sotalol are all more effective. Maintaining anti-arrhythmic levels of magnesium may not be conducive to weaning from ventilation. Extrapolating from post-myocardial infarct data would support the conversion to β-blockers if there were no contraindication.

A smaller proportion of patients develop malignant VF/VT, most often in association with poor left ventricular function and a postoperative low cardiac output state requiring catecholamine infusions. In this setting, ventricular arrhythmia is common, often initiated by short-coupling polymorphous VT (normal QT_c), due to ongoing ischaemia or reperfusion of ischaemic heart.

- High dose amiodarone may work best in combination with anti-arrhythmic levels of magnesium (1.8–2.0 mmol/l) or lignocaine
- Many of these patients need an intra-aortic balloon pump to defend coronary artery perfusion pressure not only because of the likely poor left ventricular function and low output state, but also to minimize the adverse affects of anti-arrhythmic drugs and recurrent DC shocks
- Pacing may be required to counteract bradyarrhythmia associated with escalating doses of anti-arrhythmic drugs. Pacing at faster rates (90–110 beats/min, which may be not ideal from a cardiac output point of view) may be protective against recurrent episodes by promoting homogeneity of depolarization and suppression of abnormal automaticity. The presence of epicardial or transvenous pacing wires also enables bedside programmed stimulation and overdrive pacing for termination of recurrent VT which has less deleterious effects than recurrent DC shocks

LONG QT SYNDROME[63]

The traditional criteria of prolonged QT is heart rate corrected (QT_c, Bazett's formula, QT divided by the square root of the RR interval) and is a QT_c greater than 0.44 s. This should also be adjusted for age and gender. The causes of long QT syndrome (LQTS) can be divided into acquired and idiopathic (Table 16.7). Common to all causes is a prolongation of repolarization which creates the substrate for random re-entry, giving rise to polymorphous VT (classically of the torsade de pointes type) particularly under condition of acute adrenergic arousal.

The postulated genetic basis of idiopathic LQTS is an alteration of the myocellular channel protein that regulates potassium flux during repolarization.

CLINICAL FEATURES OF IDIOPATHIC LQTS[64,65]

Thirty percent of patients with idiopathic LQTS present with unexplained syncope or aborted sudden death

Table 16.7 Causes of long QT syndrome

Acquired
  Drugs
    Class IA anti-arrhythmic drugs:
      Quinidine, procainamide
    Class III anti-arrhythmic drugs:
      Amiodarone, sotalol
    Tricyclic antidepressants
    Macrolide antibiotics
    Phenothiazines
    Anti-histamines
    Cisapride
  Myocardial ischaemia/infarction
  Hypokalaemia
  Cardiomyopathy
  Acute myocarditis
  Mitral valve prolapse
  Acute cerebral injury
  Hypothermia

Idiopathic
  Familial: 90%
    Linked to a DNA marker on the short arm of chromosome 11
    Autosomal dominant in most cases.
    Some cases linked to congenital deafness and autosomal recessive
  Sporadic: 10%
    Non-familial related to new gene mutation.

(which is often not the first episode). The majority (60%) are identified when family members are screened after syncope or cardiac arrest in a family member. Ten percent are detected on routine evaluation of ECG. The majority of episodes of syncope or sudden death (60%) are precipitated by emotions, physical activity or auditory stimuli causing acute adrenergic arousal. The degree of QT_c prolongation is not predictive of syncope or sudden death.

MANAGEMENT OF LQTS

The first line of management of polymorphous VT with shock is DC shock, with magnesium being the anti-arrhythmic of choice.[66]

- Unresponsive rhythms or recurrence despite magnesium require pharmacological intervention (isoprenaline or epinephrine depending on blood pressure) or electrical pacing
- Factors associated with acquired LQTS need to be identified and eliminated

Strategies for prevention of recurrence in idiopathic LQTS depend on the presentation. Patients who present with or have a history of syncope or aborted sudden death have a high risk of recurrence (5% per year). β-Blockers are the first line of treatment with the goal to reduce the exercise heart rate to less than 130 beats/min. Symptomatic bradycardia following adequate β-blockade requires a permanent pacemaker. Patients with recurrence despite these measures and those with an early malignant course need stellate sympathetic ganglionectomy. In 5% of these high-risk patients 'triple therapy' fails and an implantable defibrillator is required. Asymptomatic patients with incidental LQTS (<0.5% per year) and asymptomatic family members (0.5% per year) have a very low risk of syncope or sudden death. It is also very rare for the first episode to be fatal in these two groups so prophylactic measures are generally not required and close follow-up is sufficient.

Class IA, IC and III drugs may increase QT interval and should be avoided in polymorphous VT and torsade de pointes.

SUDDEN CARDIAC DEATH[67]

Arrhythmic causes of SCD can be divided into three categories:

- Primary VT or VF (most common).
- Primary supraventricular tachycardia with a very rapid ventricular rate. This is usually associated with the development of atrial fibrillation or flutter in the presence of an accessory AV connection (but can occasionally be due to enhanced conduction over the normal AV conduction system).
- Bradycardia or asystole. Usually the result of an inadequate escape pacemaker mechanism associated with either a high-degree AV block or severe sinus node dysfunction. In addition, some patients with sinus node dysfunction have paroxysmal supraventricular arrhythmia (tachycardia–bradycardia syndrome) that on termination results in an exaggerated overdrive suppression of both the sinus node and escape pacemakers such that the prolonged pause evolves into asystole or VF.

The causes of these arrhythmia can be divided into three general categories:

- Ischaemic heart disease. Acute myocardial ischaemia, AMI or old myocardial infarction scar.
- Non-ischaemic heart disease. Cardiomyopathy, valvular heart disease, congenital heart disease, ventricular hypertrophy and cardiac trauma.
- No apparent structural heart disease. Primary electrical disease, electrolyte abnormalities, prolonged QT syndromes and drugs.

Contributing factors are often multifactorial, particularly the combination of structural heart disease, pro-arrhythmic drugs and electrolyte abnormalities.

EVALUATION OF A SURVIVOR OF SCD

Primary prevention of sudden cardiac death has been disappointing due to difficulties in selecting patients at risk.

Regardless of the aetiology of the SCD, the reported recurrence rate is high, at least 30–40% at 1 year. Therefore, in-hospital assessment is critical to establish the underlying cause and to guide therapy.

CORONARY ARTERY DISEASE AND SCD

Extensive atherosclerotic coronary artery disease is the most common pathological finding in survivors and non-survivors of SCD. Less than 30% have evidence of a recent AMI. A larger proportion (up to 50%) has evidence of coronary artery thrombosis or plaque fissuring and rupture. In those patients not having an AMI, the majority (75%) have coronary artery stenosis (>50% of lumen), and 60% have three-vessel disease. Approximately 50% have evidence of an old myocardial infarction. The fact that the typical pathological background for SCD is severe epicardial coronary artery disease, with or without an old myocardial infarction and evidence of a new ischaemic syndrome, underlines the central role that coronary artery disease plays in SCD.

INVESTIGATIONS[14–16]

Chest X-ray: Cardiac size, presence of pulmonary oedema.

12-lead ECG: Acute ischaemia, previous infarction, ventricular aneurysm or left ventricular hypertrophy. Abnormalities of rate, rhythm, conduction or sinus node dysfunction. PR interval, QRS complex duration, or QT interval. Changes of electrolyte abnormalities.

Plasma electrolytes: Potassium, magnesium and calcium. Potassium levels may be difficult to interpret after a period of resuscitation.

Cardiac enzymes: Serial creatinine phosphokinase with myocardial band fractionation, tropinon and lactate dehydrogenase to establish the presence of a recent AMI.

Plasma blood levels of drugs that affect cardiac rhythm or conduction: While proarrhythmic effects of drugs are more likely at high levels, it should be emphasized that proarrhythmia can occur at normal or low plasma drug levels.

Toxicology screen: Substance abuse or drug overdose (cocaine, psychotropic drugs), particularly in patients without overt structural heart disease.

24-h Holter monitor ECG: Quantitative analysis of frequency of arrhythmia and to detect silent myocardial ischaemia.

Assessment of left ventricular function: Left ventricular ejection fraction. Gated pool scan gives a better estimate of global left ventricular systolic function, but echocardiogram will give added diagnostic information such as valvular disease and myocardial hypertrophy. Both studies will detect segmental wall motion abnormalities.

Exercise tolerance test: Standard exercise ECG or Thallium-201 scans. Echocardiogram immediately following exercise may be as informative.

Signal-average ECG: Averages between 100 and 400 heart beats, for identification of low amplitude electrical signals, such as after-depolarizations. These are found in the terminal portion of the QRS complex and cannot be seen on the 12-lead ECG. Associated with an increased risk of spontaneous and inducible ventricular arrhythmia.

Cardiac catheterization and coronary angiogram: To quantify the degree of coronary artery disease.

EPS: Virtually always indicated to document and characterize ventricular tachyarrhythmia. The initial baseline EPS should be performed in the absence of any anti-arrhythmic drugs. Inducibility of sustained ventricular arrhythmias at EPS is associated with worse outlook, with a 5-year risk of SCD of 32% versus 24% in those without inducible arrhythmia, and is an indication for an implantable defibrillator. The EPS is also important in other arrhythmic causes of SCD other than VT/VF. The inducibility of VT/F is less common in survivors of SCD (44%) than patients who present with recurrent sustained VT. In patients with sustained monomorphic haemodynamically stable VT, EPS mapping techniques are used to determine the possibility of surgical or catheter ablation. EPS is also important in other causes of SCD other than VT/F. Patients with ventricular pre-excitation (WPW syndrome) require localization of the accessory pathway. Propensity to develop complete heart block can be assessed by a His bundle electrocardiogram.

PREVENTION OF RECURRENT VENTRICULAR ARRHYTHMIA IN SURVIVORS OF SCD

MYOCARDIAL REVASCULARIZATION AND SCD

The data from the 13 476 patients in the Coronary Artery Surgery Study (CASS) registry with significant operable coronary artery disease showed an incidence of SCD of 5.2% in the medical arm compared to 1.8% in those assigned to surgery.[68] The precise mechanism of the benefit of surgery in primary prevention is unclear but is probably associated with prevention of ischaemia rather than arrhythmia control. In summary, the near universal practice of surgical coronary re-vascularization in SCD survivors with critical stenoses is based upon this primary prevention data (and the central role that ischaemia and

infarction is known to play in arrhythmia substrate) rather than data demonstrating arrhythmia control.

ANTI-ARRHYTHMIC DRUGS AND SCD[12,55–58]

The CAST study has clearly demonstrated the poor results of anti-arrhythmic drug therapy alone in the prevention of arrhythmic SCD. Data from studies in survivors of SCD using amiodarone are conflicting, but generally poor, even with EPS confirmation of lack of inducibility. Certainly patients with an ejection fraction less than 30% do poorly on amiodarone alone. The primary role of anti-arrhythmic drugs in the secondary prevention of SCD has all but disappeared, but amiodarone may be indicated if there is demonstrable suppression of inducible VT at EPS and the patient has an ejection fraction greater than 30–40%.

SURGICAL AND CATHETER ABLATION TECHNIQUES AND SCD[25]

As most sustained ventricular arrhythmias arise from a scar within the myocardium, surgical attempts were made to completely excise these areas. Catheter ablation techniques for VT are suitable for the minority of patients with haemodynamically stable VT who can withstand prolonged mapping procedures. Currently, the success rates for ablative techniques are such that a significant number still need additional preventative therapies.

IMPLANTABLE CARDIOVERTER DEFIBRILLATORS AND SCD

The reduction in SCD and overall cardiac mortality with ICD has been so spectacular and the results of previous therapies so poor that ICD were initially introduced with little randomized controlled data. More recently controlled studies have shown:

- Reduction in 3-year mortality by 31% compared to anti-arrhythmic drug therapy in SCD survivors[69]
- Reduced risk of death in patients with poor left ventricular function following myocardial infarction[70]
- Improved survival in patients with hypertrophic cardiomyopathy[71]

However, no survival benefit was shown in high-risk patients following coronary artery bypass surgery.

Representative data from several studies are shown in Table 16.8. The benefit of ICD on survival persists for at

Table 16.8 Mortality data for the various treatment regimens for SCD

	Sudden death (%)	Total mortality (%)
ICD	3.5	13.6
Empirical amiodarone	12.0	34.0
EPS-directed drug treatment	14.0	24.0
Surgery	3.7	37.0

least 8 years. Current indications are expanding, but the benefit is clear in the following groups of survivors of SCD and patients with documented VT/VF outside of the early post-infarct phase.

- Non-inducible VT/VF at EPS
- Inducible VT/VF resistant to treatment
- VT/VF in patients with left ventricular ejection fractions less than or equal to 30% regardless of results of EPS-directed drug therapy

Further developments currently taking place include:

- Transvenous catheter placement and subcutaneous patch avoiding the need for thoracotomy
- Dual chamber sensing to improve discrimination between SVT and VT that can be difficult on rate criteria alone, particularly in patients with intra-ventricular conduction delay
- Technological advances reducing size, cost and increasing battery life

While one of the proposed advantages of ICD is the avoidance of anti-arrhythmic drug side-effects, particularly the myocardial depressant effects, current practise usually combines ICD with low dose amiodarone. This enables improved arrhythmia control by reducing atrial tachyarrhythmia and slowing VT rate, and prolonging battery life by reducing the frequency of arrhythmia. The role of ICD in the management algorithms of SCD is shown in Figs 16.47 and 16.48. Given the current lack of available ICD, some advocate restriction to patients less than 75 years. With wider availability of ICD, fewer patients will be managed on drug only strategies in the future.

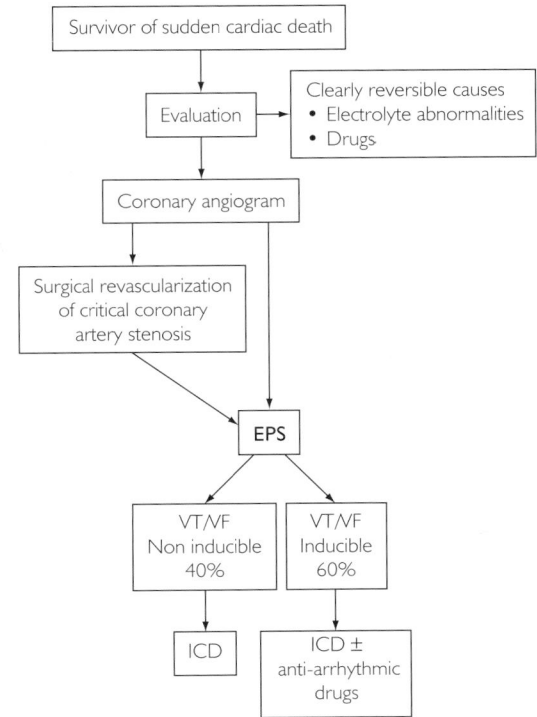

Fig. 16.47 Management algorithm of a survivor of sudden cardiac death. This algorithm does not include the option of an anti-arrhythmic drug alone in patients with intact left ventricular function who initially have inducible ventricular tachycardia/fibrillation (VT/VF) that is subsequently found to be suppressible on a drug with electrophysiological studies (EPS). (ICD, Implantable cardioverting defibrillators)

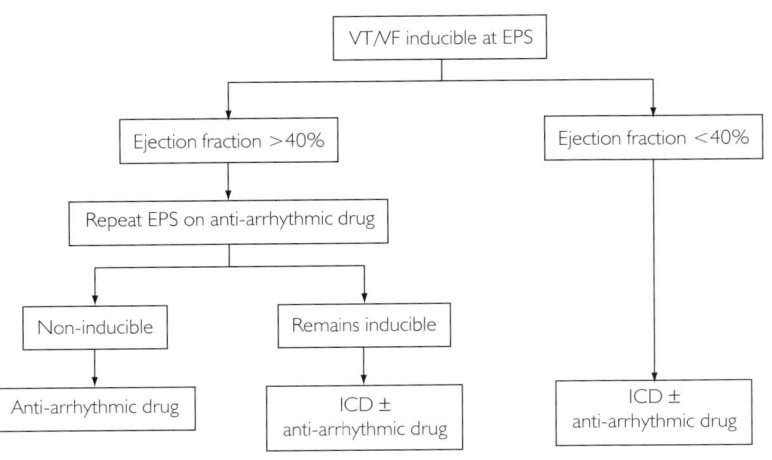

Fig. 16.48 Patients found to have inducible ventricular tachycardia (VT) or fibrillation (VF) at electrophysiological studies (EPS), with an ejection fraction >40% and subsequent drug suppression of their VT/VF can be managed on anti-arrhythmic drugs alone

CLASSIFICATION OF ANTIARRHYTHMIC DRUGS

The time-honoured physiologically based classification of anti-arrhythmic drugs is the Vaughan-Williams classification (Table 16.9), which has been modified over the years. This classification is a hybrid, with Class I and IV representing ion channel blockers, Class II representing a receptor blocker and Class III representing a change in an electrophysiological variable. The prolongation of repolarization, the defining effect of Class III agents, can be produced by a block of any one of several K^+ channels or from modification of Na^+ or Ca^+ channel function. This classification is also incomplete and does not include cholinergic agonists, digitalis, magnesium and adenosine. For this reason, an alternative classification has been advocated based upon molecular targets for drug action that include ion channels, receptors and pumps/carriers (Table 16.10).[1]

ANTIARRHYTHMIC DRUGS[53]

DIGOXIN

Digoxin is a muscurinic subtype 2 receptor (M_2) agonist and a highly potent Na^+,K^+ ATPase pump blocking agent. Digoxin exerts its anti-arrhythmic activity predominantly at the AV node where at lower doses conduction is slowed by the M_2 vagotonic effect. This effect is easily reversed by enhanced sympathetic tone in the setting of exercise, critical illness and postoperative state. At higher concentrations, digoxin has a direct effect on the AV node conduction by the Na^+,K^+ ATPase pump blockade and is more resistant to sympathomimetic effects. The decrease in $[K^+]_i$ and increase in $[Na^+]_i$ results in hyperpolarization, shortening of atrial action potential and an increase in AV nodal refractoriness. There is also increased availability of intracellular Na^+ for the Na^+–Ca^{2+} exchanger, increasing $[Ca^{2+}]_i$ which results in the positive inotropic effects of digoxin, making it an ideal agent in the setting of left ventricular dysfunction. However, the positive inotropic effects of Na/K ATPase blockade is deleterious in the setting of myocardial ischaemia and other causes of diastolic dysfunction. Digoxin also has weak vasopressor properties when administered as a slow bolus.[46] The major ECG effects of digoxin are PR prolongation and a nonspecific alteration in ventricular repolarization with characteristic reverse tick S-T segments.

INDICATIONS AND DOSE

- AF: Slowing of ventricular rate only
- Loading dose: 15 μg/kg i.v., typically administered over 30–60 min, but can be given faster
- Maintenance dose depends on renal function

PLASMA LEVELS

Oral bioavailabiliy can be reduced, especially if intestinal microflora altering antibiotics are co-administered. Therapeutic levels are 0.5–2.0 ng/ml. Plasma levels must

Table 16.9 Vaughan-Williams classification of anti-arrhythmic drugs

	Mechanism of action	Effect on action potential	Indicative drugs
Class I	Sodium channel blockade	Depresses rate of rise of phase 0	
Class IA		Prolongs repolarization	Procainamide Disopyramide Quinidine
Class IB		Shortens repolarization	Lignocaine Mexiletine Phenytoin
Class IC		Minimal effect on repolarization	Flecainide Encainide Propafenone
Class II	β-adrenergic receptor blockers		Propranolol Atenolol Metoprolol Esmolol
Class III	Potassium channel blockers	Prolongs repolarization	Amiodarone Sotalol Ibutitide Bretylium
Class IV	Calcium channel blockers		Verapamil Diltiazem

Table 16.10 Actions of anti-arrhythmic drugs on membrane channels, receptors and ionic pumps in the heart. Modified with permission from Task Force of the Working Group on Arrhythmias of the European Society of Cardiology[1]

Drug	Channels					Receptors				Pumps
	Na+			Ca^{2+}	K+	α	β	M$_2$	P	Na+,K+ ATPase
	Fast	Med	Slow							
Lignocaine	+									
Mexiletine	+									
Phenytoin	+									
Procainamide		+++			++					
Disopyramide		+++			++			+		
Quinidine		+++			++	+		+		
Propafenone		+++					++			
Flecainide			+++		+					
Encainide			+++							
Bretylium					+++	+/−	+/−			
Sotalol					+++		+++			
Amiodarone	+			+	+++	++	++			
Ibutilide					+++					
Dofetilide					+++					
Verapamil	+			+++		++				
Diltiazem				++						
Propronolol	+						+++			
Metoprolol							+++			
Esmolol							+++			
Atropine								+++		
Adenosine									A	
Digoxin								A		+++
Magnesium				+						A

Sodium channel blockers are subdivided into drugs with fast, medium, and slow time constant for recovery from block. Receptors α, β-adrenoreceptors, muscarinic subtype 2 (M$_2$) and A$_1$ purinergic (P). Relative blocking potency: low +, moderate ++, high +++. Partial agonist/antagonist: +/−. Agonist: A.

be measured during the post-distribution phase some 6–8 h after dose. The elimination half-life is 36 h with normal renal function. Difference between therapeutic and toxic levels can be reduced by hypokalaemia, hypomagnesaemia, hypercalcaemia, hypoxia, cardiac surgery and myocardial ischaemia. Many drugs increase digoxin plasma levels by competing with the renal P-glycoprotein-mediated transport, or by reducing renal blood flow or function.

CONTRAINDICATIONS

Relative contraindications include myocardial ischaemia/infarction, diastolic heart failure due to hypertrophy and ischaemia, renal failure and hyperkalaemia, planned DC shock cardioversion and tachy-bradycardia syndromes. Co-administration with other drugs that effect AV nodal conduction, typically β-adrenergic and calcium channel blockers, requires caution.

ADVERSE EFFECTS

The same increase in [Ca]$_i$ responsible for the positive inotropic effects of digoxin also forms the basis for toxicity arrhythmia. The increased inward calcium current is responsible for DAD initiated arrhythmia. Digoxin toxicity can cause virtually any arrhythmia:

- DAD related tachycardias with impairment of sinus node or AV nodal function
- Unifocal atrial tachycardia with AV block is 'classic'
- Ventricular bigeminy and various degrees of AV block occur

With advanced toxicity severe hyperkalaemia due to poisoning of Na+,K+ ATPase results. Profound bradycardia, which may be unresponsive to pacing, develops.

Any serious toxicity arrhythmia should be treated with anti-digoxin Fab fragments. Magnesium is the drug of choice for digoxin-toxic tachyarrhythmias. Digoxin, particularly if at toxic levels, increases risk of VF precipitated by DC shock. Digoxin toxicity is associated with nausea, disturbances in cognitive function and blurred or yellow vision.

β-ADRENERGIC BLOCKERS

β-Adrenergic blocking or Class II anti-arrhythmic drugs have differing properties such as relative cardioselectivity (atenolol, metoprolol), non-cardioselectivity (propranolol), intrinsic sympathomimetic activity (pindolol), lipid solubility and central activity (metoprolol, propranolol) and membrane-depressant effects (propranolol). The anti-arrhythmic properties appear to be a class effect and no agent has been shown to be superior. There are data to suggest the survival benefit of β-adrenergic blockers post-myocardial infarction may relate to some extent to the central modulation of autonomic tone of the more lipid soluble agents. The direct membrane stabilizing or 'quinidine-like' effect of propranolol requires doses far greater than those used clinically and is of negligible clinical significance. β-Adrenergic blockers competitively inhibit catecholamine binding at the β-adrenergic receptor sites, which reduces the phase 4 slope of the action potential of pacemaker cells, prolongs their refractoriness and slows conduction in the AV node. Refractoriness and conduction in the His-Purkinje system are unchanged. β-Adrenergic blockers are most effective in arrhythmia associated with increased cardiac adrenergic stimulation (postoperative states, sepsis, thyrotoxicosis, phaeochromocytoma, exercise or emotion).

INDICATIONS

Supraventricular tachycardias: β-Adrenergic blockers may terminate SVT when the AV node is an intrinsic part of the re-entry circuit (AVNRT and AVRT); adenosine is more effective. AF and Afl do not revert with β-adrenergic blockers but the ventricular rate will be slowed. β-adrenergic blockers are effective at preventing SVT following cardiac surgery. Studies involving propranolol and atenolol have produced the best results. β-Adrenergic blockers are effective in MAT, but, as this arrhythmia is most often seen in patients with severe chronic airflow limitation and cor-pulmonale, their utility is limited.[29]

Ventricular arrhythmias: ineffective for the emergency treatment of sustained VT. Empiric prophylactic administration of β-adrenergic blockers appears to be as effective in ventricular arrhythmia prevention as electrophysiologically guided drug methods. However ventricular arrhythmia most often occurs in the setting of poor left ventricular dysfunction and β-adrenergic blockers are either poorly tolerated or contraindicated.

Myocardial infarction: Survival in patients with AMI treated with thrombolytics is probably improved by early intravenous β-adrenergic blockade. There may be other benefits such as decreased incidence of VF and relief of chest pain. Long-term β-adrenergic blockade reduces mortality following myocardial infarction, the benefit being greatest in those at highest risk for sudden death. However, suppression of ventricular ectopy is not a requisite for benefit. Drugs with intrinsic sympathomimetic activity have not been shown to improve survival after AMI.

ATENOLOL

Atenolol does not have significant central action due to poor lipid solubility and is eliminated predominantly by the kidneys with an elimination half-life of 7–9 h. Care is required in patients with poor or deteriorating renal function.

- Loading dose i.v.: 5 mg every 10 min, maximum, 10 mg
- Loading dose oral: 50–100 mg
- Maintenance dose oral: 50–200 mg/day
- ISIS-1 post-MI regime: 5 mg i.v. over 5 min, repeated 10 min later if heart exceeds 60 beats/min. If heart rate exceeds 40 beats/min 10 min later, oral 50 mg and continued at 100 mg daily
- SVT prophylaxis following cardiac surgery: 5 mg i.v. within 3 h of surgery, repeated 24 h later, followed by oral 50 mg daily for 6 days

METOPROLOL

Metoprolol is lipid soluble and has significant central action. It is eliminated by the liver with an elimination half-life of 3–4 h.

- Loading dose i.v.: 1–2 mg/min, maximum dose of 15–20 mg
- Loading dose oral: 100–200 mg
- Maintenance dose oral: 50–100 mg/12 hourly

PROPRANOLOL

Propranolol has been one of the most studied β-adrenergic blockers for SVT prophylaxis following cardiac surgery

- Dose: 10 mg orally 6-hourly starting the morning after surgery

ESMOLOL

Esmolol is an ultra short-acting cardioselective β-adrenergic blocker, which is especially useful for rapid control of ventricular rate in AF or Afl. Esmolol has also been shown to prevent postoperative SVT. The distribution half-life is 2 min and the elimination half-life is 9 min. Esmolol is rapidly metabolized by hydrolysis of the ester linkage, chiefly by the esterases in the cytosol of red blood cells and not by plasma cholinesterases or red cell membrane acetyl-cholinesterase.

- Loading dose i.v.: 500 μg/kg over 1 min
- Maintenance dose i.v.: 50 μg/kg per min for 4 min, if satisfactory rate control is not achieved, the loading dose should be repeated and the maintenance dose increased to 100 μg/kg per min. If control is still not achieved after a further 4 min, then the procedure is repeated with 50 μg/kg per min increments in the maintenance infusion until 300 μg/kg per min is reached. Further increases in infusion rate are unlikely to be successful

CONTRAINDICATIONS

Reversible airways disease and poor left ventricular function are two common relative contraindications, which limit the utility of β-adrenergic blockers in patients with cardiac disease. β-Adrenergic blockers may also be poorly tolerated in diabetics and patients with severe peripheral vascular disease.

ADVERSE EFFECTS

β-Adrenergic blockers, particularly those centrally acting, are often poorly tolerated in the long term. These effects include; fatigue, hypotension, bradycardia, dry mouth, dizziness, headache and cold extremities.

CALCIUM CHANNEL BLOCKERS

Calcium channel blockers or class IV anti-arrhythmic drugs block the slow calcium channels in cardiac tissue. Verapamil and diltiazem have similar electrophysiological properties. The dihydropyridine group of calcium channel blockers, which include nifedipine, does not have any significant electrophysiological properties. Calcium channel blockers depress the slope of diastolic depolarization in the SA node cells, the rate of rise of the phase 0 and action potential amplitude in the SA and AV nodal cells. They also slow conduction and prolong the refractory period of the AV node which results in their main anti-arrhythmic actions. Refractoriness of atrial, ventricular and accessory pathway tissue is unchanged. The sinus rate usually does not change significantly because calcium channel blockers induce peripheral vasodilatation, which causes reflex sympathetic stimulation of SA node. Verapamil particularity has marked negative inotropic actions and hypotension is often seen; however, cardiac index is generally maintained because of after-load reduction. Diltiazem has less negative inotropic effect than verapamil.

INDICATIONS

- SVT: Calcium channel blockers are effective if the AV node is an integral part of the arrhythmia circuit. Verapamil has been superseded by adenosine for the first line of treatment for these AVNRT and AVRT
- AF and Afl: Slow ventricular response in AF and Afl, but termination of the arrhythmia is uncommon. Verapamil may prolong episodes of AF through a proarrhythmic effect
- MAT[29]: Effective
- SVT following cardiac surgery: Diltiazem has been shown not only to reduce, but also decrease incidence of ventricular arrhythmia and post-operative ischaemia
- AF associated with the WPW syndrome: May increase the ventricular response in and should be avoided if this suspected[26]

In general, calcium channel blockers should not be given to patients with a wide-complex tachycardia not only because of the risk of accelerating accessory pathway conduction, but also because their myocardial depressant effects can result in cardiovascular collapse in the setting of VT and pre-existing myocardial dysfunction.

VERAPAMIL

Verapamil is cleared by the liver with an elimination half-life of 3–8 h. Therapeutic plasma concentration is 0.1–0.15 mg/l. With the availability of adenosine and the better tolerance of diltiazem, the use of verapamil has fallen substantially.

- Loading dose i.v.: 1 mg per min to a maximum of 10–15 mg or 0.15 mg/kg
- Maintenance dose i.v: 5 μg/kg per min
- Maintenance dose oral: 80–120 mg 6–8-hourly

DILTIAZEM

Diltiazem is cleared by the liver with an elimination half-life of 3.5 h. There is reduced oral absorption and extensive first pass hepatic metabolism, only 40% of oral dose is available compared with i.v.

- Loading dose i.v.: 0.25 mg/kg, followed by 0.35 mg/kg if required
- Maintenance dose i.v.: 5–15 mg per h
- Maintenance dose oral: 60–120 mg 6–8-hourly
- SVT prophylaxis following cardiac surgery: 0.1 mg/kg per hour, starting at onset of bypass and continuing for 24 h. The dose can be titrated up for blood pressure control

MAGNESIUM

Magnesium is an emerging anti-arrhythmic agent with a range of indications; however, as an anti-arrhythmic agent, magnesium has largely defied classification. Magnesium has many reported electrophysiological effects, including blocking voltage dependent L-type Ca^{2+} channels. Magnesium is a necessary co-factor for the membrane enzyme Na/K ATPase that provides energy for the membrane Na/K channels.[72] The consequence of magnesium deficiency:

- Intracellular potassium falls and intracellular sodium rises leading to a reduction in resting membrane potential
- Elevated intracellular sodium increasing the availability of sodium for the Na/Ca counter transport mechanism
- The resulting elevation in intracellular calcium predisposes to DAD triggered activity

Magnesium administration reduces the availability of intracellular Na^+ and therefore this Ca^{2+} inward current. The dependency of normal membrane potassium gradients on magnesium is demonstrated by the inability to correct intracellular potassium deficiency with the administration of potassium in the setting of hypomagnesaemia. The anti-arrhythmic properties of supra-normal levels of magnesium associated with pharmacological doses of magnesium appear to be largely due to augmentation of this physiological role of magnesium.

Therefore, magnesium may be best classified as a Na/K pump agonist.

Magnesium in pharmacological doses decreases resting membrane potential resulting in a reduction in automaticity. However, once depolarization occurs, the maximum rate of depolarization and action potential amplitude is increased thereby improving conduction. Action potential duration is increased thereby increasing absolute refractory period and reducing relative refractory period. The net result is a reduction in the vulnerable period and more synchronous conduction. All of these electrophysiological effects are augmented in the setting of increased extracellular potassium. It is not surprising that the utility of magnesium appears greatest in the setting of ischaemia where loss of potassium from the cell is a major consequence. A secondary effect is the reduction in the availability of intracellular sodium to contribute to inward calcium flux producing triggered activity. Magnesium has also been shown to elevate ventricular fibrillation and ectopy threshold.[73]

INDICATIONS

- Acute rate control of AF and has been shown to be as effective as amiodarone[48]
- Prevent postoperative SVT following cardiac surgery with varying efficacy
- Acute control of MAT
- Ventricular arrhythmia associated with triggered activity, such as torsade de pointes and digoxin toxicity[66]
- Drug induced polymorphous VT, particularly that caused by Class I agents, can also be terminated with magnesium
- Appears very effective at controlling transient ventricular arrhythmia in the setting of ischaemia such as post infarct and cardiac surgery

DOSE

- AF rate and MAT control: 0.15 mmol/kg as slow i.v. push. Subsequent dose recommendation has varied from 60 mmol to 0.1 mmol/kg per h for 24 h. Magnesium levels following 0.1 mmol/kg per h were 1.92 ± 0.49 mmol/l at 24 h
- SVT prophylaxis following cardiac surgery: 20–25 mmol per day for 4 days
- Transient ventricular arrhythmia: 10 mmol as a slow i.v. push, repeated if required
- LIMIT-2 post myocardial infarction dose: 8 mmol bolus over 5 min, followed by 65 mmol over 24 h. Mean plasma level 1.55 (SD 0.44) mmol/l[50]

PLASMA LEVELS

Observational data would suggest that plasma levels of magnesium required for potent anti-arrhythmic action are at least 1.8 mmol/l.

ADVERSE EFFECTS

- When administered too rapidly can cause hypotension by excessive peripheral vasodilatation, which is associated with an unpleasant hot flush sensation
- Prolonged administration or excessive dosing can produce plasma levels associated with skeletal muscle weakness, which can be clinically significant in acute-on-chronic respiratory failure
- Excessive action can be seen if magnesium is used in the setting of hyperkalaemia resulting in bradyarrhythmia and heart block

PROCAINAMIDE

Procainamide is a class IA anti-arrhythmic drug with potent Na^+ channel blocking activity and intermediate K^+ channel blocking activity. The Na^+ channel blocking action has an intermediate time constant of recovery. Procainamide has similar electrophysiological and electrocardiographic effects to quinidine but lacks vagolytic and α-adrenergic blocking activity.

- Decreases automaticity
- Increases refractory periods
- Slows conduction.

Procainamide is metabolized to *N*-acetyl procainamide. *N*-acetyl procainamide lacks Na^+ channel blocking activity, but is equipotent in K^+ channel blockade and prolongation of action potential. The increasing effect of greater refractoriness and QT prolongation with chronic procainamide therapy relates to increased contribution of *N*-acetyl procainamide.

CLINICAL USE

Used to treat both atrial and ventricular arrhythmias.

- i.v. procainamide is more effective than lignocaine for terminating VT
- Controls ventricular rate in AF and Afl
- Effective for conversion of AVNRT, AVRT, and possibly AF and Afl
- Control of rapid ventricular rate due to accessory pathway conduction in pre-excitation syndromes and for wide-complex tachycardias that cannot be distinguished as being SVT or VT

The need to infuse slowly to avoid hypotension is the major barrier to wider use in life-threatening arrhythmia. Maintenance therapy with procainamide is not widely used due to side-effect profile.

- Loading dose i.v.: 6–17 mg/kg at 20 mg/min until arrhythmia control, hypotension ensues or QRS duration increases by more than 50%. Up to 50 mg/min has been used in urgent situations
- Maintenance dose i.v.: 1–4 mg/min

- Plasma levels: *N*-acetyl-procainamide has a longer duration of action
- Adverse effects: As with quinidine, the ventricular response may be accelerated if given for SVT. QT interval prolongation and torsade de pointes may also occur

A reversible lupus-like syndrome develops in 20–30% of patients receiving procainamide long term. Other side effects include gastrointestinal disturbances (less common than with quinidine), central nervous system (CNS) manifestations and cardiac depression.

LIGNOCAINE

Lignocaine, long considered an important anti-arrhythmic drug for ventricular tachyarrhythmia, is now relegated to lower choice options or missing from most treatment algorithms. Na^+ channel-blocking effect is increased in myocardial ischaemia and is unproven outside acute ischaemia settings. No effect on SA node automaticity, but depresses automaticity in other pacemaker tissues. Normally, lignocaine has little or no effect on conduction. The ECG shows no changes in sinus rate, PR interval, QRS width or QT interval with lignocaine.

CLINICAL USE

Lignocaine has reducing importance.

- Ineffective against SVT
- Amiodarone has taken over as the anti-arrhythmic of choice for DC shock resistant VF[43,44]
- Lignocaine increases the current required for defibrillation, increases likelihood of post DC shock asystole and therefore is detrimental during an episode of VF
- Prophylaxis to prevent VF in acute myocardial infarction can no longer be recommended

Extensive first-pass hepatic metabolism precludes oral use of lignocaine; i.v. dose should be reduced by 30–50% in severe liver disease or heart failure. The distribution half-life is about 8 min, and the elimination half-life is 1.5 h in normal patients (but may be increased >10 h in severe heart failure or shock). An initial bolus of i.v. lignocaine 1.5–2.0 mg/kg over 1–2 min, followed by an infusion of 4 mg/min for 1 h, then 2 mg/min for 2 h, and thereafter 1–2 mg/min, is recommended. Increasing the maintenance infusion rate without an additional bolus requires about 6 h (four elimination half lives) to reach a steady-state. If the initial bolus is ineffective, another bolus of 1 mg/kg may be given after 5 min. Another dosage regimen is 1.5–2.0 mg/kg initially, and 0.8 mg/kg at 8-min intervals for three doses (i.e. three distribution half-lives), and thereafter 1–2 mg/min by infusion. The half-life of lignocaine increases after 24–48 h as the drug in effect inhibits its own hepatic metabolism and dose reduction is required.

ADVERSE EFFECTS

CNS toxicity with high plasma concentrations are the most common (e.g. dizziness, paraesthesia, confusion, and coma and convulsions). Uncommonly, AV block or cardiac depression may occur. Cimetidine reduces lignocaine clearance, potentially causing toxic drug concentrations.

FLECAINIDE

Flecainide exhibits rate dependent Na^+ channel blockade with slow time constant of recovery, with marked slowing of conduction in all cardiac tissue, and little prolongation of refractoriness.

CLINICAL USE

- May revert AVNRT and AVRT, although adenosine or verapamil are more widely used
- Useful in SVT, including AF and possibly atrial flutter, particularly in the setting of accessory pathway syndromes
- Flecainide has been given in life-threatening VT

Flecainide can be administered i.v. or orally. If flecainide is deemed necessary for prophylaxis of ventricular arrhythmias, therapy should start with ECG monitoring. In CAST, suppression of VEBs after myocardial infarction with flecainide was associated with increased mortality.[12]

- Dose: i.v. loading 2 mg/kg at 10 mg/min
- Oral maintenance: 100–200 mg 12-hourly

ADVERSE EFFECTS

The drug depresses cardiac contractility and is usually contraindicated in patients with abnormal left ventricular (LV) function. It should be avoided in high-degree AV block unless a pacemaker is in–situ. Proarrhythmic events are common, especially in patients with depressed LV function, and may be life-threatening. Torsade de pointes may occur, even in patients without structural heart disease. Incessant VT may be induced, unresponsive to any therapy, including cardioversion. Although flecainide depresses intracardiac conduction, a paradoxical increase in ventricular rate may occur with atrial flutter or fibrillation. Flecainide's negative inotropic effects can worsen or precipitate heart failure. Flecainide increases pacing capture threshold. CNS effect includes visual disturbances, dizziness and nausea.

PROPAFENONE

Propafenone has a similar electrophysiological, haemodynamic and side-effect profile to flecainide and encainide. In addition, propafenone has nonselective β-blocking properties. Similar to flecainide, propafenone could be considered in both ventricular and SVT arrhythmia in the setting of normal LV function. Use of long-term propafenone should probably be limited because of its Class IC profile, even though it was not included in the CAST study.

- Dose: i.v. 2 mg/kg at 10 mg/min

AMIODARONE

Amiodarone is a potent anti-arrhythmic agent with a complex electrophysiological and pharmacological profile. The appealing broad spectrum and haemodynamic stability of amiodarone has resulted in it emerging as the most frequently used anti-arrhythmic in CIP. In this setting short-term use predominates and the formidable side-effect profile is much less significant. Amiodarone

- Prolongs action potential duration
- Increases the refractoriness of all cardiac tissue
- Na$^+$ channel blockade (Class I), anti-adrenergic (Class II), calcium-channel blockade (Class IV) and antifibrillatory effects. The Na$^+$ channel blockade of amiodarone has a fast time constant for recovery
- QT prolongation reflects a global prolongation of repolarization and is closely associated with its anti-arrhythmic effects

When given i.v., amiodarone has little immediate class III effect; the major action is on the AV node, causing a delay in intranodal conduction and a prolongation of refractoriness. This probably explains why i.v. amiodarone controls the ventricular rate in recent-onset AF, but is less effective for termination of this arrhythmia. Administration i.v. causes some cardiac depression, the magnitude depending on rate of administration and pre-existing LV function. Cardiac index is often unchanged because of its vasodilator properties.

CLINICAL USE

It is effective in suppressing both supraventricular and ventricular tachyarrhythmias.

SVT

Amiodarone is effective in terminating and suppressing recurrences of AVNRT and AVRT tachycardias, although adenosine (for acute reversion) or verapamil (acute termination and long-term prophylaxis) is superior. Amiodarone i.v. is less effective in reverting Afl or AF, but the ventricular rate will slow. Administration over a longer time span (days to weeks) may be more effective in reverting recent-onset AF. In preventing recurrence of AF after reversion, amiodarone is comparable in efficacy to quinidine and flecainide but superior to sotalol and propafenone.[37]

DOSE

- Lower doses than that required for ventricular arrhythmia are usually sufficient

- AVNRT and AVRT reversion AF and Afl rate control: 3–5 mg/kg i.v. over 10–60 min depending on blood pressure and myocardial function, followed by 0.35–0.5 mg/kg per h. Poor rate control can be improved with additional 1–2 mg/kg boluses.
- Postoperative AF prophylaxis: 200 mg orally 8-hourly for 5 days, followed by daily until hospital discharge
- Long-term SVT control or AF rate control: 100–200 mg/day orally will usually suffice

VENTRICULAR TACHYARRHYTHMIAS

Amiodarone i.v. may be effective in treating life threatening ventricular tachyarrhythmias refractory to other drugs, especially in myocardial infarction and poor LV function. Amiodarone's efficacy in DC shock resistant VF further confirms a prominent role in this setting.[43,44] Long-term oral amiodarone is useful is controlling symptomatic VT and VF, especially when other conventional anti-arrhythmics have failed. The absence of negative inotropic effect is useful in those with severely depressed LV function, but its many adverse effects limit widespread use. The Cardiac Arrest in Seattle, Conventional versus Amiodarone Drug Evaluation (CASCADE) study demonstrated that empirical amiodarone treatment was superior to guided (non-invasive Holter or invasive electrophysiology testing) Class I drugs in survivors of VF unassociated with AMI. Amiodarone prevented arrhythmia recurrence and decreased the incidence of sudden death. Amiodarone, presumably because it is better tolerated in patients with poor left ventricular function and having less proarrhythmia, can be considered as first line drug to prevent life threatening ventricular tachyarrhythmias.[56–58] The rate of arrhythmia control is often slower with ventricular arrhythmia and may take several days to achieve. This delay appears to be independent of dose. The pharmacodynamic basis for this relates to the fact that much of the Class III or K$^+$ channel blocking activity is due to the amiodarone metabolite, desethylamiodarone, whereas the predominant actions of acute administration of amiodarone are due to its Class I and Class II activity. The full potency of the Class III activity requires several days, at least, for the effects of desethylamiodarone to appear.

DOSE

- Haemodynamic stable VT: 5–7 mg/kg over 30–60 min, followed by 0.5–0.6 mg/kg per h
- DC shock resistant VF: 5 mg/kg, followed by 2.5 mg/kg if required[44]
- Long-term prevention of ventricular arrhythmia: Oral loading with 1200 mg/day for 1–2 weeks, reducing to 400–600 mg/day and then 100–400 mg/day after 2–3 months. The dose should probably not be reduced below 400 mg/day with life-threatening ventricular arrhythmia

MYOCARDIAL INFARCTION

Data are limited at present, but amiodarone may improve long-term survival in patients after myocardial infarction.

PHARMACOKINETICS

Oral bioavailabiliy of amiodarone is variable at 40–70% with a delayed onset of action (days to weeks), however loading doses reduce this interval. Initial i.v. dose recommendations were 5–7 mg/kg over 30 min, followed by 50 mg/h. The kinetics of amiodarone have been modelled to four compartments when given acutely. Following a slow intravenous bolus over 15 min, amiodarone is rapidly distributed to the active compartment ($t_{1/2}\alpha$ = 4.2 min), with demonstrable prolongation of QTc and anti-arrhythmic effect within 2–5 min. Subsequently, amiodarone is progressively re-distributed to 'deeper' compartments ($t_{1/2}\beta$ = 36.6 min, $t_{1/2}\gamma$ = 4.5 h and $t_{1/2}\delta$ = 33.6 h).[74] This is in contrast to the very prolonged terminal half-life, greater than 50 days, after long-term treatment. This re-distribution of amiodarone explains why repeated boluses are often required in the first 24–48 h of treatment. Transient loading dose hypotension due to myocardial depression or vasodilatation is dose, rate and patient dependent. A loading dose of 5 mg/kg over 20 min resulted in significant further myocardial depression and a fall in cardiac index, whereas in patients without evidence of heart failure, 5 mg/kg over 1 min resulted in hypotension due to systemic vasodilatation and an increase in cardiac index.[75,76]

MONITORING

Plasma amiodarone concentrations have poor correlation with arrhythmia control, and therapeutic levels, 1.0–2.5 mg/l have the greatest utility for avoidance of adverse effects in long-term treatment.

ADVERSE EFFECTS

Adverse effects will occur in the majority of patients if they receive amiodarone for long enough. Most are reversible when the drug is discontinued. Adverse effects include:

- Dermatological: Photosensitivity, bluish/grey skin discoloration (slate blue skin).
- Eye: Corneal micro-deposits (almost 100%) with little or no clinical significance.
- Gastrointestinal disturbances.
- Hypo- and hyperthyroidism.
- Liver dysfunction: Asymptomatic increases in liver enzymes are common, and do not require amiodarone cessation unless enzymes are 2–3 times normal; hepatitis is rare.
- Neuropathy, myopathy and cerebellar abnormalities.
- Pulmonary toxicity: Unexpected acute respiratory distress syndrome has been reported in patients on amiodarone undergoing procedures, such as uncom-plicated cardiopulmonary bypass surgery and pulmonary angiography. These observations suggest that amiodarone may predispose the lung to acute injury. Pulmonary toxicity is the most serious adverse effect, with a reported incidence of 10% at 3 years. Amiodarone pulmonary toxicity has been reported in one case after 13 days and 11.2 g cumulative dose and 11.2 g over 2 weeks in another. Patients on long term amiodarone need regular respiratory function testing and an increase in diffusion limitation of carbon monoxide 15% above baseline requires dose modification or cessation. The severe syndrome of shortness of breath, cough and fever with pulmonary crepitations and widespread pulmonary infiltrates on chest x-ray has a mortality of 10%. Immediate discontinuation is necessary. Use of steroids is controversial.

Amiodarone interacts with other drugs, potentiating warfarin, digoxin and other anti-arrhythmic agents. When administered concurrently, doses of these drugs should be reduced accordingly. On the positive side, long-term amiodarone is unlikely to precipitate or worsen heart failure and proarrhythmia are uncommon.

SOTALOL

Sotalol prolongs action potential duration, thereby prolonging the effective refractory period in the atria, ventricles, AV node and accessory AV pathways. It is also a potent non-cardioselective β-adrenergic blocker (Class II). Sotalol also has antifibrillatory actions with are superior to those of conventional β-blockers. It can worsen heart failure in patients with depressed LV function. The negative inotropic β-blocking effect is slightly offset by a weak positive inotropic effect due to prolongation of the action potential (resulting in more time for calcium influx into contracting myocardial cells).

CLINICAL USE

Higher doses of sotalol are required to prolong cardiac repolarization than to cause β-blockade. Sotalol may be administered i.v. or orally, and is excreted by the kidneys (elimination half life 15 h); i.v. dose is 0.5–1.5 mg/kg over 5–20 min. Oral therapy is initiated at 80 mg 12-hourly and increased to 160 mg 12-hourly, although doses of 320 mg 12-hourly have been administered.

SVT

- Effective in AVNRT and AVRT, although adenosine and verapamil are superior. Long-term sotalol will prevent recurrences of these arrhythmias
- Probably ineffective for reversion of AF/Afl, but is effective in preventing recurrence of AF after cardioversion. Should AF recur, heart rate is likely to be well controlled with sotalol
- Prevents postoperative SVT

VENTRICULAR ARRHYTHMIAS

Sotalol is superior to lignocaine to terminate sustained VT, and should be considered a first-line drug in patients without heart failure. Oral sotalol is more effective than class I drugs for the long-term prevention of VT or VF. Guided (Holter or electrophysiological testing) sotalol or empirical amiodarone are first line drugs to prevent recurrences of VT and VF over the long term; however, the worse outcome with sotalol in SWORD has significantly reduced the role of sotalol in this setting.[55]

ADVERSE EFFECTS

Side effects of sotalol are due mainly to β-blockade (e.g. bronchospasm, heart failure or AV conduction problems) and prolongation of QT proarrhythmia (e.g. torsade de points, similar 2% incidence as quinidine, which may occur early during drug titration or later during long-term treatment).

IBUTILIDE

Ibutilide is an I_{Kr} K^+ channel blocker, which prolongs action potential and increases the refractory period. This agent with Class III effect is recommended for acute pharmacological conversion of AF and Afl, or as an adjunct to improve success of DC shock cardioversion. The success rate for ibutilide alone is higher for Afl (50–70%) than that with AF (30–50%) and, as expected, efficacy is greatest in short-term AF/Afl without structural heart disease. The major role of ibutilide appears to be cardioversion pre-treatment to facilitate reversion to sinus rhythm from AF.[36] Ibutilide has minimal effect on blood pressure and heart rate and the major adverse effect is proarrhythmia, with torsades de pointes occurring in 3–6% of patients. For this reason, patients should be monitored for at least 6 h after administration. Ibutilide has a short duration of action and other anti-arrhythmic drugs are required for maintenance of sinus rhythm.

DOSE

For patients weighing more than 60 kg, 1 mg over 10 min, which can be repeated 10 min later if unsuccessful. In patients weighing less than 60 kg, 0.01 mg/kg as initial dose.

DOFETILIDE

Dofetilide is one of the latest Class III K^+ channel blockers being investigated in the hope of finding an anti-arrhythmic drug for long-term use with amiodarone's efficacy but without its side-effect profile. Dofetilide use in chronic AF has been associated with adequate rate control and improvement in heart failure. Consistent with its repolarization prolongation, 3.3% of patients developed torsade de pointes.[77]

ADENOSINE

Adenosine stimulates specific A_1 receptors present on the surface of cardiac cells, thereby influencing adenosine-sensitive K^+ channel cyclic adenosine monophosphate production. It slows the sinus rate and prolongs AV node conduction, usually causing transient high-degree AV block. The half-life of adenosine is usually less than 2 min as it is taken up by red blood cells and deaminated in the plasma. This ultra short half-life is a major advantage over other anti-arrhythmic drugs. The effects of adenosine, both anti-arrhythmic and haemodynamic, can be antagonized by methylxanthines, especially theophylline and caffeine. Dipyridamole, an adenosine uptake blocker, potentiates the effect of adenosine. Adenosine effects are prolonged in patients on carbamazepine and in denervated transplanted hearts.

CLINICAL USE

- AVNRT and AVRT tachycardias: the drug of choice. Expected reversion rates exceed 90%.[23] The AV nodal blocking actions of Adenosine may unmask atrial activity (e.g. flutter waves in atrial flutter).
- Diagnosis of a wide-complex tachycardia may be assisted by the use of adenosine.
- SVT with intraventricular conduction block will terminate with adenosine, whereas few VTs will revert. Whether adenosine should be used routinely to discriminate between VT and SVT with aberrancy in haemodynamically stable wide-complex tachycardia is unclear. Potential for haemodynamic collapse in VT is real and ILCOR advises against.

Adenosine will not revert AF. Ventricular rate may transiently increase AF associated with the WPW syndrome. Adenosine is given as a rapid bolus through a large peripheral or central vein followed by a saline flush, at intervals less than 60 s. The usual dose is 6 mg, followed by 12 mg if response is ineffective. Another 18 mg can be given if the last dose was well tolerated.

ADVERSE EFFECTS

Most patients experience transient side effects such as flushing, shortness of breath and chest discomfort. Adenosine should not be given to asthmatic patients as bronchospasm may result.

DIRECT CURRENT CARDIOVERSION[78]

DC cardioversion/defibrillation is an important treatment option in tachyarrhythmias. In addition to its emergency role in cardiac arrest from VF or VT, urgent DC cardioversion is indicated in haemodynamically unstable VT and sustained SVT that precipitate angina, heart failure or hypotension. More elective DC cardioversion is indicated in haemodynamically stable VT following a trial of anti-arrhythmic drug therapy. Cardioversion is most commonly used in AF/Afl once potential precipitants have been eliminated and, again, usually after anti-arrhythmic drug treatment to prevent further episodes. Digoxin toxicity is a relative contraindication to DC cardioversion, which should also be used with care in patients on digoxin.

MECHANISM OF ACTION

The exact mechanism of action is unknown. DC shocks need to produce a current density that depolarizes a critical mass of myocardium, thereby leaving insufficient myocardium to maintain the re-entrant tachycardia and prevent re-initiation. For VF and AF, the critical mass involves the entire ventricles or atria, whereas for the more organized tachyarrhythmias, VT and Afl, which involve specific re-entrant circuits, regional depolarization in the path of their circulating wave fronts is all that is required. DC shocks also prolong the refractoriness of myocardium and this effect will contribute to the arrhythmia termination and prevention of immediate recurrence.

ELECTRICAL ENERGY

Even though the goal is to achieve a certain current through the entire heart, atria or a region depending on the arrhythmia, DC shocks are prescribed as energy measured in joules or watt-seconds (J). Obviously it would make more sense to be able to deliver a set current. This would prevent delivering inappropriately low currents in patients with high impedance and excessive current flow causing myocardial damage in patients with low impedance. Clinical studies to determine current doses are underway for defibrillation and cardioversion. The optimal current for VF using monophasic damped sinusoidal (MDS) waveform appears to be 30–40 A. Current dosage for biphasic waveform is not available.

CURRENT WAVEFORM

Modern defibrillators deliver a current, the magnitude of which depends on the prescribed energy and thoracic impedance. This current can be delivered in a number of different waveforms.

Monophasic waveform defibrillators (MDS) deliver current that is in a single direction or polarity. They can be further characterized by the rate at which the current pulse returns to zero. Damped sinusoidal monophasic waveforms return to zero gradually, whereas truncated exponential return instantaneously. Recent evidence suggests that biphasic waveforms (BTE) provide equal efficacy at lower electrical energies. A sequence of two current pulses are generated, the polarity of the second in the opposite direction of the first. Biphasic waveform with lower shock energies are associated with fewer ST-segment changes and less post-resuscitation myocardial dysfunction and have an ILCOR class IIa recommendation.

THORACIC IMPEDANCE

The magnitude of current flow is dependent on the resistance to current flow or thoracic impedance. The average adult thoracic impedance is 70–80 Ω. Factors which determine thoracic impedance include:

- Energy selection
- Electrode size
- Electrode composition
- Paddle to skin coupling
- Distance between electrodes
- Number of previous shocks
- Time interval between previous and present shock
- Pressure on electrodes
- Phase of ventilation
- Patients body build
- Recent sternotomy

Conductive gel reduces impedance, while hair trapping air between skin and paddle and self-adhesive monitor/defibrillator electrode pads may increase it. There is no clear relationship between body size and energy requirements but compensation for patient–patient differences in impedance can be achieved by changes in duration and voltage of shocks, or by a process called burping which involves releasing the residual membrane charge.

PADDLE POSITION AND SIZE

ILCOR recommend standard placement of 'sternum' paddle just to the right of the upper sternal border below the clavicle and the 'apex' paddle to the left of the nipple with the center of the paddle in the mid-axillary line. Permanent pacemakers and ICD must be avoided as shock may cause malfunction or block current going to the heart. Inevitably, some current passes down the pacemaker lead and checking pacing threshold post-shock is required. Other alternative paddle placement can enable avoidance of pacemakers and ICD or perhaps improve current direction. Using self-adhesive electrodes, the 'sternum' electrode can be placed posterior to the heart on the right infrascapular region and the 'apex' on the left precordium. The use of right parasternal and left posterior infrascapular has been advocated for AF because this configuration provides an optimal vector of current delivery to the atria. Large electrodes or paddles have less impedance; however, excessively large electrodes may result in less transmyocardial current flow. The minimum recommended electrode size is 50 cm², with the sum of both electrodes exceeding 150 cm².

SYNCHRONIZED CARDIOVERSION

With cardioversion of atrial tachyarrhythmias and VT, when time permits, synchronization of DC shock with the R-wave of the QRS complex is required to reduce the possibility of inducing VF by delivering the shock during the relative refractory portion of the T-wave of the cardiac cycle. Synchronization in VT may be difficult and misleading because of the wide complex or polymorphous nature. Synchronization should not delay DC shock in pulseless VT or VT associated with unconsciousness, hypotension or severe pulmonary oedema.

DC SHOCK DOSAGE

Recommendations for energy doses are changing, as biphasic waveform generators become more widely available. Where studied, BTE shocks have been consistently as effective as higher energy MDS shocks. Recommended doses are always a balance between that energy likely to generate a critical current flow and an energy not likely to cause functional and morphological damage. Electrical energies greater than 400 J have been reported to cause myocardial necrosis.

- *VF and pulseless VT*: Escalating MDS shocks, starting at 200 J, then 200–300 J and, finally, 360 J. Evidence for sequential escalation of the energy dose is not strong and repeated shocks at the same energy result in increasing current delivery as impedance falls. Repeated non-escalating lower energy BTE shocks, in the range of 150–175 J, are as effective as escalating MDS recommendations
- *VT*: Energy dose for cardioversion of VT depends on morphology and rate. For monomorphic VT, synchronized 100 J MDS is the starting energy. For polymorphic VT, synchronized if possible, 200 J MDS is the starting energy and for both stepwise increases if the first shock fails
- *AF*: Initial energy is synchronized 100–200 J MDS and stepwise increases if first shock fails. Despite obvious concerns for myocardial injury, mega-dose energy at 720 J has been used with success in large patients with AF refractory to 360 J without evidence of myocardial injury. Constant-current, rectilinear biphasic waveforms appear to be more effective in cardioverting AF. This biphasic waveform at the low energy of 120 J was superior to 200 J MDS
- *Afl, AVNRT and AVRT*: These atrial tachyarrhythmias require least energy and the initial recommended energy is synchronized 50–100 J MDS

SEDATION

A separate doctor expert in managing the airway must perform sedation for cardioversion. The dose of the sedating agent is titrated on the basis of patient factors and type of arrhythmia. Patients with poor myocardial function not only need reduced dose, but also onset time is slower because of low cardiac output. Sensitive tachyarrhythmias such as Afl require only low doses, whereas AF is likely to need higher and repeated doses as higher energy and repeated shocks may be necessary. Cardioversions should be performed with standard resuscitation equipment available and pre-oxygenation is crucial.

DIGOXIN AND CARDIOVERSION

Digoxin toxicity results in a significant reduction in the threshold for inducing ventricular arrhythmia with DC shock. If digoxin toxicity is a possibility, then reconsideration of the need for cardioversion or at least careful titration of energy is required. Clinical experience would suggest the latter procedure of starting with 10 J MDS, and a stepwise increase thereafter increases safety of DC shock in this setting.

ANTICOAGULATION FOR CARDIOVERSION[35]

Cardioversion of AF and, to a lesser extent, Afl is associated with catastrophic thromboembolism, especially stroke. Early studies suggested an incidence of up to 6.3% without anticoagulation. It is accepted that the propensity of clots to form in the left atrium after 48 h in AF and for these to be dislodged when sinus rhythm is restored is so high that anticoagulation is indicated prior to cardioversion in AF.

Anticoagulation for 3–4 weeks before cardioversion reduced the risk of embolism by 80%. The risk of thromboembolism following cardioversion continues for a period:

- Echocardiographic findings suggestive of atrial thrombi formation, occurs in up to 35% of patients post cardioversion
- Left atrial appendage emptying velocities often decrease despite the development of coordinated electrical activity after cardioversion, presumably because of stunning of mechanical function

Prolonged AF greater than 48 h requires anticoagulation for 3 weeks prior to cardioversion and warfarin therapy for at least another 4 weeks depending on risk of recurrence of AF.

Transoesophageal echocardiography (TOE), which allows detection of thrombi in the left atrial appendage with much greater accuracy, has been found to be a safe means of expediting cardioversion. Anticoagulation with heparin for 1 day or warfarin for 5 days prior to demonstrating the left atrium to be free of thrombi by TOE, then 4 weeks of warfarin following cardioversion, was as effective in preventing emboli as the conventional longer anticoagulation regime. However, there was a significant reduction in major haemorrhagic events in the TOE-guided, shorter lead-in anticoagulation strategy.

REFERENCES

1 Task Force of the Working Group on Arrhythmias of the European Society of Cardiology. The Sicilian Gambit: a new approach to the classification of antiarrhythmic drugs based on their actions on arrhythmogenic mechanisms. *Circulation* 1991; **84**: 1831–51.

2 Hoffman BF, Rosen MR. Cellular mechanisms for cardiac arrhythmias. *Circ Res* 1981; **49**: 1–15.

3 Binah O, Rosen MR. Mechanisms of ventricular arrhythmias. *Circulation* 1992; **85** (suppl. 1): 25–31.

4 Wit AL, Cranefield PF. Reentrant excitation as a cause of cardiac arrhythmias. *Am J Physiol* 1978; **235**: H1–17.

5 Gettes LS. Electrolyte abnormalities underlying lethal and ventricular arrhythmias. *Circulation* 1992; **85** (suppl. 1): 70–6.

6 Hollifield JW. Thiazide treatment of hypertension: effects of thiazide diuretics on serum potassium, magnesium and ventricular ectopy. *Am J Med* 1986; **80**: 8–12.

7 Nordrehaug JE, Johannessen K-A, von der Lippe G. Serum potassium concentration as a risk factor of ventricular arrhythmias early in acute myocardial infarction. *Circulation* 1985; **71**: 645–9.

8 Hollifield JW. Thiazide treatment of systemic hypertension: effects on serum magnesium and ventricular ectopic activity. *Am J Cardiol* 1989; **63**: G22–5.

9 Schwartz PJ, La Rovere MT, Vanoli E. Autonomic nervous system and sudden cardiac death. *Circulation* 1992; **85** (suppl. 1): 77–91.

10 Campbell TJ. Proarrhythmic actions of antiarrhythmic drugs: a review. *Aust NZ J Med* 1990; **20**: 275–82.

11 Dhein S, Muller A, Gerwin R, Klaus W. Comparative study on the proarrhythmic effects of some antiarrhythmic agents. *Circulation* 1993; **87**: 617–30.

12 The Cardiac Arrhythmia Suppression Trial (CAST) Investigators. Preliminary report: effect of encainide and flecainide on mortality in a randomized trial of arrhythmia suppression after myocardial infarction. *N Engl J Med* 1989; **321**: 227–33.

13 Donovan KD, Power BM, Hockings BE, *et al.* Usefulness of atrial electrograms recorded via central venous catheters in the diagnosis of complex cardiac arrhythmias. *Crit Care Med* 1993; **21**: 532–7.

14 Mason JW. A comparison of electrophysiologic testing with Holter monitoring to predict antiarrhythmic drug efficacy for ventricular tachyarrhythmias. *N Engl J Med* 1993; **329**: 445–51.

15 Buxton AE, Lee KL, DiCarlo L, *et al.*, for the Multicenter Unsustained Tachycardia Trial Investigators. Electrophysiologic testing to identify patients with coronary artery disease who are at risk of sudden death. *N Engl J Med* 2000; **342**: 1937–45.

16 Gilman JK, Jalal S, Naccarelli GV. Predicting and preventing sudden cardiac death from cardiac causes. *Circulation* 1994; **90**: 1083–92.

17 Kennedy HL, Whitlock JA, Sprague MK, *et al.* Long-term follow up of asymptomatic healthy subjects with frequent and complex ventricular ectopy. *N Engl J Med* 1985; **312**: 193–7.

18 Jouven X, Zuriek M, Desnos M, *et al.* Long-term outcome in asymptomatic men with exercise-induced premature ventricular depolarizations. *N Engl J Med* 2000; **343**: 826–33.

19 Teo KK, Yusuf S, Furberg CD. Effects of prophylactic antiarrhythmic drug therapy in acute myocardial infarction: an overview of results from randomized controlled trials. *JAMA* 1993; **270**: 1589–95.

20 The American Heart Association in Collaboration with the International Liasion Committee on Resuscitation (ILCOR). Guidelines 2000 for cardiopulmonary resuscitation and emergency cardiovascular care. *Circulation* 2000; **102** (suppl. I): I172–203.

21 Ganz LI, Friedman PL. Supraventricular tachycardia. *N Engl J Med* 1995; **322**: 162–73.

22 Chauhan VS, Krahn AD Klein GJ, *et al.* Supraventricular tachycardia. *Med Clin North Am* 2001; **85**: 193–223.

23 Camm AJ, Garratt CJ. Adenosine and supraventricular tachycardia. *N Engl J Med* 1991; **325**: 1621–9.

24 The American Heart Association in Collaboration with the International Liasion Committee on Resuscitation (ILCOR). Guidelines 2000 for cardiopulmonary resuscitation and emergency cardiovascular care. *Circulation* 2000; **102** (suppl. I): I158–65.

25 Morady F. Radio-frequency ablation as treatment for cardiac arrhythmias. *N Engl J Med* 1999; **340**: 534–44.

26 Garratt C, Antoniou A, Ward D, Camm AJ. Misuse of verapamil in pre-existent atrial fibrillation. *Lancet* 1989; **1**: 367–9.

27 Scher DL, Arsura EL. Multifocal atrial tachycardia: mechanisms, clinical correlates and treatment. *Am Heart J* 1989; **118**: 574–80.

28 McCord JK, Borzak S, Davis T, Gheorghiade M. Usefulness of intravenous magnesium for multifocal atrial tachycardia in patients with chronic obstructive pulmonary disease. *Am J Cardiol* 1998; **81**: 91–3.

29 Arsura E, Lefkin AS, Scher DL, *et al.* A randomized double-blind placebo-controlled study of verapamil and metoprolol in treatment of multifocal atrial tachycardia. *Am J Med* 1988; **85**: 519–24.

30 Olshansky B, Wilber DJ, Hariman RJ. Atrial flutter – update on the mechanism and treatment. *Pace* 1992; **15**: 2308–35.

31 Falk RH. Medical progress: atrial fibrillation. *N Engl J Med* 2001; **344**: 1067–78.

32 Prichett ELC. Management of atrial fibrillation. *N Engl J Med* 1992; **326**: 1264–71.

33 Prystowski EN, Benson DW, Fuster V, *et al*. Management of patients with atrial fibrillation. A statement for healthcare professionals. From the subcommittee on electrocardiography and electrophysiology: American Heart Association. *Circulation* 1996; **93**: 1262–77.

34 Hylek EM, Skates SJ, Sheehan MA, Singer DE. An analysis of the lowest effective intensity of prophylactic anticoagulation for patients with non-rheumatic atrial fibrillation. *N Engl J Med* 1996; **335**: 540–6.

35 Klein AL, Grimm RA, Murray RD, *et al*. Assessment of cardioversion using transesophageal echocardiography investigators. Use of transesophageal echocardiography to guide cardioversion in patients with atrial fibrillation. *N Engl J Med* 2001; **344**: 1411–20.

36 Oral H, Souza JJ, Michaud GF, *et al*. Facilitating transthoracic cardioversion of atrial fibrillation with Ibutilide pre-treatment. *N Engl J Med* 1999; **340**: 1849–54.

37 Roy D, Talajie M, Dorian P, *et al*. The Canadian Trial of Atrial Fibrillation Investigators. Amiodarone to prevent recurrence of atrial fibrillation. *N Engl J Med* 2000; **342**: 913–20.

38 Wellens HJJ, Bar FWHM, Lie KL. The value of the electrocardiogram in the differential diagnosis of a tachycardia with a wide QRS complex. *Am J Med* 1978; **64**: 27–33.

39 Brugada P, Brugada J, Mont L, *et al*. A new approach to the differential diagnosis of a regular tachycardia with a wide QRS complex. *Circulation* 1991; **83**: 1649–59.

40 Antunes E, Brugada J, Steurer G, *et al*. The differential diagnosis of a regular tachycardia with a wide QRS complex on the 12-lead ECG: ventricular tachycardia, supraventricular tachycardia with aberrant intraventricular conduction, and supraventricular tachycardia with anterograde conduction over an accessory pathway. *Pacing Clin Electrophysiol* 1994; **17**: 1515–24.

41 Griffith MJ, Garratt CJ, Mounsey P, Camm AJ. Venricular tachycardia as a default diagnosis in broad complex tachycardia. *Lancet* 1994; **343**: 386–8.

42 The American Heart Association in Collaboration with the International Liasion Committee on Resuscitation (ILCOR). Guidelines 2000 for cardiopulmonary resuscitation and emergency cardiovascular care. *Circulation* 2000; **102** (suppl. I): I142–57.

43 Kudenchuk PJ, Cobb LA, Copass MK, *et al*. Amiodarone for resuscitation after out-of-hospital cardiac arrest due to ventricular fibrillation. *N Engl J Med* 1999; **341**: 871–8.

44 Dorian P, Cass D, Schwartz B, *et al*. Amiodarone as compared with lidocaine for shock-resistant ventricular fibrillation. *N Engl J Med* 2000; **346**: 884–90.

45 Artucio H, Pereira M. Cardiac arrhythmias in critically ill patients: epidemiologic study. *Crit Care Med* 1990; **18**: 1383–8.

46 Nasraway SA, Rackow EC, Astiz ME, *et al*. Inotropic response to digoxin and dopamine in patients with severe sepsis, cardiac failure and systemic hypoperfusion. *Chest* 1989; **95**: 612–5.

47 Holt AW. Hemodynamic responses to amiodarone in critically ill patients receiving catecholamine infusions. *Crit Care Med* 1989; **17**: 1270–6.

48 Moran JL, Gallagher J, Peake SL, *et al*. Parenteral magnesium sulfate versus amiodarone in the therapy of atrial tachyarrhythmias: a prospective, randomized study. *Crit Care Med* 1995; **23**: 1816–24.

49 Horner SM. Efficacy of intravenous magnesium in acute myocardial infarction in reducing arrhythmias and mortality: meta-analysis of magnesium in acute myocardial infarction. *Circulation* 1992; **86**: 774–9.

50 Woods KL, Fletcher S, Roffe C, Yasser H. Intravenous magnesium sulphate in suspected acute myocardial infarction: results of the second Leicester Intravenous Magnesium Intervention Trial (LIMIT-2). *Lancet* 1992; **339**: 1553–8.

51 Maggioni AP, Zuanetti G, Franzosi MG, *et al*., on behalf of the GISSI-2 Investigators. Prevalence and prognostic significance of ventricular arrhythmias after acute myocardial infarction in the thrombolytic era: GISSI-2 results. *Circulation* 1993; **87**: 312–22.

52 Solomon SD, Ridker PM, Antman EM. Ventricular arrhythmias in trials of thrombolytic therapy for acute myocardial infarction: a meta-analysis. *Circulation* 1993; **88**: 2575–81.

53 The American Heart Association in Collaboration with the International Liasion Committee on Resuscitation (ILCOR). Guidelines 2000 for cardiopulmonary resuscitation and emergency cardiovascular care. *Circulation* 2000; **102** (suppl. I): I112–28

54 Radford MJ, Krumholz HM. Beta-blockers after myocardial infarction – for few patients, or many? *N Engl J Med* 1998; **339**: 551–3.

55 Waldo AL, Camm AJ, de Ruyter H, *et al*. Effect of d-sotalol on mortality in patients with left ventricular dysfunction after recent or remote myocardial infarction. The SWORD Investigators. Survival with oral d-sotalol. *Lancet* 1996; **348**: 7–12.

56 Cairns JA, Connolly SJ, Roberts R, Gent M. Randomized trial of outcome after myocardial infarction in patients with frequent or repetitive ventricular premature depolarizations: CAMIAT. Canadian Amiodarone Myocardial Infarction Arrhythmia Trial Investigators. *Lancet* 1997; **349**: 675–82.

57 Julian DG, Camm AJ, Frangin G, *et al*. Randomized trial of effect of amiodarone on mortality in patients with left-ventricular dysfunction after recent myocardial infarction: EMIAT. European Myocardial Infarction Amiodarone Trial Investigators. *Lancet* 1997; **349**: 667–74.

58 Boutitie F, Boissel JP, Connolly SJ, *et al*. Amiodarone interaction with beta-blockers: analysis of merged EMIAT (European Myocardial Infarction Amiodarone Trial) and CAMIAT (Canadian Amiodarone Myocardial Infarction Arrhythmia Trial) databases. The EMIAT and CAMIAT Investigators. *Circulation* 1999; **99**: 2268–75.

59 Ommen SR, Odell JA, Stanton MS. Atrial arrhythmias after cardiothoracic surgery. *N Engl J Med* 1997; **336**: 1429–34.

60 Andrews TC, Reimold SC, Berlin JA, Antman EM. Prevention of supraventricular arrhythmias after coronary artery bypass surgery: a meta-analysis of randomized control trials. *Circulation* 1991; **84** (suppl. III): III236–44.

61 Kowey PR, Taylor JE, Rials SJ, Marinchak RA. Meta-analysis of the effectiveness of prophylactic drug therapy in preventing supraventricular arrhythmia early after coronary artery bypass grafting. *Am J Cardiol* 1992; **69**: 963–5.

62 Ferraris VA, Ferraris SP, Gilliam HS, Berry WR. Predictors of postoperative ventricular dysrrhythmias: a multivariate study. *J Cardiovasc Surg (Torino)* 1991; **32**: 12–20.

63 Moss AJ. Prolonged QT syndromes. *JAMA* 1986; **256**: 2985–7.

64 Moss AJ, Schwartz PJ, Crampton RS, *et al.* The long QT syndrome: prospective longitudinal study of 328 families. *Circulation* 1991; **84**: 1136–44.

65 Moss AJ, Robinson J. Clinical features of the idiopathic long QT syndrome. *Circulation* 1992; **85** (suppl 1): 140–4.

66 Tzivoni D, Bonai S, Schuger C, *et al.* Treatment of torsade de pointes with magnesium sulphate. *Circulation* 1988; **77**: 392–7.

67 Huikuri HV, Castellanos A, Myerburg RJ. Medical progress: sudden death due to cardiac arrhythmias. *N Engl J Med* 2001; **345**: 1473–82.

68 Holmes DR, Davis KB, Mock MB, *et al.* The effect of medical and surgical treatment on subsequent cardiac death in patients with coronary artery disease: a report from the Coronary Artery Surgery Study. *Circulation* 1986; **73**: 1254–63.

69 The Antiarrhythmics Versus Implantable Defibrillators (AVID) Investigators. A comparison of antiarrhythmic-drug therapy with implantable defibrillators in patients resuscitated from near fatal ventricular arrhythmias. *N Engl J Med* 1997; **337**: 1576–84.

70 Moss AJ, Zareba W, Hall WJ, *et al.* Multicenter Automatic Implantable Defibrillator Trial II Investigators. Prophylactic implantation of a defibrillator in patients with myocardial infarction and reduced ejection fraction. *N Engl J Med* 2002; **346**: 877–83.

71 Maron BJ, Shen W-K, Link MS, *et al.* Efficacy of implantable cardioverter-defibrillators for prevention of sudden death in patients with hypertrophic cardiomyopathy. *N Engl J Med* 2000; **342**: 365–73

72 Watanabe Y, Dreifus L. Electrophysiological effects of magnesium and its interactions with potassium. *Cardiovasc Res* 1972; **6**: 79–88.

73 Ghani MF, Rabah M. Effects of magnesium chloride on electrical stability of the heart. *Am Heart J* 1977; **94**: 600–2.

74 Mostow ND, Rakita L, Vrobel TR, *et al.* Amiodarone: intravenous loading for rapid suppression of complex ventricular arrhythmias. *J Am Coll Cardiol* 1984; **4**: 97–104.

75 Schwartz A, Shen E, Morady F, *et al.* Hemodynamic effects of intravenous amiodarone in patients with depressed left ventricular function and recurrent ventricular tachycardia. *Am Heart J* 1983; **106**: 848–55.

76 Cote P, Bourassa Mg, Delaye J, *et al.* Effects of amiodarone on cardiac and coronary hemodynamics and on myocardial metabolism in patients with coronary artery disease. *Circulation* 1954; **67**: 1347–55.

77 Torp-Pedersen C, Moller M, Bloch-Thomsen PE, *et al.*, for the Danish Investigators of Arrhythmia and Mortality on Dofetilide Study Group. Dofetilide in patients with congestive heart failure and left ventricular dysfunction. *N Engl J Med* 1999; **341**: 857–65.

78 The American Heart Association in Collaboration with the International Liasion Committee on Resuscitation (ILCOR). Guidelines 2000 for cardiopulmonary resuscitation and emergency cardiovascular care. *Circulation* 2000; **102** (suppl. I): I112–28.

17.

Cardiac pacing and implantable cardioverter defibrillators

K D Donovan and B Hockings

Cardiac pacing has rapidly evolved since its introduction by Zoll in 1952.[1] The technological knowledge gained in pacing has assisted in the even more rapidly advancing field of implantable cardioverter/defibrillators (ICDs). Although implantation and follow-up of permanent pacemakers and ICDs are in the domain of appropriately trained cardiologists, intensive care physicians should be familiar with such devices as a significant number of critically ill patients will have them *in situ*. It is also essential, when urgent pacing is required, that the intensivist is skilled in all aspects of temporary pacing, including lead insertion and testing.

Cardiac pacing repetitively delivers very low electrical energies to the heart, thus initiating and maintaining cardiac rhythm. Pacing may be temporary, with an external pulse generator, or permanent, with an implanted pulse generator. It is usually associated with the treatment of bradycardia, but rapid atrial or ventricular pacing can be used to terminate certain supraventricular tachycardias (SVTs) and ventricular tachycardias (VTs).

More recently, cardiac pacing has been used to improve haemodynamics in various conditions such as hypertrophic obstructive cardiomyopathy and dilated cardiomyopathy.

CARDIAC PACING IN BRADYARRHYTHMIAS

ELECTRODES

Unipolar (Fig. 17.1). The pacing lead has only one conducting wire and electrode. Electric current returns to the pacemaker via the body fluids. A unipolar lead is rarely used for temporary pacing, as a skin electrode is also needed for the return current pathway, which may cause muscle twitching. Unipolar systems are sometimes used for permanent pacing. Over-sensing of electromagnetic interference or skeletal muscle potentials may be a significant problem.[2]

Bipolar (Fig. 17.2). A bipolar lead has two conducting wires surrounded by a layer of insulation. Electric current travels down one wire to an electrode (usually the distal), passes through cardiac tissue to cause depolarization, and returns to the pacemaker via the second electrode. Inappropriate sensing of electromagnetic interference or myopotentials is uncommon. Bipolar pacing is the method of choice for temporary pacing. Should one limb

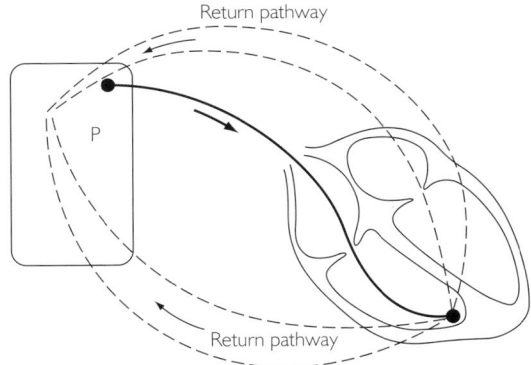

Fig. 17.1 Unipolar pacing lead. P = pacemaker.

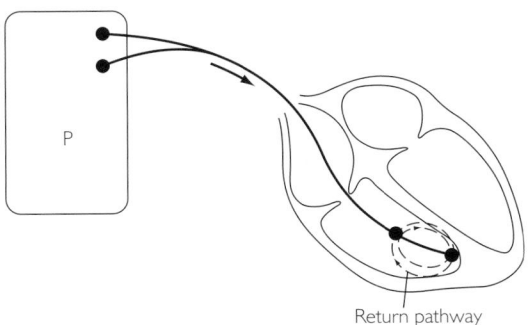

Fig. 17.2 Bipolar pacing lead. P = pacemaker.

fail, a bipolar system can be converted to a unipolar system (Fig. 17.1) by connecting the other limb to one pacemaker pole (usually positive). The other pole (usually negative) is connected to an electrocardiogram (ECG) skin electrode to complete a unipolar pacing circuit.

PACING SITES

Transvenous endocardial placement. The pacing lead is passed via a vein to the endocardial surface of the right atrium (RA), or most commonly, the right ventricle (RV). Rarely, the left atrium (LA) may be paced via the coronary sinus.

Epicardial placement. This is mainly used in conjunction with cardiac surgery, where the electrodes are attached directly to the epicardial surface of the atrium and/or ventricle.

Transcutaneous external pacing.[3] Transcutaneous pacing devices usually do not sense intrinsic ventricular rhythm. Adequate, adjustable current outputs (50–150 mA) are delivered. Some patients will experience significant pain and may need analgesics. Although transcutaneous pacing can be initiated quickly by personnel unskilled in transvenous pacing, it is only a temporizing measure until the latter can be instituted. Reliable transcutaneous pacing has rendered prophylactic temporary transvenous pacing obsolete.

Other pacing modalities such as the transoesophageal route are rarely used.

PACING LEADS

TEMPORARY PACING

Ventricular pacing (5–6 FG). Leads are relatively stiff but still flexible enough to be manipulated under fluoroscopic control to the correct position in the RV. Balloon tipped leads[4] which, in theory, float into a stable position in the RV, are occasionally used in some units when fluoroscopy is not available.

Atrial pacing. Atrial leads have a preformed J-tip to hook into the RA appendage, as this usually ensures pacing lead stability with a low pacing threshold and good sensing capacity.

PERMANENT PACING

Leads[5] for permanent pacing commonly use passive fixation with protrusions close to the tips to ensure wedging or entanglement of the electrode in the trabeculations of the RV. Alternatively, active fixation with myocardial penetration by an extendable screw at the electrode tip is used. Steroid eluting leads may reduce pacing stimulation thresholds. Pacing lead insulation problems remain a limiting factor in pacing lead longevity.

PACEMAKER MODES

The North American Society of Pacing and Electrophysiology (NASPE) and the British Pacing and Electrophysiology Group (BPEG) developed the NBG code[6] for pacing. It is a generic code used to identify different modes of pacemaker (Table 17.1). The code has five positions, but the fifth position, restricted to antitachycardia functions, is virtually never used nowadays.

Position I: refers to the chamber(s) paced (e.g. V for ventricle).

Position II: refers to the chamber(s) sensed.

Position III: refers to the response to sensing (if any). This may be:

(a) *I* (inhibition) – a pacemaker's discharge is inhibited (switched off) by a sensed signal, for example, VVI, where ventricular pacing is inhibited by spontaneous ventricular activity.

(b) *T* (triggering) – a pacemaker's discharge is triggered by a sensed signal.

(c) *D* (dual) – both *T* and *I* responses can occur, which is reserved for dual chamber systems. There is, however, a delay (the A-V interval) between the sensed atrial depolarization and triggered ventricular pacing which is similar to the normal P-R interval.

Position IV: refers to *R* or rate-adaptive (available only in permanent implantable pacemakers) – the ability to vary the pacing rate independently of intrinsic cardiac activity. A sensor,[7] in effect an artificial sinoatrial (S-A)

Table 17.1 The NBG pacemaker code

Position I	Position II	Position III	Position IV
Chamber(s) Paced	Chamber(s) Sensed	Response to Sensing	R = Rate modulation
O = None	O = None	O = None	
A = Atrium	A = Atrium	T = Triggered	
V = Ventricle	V = Ventricle	I = Inhibited	
D = Dual	D = Dual	D = Dual	
(A + V)	(A + V)	(T + I)	

node, increases or decreases the heart rate according to the body's metabolic needs. Two different sensors are widely used and dependable. (i) *Activity sensors* (piezoelectric crystal or accelerometer) have the disadvantage that they may respond to non-physiological stimuli, for example, pacing rate increase may occur when the patient is using an electrical drill. On occasions this response can be used to good effect, for example, an inappropriate bradycardia in a shocked patient with a rate-adaptive (activity sensor) permanent pacemaker can usually be speeded up by tapping the skin over the unit. (ii) *Minute-ventilation sensors* (respiratory rate times tidal volume which is estimated by measuring impedance differences between the pacing electrode and the pacemaker unit) rely on minute-volume changes to alter the pacing rate. This sensor may occasionally inappropriately accelerate the pacing rate, for example, in a mechanical ventilated patient requiring a large minute volume. Changing the 'upper rate' limit of the pacemaker or switching the rate-adaptive function 'off' will usually solve the problem. (iii) Other sensors such as ventricular paced Q-T interval systems have also been successfully used in clinical practice. Recently, rate-adaptive systems with dual sensors, where one sensor cross-checks the other and only responds if both sensors are receiving consistent data, have become available.

Position IV has in the past also referred to P or programmability (ability to change externally certain parameters of permanent pacemakers) and C or communicating (telemetry) function. Virtually all modern permanent pacemakers are both programmable and communicate with the programmer and therefore P and C terms are redundant. Thus from a practical point of view *R* (rate adaptability) is the only letter used in position IV.

SPECIFIC PACING MODES

The three-position code (Fig. 17.3) is adequate to describe emergency temporary pacing and most forms of permanent pacing in the intensive care unit (ICU) (Table 17.2).

SINGLE CHAMBER PACING

1 *AOO and VOO (asynchronous atrial and ventricular) pacing.* There is no ability to sense cardiac activity

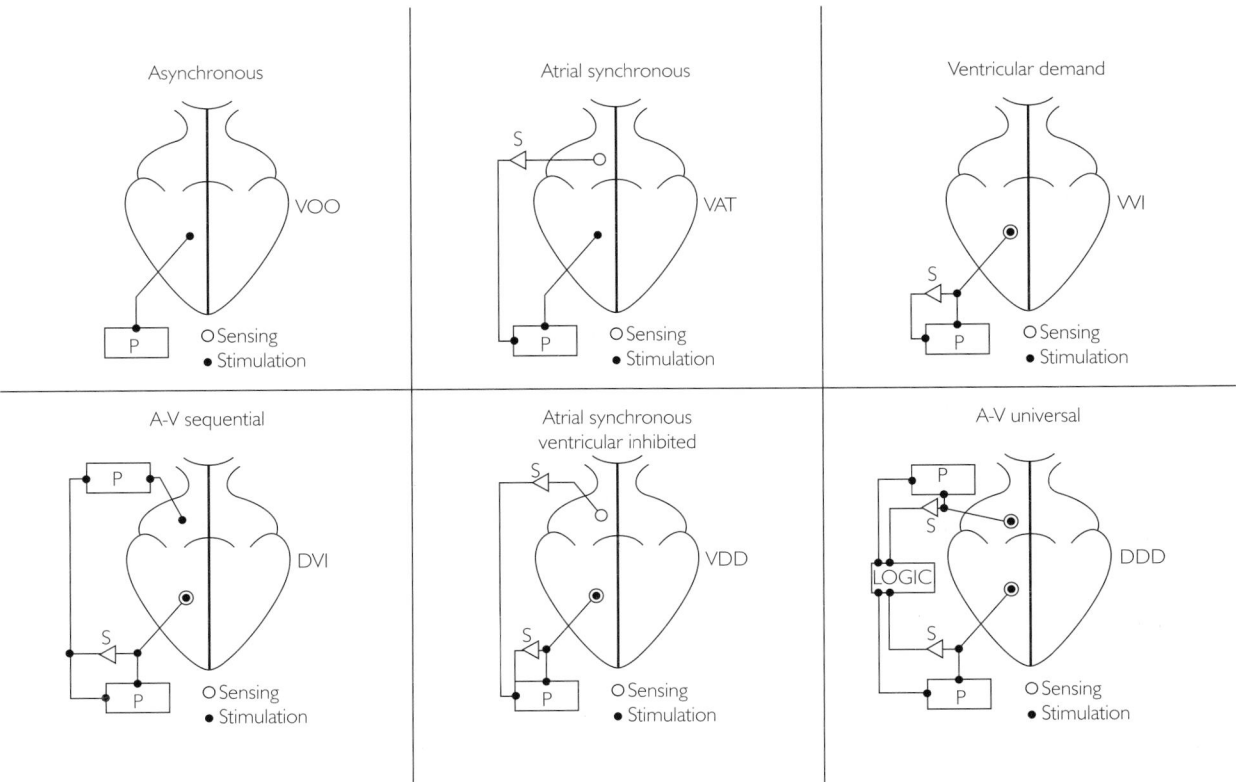

Fig. 17.3 Examples of pacemaker modes and their three position (letter) codes. P = pacemaker; S = sensing.

Table 17.2 Examples of pacemaker modes

Code		Common description	Comment
VOO	Paces the ventricle, no sensing	Fixed rate, asynchronous	Obsolete – except for pacemaker testing and 'emergency' pacing
VVI	Paces the ventricle, senses ventricular activity, ventricular activity inhibits the pacemaker	Ventricular demand	Most commonly used in life-threatening bradycardia
AAI	Paces the atrium, senses atrial activity, atrial activity inhibits the pacemaker	Atrial demand	Indicated in sinus bradycardia with intact AV conduction
VAT	Paces the ventricle, senses atrial activity, atrial activity triggers ventricular pacing	Atrial synchronized, P wave triggered	Obsolete – replaced by VDD and DDD
DVI	Paces both atrium and ventricle, senses only ventricular activity, ventricular activity inhibits atrial and ventricular pacing	A-V sequential	Commonly used dual chamber pacing mode in ICU
VDD	Paces the ventricle only, senses atrial and ventricular activity	Atrial synchronous, ventricular inhibited	May be useful when normal sinus rhythm is present with a high degree A-V block
DDD	Paces and senses both atrium and ventricle: atrial activity triggers ventricular pacing	DDD	Often ideal but more complicated
DDI	Paces and senses both atrium and ventricle. Atrial activity not tracked; thus atrial tachyarrhythmias do not trigger rapid atrial pacing	A-V sequential, non-P synchronous	Useful for sinus bradycardia with A-V block and intermittent atrial tachyarrhythmias

(Fig. 17.4). Such pacing is virtually obsolete except in some pacing emergencies (see later).

2 *AAI (atrial demand) pacing.* This is indicated for sinus bradycardia provided AV conduction is intact (to maintain A-V synchrony).

3 *VVI (ventricular demand) pacing* (Fig. 17.5). This is the most commonly used mode and the mode of choice in life-threatening bradyarrhythmias. Spontaneous cardiac rhythm is sensed, and there is minimal

danger of pacemaker induced ventricular tachyarrhythmia (Fig. 17.6). A-V synchrony is, however, lost and there is no 'speed-up for need'.

DUAL CHAMBER PACING

Two sets of electrodes are required (atrial and ventricular).

DVI (A-V sequential) pacing. Atria and ventricles are paced in sequence (Fig. 17.7). After a stimulus is delivered to the atrium, there is a delay and an impulse is then

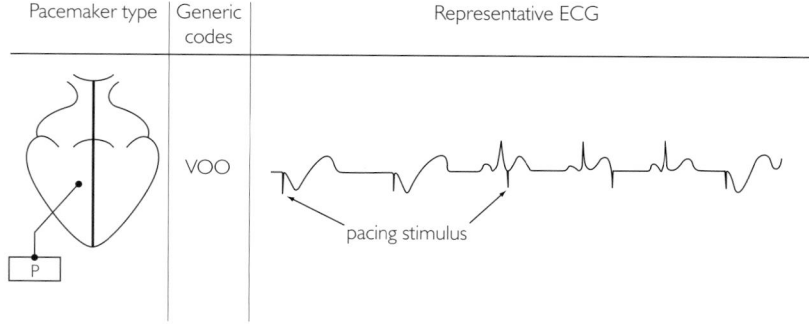

Fig. 17.4 Fixed rate ventricular pacing VOO. P = pacemaker.

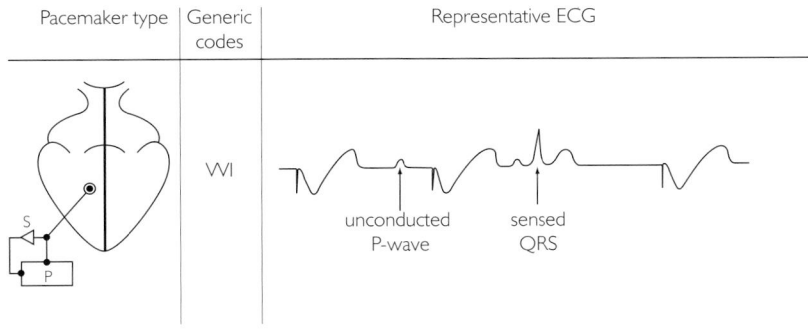

Fig. 17 5   Ventricular demand pacing VVI. P = pacemaker; S = sensing.

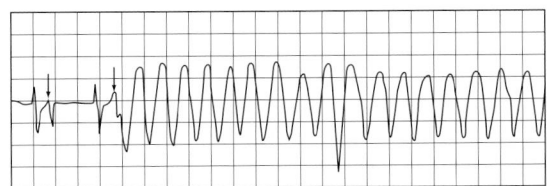

Fig. 17.6   Non-sensing of QRS (see first two beats). Pacing spikes (arrows) fall on the T wave with subsequent pacemaker induced ventricular tachycardia.

delivered after atrial stimulation, to the ventricles. If A-V conduction is successful, the ventricular output of the pacemaker is inhibited; otherwise the ventricle is paced. The advantage of this mode is that the atria and ventricles usually contract in sequence. To maintain A-V synchrony in the absence of atrial sensing, the pacemaker discharge rate must be greater than the spontaneous atrial rate; asynchronous atrial pacing can precipitate atrial fibrillation (AF). Self-inhibition ('cross talk') can occur, that is, inappropriate detection of the atrial pacing stimulus by

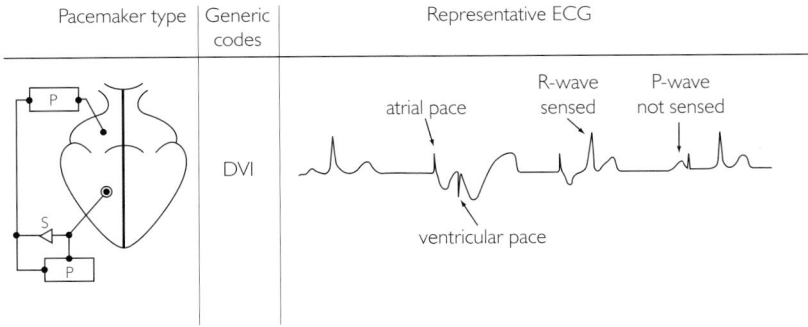

Fig. 17.7   Atrioventricular sequential demand pacing DVI. P = pacemaker; S = sensing.

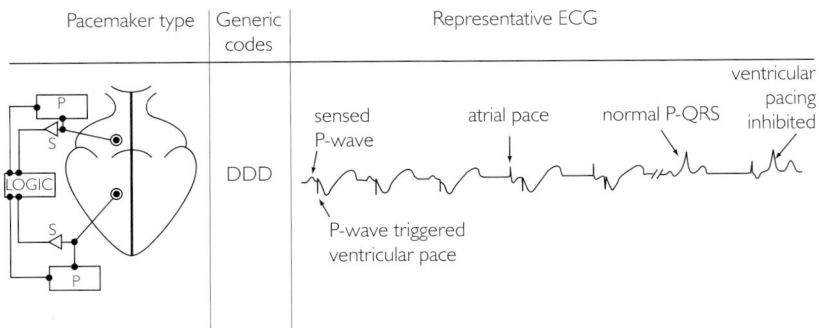

Fig. 17.8   DDD pacing. P = pacing; S = sensing.

the ventricular channel; if there is no escape rhythm, asystole may result. DVI pacing is indicated when there is impaired A-V conduction with an atrial bradycardia. It is of no value when atrial tachyarrhythmias are present.

VDD (atrial synchronous ventricular inhibited) pacing. This mode paces only the ventricle. Sensing takes place in both atrium and ventricle. A sensed P wave triggers ventricular pacing. VDD pacing is used in some permanent pacemaker systems as a single lead system capable of pacing the ventricle in response to atrial sensing (from an electrode situated in the intra-atrial part of the lead) with ventricular electrodes at the apex of the RV.

DDD pacing. There is pacing and sensing in both chambers (Fig. 17.8). An atrial impulse will trigger a ventricular output and simultaneously inhibit an atrial output. If the impulse is conducted normally to the ventricle, the ventricular output is then inhibited, as with the DVI mode. Upper rate-limiters prevent the pacemaker from following excessive atrial activity with paced ventricular responses. DDD pacemaker function depends on the underlying cardiac rhythm:

(a) Atrial bradycardia with intact A-V conduction – atrial pacing.
(b) Normal sinus rhythm with high degree A-V block – tracking of P waves with synchronized ventricular pacing.
(c) Sinus bradycardia with A-V block – pacing the atria and ventricles sequentially.
(d) Normal sinus rhythm and A-V conduction – inhibition of both atrial and ventricular pacing.

Self-inhibition can be prevented by introducing a ventricular blanking (refractory) period coinciding with the atrial pacing stimulus. With DDD and VDD pacing, re-entry pacemaker mediated 'endless-loop' tachycardias are possible.[8] These are commonly initiated by a ventricular premature beat (Fig. 17.9) conducted retrogradely to the atria, where it is sensed and ventricular pacing is triggered with an endless loop: the circuit's anterograde limb is the pacemaker, and the retrograde limb is via the A-V node. Conversion to asynchronous (non-sensing) mode or increasing the post-ventricular atrial refractory period (PVARP) will prevent endless-loop tachycardia.

DDI pacing. (A-V sequential, non-P wave synchronous). Sensing occurs in both atria and ventricle, but sensed atrial events do not trigger ventricular pacing. This mode prevents endless-loop tachycardias or tracking of supraventricular tachycardias. It is also useful in patients with S-A node dysfunction and episodes of atrial tachyarrhythmias, although DDD (R) with mode switching (ability to change to DDI with the onset of an atrial tachyarrhythmia) is preferable. During atrial tachyarrhythmias, the DDI pacemaker will simply pace the ventricle at its backup rate and not track the tachycardia.

HAEMODYNAMICS OF CARDIAC PACING

In the normal heart, cardiac output increases three- to four-fold during exercise, due mainly to increased heart rate and increases in stroke volume. Atrioventricular synchrony – the normal activation sequence of the heart in which the atria contract first and then, after an appropriate delay, the ventricles contract – contributes only about

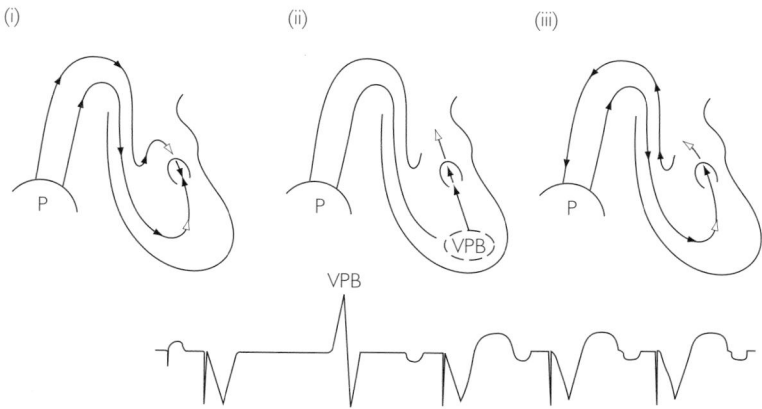

Fig. 17.9 Pacemaker mediated 'endless loop' tachycardia:
(i) Under normal conditions (first beat) there is no conduction from the ventricles to the atria because of V-A block or because the atrial and ventricular impulses collide and extinguish each other in the A-V node; (ii) if a ventricular premature beat (VPB) is conducted retrogradely to the atria (second beat) inducing an inverted 'p' wave this may be sensed by the pacemaker (P) which then triggers a ventricular paced beat (third beat); (iii) if the paced ventricular beat is then retrogradely conducted from the ventricle to the atria and sensed an 'endless loop' may occur (beats 4, 5); that is, pace ventricle → VA conduction → 'p' wave (sensed) → ventricular pace and so forth.

20% of cardiac output.[9] Thus the ability of pacemakers to increase heart rate is paramount, although A-V synchrony may on occasions be vital (e.g. low cardiac output). Many permanent pacemakers are rate adaptive. When temporary pacing is used, the arbitrary backup rate of 70–80 bpm may need to be increased if oxygen delivery is inadequate. For life-threatening bradyarrhythmias, increasing heart rate with VVI mode pacing is the treatment of choice. Permanent VVIR pacing (most commonly using an activity or respiration sensor) will allow heart rate modulation. However, in the ICU, adaptive rate changes may not occur. For example, no activity will be sensed in a patient with septic shock even when the cardiac output is low.

During VVI and VVIR pacing the atria and ventricles beat independently and A-V synchrony is lost. Sometimes, when atria contract against closed A-V valves, significant regurgitation of blood into the pulmonary and systemic circulation occurs with serious haemodynamic compromise. This 'pacemaker syndrome'[10] should be suspected whenever ventricular pacing is associated with a fall in blood pressure. The 'pacemaker syndrome' can be eliminated by restoring A-V synchrony.

Emergency and long-term haemodynamic effects of DDD or AAI pacing are generally superior to VVI pacing.[11–13] DDD, DVI pacing requires two pacing leads, one each in the RA and RV. AAI and DVI pacing under appropriate conditions provide A-V synchrony but not rate adaptation. DDD pacing will usually ensure A-V synchrony and heart rate responsiveness, provided the S-A node is normal.

Dual chamber pacemakers require the A-V interval to be set as close as possible to the normal P-R interval (140–200 ms). Traditionally, the pacing A-V interval is arbitrarily set at about 150–200 ms. If interatrial conduction time (between the RA and LA) is significantly prolonged, the LV may contract before or at the same time as the LA, causing DDD pacemaker syndrome[14] with decreased stroke volume and cardiac output (due to LA contraction against a closed mitral valve). Hence, if there is evidence of inadequate cardiac output or impaired oxygen delivery, the A-V interval may need to be increased appropriately, or optimized using thermodilution cardiac output or echocardiographic techniques at various A-V intervals.

INDICATIONS FOR CARDIAC PACING IN BRADYARRHYTHMIAS

TEMPORARY PACING

Cardiac pacing is indicated for any sustained symptomatic bradycardia that does not promptly respond to medical treatment. Pacing may also be indicated if a bradycardia predisposes to malignant ventricular arrhythmias. The decision to pace is based on bradycardia associated with haemodynamic deterioration, and not on the specific rhythm disturbance. For example, pacing is indicated in a patient with AF and a ventricular response of 50/min associated with a blood pressure of 70/40 mmHg (9.3/5.3 kPa), cardiac failure and oliguria. Pacing is not indicated in an asymptomatic, normotensive patient with an inferior infarction, complete heart block and a ventricular rate of 45/min.

Temporary pacing may be indicated prophylactically after cardiac surgery (especially valve replacement), and occasionally during cardiac catheterization and percutaneous transluminal coronary angioplasty. Asymptomatic patients with bifascicular block do not require prophylactic pacing prior to general anaesthesia, although transcutaneous pacing should be readily available. Patients with second- or third-degree A-V block should be paced prior to general anaesthesia and surgery.

Caution should be exercised in patients with acute myocardial infarction as many patients will have received thrombolytic agents; central venous cannulation should be avoided, although if necessary the femoral vein can be used. Prognosis is related to infarct size rather than the degree of A-V block. Transcutaneous pacing obviates the need for prophylactic temporary transvenous pacing leads in high-risk patients. Pacing is sometimes required for patients with anterior or inferior myocardial infarction (Table 17.3).

Table 17.3 Complete atrioventricular (A-V) block in acute myocardial infarction

Feature	Inferior	Anterior
Onset	Slow (usually via Mobitz 1)	Sudden (usually via Mobitz II)
QRS complex	Narrow	Wide
Ventricular rate	>45 bpm	<45 bpm (often 20–30 bpm)
Escape pacemaker	Stable	Unstable
Drug response (e.g. atropine)	Yes	No
Haemodynamic effects	No (usually)	Yes
Permanent pacing	No (usually)	Yes (if high degree A-V block persists)
Prognosis	Good	Very poor

PERMANENT PACING

Guidelines for permanent pacing have been published.[15]

1 **Class I**. Generally agreed indications, for example, chronic symptomatic second- or third-degree A-V block, S-A node dysfunction with documented symptomatic bradycardia, and recurrent syncope associated with hypersensitive carotid sinus.
2 **Class II**. Controversial, but often used indications, for example, asymptomatic complete A-V block with average ventricular rate $\geq$40/min in an awake patient.
3 **Class III**: Pacing is not indicated, for example, in asymptomatic first-degree heart block or reversible A-V block secondary to drug toxicity.

OTHER INDICATIONS

Recently permanent pacing has been instituted to improve haemodynamics in patients without a bradycardia. Evolving indications include the following.[16]

1 *Hypertrophic obstructive cardiomyopathy (HOCM)*. Pacing is usually reserved for symptomatic patients with a high gradient in the left ventricular outflow tract (LVOT). DDD pacing with a short A-V interval causes RV apical activation with altered septal activation thereby decreasing both the LVOT gradient and systolic anterior motion (SAM) of the mitral valve. The results of trials to date have been mixed and it is unclear whether pacing is a preferred treatment option for HOCM. Currently, it is a class IIb indication (controversial with opinion somewhat against pacing).
2 *Dilated cardiomyopathy and heart failure*. A significant number of patients with dilated cardiomyopathy have an intraventricular conduction disturbance, usually left bundle branch block (LBBB) with significant ventricular dyssynchronization and associated paradoxical septal motion and mitral regurgitation. Ventricular resynchronization using transvenous, RA, RV and LV (LV paced via branch of the coronary sinus) pacing with an optimized A-V interval has been shown to both improve haemodynamics and provide significant symptomatic improvement.[16-20] Further prospective randomized trials are in progress and will provide definitive data on safety, long-term efficacy and survival benefit in high-risk patients already receiving maximal medical therapy for cardiac failure.
3 *AF prevention*. Atrial pacing may be effective in preventing episodes of paroxysmal AF. Most trials have been performed in patients requiring permanent pacing for bradycardia who also incidentally have episodes of paroxysmal AF. Synchronous dual site pacing either RA and LA, or two different RA sites, may be superior to single site atrial pacing by virtue of decreasing dispersion of refractoriness.[16] Multiple trials are in progress. Single site RA pacing (backup rate slightly faster than intrinsic sinus rhythm, usually 80–110 bpm) decreases the incidence of AF after cardiac surgery.[21,22] Dual site, RA and LA, or 2 sites RA are more complicated but may be superior to single site RA pacing for AF prevention.[23,24]

ELECTROMAGNETIC INTERFERENCE

Any signal that can be sensed by the pacemaker, or implantable cardioverter/defibrillator (ICD), constitutes electromagnetic interference (EMI) and can cause pacing problems such as failure to pace (inappropriate sensing), asynchronous pacing ('safety pacing' when excess 'noise' detected), pacemaker reprogramming and occasionally damage to the pacemaker (DC shock, diathermy) or the heart itself.

In critically ill patients, potential EMI sources include DC shocks, diathermy and possibly mobile telephones. In general, mobile telephones, especially analogue systems, are reasonably safe. Digital telephones have a greater theoretical risk for EMI and it is recommended that telephones do not come into close contact with the pacemaker, for example the mobile telephone should not be rested on the skin over the implanted device. If there is any doubt the pacemaker (or ICD) should be checked and reprogrammed.

CARDIOVERSION/DEFIBRILLATION IN PATIENTS WITH A PERMANENT PACEMAKER (OR ICD)

Place paddles anterior–posterior position, at least 10 cm from the unit. Make sure a suitable programmer is available and check the pacemaker (or ICD) afterwards. In patients with a temporary transvenous pacemaker, keep the external unit and the leads well away from the paddles.

DIATHERMY

When electrocautery is used in pacemaker-dependent patients, it is probably safer to change the mode to asynchronous pacing. This can be achieved in permanent pacemakers by placing a magnet over the pacemaker, and in patients with temporary transvenous pacing, by switching to VOO or DOO mode. ICD devices should be switched 'off' before diathermy is used. In contradistinction to pacemakers, placing a magnet over the ICD will deactivate the unit. After surgery the pacemaker or ICD should be tested and reprogrammed appropriately.

TECHNIQUE OF TEMPORARY TRANSVENOUS PACING

VENTRICULAR PACING

A sterile technique is mandatory. In emergencies, transcutaneous pacing is used first while transvenous VVI

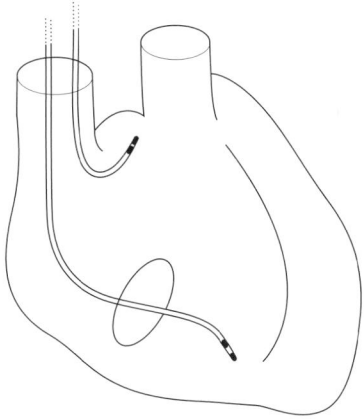

Fig. 17.10 Characteristic appearance of temporary transvenous pacing leads ideally positioned (a) in the right atrium (right atrial appendage) and (b) apex of right ventricle.

pacing is being prepared. A bipolar lead introduced under fluoroscopic control is most commonly used.

Percutaneous insertion via the right internal jugular vein probably offers least complications with ease of manipulation and stability of the lead. Antecubital veins are associated with lead instability and thrombophlebitis. The femoral vein is best avoided except in patients who have received thrombolytic agents, because of problems with sterility and increased risk of deep vein thrombosis.[25] The pacing lead is introduced using the Seldinger technique and manipulated under fluoroscopic control to the apex of the RV (Fig. 17.10). After the lead has been manipulated to a satisfactory position, a chest X-ray should be obtained to exclude pneumothorax and to

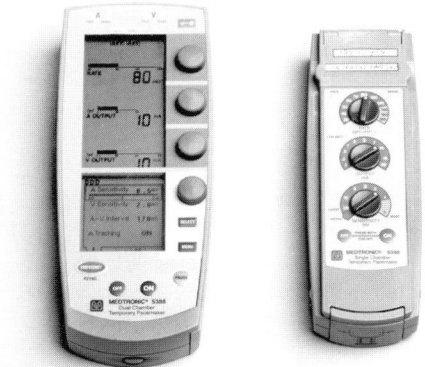

Plate 17.1 External pacemakers. Medtronic, Inc. (i) model 5388 (dual chamber); (ii) model 5348 (single chamber). Both are capable of rapid pacing for certain tachycardias (see text).

confirm adequate lead positioning. Occasionally, transvenous RV pacing may not be feasible, owing to the presence of a prosthetic tricuspid valve or a congenital anomaly.

ATRIAL PACING

Insertion of the atrial J-lead is similar to that of the ventricular lead. Correct positioning requires experience. The right atrial appendage is anterior and medial, and the tip is advanced anteriorly and to the patient's left, after passing from the superior vena cava to the RA (Fig. 17.10). The correct position can be confirmed by a lateral chest X-ray or fluoroscopy.

DUAL CHAMBER PACING

Modern external pacemakers are available (Plate 17.1) which will pace in all modes. These units are small, easy to use and can fit into a small pouch suitable for mobile patients.

TESTING THE PACING LEADS

Pacing threshold and sensing should be tested adequately using the external pacemaker.

PACING THRESHOLD

The lead is attached to the external pulse generator with the distal electrode connected to the negative pacemaker terminal. The cardiac chamber is then paced at 5–10 bpm faster than patient heart rate, while the pulse generator's output is slowly decreased until consistent capture outside the myocardial refractory period is lost. Threshold testing is always performed at an identical pulse duration, usually 0.5–1.0 ms. Ideally, ventricular pacing threshold should be ≤ 1.0 mA and the atrial threshold ≤ 2.0 mA. Pacemaker output is usually set at 2–3 times pacing threshold and always > 3 mA to allow a reasonable safety margin. After AMI the amplitude must not be set higher than necessary, as inadvertent pacing during the vulnerable period of the cardiac cycle may result in VT or VF.

SENSING

A pacemaker senses the potential difference between the two pacing electrodes. The amplitude of the ventricular signal is commonly 5–15 mV and the atrial signal 2–5 mV. Modern external pacemakers can sense signals as small as 0.8 mV for the ventricle, and 0.4 mV for atrial depolarization. Before testing the sensitivity, pacing output is set at zero, thereby avoiding potentially dangerous competition between the pacemaker and the spontaneous cardiac rhythm. Pacing rate is then set lower than the spontaneous rate of the tested cardiac chamber, and the pacemaker sensitivity is decreased until there is competition between paced and spontaneous cardiac rhythms. The pacemaker sensitivity is then set at twice that value. This involves reducing the numerical sensitivity value (e.g. changing sensitivity from 2.0 mV to 1.0 mV will double the sensitivity). Testing pacemaker sensing should not be attempted in pacemaker-dependent patients.

Assessment of sensing is important particularly in inferior infarction with RV involvement, when the intra-cardiac ventricular signal may be very small and not sensed. This resultant competition between pacemaker and spontaneous cardiac rhythm can initiate VT[26] (Fig. 17.6) or VF.[27]

COMPLICATIONS OF TEMPORARY PACING[28,29]

Temporary transvenous pacemaker insertions should have a very low complication rate. Complications may include:

- those associated with central venous line insertion, such as pneumothorax, haemothorax, arterial puncture, A-V fistula, etc. Perforation of the RV can occur, but rarely results in cardiac tamponade
- undersensing, with pacemaker-induced arrhythmias; oversensing, with pacemaker inhibition and loss of pacing stimuli; and failure to capture, due usually to device defects, unstable lead position, increasing pacing threshold and occasionally RV perforation
- extracardiac stimulation, usually diaphragmatic (may be associated with RV perforation) and local muscle stimulation can also occur
- thrombus formation and infection occasionally.

FAILURE TO PACE

A life-threatening situation may arise if the pacemaker suddenly fails. The following is an ordered approach to such an emergency.

Table 17.4 Multiprogrammable permanent dual chamber pacemakers

Parameter	Adjustment	Comments
Rate	Increase Decrease	Increase cardiac output Reduce myocardial oxygen consumption To assess underlying cardiac rhythm
Output	Increase	Increasing output may result in successful pacing when there is failure to capture
	Decrease	Increases battery life
Sensitivity	Increase	Reducing numerical value increases sensing ability. May cause oversensing occasionally.
	Decrease	Increasing numerical value decreases sensing ability. Useful in oversensing e.g. T-wave sensing.
Mode	DDD to DDI	To prevent endless-loop tachycardias and to prevent tracking of episodic atrial tachyarrhythmias. Mode switching can be automated and programmed either 'on' or 'off'.
A-V interval (AVI)	Increase/decrease	To optimize stroke volume and cardiac output. AVI can be rate adaptive, i.e. AVI shortens as the heart rate increases.
Refractory period (atrial/ventricular)	Increase	To minimize oversensing, e.g. to prevent ventricular sensing in AAI pacing.
	Decrease	To optimize sensing under certain circumstances.
Hysteresis		To preserve A-V synchrony by delaying the onset of VVI pacing until the spontaneous heart rate is significantly less than the backup ventricular pacing rate.
Polarity	Unipolar mode	To improve sensing. Occasionally to allow pacing to continue when fracture of the other conducting wire occurs.
	Bipolar mode	To prevent oversensing, e.g. muscle potentials.

1 Make sure the pacemaker is switched 'on' and connected to the pacing lead(s).
2 The pacemaker output should be increased to its maximum setting (usually 20 mA or 10 V).
3 Asynchronous DOO/VOO mode(s) is selected to prevent oversensing.
4 Connect the pacemaker directly to the pacing lead, as occasionally the connecting wires may be faulty.
5 Give consideration to replacing the pacemaker unit or the batteries.
6 External transcutaneous pacing should be immediately available and commenced while a new pacing system is being inserted.
7 Cardiopulmonary resuscitation and positive chronotropic drugs such as atropine, isoprenaline or adrenaline should be available.

PACEMAKER PROGRAMMING

An external programmer emits signals capable of changing ('programming') various pacing parameters (Table 17.4). Virtually all modern permanent pacemakers are capable of programming rate, voltage, output, pulse width, sensitivity, mode and A-V interval. Programmability is also helpful in assessing various pacemaker problems. The pacemaker format best suited to a particular patient's needs may change with time, and programmability enables optimal pacemaker function to be achieved i.e. 'prescribed'. Pacing changes may be indicated under certain circumstances, for example decreased pacing rate in a patient with angina or AMI to reduce myocardial oxygen consumption, or increased rate in a patient with haemorrhagic shock.

CARDIAC PACING IN TACHYARRHYTHMIAS

Certain tachyarrhythmias may be treated safely and effectively by rapid pacing and/or premature electrical stimulation. These include:

- A-V nodal re-entry tachycardia (AVNRT)
- A-V re-entry tachycardia (AVRT)
- atrial flutter
- unifocal atrial tachycardia
- ventricular tachycardia.

AVNRT and AVRT rarely require rapid atrial pacing as treatment with drugs such as adenosine or verapamil is usually successful. Atrial flutter, however, is often resistant to drug therapy, and rapid atrial pacing will usually convert it to sinus rhythm.[29] When unifocal atrial tachycardia is associated with an atrial re-entry circuit, rapid atrial pacing will often revert this arrhythmia; conversely, when due to automatic focus discharging at a rapid rate,

Table 17.5 Pacing versus cardioversion for the treatment of tachyarrhythmias

- Pacing may assist in rhythm diagnosis
- Pacing may be used (cautiously) in digitalis intoxication
- Pacing does not require a general anaesthetic
- Pacing avoids complications of DC shock, especially myocardial depression
- Repeated reversions are easier with pacing
- Standby pacing is immediately available should bradycardia or asystole occur after electrical reversion

Table 17.6 Pacing versus drug therapy for the treatment of tachyarrhythmias

- Pacing may aid in arrhythmia diagnosis
- Pacing avoids drug induced cardiac depression and other drug side effects
- Pacing can be used when drug therapy has failed
- Termination of the tachycardia with pacing is often immediate
- Standby pacing is immediately available

Table 17.7 Indications for rapid cardiac pacing in suitable arrhythmias

- Failure of drug therapy
- Recurrent arrhythmias
- Contraindication for cardioversion (e.g. digitalis intoxication)
- Aid to arrhythmia diagnosis (e.g. wide complex tachycardia to differentiate ventricular tachycardia from supraventricular tachycardia).

the arrhythmia is usually incessant and will respond only intermittently if at all to atrial pacing. Occasionally, dual chamber pacing with a short A-V interval can be used to prevent drug resistant AVNRT or AVRT. Rapid continuous atrial pacing can be used to slow ventricular rate during resistant SVTs associated with a rapid ventricular response,[30] by inducing AF and a high degree of A-V block. Sustained VT is responsive to rapid ventricular pacing, but this should not be used for very rapid ventricular rates (e.g. > 300/min), or when severe haemodynamic compromise is present, as immediate DC cardioversion is indicated. Rapid cardiac pacing may at times have advantages over DC cardioversion (Table 17.5) and drug therapy (Table 17.6), but is of no value in sinus tachycardia, AF and VF (Table 17.7).

SUPRAVENTRICULAR TACHYARRHYTHMIAS

The pacing lead is manipulated to a suitable position in the RA. Atrial pacing is started at a slow rate (e.g. 60–80/min) and increased slowly to about 10–20% faster than the spontaneous atrial rate. Inadvertent

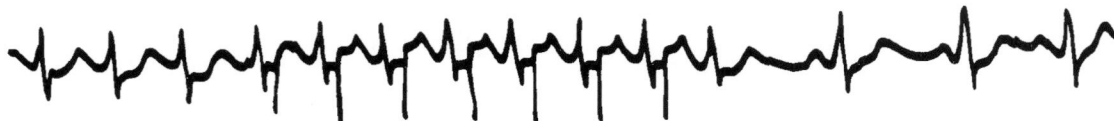

Fig. 17.11 Narrow complex tachycardia. Rapid atrial pacing with atrial capture results in sinus rhythm on cessation of pacing.

ventricular pacing, especially at rapid rates, must be avoided. The atrium is paced for about 30 seconds and the pacemaker is then switched off. Normal sinus rhythm should ensue (Fig 17.11). If not, the pacing lead is manipulated to a different position and/or a faster pacing rate is tried. A more prolonged pacing period may be effective. If sinus rhythm still does not result, AF is deliberately precipitated by rapid atrial pacing at 400–800/min. This is an unstable rhythm which usually reverts spontaneously to normal sinus rhythm. AF persists occasionally, but the ventricular rate is usually slower and more responsive to drug therapy than with SVT.[30]

VENTRICULAR TACHYCARDIA

Useful techniques to pace VT include the following.

1 Ventricular burst pacing (similar to rapid atrial pacing) is simple and effective. The ventricle is paced at a rate about 120% of the spontaneous VT rate for 5–10 beats. Normal sinus rhythm should ensue (Fig. 17.12). Potential complications include entrainment (Fig. 17.13), that is, speeding up of VT, and occasionally precipitation of VF. Trained personnel, a defibrillator and resuscitation facilities must be available.
2 Underdrive ventricular pacing at rates less than that of the tachycardia may occasionally be successful.
3 Overdrive atrial pacing may be useful if there is 1:1 A-V conduction and the ventricular rate is relatively slow (e.g. 120–180/min).

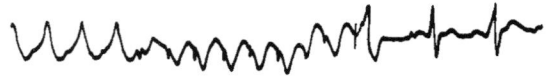

Fig. 17.12 Wide complex tachycardia. Ventricular 'burst' pacing with ventricular capture results in normal sinus rhythm on cessation of pacing.

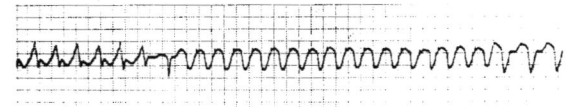

Fig. 17.13 Example of entrainment. Wide complex tachycardia is followed by ventricular 'burst' pacing. When pacing is discontinued, a wide complex tachycardia of opposite polarity is precipitated.

IMPLANTABLE CARDIOVERTER/ DEFIBRILLATOR (ICD)[31]

This is an implantable device which can recognize and automatically terminate VT and VF. Guidelines[15] have been published for ICD implantation; nevertheless, this is a rapidly evolving field with many trials in progress. ICDs are of proven survival benefit (class I) in patients who have had a cardiac arrest due to VF or VT, not due to transient or reversible cause. In other clinical situations ICD implantation may be a reasonable approach, for example, syncope with inducible VT at electrophysiology study which is poorly tolerated haemodynamically, and anti-arrhythmic drugs are ineffective and/or contraindicated. A trial[32] in over 1200 patients with recent myocardial infarction and low LV ejection fraction ($\leq$30%) has demonstrated a decrease in mortality when prophylactic ICD implantation was compared to conventional treatment. In future, ICDs may become standard therapy to prevent sudden cardiac death in such high risk patients.

Currently, most ICD devices are single chamber and are implanted pectorally with a single lead passed transvenously. This lead has defibrillator coils, one positioned in the RV, the other in the SVC. In addition to defibrillation, current devices also possess standard sensing and pacing as well as antitachycardia algorithms. Current devices continuously monitor the patient's heart rate and deliver therapy when the heart rate exceeds a predetermined limit. There is a graded response which is programmable:

1 'Slow' VT (e.g. ventricular rate 160–180/min) – antitachycardia pacing, that is, pacing at a rate faster than the intrinsic rate. If this is unsuccessful, antitachycardia pacing might be attempted at a faster rate; or
2 DC shock(s) (synchronized during VT, asynchronous during VF) initially at low energies. If unsuccessful, then high energy shocks are delivered. All shocks are biphasic as these are more efficient and require lower energies than monophasic waveforms;
3 Pacing backup (single or dual chamber) is usually available if there is a significant bradycardia after cardioversion/defibrillation.

COMPLICATIONS

As with pacemakers, EMI can potentially reprogram the ICD and care should be exercised (see before). Nerve stimulators have been sensed by an ICD. Occasionally, multiple ICD discharges occur. This is a true clinical emergency. Shocks may be appropriate or inappropriate. Frequent malignant ventricular arrhythmias may result in multiple appropriate discharges. If DC shocks are unsuccessful, the device may need to be reprogrammed to deliver higher energy shocks, conversely if the multiple shocks are successful in defibrillating the patient during an arrhythmia 'storm', then the ICD device should probably be inactivated by placing a magnet over the unit, and external transthoracic defibrillation and antiarrhythmic drug therapy should be given as required. This will save battery power and allow the patient's ICD system to be tested later. If inappropriate ICD shocks arise, the ICD device should be switched off at once. The most common reason for inappropriate shocks is AF or some other SVT. Reprogramming the device may solve the problem. Occasionally sensing of EMI may cause ICD discharge. Avoidance of the EMI source and/or reprogramming may be necessary.

REFERENCES

1 Zoll PM. Resuscitation of the heart in ventricular standstill by external electric stimulation. *N Engl J Med* 1952; **747**: 768–71.
2 Levine PA, Caplan CH, Klein MD, Brodsky SJ, Ryan JJ. Myopotential inhibition of unipolar lithium pacemakers. *Chest* 1982; **82**: 101–3.
3 Kelly JS, Royster RL. Non-invasive transcutaneous cardiac pacing. *Anesth Analg* 1989; **69**: 229–38.
4 Lang R, David D, Klein HO, *et al*. The use of the balloon-tipped floating catheter in temporary transvenous cardiac pacing. *Pace* 1981; **4**: 491–6.
5 Crossley GH. Cardiac pacing leads. *Cardiol Clin* 2000; **18**: 95–112.
6 Bernstein AD, Camm AJ, Fletcher RD, *et al*. The NASPE/BPEG generic pacemaker code for antibradyarrhythmic and adaptive rate pacing and antitachyarrhythmic devices. *Pace* 1987; **10**: 794–9.
7 Leung S-K, Lau C-P. Developments in sensor-driven pacing. *Cardiol Clin* 2000; **18**: 113–55.
8 Furman S, Fisher JD. Endless-loop tachycardia in an AV Universal (DDD) pacemaker. *Pace* 1982; **5**: 486–9.
9 Donovan KD, Dobb GJ, Lee KY. The haemodynamic importance of maintaining atrioventricular synchrony during cardiac pacing in critically ill patients. *Crit Care Med* 1991; **19**: 320–326.
10 Johnson AD, Laiken SL, Engler RL. Hemodynamic compromise associated with ventriculoatrial conduction following transvenous pacemaker placement. *Am J Med* 1978; **65**: 75–81.
11 Andersen HR, Nielsen JC, Thomsen PE, *et al*. Long term follow up of patients from a randomised trial of atrial versus ventricular pacing for sick sinus syndrome. *Lancet* 1997; **350**: 1210–16.
12 Lamas GA, Orav EJ, Stambler BS, *et al*. for the Pacemaker Selection in the Elderly Investigators. Quality of life and clinical outcomes in elderly patients treated with ventricular pacing as compared with dual chamber pacing. *N Engl J Med* 1998; **338**: 1097–104.
13 Connolly SJ, Kerr CR, Gent M, *et al*. Effects of physiologic pacing versus ventricular pacing on the risk of stroke and death due to cardiovascular causes. *N Engl J Med* 2000; **342**: 1385–91.
14 Pierantozzi A, Bocconcelli P, Sgarbi E. DDD pacemaker syndrome and atrial conduction time. *Pace* 1994; **17**: 374–6.
15 Gregoratos G, Cheitlin M, Conill A, *et al*. ACC/AHA guidelines for implantation of cardiac pacemakers and antiarrhythmia devices. A report of the American College of Cardiology/American Heart Associate Task Force on Practice Guidelines (Committee on Pacemaker Implantation). *J Am Coll Cardiol* 1998; **31**: 1175–209.
16 Bryce M, Spielman SR, Greenspan AM, Kotler MN. Evolving indications for permanent pacemakers. *Ann Intern Med* 2001; **134**: 1130–41.
17 Gras D, Mabo P, Tang T, *et al*. Multisite pacing as a supplemental treatment of congestive heart failure: preliminary results of the Medtronic Inc. InSync Study. *Pacing Clin Electrophysiol* 1998; **21**: 2249–58.
18 Auricchio A, Stellbrink C, Block M, *et al*. for the Pacing Therapies for Congestive Heart Failure Study Group and the Guidant Congestive Heart Failure Research Group. Effect of pacing chamber and atrioventricular delay on acute systolic function of paced patients with congestive heart failure. *Circulation* 1999; **99**: 2993–3001.
19 Auricchio A, Stellbrink C, Sack S, *et al*. for the PATH-CHF Study Group. The Pacing Therapies for Congestive Heart Failure (PATH-CHF) study: rationale, design, and endpoints of a prospective randomized multicenter study. *Am J Cardiol* 1999; **83**: 130D.
20 Cazeau S, Leclercq C, Lavergne T, *et al*. for the Multisite Stimulation in Cardiomyopathies (MUSTIC) Study Investigators. Effects of multisite biventricular pacing in patients with heart failure and intraventricular conduction delay. *N Engl J Med* 2001; **344**: 873–80.
21 Greenberg MD, Katz NM, Iuliano S, *et al*. Atrial pacing for the prevention of atrial fibrillation after cardiovascular surgery. *J Am Coll Cardiol* 2000; **35**: 1416–22.
22 Blommaert D, Gonzalez M, Muccumbitsi J, *et al*. Effective prevention of atrial fibrillation by continuous atrial overdrive pacing after coronary artery bypass surgery. *J Am Coll Cardiol* 2000; **35**: 1411–15.
23 Levy T, Fotopoulos G, Walker S, *et al*. Randomized controlled study investigating the effect of biatrial pacing in prevention of atrial fibrillation after coronary artery bypass grafting. *Circulation* 2000; **102**: 1382–7.
24 Daubert JC, Mabo P. Atrial pacing for the prevention of postoperative atrial fibrillation: how and where to pace? *J Am Coll Cardiol* 2000; **35**: 1423–7.
25 Pandian NG, Kosowsky BD, Gurewich V. Transfemoral temporary pacing and deep vein thrombosis. *Am Heart J* 1980; **100**: 847–80.
26 Ceuni TA, White RA, Burkart F. Pacemaker-induced ventricular tachycardia in patients with acute inferior myocardial infarction. *Int J Cardiol* 1980; **1**: 93–7.

27 Mooss AN, Ross WB, Esterbrooks DJ. Ventricular fibrillation complicating pacemaker insertion in acute myocardial infarction. *Cath Cardiol Diag* 1982; **8**: 253–9.

28 Austin R, Preis JK, Crampton WS, *et al.* Analysis of pacemaker function and complications of temporary pacing in the coronary care unit. *Am J Cardiol* 1983; **49**: 301–6.

29 Donovan KD, Lee KY. Indications for and complications of temporary transvenous cardiac pacing. *Anaesth Intensive Care* 1985; **13**: 63–70.

30 Moreira DAR, Shepard RB, Waldo AL. Chronic rapid atrial pacing to maintain atrial fibrillation: use to permit control of ventricular rate in order to treat tachycardia induced cardiomyopathy. *Pace* 1989; **10**: 519–32.

31 Gold MR. ICD therapy in the new millennium. *Cardiol Clin* 2000; **18**: 375–89.

32. Moss AJ, Zareba W, Hall WJ, *et al.* Prophylactic implantation of a defibrillator in patients with myocardial infarction and reduced ejection fraction. *N Engl J Med* 2002; **346**: 877–883.

18

Acute heart failure

D Treacher

The principal function of the heart is the generation of the energy necessary to perfuse the lungs with venous blood and to propel the oxygenated arterial blood through the systemic circulation at a rate and pressure that ensures that the fluctuating metabolic requirements of the various organs are met at rest and during exercise. This should be performed at maximum efficiency so that the work performed is not at the cost of unnecessarily high myocardial energy expenditure and the risk of myocardial ischaemia is minimized.

The heart must provide its own blood supply and if coronary blood flow does not match myocardial oxygen requirements, coronary ischaemia develops and cardiac and global circulatory failure may ensue.[1]

The pattern of heart failure seen in the community, outpatient clinics and specialist cardiac wards is dominated by the acute coronary syndromes and chronic heart failure, predominantly caused by ischaemic heart disease and hypertension.[2,3] Patients present with chest pain, fatigue, oedema and shortness of breath and will usually have single organ failure. Management focuses on myocardial salvage by minimizing cardiac work.[4–6]

Patients admitted to intensive care with heart failure may have pre-existing chronic heart failure and underlying ischaemic heart disease, but the presentation is acute and usually as part of multiple organ dysfunction. Cardiac function is assessed in the context of the wider circulation and management is focused on multiple organ support and restoring global and regional oxygen delivery, frequently with the use of drugs that stimulate rather than rest the myocardium.[7–9] If the precipitating cause is successfully treated and has not caused myocardial infarction, the acute heart failure resolves and cardiac function returns to its pre-morbid state.

This chapter addresses the assessment and principles of management of ventricular function in patients admitted to the intensive care unit with acute heart failure. This inevitably involves reference to circulatory failure and the state of the peripheral circulation but the more detailed aspects of oxygen delivery and control of the regional and micro-circulation are considered elsewhere[10] as are the acute coronary syndromes[3] and chronic heart failure.[2,11]

CIRCULATORY FAILURE OR 'SHOCK'

Failure to maintain an adequate oxygen supply to the tissues with the consequent development of anaerobic cellular metabolism defines circulatory failure or 'shock', a term that benefits from brevity but little else since it implies neither cause nor prognosis but its use is now widespread and inescapable. Table 18.1 classifies circulatory 'shock'.

In considering these causes of circulatory failure, several points require emphasis:

- Acute heart failure resulting in cardiogenic shock is not a pathological diagnosis but a collective term that embraces all causes of myocardial failure. Treatment must focus on the underlying diagnosis.
- Patients admitted to the intensive care unit (ICU) may have acute heart failure either as the primary reason for admission e.g. severe myocardial infarction or develop it as part of multiple organ failure triggered by an extracardiac cause, frequently the delayed or ineffective treatment of severe sepsis.
- Pre-existing cardiac disease, usually ischaemic heart disease, is an important factor in determining the physiological response to critical illness. Several studies investigating the effect of manipulating oxygen delivery have demonstrated the poor prognosis associated with

Table 18.1 Major categories of circulatory failure or 'shock'

Cardiogenic myocardial infarction, myocarditis, vasculitis, valve dysfunction (e.g. critical aortic stenosis, mitral regurgitation, acute endocarditis), post cardiac bypass surgery, drug overdose (β-blockers, calcium antagonists)

Hypovolaemic: haemorrhage, burns, gastrointestinal fluid loss

Obstructive pulmonary embolus, cardiac tamponade, tension pneumothorax

Anaphylactic drugs, blood transfusion, insect sting

Septic bacterial infection, non-infective inflammatory conditions e.g. pancreatitis, burns, trauma

Neurogenic intracranial haemorrhage, brainstem compression, spinal cord injury

the inability of the heart to achieve a hyperdynamic response to critical illness either spontaneously or in response to volume loading and inotropic support.[8,9,12,13]

- Although hypotension is often considered to be the cardinal sign of circulatory failure, other global features (persistent tachycardia, confusion, tachypnoea, impaired peripheral perfusion, progressive metabolic acidaemia) occur earlier since the body has powerful homeostatic mechanisms that maintain pressure at the expense of flow.
- The primary problem in hypovolaemic, cardiogenic and obstructive shock is a progressive decline in cardiac output and global oxygen delivery, which, if not corrected, leads to secondary failure of the peripheral circulation and progressive organ dysfunction. In septic, anaphylactic and neurogenic shock, however, the primary problem is the loss of control of the peripheral circulation, resulting in systemic hypotension and disordered distribution of blood flow although cardiac output and global oxygen delivery are usually increased.[14,15]
- Although a primary cause for the circulatory failure may be identified, other causes may contribute to the evolution of the final pathology. For example, in septic shock, the initial and major derangement is peripheral: it is characterized by microcirculatory chaos triggered by cytokine release, white cell activation, disruption of the coagulation cascade resulting in microthrombi that occlude the microvasculature and endothelial disruption resulting in interstitial oedema. This same process occurs in the coronary microvasculature impairing myocyte function.[16,17] There is also widespread loss of fluid from the intravascular to the extravascular space resulting in hypovolaemia. The primary peripheral circulatory failure may therefore be compounded by both cardiogenic and hypovolaemic shock.
- 'Early' and 'late' shock are terms that reflect the association between the duration and severity of the circulatory derangement and prognosis. Early intervention in circulatory shock has a major impact on survival.[15,18,19] If treatment is delayed until organ failure is established, the underlying pathological processes are frequently irreversible.

ASSESSMENT OF VENTRICULAR FUNCTION

Making the considerable assumption that the circulation can be analysed as a constant flow, fixed compliance system, six key measurements traditionally define ventricular performance:

- Right and left atrial pressures (RAP, LAP or ventricular 'preload')

- Mean systemic and pulmonary arterial pressures (MAP, PAP or ventricular 'afterload')
- Heart rate (HR)
- Cardiac output (Qt)

Table 18.2 illustrates typical values in normal subjects and in the common causes of circulatory failure with derivation of vascular resistances and oxygen delivery. The values quoted are merely examples that indicate the pattern of circulatory derangement produced by these pathologies: pre-existing cardiopulmonary disease and the severity of the condition will affect the precise figures obtained in individual cases.

Stroke volume (SV) is calculated from cardiac output and heart rate:

$$SV = Qt/HR$$

Three factors determine stroke volume:

- Preload
- Afterload
- Myocardial contractility

VENTRICULAR 'PRELOAD'

Ventricular 'preload', traditionally assessed from the atrial filling pressures, determines the end diastolic ventricular volume, which, according to Starling's law of the heart and depending on ventricular contractility, dictates the stroke work generated by each ventricle at the next cardiac contraction. The resulting stroke volume depends on the resistance or 'afterload' that confronts the ventricle.[20]

On the general ward, the jugular venous pressure is measured from the sternal angle but, in ICU, vascular pressures are measured from the mid-axillary line in the fifth intercostal space. From this reference point, in the supine position, the normal RAP is between +4 and +8 mmHg and the LAP, or 'wedge' pressure is between +8 and +12 mmHg. Relative changes in either the contractility of the two ventricles or the respective vascular resistances will change the relationship between the atrial pressures, which must then be independently assessed.[21,22]

The predominant factor determining preload is venous return which depends on the intravascular volume and venous 'tone', which is controlled by the autonomic nervous system, circulating catecholamine levels and local factors, particularly PO_2, PCO_2 and pH.

The systemic venous bed is the major intravascular capacitance or reservoir of the circulation with a compliance that can vary from 30 to over 300 ml/mmHg and which provides a buffer against the effects of intravascular volume loss. It also explains the response observed in major haemorrhage and subsequent transfusion. As volume is lost, venous tone increases preventing the large falls in atrial filling pressures and cardiac output that would otherwise occur. If the equivalent volume is returned over the subsequent few hours, the RAP

Table 18.2   Measurements in a normal 75 kg adult and in various conditions causing circulatory 'shock'

	RAP (mmHg)	LAP (mmHg)	PAP (mmHg)	MAP (mmHg)	HR (per min)	Cardiac output (l/min)	SVR*	PVR*	Stroke work (g.m) LV	RV	Venous compliance (ml/mmHg)	CaO₂ (l/100 ml)	DO₂ (ml/min)
Normal	5	10	15	90	70	5.0	17	1.0	78	10	300	20	1000
Major haemorrhage	0	3	10	80	100	3.2	25	2.2	34	4.4	40	16	510
Left ventricular failure	7	19	23	90	100	3.6	23	1.1	35	8	80	18	650
Cardiac tamponade	14	16	19	65	110	2.3	22	1.3	14	1.4	50	20	460
Major PE	10	6	35	70	110	2.6	23	11.0	21	8	40	16	420
Exacerbation of COAD	10	9	35	80	100	6.5	11	4.0	63	22	150	13	850
Septic shock:													
(i) pre-volume	2	7	17	49	130	4.2	11	2.4	18	7	350	15	630
(ii) post-volume	10	14	25	68	120	8.0	7	1.4	49	14	200	14	1120

Typical circulatory measurements in a normal adult and in various cardiorespiratory conditions that may cause shock. The severity of the condition and pre-existing cardiorespiratory disease will affect the precise figures obtained in individual cases.

Pressures referenced to zero at mid-axillary line in supine patient. Subtract vertical distance from mid-axilla to sternal angle (approximately 5–7 mmHg) if sternal angle used as reference point.

LV, Left ventricle; RV, right ventricle; CaO₂, arterial oxygen content; DO₂, global oxygen delivery; PAP/MAP, mean pulmonary artery/arterial pressure; SVR/PVR**, systemic/pulmonary vascular resistance $\times$ 80 to give SI units: $dyn \cdot s \cdot cm^{-5}$.

gradually returns to normal as the intravascular volume is restored and the reflex increase in sympathetic tone abates. However, rapid re-infusion of the same volume does not allow sufficient time for the venous and arteriolar tone to fall and may result in the LAP rising to a level that precipitates pulmonary oedema although the intravascular volume has only been returned to the pre-haemorrhage level (Fig. 18.1).

If the preload is low and either blood pressure or cardiac output is inadequate, the priority is volume loading to restore intravascular volume and venous return.

Raised preload pressures reflect either (i) high intravascular volume, (ii) impaired myocardial contractility or (iii) increased 'afterload'.

Preload may be reduced by:

- Removing volume from the circulation (diuretics, venesection, haemofiltration) or increasing the capacity of the vascular bed with venodilator therapy (e.g. glyceryl trinitrate, morphine)[23]
- Improving contractility
- Reducing afterload[24]

In assessing preload, end-diastolic volume rather than pressure is relevant and when interpreting atrial pressures as measures of preload, two points must be considered:

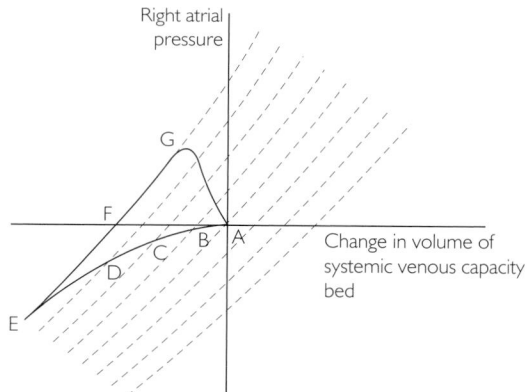

Fig. 18.1 Venous compliance curves. Each dotted line represents a line of constant venous compliance ranging from low compliance (increased 'tone') on the left to increased compliance (reduced 'tone') on the right. Line ABCDE shows the effect of progressisve haemorrhage with the reduction is venous compliance limiting the fall in atrial pressure. Line EFGI shows the effect of rapid re-infusion of the same volume that was removed but at a rate that does not allow the sympathetical mediated increase in venous 'tone' to abate. Each dotted line represents a line of constant venous compliance ranging from minimum on the left to diminished venous tone on the right

- Intravascular pressure (Pv) measurements are misleading if the intrathoracic pressure (Pt) is raised, since the true distending pressure that determines ventricular end-diastolic volume is the transmural pressure (Pv − Pt). This is particularly relevant if there is significant alveolar gas trapping as in asthma and positive-pressure ventilation with high positive end-expiratory pressure levels and an inverse inspiratory to expiratory time ratio.[25,26]
- When the ventricle is dilated and poorly compliant, the end-diastolic pressure–volume relationship is not necessarily linear and pressure will no longer reflect volume preload.

Alternative methods of assessing ventricular preload are discussed in the section on intravascular volume assessment.

VENTRICULAR 'AFTERLOAD'

The vascular resistance against which each ventricle works is calculated, by analogy with Ohm's law, as the pressure gradient across the vascular bed divided by the cardiac output (Table 18.3).

Circulatory management requires a clear understanding of this relationship between pressure, flow and resistance. If ventricular work is constant, increased vascular resistances produce higher pressures but with a lower cardiac output. A systemic dilator such as sodium nitroprusside will reduce systemic resistance and blood pressure and increase cardiac output. Although such manipulation is attractive in increasing cardiac output for the same cardiac work, it is important to maintain a blood pressure that ensures appropriate distribution of blood flow and a diastolic pressure sufficient to maintain coronary artery perfusion, particularly in patients with known ischaemic heart disease or pre-existing hypertension.

The effects of some of the commonly used vasoactive agents are shown in Table 18.4 and considered in more detail later.

VENTRICULAR CONTRACTILITY AND EFFICIENCY

The work that the ventricle performs under given loading conditions defines contractility.

It may be expressed mathematically as the gradient and intercept of the relationship between atrial filling pressure and stroke work (Fig. 18.2). The resulting stroke volume varies with the resistance of the vascular bed into which the ventricle is ejecting. Although the right ventricle generates a much smaller stroke work, the afterload (PVR) against which it ejects is correspondingly lower since the right and left ventricular stroke volumes must necessarily be the same over time.

The work output of each ventricle with each beat is the ventricular stroke work and is calculated as shown in Table 18.3.

Table 18.3 Calculation of ventricular afterload and stroke work

$$
\begin{aligned}
\text{Systemic vascular resistance (SVR)} &= [(\text{MAP} - \text{RAP})/\text{Qt}] \times 80 \text{ dyn·s·cm}^{-5} \\
&= [(90 - 5)/5] \times 80 = 1360 \text{ dyn·s·cm}^{-5} \\
\text{SVRI} &= \text{SVR} \times \text{BSA} = 1360 \times 1.65 = 2244 \text{ dyn·sec·cm}^{-9} \\
\text{Pulmonary vascular resitance (PVR)} &= [(\text{PAP} - \text{LAP})/\text{Qt} \times 80 \text{ dyn·sec·cm}^{-5} \\
&= [(15 - 5)/5] \times 80 = 160 \text{ dyn·s·cm}^{-5} \\
\text{PVRI} &= \text{PVR} \times \text{BSA} = 160 \times 1.65 = 264 \text{ dyn·sec·cm}^{-9}
\end{aligned}
$$

$$
\begin{aligned}
\text{Stroke volume (SV)} &= \text{Qt/HR} = 72 \text{ ml} \\
\text{Stroke volume index (SVI)} &= 72/1.65 = 44 \text{ ml/m}^2
\end{aligned}
$$

$$
\begin{aligned}
\text{Ventricular stroke work (VSV)} &= \text{SV} \times (\text{afterload} - \text{preload}) \\
\text{LVSW} &= \text{SV} \times (\text{MAP} - \text{LAP}) \times 0.0136 \text{ g.m} \\
&= 72 \times (90 - 10) \times 0.0136 = 78 \text{ g.m} \\
\text{LVSWI} &= 78/1.65 = 47 \text{ g.m} \\
\text{RVSW} &= \text{SV} \times (\text{PAP} - \text{RAP}) \times 0.0136 \text{ g.m} \\
&= 72 \times (15 - 5) \times 0.0136 = 10 \text{ g.m} \\
\text{RVSWI} &= 10/1.65 = 6 \text{ g.m}
\end{aligned}
$$

MAP, mean arterial pressure; PAP, mean pulmonary artery pressure.
Pressures are measured in mmHg, cardiac output (Qt) in l/min.
Values for resistance, stroke work are frequently indexed by dividing by the patient's body surface area (BSA) derived from height and weight.
In calculating ventricular stroke work, 0.0136 converts from ml.mmHg to SI units of g.m.
Example calculations assume a normal 75 kg individual with BSA 1.65 m².

Consideration of ventricular work is important since optimum circulatory management requires that the necessary pressures and flows to maintain satisfactory organ perfusion and oxygen delivery are achieved at maximum cardiac efficiency (i.e. for the minimum ventricular work to avoid myocardial ischaemia).

Left ventricular efficiency is the ratio of work output to energy input and may be less than 20% in patients with acute heart failure with over 80% of energy lost as heat. A recently described technique, based on thermodynamic principles and requiring only measurement of temperature and oxygen content difference across the left ventricular capillary bed is simpler, clinically applicable and more accurate than earlier methods. It will allow selection of therapies based on both global circulatory and myocardial metabolic considerations.[27]

If circulatory failure is due to impaired myocardial contractility as defined by a 'flattened' stroke work/filling pressure equation (Fig. 18.2), the atrial pressures are often already raised. Provided this accurately reflects volume preload, further increases are not helpful since the ventricle becomes increasingly distended with high wall tension as predicted by Laplace's law:

Wall tension = $(\text{Piv} \times \text{radius})/(\text{wall thickness} \times 2)$

This compromises myocardial blood supply, particularly epicardial to endocardial blood flow resulting in endocardial ischaemia, further impairment of ventricular contractility and the risk of pulmonary oedema developing.

The remaining therapeutic options are:

- *Reduce afterload*, using an arteriolar dilator [nitrates, α-blocker, angiotensin-converting enzyme (ACE) inhibitor] although this strategy is frequently limited by the resulting fall in systemic pressure.[28,29]
- *Increase myocardial contractility*, either by removing negatively inotropic influences (acidaemia, hyperkalaemia, drugs, e.g. β-blockers) or by using a positive inotrope, which may be defined as an agent that increases the gradient of the stroke work to filling pressure relationship resulting in a larger stroke volume for the same pre- and afterload pressures. When considering the use of an inotrope agent (Table 18.4), the adverse effects of vasoactive agents on ventricular efficiency, metabolic rate and regional distribution of flow should be considered.[30]

HEART RATE AND RHYTHM

In cardiac failure, the stroke volume is usually constant for rates up to 100 beats per min and thereafter falls as restriction of diastolic filling time limits end diastolic volume. Increasing the heart rate from 70 to 90 beats per min will increase cardiac output by almost 30%. Achieving this with a chronotrope such as the β_1 agonist isoproterenol increases myocardial work and oxygen consumption and also ventricular irritability. In patients with ischaemic heart disease, and particularly after a recent myocardial infarction, atrial or atrial-ventricular sequential pacing (which maintains co-ordinated atrial contraction in heart block) improves haemodynamics without stimulating myocardial metabolism and increasing myocardial irritability.[31]

Heart rates above 110 beats per min, particularly with an irregular rhythm, should be controlled either by drugs

Table 18.4 Circulatory effects of commonly used vasoactive drug infusions

Drug	Receptors	Cardiac contractility	Heart rate	Blood pressure	Cardiac output	Splanchnic blood flow	SVR	PVR
Dopamine								
(<5 µg/kg per min)	DA_1, $β_1$, $α$	+	0/+	0/+	+	0/+	0/+	0/+
(>5 µg/kg per min)	$β_1$, $α$, DA_1, $β_2$	++	+	+	++	0	+	+
Epinephrine	$β_1$, $α$, $β_2$	++	+	++	+++	–	+	++
Norepinephrine	$α$, $β_1$	0/+	0	++	–	– –	++	++
Isoprenaline	$β_1$, $β_2$	+	++	+/0	–	0/+	0/–	–
Dobutamine	$β_1$, $β_2$, $α$	+	+	+/0/–	++	0	–	–
Dopexamine	$β_2$, DA_1, DA_2	+	+	0	+	+	–	–
Glyceryl trinitrate	via NO	0	+	–	+	+	–	–
Nitroprusside	via NO	0	+	– –	+	+	– –	–
Milrinone	PDE	+	+	–	++	0/+	–	–
Nitric oxide (inhaled)	via NO	0	0	0	0/+	0	0	– –
Prostacyclin	via NO	0	+	– –	+	+	–	– –

+, increases; 0, no change; –, decreases.

These effects are guidelines only. The response will depend on the circulatory state of the patient when the drug is started and the differential effects on $α$, $β$, dopamine (DA_1, DA_2), phosphodiesterase (PDE) receptors and nitric oxide/cGMP with increasing dose.

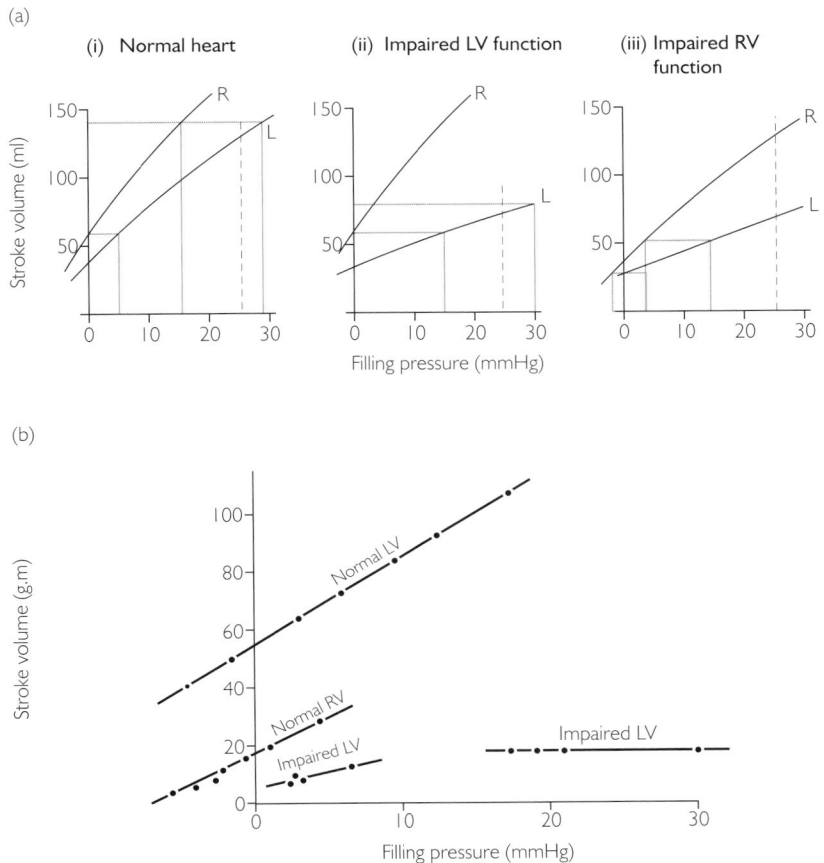

Fig. 18.2 Ventricular function curves. (a) Relationship between stroke volume (ml) and atrial filling pressure for left (L) and right (R) ventricles in patients with normal and impaired ventricular function. (b) Relationship between stroke work (g.m) and atrial filling pressure (in mmHg) for the left (L) and right (R) ventricles for a normal subject and a patient with severe left and right ventricular failure

or DC cardioversion after ensuring that plasma potassium and magnesium levels have been corrected. If the rhythm is supraventricular and unstable with intermittent periods of sinus rhythm, pharmacological control is indicated using either digoxin or amiodarone.

- Digoxin is appropriate for atrial fibrillation and has a temporary positive inotropic effect.[32]
- Amiodarone is suitable for all supraventricular rhythms and is more likely to restore sinus rhythm. A meta-analysis showed that used prophylactically it reduced the rate of arrhythmic episodes and sudden death in patients with recent myocardial infarction or congestive cardiac failure.[33] It is however a negative inotrope and this can be significant in the patient with severe heart failure.

A fixed rate of 150 beats per min suggests atrial flutter and should prompt careful inspection of the electrocardiogram and a trial of adenosine. A persistent sinus tachycardia unexplained by fever may be due to hypovolaemia, pain or anxiety.

The use of β-blockers in patients with heart failure remains controversial. Large studies have demonstrated their benefit early after acute myocardial infarction[5] and atenolol given i.v. peri-operatively produces a survival benefit for up to 2 years after non-cardiac surgery in patients deemed to be at high risk of coronary artery disease.[34] This evidence would appear to conflict with studies of 'perioperative optimization' that show benefit from increasing oxygen delivery with volume loading and the use of β-agonists.[19,35]

MONITORING CARDIAC FUNCTION

Of the six key circulatory variables that define ventricular function, three (RAP, MAP, HR) can be assessed clinically and are routinely monitored in ICU patients. However additional monitoring, traditionally using the pulmonary artery catheter, is required to measure the other variables (LAP, PAP and Qt) and answer the questions:

- Is further intravascular volume indicated?
- Is cardiac output too low and compromising global oxygen delivery?
- Is dilator, constrictor or inotropic therapy appropriate?

It is certainly not always necessary to use invasive monitoring.[36] Initial management can be based on clinical assessment of intravascular volume and cardiac output. The discipline of committing to an estimate of these key variables ensures that both the analysis of the circulation and the approach to treatment are logical. Further monitoring should be instituted if the initial management does not produce clinical improvement. Alternative, less invasive methods are available for assessing cardiac output such as transoesophageal Doppler,[37] lithium dilution,[38] echocardiography[39] and pulse contour analysis, techniques which can also provide data on the volume rather than pressure preload of the left ventricle. Table 18.5 lists some features of the techniques available for measuring cardiac output and whether they provide information on left ventricular preload. Further details of circulatory monitoring and these other techniques are described in the section on haemodynamic monitoring.

KEY POINTS RELATED TO MONITORING CARDIAC FUNCTION

- Pressure is no guarantee of flow
- Trends and changes are more important than a single observation
- Monitoring devices may be complex with many potential sources of error (e.g. 'blocked' catheters, failure to re-level the transducer after a change in the patient's position). Readings should always be interpreted with care and in conjunction with clinical assessment.
- Invasive monitoring has its own hazards (e.g. infection, trauma, immobility) and should be removed if no longer clinically indicated

ECHOCARDIOGRAPHY (see Ch. 21)

Echocardiography is an extremely valuable investigation in the management of the critically ill patient with acute heart failure. It will frequently establish the underlying cardiac pathology and can be used to monitor the response to treatment. It will identify:

- Pericardial effusions and determine whether ventricular filling is impaired (tamponade) and drainage is indicated. It will also identify obstruction to cardiac filling from other intrathoracic space occupying lesions that increase intrathoracic pressure particularly in ventilated patients (pleural effusion, alveolar gas trapping in asthma).

- Primary valvular heart disease (critical aortic stenosis, acute mitral regurgitation from papillary muscle rupture, acute endocarditis) when urgent surgery is indicated and distinguish this from functional valvular regurgitation due to primary ventricular disease for which surgery would be lethal.
- Septal defects, regional wall motion abnormalities and aneurysmal dilatation from recent or previous myocardial infarction.
- Increased end systolic and diastolic dimensions indicating ventricular contractile failure. The use of ejection fraction as an index of ventricular dysfunction can be misleading especially in patients on inotropes.
- Diastolic dysfunction when high pressure preload measurements will fail to reflect true volume preload and extra volume loading may be indicated.
- Pulmonary hypertension associated with tricuspid regurgitation when an estimate of pulmonary artery pressure can be made.

The images obtained with transthoracic echocardiography may be poor in ventilated patients but can be considerably enhanced by the injection of inert gas microbubbles.[39]

Transoesophageal echo is another advance that gives excellent views of the aorta (dissections), the atria and left heart valves. Right heart structures and the left ventricle are less well imaged.

PULMONARY ARTERY CATHETERIZATION

This remains the most widely used method for measurement of left atrial and pulmonary artery pressures and assessment of cardiac output using the thermodilution technique.[40,41] Although generally viewed as the 'gold standard' for determining cardiac output, the error is at least 10% even with fastidious attention to technical detail.

Inflation of the balloon at the end of the catheter provides a pulmonary artery occlusion or 'wedge' pressure, which reflects left atrial pressure provided that there are no significant pulmonary vascular bed abnormalities, as occur in chronic obstructive airways disease and long standing mitral valve disease. Despite obtaining a good quality 'wedge' tracing, the measurement must be interpreted with caution since increased intrathoracic pressure and diastolic dysfunction make this pressure measurement an unreliable index of true left ventricular volume preload.

The focus on 'goal directed therapy' led to the widespread use of pulmonary artery catheters but their indiscriminate use was challenged by a multicentre case controlled study which suggested that patients managed with a pulmonary artery catheter had a poorer outcome than those managed without such intervention.[42] This study probably reflected the enthusiasm for inappropriate goal directed therapy prevalent at that time, poor train-

Table 18.5 Comparison of methods for assessing cardiac output

Method	Invasion/risk	Ventricular preload assessed	Complexity	Measurement error	Cost
Indicator dilution					
Thermodilution (using PA catheter)	+++	From 'wedge' pressure	++	+	++
Fick	+++	No	+++	+	++
Indocyanine green	+++	No	++	++	++
Lithium	++	Yes	+	+	+
Respired gas					
Modified Fick	+	No	++	++	++
Inert gas rebreathing	+	Yes	+++	++	++
Doppler (transoesophageal)	+	Yes	++	+++	+++
Echocardiography	0	No	++	++	+++
Impedance cardiography	0			++	+
Pulse contour analysis	+	Yes (ITBV)	+	++	+
Clinical assessment	0	Yes	+	++	0

Table 18.6 Indications for PA catheterization in patients with heart failure

Failure to improve with initial circulatory management and uncertainty about adequacy of cardiac output and relationship between atrial filling pressures
Assessment of left ventricular preload when the relationship between RAP and LAP is uncertain due to recent myocardial infarction, valvular abnormalities or high pulmonary vascular resistance. A low 'wedge' pressure indicates that further volume is indicated but a high value does not necessarily exclude the need for further volume.
Measurement of cardiac output by thermodilution to direct appropriate choice of vasoactive drug and to manipulate therapy particularly when high doses are being used.
Need to monitor PA pressures and assess right ventricular function

ing in the use of the catheter and an inability of clinicians to respond appropriately to the data obtained.[43]

Table 18.6 lists the indications for pulmonary artery catheterization in heart failure. Other aspects of haemodynamic monitoring are discussed in Ch. 10.

ASSESSMENT OF INTRAVASCULAR VOLUME STATUS

CLINICAL

This is conventionally based on measurement of the right atrial filling pressure and the assumption that a normal relationship exists between the atrial filling pressures, which is not necessarily valid in the critically ill patient, particularly in cardiogenic shock.[21,22] Although values <12 mmHg suggest hypovolaemia, higher levels are more difficult to interpret, particularly in the ventilated patient. The RAP should therefore be interpreted carefully and in light of other clinical evidence.

Intravascular volume depletion is suggested if hypotension is precipitated by sedation, analgesia, and postural change. In the patient receiving positive-pressure ventilation respiratory fluctuation in the arterial pressure tracing also suggests relative hypovolaemia. This is confirmed if brief disconnection from the ventilator causes the blood pressure to rise and venous pressure to fall: the measurement 'off' the ventilator more accurately reflects the ventricular end-diastolic transmural pressure. This manoeuvre is relatively contra-indicated in patients with ARDS since loss of positive end-expiratory pressure may cause widespread alveolar collapse.

VALSALVA MANOEUVRE

The effect of changes in intrathoracic pressure can be used to assess intrathoracic blood volume and provide an estimate of true left ventricular preload. Figure 18.3 shows the classic Valsalva responses in a normal subject and a patient with a high intrathoracic blood volume. If a 'normal' type trace is observed on the monitor, further volume is indicated whereas a 'square wave' response indicates an adequate left ventricular volume preload.[44] This response can be quantified by calculating the ratio of the pulse pressure during phase 2 of the manoevre to the baseline value. This correlates with measurements of pulmonary artery 'wedge' pressure[45] and can be applied at the bedside in ventilated patients.[46]

FLUID CHALLENGE

If hypovolaemia is suspected, 200 ml of colloid should be administered and the impact on blood pressure, flow and preload observed. In the volume depleted patient, blood pressure and flow will increase with only a small, transient increase in filling pressure. While pulmonary gas exchange remains satisfactory, there is less anxiety about giving further colloid. Sufficient volume will have been given when either the target pressures are achieved and the evidence of poor peripheral perfusion and organ dysfunction has resolved, or when there is a sustained rise in filling pressures to a level above which there is a risk of pulmonary oedema developing.

Deciding on the 'appropriate' fluid volume to give in sepsis can be difficult and frequently represents a balance between giving sufficient volume to prevent the use of high doses of constricting inotropes and giving excessive amounts of fluid with consequent risk of tissue oedema and deterioration in pulmonary gas exchange.

If there is concern about administering even 200 ml of fluid, a 'reversible' fluid challenge can be given in sedated patients by elevating the legs to 60° from the horizontal for 2 min.

MANAGEMENT OF THE CARDIAC FUNCTION IN THE CRITICALLY ILL

Circulatory management should be regularly reviewed in the critically ill patient. Following initial assessment and in knowledge of the primary diagnosis, the need for extra monitoring should be decided, provisional targets should be set for fluid balance, ventricular preload, mean and diastolic arterial pressures and a management plan agreed on how to achieve these goals. Generally a MAP >65 mmHg with diastolic pressure >50 mmHg is acceptable but adequate cerebral, coronary, splanchnic and renal perfusion may require higher pressures particularly in the elderly patient with pre-existing hypertension or widespread atheroma.

CORRECTION OF METABOLIC FACTORS

The following metabolic factors should be promptly corrected:

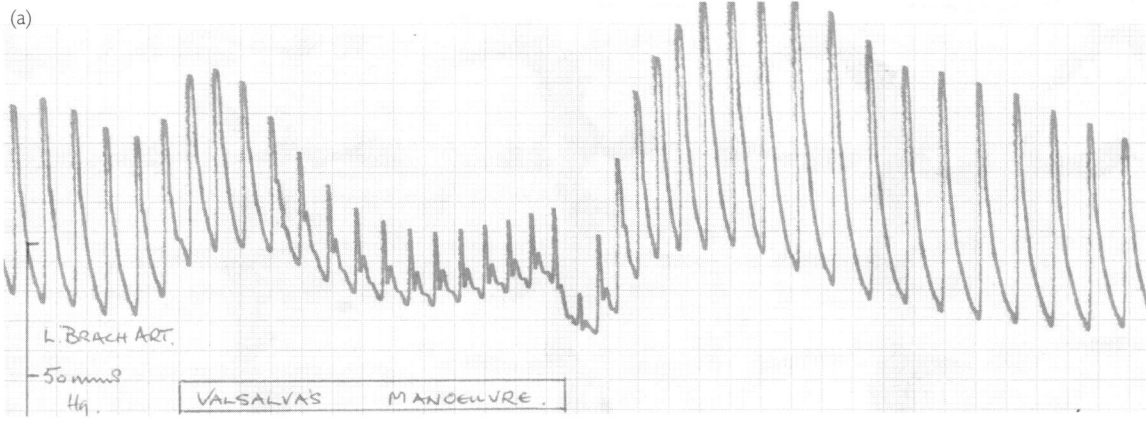

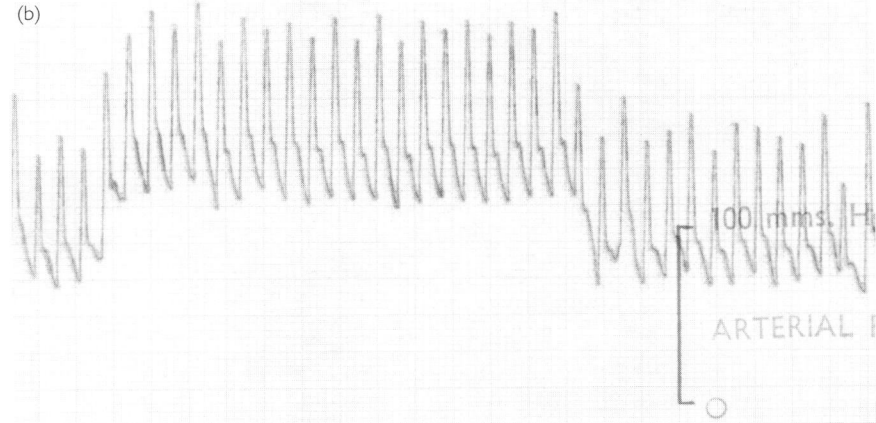

Fig. 18.3 Valsalva traces.
(a) Normal pulse pressure response to Valsalva's manoeuvre.
(b) 'Square wave' pulse pressure response to Valsalva's manoeuvre

- Hypoxaemia PO_2 < 60 mmHg (8 kPa)
- Acidaemia pH < 7.20
- Hyperkalaemia K^+ > 5.5 mmol/l
- Hypocalcaemia ionized Ca^{2+} < 1.0 mmol/l
- Hypophosphataemia PO_4^{3-} < 0.8 mmol/l
- Anaemia Hb < 9 g%
- Thiamine deficiency

Metabolic acidaemia with pH <7.20 or base deficit >10 mmol/l should be corrected since myocardial contractility increases linearly with rising pH to values >7.40. The suggestion that sodium bicarbonate produces a damaging paradoxical intracellular acidosis is misleading because the experiments demonstrating this effect were performed *in vitro* with unphysiological solutions, within a 'closed system' that allowed no correction for any rise in carbon dioxide concentration and the sodium bicarbonate was given by bolus rather than infusion.[47] The case for using bicarbonate to correct a metabolic acidaemia in the clinical setting has been recognised[48] and is supposed by studies looking at the use of bicarbonate rather than lactate as the buffer solution in haemofiltration.[49] Fig. 18.4 shows the effect of correcting a severe

metabolic academia on cardiac output by changing from lactate to bicarbonate haemofiltration.

Although a prospective randomized study demonstrated an improved survival for critically patients if haemoglobin concentration was maintained at 7–9 g% rather than at 10–12 g%, this did not apply to the elderly and those with coronary artery disease in whom the haemoglobin level should be maintained >9 g%.[50]

Patients with poor dietary thiamine intake,[51] chronic alcohol abuse and those on chronic frusemide or digoxin therapy[52] are at risk of thiamine deficiency resulting in impaired myocardial function. Oral thiamine (200mg/day) improves left ventricular function in these patients.[53]

SELECTION OF APPROPRIATE VASOACTIVE AGENTS

The choice of vasoactive agent when treating acute heart failure represents a balance between the global circulatory requirements and those of a stressed myocardium.

Properties of commonly used agents are shown in Table 18.4.

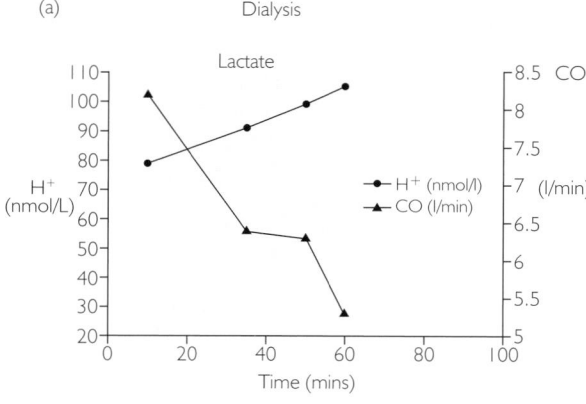

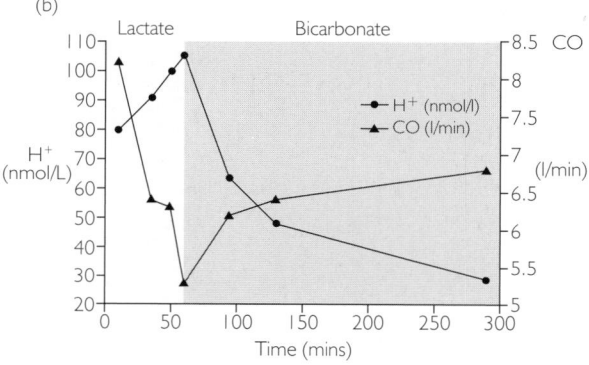

Fig. 18.4 Effect of dialysis: (a) is rising hydrogen ions and falling CO with lactate buffer dialysis; (b) change to bicarbonate buffer – there is a falling hydrogen ion concentration and a rising cardiac output

The impact of these drugs in individual patients will be influenced by the baseline state of circulation (i.e. if either intensely constricted or dilated, the same drug will potentially produce different effects on pressure, flow and its distribution). The initial choice of vasoactive agent will depend on the mean arterial pressure (MAP), cardiac output (CO) and derived systemic vascular resistance (SVR). For example:

- CO and MAP are both low with a high SVR: an inotropic and dilating (inodilator) effect is required and dobutamine would be appropriate. If CO rises but MAP falls, as may happen with dobutamine, and a more powerful inotropic effect is required, a combination of epinephrine and glyceryl trinitrate is appropriate. However, increasing doses of epinephrine risk myocardial ischaemia with ventricular irritability and splanchnic ischaemia and the development of lactic acidosis[52]
- MAP and SVR are low with high CO: this is frequently seen in sepsis: arteriolar constriction with norepinephrine is indicated after adequate volume resuscitation

- MAP is at or above target but CO is low with raised SVR: a dilating agent (nitrate e.g. GTN) or an inodilator is appropriate

When PVR and RAP are acutely raised, a pulmonary vasodilator to 'offload' the right ventricle and maintain CO is required: a nitrate or β-agonist would be appropriate but hypotension may result from arteriolar dilatation and hypoxaemia can develop due to increased ventilation-perfusion mismatch.

Dopamine has been widely used in the erroneous belief that it selectively improves renal blood flow.[55] However, if the patient has been fully volume resuscitated and a modest inotropic effect with only a small increase in SVR and a natriuretic effect are required, then a low dose dopamine infusion (<4 µmol/kg per min) is appropriate. Dopexamine is used to improve splanchnic blood flow but, despite reported benefits when used with volume loading in perioperative patients,[35] there is little evidence of outcome benefit in established shock.

When there is reduced responsiveness to β-agonists, as occurs in chronic heart failure and patients receiving long-term infusions, phosphodiesterase inhibitors, such as milrinone, by acting through different receptors increase intracellular c-AMP and improve myocardial contractility. Useful increases in CO can be achieved but these agents are powerful vasodilators and hypotension frequently limits their use or requires a norepinephrine infusion. Their effect is prolonged in renal failure.

Levosimendan is an intracellular calcium sensitizer[56] and bypasses the receptors through which other inotropic agents act. Administered as an infusion over 2 days, it has a long lasting metabolite which results in any improvement in myocardial contractility being sustained for up to 1 month.[57] It has mainly been used in chronic heart failure and its role in severe acute heart failure and cardiogenic shock following acute myocardial infarction is uncertain.

MECHANICAL SUPPORT FOR THE HEART

Continuous positive airway pressure by facemask[58] and invasive positive-pressure ventilation are the most common forms of mechanical support provided in heart failure. The benefits result from improved oxygenation and reducing or eliminating the work of breathing, which may account for up to 30% of oxygen consumption.[59] This reduction in oxygen consumption reduces left ventricular workload and alleviates myocardial ischaemia. When instituting mechanical ventilation, the clinician must be prepared to give volume and even epinephrine as the sedation, and other anaesthetic agents given for intubation will reduce endogenous levels of catecholamines, producing arteriolar and venular dilatation and potentially catastrophic hypotension.

The intra-aortic counterpulsation balloon pump (IABP) is physiologically attractive since it both improves coronary and peripheral circulatory perfusion and decreases cardiac work. This results in a more efficient cardiac performance and improved myocardial oxygenation.[60]

Left ventricular assist devices (LVAD) can temporarily take over myocardial function but are only indicated if all other treatment options have been explored and improvement in myocardial function can be anticipated.[61] There are significant problems with bleeding, infection, thromboembolism and stroke. Both IABP and LVAD should be viewed as 'bridges to recovery' after cardiac surgery or recent myocardial infarction or when there is a realistic prospect of cardiac transplantation.

CARDIOGENIC SHOCK AFTER ACUTE MYOCARDIAL INFARCTION

In patients admitted to intensive care with cardiogenic shock resulting from an acute myocardial infarction, some additional points should be noted:

- The effects on myocardial oxygenation must be considered as well as global circulatory targets.
- Although the patient may be ventilated on ICU, therapies demonstrated to improve myocardial salvage must not be overlooked or delayed. Thrombolysis may be contraindicated but the benefits of aspirin alone are significant if given in the early hours after infarction; if necessary the aspirin can be given rectally. β-blockers[5] and an ACE inhibitor[62] should be started as soon as possible but bradycardia, heart block, hypotension and impairment of renal function may cause delay. The need for urgent coronary angiography for angioplasty and stenting should be considered and the early use of an intra-aortic balloon pump[61] is preferable to escalating doses of inotropic drugs.
- It is important to recognize:
  (a) right ventricular infarction (ST elevation in lead V_4R) since further monitoring may be necessary to ensure both appropriate volume loading and to direct therapy to 'offload' the right ventricle.[64,65]
  (b) the development of either a ventricular septal defect or mitral regurgitation from papillary rupture since insertion of an intra-aortic balloon pump and urgent surgery may be indicated.[66]

REFERENCES

1 Corday E, Williams JH, DeVera LB, Gold H. Effect of systemic blood pressure and vasopressor drugs on coronary blood flow and the electrocardiogram. *Am J Cardiol* 1959; **3**: 626.

2 Packer M. Pathophysiology of chronic heart failure. *Lancet* 1992; **340**: 88–92.

3 Simoons ML, Boersma E, van der Zwaan C, Deckers JW. The challenge of acute coronary syndromes. *Lancet* 1999; **353** (suppl. II): 1–4.

4 Packer M. Treatment of chronic heart failure. *Lancet* 1992; **340**: 92–5.

5 Yusuf S, Peto R, Lewis J, *et al.*, Sleight P. Beta-blockade during and after myocardial infarction: an overview of the randomised trials. Prog Cardiovasc Dis 1985; **27**: 335–71.

6 MERIT-HF Study Group. Effect of Metoprolol CR/XL in chronic heart failure: Metoprolol CR/XL randomised intervention trial in congestive heart failure (MERIT-HF). *Lancet* 1999; **353**: 2001–7.

7 Shoemaker WC, Appel PL, Kram HB, *et al.* Prospective trial of supranormal values of survivors as therapeutic goals in high-risk surgical patients. *Chest* 1988; **94**: 1176–87.

8 Hayes MA, Timmins AC, Yau EH, *et al.* Elevation of systemic oxygen delivery in the treatment of critically ill patients. *N Engl J Med* 1994; **330**: 1717–22.

9 Gattinoni L, Brazzi L, Pelosi P, *et al.* A trial of goal-orientated haemodynamic therapy in critically ill patients. *N Engl J Med* 1995; **333**: 1025–32.

10 Leach RM, Treacher DF. Oxygen delivery and consumption in the critically ill. In Review series: The pulmonary physician in critical care. *Thorax* 2002; **57**: 170–7.

11 Packer M. How should physicians view heart failure? The philosophical and physiological evolution of three conceptual models of disease. *Am J Cardiol* 1993; **71**: 3–11.

12 Parker MM, Suffredini AF, Natanson C, *et al.* Responses of left ventricular function in survivors and non-survivors in septic shock. *J Crit Care* 1989; **4**: 19–25.

13 Shoemaker WC, Appel PL, Waxman K, *et al.* Clinical trial of survivors' cardiorespiratory patterns as therapeutic goals in critically ill postoperative patients. *Crit Care Med* 1982; **10**: 398–403.

14 Parillo JE. Pathogenetic mechanisms in septic shock. *N Engl J Med* 1993; **328**: 1471–7.

15 Astiz ME, Rackow EC, Weil MH Pathophysiology and treatment of circulatory shock. *Crit Care Clin* 1993; **9**: 183–203.

16 De Meules JE, Pigula FA, Mueller M, *et al.* Tumour necrosis factor and cardiac function. *J Trauma* 1992; **32**: 686–92.

17 Kumar A, Thota V, Dee L, *et al.* Tumour necrosis factor α and interleukin 1β are responsible for in vitro myocardial cell depression induced by human septic shock serum. *J Exp Med* 1996; **183**: 949–58.

18 Rivers E, Bguyen B, Havstad S, *et al.* Early goal directed therapy in the treatment of severe sepsis and septic shock. *N Engl J Med* 2001; **345**: 1368.

19 Lobo SMA, Salgado PF, Castillo VGT, *et al.* Effects of maximizing oxygen delivery on morbidity and mortality in high-risk surgical patients. *Crit Care Med* 2000; **28**: 3396–404.

20 Sarnov SJ, Bergland E. Ventricular function 1. Starling's law of the heart studied by means of simultaneous right and left ventricular function curves. *Circulation* 1954; **9**: 706.

21 Bradley RD. *Studies in Acute Heart Failure*. London: Edward Arnold; 1977.

22 Bradley RD, Jenkins BS, Branthwaite MA. The influence of atrial pressure on cardiac performance following myocardial infarction complicated by shock. *Circulation* 1970; **42**: 827–37.

23 Vismara LA, Leamon DM, Zelis R. The effects of morphine on venous tone in patients with acute pulmonary oedema. Circulation 1976; **54**: 335–7.

24 Ross JJ. Afterload mismatch and preload reserve: a conceptual framework for the analysis of ventricular function. *Prog Cardiovasc Dis* 1976; **18**: 255–64.

25 Cournand A, Motley H L, Werko L, Richards DW. Physiological studies of the effects of intermittent positive pressure breathing on cardiac output in man. *Am J Physiol* 1948; **152**: 162.

26 Buda AJ, Pinsky MR, Ingels NB, *et al*. Effect of intrathoracic pressure on left ventricular performance. *N Engl J Med* 1979; **301**: 453–9.

27 Stewart JT, Simpson IA. Left ventricular energetics: heat production by the human heart. *Cardiovasc Res* 1993; **27**: 1024–32.

28 Francis GS. Vasodilators in the intensive care unit. *Am Heart J* 1991; **121**: 1875–8.

29 Nelson GIC, Silke B, Ahuja RC, *et al*. Haemodynamic advantages of isosorbide dinitrate over frusemide in acute heart failure following myocardial infarction. *Lancet* 1983; **1**: 730–3.

30 Mueller H, Ayers SM, Gianelli S, *et al*. Effect of isoproterenol, l-norepinephrine and intra-aortic counterpulsation on haemodynamics and myocardial metabolism in shock following acute myocardial infarction. *Circulation* 1972; **45**: 335.

31 Chamberlain DA, Leinbach RC, Vassaux CE, *et al*. Sequential atrioventricular pacing in heart block complicating acute myocardial infarction. *N Engl J Med* 1970; **282**: 577–82.

32 Smith TW. Digoxin in heart failure. *N Engl J Med* 1993; **329**: 51–3.

33 Amiodarone Trials Meta-Analysis Investigators. Effect of prophylactic amiodarone on mortality after acute myocardial infarction and in congestive heart failure: meta-analysis of individual data from 6500 patients in randomised trials. *Lancet* 1997; **350**: 1417–24.

34 Mangano DT, Layug EL, Wallace A, Tateo I. Effect of atenolol on mortality and cardiovascular morbidity after noncardiac surgery. *N Engl J Med* 1996; **335**: 1713–20.

35 Wilson J, Woods I, Fawcett J, *et al*. Reducing the risk of major elective surgery: randomized, controlled trial of preoperative optimisation of oxygen delivery. *BMJ* 1999; **318**: 1099–103.

36 Goodwin J. The importance of clinical skills. *BMJ* 1995; **310**: 1281–2.

37 Singer M, Clarke J, Bennett ED. Continuous haemodymanic monitoring by oesophageal-doppler. *Crit Care Med* 1989; **17**: 447–52.

38 Linton RAF, Band DM, O'Brien T, *et al*. Lithium dilution cardiac output measurement: a comparison with thermodilution. *Crit Care Med* 1997; **25**: 1796–800.

39 Gmaurer G. Contrast echocardiography: clinical utility. *Echocardiography* 2000; **17**: S5–9 .

40 Steingrub JS, Celoria G, Vickers-Lahti M, *et al*. Therapeutic impact of pulmonary artery catheterisation in a medical/surgical ICU. *Chest* 1991; **99**: 1451–55.

41 Connors AF, McCaffree DR, Gray BA. Evaluation of right-heart catheterisation in the critically ill patient without myocardial infarction. *N Engl J Med* 1983; **308**: 263–7.

42 Connors A F, Speroff T, Dawson NV, *et al*. The effectiveness of right heart catheterisation in the initial care of critically ill patients. *JAMA* 1996; **276**: 889–97.

43 Iberti TJ, Fischer EP, Leibowitz AB, *et al*. A multicentre study of physicians' knowledge of the pulmonary artery catheter. *JAMA* 1990; **264**: 2928–32.

44 Sharpey-Schafer EP. Effects of Valsalva's manoeuvre on the normal and failing circulation. *BMJ* 1955; 1: 693–5.

45 McIntyre KM, Vita JA, Lambrew CT, *et al*. A non-invasive method of predicting pulmonary capillary wedge pressure. *N Engl J Med* 1992; **327**: 1715–20.

46 Marik PE. The systolic blood pressure variation as an indicator of pulmonary capillary wedge pressure in ventilated patients. *Anaesth Intens Care* 1993; **21**: 405–8.

47 Ritter JM, Doctor H, Benjamin M. Paradoxical effect of bicarbonate on cytoplasmic pH. *Lancet* 1990; **335**: 1243–6.

48 Narius RG, Cohen JJ. Bicarbonate therapy for organic acidosis: the case for its use. *Ann Intern Med* 1987; **106**: 615–618.

49 Hilton PJ, Taylor J, Formi LG, Treacher DF. Bicarbonate-based haemofiltration in the management of acute renal failure with lactic acidosis. *AJM* 1998; **91**: 279–83.

50 Hebert PC, Wells G, Blajchman MA, *et al*. A multicenter, randomized, controlled clinical trial of transfusion requirements in critical care. *N Engl J Med* 1999; **340**: 409–17.

51 Pepersack T, Garbusinski J, Robberecht J, *et al*. Clinical relevance of thiamine status amongst hospitalized elderly patients. *Gerontology* 1999; **45**: 96–101.

52 Zangen A, Botzer D, Zangen R, Shainberg A. Furosemide and digoxin inhibit thiamine uptake in cardiac cells. *Eur J Pharmacol* 1998; **361**: 151–5.

53 Leslie D, Gheorghiade M. Is there a role for thiamine supplementation in the management of heart failure? *Am Heart J* 1996; **131**: 1248–50.

54 Day NPJ, Phu NH, Bethell DP, *et al*. The effects of dopamine and adrenaline infusions on acid-base balance and systemic haemodynamics in severe infection. *Lancet* 1996; **348**: 219–23.

55 Australian and New Zealand Intensive Care Society (ANZICS) Clinical Trials Group. Low-dose dopamine in patients with early renal dysfunction: a placebo-controlled randomised trial. *Lancet* 2000; **356**: 2139–43.

56 Haikala H, Linden HB. Mechanisms of action of calcium sensitising drugs. *J Cardiovasc Pharmacol* 1995; **26**: S10–19.

57 Hasenfuss G, Pieske B, Castell M, *et al.* Influence of the novel inotropic agent levosimendan on isometric tension and calcium coupling in failing human myocardium. *Circulation* 1998; **98**: 2141–7.

58 Bersten AD, Holt AW, Vedig AE, *et al.* Treatment of severe cardiogenic pulmonary oedema with continuous positive airway pressure delivered by facemask. *N Engl J Med* 1991; **325**: 1825–30.

59 Aubier M, Trippenbach T, Roussos C. Respiratory muscle fatigue during cardiogenic shock. *J Applied Physiol Resp Environ Ex Physiol* 1981; **51**: 499–508.

60 Nanas JN, Moulopouloss D. Counterpulsation: historical background, technical improvements, hemodynamic and metabolic effects. *Cardiology* 1994; **84**: 156–67.

61 Westaby S, Katsumata T, Houel R, *et al.* Jarvik 2000 Heart: potential for bridge to myocyte recovery. *Circulation* 1998; **98**: 1568–74.

62 Pfeffer MA, Braunwald E, Moye LA, for the Save investigators. Effect of captopril on mortality and morbidity in patients with left ventricular dysfunction after myocardial infarction. Results of the survival and ventricular enlargement trial. *N Engl J Med* 1992; **327**: 669–77.

63 Mueller HS. Role of intra-aortic counterpulsation in cardiogenic shock and acute myocardial infarction. *Cardiology* 1994; **84**: 168–74.

64 Cohn JN, Guiha NH, Broder MI, Limas CJ. Right ventricular infarction, clinical and haemodynamic features. *Am J Cardiol* 1974; **33**: 209–14.

65 Zehender M, Kaspar W, Kauder E, *et al.* Right ventricular infarction as an independent predictor of prognosis after acute inferior myocardial infarction. *N Engl J Med* 1993; **328**: 981–8.

66 Hasdai D, Topol EJ, Califf RM, *et al.* Cardiogenic shock complicating acute coronary syndromes. *Lancet* 2000; **356**: 749–56.

19

Valvular and congenital heart disease

J E Sanderson

VALVULAR HEART DISEASE

Valvular heart disease is still a common cause for symptoms and disability worldwide. In most economically developed countries the main cause is no longer rheumatic heart disease, but congenital valve abnormalities such as mitral valve prolapse and bicuspid aortic valves, degenerative valve disease or infective endocarditis are more common causes.[1] However, in many parts of the world, rheumatic fever and rheumatic heart disease are still major health problems, especially in the young.[2,3] Diseases of heart valves produce stenosis, incompetence or both.

RHEUMATIC FEVER

This acute febrile illness is due to a cross-reaction following a group A β-haemolytic streptococci pharyngitis, which causes inflammatory lesions involving the joints, heart and subcutaneous tissues. It presents with polyarthritis, carditis, subcutaneous nodules, rash (erythema marginatum) and chorea. Carditis consists of:

- murmurs (most commonly mitral, aortic regurgitation or the mid-diastolic Carey–Coombs murmur)
- pericarditis
- cardiomegaly
- congestive heart failure.[4]

Chronic rheumatic heart disease occurs in about 40% of those with apical and basal diastolic murmurs, and 70% with heart failure or pericarditis during the acute attacks. It is still common in the Middle East, India, Africa and South America, and causes between 20 and 40% of all cardiovascular disease in the Third World.[2] It is rare now in North America, Western Europe, Australasia and parts of Asia.

MITRAL STENOSIS

Rheumatic fever is the main cause of mitral stenosis; rarer causes are:

- left atrial myxoma
- ball-valve thrombus
- calcification of the annulus
- systemic lupus erythematosus.

Scarring or fibrosis of the valves, especially at the edges and sometimes involving the subvalvular apparatus, causes narrowing and hence increased left atrial pressure, pulmonary venous hypertension and pulmonary arterial hypertension. Thus the lungs and right ventricle suffer the most burden. Main symptoms are breathlessness on exertion, recurrent bronchitis, fatigue, palpitations due to paroxysmal atrial fibrillation (AF), haemoptysis and stroke. The onset of AF is usually associated with marked symptomatic deterioration and increases significantly the risk for left atrial thrombus formation and embolism.

Classic signs of mitral stenosis are:

- mitral facies (peripheral cyanosis on the cheeks)
- a small-volume pulse which may be irregular (AF is common)
- right ventricular hypertrophy
- a tapping apex due to a palpable first heart sound
- a loud first heart sound, and an opening snap with a rumbling diastolic murmur.

The first clue to the diagnosis is often the loud first heart sound which should prompt a careful search for the diastolic rumble which may be soft, low-pitched and localized to the apex. An opening snap is present if the valve is not calcified and occurs between 0.04 and 0.10 s after S_2.

An electrocardiogram (ECG) shows a broad P wave in lead 2 due to left atrial hypertrophy. Chest X-ray shows an enlarged left atrium and appendage, prominent upper lobe pulmonary veins, but heart size is usually within normal limits. The diagnosis can readily be confirmed by echocardiography, which allows assessment of the valve anatomy, and estimation of valve area and gradient. Severe stenosis is considered to be present if the valve area is <1 cm^2 (Plate 19.1).

Treatment is the use of β-blockers to slow the heart rate and increase diastolic filling time diuretics, and digoxin is given if the patient is in AF. Anticoagulation is essential if there is significant mitral stenosis and AF.

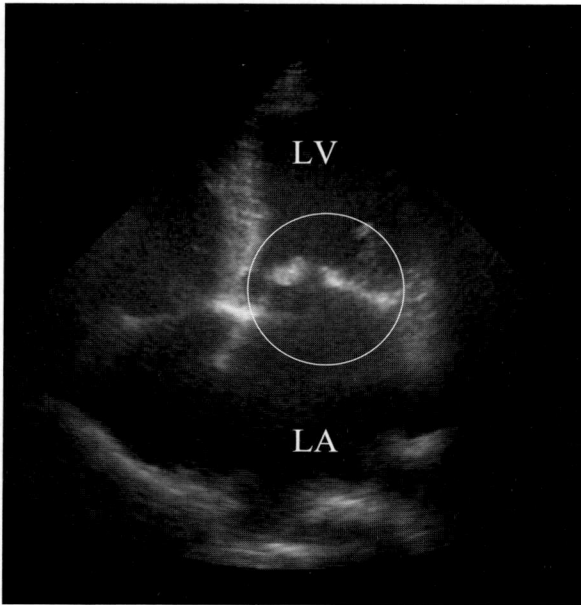

Plate 19.1　Mitral stenosis. Thickened and calcified anterior and posterior mitral valve leaflets with reduced opening.

Mitral balloon valvuloplasty has been shown to be very successful therapy with excellent long-term outcome, and compares well with surgical treatment.[5] The main contraindications to balloon valvuloplasty are significant mitral regurgitation and heavy calcification when mutual valve replacement should be done.

MITRAL REGURGITATION

There is a considerable difference between acute and chronic mitral regurgitation (Table 19.1). In chronic mitral regurgitation, there is time for the left ventricle and left atrium to adapt to the increasing regurgitation, leading to their gradual enlargement. In acute mitral regurgitation, the sudden pressure overload of the left atrium and pulmonary veins leads to severe pulmonary oedema. The treatment for acute mitral regurgitation is urgent surgery. The management of chronic mitral regurgitation is more difficult. Initially, medical therapy can be helpful, but the probability of postoperative death or persistent severe heart failure after valve replacement increases abruptly when the left ventricular (LV) end-systolic diameter exceeds 45 mm on echocardiography, or ejection fraction falls below 60%.[6] In patients without mitral stenosis, mitral valve repair is preferable to replacement, and evidence suggests that preservation of the chordae improves postoperative LV function.[7]

MITRAL VALVE PROLAPSE[8]

This is a common condition affecting 5% of the adult population, more women than men. It has a number of

Table 19.1　Mitral regurgitation

Chronic	Acute
Causes	
Mitral valve prolapse	
Rheumatic heart disease	Ruptured chordae
	Ruptured papillary muscle (Mt)
LV dilatation (IHD). cardiomyopathies, etc.)	Perforation of leaflet (tE)
Prosthetic valves	Prosthetic valves
Physiology	
LV volume overload	Sudden pressure overload of LA and pulmonary veins
LV dilatation and hypertrophy	
Increased LA size (mean pressure normal initially because of increased compliance)	No change in LV dimension
Symptoms	
Asymptomatic initially	Severe dyspnoea
Fatigue	
Dyspnoea	
Examination	
Pansystolic apical murmur radiating to axilla/lower sternal edge	Harsh pansystolic murmur radiating to axilla and back
Third heart sound	Third heart sound
ECG	
LV hypertrophy	No change (or acute MI)
LA hypertrophy	
Chest X-ray	
Increased-size LV	Normal LV and LA dimension
Increased-size LA	Pulmonary oedema
Echocardiography	
Diagnostic	Diagnostic
Treatment	
Vasodilators and ACE inhibitors (reduce afterload)	Preload and afterload reduction and prepare for urgent surgery
Diuretics and digitalis	
Surgery if symptoms and LV size increase (before LV end-systolic diameter >4.5 cm or LV ejection fraction <60%)	

MI = Myocardial infarction; LV = left ventricle/ventricular;
IHD = ischaemic heart disease; IE = infective endocarditis;
LA = left atrium/atrial; ACE = angiotensin converting enzyme.

synonyms such as Barlow and click-murmur syndrome. It is due to the myxomatous degeneration of the valve, with redundancy of the leaflets which may affect both the anterior and posterior valves. At the end of diastole, the valve closes normally, but as LV pressure rises during systole, a portion of the valve leaflet prolapses in the left atrium, with associated regurgitation. It is usually mild, but can progress and become more severe, and rarely, the chordae may rupture to produce severe acute regurgitation.

Mitral valve prolapse is usually asymptomatic, but a wide variety of symptoms have been associated, including odd chest pains, palpitations and fatigue. On examination, typical findings are a mid-systolic click and a late systolic murmur, which are separated from the first heart sound, but usually reaching the second heart sound. The murmur may have a crescendo/decrescendo quality. It is usually louder with the Valsalva manoeuvre and on standing. As the prolapse worsens with age the murmur becomes more pansystolic. Echocardiography is diagnostic, and can accurately assess the degree of severity of mitral valve prolapse (Plate 19.2). In most patients, mitral prolapse is a benign condition with a good prognosis. It poses a risk for infective endocarditis, which then leads to a substantial risk of death and need for mitral valve surgery.[9] There is a very small increased incidence of embolic neurological ischaemic events.

AORTIC STENOSIS

The commonest cause of aortic stenosis is degeneration of a bicuspid aortic valve. Valve stenosis leads to increased LV systolic pressure, LV hypertrophy and reduced LV compliance. The increased LV work may induce subendocardial ischaemia, arrhythmias and sudden death.

The main symptoms are angina, syncopy and breathlessness. Typical findings on examination are a slowly rising small-volume pulse, evidence of LV hypertrophy without an enlarged heart, and a harsh ejection systolic murmur radiating into the neck. If the valve is calcified, there is no click and the A_2 is soft.

An ECG confirms LV hypertrophy. The chest X-ray may show:

- a normal heart size
- a poststenotic dilatation in the ascending aorta
- presence of calcification.

Echocardiography is diagnostic, and allows the measurement of the aortic valve area, gradient and the degree of aortic incompetence (Plate 19.3).

Medical treatment is not effective. Valve replacement should be performed as soon as the patient is symptomatic, or if asymptomatic with left ventricular systolic dysfunction, or if the jet velocity is >4 m/s in patients undergoing coronary artery bypass surgery.[10]

AORTIC REGURGITATION

Like mitral regurgitation, the features of chronic and acute aortic regurgitation are different. *Chronic aortic regurgitation* has a number of causes, including:

- rheumatic, connective tissue disorders (e.g. ankylosing spondylitis, Reiter's syndrome and rheumatoid disease)
- syphilitic aortitis
- cystic medial necrosis (Marfan's syndrome)
- aortic root dilatation due to hypertension

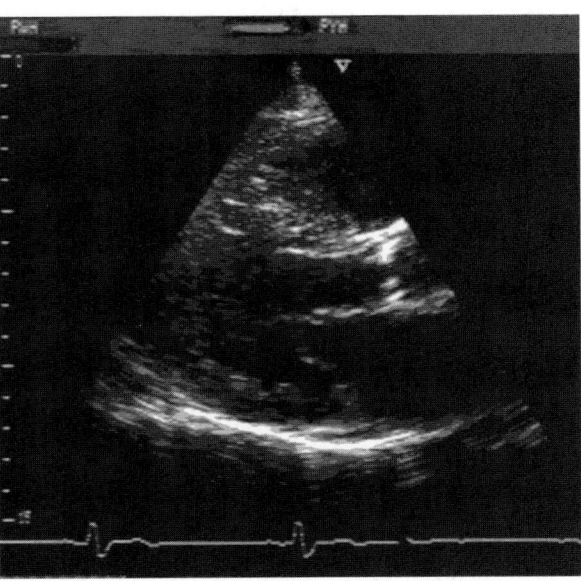

Plate 19.2 Mitral valve prolapse with bowing of the anterior mitral valve leaflet with enlargement of the left atrium but normal left ventricle size.

Plate 19.3 Aortic stenosis. A calcified thickened valve with reduced opening and the presence of left ventricular hypertrophy.

- a congenital bicuspid aortic valve
- endocarditis, which can produce aortic regurgitation in a normal valve.

The leak from the aorta increases LV volume, causing LV dilatation and LV hypertrophy. Initially, this is well tolerated but eventually LV function declines.

Main symptoms are fatigue and dyspnoea. Typical findings on examination are a large-volume, bounding, wide pulse pressure which is collapsing in nature. Other classical physical signs include Corrigans (visible carotid pulsation) and nailbed capillary pulsation (Quineke's sign), which all reflect the rapid run-off. The heart is usually enlarged with a displaced apex, and there is a high-pitched early diastolic blowing murmur which radiates from the left sternal edge to the apex. There may be a mid-diastolic murmur (Austin Flint) due to the regurgitant aortic jet hitting the anterior mitral valve leaflet.

An ECG shows LV hypertrophy, usually with a strain pattern. A chest X-ray shows an enlarged heart with a dilated aorta. Echocardiography is diagnostic and can demonstrate the degree of aortic regurgitation, LV size and function.

The decision to undertake aortic valve replacement in patients with pure aortic regurgitation is difficult. Many patients can survive despite enlarged left ventricles. In general, patients should be advised to have an operation before LV end-systolic dimension exceeds 55 mm or ejection fraction <60%. Medical therapy with vasodilators such as nefedipine or angiotensin converting enzyme inhibitors can reduce or delay the need for valve replacement.[6,11] Surgery should not be delayed for too long, otherwise irreversible LV dysfunction ensues.

Acute aortic regurgitation is a severe disease with a high mortality, usually due to endocarditis (*Staphylococcus* or *Pneumococcus*).[12] There is acute LV diastolic pressure and volume overload, which leads to severe pulmonary oedema without LV dilatation. It can be difficult to diagnose clinically, because the early diastolic murmur is very short and soft. An echocardiogram, however, is completely diagnostic, and can demonstrate severe aortic regurgitation, and more importantly, early closure of the mitral valve. The treatment is urgent surgery without delay.

TRICUSPID REGURGITATION

Tricuspid regurgitation is usually secondary to right ventricular (RV) dilatation/hypertrophy because of pulmonary hypertension. However, increasingly, infective endocarditis (usually *Staphylococcus*) in drug addicts is a common cause.[13] The diagnosis is made by the presence of large V waves in the jugular venous pressure, pansystolic murmur at the left sternal edge and echocardiography. Surgery may be necessary if the degree of valvular regurgitation is severe.

INFECTIVE ENDOCARDITIS

This is one of the most important diagnoses not to miss, because, untreated, it is lethal.[14,15] A delay in diagnosis considerably lowers the probability of survival. The old adage that 'fever + murmur = endocarditis' until proven otherwise still remains true. The pattern of infective endocarditis (IE) is changing; it may be acquired in the community but increasingly in hospital particularly as a result of procedures involving vascular catheterization. It may also affect native valves that were previously thought to be normal and increasingly is a problem associated with intravenous drug abuse.

Clinical features of chronic endocarditis may be misleading. The symptoms are vague ill health, weight loss, malaise with night sweats and mild fever, and many patients are assumed to have influenza. In more chronic cases, there may be nail and conjunctival splinter haemorrhages, clubbing, splenomegaly and anaemia. Regurgitant murmurs (aortic, mitral or tricuspid) are usually present, and heart failure is a bad prognostic sign. Emboli may occur causing strokes. Mycotic aneurysms are frequently lethal due to late rupture.

Native valve endocarditis (NVE). Most community acquired NVE is now more likely to be caused by *Staphylococcus aureus* and by coagulase negative staphylococci than the classical oral viridans streptococci. Enterococci are a less common cause but their incidence is increasing. In staphylococcal IE the skin lesion may be quite trivial. Some strains of staphylococci are particularly virulent and can attack a previously normal valve, whereas streptococci and enterococci seem to infect only previously abnormal valves. Hospital acquired NVE is almost always caused by staphylococci but occasionally coagulase-negative staphylococci and often *Staphylococcus epidermidis* may be responsible. Increasingly, more cases of MRSA endocarditis are being seen, usually from intravascular access site infections.

Prosthetic valve endocarditis (PVE). The risk of infection is always present. Preventive measures are extremely important in these patients as prosthetic PVE is a cardiological disaster. Even in the best centres, mortality remains high and reoperation is often necessary. The distinction between early IE (theatre infection) and late IE (community acquired) is artificial as bacteria acquired in the theatre (such as *S. epidermidis*) may present many months or even longer after surgery.

Intravenous drug abuse. Infection usually affects the tricuspid valve and the condition is frequently misdiagnosed as pneumonia. Vegetations from the tricuspid valve embolize into the lung causing patchy infarction with infection. The tricuspid murmur may be very soft and the degree of tricuspid regurgitation may not be severe. The diagnosis therefore is not always obvious and will always need to be considered in any i.v. drug addict with a fever.

DIAGNOSIS

The most important investigation remains the blood culture (three sets). Although echocardiography is extremely useful in IE, there is a misconception that endocarditis can be diagnosed or excluded by echocardiography. This is not true. Vegetations may be small and not visualized, and large vegetations may be old and sterile. It is not necessary to delay taking blood cultures while waiting for a spike of temperature. It is probably also not necessary to take samples from different sites. Levels of the C-reactive protein (CRP) will usually be elevated in IE. The peripheral white cell count is often very high in those infections caused by staphylococcus but may be normal in those caused by less virulent organisms. Occasionally, patients have so-called 'blood culture negative IE' despite convincing clinical and echocardiographic evidence. In these cases, it is important to look specifically for *Coxiella burnettii* (Q fever), *Chlamydia* or *Bartonella*. Echocardiography may show vegetations but only if they are >3 mm but will give useful information on the degree of regurgitation, any intramyocardial spread (abscess formation) and left ventricular function. Transoesophageal ECHO is much more useful than transthoracic, particularly for mitral valve endocarditis or PVE (Plate 19.4).[16]

TREATMENT

In acute endocarditis treatment should not be delayed while awaiting the results of blood cultures, although this may be acceptable in the patient who has been unwell for weeks or months. There are a number of guidelines for antibiotic treatment which can be consulted.[17] (See tables 19.2 and 19.3) The duration of treatment was traditionally 6 weeks. However, shorter courses with oral therapy have been successfully used for sensitive streptococcus infections.

PERSISTENT FEVER

A number of possibilities need to be considered, including infection elsewhere either in the heart or outside, such as an infection of a central line which should be removed and sent for culture. Abscesses, paravalvular or intracardiac, are an important cause of persistent or recurrent fever and require surgery. It is nearly always impossible to eradicate an abscess by medical therapy only, and it is generally better to undertake surgery earlier than later. In some patients who appear to be well controlled, an abscess may be detected by transoesophageal echocardiography, but after stopping the antibiotics the infection will recur (Plate 19.5). Extracardiac infection may be due to a myocotic aneurysm

Table 19.2 Treatment regimens for adults not allergic to the penicillins

Viridans streptococci and Streptococcus bovis
(A) Fully sensitive to penicillin (MIC 0.1 mg/l)
   Benzylpenicillin 7.2 g daily in six divided doses by intravenous bolus injection for two weeks plus intravenous gentamicin 80 g twice daily for two weeks* (table 2)
(B) Reduced sensitivity to penicillin (MIC > 0.1 mg/l)
   Benzylpenicillin 7.2 g daily in six divided doses by intravenous bolus injection for four weeks plus intravenous gentamicin 80 mg twice daily for four weeks*

Enterococci
(A) Gentamicin sensitive or low level resistant (MIC < 100 mg/l)
   Ampicillin or amoxycillin 12 g daily in six divided doses by intravenous bolus injection for four weeks plus intravenous gentamicin 80 mg twice daily for four weeks*
(B) Gentamicin highly resistant (MIC 2000 mg/l)
   Ampicillin or amoxycillin 12 g daily in six divided doses by intravenous bolus injection for a minimum of six weeks. Streptomycin can be given if strain is sensitive

Staphylococci
(A) Penicillin sensitive
   Benzylpenicillin 7.2 g daily in six divided doses by intravenous bolus injection for four week plus intravenous gentamicin 80–120 mg three times daily for one week*
(B) Penicillin resistant, methicillin sensitive
   Flucloxacillin 12 g daily in six divided doses by intravenous bolus injection for four weeks plus intravenous gentamicin 80–120 mg three times daily for one week*
(C) Penicillin and methicillin resistant
   Vancomycin initially 1 g by intravenous infusion given over at least 100 minutes twice daily. Determine blood concentration and adjust dose to achieve one hour post-infusion concentrations of about 30 mg/l and trough levels of 5–10 mg/l. Give for four weeks plus intravenous gentamicin 80–120 mg three times daily for one week*

*Gentamicin levels must be monitored.

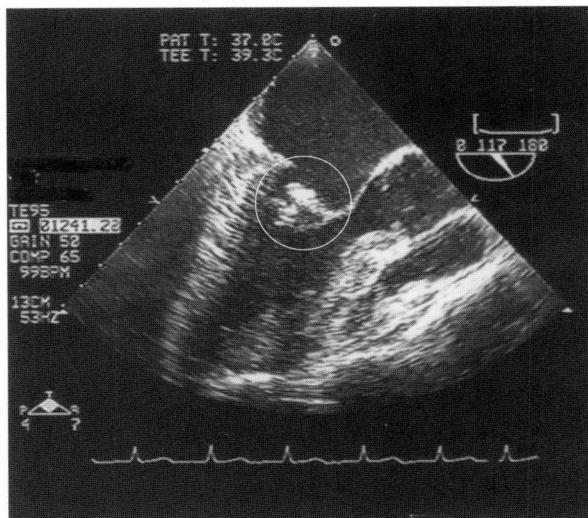

Plate 19.4 A large vegetation can be seen on the anterior mitral valve leaflet during transoesophageal echocardiography.

Table 19.3   Treatment regimens for adults allergic to the penicillins

Viridans streptococci, Strep bovis, and enterococci
    Initially **either** vancomycin 1 g by intravenous infusion given over at least 100 minutes twice daily. Determine blood concentrations and adjust dose to achieve one hour postinfusion concentrations of about 30 mg/l and trough concentrations of 5–10 mg/l **or** teicoplanin 400 mg by intravenous bolus injection 12 hourly for three doses and then a maintenance intravenous dose of 400 mg daily
    Give vancomycin or teicoplanin for four weeks **plus** intravenous gentamicin 80 mg twice daily. Viridans streptococcal and *Strep bovis* endocarditis should be treated with gentamicin for two weeks and enterococcal endocarditis for four weeks*

Staphylococci
    Vancomycin initially 1 g by intravenous infusion given over at least 100 minutes twice daily Blood concentrations should be monitored as above. Give for four weeks plus intravenous gentamicin 80–120 mg three times daily for one week*

*Gentamicin blood levels must be monitored as above.
Working Party of the British Society for Antimicrobial Chemotherapy.
Antibiotic treatment of streptococcal, enterococcal, and staphylococcal endocarditis (1998). *Heart* 79: 207–10.

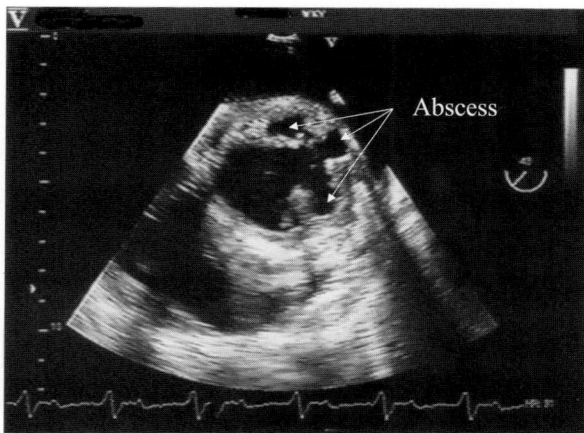

Plate 19.5   Abscess cavities seen in the aortic root during transoesophageal echocardiography.

which can cause fever or metastatic infection. Mycotic aneurysms of the brain can be a particular problem and may lead to rupture many months or even years later.

ROLE OF SURGERY

If the patient is not recovering or the fever is not under control, then surgery should always be considered. Major indications are haemodynamic deterioration with increasing aortic or mitral regurgitation and an abscess. Staphylococcal endocarditis particularly may cause rapid destruction of the valve and require urgent surgery. Infections by fungi nearly always require surgery as does

IE due to Q fever. The question of surgery to prevent embolism in a patient with a large vegetation is sometimes difficult. Vegetations >10 mm in diameter are associated with an increased risk of embolism but it has not been shown that this is a necessary indication for surgery. If there is existing severe regurgitation then the decision to operate is easier. In general, if a large vegetation is seen then it is best to operate early, as after antibiotic therapy there is a lower risk of embolism. It is a general principal that surgery should be considered early and it is not necessary to wait for antibiotic treatment to take effect. Late surgery will always be more difficult with increasing complexity of the operation, difficulty in suturing the new valve because of destruction of the valve ring, and increased complications such as renal failure.

CONGENITAL HEART DISEASE IN ADULTS

The number of adults with congenital heart disease is steadily increasing, and includes not only patients with congenital heart disease who have survived into adulthood, but an increasing number of patients who have had cardiac surgery. The commonest congenital conditions found in adults are ostium secondum atrial septal defects, pulmonary valve stenosis, patent ductus arteriosus, uncomplicated congenitally corrected transposition of the great arteries, small penmembranous ventricular septal defects and Fallot's tetralogy.

OSTIUM SECONDUM ATRIAL SEPTAL DEFECT

This is the commonest congenital cardiac abnormality in adults. It is often unrecognized because symptoms may be absent and the physical signs are subtle. Older patients may develop AF and cardiac failure. Paradoxical emboli through the defect are rare.

Examination typically shows a pulmonary ejection systolic murmur with a wide and fixed second heart sound.

ECG usually shows a right bundle branch block (and a left axis deviation with a primum defect). Chest X-ray will show pulmonary plethora.

Echocardiography, especially transoesophageal echocardiography, can demonstrate the defect and give an estimate of the pulmonary artery pressure. There is an increased risk of developing Eisenmenger's syndrome but no risk of endocarditis. Many patients can live to a good age but overall life expectancy is not normal. Closure is by surgery or by an occluder introduced percutaneously is usually recommended if the size of the shunt is >1.5:1.0, although this has been challenged.[18]

PATENT DUCTUS ARTERIOSUS (PDA)

This congenital abnormality is often asymptomatic and survival is usual. At the age of about 20, the risk of infective endocarditis increases, and at the age of about 30, patients with sizeable left-to-right shunts will begin to develop cardiac failure. Patients with significant shunts should have the PDA closed by surgery or, increasingly, by transcatheter using an umbrella device.[19]

VENTRICULAR SEPTAL DEFECTS (VSD)

These are very common at birth but are seldom found in adults. The occasional adult will survive with a persistent small perimembranous VSD which is a risk for endocarditis.

FALLOT'S TETRALOGY

This is the cyanotic malformation most frequently associated with survival to adulthood. In these patients, the pulmonary stenosis is usually sufficient to prevent excessive pulmonary blood flow, but not too severe to cause large degrees of shunting from the right to the left ventricle. An increasing number of patients who have had complete repair are surviving into adulthood, and overall outcome is excellent.[20] The 30-year actuarial survival rate is 90% of the expected, and late health status is very good.

NON-CARDIAC SURGERY

CYANOTIC CONGENITAL HEART DISEASE

These patients have an increased risk of acute cholecystitis caused by calcium bilirubinate stones, and cholecystectomy is a procedure to be anticipated. Blood taken for phlebotomy can be stored for transfusion later. Oxygen inhalation appears to be desirable. Care must be taken with all i.v. lines, infusions and drugs, so that air is not introduced because of the risk of systemic embolism. If patients with Fallot's tetralogy have a sudden fall in blood pressure because of a fall in systemic resistance, intense cyanosis and occasionally death may occur. Conversely, a sudden rise in systemic resistance may severely depress systemic blood flow. Prophylaxis is required for infective endocarditis. Cyanotic patients with elevated fixed pulmonary vascular resistance (Eisenmenger's syndrome) are not able to respond rapidly to haemodynamic changes. In these patients, a sudden fall or rise in systemic vascular resistance can be very dangerous.

OSTIUM SECONDUM ATRIAL SEPTAL DEFECT

In asymptomatic adults with this malformation and with normal pulmonary artery pressure, there is little risk during non-cardiac surgery. However, a rise in peripheral vascular resistance will increase left-to-right shunting; with hypotension, right-to-left shunting may occur. Systemic paradoxical emboli from leg veins can occur and early mobilization is recommended.

CONGENITAL COMPLETE HEART BLOCK

If the QRS is narrow and the subsidiary pacemaker is reliable with a reasonable ventricular rate, then temporary RV pacing is not required. However, all vagotonic stimuli should be minimized. If the QRS complex is wide and there is a relatively slow ventricular response, a temporary pacemaker should be inserted preoperatively.

REFERENCES

1 Soler-Soler J, Galve E. Worldwide perspective of valve disease. *Heart* 2000; **83**: 721–5.

2 Sanderson JE, Woo KS. Rheumatic fever and rheumatic heart disease – declining but not gone. *Int Cardiol* 1994; **43**: 231–2.

3 Eisenberg MJ. Rheumatic heart disease in the developing world: prevalence, prevention, and control. *Eur Heart J* 1993; **14**: 122–8.

4 Barlow JB. Aspects of active rheumatic carditis. *Aust NZ J Med* 1992; **22**: 592–600.

5 Reyes VP, Raju BS, Wynne, *et al.* Percutaneous balloon valvuloplasty compared with open surgical commissurotomy for mitral stenosis. *N Engl J Med* 1994; **331**: 961–7.

6 ACC/AHA. Guidelines for the management of patients with valvular heart disease in a report of the American College of Cardiology/American Heart Association Task Force on Practice Guidelines. *J Am Coll Cardiol* 1998; **32**: 1486–588.

7 Enriquez-Sarano M, Schaff HV, Orszulak TA, *et al.* Valve repair improves the outcome of surgery for mitral regurgitation: a mutivariate analysis. *Circulation* 1995; **91**: 1022–8.

8. Devereux RB. Recent developments in the diagnosis and management of mitral valve prolapse. *Curr Opinion Cardiol* 1995; **10**: 107–16.

9 Frary W, Devereux RB, Kramer-Fox R *et al.* Clinical and health-care cost consequences of infective endocarditis in mitral valve prolapse. *Am J Cardiol* 1994; **73**: 263–7.

10 Corabello BA. Aortic stenosis. *N Engl J Med* 2002; **346**: 677–82.

11 Scognamiglio R, Rahimtoola SH, Fasoli G, *et al.* Nifedipine in asymptomatic patients with severe aortic regurgitation and normal left ventricular function. *N Engl J Med* 1994; **331**: 689–94.

12 Benolti JR. Acute aortic insufficiency. In: Dalen JE, Alpert JS (eds) *Valvular Heart Disease,* 2nd edn. Boston: Little, Brown; 1987: pp. 319–52.

13 Robbins MJ, Sveiro R, Fishman WH and Strom JA. Right-sided valvular endocarditis: etiology, diagnosis and approach to therapy. *Am Heart J* 1986; **109**: 558–66.

14 Eykyn S. Endocarditis: basics. *Heart* 2001; **86**: 476–80.

15 Durack DT, Lukes AS, Bright DK. New criteria for diagnosis of infective endocarditis: utilization of specific echocardiographic findings. *Am J Med* 1994; **96**: 200–9.

16 Rinaldi CA, Hall RJ. Echocardiography in endocarditis. In: Izzart MB, Sanderson JE, Sutton MG. (eds) *Echocardiography in Adult Cardiac Surgery*. Oxford: ISIS Medical Media; 1999: pp. 155–6.

17 Working Party of the British Society for Antimicrobial Chemotherapy. Antibiotic treatment of streptococcal, enterococcal, and staphylococcal endocarditis. *Heart* 1998; **79**: 207–10.

18 Ward C. Secundum atrial septal defect: routine surgical treatment is not of proven benefit. *Br Heart J* 1994; **71**: 219–23.

19 Schenek MH, O'Laughlin MP, Rokey R, *et al.* Transcatheter occlusion of patent ductus arteriosus in adults. *Am J Cardiol* 1993; **72**: 591–5.

20 Murphy JG, Gersh BJ, Mair DD, *et al.* Long-term outcome in patients undergoing surgical repair of tetralogy of Fallot. *N Engl J Med* 1993; **329**: 593–9.

20.

Intensive care after cardiac surgery
R Raper

Coronary artery bypass surgery is the most frequently undertaken surgical procedure. Because of the prevalence of cardiac disease, cardiac surgery has significant health and economic implications. Intensive care may account for up to 40% of the total hospital costs for these patients and much of the short-term morbidity and mortality is based on perioperative events.

The overall mortality of cardiac surgery is low (approximately 3%). However, this ranges from less than 1% for elective coronary artery bypass grafting to in excess of 30% for more complicated surgery in patients with significant myocardial dysfunction and associated disorders.[1] Usually, intensive care post-cardiac surgery involves a short period of recovery before discharge to the ward but for a small percentage of patients, at least potentially remediable complications may require the complete intensive care armamentarium, with highly significant impact on the ICU and hospital budgets and resources.

ORGANIZATION

The convergence of large numbers of patients with very similar problems in the cardiac ICU provides an ideal environment for the standardization of care based on protocols and clinical pathways. One of the traps of postoperative cardiac care is that the sameness of the patients tends to obscure their particularity. Individual patient assessment must carefully address the multisystemic manifestations of cardiovascular and degenerative diseases.

Cardiac surgery involves a continuum of care from presentation to post-discharge management and rehabilitation. The intensive care specialist must be involved in this continuum, not functioning in isolation from surgeons, anaesthetists, cardiologists and family practitioners.

The postoperative stage is largely set by the preoperative and operative phases of management. A component of postoperative management is active participation in abstraction and, in particular, in patient selection and preparation as well as in the conduct of anaesthesia and surgery. Relevant aspects include temperature management, invasive monitoring, haemodynamic management and transport. Movement from the operating theatre to the ICU and later to the ward will only appear seamless if the management systems have been well co-ordinated in advance.

CARDIOVASCULAR MANAGEMENT

The first step in the intensive care management of the newly arrived patient who has undergone cardiac surgery involves a simple transfer of ventilation, monitoring and drug administration from transport to ICU systems. This should be structured to minimize disruption.

- Confirm integrity and position of endotracheal and gastric tubes and intravascular catheters.
- Re-establish mechanical ventilation of both lungs.
- Do early chest radiography; to assess lung expansion, pleural integrity and catheter placement.
- Carry out early 12-lead electrocardiography to exclude or identify acute ischaemia.

Management is conveniently dictated by standardized protocols, which should cover investigations, fluid and electrolyte management, vasoactive and other drug administration and mechanical ventilation. Standardization is probably more important than the particulars of the protocol, which might vary considerably among institutions. Optimal cardiovascular management requires a sound knowledge of normal and abnormal cardiovascular physiology. It also requires an understanding of the haemodynamic changes seen in the normal postoperative patient (Fig. 20.1).[2]

MONITORING

Electrocardiography and continuous invasive blood pressure and central venous pressure monitoring are standard.

Flotation pulmonary artery (PA) catheterization is controversial.[3]

- Surgery can be safely undertaken at least in low-risk patients without PA catheterization.[4]
- Collateral evidence supports PA catheter use in more complicated cases.
- It is essential that the known limitations and complications of PA catheters are considered in usage and interpretation.[3]

Continuous cardiac output measurement by impedance plethysmography, pulse contour analysis, Doppler and thermodilution is even less well established. These and continuous mixed venous saturation monitoring are, nevertheless, attractive and very useful in individual patients.

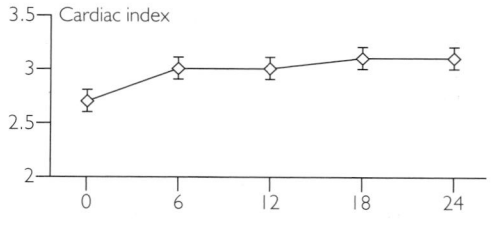

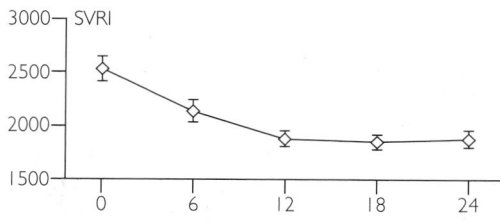

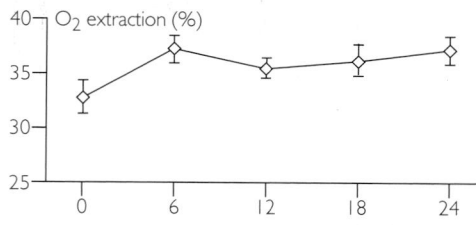

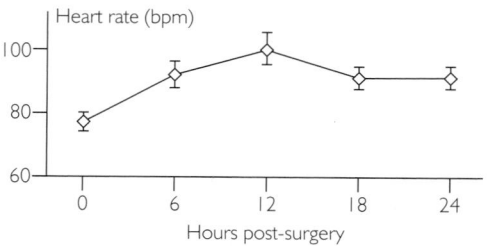

Hours post-surgery

Fig. 20.1 Haemodynamic changes following cardiac surgery. Systemic vascular resistence index (SVRI).

Transoesophageal echocardiography is commonplace, if not routine, in the operating theatre, as it enhances the accuracy of monitoring and diagnosis of cardiovascular abnormalities. The technique is less suitable for continuous monitoring in the ICU but is helpful in the diagnosis and management of cardiovascular instability in postoperative patients.

Direct, surgical cannulation of the left atrium is still occasionally recommended.[5] This procedure has a significant morbidity and has no well established benefit compared with pulmonary artery catheterization. It may provide a useful route for the administration of systemic vasoconstrictors.[6]

FLUID AND ELECTROLYTE MANAGEMENT

Despite generous intra-operative fluid administration, effective hypovolaemia is common in the early postoperative period, especially as warming with associated vasodilatation occurs.

RESUSCITATION FLUID

- Use of isotonic fluid is essential.
- No benefit for any particular resuscitation fluid has been established.
- Larger volumes of crystalloid than colloid solutions are required.

Polyuria is frequently observed in the early postoperative period, possibly related to hypothermia, haemodilution and the after effects of non-pulsatile cardiopulmonary bypass on stretch and baroreceptors. This usually settles within the first 6 hours but often necessitates considerable volume replacement in the meantime.

POTASSIUM AND MAGNESIUM HOMEOSTASIS

Hypomagnesaemia and hypokalaemia are frequent in the early postoperative stage. These are exacerbated by polyuria. Late hyperkalaemia is also quite common, especially in patients with renal impairment or prior angiotensin converting enzyme-inhibitor administration. Treatment for hyperkalaemia is rarely required in the absence of significant renal impairment. Especially in patients with atrial or ventricular ectopy or tachydysrhythmias, potassium and magnesium levels must be maintained in the high normal range.

Calcium homeostasis is generally not threatened by cardiopulmonary bypass. Massive transfusion, however, frequently causes hypocalcaemia. Ionized calcium levels are now easily monitored by ward-based blood gas machines.

HYPOTENSION

Hypotension is both a consequence and a cause of myocardial dysfunction. The major causes include:

- hypovolaemia
- vasodilation
- pericardial tamponade
- heart failure

though other causes of low cardiac output state (Table 20.1) should be considered and excluded. Whatever the cause, hypotension frequently causes myocardial ischaemia and consequent heart failure, especially if it occurs in the first 12–24 hours postoperatively. Angiography during this time almost always shows a significant reduction in the calibre of native coronary arteries, indicating increased coronary resistance and, presumably, altered coronary vasodilator reserve. Treatment of hypotension is urgent if a spiral of ischaemia and heart failure is to be averted.

MANAGEMENT

Successful management of hypotension depends on:

- rapid diagnostic assessment
- diagnosis-specific intervention.

Context is very helpful. Early hypotension in patients with well preserved ventricular function and no obvious ischaemia usually responds well to fluid administration. Patients with poor ventricular function and increasing inotrope requirement are likely to have a more sinister pathophysiology.

Table 20.1 Causes of low cardiac output in post-cardiac surgical patients.

Preload
Hypovolaemia including haemorrhage
Tamponade, pericardial constriction
LV diastolic dysfunction
hypertrophy
ischaemia
oedema
cardiomyopathy
Pulmonary hypertension
Right ventricular failure
Afterload
Excessive vasoconstriction
Aortic stenosis
Functional LV obstruction
obstructive cardiomyopathy
'SAM' of mitral valve
Myocardial function
Mechanical (VSD, valve pathology)
Cardiomyopathy
Ischaemia, post-ischaemic stunning
Metabolic, electrolyte abnormalities
Pharmacological depression

VSD = ventricular septal defect; SAM = Systolic anterior motion; LV = left ventricular.

Vasoconstrictors may be useful in breaking the cycle of hypotension–ischaemia–hypotension but must be used cautiously in patients with impaired ventricular function, and especially in patients with major vascular or aortic pathology, for whom a hypertensive overshoot may be catastrophic.

HYPERTENSION

Complications associated with hypertension include:

- bleeding
- heart failure
- vascular (especially aortic) injury
- myocardial ischaemia.

Significant postoperative hypertension is more common in patients having a history of hypertension and with cessation of β blockade, but is reasonably common in the early postoperative period. Both absolute pressure and dp/dt are important factors in vascular injury. Vascular resistance declines over the first few hours (Fig. 20.1), so that therapy during this period is best undertaken with agents with a short duration of action. Nitroglycerine is theoretically more appropriate than nitroprusside because of the possibility of coronary steal with the latter agent.[7] In practice, this is almost never apparent and nitroprusside appears to be more effective. Simple measures such as the provision of adequate analgesia and sedation should also be considered.

The target blood pressure varies with the indication. Excessive reduction of blood pressure risks reducing myocardial oxygen supply more than demand. Under most circumstances, a mean arterial pressure between 90 and 100 mmHg (12.0 and 13.5 kPa) seems optimal.[8] Much lower target pressures may be applicable for the management of heart failure or in the presence of a vulnerable aorta such as occurs with aortic dissection or aneurysms. Reduction of dp/dt with beta blockade is more important than absolute blood pressure control in the management of aortic dissection.

LOW CARDIAC OUTPUT

The aetiology of a low cardiac output following heart surgery is diverse (Table 20.1). The most common causes include:

- intravascular volume depletion
- systolic heart failure
- pericardial tamponade.

Transient reversible myocardial depression may follow an episode of acute ischaemia (preoperative or intraoperative) and is especially problematic where intraoperative myocardial protection has been difficult or suboptimal. Recognition of a low output state in the absence of invasive monitoring may be difficult. Many of the usual signs are also consequences of anaesthesia and surgery.

Tachycardia may be obscured by drugs, hypothermia and heart disease, and even lactic acidosis now seems an unreliable marker in this patient group.[2]

In the early postoperative period, a relatively low cardiac output may not warrant intervention, providing tissue oxygen delivery is adequate. Since beta blockade is beneficial in the postoperative cardiac patient, beta agonists should not be used unquestioningly. Nevertheless, optimization of cardiac function does confer some benefit[9] and intervention is clearly required when tissue oxygen delivery is inadequate.

Low cardiac output is associated with increased gastrointestinal, renal and neurological complications.

MANAGEMENT OPTIONS

1 Establish the diagnosis including aetiology. Distinguishing tamponade from heart failure may require cardiac imaging with transthoracic or transoesophageal echocardiography. This should be the first recourse when uncertainty remains following conventional haemodynamic assessment.
2 Correct all easily reversible factors including hypovolaemia, tamponade, acute myocardial ischaemia, electrolyte abnormalities and dysrhythmias.
3 Vasodilators are helpful in the presence of hypertension and ventricular dilatation. Post-surgical vasodilation after the first 4–8 hours often obviates any ongoing role for these agents.
4 Use of inotropic agents. Because of the associated vasodilatation, ino-constricting agents are frequently required, alone or in combination. Useful agents include:
   - Dobutamine, an essentially pure β_1-agonist with inotropic, lusotropic and some chronotropic effects.
   - Norepinephrine, metaraminol, vasopressin and high dose dopamine which, being predominantly vasoconstrictors, are hazardous in the presence of hypovalaemia and should probably not be used alone in the presence of a low cardiac output.
   - Epinephrine, the metabolic effects of which (especially lactic acidosis,) make usage in cardiac surgical patients problematic.[10] Epinephrine is, nevertheless, a potent ino-constrictor.
   - Milrinone,which has a long duration of action and potent vasodilating properties.These make milrinone relatively difficult to introduce and to wean. It is, however, a very effective inotropic agent, especially in patients with beta receptor down-regulation.
5 Intra-aortic balloon counterpulsation (IABC; see below).
6 Ventricular assist devices are expensive and technically far more demanding than IABC. They are effective in resting the heart while supporting organ and tissue oxygen delivery. Indications for implantation have not been well established but include intractable heart

failure, and failure to wean from cardiopulmonary bypass in spite of IABC. A combination of haemodynamic and cardiac support level criteria seem most useful and early utilization offers improved outcomes.[11,12] Usage is currently infrequent so that management expertise is difficult to acquire.
7 Delayed sternal closure has an established role in improving outcome after cardiac surgery.[13] Cardiac output is increased and inotropic requirement reduced. Subsequent sternal closure has an acceptably low complication rate. The sternum may be left open following an initial attempt at closure or reopened with later deterioration. Sternal retraction may be required.
8 Mechanical ventilation is generally continued throughout the period of low output. This reduces cardiac work-load by removing the work of breathing. Positive intra-thoracic pressure reduces left ventricular afterload which is beneficial to the dilated LV. Positive pressure may be detrimental, however, in the presence of diastolic ventricular dysfunction or hypovolaemia where the reduction in venous return may further reduce ventricular preload.

INTRA-AORTIC BALLOON COUNTERPULSATION (IABC)

IABC has an established role in support of cardiac surgery. Its two actions are: (i) augmentation of diastolic coronary perfusion pressure; and (ii) left ventricular afterload reduction. This is achieved by balloon inflation (30–50 cc capacity) within the aorta during diastole and rapid deflation of the balloon immediately before aortic valve opening. The catheter is usually inserted using a Seldinger technique, but can be placed by femoral artery cutdown or directly into the descending thoracic aorta. Timing of inflation and deflation is critical to optimal function. This is best achieved using the pressure wave form and a 1:2 ratio (Fig. 20.2).

Inflation is timed to coincide with the dicrotic notch. Deflation is timed to occur as late as possible in diastole

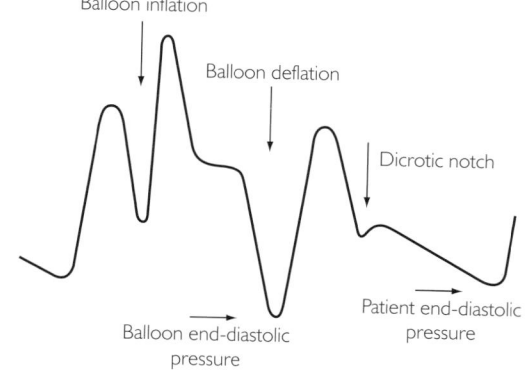

Fig. 20.2   IABC pressure waveform.

Table 20.2 Indications for intra-aortic balloon counterpulsation

- Prophylactic
  cardiac surgery
    – two of: left main >70%, LVEF <0.4, unstable angina, re-operation
  non-cardiac procedures
    – *severe* LV impairment, unstable angina
- Failure to wean from cardiopulmonary bypass
- Cardiogenic shock
  reversible myocardial depression
  support for re-perfusion, re-vascularization
  bridge to transport

LVEF = LV ejection fraction

ensuring that the IABC end-diastolic pressure is lower than the patient's end-diastolic pressure. IABC increases cardiac index and coronary perfusion and reduces left ventricular filling pressure, myocardial lactate production and oxygen extraction percentage.

Indications for IABC are summarized in Table 20.2. IABC improves:

- mortality in high risk cardiac surgery[14,15]
- clinical outcomes when used in support of infarct-related, non-surgical coronary reperfusion[16]

IABC is not helpful in the management of cardiogenic shock from irremediable causes except as a bridge to transplant. Complications are:

- limb ischaemia (6–16%)
- vascular trauma, dissection
- infection (cutdown > percutaneous)
- balloon rupture
- bleeding
- thrombocytopenia
- malposition, vascular obstruction
- malfunction, failure to unwrap.

Limb ischaemia is the most frequent complication and optimal management requires early recognition based on routine, systematic observation.

ISCHAEMIA

Postoperative myocardial ischaemia predicts a more complicated course.[17] Recognition is enhanced by automated multi lead ST analysis with confirmatory electrocardiography, although diagnosis may be difficult in the presence of preoperative ECG abnormalities.

Ischaemia may be due to graft failure. Remedial options include coronary angiography and/or re-operation. Angiography offers the potential for tailored re-operation or non-operative intervention. The surgeon knows the complete surgical story and this may influence management decisions. Close liaison among ICU personnel, cardiologists and surgeons is essential.

DIASTOLIC DYSFUNCTION

Ventricular hypertrophy is the commonest cause of diastolic dysfunction, and is exacerbated by poor myocardial protection during surgical procedures. Myocardial ischaemia, right ventricular dilatation and pericardial abnormalities (including tamponade) can also reduce left ventricular volume in spite of elevated filling pressures.[18] Recognition and management can be very difficult.

Diagnosis generally requires: (i) demonstration of small ventricular volumes (using echocardiography or other techniques); (ii) the presence of increased pressures.

MANAGEMENT

- Treatable causes should be addressed.
- Blood volume must be maintained, with blood transfusion where necessary.
- Maintenance of sinus rhythm is helpful if not essential.
- Atrial pacing is often beneficial since the stroke volume is fixed and the diastolic filling time is foreshortened.
- β agonists and milrinone improve diastolic relaxation and hence ventricular compliance.

DYSRHYTHMIAS

Ventricular and supraventricular dysrhythmias are common. Prevention and treatment of electrolyte abnormalities may be prophylactic.

New occurrence of complex ventricular dysrhythmias should stimulate a search for causal ischaemia and graft malfunction.

- Ventricular fibrillation and pulseless ventricular tachycardia require rapid defibrillation, preferably before external cardiac massage which may cause mechanical injury post-sternotomy. If haemodynamic stability cannot be rapidly restored, open cardiac massage should be instituted.
- Facilities for atrioventricular pacing are essential as transient heart block is common.

ATRIAL FIBRILLATION (AF)

AF is the most common complication of cardiac surgery.[19,20] Its incidence varies from 10 to 40% in patients undergoing coronary artery surgery and up to 50% with some valvular procedures. Predisposing factors include a history of AF, valvular heart disease (especially mitral valve pathology) increasing age and prolonged P wave duration. AF is probably less frequently observed following 'off-pump' surgery, and is most frequently encountered around the second and third postoperative days, but may occur weeks after surgery and hospital discharge.

AF is a potentially serious complication. Apart from discomfort, it may provoke or complicate haemodynamic instability. The major complication of AF, however, is stroke with an increased risk of approximately three-fold. Based on echocardiography, there is the potential for embolic stroke within 3 days of onset of AF. AF is also associated with:

- increase in inotrope usage
- increased use of IABC
- increased re-operation for bleeding
- prolonged ICU and hospital stay and
- increased costs.

Several strategies are beneficial in preventing AF:

- β blockade
- amiodarone
- sotolol
- diltiazem
- atrial pacing
- dexamethasone.

Treatment should be tempered with an understanding that spontaneous reversion to sinus rhythm is frequent. A treatment strategy is summarized in Table 20.3.

- Beta blockade is best established.
- Digitalis is not more effective than placebo at reverting AF and may not be helpful in ventricular rate control in the presence of catecholamine stimulation.
- Anticoagulation should be considered where AF persists for longer than 48 hours and in all cases where elective cardioversion is undertaken.
- Early cardioversion tends to be ineffective and potentially harmful and should only be undertaken to correct severe haemodynamic compromise.

Table 20.3 Management of atrial fibrillation (AF)

Rate control
β blockade
Calcium channel blockers
Amiodarone
Sotolol
(Digitalis)
Cardioversion
Ibuletide
Amiodarone
Magnesium
Electrical cardioversion
Anticoagulation
Always for elective cardioversion
Consider if AF persists beyond 48 hours

RIGHT VENTRICULAR (RV) DYSFUNCTION

RV failure following cardiac surgery is reasonably common. Aetiological factors include:

- direct RV ischaemia or infarction
- poor myocardial protection
- anteriorly placed RV
- bypass-related pulmonary hypertension.

Management involves:

- volume resuscitation
- maintenance of RV perfusion pressure with vasoconstrictors
- IABC as required
- inotrope administration
- RV afterload reduction.

Useful afterload reducing agents include nitric oxide[21] and prostaglandins.[6] Conventional vasodilators tend to produce excessive systemic vasodilatation. Occasionally, RV balloon counterpulsation or an RV assist device may be required. Delayed sternal closure has an established role.

EMERGENCY RE-OPERATION

Emergency re-sternotomy is indicated as part of resuscitation when haemodynamic stability cannot be rapidly re-established with conventional means.[22,23] Advantages compared to closed chest resuscitation include:

- establishment of the cause of instability
- correction of the cause (e.g. tamponade, kinked graft)
- more effective cardiac massage
- direct establishment of atrial and ventricular pacing.

Re-sternotomy also enables the re-establishment of cardiopulmonary bypass, and re-grafting or correction of mechanical abnormalities as required. Infectious complications of emergency re-sternotomy are probably increased but the incidence is not prohibitive.

RESPIRATORY MANAGEMENT

Postoperative mechanical ventilation remains routine in cardiac surgical patients. Immediate extubation appears to offer little benefit.[24] Neither is routine ventilation beyond 12 hours essential.[25] Extubation can be safely undertaken with simple protocols. Re-intubation is rarely required, but is more likely in older patients with pre-existent lung and vascular disease and impaired ventricular function. Re-operative surgery and bleeding requiring massive transfusion also increase the likelihood of early extubation failure.[26]

Hypoxia is very common in the early postoperative period. It is mostly attributable to atelectasis and responds well to simple measures such as positive end-expiratory pressure (PEEP), prolonged inspiration and simple recruitment manoeuvres. Atelectasis is a consequence of cardiopulmonary bypass and intra-operative ventilation with high inspired oxygen and without PEEP. Long-term sequelae are rare. Incentive spirometry and chest physiotherapy are commonly utilized in the postoperative period without good supportive evidence. Early mobilization appears most beneficial.

More sinister causes of hypoxia include severe heart failure and hypoxaemic respiratory failure (acute respiratory distress syndrome, ARDS). The aetiology of ARDS is diverse, but includes shock, massive blood product administration and cardiopulmonary bypass itself. Management is not particular to this group of patients. Occasionally, profound hypoxia accompanies minor atelectasis with moderate pulmonary hypertension. Patent foramen ovale (which is seen in 10–15% of the normal population) with right-to-left intracardiac shunt is the likely mechanism.

Pulmonary embolism is an uncommon complication of cardiac surgery, probably due to bypass-induced platelet dysfunction, 'routine' postoperative anti-platelet therapy and thrombo-prophylaxis.[27] The recent enthusiasm for 'off-pump' surgery may have spawned an increase in this complication and so may warrant a more aggressive prophylactic regimen.[28]

POSTOPERATIVE COMPLICATIONS

HAEMORRHAGE

Excessive postoperative bleeding is a major cause of increased morbidity and mortality.[29] Mechanisms are complex and include preoperative anticoagulation, thrombolysis and anti-platelet therapy as well as activation of haemostatic mechanisms including fibrinolysis. 'Off-pump' surgery may be associated with excessive bleeding because of administration of anticoagulant and anti-platelet therapy out of fear of early graft closure.

Most studies of pharmacological strategies to minimize postoperative blood loss have involved preoperative or intra-operative intervention. Extrapolation to the postoperative phase is intuitive rather than established. Aprotinin and the lysine analogues aminocaproic acid and tranexamic acid reduce bleeding and exposure to blood and blood products. Desmopressin is probably less effective and has been associated with an increased risk of myocardial infarction.[30]

Effective postoperative measures include reversal of residual heparin (including 'heparin rebound') and correction of coagulopathy with blood products. Application of PEEP has been shown to be effective in some studies, but not others. Retransfusion of shed blood reduces autologous transfusion requirements without apparent side effects. Controlled tamponade with discontinuation of drain suction and even clamping of drains has also been reported.[31] Finally, at least in reasonably stable patients, reduction of the transfusion threshold to at least 80 g/l reduces exposure to autologous blood transfusion[32] without adverse consequences.

RENAL FAILURE

Depending on definition and patient groups, acute renal failure is observed in 1–5% of patients undergoing cardiac surgery. Risk factors include increasing age, heart failure, prolonged bypass, diabetes, pre-existent renal impairment and postoperative shock.[33] Surgery without cardiopulmonary bypass may be relatively protective.[34] Morbidity, mortality and costs are significantly increased. Effective preventative strategies beyond careful haemodynamic management and minimization of associated nephrotoxic insults have not been established. Nevertheless, attention to urine output in the presence of known risk factors appears warranted.

SHIVERING

Shivering is frequent following cardiac surgery. Mechanisms are complex and not entirely related to core temperature. Shivering causes a significant increase in metabolic rate and hence cardiac workload.[35] This is especially important in the patient with impaired cardiac function and limited reserve. Effective preventative agents include dexamethasone, clonidine, high-dose morphine and external warming. Pethidine effectively reduces the duration of shivering. Short-term neuromuscular blockade is occasionally required.

STERNAL INFECTION

Deep sternal wound infection is uncommon (0.5–2.5%). Associated morbidity and mortality are significant. Risk factors have been variously reported but consistently include diabetes, obesity and use of internal mammary arteries, especially if bilateral. Other contributing factors include prolonged surgery, chronic lung disease, male sex, low postoperative cardiac output, blood transfusion, sternal re-opening and dialysis. Rigid control of blood sugar levels in diabetics may help prevent infection.[36]

NEUROLOGICAL COMPLICATIONS

Neurological complications of cardiac surgery include neuropsychiatric deterioration as a consequence of cardiopulmonary bypass, delirium and a range of peripheral neuropathies,[37] the most frequent of which is a unilateral phrenic nerve palsy. Paraplegia is a recognized complication of thoracic aortic surgery.

The most devastating neurological complication is cerebral infarction. The incidence varies with patient selection, but ranges from 1 to 5%. The pathophysiology is mostly embolic. Risk factors include carotid artery stenosis, hypertension, atrial fibrillation, aortic atheroma, impaired ventricular function and peripheral vascular disease.[38] 'Off pump' surgery is almost certainly protective and other operative techniques may also reduce the incidence.

GASTROINTESTINAL COMPLICATIONS

Peptic ulcer disease, pancreatitis, cholecystitis, gut ischaemia, ileus and hepatic dysfunction are uncommon (<1%) after cardiac surgery.[39] Morbidity, however, is quite high. Risk factors include increased age, more complicated surgery and postoperative shock.

LONG-TERM CONSIDERATIONS

Patients surviving cardiac surgery have a continuing risk of disease progression. It is important that effective secondary prevention strategies be considered or recommenced in the postoperative period. Initiatives with proven long term benefit in patients with ischaemic heart disease include anti-platelet therapy, beta blockade, ACE-inhibitors, lipid-lowering 'statins' and exercise. Treatment for hypertension, diabetes and other inter-current disorders should also be reinstituted.

A small percentage of patients require long-term ICU management for a variety of complications. Excellent long term survival and quality of life is possible in this group of patients, especially if the prolonged ICU stay results from pulmonary complications rather than severe heart failure or neurological dysfunction.[40]

NON-CARDIAC SURGERY

Non-cardiac surgery poses a significant risk to the patient with cardiac disease.[41,42] Postoperative cardiac complications result in a significantly increased immediate and late mortality. Simple preoperative assessment enables risk stratification which might lead to deferment or cancellation of non-essential surgery. Indications for specific investigations and treatments are probably not different in the preoperative patient. However, this might be the first time that a cardiac assessment has been undertaken and hence significant cardiac pathology identified. Risk factors are summarised in Table 20.4. Cumulative factors are more than additive. Patients undergoing vascular procedures have a high risk of associated coronary artery disease and should be carefully assessed preoperatively. Perioperative risk can be modified by anaesthetic technique and by optimal medical (or surgical) management of heart disease which might include myocardial revascularization.[41]

The principles of postoperative management are the same as those outlined for the cardiac surgical patient. The period of risk for cardiac complications extends for some days after surgery and close monitoring to identify and manage events during this time is desirable in high-risk patients. The immediate perioperative period poses risks associated with anaesthesia, bleeding, fluid and electrolyte imbalance, haemodynamic instability and temperature abnormalities. These can be effectively managed. Early re-institution of protective treatment (aspirin, beta blockers, angiotensin converting enzyme inhibition, statins, anti-hypertensive therapy) may protect against later complications.

Table 20.4 Risk factors[a] for cardiac patients undergoing non-cardiac surgery

- High-risk surgery (abdominal, thoracic, major vascular)
- History of ischaemic heart disease
- History of congestive heart failure
- History of cerebrovascular disease
- Treatment with insulin
- Renal impairment

[a] High risk = 3 or more factors.

REFERENCES

1 Society of Thoracic Surgeons *Postoperative Variables: Univariate Analysis*, 1998. http://www.ctsnet.org/doc/3033

2 Raper RF, Cameron G, Walker D, Bowey CJ. Type B lactic acidosis following cardiopulmonary bypass. *Crit Care Med* 1997; **25**: 46–51.

3 Taylor RW. Controversies in pulmonary artery catheterization. *New Horiz* 1997; **5**: 173–296.

4 Leibowitz AB, Beilin T. Pulmonary artery catheters and outcome in the perioperative period. *New Horiz* 1997; **5**: 214–21.

5 Santini F, Gatti G, Borghetti V, *et al*. Routine left atrial catheterization for the post-operative management of cardiac surgical patients: is the risk justified? *Eur J Cardiothorac Surg* 1999; **16**: 218–21.

6 Tritapepe L, Voci P, Cogliati AA, *et al*. Successful weaning from cardiopulmonary bypass with central venous prostaglandin E1 and left atrial norepinephrine infusion in patients with acute pulmonary hypertension. *Crit Care Med* 1999; **27**: 2180–3.

7 Fremes C, Weisel RD, Mickle DAG, *et al*. A comparison of nitroglycerine and nitroprusside: 1. Treatment of postoperative hypertension. *Ann Thorac Surg* 1985; **39**: 53–60.

8 Fremes C, Weisel RD, Baird RJ, *et al*. Effects of post-operative hypertension and its treatment. *J Thorac Cardiovasc Surg* 1983; **86**: 47–56.

9 Polonen P, Ruokonen E, Hippelainen M, *et al*. A prospective randomized study of goal-oriented haemodynamic therapy in cardiac surgical patients. *Anesth Analg* 2000; **90**: 1052–9.

10 Totaro RJ, Raper RF. Epinephrine-induced lactic acidosis following cardiopulmonary bypass. *Crit Care Med* 1997; **25**: 1693–9.

11 Morales DLS, Mehmet CO. Mechanical circulatory assist devices in critical care management. *New Horiz* 1999; **7**: 489–503.

12 Samuels LE, Kaufman MS, Thomas MP, *et al*. Pharmacological criteria for ventricular assist device insertion following postcardiotomy shock: experience with the Abiomed BVS system. *J Card Surg* 1999; **14**: 288–93.

13 Furnary AP, Magovern JA, Simpson KA, Magovern GJ. Prolonged open sternotomy and delayed sternal closure after cardiac operations. *Ann Thorac Surg* 1992; **54**: 233–9.

14 Dietl CA, Berkheimer MD, Woods EL, *et al*. Efficacy and cost effectiveness of preoperative IABP in patients with ejection fraction of 0.25 or less. *Ann Thorac Surg* 1996; **62**: 401–9.

15 Christenson JT, Simonet F, Badel P, Schmuziger M. Optimal timing of preoperative intraaortic balloon support in high-risk coronary patients. *Ann Thorac Surg* 1999; **68**: 934–9.

16 Ohman EM, George BS, White CJ, *et al*. Coronary heart disease/myocardial infarction/peripheral vascular disease: use of aortic counterpulsation to improve sustained coronary artery patency during acute myocardial infarction: results of a randomised trial. *Circulation* 1994; **90**: 792–9.

17 Yazigi A, Richa F, Gebara S, *et al*. Prognostic importance of automated ST-segment monitoring after coronary artery bypass graft surgery. *Acta Anaesth Scand* 1998; **42**: 532–5.

18 Raper RF, Sibbald WJ. Misled by the wedge? The Swan Ganz catheter and left ventricular preload. *Chest* 1986; **89**: 427–34.

19 Bharucha DB, Kowey PR. Management and prevention of atrial fibrillation after cardiovascular surgery. *Am J Cardiol* 2000; **85**: 20D–24D.

20 Ommen SR, Odell JA, Stanton MS. Current concepts: atrial arrhythmias after cardiothoracic surgery. *N Engl J Med* 1997; **336**: 1429–34.

21 Argenziano M, Choudhri AF, Moazami N, *et al*. Randomized, double-blind trial of inhaled nitric oxide in LVAD recipients with pulmonary hypertension. *Ann Thorac Surg* 1998; **65**: 340–5.

22 Birdi I, Chaudhuri N, Lenthall K, *et al*. Emergency reinstitution of cardiopulmonary bypass following cardiac surgery: outcome justifies the cost. *Eur J Cardiothorac Surg* 2000; **17**: 743–6.

23 Raman J, Saldanha RF, Branch J, *et al*. Open cardiac compression in the postoperative cardiac intensive care unit. *Anaesth Intensive Care* 1989; **17**: 129–35.

24 Montes FR, Sanchez SI, Giraldo JC, *et al*. The lack of benefit of tracheal extubation in the operating room after coronary artery bypass surgery. *Anesth Analg* 2000; **91**: 776–80.

25 Hickey RF, Cason BA. Timing of tracheal extubation in adult cardiac surgery patients. *J Cardiac Surg* 1995; **10**: 340–8.

26 Rady MY, Ryan T. Perioperative predictors of extubation failure and the effect on clinical outcome after cardiac surgery. *Crit Care Med* 1999; **27**: 340–7.

27 Shammas NW. Pulmonary embolus after coronary artery bypass surgery: a review of the literature. *Clin Cardiol*; **23**: 637–44.

28 Mariani MA, Gu J, Boonstra PW, *et al*. Procoagulant activity after off-pump coronary operation: is the current antocoagulation adequate? *Ann Thorac Surg* 1999; **67**: 1370–5.

29 Society of Thoracic Surgeons. *Postoperative Variables: Univariate Analysis*, 1998. http://www.ctsnet.org/doc/3036.

30 Levi M, Cromheecke ME, deJonge E, *et al*. Pharmacological strategies to decrease excessive blood loss in cardiac surgery: a meta-analysis of clinically relevant endpoints. *Lancet* 1999; **354**: 1940–7.

31 Aravot DJ, Barak J, Vidne BA. Induction of controlled tamponade in the management of massive unexplained postcardiotomy bleeding. Case report and review of the literature. *J Cardiovasc Surg* 1986; **27**: 613–17.

32 Bracey AW, Radovancevic P, Riggs SA, *et al*. Lowering the haemoglobin threshold for transfusion in coronary artery bypass procedures: effect on patient outcome. *Transfusion* 1999; **39**: 1070–7.

33 Mangano CM, Diamondstone LS, Ramsay J, *et al*. Renal dysfunction after myocardial revascularization: risk factors, adverse outcomes, and hospital resource utilization. *Ann Intern Med* 1998; **128**: 194–203.

34 Ascione R, Lloyd CT, Underwood MJ, *et al*. On-pump versus off-pump coronary revascularization: evaluation of renal function. *Ann Thorac Surg* 2000; **68**: 493–8.

35 Rodriguez JL, Weissman MC, Damask MC, *et al*. Morphine and postoperative rewarming in critically ill patients. *Circulation* 1983; **68**: 1238–46.

36 Furnary AP, Zerr KJ, Grunkemeier GL, Starr A. Continuous intravenous insulin infusion reduces the incidence of deep sternal wound infection in diabetic patients after cardiac surgical procedures. *Ann Thorac Surg* 1999; **67**: 352–60.

37 Sharma AD, Parmley CL, Sreeram G, Grocott HP. Peripheral nerve injuries during cardiac surgery: risk factors, diagnosis, prognosis and prevention. *Anesth Analg* 2000; **91**: 1358–69.

38 Das SK, Brow TD, Pepper J. Continuing controversy in the management of concomitant coronary and carotid disease: an overview. *Int J Cardiol* 2000; **74**: 47–65.

39 Halm MA. Acute gastrointestinal complications after cardiac surgery. *Am J Crit Care* 1996; **5**: 109–18.

40 Wahl GW, Swinburne AJ, Fedullo AJ, *et al*. Long-term outcome when major complications follow coronary artery bypass graft surgery. *Chest* 1996; **110**: 1394–8.

41 Eagle KA, Charanjit S, Mickel MC, *et al*. Cardiac risk of noncardiac surgery: influence of coronary disease and type of surgery in 3368 operations. *Circulation* 1997; **96**: 1882–7.

42 Lee TH, Marcantonio ER, Mangione CM, *et al*. Derivation and prospective validation of a simple index for prediction of cardiac risk of major noncardiac surgery. *Circulation* 1999; **100**: 1043–9.

21.

Echocardiography in intensive care

K D Donovan and F B Colreavy

Echocardiography refers to a group of inter-related ultrasound applications used to examine the heart and great vessels. The reflected and processed sonic waves are displayed on a monitor and the images can be stored on videotape or disk. Echocardiography includes: (1) two-dimensional (2-D) anatomical imaging; (2) M-mode echocardiography usually obtained with 2-D guidance; and (3) Doppler techniques. Echocardiography is a safe non-invasive technique which is integral to clinical cardiology. More recently, echocardiography has evolved into a powerful diagnostic and management tool in critically ill patients especially in cardiovascular emergencies of uncertain cause.[1,2]

Cardiologists, although highly skilled in echocardiography, may not appreciate the complex pathophysiology of critically ill patients in intensive care, and they have time commitments elsewhere. Echocardiography is operator dependent; optimal image acquisition requires both technical knowledge of the machine's capabilities as well as a degree of manual dexterity. As a general rule, echocardiography is not an efficient technique for monitoring haemodynamic indices over medium term (hours–days) in the intensive care unit (ICU). A pulmonary artery catheter is more suitable for repetitive trend measurements, such as stroke volume, cardiac output, pulmonary artery wedge pressure, etc., and intensive care staff are skilled and experienced in its use. As echocardiography technicians are not present in ICU, especially out of hours, intensivists must be able to act as their own sonographers as well as interpreting and reporting on the echographic images obtained. It is important that intensivists acquire all requisite skills so that echocardiography becomes more widely available.

PRINCIPLES AND TECHNICAL CONSIDERATIONS[3]

Echocardiography uses the reflection of sound waves at tissue boundaries to construct a 2-D image of cardiac structures. The human ear hears only sound waves with a frequency between 20 Hz and 20 kHz; higher frequen-cies are referred to as ultrasound. Echocardiography uses sound in the frequency 1–10 MHz. A piezo electrical crystal generates and receives the ultrasound waves.

2-D ECHOCARDIOGRAPHY

2-D echocardiography is the cornerstone of cardiac ultrasound as Doppler and M-mode are usually performed with reference to the 2-D image. Each 2-D image is defined by the position of the transducer (acoustic window) and image plane which is determined by the axis of the heart and not the spine (Table 21.1).

M-MODE ECHOCARDIOGRAPHY

Rapidly repeated transmit and receive cycle allows production of images with good resolution. M-mode echocardiography complements 2-D echocardiography.

Table 21.1 Some standard views in transthoracic and transoesophageal echocardiography

Acoustic window	Image plane
Transthoracic	
Parasternal	Long axis
	Short axis
Apical	Four-chamber
	Two-chamber
	Long axis
Subcostal	Multiple
Transoesophageal*	
Transgastric	e.g. Short axis
	Long axis
Deep transgastric	e.g. Long axis/five-chamber
Lower transoesophageal	e.g. four-chamber
	Two-chamber
	Long axis
Upper transoesophageal	e.g. Short axis of aortic valve
	Long axis of aortic valve
	RV inflow-outflow

*Multiple image planes from 0° to 180°.

The beam is not scanned but stays in a fixed position, allowing the display of structures along the beam as a function of time. The rapid sampling rate makes identification of thin moving structures, such as valve leaflets, relatively easy. The cursor is usually directed through a 2-D image giving a one dimensional slice or 'ice pick' view. Distance (depth) is on the vertical and time is on the horizontal axis (Fig. 21.1).

DOPPLER ECHOCARDIOGRAPHY

Doppler echocardiography is vital for obtaining haemodynamic information and is an integral part of every echocardiographic study.

The *Doppler effect* is based on changes in sound frequency that occur when a sound source moves towards or away from an observer. One classic example is that of an ambulance siren; as it comes toward a listener, the sound frequency increases (higher pitch) and after the ambulance moves away from the observer the sound frequency decreases (lower pitch).

The *Doppler shift* is the difference between frequencies that are transmitted and received by a transducer after striking red blood cells.

The *Doppler equation* is the mathematical relationship between the Doppler shift and the velocity of red blood cells that produce it.

$$V = C \times \Delta f / 2f_t \times \cos \theta$$

Where V = velocity of blood flow, C = speed of sound in soft tissue (1540 m/s), Δf = Doppler (frequency) shift: difference in frequency between received (f_r) and transmitted (f_t) ultrasound, θ = angle between ultrasound beam and direction of blood flow (Fig. 21.2). Echocardiographic machines contain computers that automatically calculate the Doppler shift which is then entered into the Doppler equation. Blood flow velocity (m/s) is calculated and displayed on the monitor.

It is very important that the ultrasound beam is parallel or nearly parallel with the direction of blood flow. If θ equals 0 then cosign θ equals 1, however if θ >20° then the velocity of blood flow will be significantly underestimated. Doppler data are processed and a spectral display plots instantaneous blood velocities over time. Blood flow velocity can be expressed as peak velocity or mean velocity throughout a cardiac cycle (velocity time integral, VTI) (Fig. 21.3).

The most common uses of Doppler are pulsed wave, continuous wave and colour flow Doppler.

PULSED WAVE (PW) DOPPLER

PW Doppler is usually performed with a duplex transducer (2-D and Doppler): a single ultrasound transducer transmits and receives ultrasound signals. Blood flow velocities of a small volume of blood, the 'sample volume' are obtained at a specific depth so it is useful for velocity measurements at specific sites such as the left ventricular outflow tract (LVOT). Due to technical limitations the maximum measurable velocity is usually < 2 m/s.

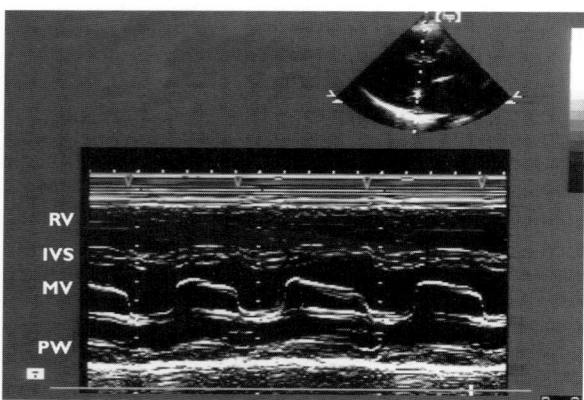

Fig. 21.1 M-mode echocardiogram guided by M-mode cursor on the 2-D image (see top). The transducer is anterior with the cursor directed through the right ventricle (RV), intraventricular septum (IVS), mitral valve (MV) and posterior wall of the left ventricle (PW). The mitral valve leaflets are thickened and there is reduced diastolic slope of the anterior leaflet and the posterior leaflet moves anteriorly during diastole due to commissural fusion

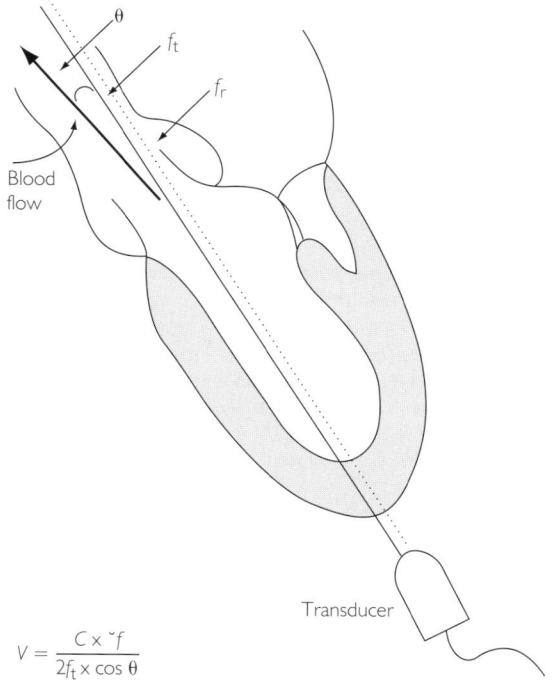

$$V = \frac{C \times \Delta f}{2f_t \times \cos \theta}$$

Fig. 21.2 The Doppler equation

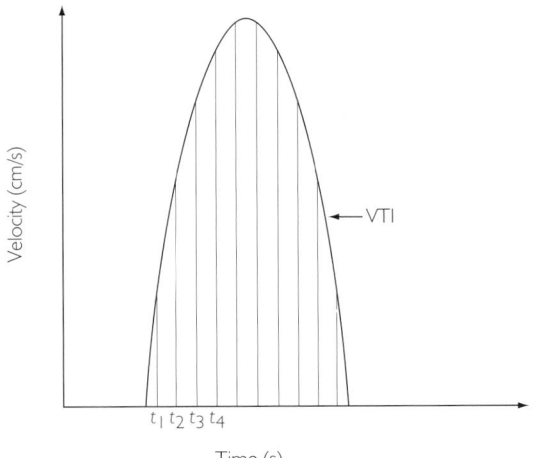

Fig. 21.3 Velocity time integral (cm/s) = area under the velocity curve: sum of velocities (cm/s) during the ejection time (s); t_1 = time one, t_2 = time two, etc.

CONTINUOUS WAVE (CW) DOPPLER

The transducer consists of two crystals, one continuously transmits and the other continuously receives ultrasound waves. It can measure high velocity blood flow, such as occurs in aortic stenosis. Unlike PW Doppler, CW Doppler measures all the frequency shifts along the beam path and it is not possible to estimate the velocity at a specific site (range ambiguity).

Blood flow velocities measured by either PW or CW Doppler can be converted to pressure gradients using the simplified Bernouilli equation, $\Delta P = 4V^2$ (where ΔP is the instantaneous pressure gradient and V is the instantaneous velocity), to provide estimates of pressure.

COLOUR FLOW DOPPLER (CFD)

This is based on PW Doppler principles. Multiple sample volumes are recorded with blood flow velocities encoded in colour (flow towards the probe is coloured red, away blue) and superimposed on 2-D images. Thus, CFD information displayed includes: (1) direction of blood flow; (2) timing of CFD signals; (3) a crude estimation of blood flow velocity; and (4) laminar flow can be differentiated from turbulent flow.

SAFETY

Ultrasound at the power levels used clinically to image cardiac structures has no known adverse biologic effects.[4] Transoesophageal echocardiography (TOE) in trained, experienced hands is a well developed and safe procedure.[5] Nevertheless, TOE is semi-invasive and serious complications and even deaths have occurred. TOE is contraindicated in the presence of oesophageal stricture

or neoplasm. Caution should be exercised in other situations such as previous oesophageal surgery or total gastrectomy. TOE should be deferred in patients with any symptoms of dysphagia until the cause has been found. Oesophageal varices, severe coagulopathy, significant cervical spine abnormalities are relative contraindications to TOE. Routine antibiotic prophylaxis does not appear to be necessary before TOE in intensive care patients.[6]

TRANSTHORACIC (TTE) AND TOE ECHOCARDIOGRAPHY

TTE and TOE are complementary ultrasound techniques, each with its own strengths and weakness (Table 21.2); for example, a vegetation imaged on the mitral valve of a septic patient will usually require a TOE to evaluate complications of endocarditis.

TTE

Recent technological advances such as harmonic imaging[7] have greatly improved transthoracic surface imaging. TTE images may be inadequate in some critically ill patients especially in intubated mechanically ventilated patients, or patients with chronic lung disease, obesity, chest trauma, or surgical wounds. Inability to appropriately position such patients is a further limiting factor.

TOE[8,9]

The transducer is mounted at the tip of a flexible gastroscope-like probe which can be manoeuvred to various positions in the oesophagus and stomach close to the heart (Fig. 21.4). The modern multiplane probes allow rotation of the ultrasound scanning plane from 0–180° which provides a mirror image orientation. Multiple tomographic imaging planes can be obtained without the necessity of further probe manipulation. Compared to TTE, TOE provides additional information in 32–100% of intensive care examinations and unexpected new diagnoses in 38–59% leading to significant changes in treatment.[10] Approximately 20% of patients with unexplained hypotension require surgery on the basis of new TOE findings.[11,12]

INDICATIONS FOR ECHOCARDIOGRAPHY

The indications for echocardiography broadly fall into three categories: (1) morphologic diagnosis of specific cardiac/great vessel pathology (usually guided by clinical suspicion); (2) haemodynamic assessment and monitoring of cardiac function; and (3) others, such as evaluation of patients with atrial fibrillation for the presence of left atrial (LA) clot prior to cardioversion. Guidelines for the use of

Table 21.2 Transthoracic echocardiography (TTE) and transoesophageal echocardiography (TOE): advantages and disadvantages

	TTE	TOE	Comments
Echocardiographic windows	'Unlimited'	'Limited'	
Time lag to diagnosis	(virtually) Instantaneous	Short (min)	
Contraindications	None	Occasional	e.g. oesophageal stricture
Invasive	No	Minimal	
Morbidity	No	Minimal	Low but measurable complication rate with TOE
Mortality	No	Minimal	TOE mortality about 1/10 000
Image quality			
Non-ventilated	Good/excellent	Excellent (usually)	TTE: poor images postop cardiac surgery, CAL, obese, etc.
Ventilated	Poor to excellent	Excellent (usually)	
Specific pathology:			
Endocarditis			
(a) Native valve	Useful if low index of suspicion	Sensitive and specific	TOE essential for diagnosis of complications, e.g. abscess, etc.
(b) Prosthetic valve	Useful in conjunction with TOE	Essential	
Aortic dissection	?	Essential	TTE occasionally useful for diagnosis. Aortic regurgitation can also be assessed
Aortic trauma	+/–	Essential	
Left atrial appendage clot	No	Essential	
Left ventricle clot	Yes	Yes	TTE more useful than TOE to image LV apical clot
Pericardial effusion	Yes	Yes	TTE essential for guiding needle pericardiocentesis
Localized tamponade (post cardiac surgery)	Occasionally useful	(Usually) essential	TOE especially useful for posterior collections

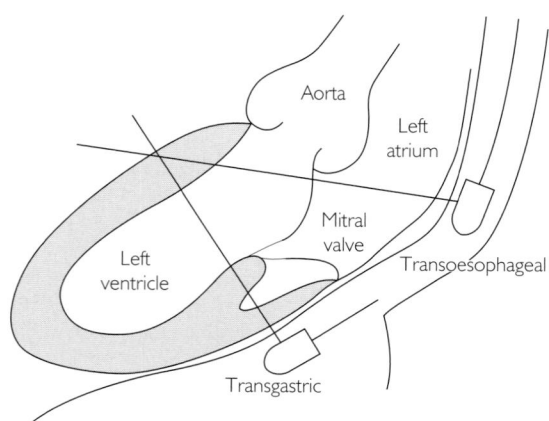

Fig. 21.4 Transducer position in transoesophageal echocardiography

echocardiography are based on expert consensus[13,14] and observational studies. There are no randomized trials that specifically test the impact of echocardiography on outcome. In intensive care practice, echocardiography is used to evaluate clinical syndrome(s) that suggest a diagnosis or, more often, a number of possible diagnoses. For example, haemodynamic instability in a patient with major blunt chest trauma suggests cardiac contusion or pericardial effusion causing tamponade. Nevertheless, the echocardiographic examination might reveal hypovolaemia with hyperdynamic LV systolic function or valvular damage with severe regurgitation.

Some common syndromes in which echocardiography is especially useful are listed in Table 21.3.

As a general rule, unless there is gross haemodynamic instability or some other overriding reason, the echocardiographic examination should be structured around a 'basic' set of 2-D views. This applies to both TTE and TOE. The focus of the TOE examination should be on the most important specific clinical question. The second priority should be other potential pathology in the differential diagnosis.

VALVULAR HEART DISEASE

Echocardiography is the 'gold standard' for evaluating valvular heart disease. 2-D echocardiography provides excellent imaging of all cardiac valves. Various Doppler techniques allow accurate haemodynamic evaluation of the valves.

Table 21.3 Indications for echocardiography in the intensive care unit according to clinical syndrome

Clinical syndrome	Findings	Comments
Hypotension		
Acute myocardial infarct		
no murmur	LV RWMA(s)	Usually severe ↓ LV systolic function
	RV RWMA	RV ↓ > LV ↓
	Hypovolaemia	'Empty' LV cavity, systolic function largely preserved
	Acute MR	Often no murmur with normal LA size
new murmur	Papillary muscle rupture/severe MR	'Good' LV function with MR
	VSD	Usually fatal
rarely	Cardiac rupture/tamponade	Often localized. There may be no 'echo free space' due to clot compressing the heart. Cardiac filling pressures may be normal
	LV pseudoaneurysm	
Cardiothoracic surgery	Cardiac tamponade	May be due to graft occlusion, air embolism
	(New) RWMA	Stunning or long standing cardiomyopathy
	Hypovolaemia	Often long standing but may be worsened by surgery e.g. ischaemia to a papillary muscle of mitral valve
	Global LV ↓	Inotropes/IABP/hypovolaemia worsen LVOT obstruction.
	Valvular dysfunction	
Dynamic LVOT obstruction	LVOT pressure gradient, SAM, MR	'Empty' LV with vigorous contraction
Trauma	Hypovolaemia	RWMA (RV > LV)
	Cardiac contusion	Most common aortic valve (AR) or mitral valve (MR), occasionally tricuspid valve (TR)
	Valvular injury	Occasionally
	VSD/ASD	More common in penetrating chest injuries
	Cardiac tamponade	Widened mediastinum (90%) at isthmus of aorta. TOE required
	Ruptured thoracic aorta	Possible global/regional LV depression
Sepsis	Often normal LV systolic function with 'empty' LV	TOE more sensitive than TTE for imaging vegetations/abscess/fistula
	Infective endocarditis – vegetations/abscess/ regurgitation	Cardiomyopathy or stunning
'Isolated' hypotension	Global LV ↓ or RWMA	Usually chronic, occasionally acute (e.g. ruptured papillary muscle of mitral valve)
('hypotension ?cause')	Valvular dysfunction	
	Dynamic LVOT obstruction	Pulmonary embolism – usually dilated right heart with depressed systolic function, sometimes with clot in a proximal pulmonary artery
	Acute cor pulmonale	

Table 21.3 *(continued)*

Clinical syndrome	Findings	Comments
Sepsis (source?)	Vegetations, regurgitation ± abscess	Infective endocarditis until proven otherwise
	Normal TOE examination	Infective endocarditis unlikely. If clinically indicated serial TOE
Systemic emboli (source?)	LA/LAA clot	Usually enlarged LA and atrial fibrillation. TOE usually required for diagnosis
	LV clot	Usually associated with RWMA or global LV decrease. TTE for apical clot
	Aortic atherosclerotic plaques	TOE essential for diagnosis
	Vegetations – aortic or mitral valve	Septic?
	Clot – prosthetic aortic or mitral valve	Associated prosthetic valve dysfunction
	Patent foramen ovale with paradoxical embolism	RA pressure > LA pressure (e.g. IPPV with high PEEP). TOE (bubble contrast) usually necessary for diagnosis
Pulmonary oedema (cause?)	Tumour (e.g. LA myxoma)	Uncommon.
	↓ LV systolic/diastolic function	Isolated LV diastolic dysfunction not uncommon
	Valvular dysfunction (MR, MS, AR, AS)	If flail leaflet/ruptured papillary muscle suspected then TOE indicated
	Intracardiac shunt	
	Normal	Suggests non-cardiac cause (e.g. ARDS)
Dyspnoea/hypoxia without pulmonary oedema (dyspnoea cause?)	Pulmonary embolism (dilated right heart chambers ± clot in pulmonary artery)	Infers moderate to large clot burden
	Cardiac tamponade	Usually other clinical signs of tamponade present
	Miscellaneous e.g. chronic cor pulmonale, RVH, constrictive pericarditis, diastolic dysfunction, intracardiac shunt, RV volume overload.	
Chest pain of uncertain aetiology (chest pain cause?)	RWMA	Infers presence of coronary artery disease
	Dissecting aortic aneurysm (intimal flap, true/false lumen)	TOE more sensitive than TTE
	Pulmonary embolism (dilated right heart chambers ± clot in pulmonary artery)	Moderate to large embolus
	Pericarditis	Effusion often too small to diagnose with echocardiography
	Aortic stenosis	Clinical signs of stenosis may be absent.

AMI, Acute myocardial infarction; AR, aortic regurgitation; AS, aortic stenosis; ASD, atrial septal defect; IABP, intra-aortic balloon pump; LA, left atrium; LAA, left atrial appendage; LV, left ventricle; LVOT, left ventricular outflow tract; MI, myocardial infarction; MR, mitral regurgitation; MS, mitral stenosis; RA, right atrium; RV, right ventricle; RWMA, regional wall motion abnormality; SAM; TR, tricuspid regurgitation; VSD, ventricular septal defect.

VALVULAR STENOSIS

Narrowing or stenosis of any heart valve obstructs blood flow, increasing velocity and causing a pressure gradient across the valve. Evaluation of valvular stenosis requires: (1) imaging of the valve to define the morphology and mobility of the valve cusps; (2) some quantification of the degree of stenosis; and (3) the effect of pressure overload on relevant cardiac chambers. Transvalvular pressure gradients (ΔP) can be estimated by Doppler techniques (see above). Note that in conditions of low cardiac output, pressure gradients will be low, thereby underestimating the severity of stenosis.

Aortic stenosis

The most common aetiology of valvular aortic stenosis is degeneration and calcification of the valve apparatus although bicuspid aortic valve and rheumatic heart disease may also cause aortic stenosis. Thickening/calcification of relatively immobile valve leaflets cause valvular obstruction and pressure overload resulting in LV hypertrophy. Severe aortic stenosis may occasionally cause sudden collapse, cardiogenic shock, or pulmonary oedema of 'unknown cause'.

Assessment of severity

Visual assessment of aortic valve cusp thickness, calcification, mobility and degree of LV hypertrophy will often indicate the physiological significance of the aortic stenosis. Doppler echocardiography is essential for assessment of severity: (1) peak aortic velocity; (2) mean transvalvular pressure gradient; (3) aortic valve area; and (4) ratio LVOT velocity/aortic valve velocity (V_1/V_2).

- *Peak aortic velocity* (normal ≤1.7 m/s) (Fig. 21.5). In the presence of thickened immobile aortic valve cusps, a peak velocity ≥4.5 m/s (i.e. peak pressure gradient 81 mmHg) almost certainly indicates severe stenosis.
- *Mean transvalvular pressure gradient.* Aortic valve velocity integrated over time is displayed on the monitor and the spectral display traced. A mean pressure gradient ≥50 mmHg suggests severe aortic stenosis. From a practical point of view, a patient with normal LV systolic function, a peak aortic velocity gradient ≤3.0 m/s and a mean pressure gradient ≤30 mmHg is extremely unlikely to have critical aortic stenosis, whereas a patient with thickened aortic leaflets, restricted movement of cusps, aortic velocity >4.5 m/s, and a mean pressure gradient ≥50 mmHg will almost certainly have critical aortic stenosis. Difficulties in assessment of aortic stenosis severity arise in patients with depressed LV function and a peak aortic velocity not greatly increased, typically about 3.0–3.5 m/s, and a transvalvular gradient of 25–30 mmHg. Such patients may have mild to moderate aortic stenosis and unrelated LV dysfunction *or* critical aortic stenosis with severe depression of LV function; dobutamine stress echocardiography

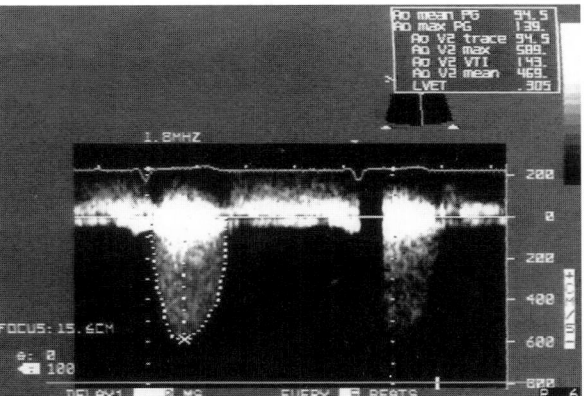

Fig. 21.5 Continuous-wave Doppler recording of an aortic stenosis jet in a patient with critical stenosis. The jet velocity is 589 cm/s (5.89 m/s). The calculated maximum pressure gradient is 139 mmHg. Mean pressure gradient is 94 mmHg

is a useful test to distinguish one condition from another.[15]

- *Aortic valve area* (normal 3–4 cm²). In severe aortic stenosis the aortic valve area is ≤0.75 cm². The aortic valve area is estimated using the *continuity equation*, which is based on the principle: if the volume of blood flow upstream from an orifice is known, then measuring the velocity of blood immediately downstream from the orifice allows calculation of its cross sectional area. According to the formula: $A_1 \times V_1 = A_2 \times V_2$, where A_1 = LVOT cross sectional area, V_1 = LVOT velocity time integral, A_2 = aortic valve cross sectional area, V_2 = aortic velocity time integral. The equation can be rearranged: $A_2 = A_1 \times V_1/V_2$.
- *Ratio of LVOT velocity/aortic valve velocity (V_1/V_2)* provides a 'dimensionless' measurement of aortic stenosis severity which is independent of cardiac output. A velocity ratio (V_1/V_2) of <0.25 implies an aortic valve area of ≤0.75 cm² (i.e. severe aortic stenosis[15]).

Accurate estimation of maximum aortic jet velocity is best obtained by TTE. However, TOE allows planimetry (tracing) of the aortic valve orifice in the short axis view which correlates well with catheter derived aortic valve area.[16] TOE planimetry may be useful in critically ill patients when other data are inconsistent or inconclusive.

Mitral stenosis

Significant mitral stenosis can occasionally contribute to haemodynamic instability in critically ill patients. Dyspnoea has usually been present for many years so that mitral stenosis has been diagnosed prior to admission to intensive care. Mitral stenosis secondary to rheumatic heart disease produces typical M-mode (Fig. 21.1) and 2-D images of thickened and fused mitral valve leaflets with diastolic doming resulting in a 'hockey stick' appearance of the anterior leaflet together with an

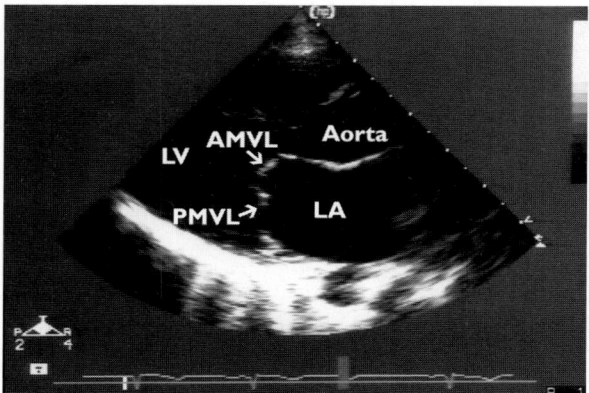

Fig. 21.6   2-D echocardiogram of a patient with mitral stenosis. The left atrium (LA) is enlarged. There is doming of both anterior (AMVL) and posterior (PMVL) leaflets with the typical 'hockey stick' appearance of the anterior leaflet (TTE parasternal long axis)

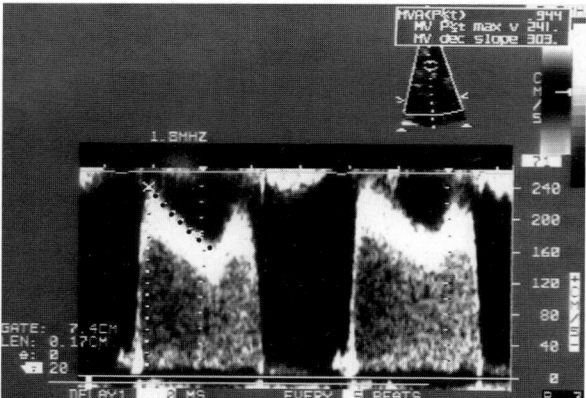

Fig. 21.8   Pressure half time ($P_t\frac{1}{2}$) measurement in a patient with mitral stenosis. The $P_t\frac{1}{2}$ corresponds to a valve area of 0.94 cm^2

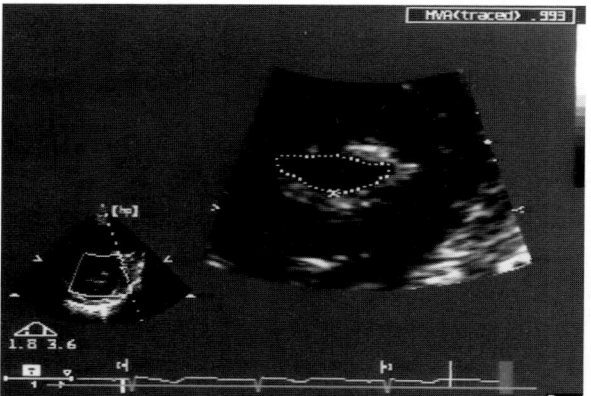

Fig. 21.7   2-D echocardiogram of a patient with mitral stenosis. There is diminished separation between the anterior and posterior leaflets with a typical 'fish mouth' appearance. The valve area by 2-D planimetry is 0.99 cm^2 (TTE parasternal short axis)

enlarged LA (Fig. 21.6). In the short axis view the mitral valve appears as a 'fish mouth' orifice the area of which can be estimated (normal 4–6 cm^2) (Fig. 21.7) using planimetry.

Assessment of severity

In addition to visualization and planimetry of the valve, accurate assessment of mitral valve stenosis requires Doppler echocardiography: (1) peak velocity ('E') across the mitral valve is increased (normal ≤1.3 m/s). In severe mitral stenosis, the 'E' velocity is usually >2 m/s; (2) transvalvular pressure gradient – the mean pressure gradient between the LA and LV is usually >10 mmHg in severe stenosis; (3) pressure half-time ($P_t\frac{1}{2}$) is the

time it takes for the peak pressure gradient to halve. The rate of pressure decline across a stenotic orifice is determined by its cross sectional area (i.e. the smaller the orifice the slower the rate of decline). Pressure half time >220 ms indicates severe mitral stenosis (mitral valve area ≤1 cm^2)[17] (Fig. 21.8). Pulmonary artery pressure should also be estimated (see below).

Tricuspid stenosis and pulmonary stenosis
These disorders can also be diagnosed and quantified using similar echocardiographic techniques.

VALVULAR REGURGITATION
Evaluation of valvular regurgitation requires: (1) assessment of the valve morphology; (2) estimation of severity of regurgitation; and (3) effects of volume overload on relevant cardiac chambers. Mild valvular regurgitation of the mitral, tricuspid and pulmonary valves is common (70–90%) and trivial aortic regurgitation is found in only about 5% of examinations; such findings have no clinical significance.

Aortic regurgitation
2-D echocardiography may show the cause of the aortic regurgitation, for example valve destruction caused by infective endocarditis or a dilated aortic root with aortic dissection or most commonly degenerative calcification disease of aortic valve.

Assessment of severity
Colour flow Doppler imaging allows some grading of severity of regurgitation by comparing the width of the regurgitant jet to the LVOT area (Fig. 21.9). If the jet occupies more than 60% of the LVOT area, then severe aortic regurgitation is probably present.

The velocity of the regurgitant jet is directly related to the pressure gradient between the aortic valve and the

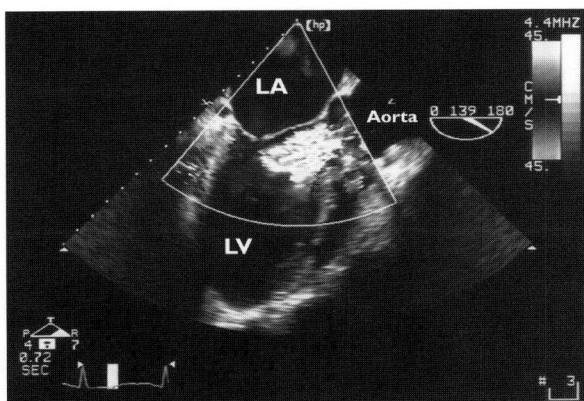

Fig. 21.9 Severe aortic regurgitation; aliased jet occupies entire left ventricular (LV) outflow tract (TOE long axis)

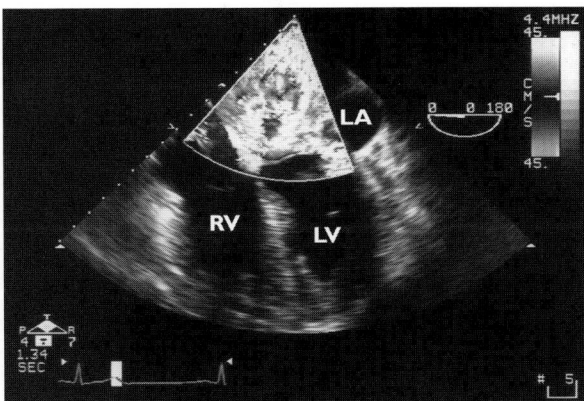

Fig. 21.10 Severe mitral regurgitation secondary to flail posterior mitral valve leaflet (TOE four-chamber)

left ventricle. In severe aortic regurgitation, especially acute, aortic diastolic pressure falls rapidly and LV end-diastolic pressure increases resulting in a rapid decay of the pressure gradient: an aortic regurgitant pressure half-time (≥ 250 m/s) suggests severe regurgitation.[15] Flow reversal downstream during diastole occurs in the descending aorta occurs when aortic regurgitation is severe.

Mitral regurgitation

As with aortic regurgitation, echocardiography is useful in detecting the aetiology and mechanism of mitral regurgitation, such as annular dilation (poor coaptation of leaflets), endocarditis (leaflet destruction/perforation) and chordal or papillary muscle rupture (inadequate leaflet support). In mitral regurgitation, the left ventricle ejects blood both into the aorta and backwards into the LA. Early in the course of mitral regurgitation the increase in stroke volume is achieved by an increase in LV ejection fraction. Thus, a hyperdynamic normal sized left ventricle with normal sized LA implies acute mitral regurgitation. Over time mitral regurgitation causes enlargement of the LA and eventually the left ventricle dilates and LV function becomes less hyperdynamic. This apparent normalization of LV function suggests impaired contractility and increased LA pressure. Pulmonary artery pressure also increases over time.

Assessment of severity

Severity of mitral regurgitation is assessed by colour Doppler imaging of the regurgitant jet. The severity of mitral regurgitation is directly proportional to the size of the regurgitant jet within the LA (Fig. 21.10). Mitral valve colour flow jet reaching the posterior wall of the LA suggests severe mitral regurgitation as does systolic flow reversal in the pulmonary veins. Colour flow mapping of the narrowest cross sectional area of a regurgitant jet (vena contracta) can estimate the severity of the mitral regur-

gitation[18] and this can be done in <1 min.[19] Combining 2-D imaging with spectral Doppler imaging can be used to quantify valvular regurgitation by measuring regurgitant volume (volume of blood that leaks through an incompetent valve) and regurgitant fraction (fraction or percentage of stroke volume that regurgitates).

Another approach for estimating the regurgitant volume is to examine the flow pattern on the LV side of the mitral valve. Proximal isovelocity surface area (PISA): PISA calculations, regurgitant volumes and fractions can be estimated.

Tricuspid regurgitation and pulmonary regurgitation

These disorders can be diagnosed and evaluated using similar principles; for example, severe tricuspid regurgitation causes systolic flow reversal in the hepatic veins.

INFECTIVE ENDOCARDITIS

Infective endocarditis should be suspected in any critically ill patient with sepsis and no obvious source of infection. The echocardiographic hallmark of endocarditis is the presence of vegetation(s) which appear as an echogenic chaotically moving mass attached to a heart valve (Fig. 21.11). The Duke criteria[20,21] integrate clinical, microbiological and echocardiographic information in suspected infective endocarditis. Echocardiographic findings consistent with vegetation or new endocardial infection (abscess, prosthetic valve dehiscence, etc.) are major diagnostic criteria. In some situations, clot, tumour or marantic vegetation may mimic endocarditis. In a patient with endocarditis, echocardiography will: (1) image the vegetation and assess its size; (2) diagnose complications such as paravalvular abscess, fistula etc.; (3) examine underlying valve morphology (e.g. bicuspid aortic valve); (4) diagnose and assess severity of associated valvular regurgitation; (5) assess cardiac function;

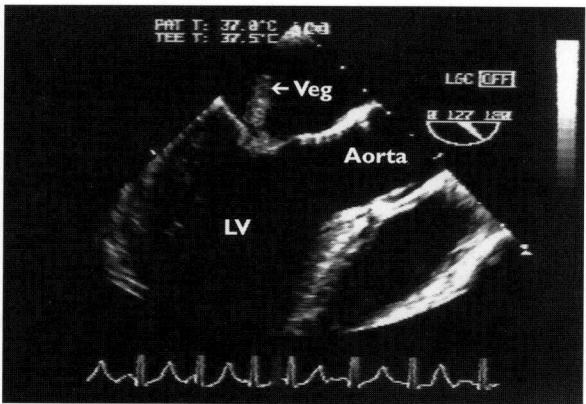

Fig. 21.11 Large vegetation (Veg) on the anterior mitral valve leaflet. The patient presented with septic shock and 'meningitis' and no obvious cardiac murmur (TOE long axis)

and (6) image other heart valves. Large vegetations (>10 mm) increase the risk of embolic events.[22] Detection of vegetations is improved with TOE compared to TTE (TOE 90–100% vs TTE 40–80%).[23] TTE may be adequate to exclude vegetations in patients when clinical suspicion for endocarditis is low[24] provided that image quality is adequate.

About 25% of patients with *Staphylococcus aureus* septicaemia have infective endocarditis even in the absence of obvious clinical signs.[25] TOE is essential for diagnosis and detection of associated complications.

PROSTHETIC VALVES

Echocardiographic examination of prosthetic valves requires knowledge of the various types of valves (bioprosthesis, homograft, mechanical). Blood velocity is nearly always increased through normal prosthetic valves and trivial regurgitation is characteristic of most mechanical valves. Such jets are always small, may be multiple and occur within the sewing ring of the valve. Paravalvular leaks are always abnormal and associated with dehiscence; infective endocarditis should always be considered. Suspected prosthetic valve endocarditis mandates TOE and serial examinations are often necessary. A characteristic rocking motion of the valve is diagnostic of dehiscence. TOE is superior to TTE for assessing mitral regurgitation in patients with prosthetic mitral valves as acoustic shadowing by the mechanical valve of the LA causes poor imaging. In many instances, adequate echocardiographic assessment of prosthetic valves requires combined transthoracic and transoesophageal imaging.

VENTRICULAR FUNCTION AND HAEMODYNAMIC ASSESSMENT

In critically ill patients, echocardiography, especially TOE, has evolved as an independent approach in the

assessment and monitoring of cardiovascular haemodynamics. Cardiac systolic function is directly visualized and other parameters can be measured.

LEFT VENTRICLE (LV)

2-D and M-mode echocardiography allow accurate measurements of LV dimensions and wall thickness.

Systolic function

Echocardiography provides global and regional estimates of LV performance.

Global LV function

In intensive care patients, the two parameters most frequently used to assess LV global systolic function are ejection fraction and cardiac output.

Ejection fraction (EF)

The EF is the percentage of the LV diastolic volume that is ejected with each heart beat (normal EF >50%). It should be appreciated that EF is the result of complex interactions between ventricular loading conditions and contractile state, and may not always reflect true ventricular contractility. Nevertheless, EF is extremely useful and can be estimated using various techniques. (1) Visual inspection of 2-D images. Although widely used, this method is subjective. (2) The American Society of Echocardiography recommends the modified *Simpson's* rule where LV volumes are measured in two orthogonal views (apical four-chamber and apical two-chamber) (Fig. 21.12a–d). The LV endocardial border is traced at end-diastole and end-systole. The ventricle is considered to be a series of discs which are summated. Calculation of LV end-diastolic and end-systolic volumes, although complicated, is easily computed using modern echocardiographic machines.

$$EF = \frac{EDV - ESV}{EDV} \times 100$$

where EDV = LV end-diastolic volume and ESV = LV end-systolic volume.

Fractional area of change (FAC)

Unlike EF, FAC measures LV area, and not volume. The measurement is performed at papillary muscle level and does not take into account regional wall motion abnormalities at LV apex and/or base. Normal FAC ≥36%. FAC may be measured (1) by visual inspection which is widely used but subjective or (2) more accurately by tracing the LV endocardial border at end-diastole (EDA) and end-systole (ESA) in the short axis view at the mid-papillary muscle level.

$$FAC = \frac{EDA - ESA}{EDA}$$

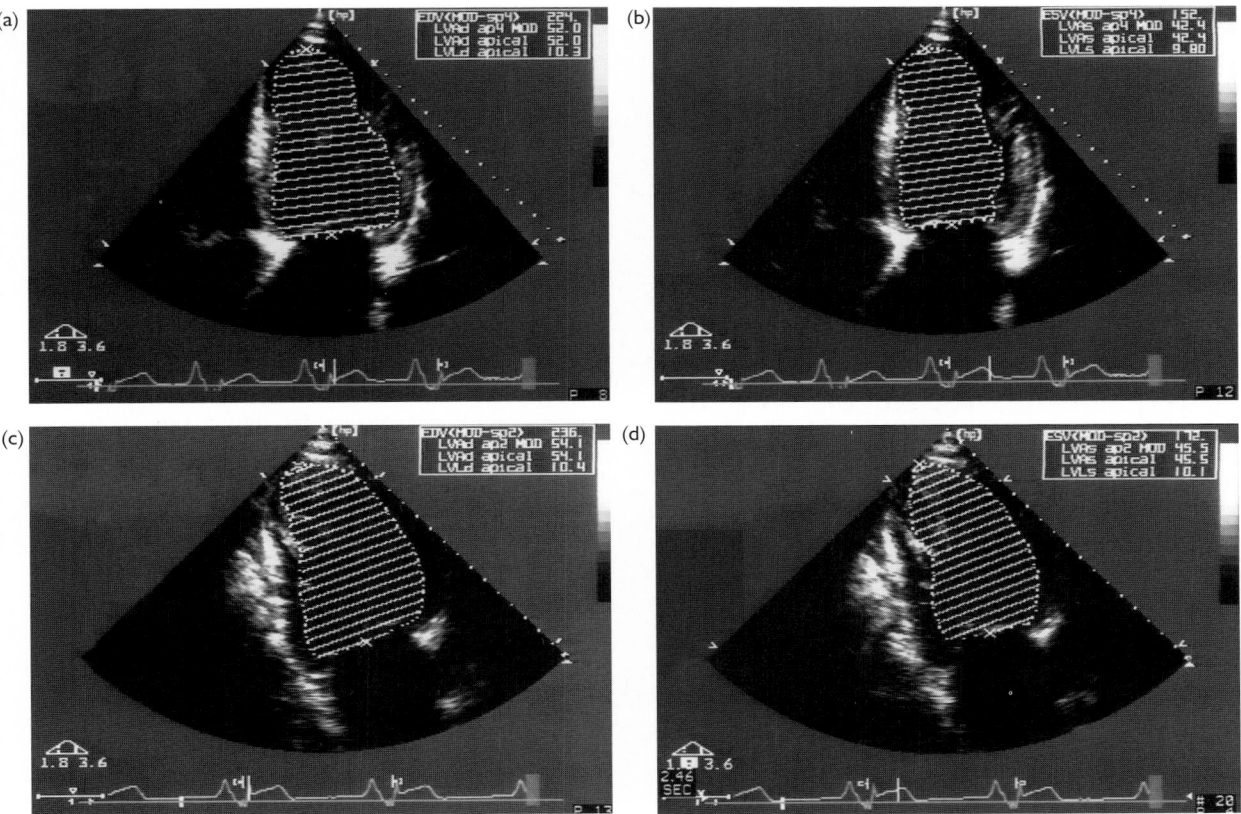

Fig. 21.12   Left ventricular (LV) ejection fraction estimation using modified Simpson's rule. The long axis of the LV is divided into a series of discs from base to apex; the LV endocardial border is traced in end-diastole (LVED) and end-systole (LVES) in two orthogonal views: apical (a) LVED, (b) LVES; four-chamber (c) LVED, (d) LVES two-chamber

Regional LV function

Assessment of LV regional wall motion analysis is based on grading the contractility of individual segments: 1 = normal, 2 = hypokinesis, 3 = akinesis, 4 = dyskinesis, 5 = aneurysmal. The American Society of Echocardiography divides the LV into 16 segments (six at the base, six at the mid-ventricular level and four at the apex) (Fig. 21.13).

Stroke volume and cardiac output

Doppler derived blood flow velocities can be used to quantify cardiac output. The technique is based on the principle that the velocity-time integral (VTI) of blood flow multiplied by the cross sectional area (CSA) of its orifice yields an estimate of stroke volume (SV = CSA × VTI) (Fig. 21.14a,b). The LVOT is the most commonly used site for stroke volume and cardiac output estimation. In general, correlation between echocardiographic and thermodilution derived cardiac output have been reasonable,[26,27] although neither method is a 'gold standard'.

Preload (LV end-diastolic volume)

The assessment of LV end-diastolic volume (LVEDV) is often important in critically ill patients. Significant hypovolaemia is inferred by LV end-systolic cavity obliteration. Although a presumptive diagnosis of hypovolaemia can often be made with such echo signs, other causes of end-systolic cavity obliteration, such as decreased systemic vascular resistance, severe mitral or aortic regurgitation, or ventricular septal defect, must be considered. Integrating the clinical picture together with colour flow Doppler and, if necessary, quantitative assessment of preload, differentiates between the various diagnoses.

LV end diastolic area (short axis at papillary muscle level: normal = 15–35 cm²)[28] assessment is a quick and relatively simple method for estimating preload.[29] Nevertheless, modified Simpson's rule technique is the most accurate echocardiographic method for measuring LVEDV/preload in clinical practice (Fig. 21.12a,c).

Afterload

End-systolic wall stress [where wall stress = (pressure × radius)/2 × wall thickness)] determined by

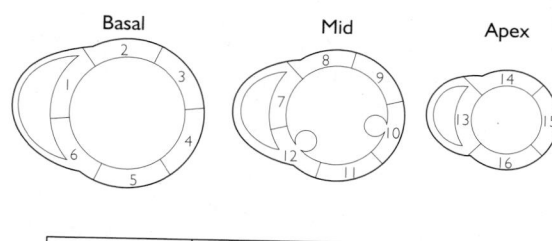

Segment level	AS	Ant	Lat	Post	Inf	Sep
Basal	1	2	3	4	5	6
Mid	7	8	9	10	11	12
Apex	13	14	15	—	16	13

Fig. 21.13 Regional wall motion analysis. AS, Anteroseptum; Ant, anterior; Lat, lateral; post, posterior; Inf, inferior; Sep, septum

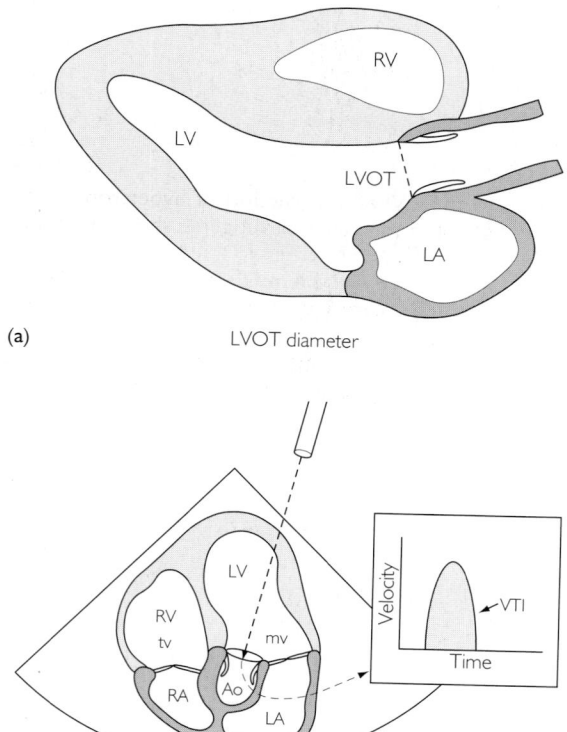

(a)   LVOT diameter

(b)

Fig. 21.14 Calculation of stroke volume (SV) using the left ventricular outflow tract (LVOT).
(a) LVOT diameter ($LVOT_d$) is measured from parasternal long axis view. $LVOT_{CSA} = 0.785 \times (LVOT_d)^2$, where $LVOT_{CSA}$ is the LVOT cross-sectional area.
(b) $LVOT_{VTI}$ measured using PW Doppler (apical five-chamber or long axis view), where $LVOT_{VTI}$ is the velocity time integral.
$SV = LVOT_{CSA} \times LVOT_{VTI}$

echocardiography, provides an index of LV afterload. This is rarely used in clinical practice.

Diastolic function

The non-invasive assessment of LV diastolic dysfunction has seen major advances in recent years.[30,31] Diastolic dysfunction is a disorder of LV filling, where the LV is unable to fill to a normal end-diastolic volume without an abnormal increase in end-diastolic pressure. All patients with LV systolic dysfunction have some degree of LV diastolic dysfunction. Some patients with congestive cardiac failure have systolic function with isolated diastolic heart failure. Recently, Gandhi *et al.*,[32] using echocardiography, demonstrated that pulmonary oedema in patients with marked systemic hypertension is commonly due to isolated diastolic dysfunction. Mitral and pulmonary inflow patterns are Doppler techniques routinely used to diagnose diastolic dysfunction and assess severity. More recently, tissue Doppler[33] which records the slower velocity within myocardial tissue, such as the mitral valve annulus, has been used as a complementary technique.

RIGHT VENTRICLE (RV)

Evaluation of right sided heart function is important in critically ill patients.

Chamber size

The normal shape of the RV is a crescent, curving in front of, and concave towards, the LV. A combination of image planes is necessary to assess RV size. Ventricular dilation may be due to right sided volume overload secondary to conditions such as tricuspid regurgitation, pulmonary regurgitation or atrial septal defect. Colour flow Doppler and occasionally i.v. injection of a contrast agent such as agitated saline will help distinguish the aetiology.

Wall thickness

RV hypertrophy (due to pressure overload) leads to increased thickness of the RV free wall.

Systolic function

Right ventricular end-diastolic volume assessment is difficult because the shape of the RV and the presence of prominent trabeculations make the endocardial border difficult to outline. TOE is essential for assessing RV dysfunction following cardiac transplantation.

Detection of regional wall motion abnormalities are sensitive and specific markers of RV ischaemia or infarction.[34] The diagnosis of cardiac contusion which occurs commonly after blunt chest trauma is often unrecognized and can be readily made by TOE.[35]

Pulmonary artery pressure

This is an important and routine part of assessing RV function. Some tricuspid regurgitation is present in >90% of the adult population. The simplified Bernoulli equation is used: RV systolic pressure is obtained by adding right atrial pressure (RAP) to the transtricuspid gradient derived from the peak tricuspid regurgitation velocity (V_{tr}) measured by Doppler (Fig. 21.15). In the absence of pulmonary stenosis, systolic RV pressure = systolic PA pressure.

CARDIOMYOPATHIES

A simple classification of the cardiomyopathies includes: dilated, hypertrophic, restrictive.

DILATED CARDIOMYOPATHY

All echocardiographic features of dilated cardiomyopathy are non-specific, but LV dilation and reduced global systolic function is characteristic. Both LV end-diastolic and LV end-systolic volumes are increased with ejection fraction and fractional area of change uniformly reduced. Mural thrombus may be present. The RV may also be affected. There may be atrial enlargement. Due to the increased LV end-diastolic volume, stroke volume and cardiac output may be preserved at rest. Significant mitral regurgitation, secondary to annular dilation and poor coaptation of the mitral leaflets, may be present. Diastolic dysfunction is invariably present and is an important prognostic feature.[35] Pulmonary hypertension estimated from tricuspid regurgitation velocity may predict a poor prognosis.

HYPERTROPHIC CARDIOMYOPATHY

In critically ill patients, the diagnosis cannot be made without the assistance of echocardiography where asym-

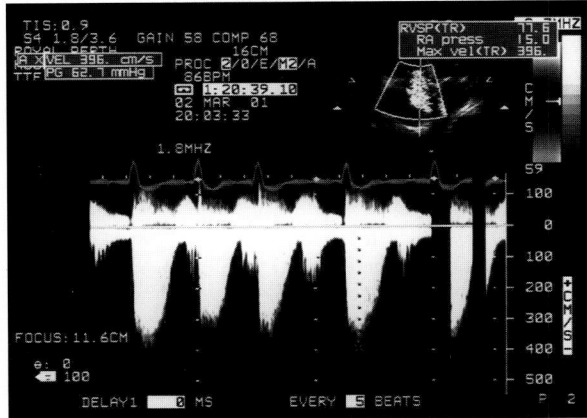

Fig. 21.15 Estimation of right ventricular systolic pressure (RVSP) and systolic pulmonary artery pressure (SPAP) in the presence of tricuspid regurgitation (TR). Peak TR velocity (V_{TR}) measured by CW Doppler is 396 cm/s (3.9 m/s). RA pressure (from CVP) = 15 mmHg. Difference in pressure between RA and RV (using Bernouilli equation) is $4 \times (V_{TR}^2)$ [i.e. $4 \times (3.9)^2 = 62$]. Therefore RVSP = 15 + 62 = 77 mmHg. In the absence of pulmonary stenosis RVSP = SPAP

metrical septal hypertrophy, the most common feature, can be readily identified and quantified, as can a variety of other hypertrophic patterns. In the elderly, a normal proximal septal bulge ('sigmoid septum') should not be confused with true hypertrophic cardiomyopathy.

Ventricular outflow tract obstruction

During systole, the anterior leaflet of the mitral valve moves anteriorly toward the interventricular septum and may obstruct the LVOT. The LVOT obstruction is dependent on loading conditions and may be absent at rest. Indeed, the dynamic nature of the LVOT obstruction is one of the hallmarks of this condition. The systolic anterior motion (SAM) of the leaflet distorts the mitral valve causing mitral regurgitation. Colour flow (and PW) Doppler not only localize the site of LVOT obstruction, but also quantify the degree of mitral regurgitation. The severity of LVOT obstruction can be estimated by CW Doppler. Although the degree of obstruction may vary, a peak gradient ≥50 mmHg indicates significant LVOT obstruction.

Dynamic LVOT obstruction without asymmetrical septal hypertrophy[36]

Dynamic LVOT obstruction with SAM can occur whenever a hyperdynamic state exists, especially in elderly patients with hypovolaemia and a septal bulge ('sigmoid' septum). The haemodynamic effects of this condition are identical to the LVOT obstruction of hypertrophic cardiomyopathy and can cause cardiogenic shock. Dynamic LVOT obstruction may be precipitated or worsened by positive inotropic or vasodilator therapy and intra-aortic balloon pumping. In hypotensive patients, a paradoxical haemodynamic response to conventional inotropic therapy is an indication for TOE. The LVOT gradient can usually be abolished by ensuring adequate volume replacement, avoiding positive inotropic agents and increasing afterload by administration of an agent such as phenylephrine (a pure α-agonist).

RESTRICTIVE CARDIOMYOPATHY

Primary restrictive cardiomyopathy is characterized by impaired LV filling secondary to idiopathic myocardial stiffening. Echocardiographic findings usually include marked biatrial enlargement with normal LV cavity size and wall thickness and normal or slightly reduced systolic function. A characteristic restrictive mitral inflow pattern is present.

Secondary restrictive cardiomyopathy has a similar abnormal diastolic filling pattern secondary to a known myocardial cause (e.g. amyloidosis).

PERICARDIAL DISEASE

PERICARDIAL EFFUSION AND TAMPONADE

Echocardiography is the accepted gold standard for both the diagnosis of pericardial effusion and its haemody-

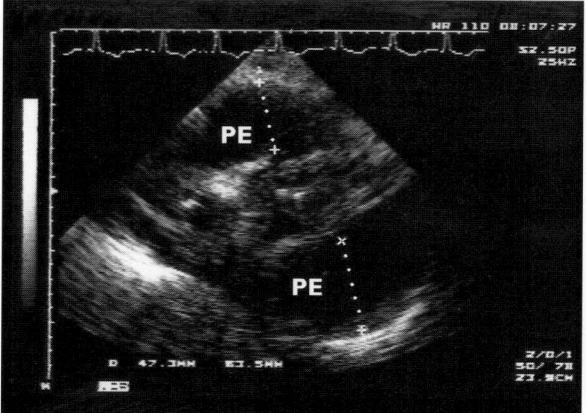

Fig. 21.16 Massive (5 cm) pericardial effusion (PE) in a patient with tamponade (TTE subcostal)

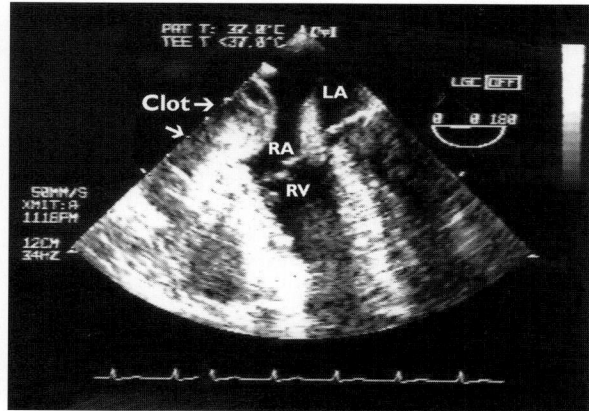

Fig. 21.17 Localized clot compressing mainly the right heart in a patient after cardiac surgery (TOE four-chamber)

namic significance. Pericardial fluid or blood can be recognized on 2-D as an 'echo free' space around the heart (Fig. 21.16). Whenever a pericardial effusion is imaged, the possibility of tamponade should be considered. When the effusion within the pericardial sac is large enough, intrapericardial pressure exceeds RV diastolic pressure and cardiac tamponade occurs causing impaired cardiac filling and low cardiac output. 2-D echocardiographic features of cardiac tamponade[3] may include: (1) moderate to large pericardial effusion (usually). However, it should be appreciated that a small rapidly accumulating effusion (50–100 ml) can increase intrapericardial pressure acutely and tamponade the heart. Conversely, a large slowly increasing effusion, sometimes over 1 l in volume, may have little effect on intrapericardial pressure and cause no haemodynamic embarrassment; (2) the heart may swing excessively in the pericardial sac. Electrocardiographically this may manifest as electrical alternans; (3) early diastolic collapse of the RV free wall is more specific (85–100%) but less sensitive (60–90%) for cardiac tamponade than (4) late diastolic atrial collapse. Sustained (≥30% of cardiac cycle) RA collapse is more likely to be significant than brief collapse; (5) respiratory variation in diastolic filling is manifested clinically by pulsus paradoxus. Doppler echocardiography demonstrates a similar phenomenon, namely exaggerated increase in tricuspid and decrease in mitral valve diastolic inflow with inspiration. The inferior vena cava is usually dilated and its diameter does not vary with respiration in patients with cardiac tamponade. Doppler examination of the hepatic veins is also very important.

Echocardiography may also be used to guide pericardiocentesis by locating the optimal site for puncture and monitoring the residual effusion after drainage.[37] As 2-D echocardiography is a tomographic imaging technique, the needle tip is often difficult to visualize.

CARDIAC TAMPONADE OCCURRING AFTER CARDIAC SURGERY

The tamponade may be localized with differential compression of the right or left sided chambers and the clot is usually 'echo dense' with little or no 'echo free' space around the heart (Fig. 21.17). Localized tamponade (e.g. of the RA or LA) is not uncommon in such patients. Not surprisingly, standard echocardiographic criteria, such as intermittent chamber collapse, are unreliable in detecting tamponade after cardiac surgery. The presence of ≥1 cm of pericardial separation (fluid/clot) in a patient with unexplained clinical deterioration (hypotension, decreased cardiac output) appears to be sensitive in detecting tamponade.[38] In the absence of tamponade, other causes of hypotension, such as unsuspected hypovolaemia, ventricular dysfunction or LVOT obstruction, may be diagnosed by echocardiography. Indeed, unnecessary reoperation may be prevented in some instances.

CONSTRICTIVE PERICARDITIS

Echocardiography is of value in the diagnosis of constrictive pericarditis. There is often thickening of the pericardium which may be imaged with 2-D echocardiography. Doppler studies of the tricuspid, mitral and pulmonary veins may show typical findings.

CARDIAC MASSES

Before any diagnosis is made of a cardiac mass, it is essential to rule out pseudo-masses (i.e. artefacts or normal cardiac structures). TOE is usually more sensitive than TTE. Intracardiac masses include thrombi, tumours and vegetations.

INTRACARDIAC THROMBUS

Thrombi can occur in any cardiac chamber but are most common in the LV (often at the apex) and the LA (usually in the LA appendage). Low flow states manifest as spontaneous echocardiographic contrast or echocardiographic 'smoke' and is a precursor of clot formation and thromboemboli. LV clot (Fig. 21.18) nearly always occurs after myocardial infarction with associated regional wall motion abnormality or in patients with dilated cardiomyopathy and severe global depression of LV systolic function. TTE is more sensitive than TOE for detection of LV apical clot. LA clot is much more common than RA clot and usually occurs in the setting of atrial fibrillation or mitral stenosis. TOE provides vastly superior images compared to TTE as LA clot is usually located in or near the LA appendage which is poorly visualized with TTE. Conventional management for patients with AF ≥ 48 h requires therapeutic anticoagulation for 3 weeks before planned cardioversion. Another approach necessitates LA clot exclusion by TOE. If there is no LA clot, then cardioversion may proceed immediately, otherwise cardioversion is delayed. This TOE based strategy has been shown to be associated with low embolic rates and a shorter time to cardioversion compared to conventional strategy.[39]

CARDIAC TUMOURS

LA myxoma is by far the most common benign cardiac tumour and can often be imaged by TTE, although superb images can be obtained with TOE. The tumour is usually attached by a pedicle to the interatrial septum. During diastole, the tumour may obstruct the mitral valve orifice. Rarely, other tumours, primary or metastatic, may be visualized.

AORTIC DISEASE

TOE is paramount for diagnosing aortic pathology in critically ill patients because of its accuracy, portability, real time imaging and low complication rate.

AORTIC DISSECTION[40]

TOE is very useful for diagnosing aortic dissection. The average time to diagnosis with TOE is 15 min.[41] The sensitivity and specificity of TOE in diagnosis of aortic dissection is equivalent to that of computed tomography (CT), magnetic resonance imaging (MRI) or angiography.[41,42] 2-D echocardiography will reveal the intimal flap (Fig. 21.19) which is the hallmark of aortic dissection. Colour flow Doppler is useful in differentiating true from false lumen: (1) the false lumen is usually larger with slower flow; (2) the intimal flap pulsates in systole towards the false lumen because of the higher pressure in the true lumen. The entry point of the tear and the presence and extent of aortic regurgitation can also be evaluated.

INTRAMURAL HAEMATOMA (IMH)[43]

Intramural haematoma represents a variant of aortic dissection with virtually identical clinical presentation. Indeed, it may be an early finding in patients who develop classical aortic dissection or rupture. IMH cannot be diagnosed by angiography as there is no

(a)

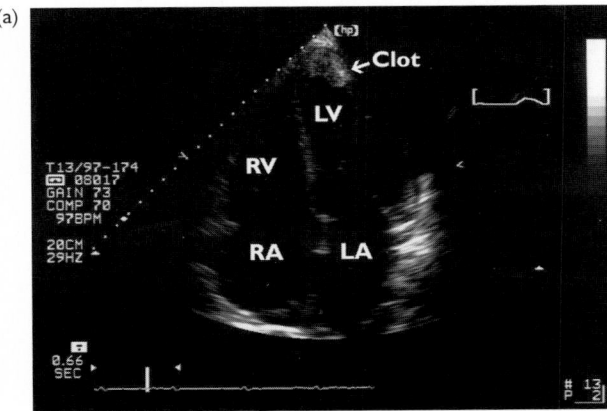

(b)

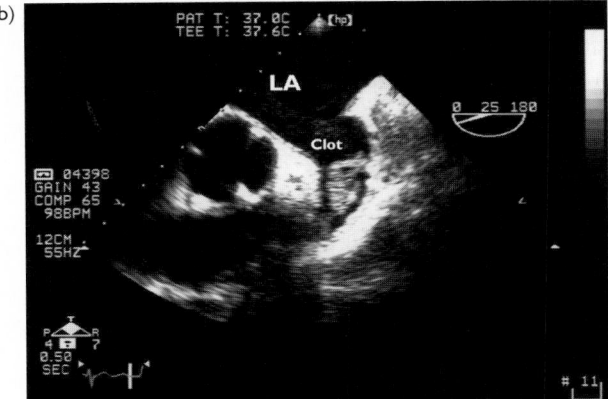

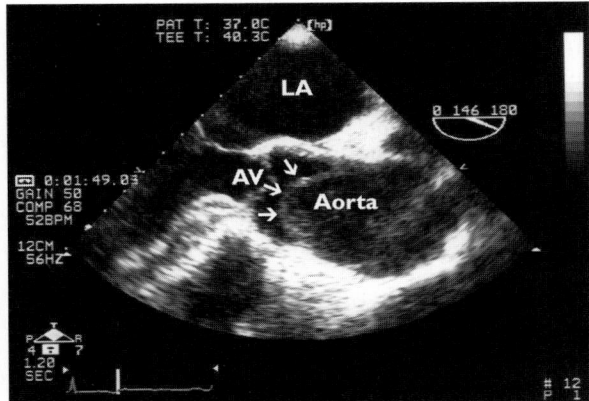

Fig. 21.18 (a) Left ventricular (LV) apical clot. There was an associated regional wall motion abnormality (TTE apical four-chamber). (b) Clot in left atrial appendage

Fig. 21.19 Aortic dissection involving the ascending aorta – the intimal flap (arrows) impinges on the aortic valve (AV) cusps during diastole (TOE)

intimal flap. 2-D echocardiography identifies IMH as a (>0.7 cm) circular or crescentric thickening of the aortic wall or an echo-lucent zone in the aortic wall. There may be a thrombus-like echo pattern of the aortic wall.

TRAUMATIC AORTIC RUPTURE

TOE is both sensitive and specific for the diagnosis of aortic trauma.[44] The echocardiographic signs of aortic injury may include an intimal flap, aortic wall haematoma, aortic occlusion and fusiform aneurysm. Echocardiographic assessment for aortic injury requires an experienced operator.

AORTIC ATHEROSCLEROSIS

TOE allows imaging of aortic plaques which may be layered and immobile or pedunculated/sessile and liable to embolize systemically. On occasions, the aetiology of stroke, renal failure or peripheral vascular ischaemia in critically ill patients may become apparent after echocardiographic examination of the aorta.

PENETRATING ATHEROSCLEROTIC ULCER

This is an ulceration of an atherosclerotic lesion which penetrates the elastic lamina, resulting in haematoma within the media of the aortic wall. It usually occurs in the descending aorta but may also occasionally occur in the ascending aorta. Aortic pseudoaneuryms or occasionally aortic rupture may be due to progressive penetration of the ulcer. TOE is usually necessary for the diagnosis.

AORTIC ANEURYSM

Aneurysms of the aorta can easily be evaluated with echocardiography. Long-term follow-up of thoracic aneurysms without dissection usually utilizes CT or MRI.

PULMONARY EMBOLISM

Pulmonary embolism causes acute obstruction of the pulmonary vasculature and haemodynamic compromise. Although there are many other potential causes of hypotension, echocardiography is extremely useful to exclude massive pulmonary embolism[45] (i.e. embolism involving two or more lobar arteries) as it invariably causes acute cor pulmonale. The RV is acutely overloaded causing distension and 'rounding' of the RV (RV to LV ratio >0.6 in four-chamber view). The RV hypokinesis is characteristic with sparing of the apex (McConnells sign).[46] The interventricular septum bulges into the LV cavity resulting in LV diastolic dysfunction. The LV cavity is usually small and appears 'undervolumed'. Significant RV hypertrophy is absent. Pulmonary hypertension is moderate and its severity can be estimated from the tricuspid regurgitant jet. Clot can also on occasions be directly imaged with TOE in the right heart cavity or proximal pulmonary arteries (Fig. 21.20).

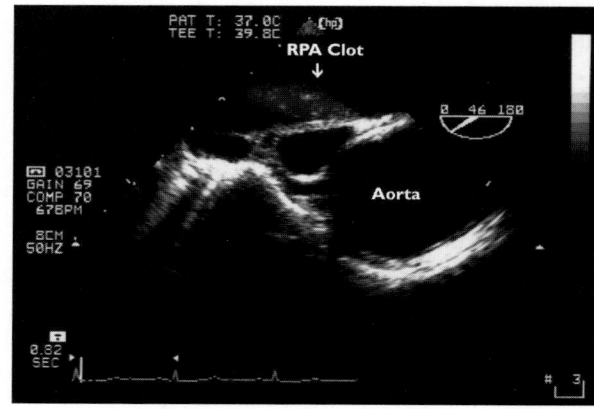

Fig. 21.20   Clot in right pulmonary artery (RPA) in a patient with massive pulmonary embolus (TOE)

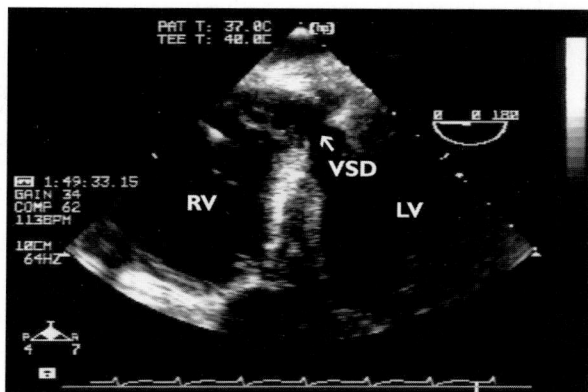

Fig. 21.21   Large ventricular septal defect (VSD) in a shocked patient with a recent myocardial infarction (TOE deep gastric)

Echocardiography is both sensitive and specific for the diagnosis of massive pulmonary embolism.[45] It should be appreciated that echocardiography is insensitive for the diagnosis of smaller pulmonary emboli where haemodynamic compromise is usually absent.

CONGENITAL HEART DISEASE

Echocardiography is essential for the evaluation of patients with known or suspected congenital heart disease. However, it is unusual for adult patients to present to intensive care with undiagnosed haemodynamically significant congenital heart disease. The transoesophageal approach is often necessary in critically ill adult patients with suspected congenital heart disease. Congenital heart abnormalities, such as patent foramen ovale atrial septal defect, ventricular septal defect, patent ductus arteriosis and coarctation of the aorta, can be diagnosed.

Non-congenital ventricular septal defect (e.g. complicating acute myocardial infarction or trauma) is easily diagnosed using either TTE or TOE (Fig. 21.21).

REFERENCES

1 Heidenreich PA. Transesophageal echocardiography (TEE) in the critical care patient. *Cardiol Clin* 2000; **18**: 789–805.

2 Colreavy F, Donovan KD, Lee KY, Weekes JW. Transoesophageal echocardiography in critically ill patients. *Crit Care Med* 2002; **30**: 989–96.

3 Otto CM. Principles of echocardiographic image acquisition and Doppler analysis. In: Otto CM (ed). *Textbook of Clinical Echocardiography*. Philadelphia: WB Saunders Company; 2000: pp. 1–29.

4 Barnett SB, Kossoff G, Edwards MJ. Is diagnostic ultrasound safe? Current international consensus on the thermal mechanism. *Med J Aust* 1994; **160**: 33–7.

5 Daniel WG, Erbel R, Kasper W, *et al.* Safety of transesophageal echocardiography. A multicentre survey of 10 419 examinations. *Circulation* 1991; **83**: 817–21.

6 Mentec H, Vignon P, Terre S, *et al.* Frequency of bacteremia associated with transesophageal echocardiography in intensive care unit patients: a prospective study of 139 patients. *Crit Care Med* 1995; **23**: 1194–9.

7 Spencer KT, Bednarz J, Rafter PG, *et al.* Use of harmonic imaging without echocardiographic contrast to improve two-dimensional image quality. *Am J Cardiol* 1998; **82**: 794–9.

8 Shanewise JS, Cheung AT, Aronson S, *et al.* ASE/SCA guidelines for performing a comprehensive intraoperative multiplane transesophageal echocardiography examination: recommendations of the American Society of Echocardiography Council for Intraoperative Echocardiography and the Society of Cardiovascular Anesthesiologists Task Force for Certification in Perioperative Transesophageal Echocardiography. *J Am Soc Echocardiogr* 1999; **12**: 884–900.

9 Flachskampf FA, Decoodt P, Fraser AG, *et al.* Guidelines from the working group: recommendations for performing transoesophageal echocardiography. *Eur J Echocardiogr* 2001; **2**: 8–21.

10 Weiss Y, Pollak A, Gilon D. The application of transesophageal echocardiography in critical care medicine. *Curr Opin Crit Care* 1997; **3**: 232–7.

11 Heidenreich PA, Stainback RF, Redberg RF, *et al.* Transesophageal echocardiography predicts mortality in critically ill patients with unexplained hypotension. *J Am Coll Cardiol* 1995; **26**: 152–8.

12 Oh JK, Seward JB, Khandheria BK, *et al.* Transesophageal echocardiography in critically ill patients. *Am J Cardiol* 1990; **66**: 1492–5.

13 Cheitlin MD, Alpert JS, Armstrong WF, *et al.* ACC/AHA guidelines for the clinical application of echocardiography. *Circulation* 1997; **95**: 1686–744.

14 Bonow RO, Carabello B, de Leon AC, *et al.* ACC/AHA practice guidelines: guidelines for the management of patients with valvular heart disease. *Circulation* 1998; **98**: 1949–84.

15 Oh JK, Seward JB, Tajik AJ. Valvular heart disease. In: Oh JK, Seward JB, Tajik AJ (eds). *The Echo Manual*. Philadelphia: Lippincott Williams & Wilkins; 1999: pp. 103–32.

16 Shively BK. Transesophageal echocardiographic (TEE) evaluation of the aortic valve, left ventricular outflow tract, and pulmonic valve. *Cardiol Clin* 2000; **18**: 711–29.

17 Hatle L, Angelsen B, Tromsdal A. Noninvasive assessment of atrioventricular pressure half-time by Doppler ultrasound. *Circulation* 1979; **60**: 1096–104.

18 Hall SA, Brickner E, Willett DL, *et al.* Assessment of mitral regurgitation severity by Doppler color flow mapping of the vena contracta. *Circulation* 1997; **95**: 636–42.

19 Thomas JD. How leaky is that mitral valve? Simplified Doppler methods to measure regurgitant orifice area. *Circulation* 1997; **95**: 548–50.

20 Durack DT, Lukes AS, Bright DK. New criteria for diagnosis of infective endocarditis: utilization of specific echocardiographic findings. Duke Endocarditis Service. *Am J Med* 1994; **96**: 200–09.

21 Bayer AS, Ward JI, Ginzton LE, Shapiro SM. Evaluation of new clinical criteria for the diagnosis of infective endocarditis. *Am J Med* 1994; **96**: 211–19.

22 Tischler MD, Vaitkus PT. The ability of vegetation size on echocardiography to predict clinical complications: a meta-analysis. *J Am Soc Echocardiogr* 1997; **10**: 562–8.

23 Shively BK, Gurule FT, Roldan CA, *et al.* Diagnostic value of transesophageal compared with transthoracic echocardiography in infective endocarditis. *J Am Coll Cardiol* 1991; **18**: 391–7.

24 Lindner JR, Case A, Dent JM, *et al.* Diagnostic value of echocardiography in suspected endocarditis. An evaluation based on pretest probability of disease. *Circulation* 1996; **93**: 730–6.

25 Fowler VG, Li J, Corey R, *et al.* Role of echocardiography in evaluation of patients with *Staphylococcus aureus* bacteremia: experience in 103 patients. *J Am Coll Cardiol* 1997; **30**: 1072–8.

26 Descorps-Declere A, Smail N, Vigue B, *et al.* Transgastric, pulsed Doppler echocardiographic determination of cardiac output. *Intensive Care Med* 1996; **22**: 34–8.

27 Muhiudeen IA, Kuecherer HF, Lee E, *et al.* Intraoperative estimation of cardiac output by transesophageal pulsed Doppler echocardiography. *Anesthesiology* 1991; **74**: 9–14.

28 Appendix A. Normal cross sectional echocardiographic measurements. In: Weyman AE (ed). *Principles and Practice of Echocardiography*. Phildelphia: Lea and Febiger; 1994: p. 1292.

29 Cheung AT, Savino JS, Weiss SJ, *et al.* Echocardiographic and haemodynamic indexes of left ventricular preload in patients with normal and abnormal ventricular function. *Anesthesiology* 1994; **81**: 376–87.

30 Appleton CP, Firstenberg MS, Garcia MJ, Thomas JD. The echo-Doppler evaluation of left ventricular dias-

tolic function: a current perspective. *Cardiol Clin* 2000; **18**: 513–46.

31 Vasan RS, Benjamin EJ. Diastolic heart failure – no time to relax. *N Engl J Med* 2001; **344**: 56–9.

32 Gandhi SK, Powers JC, Nomeir A-M, *et al.* The pathogenesis of acute pulmonary edema associated with hypertension. *N Engl J Med* 2001; **344**: 17–22.

33 Gorcsan III J. Tissue Doppler echocardiography. *Curr Opin Cardiol* 2000; **15**: 323–9.

34 Goldstein JA. Right heart ischemia: pathophysiology, natural history, and clinical management. *Progr Cardiovasc Dis* 1998; **40**: 324–41.

35 Weiss RL, Brier JA, O'Connor W, *et al.* The usefulness of transesophageal echocardiography in diagnosing cardiac contusions. *Chest* 1996; **109**: 73–7.

36 Madu EC, Brown R, Geraci SA. Dynamic left ventricular outflow tract obstruction in critically ill patients: role of transesophageal echocardiography in therapeutic decision making. *Cardiology* 1997; **88**: 292–5.

37 Tsang TS, Barnes ME, Hayes SN, *et al.* Clinical and echocardiographic characteristics of significant pericardial effusions following cardiothoracic surgery and outcomes of echo-guided pericardiocentesis for management. Mayo Clinic experience 1979–1998. *Chest* 1999; **116**: 322–31.

38 Bommer WJ, Follette D, Pollock M, *et al.* Tamponade in patients undergoing cardiac surgery: a clinical echocardiographic diagnosis. *Am Heart J* 1995; **130**: 1216–23.

39 Klein AL, Grimm RA, Murray RD. Use of transesophageal echocardiography to guide cardioversion in patients with atrial fibrillation. *N Engl J Med* 2001; **344**: 1411–20.

40 Flachskampf FA, Daniel WG. Aortic dissection. *Cardiol Clin* 2000; **18**: 807–17.

41 Erbel R, Daniel W, Visser C, *et al.*, and the European Co-operative Study Group for Echocardiography. Echocardiography in the diagnosis of aortic dissection. *Lancet* 1989; **1**: 457–61.

42 Armstrong WF, Back DS, Carey LM, *et al.* Clinical and echocardiographic findings in patients with suspected acute aortic dissection. *Am Heart J* 1998; **136**: 1051–60.

43 Mohr-Kahaly S, Erbel R, Kearney P, Puth M, *et al.* Aortic intramural hemorrhage visualized by transesophageal echocardiography: findings and prognostic implications. *J Am Coll Cardiol* 1994; **23**: 658–64.

44 Smith MD, Cassidy JM, Souther S, *et al.* Transesophageal echocardiography in the diagnosis of traumatic rupture of the aorta. *N Engl J Med* 1995; **332**: 356–62.

45 Jardin F. Dubourg O, Bourdarias J-P. Echocardiographic pattern of acute cor pulmonale. *Chest* 1997; **111**: 209–17.

46 McConnell MV, Solomon SD, Rayan ME, *et al.* Regional right ventricular dysfunction detected by echocardiography in acute pulmonary embolism. *Am J Cardiol* 1996; **78**: 469–73.

Part Four

Respiratory Failure

22

Oxygen therapy

T E Oh

Oxygen is required in aerobic metabolic pathways to produce biological energy from food fuels. With inadequate oxygenation, anaerobic metabolism leads to decreased biological energy and harmful lactic acidosis. Oxygen therapy is indicated whenever tissue oxygenation is impaired, in order to allow essential metabolic reactions to occur, and to prevent complications attributed to hypoxaemia.[1,2]

The common clinical indications are:

- Cardiac and respiratory arrest.
- Respiratory failure:
  (a) Type I: hypoxaemia without CO_2 retention (e.g. asthma, pneumonia, pulmonary oedema, and pulmonary embolism);
  (b) Type II: hypoxaemia with CO_2 retention (e.g. chronic bronchitis, chest injuries, unconscious drug overdose, postoperative hypoxaemia, and neuromuscular disease).
- Cardiac failure or myocardial infarction.
- Shock of any cause.

- Increased metabolic demands (e.g. burns, multiple injuries, and severe infections).
- Postoperative states.
- Carbon monoxide poisoning.

ARTERIAL OXYGEN TENSION (PaO$_2$)

Tissue oxygenation depends upon oxygen delivery and extraction. It is difficult to suggest a 'safe' PaO_2 value above which tissue hypoxia does not occur. PaO_2 does not reflect tissue oxygenation, and oxygen extraction mechanisms vary between organs. In general, supplementary oxygen is required when PaO_2 is 60 mmHg (8.0 kPa) or less. Profound hypoxaemia is present and death is imminent, when PaO_2 is less than 30 mmHg (4.0 kPa). The clinical significance of common PaO_2 and saturation (SaO_2) values are listed (Table 22.1).

Table 22.1 Clinical significance of some PaO_2 and SaO_2 values

PaO$_2$		SaO$_2$	
(mmHg)	(kPa)	(%)	Clinical significance
150	20.0	99	Inspired air at sea level
97	12.9	97	Young normal man
80	10.6	95	Young normal man asleep
			Old normal man awake
			Inspired air at 19 000 feet
70	9.3	93	Lower limit of normal
60	8.0	90	Respiratory failure, mild.
			Shoulder of O_2 dissociation curve
50	6.7	85	Respiratory failure, admit to hospital
40	5.3	75	Venous blood, normal
			Arterial, severe respiratory failure
			Acclimatized man at rest at 9000 feet
30	4.0	60	Unconscious if not acclimatized
26	3.5	50	P50 or 50% saturation
20	2.7	36	Acclimatized mountaineer exercising at 19 000 feet
			Hypoxic death

OXYGEN DISSOCIATION CURVE

Tissue oxygenation depends partly on the oxygen dissociation curve. A shift of the curve to the right (Table 22.2) favours Hb unloading of oxygen, and thus oxygen delivery to the tissues. Conversely, a shift to the left (Table 22.2) increases the affinity of Hb for oxygen with reduced tissue oxygenation (see Figure 22.1).

OXYGEN DELIVERY AND CONSUMPTION

Oxygen delivery ($\dot{D}O_2$) to the cells is represented by the oxygen cascade (Table 22.3). Supply of oxygen is dependent upon the Hb, SaO_2, and cardiac output (Q). $\dot{D}O_2$ (or 'oxygen flux') denotes the total amount of oxygen delivered to the body per minute and is given by the equation:

$$\dot{D}O_2 = 1.39 \times Hb \text{ in g/dl} \times \frac{SaO_2}{100} \times \frac{Q}{100} \text{ in ml/min}$$

$$= 1000 \text{ ml/min}$$

(1.39 = oxygen-carrying capacity of Hb in ml/g Hb). The amount of oxygen carried dissolved in blood is negligible.

Hence $\dot{D}O_2$ for a normal adult is approximately 1000 ml/min or 14 ml/kg per min. However, not all of this amount is available for cellular utilization. Oxygen diffuses from tissue capillaries to mitochondria in cells. Mean tissue PO_2 varies from organ to organ, and is higher near capillaries.[3] Although mitochondria in tissue cells may operate at a low PaO_2 of 8–40 mmHg (1.06–5.32 kPa), diffusion requires a capillary-tissue cell gradient. Thus tissue extraction of oxygen from blood is generally limited, and mitochondrial function jeopardized, at a PaO_2 of less than 30 mmHg (4.0 kPa) or a SaO_2 of 30%. The available oxygen/min is therefore less than the supply (by about 250–300 ml/min) and is approximately 700 ml in a normal adult.

Normal oxygen consumption ($\dot{V}O_2$) at rest is about 200–250 ml/min. The oxygen reserve (availability minus consumption) in a normal man at rest is thus about 450–500 ml/min. Some factors in the sick person

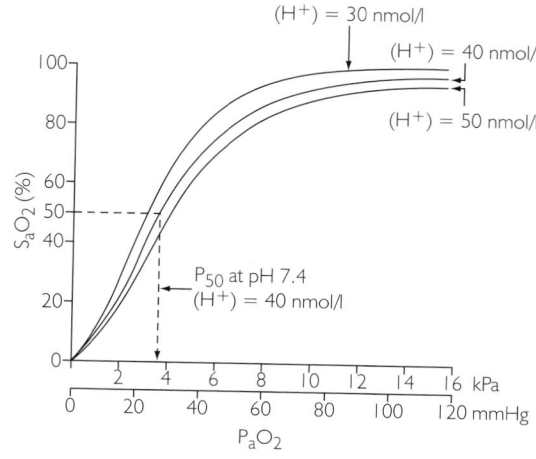

Fig. 22.1 Hb oxygen dissociation curve. Normal curve at 40 nmol/l (H^+) and shifts to left and right. P50 = tension at 50% saturation.

increase oxygen consumption greatly, for example fever, sepsis, shivering, restlessness, and hypercatabolism. When other associated factors concomitantly reduce oxygen supply and availability, oxygen reserve may be reduced to critical levels. A minimal $\dot{D}O_2$ compatible with survival at rest appears to be about 400 ml/min. Thus the use of supplemental oxygen to relieve hypoxaemia must be considered with measures to:

- reduce excessive oxygen requirements (e.g. by cooling, paralysis, and mechanical ventilation)
- increase $\dot{D}O_2$ (by correcting anaemia, low cardiac output, and adverse factors which shift the dissociation curve to the left).

OXYGEN THERAPY APPARATUS AND DEVICES

The basic requirements of apparatus or devices for oxygen therapy (see Table 22.4)[1,2,4] are:

Table 22.2 Factors Influencing the position of the oxygen dissociation curve

Factors increasing P50 (curve shifts to right)	Factors decreasing P50 (curve shifts to left)
Hyperthermia	Hypothermia
Decreased pH (acidaemia)	Increased pH (alkalaemia)
Increased PCO_2 (Bohr effect)	Decreased PCO_2
Increased 2, 3 DPG	Decreased 2, 3 DPG
	Fetal haemoglobin
	Carboxyhaemoglobin
	Methaemoglobin

P50, PaO_2 at 50% saturation; 2, 3 DPG, 2, 3 diphosphoglycerate

Table 22.3 Oxygen cascade. Pressure gradients for oxygen transfer from inspired gas to tissue cells

	mmHg	(kPa)
Inspired air	150	(20.0)
Alveolar	103	(13.7)
Arterial	100	(13.3)
Capillary	51	(6.8)
Tissue	20	(2.7)
Mitochondrial	1–20	(0.13–1.3)

- Control of fractional inspired oxygen concentration (FiO_2)
- Prevention of excessive CO_2 accumulation
- Minimal resistance to breathing
- Efficient and economical use of oxygen
- Acceptance by patients.

Anaesthesia circuits and resuscitator bags are used to pre-oxygenate patients prior to endotracheal intubation. Oxygen administration is thus achieved largely by face-masks or nasal catheters. It is important to know if the FiO_2 delivered by the apparatus will vary with the patient's ventilation. Apart from low-flow breathing circuits, some manual resuscitator bags and ventilators, no device will deliver 100% oxygen, unless the oxygen is supplied at a flow rate greater than peak inspiratory flow rate (PIFR). PIFR in adults is about 25–35 l/min at rest, increasing markedly to over 60 l/min in dyspnoeic states. The apparatus and devices for oxygen therapy are classified below.

FIXED PERFORMANCE SYSTEMS (FiO_2 IS INDEPENDENT OF PATIENT FACTORS)

HIGH-FLOW VENTURI-TYPE MASKS

Oxygen flow entrains air by the venturi principle to deliver a fixed FiO_2. Venturi masks[5] may individually offer separate oxygen concentrations, e.g. 24%, 28%, 35%, 40%. Others use a facemask with a short 'elephant trunk' hose attached to an interchangeable entrainment disc to allow a range of concentrations. The oxygen flow rate is set at 6–8 l/min depending on the FiO_2 chosen, entraining room air to give a resultant total flow rate of 40–60 l/min. Since room air is entrained, the use of a humidifier is not essential. The high-flow system also eliminates rebreathing and the need for a tight fit to the face. However, these masks may not deliver the intended FiO_2 if severe dyspnoea is present.[6,7] The large PIFR in such patients may exhaust the reservoir in smaller volume masks, leading to a lower, fluctuating FiO_2.[7] This is overcome by increasing the oxygen flow rate to 12–14 l/min (to give total entrained inspired gas flows over 60 l/min).

LOW-FLOW BREATHING CIRCUITS

These include anaesthesia circuits and circuits to deliver continuous positive airway pressure (CPAP) or spontaneous PEEP.[8] These circuits incorporate a reservoir bag to deliver an FiO_2 set by the fresh gas mixture, via an endotracheal tube, or tight face mask, or a laryngeal mask.

VARIABLE PERFORMANCE SYSTEMS (FiO_2 DEPENDS UPON OXYGEN FLOW, DEVICE FACTORS AND PATIENT FACTORS)

NO CAPACITY SYSTEM

Nasal catheters at low flow rates (less than 2 l/min; there is insufficient oxygen storage in the nasal passages during the expiratory pause to significantly affect the next inspiration. FiO_2 then depends upon the added oxygen flow rate and the peak inspiratory flow rate. In order to maintain the same FiO_2, the added oxygen flow rate will need to be altered with each change in peak inspiratory flow.

SMALL CAPACITY SYSTEM
Nasal Catheters at High Flows

Some oxygen storage occurs during the expiratory pause, and varies with the length of the pause. With the breath-to-breath variation of PIFR, FiO_2 thus varies with

Table 22.4 Apparatus/devices for oxygen therapy

Apparatus/device	Oxygen flow (l/min)	Concentrations (%)
Nasal catheters	2–6	25–40
Semi-rigid mask (e.g. MC, Edinburgh, Hudson, Harris)	4–15	35–70
Venturi-type mask		
individual concentration masks	24, 28, 35	
interchangeable entrainment discs	6–12	40, 50, 60
Soft plastic masks (e.g. Pneumask, Polymask, Oxyaire)	4–15	40–80
Ventilators	varying	21–100
Anaesthesia circuits	varying	21–100
CPAP circuits	varying	21–100
Plastic head hood	4–8	30–50
Oxygen tent/cot	7–10	60–80
Incubator	3–8	up to 40

Table 22.5 Approximate oxygen concentrations related to flow rates of semi-rigid masks

Oxygen flow rate (l/min)	Approximate FiO$_2$
4	0.35
6	0.50
8	0.55
10	0.60
12	0.65
15	0.70

ventilation. The high flow rates may cause discomfort and drying of nasal mucosa. However, nasal catheters are cheap and easy to use, and the patient is able to eat or drink with them *in situ*. CO_2 rebreathing does not occur.

Simple, Semi-rigid Plastic Masks (MC, Edinburgh, Harris, Hudson)

Since some CO_2 rebreathing occurs, especially at low flows, the oxygen flow rate should be set at 4 l/min or greater. FiO$_2$ varies with patient ventilation and the oxygen flow rate (Table 22.5). A maximum concentration of only 60–70% oxygen is achieved by these masks. Large discrepancies between the delivered FiO$_2$ and that received by the patient (i.e. intratracheal FiO$_2$) occur with increasing rate and depth of breathing (i.e. increased PIFR).[9,10]

Tracheostomy Masks

These are small, plastic masks placed over the tracheostomy tube or stoma. The patient will inspire less oxygen than delivered, as dilution by room air occurs. Otherwise, they perform similarly to simple face masks.

Laryngeal Mask and Simple Plastic Facemask

A simple plastic facemask is commonly placed over the tube connector of an inserted laryngeal mask to deliver oxygen. The inspired oxygen will be limited due to dilution by room air.

T-piece Circuit

A T-piece is a simple, large bore, non-rebreathing circuit attached directly to an endotracheal or tracheostomy tube. Humidified oxygen is delivered through one limb of the T, and expired gas leaves via the other limb. The T-piece can be a fixed performance device if the fresh gas flow rate and the circuit volume are higher than the patient's PIFR.

Face Tent

This is a large, semi-rigid plastic half-mask which wraps around the chin and cheeks. The oxygen mixture is delivered from the bottom of the mask, and gases are exhaled through the open, upper part. It is used to provide added humidification from a heated humidifier.

Otherwise it has no advantages over the simple face mask.

LARGE CAPACITY SYSTEM

Significant oxygen and CO_2 storage (i.e. rebreathing) occurs in these devices.

Soft Plastic Masks (e.g. Pneumask, Polymask, Oxyaire)

These masks have an added reservoir bag and thus a large effective dead space. FiO$_2$s greater than semi-rigid masks are possible, but considerable CO_2 rebreathing occurs if the oxygen supply fails or is reduced. They are potentially dangerous in patients without cardiopulmonary reserve, and should be used with high oxygen flow rates. Rebreathing can be eliminated, and delivered FiO$_2$ increased further, if unidirectional valves are added, but asphyxia may occur in the unconscious patient if a valve becomes faulty. These masks are obsolete but may be present in some institutions.

POSITIVE PRESSURE DEVICES

CPAP maintains a continuous positive airway pressure throughout the spontaneous breathing cycle. Oxygenation is improved mainly as a result of increased functional residual capacity. Lung compliance and work of breathing may also be improved. CPAP can be applied via an endotracheal tube, facemask, or special nasal prongs. Other CPAP modifications such as airway pressure release ventilation (APRV) and bilevel positive airway pressure (BIPAP) can also be applied.

Non-invasive positive pressure ventilation can be delivered using face or nasal masks. This may be able to provide oxygenation and ventilatory support in some patients without endotracheal intubation.

OTHER METHODS OF OXYGENATION

Extracorporeal membrane oxygenation has no benefits over ventilation modes. An intravascular blood gas exchanger (IVOX, an elongated membrane oxygenator to lie within the vena cavae)[11] has been designed, but has not been widely applied.

PAEDIATRIC OXYGEN THERAPY

The PIFR of children, because of their smaller physical size, approximates more closely with the flow rate of oxygen delivery devices. Hence, higher FiO$_2$s are achieved. However, it is difficult to retain nasal catheters and masks on children. A single nasal catheter, placed at the level of the uvula and taped to the face, is well tolerated and is useful in infants and small children.[1]

OXYGEN HEADBOX OR HOOD

Oxygen is delivered into a box encasing the child's head and neck. The FiO_2 depends on the fresh gas flow, size of box, leak around the neck, head position, and how often the box is removed. It is a useful method in infants and small children, but high flow rates should be supplied, and monitoring of oxygen concentration near the face is essential.

INCUBATOR

Incubators provide oxygen as well as a neutral thermal environment. Patient access and recovery of oxygen concentration after opening the incubator are problems. The use of a headbox inside an incubator is common to give a more stable oxygen environment.

OXYGEN COT/TENT

Oxygen cots or tents may be used to nurse larger children. Access, long recovery times for oxygen concentration, and the diffculty in achieving FiO_2s above 0.4 are problems.

HAZARDS OF OXYGEN THERAPY[12]

CO_2 NARCOSIS

When high FiO_2s are administered to patients dependent on a hypoxic (chemoreceptor) drive, e.g. those with acute exacerbation of chronic bronchitis, severe respiratory depression may occur, with loss of consciousness. If this oxygen-induced CO_2 narcosis is suspected, oxygen should not be withdrawn suddenly, as dangerous hypoxaemia will result. Such patients should be encouraged to breathe, or if unconscious, should be immediately ventilated.

OXYGEN TOXICITY

NEUROLOGICAL EFFECTS (PAUL BERT EFFECTS)

Idiopathic epilepsy occurs with exposure to oxygen at more than three atmospheres absolute.

LUNG TOXICITY

Pulmonary toxicity following exposure to high FiO_2s is a recognized clinical problem, but knowledge of the disorder remains limited. Progressive decrease in lung compliance occurs, associated with the development of haemorrhagic interstitial and intra-alveolar oedema, and ultimately, fibrosis. The exact mechanism of the toxic effects of oxygen on the lung remains unknown, but it is believed that oxygen directly effects lung tissue. A biochemical pathogenesis of toxic oxygen free radicals ('reactive oxygen species') causing lung tissue injury is suggested.[13] Normally protective antioxidants in respiratory tract lining fluids (e.g. mucin, uric acid, ascorbic acid, reduced glutathione, superoxide dismutase, and 'sacrificial' proteins) are depleted by a large or prolonged oxidative challenge. Additional indirect factors that have been suggested include increased sympathetic activity, reduced surfactant activity, and absorption collapse. Differentiation of oxygen toxicity from other conditions of lung damage is extremely difficult, and the damage may be a common response to different types of injury.

It is generally agreed that pulmonary oxygen toxicity is dependent upon the duration of exposure and the concentration. However, precise details about 'safe' periods of exposure and 'safe' concentrations are unknown. Individual susceptibility to oxygen damage may vary. Even when using high FiO_2s pulmonary toxicity does not always occur.[14] Damage in healthy lungs can occur, but whether the response is similar in lungs with pre-existing disease remains unclear. In general, clinical signs of toxicity (e.g. dyspnoea, substernal pain, deteriorating gas exchange and X-ray changes) are not usually detected with using oxygen less than 50%,[15] or 100% for short periods less than 24 h.

Bronchopulmonary dysplasia,[16] a paediatric chronic lung disease originating in the neonatal period has similar abnormalities. This is seen when the immature lung is ventilated with high FiO_2s. Pathogenetic contributions of immaturity, oxygen toxicity, and ventilatory pressure are unknown. Excessive ventilating volumes and pressures may be predisposing factors, but oxygen may accelerate the pathological process.

RETROLENTAL FIBROPLASIA[17]

Blindness occurs in premature babies under 1200 g weight (about 28 weeks) exposed to high oxygen concentrations, and relates to PaO_2 and retinal immaturity. Oxygen appears to stimulate immature retinal vessels to spasm and proliferate, resulting in obliteration, haemorrhage, fibrosis, retinal detachment, and blindness. FiO_2 should be restricted to keep PaO_2 between 60–80 mmHg (6.6–10.6 kPa). Oxygen therapy must be closely monitored.

BAROTRAUMA[18]

Alveolar rupture with interstitial and mediastinal emphysema is a disastrous consequence when oxygen flow is inadvertently delivered at wall outlet or cylinder pressure, directly to the patient's airway.

CLINICAL APPLICATION OF OXYGEN

Oxygen is a drug and has to be used correctly. It is given usually as a temporary measure to relieve hypoxaemia, but does not replace definitive treatment of the underlying condition. Oxygen therapy must be assessed by indices of oxygenation (e.g. pulse oximetry SpO_2, arterial blood gases, mixed venous PO_2, and shunt equations. PaO_2 must always be related to FiO_2 and the ventilation pattern; a quoted PaO_2 value by itself is meaningless. Oxygen therapy must be continuous. Intermittent oxygen is harmful, as PaO_2 falls (possibly profoundly) when oxygen is withheld.

Oxygen therapy will correct hypoxaemia from hypoventilation or ventilation:perfusion mismatch. Hypoxaemia due to right-to-left shunting is less responsive, and will usually perisist despite 100% oxygen if the shunt fraction exceeds 20–25%. The lowest FiO_2 to provide adequate oxygenation should be given. However, in profound life-threatening hypoxaemia, high concentrations (even 100%) should never be withheld.

MILD HYPOXAEMIA

Nasal catheters at 2–4 l/min or a simple mask at 4 l/min are suitable.

MODERATE HYPOXAEMIA WITH NORMAL OR LOW PaCO$_2$ (TYPE I RESPIRATORY FAILURE)

A simple mask is used with a flow rate of 4–15 l/min according to the PaO_2 and patient requirements. Extremely dyspnoeic patients with large PIFR will require oxygen delivered as high a flow as possible. The standard oxygen flow meter has a maximum flow rate of only 15 l/min, and may not deliver adequate inspired oxygen. Special high-flow flowmeters or two flowmeters linked by a Y-connector can be used. Oxygen must never be rationed ('asphyxia therapy') in acute asthma[19] and shock.

HYPOXAEMIA WITH INCREASED PaCO$_2$ (TYPE II RESPIRATORY FAILURE)

HYPOVENTILATORY CAUSES

Hypoventilatory causes (e.g. central depression, neuro-muscular dysfunction, head injury, and chest wall abnormalities). A high FiO_2 by simple face mask may be sufficient. Endotracheal intubation may be indicated to protect the airway, and mechanical ventilation is insti-

tuted if ventilatory efforts are inadequate. Restricting oxygen to these patients is illogical and dangerous.

CHRONIC OBSTRUCTIVE AIRWAYS DISEASE

Controlled oxygen therapy with a venturi-type mask is used. A concentration of 24% is started, and blood gases are measured after 30–60 min. If $PaCO_2$ increases less than 10 mmHg (1.3 kPa) and is below 75 mmHg (10 kPa), FiO_2 is increased to 0.28. Since these patients lie on the steep part of the oxygen dissociation curve, a small rise in PaO_2 will result in a relatively large increase in oxygen available to tissues. FiO_2 may be increased further in the same way if hypoxaemia persists. Nasal catheters at low flows may be used but are not ideal. At higher flows, controlled oxygen therapy cannot be achieved with nasal catheters. The concept of limiting FiO_2 for fear of depressing the hypoxic drive to breathe is based on little scientific evidence. In many patients, the danger of hypercarbia is overstressed, and severe hypoxaemia is undertreated.[4,20]

PROFOUND HYPOXAEMIA

Mechanical ventilatory support is indicated. CPAP by mask, or non invasive pressure ventilation may be tried initially in awake patients to avoid intubation. PEEP may be used to help reduce FiO_2.

'SUPRANORMAL' OXYGEN SUPPLY

In normal humans and animals, $\dot{V}O_2$ remains relatively constant over a wide range of $\dot{D}O_2$. This $\dot{V}O_2$ autoregulation is due to increased oxygen extraction as $\dot{D}O_2$ decreases. However, if $\dot{D}O_2$ decreases below a 'critical $\dot{D}O_2$' of 5–10 ml/kg per min, $\dot{V}O_2$ then becomes dependent on $\dot{D}O_2$, denoting inadequate oxygen supply to tissues. Some workers have reported that critical $\dot{D}O_2$ is increased in sepsis and systemic inflammatory response syndrome (to 16–22 ml/kg per min) due to impaired oxygen extraction and increased $\dot{V}O_2$.[21,22] Thus, some workers advocate using 'supranormal' $\dot{D}O_2$ and haemodynamic values (Table 22.6) by increasing FiO_2, haemoglobin, and cardiac output, to achieve adequate tissue oxygenation in these patients. Using this objective, lower mortality figures were reported.[23–25] However, this

Table 22.6 'Supranormal' oxygen delivery end-points

Variable	End-point	(Normal values)
Cardiac index	>4.5 l/min per m^2	(2.5–3.5)
Oxygen delivery index	>650 ml/min per m^2	(400–700)
Systemic vascular resistence	>800 dyne.s/cm^5	(770–1500)
Oxygen consumption index	>170 ml/min per m^2	(130–150)
Pulmonary occlusion pressure	>18 mmHg	(15)

'pathological supply dependency' concept is not universally accepted. In earlier studies, $\dot{V}O_2$ was calculated rather than measured, and a resultant $\dot{V}O_2/\dot{D}O_2$ relationship was possible from mathematical coupling.[26–28] Data from too few patients were often pooled, and the calorigenic effect of inotropes used was ignored.[29] Evidence of a pathological critical $\dot{D}O_2$ with plateau has never been demonstrated clinically. More recent studies have not shown a pathological $\dot{V}O_2/\dot{D}O_2$ relationship nor better patient outcome with 'supranormal' therapy.[26,27,30–32] Therefore, while it is worthwhile to improve $\dot{D}O_2$ in critically ill patients, the intensivist should not blindly apply 'supranormal' end-points to all patients, as attempting this objective may be detrimental.[32] The concept does not enjoy wide support.

HYPERBARIC OXYGEN THERAPY

Hyperbaric oxygen (HBO) therapy delivers 100% oxygen at a pressure above atmospheric, in a pressurized multi- or one-man chamber. Oxygen inhaled at pressure dissolves in plasma, for example PaO_2 approaches 1500 mmHg (200 kPa) at two atmospheres absolute. Increases in oxygen tensions of tissues vary widely, depending on local perfusion and metabolic conditions. HBO therapy is the treatment for decompression sickness or 'bends'. It has been used in the treatment of carbon monoxide poisoning,[33,34] burns,[35] gas gangrene,[36–38] osteomyelitis, osteoradionecrosis, crush injuries, and ischaemic skin grafts. While favourable clinical results have been claimed for each of these conditions, no proper trials have demonstrated benefits of HBO therapy over conventional treatment.[33,38] Complications of HBO therapy include barotrauma to ears, sinuses, and lung, oxygen toxicity, grand mal fits, and changes in visual acuity. Patient selection for HBO therapy is probably important.[34]

REFERENCES

1 Oh TE, Duncan AW. Oxygen therapy. *Med J Aust* 1988; **149**: 141–6.
2 Leigh JM. Oxygen therapy: physiological principles, monitoring and administration technique. *Crit Care Int* 1984; **3**: 4–7.
3 Nunn JF. *Applied Respiratory Physiology*, 3rd edn. London: Butterworths; 1987, p. 201.
4 Leach RM, Bateman NT. Acute oxygen therapy. *Br J Hosp Med* 1993; **49**: 637–44.
5 Goddard JM. Concentrations of oxygen delivered by air entrainment oxygen masks. *Ann R Coll Surg Engl* 1985; **67**: 366–7.
6 Editorial. Oxygen behind the mask. *Lancet* 1982; **2**: 1197–8.
7 Campbell EJM. How to use the venturi mask. *Lancet* 1982; **2**: 1206.
8 Duncan AW, Oh T E, Hillman DR. PEEP and CPAP. *Anaesth Intens Care* 1986; **14**: 236–50.
9 Wexler HR, Levy H, Cooper JD, Aberman A. Measurement of intratracheal oxygen concentrations during face mask administration of oxygen. *Canad Anaesth Soc J* 1975; **22**: 417–31.
10 Goldstein RS, Young J, Rebuck AS. Effect of breathing pattern on oxygen concentration received from standard face masks. *Lancet* 1982; **2**: 1188–90.
11 Mortenson JD. Augmentation of blood gas transfer by means of an intravascular blood gas exchanger (IVOX). In: Marini JJ, Roussos C, (eds) *Ventilatory Failure*. Berlin: Springer-Verlag; 1991: pp. 318–46.
12 Coates JE. Lung Function. *Assessment and Application in Medicine*, 5th edn. London: Blackwell Scientific Publications; 1993: pp. 629–33.
13 Cross CE, van der Vliet A, O'Neill CAO, Eiserich JP. Reactive oxygen species and the lung. *Lancet* 1994; **344**: 930–3.
14 Gibbs PS, Moorthy SS, Losasso AM. Sustained high inspired PaO_2 without toxic sequelae. *Anesth Analg* 1976; **55**: 588–9.
15 Klein J. Normobaric pulmonary oxygen toxicity. *Anesth Analg* 1990; **70**: 195–207.
16 Martin R, Bruce M, Fanaroff A. Bronchopulmonary dysplasia. In: Nussbaum E (ed.) *Pediatric Intensive Care*. New York: Futura Publishing; 1989: pp. 469–81.
17 Phelps DL. Retinopathy of prematurity. *N Eng J Med* 1992; **326**: 1078–80.
18 Newton NI. Supplementary oxygen – potential for disaster. *Anaesthesia* 1991; **46**: 905–6.
19 Elder AT, Crompton GK. Misleading guidelines on oxygen treatment in asthma. *Br Med J* 1985; **291**: 823.
20 Schmidt GA, Hall JB. Acute on chronic respiratory failure. Assessment and management of patients with COPD in the emergency setting. *JAMA* 1989; **261**: 3444–53.
21 Mohensifar Z, Goldbach P, Tashkin DP, *et al.* Relationship between O_2 delivery and O_2 consumption in the adult respiratory distress syndrome. *Chest* 1983; **84**: 267–71.
22 Danek SJ, Lynch JP, Weg JG, Dantzker DR. The dependence of oxygen uptake on oxygen delivery in the adult respiratory distress syndrome. *Am Rev Respir Dis* 1980; **122**: 387–95.
23 Shoemaker WC, Appel PL, Kram HB. Hemodynamic and oxygen transport responses in survivors and non-survivors of high-risk surgery. *Crit Care Med* 1993; **21**: 977–90.
24 Edwards JD, Brown GCS, Nightingale P. Use of survivors' cardiorespiratory values as therapeutic goals in septic shock. *Crit Care Med* 1989; **17**: 1098–1103.
25 Tuschmidt J, Fired J, Astiz M, Rackow E. Elevation of cardiac output and oxygen delivery improves outcome in septic shock. *Chest* 1992; **102**: 216–20.
26 Ronco JJ, Phang PT, Walley KR *et al.* Oxygen consumption is independent of changes in oxygen delivery in severe adult respiratory distress syndrome. *Am Rev Respir Dis* 1991; **143**: 1267–73.

27 Wysocki M, Bebes M, Roupie E, Brun-Buisson C. Modification of oxygen extraction ratio by change in oxygen transport in septic shock. *Chest* 1992; **102**: 221–6.

28 Hanique G, Dugernier T, Laterre PF *et al*. Significance of pathologic oxygen supply dependency in critically ill patients: comparison between measured and calculated methods. *Intensive Care Med* 1994; **20**: 12–18.

29 Bhatt SB, Hutchinson RC, Tomlinson B, Oh TE. Effect of dobutamine infusion on oxygen supply and uptake in healthy volunteers. *Br J Anaesth* 1992; **69**: 298–303.

30 Vermeij CG, Feenstra BWA, Adrichem WJ, Bruning HA. Independent oxygen uptake and oxygen delivery in septic and postoperative patients. *Chest* 1991; **99**: 1438–43.

31 Ronco JJ, Fenwick JC, Wiggs BR *et al*. Oxygen consumption is independent of increases in oxygen delivery in septic patients who have normal or increased plasma lactate. *Am Rev Respir Dis* 1993; **147**: 25–31.

32 Hayes MA, Timmins AC, Yau EH *et al*. Elevation of systemic oxygen delivery in the treatment of critically ill patients. *N Engl J Med* 1994; **330**: 1717–22.

33 Tibbles PM, Perrotta PL. Treatment of carbon monoxide poisoning: A critical review of human outcome studies comparing normobaric oxygen with hyperbaric oxygen. *Ann Emerg Med* 1994; **24**: 269–76.

34 Gorman DF, Runciman WB. Carbon dioxide poisoning. *Anaesth Intens Care* 1991; **19**: 506–11.

35 Cianci P, Sato R. Adjunctive hyperbaric oxygen therapy in the treatment of thermal burns: A review. *Burns* 1994; **20**: 5–14.

36 Thom S. A role for hyperbaric oxygen in clostridial myonecrosis. *Clin Infect Dis* 1993; **17**: 238.

37 Brown DR, Davis NL, Lepawsky M *et al*. A multicenter review of the treatment of major truncal necrotizing infections with and without hyperbaric oxygen therapy. *Am J Surg* 1994; **167**: 485–9.

38 Heimbach D. Use of hyperbaric oxygen. *Clin Infect Dis* 1993; **17**: 239–40.

23

Airway management and acute upper airway obstruction

G M Joynt

The primary objective of airway management is to clear or bypass the obstructed airway, assist or replace spontaneous ventilation and protect the lungs from soiling. Acute upper airway obstruction is a life-threatening emergency, resulting from a wide range of pathophysiological processes. Rapid assessment and establishment of a patent airway are vital, often in the absence of a specific diagnosis. As no single treatment modality is universally applicable, the ICU physician must be capable of instituting a variety of airway management techniques (Figure 23.1).

AIRWAY MANAGEMENT TECHNIQUES

Airway management techniques can be considered non-invasive or invasive, depending on whether instrumentation occurs above or below the glottis, and is surgical or non-surgical (Table 23.1). Definitive techniques secure the trachea and provide some protection from aspiration and soiling. While most airway management in ICU is still achieved by bag-and-mask ventilation and direct laryngoscopic tracheal intubation, the use of fibreoptic bronchoscopy has become routine, especially in special circumstances. Management of failed intubation and ventilation by various alternative techniques (e.g. laryngeal mask airway and cricothyroidotomy) is now well described.[1,2]

The technique of choice will depend on each situation and is a consequence of the interaction of patient factors and the clinician's experience (Table 23.2). Other factors include availability of help, levels of training and supervision, and accessibility of equipment. A portable storage unit with a wide choice of equipment appropriate for difficult airway management is necessary in the ICU (Table 23.3).[1]

Table 23.1 Characteristics of airway management techniques

Technique	Experience required	Time	Definitive
Non-invasive			
Bag-and-mask	+	seconds	–
LMA	–	<1 min	–
Combitube	–	<1 min	+
Invasive (non-surgical)			
Endotracheal intubation			
Direct laryngoscopy	+	variable	+
Bronchoscopic	+	minutes	+
Retrograde	–	minutes	+
Invasive (surgical)			
Jet ventilation	–	<1 min	–
Cricothyroidotomy			
Percutaneous	–	variable	±
Surgical	+	minutes	+
Tracheostomy			
Percutaneous	+	minutes	+
Surgical	+	minutes	+

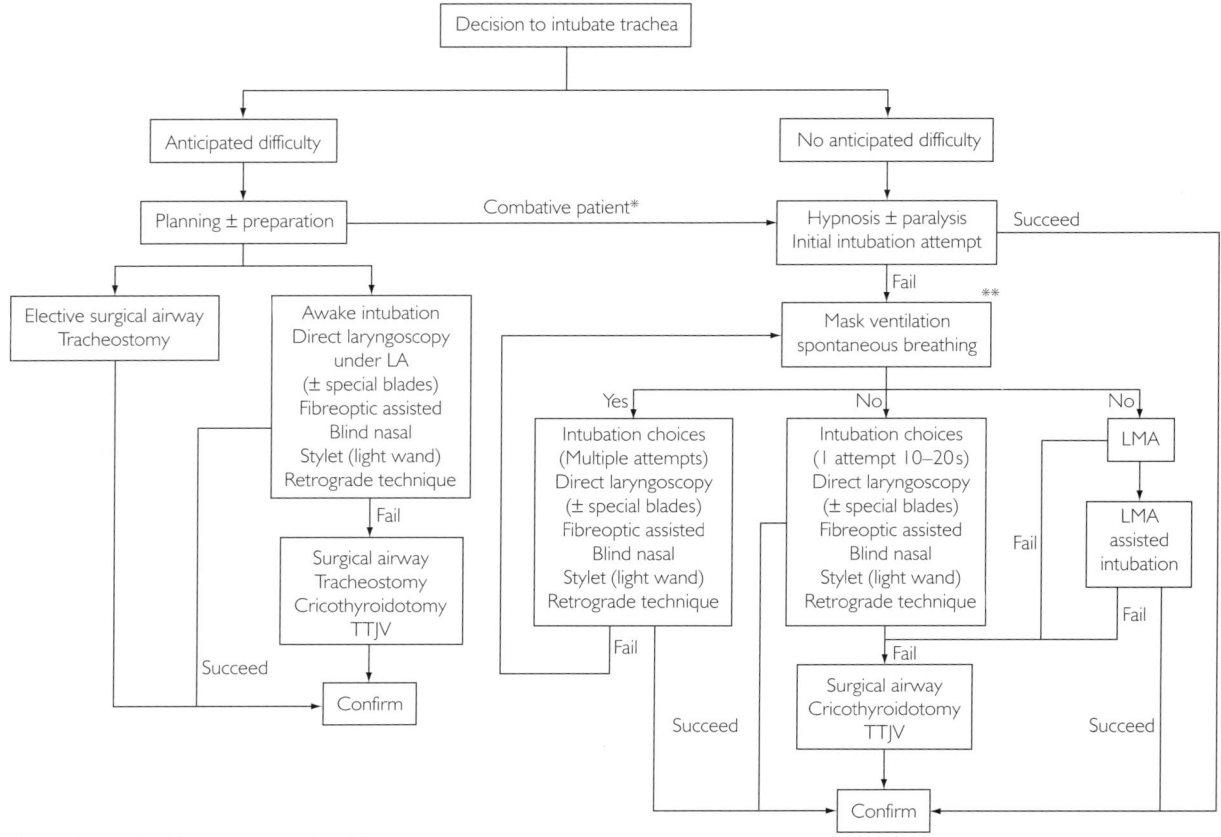

* Consider maintaining spontaneous breathing
** Consider allowing patient to wake up if immediate intubation is not essential

Fig. 23.1 Difficult airway algorithm (see text). LMA laryngeal mask airway, TTJV Trans tracheal jet ventilation.

Table 23.2 Application of airway management techniques

	Difficult direct laryngoscopic intubation +	**Difficult mask ventilation**
Awake	Fibreoptic bronchoscopic intubation	Percutaneous cricothyroidotomy*
	Blind nasal intubation	Surgical tracheostomy*
	Retrograde intubation	Transtracheal jet ventilation
	Laryngeal mask airway	
Anaesthetized	Bag-and-mask ventilation	Laryngeal mask airway
Comatose	Direct laryngoscopic intubation	Transtracheal jet ventilation
(empty stomach)	Different blade	Rigid ventilating bronchoscope
	Bougie/stylet	Percutaneous cricothyroidotomy
	Lighted stylet	Surgical tracheostomy
	Blind nasal intubation	
	Laryngeal mask airway	
	Fibreoptic bronchoscopic intubation	
(full stomach)	Bag-and-mask with cricoid pressure	Percutaneous cricothyroidotomy
	Combitube	Surgical tracheostomy
		Combitube

Examples of common alternatives are given. The technique(s) chosen will depend on the clinician.
*Under local anaesthesia.

Table 23.3 Suggested contents of a portable kit for difficult airway management

Masks
  Face and nasal masks
  Patil endoscopic mask for oral endoscopic intubation
Airways
  Oropharyngeal airways
  Nasopharyngeal airways
  Airway intubator guide for oral endoscopic intubation
Rigid laryngoscope with a variety of designs and sizes
  Short handle or variable angle (Patil-Syracuse) laryngoscope
  Curved blades: Macintosh, Bizarri-Guiffrida
  Straight blades: Miller
  Bent blade: Belscope
  Articulating tip blade: McCoy
  Fibreoptic stylet laryngoscope or Bullard laryngoscope
Endotracheal tubes of assorted size
  Murphy tubes
  Microlaryngoscopy tubes
Endotracheal tube stylets
  Gum elastic bougie (Eschmann stylet)
  Malleable stylet
  Tube changer, hollow tube changer (jet stylet)
  Lighted stylet (light wand)
Fibreoptic intubation equipment
  Fibreoptic endoscopes with light source, adult and paediatric-sized
  Device for emergency non-surgical airway ventilation
  Laryngeal mask airway (including intubating laryngeal mask)
  Combitube
Emergency surgical airway access
  Percutaneous cricothyroidotomy set
  Transtracheal jet ventilation – cannula and high-pressure O_2 source connectors
Exhaled carbon dioxide monitor
  Capnometer/Capnograph
  Chemical indicators
High-pressure O_2 source should be available at the airway management location
  Regulated central wall O_2 pressure (Sanders-type injector)
  Unregulated central wall O_2 pressure
  Anaesthesia machine fresh gas outlet and O_2 flush valve

NON-INVASIVE TECHNIQUES

BAG-MASK VENTILATION

As with most airway management techniques, mask ventilation is a basic skill that requires time and experience to master. It should be learned using mannequins, simulators and practice in the controlled environment of the operating theatre so that in the emergency setting the skill is well established. The bag may be a self-inflating resuscitator or one attached to an anaesthetic circuit. Most resuscitators require a reservoir bag in series to deliver a consistent oxygen concentration. The addition of positive end-expiratory pressure (PEEP) may overcome airway obstruction due to laryngospasm, and

improve arterial oxygenation. Many designs of facemask are available, including the anatomical mask, Trimar mask, Ambu transparent mask and Laerdal mask. Transparent masks are recommended. Artificial airways are used to assist mask ventilation.

Some considerations when performing of mask ventilation include the following:

● *Inadequate ventilation*: The seal of the mask against the face may be inadequate and good hand position is essential. A beard may be covered with a large adhesive plastic dressing with a hole cut out for the mouth, or smeared with petroleum jelly or water-based lubricant. Ventilation of edentulous patients may be aided by improving hand position or special masks. Two operators are recommended if a mask-face leak is excessive, one to hold the mask and the other to manipulate the bag.
● *Gastric insufflation* increases the risk of vomiting and aspiration. Severe distension may cause cardiovascular compromise. Carefully applied cricoid pressure may prevent gastric gas insufflation.
● *Pulmonary aspiration*: In the emergency situation with a full stomach, mask ventilation with cricoid pressure may be necessary until the airway can be secured. Passage of a nasogastric tube to aspirate gastric contents may be reasonable, but complete emptying of gastric contents cannot be guaranteed, and vomiting may be induced.

ORO- AND NASOPHARYNGEAL AIRWAYS

In the unconscious patient, functional obstruction may occur due to loss of pharyngeal tone and inspiratory airway narrowing at the levels of the soft palate, epiglottis and base of tongue. An oropharyngeal airway may establish an adequate airway for spontaneous or bag-mask ventilation when proper head positioning is insufficient. It is inserted with the concavity facing the palate and then rotated 180° into the proper position as it is advanced. Complications include mucosal trauma, worsening the obstruction by pressing the epiglottis against the laryngeal outlet or displacing the tongue more posteriorly. The following sizes (length measured from flange to tip) are recommended: large adult: 100 mm (Guedel size 5); medium-sized adult: 90 mm (Guedel size 4); small adult; 80 mm (Guedel size 3).

A nasopharyngeal airway is a soft rubber or plastic tube inserted into the nostril and advanced along the floor of the nose into the posterior pharynx. It is better tolerated by semi-conscious patients than the oropharyngeal airway. Complications include epistaxis, aspiration, laryngospasm and oesophageal placement.

LARYNGEAL MASK AIRWAY (LMA)

The LMA is a reusable device designed as an intermediate between facemask ventilation and endotracheal intubation. It consists of a silicone rubber tube connected to a distal elliptical spoon-shaped mask with an inflatable rim, which is positioned blindly into the pharynx to form a low-pressure seal against the laryngeal inlet.[3] There are a variety of sizes for use in children and adults. LMAs are widely used in elective general anaesthesia, enabling spontaneous breathing and limited positive-pressure ventilation. LMAs are useful to achieve non-definitive airway patency in many emergency situations (Figure 23.1). Once positioned it can be used to guide the passage of stylets, bougies, the bronchoscope or even the endotracheal tube itself into the trachea.[4,5] The FasTrach or intubating LMA has several features to facilitate intubation once the LMA is placed. There is a guiding ramp and epiglottic elevating bar at the aperture to direct the endotracheal tube to the glottis. It also has an anatomically curved, rigid shaft and handle to allow easy and firm manipulation during placement and when the endotracheal tube is passed.[6]

An LMA is prepared for insertion by deflating and smoothing out the cuffed rim to be wrinkle-free, and the posterior surface is lubricated with water soluble jelly. The patient is positioned as for endotracheal intubation, with slight flexion of the neck and extension of the atlanto-occipital joint (sniffing the morning air position). The LMA is inserted with the tip of the cuff continuously applied to the hard palate, and with the right index finger guiding the tube to the back of the tongue until a firm resistance is encountered. The cuff is then inflated with 20–40 ml of air (adult sizes) before attachment of the breathing circuit.

Contraindications for using an LMA include inability to open the mouth, pharyngeal pathology, airway obstruction at or below the larynx, low pulmonary compliance or high airway resistance and increased risk of regurgitation. Complications include aspiration, gastric insufflation, partial airway obstruction, coughing, laryngospasm, postextubation stridor and kinking of the shaft of the LMA.

COMBITUBE (OESOPHAGEAL-TRACHEAL DOUBLE-LUMEN AIRWAY)

The oesophageal-tracheal combitube is a double-lumen tube that is blindly inserted into the oropharynx up to the indicated markings.[7] The oesophageal lumen has a stopper at the distal end and side perforations at the pharyngeal level while the tracheal lumen has a hole at the distal end. It has two cuffs, a distal one and a proximal pharyngeal balloon. The patient is ventilated through the oesophageal lumen initially as the combitube usually enters the oesophagus,[7] with the distal cuff sealing the oesophagus and the proximal balloon sealing the pharynx. Gas exits the perforations and enters the pharynx and larynx. In the event of failure of ventilation, the tracheal lumen is ventilated and the distal cuff now seals the trachea. While demonstrated to be useful in the pre-hospital setting, its role in resuscitation and management of the difficult airway in the ICU environment is yet to be established. Barotrauma, especially oesophageal rupture, has been reported.

INVASIVE TECHNIQUES

ENDOTRACHEAL INTUBATION

Endotracheal intubation remains the 'gold standard' of airway management, allowing for spontaneous and positive-pressure ventilation, with good (though not absolute) protection from aspiration. Indications include acute airway obstruction, facilitation of tracheal suctioning, protection of the airway in those without protective reflexes, and respiratory failure requiring ventilatory support and high inspired concentrations of oxygen.

Prior to proceeding with any attempts at intubation, regardless of the technique chosen, preparation and checking of all relevant equipment is essential. Difficult airway management equipment (Table 23.3) should also be accessible within a few minutes. Food, vomitus, blood or sputum may obstruct the airway and suction should always be available. Suction apparatus should be able to generate at least 300 mmHg (40 kPa) and 30 l/min. Potential complications of vigorous suctioning include laryngospasm, vagal stimulation producing bradycardia and hypotension, mucosal injury and bleeding.

Direct Laryngoscopy

Although essential for all intensivists, direct laryngoscopy is a difficult skill to master.[8] Tracheal intubation should be preceded by adequate preoxygenation of the patient. If multiple intubation attempts are required the maximum interruption to ventilation should be about 30 s. Adequate ventilation and oxygenation must be provided between attempts. Minimum monitoring should consist of continuous pulse oximetry and ECG. The BURP (Backward, Upward, Rightward Pressure) technique may be helpful to bring the vocal cords into the field of vision. Endotracheal tube size describes the internal diameter, and in the absence of obstruction, 8.0–9.0 mm in adult males and 7.0–8.0 mm in adult females are generally used. A great variety of tubes are available, the most common being a disposable Murphy type made of polyvinyl chloride with a high-volume/low-pressure cuff. Special-purpose tubes include double-lumen tubes for lung isolation, spiral embedded tubes and laser-resistant tubes.

The route of intubation may be orotracheal or nasotracheal. Nasotracheal intubation has potential long-term advantages like greater patient comfort and better tolerance, easier tube fixation, and avoidance of tube occlusion from biting. Immediate complications include possible epistaxis, turbinate cartilage or nasal septal damage, and submucosal dissection. It is contraindicated in the presence of base of skull fracture. The risk of sinusitis is increased and the requirement for a smaller diameter tube may increase airway resistance, difficulty of tracheal suctioning and risk of tube obstruction.

Stylet Guide (Introducer)

Direct laryngoscopic intubation can be difficult if the glottis cannot be well visualized. The 'anterior larynx' can often be more easily intubated if a guide is first advanced in the midline and directed anteriorly into the trachea. The endotracheal tube is then advanced over the guide. Clinical signs of tracheal placement of the guide include coughing, a resistance felt before the guide is fully advanced (due to the carina or bronchus), and a sensation of clicks from the tracheal rings. A number of guides are available, including the gum elastic bougie, tube changer and hollow tube changer. The hollow tube changer can be attached to a side-stream capnometer, or to an oxygen source. The lighted stylet has a light at the distal end that results in a characteristic midline transillumination appearance when the light enters the larynx.[9]

Rigid Indirect Fibreoptic Instruments

The Bullard laryngoscope is a rigid, indirect fibreoptic instrument that is shaped like the hard palate. The learning curve appears reasonable and it has been shown to be a viable alternative for intubation in the difficult airway and reduces cervical spine movement during laryngoscopy compared with the Macintosh or Miller laryngoscope.[10] The utility of other rigid scopes like the Wu and Upsher scopes is unclear.

Fibreoptic Bronchoscopic Intubation

This technique offers advantages of direct visualization, immediate diagnosis (and treatment) of upper airway obstruction and immobility of the neck during the procedure.[11] It also allows reasonably comfortable intubation of a cooperative, awake patient and use of the sitting position. Experience and skill are necessary, especially for dealing with emergent situations, but success rates of up to >96% are expected.[12] Fibreoptic intubation may also be performed in anaesthetized patients, using a mouth mask for nasal intubation or a modified facemask with diaphragm for oral intubation. Nasal intubation is usually performed through the endotracheal tube placed in the nasopharynx, with the tip just above the glottis. The fibreoptic bronchoscope is placed the trachea and the tube is advanced over the bronchoscope. Correct placement is visually checked before the scope is removed. In ICU the fibreoptic bronchoscope can be used to improve the safety of airway procedures such as endotracheal tube changes and percutaneous tracheostomy.[13,14] A number of specially designed oral airways are available to assist oral fibreoptic intubation. The most common cause of failure is obstructed vision from blood or secretions.

Blind Nasal Intubation

Blind nasal intubation offers the patient a nasopharyngeal airway prior to intubation and is sometimes considered in spontaneously breathing patients. Possible indications include inability to open the mouth (e.g. mandibular fracture or temporomandibular joint pathology), cervical spine injury and faciomaxillary surgery. Contraindications include bleeding disorders, nasal airway obstruction or distortion, fractured base of skull and pre-existing sinusitis. The technique requires operator proficiency.

Retrograde Intubation

A J-tip guide wire is introduced percutaneously through the cricothyroid membrane, and advanced into the retropharynx. The tip is retrieved from the oral cavity, and the wire is used to guide an oral endotracheal tube past the obstruction and into the trachea.[15] The procedure is a relatively simple and safe alternative if other techniques fail or are not possible. Commercial kits are available.

Confirmation of Tracheal Tube Placement

Confirming correct intratracheal tube placement is essential. Direct visualization and measurement of expired CO_2 by capnography are the most reliable methods.[16] Capnography may produce false-positive results with the first few breaths after oesophageal intubation (i.e. detectable $PE'CO_2$), if gastric insufflation from mask ventilation has occurred. A false-negative (decreased $PE'CO_2$, despite correct position) may occur with cardiac arrest and low cardiac output states. Other clinical signs such as auscultation of breath sounds over the chest and epigastrium, visualization of condensed water vapour in the tube and chest wall movement are less reliable.

Complications of Endotracheal Intubation

These may be classified into those occurring during intubation (e.g. incorrect tube placement, laryngeal trauma, cardiovascular response to laryngoscopy and intubation, increase in intra-cranial pressure (ICP), hypoxaemia and aspiration), while the tube is in place (e.g. blockage, dislodgment, tube deformation, damage to larynx and complications of mechanical ventilation), and following extubation (e.g. aspiration and post-extubation airway obstruction, laryngeal and tracheal stenosis). Specific techniques should be used to minimize certain side effects such as cardiovascular responses and increases in intra-cranial pressure.

TRANSTRACHEAL JET VENTILATION

Percutaneous TTJV, using a large-bore intravenous catheter inserted through the cricothyroid membrane can be used to provide temporary ventilation when other techniques have failed.[17] Ventilation through the cannula with a standard manual resuscitator bag is inadequate, and a jet ventilation system is necessary. A high-pressure (up to 50 psi or 344 kPa) oxygen source is required for adequate ventilation through a 14 FG i.v. cannula. The method of ventilation is usually manually regulated breaths (with a jet injector or anaesthesia machine flush button). Expiratory gases must be able to escape via the glottis. Appropriate chest movements during expiration must be noted. The consequence of expiratory obstruction is severe and potentially fatal barotrauma.

Complications may be caused by insertion of the i.v. cannula (e.g. bleeding and oesophageal perforation), use of high pressure gases (e.g. hyperinflation, barotrauma), catheter displacement (i.e. subcutaneous emphysema) and failure to protect the airway (i.e. aspiration).

CRICOTHYROIDOTOMY

Cricothyroidotomy, by surgery or percutaneously, is a reliable, safe, and relatively easy way of providing an emergency airway.[18] It is the method of choice if severe to complete upper airway obstruction exists. The simplest and fastest method uses a horizontal incision over and through the cricothyroid membrane and (with the space held wide open by the scalpel handle) followed by insertion of a small tracheostomy or endotracheal tube (Figure 23.2). Commercial cricothyroidotomy sets using the Seldinger technique are available. A tube with internal diameter of 2.5 and 3.0 mm will allow adequate gas flow for self-inflating bag ventilation and spontaneous breathing respectively, provided supplemental oxygen is used. Since the diameter of the cricothyroid space is 9 by 30 mm, tubes of 8.5 mm outer diameter or less should avoid laryngeal and vocal cord damage. Commercially available percutaneous tracheostomy sets that meet the above requirements are available. Complications such as subglottic stenosis (1.6%), thyroid fracture, haemorrhage and pneumothorax are acceptably low. It is generally contraindicated in complete laryngotracheal disruption and age <12 years.

TRACHEOSTOMY

There is little agreement on the indications, best technique, or optimal timing of tracheostomy in ICU patients. Suggested indications for tracheostomy include

- bypass of glottic and supraglottic obstruction
- access for tracheal toilet
- provision of a more comfortable airway for prolonged ventilatory support and
- protection of the airways from aspiration.[19]

In uncomplicated patients, percutaneous tracheostomy performed by an intensivist at the bedside is at least as safe as surgical tracheostomy performed in the operating room.[20] Convenience and cost savings have made percutaneous tracheostomy the procedure of choice in many institutions. Ciaglia's percutaneous technique was described in 1985.[21] After making an adequate skin incision and using blunt dissection with forceps, the endotracheal tube is first withdrawn so that its cuff lies just above the vocal cords. The operator confirms tube position to be above the stoma site by palpation of the trachea. A J-wire is placed in the trachea through a needle inserted through the membrane above or below the second tracheal ring. A series of curved dilators to progressively enlarge the stoma. A tracheostomy tube is then inserted into the trachea and the endotracheal tube removed. Ciaglia later introduced a modified tapered dilator to avoid the use of multiple dilators. While quicker, the single dilator may cause more tracheal wall injuries and ring fractures.[22] The Griggs technique utilizes a Kelly forceps, modified to allow it to be guided by the J-wire, to dilate the tract before insertion of tracheostomy tube.[23] The speed and safety of the Ciaglia and Griggs techniques is similar, although the Griggs technique may cause more bleeding and cannula insertion may be difficult.[24,25] Fibreoptic bronchoscopy during percutaneous tracheostomy may help to prevent incorrect guidewire placement and tracheal ring rupture or herniation, but definitive evidence supporting its routine use is lacking. Definitive identification of the best techniques will require further investigation and long-term follow-up.

Mini-tracheostomy describes the percutaneous insertion of a small 4-mm non-cuffed tracheostomy tube through the cricothyroid membrane or trachea, mainly to facilitate suctioning in patients with poor cough ability.

Complications of tracheostomy are listed in Table 23.4.

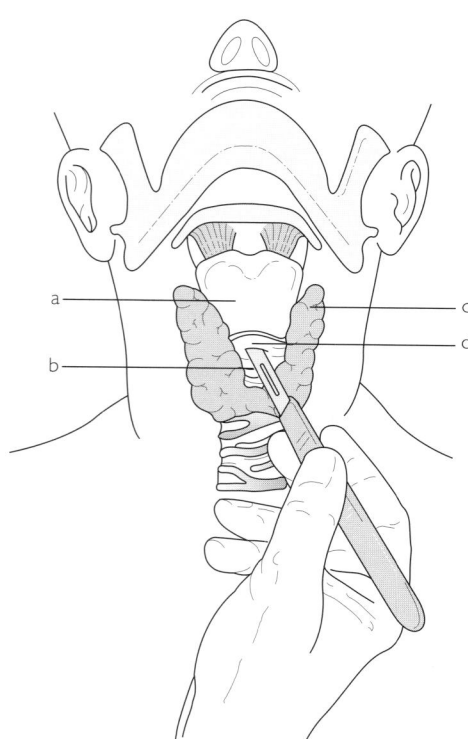

Fig. 23.2 Cricothyroidotomy performed with a scalpel. (a) thyroid cartilage; (b) cricoid cartilage; (c) thyroid gland; (d) cricoid membrane, usually easily palpable subcutaneously.

LOCAL ANAESTHESIA

Instrumentation of the upper airway in awake patients requires good local anaesthesia to increase comfort, improve cooperation, attenuate cardiovascular responses and reduce the risk of laryngospasm. Rapid trans-cricoid injection and either sprayed or nebulized lignocaine to the nares, posterior pharynx and tongue is effective (Table 23.5).[26] Nerve block techniques may improve analgesia but are not essential. Cocaine has been a popular choice for its vasoconstrictor properties, but it is toxic and its supply is regulated. Systemic absorption of topically applied lignocaine (maximum dose 4 mg/kg) is variable, and the clinician should be alert for signs and symptoms of toxicity.

THE DIFFICULT AIRWAY

The difficult airway has been described as one in which a conventionally trained anaesthesiologist experiences difficulty with mask ventilation, tracheal intubation or both. Difficult intubations may be expected in 1–3% of patients presenting for general anaesthesia, and the incidence is likely to be to be considerably higher in ICU patients.

More than 85% of difficult intubations can be managed successfully by experienced clinicians without resorting to a surgical solution. The experience of the operator is probably the most important factor determining success or failure. Experience implies greater manual skills, better anticipation of problems, pre-formulation of strategies, and familiarity with multiple techniques. Thus training of intensivists must specifically include a variety of airway management skills.

ASSISTANCE AND ENVIRONMENT

The patient's condition may rapidly deteriorate as a consequence of a poorly managed airway emergency. The most senior help available should be immediately summoned. If the situation allows, the patient should be moved to the best location for emergency airway interventions, usually the operating theatre or ICU. A senior assistant can help in gaining i.v. access, administering drugs, setting up equipment and managing the airway. A

Table 23.4 Complications of tracheostomy

Immediate
  Procedural complications
    Haemorrhage
    Surgical emphysema, pneumothorax, air embolism
    Cricoid cartilage damage
  Misplacement in pretracheal tissues or right main bronchus
  Compression of tube lumen by cuff herniation
  Occlusion of the tip against the carina or tracheal wall
Delayed
  Blockage with secretions
  Infection of the tracheostomy site, tracheobronchial tree, and larynx
  Pressure on tracheal wall from the tracheostomy tube or cuff
    Mucosal ulceration and perforation
    Deep erosion into the innominate artery
    Tracheo-oesophageal fistula
Late
  Granulomata of the trachea
  Tracheal and laryngeal stenosis
  Persistent sinus at tracheostomy site
  Tracheomalacia and tracheal dilatation

Table 23.5 Local anaesthesia of the upper airway in adults

Technique	Drug dosage
Nerve block	
Internal branch of superior laryngeal nerve	Lignocaine 1–2% (2 ml/side)
Glossopharyngeal nerve	Lignocaine 1–2% (3 ml/side)
Topical anaesthesia of the tongue and oropharynx	
Gargle	Lignocaine viscous 4% (5 ml)
Spray	Lignocaine 10% (5–10 sprays = 50–100 mg)
Nebulized	Lignocaine 4%
Topical anaesthesia of the nasal mucosa	
Cocaine spray or paste	Cocaine 4–5% (0.5 – 2 ml)
Gel	Lignocaine 2% gel (5 ml)
Lignocaine spray	Lignocaine 10% (10 sprays = 100 mg)
Lignocaine + phenylephrine spray	Lignocaine 3% + phenylephrine 0.25% (0.5 ml)
Topical anaesthesia of glottis and trachea	
Spray-as-you-go through bronchoscope	Lignocaine 1–4% (3 mg/kg)
Cricothyroid membrane puncture	Lignocaine 2% (5 ml)
Nebulized	Lignocaine 4% (4 ml) ± phenylephrine 1% (1 ml)

skilled intensivist or ENT surgeon (gowned and standing by) can help to provide a surgical airway or perform rigid bronchoscopy to remove foreign bodies.

ANTICIPATING AND GRADING A DIFFICULT AIRWAY

Intubation difficulty can be anticipated or predicted by the following (although the sensitivity and specificity of individual features and classifications tends to be low):

1 Anatomical or pathological features of difficult intubation in subjects who otherwise appear normal:
    (a) short neck, especially if obese or muscular (thyromental distance <6 cm)
    (b) limited neck and jaw movements (e.g. as a result of trismus, osteoarthritis, ankylosing spondylitis, rheumatoid arthritis or perioral scarring)
    (c) protruding teeth, small mouth, long high curved palate, or receding lower jaw
    (d) space-occupying lesions of the oropharynx and larynx
    congenital conditions with any of the above features (e.g. Marfan's syndrome).
2 Mallampatti classification[27] of visualizing the oropharyngeal structures (a co-operative sitting patient is required for this assessment):
    (a) Class 1: visible soft palate, uvula, fauces and pillars
    (b) Class 2: visible soft palate, uvula and fauces
    (c) Class 3: visible soft palate and base of uvula
    (d) Class 4: soft palate is not visible
3 The degree of difficulty experienced visualizing the larynx by direct laryngoscopy should be recorded and is commonly graded by the classification of Cormack and Lehane[28]:
    (a) Grade I: complete glottis is visible
    (b) Grade II: anterior glottis is not visible
    (c) Grade III: epiglottis but not glottis is visible
    (d) Grade IV: epiglottis is not visible

FAILED INTUBATION AND VENTILATION ALGORITHMS

A pre-formulated plan in the event of failed intubation and/or ventilation is essential and a number have been described.[1,2] The algorithm shown here is an example, (Figure 23.1), however effective implementation depends on the appropriate use of the techniques described above.

If the initial attempt at intubation fails, repeated attempts at direct laryngoscopy should be avoided unless a more experienced operator intervenes, or a potentially helpful maneuver has been carried out (e.g. repositioning, externally applied laryngeal pressure or change of laryngoscope blade). Hypoxia will quickly result if the patient is inadequately ventilated between attempts. In addition, the oedema and bleeding caused

may impair mask ventilation and the use of alternative techniques such as fibreoptic intubation. When indicated to prevent hypoxia a surgical airway should not be delayed (Figures 23.1 and 23.2).

UPPER AIRWAY OBSTRUCTION

ANATOMY AND PATHOPHYSIOLOGY

The upper airway begins at the nose and mouth, and ends at the carina. Obstruction is likely to occur at sites of anatomical narrowing, such as the hypopharynx at the base of the tongue, and the false and true vocal cords at the laryngeal opening. Sites of airway obstruction are classified as supraglottic (above the true cords), glottic (involving the true vocal cords) or infraglottic (below the true cords and above the carina).

The upper airway can also be divided into intrathoracic and extrathoracic portions, which behave differently during inspiration and expiration. The intrathoracic airway dilates during inspiration, that is, it is 'pulled outwards' by negative intrapleural pressure. Positive intrapleural pressure during expiration causes compression and narrowing. Conversely the compliant extrathoracic airway, unexposed to intrapleural pressure, collapses during inspiration, and expands during expiration. Recalling this phenomenon improves the understanding of typical clinical signs, radiographs and flow-volume loops.

AETIOLOGY

Acute upper airway obstruction may result from functional or mechanical causes (Table 23.6). Functional causes involve central nervous system and neuromuscular dysfunction. Mechanical causes may occur within the lumen, in the wall or extrinsic to the airway.

CLINICAL PRESENTATION

The signs of sudden complete upper airway obstruction are characteristic and progress rapidly. The victim cannot breathe, speak or cough, and may hold the throat between the thumb and index finger – the universal choking sign.[29] Agitation, panic and vigorous breathing efforts are rapidly followed by cyanosis. Respiratory efforts diminish as consciousness is lost, and death results within 2–5 min if obstruction is not relieved.

Signs of partial airway obstruction include choking, drooling, gagging, coughing, inspiratory stridor with noisy respiration and dysphonia. Paradoxical chest wall movements and intercostal and supraclavicular retractions may be marked. Powerful respiratory efforts may produce dermal ecchymoses and subcutaneous emphysema. Respiratory decompensation may be rapid in onset, and progress to complete obstruction. Lethargy, diminishing respiratory efforts and loss of consciousness are late signs of hypoxaemia and hypercarbia. Bradycardia and hypotension herald impending cardiac arrest.

SPECIAL EVALUATION OR INVESTIGATIONS

If the patient remains stable, specific diagnostic evaluation may be undertaken, provided airway management facilities are immediately available.

LARYNGOSCOPY AND BRONCHOSCOPY

Indirect laryngoscopy, in a stable, cooperative patient is useful to diagnose foreign bodies, retropharyngeal or laryngeal masses and other glottic pathology.[30]

Assessment with a flexible fibreoptic bronchoscope or laryngoscope enables direct visualization of upper airway anatomy and function. The procedure can be performed in the Emergency Department without transporting the patient and risking complete obstruction. It can be applied to an awake, spontaneously breathing patient and, with care, should not worsen the obstruction. Definitive airway control by intubation can usually be achieved at the end, by advancing an endotracheal tube over the bronchoscope into the trachea. Disadvantages are the need for a skilled operator and a cooperative patient, and a poor visual field if blood and secretions are copious.

Direct laryngoscopy will enable forceps removal of foreign bodies and high volume suctioning of blood, vomitus and secretions. Endotracheal intubation can rapidly be achieved under direct vision. Disadvantages are the need for general anaesthesia or good local analgesia (often difficult in the emergency setting). Direct laryngoscopy can be traumatic, and may worsen soft-tissue bleeding and oedema.

RADIOGRAPHIC IMAGING

Patients with potentially unstable airways should not be transported from a 'safe' environment like the emergency room, operating theatre or ICU for radiological investigation until the airway is secure. Anterior-posterior and lateral plain neck X-rays are useful to detect radiopaque foreign bodies, retropharyngeal masses and epiglottitis. The lateral view in the upright position is obtained in inspiration with the neck fully extended. Swelling of the epiglottis and supraglottic tissues, and ballooning of the hypopharynx, are classical signs of epiglottitis, but are not always present. A computed tomography (CT) scan can assess the thyroid, cricoid and arytenoid cartilages and the airway lumen in stable patients, or in those in whom the airway has been secured.[31] Although magnetic resonance imaging (MRI) has been used to image the upper airway, its use in acute airway obstruction is unproven.

GAS FLOW MEASUREMENT

Flow-volume loop measurement reveals characteristic patterns corresponding to different types and position of pathological lesions (Figure 23.3).[32]

MANAGEMENT

Simplified algorithms to manage partial and complete upper airway obstruction are shown in Figures 23.4 and 23.5. Improvization may be required for certain difficult problems. The chosen technique should be an appropriate one in which the clinician has the reasonable skill and experience. Special techniques in patients with suspected cervical spine instability are discussed in Chapter 68.

1 Supplemental oxygen (100%) is immediately administered.

Table 23.6 Clinical conditions associated with acute upper airway obstruction

Functional causes
  Central nervous system depression
    Head injury, cerebrovascular accident, cardiorespiratory arrest, shock, hypoxia, drug overdose, metabolic encephalopathies
  Peripheral nervous system and neuromuscular abnormalities
    Recurrent laryngeal nerve palsy (postoperative, inflammatory or tumour infiltration), obstructive sleep apnoea, laryngospasm, myasthenia gravis, Guillain–Barré polyneuritis, hypocalcaemic vocal cord spasm
Mechanical causes
  Foreign body aspiration
  Infections
    Epiglottitis, retropharyngeal cellulitis or abscess, Ludwig's angina, diphtheria and tetanus, bacterial tracheitis, laryngotracheobronchitis
  Laryngeal oedema
    Allergic laryngeal oedema, angiotensin converting enzyme inhibitor associated, hereditary angioedema, acquired C1 esterase deficiency
  Haemorrhage and haematoma
    Postoperative, anticoagulation therapy, inherited or acquired coagulation factor deficiency
  Trauma
  Burns
    Inhalational thermal injury, ingestion of toxic chemical and caustic agents
  Neoplasm
    Pharyngeal, laryngeal and tracheobronchial carcinoma, vocal cord polyposis
  Congenital
    Vascular rings, laryngeal webs, laryngocele
  Miscellaneous
    Cricoarytenoid arthritis, achalasia of the oesophagus, hysterical stridor, myxoedema

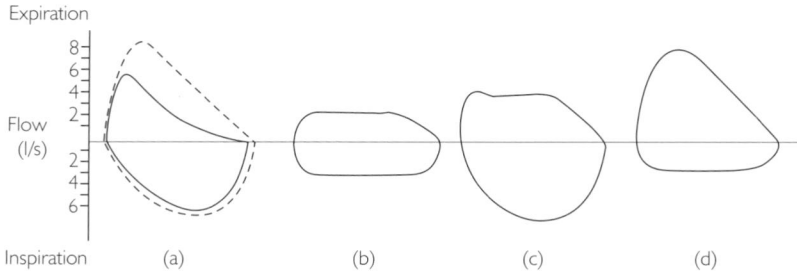

Fig. 23.3 Flow-volume loops. Patterns resulting from different pathological lesions: (a) lower airway obstruction (e.g. chronic obstructive pulmonary disease or asthma); (b) fixed, non-variable upper airway obstruction (e.g. fibrous ring in trachea); (c) variable upper airway obstruction, intrathoracic (e.g. tumour in the lower trachea); (d) variable upper airway obstruction, extrathoracic (e.g. vocal cord tumour or paralysis).

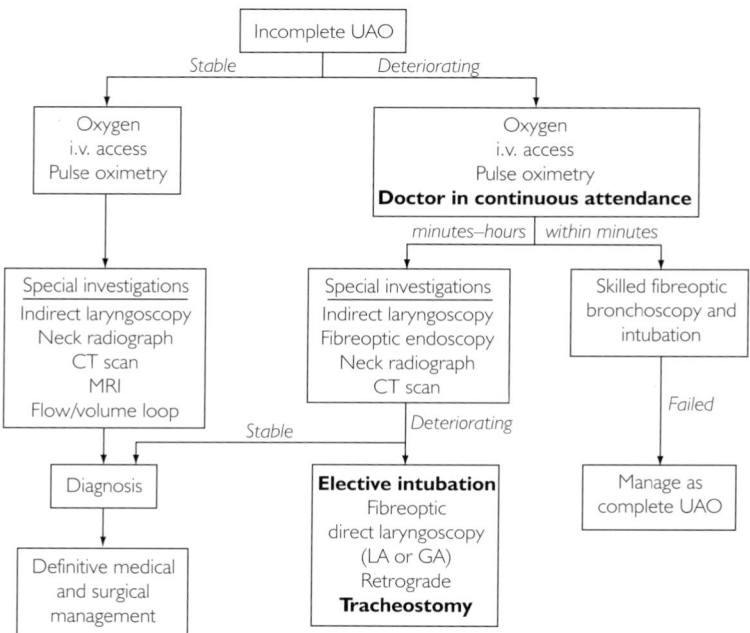

Fig. 23.4 Management of partial upper airway obstruction (UAO). i.v., intravenous; CT, computerized tomography; MRI, magnetic resonance imaging; LA, local anaesthesia; GA, general anaesthesia.

2 A choice of equipment for definitive airway control must be available and ready for use (Table 23.3).[3]
3 In adults intravenous access should be secured.
4 Initiate continuous monitoring of vital signs and pulse oximetry.
5 Patient transport before securing the airway must be carefully considered. It is difficult to provide safe conditions during transport.[30]

AIRWAY MANAGEMENT TECHNIQUES IN AIRWAY OBSTRUCTION

THE UNCONSCIOUS PATIENT

If the upper airway is obstructed by the tongue in an unconscious patient, airway patency is initially achieved by using standard airway maneuvers[33] and oropharyngeal or

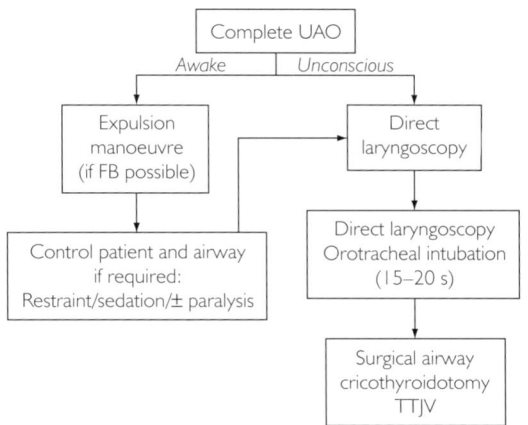

Fig. 23.5 Management of complete upper airway obstruction (UAO). Attempts at orotracheal intubation should not take longer than 10–20 s. FB, foreign body; TTJV, transtracheal jet ventilation.

nasopharyngeal airways. Definitive airway control should follow if consciousness does not immediately return.

ENDOTRACHEAL INTUBATION

1 *Direct laryngoscopic intubation* is the method of choice for the unconscious, apnoeic patient as it allows rapid evaluation of any supraglottic problem and immediate airway security. It can also be attempted in an awake patient after careful application of local anaesthesia. Although there is some risk of loss of the airway after local anaesthesia, complete loss of the airway *under general anaesthesia* is common and may be catastrophic.

2 *Awake fibreoptic intubation* in a spontaneously breathing patient is usually safe, but requires a skilled operator. The procedure will take 2–10 min or longer,[34] and urgency of the case must be assessed beforehand with this time frame in mind. Alternatives should be initiated if the obstruction progresses or if intubation fails after a reasonable time. The following points may assist visualization in acute upper airway obstruction:
 (a) The procedure is clearly explained to the patient.
 (b) Good local anaesthesia and mucosal vasoconstrictors are important. Failure is most commonly due to excessive secretions and bleeding.
 (c) If desired, the suction port of the fibrescope can be used to insufflate 100% oxygen or apply local anaesthetic. This also clears the fibrescope tip of secretions. Additional large bore suction catheters may help.

3 *Blind nasotracheal intubation* provides a patent nasopharyngeal airway during the procedure, but is less useful when fibreoptic laryngoscopy is available.

4 *Retrograde tracheal intubation* is a less invasive alternative to cricothyroidotomy in proximal obstructions.

Once endotracheal intubation is safely accomplished secure fixation of the endotracheal tube is mandatory. The patient's upper limbs may need to be restrained to avoid self-extubation.

SURGICAL AIRWAYS

A surgical airway is indicated when endotracheal intubation is not possible, or when an unstable cervical spine is threatened by available airway techniques. It is the last line of defence against hypoxia. In airway obstruction options include:

1 *Cricothyroidotomy* is the method of choice if severe or complete upper airway obstruction exists.

2 *Percutaneous transtracheal jet ventilation.* In complete upper airway obstruction, the technique must *not* be used because expiratory obstruction can cause severe and potentially fatal barotrauma.

3 *Tracheostomy* in the emergency setting is rarely required, although surgical tracheostomy under local anaesthesia may be reasonable under some controlled conditions (Figure 23.4).

COMMON CLINICAL CONDITIONS AND THEIR MANAGEMENT

FOREIGN BODY OBSTRUCTION

Foreign body obstruction is the most common cause of acute airway obstruction. The elderly, especially those in institutions, are at risk. The use of dentures, alcohol and depressant drugs also increase risk. Fatal food asphyxiation or 'cafe coronary' has an incidence of 0.66 per 100 000 population.[35] The diagnosis should be considered in any acute respiratory arrest where the victim can not be ventilated.

Expulsion of the foreign body can be attempted with the Heimlich manoeuvre.[29] From behind, the rescuer encircles the arms around the victim, placing the thumb of one fist between the umbilicus and xiphisternum. The fist is gripped by the other hand, and an inward, upward thrust is applied. Chest thrusts (rescuer's arms should encircle the chest, and a fist placed over mid-sternum) for use in pregnancy and obesity have been described. The technique is not without controversy. Unwanted effects such as vomiting, aspiration, fractured ribs, barotrauma and ruptured organs have been reported. Extract solid material with a hooked finger.[33] If these maneuvers fail, management immediately proceeds as shown in Figures 23.4 and 23.5.

EXTRINSIC AIRWAY COMPRESSION

Extrinsic space-occupying lesions can cause upper airway obstruction. Compression from haematomas may be associated with trauma, neck surgery, central venous catheterization, anticoagulants and congenital or acquired coagulopathies. Haematomas following surgery should immediately be evacuated by removing skin and subcutaneous sutures. If this fails, an artificial airway must be secured. In patients with coagulation abnormalities, intubation is preferred over a surgical airway. Most haematomas secondary to coagulopathy do not require surgical intervention, and resolve with conservative therapy (i.e. vitamin K and blood component therapy).

Partial airway obstruction caused by retropharyngeal abscess is best managed by drainage under local anaesthesia. Gentle fibreoptic examination and intubation or direct laryngoscopy and intubation in the lateral, head-down position is favored by some.[30] Risks are related to inadvertent rupture of the abscess, with subsequent flooding of the airway. Ludwig's angina is a mixed infection of the floor of the mouth. An inflammatory mass develops in the space between the tongue and the muscles and fascia of the anterior neck. The supraglottic airway is compressed and becomes narrowed.[36] Direct laryngoscopy is difficult, as the tongue cannot be anteriorly displaced. Awake fibreoptic bronchoscopy or a surgical airway, along with antibiotic therapy are management options.

INTRINSIC AIRWAY COMPRESSION
Burn Injury: Inhalation and Ingestion

Patients with large burn area, facial burns or inhalation injuries develop progressive supraglottic oedema, usually within 24–48 h. Such patients may require early, prophylactic tracheal intubation. Assessment of the injury and need tracheal intubation can best be achieved by frequently repeated awake fibreoptic laryngoscopy.[37] If considered safe, inspection by direct lanyngoscopy with or without intubation under general anaesthesia is an alternative. Ingestion of hot fluids or corrosive agents can also cause delayed oedema and airway swelling.[38] See Chapter 71.

Adult Epiglottitis
Epiglottitis is an uncommon but increasingly recognized infectious disease in adults.[39] It involves the epiglottis and supraglottic larynx, causing swelling with consequent airway obstruction. *Haemophilus influenzae,* and *H. parainfluenzae, Streptococcus pneumoniae,* haemolytic Steptococci, and *Staphylococcus aureus* are common causative organisms. Mortality is varied in adults (0%–7%), due to difficult diagnosis and non-standardized treatment.[40] Clinical features are sudden onset of sore throat (pain often greater than suggested by clinical findings), muffled voice, dysphagia, stridor, dyspnoea and respiratory distress. Systemic toxaemia is common. Gentle indirect laryngoscopy, fibreoptic laryngoscopy or lateral neck X-ray confirms the diagnosis.

Airway management is controversial.[39–41] Some recommend securing a definitive airway on presentation while others suggest close observation in ICU. However, there are reports of sudden obstruction and death with the latter approach.[40] Dyspnoea may predict the need for intubation. Tracheal intubation and tracheostomy are acceptable, but tracheal intubation may result in better long-term outcome. Patient positioning is important, and changing from a sitting to supine position may induce complete obstruction. In more stable patients, awake fibreoptic intubation is possible if a skilled operator is available. Endotracheal intubation under general anaesthesia using a gaseous induction is frequently recommended. Obstruction can occur, even when this procedure is undertaken by a skilled anaesthetist[41] in the operating room. A skilled assistant, scrubbed and ready to secure a surgical airway may prevent disaster. Rapid-sequence induction using muscle relaxants is dangerous. Tracheostomy under local anaesthesia is a safe alternative.

Airway management is followed by appropriate antibiotics and supportive care. Cefotaxime 2 g i.v. 6-hourly or ampicillin 1–2 g i.v. 6-hourly *plus* chloramphenicol 50 mg/kg per day, are empiric regimens. Patient factors, local bacterial sensitivities, and cultures of epiglottal swabs and blood will influence the antibiotic choice. Supportive care includes adequate sedation and tracheobronchial toilet. Abscesses should be surgically drained. There is no good evidence supporting the use of steroids.

Angioedema
Allergic responses involving the upper airway may be localized or part of a systemic anaphylactic reaction. Angioedema is characterized by subepithelial swelling. Angioedema of the lips, supraglottis, glottis and infraglottis may result in airway obstruction. The systemic reaction consists of variable combinations of urticaria (79%), bronchospasm (70%), shock, cardiovascular collapse and abdominal pain.[42] Common causative agents are Hymenoptera stings, shellfish ingestion and drugs. Treatment consists of immediately ensuring an adequate airway (Figures 23.4 and 23.5), and administration of oxygen, epinephrine and steroids. As it is likely to recur, the patient should be followed up and fully investigated.

Hereditary angioedema is a rare, inherited disorder of the complement system, caused by functionless or low levels of C1 esterase inhibitor.[43] Non-pruritic, non-painful angioedema involving skin and subcutaneous tissue occurs in various locations, including the upper airway. Precipitating causes include stress, physical exertion and localized trauma (including dental or maxillofacial surgery and laryngoscopy). Acute attacks do not respond to epinephrine, antihistamines or corticosteroids. Management consists of establishing a secure airway and infusion of C1 esterase inhibitor concentrate (25 U/kg) which has an onset of action of 30–120 minutes.[44,45] If not available, fresh frozen plasma (2–4 U) may be considered. Stanozolol 1–4 mg daily or danazol 50–600 mg daily have been shown to be effective in decreasing frequency and severity of attacks.[46] Antifibrinolytic agents (e.g. tranexamic acid) are less effective. Danazol, C1 esterase inhibitor and fresh frozen plasma (2–4 units) can be used as pre-operative prophylaxis.[45]

Angiotensin-converting enzyme (ACE) inhibitor-related angioedema is increasingly seen and is possibly the result of reduced bradykinin metabolism.[47] Treatment focuses on airway support.

Post-extubation Laryngeal Oedema

Laryngeal oedema following extubation occurs in about 20% of adults, but need for re-intubation is uncommon.[48] It may occur after airway manipulation, traumatic or prolonged tracheal intubation, and if high cuff pressures are used. Treatment in adults is conservative, with close observation and humidified oxygen therapy. Nebulized plain epinephrine (1–2 ml 1:1000 solution diluted with 2 ml saline or undiluted 1:1000 solution 4–5 ml) or racemic epinephrine (0.25–0.5 ml 2.25% solution in 2–4 ml saline) has been used. Nebulization may need to be repeated every 30–60 min. Steroids do not appear to be useful.[48]

POSTOBSTRUCTION PULMONARY OEDEMA

Postobstruction pulmonary oedema may occur in up to 11% of cases.[49] This appears to be related to the markedly decreased intrathoracic pressure caused by forced inspiration against a closed upper airway, resulting in transudation of fluid from pulmonary capillaries to the interstitium. In addition, increased venous return may increase pulmonary blood flow, further worsening oedema. Hypoxia and the hyperadrenergic stress state may also affect capillary hydrostatic pressure, although pulmonary capillary wedge pressure is usually normal. The oedema usually occurs within minutes after the relief of the obstruction, but may be delayed up to 2.5 h.[50] Management includes maintenance of airway patency, oxygen therapy, diuretics, morphine and fluid restriction. Application of continuous positive airway pressure or ventilation with positive end-expiratory pressure may be necessary in severe cases. Pulmonary artery catheterization should be reserved only for complicated cases.

REFERENCES

1 Task Force on Guidelines for Management of the Difficult Airway. Practice guidelines for management of the difficult airway. *Anesthesiology* 1993; **78**: 597–602.
2 Benumof JL. Laryngeal mask airway and the ASA difficult airway algorithm. *Anesthesiology* 1996; **84**: 686–99.
3 Brain AIJ. The laryngeal mask: a new concept in airway management. *Br J Anaesth* 1983; **55**: 801–05.
4 McNamee CJ, Meyns B, Pagliero KM. Flexible bronchoscopy via the laryngeal mask: a new technique. *Thorax* 1991; **46**: 141–42.
5 Pennant JH, Walker MB. Comparison of the endotracheal tube and laryngeal mask in airway management by paramedical personnel. *Anesth Analg* 1992; **74**: 531–34.
6 LMA. *FasTrach Instruction Manual*. San Deigo, CA: LMA North America; 1998.
7 Frass M, Frenzer R, Rauscha F, *et al.* Evaluation of esophageal tracheal combitube in cardiopulmonary resuscitation. *Crit Care Med* 1986; **15**: 609–11.

8 Konrad C, Schupfer G, Witlisbach M, *et al.* Learning manual skills in anesthesiology: is there a recommended number of cases for anesthetic procedures? *Anesth Analg* 1998; **86**: 635–39.
9 Hung O, Pytka S, Morris I, *et al.* Lightwands intubation: Clinical trial of a new lightwand for tracheal intubation in patients with difficult airways. *Can J Anesth* 1995; **42**: 826–30.
10 Hastings R, Vigil CA, Hanna R, *et al.* Cervical spine movement during laryngoscopy with the Bullard, Macintosh, and Miller laryngoscopes. *Anesthesiology* 1995; **82**: 859–69.
11 Giudice JC, Komansky H, Gordon R, Kaufman JL. Acute upper airway obstruction – fibreoptic bronchoscopy in diagnosis and therapy. *Crit Care Med* 1981 **9**: 878–79.
12 Ovassapian A. Fibreoptic assisted airway management. *Acta Anaesthesiol Scand* 1997; **110**(**Suppl**): 46–7.
13 Bapat P. Use of a fibreoptic bronchoscope to change endotracheal tubes. *Anesthesiology* 1997; **86**: 509.
14 Reilly PM, Schapiro MB, Malcynski JT. Percutaneous dilation tracheostomy under the microscope: justification for intra-procedural bronchoscopy? *Intensive Care Med* 1999; **25**: 3–4.
15 McNamara RM. Retrograde intubation of the trachea. *Ann Emerg Med* 1987; **16**: 680–2.
16 Tinker JH, Dull DL, Caplan RA. Role of monitoring devices in prevention of anesthetic mishaps: a closed claim analysis. *Anesthesiology* 1989; **71**: 541.
17 Benumof JL, Scheller MS. The importance of transtracheal jet ventilation in the management of the difficult airway. *Anesthesiology* 1989; **71**: 769–78.
18 Kress TD, Balasubramaniam S. Cricothyroidotomy. *Ann Emerg Med* 1982; **11**: 197–201.
19 Pryor JP, Reilly, PM, Schapiro MB. Surgical airway management in the intensive care unit. *Crit Care Clin* 2000; **16**: 473–88.
20 Cheng E, Fee WE. Dilatational versus standard tracheostomy: a meta-analysis. *Ann Otol Rhinol Laryngol* 2000; **109**: 803–7.
21 Ciaglia P, Firsching R, Syniec C. Elective percutaneous dilatational tracheostomy. *Chest* 1985; **87**: 715–19.
22 Byahn C, Wilke HJ, Halbig S, *et al.* Percutaneous tracheostomy: Ciaglia Blue Rhino versus the basic Ciaglia technique of percutaneous tracheostomy. *Anesth Analg* 2000; **91**: 882–6.
23 Griggs WM, Worthley LIG, Gilligan JE, *et al.* A simple percutaneous tracheostomy technique. *Surg Gynecol Obstet* 1990; **170**: 543–5.
24 Van Heurn LW, Mastboom WB, Scheeren CI, *et al.* Comparative clinical trial of progressive dilatational and forceps dilatational tracheostomy. *Intensive Care Med* 2001; **27**: 292–5.
25 Nates JL, Cooper DJ, Myles PS, *et al.* Percutaneous tracheostomy in critically ill patients: a prospective, randomized comparison of two techniques. *Crit Care Med* 2000; **28**: 3734–9.
26 Gross JB, Hartigan M, Schaffer DW. A suitable substitute for 4% cocaine before blind nasotracheal

intubation: 3% lidocaine–0.25% phenylephrine nasal spray. *Anesth Analg* 1984; **63**: 915–18.

27 Mailampati SR, Gugino LD, Desai SP, Freiberger D. A clinical sign to predict difficult tracheal intubation: a prospective study. *Can J Anaesth* 1985; **32**: 429–34.

28 Cormack RS, Lehane J. Difficult tracheal intubation in obstetrics. *Anaesthesia* 1984; **39**: 1105–11.

29 Heimlich HJ. A life saving maneuver to prevent food-choking. *J Am Med Assoc* 1975; **234**: 398–401.

30 Bogdonoff DL, Stone DJ. Emergency management of the airway outside the emergency room. *Can J Anaesth* 1992; **39**: 1069–89.

31 Angood PB, Attia EL, Brown RA, Mulder DS. Extrinsic civilian trauma to the larynx and cervical trachea – important predictors of long term morbidity. *J Trauma* 1986; **26**: 869–73.

32 Miller RD, Hyatt RE. Evaluation of obstructing lesions of the trachea and larynx by flow volume loops. *Am Rev Respir Dis* 1973; **108**: 475–81.

33 The American Heart Association in collaboration with the International Liaison Committee on Resuscitation. Guidelines 2000 for cardiopulmonary resuscitation and emergency cardiovascular care. Part 3: adult basic life support. *Circulation* 2000; **102**(**Suppl 8**): I22–59.

34 Afilalo M, Guttman A, Stern E, *et al.* Fibreoptic intubation in the emergency department: a case series. *J Emerg Med* 1993; **11**: 387–91.

35 Mittleman RE, Wetli CV. The fatal café coronary: foreign body airway obstruction. *J Am Med Assoc* 1982; **247**: 1285–8.

36 Barakate MS, Jensen MJ, Hemli JM, Graham AR. Ludwig's angina: report of a case and review of management issues. *Ann Otol Rhinol Laryngol* 2001; **110**(5 Pt 1): 453–6.

37 Muehlberger T, Kunar D, Munster A, Couch M. Efficacy of fibreoptic laryngoscopy in the diagnosis of inhalation injuries. *Arch Otolaryngol Head Neck Surg* 1998; **124**: 1003–7.

38 Joynt GM, Ho KM, Gomersall CD. Delayed upper airway obstruction. A life-threatening complication of Dettol poisoning. *Anaesthesia* 1997; **52**: 261–3.

39 Park KW, Darvish A, Lowenstein E. Airway management for adult patients with acute epiglottitis: a 12-year experience at an academic medical center (1984–1995). *Anesthesiology* 1998; **88**: 254–61.

40 Mayo-Smith M. Fatal respiratory arrest in adult epiglottitis in the intensive care unit. *Chest* 1993; **104**: 964–5.

41 Ames WA, Ward VM, Tranter RM, Street M. Adult epiglottitis: an under-recognized, life-threatening condition. *Br J Anaesth* 2000; **85**: 795–7.

42 Corren J, Schocket AL. Anaphylaxis: a preventable emergency. *Postgrad Med* 1990; **87**: 167–78.

43 Donaldson VH, Evans RR. A biochemical abnormality in hereditary angioneurotic edema: absence of serum inhibitor of C'1–esterase. *Am J Med* 1963; **35**: 37–44.

44 Joynt GM, Abdullah V, Wormald PJ. Hereditary Angioedema: report of a case. *Ear Nose Throat J* 2001; **80**: 321–4.

45 Bork K, Barnstedt SE. Treatment of 193 episodes of laryngeal edema with C1 inhibitor concentrate in patients with hereditary angioedema. *Arch Intern Med* 2001; **161**: 714–18.

46 Niels JF, Weiler JM. C1 esterase inhibitor deficiency, airway compromise, and anesthesia. *Anesth Analg* 1998; **87**: 480–8.

47 Agostoni A, Cicardi M, Cugno M, *et al.* Angioedema due to angiotensin-converting enzyme inhibitors. *Immunopharmacology* 1999; **44**: 21–5.

48 Ho LI, Harn HJ, Lien TC, *et al.* Postextubation laryngeal edema in adults. Risk factor evaluation and prevention by hydrocortisone. *Intensive Care Med* 1996; **22**: 933–6.

49 Tami TA, Chu F, Wildes TO, Kaplan M. Pulmonary edema and acute upper airway obstruction. *Laryngoscope* 1986; **96**: 506–9.

50 Willms D, Shure D. Pulmonary edema due to upper airway obstruction in adults. *Chest* 1988; **94**: 1090–2.

24.

Acute respiratory failure in chronic obstructive pulmonary disease

M T Naughton and D V Tuxen

The terms chronic obstructive pulmonary or airways disease (COPD or COAD) are applied to patients with chronic bronchitis and/or emphysema. COPD affects 5% of the adult population, is the fifth most common cause of death world-wide, and is the only major cause of death that is increasing in prevalence.[1] Despite this, when an acute deterioration occurs, most precipitating factors are reversible and the outcome is usually good.[2] This justifies aggressive management in the majority of patients.

AETIOLOGY OF COPD

The causes of COPD can be divided into environmental and host factors. Environmental factors include tobacco smoke, air pollution, indoor fumes (e.g. indoor cooking with solid biomass fuel) and poor socio-economic status. The biggest single factor in over 95% of patients with COPD is tobacco smoking (Figure 24.1). However, only approximately 15% of smokers develop COPD. Host factors are the balance between circulating proteases and antiproteases (e.g. alpha 1 antitrypsin deficiency) and the intake of antioxidant vitamins (A, C, E).[3]

PATHOPHYSIOLOGY

Reduced expiratory airflow in COPD is due to both increased airway resistance and reduced lung elastic recoil. Airway resistance is increased by mucosal oedema and hypertrophy, secretions, bronchospasm, airway tortuosity and airflow turbulence, and loss of lung parenchymal elastic tissues that normally support the small airways. Loss of lung elastic recoil pressure is due both to loss of lung elastin and loss of alveolar surface tension from alveolar wall destruction.

Reduced lung elastic recoil decreases expiratory airflow by reducing the alveolar pressure driving expiratory airflow and by reducing the intraluminal airway pressure, which normally distends small airways during expiration. Forced expiration increases alveolar driving pressure but also causes dynamic airway compression resulting in no improvement or sometimes reduction in expiratory airflow. These factors are present in varying proportions, depending on the degree of chronic bronchitis and emphysema and the individual patient.

Airflow limitation results in prolonged expiration, pulmonary hyperinflation, inspiratory muscle disadvantage, increased work of breathing and the sensation of dyspnoea. All these factors are worsened during an exacerbation of COPD.

Pulmonary hyperinflation has both static and dynamic components. The static component is that which would remain at the end of an expiratory period long enough for all expiratory airflow to cease (30–120 s) enabling the lungs and chest wall to reach their static functional residual capacity (FRC). This component of hyperinflation is due to loss of parenchymal elastic recoil, chest wall adaptation[4] and airway closure that occurs throughout expiration. Dynamic pulmonary hyperinflation is the further increase in hyperinflation due to slow expiratory airflow not

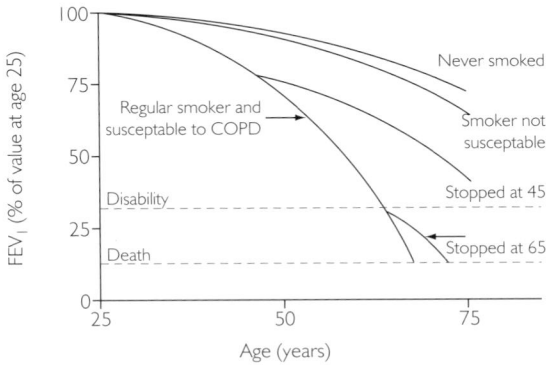

Fig. 24.1 Decline in lung function with age in different smoking categories.

Table 24.1   Decline in lung function with age in different smoking categories

Normocapnic (PaCO$_2$ 35–45 mmHg)	Hypercapnic (PaCO$_2$ >45 mmHg)
(emphysema > chronic bronchitis)	(chronic bronchitis > emphysema)
thin	obese
pursed lip breathing	CNS depression consider the role of oxygen therapy
accessory muscle use	alcohol, sedatives, analgesics
hyperinflated	sleep related hypoventilation
right heart failure late	right heart failure early

allowing completion of expiration before the arrival of the next breath. The extent of dynamic hyperinflation depends on the severity of airflow obstruction, the amount inspired (tidal volume) and the expiratory time.[5] Thus, the degree of hyperinflation may vary in a patient with changes in minute ventilation due to changes in CO_2 production (depending on exercise, diet or the metabolic response illness) or dead space, as well as with changes in airflow obstruction during an exacerbation.

Chest wall hyperinflation leads to sub-optimal muscle length–tension relationships and mechanical disadvantage, thereby predisposing patients to respiratory muscle fatigue, as the work of breathing increases, particularly if associated with myopathic situations (steroids, electrolyte disturbances). Minor reductions in lung function due to infection, mild cardiac failure or atelectasis, increase the work of breathing both due to increases in respiratory impedance and increases in dead space. With acute changes in work-load, rapid decompensation with ventilatory failure and acute hypercapnia may occur.

Central respiratory drive may also be impaired, or poorly responsive to physiological triggers – hypoxaemia or hypercapnia, and lead to chronic hypercapnia. This may occur in the setting of sleep (i.e. obstructive sleep apnoea), obesity or drugs (sedatives, antiepileptics, alcohol).

Hypoxia and vascular wall changes leads to pulmonary vasoconstriction, pulmonary hypertension, cor pulmonale, $\dot{V}/\dot{Q}$ mismatching and the development of shunts.

CHRONIC BRONCHITIS OR EMPHYSEMA?

The value of labelling patients as chronic bronchitis or emphysema is uncertain as the two disease processes usually co-exist and the principles of management are similar. Five pathophysiologic processes may be present to varying degrees in each patient with COPD – inflammatory airway narrowing (bronchiolitis), loss of connective tissues tethering airways, loss of alveoli and capillaries, hyperinflation, and increased pulmonary vascular resistance. Early/mild COPD tends to be dominated by bronchiolitis with a minimal component of

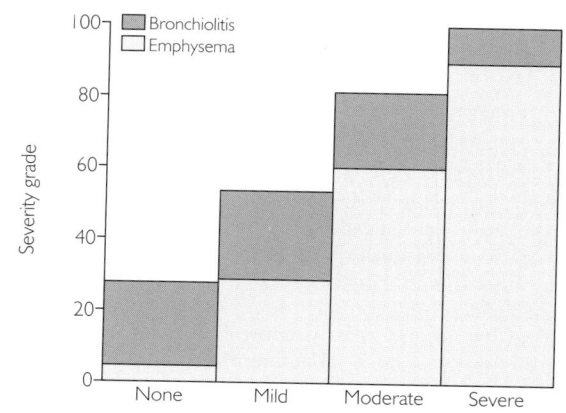

Fig. 24.2   Proportional contributions of bronchiolitis and emphysema at different levels of severity of lung disease.

emphysema (Figure 24.2) whereas when COPD becomes severe, the reverse is true. However, recognition that COPD is dominated by one of these patterns is helpful with regard to clinical pattern and prognosis.

CLINICAL FEATURES OF ARF IN COPD

Acute respiratory failure (ARF) in COPD can present with two distinct clinical patterns.[6] (See Table 24.1.)

PRECIPITANTS OF ACUTE RESPIRATORY FAILURE

In approximately 50% of patients, there is an infective cause, in 25% heart failure and in the remaining 25% retained secretions, air pollution, co-existent medical problems (e.g. pulmonary embolus, medication compliance or side effects) or no cause can be identified.[7] (See Table 24.2.)

The most common bacterial isolates are *Strep. pneumoniae* and *Haemophilus influenzae* in 80% of exacerbations,[8] *Strep viridans*,[9] *Moraxella* (previously Branhamella) *catarrhalis*,[10] *Mycoplasma pneumoniae*[11] and *Pseudomonas*

Table 24.2 Proportional contributions of bronchiolitis and emphysema at different levels of severity of lung disease

> Infective (including aspiration)
> Left ventricular failure (systolic and diastolic failure)
> Sputum retention (post operative, traumatic)
> Pulmonary embolism
> Pneumothoraces and bullae
> Uncontrolled oxygen
> Sedation
> Medication – non-compliance or side-effects
> Nutritional (K, PO_4, Mg deficiency, CHO excess)
> Sleep apnoea

aeruginosa may be found. Viruses can be isolated in 20–30% of exacerbations[12] and include *rhinovirus*, *influenza* and *parainfluenza* viruses, *corona* viruses and occasionally *adenovirus*, and *respiratory syncitial* virus. Whether these organisms are pathogens or colonizers is often unclear.

PNEUMONIA

Pneumonia has been estimated to account for 20% of presentations requiring mechanical ventilation.[12] It is most commonly caused by *Strep. pneumoniae* and *Haemophilus influenzae* but *mycoplasma*, *legionella*, enteric Gram negatives and viruses are occasional causes.

LEFT VENTRICULAR FAILURE

Left ventricular systolic failure may result from coexisting ischaemic heart disease, fluid overload, tachyarrhythmias or biventricular failure secondary to cor pulmonale. Left ventricular diastolic failure occurs commonly and is precipitated by hypoxemia, tachycardia,[13] pericardial constraint due to intrinsic PEEP (PEEPi) or right ventricular (RV) dilation. Increased work of breathing related to COPD will also increase by up to 10 fold the amount of blood flow to the respiratory pump muscles[14] thereby causing an increased demand upon the overall cardiac output. In patients with borderline cardiac status, this may precipitate heart failure. The components of right and left ventricular failure can be accurately distinguished by Doppler echocardiography. Pulmonary congestion can be difficult to diagnose because of the abnormal breath sounds and chest X-ray appearance, which are commonly present in COPD.

UNCONTROLLED OXYGEN ADMINISTRATION

This may precipitate acute hypercapnia in patients with more severe COPD, due to (i) shunting blood to low $\dot{V}/\dot{Q}$ lung units and increasing dead space, (ii) loss of hypoxic drive, (iii) dissociation of CO_2 from Hb molecule (Haldane effect), (iv) anxiolysis and reduction in tachypnoea.

DIAGNOSIS AND ASSESSMENT

DIAGNOSIS OF COPD

The clinical examination findings of COPD depend upon severity.

In mild stable disease (e.g. FEV_1 50–70% predicted normal), an expiratory wheeze on forced expiration and mild exertional dyspnoea may be the only symptoms.

In moderate severity COPD (e.g. FEV_1 30–50% predicted normal), modest to severe exertional dyspnoea is associated with clinical signs of hyperinflation (ptosed upper border of liver beyond the level of nipple and loss of cardiac percussion) and signs of increased work of breathing (use of accessory muscles and tracheal tug).

In severe stable COPD (e.g. FEV_1 <30% predicted normal), marked accessory muscle use is associated with tachypnoea at rest, pursed lip breathing, hypoxemia and signs of pulmonary hypertension (right ventricular heave, loud and palpable pulmonary second sound and elevated 'a' wave in JVP) and cor pulmonale (elevated JVP, hepatomegaly, ankle swelling).

In severe unstable COPD, there is marked tachypnoea at rest, hypoxemia and tachycardia, and, in some, signs of hypercapnia (dilated cutaneous veins, blurred vision, headaches, obtunded mentation, confusion).

Clinical examination may also identify associated medical conditions that might have precipitated the exacerbation such as crepitations and bronchial breathing due to infection, crepitations and cardiomegaly related to heart failure or mediastinal shift related to a pneumothorax.

Basic investigations such as spirometry are very useful in confirming a clinical diagnosis and determining severity of disease. The severity of COPD may be best judged by the reduction in FEV_1 compared with predicted values. Vital capacity (VC) is initially normal and decreases later in the course of the disease but to a lesser degree than the FEV_1.

An FEV_1/VC ratio <70% with an FEV_1 of 50–80% predicted normal without a bronchodilator response usually indicates mild COPD. A significant bronchodilator response, which implies asthma, is regarded as a 12% or greater increase and 200 ml increase in either FEV_1 or VC. An FEV_1 30–50% predicted normal indicates moderately severe COPD and FEV_1 <30% predicted normal indicates severe COPD.

Although the diagnosis may be based on spirometry alone further lung function testing may be useful to characterize the disease. Flow volume curves demonstrate reduced expiratory flow rates at various lung volumes and show the characteristic 'concave' expiratory flow pattern. Lung volumes measured either by helium dilution or plethysmography show elevated total lung capacity, functional residual capacity and residual volume. Characteristically, the residual volume/total lung capacity ratio is >40% in COPD and represents intra-thoracic gas trapping. The total lung carbon monoxide (TLCO) uptake is a measurement of alveolar surface area and its reduction approximates the amount of emphysema present (usually <80% predicted normal).

A chest X-ray will commonly show hyperinflated lung fields as suggested by 10 ribs visible posteriorly, six ribs visible anteriorly or large airspace anterior to heart (>1/3 of the length of the sternum), flattened diaphragms (best seen on lateral CXR) and a paucity of lung markings. Pulmonary hypertension is manifest by enlarged proximal and attenuated distal vascular markings and by RV and atrial enlargement. Lung bullae may be evident.

A high resolution CT scan of the chest (1–2 mm slices) can demonstrate characteristic appearance and regional distribution of emphysema. It can also assess for coexistent bronchiectasis, left ventricular failure[15] and pulmonary fibrosis. Such scans are less sensitive than standard chest CT scans (1 cm slice) for detecting pulmonary lesions (e.g. neoplasms). Nuclear ventilation perfusion scans can also provide a characteristic appearance of COPD.

An ECG is commonly normal but may show features of right atrial or RV hypertrophy and RV strain, including P pulmonale, right axis deviation, dominant R waves in V_{1-2}, right bundle branch block and ST depression and T wave flattening or inversion in V_{1-3}. These changes may be chronic or may develop acutely if there is significant increase in pulmonary vascular resistance during the illness. The electrocardiogram may also show co-existent ischaemic heart disease, tachycardia and atrial fibrillation. Occasionally, continuous ECG monitoring is required to identify transient arrhythmias, which may also precitiate acute deterioration.

DIFFERENTIAL DIAGNOSIS OF COPD

Chronic asthma: the history of chronic asthma is one of long term dyspnoea, wheeze and cough usually at night or upon exercise beginning in childhood with clear cut precipitating agents (e.g. weather, dust, pets, drugs) and a favourable response to either steroids or inhaled β agonists. Late onset asthma (>40 years of age) is not uncommon and is often associated with recurrent gastro-oesophageal reflux. In both forms of asthma, carbon monoxide diffusing capacity (TLCO) is normal. There is usually a bronchodilator response in the FEV_1 if the patient has unstable but lung function tests are normal, the FEV_1 response to an inhalational challenge (e.g. methacholine or hypertonic saline) may assist in discriminating asthma from other causes of dyspnoea.

Bronchiolitis obliterans is a condition which presents as a fixed airflow obstruction following a viral illness, inhalation of toxic fumes, following bone marrow or heart/lung transplantation or related to drugs (e.g. penicillamine). It generally begins as a cough some weeks after insult and insidious onset of dyspnoea. There is a broad spectrum of radiological appearances from normal to reticulonodular to diffuse nodular. Lung tissue via bronchoscopy or by thoracoscopy is required for diagnosis. Histologically, there is a characteristic chronic bronchiolar inflammation appearance, and if granulation tissue extends into the alveloii, it is referred to as bronchiolitis obliterans or organising pneumonia. Removal of the offending agent and instigation of steroids is generally associated with a favourable prognosis.

Bronchiectasis is often associated with fixed mild to moderate airflow obstruction. A chronic productive cough (daily for two consecutive years) is characteristic. Clinical features such as clubbing, localized pulmonary crepitations and a characteristic appearance on HRCT (dilated or plugged small airways at least twice the size of accompanying blood vessel) assist in the diagnosis.

Congestive heart failure may be a differential diagnosis of COPD, or simply co-exist, as both disorders are common in smokers.[13] Orthopnoea and paroxysmal nocturnal dyspnoea are features which correlate with heart failure severity. A past history of myocardial ischaemia or atrial fibrillation should alert one to the possibility of heart failure. An echocardiogram and high resolution CT (HRCT) (looking for shift in interstitial oedema with changes in posture from supine to prone)[15] are sensitive markers of congestive heart failure (CHF).

DIAGNOSIS OF RESPIRATORY FAILURE

An exacerbation of COPD is usually clinically obvious. However, it is important to diagnose the extent of deterioration. The following may be useful.

BLOOD GASES

Blood gases are mandatory to assess hypoxia, hypercapnia and acid-base status. Chronic hypercapnia may be recognized by a bicarbonate level >30 mmol/l and a base excess >4 mmol/l indicating renal compensation. However, other causes of a high serum bicarbonate need to be excluded (e.g. diuretic therapy, high dose steroids or high volume gastric fluid loss) or chronic hypercapnia may be incorrectly assumed and the severity of COPD overestimated. Renal compensation for chronic hypercapnia will increase the serum bicarbonate by approximately 4 mmol/l for each 10 mmHg (1.33 kPa) of chronic PCO_2 rise above 40 mmHg (5.3 kPa), in order to return pH to the low normal range. Irrespective of the COPD patients usual $PaCO_2$ level an acute increase in $PaCO_2$ a decreased arterial pH. This indicates that compensatory mechanisms are exhausted and an increased risk of respiratory collapse.

NON-VENTILATORY MANAGEMENT OF COPD

OXYGEN THERAPY

Oxygen given by low-flow intranasal cannulae or 24% to 35% Venturi mask should be titrated to achieve a saturation (SaO_2) of $90\pm2\%$ as these levels will avoid significant increases in $PaCO_2$ in the majority of COPD patients with ARF. Increases in $PaCO_2$ are most common in patients with initial $PaCO_2$ >50 mmHg and pH <7.35.[16] If the rise in $PaCO_2$ is excessive (>10 mmHg or 1.33 kPa) then FiO_2 should be reduced, titrating SaO_2 to 2–3% below the previous value and ABGs repeated. If no $PaCO_2$ rise occurs with oxygen therapy then a higher SaO_2 may be targeted with repeat blood gases.

Inadequate reversal of hypoxia (e.g. SaO_2 <85%) is suggestive of an additional problem such as pneumonia, pulmonary oedema or embolus, or a pneumothorax. Investigation of this should commence and a higher O_2 delivery system should be used. (See the Chapter 22 on Oxygen Therapy.) While high levels of O_2 should be avoided, reversal of hypoxia is important and O_2 should not be withheld in the presence of hypercapnia nor withdrawn if it worsens.

BRONCHODILATORS

Bronchodilators are routinely given in all exacerbations of COPD because a small reversible component of airflow obstruction is common, and bronchodilators improve mucociliary clearance of secretions.[17]

ANTICHOLINERGIC AGENTS

Anticholinergic agents, such as ipratropium bromide, have been shown to have a similar or greater bronchodilator action than β-agonists in COPD,[18,19] and also to have fewer side-effects and no tachyphylaxis. Anticholinergic agents should be used routinely in COPD with ARF and many now believe them to be the agent of first choice.[1] An ipratropium bromide nebule of 0.5 mg in 2 ml should be nebulized initially 2-hourly, then every 4–6 hours. Long-term use of ipratropium bromide has been shown to reduce the incidence of exacerbations[20] and is therefore recommended for chronic use in COPD. Long acting anticholinergics (e.g. tiotropium) offer potential of once daily dosing.

NEBULIZED β-AGONISTS

Nebulized β-agonists are also effective bronchodilators in COPD,[18,19] although they may cause tachycardia, tremor, mild reductions in potassium and PaO_2 (due to pulmonary vasodilatation), and tachyphylaxis. Nebulized β-agonists (e.g. salbutamol, terbutaline, or fenoterol) given 2- to 4-hourly should be used routinely in combination with ipratropium. This combination has been shown to be more effective than either agent alone.[1] Parenteral sympathomimetic agents are rarely indicated and not recommended for routine use. In stable patients, long term use of β-agonists may improve symptoms of dyspnoea, particularly in the subgroup of COPD with an objective bronchodilator response. Long acting β-agonists may also have a beneficial effect on symptoms, quality of life and exercise capacity in COPD.[21]

AMINOPHYLLINE

Aminophylline is a weak bronchodilator in COPD. It improves diaphragm contractility,[22] stimulates respiratory drive,[23] improves mucociliary transport,[24] right heart function,[25] is anti-inflammatory[26] and is a weak diuretic. Some studies have shown no benefit and significant side-effects,[27] whereas others have shown small benefit[28] in stable COPD. Theophylline has a number of additional effects that may also be of benefit in COPD although the clinical importance of these is not yet established. For an exacerbation aminophylline (loading dose 5–6 mg/kg i.v. over 30 min, followed by an infusion of 0.5 mg/kg per h) is commonly also given despite doubt about its overall benefit. Serum theophylline levels must be monitored regularly to reduce risk of toxicity. The low therapeutic range should be targeted (55–85 μmol/l) for the best effect to side-effect ratio.[29] The high therapeutic range (85–110 μmol/l) has little additional benefit and a significant increase in side-effects,[29] but is thought necessary for diaphragm contractility and respiratory stimulation effects. There is some evidence in favour of theophylline use in the long-term management[30] of COPD but due to its narrow therapeutic window, it should be used with caution.

STEROIDS

In acute exacerbations of COPD, short-term steroids have been shown to improve airflow obstruction[31] including those patients requiring mechanical ventilation for COPD.[32] Doses similar to those for acute asthma should be used. Methylprednisolone 0.5 mg/kg, given 6-hourly for 72 h was used in the study by Albert *et al.*[31] demonstrating benefit in patients with an exacerbation of COPD. Current American Thoracic Society guidelines recommend the equivalent to oral prednisolone at 0.5 mg/kg body weight for 10 d, then ceasing; however, this will depend upon the response to treatment, and their pre-morbid use.[1] Steroids should be avoided if the deterioration is clearly due to bacterial pneumonia without bronchospasm.

Longer-term oral steroids in COPD are associated with a substantial increased risk of side-effects (osteoporosis, diabetes, peptic ulcer, myopathy, systemic hypertension, fluid retention, weight gain), which are likely to impair quality of life and precipitate readmission and are therefore not recommended.[1] A small group of patients (15%) may demonstrate a significant bronchodilator response, in whom co-existent asthma is likely and longer-term high dose (oral or inhaled) steroids may be necessary. However, in the majority of patients, long-term inhaled steroids do not improve lung function or survival, however they do improve quality of life and reduce admissions and are therefore recommended long term treatment at low to medium dose.[1]

ANTIBIOTICS

Antibiotics have an accepted role in the treatment of infection-induced exacerbations of COPD. Amoxycillin is a suitable first line agent against *Haemophilus influenzae* and *Streptococcus pneumoniae* for outpatient exacerbations.[33] Serious exacerbations requiring hospital admission require newer agents such as ciprofloxacin or a third generation cephalosporin.[34] Antibiotics for pneumonia are discussed elsewhere in this volume.

SECRETION CLEARANCE TECHNIQUES

Clearance of lower respiratory secretions is of crucial importance.

CHEST PHYSIOTHERAPY

Chest physiotherapy should be initiated and regularly repeated as both a curative and preventative measure. Encouragement of coughing and deep breathing are the two most important factors.

NEBULIZED MUCOLYTIC AGENTS

Nebulized mucolytic agents, such as acetylcysteine continue to be proposed although their benefit has never been established in acute exacerbations of COPD.[35] Oral mucolytics have been shown to reduce cough frequency and severity in stable COPD.[36]

OROPHARYNGEAL/NASOPHARYNGEAL SUCTIONING

Oropharyngeal/nasopharyngeal suctioning with or without a nasopharyngeal airway. It is desirable but uncommon for the suctioning catheter to enter the trachea, but the technique is useful in clearing pharyngeal secretions, stimulating coughing and clearing lower respiratory secretions coughed only as far as the hypopharynx in patients with suppressed conscious states.

Fibreoptic Bronchoscopy

Fibreoptic bronchoscopy is occasionally used in COPD with ARF. Although effective in clearing sputum, it is labour intensive and may be poorly tolerated by a patient with marginal respiratory function. Indications are lobar consolidation where sputum plug obstruction is suspected, for bronchoalveolar lavage to diagnose pneumonia or to assist difficult secretion clearance.

OTHER MEASURES

Other adjunctive measures are applicable to some patients.

HYDRATION, DIURETICS, DIGOXIN AND VASODILATORS

COPD patients are sensitive to changes in fluid status and intravenous hydration should be undertaken with care and minimized. Diuretics and digoxin are of benefit if LV failure is present. Even if evidence of LV failure is minimal, a trial of diuresis is worthwhile in patients refractory to usual treatment. Digoxin has been shown to improve LV function in patients with cor pulmonale.[37]

Diuretics will reduce fluid overload in cor pulmonale, however care should be taken with severe pulmonary hypertension where a decrease in RV filling pressure may result in a low output state. Digoxin is of no established benefit to RV function in cor pulmonale where the primary problem is increased afterload.[38] Pulmonary hypertension is commonly present in severe COPD and is associated with a poor prognosis. In stable COPD pulmonary vasodilators may have acutely beneficial effects[39] but have not yet been shown to improve outcome.[40] In ARF, pulmonary hypertension invariably increases and may precipitate acute cor pulmonale. Although not clinically proven, pulmonary vasodilators have a rational basis in this setting. Numerous agents have been shown to reduce pulmonary hypertension but calcium channel blockers appear to be the most promising agents[39] at present. Side effects include systemic hypotension, tachycardia, worsening of hypoxia and failure to improve haemodynamics. A trial of vasodilators appears reasonable if cor pulmonale is present with ARF, provided that response to therapy is carefully monitored. The diagnosis and response to treatment of pulmonary hypertension may require a right heart catheter.

ANTICOAGULANTS

Subcutaneous heparin (e.g. 5000 units b.d.) is recommended as a prophylactic measure against venous thromboembolism. There is no evidence for warfarinization in COPD patients with pulmonary hypertension.

ELECTROLYTE CORRECTION

Electrolyte correction is important. Hypophosphataemia is common and may cause respiratory muscle weakness.[41] Hypomagnesaemia,[42] hypocalcaemia[43] and hypokalaemia may also be present and also may impair respiratory muscle function. Hyponatraemia may occur with inappropriate anti-diuretic hormone release or with excess use of diuretics and inappropriate intravenous fluids.

Hypothyroidism

Hypothyroidism is an important condition to be recognized, particularly in the hypercapnic patient group.

Intercostal Drainage

Intercostal drainage is indicated for pneumothorax and pleural effusions of sufficient volume to compromise respiratory function. Formal intercostal catheter insertion may be required but mandates hospital admission and is associated with infection and discomfort. Simple aspiration of pneumothoraces has been shown to result in few complications, a reduced admission rate and reduced hospital stay.

RESPIRATORY STIMULANTS
Many drugs have been shown to increase respiratory drive and lower $PaCO_2$. These include acetazolamide, medroxyprogesterone, naloxone, doxapram and almitrine. Use of such agents presupposes that the limiting factor is reduced respiratory drive, whereas the majority of ARF is limited by a reduced capacity to deal with an increased load to breathing. Side effects include increased dyspnoea and fatigue, impaired sleeping, with almitrine, and increased pulmonary hypertension. Respiratory stimulants have not been shown to improve either short-term or long-term outcome. As a result respiratory stimulants are not recommended or used in ARF. Narcotic or benzodiazepine induced respiratory depression is best managed with the appropriate antagonist, naloxone or flumazenil.

NUTRITION
Nutrition is important, as patients with severe COPD are often undernourished and suffer a deterioration in nutritional status when hospitalized. This poor nutritional state is associated with decreased respiratory muscle mass and strength, increased risk of fatigue, ARF and death. Enteral feeding is preferred, but parenteral nutrition should be considered if enteral feeding is not tolerated. Excessive carbohydrate calories should be avoided as this increases CO_2 production (by ~15%) and may worsen respiratory failure. Low carbohydrate/high fat combinations are preferred in ARF during spontaneous ventilation.

NON-INVASIVE VENTILATION

Non-invasive ventilation (NIV) is a technique in which ventilatory support is provided via a nasal or facial mask without endotracheal intubation. There have been several randomized controlled trials of NIV in COPD patients with acute hypercapnic respiratory failure which have demonstrated improved respiratory physiology, reduced mortality (up to 12 months), reduced iatrogenic complications, reduced need for intubation and mechanical ventilation and reduced length of stay in hospital.[44–47] All studies have shown good tolerance of the technique (~80% of patients) with few side-effects, improvements in both oxygenation and $PaCO_2$ compared with medically treated control patients.[48,49]

The goal of this technique is to (i) unload respiratory muscles and augment ventilation, oxygenation, reduce CO_2 and correct acidosis until the underlying problem can be reversed, (ii) when applied intermittently, to offset the adverse effects of sleep or position induced adverse changes to ventilation, increased upper airway resistance and lung volume.

Indications for NIV are a deterioration of COPD with (i) acute dyspnoea, (ii) respiratory rate >28/min, (iii) $PaCO_2$ >45 mmHg with a pH <7.35, despite optimal medical treatment and not related to excessive supplemental oxygen. Although these indications are for mild exacerbations, most randomized studies have used these as entry guidelines.[44–47] Included in the indications are recently extubated patients in whom NIV has been shown to significantly reduce reintubation rates.[50] Recently NIV has been advocated for use in patients with hypoxic respiratory failure,[51] but success is significantly less in the setting of hypoxemia and either normocapnia or hypocapnia[52] NIV may also have a role in some patients where mechanical ventilation is considered inappropriate.

Side-effects of NIVS have included discomfort, intolerance, skin necrosis, gastric distension and aspiration. Pressure support has been reported as better tolerated than assist/control.[48]

INVASIVE MECHANICAL VENTILATION

OUTCOME OF ARF AND THE DECISION TO INVASIVELY VENTILATE

When respiratory failure progresses or fails to resolve despite aggressive conservative management including NIV, mechanical ventilatory support may be necessary. The decision to ventilate requires careful consideration in some patients who may have near end-stage lung disease and whose quality of life may not justify aggressive treatment. This decision requires consideration of the outcome of ARF.

Patients with COPD have a reduced life expectancy compared with an age matched general population group and this life expectancy decreases in proportion with severity of COPD as assessed by FEV_1 (Figure 24.3).

An episode of ARF further decreases survival (Figure 24.3). ARF precipitated only by bronchitis has a better outcome[2] whereas ARF due to more serious causes such as pneumonia, left ventricular failure and pulmonary embolus have a worse outcome[53] and studies including all such outcomes have lower survival rates (Figure 24.3).

If ARF requires invasive mechanical ventilation survival decreases further still (Figure 24.3). Although the majority of patients do not require mechanical ventilation, the short-term survival in this more severe subset is still good, with a hospital survival rate in some series as high as 80%[54] but 2- and 3-year survival is significantly lower (Figure 24.3).[55,56] The severity of ARF and the severity of underlying COPD based on FEV_1, lifestyle score and dyspnoea score are also predictors of outcome.[12,53] Lifestyle[12] and dyspnoea[57] categories may be the most useful factors in the decision to withhold mechanical ventilation. Lifestyle categories '3' (housebound and at least partly dependent) and '4'

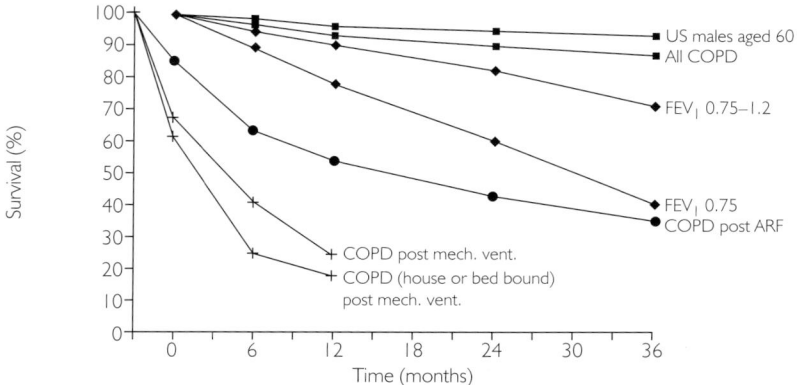

NB: These are approximations only, based on references 16, and 77 with different patient numbers
criteria, and study periods

Fig. 24.3 Survival curves for various patient groups with COPD. Note: These are approximations only, based on other studies,[16,77] with different patient numbers, criteria, and study periods.

(bed- or chair-bound) indicate both a poor outcome (Figure 24.3),[12] and quality of life that may not justify aggressive treatment.

Thus invasive mechanical ventilation may be withheld in endstage lung disease, when low survival, poor quality of life or permanent ventilator dependence is likely. This decision should be based on the following criteria. In general, patients must fulfil all the following criteria for invasive mechanical ventilation to be withheld:

- Known severe COPD, which has been assessed and failed to respond to adequate therapy.
- Severe limitation of lifestyle by dyspnoea with a poor prior 'quality of life'.
- No identifiable reversible factors (e.g. pneumonia, sputum retention, left ventricular failure).

If endstage lung disease is suspected but there is insufficient information, then a trial of aggressive therapy including invasive mechanical ventilation should be undertaken and subsequently withdrawn if unsuccessful. Despite this, most patients with COPD who present with ARF do not have endstage disease and although their immediate problems may be life threatening their short term outcome is sufficiently good to justify full active treatment.

INDICATIONS FOR INVASIVE MECHANICAL SUPPORT

- The clinical appearance of fatigue and impending respiratory collapse despite non-invasive ventilatory support.
- Deteriorating conscious state due to fatigue or hypercapnia or both.
- Hypoxia refractory to high levels of inspired O_2.
- Deterioration due to failure of secretion clearance.
- Respiratory arrest.

MECHANICAL VENTILATION TECHNIQUE

The goals of mechanical ventilation in COPD are to support ventilation while reversible components improve, to allow respiratory muscle to rest and recover whilst preventing wasting from total inactivity, and to minimize dynamic hyperinflation. This is usually best accomplished with low level ventilatory support. Patients requiring low level support may be commenced on 8–15 cmH$_2$O pressure support, with 3–8 cmH$_2$O PEEP. Patients who are completely exhausted, post arrest, comatose or not tolerating pressure support alone, should be commenced or transferred to SIMV mode.

Excessive dynamic hyperinflation must be avoided by using a low minute ventilation: 115/ml per kg is a guideline,[5] and allowing adequate time for expiration. This should be achieved by the use of a small tidal volume (8 ml/kg) and a ventilator rate <14 breaths/min.[5,58] Dynamic hyperinflation can be assessed clinically, by visualizing the expiratory flow-time curve, and by measuring Pplat or PEEPi. Plateau airway pressure should be measured by applying an end-inspiratory pause of 0.5 s. This should only be applied following a single breath as it shortens expiratory time and if it is applied to a series of breaths it increases dynamic hyperinflation resulting in an increased Pplat level and increased risk to the patient. If Pplat is >25 cmH$_2$O, there is likely to be dynamic hyperinflation, and the ventilator rate should be reduced. However, Pplat may be high without dynamic hyperinflation if chest wall compliance is low. Intrinsic PEEP measured as a prolonged end-expiratory pause more directly assesses dynamic hyperinflation. Provided PEEPi is accurately measured, it is a useful tool to follow dynamic hyperinflation. In severe airflow limitation it may be necessary to accept low levels of PEEPi, but as PEEPi rises above 8–10 cmH$_2$O further prolongation of expiratory time must be considered. Although still controversial, the use of a high inspiratory flow rate is recommended[5,59] as it results in a shorter inspiratory time and hence a longer expiratory time for a given ventilatory rate. It has been shown to further reduce dynamic hyperinflation and alveolar pressure[5] and to improve gas exchange.[59]

If dynamic hyperinflation is excessive and causing circulatory compromise or risk of barotrauma, then minute ventilation should be decreased, hypercapnic acidosis accepted and spontaneous ventilation, which will only increase dynamic hyperinflation, should be discouraged by sedation. Muscle relaxants should be avoided unless essential. When dynamic hyperinflation is critical during controlled mechanical ventilation, extrinsic positive end expiratory pressure (PEEPi) increases pulmonary hyperinflation and should not be applied.[60]

If dynamic hyperinflation is not excessive then spontaneous ventilation should be encouraged to promote ongoing respiratory muscle activity and to minimize wasting. Flow-by, pressure support and low level CPAP may all reduce the work of spontaneous breathing and promote a better ventilatory pattern. CPAP approximately equal to the level of PEEPi is most commonly recommended.[61] Care must be taken with all of these supports as each can increase dynamic hyperinflation by a different mechanism, leading to circulatory compromise or risk of barotrauma. Flow-by increases resistance through the expiratory valve, pressure support increases tidal volume and may increase inspiratory time, and CPAP increases functional residual capacity.

WEANING FROM INVASIVE MECHANICAL VENTILATION

Weaning a patient with severe COPD from ventilatory support can be difficult and prolonged. Numerous criteria have been proposed to assess the capacity of the patient to wean;[62] however, the predictive value of any of these individual criteria is limited. The simple criterion of patient respiration rate/tidal volume <100 breaths per min/l had the best predictive value for weaning success, but the advantage of this over simple clinical assessment during weaning is uncertain.[62] Weaning or withdrawal of ventilation is further discussed elsewhere in this volume.

TRACHEOSTOMY

In a small group of patients who have failed extubation despite NIV or who have required long-term ventilatory support, tracheostomy may be beneficial. After 10 days of endotracheal intubation, the risk of trauma and sepsis increases.

A tracheostomy allows long-term ventilatory support, sputum clearance, protection of the upper airway from oral secretions and, off mechanical ventilation, reduced dead space and upper airway resistance. Compared with naso/oro tracheal intubation, tracheostomy is much less intrusive and therefore less sedation is required. Also, it allows direct access to the large airways for the purpose of suctioning and bronchoscopy. Usually nasoenteric feeding tube is required. Consider percutaneous endoscopic gastrostomy (PEG) tube feeding if long-term tracheostomy is being considered to avoid nasal trauma, infection and to reduce oesophagitis. Minimal occlusion tracheostomy cuff pressures (usually <20 cmH$_2$O) should be checked 8-hourly.

Consider removing the tracheostomy when:

1 there is an absence of upper airway obstruction (e.g. no granulation tissue or tracheal stenosis)
2 suctioning is becoming less frequent (<2–4-hourly)
3 the patient is co-operative and has a good capacity to cough, for example good respiratory muscle strength
4 the patient is able to protect their upper airway from aspiration
5 the patient is less dependent on invasive ventilatory support (e.g. not continuous) and non-invasive ventilatory support is available and
6 there is a decreasing oxygenation requirement (e.g. FiO$_2$ <40%).

FAILED WEANING

A small group of patients with endstage lung disease will be unable to successfully wean from ventilator support despite optimization of all reversible factors. A number of options now exist for such patients:

● Long-term institutional or home ventilatory support.
● Withdrawal of support. Permanent institutional mechanical ventilation for a patient with low general health status represents a poor quality of life and withdrawal of support may be a preferable alternative.

POST INTENSIVE UNIT CARE

REHABILITATION

Rehabilitation should be considered for all patients with COPD, particularly those following ARF. There are numerous randomized controlled trials showing improvements in exercise physiology, lung function, quality of life and reduced hospitalization rates.[63,64] Such programmes include extensive education and aerobic upper and lower limb and respiratory muscle exercise usually three times per week over a 6-week period. Patients are recommended to continue with exercises regularly and independently thereafter.

VACCINATION

Vaccination should be considered in all patients with COPD when stable. Annual influenza and 5-yearly pneumococcal vaccination is recommended.[1]

LUNG VOLUME REDUCTION SURGERY

Lung volume reduction surgery is a palliative surgical procedure for patients aged <75 years, with advanced disabling emphysema. Poorly perfused and poorly ventilated areas of one or both lungs, thought to compress relatively preserved areas of well functioning lung tissue, are excised by either midline sternotomy or endoscopically, with video assistance.[65] Such areas in the lung, usually apically placed, are determined by $\dot{V}/\dot{Q}$ scans and high resolution CT scans. Suitable patients must have undergone a pulmonary rehabilitation programme, be on optimal medical treatment, have disabling dyspnoea and anatomically suitable (apical bullous) emphysema. Patients with profoundly severe emphysema (e.g. FEV_1 or TLCO <20% predicted are unlikely to benefit.[65] Group mean data suggest that the mean FEV_1 increases from 0.5 to 0.91 l, and the mean 6-min walk distance increases from 205 to 290 metres, both associated with significant improvement in quality of life. The peak improvements in physiology occur at 1–2 years and thereafter decline to presurgical levels. Improvements in survival are yet to be determined.[65]

LUNG TRANSPLANTATION

Lung transplantation is another palliative surgical procedure for patients with advanced disabling COPD who are aged <65 years, are not ventilator dependent, are on less than 10 mg prednisolone/d and are free of significant co-existent disease. It may be used following lung volume reduction surgery. The current 1, 2 and 5-year international survival figures are 75, 66 and 50% respectively.[66] Common complications are systemic hypertension, bronchiolitis obliterans, acute rejection, viral infection with CMV and neoplasms.[66] Its widespread application in COPD is in doubt because of the very limited supply of donor lungs.[67]

REFERENCES

1 Pauwels RA, Buist AS, Ma P, et al. Global strategy for the diagnosis, management, and prevention of chronic obstructive pulmonary disease. NHLBI/WHO global initiative for chronic obstructive lung disease (GOLD) workshop summary. *Am J Respir Crit Care Med* 2001; **163**: 1256–76.

2 Martin T, Lewis S, Albert R. The prognosis of patients with chronic obstructive pulmonary disease after hospitalization for acute respiratory failure. *Chest* 1982; **82**: 310–4.

3 Britton JR, Pavord ID, Richards KA, et al. Dietary antioxidant vitamin intake and lung function in the general population. *Am J Respir Crit Care Med* 1995; **151**: 1383–7.

4 Burrows B, Fletcher C, Heard B. The emphysematous and bronchial types of chronic airways obstruction. A clinicopathological study of patients in London and Chicago. *Lancet* 1966; 1830–6.

5 Tuxen D, Lane S. The effects of ventilatory pattern on hyperinflation, airway pressures, and circulation in mechanical ventilation of patients with severe airflow obstruction. *Am Rev Respir Dis* 1987; **136**: 872–9.

6 Fahey P, Hyde R. 'Won't breathe' versus 'can't breathe'. Detection of depressed ventilatory drive in patients with obstructive pulmonary disease. *Chest* 1983; **84**: 19–25.

7 Connors AF Jr, Dawson NV, Thomas C, et al. Outcomes following acute exacerbations of severe chronic obstructive lung disease. *Am J Respir Crit Care Med* 1996; **154**: 959–67.

8 Schreiner A, Bjerkestrand G, Digrannes A. Bacteriologic findings in the transtracheal aspirate from patients with acute exacerbations of chronic bronchitis. *Infection* 1978; **6**: 54–6.

9 Irwin R, Erickson A, Pratter M. Prediction of tracheobronchial colonization in current cigarette smokers with chronic obstructive bronchitis. *J Infect Dis* 1982; **145**: 234–41.

10 Christensen J, Gadeberg O, Bruvn B. Branhamella catarrhalis: significance in pulmonary infections and bacteriological features. *Acta Pathol Microbiol Immunol Scand* 1986; **94**: 89–95.

11 Smith CB, Golden CA, Kanner RE, Renzetti AD Jr. Association of viral and *Mycoplasma pneumoniae* infections with acute respiratory illness in patients with chronic obstructive pulmonary disease. *Am Rev Respir Dis* 1980; **121**: 225–32.

12 Menzies R, Gibbons W, Goldberg P. Determinants of weaning and survival among patients with COPD who require mechanical ventilation for acute respiratory failure. *Chest* 1989; **95**: 398–405.

13 Baum GL, Schwartz A, Llamas R, Castillo C. Left ventricular function in chronic obstructive lung disease. *N Engl J Med* 1971; **285**: 361–5.

14 Robertson C, Foster G, Johnson R. The relationship of respiratory failure to the oxygen consumption of, lactate production by, and distribution of blood flow among respiratory muscles during increasing inspiratory resistance. *J Clin Invest* 1977; **59**: 31–42.

15 Kato S, Nakamoto TK, Iizuka M, Early diagnosis and estimation of pulmonary congestion and edema in patients with left-sided heart disease from histogram of pulmonary CT number. *Chest* 1996; **109**: 1439–45.

16 Bone R, Pierce A, Johnson R. Controlled oxygen administration in acute respiratory failure in chronic obstructive pulmonary disease. *Am J Med* 1978; **65**: 896–902.

17 Mossberg B, Strandberg K, Philipson K, Camner P. Tracheobronchial clearance and beta-adrenoceptor stimulation in patients with chronic bronchitis. *Scand Respir Dis* 1976; **57**: 281–9.

18 Braun SR, McKenzie WN, Copeland C, et al. A comparison of effect of ipratropium and albuterol (salbutamol) in chronic obstructive airway disease. *Arch Intern Med* 1989; **149**: 544–7.

19 Karpel JP, Schacter EN, Fanta C, et al. A comparison of ipratropium and albuterol vs albuterol alone for the treatment of acute asthma. *Chest* 1996; **110**: 611–6.

20 Friedman M, Serby CW, Menjoge SS, *et al.* Pharmacoeconomic evaluation of a combination of ipratropium plus albuterol compared with ipratropium alone and albuterol alone in COPD. *Chest* 1999; **115**: 635–41.

21 Boyd G, Morice A, Pounsford J. An evaluation of salmeterol in the treatment of chronic obstructive pulmonary disease. *Eur Respir J* 1997; **10**: 815–21.

22 Aubier M, De Troyer A, Sampson M, *et al.* Aminophylline improves diaphragmatic contractility. *N Engl J Med* 1981; **305**: 249–52.

23 Berry RB, Desa MM, Branum JP, Light RW. Effect of thoephylline on sleep and sleep-disordered breathing in patients with chronic obstructive pulmonary disease. *Am Rev Respir Dis* 1991; **143**: 245–50.

24 Wanner A. Effects of methyxanthines on airway mucociliary function. *Am J Med* 1985; **79**: 16–21.

25 Matthay RA, Berger HJ, Davies R. Improvement in cardiac performance by oral long-acting theophylline in chronic obstructive pulmonary disease. *Am Heart J* 1982; **104**: 1022–6.

26 Pauwels R. New aspects of the therapeutic potential of theophylline in asthma. *J Allergy Clin Immunol* 1989; **83**: 548–53.

27 Rice KL, Leatherman JW, Duane PG, *et al.* Aminophylline for acute exacerbations of chronic obstructive pulmonary disease. *Ann Intern Med* 1987; **107**: 305–9.

28 Guyatt GH, Townsend M, Pugsley SO, *et al.* Bronchodilators in chronic air-flow limitation. Effects on airway function, exercise capacity, and quality of life. *Am Rev Respir Dis* 1987; **135**: 1069–74.

29 Rogers R, Owens G, Pennock B. The pendulum swings again: toward a rational use of theophylline. *Chest* 1985; **87**: 280–2.

30 Chrystyn H, Mulley B, Peake M. Dose response relation to oral theophylline in severe chronic obstructive airways disease. *BMJ* 1988; **297**: 1506–10.

31 Albert R, Martin T, Lewis S. Controlled clinical trial of methylprednisolone in patients with chronic bronchitis and acute respiratory insufficiency. *Ann Intern Med* 1980; **92**: 753–8.

32 Rubini S, Rampullua C, Nava S. Acute effect of corticosteroids on respiratory mechanics in mechanically ventilated patients with chronic airflow obstruction and acute respiratory failure. *Am J Respir Crit Care Med* 1994; **149**: 306–10.

33 Hosker H, Cooke N, Hawkey P. Antibiotics in chronic obstructive pulmonary diesease. *BMJ* 1994; **308**: 871–2.

34 Basran GS, Joseph J, Abbas AM, *et al.* Treatment of acute exacerbations of chronic obstructive airways disease – a comparison of amoxycillin and ciprofloxacin. *J Antimicrob Chemother* 1990; **26(Suppl F)**: 19–24.

35 Siafakas NM, Vermeire P, Pride NB, *et al.* Optimal assessment and management of chronic obstructive pulmonary disease (COPD). *Eur Respir J* 1995; **8**: 1398–1420.

36 Petty T. The National Mucolytic Study. Results of a randomized, double-blind, placebo-controlled study of iodinated glycerol in chronic obstructive bronchitis. *Chest* 1990; **97**: 75–83.

37 Mathur P, Pugsley S, Powles A. Effect of digitalis on left ventricular function in chronic cor pulmonale. *Am Rev Respir Dis* 1980; **121**: 163.

38 Green L, Smith T. The use of digitalis in patients with pulmonary disease. *Ann Intern Med* 1977; **87**: 459–65.

39 Sajkov D, McEvoy R, Cowie R. Felodipine improves pulmonary hemodynamics in chronic obstructive pulmonary disease. *Chest* 1993; **103**: 1354–61.

40 Salvaterra C, Rubin L. Investigation and management of pulmonary hypetension in chronic obstructive pulmonary disease. *Am Rev Respir Dis* 1994; **148**: 1414–17.

41 Aubier M, Murciano D, Lecocguic Y. Effect of hypophosphatemia on diaphragmatic contractility in patients with acute respiratory failure. *N Engl J Med* 1985; **313**: 420–4.

42 Dhingra S, Solven F, Wilson A, McCarthy DS. Hypomagnesemia and respiratory muscle power. *Am Rev Respir Dis* 1984; **129**: 497–8.

43 Aubier M, Viires N, Piquet J. Effects of hypocalcemia on diaphragmatic strength generation. *J Appl Physiol* 1985; **58**: 2054–61.

44 Brochard L, Mancebo J, Wysocki M, *et al.* Noninvasive ventilation for acute exacerbations of chronic obstructive pulmonary disease. *N Engl J Med* 1995; **333**: 817–22.

45 Bott J, Carroll MP, Conway JH, *et al.* Randomised controlled trial of nasal ventilation in acute ventilatory failure due to chronic obstructive airways disease. *Lancet* 1993; **341**: 1555–7.

46 Kramer N, Meyer TJ, Meharg J, *et al.* Randomised prospective trial of noninvasive positive pressure ventilation in acute respiratory failure. *Am J Respir Crit Care Med* 1995; **151**: 1799–806.

47 Plant P, Owen J, Elliott M. Early use of noninvasive ventilation for acute exacerbations of chronic obstructive pulmonary disease on general respiratory wards: a multicentre randomised controlled trial. *Lancet* 2000; **355**: 1931–5.

48 Mehta S, Hill NS. Noninvasive ventilation. *Am J Respir Crit Care Med* 2001; **163**: 540–77.

49 Hillberg RE, Johnson DC. Noninvasive ventilation. *N Engl J Med* 1997; **337**: 1746–52.

50 Nava S, Ambrosino N, Clini E, *et al.* Noninvasive mechanical ventilation in the weaning of patients with respiratory failure due to chronic obstructive pulmonary disease. A randomized controlled trial. *Ann Intern Med* 1998; **128**: 721–8.

51 Antonelli M, Conti G, Rocco M, *et al.* A comparison of noninvasive positive-pressure ventilation and conventional mechanical ventilation in patients with acute respiratory failure. *N Engl J Med* 1998; **339**: 429–35.

52 Wysocki M, Tric L, Wolff MA, *et al.* Noninvasive pressure support ventilation in patients with acute respiratory failure. *Chest* 1993; **103**: 907–13.

53 Hudson L. Survival data in patients with acute and chronic lung disease requiring mechanical ventilation. *Am Rev Respir Dis* 1989; **140**: S19–S24.

54 Petty T. Acute respiratory failure in chronic obstructive pulmonary disease. In: Sheomaker W, Thompson W, Holbrook P (eds) *Textbook of Critical Care*. Sydney: WB Saunders; 1984: pp. 264–72.

55 Burk R, George R. Acute respiratory failure in chronic obstructive pulmonary disease (immediate and long term prognosis). *Arch Intern Med* 1972; **132**: 865–8.

56 Admandsson T, Kilburn K. Survival after respiratory failure (145 patients observed 5 to 8.5 years). *Ann Intern Med* 1974; **80**: 54–9.

57 Ferris B. Epidemiology standardization project. *Am Rev Respir Dis* 1978; **118**(**Suppl**): 1–120.

58 Curtis J, Hudson L. Emergent assessment and management of acute respiratory failure in COPD. *Clin Chest Med* (Respir Emergencies II) 1994; **15**: 481–500.

59 Connors A, McCaffree D, Gray B. Effect of inspiratory flow rate on gas exchange during mechanical ventilation. *Am Rev Respir Dis* 1981; 124: 537–43.

60 Tuxen D. Detrimental effects of positive end-expiratory pressure during controlled mechanical ventilation of patients with severe airflow obstruction. *Am Rev Respir Dis* 1989; 140: 5–9.

61 Biagorri F, De Monte A, Blanch L. Hemodynamic response to external counterbalancing of auto-positive end expiratory pressure in mechanically ventilated patients with chronic obstructive pulmonary disease. *Crit Care Med* 1994; **22**: 1782–91.

62 Esteban A, Frutos F, Tobin MJ, *et al*. A comparison of four methods of weaning patients from mechanical ventilation. *N Engl J Med* 1995; **332**: 345–50.

63 Lacasse Y, Ferreira I, Brooks D, *et al*. Critical appraisal of clinical practice guidelines targeting chronic obstructive pulmonary disease. *Arch Intern Med* 2001; **161**: 69–74.

64 Goldstein RS, Gort EH, Stubbing D, *et al*. Randomised controlled trial of respiratory rehabilitation. *Lancet* 1994; **344**: 362–8.

65 Stirling GR, Babidge WJ, Peacock MJ, *et al*. Lung volume reduction surgery in emphysema: a systematic review. *Ann Thoracic Surg* 2001; **72**: 641–8.

66 Hosenpud JD, Bennett LE, Keck BM, *et al*. The registry of the International Society for Heart and Lung Transplantation: seventeenth official report-2000. *J Heart Lung Transplant* 2000; **19**: 909–31.

67 Snell GI, Griffiths A, Macfarlane L, *et al*. Maximising thoracic organ transplant opportunities: the importance of efficient co-ordination. *J Heart Lung Transplant* 2000; **19**: 410–7.

25

Mechanical ventilation

A D Bersten

Mechanical ventilation for acute respiratory failure (ARF) is now a routine aspect of patient management in the ICU. The 1952 Copenhagen polio epidemic introduced the notion of organized areas (ICU) for the provision of positive pressure ventilation,[1] which was usually applied through a tracheostomy that had been inserted to allow suction of secretions. However, methods of ventilatory assistance without intubation had proliferated prior to the polio epidemic (both negative pressure chest wall devices and positive pressure face mask devices), and current trends are to an increased use of non-invasive ventilation (NIV) in patients with respiratory failure.[2]

Almost all of the ventilatory modes that are conventionally applied during *intubated* ventilation (IV), can be applied *non-invasively*; however, IV remains the primary mode of respiratory assistance in critically ill patients. There are also an increasing number of patients receiving chronic ventilatory assistance; but, since the majority of these use chronic NIV, this chapter is primarily directed at intubated mechanical ventilation for both ARF and acute-on-chronic respiratory failure.

A PHYSIOLOGICAL APPROACH

During normal spontaneous breathing contraction of the respiratory muscles overcomes both the elastic recoil and resistance of the respiratory system (lung and chest wall). A fall in regional pleural pressure results in alveolar inflation as gas is forced in under the resultant pressure gradient. Expiration is usually passive but the expiratory muscles may assist the elastic recoil of the respiratory system.

The work (W) performed by the respiratory muscles (Wmus) can be measured from the pressure (P)-volume (V) loop, and partitioned into elastic (Wel) and resistive (Wres) work:

$$Wmus = Wel + Wres \qquad (1)$$

Inertial work is negligible, and usually ignored, and Equation (1) does not include the threshold work (Wthres) required to initiate inspiration when intrinsic PEEP (PEEPi) is present.

Because volume is constant in Equation (1) it can be simplified to:

$$Pmus = Pel + Pres \qquad (2)$$

It follows that during positive pressure ventilatory assistance, where Pao is the ventilatory pressure applied at the airway:

$$Pao + Pmus = Pel + Pres \qquad (3)$$

and that when the work is solely applied by the ventilator with no respiratory muscle contraction (controlled mechanical ventilation), that

$$Pao = Pel + Pres \qquad (4)$$

This nomenclature allows physiologic discussion of the different ventilatory modes from controlled ventilation to spontaneous, unassisted ventilation, and introduces the Equation of Motion which is used in the estimation of respiratory mechanics:

$$Pao = Ers\ V + Rrs\ \dot{V} + Po \qquad (5)$$

where Ers is the respiratory system (lung and chest wall) elastance (the inverse of compliance), Rrs is the respiratory system resistance, $\dot{V}$ is the gas flow rate, and Po is the total PEEP (the sum of extrinsic PEEP [PEEPe] and PEEPi). PEEPi imposes Wthres, as inspiratory muscle contraction must occur without $\dot{V}$ until Pao falls below atmospheric pressure (see below, in 'Patient–Ventilator Interaction').

MODES OF VENTILATION

CONTROLLED MECHANICAL VENTILATION

The simplest form of positive pressure breath occurs in a relaxed subject, and the ventilator provides a constant

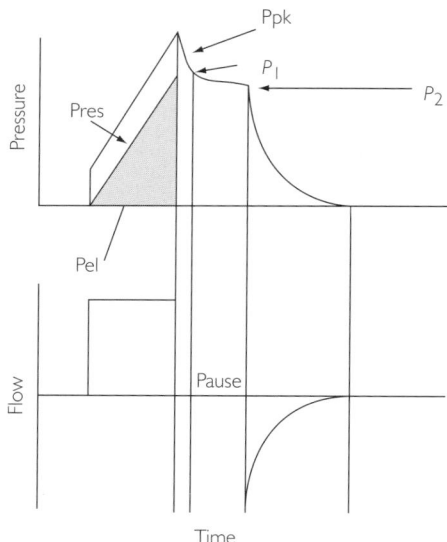

Fig. 25.1 Schematic diagram of a volume controlled breath with constant inspiratory flow. A period of no inspiratory gas flow has been interposed before expiration (pause) to illustrate dissipation of lung resistance as airways resistance (fall from Ppk to P_1) and tissue resistance (fall from P_1 to P_2). The inspiratory pressure due to the elastic properties of the respiratory system is illustrated as the filled area, Pel), and the lung resistive pressure is labelled as Pres. See text for more detail.

gas flow during inspiration. The volume delivered will depend upon the inspiratory time (Ti), and Pao during inspiration will reflect Ers and Rrs (Figure 25.1). Expiration is a passive, and usually exponential, decline in volume to the relaxation volume of the respiratory system, equal to the functional residual capacity (FRC).

CMV is the most basic form of mechanical ventilation; however, it is an extremely useful baseline, and is still commonly used. A preset minute ventilation is made up from a fixed respiratory rate (f) and tidal volume (V_T). Provided that there are not large variations in alveolar dead space, this maintains a preset alveolar ventilation (V_A) and CO_2 clearance. Consequently, CMV is useful in conditions where there is alveolar hypoventilation (e.g. respiratory muscle weakness), when $PaCO_2$ needs to be maintained in a fixed range (e.g. raised intracranial pressure), or when the work of breathing must be minimized (e.g. severe cardiorespiratory failure). Because CMV may not match respiratory drive, and spontaneous, supported or assisted breaths are not possible during CMV, sedation, and sometimes muscle paralysis, may be needed. CMV is usually combined with PEEPe, which can recruit collapsed lung and reduce intrapulmonary shunt. The components are discussed below.

TIDAL VOLUME (V_T)

Although traditional CMV V_T has been 12–15 ml/kg, this may result in excessive lung stretch, particularly in patients with acute lung injury (ALI), leading to ventilator-induced (VILI) or ventilator-associated lung injury (VALI).[3] The basis for this larger V_T can be traced back to progressive atelectasis and intra-pulmonary shunt when physiologic V_T were used during general anaesthesia. This could be reversed by larger V_T ventilation or intermittent sigh breaths.[4] In patients with ALI, V_T of 6 ml/kg vs 12 ml/kg predicted body weight (i.e. often 4–5 ml/kg vs 9–10 ml/kg true weight) reduced mortality from 40% to 31%.[5] Consequently, lower V_T should be strongly considered during CMV, and other forms of ventilatory assistance, in patients with ALI. However, greater levels of PEEP are usually required, and similar data are not available for other respiratory diseases. Indeed, while the reduction in V_T is particularly applicable to ALI, excessive lung stretch will be less likely in other patient cohorts that are able to ventilate a greater proportion of the lung (see Chapter 27 on Acute Respiratory Distress Syndrome).

RESPIRATORY RATE (f)

The desired minute ventilation can be selected from the product of V_T and f. Common CMV rates are 10–20 breaths/min in adults. Sufficient expiratory time (Te) must be allowed to minimize dynamic hyperinflation and PEEPi. Although high f (up to 35 breaths/min) were allowed in the ARDS Network protocol, and the low V_T, low mortality group had a mean f of ~30 breaths/min,[5] laboratory data suggest a possible additive role of high f in VILI.[6]

INSPIRATORY FLOW PATTERN

The simplest form of CMV uses a constant inspiratory $\dot{V}$ ($\dot{V}_I$), and in combination with Ti, a preset volume is delivered. This is also called volume controlled ventilation (VC), and some ventilators use V_T and Ti to set $\dot{V}_I$. Alternative $\dot{V}_I$ patterns that are commonly available with VC include a ramped descending flow pattern and a sine pattern. When a time preset inspiratory pressure is delivered this is termed pressure controlled ventilation (PCV).

There are no convincing outcome data differentiating these different modes of CMV and PCV. Although the peak airway pressure (Ppk) is lower with PCV than constant flow CMV, the alveolar distending pressure, which is usually inferred from the plateau pressure (Pplat), is no different provided that Ti and V_T are the same.[7] During PCV, Pres is dissipated during inspiration so Ppk and Pplat are equal, and during CMV, Pres accounts for the difference between Ppk and Pplat (Figure 25.2). Similarly, different CMV ($\dot{V}_I$ $\dot{V}_I$ patterns will alter Ppk without changing Pplat or mean airway pressure (Pmean) when Ti and V_T are constant. In ARDS patients there is no difference in haemodynamics, oxygenation, or recruited lung volume;[7,8] however, PCV may reduce non-linear behaviour.[8]

Pressure-regulated volume control (PRVC) is a form of CMV where the V_T is preset, and achieved at a minimum pressure using a decelerating flow pattern.

INSPIRATORY PAUSE

An end-inspiratory pause allows examination of the decay in Ppk, and measurement of Pplat. If Ti and V are maintained constant there is no improvement in oxygenation, and a more rapid $\dot{V}_I$ will be needed. This may alter the distribution of ventilation. Theoretically, an end-inspiratory pause will allow a 32% dissipation of the total energy loss within the respiratory system,[9] which may significantly reduce the forces driving expiration,

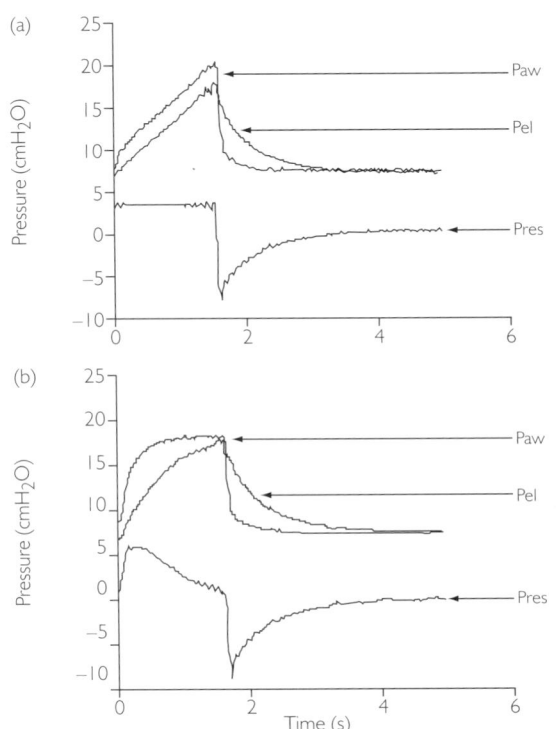

and this could exacerbate gas trapping in patients with severe airflow limitation.

INSPIRATORY TIME, EXPIRATORY TIME, I:E RATIO

The combination of V_T and inspiratory $\dot{V}$ will determine Ti, which in combination with f sets Te. A typical Ti is 0.8–1.2 s; with a V_T of 500 ml and inspiratory $\dot{V}$ of 0.5 l/s the Ti is 1.0 s. During spontaneous ventilation, the distribution of ventilation at low $\dot{V}$ is determined by regional E, and at high inspiratory $\dot{V}$ by regional R leading to greater ventilation of non-dependent lung. In patients with severe airflow limitation high inspiratory flow rates may be used in order to prolong Te and minimize dynamic hyperinflation.[10]

The I:E ratio is usually set at or below 1:2 to allow an adequate Te for passive expiration. During inverse ratio ventilation (IRV) the I:E ratio is greater than 1:1. The putative benefits of a prolonged Ti include recruitment of long time constant alveoli, and a short Te results in gas trapping and PEEPi. Early reports of clinical benefit did not control for PEEPi, and when total PEEP, f and V_T are constant,[7,8] PCIRV tends to reduce $PaCO_2$ but does not improve oxygenation, and may have deleterious haemodynamic effects and exaggerate regional over-inflation.[8]

POSITIVE END-EXPIRATORY PRESSURE

Positive end-expiratory pressure (PEEP) is an elevation in the end-expiratory pressure upon which all forms of mechanical ventilation may be imposed. When PEEP is maintained throughout the respiratory cycle in a spontaneously breathing subject, the term constant positive airway pressure (CPAP) is used. The primary role of PEEP is to recruit collapsed lung, increase FRC and minimize intrapulmonary shunt. PEEP may also improve oxygenation by redistributing lung water from the alveolus to the interstitium, and although there is no direct effect of PEEP to reduce extravascular lung water, this may occur in patients with left ventricular failure due to a reduction in venous return and left ventricular afterload. Further, inadequate PEEP may contribute to VILI by promoting tidal opening and closing of alveoli.[3] PEEP levels of 5–15 cmH_2O are commonly used, and levels up to 25 cmH_2O may be required in patients with severe ARDS. PEEP titration in ARDS is complex (see the chapter on Acute Respiratory Distress Syndrome), and should aim to improve oxygenation and minimize VILI. Since PEEP reduces venous return, cardiac output and O_2 delivery may fall despite an improvement in PaO_2; indeed this concept has been used to optimize PEEP in ARF.[11] However, in addition to recruitment, increasing PEEP may lead to overinflation of non-dependent alveoli, which are already aerated at end-expiration.[12,13] This will be less likely if alveolar distending pressure is kept <30–35 cmH_2O, or the change in driving pressure is <2 cmH_2O when V_T is constant.[14]

Fig. 25.2 Actual pressure-time data from a patient with acute lung injury ventilated with volume controlled ventilation (a), and then with pressure controlled ventilation (b); tidal volume, I:E ratio and respiratory rate are constant. The airway pressure (Paw, bold line) has been broken down to its components, Pel and Pres (see Figure 25.1). Although there is no inspiratory pause, there is marked similarity between (a) and Figure 25.1, with the inspiratory difference between Paw and Pel due to a constant Pres. In (b), the decelerating inspiratory flow pattern seen with pressure controlled ventilation results in dissipation of Pres by end-inspiration. Consequently, during pressure controlled ventilation Paw = Pplat obtained during volume controlled ventilation. In other words for the same ventilator settings there is no difference in the static elastic distending pressure.

PEEPe is applied by placing a resistance in the expiratory circuit (Figure 25.3), with most ventilators using a solenoid valve. Independent of the technique, a threshold resistor is preferred, since it offers minimal resistance to flow once its opening P is reached. This will minimize expiratory work, and avoid barotrauma during coughing or straining.

PEEPi is an elevation in the static recoil pressure of the respiratory system at end-expiration. PEEPi arises due to an inadequate Te, usually in the setting of severe airflow obstruction. However, it may be a desired endpoint during IRV. The sum of PEEPe and PEEPi is the total PEEP (PEEPtot). The distribution of PEEPi is likely to be less uniform than an equivalent PEEPe, and this may not have the same physiological effects. When patients with severe airflow obstruction are triggering ventilation PEEPe, less than PEEPi may be applied to reduce Wthres (see below, 'Patient-Ventilator Interaction').

FRACTIONAL INSPIRED OXYGEN CONCENTRATION (FiO$_2$)

Adequate arterial oxygen saturation is achieved through a combination of minute ventilation, PEEP and FiO$_2$ adjustment. Even patients with normal respiratory systems usually need an FiO$_2$ >0.21, due to ventilation-perfusion mismatch secondary to positive pressure ventilation. In patients with ARF it is common to start with an FiO$_2$ of one and titrate down as PEEP and minute ventilation are adjusted. Because high FiO$_2$s are damaging to the lung, and nitrogen washout may exacerbate atelectasis, it is reasonable to aim at an FiO$_2$ ≤0.6.

SIGH

Many ventilators have the ability to intermittently deliver a breath at least twice V$_T$. Sighs may reduce atelectasis, in part, through release of pulmonary surfactant,[15] resulting in recruitment and improved oxygenation in ARDS.[16] However, if sighs or recruitment manoeuvres are used, care must be taken to avoid recurrent excessive lung stretch.

ASSIST-CONTROL VENTILATION

During assist-control ventilation (ACV), in addition to the set f, patient effort can trigger a standard CMV breath (Figure 25.4). This allows greater patient comfort; however, there may be little reduction in respiratory work compared with an unassisted breath at low inspiratory V̇, because the respiratory muscles continue to contract through much of the breath.[17] The equivalent PCV breath is termed pressure assist-control ventilation (PACV). Differences between triggering modes are discussed below (Patient–ventilator interaction).

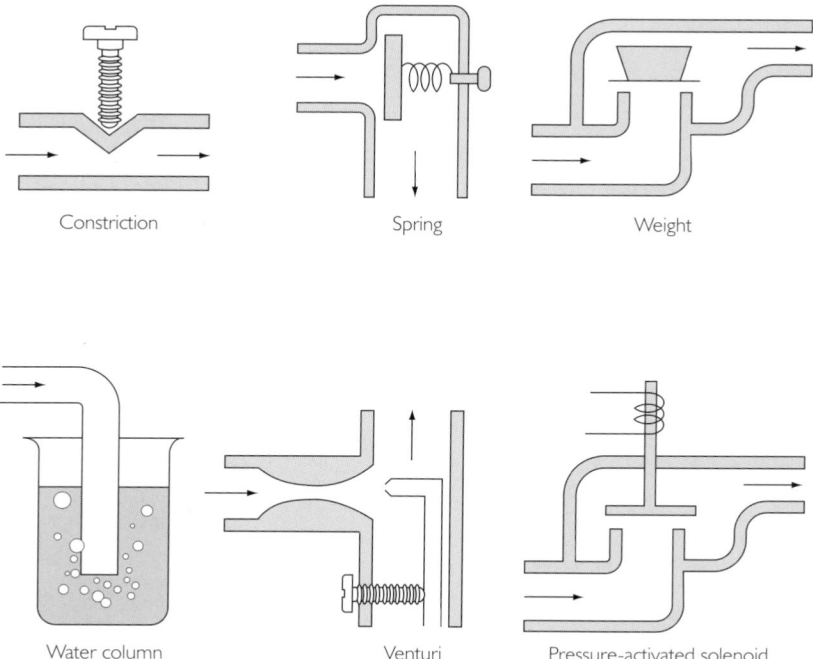

Constriction   Spring   Weight

Water column   Venturi   Pressure-activated solenoid

Fig. 25.3 Positive end-expiratory pressure valves.

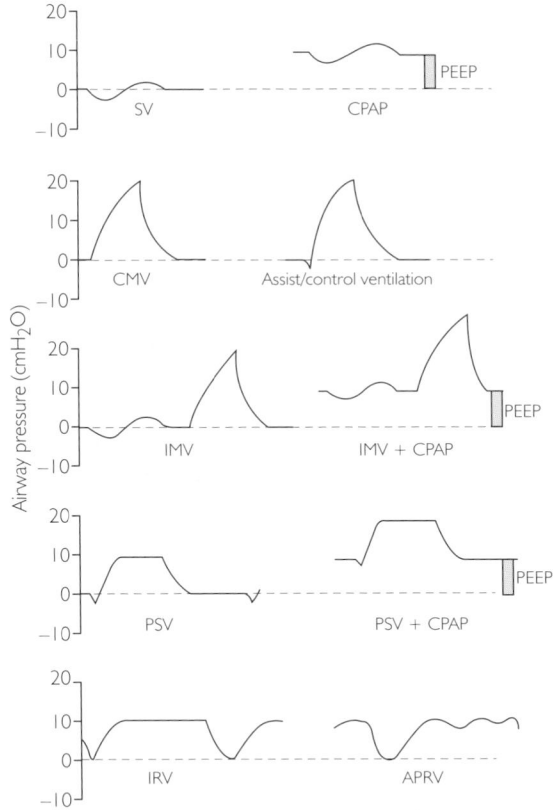

Fig. 25.4 Schematic representation of airway pressure versus time for a variety of forms of ventilatory assistance. SV, spontaneous ventilation; CPAP, continuous positive airway pressure; PEEP, positive end-expiratory pressure; CMV, conventional mechanical ventilation; IMV, intermittent mandatory ventilation; PSV, pressure support ventilation; IRV, inverse ratio ventilation; APRV, airway pressure release ventilation.

INTERMITTENT MANDATORY VENTILATION, SYNCHRONIZED IMV

Intermittent mandatory ventilation (IMV) was introduced in the 1980s to aid weaning from CMV by allowing the patient to take 'unimpeded' breaths while still receiving a background of controlled breaths. Proposed advantages include a reduction in sedation, lower mean intrathoracic pressure with less barotrauma and adverse haemodynamic consequences, improved intrapulmonary gas distribution, continued use of respiratory muscles and faster weaning. During SIMV Ti is partitioned into patient-initiated and true spontaneous breaths to avoid breath stacking. However, during spontaneous breaths the work of breathing imposed by the endotracheal tube, circuit and ventilator must be overcome.[18] In weaning

studies comparing SIMV with T-piece trials and pressure support ventilation (PSV), SIMV appears to be the least efficient.[19] Many clinicians add PSV during gradual reduction in respiratory rate with SIMV to overcome the added respiratory work imposed by the circuit and endotracheal tube, however, this approach has not been formally compared with other weaning techniques.

PRESSURE SUPPORT VENTILATION

During pressure support ventilation (PSV), each patient-triggered breath is supported by gas flow to achieve a preset pressure, usually designated to be above the PEEPe. This can be explained by referring to the equation of motion where:

$$Pmus + Pao = Ers\ V + Rrs\ \dot{V} + Po \qquad (6)$$

During PSV, Pao is the targeted variable by the ventilator, which leads to a significant and important reduction in Pmus and work of breathing.[20] The detection of neural expiration varies between ventilators, but commonly relies upon a fall in the inspiratory $\dot{V}$ to either 25% of the initial flow rate or to less than 5 l/min. PSV may also be titrated to offset the work imposed by the circuit and endotracheal tube. The absolute level required to offset this will vary with endotracheal tube size and inspiratory $\dot{V}$,[21] but is commonly 5–10 cmH$_2$O.[22] PSV can be used during weaning, or as a form of variable ventilatory support with pressures of 15–20 cmH$_2$O commonly used. Disadvantages include variable V$_T$, and hence minute ventilation, the potential to deliver an excessive V$_T$, and patient-ventilator asynchrony (see below).

Volume-assured pressure support (VAPS) is a mode of adaptive PSV where breath-to-breath logic achieves a preset V$_T$.

PROPORTIONAL ASSIST VENTILATION

Proportional assist ventilation (PAV) is a form of partial ventilatory support where inspiratory P is applied in proportion to patient effort. Because this allows the breathing pattern and minute ventilation to be matched to patient effort it is only suitable if respiratory drive is normal or elevated. In concept this should optimize the patient–ventilator interaction; however, the prescription of PAV requires a greater level of physiological understanding than similar forms of partial ventilatory support such as PSV, since there is no target P, V, or $\dot{V}$. PAV is usually prescribed using volume assist (VA) and flow assist (FA), with V and $\dot{V}$ measured continuously. VA generates greater P as V increases leading to elastic unloading, and FA generates greater P as $\dot{V}$ increases leading to resistive unloading. Not surprisingly, the units of VA are cmH$_2$O/l (i.e. an elastance term) and those for FA are cmH$_2$O/l per s (i.e. a resistance term). This can be illustrated by referring to Equation (6):

Pmus + Pao = Ers V + Rrs V̇ + Po

Where Pao is determined by PAV, where PAV = VA + FA, so:

Pmus + VA × V + FA V̇ = Ers V + Rrs V̇ + Po   (7)

consequently:

Pmus = (Ers − VA) V + (Rrs − FA) V̇ + Po   (8)

If Ers and Rrs are known, PAV can, at least in principle, be targeted to reduce a specified proportion of either, or both, elastic and resistive respiratory work. For example, when VA and FA are adjusted to counterbalance Ers and Rrs, so as to achieve normal values, minute ventilation increases, and respiratory drive and work decrease; if PEEPi is present, work can be further reduced by applying PEEPe.[23] However, estimates of respiratory mechanics are often not known, and are relatively hard to measure in spontaneously breathing patients. Consequently, PAV is often titrated to patient comfort. Despite a growing body of data demonstrating reduced work of breathing, and improved patient-ventilator synchrony with PAV, it is a more difficult technique to use, and definitive studies showing a clinically important outcome difference are awaited.

BILEVEL VENTILATION

Also described as biphasic positive airway pressure (BIPAP), this describes ventilatory modes where two levels of airway pressure are provided. The patient may cycle between these two levels as triggered by their ventilatory effort, in which case inspiratory positive airway pressure (IPAP) and expiratory positive airway pressure (EPAP) are set. However, another use of bilevel ventilation is to allow spontaneous breathing at both levels of airway pressure, with time cycling between both pressure levels (high and low CPAP). An example of this is airway pressure release ventilation (APRV), where minute ventilation, and CO_2 excretion, are augmented by brief (1–1.5 s) periodic cycling to the lower level of CPAP. APRV without spontaneous breathing has a similar pressure profile to PCIRV.

Adequate ventilatory support can be supplied by both of these forms of bilevel ventilation. Patient triggered bilevel ventilation is most commonly used during non-invasive ventilation (NIV), but the role of bilevel ventilation in intubated patients needs further delineation.

HIGH FREQUENCY VENTILATION

HFV encompasses techniques where small V_T (1–3 ml/kg) are delivered at high f (100–300/min). Hazards include inadequate humidification and gas trapping in patients with severe airflow limitation. High frequency jet ventilation (HFJV) utilizes dry gas from a high-pressure source delivered into an intra-tracheal catheter or specifically manufactured endotracheal tube. High frequency oscillation (HFO) uses oscillatory flow within the airway to provide active inspiration and expiration at rates of 3–20 Hz. HFO offers benefit over conventional ventilation in neonates and children with respective infant and acute respiratory distress syndrome. HFJV has been used with improvement in gas exchange in adults with ARDS,[24] but no definitive comparisons with HFJV or HFO are available.

LIQUID VENTILATION

Perfluorocarbons have a high solubility for both O_2 and CO_2, and reduce surface tension somewhat analogous to pulmonary surfactant. These properties may prove to be beneficial in ARF. Partial liquid ventilation is now the most common method of administration, with perfluorocarbon equal to the functional residual capacity administered via the endotracheal tube. The non-dependent lung is still ventilated, and may have increased blood flow due to compression of the pulmonary circulation in the dependent lung by the perfluorocarbon. Together with the perfluorocarbon-mediated reduction in surface tension, alveoli are recruited and oxygenation improved. However, when PEEP is applied the perfluorocarbon may be pushed distally and overdistend dependent alveoli.

Small clinical studies have reported improved gas exchange and respiratory mechanics after administration of perfluorocarbons,[25] however, they have been inadequately powered, and improved survival or ventilator-free days have not accompanied these effects. Further studies are awaited, particularly combining partial liquid ventilation with ventilatory strategies aimed at reducing VILI.

INDICATIONS AND OBJECTIVES OF MECHANICAL VENTILATION

Institution of mechanical ventilation is a clinical decision,[26] it can only be supported by parameters such as blood gases or measures of respiratory muscle function. Even then, the decision to choose IV over NIV will be influenced by numerous factors including the likely course of the ARF and its response to treatment. Often there will be an indication for intubation (Table 25.1) and mechanical ventilation; however, if intubation is required to overcome upper airway obstruction no ventilatory assistance may be needed despite the increase in respiratory work imposed by the endotracheal or tracheostomy tube.[18] Once the decision has been made to proceed to ventilatory support the choice of mode should be based on a physiological approach, local expertise, and simplicity.

Patients who are likely to need ventilatory assistance (e.g. acute severe asthma) should be considered for early ICU admission since this will allow faster responses and avoid cardiorespiratory arrest. Specific issues and methods of ventilatory assistance are dealt with in the chapters on ARDS, asthma and non-invasive ventilation. In patients with traumatic brain injury IV is commonly required to protect the airway and control ICP, similarly patients with severe pancreatitis or serious abdominal infection may need prolonged IV to maintain an adequate FRC, reduce work of breathing, protect their airway and allow suctioning of secretions.

INITIATION OF INTUBATED MECHANICAL VENTILATION

A manual resuscitation circuit, mechanical ventilator and equipment for safe endotracheal intubation should be available. Initial ventilator settings are commonly set to achieve adequate oxygenation and V_A; however, this will depend upon the patients condition. Common settings are: V_T 6–10 ml/kg, f 10–20 breaths/min, PEEP 5 cmH$_2$O, and FiO$_2$ 1.0, and these will need to be adjusted according to the specific patients pathophysiology and response.

MANUAL RESUSCITATION CIRCUITS

Manual resuscitation circuits are primarily used to provide emergency ventilation when spontaneous effort is absent or inadequate. They may be used with a face or laryngeal mask, or an endotracheal tube. Occasionally they are used to provide a high inspired O_2 concentration during spontaneous breathing; however, this may impose significant additional respiratory work.[27] In the ICU they are commonly used for pre-oxygenation and manual lung inflation.

Their basic design includes a fresh gas flow of O_2, a reservoir bag and valves to allow spontaneous or positive pressure breathing. Most manual resuscitation circuits use a self inflating reservoir bag since this allows the circuit to be used by unskilled personnel and does not require a fresh gas flow. However, circuits using reservoir bags that are not self inflating are still used in some institutions since they allow a better manual assessment of the respiratory mechanics, the 'educated hand', and it is clear when there is an inadequate seal with a mask. Oxygen powered manually triggered devices have been used for many years; however, this has declined markedly since high $\dot{V}$ and P may lead to barotrauma or gastric inflation.

Self inflating reservoir bags use a series of one-way valves to allow fresh gas flow oxygen and entrained air to fill the bag. Inspired oxygen fractions as high as 0.8 may be achieved with neonatal or paediatric bags when an additional reservoir bag is used to allow fresh gas flow filling during expiration, after the bag has re-filled.[28] However, lower FiO$_2$s (~0.6) will be obtained with conventional O_2 flow rates of 8–15 l/min, V_T and f, with an adult bag. Generally the valves are simple flap or duckbill in nature, and both positive pressure and spontaneous ventilation are possible. The reservoir bag volume in adults is typically 1600 ml, and V_T can be judged from chest wall movement. It is essential these devices use standard 15/22 mm connectors to allow rapid connection to standard endotracheal tubes and ventilator circuits.

COMPLICATIONS OF MECHANICAL VENTILATION

Although mechanical ventilation may be vital, it also introduces numerous potential complications (Table 25.2).[26] Monitoring includes a high nurse:patient ratio (usually 1:1), ventilator alarms, and pulse oximetry. Capnography is often recommended to confirm endotracheal tube placement, and may be used to monitor the adequacy of V_A; however, expired CO_2 is strongly influenced by factors that alter alveolar dead space such as cardiac output. Intermittent blood gases, PEEPi, airway pressures in volume-preset modes and V_T in pressure-preset modes should be recorded. Individual patients may benefit from more extensive monitoring of their respiratory mechanics or tissue oxygenation.

The patients airway (i.e. patency, presence of leaks and nature and amount of secretions), breathing (i.e. rate, volume, oxygenation), and circulation (i.e. pulse, blood pressure and urine output) must be monitored. Ventilatory and circuit alarms should be adjusted to monitor an appropriate range of V, P, and temperature. This should alert adjacent staff to changes in P and or V that may be caused by an occluded endotracheal tube, tension pneumothorax or circuit disconnection. These alarms may be temporarily disabled while the cause is detected, but never permanently disabled. Sudden difficulties with high P during volume-preset ventilation, or oxygenation must initiate an immediate search for the cause. This should start with the patency of the airway,

Table 25.1 Indications and objectives of intubated mechanical ventilation

Endotracheal intubation or tracheostomy
For airway protection (e.g. coma)
For suction of secretions
To assist sedation and neuromuscular paralysis (e.g. to ↓ VO$_2$, ↓ respiratory distress)
To overcome upper airway obstruction
Mechanical ventilation
To manipulate alveolar ventilation (V_A) and PaCO$_2$ (e.g. reverse respiratory acidosis, ↓ cerebral blood flow and ICP)
To ↑ SaO$_2$ and PaO$_2$ (by ↑ FRC, ↑end-inspiratory lung volume, ↑ V_A, ↑ FiO$_2$)
To ↓ work of breathing (e.g. to overcome respiratory muscle fatigue)
To ↑ FRC (e.g. ↑ PaO$_2$, ↓ VILI)
To stabilize the chest wall in severe chest injury

Table 25.2 Complications of intubation and mechanical ventilation

Equipment
Malfunction or disconnection
Incorrectly set or prescribed
Contamination
Pulmonary
Airway intubation (e.g. damage to teeth, vocal cords, trachea)
Ventilator-associated pneumonia (reduced lung defence)
VILI (e.g. diffuse lung injury due to regional overdistension or tidal recruitment recruitment of alveoli)
Overt barotrauma (e.g. pneumothorax)
O_2 toxicity
Patient–ventilator asynchrony
Circulation
↓RV preload → ↓cardiac output
↑RV afterload (if the lung is overdistended)
↓splanchnic blood flow with high levels of PEEP or mean Paw
↑ICP with high levels of PEEP or mean Paw
Fluid retention due to ↓cardiac output→ ↓renal blood flow
Other
Gut distension (air swallowing, hypomotility)
Mucosal ulceration and bleeding
Peripheral and respiratory muscle weakness
Sleep disturbance, agitation and fear (which may be prolonged after recovery)
Neuropsychiatric complications

followed by a structured approach both to the circuit and ventilator, and to factors altering the E and R of the lung and chest wall such as bronchospasm, secretions, pneumothorax, and asynchronous breathing. In addition to careful clinical examination an urgent chest radiograph and bronchoscopy may be required.

Mechanical ventilation is also associated with a marked increase in the incidence of nosocomial pneumonia, due to a reduction in the natural defence of the respiratory tract, and this represents an important advantage offered by NIV. In patients successfully managed with NIV, Girou and colleagues reported a reduction in the incidence of nosocomial pneumonia, associated with improved survival, compared with IV.[29] Erect vs semi-recumbent posture[30] also reduces the incidence of ventilator-associated pneumonia.

While lung overdistension may result in alveolar rupture leading to pulmonary interstitial air, pneumomediastinum or pneumothorax, it may also lead to diffuse alveolar damage similar to that found in ALI and ARDS. Both are termed VILI, and V_T reduction leads to a marked decrease in ALI mortality, due to a reduction in multiple organ dysfunction.[5] There is also laboratory data suggesting that inadequate PEEP with tidal recruitment and derecruitment of alveoli also leads to VILI; however, this has not been proven in a clinical trial. Finally, patient-ventilator asynchrony may result in wasted respiratory work, impaired gas exchange and respiratory distress (see below).

Positive pressure ventilation elevates intrathoracic pressure which reduces venous return, right ventricular preload, and cardiac output. The impact is reduced by hypervolaemia, and partial ventilatory support where patient effort and a reduction in pleural pressure augments venous return. Secondary effects include a reduction in regional organ blood flow leading to fluid retention by the kidney, and possibly impaired hepatic function. This latter effect is only seen at high levels of PEEP where an increase in resistance to venous return and a reduction in cardiac output may combine to reduce hepatic blood flow.

Sleep disturbance, and agitation and discomfort are common in mechanically ventilated patients. These effects may be reduced with sedation until weaning is planned; however, it is important not to prolong mechanical ventilation due to excessive use of sedatives, which may also depress blood pressure and spontaneous respiratory effort. Finally, complex neuropsychological sequelae have been described in recovering ARDS patients.[31,32] These do not appear to reflect the severity of the acute illness since ARDS patients have a poorer quality of life than patients with a similar severity of illness without ARDS.[33] However, they do correlate with their duration of hypoxaemia. Clearly, this is an important issue that needs further research.

WITHDRAWAL (WEANING) FROM MECHANICAL VENTILATION

Once the underlying process necessitating mechanical ventilation has started to resolve, withdrawal of ventilatory support should be considered. However, other important parameters that must be considered include the neuromuscular state of the patient (ability to cooperate, muscle strength) and their cardiovascular stability. Many patients can rapidly make the transition from mechanical ventilation to extubation, but, ~20% of patients fail weaning despite meeting clinical criteria.[19] Advanced age, prolonged mechanical ventilation and chronic obstructive pulmonary disease all increase the likelihood that weaning will be difficult.[19]

Although numerous indices have been proposed to be predictive of weaning, simple clinical assessment is usually adequate, yielding a reintubation rate as low as 3%,[34] and none of these indices assess airway function following extubation. One simple, and recently proposed index, an f/V_T ratio >100, was initially shown to be highly predictive of weaning failure, however, subsequent studies have reported varying results.[19] Consequently, weaning indices should not necessarily delay extubation or a weaning trial. However, they may quantitate important issues in the general clinical assessment, and may be directly relevant for a given patient. For example frequent small V_T, an inadequate vital capacity (less than 8–12 ml/kg), large minute ventilation (>10 l/min), depressed respiratory drive, and reduced respiratory muscle strength (maximum inspiratory P <-20 cmH$_2$O), or drive should be strongly factored into deciding whether a patient is ready to safely undergo a trial of weaning.

Direct comparisons between T-piece trials, PSV and SIMV as weaning techniques have been performed in patients showing respiratory distress during a two hour trial of spontaneous breathing. In the study by Brochard and colleagues,[35] PSV led to fewer failures and a shorter weaning period. In contrast Esteban and co-workers[36] found that a once daily trial of spontaneous breathing resulted in the shortest duration of mechanical ventilation; however, a relatively high proportion of patients required reintubation (22.6%). Viewed together, these studies suggest that weaning was slower with SIMV,[19] but SIMV with PSV was not studied. Since low levels of PSV can help compensate for the additional work of breathing attributable to the endotracheal tube and circuit, assessment of respiratory work can be done 'as if' the patient were extubated. Consequently, low levels of PSV or T-piece trials are often recommended prior to extubation.[19]

Reintubation is associated with a 7–11-fold increased risk of hospital death.[19] A number of factors may account for this including selection of previously unaccounted for severity of illness, and the development of complications which may (pneumonia, heart failure) or may not be attributable to extubation. Hence, an important goal during mechanical ventilation will be to proceed to early and expeditious extubation with a low reintubation rate.

PATIENT–VENTILATOR INTERACTION

This is an extremely important issue in patients with either partial ventilatory support, or those breathing spontaneously through the ventilator. For simplicity the discussion of patient–ventilator interaction will be subdivided into (i) triggering of inspiration, (ii) inspiration and (iii) cessation of inspiration; however, difficulties at each of these phases will lead to changes in respiratory drive and effort that may be expressed throughout the respiratory cycle. Importantly, major problems with patient–ventilator dyssynchrony can be identified by carefully observing respiratory effort and ventilator cycling at the bedside and this may be assisted by observing P, V and $\dot{V}$ waveforms displayed by the ventilator.

TRIGGERING OF INSPIRATION

1 PEEPi is an important hindrance to the triggering of inspiration in patients with severe airflow limitation, since their inspiratory muscles must first reduce Pao below ambient pressure.[37] Consequently Pmus must exceed PEEPi prior to triggering an assisted breath by either reducing airway pressure (pressure trigger) or by reducing circuit flow (flow trigger). This inspiratory threshold load may be up to 40% of the total inspiratory work in acute respiratory failure with dynamic hyperinflation, and commonly results in ineffective triggering. Triggering can be markedly improved and respiratory work reduced by low levels of CPAP;[37,38] commonly 80–90% of dynamic PEEPi.[39]

2 A fall in Pao has been the most common form of triggering. Pressure is usually sensed at the expiratory block of the ventilator. Sensing at the Y-piece is not superior since there is a similar delay in sensing as the transducer is usually sited in the ventilator. Flow triggering senses a fall in continuous circuit flow, and was introduced as a method of reducing inspiratory work. However, there has been a marked improvement of both pressure and flow triggering in modern ventilators with the trigger time delay falling from ~400 ms to ~100 ms, and a similar improvement in the maximum fall in airway pressure.[40] Attempts to improve the trigger function by oversetting the pressure sensitivity (>-0.5 cmH$_2$O) may lead to autocycling, which may also occur with overset flow triggering. This is due to the P and $\dot{V}$ effects of cardiac oscillations, and has been reported as a cause of apparent respiratory effort in brain dead patients.[41] Flow triggering reduces the risk of autocycling at a given trigger sensitivity, and reduces respiratory effort a small amount compared to pressure triggering; however, it does not alter the frequency of ineffective efforts,[42] or patient effort following triggering.[40]

INSPIRATION

Once inspiration is triggered or sensed by the ventilator, $\dot{V}$ is determined by P, Ti or $\dot{V}$. For example, during PSV ventilation a target P is held until expiration is sensed, and during ACV $\dot{V}$ is held for a set Ti. During ACV there may be continued inspiratory effort, and since inspiratory $\dot{V}$ is fixed, this will be reflected by a scalloping of the Pao-T graph if $\dot{V}$ is inadequate. Again this may be illustrated using the Equation (6) of motion:

$$\text{Pmus} + \text{Pao} = \text{Ers V} + \text{Rrs } \dot{V} + \text{Po}$$

Pmus will reflect the difference between Pao due to E, R and Po and the observed Pao. In contrast, during P cycled ventilation (PACV) greater patient effort is rewarded, and inspiratory work is lower than during equivalent ACV.[43]

Modern ventilators allow adjustment of inspiratory $\dot{V}$ and V pattern, and the rate of rise of Pao. Low inspiratory $\dot{V}$ rates during ACV results in significant inspiratory work, but this may be markedly reduced by increasing inspiratory $\dot{V}$ to 65 l/min.[44] However, these issues are quite complex, and f increases (probably due to a lower respiratory tract reflex) as $\dot{V}_I$ increases,[45] reducing Te, which may contribute to dynamic hyperinflation in patients with severe airflow obstruction. During PSV and PACV, many ventilators allow adjustment of the rate of rise of P to its target. A steeper P ramp, leads to earlier attainment of the P target, greater early $\dot{V}$ rates and reduction of inspiratory drive and work.[46,47]

CESSATION OF INSPIRATION

During PSV, an increase in airways resistance will result in a delayed fall in $\dot{V}_I$. Since this is the trigger for cycling to expiration, the ventilator may continue to provide $\dot{V}_I$ while the patient desires to exhale. This commonly leads to recruitment of expiratory muscles, detected both clinically and as a transient rise in the end-inspiratory Pao.[48] High levels of PSV (≥ 20 cmH$_2$O), weak respiratory muscles and mask leak with NIV are other common causes of asynchrony at the termination of inspiration. In this last group, PACV, which is time cycled, allows improved patient-ventilator synchrony at end-inspiration compared with PSV.[49]

REFERENCES

1 Lassen HC. A preliminary report on the 1952 epidemic of poliomyelitis in Copenhagen with special reference to the treatment of acute respiratory insufficiency. *Lancet* 1953; **3**: 37–41.
2 Mehta S, Hill NS. Noninvasive ventilation. *Am J Respir Crit Care Med* 2001; **163**: 540–7.
3 International Consensus Conference in Intensive Care Medicine. Ventilator-associated lung injury in ARDS. *Am J Respir Crit Care Med* 1999; **160**: 2118–24.
4 Bendixen HH, Hedley-White J, Laver MB. Impaired oxygenation in surgical patients during general anesthesia with controlled ventilation: A concept of atelectasis. *N Engl J Med* 1963; **269**: 991–6.
5 Ventilation with lower tidal volumes as compared with traditional volumes for acute lung injury and the acute respiratory distress syndrome. *N Engl J Med* 2000; **342**: 1301–8.
6 Hotchkiss JR, Blanch L, Murias G, *et al.* Effects of decreased respiratory frequency on ventilator-induced lung injury. *Am J Respir Crit Care Med* 2000; **161**: 463–8.
7 Lessard MR, Guerot E, Lorino H, *et al.* Effects of pressure-controlled with different I:E ratios versus volume-controlled ventilation on respiratory mechanics, gas exchange, and hemodynamics in patients with adult respiratory distress syndrome. *Anesthesiology* 1994; **80**: 983–91.
8 Edibam C, Rutten AJ, Collins DV, Bersten AD. Effect of inspiratory flow pattern and inspiratory to expiratory ratio on non-linear elastic behavior in patients with acute lung injury. *Am J Respir Crit Care Med* (2003, in press)
9 Jonson B, Beydon L, Brauer K, *et al.* Mechanics of respiratory system in healthy anesthetized humans with emphasis on viscoelastic properties. *J Appl Physiol* 1993; **75**: 132–40.
10 Tuxen DV, Lane S. The effects of ventilatory pattern on hyperinflation, airway pressures, and circulation in mechanical ventilation of patients with severe airflow obstruction. *Am Rev Respir Dis* 1987; **136**: 872–9.
11 Suter PM, Fairley B, Isenberg MD. Optimum end-expiratory airway pressure in patients with acute pulmonary failure. *N Engl J Med* 1975; **292**: 284–9.
12 Gattinoni L, Pelosi P, Crotti S, *et al.* Effects of positive end-expiratory pressure on regional distribution of tidal volume and recruitment in adult respiratory distress syndrome. *Am J Respir Crit Care Med* 1995; **151**: 1807–14.
13 Vieira SRR, Puybasset L, Richecoeur J, *et al.* A lung computed tomographic assessment of positive end-expiratory pressure-induced lung overdistension. *Am J Respir Crit Care Med* 1998; **158**: 1571–7.
14 Bersten AD. Measurement of overinflation by multiple linear regression analysis in patients with acute lung injury. *Eur Respir J* 1998; **12**: 526–32.
15 Nicholas TE, Power JHT, Barr HA. The pulmonary consequences of a deep breath. *Respir Physiol* 1982; **49**: 315–24.
16 Pelosi P, Cardringher P, Bottino N, *et al.* Sigh in acute respiratory distress syndrome. *Am J Respir Crit Care Med* 1999; **159**: 872–80.
17 Marini JJ, Rodriguez M, Lamb V. The inspiratory workload of patient-initiated mechanical ventilation. *Am Rev Respir Dis* 1986; **134**: 902–9.
18 Bersten AD, Rutten AJ, Vedig AE, *et al.* Additional work of breathing imposed by endotracheal tubes, breathing circuits and intensive care ventilators. *Crit Care Med* 1989; **17**: 671–80.
19 Esteban A, Alia I. Clinical management of weaning from mechanical ventilation. *Intensive Care Med* 1998; **24**: 999–1008.
20 Brochard L, Harf A, Lorino H, *et al.* Inspiratory pressure support prevents diaphragmatic fatigue during weaning from mechanical ventilation. *Am Rev Respir Dis* 1989; **139**: 513–21.
21 Bersten AD, Rutten AJ, Vedig AE. Efficacy of presure support ventilation in compensating for apparatus work. *Anaesth Intens Care* 1993; **21**: 67–71.
22 Brochard L, Rua F, Lorino H, *et al.* Inspiratory pressure support compensates for the additional work of breathing caused by the endotracheal tube. *Anesthesiology* 1991; **75**: 739–45.
23 Appendini L, Purro A, Gudjonsdottir M, *et al.* Physiologic response of ventilator-dependent patients with chronic obstructive pulmonary disease to proportional assist ventilation and continuous positive airway pressure. *Am J Respir Crit Care Med* 1999; **159**: 1510–7.
24 Gluck E, Heard S, Patel C, *et al.* Use of ultrahigh frequency ventilation in patients with ARDS: A preliminary report. *Chest* 1993; **103**: 1413–20.
25 Hirschl RB, Pranikoff T, Wise C, *et al.* Initial experience with partial liquid ventilation in adult patients with the acute respiratory distress syndrome. *JAMA* 1996; **275**: 383–9.
26 Slutsky AS. Mechanical ventilation. Chest 1993; **104**: 1833–59.
27 Hess D, Hirsch C, Marquis-D'Amico C, *et al.* Imposed work and oxygen delivery during spontaneous breathing with adult disposable manual ventilators. Anesthesiology 1994; **81**: 1256–63.
28 Agarwal KS, Puliyel JM. A simple strategy to improve first breath oxygen delivery by self inflating bag. *Resuscitation* 2000; **45**: 221–4.

29 Girou E, Schortgen F, Delclaux C, *et al*. Association of noninvasive ventilation with nosocomial infections and survival in critically ill patients. *JAMA* 2000; **284**: 2361–7.

30 Drakulovic MB, Torres A, Bauer TT, *et al*. Supine body position as a risk factor for nosocomial pneumonia in mechanically ventilated patients: a randomised trial. *Lancet* 1999; **354**: 1851–8.

31 Hopkins RO, Weaver LK, Opep D, *et al*. Neuropsychological sequelae and impaired health status in survivors of severe acute respiratory distress syndrome. *Am J Respir Crit Care Med* 1999; **160**: 50–6.

32 Rothenhausler H, Ehrentraut S, Stoll C, *et al*. The relationship between cognitive performance and employment and health status in long-term survivors of the acute respiratory distress syndrome: results of an exploratory study. *Gen Hosp Psychiatry* 2001; **23**: 90–6.

33 Davidson TA, Caldwell ES, Curtis JR, *et al*. Reduced quality of life in survivors of acute respiratory distress syndrome compared with critically ill control patients. *JAMA* 1999; **281**: 354–60.

34 Leitch EA, Moran JL, Grealy B. Weaning and extubation in the intensive care unit. Clinical or index-driven approach? *Intensive Care Med* 1996; **22**: 752–9.

35 Brochard L, Rauss A, Benito S, *et al*. Comparison of three methods of gradual withdrawal from ventilatory support during weaning from mechanical ventilation. *Am J Respir Crit Care Med* 1994; **150**: 896–903.

36 Esteban A, Frutos F, Tobin MJ, *et al*. A comparison of four methods of weaning patients from mechanical ventilation. *N Engl J Med* 1995; **332**: 345–50.

37 Smith TC, Marini JJ. Impact of PEEP on lung mechanics and work of breathing in severe airflow obstruction. *J Appl Physiol* 1988; **65**: 1488–99.

38 Petrof BJ, Legare M, Goldberg P, *et al*. Continuous positive airway pressure reduces work of breathing and dyspnea during weaning form mechanical ventilation in severe chronic obstructive pulmonary disease. *Am Rev Respir Dis* 1990; **141**: 281–9.

39 Ranieri VM, Giuliiani R, Cinnella G, *et al*. Physiologic effects of positive end-expiratory pressure in patients with chronic obstructive pulmonary disease during acute ventilatory failure and controlled mechanical ventilation. *Am Rev Respir Dis* 1993; **147**: 5–13.

40 Alsanian P, El Atrous S, Isabey D, *et al*. Effects of flow triggering on breathing effort during partial ventilatory support. *Am J Respir Crit Care Med* 1998; **157**: 135–43.

41 Willatts SM, Drummond G. Brainstem death and ventilator trigger settings. *Anaesthesia* 2000; **55**: 676–7.

42 Sassoon CSH, Foster GT. Patient–ventilator asynchrony. *Current Opinion in Critical Care* 2001; **7**: 28–33.

43 Cinnella G, Conti G, Lofaso F, *et al*. Effects of assisted ventilation on the work of breathing: volume controlled versus pressure-controlled ventilation. *Am J Respir Crit Care Med* 1996; **153**: 1025–33.

44 Ward ME, Corbeil C, Gibbons W, *et al*. Optimization of respiratory muscle relaxation during mechanical ventilation. *Anesthesiology* 1988; **69**: 29–35.

45 Corne S, Gillespie D, Roberts D, *et al*. Effect of inspiratory flow rate on respiratory rate in intubated ventilated patients. *Am J Respir Crit Care Med* 1997; **156**: 304–8.

46 Bonmarchand G, Chevron V, Chopin CC, *et al*. Increased initial flow rate reduces inspiratory work of breathing during pressure support ventilation in patients with exacerbation of chronic obstructive pulmonary disease. *Intensive Care Med* 1996; **22**: 1147–54.

47 Bonmarchand G, Chevron V, Menard JF, *et al*. Effects of pressure ramp slope values on the work of breathing during pressure support ventilation in restrictive patients. *Crit Care Med* 1999; **27**: 715–22.

48 Parthasarathy S, Jubran A, Tobin MJ. Cycling of inspiratory and expiratory muscle groups with the ventilator in airflow limitation. *Am J Respir Crit Care Med* 1998; **158**: 1471–8.

49 Calderinin E, Confalonieri M, Puccio PG, *et al*. Patient-ventilator asynchrony during noninvasive ventilation: the role of expiratory trigger. *Intensive Care Med* 1999; **25**: 662–7.

26

Humidification and inhalation therapy

A D Bersten

The upper airway normally warms, moistens and filters inspired gas. When these functions are impaired by disease, or when the nasopharynx is bypassed by endotracheal intubation, artificial humidification of inspired gases must be provided.

PHYSICAL PRINCIPLES

Humidity, the amount of water vapour in a gas, may be expressed as:

1 *Absolute humidity* (AH): the total mass of water vapour in a given volume of gas at a given temperature (g/m^3).
2 *Relative humidity* (RH): the actual mass of water vapour (per volume of gas) as a percentage of the mass of saturated water vapour, at a given temperature. Saturated water vapour exerts a saturated vapour pressure (SVP). As the SVP has an exponential relation with temperature (Table 26.1), addition of further water vapour to the gas can only occur with a rise in temperature.
3 *Partial pressure.*

Table 26.1 Relationship of temperature and saturated vapour pressure

Temperature (°C)	Saturated vapour pressure		Absolute humidity (g/m^3)
	(mmHg)	(kPa)	
0	4.6	0.6	4.8
10	9.2	1.2	9.3
20	17.5	2.3	17.1
30	31.3	4.2	30.4
34	39.9	5.3	37.5
37	47.1	6.3	43.4
40	55.3	7.4	51.7
46	78.0	10.4	68.7

PHYSIOLOGY

Clearance of surface liquids and particles from the lung depends on beating cilia, airway mucus and transepithelial water flux. Airway mucus is derived from secretions from goblet cells, submucosal glands and Clara cells, and from capillary transudate. Conducting airways are lined with pseudostratified, ciliated columnar epithelium and numerous fluid-secreting glands. As the airway descends, the epithelium becomes stratified, and then cuboidal and partially ciliated, with very few secretory glands at the terminal airways. The cilia beat in a watery (sol) layer over which is a viscous mucus layer (gel), and move a superficial layer of mucus from deep within the lung toward the glottis (at a rate of 10 mm/min at 37°C and 100% RH). Both cilia function and mucus composition are influenced by temperature and adequate humidification.

The nasal mucosa has a large surface area with an extensive vascular network which humidifies and warms inhaled gas more effectively than during mouth-breathing. Heating and humidification of dry gas are progressive down the airway, with an isothermic boundary (i.e. 100% RH at 37°C or AH of 43 g/m^3) just below the carina.[1] Under resting conditions, approximately 250 ml of water and 1.5 kJ (350 kcal) of energy is lost from the respiratory tract in a day. A proportion (10–25%) is returned to the mucosa during expiration due to condensation.

The minimal moisture level to maintain ciliary function and mucus clearance is uncertain. Although reproducing an isothermic boundary at the carina may be ideal, it does not seem essential in all situations. Mucus flow is markedly reduced when RH at 37°C falls below 75% (AH of 32 g/m^3), and ceases when RH is 50% (AH of 22 g/m^3).[2] This suggests that an AH exceeding 33 g/m^3 is needed to maintain normal function. At this AH level, inspired gas temperature does not appear to be important unless excessive.[3] Mucociliary function is also impaired by upper respiratory tract infection, chronic bronchitis, cystic fibrosis, bronchiectasis, immotile cilia syndrome (including Kartagener's syndrome), dehydration, hyperventilation, general anaesthetics, opioids, atropine, and exposure to noxious gases. High fractional inspired oxygen concentrations (FiO_2) may lead to acute tracheobronchitis, with depressed tracheal mucus velocity within 3 h.[4] Inhaled β_2-adrenergic agonists increase mucociliary clearance by augmenting ciliary beat frequency, and mucus and water secretion.[5]

CLINICAL APPLICATIONS OF HUMIDIFICATION

TRACHEAL INTUBATION

The need for humidification during endotracheal intubation and tracheostomy is unquestioned. As the upper airway is bypassed, RH of inspired gas falls below 50% with adverse effects including:[6]

- increased mucus viscosity
- depressed ciliary function
- cytological damage to the tracheobronchial epithelium, including mucosal ulceration, tracheal inflammation and necrotizing tracheobronchitis[7]
- microatelectasis from obstruction of small airways
- airway obstruction due to tenacious or inspissated sputum.

Metaplasia of the tracheal epithelium occurs over weeks to months in patients with a permanent tracheostomy. These patients do not usually require humidified gas, suggesting that humidification occurs lower down the respiratory tree. None-the-less, humidification of inspired gas may be needed during an acute respiratory tract infection.

HEAT EXCHANGE

The respiratory tract is an important avenue to adjust body temperature by heat exchange. Humidification of gases reduces the fall in body temperature associated with anaesthesia and surgery.[6] In this setting, active humidifiers are of no benefit over heat and moisture exchangers (HMEs).[8] Excessive heat from humidification may produce mucosal damage, hyperthermia and over-humidification.[9] However, if water content is not excessive, mucociliary clearance is unaffected up to temperatures of 42°C.[3] Over-humidification may increase secretions and impair mucociliary clearance and surfactant activity, resulting in atelectasis.[9]

IDEAL HUMIDIFICATION

The basic requirements of a humidifier should include the following features:[10]

- The inspired gas is delivered into the trachea at 32–36°C with a water content of 30–43 g/m[3].
- The set temperature remains constant and does not fluctuate.

- Humidification and temperature remain unaffected by a large range of fresh gas flows, especially high flows.
- The device is simple to use and to service.
- Humidification can be provided for air, oxygen or any mixture of inspired gas, including anaesthetic agents.
- The humidifier can be used with spontaneous or controlled ventilation.
- There are safety mechanisms, with alarms, against overheating, overhydration and electrocution.
- The resistance, compliance and dead-space characteristics do not adversely affect spontaneous breathing modes.
- The sterility of the inspired gas is not compromised.

METHODS AND DEVICES

WATER BATH HUMIDIFIERS

Inspired gas is passed over or through a water reservoir to achieve humidification. Their efficiency is dependent on ambient temperature and the surface area available for gas vaporization.

COLD WATER HUMIDIFIERS

These units are simple and inexpensive, but are inefficient, with a water content of around 9 g/m[3] (i.e. about 50% RH at ambient temperatures). They are also a potential source of microbiological contamination. Routine use of cold-water humidifiers to deliver oxygen with simple facemasks is unnecessary.

HOT WATER HUMIDIFIERS

Inspired gas is passed over (i.e. blow-by humidifier, e.g. Fisher-Paykel, Fisher and Paykel Medical, New Zealand) or through (i.e. bubble or cascade humidifier, e.g. Bennett Cascade, Bennett Medical Equipment, USA) a heated water reservoir (see Figures 26.1 and 26.2). Gas leaving the reservoir contains a high water content, often more than 43 g/m[3]. The water bath temperature is thermostatically controlled (e.g. at 45–60°C) to compensate for cooling along the inspiratory tubing targeting an inspired RH of 100% at 37°C. A heated wire may be sited in the inspiratory tubing to maintain preset gas temperature and humidity (e.g. Fisher-Paykel humidifier). It is commonly believed that hot-water humidifiers (HH) do not produce aerosols, but micro-droplets (mostly less than 5 μm diameter) have been reported with bubble humidifiers,[11] and this may be a potential source of infection.

Fisher-Paykel Humidifier

This is a commonly used blow-by humidifier. Reservoir temperature is variable for flows 3–25 l/min. The delivery hose is heated by an insulated heating wire to achieve a manual preset inspired temperature. An additional servo-control unit is available, while more recent models have a dual servo unit which combines this function in the heater base. Audible alarms indicate disconnection and variations over 2°C from the set delivery temperature. The heater base is protected from overheating by a thermostat set at 47°C. If this fails, another safety thermostat operates at 70°C. The heated wire avoids or minimizes 'rainout', which is a problem in recent models (series 600 and 700). These models are used with a disposable humidification chamber that is filled manually with water or by a gravity-feed set. To minimize rainout, the chamber outlet can be set at a temperature below the delivery hose outlet temperature: −2°C is usually adequate and does not compromise RH. Temperature alarms are fixed at 41°C and 29.5°C, with a back-up safety set at 66°C for the delivery chamber.

HEAT AND MOISTURE EXCHANGERS

Modern HMEs are popular ICU humidifiers due to their simplicity and increased efficiency. They all work on the basic principle of heat and moisture conservation during expiration, allowing inspired gas to be heated and humidified. HMEs may be hydrophobic or hygroscopic, and may also act as a microbial filter (HMEF). However, since nosocomial pneumonia is primarily due to aspiration of oropharyngeal secretions followed by secondary ventilator tubing colonization HMEFs have not been shown to reduce the frequency of nosocomial pneumonia, and the incidence is similar when HMEs and HHs are compared during prolonged ventilation.[12,13]

Modern HMEs are light with a small dead space, but are varied in their level of humidification. Hygroscopic HMEs adsorb moisture on to a foam or paper-like material that is chemically coated (often calcium chloride or lithium chloride), and this tends to increase their efficiency (i.e. AH around 30 g/m³) compared with hydrophobic HMEs (i.e. AH 20–25 g/m³).[14–19] The efficiency of older HMEs decreases with time;[13] however, modern HMEs may retain their ability to humidify for at least 4 d, with minimal change in resistance.[20] Consequently, HMEs that achieve relatively high AH may be suitable for long-term mechanical ventilation in selected patients, particularly as the majority of reported HME complications (e.g. thick secretions and endotracheal tube occlusion) occurred with units of lower humidification levels.[21–23] Nevertheless, HMEs cannot match the humidification offered by hot-water humidifiers, which remain the 'gold standard', particularly if secretions are thick or bloody, minute ventilation is high,[15,19] humidification is necessary for more than 4 d,[24] or if used in children and neonates.

COMPLICATIONS OF HUMIDIFICATION

INADEQUATE HUMIDIFICATION

An AH exceeding 30 g/m³ is recommended in respiratory care.[24] Inadequate humidification is usually only a problem with HMEs. With hot-water humidifiers, however, efficiency is reduced by increasing gas flow rates and rainout. A decrease of about 1°C occurs for each 10 cm tubing beyond the end of the delivery hose (i.e. the Y-connector and right-angled connector), and should be catered for. Inadequate humidification in high-frequency ventilation can be overcome by using superheated humidification of the entrained gas with a temperature thermistor built into the endotracheal tube.[23–25]

OVERHUMIDIFICATION

Overheating malfunction of hot-water humidifiers may cause a rise in core temperature, water intoxication, impaired mucociliary clearance and airway burns.[9]

Fig. 26.1 Hot water 'blow-by' humidifier.

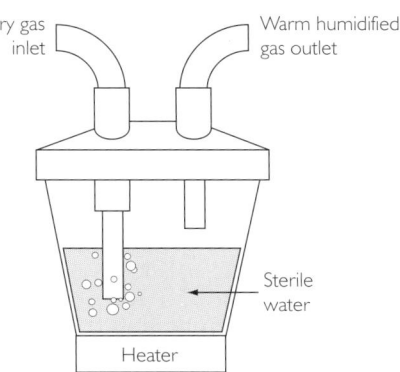

Fig. 26.2 Hot water 'cascade' or 'bubble' humidifier.

IMPOSED WORK OF BREATHING

The work of breathing imposed by a humidifier, primarily resistive work, is an important additional respiratory load in ICU patients. Consequently their imposed work increases with inspiratory flow rate, and the progressive increase in water content of HMEs is also associated with increased resistance.[26] The Fisher-Paykel humidifier imposes relatively low work compared to the Bennett cascade,[27] and HMEs typically have a resistance of 2.5 cmH$_2$O/l per s.[19]

INFECTION

Current evidence argues against humidifiers as important factors in nosocomial respiratory tract infection. Although water reservoirs represent a good culture medium for bacteria such as *Pseudomonas* species, it is rare to culture bacteria from humidifiers. Any such positive finding is usually preceded by colonization of the circuit by the patient's own flora within the first 24 h of use.[28,29] Indeed, the incidence of nosocomial pneumonia is reported to be higher (due to outside contamination) if the circuit is changed too frequently (every 24 h[30] or 48 h[29]).

Many HMEs are also effective bacterial filters, with efficiencies usually greater than 99.9977%,[15] i.e. less than 23 out of 1 million bacteria will pass through (filters that can exclude all virus particles are not currently available). However, provided that fresh circuits are used for each new patient, filtration does not alter the incidence of nosocomial pneumonia.

ELECTRICAL HAZARDS

See Chapter 73.

INHALATION THERAPY

Therapeutic aerosols are particles suspended in gas that are inhaled and deposited within the respiratory tract. Numerous factors, including particle size, inertia and physical nature, gravity, volume and pattern of ventilation, temperature and humidity, airway geometry, lung disease and the delivery system alter aerosol deposition. In general, particles of diameter 40 μm deposit in the upper airway, 8–15 μm deposit in bronchi and bronchioles, 3–5 μm deposit in peripheral conducting airways, and 0.8–3.0 μm settle in lung parenchyma. Optimal particle size will depend on the clinical indication and agent used (e.g. β_2-adrenergic agonists, anticholinergics, corticosteroids, antibiotics, anti-virals, surfactant therapy, sputum induction and water). Obviously, if an HME with filtration characteristics is being used, the aerosol needs to be delivered proximal to the filter.

AEROSOL DELIVERY

Therapeutic aerosols may be delivered by nebulizer (jet or ultrasonic), metered dose (MDI) or dry particle inhaler (DPI). Although each of these methods tend to be less efficient in ventilated patients, provided that care is taken to optimize their performance, each can provide equivalent clinical effect.

NEBULIZERS

The most common jet nebulizers are sidestream nebulizers.[31] These use an extrinsic gas flow through a narrow orifice, to create a presure gradient that draws the drug mixture from a liquid reservoir (i.e. Bernoulli's principle; see Figure 26.3). The gas is then directed at a baffle to reduce the mean particle size. This extrinsic gas flow (usually 3–10 l/min) adds to the inspiratory flow, and may increase patient tidal volume unless the ventilator automatically compensates, or the preset tidal volume is adjusted. Further, this additional gas flow may impair ventilator triggering since it may prevent the development of a negative pressure or necessary reduction in continuous flow needed. Mainstream nebulizers employ inspiratory gas flow to actuate nebulization. These are commonly large-volume water nebulizers that entrain air to achieve fresh gas flow rates of 20–30 l/min.

Ultrasonic nebulizers use high-frequency sound waves (typically 1 MHz) to create an aerosol above a liquid reservoir, to produce small uniform droplets (<5 μm) and a high mist density (i.e. 100–200 g/m^3). Tidal volume is not altered; however, ultrasonic nebulizers may cause overhydration, and increased airway resistance.

Nebulizer aerosol deposition is typically 1–3% with the remainder 'raining out' in the ventilatory circuit, endotracheal tube (ETT) and large conducting airways. Numerous factors have been shown to improve aerosol deposition; but, only some of these are commonly practiced. For example although heating and humidification reduces aerosol deposition by ~40%, regular circuit disconnection and exclusion of humidification prior to nebulization is not practical. However, placement of the nebulizer in the inspiratory limb of the circuit less than 30 cm from the ETT allows this tubing to act as a spacer or aerosol holding chamber. This reduces aerosol velocity and losses due to impaction. Inspiratory activation of the nebulizer, use of a large chamber fill, and minimization of turbulent inspiratory flow (low flow rate, prolonged inspiratory time) also augment aerosol delivery.[31,32]

MDIs suspend micronized crystals of drug in a propellant gas under high pressure, allowing a relatively fixed volume (i.e. dose) to be delivered with each actuation (e.g. 90 μg for salbutamol and 18 μg for ipratropium).[33] Aerosol delivery is approximately 4–6% in ventilated adults which is one quarter of that found in

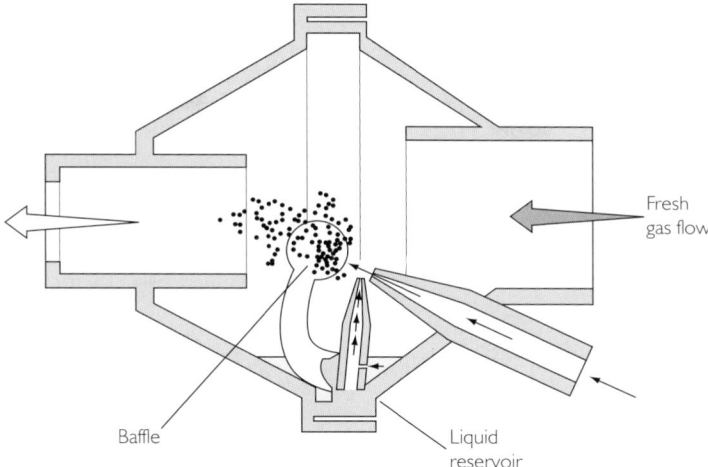

Fig. 26.3 Sidestream nebulizer.

ambulatory studies. Similar to nebulizers, absence of humidification, inspiratory limb position, inspiratory activation and minimization of turbulence by lowering inspiratory flow rate and prolonging inspiratory time will increase aerosol delivery. However, the greatest improvement in aerosol delivery can be achieved with use of a spacer or aerosol holding chamber. It is important to avoid use of an elbow adapter, because this has been associated with dramatic reductions in aerosol delivery and efficacy. Further hazards of MDIs include a low risk of reaction to chloroflourocarbons (CFCs), and the risk of necrotizing inflammation of the airway mucosa when large doses of drug are administered with a MDI and catheter system due to oleic acid which is present in some MDI formulations.[34]

CLINICAL APPLICATIONS OF INHALATION THERAPY

HUMIDIFICATION

Humidifiers produce gas with a water content dictated by temperature and water vapour pressure, whereas nebulizers produce gas with a water content determined by the aerosol content. The latter can provide water to the respiratory tract, particularly if the water reservoir is heated to increase mist density. However, the risk of infection is increased, as droplets can carry bacteria to the alveoli. Consequently, only sterile water should be used to fill the reservoir, and all units should be regularly changed and sterilized. Acetylcysteine has been used as a mucolytic, but may cause bronchospasm, and benefits are not supported by clinical data.[33]

BRONCHODILATOR THERAPY

Optimal aerosol delivery and bronchodilator response is extremely important in critically ill patients with severe airflow limitation, and this can be achieved using either a nebulizer or MDI technique provided that care is taken to optimize performance. The response can be judged clinically, and in ventilated patients monitored by changes in peak-to-plateau airway pressure gradient, calculated airways resistance, and intrinsic-PEEP. Numerous studies show effective bronchodilatation with β_2-agonists and ipratropium in ventilated patients,[31] but it is uncertain whether additional nebulized steroids are useful.[33] Although entrainment of nebulized drug in a high-gas-flow CPAP circuit can be expected to reduce drug delivery, good bronchodilator response with salbutamol has been reported in this setting.[35]

DELIVERY OF ANTIBIOTICS AND ANTIVIRAL AGENTS

Aerosolized antibiotics have been contentious for many years; however, the potential to achieve high concentrations of antibiotics at the site of infection remains appealing. Numerous studies in patients with cystic fibrosis have shown a reduction in sputum volume and density of bacteria, and improved lung function with reduced risk of hospitalization when inhaled aminoglycosides are used.[36,37] Similar results, including a reduction of markers of airway inflammation, have been reported with bronchiectasis,[38,39] and in mechanically ventilated patients with chronic respiratory failure.[40] Although there has been concern that aerosolized antibiotics will promote the development of resistant organisms,[41] this study examined whole ICU prophylaxis with polymyxin, rather than treatment, and other studies using amino-glyocides have not reported the development of resistance.[39,42] Other antimicrobials that have been safely nebulized include vancomycin, amphotericin B and pentamidine for *Pneumocystis carinii* pneumonia. However, inhaled amphotericin may result in bronchospasm, and no study has demonstrated major clinical benefit in the treatment of pneumonia in critically ill patients. Consequently, if these drugs are used as an aerosol this should be done cautiously, and treatment of pneumonia should include standard intravenous therapy. Aerosolized ribavarin is effective for respiratory syncytial virus infection, resulting in a shorter period of ventilation and hospitalization.[43] However, ribavarin deposition in the circuit may cause valve malfunction, and concerns of teratogenicity in health care personnel have dictated its use with care.[43]

SPUTUM INDUCTION

Nebulized 3% saline is effective in sputum induction for diagnosing *P. carinii* pneumonia in patients with the acquired immunodeficiency syndrome, thereby often obviating the need for bronchoscopy.[44] Sputum induction has been used to diagnose a number of other infections, and appears to be safe in patients with severe airflow limitation.[45]

SURFACTANT THERAPY

Surfactant preparations have been delivered by instillation and as an aerosol in neonates with respiratory distress syndrome, and in adults with the acute respiratory distress syndrome. Aerosolized surfactant achieves a more uniform distribution and avoids problems of instilling liquid into injured lungs. However, large amounts are needed for lung deposition, and preferential distribution occurs to less damaged lung areas that receive better ventilation.[46]

REFERENCES

1 Hedley RM, Allt-Graham J. Heat and moisture exchangers and breathing filters. *Br J Anaesth* 1994; **73**: 227–36.
2 Forbes AR. Humidification and mucus flow in the intubated trachea. *Br J Anaesth* 1973; **45**: 874–8.
3 Forbes AR. Temperature, humidity and mucus flow in the intubated trachea. *Br J Anaesth* 1974; **46**: 29–34.
4 Sackner MA, Landa J, Hirsch J, *et al.* Pulmonary effects of oxygen breathing: a six-hour study in normal man. *Ann Intern Med* 1975; **82**: 40–3.
5 LaFortuna CL, Fazio F. Acute effect of inhaled salbutamol on mucociliary clearance in health and chronic bronchitis. *Respiration* 1985; **45**: 111–3.
6 Chalon J, Patel C, Ali M, *et al.* Humidity and the anesthetized patient. *Anesthesiology* 1974; **50**: 195–8.
7 Circeo LE, Heard SO, Griffiths E, *et al.* Overwhelming necrotizing tracheobronchitis due to

inadequate humidification during high-frequency jet ventilation. *Chest* 1991; **100**: 268–9.
8 Linko K, Honkavaara P, Niemenen MT. Heated humidification after major abdominal surgery. *Eur J Anaesthesiol* 1984; **1**: 285–91.
9 Shelley MP, Lloyd GM, Park GR. A review of the mechanisms and methods of humidification of inspired gases. *Intens Care Med* 1988; **14**: 1–9.
10 Chamney AR. Humidification requirements and techniques. *Anaesthesia* 1969; **24**: 602–17.
11 Rhame FS, Streifel A, McComb C, *et al.* Bubbling humidifiers produce microaerosols which can carry bacteria. *Infection Control* 1986; 7: 403–7.
12 Dreyfuss D, Djedaini K, Gros K, *et al.* Mechanical ventilation with heated humidifiers or heat and moisture exchangers: effects on patient colonization and incidence of nosocomial pneumonia. *Am J Respir Crit Care Med* 1995; **151**: 986–92.
13 Kollef M, Shapiro S, Boyd V, *et al.* A randomized clinical trial comparing an extended-use hygroscopic condenser humidifier with heated-water humidification in mechanically ventilated patients. *Chest* 1998; **113**: 759–67.
14 Jackson C, Webb AR. An evaluation of the heat and moisture exchange performance of four ventilator circuit filters. *Intensive Care Med* 1992; **18**: 246–68.
15 Mebius C. Heat and moisture exchangers with bacterial filters: a laboratory evaluation. *Acta Anaesthesiol Scand* 1992; **36**: 572–6.
16 Martin C, Papazian L, Perrin G, *et al.* Performance evaluation of three vaporizing humidifiers and two heat and moisture exchangers in patients with minute volumes > 10 l/min. *Chest* 1992; **102**: 1347–50.
17 Shelley M, Bethune DW, Latimer RD. A comparison of five heat and moisture exchangers. *Anaesthesia* 1986; **41**: 527–32.
18 Sottiaux T, Mignolet G, Damas P, *et al.* Comparative evaluation of three heat and moisture exchangers during short-term postoperative mechanical ventilation. *Chest* 1993; **104**: 220–4.
19 Unal N, Kanhai JKK, Buijk SLCE, *et al.* A novel method of evaluation of three heat-moisture exchangers in six different ventilator settings. *Intensive Care Med* 1998; **24**: 138–46.
20 Thomachot L, Boisson C, Arnaud S, *et al.* Changing heat and moisture exchangers after 96 hours rather than 24 hours: A clinical and microbiological evaluation. *Crit Care Med* 2000; **28**: 714–20.
21 Misset B, Escudier B, Rivara D, *et al.* Heat and moisture exchanger vs heated humidifier during long-term mechanical ventilation: a prospective randomized study. *Chest* 1990; **100**: 160–63.
22 Martin C, Perrin G, Gevaudan MJ, *et al.* Heat and moisture exchangers and vaporizing humidifiers in the intensive care unit. *Chest* 1990; **97**: 144–9.
23 Cohen IL, Weinberg PF, Fein IA, *et al.* Endotracheal tube occlusion associated with the use of heat and moisture exchangers in the intensive care unit. *Crit Care Med* 1988; **16**: 277–9.
24 AARC clinical practice guideline. Humidification during mechanical ventilation. *Respir Care* 1992; **37**: 887–90.

25 Gluck E, Heard S, Patel C, *et al*. Use of high frequency ventilation in patients with ARDS: a preliminary report. *Chest* 1993; **103**: 1413–20.

26 Ploysongsang Y, Branson R, Rashkin MC, *et al*. Pressure flow characteristics of commonly used heat-moisture exchangers. *Am Rev Respir Dis* 1988; **138**: 675–8.

27 Oh TE, Lin ES, Bhatt S. Resistance of humidifiers, and inspiratory work imposed by a ventilator-humidifier circuit. *Br J Anaesth* 1991; **66**: 258–63.

28 Craven DE, Goularte TA, Make BJ. Contaminated condensate in mechanical ventilator circuits: a risk factor for nosocomial pneumonia. *Am Rev Respir Dis* 1984; **129**: 625–8.

29 Dreyfuss D, Djedaini K, Weber P, *et al*. Prospective study of nosocomial pneumonia and of patient and circuit colonisation during mechanical ventilation with circuit changes every 48 hours versus no change. *Am Rev Respir Dis* 1991; **143**: 738–43.

30 Craven DE, Connolly MG, Lichtenberg DA, *et al*. Contamination of mechanical ventilators with tubing changes every 24 or 48 hours. *N Engl J Med* 1982; **306**: 1505–9.

31 O'Doherty MJ, Thomas SHL. Nebuliser therapy in the intensive care unit. *Thorax* 1997; **52(Suppl 2)**: S56–9.

32 Dhand R, Tobin MJ. Inhaled bronchodilator therapy in mechanically ventilated patients. *Am J Respir Crit Care Med* 1997; **156**: 3–10.

33 Manthous CA, Hall JB. Administration of therapeutic aerosols to mechanically ventilated patients. *Chest* 1994; **106**: 560–71.

34 Spahr-Schopfer IA, Lerman J, Cutz E, *et al*. Proximate delivery of a large experimental dose from salbutamol MDI induces epithelial airway lesions in intubated rabbits. *Am J Respir Crit Care Med* 1994; **150**: 790–4.

35 Parkes SN, Bersten AD. Aerosol delivery and bronchodilator efficacy during continuous positive airway pressure delivered by face mask. *Thorax* 1997; **52**: 171–5.

36 Ramsey BW, Dorkin HL, Eisenberg JD, *et al*. Efficacy of aerosolized tobramycin in patients with cystic fibrosis. *N Engl J Med* 1993; **328**: 1740–6.

37 Ramsey BW, Pepe MS, Quan JM, *et al*. Intermittent administration of inhaled tobramycin in cystic fibrosis. Cystic fibrosis inhaled tobramycin study group. *N Engl J Med* 1999; **340**: 23–30.

38 Lin H-C, Cheng H-F, Wang C-H, *et al*. Inhaled gentamicin reduces airway neutrophil activity and mucus secretion in bronchiectasis. *Am J Respir Crit Care Med* 1997; **155**: 2024–9.

39 Barker AF, Couch L, Fiel SB, *et al*. Tobramycin solution for inhalation reduces sputum *Pseudomona aeruginosa* density in bronchiectasis. *Am J Respir Crit Care Med* 2000; **162**: 481–5.

40 Palmer LB, Smaldone GC, Simon SR, *et al*. Aerosolized antibiotics in mechanically ventilated patients: delivery and response. *Crit Care Med* 1998; **26**: 31–9.

41 Feeley TW, DuMoulin GC, Hedley-White J, *et al*. Aerosol polymyxin and pneumonia in seriously ill patients. *N Engl J Med* 1975; **293**: 471–5.

42 Burns JL, Van Dalfsen JM, Shawar RM, *et al*. Effect of chronic intermittent administration of inhaled tobramycin on respiratory microbial flora in patients with cystic fibrosis. *J Infect Dis* 1999; **179**: 1190–6.

43 Committee on infectious diseases. Use of ribavarin in the treatment of respiratory syncytial virus infection. *Pediatrics* 1993; **92**: 501–4.

44 Bigby TD, Margolskee D, Curtis JL, *et al*. The usefulness of induced sputum in the diagnosis of *Pneumocystis carinii* pneumonia in patients with the acquired immunodeficiency syndrome. *Am Rev Respir Dis* 1986; **133**: 515–8.

45 Vlachos-Mayer H, Leigh R, Sharon RF, *et al*. Success and safety of sputum induction in the clinical setting. *Eur Respir J* 2000; **16**: 997–1000.

46 Lewis JF, Jobe AH. Surfactant and the adult respiratory distress syndrome. *Am Rev Respir Dis* 1993; **147**: 218–33.

27

Acute respiratory distress syndrome

A D Bersten

The acute respiratory distress syndrome (ARDS) was first described in 1967 when Ashbaugh and colleagues described 12 patients with 'acute onset of tachypnea, hypoxemia and loss of compliance after a variety of stimuli'.[1] Since then, a large amount of research has examined the underlying mechanisms and management strategies. However, until recently, this had failed to translate into improvements in outcome.

DEFINITIONS

Acute lung injury (ALI) and its more severe subset ARDS are the result of bilateral and diffuse alveolar damage due to an acute insult. When this is manifest as acute hypoxaemic respiratory failure not due to elevated pulmonary capillary pressure, ALI and ARDS are diagnosed. The most common criteria are the 1994 American-European Consensus Conference definitions[2] (Table 27.1), which have allowed a more uniform approach to research. However, these fail to specify an acute cause, use a PaO_2/FiO_2 ratio independent of respiratory support, and are not specific about the radiographic criteria. Consequently, some of these issues will be addressed by forthcoming modifications of these definitions, but some investigators use the lung injury score (LIS) which encompasses many of these issues.[3] This consists of a four point lung injury score attributed to ranges of PaO_2/FiO_2 ratio, PEEP, respiratory system compliance and the number of quadrants involved on chest radiograph. The final

score is the sum of these components divided by the number measured, and a LIS >2.5 is defined as severe lung injury.

CHEST RADIOGRAPH AND CHEST CT IN ACUTE LUNG INJURY

The interpretation of the chest radiograph is central to these definitions of ALI and ARDS, however, there is both considerable inter-observer variability in chest radiograph interpretation, and in the definition of an infiltrate. In the American-European Consensus Conference definition the infiltrate must be bilateral and consistent with pulmonary oedema,[2] whereas the LIS rates the number of quadrants with alveolar consolidation.[3] The intention of these two descriptions is fairly clear and excludes opacity due to pleural effusion, nodules, masses, collapse and pleural thickening. However, it is desirable to improve interobserver agreement and this will require training and more specific definitions.

Chest CT[4] has proved extremely helpful in pathophysiologic studies of ALI, has demonstrated the heterogeneity of lung inflation, and is commonly used to assist clinical management. Autopsy and chest radiographs of ALI show a uniform process effecting both lungs, however, chest CT early in the course of ALI in supine patients demonstrated that there was a dorsal, dependent increase in lung density, and that the ventral lung was relatively normal. In addition, CT frequently showed previously undiagnosed pneumothorax, pneumomediastinum and pleural effusion. After

Table 27.1 Definition of acute lung injury (ALI) and acute respiratory distress syndrome (ARDS)[2]

Condition	Timing	PaO₂/FiO₂	Chest radiograph	PAoP
ALI	Acute	≤300 mmHg	Bilateral infiltrates	≤18 mmHg or no clinical evidence of elevated left atrial pressure
ARDS	Acute	≤200 mmHg	Bilateral infiltrates	≤18 mmHg or no clinical evidence of elevated left atrial pressure

the second week of mechanical ventilation CT scans may demonstrate altered lung architecture and emphysematous cysts or pneumatoceles.

CT numbers or Hounsfield units can be assigned to each voxel (~2000 alveoli in a standard 10 mm slice).[4] These data can then be used to assess what proportion of a region of interest is non-aerated, poorly aerated, normally aerated, or hyperinflated. Initially a single basal lung slice was studied, but it is clear that far more information can be obtained by studying the whole lung. This allows (i) reconstruction of the upper and lower lobes (the middle lobe is difficult to separate), (ii) the same section of lung to be studied at different levels of inflation or PEEP (the lung also moves in a cepahalo-caudad direction with respiration) and (iii) a broader picture of the lung to be obtained (lung damage is heterogenous in ALI). However, whole lung CT demands considerable exposure to ionizing radiation, and different information, perhaps more pertinent to mechanical ventilation is obtained from dynamic CT.

Clinical assessment of chest CT is discussed in Chapter 32 and CT findings in ALI are discussed below under 'clinical management'.

EPIDEMIOLOGY

Estimates of the incidence and outcome from ALI and ARDS vary widely. In part, this has been due to differences in the definitions used, but it also appears likely that case-mix and local factors also influence outcome and incidence. A recent Australian study[5] using the 1994 consensus definition reported an incidence of 34 per 100 000 for ALI and 28 per 100 000 for ARDS, which is much greater than many previous estimates, but consistent with the early NIH estimate of 75 per 100 000.[6] The Australian data equates to one in ten non-cardiothoracic ICU patients developing ARDS, which reflects the tendency for clinicians to underestimate the incidence of ALI and ARDS.

Reported mortality rates are also influenced by the definitions used. For many years the mortality for ARDS was reported to be ~60%, but single centre studies from the USA[7] and UK[8] have reported reductions to 36% and 34% respectively by the mid-1990s. Similarly the Australian multi-centre data reported mortality rates of 32% for ALI, and 34% for ARDS.[5] However, particular diagnostic groups such as multiple trauma have lower mortality rate than other causes of ARDS, and patients with ALI who have chronic liver disease, non-pulmonary organ dysfunction, sepsis or age greater than 70 years (hazard ratio 2.5)[9] have a higher risk of death. Consequently, many factors need to be considered when assessing outcome prediction.

PULMONARY FUNCTION IN SURVIVORS

Respiratory function is most abnormal soon after discontinuation of mechanical ventilation, but usually returns towards normal by 6–12 months. Although a variety of abnormal pulmonary function tests may be found, the most common are abnormal diffusing capacity and mild-to-moderate restrictive lung disease. This is rarely symptomatic, but occasional patients have severe restrictive disease, and this is correlated with their cumulative LIS.[10]

QUALITY OF LIFE IN SURVIVORS

Compared with disease-matched ICU patients who do not develop ARDS, patients with ARDS have a more severe reduction in both pulmonary and general health-related quality of life.[11] Even more provocative, most survivors have cognitive impairments such as slowed mental processing, or impaired memory or concentration, and these correlate with the period and severity of desaturation <90%.[12] Although these data suggest that ARDS confers a specific risk of impaired quality of life, the mechanism is unclear. However, they do caution against permissive hypoxaemia as a strategy to reduce ventilator-induced lung injury (VILI).

PATIENTS AT-RISK FOR ALI AND ARDS

Clinical risk factors for the development of ALI and ARDS can be classified as either direct or indirect (Table 27.2). These identify over 80% of patients who develop ARDS, and the most common risk factors are sepsis, pneumonia and aspiration of gastric contents. Multiple risk factors, low pH, chronic alcohol abuse or chronic lung disease substantially increase the incidence of ALI in at-risk patients.[6]

BIOLOGICAL MARKERS AS PREDICTORS OF ALI

In addition to identifying these clinical risk groups, there has been considerable interest in identifying possible

Table 27.2   Clinical risk factors for acute lung injury (ALI) and acute respiratory distress syndrome (ARDS)

Direct	Indirect
Pneumonia (46%)*	Non-pulmonary sepsis (25%)
Aspiration of gastric contents (29%)	Multiple trauma (41%)
	Massive transfusion (34%)
Lung contusion (34%)	Pancreatitis (25%)
Fat embolism	Cardiopulmonary bypass
Near drowning	
Inhalational injury	
Reperfusion injury	

*Denotes the percentage of ICU at-risk cases that developed ALI.[13]

biological markers that could be used to predict the development of ALI. Although greater specificity may be gained from sampling the epithelial lining fluid (e.g. using bronchoalveolar lavage fluid), an ideal biological marker would be more simply sampled, such as plasma. While numerous proteins, such as the cytokines IL-1, TNF-α, and IL-10, and von-Willebrand's factor antigen are elevated in at-risk patients and patients with ALI and ARDS, they are not predictive. However, in relatively small studies both ferritin[14] and surfactant protein-B (SP-B)[15] have been shown to be predictive of ARDS. While ferritin likely represents a non-specific oxygen free-radical response, the leakage of SP-B from the alveolus into the blood is lung specific.

PATHOGENESIS

Although it is well accepted that diffuse alveolar damage with (i) pulmonary oedema due to damage of the alveolocapillary barrier, (ii) a complex inflammatory infiltrate and (iii) surfactant dysfunction, are essential components of ALI, the sequence of events is uncertain and probably depends upon the precipitating insult and host response. For example in endotoxin-induced lung injury hypoxaemia and reduced lung compliance occur well before recruitment of neutrophils or an increase in lung weight due to an increase in permeability.[16] In addition, surfactant turnover is dramatically increased prior to these changes often thought to be typical of early ALI. Further, epithelial lining fluid sampled immediately following intubation in patients with ALI has markedly increased concentrations of type III procollagen peptide, suggestive of fibrosing alveolitis extremely early in the course of lung damage.

THE ALVEOLOCAPILLARY BARRIER

The normal lung consists of 300 million alveoli with alveolar gas separated from the pulmonary microcirculation by the extremely thin alveolocapillary barrier (0.1–0.2 μm thick). Since the endothelial pore size is 6.5–7.5 nm, and the epithelial pore size is almost one tenth that at 0.5–0.9 nm, the epithelium is the major barrier to protein flux.[17] The surface area of the alveoli is estimated to be 50–100 m^2, which is made up predominantly of alveolar type I cells, with the metabolically active type II cells accounting for ~10% of the surface area. In turn, these cells are covered by the epithelial lining fluid with an estimated volume of 20 ml, ~10% of which is surfactant with the remained filtered plasma water and low molecular weight proteins, and a small number of cells mainly alveolar macrophages and lymphocytes.

In ALI the alveolocapillary barrier is damaged with bidirectional leakage of fluid and protein into the alveolus and leakage of surfactant proteins and alveolar cytokines into the plasma, disruption of the epithelial barrier, surfactant dysfunction, and proliferation of alveolar type II cells as the progenitor of type I cells. The outcome of this process must reflect a balance between repair and fibrosing alveolitis. As discussed above the precise sequence of events causing and maintaining damage of the alveolocapillary barrier is complex and uncertain, and likely varies depending on the underlying cause. For example indirect causes of ALI may initially cause pulmonary endothelial injury followed by recruitment of inflammatory cells and epithelial damage, while direct causes of ALI may initially cause epithelial injury and secondary recruitment of inflammatory cells.

NEUTROPHILS IN ALI

Neutrophils are the most abundant cell type found in both the epithelial lining fluid (e.g. bronchoalveolar lavage fluid), and alveoli in histologic specimens from early in the course of ALI. Although neutrophil migration across the endothelium or epithelium does not cause injury, when activated they release reactive oxygen species, cytokines, eicosanoids and a variety of proteases that may make an important contribution to tissue damage in ALI. Following bone marrow demargination, activated neutrophils adhere to the endothelium on their passage to the alveolus, and this may be accompanied by an early, transient leukopenia. While neutrophils have an important role in host defence due to their bactericidal activity; there is a marked (50–1000-fold) increase in the release of cytotoxic compounds when they are activated by adherence to the endothelium, epithelium or contact with interstitial extracellular matrix proteins.[18] The factors involved in adhesion of neutrophils are complex and involve the integrin family of proteins, selectins and a number of adhesion molecules.

In models of ALI, antibodies to adhesion molecules (e.g. CD11b/CD18 antibodies) ameliorate lung injury, suggesting a crucial and central role of this cell type. However, ALI occurs in neutropenic patients, and was not more common when granulocyte colony-stimulating factor was administered to patients with pneumonia.[19] Clearly, other cell types play an important role, and neutrophil chemoattractants such as IL-8 must be present in the lung prior to neutrophil accumulation.

OTHER CELL TYPES INVOLVED IN ALI

Pulmonary endothelial cells, platelets, interstitial and alveolar macrophages and alveolar type II cells also play important roles in alveolar inflammation. Pulmonary endothelial cells express a variety of adhesion molecules and COX-2, secrete endothelin and cytokines including IL-8,[20] stimulate procoagulant activity and 'cross talk' with the alveolar macrophages and type II cells. They will be involved in generalized endothelial activation, and are subject to mechanical stress both secondary to vascular pressure, and to their close association with the alveolus. Von Willebrand's factor antigen is synthesized by vascular endothelial cells, and while this may explain its lack of specificity for ALI, its plasma levels are a good marker of endothelial injury.[21]

Microvascular thrombosis is common in ALI, and contributes to pulmonary hypertension and wasted ventilation. Although platelet aggregation may contribute to ALI through release of thromboxane A_2, serotonin, lysosomal enzymes, and platelet activating factor, they are less important than the other cell types.

Alveolar macrophages are the most common cell type normally found in bronchoalveolar lavage fluid, and together with interstitial macrophages play an important role in host defence and modulation of fibrosis. They are capable of releasing IL-6 and a host of mediators, similar to the activated neutrophil, including TNF-α and IL-8 in response to stretch,[22] and may amplify lung injury. However, depletion of alveolar macrophages does not reduce neutrophil recruitment or outcome from tracheal instillation of *Pseudomonas aeruginosa*,[23] again questioning the central role of this cell type. Macrophages also release a number factors such as TGF-α and PDGF that stimulate fibroblast proliferation, deposition of collagen and glycosaminoglycans, angiogenesis and lung fibrosis.

Alveolar epithelial type II cells are extremely metabolically active; they manufacture and release surfactant, control alveolar water clearance using ion pumps, express cytokines, which in turn interact with surfactant production, and are the progenitor of type I cells following injury. In response to both stretch and endotoxin, type II cells express IL-8 and TNF-α, with the latter cytokine augmenting Na^+, and hence water, egress from the alveolus.[24]

CHEMOKINES IN ALI

The expression and secretion of chemokines (chemoattractant cytokines) at sites of inflammation is probably the key proximal step in initiating the inflammatory cascade. IL-8 appears particularly important in initiating ALI because of its ability to induce chemotaxis and activation of neutrophils. IL-8 is elevated in ALI bronchoalveolar lavage fluid within hours of the initiating insult and before recruitment of neutrophils, and in a manner that reflects subsequent morbidity and mortality. In animal models of sepsis and acid aspiration instillation of antibodies against IL-8 prevents the recruitment of neutrophils and protects the lung. Indeed, the recruitment and retention of neutrophils requires the generation and maintenance of a localized chemotactic/haptotactic gradient.[25]

MEDIATORS IN ALI

From the discussion above it is clear that numerous mediators, derived from a number of different cell types, play important roles in the pathophysiology of ALI. These include cytokines, chemokines, complement, reactive oxygen species, eicosanoids, platelet activating factor, nitric oxide, proteases, growth factors and lysosomal enzymes. As the alveolocapillary barrier becomes injured these are no longer compartmentalized in the alveolus, and many mediators have been measured in blood as well as in the epithelial lining fluid. Care must be taken when interpreting these data as immunologic levels may not reflect biologic activity, inhibitors or binding proteins may complex with the active protein or epitope and interfere with immunologic detection, and the ultimate biologic effect will depend upon a balance of pro-inflammatory and anti-inflammatory effects.

Although many of the over 40 biologically active cytokines are implicated in ALI, TNF-α, IL-1β, IL-6 and IL-8 are the most important. However, even greater increases are found in their cognate receptors or antagonists such as the counter-regulatory cytokine IL-10, so that their biological impact is markedly reduced.[26] Despite numerous studies measurement of cytokines in blood or epithelial lining fluid have not proven predictive of the development of ALI or of mortality.

RESOLUTION OF ALI AND THE DEVELOPMENT OF FIBROSING ALVEOLITIS

Although elevated levels of type III procollagen peptide are found in the epithelial lining fluid soon after diagnosis, histologic evidence of fibrosing alveolitis (mesenchymal cells and new vessels in alveoli) is not usually found until at least five days following the onset of ALI. In the majority of patients there is clinical resolution of ALI provided that the underlying cause is promptly and effectively treated. Alveolar oedema resolves with active transport of Na^+ by the type II cells followed by passive clearance of water through transcellular aquaphorin channels, and repair of the alveolocapillary barrier is associated with improved outcome. Type II cells proliferate and cover the denuded epithelium before differentiating into type I cells. Both pro-apoptotic and anti-apoptotic (G-CSF and GM-CSF) factors are found in the alveolus during this phase, however, little is known regarding control over the delicate balance between repair and fibrosis.

CLINICAL MANAGEMENT OF ALI

The factors leading to ALI must be promptly and appropriately treated. This includes diagnosis and appropriate treatment of infection with drainage of collections and appropriate anti-microbial agents, recognition and rapid resuscitation from shock, splinting of fractures, and careful supportive care. Prevention of deep venous thrombosis, stress ulceration, and nosocomial infection are important in all critically ill patients. Adequacy of nutrition, often enteral nutrition, must also be considered.

Table 27.3   Pathophysiology of acute lung injury (ALI) and acute respiratory distress syndrome (ARDS)

Feature	Cause(s)
Hypoxaemia	True shunt (perfusion of non-ventilated airspaces)[28]
	Impaired hypoxic pulmonary vasoconstriction
	$\dot{V}/\dot{Q}$ mismatch is a minor component
↑ Dependent densities (CT)	Surfactant dysfunction → alveolar instability
(Collapse/consolidation)	Exaggeration of normal compression of dependent lung due to ↑ weight (↑ lung water, inflammation)
↑ Elastance (↓ Compliance)	Surfactant dysfunction (↑ specific elastance)
	↓ lung volume ('baby lung')
	↑ chest wall elastance
	Fibrosing alveolitis (late)
↑ Minute volume requirement	↑ Alveolar dead space (V_{Dphys}/V_T often 0.4–0.7)
	↑ $\dot{V}_{CO2}$
↑ Work of breathing	↑ elastance
	↑ minute volume requirement
Pulmonary hypertension	Pulmonary vasoconstriction (T_XA_2, endothelin)
	Pulmonary microvascular thrombosis
	Fibrosing alveolitis
	PEEP

MECHANICAL VENTILATION

Patients present with acute hypoxaemic respiratory failure, and an increase in the work of breathing, usually requiring mechanical ventilation (Table 27.3). The role of non-invasive ventilation in ALI is uncertain, with a recent study suggesting a greater complication rate, perhaps due to delayed intubation.[27] However, non-invasive ventilation is worth considering in particular circumstances.

The method and delivery of ventilatory support must take into account the pathophysiology of ALI and ARDS. For many years laboratory studies have described ventilator-induced lung injury (VILI), and recent clinical studies have found that mortality is influenced by mechanical ventilation. The most important of these was the ARDS Network study where 861 ALI patients from 75 ICUs were randomized to receive either a tidal volume (V_T) of 12 or 6 ml/kg predicted body weight.[29] Mortality was reduced by 22% from 40% to 31% in the lower V_T group. There was a strict PEEP and FiO_2 protocol, and patients were ventilated with assist-control ventilation to avoid excessive spontaneous V_T. Despite the importance of this study, and that this protocol has become the baseline for current pharmacological studies in this area, this and other recent studies represent the beginning of clinical investigation into protective ventilation strategies in ALI and ARDS.

AVOIDANCE OF OVERSTRETCH AND INADEQUATE RECRUITMENT

The increase in dependent lung density found on chest CT, due to non-aerated and poorly aerated lung, reduces the volume of aerated lung. Both PEEP and tidal recruit-ment will increase aeration of some of these airspaces, but a V_T that is not reduced in proportion to the reduction in aerated lung will lead to over stretch of that lung parenchyma in turn leading to diffuse alveolar damage. Studies using increased chest wall compliance to increase airway pressure (Paw) have clearly shown that it is lung stretch, not increased Paw that causes injury;[30] consequently this has been termed 'volutrauma'. In addition, repeated opening and closing of airspaces by tidal recruitment results in diffuse alveolar damage ('atelectrauma'). There is considerable data supporting both as important mechanisms of VILI, and both result in alveolar inflammation with high levels of alveolar cytokines ('biotrauma'),[30] which may 'spill' into the systemic circulation.[31]

OVERSTRETCH

The normal lung is fully inflated at a transpulmonary pressure of ~30 cmH_2O. Consequently, maximum plateau pressures (Pplat), the elastic distending pressure, of 30–35 cmH_2O have been recommended to avoid overstretch, and the ARDS Network study targetted Pplat ≤30 cmH_2O.[29] The transpulmonary pressure may be lower than expected for a given Pplat in patients with a high chest wall elastance (e.g. obesity, abdominal compartment syndrome, post-abdominal or thoracic surgery). It is also common for individual patients to show evidence of overinflation at much lower elastic distending pressures (18–25 cmH_2O).[32] Finally, inspiratory effort will lower Pplat by reduction of intrapleural pressure, potentially avoiding detection of an excessive transpulmonary pressure. This is particularly common when pressure support ventilation is used as a primary mode of ventilatory support; V_T that would produce an unacceptably high Pplat during mechanical ventilation will produce the same volutrauma during a spontaneous or supported mode of ventilation, and should be avoided. None of these issues are easily overcome. While placement of an oesophageal balloon allows measurement of the transpulmonary pressure, it must be correctly placed, have an adequate occlusion pressure ratio, and measurements are preferably performed in a semi-sitting position in order to lift the mediastinum off the oesophagus. Similarly, static or dynamic volume-pressure curves or quantitative chest CT can be used to determine overinflation, though chest CT cannot determine over-stretch.[4] Consequently, unless particular expertise is available, V_T limitation at ~6 ml/kg predicted body weight is currently the most practical approach.

ADEQUATE PEEP

PEEP improves PaO_2 by increasing functional residual capacity, and recruiting alveoli. Because PEEP may reduce cardiac output by impairing venous return, Suter and co-workers suggested that maximum oxygen delivery (oxygen content × flow) be used to optimize PEEP.[33] Other end-points, such as titrating PEEP to a particular PaO_2/FiO_2 ratio have been suggested, however, prevention of repeated opening and closing of alveoli with the development of lung injury secondary to high local shear forces (atelectrauma) is now regarded as an important target end-point for PEEP.

The lower inflection point of a volume-pressure curve has been used to set PEEP, because early studies suggested that this reflected recruitment of collapsed alveoli. However, in patients with ALI recruitment occurs well above the lower inflection point, along the entire volume-pressure curve and above the upper inflection point.[34,35] Concurrently, there is frequently evidence of over stretching and hyperinflation on CT scans[36] or dynamic volume-pressure analysis.[32] Consequently, PEEP titration is often a compromise aiming to minimize both atelectrauma and volutrauma.[37]

In patients at-risk for ARDS prophylactic PEEP (8 cmH$_2$O) was not protective.[38] In ALI or ARDS patients, no published study has specifically looked at different PEEP strategies. Although a protective ventilation strategy using the 'open lung' approach with PEEP levels above the lower inflection point did report a reduction in mortality, the treatment arm also included low V_T and recruitment manoeuvres.[39] Reasonable approaches to PEEP titration include (i) the use of a scale similar to the ARDS Network trial which will result in relatively conservative PEEP levels, (ii) titration of PEEP to PaO_2 aiming for a PEEP of ~15 cmH$_2$O, or (iii) measuring elastic mechanics at the bedside. The delta-PEEP technique is a simple technique that indirectly assesses overstretch, as PEEP is changed at a constant V_T.[32]

Recruitment Manoeuvres

It is unclear whether additional recruitment manoeuvres are of additional benefit once an adequate level of PEEP is applied. Typically, a high level of CPAP (30–40 cmH$_2$O) is applied for 30–40 s in an apnoeic patient, followed by return to a lower level of PEEP and controlled ventilation. This may be followed by a marked improvement in oxygenation, however, this is not a consistent finding. Although a recruitment manoeuvre was applied by Amato and colleagues and associated with an improvement in outcome, they also applied a higher level of PEEP and lower V_T in the protective lung strategy group.[39]

In addition to physical recruitment of alveoli, lung stretch above resting V_T is the most powerful physiological stimulus for release of pulmonary surfactant from type II cells. This is associated with a decrease in lung elastance and improved PaO_2 in the isolated perfused lung,[40] and is a possible explanation for the improvement in oxygenation, recruited lung volume and elastance reported with addition of three sigh breaths in patients with ARDS.[41] Similarly, in models of lung injury biologically variable or fractal V_T is associated with less lung damage with lower alveolar levels of IL-8,[42] improved oxygenation and lung elastance with greater surfactant release.[43] Again, these data caution against monotonous low V_T ventilation, and suggest that intermittent or variable lung stretch may reduce lung injury. Along with data examining recruitment manoeuvres, consistent clinical data is awaited.

MODE OF VENTILATION

The role of non-invasive ventilation is uncertain in ALI and ARDS and most patients require intubated mechanical ventilation. Following intubation, controlled ventilation allows immediate reduction in the work of breathing and application of PEEP and a high fractional inspired concentration of oxygen (FiO_2). Later in the clinical course, assisted or supported modes of ventilation may allow better patient-ventilator interaction and possibly improved oxygenation through better $\dot{V}/\dot{Q}$ mismatch as a result of diaphragmatic contraction.[44] Withdrawal or weaning from mechanical ventilation is discussed elsewhere.

An advantage of assist-control ventilation (as used in the ARDS Network study) is that spontaneous effort cannot generate a greater volume than V_T. Care should be taken with synchronized intermittent mandatory ventilation (SIMV), particularly if pressure support is added to SIMV, as excessive V_T may occur during supported breaths. There is an increasing tendency to use pressure-controlled ventilation (PC) or pressure regulated volume control (PRVC) as Ppk is lower than volume controlled (VC) ventilation with a constant inspiratory flow pattern. However, the decelerating flow pattern of PC or PRVC means that most of the resistive pressure (Pres) during inspiration is dissipated by end-inspiration, which is in contrast to VC with a constant inspiratory flow pattern where Pres is dissipated at end-inspiration (see Ch. 25, Figure 25.2). Consequently, with PC and PRVC Ppk ≈Pplat, which is the same as Pplat during VC.[45] In addition oxygenation, haemodynamic stability and mean airway pressure are no different between PC and VC, and a moderate sized randomized study found no difference in outcome.[46] However, there may be differences in the regional distribution of gas with a tendency to greater hyperinflation with VC.[47]

Inverse ratio ventilation, often together with PC, has been used in ARDS. However, when PEEPi and total PEEP is taken into account, apart from a small decrease in $PaCO_2$, there are no advantages with inverse ratio ventilation. Mean airway pressure is higher with a greater risk of both haemodynamic consequences,[45] and regional hyperinflation as found on dynamic volume-pressure analysis,[47] and dynamic CT scans. Consequently, an inspiratory to expiratory ratio greater than 1:1 is recommended.

A number of other modes of ventilation (see Ch. 25) including airway pressure release ventilation and high frequency oscillation have been proposed for use in ARDS, but without new data there do not appear to be any major advantages over optimal conventional ventilation.

TARGET BLOOD GASES

As discussed above, there are many variables that need to be considered when choosing target blood gases in ARDS. For example if a patient also has a traumatic brain injury, it may be inappropriate to accept hypercapnia.

Oxygenation Targets and FiO₂

There must be a compromise between the major determinants of oxygenation including the extent of poorly or non-aerated lung, hypoxic pulmonary vasoconstriction, and mixed venous oxygen saturation, and the target PaO_2. The association between cognitive impairment and arterial saturation (SaO_2) <90%,[12] suggest that a SaO_2 ≥90%, usually a PaO_2 >60 mmHg, is a reasonable target. Because positive pressure ventilation may reduce cardiac output it is also important to consider tissue oxygenation in this decision process.

In addition to PEEP, increased FiO_2 is used to improve SaO_2. However, high FiO_2 may also cause tissue injury including diffuse alveolar damage. The balance between increased airway pressure and FiO_2 is unknown, but high FiO_2 is generally regarded as being less damaging.[48] In part this is because diffuse alveolar damage itself protects the lung against hyperoxia, perhaps through prior induction of scavengers for reactive oxygen species.[49] A reasonable compromise is to start ventilation at a FiO_2 of one and to titrate down aiming for an FiO_2 ≤0.6. In patients with extreme hypoxaemia, additional measures such as inhaled nitric oxide (iNO), and prone positioning may be tried, along with a lower SaO_2 target.

Carbon Dioxide Target

Low V_T strategies will result in elevations in $PaCO_2$ unless minute ventilation is augmented by an increase in respiratory rate. The ARDS Network protocol aimed at normocapnia, with a maximum respiratory rate of 35, to minimize respiratory acidosis.[29] This exposes the lung to more repeated tidal stretch, and may result in dynamic hyperinflation due to a shortened expiratory time (although this did not appear to occur in the ARDS Network study). In addition, allowing the $PaCO_2$ to rise above normal may not be harmful in many patients.

If hypercapnic acidosis occurs slowly, intracellular acidosis is well compensated, and the associated increase in sympathetic tone may augment cardiac output and blood pressure. Although the respiratory acidosis may worsen pulmonary hypertension, and induce myocardial arrhythmias these effects are often small, particularly if there has been time for metabolic compensation. In addition, in an ischaemia-reperfusion model of ALI, therapeutic hypercapnia reduced lung injury and apoptosis.[50] However, clinical studies of permissive hypercapnia must be undertaken before therapeutic hypercapnia is considered. Hypercapnia should be avoided in patients with or at-risk from raised intracranial pressure.

ADDITIONAL MEASURES TO IMPROVE OXYGENATION

PRONE POSTURE

In ~70% of patients with ARDS, prone positioning will result in a significant increase in PaO_2, with a modest increase in PaO_2 sustained in the supine position.[51] The mechanisms involved include recruitment of dorsal lung, with concurrent collapse of ventral; however, perfusion is more evenly distributed leading to better $\dot{V}/\dot{Q}$ matching. Although mortality clinical studies have not found an improvement in mortality, *post-hoc* analysis suggests that mortality may be reduced in the most hypoxaemic patients.[51] While further data are awaited, prone positioning may be used as rescue therapy in life-threatening hypoxaemia.

MANIPULATION OF THE PULMONARY CIRCULATION

Inhaled nitric oxide (iNO) and prostacyclin (PGI_2) may be used to reduce pulmonary shunt and right ventricular afterload by reducing pulmonary artery impedance. When hypoxic pulmonary vasoconstriction is active, there is redistribution of pulmonary blood flow away from the poorly ventilated dependent areas to more normally ventilated lung leading to an increase in PaO_2. Both iNO and PGI_2 are potent vasodilators, and since they are delivered as part of the gas mix (iNO) or inhaled (PGI_2), they are delivered to well ventilated lung. Both act to vasodilate the local pulmonary circulation and increase the redistribution of pulmonary blood flow away from poorly ventilated lung, reducing pulmonary shunt and improving oxygenation. Intravenous almitrine is a selective pulmonary vasoconstrictor that reinforces hypoxic pulmonary vasoconstriction, and although this may improve oxygenation alone, there is a synergistic effect with iNO.

Inhaled NO or PGI$_2$ may also be used to reduce right ventricular afterload; however a consequent increase in cardiac output is rare in ARDS. Intravenous PGI$_2$ will improve cardiac output in ARDS, however, there is non-specific pulmonary vasodilation with increased blood flow through poorly ventilated lung zones, resulting in a deterioration in oxygenation.

Inhaled Nitric Oxide

Nitric oxide is an endothelium-derived smooth muscle relaxant. It also has other important physiological roles including neurotransmission, host defence, platelet aggregation leukocyte adhesion, and bronchodilation. Doses as low as 60 parts per billion iNO may improve oxygenation, however, commonly used doses in ARDS are 1–40 parts per million, with the higher doses required for reduction in pulmonary artery pressure. A rise in PaO$_2$ exceeding 20% is generally regarded as a positive response, and iNO should be continued at the minimum effective dose.

Inhaled NO may be delivered continuously or using intermittent inspiratory injection. Delivery is usually in the form of medical grade NO/N$_2$, and this should be adequately mixed to avoid delivery of variable NO concentrations. It is recommended that inspiratory NO and NO$_2$ concentrations are measured, either by an electro-chemical method or by chemiluminescence. The electro-chemical method is accurate to 1 ppm, which is adequate for clinical use, and is less expensive. Local environmental levels of NO and NO$_2$ are low and predominantly influenced by atmospheric concentrations, however, it is still common practice to scavenge expired gas. Binding to haemoglobin in the pulmonary circulation rapidly inactivates NO, and systemic effects are only reported following high concentrations of iNO. Systemic methaemoglobin levels may be monitored, and are generally less than 5% during clinical use of iNO, but they should be compared with a baseline level. Nitric oxide may cause lung toxicity through combination with oxygen free radicals, and through metabolism of NO to NO$_2$, however, these do not appear to be major clinical problems.

Only 40–70% of patients with ARDS have improved oxygenation with iNO (responders), and this is likely due to active hypoxic pulmonary vasoconstriction in the remainder. Addition of i.v. almitrine can have an additive effect on oxygenation, and may improve the number of responders. Two large trials of iNO[52,53] have shown no improvement in mortality or reversal of ALI. However, iNO was safe and did significantly improve oxygenation initially (compared with placebo or no iNO), but this was not sustained beyond 12–24 h, and some patients receiving placebo had an increase in PaO$_2$ ≥20% at 4 h. Consequently, the role of iNO in patients with ARDS remains uncertain. In some patients with severe hypox-

aemia, perhaps in combination with almitrine, iNO will provide temporary rescue.

Inhaled Prostacyclin

PGI$_2$ (up to 50 ng/kg per min) improves oxygenation as effectively as iNO in ARDS patients. It is continuously jet nebulized due to its short half-life (2–3 min). Potential advantages include increased surfactant release from stretched type II cells, avoidance of the potential complications of iNO, and minimal toxicity. However, PGI$_2$ is dissolved in an alkaline glycine buffer, which alone can result in airway inflammation. Iloprost is a derivative of PGI$_2$ with similar activity, a longer duration of action, without an alkaline buffer. However, neither agent has been shown to improve outcome in ARDS patients.

PHARMACOLOGICAL THERAPY

Apart from improved mortality in sepsis following activated protein-C,[54] there are no proven pharmacological therapies for ALI or ARDS despite numerous studies. However, the lack of a protective ventilation strategy in many of these studies may have masked a drug effect.

SURFACTANT REPLACEMENT THERAPY

Surfactant dysfunction is an important and early abnormality contributing to lung damage in ALI.[37] Pulmonary surfactant reduces surface tension promoting alveolar stability, reducing work of breathing and lung water. In addition surfactant has important roles in lung host defence. Reactive oxygen species, phospholipases and increased protein permeability lead to inhibition of surfactant function, composition is abnormal, and turnover markedly increased. Ventilator-induced lung injury is difficult to demonstrate without surfactant dysfunction.[55] Consequently, there has been considerable interest in exogenous surfactant replacement therapy.

Despite encouraging laboratory data and small studies, exogenous surfactant replacement cannot be recommended without more data. Although a large study of aerosolized surfactant failed to alter outcome or show any physiological effect,[56] it is doubtful whether any surfactant reached the distal lung due to a low dose and 'rain out' of the aerosol. In addition, the preparation used is sensitive to protein inhibition and does not contain surfactant proteins, which markedly reduce surface tension. More promising results have been found with surfactant protein containing preparations administered by instillation; however, definitive data are awaited.

GLUCOCORTICOIDS

These agents may be used to reduce fibrosing alveolitis, however, this is based on a small study, with cross-over, showing a reduction in mortality.[57] Larger studies will be reported soon. It is crucial to have excluded infection prior to starting steroids, and to continue with aggressive surveillance. This may include bronchoalveolar lavage to exclude ventilator-associated pneumonia.

KETOCONAZOLE

Ketoconazole is an anti-fungal drug that also inhibits thromboxane synthase and 5-lipooxygenase. However, promising results from small studies in at-risk patients have not been confirmed in a larger trial.[58]

OTHER PHARMACOLOGIC THERAPIES

Numerous other therapies including cytokine antagonism, non-steroidal anti-inflammatory drugs, scavengers of reactive oxygen species, and lisofylline[59] have been trialled without success. The complex balance of inflammation and repair in ALI, and the critical additional damage secondary to VILI may explain these results. However, studies in less heterogeneous groups with minimization of VILI using standardized ventilation protocols, together with a growing understanding of ALI and ARDS offers potential pharmacologic therapies.

REFERENCES

1 Ashbaugh DG, Bigelow DB, Petty TL, Levine BE. Acute respiratory distress in adults. *Lancet* 1967; **ii**: 319–23.

2 Bernard GR, Artigas A, Brigham KL, *et al.* The American-European Consensus Conference on ARDS: definitions, mechanisms, relevant outcomes, and clinical trial coordination. *Am J Respir Crit Care Med* 1994; **149**: 818–24.

3 Murray JF, Matthay MA, Luce JM, Flick MR. An expanded definition of the adult respiratory distress syndrome. *Am Rev Respir Dis* 1988; **138**: 720–3. [Erratum, *Am Rev Respir Dis* 1989; **139**: 1065].

4 Gattinoni L, Caironi P, Pelosi P, Goodman LR. What has computed tomography taught us about the acute respiratory distress syndrome. *Am J Respir Crit Care Med* 2001; **164**: 1701–11.

5 Bersten AD, Edibam C, Hunt T, *et al.* Incidence and mortality from acute lung injury and the acute respiratory distress syndrome in three Australian states. *Am J Respir Crit Care Med* 2002; **165**: 443–8.

6 Ware LB, Matthay MA. The acute respiratory distress syndrome. *N Engl J Med* 2000; **342**: 1334–49.

7 Milberg JA, Davis DR, Steinberg KP, Hudson LD. Improved survival of patients with acute respiratory distress syndrome (ARDS): 1983–1993. *JAMA* 1995; **273**: 306–9.

8 Abel SJC, Finney SJ, Brett SJ, *et al.* Reduced mortality in association with the acute respiratory distress syndrome (ARDS). *Thorax* 1998; **53**: 292–4.

9 Ely EW, Wheeler AP, Thompson BT, *et al.* Recovery rate and prognosis in older persons who develop acute lung injury and the acute respiratory distress syndrome. *Ann Internal Med* 2002; **136**: 25–36.

10 McHugh LG, Milberg JA, Whitcomb ME, *et al.* Recovery of function in survivors of the acute respiratory distress syndrome. *Am J Respir Crit Care Med* 1994; **250**: 90–4.

11 Davidson TA, Caldwell ES, Curtis SR, *et al.* Reduced quality of life in survivors of acute respiratory distress syndrome compared with other critically ill control patients. *JAMA* 1999; **281**: 354–60.

12 Hopkins RO, Weaver LK, Pope D. Neuropsychological sequelae and impaired health status in survivors of severe acute respiratory distress syndrome. *Am J Respir Crit Care* 1999; **160**: 50–6.

13 Bersten AD, Hunt T, Nicholas TE, Doyle IR. Plasma surfactant proteins (SP) as predictors of ARDS: Patient demographics from an Australian multicentred study. *Am J Respir Crit Care Med* 2002; **165**: A476.

14 Connelly KG, Moss M, Parsons PE, *et al.* Serum ferritin as a predictor of the acute respiratory distress syndrome. *Am J Respir Crit Care Med* 1997; **155**: 21–5.

15 Bersten AD, Hunt T, Nicholas TE, Doyle IR. Elevated plasma surfactant protein-B predicts development of acute respiratory distress syndrome in patients with acute respiratory failure. *Am J Respir Crit Care Med* 2001; **164**: 648–652.

16 Davidson KG, Bersten AD, Barr HA, *et al.* Endotoxin induces respiratory failure and increases surfactant composition and respiration independent of alveolocapillary injury in rats. *Am J Respir Crit Care Med* 2002; **165**: 1516–25.

17 Doyle IR, Nicholas TE, Bersten AD. Partitioning lung and plasma proteins: circulating surfactant proteins as biomarkers of alveolocapillary permeability. *Clin Exp Pharmacol Physiol* 1999; **26**: 185–97.

18 Downey GP, Dong Q, Kruger J, *et al.* Regulation of neutrophil activation in acute lung injury. *Chest* 1999; **116**: 46S-54S.

19 Nelson S, Belknap SM, Carlson RW, *et al.* A randomized controlled trial of figastrim as an adjunct to antibiotics for treatment of hospitalized patients with community-acquired pneumonia. *J Infect Dis* 1998; **178**: 1075–80.

20 Zimmeraman GA, Albertine KH, Carveth HJ, *et al.* Endothelial activation in ARDS. *Chest* 1999; **116**: 18S-24S.

21 Pittet JF, Mackersie RC, Martin TR, Matthay MA. Biological markers of acute lung injury: Prognostic and pathogenetic significance. *Am J Respir Crit Care Med* 1997; **155**: 1187–1205.

22 Pugin J, Dunn I, Jolliet P, *et al.* Activation of human macrophages by mechanical ventilation in vitro. *Am J Physiol* 1998; **275**: L1040–50.

23 Cheung DO, Halsey K, Speert DP. Role of pulmonary alveolar macrophages in defense of the lung against *Pseudomonas aeruginosa*. *Infect Immun* 2000; **68**: 4585–92.

24 Rezaiguia S, Garat C, Declauc C, *et al.* Acute bacterial pneumonia in rats increases alveolar epithelial fluid clearance by a tumor necrosis-factor-alpha dependent mechanism. *J Clin Invest* 1997; **99**: 325–35.

25 Modelska K, Pittet JF, Folkesson HG, *et al.* Acid-induced lung injury. Protective effect of anti-interleukin-8 pretreatment on alveolar epithelial barrier function in rabbits. *Am J Respir Crit Care Med* 1999; **160**: 1450–6.

26 Park WY, Goodman RB, Steinberg KP, *et al*. Cytokine balance in the lungs of patients with acute respiratory distress syndrome. *Am J Respir Crit Care Med* 2001; **164**: 1896–903.

27 Delclaux C, L'Her E, Alberti C, *et al*. Treatment of acute hypoxemic nonhypercapnic respiratory insufficiency with continuous positive airway pressure delivered by a face mask. A randomized controlled trial. *JAMA* 2000; **284**: 2352–60.

28 Dantzker DR, Brook CJ, Demart P, *et al*. Ventilation-perfusion distributions in the adult respiratory distress syndrome. *Am Rev Respi Dis* 1979; **120**: 1039–52.

29 Ventilation with lower tidal volumes as compared with traditional tidal volumes for acute lung injury and the Acute respiratory distress syndrome. *N Engl J Med* 2000; **342**: 1301–8.

30 Dreyfuss D, Saumon G. Ventilator-induced lung injury: Lessons from experimental studies. *Am J Respir Crit Care Med* 1998; **157**: 294–323.

31 Chiumello D, Pristine G, Slutsky AS. Mechanical ventilation affects local and systemic cytokines in an animal model of acute respiratory distress syndrome. *Am J Respir Crit Care Med* 1999; **160**: 109–16.

32 Bersten AD. Measurement of overinflation by multiple linear regression analysis in patients with acute lung injury. *Eur Respir J* 1998; **12**: 526–32.

33 Suter PM, Fairley B, Isenberg MD. Optimum end-expiratory airway pressure in patients with acute pulmonary failure. *N Engl J Med* 1975; **292**: 284–9.

34 Jonson B, Richard J-C, Straus R, *et al*. Pressure-volume curves and compliance in acute lung injury: Evidence for recruitment above the lower inflection point. *Am J Respir Crit Care Med* 1999; **159**: 1172–8.

35 Crotti S, Mascheroni D, Caironi P, *et al*. Recruitment and derecruitment during acute respiratory failure: A clinical study. *Am J Respir Crit Care Med* 2001; **164**: 131–40.

36 Malbouisson LM, Muller J-C, Constantin J-M, *et al*. Computed tomography assessment of positive end-expiratory pressure-induced alveolar recruitment in patients with acute respiratory distress syndrome. *Am J Respir Crit Care Med* 2001; **163**: 1444–50.

37 Rouby JJ, Lu Q, Goldstein I. Selecting the right level of positive end-expiratory pressure in patients with acute respiratory distress syndrome. *Am J Respir Crit Care Med* 2002; **165**: 1182–6.

38 Pepe PE, Hudson LD, Carrico CJ. Early application of positive end-expiratory pressure in patients at-risk for adult respiratory distress syndrome. *N Engl J Med* 1984; **311**: 281–6.

39 Amato MBP, Barbas CSV, Medeiros DM, *et al*. Effect of a protective ventilation strategy on mortality in the acute respiratory distress syndrome. *N Engl J Med* 1998; **338**: 347–54.

40 Nicholas TE, Power JHT, Barr HA. The pulmonary consequences of a deep breath. *Respir Physiol* 1982; **49**: 315–24.

41 Pelosi P, Cadringher P, Bottino N, *et al*. Sigh in acute respiratory distress syndrome. *Am J Respir Crit Care Med* 1999; **159**: 872–80.

42 Boker A, Ruth Graham M, Walley KR, *et al*. Improved arterial oxygenation with biologically variable or fractal ventilation using low tidal volumes in a porcine model of acute respiratory distress syndrome. *Am J Respir Crit Care Med* 2002; **165**: 456–62.

43 Ingenito EP, Arold S, Lutchen K, Suki B. Effects of noisy ventilation (NV) and open lung ventilation (OLV) on lung mechanics, gas exchange, and surfactant content and properties (abstract). *Am J Respir Crit Care Med* 2001; **163**: A483.

44 Zinserling J, Wrihhe H, Neumann P, *et al*. Effect of spontaneous breathing during ventilatory support on CT lung density and atelectasis formation in pigs. *Am J Respir Crit Care Med* 2001; **163**: A682.

45 Lessard MR, Guerot E, Lorino H, *et al*. Effects of pressure-controlled with different I:E ratios versus volume-controlled ventilation on respiratory mechanics, gas exchange, and hemodynamics in patients with adult respiratory distress syndrome. *Anesthesiology* 1994; **80**: 983–91.

46 Esteban A, Alia I, Gordo F, *et al*. Prospective randomized trial comparing pressure-controlled ventilation and volume-controlled ventilation in ARDS. For the Spanish Lung Failure Collaborative Group. *Chest* 2000; **117**: 1690–6.

47 Edibam C, Rutten AJ, Collins DV, Bersten AD. Effect of inspiratory flow pattern and Inspiratory to expiratory ratio on non-linear elastic behavior in patients with acute lung injury. *Am J Respir Crit Care Med* (2003, in press)

48 Slutsky AS. Mechanical ventilation. *Chest* 1993; **104**: 1833–59.

49 Frank L, Yam J, Roberts RJ. The role of endotoxin in protection of adult rats from oxygen-induced lung injury. *J Clin Invest* 1978; **61**: 269–75.

50 Laffey JG, Tanaka M, Engelberts D, *et al*. Therapeutic hypercapnia reduces pulmonary and systemic injury following *in vivo* lung reperfusion. *Am J Respir Crit Care Med* 2000; **162**: 2287–94.

51 Gattinoni L, Tognoni G, Pesenti A, *et al*. Effect of prone positioning on the survival of patients with acute respiratory failure. *N Engl J Med* 2001; **345**: 568–73.

52 Dellinger RP, Zimmerman JL, Taylor RW, *et al*. Effects of inhaled nitric oxide in patients with acute respiratory distress syndrome: Results of a randomized phase II trial. *Crit Care Med* 1998; **26**: 15–23.

53 Lundin S, Mang H, Smithies M *et al*. for the European Study Group of Inhaled Nitric Oxide. Inhalation of nitric oxide in acute lung injury: results of a European multicentre study. *Intensive Care Med* 1999; **25**: 911–19.

54 Bernard GR, Vincent J-L, Laterre P-F, *et al* for the PROWESS Study Group. Efficacy and safety of recombinant human activated protein C for severe sepsis. *N Engl J Med* 2001; **344**: 699–709.

55 Bersten AD, Davidson K, Nicholas TE, Doyle IR. Respiratory mechanics and surfactant in the acute

respiratory distress syndrome. *Clin Exp Pharmacol Physiol* 1998; **25**: 955–63.

56 Anzueto A, Baughman RP, Guntupalli KK, *et al*. Aerosolized surfactant in adults with sepsis-induced acute respiratory distress syndrome. Exosurf acute respiratory distress syndrome study group. *N Engl J Med* 1996; **334**: 1417–21.

57 Meduri GU, Headley AS, Golden E, *et al*. Effect of prolonged methylprednisolone therapy in unresolving acute respiratory distress syndrome: a randomized controlled trial. *JAMA* 1998; **280**: 159–65.

58 Ketoconazole for early treatment of acute lung injury and acute respiratory distress syndrome. *JAMA* 2000; **283**: 1995–2002.

59 Randomized placebo-controlled trial of lisofylline for early treatment of acute lung injury and acute respiratory distress syndrome. *Crit Care Med* 2002; **30**: 1–6.

28

Respiratory monitoring

A D Bersten

Clinical examination and the trend of vital signs such as respiratory rate (f), and quantity and nature of sputum are extremely important in managing patients with respiratory disease. In particular, clinical examination should look for evidence of excessive inspiratory and/or expiratory pleural pressure changes and effort such as accessory muscle use, tracheal tug, supraclavicular and intercostal indrawing, paradoxical abdominal movement (which is suggestive of diaphragmatic fatigue),[1] and pulsus paradoxus. During spontaneous ventilation an excessive fall in blood pressure during inspiration (>10 mmHg) is found in a number of conditions such as cardiac tamponade, cardiogenic shock, pulmonary embolism, hypovolaemic shock and acute respiratory failure. A curvilinear relationship exists between the fall in blood pressure and the change in pleural pressure during inspiration, however, there is marked variation between individuals.[2] Consequently, pulsus paradoxus is most useful in following trends, and a reduction in the degree of paradox may be due to improvement and a fall in the negative pleural pressure needed for ventilation, or due to respiratory muscle insufficiency, and an inability to generate the same negative pleural pressure.

Additional information can be gained from blood gases and pulse oximetry (see Ch. 11), capnography, ventilatory pressures, and waveform analysis in patients receiving respiratory assistance. This chapter will focus on tests of respiratory function that are directly relevant to critically ill patients.

MONITORING GAS EXCHANGE

OXYGENATION

This is reviewed in Chapter 11 and will only be briefly discussed here. Hypoxaemia may be due to a low partial pressure of inspired O_2 (rare), hypoventilation, diffusion impairment (rare), ventilation-perfusion ($\dot{V}/\dot{Q}$ mismatch) and shunt. Inert gas analysis has been used to quantitate $\dot{V}/\dot{Q}$ mismatch, and has demonstrated that hypoxaemia in ARDS is predominantly due to alveoli that are perfused but not ventilated,[3] consistent with CT scan evidence of increased dependent lung density. However, inert gas analysis remains a research tool, and less direct methods, such as the alveolar gas equation, are used to assess hypoxaemia:

$$PAO_2 = \text{inspired } PO_2 - PaCO_2/\text{respiratory quotient} \quad (1)$$

where PAO_2 is the alveolar PO_2, and this is usually simplified to:

$$PAO_2 = (760 - 47) \times FiO_2 - PaCO_2/0.8 \quad (2)$$

Where 760 is atmospheric pressure in mmHg, and 47 is the saturated vapour pressure of water at 37°C since gas at the alveolus is fully humidified. The normal PAO_2 to PaO_2 gradient is less than 15 mmHg, but increases to 25 mmHg in the elderly. This normal A-a gradient is due to some venous admixture through the lungs, and a small right-to-left shunt through both the bronchial veins, and the Thebesian veins of the coronary circulation. This equation removes hypercarbia as a direct cause of hypoxaemia, and an increase in the A-a gradient will usually be due to $\dot{V}/\dot{Q}$ mismatch or right-to-left shunt. A commonly used alternative measure of hypoxaemia is the PaO_2/FiO_2 ratio. However, this does not account for the effect of a raised $PaCO_2$, and both measures are influenced by a number of factors (e.g. cardiac output, Hb, FiO_2) in addition to the extent of venous admixture, which may be estimated from the intrapulmonary shunt equation:

$$\frac{\dot{Q}s}{\dot{Q}t} = Cc'O_2 - CaO_2/Cc'O_2 - CvO_2 \quad (3)$$

where $\dot{Q}s$ is the intrapulmonary shunt blood flow, $\dot{Q}t$ is the total pulmonary blood flow, $Cc'O_2$ is the end-capillary O_2 content calculated from the PAO_2, and CaO_2 and CvO_2 are the O_2 contents of arterial and mixed venous blood respectively.

CARBON DIOXIDE

$PaCO_2$ is determined by alveolar ventilation ($\dot{V}_A$), and CO_2 production ($\dot{V}CO_2$):

$$PaCO_2 \text{ (mmHg)} =$$
$$\dot{V}CO_2 \text{(ml/min STPD)} \times 0.863/\dot{V}_A \quad \text{(l/min BTPS)} \quad (4)$$

where $\dot{V}_A$ is the minute ventilation ($\dot{V}_E$) minus the wasted or dead space ventilation ($\dot{V}_D$). The modified Bohr equation (assuming $PACO_2 = PaCO_2$) calculates the proportion of the V_T which is wasted ventilation (i.e. physiological dead space; V_{Dphys}):

$$V_{Dphys}/V_T = PaCO_2 - PE'CO_2/PaCO_2 \quad (5)$$

where $PE'CO_2$ is the mixed expired PCO_2, and V_{Dphys} is composed of anatomical dead space (V_{Danat}) and alveolar dead space (V_{Dalv}) – notionally due to alveoli that are ventilated but not perfused. Normally V_{Dalv} is minimal and V_{Danat} comprises 30% of V_T. Since the volume of an endotracheal tube is less than the mouth or nose, and pharynx, intubation may reduce V_{Danat}; however, when the connection from the endotracheal tube is taken into account there is little change in dead space. Positive pressure ventilation increases dead space by distension of the airways increasing V_{Danat}, and through a tendency to increase alveoli that are ventilated but not perfused. In patients with respiratory failure, marked increases in V_{Dalv} lead to V_{Dphys}/V_T ratios exceeding 0.6, and this will be exacerbated by V_T reduction.

CAPNOGRAPHY

Capnography measures and displays exhaled CO_2 throughout the respiratory cycle, with sampling usually by a mainstream sensor since sidestream systems tend to become blocked by secretions. However, when capnography is used in unintubated patients, sidestream sampling is commonly used (e.g. modified nasal cannulae). Infrared spectroscopy measures the fraction of energy absorbed and converts this to a percentage of CO_2 exhaled. During expiration the capnogram initially reads no CO_2, but as anatomical dead space is exhaled there is a rise in the exhaled CO_2 to a plateau which falls to 0% CO_2 with the onset of inspiration. In patients with significant respiratory disease a plateau may never be achieved. The end-tidal CO_2 ($PE'CO_2$) is the value at the end of the plateau, and is normally only slightly less than the $PaCO_2$. However, this gradient will increase when alveolar dead space (V_{Dalv}) increases, such as low cardiac output, pulmonary embolism and elevated alveolar pressure. Consequently the $PE'CO_2$ may not reflect $PaCO_2$ in critically ill patients. Nevertheless, in a stable patient the gradient will be fairly constant, and can be used to guide $\dot{V}_E$ during transport,[4] and when other factors including the adequacy of minute ventilation are unchanged, sudden changes in the $PE'CO_2$ may provide an early signal. Indeed, $PE'CO_2$ directly correlates with cardiac output, and $PE'CO_2$ monitoring has been used to assess adequacy of cardiopulmonary resuscitation, and its prognosis.[5]

The presence of exhaled CO_2 is secondary confirmation of endotracheal tube placement, and is commonly recommended even when the tube is seen to pass through the vocal cords,[6] since clinical assessment is not always reliable. Simple colorimetric devices may be used for this purpose. False positives can rarely occur following ingestion of carbonated liquids, and false negatives may be due to extremely low pulmonary blood flow, or very large alveolar dead space such as pulmonary embolus or severe asthma. Monitoring with capnography has also been recommended for transport[7] and respiratory monitoring[8] in critically ill patients, and should be available for every anaesthetized patient.[9]

GAS TRANSFER (DIFFUSING CAPACITY)

This is a test of the transfer of a gas, typically carbon monoxide (CO), across the alveolocapillary barrier. The transfer factor is calculated as:

$$\text{Volume of CO taken up}/(PACO - PcCO) \quad (6)$$

and since CO is so completely taken up by Hb, PcCO is taken as zero. This test is usually performed as an outpatient, is not usually measured in ICU, and diffusion abnormality is rarely a cause of hypoxaemia. The transfer factor is often corrected for lung volume since diseases such as emphysema and pulmonary fibrosis may effect both lung volume and diffusion.

LUNG VOLUME AND CAPACITIES

The tidal volume (V_T) is the volume of gas inspired and expired with each breath, with the volume at end-expiration termed the functional residual capacity (FRC) (see Figure 28.1). If a forced expiration is performed the expiratory reserve volume (ERV) is expired down to the residual volume (RV). If a maximum inspiratory effort is made from FRC this is termed a vital capacity (VC) manoeuvre when the total lung capacity (TLC) is reached. Clinically, the most important of these are the FRC, V_T, and VC, and the latter two are easily measured using a spirometer or integrated from flow.

TIDAL VOLUME

Minute volume is composed of f and V_T; normally ~17 breaths/min and ~400 ml respectively in adults.[10] Rapid shallow breathing is common in patients with respiratory distress, and in those failing weaning. Although a proposed index, an f/V_T ratio >100, was initially shown to be highly predictive of weaning failure,[11] subsequent studies have reported varying results.

VITAL CAPACITY

At TLC the forces due to the inspiratory muscles are counterbalanced by elastic recoil of the lung and chest

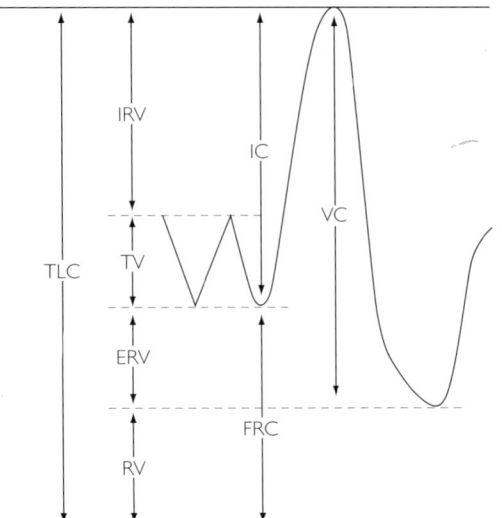

Fig. 28.1 Lung volumes and capacities. TLC, total lung capacity; IRV, inspiratory reserve volume; TV, tidal volume; ERV, expiratory reserve volume; RV, residual volume; IC, inspiratory capacity; FRC, functional residual capacity; VC, vital capacity.

Table 28.1 Factors that decrease vital capacity

Decreased muscle strength
Myopathy
Neuropathy
Spinal cord injury
Increased lung elastance
Pulmonary oedema
Atelectasis
Pulmonary fibrosis
Loss of lung tissue
Increased chest wall elastance
Pleural effusion
Haemothorax
Pneumothorax
Kyphoscoliosis
Obesity
Ascites
Reduced FRC
Atelectasis
Premature airway closure (e.g. COPD)

wall. Consequently, the TLC is determined by the strength of the inspiratory muscles, the mechanics of the lung and chest wall, and the size of the lung which varies with body size and gender (Table 28.1). Since the VC is the difference between TLC and FRC, factors that reduce FRC, such as increased abdominal chest wall elastance and premature airway closure in COPD will also reduce it. The normal VC is ~70 ml/kg and reduction to 12–15 ml/kg has previously indicated a probable need for mechanical ventilation. However, many other factors need to be considered including the patient's general condition, the strength of their expiratory muscles, glottic function, and the use of non-invasive ventilation. Indeed, many chronically weak patients are able to manage at home with extremely low VC with the assistance of non-invasive ventilation.

FUNCTIONAL RESIDUAL CAPACITY

Apart from research purposes,[12] FRC is rarely measured in the ICU. However, when FRC is less than the closing volume, the lung volume at which airway closure collapse is present during expiration, there is a marked increase in $\dot{V}/\dot{Q}$ mismatch. Consequently, PEEP is commonly used to elevate FRC. Increases in lung volume above FRC can be directly measured from a prolonged expiration to atmospheric pressure using either a spirometer or integration of flow.[13] FRC is decreased in ARDS and pulmonary oedema, in patients with abdominal dis-

tension, and following abdominal and thoracic surgery. An increase in FRC places the diaphragm at a mechanical disadvantage, and is seen with severe airflow limitation and dynamic overinflation, and when there is loss of elastic recoil (e.g. emphysema).

MEASUREMENT OF LUNG MECHANICS

This describes the forces the respiratory muscles must overcome during breathing, which are the elastic recoil of the lung and chest wall, and airway and tissue resistance. During controlled mechanical ventilation the ventilatory pressures reflect the work done to overcome these forces; however during partial ventilatory support the pressure at the airway opening reflects both these forces and those generated by the respiratory muscles. Estimates of respiratory mechanics are often readily available, and can assist titration of ventilatory support.

ELASTIC PROPERTIES OF LUNG AND CHEST WALL

The respiratory system (RS) is composed of the lung (L), and chest wall (CW) which is comprised of the rib cage and abdomen. Although it is often convenient to consider respiratory system mechanics as implying information about the lung, abnormal chest wall compliance can markedly influence these measurements.[14–17]

The pressure gradient across the lung (P_L) that generates gas flow, is equal to the difference between the pressure at the airway opening (Pao) and the oesophageal pressure (Pes): P_L = Pao – Pes. Although the oesophageal pressure is not always an accurate measure of the absolute pleural pressure, the change in the oesophageal pressure does reflect the change in pleural pressure. However, this requires an appropriately positioned and functioning oesophageal balloon. In spontaneously breathing subjects a thin latex balloon sealed over a catheter is introduced into the lower third of the oesophagus and Pes and Pao measured simultaneously during an end-expiratory airway occlusion. A well-positioned oesophageal balloon will have a ratio of ΔPes/ΔPao of ~1.[18] This technique is reliable in supine, intubated spontaneously breathing patients,[19] and in paralysed subjects it appears that a similar pressure change, induced by manual rib cage pressure,[20] can be used to verify oesophageal balloon function.

Chest wall mechanics are derived from Pes referenced to atmospheric pressure, and in ventilated relaxed subjects respiratory system mechanics are derived from Pao referenced to atmospheric pressure. It is not surprising then that $P_{RS} = P_L + P_{CW}$. Finally, abdominal mechanics can be measured using an intragastric balloon. However, despite these provisos, useful information can be obtained from respiratory system mechanics.

Measuring the slope of the V–P relationship of the lung or respiratory system allows a simple estimate of the elastic properties of the lung. This is termed the elastance, which is the inverse of the compliance. The E_{RS} is directly related to its components ($E_{RS} = E_L + E_{CW}$, and $1/C_{RS} = 1/C_L + 1/C_{CW}$. The normal E_{RS} is 10–15 cmH$_2$O/l and the normal C_{RS} is 60–100 ml/cmH$_2$O in ventilated patients. Since elastance directly refers to the elastic properties of the lung and respiratory system mechanics will be described in terms of elastance rather than compliance.

MEASUREMENT OF ELASTANCE

Elastance and resistance are frequency dependent and respiratory mechanics depend upon the volume and volume history of the lung.[21] With increasing frequency of breathing, total respiratory system resistance falls and elastance increases, and this is particularly obvious in patients with airflow obstruction.[22,23] Consequently, these factors must be taken into account when interpreting respiratory mechanics. In a passively ventilated subject Pao is the sum of (i) the pressure required to overcome airway, endotracheal tube and circuit resistance (Pres), (ii) the elastic pressure required to expand the lung and chest wall (Pel), (iii) the elastic recoil pressure at end-expiration or total PEEP (Po), and (iv) the inertial pressure required to generate gas flow (Pinert):

$$Pao = Pel + Pres + Po + Pinert \qquad (7)$$

Since the elastance (E), is equal to $\Delta P/\Delta V$, with the resistance (R) equal to $\Delta P/\Delta \dot{V}$, and ignoring the inertance,[24] this can be rewritten as the single-compartment equation of motion:

$$Pao = E_{RS}V + R_{RS}\Delta\dot{V} + Po \qquad (8)$$

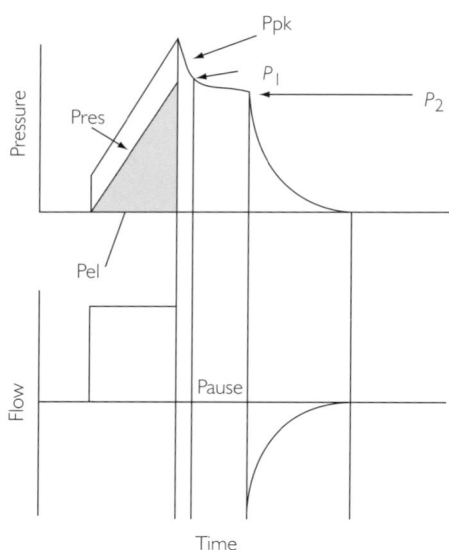

Fig. 28.2 Schematic diagram of a volume controlled breath with constant inspiratory flow. A period of no inspiratory gas flow has been interposed before expiration (pause) to illustrate dissipation of lung resistance as airways resistance (fall from Ppk to P$_1$) and tissue resistance (fall from P$_1$ to P$_2$). The inspiratory pressure due to the elastic properties of the respiratory system is illustrated as the filled area, Pel), and the lung resistive pressure is labelled as Pres (see text for more detail).

Elastance can then be measured using either static techniques where cessation of gas flow allows dissipation of Pres, or using dynamic techniques where flow is not interrupted.

END-INSPIRATORY OCCLUSION METHOD
The simplest estimate of E_{RS} can be made using a rapid end-inspiratory airway occlusion during a constant flow breath, provided that the respiratory muscles are relaxed (Figure 28.2). If a plateau is introduced at end-inspiration there is a sudden initial pressure drop due to dissipation of flow resistance (Ppk – P$_1$) followed by a slower, secondary pressure drop to a plateau (Pdif = P$_1$ – P$_2$) due to stress relaxation. At least 1–2 s are taken for this plateau to be achieved, and P$_2$ is often called the plateau pressure; however, if Pplat is measured too soon it will lie somewhere between P$_1$ and P$_2$.

Stress Adaptation
Stress relaxation of the respiratory system is due to both tissue viscoelasticity and time constant inequalities of the respiratory system (pendelluft). In the normal lung pendelluft has a minimal contribution to stress relaxation,[25] however, heterogeneity of regional resistance and elastance can markedly influence stress relaxation.[26]

Pulmonary surfactant and its contribution to changes in surface tension, parenchymal factors including elastic fibres in the lung, contractile elements such as the alveolar duct muscle and changes in pulmonary blood volume have all been implicated in the viscoelastic properties of the lung. However, it is not possible to separate either of these factors or the role of pendelluft in stress adaptation.

Calculation of Respiratory Mechanics

Returning to Figure 28.2, it is now simple to estimate respiratory system resistance and elastance from Pao. The static elastance (Ers,st) and the dynamic elastance (Ers,dyn) are calculated as:

$$Ers,st = (P_2 - Po)/V_T$$
$$Ers,dyn = (P_1 - Po)/V_T$$

where Po is the total PEEP (extrinsic plus intrinsic PEEP). This embodies the concept that Pel,dyn not Pel,st is the effective recoil pressure of the respiratory system during mechanical ventilation. Consequently, additional work is performed during inspiration to overcome stress adaptation, and this is stored and dissipated during expiration. This contributes to the hysteresis seen in dynamic volume–pressure curves during mechanical ventilation, and to the generation of expiratory flow. This latter component may be important in patients with airflow obstruction since the imposition of a pause at end-inspiration results in a 32% dissipation of the total energy loss within the respiratory system.[27]

THE STATIC VOLUME–PRESSURE CURVE

The quasistatic volume–pressure (V–P) curve has become the *de facto* 'gold standard' for the measurement of respiratory elastance. However, it is infrequently performed, and the relevance of a measurement performed on a single occasion is questionable when lung mechanics are not constant. Various techniques have been described, but the overall concept is that incremental volume and pressure points are made after a sufficient period of no-flow has allowed Pres to be dissipated. This allows definition of a sigmoidal shaped curve with upper and lower inflection points, and a mid-section with relatively linear V–P relations, allowing inflation elastance to be measured as this slope at a given lung volume. If similar measures are made during deflation a deflation curve and its hysteresis can also be described.

The V–P curve provides an advantage over an end-inspiratory elastance since, with the latter, it is not possible to know which part of the V–P curve is being measured. Consequently this 'chord' elastance may span either inflection point, yielding a falsely high figure. The upper inflection point represents a sudden decrease in elastance with increasing volume, and this has been interpreted as lung overinflation. The lower inflection point represents a sudden decrease in elastance with increased volume, and this has been interpreted as recruitment of atelectatic airspaces. Ventilation between these two inflection points should minimize both shearing forces secondary to repetitive collapse and reopening of alveoli, and overstretch of alveoli. However, this interpretation of the V–P curve has been questioned. In patients with ALI recruitment occurs well above the lower inflection point, along the entire V–P curve and above the upper inflection point.[28,29] An alternative interpretation of these inflection points is that the lower inflection point represents a zone of rapid recruitment, and that the upper inflection point is due to a reduced rate of recruitment.[30]

Conventionally the static V–P curve has been measured in ventilated patients with the 'super-syringe' method.[31] In a paralysed patient the respiratory system is progressively inflated from FRC in 100 ml steps up to ~1700 ml or a predefined pressure limit. After each step sufficient time is allowed for a well-defined plateau to become apparent (using a pause of 3–6 s). The effects of temperature, humidity, gas compression and ongoing gas exchange during the maneuver need to be taken into account,[32,33] and the volume history standardized before it is performed. Since this technique is cumbersome and many patients become hypoxaemic following disconnection from the ventilator and the 60 s or so without PEEP, other techniques have been developed. The static V–P curve can also be measured by randomly inserting a range of single volume inflations, followed by a prolonged pause,[34] during normal mechanical ventilation. This is performed in the paralysed state at 0 cmH$_2$O PEEP. This technique has a number of advantages including its simplicity, the patient is not disconnected from the ventilator, the volume history is the same for each measurement and gas exchange during the measurement is negligible. However, again, many patients will become hypoxaemic due to prolonged periods without PEEP (this procedure may take ~15 min), particularly following a small volume breath. Finally, an automated low flow V–P curve method allowing subtraction of Pres has been described which takes around 20 s to perform, and this seems to correlate well with the static occlusion technique.[35,36]

THE DYNAMIC V–P CURVE

Dynamic Pao, $\dot{V}$ and V are displayed by many ventilators, but the volume signal is not referenced to FRC and the signals are not readily available for quantitative analysis. However, $\dot{V}$ is readily measured with a heated pneumotachograph, and volume can then be derived by simple integration if the signal is collected after analogue-to-digital conversion. If Pao is also collected it is relatively simple to measure dynamic mechanics.

The dynamic V–P curve always shows hysteresis, mainly due to the effects of airway and tissue resistance, and it is unlikely that hysteresis of the static V–P occurs during tidal breathing.[37] In contrast to static V–P relations, dynamic mechanics are collected during normal ventilation so they do not interfere with patient care, and they provide a 'functional' description of respiratory mechanics. Indeed the 'effective' alveolar distending pressure is more accurately Pel,dyn, not Pel,st. Since dynamic mechanics are potentially continuous they could also be used to servo-control ventilatory strategies.

There a number of ways to analyse dynamic V–P data. A line can be drawn between no-flow points at end-inspiration and end-expiration to determine elastance, however, this is relatively inaccurate as it is based on two points that can be hard to exactly identify. Multiple linear regression analysis is now the technique most commonly employed. The patient does not need to be paralysed[38] provided the respiratory muscles are not active during ventilation, and the signal can be split to allow analysis of inspiratory and expiratory mechanics.

Provided the model fit is acceptable, elastance and resistance is accurately and reproducibly calculated using the single compartment equation of motion:

$$Pao = E_{RS}V + R_{RS}\Delta\dot{V} + Po \qquad (9)$$

Static PEEPi is accurately calculated, as Po–PEEPe, when compared with either an end-expiratory airway occlusion method,[39] or by direct measurement of end-expiratory alveolar pressure.[40] However, the single compartment model only approximates the respiratory system, and frequency and volume dependence of the derived mechanics are observed. Provided these factors are recognised and accounted for, it is sound to compare data within and between patients.

A number of techniques have been used to further analyse dynamic V–P data. The most promising of these are polynomial curve analysis ($\Delta V = a + bP + cP^2$)[41,42] and addition of a volume-dependent term to the equation of motion:[13,43]

$$Pao = (E_1 + E_2V)V + R_{RS}\Delta\dot{V} + Po$$
$$Ers = E_1 + E_2V$$

Since polynomial curve analysis requires a constant inspiratory $\dot{V}$ pattern to discount resistive effects, it is not as versatile as the volume-dependent technique, which improves model fit in some patients ($R^2 \sim 99\%$), and allows conceptual placement of tidal breathing on a dynamic V–P curve. If the $\%E_2$ is calculated as:

$$\%E_2 = 100E_2V/Ers \qquad (10)$$

then a $\%E_2 > 30\%$ quantitates overinflation, and a negative volume dependence (negative $\%E_2$) suggests signficant atelectasis during tidal beathing. During constant $\dot{V}$ ventilation, and provided V_T is also constant, the change in either Ppk – PEEPtot or P_1 – PEEPtot (the delta pressure; ΔP) 20–30 min following a change in PEEP is highly correlated with $\%E_2$.[13] Using the 95% predictive interval for this data, an increase in $\Delta P > 2$ cmH$_2$O indicates overinflation, a $\%E_2 > 30\%$.

INTERPRETATION OF ELASTANCE

Elastance may be increased due to a reduction in lung volume or to an increase in specific elastance, the product of E and FRC. Small body size, female gender, lung resection, and reduced aerated lung volume are important factors reducing effective lung volume, and this final factor is one important reason for the elevated elastance seen in ARDS. Specific elastance is increased with pulmonary oedema, pulmonary fibrosis, and reduced or dysfunctional surfactant.

MEASRUREMENT OF THE RESISTANCE OF THE LUNG AND CHEST WALL

Lung resistance (R_L) is the sum of airway (Raw) and tissue resistance (Rti). Resistance is flow, volume and frequency dependent, and R_L decreases as f increases. It is also important to compare measurements at similar lung volumes since there is a hyperbolic relation between lung volume and R. This is particularly obvious in ARDS where the incremental administration of PEEP can result in a decrease in Raw due to concurrent recruitment and an increase in lung volume. Indeed, although the absolute values are increased, when corrected for end-expiratory lung volume R_L, Raw + Rti are unchanged in ARDS.[14] Finally, since gas flow may be a mixture of laminar and turbulent flow, resistance is often flow dependent.

END-INSPIRATORY OCCLUSION TECHNIQUE

The total inspiratory airways resistance, including the endotracheal tube and associated ventilatory apparatus, can be calculated in a relaxed patient following an inspiratory pause (see Figure 28.2) as:

$$Raw = (Ppk - P_1)/\dot{V} \qquad (11)$$

and R_L calculated by using P_2 instead of P_1. Since the endotracheal tube and apparatus will make a significant contribution to Raw it is best to measure Pao distal to the endotracheal tube with an intra-tracheal catheter. An alternative approach is to calculate and subtract endotracheal tube resistance using the Rohrer equation ($R = K_1 + K_2\dot{V}$),[44] and this is now automatically included in some ventilators. However, in vivo endotracheal tube resistance is often greater than in vitro resistance[45] due to the effect of secretions and interaction with the tracheal wall, so that these corrections may be inaccurate. Despite these provisos, this simple measure of resistance, or the Ppk to Pplat difference at a constant $\dot{V}$, can be clinically useful both in the diagnosis and monitoring of airflow obstruction.[46]

DYNAMIC TECHNIQUES

Total, inspiratory and expiratory R can also be made, using either multiple linear regression analysis or from linear interpolation of the V–P curve at a constant volume. However, this latter technique assumes a constant elastance during tidal inflation, and may be inaccurate because it relies on only two measurements. Finally, an average expiratory R can be calculated from the time constant (τ) derived from passive expiration if the E is known, since:

$$\tau = R/E \qquad (12)$$

However, the lung does not empty as a single compartment in patients with airflow obstruction, and E is assumed to be constant over the tidal expiration.

OTHER MEASUREMENT TECHNIQUES

The interrupter technique consists of a series of short (100–200 ms) interruptions to relaxed expiration by a pneumatic valve.[47] This results in an expiratory plateau in P_{ao} following equilibration with alveolar pressure. From the V, P and $\dot{V}$ data expiratory elastance and the expiratory P–$\dot{V}$ relationship is measured. This technique does not make assumptions about the behaviour of the respiratory system and can identify dynamic airflow limitation.

Assuming that the respiratory system behaves linearly, it can be analysed following a forced flow oscillation at the airway opening.[48] The resultant pressure waveform depends upon the impedance of the respiratory system, which can be analysed following Fourier analysis of the P and $\dot{V}$ waveforms into resistance and reactance. This will then allow measurement of Raw, Rti, Ers and inertance, and information can be gained regarding small airways disease by examining Raw at different oscillatory frequencies.

FORCED EXPIRATORY FLOW

Maximum expiratory flow rates from TLC, the forced vital capacity (FVC), the forced expiratory volume in the first second of expiration (FEV_1) and the peak expiratory flow rate (PEFR) are commonly measured in cooperative subjects with a spirometer or flow meter. The PEFR is cheap but is relatively effort dependent, and is less specific and reliable than the FEV_1. It is most useful for office or home use. The normal PEFR is 450–700 l/min in males and 300–500 l/min in females. It is reduced with obstructive diseases, and gross muscle weakness.

The FEV_1 is usually expressed as a ratio of the FVC since both may be reduced in restrictive disease, with a normal ratio. The FEV_1 is normally 50–60 ml/kg and 70–83% of FVC. In asthma and COPD the FEV_1 is reduced out of proportion to the FVC and the ratio is less than 70%.

MEASUREMENT OF INTRINSIC PEEP

This is an important measurement in critically ill patients. PEEPi (i) may have unrecognized haemodynamic consequences,[49] (ii) adds a threshold load to inspiratory work during partial ventilatory modes, which may be reduced by application of small amounts of PEEPe,[50] and (iii) reflects dynamic hyperinflation with the consequent risks of barotrauma[51] and right heart failure. If PEEPi is not taken into account during calculation of chord compliance an incorrect denominator is used which may markedly alter the result.[52]

The two most commonly described techniques for measuring PEEPi are end-expiratory airway occlusion in a relaxed subject, and the fall in oesophageal pressure during inspiration prior to initiation of inspiratory $\dot{V}$. However, these are not really comparable measures since static and dynamic PEEPi respectively are measured. Static PEEPi is measured as the plateau Pao that is reached after ~5 s following an end-expiratory occlusion. With the cessation of gas flow alveolar pressure equilibrates with Pao. Since the lung is composed of non-homogeneous units this will represent the average static PEEPi. All respiratory effort must be absent since they may independently influence end-expiratory Pao, and end-expiration must be accurately identified. This is most easily done by the ventilator itself either using an end-expiratory hold manoeuvre or by using the next inspiration, the onset of which is concurrent with expiratory valve closure, to close a valve that directs inspiratory flow to atmosphere and seals the circuit. Static PEEPi is a surrogate measure of dynamic hyperinflation, and this volume may be directly measured using a spirometer[51] or a pneumotachograph[13] during a prolonged expiration.

Dynamic PEEPi is measured as the pressure change required to initiate inflation. In ventilated subjects this will be the change in Pao prior to initiation of inspiratory $\dot{V}$,[52] and in spontaneously breathing subjects the change in oesophageal[50] or trans-diaphragmatic[53] pressure from their end-expiratory relaxation values prior to inspiratory $\dot{V}$. Measurement of dynamic PEEPi in spontaneously breathing subjects is not particularly straightforward. The changes in pressure are small and influenced by cardiogenic oscillations which are preferably filtered out.[54] Further dynamic PEEPi is not constant, with breath-to-breath variation probably due to variation in the extent of dynamic hyperinflation, and many patients with airflow obstruction have an active expiration. This 'falsely' increases PEEPi, at least with respect to its threshold load since cessation of active expiration does not require work, with part of the measured threshold load suddenly dissipated.[55] Consequently, it is preferable to concurrently measure intra-gastric pressure as a measure of active expiration.

Finally, PEEPi can be measured as Po from dynamic P, V and $\dot{V}$ data in ventilated subjects. This is thought to be a measure of dynamic PEEPi since static PEEPi systematically yields a slightly greater result,[39] with similar discrepancies reported between other dynamic measures of PEEPi and static PEEPi.[56,57] This systematic difference correlates with, and is thought to be due to the viscoelastic properties and regional time constant inequalities of the respiratory system.[56] This has clinical significance since although matching dynamic PEEPi with PEEPe reduces respiratory work through a decrease in threshold inspiratory load,[50] it does not counterbalance these forces which represent an additional threshold load to inspiration.

MONITORING NEUROMUSCULAR FUNCTION

INSPIRATORY OCCLUSION PRESSURE

The pressure 100 ms (P_{100} or $P_{0.1}$) after a random occlusion timed at the beginning of inspiration is a measure of respiratory drive. There is a large range of normal values (1.5–5 cmH$_2$O), but it is reproducible in an individual patient. In ventilated patients the $P_{0.1}$ correlates with the work of breathing during pressure support ventilation, and changes in the same direction as PEEPe is increased and work is reduced.[58] Consequently, $P_{0.1}$ may prove to be a useful method of titrating PEEPe in patients with dynamic hyperinflation; however, this is not valid when flow triggering is used.

MAXIMUM MOUTH PRESSURES

Maximum inspiratory (MIP) and expiratory (MEP) mouth pressures can be used to estimate the power of the respiratory muscles. MIP is usually measured in ventilated patients using a unidirectional expiratory valve for ~20 s.[59] This ensures the procedure is performed from a low lung volume and does not require patient cooperation. However, despite this, the results are quite variable.[60] Normal values vary with age and gender; young females may exceed ~–90 cmH$_2$O, and young males ~–130 cmH$_2$O. A MIP <–20 cmH$_2$O is predictive of weaning failure; however, this is associated with too many false positives and negatives to be useful.[11] MEP may be useful in myopathic patients with expiratory muscle weakness. Transdiaphragmatic pressure is assessed using an oesophageal and gastric balloon to measure the pressure in these two cavities.

WORK OF BREATHING

The work of breathing (W_B) is the sum of elastic work (Wel), flow resistive work (Wres) and inertial work (negligible), and can be estimated from V–P data during spontaneous or assisted ventilation. An oesophageal balloon is used to examine changes in pleural pressure, $\dot{V}$ is measured with a pneumotachograph, and volume is derived as its integral. Although conceptually W_B is the inspiratory area of a V–P loop, this needs to be referenced to the chest wall V–P curve, and the appropriate area measured from a Campbell diagram.[61]

The normal W_B is ~0.5 J/L of $\dot{V}_E$, and this may be significantly increased in patients with acute respiratory failure, and by additional work imposed by ventilatory apparatus including the endotracheal tube and connector, humidifier and ventilator circuit.[62] The consequences of a large increase in W_B may include an increase in the $\dot{V}O_2$ attributable to breathing ($\dot{V}O_{2\,resp}$), respiratory muscle insufficiency, CO_2 retention and acute respiratory failure. However, W_B is rarely measured outside of research projects since the Campbell diagram is a relatively tedious approach. Simplifications have been used, but these are not as accurate, and W_B only estimates energy expenditure during muscle shortening with relatively poor correlation with $\dot{V}O_{2\,resp}$.[63] Consequently, the pressure-time product (PTP), which does correlate with $\dot{V}O_{2\,resp}$,[64] is more commonly measured.[10]

PRESSURE–TIME PRODUCT

PTP is usually calculated from the esophageal pressure-time integral during inspiration. In mechanically ventilated patients the oesophageal pressure during assisted breathing is compared with that during a controlled breath, or that pressure calculated from the chest wall elastance and lung volume.[10] However, the early correlation of $\dot{V}O_{2\,resp}$ with PTP used the transdiaphragmatic pressure is spontaneously breathing subjects.[64] Using either technique, importantly, the effort expended before $\dot{V}$ occurs due to PEEPi is measured, probably accounting for the better correlation of $\dot{V}O_{2\,resp}$ with PTP than W_B.[64] Although incremental pressure support ventilation may reduce PTP in COPD patients, the effect can be variable with some patients also showing evidence of expiratory muscle activity due to delayed sensing of neural expiration.[10]

REFERENCES

1 Cohen CA, Zagelbaum G, Gross D, *et al.* Clinical manifestations of inspiratory muscle fatigue. *Am J Med* 1982; **73**: 308–16.

2 Martin J, Jardim J, Sampson M, *et al.* Factors influencing pulsus paradoxus in asthma. *Chest* 1981; **80**: 543–9.

3 Dantzker DR, Brook CJ, Dehart P, *et al.* Ventilation-perfusion distributions in the adult respiratory distress syndrome. *Am Rev Respir Dis* 1979; **120**: 1039–52.

4 Palmon SC, Liu M, Moore LE, *et al.* Capnography facilitates tight control of ventilation during transport. *Crit Care Med* 1996; **24**: 608–11.

5 Levine RL. End-tidal CO$_2$: physiology in pursuit of clinical applications. *Intensive Care Med* 2000; **26**: 1595–7.

6 ECC Guidelines. Part 6: Advanced cardiovascular life support; Section 3: Adjuncts for oxygenation, ventilation, and airway control. *Circulation* 2000; **102**: I–95.

7 ANZCA. Intrahospital transport of critically ill patients. *Faculty of Intensive Care, Australian and New Zealand College of Anaesthetists Review*; 2000: PS39.

8 ANZCA. Minimum standards for intensive care units. *Faculty of Intensive Care, Australian and New Zealand College of Anaesthetists Review*; 1996: IC-10.

9 ANZCA. Monitoring during anaesthesia. *Australian and New Zealand College of Anaesthetists Review*; 1995: P18.

10 Jubran A. Advances in respiratory monitoring during mechanical ventilation. *Chest* 1999; **116**: 1416–25.

11 Yang K, Tobin MJ. A prospective study of indices predicting outcome of trials of weaning from mechanical ventilation. *N Engl J Med* 1991; **324**: 1445–50.

12 Wrigge H, Sydow M, Zinserling J, *et al.* Determination of functional residual capacity (FRC) by multibreath nitrogen washout in a lung model and in mechanically ventilated patients. Accuracy depends on continuous dynamic compensation for changes of gas sampling delay time. *Intensive Care Med* 1998; **24**: 487–93.

13 Bersten AD. Measurement of overinflation by multiple linear regression analysis in patients with acute lung injury. *Eur Respir J* 1998; **12**: 526–532.

14 Pelosi P, Cereda M, Foti G, *et al.* Alterations of lung and chest wall mechanics in patients with acute lung injury: effects of positive end-expiratory pressure. *Am J Respir Crit Care Med* 1995; **152**: 531–7.

15 Mergoni M, Martelli A, Volpi A, *et al.* Impact of positive end-expiratory pressure on chest wall and lung pressure-volume curve in acute respiratory failure. *Am J Respir Crit Care Med* 1997; **156**: 846–54.

16 Ranieri VM, Brienza N, Santostasi S, *et al.* Impairment of lung and chest wall mechanics in patients with acute respiratory distress syndrome: role of abdominal distension. *Am J Respir Crit Care Med* 1997; **156**: 1082–91.

17 Gattinoni L, Pelosi P, Suter PM, *et al.* Acute respiratory distress syndrome caused by pulmonary and extra-pulmonary disease. Different syndromes? *Am J Respir Crit Care Med* 1998; **158**: 3–11.

18 Baydur A, Behrakis PK, Zin WA, *et al.* A simple method for assessing the validity of the esophageal balloon technique. *Am Rev Respir Dis* 1982; **126**: 788–91.

19 Higgs BD, Behrakis PK, Bevan DR, Milic-Emili J. Measurement of pleural pressure with esophageal balloon in anesthetized humans. *Anesthesiology* 1983; **59**: 340–3.

20 Lanteri CJ, Kano S, Sly PD. Validation of esophageal pressure occlusion test after paralysis. *Pediatr Pulmonol* 1994; **17**: 56–62.

21 Fredberg JJ, Stamenovic D. On the imperfect elasticity of lung tissue. *J Appl Physiol* 1989; **67**: 2408–19.

22 Grimby G, Takishima T, Graham W, *et al.* Frequency dependence of flow resistance in patients with obstructive lung disease. *J Clin Invest* 1968; **47**: 1455–65.

23 Woolcock AJ, Vincent NJ, Macklem PT. Frequency dependence of compliance as a test for obstruction in the small airways. *J Clin Invest* 1969; **48**: 1097–106.

24 Mead J. Measurement of inertia of the lungs at increased ambient pressure. *J Appl Physiol* 1956; **9**: 208–12.

25 Bates JH, Rossi A, Milic-Emili J. Analysis of the behavior of the respiratory system with constant inspiratory flow. *J Appl Physiol* 1985; **58**: 1840–8.

26 Otis AB, McKerrow CB, Bartlett RA, *et al.* Mechanical factors in distribution of pulmonary ventilation. *J Appl Physiol* 1956; **8**: 427–43.

27 Jonson B, Beydon L, Brauer K, *et al.* Mechanics of respiratory system in healthy anesthetized humans with emphasis on viscoelastic properties. *J Appl Physiol* 1993; **75**: 132–40.

28 Jonson B, Richard J-C, Straus R, *et al.* Pressure-volume curves and compliance in acute lung injury: Evidence for recruitment above the lower inflection point. *Am J Respir Crit Care Med* 1999; **159**: 1172–8.

29 Crotti S, Mascheroni D, Caironi P, *et al.* Recruitment and derecruitment during acute respiratory failure: A clinical study. *Am J Respir Crit Care Med* 2001; **164**: 131–40.

30 Hickling KG. The pressure-volume curve is greatly modified by recruitment. A mathematical model of ARDS lungs. *Am J Respir Crit Care Med* 1998; **158**: 194–202.

31 Matamis D, Lemaire F, Harf A, *et al.* Total respiratory pressure-volume curves in the adult respiratory distress syndrome. *Chest* 1984; **86**: 58–66.

32 Gattinoni L, Mascheroni D, Basilico E, *et al.* Volume/pressure curve of total respiratory system in paralysed patients: artefacts and correction factors. *Intensive Care Med* 1987; **13**: 19–25.

33 Dall'ava-Santucci J, Armaganidis A, Brunet F, *et al.* Causes of error of respiratory pressure-volume curves in paralyzed subjects. *J Appl Physiol* 1988; **64**: 42–9.

34 Levy P, Similowski T, Corbeil C, *et al.* A method for studying volume-pressure curves of the respiratory system during mechanical ventilation. *J Crit Care* 1989; **4**: 83–9.

35 Servillo G, Svantesson C, Beydon L, *et al.* Pressure-volume curves in acute respiratory failure: automated low flow inflation versus occlusion. *Am J Respir Crit Care Med* 1997; **155**: 1629–36.

36 Lu Q, Vieira SRR, Richecoeur J, *et al.* A simple automated method for measuring pressure-volume curves during mechanical ventilation. *Am J Respir Crit Care Med* 1999; **159**: 275–82.

37 Beydon L, Svantesson C, Brauer K, *et al.* Respiratory mechanics in patients ventilated for critical lung disease. *Eur Respir J* 1996; **9**: 262–73.

38 Peslin R, da Silva JF, Chabot F, *et al.* Respiratory mechanics studied by multiple linear regression in unsedated ventilated patients. *Eur Respir J* 1992; **5**: 871–8.

39 Eberhard L, Guttmann J, Wolff G, *et al.* Intrinsic PEEP monitored in the ventilated ARDS patient with a mathematical method. *J Appl Physiol* 1992; **73**: 479–85.

40 Nicolai T, Lanteri C, Freezer N, *et al.* Non-invasive determination of alveolar pressure during mechanical ventilation. *Eur Respir J* 1991; **4**: 1275–83.

41 Ranieri VM, Giuliani R, Fiore T, *et al.* Volume-pressure curve of the respiratory system predicts effects of PEEP in ARDS: 'occlusion' versus 'constant flow' technique. *Am J Respir Crit Care Med* 1994; **149**: 19–27.

42 Neve V, de la Roque ED, Leclerc E, *et al.* Ventilator-induced overdistension in children: Dynamic versus low-flow inflation volume-pressure curves. *Am J Respir Crit Care Med* 2000; **162**: 139–47.

43 Kano S, Lanteri CJ, Duncan AW, *et al.* Influence of nonlinearities on estimates of respiratory mechanics using multilinear regression analysis. *J Appl Physiol* 1994; **77**: 1185–97.

44 Sullivan M, Paliotta J, Saklad M. Endotracheal tube as a factor in measurement of respiratory mechanics. *J Appl Physiol* 1976; **41**: 590–2.

45 Wright PE, Marini JJ, Bernard GR. In vitro versus in vivo comparison of endotracheal tube airflow resistance. *Am Rev Respir Dis* 1989; **140**: 10–16.

46 Manthous CA, Hall JB, Schmidt GA, *et al.* Metered-dose inhaler versus nebulized albuterol in mechanically ventilated patients. *Am Rev Respir Dis* 1993; **148**: 1567–70.

47 Gottfried SB, Rossi A, Higgs BD, *et al.* Noninvasive determination of respiratory system mechanics during mechanical ventilation for acute respiratory failure. *Am Rev Respir Dis* 1985; **131**: 414–20.

48 Peslin R, Fredberg JJ. Oscillation mechanics of the respiratory system. *Handbook of Physiology: Respiratory System*, Bethesda, Maryland: American Physiological Society; 1986: pp. 145–77.

49 Pepe PE, Marini JJ. Occult positive end-expiratory pressure in mechanically ventilated patients with airflow obstruction: the auto-PEEP effect. *Am Rev Respir Dis* 1982; **126**: 166–70.

50 Petrof BJ, Legare M, Goldberg P, *et al.* Continuous positive airway pressure reduces work of breathing and dyspnea during weaning from mechanical ventilation in severe chronic obstructive pulmonary disease. *Am Rev Respir Dis* 1990; **141**: 281–9.

51 Tuxen DV, Lane S. The effects of ventilatory pattern on hyperinflation, airway pressures, and circulation in mechanical ventilation of patients with severe air-flow obstruction. *Am Rev Respir Dis* 1987; **136**: 872–9.

52 Rossi A, Gottfried SB, Zocchi L, *et al.* Measurement of static compliance of the total respiratory system in patients with acute respiratory failure during mechanical ventilation. The effect of intrinsic positive end-expiratory pressure. *Am Rev Respir Dis* 1985; **131**: 672–7.

53 Lessard MR, Lofaso F, Brochard L. Expiratory muscle activity increases intrinsic positive end-expiratory pressure independently of dynamic hyperinflation in mechanically ventilated patients. *Am J Respir Crit Care Med* 1995; **151**: 562–9.

54 Schuessler TF, Gottfried SB, Goldberg P, *et al.* An adaptive filter to reduce cardiogenic oscillations on esophageal pressure signals. *Biomed Eng* 1998; **26**: 260–7.

55 Ninane V, Yernault JC, de Troyer A. Intrinsic PEEP in patients with chronic obstructive pulmonary disease. Role of expiratory muscles. *Am Rev Respir Dis* 1993; **148**: 1037–42.

56 Maltais F, Reissmann H, Navalesi P, *et al.* Comparison of static and dynamic measurements of intrinsic PEEP in mechanically ventilated patients. *Am J Respir Crit Care Med* 1994; **150**: 1318–24.

57 Yan S, Kayser B, Tobiasz M, *et al.* Comparison of static and dynamic intrinsic positive end-expiratory pressure using the Campbell diagram. *Am J Respir Crit Care Med* 1996; **154**: 938–44.

58 Mancebo J, Albaladejo P, Touchard D, *et al.* Airway occlusion pressure to titrate positive end-expiratory pressure in patients with dynamic hyperinflation. *Anesthesiology* 2000; **93**: 81–90.

59 Caruso P, Friedrich C, Denari SDC, *et al.* The unidirectional valve is the best method to determine maximal inspiratory pressure during weaning. *Chest* 1999; **115**: 1096–1101.

60 Multz AS, Aldrich TK, Prezant DJ, *et al.* Maximal inspiratory pressure is not a reliable test of inspiratory muscle strength in mechanically ventilated patients. *Am Rev Respir Dis* 1990; **142**: 529–32.

61 Banner MJ, Jaeger MJ, Kirby RR. Components of the work of breathing and implications for monitoring ventilator-dependent patients. *Crit Care Med* 1994; **22**: 515–23.

62 Bersten AD, Rutten AJ, Vedig AE, *et al.* Additional work of breathing imposed by endotracheal tubes, breathing circuits and intensive care ventilators. *Crit Care Med* 1989; **17**: 671–80.

63 Annat G, Viale J-P. Measuring the breathing workload in mechanically ventilated patients. *Intensive Care Med* 1990; **16**: 418–21.

64 Field S, Sanci S, Grassino A. Respiratory muscle oxygen consumption estimated by the diaphragmatic pressure-time index. *J Appl Physiol* 1984; **57**: 44–51.

29

Pulmonary embolism

A R Davies

Pulmonary embolism (PE) is a commonly considered, but relatively uncommonly diagnosed condition. It is important to have an adequate understanding of the pathophysiology, as well as a rapid and reliable strategy of investigation and management. This is particularly important in critically ill patients, where diagnosis can be difficult, and PE may be life-threatening.

AETIOLOGY

Deep venous thrombosis (DVT) and PE are components of a single disease, termed venous thromboembolism (VTE). Embolization of DVT to the pulmonary arteries, leads to PE, which is the most severe and life-threatening manifestation. VTE occurs in the population at a rate of about 1 in 1000 per year (half of whom develop PE), and is more common both with advancing age, and in males.[1]

Most PE results from DVT of the lower limbs, pelvic veins or inferior vena cava, although DVT of the upper limbs, right atrium or ventricle does also occur. Up to 40% of patients with DVT develop PE,[2] although if the DVT is isolated to below the knee, clinically obvious PE is rare.

Predisposing risk factors for thrombosis involve one or more components of Virchow's triad: (1) venous stasis, (2) vein wall injury and (3) hypercoagulability of blood. The main factors are immobility (from any cause), surgery, trauma, malignancy, pregnancy, and thrombophilia (see Table 29.1).

VTE can be recurrent which should prompt investigation for thrombophilia, which describes a group of conditions which are inherited and associated with a high incidence of VTE. The most important of these is activated protein C resistance, which has been discovered recently and is known to be mediated by a factor V Leiden mutation. Up to 50% of patients with recurrent VTE episodes (as well as 20% of patients with a single episode) have this condition.[3]

PATHOPHYSIOLOGY

The effects of PE range from being incidental and clinically irrelevant to causing severe obstruction to the pulmonary circulation and sudden death. Pulmonary arterial obstruction, and the subsequent release of vasoactive agents such as serotonin and thromboxane A_2 from platelets, leads to elevated pulmonary vascular resistance and acute pulmonary hypertension.

Acute pulmonary hypertension increases right ventricular (RV) afterload and RV wall tension which lead to RV dilatation and dysfunction,[4] with coronary ischaemia being a major contributing mechanism.[5] In massive PE, the combination of coronary ischaemia,[6] RV systolic failure, paradoxical interventricular septal

Table 29.1 Risk factors for VTE

Primary hypercoagulable states (thrombophilia)
Antithrombin III deficiency
Protein C deficiency
Protein S deficiency
Resistance to activated protein C (inherited factor V Leiden mutation)
Hyperhomocysteinaemia
Lupus anticoagulant (antiphospholipid antibody)
Secondary hypercoagulable states
Immobility
Surgery
Trauma
Malignancy
Pregnancy and the puerperium
Obesity
Smoking
Oral contraceptive pill
Indwelling catheters in great veins and the right heart
Burns
Patients with limb paralysis (e.g. spinal injuries)
Heart failure

shift and pericardial constraint leads to LV dysfunction and a 'low cardiac output' shock state. In patients with underlying cardiorespiratory disease, a small PE has disproportionate consequences.

Pulmonary arterial obstruction causes a mismatch between lung ventilation and perfusion, which leads to hypoxaemia. Alveolar hyperventilation also occurs leading to hypocapnia.[7]

Increased right atrial pressure can open a patent foramen ovale, which often results in right to left shunting, manifested as either profound hypoxaemia or paradoxical (arterial) embolization, which commonly presents as a cerebral infarct.

CLINICAL PRESENTATION

PE is relatively uncommon in critically ill patients despite the frequent presence of risk factors for VTE. However, when PE does occur, the diagnosis is frequently overlooked or is difficult to confirm, because of the presence of coexistent cardio-respiratory disease. Clinical assessment raises the suspicion of PE but is neither sensitive nor specific. The differential diagnosis is listed in Table 29.2.

SYMPTOMS

Dyspnoea, pleuritic chest pain, and haemoptysis are the classic symptoms of PE. Most patients will have at least one of these symptoms, with dyspnoea being the most common.[8] The combination of pleuritic chest pain and haemoptysis reflects a late presentation where pulmonary infarction has occurred. If syncope occurs there is a high likelihood that a massive PE has occurred. A family history of venous thrombosis raises the possibility of inherited thrombophilia.

PHYSICAL SIGNS

Physical signs can be absent, but the most frequent sign is tachypnoea.[8] Others include tachycardia, fever, and

Table 29.2 Differential diagnosis of pulmonary embolism

Acute myocardial infarction
Acute pulmonary oedema
Pneumonia
Asthma or exacerbation of chronic obstructive pulmonary disease
Pericardial tamponade
Pleural effusion
Fat embolism
Pneumothorax
Aortic dissection
Rib fracture
Musculoskeletal pain
Anxiety

signs of RV dysfunction (raised jugular venous pressure, parasternal heave, loud pulmonary component of the second heart sound). If massive PE is present, signs include hypotension, pale mottled skin and peripheral or even central cyanosis. It is important to also examine for signs of DVT in the legs and arms.

INVESTIGATIONS

The diagnosis of PE requires a high level of clinical suspicion and the appropriate use of investigations. The optimal investigation strategy depends upon the individual patient and institution, as there are a number of investigations available. Many tests are helpful when positive in cases of suspected PE, however pulmonary angiography, which has been the gold standard for many years, is the only test that satisfactorily excludes PE. This dogma has been recently challenged by the use of spiral CT, although a diagnostic algorithm which ends with pulmonary angiography is preferable.

D-DIMER

The serum D-dimer level is useful for exclusion of pulmonary embolism in some patients. Patients with PE often have an elevated D-dimer, however this also occurs in patients with as diverse conditions as trauma, surgery, diffuse intravascular coagulation, malignancy, acute myocardial infarction, pneumonia and heart failure. The most useful D-dimer result is a normal level in a patient in the emergency or outpatient department who has a low clinical likelihood of PE and no other systemic illness, as this excludes PE.[9] The combination of a normal D-dimer with the absence of hypoxaemia is even more reliable in excluding PE.[10]

ARTERIAL BLOOD GASES

A normal arterial blood gas profile does not rule out the diagnosis,[11] however hypoxaemia (with a widened alveolar-arterial oxygen gradient) and hypocapnia should raise the suspicion of PE. Metabolic acidosis may be present if shock from a large PE occurs.

ELECTROCARDIOGRAPH

A normal electrocardiograph (ECG) is found in about one-third of patients. Apart from sinus tachycardia (which is non-specific), the most frequent ECG abnormalities are non-specific S-T depression and T-wave inversion in the anterior leads reflecting right heart strain.[12] The pattern of a deep S wave in lead I, and a Q wave and inverted T wave in lead III ($S_1Q_3T_3$) is classical but is infrequently present.[8] Other possible abnormalities include left or right axis deviation, P pulmonale, right bundle branch block and atrial arrythmias. The ECG is also useful in excluding acute myocardial infarction and pericarditis.

CHEST X-RAY

The chest X-ray is often normal or only slightly abnormal with non-specific signs such as cardiac enlargement, pleural effusion, elevated hemidiaphragm, atelectasis and localized infiltrates.[13] More specific findings, including focal oligaemia, a peripheral wedge-shaped density above the diaphragm or an enlarged right descending pulmonary artery,[14] are uncommon and difficult for non-radiologists to identify. The chest X-ray is also useful in identifying an alternative diagnosis such as pneumothorax, pneumonia, acute pulmonary oedema, rib fracture and pleural effusion.

VENTILATION/PERFUSION SCANNING

The lung ventilation/perfusion ($\dot{V}/\dot{Q}$) scan remains an important investigation for PE. The perfusion scan identifies defects in perfusion which may be classified as single or multiple, and as subsegmental, segmental or lobar. By combining this with ventilation scanning, these perfusion defects can then be labelled as mismatched (normal ventilation in a zone of perfusion defect) or matched defects (ventilation defect corresponds to perfusion defect). The probability of PE is then classified as high, intermediate or low probability for PE, or normal[15] (see Table 29.3).

A normal lung scan effectively excludes PE and treatment can be safely withheld.[16] A high probability scan is considered diagnostic for PE.[15] The majority of patients do not have such clear-cut scan results, and even a low probability scan cannot satisfactorily exclude PE, as a patient with a low probability scan but with a high level of clinical suspicion has a 40% chance of having a PE. For this reason all low and intermediate probability scans should be considered non-diagnostic and further investigation is obligatory.

SPIRAL COMPUTED TOMOGRAPHY

A recent alternative to the $\dot{V}/\dot{Q}$ scan or pulmonary angiography is spiral (or helical) computed tomography (CT) of the chest, where a rapid scan using contrast medium can identify proximal PE with a high rate of accuracy. RV size can be estimated, which may assist in prognostication, and it is also possible to scan the veins of the legs, pelvis, and abdomen to identify the causative DVT. Alternative diagnoses such as a pulmonary mass, pneumonia, emphysema, pleural effusion and mediastinal adenopathy can also be identified.

A recent meta-analysis of spiral CT found that the sensitivity and specificity were 88% and 92% respectively and that withholding treatment when it is normal has an

acceptable morbidity.[17] Spiral CT may eventually replace the $\dot{V}/\dot{Q}$ scan as the initial screening test.[18]

When spiral CT is used as a confirmatory test for a non-diagnostic $\dot{V}/\dot{Q}$ scan with a high level of clinical suspicion, it significantly reduces the conventional angiography rate and has a very high negative predictive value.[19]

ECHOCARDIOGRAPHY

Because of its portability, echocardiography has become increasingly useful in critically ill patients with possible PE. Many patients with PE have an abnormality in RV size, RV function or tricuspid flow velocity,[20] and the pattern of RV hypokinesis with apical sparing is considered pathognomonic for PE.[21] Echocardiography is poor at excluding PE, as a negative echocardiogram can miss up to 50% of PEs.[22]

Transthoracic echocardiography will also allow estimation of pulmonary arterial pressure, identification of

Table 29.3 Interpretation of lung $\dot{V}/\dot{Q}$ scan result, based on PIOPED criteria[15]

High probability

≥2 large (>75% of a segment) segmental perfusion defects without corresponding ventilation or chest X-ray abnormalities or substantially larger segmental perfusion defects than either matching ventilation or chest X-ray abnormalities

≥2 moderate segmental (25–75% of a segment) perfusion defects without matching ventilation or chest X-ray abnormalities and one large mismatched segmental defect

≥4 moderate segmental perfusion defects without ventilation or chest X-ray abnormalities

Intermediate probability

Not falling into normal, very low, low or high probability categories

Borderline high or borderline low

Difficult to categorize as high or low

Low probability

Non-segmental perfusion defects

Single moderate mismatched segmental perfusion defect with normal chest X-ray

Any perfusion defect with a substantially larger chest X-ray abnormality

Large or moderate segmental perfusion defects involving no more than four segments in one lung and no more than three segments in one lung region with matching ventilation defects either equal to or larger in size and chest X-ray either normal or with abnormalities substantially smaller than perfusion defects

≥3 small segmental perfusion defects (<25% of a segment) with a normal chest X-ray

Very low probability

≤3 small segmental perfusion defects with a normal chest X-ray

Normal

No perfusion defects

intracardiac thrombi (which usually requires surgical embolectomy) and aids in differential diagnosis by excluding aortic dissection and pericardial tamponade. Transoesophageal echocardiography has the additional benefit of directly identifying embolus in the proximal pulmonary arteries which is common in patients with haemodynamically significant pulmonary embolism.[23]

Echocardiography has its best application in haemodynamically unstable patients, where it can be rapidly brought to the patient. If the patient has RV dilatation and hypokinesis in the right clinical setting, PE is extremely likely.

MAGNETIC RESONANCE IMAGING

Gadolinium-enhanced magnetic resonance pulmonary angiography is promising,[24] although clearly its use is limited in most hospitals and takes longer to perform than other tests.

PULMONARY ANGIOGRAPHY

The pulmonary angiogram is regarded as the only test which can exclude PE with relative certainty, and is safe even in the high risk patient.[25] However, it is unavailable in many centres.

One of the potential drawbacks of standard pulmonary angiography is that patients who then have thrombolytic agents have a greater risk of bleeding. It appears that a gradual shift is underway to less invasive angiography (via spiral CT).

SEARCH FOR DVT

Doppler ultrasound has been recommended to search for DVT in the leg veins, from where over 90% of emboli originate. If a leg DVT is confirmed, anticoagulation is required unless the DVT is entirely popliteal, where the associated morbidity is low. Ultrasound is highly accurate in symptomatic DVT, although in asymptomatic patients, ultrasound is much less likely to find DVT, meaning that the absence of a DVT does not exclude PE.

Leg venography is a more sensitive test however it is invasive and now uncommonly performed.

INVESTIGATION STRATEGY IN HAEMODYNAMICALLY STABLE PATIENTS

1 If there are obvious clinical signs of DVT, then an ultrasound should be performed. If a DVT is confirmed, the patient should be anticoagulated.
2 If there are no signs of DVT, a $\dot{V}/\dot{Q}$ scan or a spiral CT should be performed.
   (a) If the $\dot{V}/\dot{Q}$ scan result is high probability of PE or the spiral CT is positive, PE is confirmed.

(b) If the $\dot{V}/\dot{Q}$ scan is normal, then PE is excluded.
3 If there is a high clinical suspicion of PE and the $\dot{V}/\dot{Q}$ scan is low or intermediate probability or the spiral CT is negative, a pulmonary angiogram is required to exclude PE.

INVESTIGATION STRATEGY IN HAEMODYNAMICALLY UNSTABLE PATIENTS

1 Echocardiography (preferably transoesophageal) should be the first test performed.
   (a) If the patient has acute RV dilatation and visible embolus, PE is confirmed.
   (b) If there is RV dilatation but no visible embolus, then depending on how unstable the patient is, either a spiral CT or a pulmonary angiogram should be performed.
   (c) If there is no RV dilatation, it is unlikely that the haemodynamic instability is caused by PE (although this cannot be excluded completely). Efforts towards finding an alternative diagnosis are the priority.
2 If echocardiography is not readily available, a spiral CT should be performed.

MANAGEMENT

MANAGEMENT PRINCIPLES

To assist in planning management, it is worth grading the severity of PE as follows:

MASSIVE PE (HAEMODYNAMICALLY UNSTABLE)

Patients with PE and hypotension have a 30% mortality rate despite treatment. These patients will benefit most from a strategy that includes attempts at urgent removal of embolus (by a thrombolytic agent or embolectomy), concurrent haemodynamic support, and prevention of further embolization.

MODERATE PE (HAEMODYNAMICALLY STABLE BUT EVIDENCE OF RIGHT VENTRICULAR DYSFUNCTION)

Patients with PE and evidence of RV dysfunction have higher mortality and recurrence rates[26] than those with normal RV function. These patients require prevention of further embolization, and although controversial, removal of embolus (using thrombolysis) appears to improve outcome at the expense of a slightly higher bleeding complication rate.[27]

Unless echocardiography is performed, many patients with RV dysfunction due to PE will be overlooked for such a treatment strategy. However, RV dysfunction can be inferred without echocardiography if the perfusion defect on $\dot{V}/\dot{Q}$ scanning is large.[28]

MILD PE (HAEMODYNAMICALLY STABLE WITH NO RIGHT VENTRICULAR DYSFUNCTION)

Patients with PE who have normal blood pressure and normal RV function have a low risk of death or recurrence. Methods to remove embolus will therefore be unlikely to confer benefit. Prevention of recurrent embolization is the major goal.

Therefore the major principles of management are:

- Prevention of further embolization (massive, moderate or mild PE)
- Removal of emboli (massive or moderate PE)
- Concurrent haemodynamic support (massive PE)

A basic management strategy is outlined in Figure 29.1.

PREVENTION OF FURTHER EMBOLIZATION

ANTICOAGULATION

Heparin has been known to prevent recurrence and reduce mortality of PE for over 30 years. Heparin should be the standard for all patients who are haemodynamically stable as well as immediately after a patient has a thrombolytic agent. Heparin is effectively secondary prevention rather than primary treatment. Endogenous fibrinolysis will remove the embolus, whilst heparin prevents new thrombus formation.

Heparin should be administered by intravenous infusion with a bolus and initial monitoring should be with 6-hourly activated partial thromboplastin time (APTT) testing. Since sub-therapeutic levels of anticoagulation over the first 24 hours increase the risk of recurrence, it is important to rapidly achieve therapeutic heparinization. Weight-based dosing of heparin should be used, as target anticoagulation levels are reached sooner[29] (see Table 29.4).

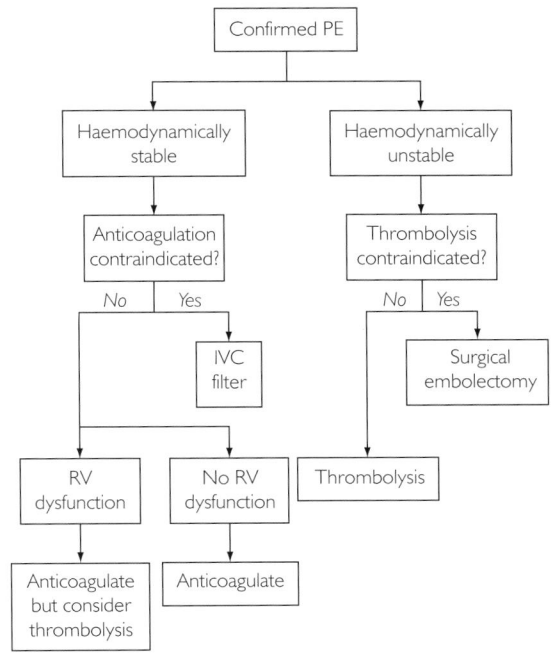

Fig. 29.1 General management algorithm for pulmonary embolism (PE).

The predominant complications of heparin are haemorrhagic including bleeding peptic ulcer, stroke, retroperitoneal haematoma and post-surgical wound haemorrhage. Heparin-induced thrombotic thrombocytopaenia syndrome (HITTS) can also occur.

Low molecular weight heparins (LMWH) are as effective and safe as unfractionated heparin,[30,31] and may even be better.[32] There is no satisfactory evidence for LMWH in patients with massive PE or after thrombolysis, and as they are more expensive than heparin, they are not commonly used. Monitoring (by measuring the level of anti-factor Xa) is only required in patients with renal

Table 29.4 Weight-based dosing of intravenous heparin (adapted from Raschke *et al.*[29])

Initial dosing	Loading 80 U/kg
	Maintenance infusion 18 U/kg per h
	Perform APTT in 6 h

Susequent dose adjustments:			
APTT	**Dose change (U/kg per h)**	**Additional action**	**Next APTT (hours)**
<35	+4	Rebolus of 80 U/kg	6
35–45	+2	Rebolus of 40 U/kg	6
46–70	0	Nothing	6
71–90	−2	Nothing	6
>90	−3	Stop infusion for 1 h	6

impairment. Haemorrhagic complications are similar in nature to standard heparin.

Oral anticoagulants should be started as soon as possible, so that heparin can be ceased when the international normalized ratio (INR) is >2.0.

There are a number of conditions which are considered to be relative contra-indications to anticoagulant therapy, the major ones being active peptic ulceration, recent surgery, recent trauma and recent cerebral haemorrhage, although in each individual patient the risk-benefit ratio (taking into account the severity of the PE) should be considered before anticoagulation is withheld from the patient.

INFERIOR VENA CAVA FILTER

Another mechanism to prevent further embolization is the placement of an inferior vena cava filter. This is usually performed percutaneously in the radiology department. Early recurrence rates are low, however the long-term DVT recurrence rate is greater.[33] Complication rates are low, although device migration can be life-threatening.

Firm indications include:

- new or recurrent PE despite anticoagulation
- contra-indications to anticoagulation
- complications resulting from anticoagulation.

Relative indications include:

- patients with extensive DVT
- patients following a surgical embolectomy
- patients with massive PE.

REMOVAL OF EMBOLI

THROMBOLYTIC AGENTS

Thrombolytic agents lead to dramatic and immediate haemodynamic improvement in some patients by dissolving the embolus and reducing pulmonary arterial obstruction. The commonly used agents include streptokinase, urokinase, recombinant tissue plasminogen activator (TPA) and reteplase, all of which activate plasminogen to form plasmin which degrades both fibrin and fibrinogen. All of the thrombolytic agents lead to early resolution of PE (in the first few hours), although after a few days, patients receiving heparin have similar degrees of embolus resolution.

There has been no randomized comparative study of a thrombolytic agent with standard anticoagulation which has been large enough to detect a mortality difference, however in a large multicentre patient registry, patients receiving thrombolysis (in a non-randomized fashion) had lower rates of mortality and recurrence than patients receiving heparin.[27] One group of patients who appear to have a more substantial benefit from thrombolysis is those with recognized RV dysfunction at presentation.[27]

Although there may be slight differences between thrombolytic agents, the choice of agent is less important

Table 29.5 Recommended doses of thrombolytic agents for PE

TPA	10 mg bolus followed by 90 mg over 2 h
Urokinase	4400 U/kg bolus (10 min) followed by 4400 U/kg per h for 12 h
Streptokinase	250 000 to 500 000 U bolus (15 min) followed by 100 000 U/h for 24 h
Reteplase	10 U boluses 30 min apart

than the choice to give thrombolysis at all. One should be given in the doses recommended in Table 29.5, and this can be administered through either a peripheral or a central venous catheter. Contrary to the use of thrombolysis in acute myocardial infarction, in PE thrombolysis is useful when given up to 14 days after symptoms begin.[34] Once the thrombolytic agent has been ceased, heparin should be commenced.

Haemorrhagic complications are not uncommon and can significantly affect patient morbidity, however it is difficult to predict those patients who are at the highest risk for bleeding. Fortunately, major clinically significant bleeding is uncommon with a cerebral haemorrhage rate of 1–2%,[27] and even in patients following recent surgery, acceptable safety has been demonstrated.[35] Individual patient presentation necessitates weighing the risks and the benefits, however in shocked patients with PE, the balance appears to be in favour of thrombolytic agents for most.

Should bleeding occur, thrombolysis should be ceased, fresh frozen plasma should be given to replace coagulation factors, and an antifibrinolytic agent (such as aprotinin) should be commenced.

SURGICAL EMBOLECTOMY

The merit of surgical embolectomy, which has traditionally been seen as a life-saving option for moribund patients with massive PE, has been questioned in the era of increasingly effective thrombolysis. Results of embolectomy surgery vary widely and there is an associated 25–50% peri-operative mortality. There is little evidence to reliably compare embolectomy and thrombolysis.

Nevertheless, shocked patients with PE who are in a centre where cardiothoracic surgery is available should have urgent consideration regarding embolectomy, although if there are no contra-indications, thrombolysis is preferred.

Indications for embolectomy in patients with PE include:

- massive PE with shock
- patients where thrombolytic agents are contra-indicated
- patients who appear to fail thrombolysis
- patients with free-floating cardiac thrombus.

PERCUTANEOUS EMBOLECTOMY

Percutaneous (or catheter device) methods of embolectomy (where the embolus is either extracted or disrupted) are now performed in some specialized centres. Successful embolectomy does not occur in all patients and mortality is still about 20–30%. Methods described include the use of suction to remove the embolus, mechanical fragmentation, rotatable pigtail catheters and rheolytic thrombectomy. The combination of mechanical disruption with thrombolysis is promising.

CONCURRENT HAEMODYNAMIC SUPPORT

Shocked patients with PE need urgent haemodynamic support in addition to the definitive measures mentioned above. Resuscitation of the circulation is the most important, although other aspects of resuscitation including administration of oxygen, and intubation and mechanical ventilation should not be overlooked.

INTRAVENOUS FLUIDS

In patients with moderate or massive PE, volume loading can improve haemodynamic status,[36] although if excessive, fluid therapy worsens RV function, which can be detrimental. For this reason cautious amounts of intravenous fluid should be given.

INTRAVENOUS VASOACTIVE AGENTS

Coronary ischaemia is an important component of the pathogenesis of haemodynamic instability in massive PE. A focus on reducing this ischaemia requires elevation of the blood pressure, whilst attempts are being made to lower the pulmonary and RV pressure by removing the embolus (with thrombolysis or embolectomy).

An important concept to consider is the right ventricular coronary perfusion pressure (RVCPP), which is estimated by the formula:

$$RVCPP = MAP - RVP_m$$

where

$$RVP_m = CVP + 1/3 (PAP_s - CVP)$$

(MAP is the mean arterial pressure, RVP_m is the mean RV pressure, CVP is the central venous pressure and PAP_s is the systolic pulmonary arterial pressure, all in mmHg).

When the RVCPP falls as low as 30 mmHg, RV myocardial blood flow falls substantially leading to severe RV failure and shock.[5] Efforts to elevate the MAP and reduce the PAP_s will clearly raise this RVCPP. Therefore, vasopressor agents are the most important initial therapy in the shock state due to PE as they will predominantly increase MAP, and therefore RVCPP.

Noradrenaline is the most appropriate vasopressor, because of its α-adrenoceptor agonist activity. Noradrenaline is preferred to a pure α-agonist, such as phenylephrine, as cardiac output and RV myocardial

blood flow effects are greater due to the added β-adrenoceptor agonist action. Dopamine and epinephrine seem appropriate alternatives to norepinephrine, however, there is little evidence to support these drugs.

Systemic vasodilators can be harmful in the setting of massive PE, as although cardiac output improves, MAP either remains the same or falls, and therefore RVCPP is not improved. Therefore isoprenaline, dobutamine, nitroglycerin, nitroprusside or milrinone should only be considered if MAP is adequate and treatment is focussed on cardiac output or pulmonary artery pressure.

Beneficial effects have been shown with intra-aortic balloon counterpulsation in animal studies,[6] and in patients apparently dying of PE despite thrombolysis and ongoing resuscitative efforts. This appears a reasonable approach as a method of augmenting RVCPP, as long as it is in association with the use of pressor agents.

SELECTIVE PULMONARY VASODILATORS

Inhaled nitric oxide has been used in patients with massive PE based on animal studies and case series,[37] because it selectively decreases pulmonary arterial pressure without influencing systemic haemodynamics, as well as inhibiting platelet aggregation.[38] It may have dramatic haemodynamic effects, but should be adjunctive to other resuscitative efforts including elevation of the systemic blood pressure. Inhaled prostacyclin is an alternative, but has limited supporting evidence.[39]

OTHER MANAGEMENT ISSUES
Oxygen Therapy

Oxygen should be given to keep an adequate oxygen saturation. High flows may be required because of hyperventilation and the increased dead space. Intubation and mechanical ventilation may become necessary.

Pain
If chest pain is prominent, morphine should be given.

Monitoring
To guide resuscitation, it is useful to have at least a central venous catheter, particularly before a thrombolytic agent is given. Whilst not essential, if a patient is severely shocked, a pulmonary artery (PA) catheter is recommended to assist in the titration of vasoactive agents and measure the pulmonary artery pressure. The PA catheter also assists in the estimation of the RVCPP, either through direct measurement of the mean RV pressure using the 20 cm lumen of a 'pacing' pulmonary artery catheter, or by calculation using the formula above. While there is increased risk of bleeding due to the concurrent administration of thrombolytic agents and/or anticoagulants in these patients, this is probably outweighed by the importance of secure venous access and monitoring of the circulation

Table 29.6 Prophylaxis of VTE (adapted from Geerts, et al.[49])

Category of patient	Recommended	Alternatives
Low risk surgery	Aggressive mobilization	
Moderate risk surgery	Heparin b.d.	LMWH
		or GCS
		or IPC
High risk surgery	Heparin t.d.s.	LMWH
		or IPC
Highest risk surgery	LMWH	Warfarin
		or IPC + heparin/LMWH
		or GCS + heparin/LMWH
		or adjusted dose heparin
Neurosurgery	IPC ± GCS	IPC with heparin/LMWH
		or Heparin
		or LMWH
Trauma	LMWH	GCS
		or IPC
Spinal cord injury	LMWH	IPC with heparin/LMWH
		or GCS with heparin/LMWH
Medical patients		
AMI	Heparin b.d.	
Ischaemic stroke	Heparin b.d.	LMWH
Other (if risk factors)	Heparin b.d.	LMWH

Heparin b.d., 5000 units subcutaneously twice daily; Heparin t.d.s., 5000 units subcutaneously three times daily; LMWH, low molecular weight heparin; GCS, graduated compression stockings; IPC, intermittent pneumatic compression device.
Low risk surgery = minor surgery in patients <40 years old, with no risk factors.
Moderate risk surgery = minor procedures in patients with risk factors.
Non-major surgery = in patients who are 40–60 years old, with no risk factors.
Major surgery in patients = <40 years old with no risk factors.
High risk surgery = non-major surgery in patients >60 years old, with risk factors.
Major surgery = in patients >40 years old with no risk factors.
Major surgery = in patients <40 years old with risk factors.
Highest risk surgery = major surgery in patients >40 years old, with prior VTE, or thrombophilia, or hip or knee arthroplasty, or hip fracture surgery, or spinal cord injury.

in patients with haemodynamic compromise due to PE, who have a high mortality rate.

PREVENTION

Prophylaxis is the most important management aspect of VTE. All ICU patients should have an adequate assessment as to whether prophylaxis is warranted. The specific regimen chosen is probably less important than ensuring that the patient receives prophylaxis, as in the majority of ICU patients, it appears that the benefits outweigh the risks. Omission of prophylaxis,[40] as well as failure of prophylaxis[41] both contribute to increasing the morbidity of VTE.

Prophylaxis has traditionally been fixed, low doses of subcutaneous unfractionated heparin. Various low molecular weight heparin agents are now used frequently in place of heparin, because of improved results, as well as less need for monitoring.[42] LMWH is also appropriate

prophylaxis for medical[43] and trauma patients,[44,45] although cost-effectiveness is an issue.[46,47]

Aspirin has recently been shown to significantly reduce VTE rate and mortality in high risk patients[48] although other measures are more efficacious.[49]

Mechanical approaches include graduated-compression stockings and intermittent pneumatic compression devices. These are best utilized in low risk patients, patients with a contra-indication to anticoagulation, or in addition to anticoagulation in high risk patients.

A recommended approach to prophylaxis is included in Table 29.6.[49]

REFERENCES

1 Silverstein MD, Heit JA, Mohr DN, *et al.* Trends in the incidence of deep vein thrombosis and pulmonary embolism: a 25-year population-based study. *Arch Intern Med* 1998, **158**: 585–93.

2 Moser KM, Fedullo PF, LitteJohn JK, Crawford R. Frequent asymptomatic pulmonary embolism in

patients with deep venous thrombosis. *JAMA* 1994, **271**: 223–5.

3 Price DT, Ridker PM. Factor V Leiden mutation and the risks for thromboembolic disease: a clinical perspective. *Ann Intern Med* 1997, **127**: 895–903.

4 Lualdi JC, Goldhaber SZ. Right ventricular dysfunction after acute pulmonary embolism: pathophysiologic factors, detection, and therapeutic implications. *Am Heart J* 1995, **130**: 1276–82.

5 Vlahakes G J, Turley K, Hoffman JI. The pathophysiology of failure in acute right ventricular hypertension: hemodynamic and biochemical correlations. *Circulation* 1981, **63**: 87–95.

6 Darrah WC, Sharpe MD, Guiraudon GM, Neal A. Intraaortic balloon counterpulsation improves right ventricular failure resulting from pressure overload. *Ann Thorac Surg* 1997, **64**: 1718–23.

7 Santolicandro A, Prediletto R, Fornai E, *et al.* Mechanisms of hypoxemia and hypocapnia in pulmonary embolism. *Am J Respir Crit Care Med* 1995, **152**: 336–47.

8 Stein PD, Terrin ML, Hales CA, *et al.* Clinical, laboratory, roentgenographic, and electrocardiographic findings in patients with acute pulmonary embolism and no pre-existing cardiac or pulmonary disease. *Chest* 1991, **100**: 598–603.

9 Ginsberg JS, Wells PS, Kearon C, *et al.* Sensitivity and specificity of a rapid whole-blood assay for D-dimer in the diagnosis of pulmonary embolism. *Ann Intern Med* 1998, **129**: 1006–11.

10 Egermayer P, Town GI, Turner JG, *et al.* Usefulness of D-dimer, blood gas, and respiratory rate measurements for excluding pulmonary embolism. *Thorax* 1998, **53**: 830–4.

11 Stein PD, Goldhaber SZ, Henry JW, Miller AC. Arterial blood gas analysis in the assessment of s uspected acute pulmonary embolism. *Chest* 1996, **109**: 78–81.

12 Ferrari E, Imbert A, Chevalier T, *et al.* The ECG in pulmonary embolism: predictive value of negative T waves in precordial leads – 80 case reports. *Chest* 1997, **111**: 537–43.

13 Elliott CG, Goldhaber SZ, Visani L, DeRosa M. Chest radiographs in acute pulmonary embolism: results from the International Cooperative Pulmonary Embolism Registry. *Chest* 2000, **118**: 33–8.

14 Goldhaber SZ. Pulmonary embolism. *N Engl J Med* 1998, **339**: 93–104.

15 The PIOPED Investigators. Value of the ventilation/perfusion scan in acute pulmonary embolism: results of the prospective investigation of pulmonary embolism diagnosis (PIOPED). *JAMA* 1990, **263**: 2753–9.

16 van Beek EJ, Kuyer PM, Schenk BE, *et al.* A normal perfusion lung scan in patients with clinically suspected pulmonary embolism: frequency and clinical validity. *Chest* 1995, **108**: 170–3.

17 van Beek EJ, Brouwers EM, Song B, *et al.* Lung scintigraphy and helical computed tomography for the diagnosis of pulmonary embolism: a meta-analysis. *Clin Appl Thromb Hemost* 2001, 7: 87–92.

18 Cross JJ, Kemp PM, Walsh CG, *et al.* A randomized trial of spiral CT and ventilation perfusion scintigraphy for the diagnosis of pulmonary embolism. *Clin Radiol* 1998, **53**: 177–82.

19 Ost D, Rozenshtein A, Saffran L, Snider A. The negative predictive value of spiral computed tomography for the diagnosis of pulmonary embolism in patients with nondiagnostic ventilation-perfusion scans. *Am J Med* 2001, **110**: 16–21.

20 Come PC. Echocardiographic evaluation of pulmonary embolism and its response to therapeutic interventions. *Chest* 1992, **101**: 151S–162S.

21 McConnell MV, Solomon SD, Rayan ME, *et al.* Regional right ventricular dysfunction detected by echocardiography in acute pulmonary embolism. *Am J Cardiol* 1996, **78**: 469–73.

22 Miniati M, Monti S, Pratali L, *et al.* Value of transthoracic echocardiography in the diagnosis of pulmonary embolism: results of a prospective study in unselected patients. *Am J Med* 2001, **110**: 528–35.

23 Pruszczyk P, Torbicki A, Kuch-Wocial A, *et al.* Diagnostic value of transoesophageal echocardiography in suspected haemodynamically significant pulmonary embolism. *Heart* 2001, **85**: 628–34.

24 Meaney JF, Weg JG, Chenevert TL, *et al.* Diagnosis of pulmonary embolism with magnetic resonance angiography. *N Engl J Med* 1997, **336**: 1422–7.

25 Stein PD, Athanasoulis C, Alavi A, *et al.* Complications and validity of pulmonary angiography in acute pulmonary embolism. *Circulation* 1992, **85**: 462–8.

26 Grifoni S, Olivotto I, Cecchini P, *et al.* Short-term clinical outcome of patients with acute pulmonary embolism, normal blood pressure, and echocardiographic right ventricular dysfunction. *Circulation* 2000, **101**: 2817–22.

27 Konstantinides S, Geibel A, Olschewski M, *et al.* Association between thrombolytic treatment and the prognosis of hemodynamically stable patients with major pulmonary embolism: results of a multicenter registry. *Circulation* 1997, **96**: 882–8.

28 Wolfe MW, Lee RT, Feldstein ML, *et al.* Prognostic significance of right ventricular hypokinesis and perfusion lung scan defects in pulmonary embolism. *Am Heart J* 1994, **127**: 1371–5.

29 Raschke RA, Reilly BM, Guidry JR, *et al.* The weight-based heparin dosing nomogram compared with a 'standard care' nomogram: a randomized controlled trial. *Ann Intern Med* 1993, **119**: 874–81.

30 The Columbus Investigators. Low-molecular-weight heparin in the treatment of patients with venous thromboembolism. *N Engl J Med* 1997, **337**: 657–62.

31 Simonneau G, Sors H, Charbonnier B, *et al.* A comparison of low-molecular-weight heparin with unfractionated heparin for acute pulmonary embolism: the THESEE Study Group. *N Engl J Med* 1997, **337**: 663–9.

32 Hull RD, Raskob GE, Brant RF, *et al.* Low-molecular-weight heparin vs heparin in the treatment of patients with pulmonary embolism: American-Canadian

Thrombosis Study Group. *Arch Intern Med* 2000, **160**: 229–36.

33 Decousus H, Leizorovicz A, Parent F, *et al.* A clinical trial of vena caval filters in the prevention of pulmonary embolism in patients with proximal deep-vein thrombosis. *N Engl J Med* 1998, **338**: 409–15.

34 Daniels LB, Parker JA, Patel SR, *et al.* Relation of duration of symptoms with response to thrombolytic therapy in pulmonary embolism. *Am J Cardiol* 1997, **80**: 184–8.

35 Molina JE, Hunter DW, Yedlicka JW, Cerra FB. Thrombolytic therapy for postoperative pulmonary embolism. *Am J Surg* 1992, **163**: 375–80.

36 Mercat A, Diehl JL, Meyer GT, *et al.* Hemodynamic effects of fluid loading in acute massive pulmonary embolism. *Crit Care Med* 1999, **27**: 540–4.

37 Capellier G, Jacques T, Balvay P, *et al.* Inhaled nitric oxide in patients with pulmonary embolism. *Intensive Care Med* 1997, **23**: 1089–92.

38 Gries A, Bottiger BW, Dorsam J, *et al.* Inhaled nitric oxide inhibits platelet aggregation after pulmonary embolism in pigs. *Anesthesiology* 1997, **86**: 387–93.

39 Webb SA, Stott S, van Heerden PV. The use of inhaled aerosolized prostacyclin (IAP) in the treatment of pulmonary hypertension secondary to pulmonary embolism. *Intensive Care Med* 1996, **22**: 353–5.

40 Stratton MA, Anderson FA, Bussey HI, *et al.* Prevention of venous thromboembolism: adherence to the 1995 American College of Chest Physicians consensus guidelines for surgical patients. *Arch Intern Med* 2000, **160**: 334–40.

41 Goldhaber SZ, Dunn K, MacDougall RC. New onset of venous thromboembolism among hospitalized patients at Brigham and Women's Hospital is caused more often by prophylaxis failure than by withholding treatment. *Chest* 2000, **118**: 1680–4.

42 van Den Belt AG, Prins MH, Lensing AW, *et al.* Fixed dose subcutaneous low molecular weight heparins versus adjusted dose unfractionated heparin for venous thromboembolism. *Cochrane Database Syst Rev* 2000, 2.

43 Samama MM, Cohen AT, Darmon JY, *et al.* A comparison of enoxaparin with placebo for the prevention of venous thromboembolism in acutely ill medical patients: Prophylaxis in Medical Patients with Enoxaparin Study Group. *N Engl J Med* 1999, **341**: 793–800.

44 Geerts WH, Jay RM, Code KI, *et al.* A comparison of low-dose heparin with low-molecular-weight heparin as prophylaxis against venous thromboembolism after major trauma. *N Engl J Med* 1996, **335**: 701–7.

45 Norwood SH, McAuley CE, Berne JD, *et al.* A potentially expanded role for enoxaparin in preventing venous thromboembolism in high risk blunt trauma patients. *J Am Coll Surg* 2001, **192**: 161–7.

46 Cook D, Attia J, Weaver B, *et al.* Venous thromboembolic disease: an observational study in medical-surgical intensive care unit patients. *J Crit Care* 2000, **15**: 127–32.

47 Velmahos GC, Oh Y, McCombs J, Oder D. An evidence-based cost-effectiveness model on methods of prevention of posttraumatic venous thromboembolism. *J Trauma* 2000, **49**: 1059–64.

48 Pulmonary Embolism Prevention (PEP) Trial Collaborative Group. Prevention of pulmonary embolism and deep vein thrombosis with low dose aspirin: Pulmonary Embolism Prevention (PEP) trial. *Lancet* 2000, **355**: 1295–302.

49 Geerts WH, Heit JA, Clagett GP, *et al.* Prevention of venous thromboembolism. *Chest* 2001, **119**: 132S–175S.

30

Acute severe asthma

D V Tuxen and J Leong

Acute severe asthma is a medical emergency requiring prompt careful assessment and management. World-wide prevalence of asthma in a 1998 survey of children aged 13 to 14 years varied between 1.6% and 36.8%, with the top three countries being the United Kingdom, New Zealand and Australia.[1] Overall, the prevalence of asthma appears to be increasing[2] with life-threatening episodes affecting 0.5% of asthmatics per year.[3] Asthma is a significant problem in Australia with 1 in 11 Australians reporting having asthma as a long-term condition[4] and up to 40% of Australian children have some form of asthma.[5] The reported rate of death from asthma in the United States has always been low but has doubled in the 1980s and early 1990s.[6] More recently, mortality from asthma in Australia has declined from 2.32 per 100 000 in 1980 to 1.36 per 100 000 in 1996.[4] This decline has been associated with the introduction of a National Asthma Campaign which included a formalized 'Asthma Management Plan'[7] and increased use of inhaled steroids.[8] The decline is mirrored in a reduction in hospital readmission rate.[7]

CLINICAL DEFINITION

Asthma has been defined as a lung disease with the following characteristics:[9]

- Airway obstruction that is reversible (completely or partially), either spontaneously or with treatment
- Airway inflammation
- Increased airway responsiveness to a variety of stimuli.

Status asthmaticus has had varying definitions. However for practical purposes, any patient not responding to initial doses of nebulized broncho-dilating agents should be considered to have status asthmaticus.[10]

AETIOLOGY

The pathogenesis of asthma is complex with contribution from both genetic factors and environmental influences. The increase in asthma prevalence may be accounted for by the 'hygiene hypothesis' which suggests that exposure to antibiotics early in life promotes an imbalance in T cell phenotype leading to inflammatory cytokine overproduction. IgE dependent mechanisms appear to be particularly important in generating the characteristic state of airway inflammation and bronchial hyperresponsiveness with the allergens in the local environment dictating the specificity of the antibody response.[11] Triggers of acute asthma can be non-specific (cold air, exercise, atmospheric pollutants) or specific allergens (housemite, pollen, animal danders) or modifiers of airway control (aspirin, β-blockers). No precipitant can be identified in over 30% of patients.

PATHOPHYSIOLOGY

The post-mortem airway pathology of patients who die from acute asthma includes bronchial wall thickening from oedema and inflammatory cell infiltrate, hypertrophy and hyperplasia of bronchial smooth muscle and submucosal glands, deposition of collagen beneath the epithelial basement membrane and prominent intraluminal secretions.[12] These secretions may reduce the cross-sectional area or completely occlude the small airways. In some deaths bronchial mucus is absent; in these cases airway obstruction may be mainly due to intense smooth muscle contraction.[13]

This observation may account for two patterns of progression of asthma:

1 Hyperacute fulminating asthma: where the interval between onset of symptoms and intubation is less than 3 h. This pattern typically responds quickly to bronchodilators and is thought to be mainly due to bronchial smooth muscle contraction. This tends to

occur in younger patients with relatively normal lung function but high bronchial reactivity.[14,15] This presentation is less common (approximately 30% of life threatening presentations) and the majority of patients are male.

2 Acute severe asthma: the more common group, with progression of symptoms over many hours or days which may occur on a background of recurrent presentations. It responds more slowly to treatment; this may reflect greater contribution from mucous inspissation and bronchial wall inflammation.[15] The majority of patients are female.

The characteristic pathology of asthma leads to increased airway resistance and dynamic hyperinflation. This has the following consequences.

INCREASED WORK OF BREATHING

Increased work of breathing results from increased airway resistance, PEEPi, and increased elastic recoil generated by gas trapping. When asthma is severe, dynamic hyperinflation may bring the lung volume close to total lung capacity.[16] This causes a severe mechanical disadvantage of inspiratory muscles with diaphragm flattening and results in a large inspiratory muscle effort affecting a small change in inspiratory pressure. The final outcome is respiratory muscle failure with insufficient alveolar ventilation and consequent hypercapnia.

VENTILATION-PERFUSION MISMATCH

Ventilation-perfusion mismatch is the result of airway narrowing and closure. This leads to hypoxemia and forces minute ventilation to rise, adding to the work of breathing.

ADVERSE CARDIOPULMONARY INTERACTIONS

Adverse cardiopulmonary interactions are seen when the marked changes in lung volume and pleural pressure impact on the function of both left and right ventricles. Spontaneous breathing during acute asthma can generate inspiratory pressures as low as −35 cmH$_2$O.[17] Negative intrapleural pressure causes increased left ventricular afterload[18] and promotes egress of fluid into the alveolar airspace. Right ventricular afterload is increased by hypoxic pulmonary vasoconstriction, acidosis and increased lung volume.[19] Pulsus paradoxus is a result of the cardiopulmonary interaction in severe asthma. It describes an increase in the normal inspiratory drop in systolic blood pressure (normal <5 mmHg) to greater than 10 mmHg.[20] This is a consequence of the marked drop during inspiration in left-sided cardiac output caused by decreased left atrial return (as a result of increased pulmonary capacitance) and increased left ventricular afterload. The degree of pulsus paradoxus may not correlate with the severity of asthma as the patient may be too fatigued or compromised by hyperinflation to generate the necessary negative inspiratory pressure.

CLINICAL FEATURES AND ASSESSMENT OF SEVERITY

The symptoms of asthma are well known and will typically include wheeze, cough and dyspnoea. Chest pain or tightness may be present. Triage and assessment of severity of the acute asthma attack are crucial. Underestimation or non-measurement of asthma severity is associated with increased mortality.[21]

HISTORY

Any history of prior intubation and mechanical ventilation for asthma is a predictor for life-threatening asthma.[22] A history of poor asthma control and multiple recent medical presentations for asthma are recognized risk factors.[23]

PHYSICAL EXAMINATION

Use of accessory muscles, markedly diminished breath sounds or a silent chest, central cyanosis, inability to speak, a disturbance in the level of consciousness, upright posture and diaphoresis all suggest a severe attack.[21] A respiratory rate >30/min, pulse rate >120/min and pulsus paradoxus of >15 mmHg are associated with severe asthma though their absence does not preclude life-threatening asthma.

VENTILATORY FUNCTION TESTS

The patient may not be able to perform these due to breathlessness. However, FEV$_1$ and peak expiratory flow rate (PEFR) are useful indicators of severity and response to treatment when done serially. An FEV$_1$ <1.0 l, or PEFR <100 l/min indicate very severe asthma at significant risk of requiring mechanical ventilation. In some patients forced expiration may worsen symptoms; these measurements should cease should this be the case.

ARTERIAL BLOOD GASES

Arterial hypoxemia is almost invariably present in a patient with severe asthma breathing room air though it responds well to oxygen supplementation.[24] The arterial PaCO$_2$ is an important measure of severity. Ventilation is initially increased in an acute attack leading to hypocarbia and a respiratory alkalosis. As the asthmatic attack worsens, the downward spiral of increased work of breathing, $\dot{V}/\dot{Q}$ mismatch and adverse cardiopulmonary interactions continues. The minute ventilation required to maintain the same alveolar ventilation and $PaCO_2$ increases; eventually the patient is incapable of meeting this demand and the $PaCO_2$ rises. Thus a $PaCO_2$ rising towards normal may represent deterioration rather than improvement. The presence of hypercarbic acidosis is associated with a FEV_1 of <20% predicted[21] and reliably indicates that asthma is severe. A metabolic acidosis may also be present, ranging from a mild normal anion gap acidosis due to renal compensation for hypocarbia to a severe raised anion gap acidosis due to lactic acidosis.[25]

CHEST X-RAY

Although not generally helpful in assessing severity, a chest X-ray should be performed when asthma is severe or refractory to treatment, when barotrauma or infection is suspected or when the diagnosis is in doubt. It is not required in milder attacks that respond well to treatment.

PATIENT PROGRESS

Repeated evaluation of the patient's response to treatment is a valuable tool in assessing severity of acute asthma. The response to the first 2 h of treatment is an important predictor of outcome.[26] Admission to intensive care is preferred if the patient fulfils the above criteria for severe asthma. Other indications for immediate admission to intensive care include respiratory arrest, altered mental status, dysrhythmias and associated myocardial ischaemia.[27]

DIFFERENTIAL DIAGNOSIS

The diagnosis of asthma is usually obvious. However, wheeze and dyspnoea may be caused by other illnesses such as left ventricular failure, aspiration, upper airway obstruction, inhaled foreign body and pulmonary embolism. Wheeze and dyspnoea arising in hospitalized patients who were not admitted with asthma are less likely to be due to asthma.

MANAGEMENT

ESTABLISHED TREATMENTS

Initial pharmacotherapy of acute severe asthma should include the following:

OXYGEN

Hypoxemia contributes to life-threatening events that complicate acute severe asthma. Humidified supplemental oxygen should be administered and titrated to achieve a SaO_2 >96%. If there is concern about oxygen-induced hypercarbia with co-existing chronic airflow limitation then oxygen can be titrated to a lower SaO_2, for example, 90–92%. In the absence of pre-existing chronic pulmonary disease there is no evidence that oxygen will suppress the respiratory drive.[28]

β-AGONISTS

β-agonists remain the 1st-line bronchodilator therapy. Agents include salbutamol (albuterol), terbutaline, isoprenaline and epinephrine. Salbutamol is generally the agent of first choice as it has relative β_2 selectivity, with decreased β_1-mediated cardiac toxicity.[29] Long-acting β-agonists such as salmeterol have no role in status asthmaticus due to slow onset of action and association with fatalities in this setting.[10] β-agonists cause bronchodilatation by stimulation of β_2 receptors on airway smooth muscle and may reduce bronchial mucosal oedema.

The standard approach is to start with nebulized salbutamol. The typical adult dose is 5–10 mg (in 2.5 to 5.0 ml diluent volume) every 2–4 h, but more frequent doses with a higher total dose are often required in severe asthma. It should be noted that less than 10% of the nebulized drug reaches the lung even under ideal conditions. Continuous nebulization appears to be superior to intermittent doses and is commonly used at the beginning of treatment in severe asthma.[10,30] The nebulizer should be driven by oxygen with the flow at 10–12 l/min with a reservoir volume of 2–4 ml, so as to produce particles in the desired 1–3 μm range. The total dose should be modulated by response to treatment and the level of toxic side-effects.

β-agonists can also be delivered by metered dose inhaler (MDI). There is data to suggest that in non-intubated patients, MDIs combined with a spacing device are as effective as nebulizers and are cheaper to use.[31] In intubated patients both nebulizers and MDIs have been used though there is some doubt as to the effectiveness of MDI drug delivery when used via a simple inspiratory limb adapter.[32]

Intravenous β-agonists should be considered if the patient is not responding to continuous nebulization. Increasing airway obstruction may prevent nebulized drug delivery; some studies have demonstrated improved response when intravenous β-agonist is used.[33] The typical dose is 5–20 μg/min. Side-effects should be monitored closely. Salbutamol 100–300 μg may also be given intravenously to non-intubated patients in extremis or delivered down an endotracheal tube should there be no time to gain i.v. access.

Side-effects of β-agonists include tachycardia, dysrhythmias, hypertension, hypotension, tremor, hypokalemia, worsening of ventilation-perfusion mismatch and hyperglycemia. The most common side-effect of parenteral β-agonist, and occasionally seen with continuous nebulized β-agonists, is lactic acidosis. This occurs in over 70% of patients, has an onset within 2–4 h of commencing an infusion or following intravenous statim doses, levels may reach 4–12 mmol/l and may significantly add to a respiratory acidosis and respiratory distress. Parenteral infusions should be initially limited to 10 μg/min and statim doses should not exceed 250 μg. Serum bicarbonate and lactate should be regularly monitored. If lactic acidosis becomes significant, the salbutamol infusion should be reduced or ceased. Lactic acidosis will generally resolve within 4–6 h of infusion cessation and is seldom a problem with infusions in place for more than 24 h.

Long-term, high-dose β-agonist use has been associated with increased mortality,[34] but whether high-dose β-agonists are a marker of disease severity, an indicator of suboptimal inhaled steroids or a direct cause of death is unclear. These concerns do not apply in the treatment of the acute asthma attack.

ANTICHOLINERGICS

Anticholinergics cause bronchodilatation by decreasing parasympathetic mediated cholinergic bronchomotor tone. Ipratropium bromide is the most commonly used anticholinergic for asthma and is a quaternary derivative of atropine. It should not be considered first line therapy for acute asthma but has an accepted place as an adjunct to β-agonist therapy. Several studies and meta-analyses suggest that pulmonary function is improved when ipratropium bromide is added to the β-agonist regimen.[35,36] Preservative-induced bronchoconstriction has been reported in a few patients and can be prevented by using preservative-free solutions. The bronchodilatation effect of ipratropium bromide appeared to be maximal with a dose of 250 μg when studied in children between 9 and 17 years of age.[37] The optimal dose is not known in adults; a reasonable regimen would be to add 500 μg of ipratropium bromide to the salbutamol nebulizer every 2 to 6 h. Ipratropium bromide is not absorbed into the bloodstream and has minimal cardiovascular side-effects.

CORTICOSTEROIDS

The role of corticosteroids in the acute asthma attack is well established;[38] they will usually start taking effect within 6 to 12 h of administration. Their benefits include increased β-responsiveness of airway smooth muscle, decreased inflammatory cell response and decreased mucus secretion. Early treatment with corticosteroids has been shown to decrease the likelihood of hospitalization[39] and probably decrease the mortality rate from acute asthma.[40]

Hydrocortisone or methylprednisolone are the most commonly used parenteral corticosteroids. The optimal dose is unclear; a reasonable regimen is 2–4 mg/kg of hydrocortisone every 6 h, or 0.5–1 mg/kg of methylprednisolone every 4–6 hours. Corticosteroids are usually given for 1–3 d before dose reduction and should be adjusted according to the severity of the attack, the degree of chronic inflammation and the response to treatment. A course of oral prednisolone starting at 40–60 mg/d usually replaces the parenteral regimen. If treatment is required for longer than 5–10 d, a slow reduction in dose is recommended.

Side-effects of corticosteroids include hyperglycaemia, hypokalaemia, hypertension, acute psychosis and myopathy, though they are usually well tolerated acutely. The immunosuppressive effects can increase the risk of infections including Legionella, *Pneumocystis carinii* and varicella[41,42] especially when the patient is on long term corticosteroids. Allergic reactions including anaphylaxis have been reported with the use of most corticosteroid preparations.

Inhaled steroids have established long-term benefit and are believed to be a major factor in asthma mortality reduction.[7,8] Their role during an acute attack is not established but they may be used to enable more rapid dose reduction of parenteral steroids, thus potentially reducing side-effects.

AMINOPHYLLINE

The role of aminophylline in acute asthma remains controversial. The mechanism of effect of aminophylline is unclear. The postulated actions include inhibition of phosphodiesterase, β-agonism, augmentation of diaphragmatic contractility and increased binding of cyclic-AMP.

There are conflicting studies regarding the efficacy of aminophylline in acute asthma. Some studies show no benefit when aminophylline is added to β-agonist therapy and an increased incidence of adverse side-effects.[43] A meta-analysis of randomized controlled trials of aminophylline in mild to moderate acute asthma in children showed no benefit.[44] However, other studies show an improvement in ventilatory function with aminophylline.[45] A recent double-blind placebo-controlled trial of aminophylline in children with severe status asthmaticus showed improved oxygen saturation and pulmonary function testing and a significant reduction in intubation requirement though no difference in intensive care length of stay.[46] Against this must be weighed the narrow therapeutic range with side-effects of headache, nausea, vomiting and restlessness. Cardiac dysrhythmias and convulsions can occur at serum levels above 200 μmol/l (40 mg/l).

With this in mind, aminophylline is not a first line treatment but is most commonly given to patients with acute asthma who are not showing a favourable response to initial treatment with β-agonists and corticosteroids. Careful administration and monitoring is required with an initial loading dose of 3 mg/kg (omitted if the patient is already taking oral theophylline) and an infusion of 0.5 mg/kg per h. This should be reduced in patients with cirrhosis, cardiac failure or chronic obstructive airways disease and in patients taking cimetidine, erythromycin or antiviral vaccines. Drug levels should be taken after a loading dose (if given), and then 24 h later, aiming for a level of 30–110 μmol/l (5–20 mg/l).

Levels should be repeated daily thereafter until stability has been achieved. The duration should be based on the response to treatment.

NON-ESTABLISHED TREATMENTS

Many other therapies have been proposed in acute severe asthma. Most have some evidence of benefit but as it has not been clearly established these agents are not advocated for routine use nor widely accepted. However, these modes of therapy can be considered in the patient who is not responding to conventional treatment.

EPINEPHRINE

Epinephrine has some theoretical advantages over pure β_2-agonists in that its α-agonist actions of vasoconstriction and mucosal shrinkage may improve bronchodilatation. However, in practice, nebulized or subcutaneous epinephrine has not been conclusively shown to confer any advantage over nebulized β_2-agonists.[47] Epinephrine may be tried in the patient who is failing to respond to conventional treatment. The nebulized dose is 2–4 mg in 2–4 ml (1% solution, 0.05 ml/kg), 1–4-hourly. The subcutaneous dose is 0.2–0.5 mg (0.2–0.5 ml of 1:1000 epinephrine), repeated if necessary 2–3 times at 30 min intervals. Epinephrine by infusion may avert mechanical ventilation in very severe cases, but should be used with caution with ECG monitoring and preferably with central venous access. An initial i.v. dose of 0.2–1.0 mg (2–10 ml of 1:10 000 epinephrine) is given slowly over 3–5 min. This may be followed by a continuous infusion of 1–20 μg/min, which is weaned when the acute attack subsides.[48]

MAGNESIUM SULPHATE

Magnesium sulphate is postulated to block calcium channels thereby mediating smooth muscle relaxation and bronchodilatation.[49] It may also inhibit acetylcholine release at the neuromuscular junction. It appears to be well tolerated in studies published to date[50] though its efficacy is unclear. Two randomized, double-blind, prospective trials showed no benefit in adding magnesium sulphate to conventional therapy in adults with acute asthma.[51,52] Conversely two small, randomized trials in children and one in adults found that pulmonary function was improved in the magnesium sulphate group compared with placebo.[53,54] Magnesium is not generally recommended for acute asthma. If given, recommended doses are 5–10 mmol (1.25–2.5 g, 2.5–5.0 ml of 50% solution) given slowly over 20 min, but doses up to 40–80 mmol (10–20 g) have been given.[50] Side-effects include hypotension, flushing, sedation, weakness, areflexia, respiratory depression and cardiac arrhythmias seen at higher serum levels (>5 mmol/dl or 12 mg/dl). Serum concentrations should be measured if repeated or high doses are used.

HELIOX

Inhalation of a helium:oxygen mixture (heliox, most commonly 60:40) reduces gas density and turbulence with reduced airflow resistance. Work of breathing is decreased and pulmonary access of inhaled bronchodilators may be improved. Small case-series and case reports suggest some benefit to the use of heliox.[55,56] The results of randomized prospective trials are conflicting with both positive and negative results. The best improvements in flow dynamics occur with helium as 60–80% of the gas mixture; patients with a high FiO_2 requirement may not tolerate this mixture. It otherwise appears safe and may be tried in critical asthma to avert intubation or during difficult mechanical ventilation.

ANAESTHETIC AGENTS

Ketamine, a dissociative anaesthetic agent, has been used in severe asthma. It may cause bronchodilatation by both sympathomimetic potentiation and a direct effect on airway smooth muscle. Small case-series suggest some benefit[57] although a small randomized controlled trial found no benefit with ketamine in the treatment of acute severe asthma.[58] Ketamine may be a useful induction agent for endotracheal intubation (dose 1–2 mg/kg) as it may ameliorate the bronchoconstrictor response to intubation.[59] It has been used as a continuous infusion in the dose range of 0.5–2 mg/kg per h to treat refractory asthma. Side-effects include increased bronchial secretions, a hyperdynamic cardiovascular response and hallucinations; the hallucinations can be reduced with concomitant benzodiazepines.

The volatile inhalational agents including halothane, isoflurane and enflurane have been used in mechanically ventilated patients with severe asthma. Clinical data is limited to small case-series.[60] Side-effects include direct myocardial depression, arrhythmias and hypotension.[56] The volatile anaesthetic agents should be used with great care and only as a prelude to or during invasive ventilation. An anaesthetic machine or custom-fitted ventilator is required for safe administration.

BRONCHOALVEOLAR LAVAGE

Bronchoalveolar lavage has been used in severe refractory asthma to clear mucous plugging. It may however, transiently worsen bronchospasm and hypoxemia and aggravate dynamic hyperinflation during mechanical ventilation. It may have a role in ventilated patients without critical hyperinflation, whose recovery is delayed by resistant mucus impaction, but it is rarely used.

HYDRATION

Patients with more prolonged severe attacks prior to presentation may develop mild dehydration because of poor fluid intake. A positive fluid balance of 1–3 l is commonly required during the first 24 h of mechanical ventilation for asthma. Although this requirement is traditionally attributed to dehydration, most of it is due to the vasodilatory effects of sedation, hypercapnia and the circulatory depressant effects of dynamic hyperinflation in association with mechanical ventilation, with elimination of this fluid load on recovery.

THERAPIES NOT RECOMMENDED

Antibiotics are not indicated unless there is clear evidence of infection. Antihistamines and mucolytics are not considered to be effective. No sedative is safe in acute asthma. Patients with severe asthma should not be sedated unless being intubated and ventilated.

MONITORING PROGRESS

Patients with severe asthma must not be left unattended. Their progress should be closely monitored after initiation of treatment. Major contributors to deterioration and mortality are inadequate observation and measurement.

- The patient should be observed for changes in their clinical state and their degree of respiratory distress.
- Severity of airflow obstruction should be measured with the use of a peak flow meter or spirometer repeated at 2–4 h intervals to assess severity and monitor progress. Patients with severe respiratory distress may be unable or unwilling to perform this manoeuvre. Oxygenation should be assessed with pulse oximetry; serial arterial blood gases should be performed if the patient presents with severe asthma.
- Treatment effects should be monitored including titration of β-agonist therapy according to clinical state and observed side-effects and measurement of aminophylline levels.

NON-INVASIVE VENTILATORY ASSISTANCE

Non-invasive positive pressure ventilation (NIV) has been used for a number of years in severe asthma. To date there have been no randomized controlled trials in asthma. A case-series of 17 patients with asthma treated with NPPV has been reported;[61] the authors report significant improvement in respiratory acidosis and respiratory rate following the introduction of NIV. Only two patients subsequently required invasive ventilation. The trial used a pressure support ventilation mode of NIV with initial settings of 4 ± 2 cmH$_2$O of PEEP and 14 ± 5 cmH$_2$O of pressure support aiming at a respiratory rate of less than 25 breaths/min and an exhaled tidal volume of 7 ml/kg.

There are as yet no clear guidelines for the use of NPPV in severe asthma. A trial of NPPV is reasonable once patients are screened for contra-indications and are willing to cooperate. Selection criteria may include

Table 30.1 Cause of death in 99 patients requiring mechanical ventilation for acute severe asthma

	n
Cerebral ischaemia/hypoxia	40
Hypotension	15
Pneumonia or sepsis with hypotension	10
Tension pneumothorax	6
Technical complications with ventilation	6
Arrhythmia	4
Respiratory complication (aspiration, tracheostomy, sputum plug)	3
Gastrointestinal complication	3
Suspected pulmonary embolus	3
Arrest post extubation	3
Arrest post ICU	2
Treatment withdrawn (endstage)	2
Unknown	3
TOTAL	99

moderate to severe dyspnoea, a respiratory rate of >24 breaths/min, accessory muscle use or paradoxical breathing,[62] or the presence of hypercapnic acidosis. Patients should be admitted to intensive care and monitored closely for deterioration.

INVASIVE VENTILATION

Invasive mechanical ventilation in acute severe asthma may be life-saving, but can be associated with significant morbidity and mortality (Table 30.1).[63] Institution of invasive ventilation with endotracheal intubation carries the risk of inadvertent pulmonary hyperinflation[63–65] (see below) and potential aggravation of bronchospasm.[60] In addition, the usual caveats to invasive ventilation are also present; these include failed intubation, damage to the airway, aspiration and increased risk of stress ulceration and nosocomial pneumonia.

Absolute indications for intubation include cardiac or respiratory arrest, severe hypoxia or rapid deterioration of conscious state.[10,27] Progressive patient fatigue and hypercapnia are relative indications and must be balanced against the risks of intubation. Patients are often able to tolerate hypercapnia without requiring invasive ventilation.[66]

Hyperacute asthma may present with marked hypercapnia (PaCO$_2$ >60 mmHg) due to mechanical limitations to ventilation as a result of dynamic hyperinflation. Such patients may not initially be fatigued and may respond rapidly to treatment, thereby avoiding mechanical ventilation. Acute severe asthma that has been progressing for days may have less hypercapnia but will often respond poorly to treatment. The PaCO$_2$ may rise despite maximal treatment due to fatigue and the patient may in fact require intubation at a lower PaCO$_2$. The assessment of need for invasive ventilation will be influenced by the pattern of presentation, the degree of hypercapnia and most importantly, recognition of patient deterioration and distress despite maximal medical therapy by an experienced clinician.

There are numerous possible approaches to intubation. A safe option is to perform rapid sequence intubation using the orotracheal approach. Once the endotracheal tube is in place, slow hand ventilation (8–10 breaths/min) should maintain oxygenation until the ventilator can be connected.[67]

DYNAMIC HYPERINFLATION

Gas trapping occurs in asthma as a consequence of airflow obstruction. Incomplete exhalation of each breath results in progressive dynamic hyperinflation (DHI). This continues until an equilibrium point is reached where the exhaled volume increases to match the inspired volume (Figure 30.1).[64] This equilibrium occurs because increasing lung volume increases small airway calibre and lung elastic recoil pressure, both of which improve expiratory airflow and allow the inspired tidal volume to be exhaled in the expiratory time available. Gas trapped at the end of expiration exerts a positive pressure on the alveoli (PEEPi or auto-PEEP).[64,65] During expiration, sequential closure of the most severely obstructed airways occurs with only the less obstructed airways remaining in communication with the central airway at the end of tidal expiration.[68] As a consequence, measured PEEP$_i$ underestimates the true magnitude of PEEP$_i$ and is recognized as being insensitive to changes in severity.[68]

In severe asthma, the minute ventilation required to maintain normocapnia would cause hyperinflation beyond normal total lung capacity.[16] The spontaneously breathing asthmatic patient is unable to generate the inspiratory force required to achieve such end-inspiratory volume and consequently becomes hypercapnic.[10]

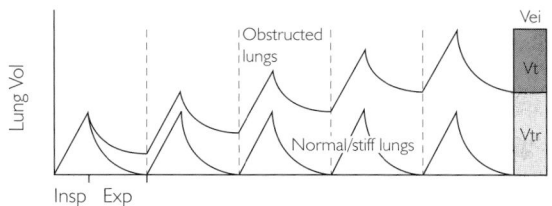

Fig. 30.1 Dynamic hyperinflation. The volume history of normal or acutely injured lungs compared with that of obstructed lungs when commenced on controlled mechanical ventilation. This figure shows initial lung volume to be at the passive relaxation volume of the respiratory system or functional residual capacity (FRC). (Vt, tidal volume; Vtr, trapped gas volume; Vei, end-inspiratory lung volume.)

Conversely, the mechanical ventilator is able to increase the degree of DHI well beyond normal total lung capacity. Increasing minute ventilation to correct hypercapnia by increasing tidal volume or respiratory rate is the factor most likely to increase hyperinflation.[64] The consequences of hyperinflation above a safe level are hypotension (due to increased intrathoracic pressure and decreased venous return) and barotrauma (Figure 30.2).

INITIAL VENTILATOR SETTINGS

The place of volume controlled ventilation is clearly established in asthma. Pressure controlled or assisted modes have been used[69] without adverse consequences. The theoretical advantage of a safe pressure limit in pressure modes is offset by the fact that equilibrium with the set safe pressure cannot be reached during the short inspiratory times required and thus either a higher pressure must be set or more than necessary hypoventilation may occur. It is not clear if one mode is superior to the other.

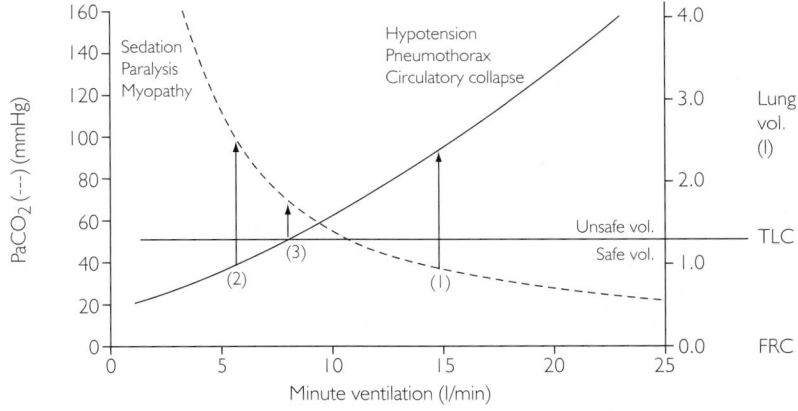

Fig. 30.2 The effects of minute ventilation on PaCO$_2$ and end-inspiratory lung volume above FRC in a typical patient with severe asthma. (1) The minute ventilation required for normocapnia, (2) profound hypoventilation, (3) optimal hypoventilation.

The principles are nonetheless the same with small tidal volumes, long expiratory time and slow respiratory rate. A typical volume-controlled setting would aim to achieve a minute ventilation of <115 ml/kg or <8 l/min in a 70 kg patient. Initial settings would include a tidal volume of 6–8 ml/kg, a respiratory rate of 8–10 breaths/min and a high inspiratory flow rate of 80 l/min. The peak inspiratory pressure (PIP) is likely to be high with these settings but there does not appear to be a correlation between high PIPs and barotrauma in ventilated patients with asthma.[63] No PEEP is set initially. The FiO_2 is titrated to achieve a SaO_2 of >94%. This level of ventilation will usually result in respiratory acidosis that usually requires initial sedation and, in some patients, transient neuromuscular blockade. If significant hypotension occurs this should be treated by reducing the respiratory rate, (thereby reducing dynamic hyper-inflation) and volume loading.

ASSESSMENT OF VENTILATION

Once mechanical ventilation has started, the degree of DHI should be assessed by measurement of:

- Plateau airway pressure is measured by occluding the expiratory valve at the end of inspiration and recording the pressure after a 0.5 s pause applied after one breath only (application for several breaths in a row will decrease expiratory time and increase dynamic hyperinflation). This is the most easily measured estimate of alveolar pressure at the end of inspiration and is affected by the degree of hyperinflation. Ideally this should be maintained at <25 cmH_2O.[63,64]
- Intrinsic PEEP ($PEEP_i$) can be detected (but not quantified) from the ventilator expiratory flow curve that does not reach zero at the end of the expiratory period. It can be measured by occluding the exhalation valve of the ventilator at end-expiration and recording the pressure; this is an automated manoeuvre on most modern ventilators.[67] It should be noted that this may underestimate true intrinsic PEEP, as a consequence of small airway closure during expiration.[68] Ideally $PEEP_i$ should be <12 cmH_2O though the exact safe level is unknown.
- End-inspiratory lung volume (V_{EI}) (Figure 30.2) above functional residual capacity (FRC) has been shown to be a good predictor of complications during mechanical ventilation[63] and to cor-relate with total lung volume.[16] It is assessed in a paralysed patient by measuring the total exhaled volume during a period of apnoea (30–60 s), so that the lungs return to FRC. V_{EI} below 20 ml/kg (1.4 l in a 70 kg patient) has been shown to be safe by maintaining total lung volume below total lung capacity (TLC).[63] This manoeuvre is not routinely used as it requires paralysis and is complex and labour-intensive.

ADJUSTMENT OF VENTILATION

Ventilatory patterns with an excessive minute ventilation risk hypotension and barotrauma are associated with a high mortality. Using profound hypoventilation will guarantee avoidance of these complications but usually necessitates heavy sedation and neuromuscular blockade (Figure 30.2). This, in association with parenteral steroids, has a high probability of myopathy,[70] which may cause severe prolonged disability. To minimize the risk of both these complications, DHI should be carefully assessed and the minimum amount of hypoventilation used to achieve a safe level of DHI (Figure 30.2).

Hypercapnia is usually present but is well tolerated[71] and does not appear to depress cardiac function.[72] There is no evidence of benefit from sodium bicarbonate but it may reduce acidemia induced respiratory distress, and may be given if pH <7.1.

Pressure support ventilation has been used after stabilization and resolution of neuromuscular blockade. A case-series in children used pressure support of between 22 and 37 cmH_2O and PEEP of 3 cmH_2O.[73] This mode allows the patient to breathe spontaneously, often with improved patient–ventilator synchrony. Additional theoretical benefits are less neuromuscular blockade and sedation. It is not known whether this approach improves patient outcome. We believe a starting pressure of 10–15 cmH_2O is reasonable in an adult. If pressure support ventilation is used patients should still be carefully assessed for dynamic hyperinflation.

COMPLICATIONS OF INVASIVE VENTILATION IN ASTHMA

HYPOTENSION

Hypotension may be caused by sedation, DHI, pneumothoraces or arrhythmias.[63,64] Hypovolaemia may be a contributory factor but is rarely a cause. Hypotension may be mild or life-threatening.[74] Hypotension due to DHI may be diagnosed by recovery of blood pressure during apnoea of 60 s (the 'apnoea test'). If this occurs, ventilation should be recommenced at a lower rate.

CIRCULATORY ARREST WITH APPARENT ELECTROMECHANICAL DISSOCIATION

Circulatory arrest with apparent electromechanical dissociation (EMD) is a recognized complication that may occur within 10 min of intubation and can lead to death or severe cerebral ischemic injury if not managed correctly.[74,75] Standard mechanical ventilation recommendations (minute ventilation 115 ml/kg per min) have been estimated to be safe for 80% of patients requiring mechanical ventilation for acute severe asthma with the remaining 20% requiring a small to moderate reduction in minute ventilation to return DHI to a safe level.[63] A small percentage of patients with unusually severe asthma can rapidly develop excessive DHI during initial uncontrolled mechanical ventilation leading to EMD, sometimes despite 'safe' levels of minute ventilation. If the cause of this is not immediately recognized, it can lead to prolonged and unnecessary CPR, unsafe procedures such as intercostal insertion of a needle or pericardial aspiration and risk cerebral injury and death. When this occurs immediate disconnection from ventilation for 60–90 s (the 'apnoea test', above) or profound hypoventilation (2–3 breaths/min)[27] will diagnose and improve this situation. An even smaller percentage of patients may remain hypotensive despite profound hypoventilation with marked hypercapnia, fluid loading and inotropes. These patients may require Heliox delivered by the mechanical ventilator or extra-corporeal membrane oxygenation.

PNEUMOTHORACES

Pneumothoraces were common before the advent of protective ventilatory strategies; DHI during mechanical ventilation was probably the major factor involved.[63,64] The airflow obstruction favours gas loss through the ruptured alveoli, increasing the chance of tension pneumothorax. Once a unilateral tension pneumothorax is present the degree of hyperinflation in the contralateral lung is increased and bilateral pneumothoraces may result.

ACUTE MYOPATHY

Acute myopathy is a common complication seen in patients who are invasively ventilated for asthma.[70,76,77] It is characterized by weakness with electromyographic evidence of myopathy and increased serum creatine kinase levels. Muscle biopsy reveals two patterns; myonecrosis with muscle cell vacuolization or predominant type II fibre atrophy.[77,78] Recovery is slow with often prolonged weaning from mechanical ventilation; incomplete recovery after 12 months has been reported in a few patients. The aetiology of the myopathy appears to be a combination of the effects of corticosteroids and neuromuscular blocking agents (NMBA) with the duration of paralysis a strong predictor of myopathy.[76] The type of NMBA used seems to make no difference to the incidence of myopathy.[78] The relative contributions of corticosteroids versus NMBAs in the causation of myopathy is unclear; it seems wise to minimize the dose of parenteral corticosteroids with early introduction of nebulized agents and preferable to avoid NMBAs if at all possible.

MORTALITY AND LONG-TERM OUTCOME

There are encouraging signs that mortality from asthma is on the decline.[7,8] Changes in practice in the last 10 years of the 20th century include better primary treatment with formalized asthma management approaches and increased inhaled corticosteroid use. This era has also coincided with changed ventilator practice; most notably awareness of dynamic hyperinflation and permissive hypercapnia.[63]

Slightly fewer than half of the deaths occur in hospital and in nearly 85% of deaths, the final episode lasted at least 12 h, suggesting some component of treatment failure.[79] There is some suggestion that inadequate assessment and treatment remain problems.[79,80] The need for invasive ventilation increases the risk of death[81] and the mortality following a near-fatal attack of asthma is 10% in the first year.[79] Patients who have had respiratory failure with one episode of asthma tend to have respiratory failure with subsequent episodes.

For these reasons, patients who have an episode of asthma severe enough to require hospitalization, particularly intensive care admission, need careful follow-up. This should include active identification and avoidance of precipitants, aggressive bronchodilator therapy including inhaled steroids, regular medical review, regular measurement of lung function, management plans for a deteriorating status, and ready access to emergency services.

REFERENCES

1 The International Study of Asthma and Allergies in Childhood (ISAAC). Worldwide variation in prevalence of symptoms of asthma, allergic rhinoconjunctivitis, and atopic eczema. ISAAC Steering Committee. *Lancet* 1998; **351**: 1225–32.
2 Sly RM. Changing prevalence of allergic rhinitis and asthma. *Ann Allergy Asthma Immunol* 1999; **82**: 233–48.
3 Seale JP. Asthma deaths: where are we now? *Aust N Z J Med* 1991; **21**: 678–9.
4 Strong K, de Looper M, Magnus P. Asthma mortality in Australia, 1980–1996. *Aust Health Rev* 1998; **21**: 255–63.
5 Pearce N, Weiland S, Keil U, et al. Self-reported prevalence of asthma symptoms in children in Australia, England, Germany and New Zealand: an international comparison using the ISAAC protocol. *Eur Respir J* 1993; **6**: 1455–61.
6 Mannino DM, Homa DM, Pertowski CA, et al. Surveillance for asthma – United States, 1960–1995. *Mor Mortal Wkly Rep CDC Surveill Summ* 1998; **47**: 1–27.
7 McCaul KA, Wakefield MA, Roder DM, et al. Trends in hospital readmission for asthma: has the Australian National Asthma Campaign had an effect? *Med J Aust* 2000; **172**: 62–6.
8 Suissa S, Ernst P. Inhaled corticosteroids: impact on asthma morbidity and mortality. *J Allergy Clin Immunol* 2001; **107**: 937–44.
9 Guidelines for the diagnosis and management of asthma. National Heart, Lung, and Blood Institute. National Asthma Education Program. Expert Panel Report. *J Allergy Clin Immunol* 19911; **88**: 425–534.
10 Werner HA. Status asthmaticus in children: a review. *Chest* 2001; **119**: 1913–29.

11 Busse WW, Lemanske RF Jr. Asthma. *N Engl J Med* 2001; **344**: 350–62.

12 Dunnill M. The pathology of asthma with special reference to the changes in the broncial mucosa. *J Clin Pathol* 1960; **13**.

13 Reid LM. The presence or absence of bronchial mucus in fatal asthma. *J Allergy Clin Immunol* 1987; **80**: 415–6.

14 Kallenbach JM, Frankel AH, Lapinsky SE, *et al.* Determinants of near fatality in acute severe asthma. *Am J Med* 1993; **95**: 265–72.

15 Wasserfallen JB, Schaller MD, Feihl F, *et al.* Sudden asphyxic asthma: a distinct entity? *Am Rev Respir Dis* 1990; **142**: 108–11.

16 Tuxen DV, Williams TJ, Scheinkestel CD, *et al.* Use of a measurement of pulmonary hyperinflation to control the level of mechanical ventilation in patients with acute severe asthma. *Am Rev Respir Dis* 1992; **146**: 1136–42.

17 Stalcup SA, Mellins RB. Mechanical forces producing pulmonary edema in acute asthma. *N Engl J Med* 1977; **297**: 592–6.

18 Buda AJ, Pinsky MR, Ingels NB Jr, *et al.* Effect of intrathoracic pressure on left ventricular performance. *N Engl J Med* 1979; **301**: 453–9.

19 Dawson CA, Grimm DJ, Linehan JH. Lung inflation and longitudinal distribution of pulmonary vascular resistance during hypoxia. *J Appl Physiol* 1979; **47**: 532–6.

20 Rebuck AS, Pengelly LD. Development of pulsus paradoxus in the presence of airways obstruction. *N Engl J Med* 1973; **288**: 66–9.

21 Rebuck AS, Read J. Assessment and management of severe asthma. *Am J Med* 1971; **51**: 788–98.

22 Rea HH, Scragg R, Jackson R, *et al.* A case-control study of deaths from asthma. *Thorax* 1986; **41**: 833–9.

23 Strunk R. Identification of the fatality-prone subject with asthma. *J Allergy Clin Immunol* 1989; **83**: 477–85.

24 McFadden ER, Jr., Lyons HA. Arterial-blood gas tension in asthma. *N Engl J Med* 1968; **278**: 1027–32.

25 Mountain RD, Heffner JE, Brackett NC Jr, *et al.* Acid-base disturbances in acute asthma. *Chest* 1990; **98**: 651–5.

26 Rodrigo G, Rodrigo C. Assessment of the patient with acute asthma in the emergency department. A factor analytic study. *Chest* 1993; **104**: 1325–8.

27 Corbridge TC, Hall JB. The assessment and management of adults with status asthmaticus. *Am J Respir Crit Care Med* 1995; **151**: 1296–316.

28 Schiff M. Control of breathing in asthma. *Clin Chest Med* 1980; **1**: 85–9.

29 Paterson JW, Evans RJ, Prime FJ. Selectivity of bronchodilator action of salbutamol in asthmatic patients. *Br J Dis Chest* 1971; **65**: 21–38.

30 Papo MC, Frank J, Thompson AE. A prospective, randomized study of continuous versus intermittent nebulized albuterol for severe status asthmaticus in children. *Crit Care Med* 1993; **21**: 1479–86.

31 Idris AH, McDermott MF, Raucci JC, *et al.* Emergency department treatment of severe asthma. Metered-dose inhaler plus holding chamber is equivalent in effectiveness to nebulizer. *Chest* 1993; **103**: 665–72.

32 Manthous CA, Hall JB, Schmidt GA, *et al.* Metered-dose inhaler versus nebulized albuterol in mechanically ventilated patients. *Am Rev Respir Dis* 1993; **148**: 1567–70.

33 Browne GJ, Penna AS, Phung X, *et al.* Randomised trial of intravenous salbutamol in early management of acute severe asthma in children. *Lancet* 1997; **349**: 301–5.

34 Spitzer WO, Suissa S, Ernst P, *et al.* The use of beta-agonists and the risk of death and near death from asthma. *N Engl J Med* 1992; **326**: 501–6.

35 Rodrigo G, Rodrigo C, Burschtin O. A meta-analysis of the effects of ipratropium bromide in adults with acute asthma. *Am J Med* 1999; **107**: 363–70.

36 Stoodley RG, Aaron SD, Dales RE. The role of ipratropium bromide in the emergency management of acute asthma exacerbation: a metaanalysis of randomized clinical trials. *Ann Emerg Med* 1999; **34**: 8–18.

37 Davis A, Vickerson F, Worsley G, *et al.* Determination of dose-response relationship for nebulized ipratropium in asthmatic children. *J Pediatr* 1984; **105**: 1002–5.

38 Rowe BH, Keller JL, Oxman AD. Effectiveness of steroid therapy in acute exacerbations of asthma: a meta-analysis. *Am J Emerg Med* 1992; **10**: 301–10.

39 Littenberg B, Gluck EH. A controlled trial of methylprednisolone in the emergency treatment of acute asthma. *N Engl J Med* 1986; **314**: 150–2.

40 Benatar SR. Fatal asthma. *N Engl J Med* 1986; **314**: 423–9.

41 Kasper WJ, Howe PM. Fatal varicella after a single course of corticosteroids. *Pediatr Infect Dis J* 1990; **9**: 729–32.

42 Abernathy-Carver KJ, Fan LL, Boguniewicz M, *et al.* Legionella and Pneumocystis pneumonias in asthmatic children on high doses of systemic steroids. *Pediatr Pulmonol* 1994; **18**: 135–8.

43 Murphy DG, McDermott MF, Rydman RJ, *et al.* Aminophylline in the treatment of acute asthma when beta 2-adrenergics and steroids are provided. *Arch Intern Med* 1993; **153**: 1784–8.

44 Goodman DC, Littenberg B, O'Connor GT, *et al.* Theophylline in acute childhood asthma: a meta-analysis of its efficacy. *Pediatr Pulmonol* 1996; **21**: 211–8.

45 Pierson WE, Bierman CW, Stamm SJ, *et al.* Double-blind trial of aminophylline in status asthmaticus. *Pediatrics* 1971; **48**: 642–6.

46 Yung M, South M. Randomised controlled trial of aminophylline for severe acute asthma. *Arch Dis Child* 1998; **79**: 405–10.

47 Spiteri MA, Millar AB, Pavia D, *et al.* Subcutaneous adrenaline versus terbutaline in the treatment of acute severe asthma. *Thorax* 1988; **43**: 19–23.

48 Tirot P, BG, Varache N. Use of intravenous adrenaline in severe acute asthma. *Rev Mal Respir* 1993; 9: 319–323.

49 Lindeman KS, Hirshman CA, Freed AN. Effect of magnesium sulfate on bronchoconstriction in the lung periphery. *J Appl Physiol* 1989; 66: 2527–32.

50 Sydow M, Crozier TA, Zielmann S, *et al.* High-dose intravenous magnesium sulfate in the management of life-threatening status asthmaticus. *Intensive Care Med* 1993; 19: 467–71.

51 Tiffany BR, Berk WA, Todd IK, *et al.* Magnesium bolus or infusion fails to improve expiratory flow in acute asthma exacerbations. *Chest* 1993; 104: 831–4.

52 Green SM, Rothrock SG. Intravenous magnesium for acute asthma: failure to decrease emergency treatment duration or need for hospitalization. *Ann Emerg Med* 1992; 21: 260–5.

53 Skobeloff EM, Spivey WH, McNamara RM, *et al.* Intravenous magnesium sulfate for the treatment of acute asthma in the emergency department. *JAMA* 1989; 262: 1210–3.

54 Ciarallo L, Brousseau D, Reinert S. Higher-dose intravenous magnesium therapy for children with moderate to severe acute asthma. *Arch Pediatr Adolesc Med* 2000; 154: 979–83.

55 Manthous CA, Hall JB, Caputo MA, *et al.* Heliox improves pulsus paradoxus and peak expiratory flow in nonintubated patients with severe asthma. *Am J Respir Crit Care Med* 1995; 151: 310–4.

56 Tobias JD, Garrett JS. Therapeutic options for severe, refractory status asthmaticus: inhalational anaesthetic agents, extracorporeal membrane oxygenation and helium/oxygen ventilation. *Paediatr Anaesth* 1997; 7: 47–57.

57 Nehama J, Pass R, Bechtler-Karsch A, *et al.* Continuous ketamine infusion for the treatment of refractory asthma in a mechanically ventilated infant: case report and review of the pediatric literature. *Pediatr Emerg Care* 1996; 12: 294–7.

58 Howton JC, Rose J, Duffy S, *et al.* Randomized, double-blind, placebo-controlled trial of intravenous ketamine in acute asthma. *Ann Emerg Med* 1996; 27: 170–5.

59 L'Hommedieu CS, Arens JJ. The use of ketamine for the emergency intubation of patients with status asthmaticus. *Ann Emerg Med* 1987; 16: 568–71.

60 O'Rourke PP, Crone RK. Halothane in status asthmaticus. *Crit Care Med* 1982; 10: 341–3.

61 Meduri GU, Cook TR, Turner RE, *et al.* Noninvasive positive pressure ventilation in status asthmaticus. *Chest* 1996; 110: 767–74.

62 Mehta S, Hill NS. Noninvasive ventilation. *Am J Respir Crit Care Med* 2001; 163: 540–77.

63 Williams TJ, Tuxen DV, Scheinkestel CD, *et al.* Risk factors for morbidity in mechanically ventilated patients with acute severe asthma. *Am Rev Respir Dis* 1992; 146: 607–15.

64 Tuxen DV, Lane S. The effects of ventilatory pattern on hyperinflation, airway pressures, and circulation in mechanical ventilation of patients with severe air-flow obstruction. *Am Rev Respir Dis* 1987; 136: 872–9.

65 Pepe PE, Marini JJ. Occult positive end-expiratory pressure in mechanically ventilated patients with airflow obstruction: the auto-PEEP effect. *Am Rev Respir Dis* 1982; 126: 166–70.

66 Mountain RD, Sahn SA. Clinical features and outcome in patients with acute asthma presenting with hypercapnia. *Am Rev Respir Dis* 1988; 138: 535–9.

67 Jain S, Hanania NA, Guntupalli KK. Ventilation of patients with asthma and obstructive lung disease. *Crit Care Clin* 1998; 14: 685–705.

68 Leatherman JW, Ravenscraft SA. Low measured auto-positive end-expiratory pressure during mechanical ventilation of patients with severe asthma: hidden auto-positive end-expiratory pressure. *Crit Care Med* 1996; 24: 541–6.

69 Mansel JK, Stogner SW, Petrini MF, *et al.* Mechanical ventilation in patients with acute severe asthma. *Am J Med* 1990; 89: 42–8.

70 Nates J, CD, Tuxen D. Acute weakness syndromes in critically ill patients – a reappraisal. *Anaesth Intensive Care* 1997; 25: 502–513.

71 Bellomo R, McLaughlin P, Tai E, *et al.* Asthma requiring mechanical ventilation. A low morbidity approach. *Chest* 1994; 105: 891–6.

72 Cooper D. Acute severe asthma and acidosis – effect of bicarbonate on cardiac and respiratory function. *Anaesth Intensive Care* 1994; 22: 212–13(Abstract).

73 Wetzel RC. Pressure-support ventilation in children with severe asthma. *Crit Care Med* 1996; 24: 1603–5.

74 Rosengarten PL, Tuxen DV, Dziukas L, *et al.* Circulatory arrest induced by intermittent positive pressure ventilation in a patient with severe asthma. *Anaesth Intensive Care* 1991; 19: 118–21.

75 Kollef M. Lung hyperinflation caused by inappropriate ventilation resulting in electromechanical dissociation: a case report. *Heart Lung* 1992; 21: 74–77.

76 Behbehani NA, Al-Mane F, D'Yachkova Y, *et al.* Myopathy following mechanical ventilation for acute severe asthma: the role of muscle relaxants and corticosteroids. *Chest* 1999; 115: 1627–31.

77 Douglass JA, Tuxen DV, Horne M, *et al.* Myopathy in severe asthma. *Am Rev Respir Dis* 1992; 146: 517–9.

78 Leatherman JW, Fluegel WL, David WS, *et al.* Muscle weakness in mechanically ventilated patients with severe asthma. *Am J Respir Crit Care Med* 1996; 153: 1686–90.

79 McFadden ER Jr, Warren EL. Observations on asthma mortality. *Ann Intern Med* 1997; 127: 142–7.

80 Hartert TV, Windom HH, Peebles RS Jr, *et al.* Inadequate outpatient medical therapy for patients with asthma admitted to two urban hospitals. *Am J Med* 1996; 100: 386–94.

81 Marquette CH, Saulnier F, Leroy O, *et al.* Long-term prognosis of near-fatal asthma. A 6-year follow-up study of 145 asthmatic patients who underwent mechanical ventilation for a near-fatal attack of asthma. *Am Rev Respir Dis* 1992; 146: 76–81.

31

Lung infections

C D Gomersall

PNEUMONIA

The management of pneumonia is based on four findings and premises:

1 Pneumonia is associated with a wide range of largely non-specific clinical features.[1]
2 Pneumonia can be caused by over 100 organisms.[2]
3 The relationship between specific clinical features and the aetiological organism is insufficiently strong to allow a clinical diagnosis of the causative organism.[3–6]
4 Early administration of appropriate antibiotics is important.[5,7]

Although the differential diagnosis is wide, treatment should be started before the aetiological agent is identified. The differential diagnosis and the likely causative organisms can be narrowed by using epidemiological clues, the most important of which are whether the pneumonia is community or hospital acquired, and whether the patient is immunocompromised. Note that the flora and antibiotic resistance patterns vary from country to country,[8] hospital to hospital, and even ICU to ICU within a hospital,[9] and this must be taken into account.

COMMUNITY ACQUIRED PNEUMONIA

Recent evidence-based guidelines have been issued by the Canadian Infectious Diseases Society and Canadian Thoracic Society,[2] the Infectious Diseases Society of America (IDSA)[10] (http://www.journals.uchicago.edu/IDSA/guide/MY56_1042.pdf) and the American Thoracic Society (ATS)[5] (http://www.thoracic.org/adobe/statements/commacq1-25.pdf).

DEFINITION

An acute infection of the pulmonary parenchyma that is associated with at least some symptoms of acute infection, accompanied by an acute infiltrate on a chest radiograph (CXR) or auscultatory findings consistent with pneumonia (e.g. altered breath sounds, localized crackles) in a patient not hospitalized or residing in a long-term care facility for ≥14 d prior to the onset of symptoms.[10]

AETIOLOGY

Table 31.1 lists possible aetiological agents based on epidemiological clues. *Strep. pneumoniae* is the most commonly isolated organism. Other less commonly isolated agents include *Haemophilus influenzae, Mycoplasma pneumoniae, Chlamydia pneumoniae, Staphylococcus aureus, Streptococcus pyogenes, Neisseria meningitides, Moraxella catarrhalis, Klebsiella pneumoniae* and other gram negative bacilli.[2,5,10]

CLINICAL PRESENTATION

Pneumonia produces both systemic and respiratory manifestations. Common clinical findings include fever, sweats, rigors, cough, sputum production, pleuritic chest pain, dyspnoea, tachypnoea, pleural rub and inspiratory crackles. Classic signs of consolidation occur in less than 25% of cases. Multi-organ dysfunction or failure may occur depending on the type and severity of pneumonia.

The diagnosis of pneumonia may be more difficult in the elderly. Although the vast majority of elderly patients with pneumonia have respiratory symptoms and signs, over 50% may also have non-respiratory symptoms, and over one third may have no systemic signs of infection.[11,12]

INVESTIGATIONS[2,5,10]

Investigations should not delay administration of antibiotics. Delays of as little as 8 h are associated with an increase in mortality.[5] Important investigations include:

Chest X-ray
Arterial blood gases or oximetry
Full blood count
Serum creatinine, urea and electrolytes

Table 31.1 Possible aetiological agents based on epidemiological clues[2,5,10]

Exposure	Organism
Exposure to animals	
Handling turkeys, chickens, ducks or psittacine birds or their excreta	*Chlamydia psittaci*
Handling infected parturient cats, cattle, goats or sheep or their hides	*Coxiella burnetii*
Handling infected wool	*Bacillus anthracis*
Handling infected cattle, pigs, goats or sheep or their milk	*Brucella* spp
Insect bite. Transmission from rodents and wild animals to laboratory workers, farmers and hunters	*Francisella tularensis*
Insect bites or scratches. Transmission from infected rodents or cats to laboratory workers and hunters	*Yersinia pestis*
Contact with infected horses (very rare)	*Pseudomonas mallei*
Exposure to mice or mice droppings	Hantavirus
Travel history	
Immigration from countries with high prevalence of TB	*M. tuberculosis*
N. America. Contact with infected bats or birds or their excreta. Excavation in endemic areas	*Histoplasma capsulatum*
South-west USA	*Coccidiodes* species
USA. Inhalation of spores from soil	*Blastomyces dermatitidis*
Asia, Pacific, Caribbean, N. Australia. Contact with local animals or contaminated skin abrasions	*Pseudomonas pseudomallei*
Host factors	
Diabetic ketoacidosis	*Strep. pneumoniae, S. aureus*
Alcoholism	*Strep. pneumoniae, S. aureus, Klebsiella pneumoniae, anaerobes*
Chronic obstructive lung disease	*Strep. pneumoniae, Haemophilus influenzae, Moraxella catarrhalis, Chlamydia pneumoniae, Legionella* spp.
Sickle cell disease	*Strep. pneumoniae*
Pneumonia complicating whooping cough	*Bordatella pertussis*
Pneumonia complicating influenza	*Strep. pneumoniae, S. aureus*
Pneumonia severe enough to necessitate artificial ventilation	*Strep. pneumoniae, Legionella* spp., *S. aureus, Haemophilus influenzae, Mycoplasma pneumoniae,* enteric gram negative bacilli, *Chlamydia pneumoniae, Mycobacterium tuberculosis,* viral infection, endemic fungi
Nursing home residency	Gram negative bacilli, *Strep. pneumoniae, H. influenzae, S. aureus,* anaerobes, *Chlamydia pneumoniae*
Poor dental hygiene	Anaerobes
Suspected large volume aspiration	Anaerobes
Structural disease of lung (e.g. bronchiectasis, cystic fibrosis)	*Pseudomonas aeruginosa, Burkholderia cepacia, S. aureus*
Intravenous drug addict	*S. aureus,* anaerobes, *M. tuberculosis, Strep. pneumoniae*
Others	
Epidemic	*Mycoplasma pneumoniae,* influenza virus
Air-conditioning cooling towers, hot tubs	*Legionella pneumophilia*

Liver function tests
Blood cultures (×2)
Sputum

Sputum (if immediately available) for urgent gram stain, culture and pneumococcal antigen. The usefulness of sputum tests remains debatable because of contamination by upper respiratory tract commensals. However, a single or predominant organism on a gram stain of a fresh sample or a heavy growth on culture of purulent sputum is likely to be the organism responsible. The finding of many polymorphonuclear cells (PMN) with no bacteria in a patient who has not already received antibiotics can reliably exclude infection by most ordinary bacterial pathogens.

Specimens should be obtained by deep cough and be grossly purulent. Ideally, the specimen should be obtained before treatment with antimicrobials, and be transported to the laboratory immediately for prompt processing to minimize the chance of missing fastidious organisms (e.g. *Strep. pneumoniae*). Acceptable specimens (in patients with normal or raised white blood cell counts) should contain >25 PMN per low power field (LPF) and <10–25 squamous epithelial cells (SEC)/LPF or >10 PMN per SEC. These criteria should not be used for *Mycobacteria* and *Legionella* infection.

Certain organisms are virtually always pathogens when recovered from respiratory secretions (Table 31.2).

Patients with risk factors for tuberculosis (TB) (see Table 31.6) and particularly those with cough for more than a month, other common symptoms of TB and suggestive radiographic changes should have sputum examined for acid-fast bacilli.

Sputum cannot be processed for culture for anaerobes due to contamination by the endogenous anaerobic flora of the upper respiratory tract. In addition to the factors listed in Table 31.1, foul smelling sputum, lung abscess and empyema should raise suspicion of anaerobic infection.

Table 31.2 Organisms which are virtually always pathogens when recovered from respiratory secretions[10]

Legionella
Chlamydia
TB
Influenza, para-influenza virus, RSV, adenovirus, Hantavirus
Stronglyoides stercoralis
Toxoplasma gondii
Pneumocystis carinii
Histoplasma capsulatum
Coccidiodes immitis
Blastomycoses dermatitidis
Cryptococcus neoformans

ASPIRATION OF PLEURAL FLUID

Aspiration of pleural fluid for gram stain, culture, pH and leukocyte count if there is a pleural effusion >1 cm thick on a lateral decubitus CXR.

URINARY *LEGIONELLA* ANTIGEN

This test is specific (>95%) but only moderately sensitive (50–60%) for detection of *L. pneumophilia* serogroup 1 (the most commonly reported cause of legionella infection). Thus a positive result is virtually diagnostic of *Legionella* infection but a negative result does not exclude it.

HIV SEROLOGICAL STATUS
FIBREOPTIC BRONCHOSCOPY

Fibreoptic bronchoscopy with quantitative culture of samples retrieved by bronchoalveolar lavage or protected specimen brushing is a useful technique (Table 31.3), but its exact role is not well defined. Its use has been recommended for patients with a fulminant course, who require ICU admission or have complex pneumonia unresponsive to antimicrobial therapy.

MANAGEMENT

GENERAL SUPPORTIVE MEASURES

Give intravenous fluids to correct dehydration and provide maintenance fluid. Provide organ support with an emphasis on correcting hypoxia.

ANTIMICROBIAL REGIMES

Ideally each ICU should have its own regimens tailored to the local flora and antibiotic resistance patterns. In the absence of such regimes, those in Tables 31.4 and 31.5 may be helpful. These should be modified in the light of risk factors (Table 31.1). There is controversy regarding the appropriate change to empiric therapy based on the sputum gram stain findings. The ATS recommends broadening antimicrobial cover while the IDSA recommends narrowing it.[5,10] There is also controversy regarding the treatment of drug resistant *Streptococcus pneumoniae* (DRSP).[5,13] For isolates with a penicillin MIC ≤2 mg/l, the regimens in Table 31.4 are probably suitable. If the MIC is 4 mg/l or greater an antipneumococcal fluoroquinolone or clindamycin should be given with vancomycin reserved for patients who are failing other therapies. Linezolid, a new oxazoldinone antibacterial, and quinupristin-dalfopristin, a new streptogramin combination, are also active against DRSP.[14,15]

The role of the newer anti-virals (zanamivir, oseltamivir) in severe influenza pneumonia is not clear. Treatment of patients with less severe symptoms results in a reduction of the duration of symptoms if treatment is started within 48 h from onset.[16]

Table 31.3 Procedure for obtaining microbiological samples using bronchoscopy and protected specimen brushing and/or bronchoalveolar lavage[12]

General recommendations	Suction through the endotracheal tube should be performed before bronchoscopy
	Avoid suction through the working channel of the bronchoscope
	Perform protected specimen brushing before bronchoalveolar lavage
Ventilated patients	Set FiO$_2$ at 1.0
	Set peak pressure alarm at a level that allows adequate ventilation
	Titrate ventilator settings against exhaled tidal volume
	Consider neuromuscular blockade in addition to sedation in patients at high risk of complications who are undergoing prolonged bronchoscopy
Protected specimen brushing (PSB)	Sample the consolidated segment of lung at subsegmental level
	If purulent secretions are not seen advance the brush until it can no longer be seen but avoid wedging it in a peripheral position
	Move brush back and forth and rotate it several times
Bronchoalveolar lavage (BAL)	Wedge tip of bronchoscope into a subsegment of the consolidated segment of lung. If there is no obvious target area, choose non-dependent lung (e.g. upper lobe) for better return of BAL fluid.
	Inject, aspirate and collect 20 ml of sterile isotonic saline. Do not use this sample for quantitative microbiology or identification of intracellular organisms. It can be used for other microbiological analysis
	Inject, aspirate and collect additional aliquots of 20–60 ml
	The total volume of saline injected can be 60–200 ml
Complications	Hypoxaemia (possibly less with smaller BAL volumes)
	Arrhythmia
	Transient worsening in pulmonary infiltrates
	Bleeding (particularly following PSB)
	Fever (more common after BAL)
Positive results	>5% of cells in cytocentrifuge preparations of BAL fluid contain intracellular bacteria OR
	$\geq 10^3$ colony forming units/ml in PSB specimen OR
	$\geq 10^4$ colony forming units/ml in BAL fluid

DURATION OF THERAPY

There are no clinical trials that have specifically addressed this issue. *Strep. pneumoniae* pneumonia should probably be treated until the patient has been afebrile for 72 h. Pneumonia due to organisms that cause pulmonary necrosis (e.g. *S. aureus, P. aeruginosa, Klebsiella* and anaerobes), *M. pneumoniae, C. pneumoniae* or *Legionella* should probably be treated for at least 2 weeks.

RESPONSE TO THERAPY[10,17]

This can be assessed subjectively (a response is usually seen within 1–3 d of starting therapy) or objectively on the basis of respiratory symptoms, fever, oxygenation, WBC count, bacteriology and CXR changes. The average time to defeverscence varies with organism, severity and patient age. It is 7 d in elderly patients, 2.5 d in young patients with pneumococcal pneumonia, 6–7 d in bacteraemic patients with pneumococcal pneumonia, 1–2 d in patients with *M. pneumoniae* pneumonia and 5 d in patients with *Legionella* pneumonia. Both blood

and sputum cultures are usually negative within 24–48 h of treatment, although *P. aeruginosa* and *M. pneumoniae* may persist in the sputum despite effective therapy. CXR changes lag behind clinical changes with the speed of change depending on the organism, the age of the patient and the presence and absence of comorbid illnesses. The CXR changes of most young or middle-aged patients with bacteraemic pneumococcal pneumonia have resolved by 4 weeks, but the percentage of elderly patients or patients with underlying illness or patients with extensive pneumonia on presentation who have CXR resolution by 4 weeks is only 20–30%. Only 55% of patients with *Legionella pneumophilia* pneumonia have CXR resolution by 12 weeks.

If the patient fails to respond consider the following questions:

- Has the patient got pneumonia?
- Are there host factors which explain the failure (e.g. obstruction of bronchus by a foreign body or tumour, inadequate host response)?

Table 31.4 Antibiotic regimens for treatment of community acquired pneumonia in hospitalized patients[5]

Type of patient	Recommended antibacterials
General medical ward	Extended spectrum cephalosporin (e.g. cefotaxime, ceftriaxone) plus macrolide (e.g. erythromycin or clarithromycin) OR
	β-lactam/β-lactamase inhibitor (e.g. ampicillin/sulbactam) plus macrolide OR
	antipneumococcal fluoroquinolone (e.g. levofloxacin)
Intensive care unit	
No special risk factors	Dual therapy with one of: extended spectrum cephalosporin or β-lactam/β-lactamase inhibitor plus: macrolide or antipneumococcal fluoroquinolone
Risk of *P. aeruginosa* infection: bronchiectasis, >7 d of broad spectrum antibiotics in past month, malnutrition, diseases/therapies associated with neutrophil dysfunction (e.g. >10 mg/day prednisolone)	Antipseudomonal β-lactam (e.g. piperacillin, carbapenem or cefepime) plus antipseudomonal fluoroquinolone (e.g. ciprofloxacin) OR
	Antipseudomonal β-lactam plus aminoglycoside plus macrolide or intravenous non antipseudomonal fluoroquinolone
β-lactam allergy	Antipneumococcal fluoroquinolone ± clindamycin
Suspected aspiration	Antipneumococcal fluoroquinolone ± clindamycin OR
	Metronidazole OR
	β-lactam/β-lactamase inhibitor
Risk of *S. aureus* infection	Add flucloxacillin/cloxacillin

- Has a complication developed (e.g. empyema, superinfection)?
- Is the right drug being given in an adequate dose by the right route?
- Is the organism resistant to the drug being given?
- Are there other organisms?

ADMISSION TO ICU

This will largely be determined by the need for organ support, however, the presence of two of the following should also prompt admission: systolic blood pressure ≤90 mmHg, multilobar disease, PaO_2/FiO_2 ratio <250 (PaO_2 in mmHg).[18]

HOSPITAL ACQUIRED PNEUMONIA

This occurs in 0.5–5% of hospital patients, with a higher incidence in certain groups, e.g. postoperative patients and patients in ICU. Diagnosis may be difficult: the clinical features of pneumonia are nonspecific and many non-infectious conditions (e.g. atelectasis, pulmonary embolus, aspiration, congestive heart failure and cancer) can cause infiltrates on a CXR. Identification of the organism responsible is even more difficult than in patients with community acquired pneumonia due to the high incidence of colonization of the oropharynx by gram negative bacteria. Approximately 30–40% of non-critically ill patients become colonized within 48 h, while the figure for moribund and chronically ill patients is

about 70–75%. Blood cultures are only positive in about 6% of cases of nosocomial pneumonia. Ventilator associated pneumonia is nosocomial pneumonia occurring in a mechanically ventilated patient.[19] It is associated with a higher incidence of *P. aeruginosa* and *Acinetobacter* spp. infection.[1]

PATHOGENESIS

Nosocomial pneumonia is thought to result from micro-aspiration of bacteria colonizing the upper respiratory tract. The upper airway of 75% of critically ill patients is colonized by enteric gram negative bacilli,[1] and micro-aspiration occurs in 45% of humans when asleep.[20] Other routes of infection include macro-aspiration of gastric contents, inhaled aerosols, haematogenous spread, spread from pleural space and direct innoculation from ICU personnel.

CLINICAL DIAGNOSIS

Hospital acquired pneumonia is defined on the basis of time of onset (developing more than 2–3 d after admission to hospital),[1] CXR changes (new or progressive infiltrates) and either clinical features and simple laboratory investigations or the results of quantitative microbiology. Using a clinical approach, pneumonia is diagnosed by the finding of a new infiltrate or a change in an infiltrate on CXR and growth of pathogenic organisms from sputum plus one of the following: WBC count

Table 31.5 Recommendations for empiric antimicrobial treatment of hospital acquired pneumonia (HAP). (MRSA, methicillin resistant *S. aureus*; MSSA, methicillin sensitive *S. aureus*)

Situation	Likely organisms	Antibiotics	Comments
Mild/moderate HAP (with no unusual risk factors, onset at any time) OR **Severe HAP** (early onset)	Core organisms: enteric gram negative bacteria (excluding *Pseudomonas aeruginosa*), *Haemophilus influenzae*, MSSA, *Strep. pneumoniae*	Core antibiotics (2nd or non-pseudomonal 3rd generation cephalosporin or β-lactam/β-lactamase inhibitor) Fluoroquinolone (e.g. mofifloxacin) can be used for penicillin-hypersensitive patients.	If likely organism is *Enterobacter* spp. and a 3rd generation cephalosporin is used, it should be combined with another agent because of risk of *in vivo* β-lactamase production, regardless of *in vitro* results.
Mild/moderate HAP, (risk factors, onset at any time)	Core organisms plus	Core antibiotics plus	
Abdominal surgery or witnessed aspiration	Anaerobes	Clindamycin or β lactam/ β lactamase inhibitor alone	
DM, head trauma, coma, renal failure	*S. aureus*	± Vancomycin until MRSA excluded	
High dose steroids, patient not intubated at onset of HAP	*Legionella*	Macrolide ± rifampicin	
Prolonged ICU stay, steroids, antibiotics, structural lung disease	*P. aeruginosa*	Treat as severe HAP	
Severe HAP (late onset or early onset with risk factors)	Core organisms plus *P. aeruginosa*, *Acinetobacter* ± MRSA	Aminoglycoside or ciprofloxacin ± vancomycin + anti-Pseudomonal penicillin OR β lactam/β lactamase inhibitor OR ceftazidime/ cefoperazone OR imipenem	Initially treat with combination therapy. Review after 2–3 days. If patient improving and cultures do not grow Pseudomonas, resistant Acinetobacter or MRSA it may be reasonable to switch to monotherapy

greater than $12 \times 10^5/l$, core temperature $\geq 38.3°C$, or a positive sputum gram stain with a PMN score of more than two out of four.

INVESTIGATIONS

These are broadly similar to those required in community acquired pneumonia

1 *CXR*: although studies using a histological diagnosis as the gold standard have demonstrated that pneumo-nia may be present despite a normal CXR,[21] most definitions of nosocomial pneumonia require the presence of new persistent infiltrates on a CXR.

2 *Respiratory secretions*: considerable controversy surrounds the need for invasive bronchoscopic sampling (Table 31.3) of respiratory secretions. A randomized controlled trial has demonstrated a reduced 14 d mortality among patients with ventilator associated pneumonia who underwent invasive bronchoscopic sampling, compared with those who were treated using

a non-invasive management strategy.[22] However, the important difference between the two groups may have been the use of quantitative microbiological techniques in the former rather than the use of invasive sampling.[23] Previous data have demonstrated a high correlation between the results of quantitative culture of invasive samples and quantitative culture of tracheal aspirates.[24]

Although tracheal aspirates may predominantly reflect the organisms colonizing the upper airway, they may be useful in indicating which organisms are not responsible for the pneumonia, thus allowing the antimicrobial cover to be narrowed.[1] This interpretation is based on the premise that the predominant route of infection is via the upper respiratory tract. From this it can be assumed that if the organism is not present in the upper respiratory tract, the probability of it being present in the lung parenchyma is low. Certain organisms are virtually always pathogens when recovered from respiratory secretions (Table 31.2).

3 *Blood cultures* identify the aetiological agent in 8–20% of patients. Bacteraemia is associated with a worse prognosis. In 50% of patients with severe hospital acquired pneumonia and positive blood cultures there is another source of sepsis.

MANAGEMENT

Early treatment with antimicrobials that cover all likely pathogens results in a reduction in morbidity and mortality.[7] Until quantitative microbiology is available, the initial selection of antimicrobials is made on the basis of epidemiological clues. The results of microbiological investigations are used to narrow antimicrobial cover later (Table 31.5, Figure 31.1).

DURATION OF THERAPY

Again there are no good data to support any particular recommendation. However, the ATS recommend 14–21 d treatment for *P. aeruginosa or Acinetobacter* spp. pneumonia, multilobar involvement, cavitation or necrotizing gram negative pneumonia and for patients who are malnourished or severely debilitated.[1]

RESPONSE TO THERAPY

Clinical improvement is usually not apparent for 48–72 h and therapy should not be changed in this time. The CXR is of limited value for assessing response: initial deterioration is common and improvement often lags behind clinical response. However, a rapidly deteriorating CXR pattern with a >50% increase in size of infiltrate in 48 h, new cavitation or a significant new pleural

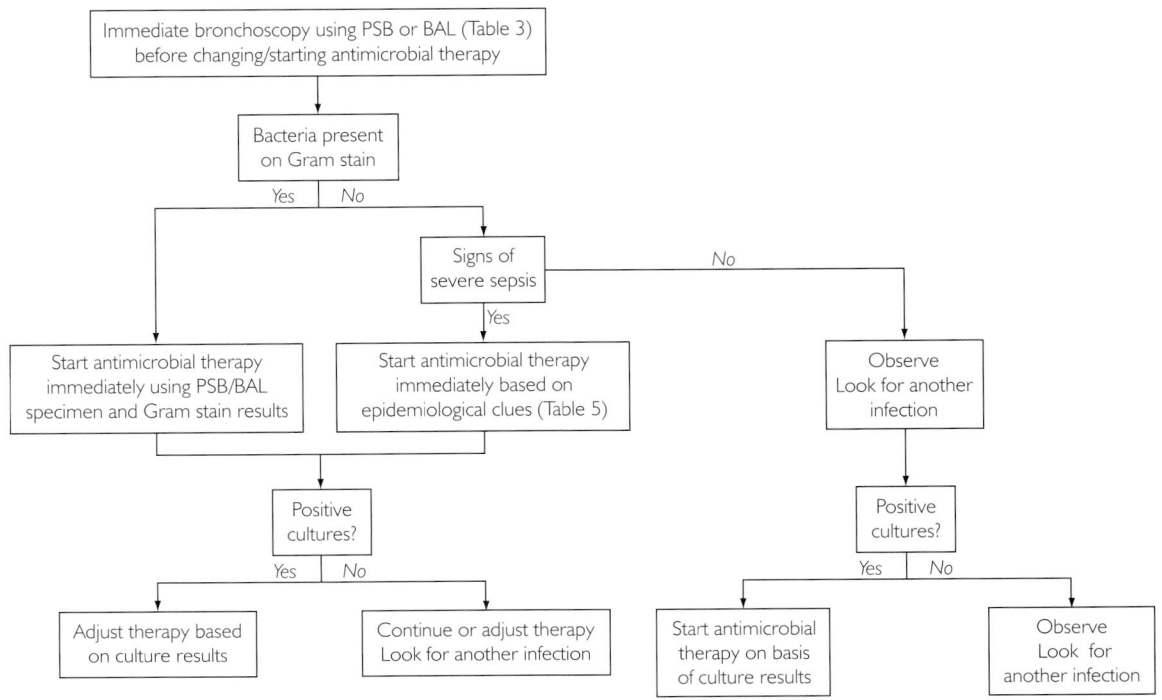

Fig. 31.1 Management of suspected nosocomial pneumonia based on invasive sampling of respiratory secretions.

effusion should raise concern. If a patient fails to respond consider the diagnosis, host factors (e.g. immunosuppressed, debilitated), bacterial factors (e.g. virulent organism) and therapeutic factors (e.g. wrong drug, inadequate dose). Review the antibiotics and repeat cultures. Consider invasive sampling of respiratory secretions, computerized tomography or ultrasound of the chest (to look for an empyema or abscess), another source of infection, open lung biopsy to establish diagnosis and aetiology, or administration of steroids.

PREVENTION

Measures that reduce the incidence of ventilator associated pneumonia include hand washing, nursing patients in a 30° head up position,[25] selective gut decontamination,[26-28] non-invasive ventilation[29,30] and use of sucralfate instead of H_2 antagonists.[31] Measures that are less clearly demonstrated to be beneficial include subglottic aspiration of secretions, use of closed suction systems, lateral rotational bed therapy and use of heat and moisture exchangers, instead of heated water humidifiers.[32-34] (The Centers for Disease Control (CDC) guidelines for prevention of nosocomial pneumonia can be found at: http://aepo-xdv-www.epo.cdc.gov/wonder/prevguid/m0045365/m0045365.asp.)

TUBERCULOSIS

The main risk factors are listed in Table 31.6. Typical clinical features include fever, sweating, weight loss, lassitude, anorexia, cough productive of mucoid or purulent sputum, haemoptysis, chest wall pain, dyspnoea, localized wheeze and apical crackles. Patients may also present with unresolved pneumonia, pleural effusions, spontaneous pneumothorax and hoarseness or with enlarged cervical nodes or other manifestations of extrapulmonary disease. Clinical disease is seldom found in

Table 31.6 Risk factors for pulmonary tuberculosis

Living in or originating from a developing country
Age (<5 years, middle-aged and elderly men)
Alcoholism and/or drug addiction
HIV infection
Diabetes mellitus
Lodging house dwellers
Immunosuppression
Close contact with smear positive patients
Silicosis
Poverty and/or malnutrition
Previous gastrectomy
Smoking

asymptomatic individuals, even those with strongly positive tuberculin test (Heaf grade III or IV). Older patients, who may have co-existent chronic bronchitis, can be missed unless a CXR is taken. The outlook of patients with tuberculosis who require ICU admission is poor. In one retrospective study, the in-hospital mortality for all patients with tuberculosis requiring ICU admission was 67%, but in those with acute respiratory failure it rose to 81%.[35] The presentation and management of TB in HIV positive patients is different (see below).

INVESTIGATION OF PULMONARY TUBERCULOSIS

ISOLATION OF MYCOBACTERIA[36]

Multiple (3–6) sputum samples should be collected, preferably on different days, for microscopy for acid-fast bacilli and culture. If sputum is not available bronchial washings taken at bronchoscopy and gastric lavage or aspirate samples should be obtained. Gastric aspirates need to be neutralized immediately on collection. Bronchoscopy and transbronchial biopsy may be useful in patients with suspected TB but negative sputum smear. Pleural biopsy is often helpful and mediastinoscopy is occasionally needed in patients with mediastinal lymphadenopathy. Part of any biopsy specimen should always be sent for culture. (Further details of the collection and processing of specimens can be obtained from http://www.cdc.gov/nchstp/tb/pubs/1376.pdf.)

CXR

A normal CXR almost excludes TB (except in HIV infected patients), but endobronchial lesions may not be apparent and early apical lesions can be missed. Common appearances include patchy/nodular shadowing in the upper zones (often bilateral), cavitation, calcification, hilar or mediastinal lymphadenopathy (which may cause segmental or lobar collapse), pleural effusion, tuberculomas (dense round or oval shadows) and diffuse fine nodular shadowing throughout the lung fields in miliary TB. Inactivity of disease cannot be inferred from the CXR alone. This requires three negative sputum samples *and* failure of any lesion seen on CXR to progress. CXR appearances in HIV positive patients with TB differ from non-HIV infected patients.

TREATMENT OF PULMONARY TB[37,38]

The most commonly used regimen consists of a 6-month course of rifampicin, 600 mg daily (450 mg for patients <50 kg) and isoniazid 300 mg daily plus a 2-month course of pyrazinamide 2 g daily (1.5 g for patients <50 kg) and ethambutol 15 mg/kg daily (streptomycin can be substituted for ethambutol). Ethambutol should only be used in patients who have reasonable visual acuity, and who are able to appreciate and report visual disturbances. Visual acuity and colour perception must be assessed (if ethambutol is to be used) and liver and renal function checked before treatment is started. Steroids are recommended for children with endobronchial disease and, possibly, for patients with tuberculous pleural effusions. Pyrazinamide 10 mg daily should be given to prevent isoniazid induced neuropathy to those at increased risk (e.g. patients with diabetes mellitus, chronic renal failure, malnutrition, or alcoholic or HIV positive patients). (Further details and recommendations for managing adverse reactions can be obtained from http: //www.brit-thoracic.org.uk/ pdf/ Chemotherapy.pdf.)

INFECTION CONTROL

The CDC recommend that patients with infectious TB or suspected of having active pulmonary TB should be managed in an isolation room with special ventilation characteristics, including negative pressure. Patients should be considered infectious if they are coughing or undergoing cough-inducing procedures, or if they have positive AFB smears and they are not on or have just started chemotherapy or have a poor clinical or bacteriologic response to chemotherapy. Hospitalized patients with active TB should be monitored for relapse by having sputum AFB smears examined every 2 weeks.[39] The United Kingdom guidelines recommend isolation of patients who are sputum smear positive. Patients whose bronchial washings are smear positive should also be isolated if they are on a ward with immunocompromised patients or if they are known/suspected of having multi-drug resistant tuberculosis. Patients with non-drug resistant TB should be non-infectious after 2 weeks of treatment which includes rifampicin and isoniazid.[40] As TB is spread through aerosols it is probably appropriate to isolate patients who are intubated even if only their bronchial washings are smear positive. Staff who have undertaken mouth-mouth resuscitation without appropriate protection, prolonged care of a high dependency patient or repeated chest physiotherapy on a patient with undiagnosed respiratory tuberculosis should be managed as close close contacts.[40] (For details see http: //www.brit-thoracic.org.uk/pdf/TB.pdf.)

PNEUMONIA IN THE IMMUNOCOMPROMISED SUBJECT

The lungs are among the most frequent target organs for infectious complications in the immunocompromised subject, and pneumonia is highest among patients with haematological malignancies, bone marrow transplant (BMT) recipients and patients with AIDS.

The speed of progression of pneumonia, the CXR changes (Table 31.7) and the type of immune defect provide clues to the aetiology. Bacterial pneumonias progress rapidly (1–2 d), while fungal and protozoal

Table 31.7 Likely aetiology of pneumonia in the immunocompromised subject based on CXR features

Causes of focal infiltrates:	Gram negative rods
	Staph. aureus
	Aspergillus
	Malignancy
	Non-specific interstitial pneumonitis
	Cryptococcus
	Nocardia
	Mucormycosis
	Pneumocystis carinii (uncommon)
	Tuberculosis
	Legionella or legionella-like organisms
	Radiation pneumonitis.
Causes of diffuse infiltrates:	CMV and other herpes viruses
	Pneumocystis carinii
	Drug reaction
	Non-specific interstitial pneumonitis
	Bacteria (uncommon)
	Aspergillus (advanced)
	Cryptococcus (uncommon)
	Radiation pneumonitis (uncommon)
	Malignancy
	Leucoagglutinin reaction

pneumonias are less fulminant (several days to a week or more). Viral pneumonias are usually not fulminant but on occasions may develop quite rapidly. Bronchoscopy is a major component of the investigation of these patients.[41] Empiric management based on CXR appearances is outlined in Table 31.8. There is some evidence that early non-invasive ventilation may improve outcome amongst immuncompromised patients with fever and bilateral infiltrates.[42]

PNEUMOCYSTIS CARINII PNEUMONIA

The classical appearance of the CXR is diffuse bilateral perihilar interstitial shadowing, but in the early stages this is very subtle and easily missed. The initial CXR is normal in 10%. In a further 10% the changes are atypical with focal consolidation or coarse patchy shadowing. None of the changes are specific for PCP and may be seen in other lung diseases asssociated with AIDS. Pleural effusions, hilar or mediastinal lymphadenopathy are unusual in PCP but common in mycobacterial infection or Kaposi's sarcoma or lymphoma.

Treatment should be started as soon as the diagnosis is suspected. Azidothymidine should be stopped as both it and anti-PCP treatment are myelotoxic. Treatment of choice is trimethoprim plus sulphamethoxazole (co-trimoxazole) 20 mg/kg per day + 100 mg/kg per day for 3 weeks plus prednisolone 40 mg orally twice daily for 5 d, followed by 20 mg twice daily for 5 d and then 20 mg/d until the end of anti-pneumocystis treatment. Side-effects of cotrimoxazole are common in HIV patients (nausea, vomiting, skin rash, myelotoxicity). The dose should be reduced by 25% if the WBC count falls. Patients who are intolerant of cotrimoxazole should be treated with pentamidine 4 mg/kg per day i.v. plus prednisolone for 3 weeks. Pentamidine has more severe side-effects than co-trimoxazole (hypoglycaemia, hyperglycaemia, pancreatitis, nephrotoxicity, hepatotoxicity). Response to treatment is usually excellent, with a response time of 4–7 d. If the patient deteriorates or fails to improve: consider (re-)bron-choscopy looking for other pathogens, treat co-pathogens and consider a short course of high dose i.v. methylpred-nisolone and/or diuretics (these patients are often fluid overloaded).

Approximately 40% of patients with HIV related PCP who require mechanical ventilation survive to hospital discharge.[43]

BACTERIAL PNEUMONIA

This is the most common cause of acute respiratory failure in HIV positive patients. Bacterial pneumonia is more common in HIV infected patients than in the general population and tends to be more severe. *Strep. pneumoniae*, *H. influenza*, *Branhamella catarrhalis* and *S. aureus* are the common organisms. *Nocardia* and gram negatives should also be considered. Response to appropriate antibiotics is usually good but may require

Table 31.8 Empiric treatment of pneumonia in the immunocompromised subject

Diffuse infiltrate	Broad spectrum antibiotics for at least 48 h (e.g. 3rd generation cephalosporin and aminoglycoside) plus cotrimoxazole. Lung biopsy or lavage within 48 h or full 2-week course of cotrimoxazole (depends on patient tolerance of invasive procedure).
Focal infiltrate	Broad spectrum antibiotics. If response seen continue treatment for 2 weeks. If disease progresses lung biopsy/aspirate within 48–72 h, or empiric trial of amphotericin B (or fluconazole) ± erythromycin.

protracted courses of antibiotics because of a high tendency to relapse.

TUBERCULOSIS

TB may be the initial presentation of AIDS, particularly in sub-Saharan Africa. The pattern of TB in HIV positive patients is more commonly lymphatic or disseminated, and pulmonary disease is more commonly non-cavitatory and sputum smear-negative. It often presents with unusual features and the more immunosuppressed the patient the more atypical the presentation. The CXR often shows atypical features and the tuberculin test may be negative. Response to treatment is usually rapid. Complex interactions occur between rifamycins (e.g. rifampicin and rifabutin) and protease inhibitors and nonnucleosidase reverse transcriptase inhibitors used to treat patients infected with HIV. The choice of rifampicin or rifabutin depends on a number of factors including the unique and synergistic adverse effects for each individual combination of rifamycin and anti-HIV drugs and consultation with a physician with experience in treating both TB and HIV is advised.[44] (Information regarding the various interactions can be obtained from http://www.cdc.gov/mmwr/PDF/wk/mm4909.pdf (pp. 13–16)). The UK recommendations (1998) state that patients with HIV-related TB should be given standard therapy unless multi-drug resistant TB is suspected,[37] however, these guidelines pre-date the CDC recommendations.[44]

CYTOMEGALOVIRUS PNEUMONITIS

Risk of infection is highest following allogeneic stem cell transplantation, followed by lung transplantation, pancreas transplantation and then liver, heart and renal transplantation, and advanced AIDS.[45,46] If both the recipient and the donor are seronegative, then the risk of both infection and disease are negligible. If the recipient is seropositive the risk of infection is approximately 70%, but the risk of disease is only 20%, regardless of the serostatus of the donor. However, if the recipient is seronegative and the donor is seropositive the risk of disease is 70%. If steroid pulses and anti-lymphocyte globulin are given for treatment of acute rejection the risk of developing disease is markedly increased. Infection may be the result of primary infection or reactivation of latent infection. It is clinically important, but often difficult, to distinguish between CMV infection and CMV disease and a definitive diagnosis can only be made histologically. Detection of CMV-pp65 antigen in peripheral white blood cells (WBC) and detection of CMV DNA or RNA in the blood by quantitative polymerase chain reaction are the most useful tests for demonstrating CMV disease. Varying thresholds (10/50 000–100/200 000 positive circulating peripheral WBC) are used for CMV-pp65. Treatment consists of intravenous ganciclovir for at least 14 d. Foscarnet can be used if ganciclovir fails.

FUNGAL PNEUMONIA

Fungi are rare but important causes of pneumonia. They can be divided into two main groups, based on the immune response required to combat infection with these organisms. Histoplasma, blastomycosis, coccidioidomycosis, paracoccidioidomycosis and cryptococcus require specific cell-mediated immunity for their control and thus, in contrast to infections which are controlled by phagocytic activity, the diseases caused by these organisms can occur in otherwise healthy individuals although they cause much more severe illness in patients with impaired cell mediated immunity (e.g. patients infected with HIV and organ transplant recipients). With the exception of cryptococcus these organisms are rarely seen outside North America. Aspergillus and mucormycosis spores are killed by non-immune phagocytes and as a result these fungi rarely result in clinical illness in patients with normal neutrophil numbers and function.

CANDIDIASIS

This is effectively a combination of the two types of fungal infection in that impaired cell-mediated immunity predisposes to mucosal overgrowth with Candida but impaired phagocytic function or numbers is usually required before deep invasion of tissues occurs. Primary Candida pneumonia (i.e. isolated lung infection) is uncommon[41,45,47] and more commonly pulmonary lesions are only one manifestation of disseminated candidiasis. Even more common is benign colonization of the airway with *Candida*. In most reported cases of primary *Candida* pneumonia amphotericin B has been used. In disseminated candidiasis treatment should be directed to treatment of disseminated disease rather than *Candida* pneumonia *per se*.[47]

INVASIVE ASPERGILLOSIS

This is a highly lethal condition in the immunocompromised, despite treatment; therefore investigation and treatment should be prompt and aggressive.[48] Definitive diagnosis requires both histological evidence of acute-angle branching, septated non-pigmented hyphae, measuring 2–4 μm in width, and cultures yielding *Aspergillus* species from biopsy specimens of involved organs. In immunocompromised, but not immunocompetent, patients recovery of *Aspergillus* species from respiratory secretions may indicate inva-

sive disease with a positive predictive value as high as 80–90% in patients with leukaemia or bone marrow transplant recipients. Bronchoalveolar lavage with smear, culture and antigen detection has excellent specificity and reasonably good positive predictive value for invasive aspergillosis in immunocompromised patients. Although radiological features may give a clue to the diagnosis they are not sufficiently specific to be diagnostic. Characteristic CXR features (wedge-shaped, pleural-based densities or cavities) occur late. The 'halo sign' (area of low attenuation surrounding a nodular lung lesion) is an early CT finding while the 'crescent sign' (an air crescent near the periphery of a lung nodule), is a late feature.

In acutely ill immunocompromised patients, intravenous therapy should be initiated if there is suggestive evidence of invasive aspergillosis while further investigations to confirm or refute the diagnosis are carried out. Standard therapy consists of amphotericin B at maximum tolerated doses (1–1.5 mg/kg per d). This should be continued, even in the face of moderate rises in serum creatinine. Lipid formulations of amphotericin are indicated for those patients who have impaired renal function or who develop nephrotoxicity while receiving the standard formulation.

PARAPNEUMONIC EFFUSION

Parapneumonic effusion[49] may be an uncomplicated effusion which resolves with appropriate treatment of the underlying pneumonia or a complicated effusion which develops into an empyema, unless drained. Complicated effusions tend to develop 7–14 d after initial fluid formation. They are characterized by increasing pleural fluid volume, continued fever and pleural fluid of low pH (<7.3), which contains a large number of neutrophils and may reveal organisms on Gram staining or culture. An outline of management is given in Figure 31.2.

EMPYEMA

DEFINITION

The common definition of empyema[50] is the collection of pus in the pleural space.

AETIOLOGY

Aetiology follows infection of the structures surrounding the pleural space, including subdiaphragamatic structures, and chest trauma or may be associated with malignancy. Anaerobic bacteria, usually streptococci or gram negative rods are responsible for 76% of cases.

DIAGNOSIS

The diagnosis is usually simple. The patient is usually 'toxic' and may have a productive cough and chest pain. The chest X-ray may show features suggestive of a pleural effusion and underlying consolidation, but may also show an abscess cavity with a fluid level in which case CT scanning will be required to distinguish between an abscess and an empyema. Ultrasound can be useful to confirm the presence of fluid in the pleural space and to determine whether it can be drained by needle aspiration or, if there is debris within the fluid, requires drainage using an intercostal drain. The diagnosis is confirmed by aspiration of pus.

TREATMENT

The mainstay of treatment is drainage, either by intercostal drain or by surgical intervention. Patients who present before the pus is loculated and a fibrinous peel has formed on the lung can usually be treated by simple drainage. Optimal surgical management, which consists of decortication (open or thoracoscopic), is indicated if the empyema is more advanced, or if simple drainage fails. This is a major procedure and many patients with cardiac or chronic respiratory disease will not tolerate it. Alternatives for these patients are instillation of thrombolytics into the pleural space or thoracostomy. Antibiotics have only an adjunctive role. Broad spectrum antibiotic regimes with anaerobic cover should be used until the results of microbiological analysis of the aspirated pus are available.

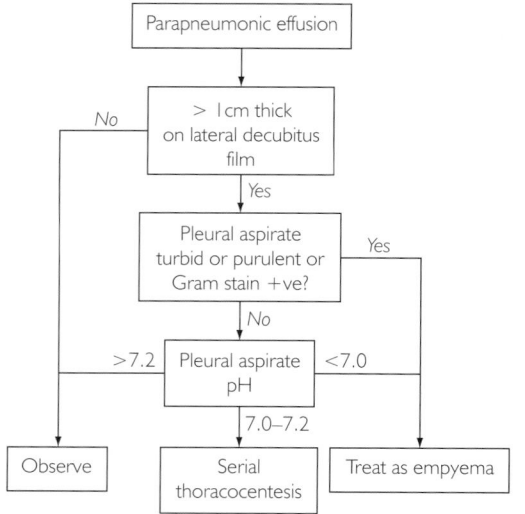

Fig. 31.2 An approach to the management of parapneumonic effusions.[49]

REFERENCES

1 American Thoracic Society. Hospital-acquired pneumonia in adults: diagnosis, assessment of severity, initial antimicrobial therapy, and preventative strategies. A consensus statement. *Am J Respir Crit Care Med* 1995; **153**: 1711–25.

2 Mandell LA, Marrie TJ, Grossman RF, *et al*. Canadian guidelines for the initial management of community-acquired pneumonia: an evidence-based update by the Canadian Infectious Diseases Society and the Canadian Thoracic Society. *Clin. Infect Dis* 2001; **31**: 383–421.

3 Farr BM, Kaiser DL, Harrison BD, *et al*. Prediction of microbial aetiology at admission to hospital for pneumonia from the presenting clinical features. British Thoracic Society Pneumonia Research Subcommittee. *Thorax* 1989; **44**: 1031–5.

4 Woodhead MA, MacFarlane JT. Comparative clinical and laboratory features of legionella with pneumococcal and mycoplasma pneumonias. *Brit J Dis Chest* 1987; **81**: 133–9.

5 American Thoracic Society. Guidelines for the management of adults with community-acquired pneumonia. *Am J Respir Crit Care Med* 2001; **163**: 1730–54; http://www.thoracic.org/adobe/statements/commacq1-25.pdf.

6 Fang GD, Fine M, Orloff J, *et al*. New and emerging etiologies for community-acquired pneumonia with implications for therapy. A prospective multicenter study of 359 cases. *Medicine* (Baltimore) 1990; **69**: 307–16.

7 Dupont H, Mentec H, Sollet JP, *et al*. Impact of appropriateness of initial antibiotic therapy on the outcome of ventilator-associated pneumonia. *Intensive Care Med* 2001; **27**: 355–362; http://link.springer.de/link/service/journals/00134/papers/1027002/10270355.pdf

8 Rello J, Sa-Borges M, Correa H, *et al*. Variations in etiology of ventilator-associated pneumonia across four treatment sites. Implications for antimicrobial prescribing practices. *Am J Respir Crit Care Med* 1999; **160**: 608–13.

9 Namias N, Samiian L, Nino D, *et al*. Incidence and susceptibility of pathogenic bacteria vary between intensive care units within a single hospital: implications for empiric antibiotic strategies. *J Trauma* 2001; **49**: 638–46.

10 Bartlett JG, Dowell SF, Mandell LA, *et al*. Practice guidelines for the management of community-acquired pneumonia in adults. *Clin Infect Dis* 2000; **31**: 347–82; http://www.journals.uchicago.edu/IDSA/guide/MY56_1042.pdf

11 Venkatesan P, Gladman J, MacFarlane JT, *et al*. A hospital study of community acquired pneumonia in the elderly. *Thorax* 1990; **45**: 254–8.

12 Meduri GU, Chastre J. The standardization of bronchoscopc techniques for ventilator-associated pneumonia. *Chest* 1992; **102**: 557S–64S.

13 Heffelfinger JD, Dowell SF, Jorgensen JH, *et al*. Management of community-acquired pneumonia in the era of pneumococcal resistance: a report from the

Drug-Resistant *Streptococcus pneumoniae* Therapeutic Working Group. *Arch Intern Med* 2000; **160**: 1399–1408; http://archinte.ama-assn.org/issues/v160n10/rpdf/isa90008.pdf

14 Lamb HM, Figgitt DP, Faulds D. Quinupristin/Dalfopristin. A review of its use in the management of serious Gram-positive infections. *Drugs* 1999; **58**: 1061–97.

15 Clemett D, Markham A. Linezolid. *Drugs* 2000; **59**: 815–27.

16 Jefferson T, Demicheli V, Deeks J, *et al.* Neuraminidase inhibitors for preventing and treating influenza in healthy adults (Cochrane Review). In: *The Cochrane Library*. Oxford: Update Software; 2001: Issue 3.

17 O'Grady NP, Barie PS, Bartlett JG, *et al.* Practice guidelines for evaluating new fever in critically ill adult patients. *Clin Infect Dis* 1998; **26**: 1042–59.

18 Ewig S, Ruiz M, Mensa J, *et al.* Severe community-acquired pneumonia: assessment of severity criteria. *Am J Respir Crit Care Med* 1998; **158**: 1102–8.

19 Pingleton GU, Fagon JY, Leeper KV. Patient selection for clinical investigation of ventilator-associated pneumonia; criteria for evaluating diagnostic techniques. *Chest* 1992; **102**: 553S–4S.

20 Huxley EJ, Viroslav J, Gray WR, *et al.* Pharyngeal aspiration in normal adults and patients with depressed consciousness. *Am J Med* 1973; **64**: 564–8.

21 Fàbregas N, Torres A, el-Ebiary M, *et al.* Histopathologic and microbiologic aspects of ventilator-associated pneumonia. *Anesthesiology* 1996; **84**: 760–71.

22 Fagon JY, Chastre J, Wolff M, *et al.* Invasive and non-invasive strategies for management of suspected ventilator-associated pneumonia. A randomized trial. *Ann Intern Med* 2000; **132**: 621–30.

23 Ruiz M, Torres A, Ewig S, *et al.* Noninvasive versus invasive microbial investigation in ventilator-associated pneumonia: evaluation of outcome. *Am J Respir Crit Care Med* 2000; **162**: 119–25.

24 Kirtland SH, Corley DE, Winterbauer RH, *et al.* The diagnosis of ventilator-associated pneumonia. A comparison of histologic, microbiologic, and clinical criteria. *Chest* 1997; **112**: 445–57.

25 Drakulovic MB, Torres A, Bauer TT, *et al.* Supine body position as a risk factor for nosocomial pneumonia in mechanically ventilated patients: a randomised trial. *Lancet* 1999; **354**: 1851–8.

26 Bonten MJ, Kullberg BJ, Van Dalen R, *et al.* Selective digestive decontamination in patients in intensive care. *J Antimicrob Chemother* 2000; **46**: 351–62.

27 Liberati A, D'Amico R, Pifferi S, *et al.* Antibiotics for preventing respiratory tract infections in adults receiving intensive care (Cochrane Review). *The Cochrane Library*. Oxford: Update Software; 2001: Issue 2.

28 Nathens AB, Marshall JC. Selective decontamination of the digestive tract in surgical patients: a systematic review of the evidence. *Arch Surg* 1999; **134**: 170–6.

29 Nourdine K, Combes P, Carton MJ, *et al.* Does noninvasive ventilation reduce the ICU nosocomial infection risk? A prospective clinical survey. *Intensive Care Med* 1999; **25**: 567–73.

30 Guerin C, Girard R, Chemorin C, *et al.* Facial mask noninvasive mechanical ventilation reduces the incidence of nosocomial pneumonia. A prospective epidemiological survey from a single ICU. [erratum appears in *Intensive Care Med* 1998; **24**: 27]. *Intensive Care Med* 1997; **23**: 1024–32.

31 Cook DJ, Reeve BK, Guyatt GH, *et al.* Stress ulcer prophylaxis in critically ill patients. Resolving discordant meta-analyses. *JAMA* 1996; **275**: 308–14.

32 Cook D, De Jonghe B, Brochard L, *et al.* Influence of airway management on ventilator-associated pneumonia: evidence from randomized trials. *JAMA* 1998; **279**: 781–7.

33 Combes P, Fauvage B, Oleyer C. Nosocomial pneumonia in mechanically ventilated patients, a prospective randomised evaluation of the Stericath closed suctioning system. *Intensive Care Med* 2000; **26**: 878–82.

34 Valles J, Artigas A, Rello J, *et al.* Continuous aspiration of subglottic secretions in preventing ventilator-associated pneumonia. *Ann Intern Med* 1995; **122**: 179–86.

35 Frame RN, Johnson MC, Eichenhorn MS, *et al.* Active tuberculosis in the medical intensive care unit: a 15-year retrospective analysis. *Crit Care Med* 1987; **15**: 1012–14.

36 American Thoracic Society and Centers for Disease Control. Diagnostic standards and classification of tuberculosis in adults and children. *Am J Respir Crit Care Med* 2000; **161**: 1376–95; http://www.cdc.gov/nchstp/tb/pubs/1376.pdf

37 Joint Tuberculosis Committee of the British Thoracic Society. Chemotherapy and management of tuberculosis in the United Kingdom: recommendations 1998. *Thorax* 1998; **53**: 536–48; http://www.brit-thoracic.org.uk/pdf/Chemotherapy.pdf

38 Small PM, Fujiwara PI. Management of tuberculosis in the United States. *N Engl J Med* 2001; **345**: 189–200.

39 Centers for Disease Control. Guidelines for preventing the transmission of *Mycobacterium tuberculosis* in health-care facilities, 1994. *Morbidity and Mortality Weekly Report* 1994; **43**: 1–141.

40 Joint Tuberculosis Committee of the British Thoracic Society. Control and prevention of tuberculosis in the United Kingdom: Code of practice 2000. *Thorax* 2000; **55**: 887–901; http://www.brit-thoracic.org.uk/pdf/TB.pdf

41 Baughman RP. The lung in the immunocompromised patient. Infectious complications, Part 1. *Respiration* 1999; **66**: 95–109.

42 Hilbert G, Gruson D, Vargas F, *et al.* Noninvasive ventilation in immunosuppressed patients with pulmonary infiltrates, fever, and acute respiratory failure. *N Engl J Med* 2001; **344**: 481–7.

43 Randall CJ, Yarnold PR, Schwartz DN, *et al.* Improvements in outcomes of acute respiratory failure for patients with human immunodeficiency virus-related Pneumocystis carinii pneumonia. *Am J Respir Crit Care Med* 2000; **162**: 393–8.

44 Centers for Disease Control. Updated guidelines for the use of rifabutin or rifampicin for the treatment and prevention of tuberculosis among HIV-infected patients taking protease inhibitors or nonnucleoside reverse transcriptase inhibitors. *Morbidity and Mortality Weekly Report* 2000; **49**: 185–9.

45 Tamm M. The lung in the immunocompromised patient. Infectious complications, Part 2. *Respiration* 1999; **66**: 199–207.

46 van der Bij W, Speich R. Management of cytomegalovirus infection and disease after solid-organ transplantation. *Clin Infect Dis* 2001; **33**(Suppl 1): S32–S37.

47 Rex JH, Walsh TJ, Sobel JD, *et al*. Practice guidelines for the treatment of candidiasis. Infectious Diseases Society of America. *Clin Infect Dis* 2000; **30**: 662–78.

48 Stevens DA, Kan VL, Judson MA, *et al*. Practice guidelines for diseases caused by *Aspergillus*. *Clin Infect Dis* 2000; **30**: 696–709; http://www.idsociety.org/pg/Asper.pdf

49 Hamm H, Light RW. Parapneumonic effusion and empyema. *Eur Respir J* 1997; **10**: 1150–6.

50 Peek GJ, Morcos S, Cooper G. The pleural cavity. *BMJ* 2000; **320**: 1318–21.

32

Imaging the chest
S P G Padley

RADIOLOGICAL TECHNIQUES

Of the imaging techniques available for investigating patients in the intensive care unit the chest radiograph remains the most important, with ultrasound (US) being utilized in a selected group of patients. High resolution and spiral computed tomography allow further investigation of these patients in certain situations.

CONVENTIONAL CHEST RADIOGRAPHY

The views of the chest most frequently performed in the ambulant patient are the erect postero-anterior (PA) and lateral projections, taken with the patient breath-holding at total lung capacity. While portable or mobile chest radiography, as undertaken on an ICU, has the obvious advantage that the examination can be done without moving the patient from the ward, there are many disadvantages. These include:

- shorter focus-film distance causing magnification
- limited X-ray output necessitating long exposure times with resultant movement blurring
- difficulties with satisfactory patient positioning.

DIGITAL CHEST RADIOLOGY

In the ICU, digital chest radiographs may be obtained utilizing conventional X-ray generators, but the image is captured on a re-usable photostimulable plate instead of conventional film. The digital information is then manipulated, displayed and stored in whatever format is desired. Traditional systems suffer greatly from the large day-to-day variations in the density of the radiograph due to small differences in exposure. Digital radiographic systems are able to capture and display a standard density image from a much wider range of exposures (Figure 32.1).

COMPUTED TOMOGRAPHY

Computed tomography relies on differing absorption of X-rays by tissues with constituents of differing atomic number, so slight differences in X-ray absorption can be interpreted to produce a cross-sectional image. The components of a CT scanner are an X-ray tube, which rotates around the patient, and an array of X-ray detectors opposite the tube. The speed with which a CT scanner acquires an image depends upon the time it takes to rotate the anode around the patient. Modern CT machines have scan times of below 0.5 s.

Spiral (also known as volume or helical) scanning entails sustained patient exposure by the rotating X-ray tube during continuous movement of the examination couch through the CT gantry aperture. In this way, a continuous data set or 'spiral' of information may be acquired in a single breath hold. The information is reconstructed into axial sections, perpendicular to the long axis of the patient, identical to conventional CT sections. Three-dimensional reconstructions of complex anatomical areas can also be produced.

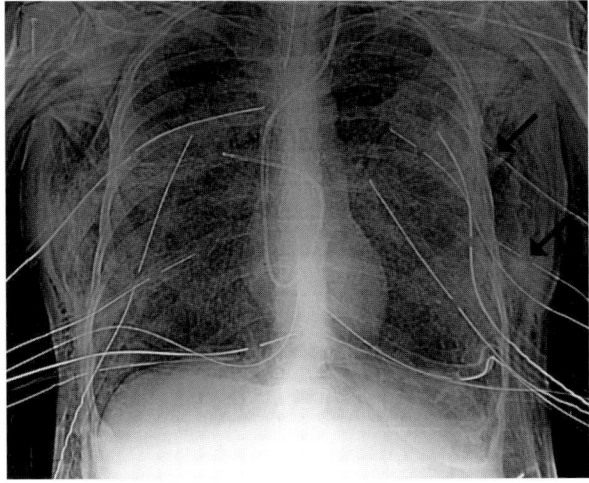

Fig. 32.1 Digital radiograph. The image has been edge enhanced, which makes the multiple chest drains, Swan Ganz catheter and ET tube position more conspicuous. Note that two of the chest drain side holes lie within the soft tissues of the chest wall.

INTRAVENOUS CONTRAST ENHANCEMENT

Because of the high contrast on CT between vessels and surrounding air in the lung, and vessels and surrounding fat within the mediastinum, intravenous contrast enhancement only needs to be given in specific instances, for example to aid the distinction between hilar vessels and a soft tissue mass. The exact timing of the injection of contrast media depends most on the time the CT scanner takes to scan the thorax. Rapid scanning protocols with automated injectors tend to improve contrast enhancement of vascular structures at the expense of enhancement of solid lesions because of the rapidity of scanning. With spiral CT, it is possible to achieve good opacification of all the thoracic vascular structures with small volumes of contrast media. Optimal contrast enhancement of the pulmonary arteries occurs 10–15 s after the start of contrast injection, usually at 3–5 ml/s by a power injector. Timing of image acquisition is vital for accurate diagnosis of pulmonary embolism. However when examining inflammatory lesions, such as the reaction around an empyema, it may be necessary to delay scanning by 30–40 s to allow contrast to diffuse into the extra-vascular space.

HIGH RESOLUTION COMPUTED TOMOGRAPHY

HRCT images of the lung correlate closely with the macroscopic appearances of pathological specimens. In diffuse lung disease, HRCT allows a substantial improvement in diagnostic accuracy compared with chest radiography. Three factors significantly improve the spatial resolution of CT and so confer the description 'high resolution' CT: narrow beam collimation (1.5 mm), a high spatial frequency reconstruction algorithm and a small field of view. The relatively high radiation dose to the patient inherent in all CT scanning needs to be appreciated. However the radiation burden to the patient is considerably less with HRCT than with conventional CT scanning.

CLINICAL APPLICATIONS OF HRCT IN THE ICU PATIENT

HRCT is increasingly being used to confirm the impression of an abnormality seen on a chest radiograph. HRCT may also be used to achieve a histospecific diagnosis in some patients with obvious but non-specific radiographic abnormalities. Furthermore, HRCT has provided a number of useful insights into chest disease in the severely ill patient in an ICU setting.

HRCT IN UNCOMPLICATED ARDS[1]

Reveals that the apparently homogeneous opacification on the chest radiograph has an anterior to posterior graded increase in density – an appearance referred to as a gravitational gradient (Figure 32.2).

Demonstrates early dilatation of the smaller airways within areas of ground glass density, an appearance that

suggests development of fibrosis, and may prompt anti-inflammatory treatment.

Demonstrates that a shift from the supine to the prone position results in redistribution of the previously dependent dense parenchymal opacification to the now dependent anterior lung, a phenomenon that may be accompanied by improvements in patient oxygenation.

HRCT OF COMPLICATIONS OF ARDS[2]

Infection: this is common in ARDS. Diagnosis may be difficult. Radiographically, there may be a lack of specific findings, often due to superimposition of changes attributable to ARDS. This is a particular problem in the critically ill patient when the usual indicators of pneumonia are also unreliable. Although the diagnosis may still be in question following HRCT, associated pneumonic changes such as abscess formation, empyema and mediastinal disease, as well as development of non-dependent areas of consolidation are all useful pointers to super-added infection (Figure 32.2).

Barotrauma: mediastinal and interstitial emphysema, as well as pneumothorax, are all increasingly common at higher levels of peak end-expiratory pressure (PEEP) ventilation.[3] HRCT delineates early change and allows exact location of loculated air collections to be defined.

NORMAL RADIOGRAPHIC ANATOMY

THE MEDIASTINUM, CENTRAL AIRWAYS AND HILAR STRUCTURES

Appreciation of abnormality requires a sound grasp of normal radiological anatomy. The mediastinum is delimited by the lungs on either side, the thoracic inlet

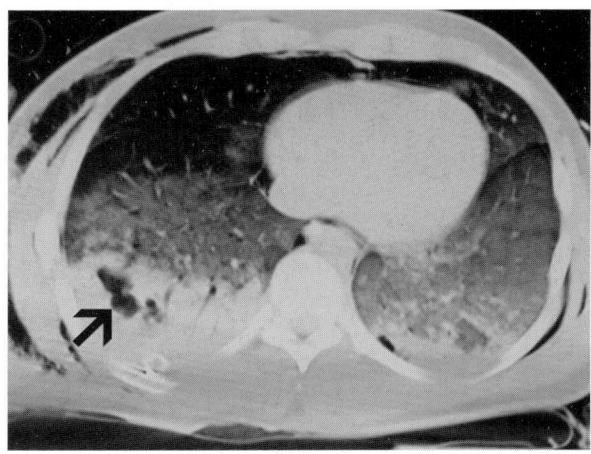

Fig. 32.2   CT of a patient with ARDS. Note the marked anterior to posterior density gradient. There is an area of consolidation posteriorly on the right side and cavitation had developed due to abscess formation (arrow).

above, the diaphragm below and the vertebral column posteriorly. Because the various structures that make up the mediastinum are superimposed on each other on the chest radiograph, they cannot be separately identified. Nevertheless, because a chest radiograph is usually the first imaging investigation, it is necessary to have an appreciation of the normal appearances of the mediastinum, together with variations due to the patient's body habitus and age. Key points include:

- Only the outline of the mediastinum and the air-containing trachea and bronchi (and sometimes oesophagus) are clearly seen on a normal chest radiograph.
- The right superior mediastinal border is formed by the right brachiocephalic vein and superior vena cava, and becomes less distinct as it reaches the thoracic inlet. The right side of the superior mediastinum can appear to be considerably widened in patients with an abundance of mediastinal fat.
- The left mediastinal border above the aortic arch is the result of summation of the left carotid and left subclavian arteries together with the left brachiocephalic and jugular veins.
- The left cardiac border comprises the left atrial appendage which merges inferiorly with the left ventricle. The silhouette of the heart should always be sharply outlined. Any blurring of the border is due to loss of immediately adjacent aerated lung, usually by collapse or consolidation.
- The density of the heart shadow to the left and right of the vertebral column should be identical and any difference indicates pathology (for example, an area of consolidation or a mass in a lower lobe).
- The trachea and main bronchi should be visible through the upper and middle mediastinum.
- In older individuals, the trachea may be displaced by a dilated aortic arch. In approximately 60% of normal subjects, the right wall of the trachea (the right paratracheal stripe) can be identified as a line of uniform thickness (less than 4 mm in width); when it is visible it excludes the presence of an adjacent space occupying lesion, most usually lymphadenopathy.
- The carinal angle is usually less than 80°. Splaying of the carina is an insensitive sign of subcarinal disease, either in the form of massive sub-carinal lymphadenopathy, or a markedly enlarged left atrium.
- The origins of the lobar bronchi, where they are projected over the mediastinal shadow, can usually be identified but the segmental bronchi within the lungs are not generally seen on plain radiography.
- Normal hilar shadows on a chest radiograph represent the summation of the pulmonary arteries and veins.
- The hila are approximately the same size and the left hilum normally lies between 0.5 cm and 1.5 cm above the level of the right hilum. The size and shape of the hila show remarkable variation in normal individuals, making subtle abnormalities difficult to identify.

THE PULMONARY FISSURES, VESSELS AND BRONCHI

The two lungs are separated by the four layers of pleura behind and in front of the mediastinum. The resulting posterior and anterior junction lines are often visible on chest radiographs as nearly vertical stripes, the posterior junction line lying higher than the anterior. The junction lines are not invariably seen and their presence or absence is not usually of significance (Figures 32.3a,b).

The upper and lower lobes of the left lung are separated by the major (or oblique) fissure. The upper, middle and lower lobes of the right lung are separated by the major fissure and the minor (horizontal or transverse) fissure. The minor fissure is visible in over half of normal PA chest radiographs. The major fissures are not visible on a frontal radiograph and are inconstantly identifiable on lateral radiographs. In a few individuals, fissures are incompletely developed; a point familiar to thoracic surgeons performing a lobectomy, because of incomplete cleavage between lobes. Accessory fissures are occasionally seen.

All of the branching structures seen within normal lungs on a chest radiograph represent pulmonary arteries or veins. It is often impossible to distinguish arteries from veins in the lung periphery. On a chest radiograph taken in the erect position, there is a gradual increase in the diameter of the vessels, at equidistant points from the hilum, travelling from lung apex to base; this gravity-dependent effect disappears if the patient is supine or in cardiac failure.

THE DIAPHRAGM AND THORACIC CAGE

The interface between aerated lung and the hemidiaphragms is sharp and the highest point of each dome is normally medial to the mid-clavicular line. The right dome of the diaphragm is higher than the left by up to 2 cm in the erect position unless the left dome is elevated by air in the stomach (Figure 32.4).

Filling in or blunting of these costophrenic angles usually represents pleural disease, either pleural thickening or an effusion.

POSITIONING OF TUBES AND LINES[4]

CENTRAL VENOUS PRESSURE CATHETERS

The end of a CVP line needs to be intrathoracic, and is ideally in the superior vena cava. CVP lines may be introduced via an antecubital, subclavian or jugular vein. Subclavian venous puncture carries a risk of pneumothorax and mediastinal hematoma. Rarely, perforation of the subclavian vein leads to fluid collecting in the mediastinum or pleura. All catheters have a potential risk of coiling, misplacement, knotting and fracture (Figure 32.5). The tip should not abut the vessel wall at an obtuse angle.

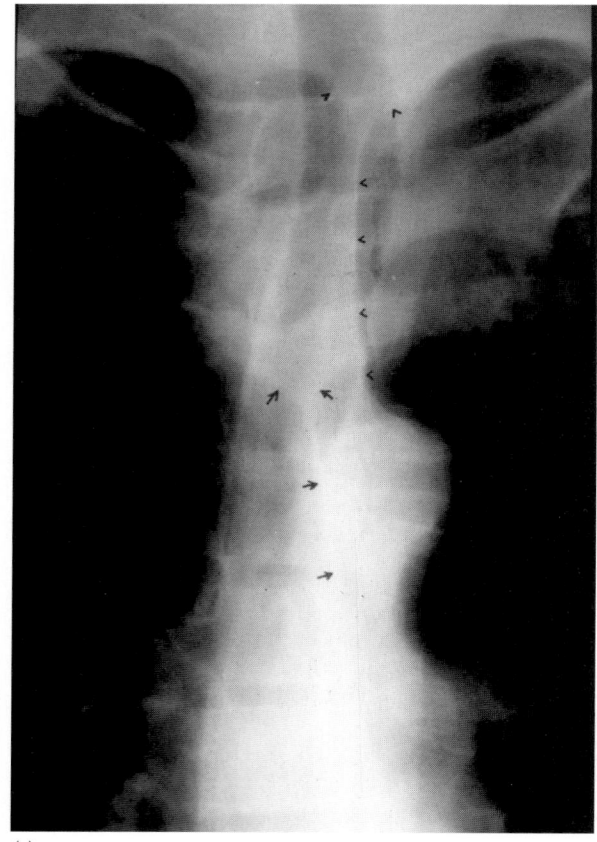

(a)

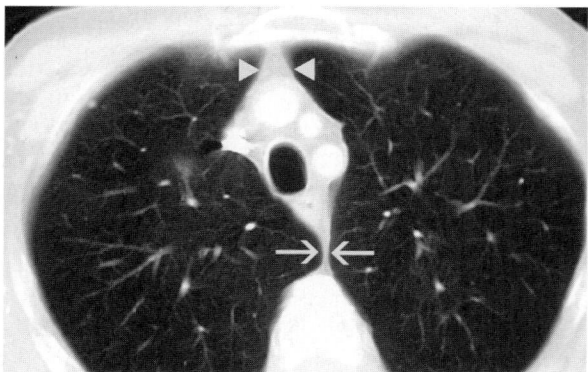

(b)

Fig. 32.3 (a) Close up of the mediastinum of a patient in whom both the anterior and posterior junction lines are evident. The anterior junction line is more inferior and slants from right to left (short arrows), while the posterior junction line is more vertical, superior and is delineated by the arrowheads. (b) CT scan through the upper mediastinum demonstrating the anterior (arrowheads) and posterior (arrows) junction lines in a different patient.

SWAN–GANZ CATHETERS (PULMONARY ARTERY FLOTATION CATHETERS)

Ideally the end of the catheter should be maintained 5–8 cm (2–3 in) beyond the bifurcation of the main pulmonary artery in either the right or left pulmonary artery (Figure 32.5). When the pulmonary wedge pressure is measured the balloon is inflated, and the flow of blood carries the catheter tip peripherally, to a wedged position. After the measurement has been made the balloon is deflated and the catheter returns to a central position, otherwise there is a risk of pulmonary infarction. The inflation balloon is radiolucent. The balloon should normally be kept deflated.

NASOGASTRIC TUBES

These should reach the stomach but may coil in the oesophagus or occasionally are inserted into the tracheobronchial tree (Figure 32.6a,b,c).

ENDOTRACHEAL TUBES

Extension and flexion of the neck may make the tip of an endotracheal tube move by as much as 5 cm. With the neck in neutral position the tip of the tube should

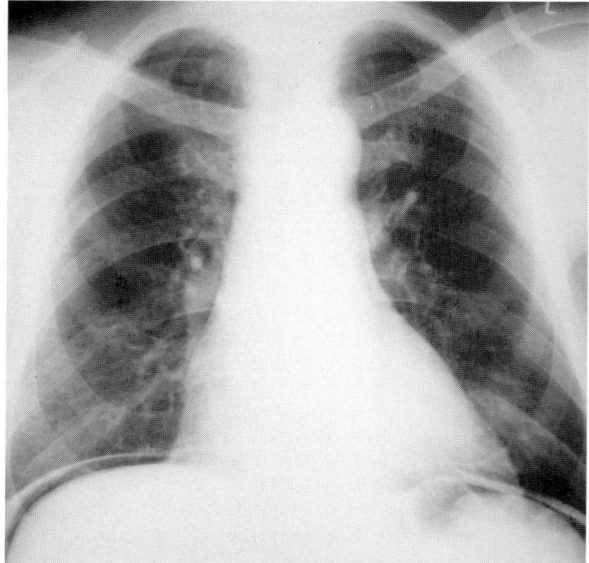

Fig. 32.4 Erect chest radiograph of a patient with a pneumoperitoneum demonstrating the normal thickness in position of the hemidiaphragms. The right lies slightly higher than the left.

ideally be about 5–6 cm above the carina. A tube that is inserted too far usually passes into the right bronchus, with the risk of non-ventilation or collapse of the left lung (Figure 32.7).

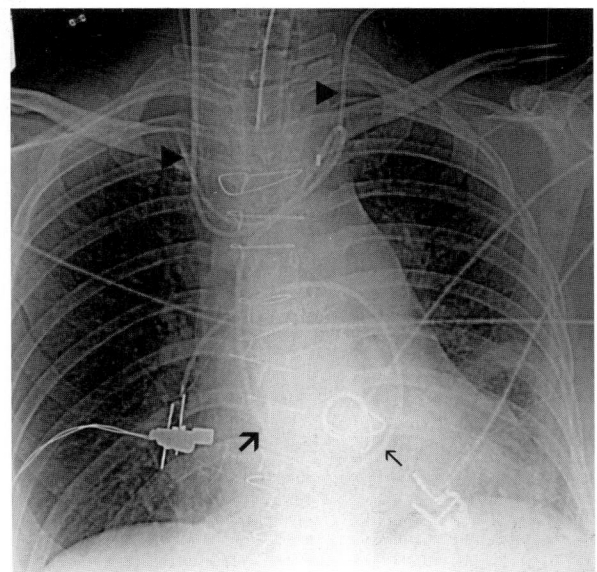

Fig. 32.5 ICU patient with multiple tubes and lines in place. The ET tube tip position is satisfactory, there are sternotomy wires, an intra-aortic balloon pump (radio-opaque tip) and a prosthetic heart valve. The central line inserted into the left internal jugular vein passes into the right internal jugular vein. The Swan Ganz catheter, which has been inserted via the right internal jugular vein, loops into the left brachio-cephalic vein, before taking a satisfactory course through the cardiac chambers (black arrows).

TRACHEOSTOMY TUBES

The tube tip should be situated centrally in the airway at the level of T3. Acute complications of tracheostomy include pneumothorax, pneumomediastinum and subcutaneous emphysema. Long-term complications include tracheal ulceration, stenosis and perforation.

PLEURAL TUBES

These are used to treat pleural effusions and pneumothoraces. A radiopaque line usually runs along pleural tubes, and is interrupted where there are side holes. It is important to check that all the side holes are within the thorax. Tracks may remain on the chest X-ray following removal of chest tubes, causing tubular or ring shadows. When doubt remains about tube position then CT scanning should be considered (Figures 32.1 and 32.8).

MEDIASTINAL DRAINS

These are usually present following sternotomy. Apart from their position, they look like pleural tubes.

INTRA-AORTIC BALLOON PUMP

These are used in patients with cardiogenic shock, often following cardiac surgery. The ideal position of the catheter tip is just distal to the origin of the left subclavian artery (Figure 32.9). If the catheter tip is advanced too far it may occlude the left subclavian artery, and if it is too distal the balloon may occlude branches of the abdominal aorta. The IABP may only be visible by its radio-opaque tip (Figure 32.5).

PACEMAKERS

These may be permanent or temporary (Figure 32.10). Temporary epicardial wires are sometimes inserted during cardiac surgery, and may be seen as thin, almost hair-like metallic opacities overlying the heart. Temporary pacing electrodes are usually inserted transvenously via a subclavian or jugular vein. If a patient is not pacing properly, a chest X-ray may reveal that the position of the electrode tip is unstable, or a fracture in the wire may be seen.

RADIOGRAPHIC SIGNS OF PATHOLOGY

CONSOLIDATION

Consolidation, or synonymously air space shadowing, is due to opacification of the air-containing spaces of the lung, usually without a change in volume of the affected area. It is not possible to tell what the airspace filling is due to in the absence of a clinical history, except perhaps for shadowing due to cardiogenic alveolar oedema, when there will be associated signs of congestive cardiac failure. Typical features of all forms of consolidation (Figure 32.11) include:

- ill-defined margins, except where it directly abuts a pleural surface
- sharply demarcated by fissures
- loss of vascular markings
- air bronchograms – the bronchi, usually invisible, may become apparent in negative contrast to the air space opacification
- acinar opacities, due to individual acini or secondary pulmonary lobules being opacified but still surrounded by normally aerated lung, usually seen at the periphery of a more confluent area of consolidation, and 0.5–1 cm in diameter
- ground glass opacification, when consolidation has caused only partial filling of the air spaces
- silhouette sign – consolidation abutting a soft tissue structure causes the silhouette of that structure to be lost.

When an area of consolidation undergoes necrosis, either due to infection or infarction, then liquefaction may result, and if there is either a gas forming organism or communication with the bronchial tree, then an air-fluid level may develop in addition to cavity formation.

COLLAPSE

When there is partial or complete volume loss in a lung or lobe this is referred to as collapse or atelectasis, implying a diminished volume of air in the lung with associ-

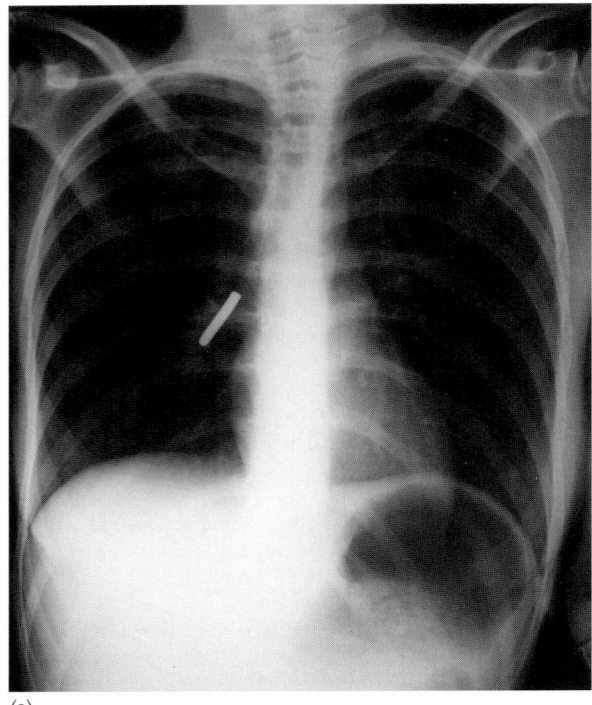

(a)

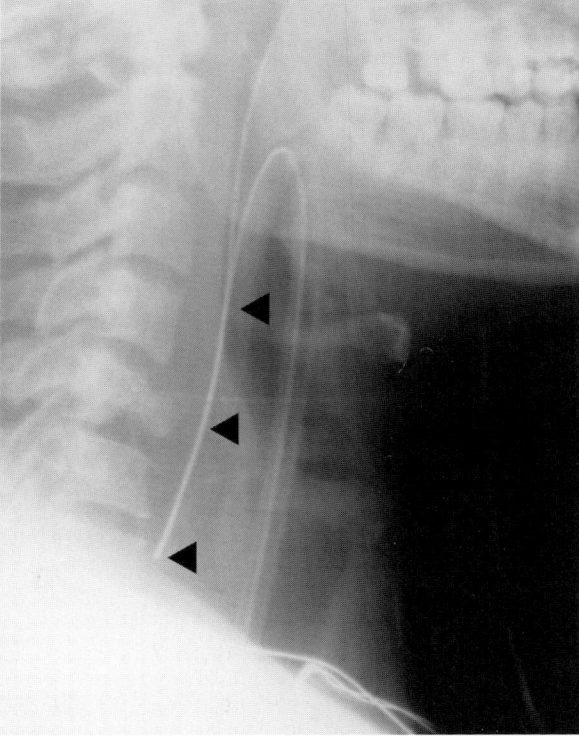

(b)

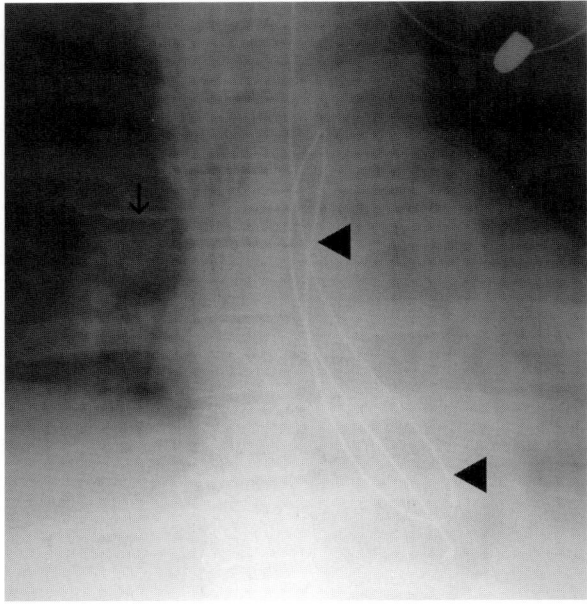

(c)

Fig. 32.6 Misplaced nasogastric tube. (a) The tip of the tube is in the bronchus intermedius. (b) The tube is looped in the oesophagus (black arrowheads) before passing into the trachea as demonstrated on this lateral spine view. Note the anterior wedge fracture of C5. (c) The tube is coiled in the oesophagus without passing into the stomach. Note the bullet projected over the left upper zone and the adequately positioned Swan Ganz catheter (black arrowheads).

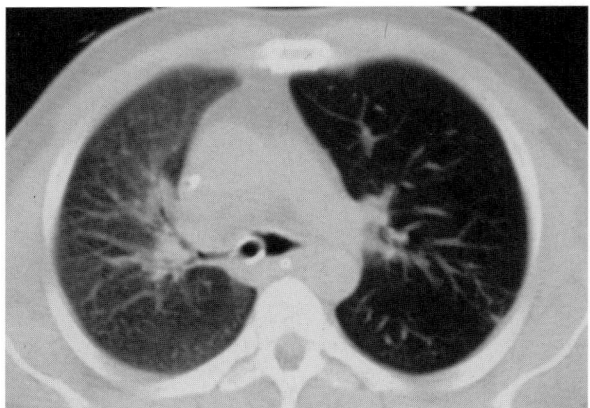

Fig. 32.7 Endotracheal tube inserted into the right main bronchus as demonstrated on CT. This image, obtained in expiration, demonstrates air trapping in the left lung.

ated reduction of lung volume. There are several different mechanisms for lung or lobar collapse, for example *relaxation* or *passive collapse* when fluid or air accumulates in the pleural space, *cicatrization collapse* when volume loss is associated with pulmonary fibrosis,

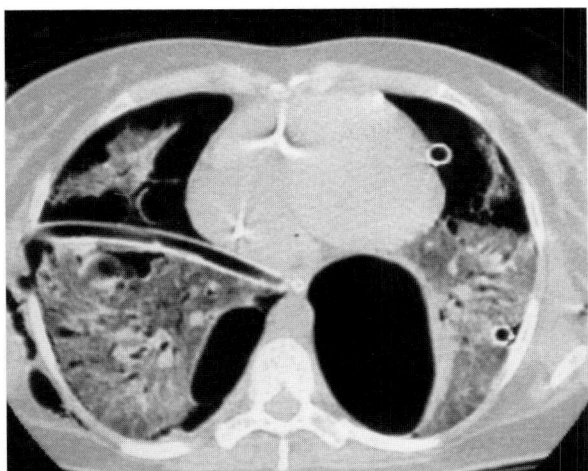

Fig. 32.8 CT scan demonstrating loculated pneumothoraces in a patient with acute lung injury. The postero-medial pneumothorax on the left is not being drained by the multiple chest tubes.

adhesive collapse as in ARDS, or resorption collapse, as in bronchial obstruction.

The radiographic appearance in pulmonary collapse depends upon a number of factors. These include the mechanism of collapse, the extent of collapse, the presence or absence of consolidation in the affected lung, and the pre-existing state of the pleura. This latter factor includes the presence of underlying pleural tethering or thickening and the presence of pleural fluid.

The direct signs of collapse include:

- displacement of interlobar fissures
- loss of aeration resulting in increased density or the presence of the silhouette sign
- crowding of vessels and bronchi.

The indirect signs of collapse include:

- elevation of the hemidiaphragm especially with lower lobe collapse
- mediastinal displacement, especially in upper lobe collapse
- hilar displacement, where the hilum is elevated in upper lobe collapse, and depressed in lower lobe collapse
- compensatory hyperinflation of remaining normal lung, resulting in increased transradiancy or herniation across the midline from the normal side
- crowding of the ribs reflecting diminished overall volume of the affected hemithorax.

COMPLETE LUNG COLLAPSE

Complete collapse (Figure 32.12) will cause complete opacification of the hemithorax, with displacement of the mediastinum to the affected side and elevation of the hemi-diaphragm. Compensatory hyperinflation of the

contralateral lung with herniation across the midline may be apparent. Herniation may occur in the retrosternal space, anterior to the ascending aorta or may be posterior to the heart.

INDIVIDUAL OR COMBINED LOBAR COLLAPSE

In any situation, some or all of the signs may be present.

Right Upper Lobe Collapse (Figure 32.13)

- horizontal fissure moves upwards and medially towards the superior mediastinum
- trachea deviates to the right
- compensatory hyperinflation of the right middle and lower lobes.

Middle Lobe Collapse (Figure 32.14)

- horizontal fissure and lower half of the oblique fissure move towards each other, best seen on the lateral projection
- frontal radiograph changes may be subtle with obscuration of the right heart border
- indirect signs of volume loss are rarely obvious.

Right Lower Lobe Collapse

- partial depression of the horizontal fissure
- triangular opacity of the collapsed lower lobe on the frontal projection, usually obscuring the diaphragm but preserving the right heart border
- eventually a completely collapsed lower lobe may be so small that it flattens and merges with the mediastinum, producing a thin, wedge-shaped shadow.

Left Lower Lobe Collapse (Figure 32.15)

- collapsed lobe may be obscured by the heart and a penetrated view may be required
- mediastinal structures and the diaphragm adjacent to the non-aerated lobe are obscured
- extreme volume loss may cause the lobe to be so small as to be invisible as a separate opacity
- loss of lower lobe artery silhouette at the hilum.

Lingula Collapse

- often involved in collapse of the left upper lobe
- may collapse individually
- radiographic features are similar to those of middle lobe collapse.

Left Upper Lobe Collapse (Figure 32.16)

- lateral view demonstrates anterior displacement of the entire oblique fissure, oriented almost parallel to the anterior chest wall, demarcating the posterior surface of the upper lobe as an elongated opacity extending from the apex almost reaching the diaphragm and lying anterior to the hilum

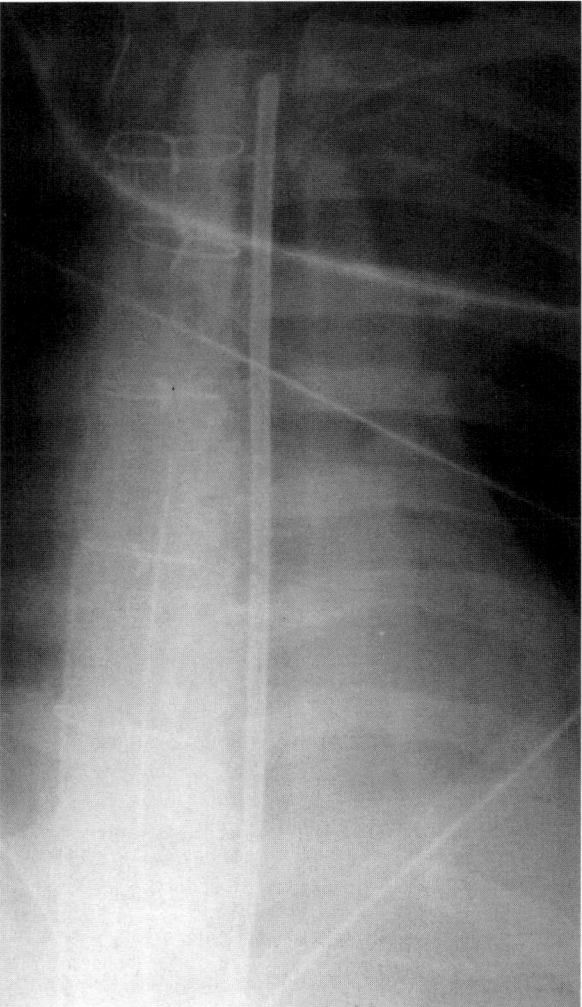
(a)

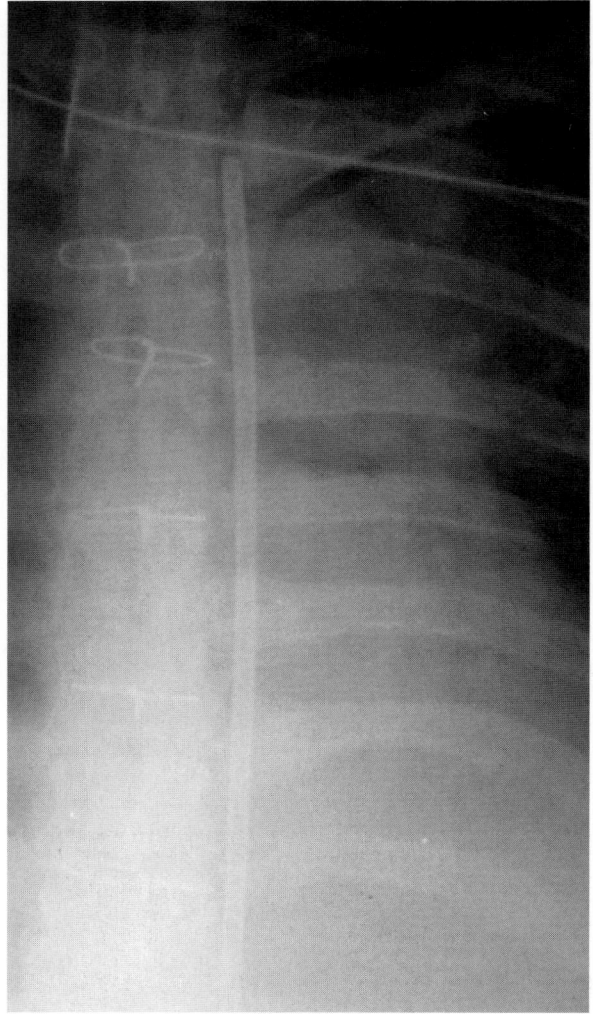
(b)

Fig. 32.9 Intra-aortic balloon pump. Two chest radiographs in the same patient demonstrating the balloon pump during the inflated (a) and deflated (b) phases. The tip of this balloon pump will be impinging upon the origin of the left subclavian artery and is slightly too high.

- eventually the upper lobe retracts posteriorly and loses contact with the anterior chest wall
- frontal radiograph demonstrates an ill-defined hazy opacity in the upper, mid and sometimes lower zones, with loss of hilar clarity
- hilum is often elevated, and the trachea deviated to the left.

COMBINED COLLAPSE

Right lower and middle lobe collapse is the most common pairing since a lesion may occur in the bronchus intermedius. The appearances are similar to right lower lobe collapse except that the horizontal fissure is not apparent, and the opacification reaches the lateral chest wall on the frontal radiograph, and similarly extends to the anterior chest wall on the lateral view.

Right upper and middle lobe collapse is much less common because of the distance between the origins of their bronchi, and can generally be taken to imply the presence of more than one lesion. This combination will produce appearances almost identical to those of left upper lobe collapse (Figure 32.16). On occasion isolated right upper lobe collapse will also produce appearances that are identical to left upper lobe collapse.

UNILATERAL INCREASED TRANSRADIANCY

The commonest causes are technical and include:

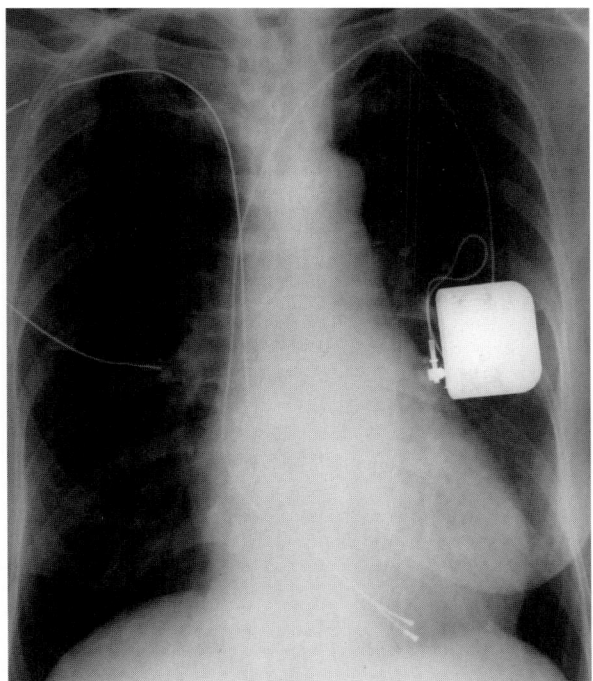

Fig. 32.10 There is a fracture in the now redundant pacing wire on the right side. The functioning pacing wire is sharply kinked as it passes over the first rib and is of increased risk of subsequent fracture.

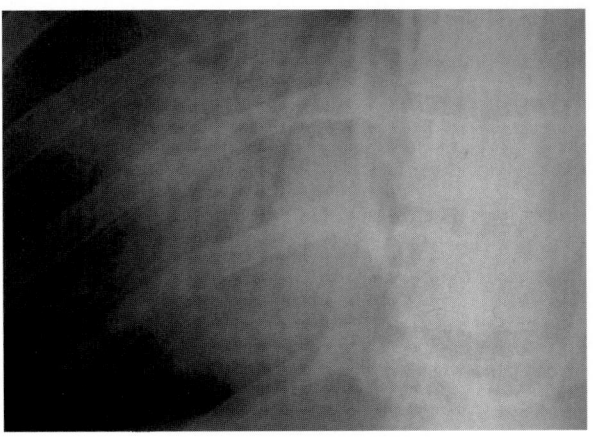

Fig. 32.11 Close up view of an area of consolidation adjacent to the right heart border, which is obscured. Air bronchograms can be identified passing through this area, which fades out peripherally having an ill-defined margin.

- patient rotation
- poor beam centring
- offset grid.

Pathological causes include:

- chest wall changes

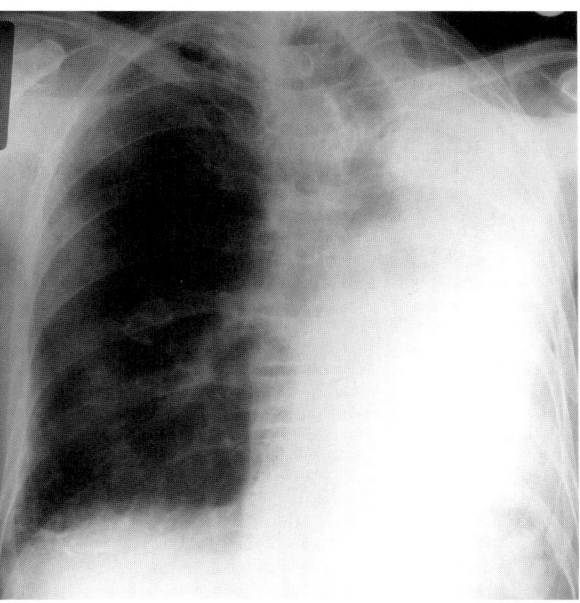

Fig. 32.12 Complete lung collapse. The left hemithorax is opaque and the mediastinum has shifted to that side, together with deviation of the trachea. There was an obstructing tumour in the left main stem bronchus.

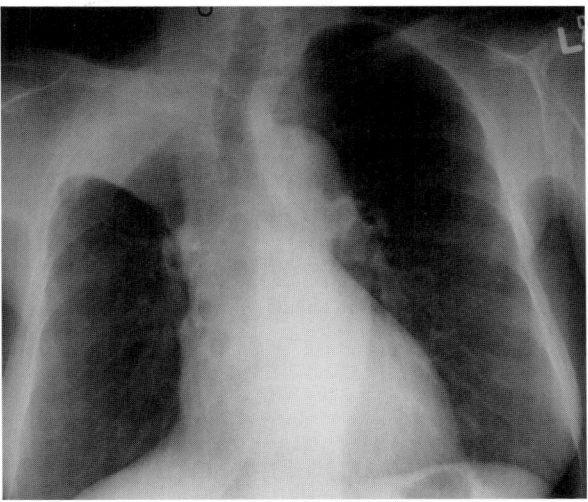

Fig. 32.13 Right upper lobe collapse. The horizontal fissure has become elevated and the right upper lobe has become a wedge-shaped density extending from the hilum to the right lung apex. There is evidence of volume loss with shift of the trachea to the right side.

(a) mastectomy
(b) congenital unilateral absence of pectoral muscles, known as Poland's syndrome
- reduced vascularity when interruption or significant reduction in the blood supply to one lung may cause that lung to be of increased transradiancy

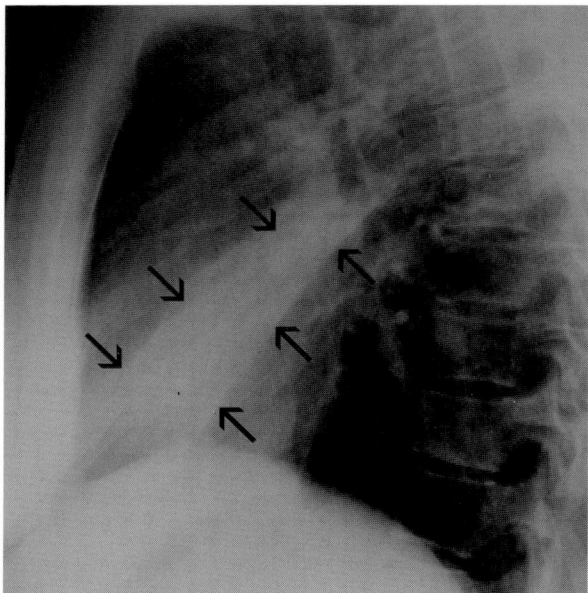

Fig. 32.14 Middle lobe collapse. The horizontal fissure is depressed and demarcates the collapsed middle lobe as a wedge-shaped density best demonstrated on the lateral (arrows).

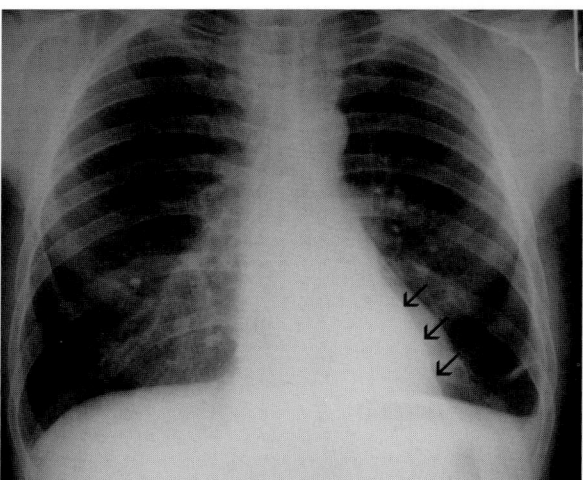

Fig. 32.15 Left lower lobe collapse. The left lower lobe has become a wedge shaped density behind the heart forming a double left heart border (arrows). The left hilar vessel to the lower lobe has disappeared as a result of collapse.

- lung hyperexpansion due to air trapping or asymmetric emphysema.

When there is relative increased transradiancy of one hemithorax for which there is no obvious cause then the possibility of generalized increase in radio-opacity of the opposite side should be considered, for example, the posterior layering of a pleural effusion in a supine patient. Usually hypertransradiancy due to technical factors can be identified by comparison of the soft tissues around the shoulder girdle, and particularly over the axillae.

ABNORMALITIES OF THE MEDIASTINUM

Pneumomediastinum or *mediastinal emphysema* is the presence of air between the tissue planes of the mediastinum (see 'Injuries to the Mediastinum' below). Chest radiography may show vertical, translucent streaks in the mediastinum, representing air separating the soft tissue planes. The air may extend up into the neck and over the chest wall causing subcutaneous emphysema, and also over the diaphragm. The mediastinal pleura may be displaced laterally and then be visible as a thin stripe alongside the mediastinum.

Acute mediastinitis is usually due to perforation of the oesophagus, pharynx or trachea and chest radiograph usually shows widening of the mediastinum and pneumomediastinum is often apparent.

Mediastinal haemorrhage may occur from venous or arterial bleeding (Figure 32.17a,b). The mediastinum

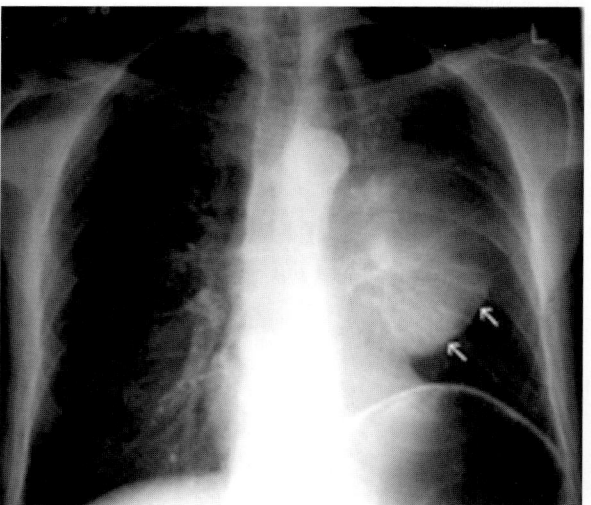

Fig. 32.16 Left upper lobe collapse. A hazy opacity extends from the hilum towards the left lung apex. It is sharply demarcated inferiorly and laterally (white arrows) due to the presence of a large tumour at the left hilum which is obstructing the left upper lobe bronchus. Note the signs of volume loss, particularly the elevation of the left

appears widened, and blood may be seen tracking over the lung apices. It is obviously imperative to identify a life-threatening cause such as aortic rupture.

PLEURAL FLUID

The most dependent recess of the pleural space is the posterior costophrenic angle and this is where a small

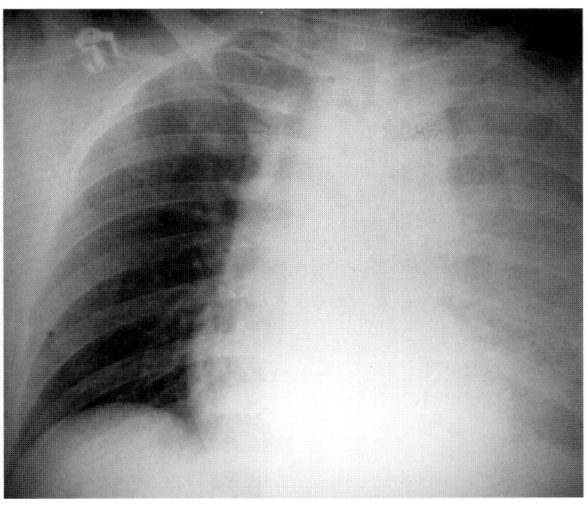

(a)

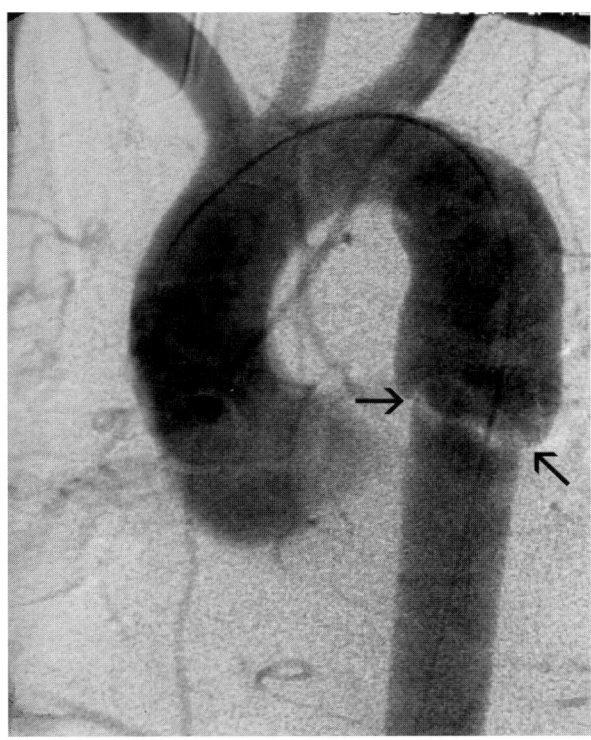

(b)

Fig. 32.17 Aortic rupture. (a) Demonstrated opacification of the left hemithorax due to a large haemothorax which is layering posteriorly in this supine patient. There is widening of the mediastinum due to mediastinal haemorrhage. (b) Arch aortogram demonstrating widening of the descending thoracic aorta due to the aortic wall rupture. The point of return to normal calibre is demarcated by the arrows.

effusion will tend to collect. As little as a few millilitres of fluid may be detected using decubitus views with a horizontal beam, ultrasound or CT. Larger volumes of fluid eventually fill in the costophrenic angle on the frontal view, and with increasing fluid a homogeneous opacity spreads upwards, obscuring the lung base (Figure 32.18). The fluid usually demonstrates a concave upper edge, higher laterally than medially, and obscures the diaphragm. Fluid may track into the fissures. A massive effusion may cause complete opacification of a hemithorax with passive atelectasis. The space-occupying effect of the effusion may push the mediastinum towards the opposite side especially when the lung does not collapse significantly. Effusions in a supine patient redistribute into the paravertebral sulcus and produce an even increased density throughout that hemithorax.

Lamellar effusions are shallow collections between the lung surface and the visceral pleura, sometimes sparing the costophrenic angle, and occur early in heart failure.

Sub-pulmonary effusions accumulate between the diaphragm and undersurface of a lung, mimicking elevation of the hemidiaphragm, altering the diaphragmatic contour so the apex moves more laterally than usual. When left sided, there is increased distance between the gastric air-bubble and lung base.

Fluid may become loculated in the interlobar fissures and is most frequently seen in heart failure. Loculated interlobar effusions may disappear rapidly and are sometimes known as pulmonary pseudotumours.

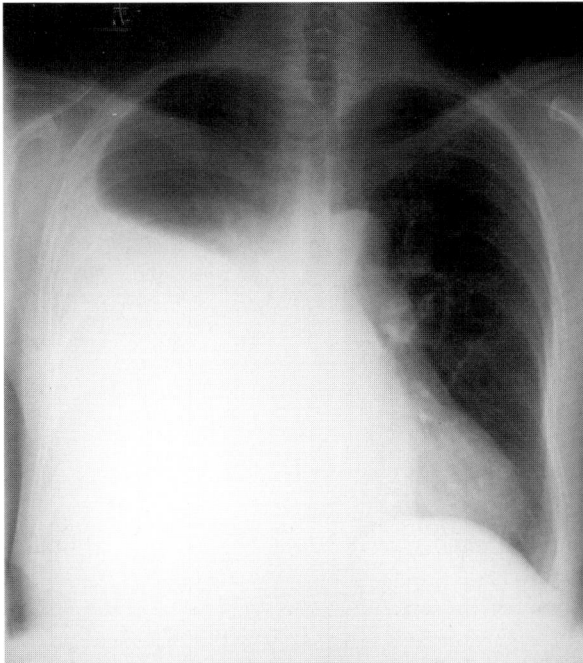

Fig. 32.18 A large right pleural effusion is present in this patient with a typical configuration of its upper border, a meniscus extending up the lateral chest wall.

Differentiation between a simple effusion and a complicated para-pneumonic effusion or an empyema usually requires thoracentesis. Loculation is best demonstrated with ultrasound.

PNEUMOTHORAX

In an erect patient, air will usually collect at the apex (Figure 32.19a,b). The lung retracts towards the hilum and on a frontal chest film the sharp white line of the visceral pleura will be visible, separated from the chest wall by the radiolucent pleural space, which is devoid of lung markings. This should not be confused with a skin fold, which mostly occur in supine or recumbent patients. The lung usually remains aerated although perfusion is reduced in proportion to ventilation and therefore the radiodensity of the partially collapsed lung remains relatively normal. A large pneumothorax may lead to complete relaxation and retraction of the lung, with some mediastinal shift towards the normal side. Because it is a medical emergency, tension pneumothorax is often treated before a chest radiograph is obtained. However if a radiograph is taken in this situation it will show marked displacement of the mediastinum. Radiographically the lung may be squashed against the mediastinum, or herniate across the midline, and the ipsilateral hemi-diaphragm may be depressed. A supine pneumothorax may produce increased transradiancy towards the diaphragm, and a deep-sulcus sign.

COMPLICATIONS OF PNEUMOTHORAX

Pleural adhesions may limit the distribution of a pneumothorax and result in a loculated or encysted pneumothorax (Figure 32.8). The usual appearance is an ovoid air collection adjacent to the chest wall, and it may be radiographically indistinguishable from a thin-walled sub-pleural pulmonary cyst or bulla. Pleural adhesions are occasionally seen as line shadows stretching between the two pleural layers, preventing relaxation of the underlying lung. Rupture of an adhesion may produce a haemo-pneumothorax. Collapse or consolidation of a lobe or lung in association with a pneumothorax is important because they may delay re-expansion of the lung.

Since the normal pleural space contains a small volume of fluid, blunting of the costophrenic angle by a short fluid level is commonly seen in a pneumothorax. In a small pneumothorax this fluid level may be the most obvious radiological sign. A larger fluid level usually signifies a complication and represents exudate, pus or blood, depending on the aetiology of the pneumothorax. A hydro-pneumothorax is a pneumothorax containing a significant amount of fluid (Figure 32.20). On a radiograph obtained with a horizontal beam, a fluid level is evident. A hydro- or pyo-pneumothorax may arise as a result of a broncho-pleural fistula, and may be a complication of surgery, tumour or infection.

PULMONARY EMBOLISM

CT diagnosis of PE is becoming routinely available, and depends upon the ability to acquire, within a single breath-hold, a volume of data large enough to include the entire thorax. This rapid acquisition allows excellent contrast opacification of the pulmonary arterial tree for the duration of the scan, so revealing any thrombus

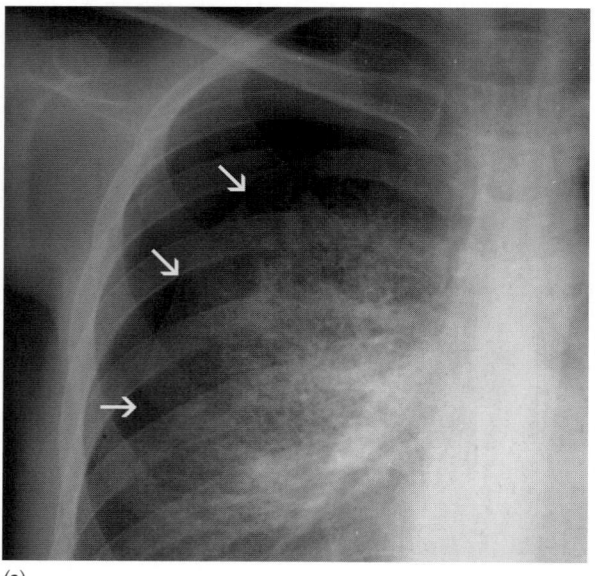

(a)

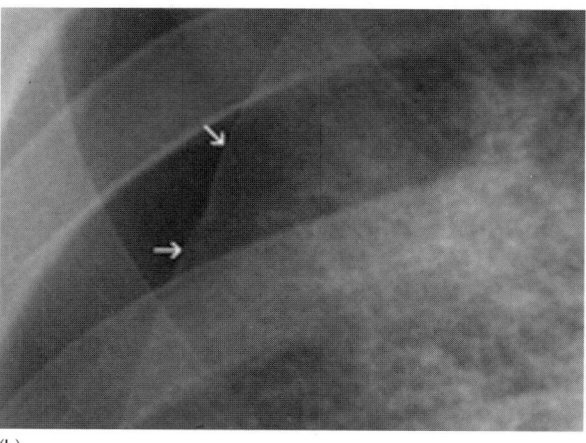

(b)

Fig. 32.19 Pneumothorax. (a) This patient, with underlying lung abnormality, has developed a pneumothorax. The fine white line that represents the visceral pleura delineates the edge of the lung. (b) Close up of the pleural line. Note how there are no vascular markings beyond this point.

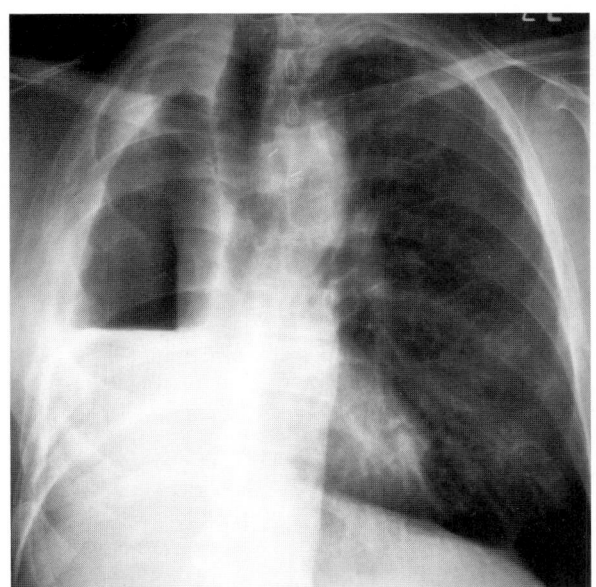

Fig. 32.20 Hydropneumothorax developing in a patient who has had a previous pneumonectomy on the right for carcinoma. Spontaneous development of a broncho-pleural fistula has occurred.

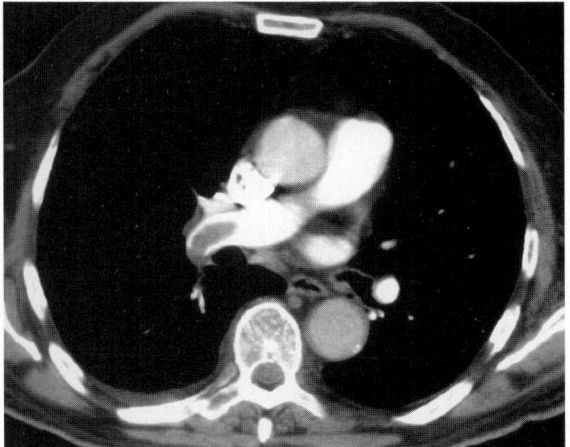

Fig. 32.21 Large pulmonary embolus in the right main pulmonary artery demonstrated by spiral CT scanning. Both pulmonary arteries are outlined by contrast except for the embolus itself.

within the central pulmonary vessels (Figure 32.21). There are numerous studies evaluating helical and electron beam CT in the diagnosis of acute pulmonary embolus, with excellent reported sensitivity and specificity for the detection of clot down to the segmental level.[5-8] Most of these studies also allow other diagnoses to be made that explain the symptoms of chest pain or dyspnoea, even when no PE is present.

TRAUMA AND THE ICU PATIENT

SKELETAL INJURY[9]

Following trauma rib fractures are common and may be single, multiple, unilateral or bilateral. In cases of chest trauma, the chest X-ray is more important in detecting a complication of rib fracture than the fracture itself. Fracture of one of the first three ribs is often associated with major intrathoracic injury, and fracture of the lower three ribs may be associated with important hepatic, splenic or renal injury. Complications of rib fracture include a flail segment, pneumothorax, haemothorax and subcutaneous emphysema. A flail segment is usually apparent clinically and radiologically. The fractured ends of ribs may penetrate underlying pleura and lung and cause a pneumothorax, haemothorax, haemopneumothorax or intrapulmonary haemorrhage. Air may also escape into the chest wall and cause subcutaneous emphysema. Fractures of the sternum usually require a

lateral film or CT for visualization. Fractures of the thoracic spine may be associated with a paraspinal shadow, which represents haematoma. Fractures of the clavicle may be associated with injury to the subclavian vessels or brachial plexus, and posterior dislocation of the clavicle at the sternoclavicular joint may cause injury to the trachea, oesophagus, great vessels or nerves of the superior mediastinum.

DIAPHRAGMATIC INJURY[10]

Laceration of the diaphragm may result from penetrating or non-penetrating trauma to the chest or abdomen. Ruptures of the left hemidiaphragm are encountered more frequently in clinical practice than ruptures on the right (Figure 32.22). The typical plain film appearance is of obscuration of the affected hemidiaphragm and increased shadowing in the ipsilateral hemithorax due to herniation of stomach, omentum, bowel or solid viscera, although such herniation may be delayed. Ultrasound may demonstrate diaphragmatic laceration and free fluid in both the pleura and peritoneum. Barium studies may be useful to confirm herniation of stomach or bowel into the chest.

PLEURAL INJURY[9,11]

Pneumothorax may be a complication of rib fracture, and is then usually associated with a haemothorax. If no ribs are fractured, pneumothorax is secondary to a pneumomediastinum, pulmonary laceration or penetrating chest injury. Pneumothorax due to a penetrating injury is liable to develop increased pressure, resulting in a tension pneumothorax, which may require emergency decompression.

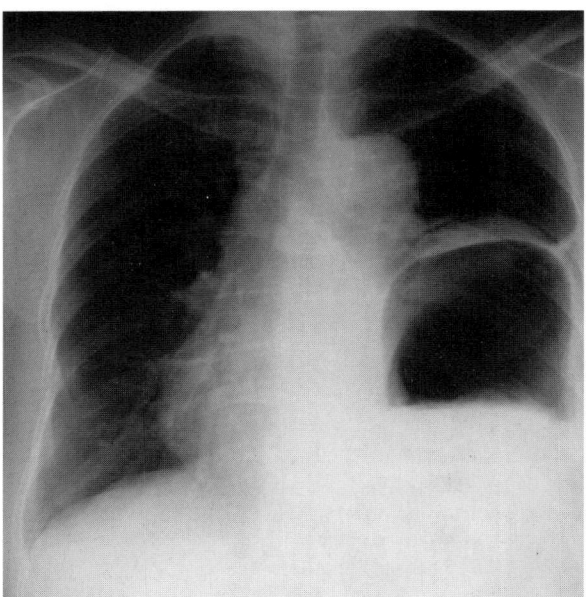

Fig. 32.22 Ruptured left hemidiaphragm. Previous trauma resulted in rupture of the hemidiaphragm. A chest radiograph obtained some months later demonstrates herniation of the stomach into the left hemithorax.

Haemothorax may also occur with or without rib fractures, and is due to laceration of intercostal or pleural vessels. If a pneumothorax is also present a fluid level will be seen on a horizontal-beam film. Pleural effusion may also result from trauma. Open injuries to the pleura are prone to infection and development of an empyema.

INJURIES TO THE LUNG[12–14]

Pulmonary contusion is due to haemorrhagic exudation into the alveoli and interstitial spaces and appears as patchy, non-segmental consolidation within the first few hours of penetrating or non-penetrating trauma. There is usually improvement within 2 days and clearance within 3–4 days. Pulmonary lacerations may be obscured by pulmonary contusion, but as this resolves, the laceration will become evident. If filled with blood it appears as a homogenous round opacity, and if partly filled with blood it may show a fluid level. Such pulmonary haematomas or blood cysts gradually decrease in size, but may take a few months to resolve completely. *Fat embolism* is a rare complication of multiple fractures, with poorly defined nodular opacities throughout both lungs, which resolve within a few days.

INJURIES TO THE TRACHEA AND BRONCHI[13,15]

Laceration or rupture of a major airway is an uncommon result of severe chest trauma. Fracture of the first three ribs and mediastinal emphysema and pneumothorax may also be evident. The injury is usually in the *trachea* just above the carina, or in a *main bronchus* just distal to the carina. If the bronchial sheath is preserved there may be no immediate signs or symptoms, but tracheostenosis or bronchiectasis may occur later. Computed tomography may be helpful in diagnosis, but bronchoscopy is the best diagnostic method in the acute stage.

INJURIES TO THE MEDIASTINUM[16]

Pneumomediastinum and mediastinal emphysema, discussed above, is the presence of air between the tissue planes of the mediastinum. Air may reach here as a result of pulmonary interstitial emphysema, perforation of the oesophagus, trachea or bronchus, or from a penetrating chest injury. Pulmonary interstitial emphysema is a result of alveolar wall rupture due to high intra-alveolar pressure, and may occur during violent coughing, asthmatic attacks or severe crush injuries, or be due to positive pressure ventilation. Air dissects centrally along the perivascular sheath to reach the mediastinum. Rarely, air may dissect into the mediastinum from a pneumoperitoneum. A pneumomediastinum may extend beyond the thoracic inlet into the neck, and over the chest wall. Pneumothorax is a common complication of pneumomediastinum, but the converse rarely occurs. Pneumomediastinum usually produces vertical translucent streaks in the mediastinum. This represents gas separating and outlining the soft-tissue planes and structures of the mediastinum. Gas shadows may extend up into the neck, or dissect extrapleurally over the diaphragm, or extend into the soft-tissue planes of the chest wall, causing subcutaneous emphysema. The mediastinal pleura may be displaced laterally, and become visible as a linear soft-tissue shadow parallel to the mediastinum. If mediastinal air collects beneath the pericardium the central part of the diaphragm may be visible, producing the 'continuous diaphragm' sign. Mediastinal haemorrhage may result from penetrating or non-penetrating trauma, and be due to venous or arterial bleeding. Many cases are probably unrecognized, as clinical and radiographic signs are absent. Important causes include automobile accidents, aortic rupture and dissection, and introduction of central venous catheters. There is usually bilateral mediastinal widening, but a localized haematoma may occur.

ACUTE AORTIC INJURY

Aortic rupture (Figure 32.17)[17] is usually the result of an automobile accident. Most non-fatal aortic tears occur at the aortic isthmus, the site of the ligamentum arteriosum. Only 10–20% of patients survive the acute episode, but a small number may develop a chronic aneurysm at the site of the tear. The commonest acute radiographic signs are widening of the superior mediastinum, and obscuration of the aortic knuckle. Other radiographic signs include deviation of the left main bronchus anteriorly, inferiorly and to the right, and rightward displacement of the trachea, a nasogastric tube or the right parasternal line. A left apical extrapleural cap or a left haemothorax may be visible. While aortography is the definitive investigation, CT, transoesophageal echocardiography or MRI may be diagnostic. In everyday practice, many departments will have emergency access to a CT scanner, but will not be centres of cardiothoracic surgery. A properly conducted CT scan demonstrating a normal mediastinum has a very high negative predictive value for aortic rupture. However, if CT is equivocal or shows a mediastinal haematoma then generally angiography will be required prior to surgery.

CARDIAC INJURY[18]

This is rare but may result from penetrating or blunt trauma. Penetrating injuries are usually rapidly fatal but may cause tamponade, ventricular aneurysm or septal defects. Blunt trauma may cause myocardial contusion and infarction and may be associated with transient or more permanent rhythm disturbance.

OESOPHAGEAL RUPTURE[19]

This is usually the result of instrumentation or surgery, but occasionally occurs in penetrating trauma, and is rarely spontaneous and due to sudden increase of intraoesophageal pressure (Boerhaave syndrome). Clinically there is acute mediastinitis; radiographically there are signs of pneumomediastinum, with or without a pneumothorax or hydropneumothorax, which is usually left-sided. The diagnosis should be confirmed by a swallow. This should initially be with water-soluble contrast medium in order to avoid the small risk of granuloma formation in the mediastinum that has been described following barium leakage. *Chylothorax* due to damage to the thoracic duct may become apparent hours or days after trauma. Thoracic surgery is the commonest cause.

THE POSTOPERATIVE CHEST

THORACIC COMPLICATIONS OF GENERAL SURGERY

ATELECTASIS

Atelectasis is the commonest pulmonary complication of thoracic or abdominal surgery. The chest X-ray usually shows elevation of the diaphragm, due to a poor inspiration. Linear opacities are present in the lower zones, and represent a combination of subsegmental volume loss

and consolidation. The shadows usually appear about 24 h postoperatively and resolve within 2 or 3 days.

PLEURAL EFFUSIONS

Pleural effusions are common immediately following abdominal surgery and usually resolve within 2 weeks. They may be associated with pulmonary infarction. Effusions due to subphrenic infection usually occur later.

PNEUMOTHORAX

Pneumothorax, when it complicates extrathoracic surgery, is usually a complication of positive pressure ventilation or central venous line insertion. It may complicate nephrectomy.

ASPIRATION PNEUMONITIS

Aspiration pneumonitis is common during anaesthesia, but fortunately is usually insignificant. When significant, patchy consolidation appears within a few hours, usually basally or around the hila. Clearing occurs within a few days, unless there is superinfection.

PULMONARY OEDEMA

In the postoperative period oedema may be cardiogenic or non-cardiogenic.

PNEUMONIA

Postoperative atelectasis and aspiration pneumonitis may be complicated by pneumonia. Postoperative pneumonias, therefore, tend to be associated with bilateral basal shadowing.

SUBPHRENIC ABSCESS

Subphrenic abscess usually produces elevation of the hemidiaphragm, pleural effusion and basal atelectasis. Loculated gas may be seen below the diaphragm, and fluoroscopy may show splinting of the diaphragm. Subphrenic abscess can be demonstrated by CT or ultrasound.

PULMONARY EMBOLISM

Pulmonary embolism may produce pulmonary shadowing, pleural effusion or elevation of the diaphragm, but is not excluded by a normal radiograph. In the ICU setting the radiological investigation of choice is spiral CT scanning.

THORACIC COMPLICATIONS OF CARDIAC SURGERY

Most cardiac operations are performed through a *sternotomy* incision, and wire sternal sutures are often seen on the postoperative films. Mitral valvotomy is now rarely performed via a *thoracotomy* incision, but this route is still used for surgery of coarctation of the aorta, patent ductus arteriosus, Blalock–Taussig shunts and pulmonary artery banding.

Widening of the cardiovascular silhouette is usual, and represents bleeding and oedema. Marked or progressive

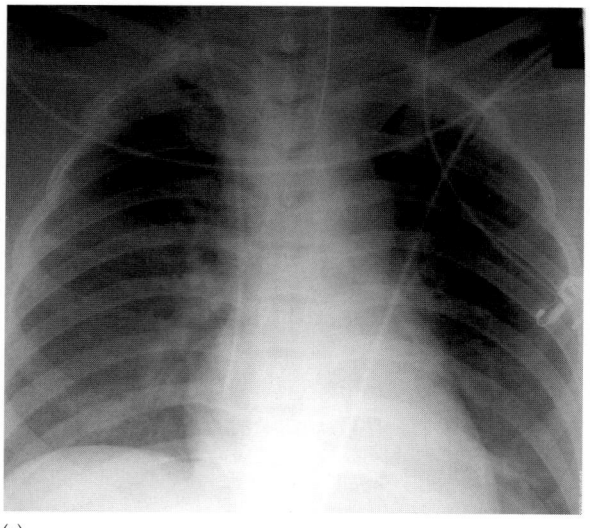

(a)

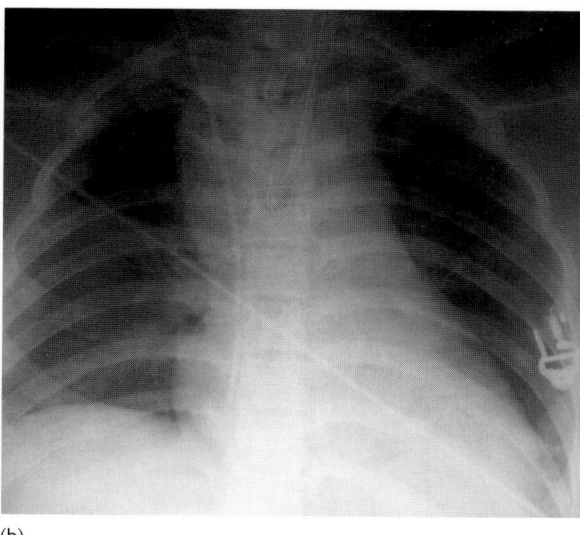

(b)

Fig. 32.23 Following cardiac surgery (a) the postoperative chest radiograph appears satisfactory. A few hours later (b) the mediastinum has widened considerably, due to mediastinal haemorrhage.

widening of the mediastinum suggests significant haemorrhage (Figure 32.23). Some air commonly remains in the pericardium following cardiac surgery, so that the signs of pneumopericardium may be present.

Left basal shadowing is almost invariable, representing atelectasis. This shadowing usually resolves over a week or two. Small pleural effusions are also common in the immediate postoperative period.

Pneumoperitoneum is sometimes seen, due to involvement of the peritoneum by the sternotomy incision. It is of no pathological significance (Figure 32.4).

Violation of left or right pleural space may lead to a pneumothorax. Damage to a major lymphatic vessel may lead to a chylothorax or a more localized chyloma.

Phrenic nerve damage may cause paresis or paralysis of a hemidiaphragm.

Surgical clips or other metallic markers have sometimes been used to mark the ends of coronary artery bypass grafts. Prosthetic heart valves are usually visible radiographically, but they may be difficult to see on an underpenetrated film.

Sternal dehiscence may be apparent radiographically by a linear lucency appearing in the sternum and alteration in position of the sternal sutures on consecutive films. The diagnosis is usually made clinically and may be associated with osteomyelitis. A first or second rib may be fractured when the sternum is spread apart. The importance of this observation is that it may explain chest pain in the postoperative period.

Acute mediastinitis may complicate mediastinal surgery although it is more commonly associated with oesophageal perforation or surgery. Radiographically there may be mediastinal widening or pneumomediastinum, and these features are best assessed by CT scan.

REFERENCES

1 Desai SR, Hansell DM. Lung imaging in the adult respiratory distress syndrome: current practice and new insights. *Intensive Care Med* 1997; **23**: 7–15.

2 Chastre J, Trouillet J-L, Vuagnat A, *et al.* Nosocomial pneumonia in patients with acute respiratory distress syndrome. *Am J Respir Crit Care Med* 1998; **157**: 1165–72.

3 Gillette MA, Hess DR. Ventilator-induced lung injury and the evolution of lung-protective strategies in acute respiratory distress syndrome. *Respir Care* 2001; **46**: 130–48.

4 Manzar S. Percutaneous central venous catheter placement. *Hosp Med* 1999; **60**: 914.

5 Task force report. Guidelines on the diagnosis and management of acute pulmonary embolism. *European Heart Journal* 2000; **21**: 1301–36.

6 Remy-Jardin M, Remy J, Deschildre F, *et al.* Diagnosis of pulmonary embolism with spiral CT: comparison with pulmonary angiography and scintigraphy. *Radiology* 1996; **200**: 699–706.

7 Baile EM, King GG, Muller NL, *et al.* Spiral computed tomography is comparable to angiography for the diagnosis of pulmonary embolism. *Am J Respir Crit Care Med* 2000; **161**: 1010–5

8 Goodman LR, Lipchik RJ. Diagnosis of acute pulmonary embolism: time for a new approach. *Radiology* 1996; **199**: 25–7.

9 Wicky S, Wintermark M, Schnyder P, *et al.* Imaging of blunt chest trauma. *Eur Radiol* 2000; **10**: 1524–38.

10 Shanmuganathan K, Killeen K, Mirvis SE, White CS. Imaging of diaphragmatic injuries. *J Thorac Imaging* 2000; **15**: 104–11.

11 Collins J. Chest wall trauma. *J Thorac Imaging* 2000; **15**: 112–9.

12 Nelson LD. Ventilatory support of the trauma patient with pulmonary contusion. *Respir Care Clin N Am* 1996; **2**: 425–47.

13 Haenel JB, Moore FA, Moore EE. Pulmonary consequences of severe chest trauma. *Respir Care Clin N Am* 1996; **2**: 401–24.

14 Cohn SM. Pulmonary contusion: review of the clinical entity. *J Trauma* 1997; **42**: 973–9.

15 Kiser C, O'Brien SM, Detterbeck FC. Tracheobronchial injuries: treatment and outcomes. *Ann Thorac Surg* 2001; **71**: 2059–65.

16 Ketai L, Brandt MM, Schermer C. Nonaortic mediastinal injuries from blunt chest trauma. *J Thorac Imaging* 2000; **15**: 120–7.

17 Esterra A, Mattox KL, Wall MJ. Thoracic aortic injury. *Semin Vasc Surg* 2000; **13**: 345–52.

18 May K, Patterson MA, Rue LW, *et al*. Combined blunt cardiac and pericardial rupture: review of the literature and report of a new diagnostic algorithm. *Am Surg* 1999; **65**: 568–74.

19 Younes Z, Johnson DA. The spectrum of spontaneous and iatrogenic esophageal injury: perforations, Mallory-Weiss tears, and hematomas. *J Clin Gastroenterol* 1999; **29**: 306–17.

33

Non-invasive ventilation

G Duke and A D Bersten

Non-invasive ventilation (NIV) is a valuable therapeutic option in the management of acute and chronic respiratory failure. Successful use of NIV in acute respiratory failure was first published in 1936,[1] and the use of NIV predates the introduction of laryngoscopy (early 1900s) and the widespread use of positive-pressure mechanical ventilation via an endotracheal tube (1950s).[2]

NIV is defined as ventilatory support without an endotracheal airway. This may be achieved through the delivery of positive airway pressure (Pao) or the application of a negative pressure generator to the chest ('chest box') or body ('iron lung'). This chapter deals primarily with the use of positive pressure NIV to treat acute respiratory failure (ARF). Major limitations to the use of negative pressure generators include the induction of obstructive sleep apnoea, lack of FiO_2 control, equipment bulk and size. However, external negative pressure generators suit some patients with chronic respiratory failure, particularly as there is no oral or nasal prosthesis.

The clinical application of NIV support depends upon the mode used and the nature and severity of the underlying respiratory disorder. An understanding of the physiologic rationale for NIV will assist the clinician predict the indications, the benefits, and the side-effects of the various NIV modes.[3,4] (Many of the general issues regarding ventilation are discussed in Ch. 25 (Mechanical Ventilation), and this chapter will focus on those issues specific to NIV.)

PHYSIOLOGY OF NON-INVASIVE VENTILATION

The application of NIV can reverse many of the physiologic and mechanical derangements associated with respiratory failure through:

- augmentation of alveolar ventilation (V_A) to reverse respiratory acidosis and hypercarbia
- alveolar recruitment and increased FiO_2 to reverse hypoxia

- reduction in work of breathing (Wmus) to reduce or prevent respiratory muscle insufficiency
- stabilization of the chest wall in the presence of severe chest injury
- reduction in left ventricular afterload which may lead to an improved cardiac output.

The respiratory effort (pressure-volume work) required to achieve a desired minute volume (V_E) may be viewed as the summation of the individual forces that must be overcome to generate inspiratory flow, namely: elastic work (or 'stretch'; Wel), flow-resistive work (airflow obstruction; Wres), and threshold work (Wthres.) Since the volume component is constant, the equation of motion can be written as:

$$Pmus = Pel + Pres + Pthres$$

(see Ch. 25 for more detailed explanation.)

With the addition of a device for ventilatory support, the respiratory muscle effort (Pmus) required by the patient is equivalent to the difference between the applied Pao and the total work required.

$$Pmus = (Pel + Pres + Pthres) - Pao$$

This relationship may be rearranged into its individual components, as follows:

$$Pmus + Pao = EV + R\dot{V} + PEEPi$$

Where E is the respiratory elastance (inverse of compliance); V is the volume of gas; R is the respiratory and circuit flow-resistance; $\dot{V}$ is the inspiratory flow rate; and PEEPi the intrinsic PEEP ($\approx$Pthres).

It is important to remember that breathing via a circuit will create additional airflow resistance (R) adding to breathing work (Pmus), and thus attention to circuit design is important (see below.)

PEEPi is absent in the healthy lung, but common in the presence of airflow obstruction and dynamic hyperinflation. This threshold load must be counterbalanced by an equivalent amount of inspiratory effort before inspiratory flow can commence. Since threshold load impedes inspiration it will also impede the onset (triggering) of inspiratory support modes, such as pressure support ventilation (PSV).

Although all invasive mechanical ventilation (MV) modes may be delivered non-invasively, four are commonly described: continuous positive airway pressure (CPAP); PSV; bilevel or biphasic positive airway pressure (BIPAP); and pressure- or volume-limited intermittent positive pressure ventilation (NIPPV). Other modes under investigation include high frequency and proportional assist ventilation.

All NIV modalities utilize closed (or semi-closed) circuits and are thus capable of controlling and delivering high inspired oxygen (FiO_2.) This is an important mechanism by which NIV improves oxygenation, independent of other mechanisms.

CPAP

This mode can address a number of objectives of ventilatory support, namely:

- Reduction in the work of breathing by:
  (a)   Alveolar recruitment leading to reduction in elastic work
  (b)   Reducing threshold load created in the presence of $PEEP_i$.
- Reversing hypoxia through alveolar recruitment and reduction of intrapulmonary shunt.
- Reduction of left ventricular (LV) transmural pressure (afterload).[5,6]

INSPIRATORY POSITIVE AIRWAY PRESSURE AND PSV

Positive inspiratory airway pressure, without expiratory pressure (e.g. PSV or IPAP), provides respiratory support by reducing both the elastic and resistive components of respiratory work. This may result in:

- augmentation of tidal volume (V_E) and reduction in $PaCO_2$
- reduction in Pmus with reduction or prevention of respiratory muscle insufficiency
- induction of pulmonary surfactant release through alveolar inflation above resting tidal volume.[7]

BIPAP

BIPAP allows separate settings for inspiratory (IPAP) and expiratory (EPAP) airway pressure levels, and is conceptually similar, but not identical, to PSV plus CPAP. Respiratory frequency is usually determined by the spontaneous rate but may be time-cycled and independent of patient effort. In some patients, BIPAP may not be as effective in reducing Pmus as the combination of PSV plus CPAP.[2,8]

NIPPV

NIPPV may be considered as volume- or pressure-limited mechanical ventilation applied via a mask (instead of an endotracheal airway).

PATIENT–VENTILATOR INTERACTION

This is discussed in Chapter 25 and is subdivided into (a) triggering of inspiration, (b) inspiration, and (c) cessation of inspiration. The only aspect that is specific to NIV arises from mask leaks which may interfere with the ability to sense the end of expiration because there is continued 'expiratory' gas flow.

NIV EQUIPMENT

Equipment design varies according to NIV mode and purpose (e.g. critical care or domiciliary setting), and significant variation in performance characteristics have been documented.[2,9] The important characteristics of an efficient NIV circuit include:

- High gas flow that can match the peak inspiratory airflow. Mechanisms to generate high flows include a pressurized gas supply, a gas turbine, or a jet venturi mechanism. A continuous flow device often imposes less circuit work than a demand flow device.
- An expiratory resistor capable of maintaining the desired PEEP, yet offering a low resistance to expiratory flow to reduce fluctuations in the desired Pao. This may be a threshold resistor or flow resistor. The optimal position for the expiratory valve is as close to the patient's airway as possible.
- Minimal length, wide bore, tubing to reduce turbulence and flow resistance.
- A flow or pressure sensor for identifying inspiratory effort, and triggering positive inspiratory pressure support (e.g. PSV or IPAP.)
- Ability to control and deliver a wide range of FiO_2.
- Other desirable features include the facility to humidify inspired gases and nebulize drugs, and the provision for pressure-relief safety valves, battery-backup, apnoea backup support, acoustic suppression and monitoring of volume and Pao. These features are less important for domiciliary (long-term) NIV equipment.

Many mask designs are also available and the optimal design depends upon the purpose and mode of NIV and patient preference. These include intra-nasal, nasal, and oro-nasal (full-face) masks. Desirable features of a nasal- or face-mask include lightweight and transparent materials providing a comfortable air-tight seal with minimal dead-space and separate inspiratory and expiratory ports to minimize airflow turbulence and rebreathing.[9,10]

Mask discomfort is a common cause of poor compliance with NIV, and often associated with full-face masks.

On the other hand full-face masks tend to produce more reliable and constant Pao because they are unaffected by mouth breathing, a common problem in the critically ill patient. Nasal masks are less restrictive on the patient's ability to talk, eat/drink, and expectorate and have a higher compliance in longer-term and domiciliary applications. To effectively compensate for air leaks, nasal masks should be used with circuits capable of rapidly augmenting and delivering high flows >100 l/min.

Fibreoptic bronchoscopy can be easily, and often safely, performed during NIV. In addition to the usual precautions regarding fibreoptic bronchoscopy a full-face mask with at least two ports is required. One of these can be modified to allow a simple valve for insertion of the bronchoscope, and the other used for NIV. Provided there is adequate NIV flow-reserve during suction, this can be performed during all modes of NIV. This technique may allow both diagnostic and therapeutic bronchoscopy without intubation in critically ill patients.

COMPLICATIONS AND ASSESSMENT OF EFFICACY

Contraindications and complications specific to NIV are listed in Table 33.1.

Although reversal of hypoxia is an important goal of respiratory support it is a poor guide to the efficacy of NIV. However, reduction of $PaCO_2$ in hypercarbic ARF is often a guide to the success of NIV. Efficacy of NIV should be measured using outcomes such as compliance, intubation rate, nosocomial pneumonia, or mortality.

Most patients requiring NIV should be managed in a critical care ward with appropriately trained medical and nursing staff. Although the development of sophisti-

Table 33.1   Contraindications and complications of NIV

Contraindications	Respiratory arrest
	Unprotected airway (coma, sedation)
	Upper airway obstruction
	Inability to clear secretions
	Untreated pneumothorax
	Marked haemodynamic instability
Complications	Mask discomfort, patient intolerance
	Facial or ocular abrasions
	Nasal congestion, sinus pain
	Oronasal dryness
	↑ intraocular pressure (particularly in patients with glaucoma)
	↑ intracranial pressure (particularly in patients with neurotrauma)
	↓ blood pressure (if hypovolaemic)
	Aspiration pneumonitis (rare)
	Aerophagy and gastric distension (uncommon; routine gastric decompression is unnecessary)

cated, portable non-invasive ventilators make it easy to provide NIV in any environment, its benefits have not been proven outside the critical care environment.[11]

NIV AND ACUTE RESPIRATORY FAILURE[2,11,12]

CARDIOGENIC PULMONARY OEDEMA

CPO is a common cause of severe reversible acute respiratory failure (ARF). Since the 1930s, a number of investigators have documented the therapeutic benefits of all modes of NIV, but particularly CPAP, in the treatment of CPO. CPAP reverses hypoxia, recruits alveoli, and reduces intrapulmonary shunt and LV afterload. Redistribution of extravascular lung water from alveoli to the interstitial space is aided by recruitment of alveoli and surfactant production.

A number of prospective randomized controlled trials of NIV in CPO[2-4] have demonstrated physiologic improvements in hypoxic and hypercapnic respiratory failure, and a significant reduction in the need for invasive ventilation, and a reduction in hospital length of stay. Even though the majority of these patients were managed in a critical care setting the average duration of respiratory support was much shorter for NIV (9 ± 11 h) than those who required MV.[13]

The optimal mode of NIV in CPO appears to be CPAP alone. Although BIPAP and PSV/CPAP are effective there is no evidence of improved outcomes from the additional inspiratory Pao, while one study found a higher rate of myocardial infarction with BIPAP.[2] The optimal Pao level remains to be resolved, although 10 cmH_2O appeared to be safe and effective in the majority of subjects.

Current evidence supports the routine use of mask-CPAP in moderate or severe CPO as standard therapy and as the first-line option for respiratory support.[11]

ACUTE RESPIRATORY FAILURE IN CHRONIC OBSTRUCTIVE PULMONARY DISEASE

Chronic obstructive pulmonary disease (COPD) patients have an elevated resistive work, often coupled with an elevated basal V_E as a result of the pre-existing parenchymal damage. Threshold load is frequently present as a result of airflow obstruction, and is exacerbated during ARF by further increased resistive work and respiratory rate. Reversible ARF is a common complication of COPD.

Both CPAP and PSV have been shown to reduce Pmus in intubated COPD patients weaning from MV. Numerous uncontrolled reports advocating NIV in hypercapnic ARF have now been supported by prospective randomized controlled studies.[12,14-16] Most investigators have demonstrated a low incidence of side-effects and a significant decrease in intubation rates and in-hospital mortality.[16] The incidence of nosocomial pneumonia may also be lower with NIV.[17] Nevertheless, mask intolerance, nursing workload, and failure rates are greater than those reported with NIV in CPO.[2]

Current evidence supports the use of NIV in hypercapnic ARF as a component of standard therapy in COPD subjects. The American Thoracic Society Consensus Statement[11] concludes that: 'patients hospitalized for exacerbations of COPD with rapid clinical deterioration should be considered for non-invasive positive pressure (ventilatory support) to prevent further deterioration in gas exchange, respiratory workload and the need for endotracheal intubation.'

All modes of NIV have been shown to be effective but there are no comparative trials that address the question of optimal mode or pressure level.[11] Patients with ARF arising predominantly from airflow obstruction (Pres) and/or threshold load are likely to respond to CPAP. Those with reduced alveolar ventilation, marked hypercapnia, or respiratory muscle insufficiency are likely to benefit from the addition of inspiratory support, i.e. PSV, IPAP, or NIPPV.

The level of inspiratory support should be titrated to improve V_A as indicated by improvement in tidal volume and reductions in respiratory rate and $PaCO_2$. Low levels of CPAP should be titrated to minimize the patient effort required to trigger inspiratory assistance (Pthres), and FiO_2 titrated to reverse hypoxia. Inspiratory pressures of 5–15 cmH_2O and expiratory pressures (EPAP or CPAP) of 2–5 cmH_2O are usually required.

Early predictors of NIV response in COPD patients have not been identified, but it has been suggested that positive responders show clinical improvement within the first 2 h of NIV support. Prior to the commencement of NIV, the clinician should develop a clear management strategy for those patients who fail a trial of NIV. These patients should be managed in a critical care setting where appropriate equipment and skill is available.[2]

ASTHMA

Mask-CPAP has been shown in uncontrolled laboratory[18] and clinical[19] studies to reduce the work of breathing and dyspnoea associated with airflow obstruction. The clinical role, if any, for NIV in the management of acute asthma remains to be identified. We have found 5 cmH_2O CPAP to be effective in the management of patients with moderate to severe asthma who do not respond to continuous inhaled bronchodilators. Nebulized drugs can be effectively delivered even in the presence of a high-flow NIV circuit.[20] Controlled clinical studies with robust endpoints are awaited.

ACUTE LUNG INJURY AND ACUTE RESPIRATORY DISTRESS SYNDROME

In contrast to CPO, there is little supportive evidence for NIV in non-cardiogenic pulmonary oedema such as acute lung injury (ALI) and acute respiratory distress syndrome (ARDS). Even though the addition of PEEP is important during MV for ALI or ARDS, current data does not support the routine use of NIV.

Despite numerous reports of successful use of NIV in the setting of community-acquired pneumonia (without COPD) and other forms of ALI, the failure rate remains high.[16,21-23] This may reflect the differences in duration, severity, and the pathophysiology of ALI and ARDS compared with CPO. Some studies showing apparent benefit have failed to exclude patients with cardiogenic pulmonary oedema[24] or COPD-specific subgroups known to benefit from NIV.[25,26]

However, immunocompromised patients with pneumonia and ARF appear to benefit from NIV.[26,27] Whether NIV avoids a high morbidity therapy (MV),[17] or NIV simply selects those who have a more readily reversible form of ARF, and thus more likely to survive, is unclear. Nevertheless, it seems reasonable, based on the current data, to offer NIV to these patients.[11] Once again, clear guidelines need to be established for the management of those patients who fail a trial of NIV.

POST-OPERATIVE AND POST-TRAUMATIC ACUTE RESPIRATORY FAILURE

ARF in post-operative and trauma patients may arise from a number of pathological processes, including dependent atelectasis, impaired chest-wall mechanics, poor cough, nosocomial infection, aspiration pneumonitis, and non-respiratory trauma or sepsis.

Although mask CPAP improves physiological parameters (e.g. oxygenation and respiratory rate) in general surgical and cardiothoracic patients with hypoxic respiratory failure, controlled trials have not demonstrated a reduction in morbidity.[28] Other modes of NIV have been not been studied and it is possible that modes with inspiratory support (PSV or BIPAP) may be beneficial.

Mask CPAP together with regional analgesia has been shown to be superior to MV and morphine infusion in patients with isolated severe chest trauma,[29] but the benefit of NIV alone is unclear. NIV is contraindicated in the presence of other significant injuries such as neurotrauma and intracranial hypertension and in the presence of an untreated pneumothorax.

NIV-ASSISTED WEANING

As a result of the demonstrable benefits of NIV in COPD and the widespread use of invasive-PSV to assist weaning from MV, NIV has also been recommended to expedite weaning from MV by allowing early extubation, and to treat failed or accidental extubation. The putative advantages relate to reduction in the duration and the risks of MV (e.g. nosocomial pneumonia). However, evidence from controlled studies does not support an overall benefit,[11] and this suggests that NIV is not a substitute for strategies to improve weaning from MV and reduce accidental extubation.

NIV AND CHRONIC RESPIRATORY FAILURE

NIV is an important modality in the treatment of severe chronic respiratory failure associated with obstructive and central sleep apnoea syndromes,[11,30] and chronic hypoventilation syndromes associated with neuromuscular disease, pulmonary fibrosis, or thoracic deformities.[31]

These patients may require short-term MV or NIV in a critical care environment for respiratory support during an acute illness or as an aid to peri-operative care. Alternatively these conditions may be first diagnosed during admission for treatment of severe ARF and, following recovery, will require assessment for long-term NIV.

NIV AND SLEEP APNOEA SYNDROMES

Moderate or severe obstructive sleep apnoea results in nocturnal hypoventilation and episodic hypoxia that can lead to pulmonary and systemic hypertension, cardiac failure, and daytime hypercapnia and somnolence. Many of these complications can be arrested or reversed through the appropriate use of nocturnal CPAP.[11,30,32] Patients with suspected sleep apnoea require accurate assessment by a respiratory physician, including sleep studies, prior to the routine use of domiciliary CPAP. Occasionally BIPAP or NIPPV will be needed when there is inadequate central respiratory drive. In many patients respiratory drive will improve, and they can then be managed with CPAP after a period of BIPAP or NIPPV.

Intercurrent illness, surgery, or the use of sedatives and opioid analgesics will increase the frequency and duration of apnea and hypoxia. CPAP should be available even for those patients who do not require admission to a critical care ward.

NIV AND CHRONIC HYPOVENTILATION SYNDROMES[31]

Domiciliary NIV (predominantly using inspiratory support modes or NIPPV) should be considered in all patients presenting with severe chronic respiratory failure from restrictive lung disease or neuromuscular disease. However, there is little or no benefit of domiciliary NIV in the presence of chronic obstructive lung disease, unless one of the former conditions co-exists.

Assessment of these patients includes respiratory function tests, blood gas analysis, sleep studies, together with trials of NIV modes and pressure settings. In general, indications for long-term NIV include the demonstration of symptomatic respiratory failure, daytime hypercapnia, and a significantly reduced (<20% predicted) vital capacity. The use of nocturnal or intermittent NIV has been shown to improve daytime respiratory and cardiac function, to improve exercise endurance, to slow the progression of respiratory dysfunction, and to reduce the frequency of hospitalization.

REFERENCES

1 Poulton EP. Left-sided heart failure with pulmonary oedema. Its treatment with the 'pulmonary plus pressure' machine. *Lancet* 1936; **231**: 981–3.
2 Mehta S, Hill NS. Noninvasive ventilation. State of the Art. *Am J Respir Crit Care Med* 2001; **163**: 540–77.
3 Duke GJ, Bersten AD. Noninvasive ventilation for acute respiratory failure. Part 1. *Crit Care Resus* 1999; 1: 187–98.
4 Duke GJ, Bersten AD. Non-invasive ventilation for adult acute respiratory failure. Part 2. *Crit Care Resus* 1999; **1**: 199–210.
5 Buda AJ, Pinsky MR, Ingels NB, *et al*. The effect of intrathoracic pressure on left ventricular performance. *N Engl J Med* 1979; **301**: 453–9.
6 Naughton MT, Rahman A, Hara K, *et al*. Effect of continuous positive airway pressure on intrathoracic and left ventricular transmural pressures in patients with congestive heart failure. *Circulation* 1995; **91**: 1725–31.
7 Nicholas TE, Power JH, Barr HA. The pulmonary consequences of a deep breath. *Respir Physiol* 1982; **49**: 315–24.
8 Calzia E, Lindner KH, Witt S, *et al*. Pressure-time product and work of breathing during biphasic continuous positive airway pressure and assisted spontaneous breathing. *Am J Respir Crit Care Med* 1994; **150**: 904–10.
9 Lofaso F, Brochard L, Hang T, *et al*. Home versus intensive care pressure support devices. *Am J Respir Crit Care Med* 1996; **153**: 1591–9.
10 Ferguson GF, Gilmartin M. CO_2 rebreathing during BiPAP ventilatory assistance. *Am J Respir Crit Care Med* 1995; **151**: 1125–35.
11 American Thoracic Society. International Consensus Conferences in Intensive Care Medicine: Noninvasive positive pressure ventilation in acute respiratory failure. *Am J Resp Crit Care* 2001; **163**: 283–91.
12 Meduri GU, Turner RE, Abou-Shala N, *et al*. Noninvasive positive pressure ventilation via face mask. First line intervention in patients with acute hypercapnic and hypoxemic respiratory failure. *Chest* 1996; **109**: 179–93.
13 Bersten AD, Holt AW, Vedig AE, *et al*. Treatment of severe cardiogenic pulmonary oedema with continuous positive airway pressure delivered by face mask. *N Engl J Med* 1991; **325**: 1825–30.

14 Bott J, Carroll MP, Keilty SEJ, *et al.* Randomised controlled trial of nasal ventilation in acute ventilatory failure due to chronic obstructive airways disease. *Lancet* 1993; **341**: 1555–7.

15 Brochard L, Mancebo J, Wysocki M, *et al.* Non-invasive ventilation for acute exacerbations of chronic obstructive pulmonary disease. *N Engl J Med* 1995; **333**: 817–22.

16 Keenan SP, Kernerman PD, Cook DJ, *et al.* Effect of noninvasive positive pressure ventilation on mortality in patients admitted with acute respiratory failure: a meta-analysis. *Crit Care Med* 1997; **25**: 1685–92.

17 Girou E, Schortgen F, Declaux C, *et al.* Association of noninvasive ventilation with nosocomial infections and survival in critically ill patients. *JAMA* 2000; **284**: 2361–7.

18 Martin JG, Shore S, Engel LA, *et al.* Effect of continuous positive airway pressure on respiratory mechanics and pattern of breathing in induced asthma. *Am Rev Resp Dis* 1982; **126**: 812–7.

19 Shivaram U, Miro AM, Cash ME, *et al.* Cardiopulmonary responses to continuous positive airway pressure in acute asthma. *J Crit Care* 1993; **8**: 87–92.

20 Parkes SN, Bersten AD. Aerosol kinetics and bronchodilator efficacy during continuous positive airway pressure delivered by face mask. *Thorax* 1997; **52**: 171–5.

21 Abou-Shala N, Meduri GU. Noninvasive ventialtion in patients with acute respiratory failure. *Crit Care Med* 1996; **24**: 705–15.

22 Jolliet P, Abajo B, Pasquina P, *et al.* Non-invasive respiratory support ventilation in severe community-acquired pneumonia. *Intensive Care Med* 2001; **27**: 812–21.

23 Delclaux C, L'Her E, Alberti C, *et al.* Treatment of acute hypoxemic nonhypercapnic respiratory insufficiency with continuous positive airway pressure delivered by a face mask. A randomized controlled trial. *JAMA* 2000; **284**: 2352–60.

24 Kramer N, Meyer TJ, Meharg J, *et al.* Randomized prospective trial of non-invasive positive pressure ventilation in acute respiratory failure. *Am J Respir Crit Care Med* 1995; **151**: 1799–806.

25 Confalonieri M, Potena A, Carbone G, *et al.* Acute respiratory failure in patients with severe community acquired pneumonia. *Am J Respir Crit Care Med* 1999; **160**: 1585–91.

26 Hilbert G, Gruson D, Vargas F, *et al.* Noninvasive ventilation in immunosuppressed patients with pulmonary infiltrates, fever and acute respiratory failure. *N Engl J Med* 2001; **344**: 481–7.

27 Antonelli M, Conti G, Bufi M, *et al.* Noninvasive ventilation for treatment of acute respiratory failure in patients undergoing solid organ transplantation: a randomized trial. *JAMA* 2000; **283**: 235–41.

28 Richter-Larsen K, Ingwersen U, Thode S, *et al.* Mask physiotherapy in patients after heart surgery: a controlled study. *Intensive Care Med* 1995; **21**: 469–74.

29 Bolliger CT, Van Eeden SF. Treatment of multiple rib fractures. Randomised controlled trial comparing ventilatory with non-ventilatory management. *Chest* 1990; **97**: 943–8.

30 American Thoracic Society. Indications and standards for use of nasal continuous positive airway pressure (CPAP) in sleep apnoea syndromes. *Am J Respir Crit Care Med* 1994; **150**: 1738–45.

31 National Association for Medical Direction of Respiratory Care. Clinical indications for non-invasive positive pressure ventilation in chronic respiratory failure due to restrictive lung disease, COPD, and nocturnal hypoventilation – a consensus conference report. *Chest* 1999; **116**: 521–34.

32 Granton JT, Naughton MT, Benard DC, *et al.* CPAP improves respiratory muscle strength in patients with heart failure and central sleep apnoea. *Am J Resp Crit Care Med* 1996; **153**: 277–87.

Part Five

Gastroenterological Emergencies

34

Acute gastrointestinal bleeding

J J Y Sung

Acute gastrointestinal (GI) bleeding is a common admission to the ICU and a major cause of morbidity and mortality. Peptic ulcer disease accounts for 75% of upper GI bleeding.[1] Bleeding from varices, oesophagitis, duodenitis and Mallory–Weiss syndrome each account for between 5% and 15% of cases. About 20% of GI bleeding arises from the lower GI tract. Common aetiological causes for GI bleeding are listed in Table 34.1. Mortality from upper GI bleeding has remained at approximately 10% for decades,[1] but recent reports suggest that mortality from bleeding ulcers has fallen substantially to about 5%.[2] On the other hand, variceal bleeding has a much higher mortality of about 30%. Risk factors for mortality include old age, associated medical problems, coagulopathy and magnitude of bleeding.[3]

UPPER GASTROINTESTINAL BLEEDING

CLINICAL PRESENTATION

The patient may or may not present a history of upper GI problems. There may be pain but bleeding ulcers can be painless, especially in elderly patients and users of non-steroidal anti-inflammatory drugs. Frequently, the symptoms of hypovolaemia such as tachycardia, pallor,

Table 34.1 Common causes of acute gastrointestinal bleeding

Upper gastrointestinal bleeding
Peptic ulcers (DU:GU ≈ 3:1)
Varices (oesophageal varices:gastric varices ≈ 9:1)
Portal hypertensive gastropathy
Mallory–Weiss syndrome
Gastritis, duodenitis and oesophagitis

Lower gastrointestinal bleeding
Diverticular bleeding
Angiodysplasia and arteriovenous malformation
Colonic polyps or tumours
Meckel's diverticulum
Inflammatory bowel diseases

DU = Duodenal ulcer; GU = gastrointestinal ulcer.

sweating, cyanosis, mental confusion and oliguria may be present, especially in massive GI bleeding. A history of vomiting and retching preceding haematemesis suggests Mallory–Weiss syndrome.

Haematemesis and melaena are the most common presentations of acute upper GI bleeding. Haematochezia is the passage of bright red or maroon blood from the rectum, in the form of pure blood or admixed with stool. It usually represents a lower intestinal source of bleeding, but can also be a feature of massive upper GI bleeding.

INVESTIGATION

ENDOSCOPY OR BARIUM STUDY

As history and physical examination are seldom useful in identifying the source of bleeding, investigations are necessary in most cases of GI bleeding. Endoscopy has replaced barium studies as the investigation of choice. It should be performed as soon as the patient is haemodynamically stabilized, and adequate supportive personnel are available. Endoscopy is preferred to barium X-rays for the following reasons:

- Endoscopy allows more precise identification of the site and nature of bleeding.
- Endoscopic appearance often predicts the risk of recurrent bleeding from ulcer and varices (see below).
- Lesions such as gastritis, portal hypertensive gastropathy and duodenitis are difficult to diagnose by barium X-ray.
- Treatments such as injecting ulcers may be instigated during endoscopy (see below).
- Barium X-ray is notoriously unreliable in patients with previous gastric surgery.

However, endoscopy can induce serious hypoxia in patients with cardiorespiratory diseases. Continuous monitoring of blood pressure, pulse and oxygen saturation with a pulse oximeter is mandatory. Oxygen should be administered by nasal cannula when necessary.

ANGIOGRAPHY

Angiography is seldom used for the diagnosis of upper GI bleeding. Theoretically, when the bleeding is very brisk and obscures the endoscopic view, angiography may help to identify the sources of bleeding and may sometimes be used to embolize the bleeding point. In practice, however, most patients with this degree of haemorrhage should be considered for emergency laparotomy.

MANAGEMENT OF NON-VARICEAL UPPER GI BLEEDING

The goals of managing a patient with acute GI bleeding are first to resuscitate; second, to control active bleeding; and third, to prevent recurrence of haemorrhage.

RESUSCITATION

Blood and plasma expanders should be given through large-bore intravenous cannulae. Vital signs should be closely monitored. In patients with hypovolaemic shock, central venous pressure and hourly urine output should also be observed (see Ch. 9). Following adequate resuscitation, management is directed to identify the lesion and distinguish the high-risk patient, who is likely to require early endoscopic or surgical treatment.

THE HIGH-RISK PATIENT

Significant GI bleeding is indicated by syncope, haematemesis, systolic blood pressure below 100 mmHg (13.3 kPa), postural hypotension and, if more than 4 units of blood have to be transfused in 12 hours, to maintain blood pressure. Patients over 60 years old and with multiple underlying diseases are of even higher risk.[3] Those admitted for other medical problems (e.g. heart or respiratory failure, or cerebrovascular bleed) and who have GI bleeding during hospitalization also have a higher mortality.

THE HIGH-RISK ULCER

Peptic ulcers that are actively bleeding or have bled recently may show stigmata of haemorrhage on endoscopy. These include localized active bleeding (i.e. pulsatile, arterial spurting or simple oozing), an adherent blood clot, a protuberant vessel or a flat pigmented spot on the ulcer base. Stigmata of haemorrhage are important predictors of recurrent bleeding (Table 34.2).[4-6] The proximal posteroinferior wall of the duodenal bulb and the high lesser curve of the stomach are common sites for severe recurrent bleeding, due probably to their respective large arteries (gastroduodenal and left gastric arteries).

TREATMENT
Pharmacological control

Acid-suppressing drugs such as H_2-receptor antagonists and proton-pump inhibitors are very effective drugs to promote ulcer healing. An acidic environment impairs platelet function and haemostasis. Therefore, reducing the secretion of gastric acid should reduce bleeding and encourage ulcer healing. Recent study has shown that potent acid suppression using intravenous proton pump inhibitors reduces recurrent bleeding after endoscopic therapy.[7] Proton pump inhibitors should be recommended in high-risk peptic ulcer bleeding patients as an adjuvant to endoscopic therapy. On the contrary, antifibrinolytic agents such as tranexamic acid have not been effective in reducing the operative rate and mortality of acute GI haemorrhage.

Endoscopic therapy

Most patients with acute upper GI haemorrhage stop bleeding spontaneously and have an uneventful recovery. No specific intervention is required in these patients. Endoscopic haemostasis should be used in patients with a high risk of persistent or recurrent bleeding.[8] In the last two decades, endoscopic haemostasis, with its high efficacy and low morbidity, has resulted in a dramatic decrease in emergency surgery, and has reduced the mortality of ulcer bleeding. The three most popular methods of haemostasis are as follows.

Adrenaline injection. Endoscopic injection of adrenaline (1:10 000 dilution) at 0.5–1.0 ml aliquots (up to 10–15 ml) into and around the ulcer bleeding point has achieved successful haemostasis in over 90% of cases.[9] Debate exists as to whether the haemostatic effect is a result of local tamponade by the volume injected, or vasoconstriction by adrenaline. Absorption of adrenaline into the systemic circulation has been documented, but without any significant effect on the haemodynamic status of the patient.[10] Adrenaline injection is an effective, cheap, portable and easy-to-learn method of haemostasis, and has acquired a world-wide popularity.

Coaptive coagulation. This method uses direct pressure and heat energy (heater probe) or electrocoagulation (BICAP probe) to control ulcer bleeding. The depth of tissue injury induced by these devices is minimized, as the bleeding vessel is tamponaded prior to coagulation. The overall efficacy of the adrenaline injection, heater probe and BICAP probe methods is comparable.[11-13] Occasionally, it is not possible to obtain a view *en face* of the bleeding ulcers, particularly those on the lesser curve or on the posterior wall of the duodenal bulb. In these situations, direct pressure cannot be applied, and the failure rate of coaptive coagulation in these situations is expected to be higher.

Table 34.2 Stigmata of haemorrhage and risk of recurrent bleeding in peptic ulcers

Stigmata of haemorrhage	% recurrent bleeding
Spurter or oozer	85–90
Protuberant vessel	35–55
Adherent clot	30–40
Flat spot	5–10
None	<5

Haemoclips. Endoscopic clipping of a bleeding vessel is an appealing alternative treatment which has gained popularity in recent years. The advantage of haemoclips over thermocoagulation is that there is no tissue injury induced and hence reduced risk of perforation. Studies comparing haemoclips against injection[14] and thermocoagulation[15] have shown favourable results. However, the application of haemoclips in certain sites, for example lesser curve, gastric fundus and posterior wall of the duodenum, is technically difficult. Loading of clip on the application device is cumbersome and time-consuming and transfer of torque from the handle to the tip of the device is limited.

SURGERY

Surgery remains the most definitive method of stopping haemorrhage. However, there is little agreement on the exact indications and best timing for surgical intervention. These issues are even less clear now that endoscopic treatment is so effective. Accordingly, good co-operation among intensivists, gastroenterologists and surgeons is essential. Indications for surgery can be:

- arterial bleeding that cannot be controlled by endoscopic haemostasis;
- massive transfusion (i.e. total of 6–8 units of blood) required to maintain blood pressure;
- recurrent clinical bleeding after initial success with endoscopic therapy or retreatment;
- evidence suggestive of GI perforation.

Surgical procedures include under-running of the ulcer, under-running plus vagotomy and drainage, and various types of gastrectomy. The overall mortality of emergency surgery for GI bleeding is about 15–20%. In a recent study investigating the best salvage treatment for patients with recurrent bleeding after endoscopic therapy, surgery was found to be comparable to repeating endoscopic treatment in securing hemostasis.[17] However, morbidity is significantly higher in surgical patients than in endoscopic patients. Early surgery should be considered in patients with hypovolemic shock and/or large peptic ulcer with protuberant vessels. A protocol to manage bleeding peptic ulcer is shown in Fig. 34.1.

ACUTE STRESS ULCERATION

Acute stress ulceration is associated with shock, sepsis, burns, multiple trauma, head injuries, spinal injuries and respiratory, renal and hepatic failure. Lesions are most commonly seen in the gastric fundus, and range from mild erosions to acute ulcerations. The exact mechanism leading to acute mucosal erosion/ulceration in critically ill patients is still unclear. Hypoxia and hypoperfusion of the gastroduodenal mucosa are probably the most important factors. Besides haemodynamic instability, respiratory failure and coagulopathy are also strong inde-

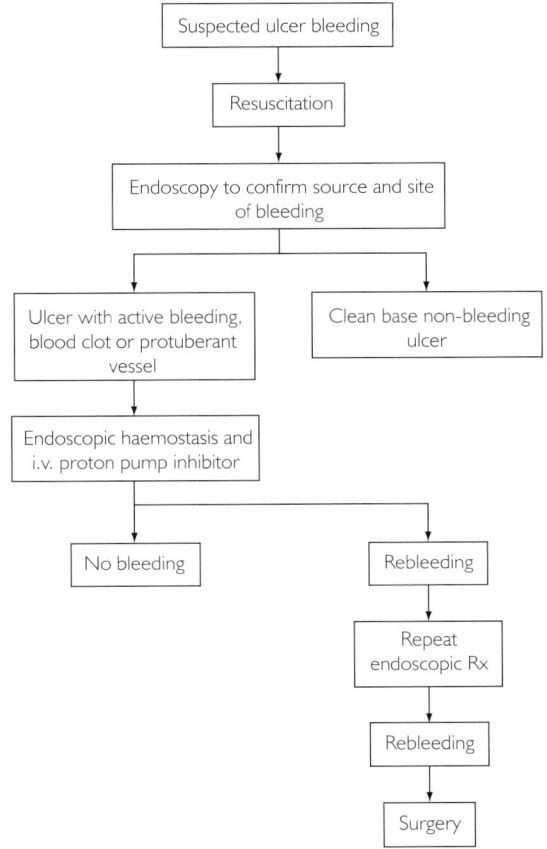

Fig. 34.1 Management of peptic ulcer bleeding.

pendent factors in critically ill patients.[17] The incidence of stress-related mucosal bleeding in ICU patients was reported to be ranging from 8 to 45%.[17] It has been declining in the last decade as a result of highly effective management of hypotension and hypoxaemia. Bleeding may be occult or overt, from 'coffee grounds' aspirates to frank haemorrhage.

PROPHYLAXIS AND TREATMENT

Significant ulcerations are managed as above. Minor bleeding and *prophylactic* treatment are considered together. Prophylactic treatment aims for gastric alkalinization (gastric pH > 3.5), on the rationale that gastric acidity is the main cause of stress ulceration. The incidence of stress ulcerations appears to be lower with prophylactic gastric alkalinization than with placebos, although an improvement in survival has not been shown.[18] Gastric bacterial overgrowth and the associated nosocomial pneumonia has been a concern but not substantiated by existing data.[19] On balance, prophylactic treatment should probably be reserved only for at-risk patients. Scoring systems to estimate the risk of stress-ulcer bleeding have been proposed, for example Zinner[20] and Tryba scores.[21] The mainstay of prophylaxis and treatment for minor bleeding remain supportive – optimize oxygenation and tissue perfusion and control of infection. There is little consensus among critical care experts in the choice of prophylactic treatment used.[22] Drugs given include the following:

Antacids

Antacids given hourly via a nasogastric tube can maintain gastric alkalinization. Gastric pH monitoring is necessary. Antacids contain magnesium, aluminium, calcium or sodium, and complications may arise from excessive intake of these minerals. Bowel stasis and diarrhoea can also be problems. They are used less commonly now.

Sucralfate

This is a basic aluminium salt of sucrose octasulphate. It is effective in healing ulcers by increasing mucus secretion, mucosal blood flow and local prostaglandin production. These effects promote mucosal resistance against acid and pepsin (i.e. they are cytoprotective). As it does not alter gastric pH, Gram-negative bacterial colonization of gastric juice is less likely. The incidence of nosocomial pneumonia may be less with sucralfate than with antacids or H_2-receptor antagonists, but this is debatable.[20,23] Sucralfate is given via the nasogastric tube as 1.0 g every 4–6 h. Constipation is a side-effect, and aluminium toxicity may arise from renal dysfunction.

H_2-receptor antagonists

These drugs suppress acid secretion by competing for the histamine receptor on the parietal cell. Cimetidine is less potent and has interactions with anticonvulsants, theophyllines and warfarin. Famotidine and nizatidine are newer agents but have no particular advantage over ranitidine. The problem of H_2-receptor antagonists is the development of tachyphylaxis after the first day of administration, leading to reduction of effectiveness in acid suppression. Recent meta-analysis showed that ranitidine did not confer any protection against stress ulcer in the intensive care patients.[23]

Proton-pump inhibitors

These are potent acid-suppressing agents as they block the final common pathway of acid secretion by the parietal cell, namely the proton pump. All proton pump inhibitors (omeprazole, lansoprazole, pantoprazole and rabeprazole) can be given as oral medication. Omeprazole and pantoprazole are also available in intravenous form for those who cannot be fed orally. In two non-randomized studies, intravenous omeprazole has been shown to protect critically ill patients who required ventilation from the development of stress-related mucosal bleeding from the upper GI tract.[24,25] Yet, there are no prospective data indicating which are the high-risk patients who might benefit from this treatment.

VARICEAL BLEEDING

Acute variceal bleeding is a serious complication of portal hypertension, with a high mortality. About 50% of patients with bleeding varices have had an earlier bleed during hospitalization. The degree of liver failure, that is, Child–Pugh's classification (see Ch. 36) is the most important prognostic factor for early rebleeding and survival.

RESUSCITATION

Immediate resuscitation with whole blood and fluid is mandatory. Overtransfusion may cause a rebound increase in portal pressure (with a consequent increased risk of rebleeding) and must be avoided. Fresh frozen plasma and platelet concentrates transfusion may be indicated. A nasogastric cannula is often inserted for the removal of blood (and also drug administration). Forceful aspiration through the nasogastric tube should be discouraged as bleeding may be induced. Lactulose (15–30 ml every 4–6 h) should be given to prevent or correct hepatic encephalopathy. A colonic wash-out can be used, but a magnesium-containing enema should be avoided in the presence of renal failure. Close attention must be given to haemodynamic monitoring.

When the patient is haemodynamically stable, upper endoscopy should be performed to identify the source of bleeding. Patients with portal hypertension could bleed from oesophageal or gastric varices, peptic ulcers and portal hypertensive gastropathy.

PHARMACOLOGICAL CONTROL

Vasopressin (0.2–0.4 U/min) used to be the most widely used agent to reduce portal blood pressure and control variceal bleeding. Adverse effects of vasopressin such as cardiac ischaemia (in about 10% of patients) and worsening coagulopathy (by release of plasminogen activator) have discouraged the use of this drug in recent years. Terlipressin, a triglycyl synthetic analogue of vasopressin, has a longer half-life and fewer cardiac side-effects and appears more effective and safe when used in combination with glyceryl trinitrate.[26] Infusion of somatostatin and its analogue (octreotide, vapreotide) reduces portal blood pressure and azygous blood flow. They are safe and effective vasoactive agents to be used in acute variceal bleeding.[27,28] The benefit is more prominent if these vasoactive agents are given early, even before endoscopy.[29–31] Octreotide has also been shown to be effective when used as an adjuvant therapy in combination with endoscopic therapy.[32,33] Recurrent bleeding episodes and hence requirement of transfusion are significantly reduced.

ENDOSCOPIC SCLEROTHERAPY

Endoscopic injection sclerotherapy is the mainstay of treatment. At endoscopy, sclerosants can be injected directly into the variceal columns (intravariceal injection) or into the mucosa adjacent to the varices (paravariceal injection) to cause venous thrombosis, inflammation, and tissue fibrosis. Commonly used sclerosants are ethanolamine oleate, sodium tetradecyl sulphate (1–3%), polidocanol and ethyl alcohol. None has appreciable advantage over the others and the choice is very much a personal preference of the endoscopist, and depends also on availability. Endoscopic sclerotherapy controls 80–90% of acute variceal bleeding. Complications such as ulcer formation, fever, chest pain and mediastinitis are common. Bleeding from gastric varices is more difficult to control by injection sclerotherapy because of difficult access. Butylcyanoacrylate (Histoacryl) has been used recently for gastric variceal injections, with a claimed superior haemostatic effect.[34] It is mixed with lipiodol to delay the rate of polymerization and allow radiological monitoring of the injection.

ENDOSCOPIC VARICEAL LIGATION

Endoscopic variceal ligation was introduced in the late 1980s as a mechanical method to control bleeding from varices. Rubber bands mounted on the banding device at the tip of the endoscope are released to strangulate the bleeding varices. Numerous studies comparing endoscopic variceal ligation with endoscopic sclerotherapy showed that the technique is as effective as injection sclerotherapy in acute bleeding.[35] Procedure-related complications are significantly fewer, as there is no tissue chemical irritation. An overtube to facilitate banding avoids aspiration during the procedure, but may result in serious oesophageal injury if used improperly. The tunnel vision produced by the banding device as originally designed restricts visibility, and thus makes the procedure technically difficult when bleeding is heavy. With the introduction of multiple banding devices which are loaded with 5–10 rubber bands, and the use of transparent caps, the problems of overtube injury and tunnel vision have been overcome. Endoscopic variceal ligation, in many centres, has replaced injection sclerotherapy as the first choice for variceal hemorrhage. Many have combined the two endoscopic treatments together in an attempt to improve the outcome. Existing data so far do not support this combined therapy to be better. Combined endoscopic therapy cannot be recommended.

BALLOON TAMPONADE

Variceal bleeding can be controlled by exerting pressure directly on the bleeding point using a balloon. The Sengstaken–Blackmore tube has been replaced by the four-lumen Minnesota tube which allows aspiration of gastric and oesophageal contents. Inflation of the gastric balloon (by 250–350 ml of water) is often sufficient to stop the bleeding by occluding the feeding veins to the oesophageal varices. If bleeding continues, the oesophageal balloon can be inflated by air and kept at a pressure of 50–60 mmHg (6.7–8.0 kPa). Duration of using balloon tamponade should be limited to 24 hours to avoid tissue pressure necrosis. Because of available effective pharmacological and endoscopic therapies, balloon tamponade should only be used in the exceptional cases when these therapies fail to effect control of bleeding.

TRANSJUGULAR INTRAHEPATIC PORTOSYSTEMIC SHUNT (TIPS)

Using a transjugular approach, a catheter is inserted into the hepatic vein, and advanced under fluoroscopic guidance into a branch of the portal vein.[36] By means of a guide wire and dilators, a self-expandable metal stent is introduced to create an intrahepatic portosystemic shunt. In good hands, success can be achieved in over 90% of cases. This procedure significantly reduces portal blood pressure and thus bleeding from varices. Major complications include intra-abdominal haemorrhage and stent occlusion. Hepatic encephalopathy has been reported in 25–60% of patients. Nevertheless, this is an effective salvage treatment for uncontrolled variceal bleeding. Meta-analysis comparing TIPS against endoscopic therapy showed that the former has secure haemostasis but at the cost of increasing risk of hepatic encephalopathy.[37]

A number of markers of outcome after TIPS have been under investigation, including the APACHE score, presence of hyponatremia and Child C liver disease, hepatic encephalopathy before TIPS, presence of ascites and serum albumin. Before a reliable marker of outcome can be identified, TIPS should be reserved for the subset of patients who continue to bleed or develop recurrent bleeding after endoscopic therapy. Unlike shunt surgery, TIPS will not reduce the chance of future liver transplantation.

SURGERY

Surgical treatments for variceal bleeding include direct devascularization of the lower oesophagus plus the proximal stomach and a variety of surgical shunts. The role of surgery has diminished since the advent of endoscopic treatment and TIPS.[38] Surgery is now used as a second-line treatment, when bleeding continues or recurs after two sessions of injection sclerotherapy or banding ligation. Both staple transection of the oesophagus and portocaval shunt surgery are highly effective emergency measures. Despite successful control of bleeding, long-term survival is not significantly improved. Hepatic encephalopathy is one of the major complications of shunting operations. Expectations that the Warren distal splenorenal shunt will preserve antegrade portal flow and avoid accelerated deterioration of liver function have not been realized.[39,40] The Warren shunt is technically more difficult, especially if per-formed as an emergency. Choice of surgery should be carefully made in those who are potential transplant candidates, as it may complicate subsequent surgery. A protocol to manage variceal bleeding is shown in Fig. 34.2.

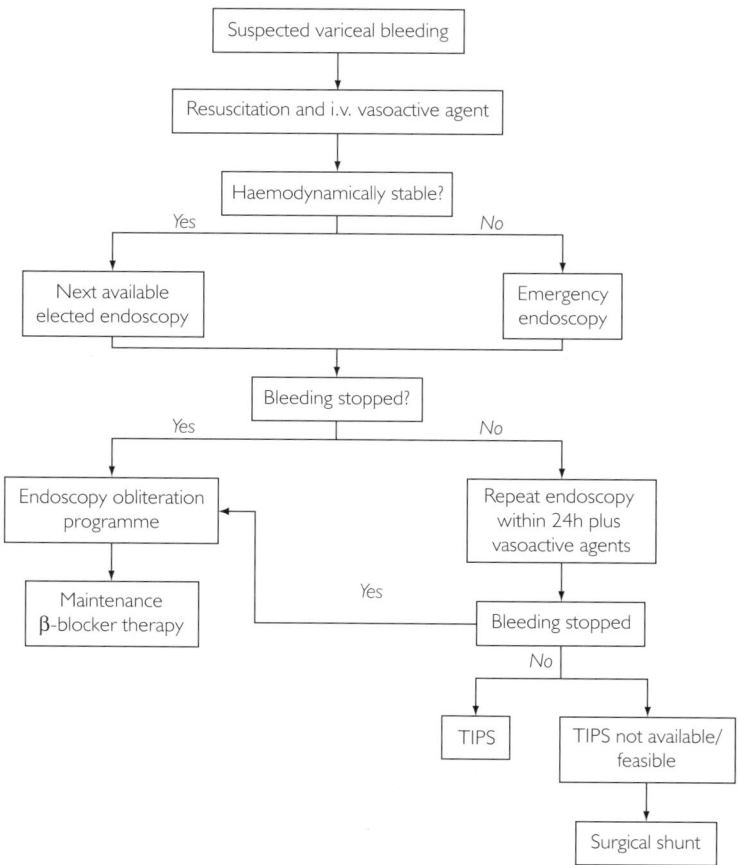

Fig. 34.2 Management of variceal haemorrhage. Transjugular intrahepatic portosystemic shunt (TIPS)

LOWER GASTROINTESTINAL BLEEDING

Lower GI bleeding arises from a source distal to the ligament of Treitz. It accounts for 10–20% of acute GI bleeding. Common causes of colonic bleeding include diverticular haemorrhage and angiodysplasia (both occur on the right-sided colon), colonic polyps and carcinoma, and inflammatory bowel diseases.[41,42]

CLINICAL PRESENTATION

Haematochezia (bright red blood) is the most common presentation of lower GI bleeding. However, bleeding from small intestine and right colon may also present as melaena. Abdominal pain preceding a massive bleeding episode suggests either ischaemia or inflammatory bowel disease. Painless massive bleeding is common in diverticulosis, angiodysplasia or from a Meckel's diverticulum. In a patient with portal hypertension, haemorrhoids may present with massive haematochezia.

INVESTIGATIONS

Haemorrhoids and rectal tumour can easily be identified by proctosigmoidoscopy, which should always be performed. Since upper GI bleeding is about five times as common as lower GI bleeding, the former should be excluded. When both proctosigmoidoscopy and gastroscopy are negative, the lower GI tract should be examined by colonoscopy, angiography or radio-nucleotide scan. Barium enema plays no role in the management of acute rectal bleeding.

COLONOSCOPY

Patients with mild-to-moderate haematochezia can be examined safely by colonoscopy. Colonoscopy is difficult in an actively bleeding patient, and may carry an increased risk of perforation. Visualization is often unsatisfactory due to the dark discoloration of blood.[43] Colonoscopy yields much better results with adequate bowel preparation once bleeding has stopped.

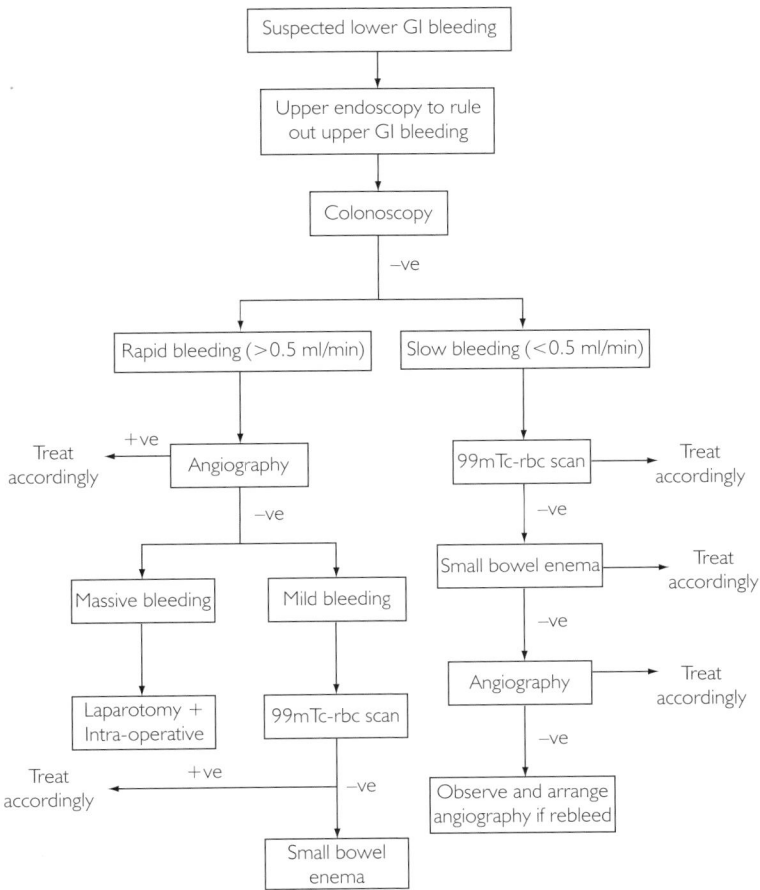

Fig. 34.3 Management of lower gastrointestinal bleeding.

ANGIOGRAPHY OR RADIONUCLIDE SCAN

The diagnostic efficacy of radionuclide scan and angiography varies in different studies. [99m]Tc sulphur colloid is quickly removed from the blood stream after injection. Its diagnostic yield is low because of its short circulatory half-life. [99m]Tc labelling of red cells prolongs the duration of radioactivity in the body. Red cell scan has been reported to detect the source of active bleeding in over 80% of cases.[44]

Diagnostic angiography is helpful in two situations: (i) when the view of endoscopy is completely obscured by active haemorrhage; (ii) in defining abnormal vasculatures, where angiography is more sensitive even if extravasation of contrast material is not seen. These lesions include angiodysplasia, arteriovenous malformation and various inherited vascular anomalies (e.g. Rendu–Osler–Weber syndrome, pseudoxanthoma elasticum and Ehlers–Danlos syndrome). Angiography may localize the site of bleeding in 80–85% of patients when the bleeding rate is more than 0.5 ml/min.[45] Both

superior and inferior mesenteric angiograms are often needed.

MANAGEMENT

ENDOSCOPY

Bleeding from vascular anomalies can be treated by electro-coagulation, heater probe and laser photocoagulation, unless they are too large or too diffuse.[46] Bleeding colonic polyps can be removed by polypectomy or coagulated by hot biopsy forceps. Bleeding from colonic diverticuli can also been controlled with thermocoagulation through colonoscopy.[47]

ANGIOGRAPHY

Angiographic intra-arterial infusion of vasopressin or occlusion of the bleeding artery with embolic agents such as an absorbable gelatin sponge (Gelfoam) may be used in lower GI bleeding pathologies.[48] Both diverticular bleeding and bleeding from angiodysplasia can be stopped by vasopressin infusion during angiography, but recurrence of bleeding occurs frequently with diverticular disease.

SURGERY

Diverticular bleeding usually arises from a relatively large vessel, and may be difficult to control with endoscopic or angiographic therapy. Partial resection of the colon is warranted after localization of the bleeding site. Surgery is also indicated in vascular anomalies when endoscopic treatment fails. When an obvious and refractory massive lower GI bleeding is not identified by endoscopic or angiographic examinations, immediate laparotomy with possible subtotal colectomy should be offered. A protocol to manage lower GI bleeding is shown in Fig. 34.3.

REFERENCES

1 Silverstein FE, Gilbert DA, Tedesco FJ, *et al.* The National ASGE survey on upper gastrointestinal bleeding. I. Study design and baseline data. *Gastrointest Endosc* 1981; **27**: 73–9.
2 Holman RAE, Davis M, Gough KR, *et al.* Value of a centralized approach in the management of haematemesis and melaena: experience in a district general hospital. *Gut* 1990; **31**: 504–8.
3 Silverstein FE, Gilbert DA, Tedesco FJ, *et al.* The National ASGE survey on upper gastrointestinal bleeding. II. Clinical prognostic factors. *Gastrointest Endosc* 1981; **27**: 80–93.
4 Swain CP, Storey DW, Bown SG, *et al.* Nature of bleeding vessel in recurrently bleeding gastric ulcers. *Gastroenterology* 1986; **90**: 595–608.
5 Foster DN, Miloszewski K, Losowsky MS, *et al.* Stigmata of recent haemorrhage in diagnosis and prognosis of upper gastrointestinal bleeding. *BMJ* 1978; **1**: 1173–7.
6 Griffiths WJ, Neumann DA, Welsh JD. The visible vessel as an indicator of uncontrolled or recurrent gastrointestinal haemorrhage. *N Engl J Med* 1979; **300**: 1411–13.
7 Lau JYW, Sung JJY, Lee KKC, *et al.* A comparison of high-dose omeprazole infusion to placebo after endoscopic hemostasis to bleeding peptic ulcer. *N Engl J Med* 2000; **343**: 310–16.
8 NIH Consensus Conference. Therapeutic endoscopy and bleeding ulcers. *JAMA* 1989; **262**: 1369–72.
9 Chung SCS, Lau JYW, Sung JJY, et al A randomized comparison between adrenaline injection alone and injection combined with heat probe for peptic ulcer bleeding *BMJ* 1997; **314**: 1307–10.
10 Sung JY, Chung SCS, Low JM, *et al.* Systemic absorption of epinephrine after endoscopic submucosal injection in patients with bleeding peptic ulcers. *Gastrointest Endosc* 1993; **39**: 20–22.
11 Chung SCS, Leung JWC, Sung JY, *et al.* Injection or heat probe for bleeding ulcer. *Gastroenterology* 1991; **100**: 33–7.

12 Jensen DM, Machicado GA, Kovacs TG, *et al.* Controlled, randomized study of heater probes and BICAP for haemostasis of severe ulcer bleeding. *Gastroenterology* 1988; **94**: A208. [Abstr]
13 Laine L. Multipolar electrocoagulation in the treatment of active upper gastrointestinal haemorrhage: a prospective controlled trial. *N Engl J Med* 1987; **316**:1613–17.
14 Chung IK, Ham JS, Kim HS, *et al.* Comparison of the hemostatic efficacy of the endoscopic hemoclip method with hypertonic saline–epinephrine injection and a combination of the two for the management of bleeding peptic ulcers. *Gastroint Endosc* 1999; **49**: 13–18.
15 Cipolletta L, Bianco MA, Marmo R, *et al.* Endoclip versus heater probe in preventing early rebleeding from peptic ulcers: a prospective randomized trial. *Gastroint Endosc* 2001; **53**: 147–51.
16 Cook DJ, Fuller HO, Guyatt GH, *et al.* Risk factors for gastrointestinal bleeding in critically ill patients. *N Engl J Med* 1994; **330**: 377–81.
17 Lau JYW, Sung JJY, Lam YH, *et al.* Endoscopic retreatment versus surgery in patients rebleeding after initial endoscopic ulcer hemostasis: a prospective randomized controlled trial. *N Engl J Med* 1999; **340**: 751–6.
18 Cook DJ, Witt LJ, Guyatt GH. Stress ulcer prophylaxis in the critically ill: a meta-analysis. *Am J Med* 1991; **91**: 519–27.
19 Zandstra DF, Stoutenbeek CP. The virtual absence of stress-ulceration related bleeding in ICU patients receiving prolonged mechanical ventilation without any prophylaxis – a prospective cohort study. *Intensive Care Med* 1994; **20**: 335–40.
20 Zinner MJ, Zuidema GD, Smith PL, Mignosa M. The prevention of upper gastrointestinal tract bleeding in patients in an intensive care unit. *Surg Gynecol Obstet* 1981; **153**: 214–20.
21 Tryba M Risk of acute stress bleeding and nosocomial pneumonia in ventilated intensive care patients: sucralfate versus antacids. *Am J Med* 1987; **83**(Suppl 3B): 117–24.
22 Lam NP, Le PD, Crawford SY, *et al.* National survey of stress ulcer prophylaxis. *Crit Care Med* 1999; **27**: 98–103.
23 BenMessori A, Trippoli M, Vaiani M *et al.* Bleeding and pneumonia in intensive care patients given ranitidine and sucralfate for prevention of stress ulcer: meta-analysis of randomized controlled trials. *BMJ* 2000; **321**: 1103–6.
24 Phillips JO, Metzler MH, Palmieri MT, *et al.* A prospective study of simplified omeprazole for the prophylaxis of stress-related mucosal damage. *Crit Care Med* 1996; **24**: 1793–800.
25 Lasky MR, Metzler MH, Phillips JO. A prospective study of omeprazole suspension to prevent clinically significant gastrointestinal bleeding from stress ulcers in mechanically ventilated trauma patients. *J Trauma.* 1998; **44**: 527–33.

26 Levacher S, Letoumelin P, Pateron D, *et al*. Early administration of terlipressin and glyceryl trinitrate to control acute upper gastrointestinal bleeding in cirrhotic patients. *Lancet* 1995; **346**: 865–8.

27 Burroughs AK, McCormick PA, Hughes MD, *et al*. Randomized, double-blind, placebo-controlled trial of somatostatin for variceal bleeding: emergency control and prevention of early variceal bleeding. *Gastroenterology* 1990; **99**: 1388–95.

28 D'Amico G, Politi F, Morabito A, *et al*. Octreotide compared with placebo in a treatment strategy for early rebleeding in cirrhosis. A double blind, randomized pragmatic trial. *Hepatology* 1998; **28**: 1206–14.

29 Averginos A, Nevens F, Raptis S, *et al*. Early administration of somatostatin and efficacy of sclerotherapy in acute esophageal variceal bleeds: the European Acute Bleeding Oesophageal Variceal Episodes (ABOVE) randomised trial. *Lancet* 1997; **350**: 1495–9.

30 Levacher S, Letoumelin P, Pateron D, *et al*. Early administration of terlipressin and glyceryl trinitrate to control acute upper gastrointestinal bleeding in cirrhotic patients. *Lancet* 1995; **346**: 865–8.

31 Sung JJY, Chung SCS, Lai CW, *et al*. Octreotide infusion or emergency sclerotherapy for variceal haemorrhage. *Lancet* 1993; **342**: 637–41.

32 Sung JJY, Chung SCS, Yung MY, *et al*. Prospective randomised study of effect of octreotide on rebleeding from oesophageal varices after endoscopic banding ligation. *Lancet* 1995; **346**: 1666–9.

33 Besson I, Ingrand I, Person B, *et al*. Sclerotherapy with or without octreotide for acute variceal bleeding. *N Engl J Med* 1995; **333**: 555–60.

34 Soehendra N, Grimm H, Nam VC, *et al*. N-butyl-2-cyanoacrylate: a supplement to endoscopic sclerotherapy. *Endoscopy* 1987; 19: 221–24.

35 Laine L, Cook D. Endoscopic ligation compared with sclerotherapy for treatment of esophageal variceal bleeding. A meta-analysis. *Ann Intern Med* 1995; **123**: 280–7.

36 Rossle M, Haag K, Ochs A, *et al*. The transjugular intrahepatic portosystemic stent-shunt procedure for variceal bleeding. *N Engl J Med* 1994; **330**: 165–71.

37 Papatheodoridis GV, Goulis J, Leandro G, *et al*. Transjugular intrahepatic portosystemic shunt compared with endoscopic treatment for prevention of variceal rebleeding: a meta-analysis. *Hepatology* 1999; **30**: 612–22.

38 Bornman PC, Krige JEJ, Terblanche J. Management of esophageal varices. *Lancet* 1994; **343**: 1079–1084.

39 Millikan WJ, Warren WD, Henderson JM, *et al*. The Emory prospective randomized trial: selective versus nonselective shunt to control variceal bleeding. *Ann Surg* 1985; **201**: 712–22.

40 Langer B, Taylor BR, MacKenzie DR, *et al*. Further report of a prospective randomized trial comparing distal splenorenal shunt with end-to-side portacaval shunt: an analysis of encephalopathy; survival, and quality of life. *Gastroenterology* 1985; **88**: 424–9.

41 Boley SJ, Brandt LJ, Frank MS. Severe lower intestinal bleeding: diagnosis and treatment. *Clin. Gastroenterol* 1981; **10**: 65–91.

42 Leitman IM, Paull DE, Shires GT. Evaluation and management of massive lower gastrointestinal haemorrhage. *Ann Surg* 1989; **209**: 175–80.

43 Jensen DM, Machicado GA. Diagnosis and treatment of severe haematochezia: the role of urgent colonoscopy after purge. *Gastroenterology* 1988; **95**:1569–74.

44 Bunker SR, Lull RJ. Scintigraphy of gastrointestinal bleeding: superiority of ^{99m}Tc red blood cells over ^{99m}Tc sulfur colloid. *Am J Radiol* 1984; **143**: 543–8.

45 Wright HK. Massive colonic haemorrhage. *Surg Clin North Am* 1980; **60**: 1297–304.

46 Rutgeerts P, Van Gompel F, Geboes K, *et al*. Long term results of treatment of vascular malformations of the gastrointestinal tract by neodymium YAG laser photocoagulation. *Gut* 1985; **26**: 586–93.

47 Jensen DM, Machicado GA, Jubata R, *et al*. Urgent colonoscopy for the diagnosis and treatment of severe diverticular hemorrhage. *N Engl J Med* 2000; **342**: 78–82.

48 Sherman LM, Shenoy SS, Cerra FB. Selective intra-arterial vasopressin: clinical efficacy and complications. *Ann Surg* 1979; **189**: 298–302.

35

Severe acute pancreatitis

D L A Wyncoll

Acute inflammation of the pancreas produces a spectrum of symptoms, which may be mild and self-limiting, or reflect severe disease that leads rapidly to multiple organ failure and death. In a majority of patients a treatable underlying cause is not identified. Mild, interstitial, oedematous pancreatitis is relatively common. The severe form, acute necrotizing pancreatitis (ANP) is less common, but is associated with a mortality of 27–45%.[1] Management of patients with severe ANP is time-consuming, and labour and resource intensive. Long-term follow-up suggests that those who do survive maintain a good quality of life, although some suffer permanent exocrine and endocrine insufficiency.[2]

In the last 20 years there has been a gradual move towards aggressive supportive therapy for ANP. Numerous putative therapeutic interventions have been tried, but few have provided any objective evidence of clinical benefit. Thus clear treatment guidelines based on compelling data do not exist.

AETIOLOGY

Biliary disease and alcohol remain the two commonest causes of acute pancreatitis world-wide, accounting for 70% of cases. Although no discernible cause is found in many of the remaining cases, there are well-established associations with a number of infections, certain drugs, hyperlipidaemias and trauma (see Table 35.1 for a more exhaustive list).

RANSON'S CRITERIA

Although the overall mortality rate for acute pancreatitis is approximately 10% of patients, the vast majority of deaths occur in the 25% who suffer the severe form of the disease. Since 1974, the standard means of documenting the severity of disease and risk of mortality has been by Ranson's criteria (Table 35.2).[3] These

Table 35.1   Aetiology of acute pancreatitis

Excess alcohol ingestion
Biliary tract disease
Idiopathic
Metabolic
   Hyperlipidaemia
   Hyperparathyroidism
   Diabetic ketoacidosis
   End-stage renal failure
   Pregnancy
   Post renal transplant
Mechanical disorders
   Post-traumatic, postoperative, post-ERCP
   Penetrating duodenal ulcer
   Duodenal obstruction
Infections
   HIV, mumps, EBV, *Mycoplasma, Legionella, Campylobacter,* Ascariasis
Vascular
   Necrotizing vasculitis – SLE, TTP
   Atheroma
   Shock
Drugs
   Azathioprine, thiazides, furosemide (frusemide), tetracyclines, oestrogens, valproic acid, metronidazole, pentamidine, nitrofuration, erythromycin, methydopa, ranitidine, nucleoside reverse transcriptase inhibitors (didanosine) and hydroxyurea.
Toxins
   Scorpion venom, organophosphates, methyl alcohol

factors were determined following the analysis of 100 patients with predominantly alcohol-induced pancreatitis using clinical and laboratory data obtained on admission and after 48 hours, and were based on the assertion that the number of positive criteria should predict outcome. A decade later these criteria were re-evaluated and the first eight were found to be most predictive; these are now known as the Glasgow criteria, or Imrie score.[4]

Table 35.2   Adverse prognostic factors in acute pancreatitis: Ranson's score[3]

On admission	Age >55 years
	White cell count >16 000/mm³
	Glucose >11 mmol/l
	LDH >400 IU/l
	AST >250 IU/l
Within 48 hours of hospitalization	Decrease in Hct >10%
	Increase in blood urea >1.8 mmol/l
	Calcium <2 mmol/l
	PaO₂ <8 kPa
	Base deficit >4 mmol/l
	Fluid deficit >6 l

Risk factors	Mortality rate
0–2	<1%
3–4	≅15%
5–6	≅40%
>6	≅100%

Blamey et al[4] found only eight variables (not LDH, base deficit & fluid deficit) were predictive and are often referred to as the Glasgow criteria or Imrie score.

SCORING

The Acute Physiology and Chronic Health Evaluation (APACHE) II scoring system has also been used in predicting the severity of pancreatitis, and can be used daily throughout the patient's hospital admission and rather than solely within the first 48 hours, thus potentially documenting progress or deterioration. However, such scoring systems are complex to perform and have only been evaluated prospectively 24–48 hours after the onset of pancreatitis, which means that the criteria may not be valid for patients admitted to the ICU subsequently. Those factors with most predictive value for mortality include advanced age, presence of renal or respiratory insufficiency, and presence of shock.

The scoring of patients with acute pancreatitis is important for a number of reasons. First, the clinician can be alerted to the presence of potentially severe disease. Second, comparisons of severity can be made both within and between patient series; and third, rational selection of patients can be made for inclusion in trials of potential new treatments or interventions. Unfortunately, the scoring systems used at present are often inadequate in patients with severe ANP, which is characterized by rapidly progressive multiple system organ dysfunction. In this setting, the Ranson criteria and APACHE score do not take account of the effects of treatment upon measured parameters. The way forward may be to use a combination of the Ranson score, the radiological scoring systems (see below) and a descriptive organ failure score such as the Sepsis-related Organ Failure Assessment (SOFA).[5]

MANAGEMENT OF SEVERE PANCREATITIS

IMAGING

Dynamic contrast-enhanced computed tomography (CT) provides the best means of accurately visualizing the pancreas and diagnosing pancreatitis and its local complications. It also may be used for guiding percutaneous catheter drainage. Guidelines have been suggested for the efficacious use of CT scanning and are shown in Table 35.3.[6]

In severe acute pancreatitis, there is lack of normal enhancement to contrast of the gland or a portion thereof. This is consistent with pancreatic necrosis, defined as diffuse or focal areas of non-viable parenchyma (Table 35.4). Microscopically, there is evidence of damage to the parenchymal network, acinar cells and pancreatic ductal system and necrosis of perilobular fat. Areas of necrosis are often multifocal and rarely involve the whole gland, and may be confined to the periphery with preservation of the core. Necrosis develops early in the course of the disease and is usually established 96 hours after the onset of symptoms.[7] The extent of pancreatic necrosis and the degree of peripancreatic inflammation have been used to determine outcome. A grading system combining the two CT prognostic indicators (the extent of necrosis and the grade of peripancreatic inflammation) has been developed to give the 'CT severity index'. Most complications of acute pancreatitis occur in patients in whom the initial diagnosis is based upon peripancreatic fluid collections, and an excellent correlation

Table 35.3   Guidelines for efficacious use of CT scanning in suspected acute pancreatitis[6]

- Patients in whom the clinical diagnosis is in doubt
- Patients with hyperamylasaemia and severe clinical pancreatitis, abdominal distension, tenderness, high fever (>39°C), and leukocytosis
- Patients with Ranson score >3 or APACHE II >8
- Patients showing lack of improvement after 72 hours of initial conservative therapy
- Acute deterioration following initial clinical improvement

Table 35.4   Grades of peripancreatic inflammation by CT scanning

A	Normal pancreas
B	Focal or diffuse enlargement of the pancreas
C	Pancreatic gland abnormalities associated with peripancreatic inflammation
D	Fluid collection in a single location
E	Two or more fluid collections and/or the presence of gas in or adjacent to the pancreas

has been established between the CT depiction of necrosis and the development of complications and death.[8]

For patients with necrosis in the pancreatic head, the outcome is as severe as when the entire pancreas is affected. By contrast, for patients with necrosis in only the distal portion of the gland, the outcome is favourable with few complications.[9] The mechanism may be that necrosis in the pancreatic head causes obstruction of the pancreatic duct and produces a rise in pressure in the acinar cells, leading to damage and leakage of activated destructive proteases.

After the initial CT scan, additional scanning is only indicated if the patient's clinical condition deteriorates, usually through the development of pancreatic necrosis, abscess or pancreatic pseudocyst, haemorrhage, colonic ischaemia or perforation.

Ultrasonography in acute pancreatitis is less useful, since visualization of the gland may be obscured by 'gas filled' bowel. Moreover, the degree of necrosis, which determines prognosis, cannot be assessed. However, there may be a role for this mode of imaging in demonstrating gallstones, or in the subsequent management, when ultrasound-guided fine-needle aspiration of the pancreas or surrounding tissue may help to establish the presence of infection.

SURGERY

The role of surgery remains the most controversial area in the management of severe ANP. Early in the 20th century most patients with acute pancreatitis of even moderate severity underwent operative intervention. The results were poor, with mortality rates in excess of 50%, although this was without ICU facilities. In 1972, this feeling was summarized in a cynical comment that a '10 minute surgical discussion of acute pancreatitis should probably include 9 minutes of silence'.[10] The conservative, non-surgical approach to severe pancreatitis persisted for many years. During the past decade, however, it has become clear that certain patients with severe pancreatitis do benefit from operative intervention, and that they will not survive without it.[11] Nevertheless, the decision regarding whether to and when to operate is often difficult, and requires careful clinical judgement.

A laparotomy for an acute abdomen is essential when the diagnosis of pancreatitis is in doubt. Surgery may increase the incidence of subsequent infection, but this risk is outweighed by the dangers of delaying the diagnosis and treatment of other serious intra-abdominal conditions. Indications for surgery in severe ANP have been proposed (Table 35.5).[12] If severe acute pancreatitis is an unsuspected 'chance' finding at laparotomy, a T-tube should be inserted into the common bile duct, particularly if it has been explored and the opportunity taken for placement of a feeding jejunostomy tube.[13] Others oppose this approach on the basis that opening a hollow viscus risks peritonitis.

Table 35.5 Indications for surgery in severe acute pancreatitis[12]

Accepted	Controversial
Differential diagnosis	>50% Sterile pancreatic
Persistent biliary pancreatitis	necrosis
Infected pancreatic necrosis	Stable but persistent necrosis
Pancreatic abscess	Deterioration in clinical course
	Organ system failure

INFECTED PANCREATIC NECROSIS

The presence of infected pancreatic necrosis seems to be an undisputed indication for urgent surgery. Contrast-enhanced CT scan documents necrosis, and infection is proven by percutaneous aspiration of localized fluid collections or of the necrotic tissue. All such patients require some form of surgical treatment, although whether this should consist of debridement and gravity drainage, continuous closed lavage of the lesser sac, staged repeated laparotomy, or open packing, remains to be established. Non-operative methods for the treatment of infected pancreatic necrosis, such as radiological placement of drainage tubes are doomed to failure because of repeated blockage due to the viscid nature of the infected material.

STERILE PANCREATIC NECROSIS

The observation that some patients with severe ANP survive without becoming infected and avoid surgery is well known. Moreover, operating upon such patients hypothetically may increase the risk of subsequent infection and of its associated mortality. This is the basis of the critical decision as to whether patients with sterile ANP should undergo operative intervention; the question remains unanswered.

PANCREATIC ABSCESSES

Pancreatic abscesses are circumscribed collections of pus containing little or no pancreatic necrosis, which arise as a later consequence of acute pancreatitis or pancreatic trauma. They commonly occur four weeks or more after the onset of severe pancreatitis, and CT scan most accurately makes the diagnosis. If the appropriate expertise is available, percutaneous catheter drainage may be successful, although the most recent series still reports a 40% failure rate.[14] Consequently, proceeding to open surgical drainage is often used as the initial procedure.

ENDOSCOPIC RETROGRADE CHOLANGIOPANCREATOGRAPHY (ERCP)

ERCP represents an alternative approach particularly for patients with severe biliary pancreatitis. Three prospective randomized studies have been carried out to compare early ERCP with conservative treatment in acute biliary pancreatitis.[15–17] Although the studies are not entirely consistent, ERCP and papillotomy seem to be beneficial in severe biliary pancreatitis if undertaken by a skilled operator, whereas in mild pancreatitis the risks of intervention probably outweigh the benefits.

TREATMENT WITH PHARMACOLOGICAL AGENTS

Theories regarding the pathogenesis of acute pancreatitis have promoted the concept that autodigestion of the gland and peri-pancreatic tissue by activated pancreatic enzymes is a central component. This has led to the suggestion that the reduction of pancreatic exocrine secretion, thereby 'resting the pancreas', might improve outcome. The problem is that the secretory status of the pancreas in severe ANP is not known. Consequently, it is not clear whether inhibition of secretion actually occurs or whether this is beneficial. Therapies designed to inhibit pancreatic secretion, such as cimetidine, atropine, calcitonin, glucagon, and fluorouracil do not alter the course of the disease. However, other pharmacological therapies such as aprotonin and gabexate mesilate, both protease inhibitors, and somatostatin and octreotide are in widespread use in the hope of improving the outcome.

SOMATOSTATIN AND OCTREOTIDE

Somatostatin and its long-acting analogue octreotide are potent inhibitors of pancreatic secretion. They also stimulate activity of the reticuloendothelial system and play a regulatory role, mostly inhibitory, in the modulation of the immune response via autocrine and neuroendocrine pathways. Both are cytoprotective with respect to the pancreas.[18] Other effects include:

- Somatostatin blocks the release of tumour necrosis factor and interferon-γ by peripheral mononuclear cells.
- Octreotide increases the phagocytotic activity of monocytes.[19]

These actions may be important in the modulation of the pathogenesis of adult respiratory distress syndrome (ARDS) and septic shock, both of which can complicate severe ANP. Both agents are effective in experimental pancreatitis,[20] and in the prevention of complications in patients undergoing surgery for chronic pancreatitis.[21] Potential difficulties include:

- Pre-emptive administration is not possible in the acute situation.
- Both agents are powerful splanchnic vasoconstrictors.

The development of pancreatic necrosis has been linked to hypoperfusion of the gland and vasoconstrictors worsen the histological severity of experimental pancreatitis.[22] Consequently, these agents have both beneficial and detrimental effects.

Systematic evaluation of this therapy suggests that there is insufficient evidence at present to support the use of octreotide or somatostatin in the treatment of patients with moderate-to-severe acute pancreatitis.[23]

Additionally, the therapeutic effect of octreotide, if present at all, is probably very small and therefore unlikely to make any significant impact in the management of acute pancreatitis.

PROTEASE INHIBITORS

A further pathogenic mechanism involved in acute pancreatitis is autodigestion of the pancreas by the activation of proteases. More accurately, there is an imbalance between proteases and anti-proteases. Aprotinin and gabexate mesilate are proteolytic enzyme inhibitors that act on serine-proteases such as trypsin, phospholipase A_2, kallikrein, plasmin, thrombin and C1r and C1s esterases.

The largest randomized study of a protease inhibitor included 223 patients with moderate or severe pancreatitis who received gabexate mesilate for 7 days or placebo.[24] There was no difference between the groups with regard to mortality (16 versus 15%), complications or the need for surgery.

The reason why these agents, in clinical practice, do not have the expected beneficial effect on outcome may be the lag time between the onset of pancreatitis and administration. Additionally, derangement to the microvascular control of the pancreas combined with increased vascular permeability may be contributory. Continuous regional arterial infusion or intraperitoneal administration may be more advantageous, but so far trials using these modes of administration have only involved small numbers of patients. At present, there is insufficient evidence to recommend protease inhibitors in acute pancreatitis.

PROPHYLACTIC ANTIBIOTICS

Bacterial infection of necrotic pancreatic tissue occurs in approximately 40–70% of patients with ANP, and infection is the major cause of morbidity and mortality.[25] Early studies investigating the role of antibiotics in acute pancreatitis showed no benefit, but most included patients with mild disease and employed agents (e.g. ampicillin) with inefficient penetration of pancreatic tissue. Subsequent studies are more encouraging.

Imipenem has exceptional penetration into pancreatic tissues and broad activity against most of the common pathogens encountered in this disease. One study compared imipenem with placebo in patients with early necrotizing pancreatitis.[26] The incidence of septic complications was significantly reduced in the treated group (12.2 versus 30.3%), although there was only a trend towards decreased mortality (7 versus 12%).

In another study of ethanol-induced ANP, cefuroxime was compared to placebo.[27] There were more infectious complications in the non-antibiotic group (mean per patient 1.8 versus 1.0; $p < 0.01$) and mortality was also higher (7 versus 1 death; $p = 0.03$).

The evidence at present suggests that administration of an i.v. antibiotic such as high dose cefuroxime, a quinolone or a carbapenem to patients with ANP is beneficial. Patients with mild pancreatitis do not benefit from antibiotics.

SELECTIVE DECONTAMINATION OF THE GUT

The original selective digestive decontamination (SDD) strategy contained three components: oropharyngeal and gastric decontamination with polymyxin E, tobramicin, and amphotericin B and intravenous cefotaxime for 4 days.[28] There is ongoing debate as to the effectiveness of this strategy and results are conflicting regarding any reduction in mortality, particularly when applied to a general critically ill population. However, more promising results have been seen in specific patient populations.

Severe acute pancreatitis may be one clinical situation which supports the hypothesis that gut hypoperfusion promotes bacterial translocation, leading to infection of the inflamed pancreas and peripancreatic tissue.[29] The only controlled trial of SDD in pancreatitis was performed in 102 patients,[30] who were randomized to receive control teatment or SDD: oral colistin, amphoteracin and norfloxacin with addition of a daily dose of the three drugs were given as a rectal enema and systemic cefotaxime until Gram-negative bacteria were successfully eliminated from the oral cavity and rectum. Surveillance samples were taken regularly to assess whether any subsequent infection was of exogenous or endogenous origin. There were 18 deaths (35%) in the control group, compared with 11 (22%) in the SDD group ($p < 0.05$). This difference was caused by a fall in late mortality due to significant reduction in the incidence of Gram-negative pancreatic infection. There was also a reduction in the mean number of laparotomies in the SDD patients. Since the SDD regimen used in this study incorporated i.v. cefotaxime it could be argued that the improvement in outcome was not due to the colistin, amphoteracin, norfloxacin components, but merely due to a systemic antibiotic effect.

Meta-analyses of SDD suggest that there are clear trends towards a reduction in mortality in critically ill patients.[31] However, fear of the emergence of resistant Gram-positive cocci prevents widespread institution of this strategy.

NUTRITIONAL SUPPORT

The provision of nutritional support for the patient with ANP is an essential component of supportive therapy, especially since many patients with pancreatitis are nutritionally depleted prior to their illness and face increased metabolic demands throughout the course of their disorder. Failure to reverse or prevent malnutrition, and a prolonged negative nitrogen balance, increases mortality rates. The route by which nutrition is administered is, none the less, still hotly debated. In the last decade there has been a trend away from the use of total parenteral nutrition (TPN) in favour of enteral nutrition (EN) in

supporting the critically ill. Studies suggest that early EN started within 24 hours of admission to ICU, compared with TPN or delayed EN, is associated with improved wound healing and decreased septic morbidity.[32] Additionally, there is increasing evidence of negative effects of TPN,[33] such as increased gut permeability, increased catheter-related sepsis, an immunosuppressive effect,[34] increased incidence of septic complications and greatly increased costs.

TOTAL PARENTERAL NUTRITION

Severe pancreatitis is often quoted as an absolute contraindication to EN, and TPN is considered 'standard' therapy in most recently reported trials. This is largely because it is regarded as a way of 'resting the pancreas', based on the assumption that the necrotic pancreas is still a secretor of activated enzymes. In fact, the secretory state of the pancreas has never been prospectively studied in severe necrosis. Several retrospective and prospective evaluations of TPN in acute pancreatitis have failed to demonstrate conclusively an effect on survival, or on the incidence and severity of organ failure.[35,36]

ENTERAL NUTRITION

An increasing number of studies report on the use of EN in severe ANP, challenging the persisting dogma regarding the use of TPN in this condition. When EN is given it has been suggested that it should be delivered distal to the ligament of Treitz, below the area of the cholecystokinin (CCK) cells distal to the third part of the duodenum, as CCK stimulation of this region may worsen the course of the disease.[37] Intragastric delivery of nutrients results in an increased volume of pancreatic protein and bicarbonate secretion. By contrast, jejunal nutrient delivery is not associated with any increase in pancreatic exocrine secretion.

Consequently, jejunal tube feeding as far distally as possible in the upper gastrointestinal tract conforms to the concept of 'pancreatic rest'. A number of comparisons of EN with TPN have been made in mild and severe acute pancreatitis, all suggesting that EN is well tolerated without adverse effects on the course of the disease.[38] Patients who received EN experienced fewer total complications and were at lower risk of developing septic complications than those receiving TPN.[39] EN seems to beneficially modulate the inflammatory and sepsis response, and if tolerated, may be superior to TPN.[40]

The following recommendations can be made:

1   Most patients with mild uncomplicated pancreatitis do not benefit from nutritional support.
2   In moderate to severe pancreatitis, let hyperacute inflammation settle, then start a trial of EN via a jejunal tube.
3   In patients who require surgery for diagnosis or treatment, a jejunal tube should be placed, either pulled down from the stomach,[41] or a separate jejunostomy.
4   TPN is only indicated if an adequate trial of EN is not tolerated.

CONCLUSIONS

Clearly the main determinant of outcome in severe acute pancreatitis is the extent of pancreatic necrosis and the subsequent risk for the development of infected necrosis. A thorough assessment using appropriate scoring systems and the early use of dynamic contrast-enhanced CT will highlight those patients likely to benefit from early critical care. Despite numerous suggested specific therapies, there is still no incontrovertible evidence that any one confers a significant mortality benefit. However, general supportive measures should include vigorous replacement of fluid losses to correct circulating volume, correction of electrolyte and glucose abnormalities, and respiratory, cardiovascular and renal support as necessary. Those patients with infected pancreatic necrosis or deteriorating organ systems should undergo surgery. Patients with sterile necrosis should receive a broad-spectrum prophylactic antibiotic that adequately penetrates pancreatic tissue. Due attention should also be paid to nutritional support, for which a jejunal feeding tube with EN is recommended prior to initiation of TPN.

REFERENCES

1 Banerjee AK, Kaul A, Bache E, *et al.* An audit of fatal acute pancreatitis. *Postgrad Med J* 1995; **71**: 472–5.
2 Broome AH, Eisen GM, Harland RC, *et al.* Quality of life after treatment for pancreatitis. *Ann Surg* 1996; **223**: 665–70.
3 Ranson JHC, Rifkind KM, Roses DF, *et al.* Prognostic signs and the role of operative management in acute pancreatitis. *Surg Gynecol Obstet* 1974; **139**: 69–81.
4 Blamey SL, Imrie CW, O'Neill J *et al.* Prognostic factors in acute pancreatitis. *Gut* 1984; **25**: 1340–6.
5 Vincent JL, Moreno R, Takala J, *et al.* The SOFA (Sepsis-related Organ Failure Assessment) score to describe organ dysfunction/failure. *Intensive Care Med* 1996; **22**: 707–10.
6 Balthazar E, Freeny P, vanSonnenberg E. Imaging and intervention in acute pancreatitis. *Radiology* 1994; **193**: 297–306.
7 Isenmann R, Buchler M, Uhl W, *et al.* Pancreatic necrosis: an early finding in severe acute pancreatitis. *Pancreas* 1993; **8**: 358–61.
8 Balthazar E, Robinson D, Megibow A, Ranson J. Acute pancreatitis: value of CT in establishing prognosis. *Radiology* 1990; **174**: 331–6.
9 Kemppainen E, Sainio V, Haapianen L, *et al.* Early localization of necrosis by contrast-enhanced computed tomography can predict outcome in severe acute pancreatitis. *Br J Surg* 1996; **83**: 924–9.
10 Geokas MC, Vanlacker JL, Kadell BM, Machleder HI. acute pancreatitis. *Ann Intern Med* 1972; **76**: 105–12.
11 Martin JK, van Heerden JA, Bess MA. Surgical management of acute pancreatitis. *Mayo Clin Proc* 1984; **59**: 259–70.
12 McFadden DW, Reber HA. Indications for surgery in severe acute pancreatitis. *Int J Pancreatol* 1994; **15**: 83–90.
13 Poston GJ, Williamson RCN. Surgical management of acute pancreatitis. *Br J Surg* 1990; **77**: 5–12.
14 Lee M, Ratner D, Legmate D, *et al.* Acute complicated pancreatitis: redefining the role of interventional radiology. *Radiology* 1992, **183**: 171–4.
15 Neoptolemos JP, Carr-Locke DL, London NJ, *et al.* Controlled trial of urgent endoscopic retrograde cholangiopancreatography and endoscopic sphincterotomy versus conservative treatment due to gallstones. *Lancet* 1988; **2**: 979–83.
16 Fan ST, Lai ECS, Mok FPT, *et al.* Early treatment of acute biliary pancreatitis by endoscopic papillotomy. *N Engl J Med* 1993; **328**: 228–33.
17 Folsch UR, Nitsche R, Ludtke R, *et al.* Early ERCP and papillotomy compared with conservative treament for acute biliary pancreatitis. *N Engl J Med* 1997; **336**: 237–42.
18 Van Hagen PM, Krenning EP, Kwekkeboom DJ, *et al.* Somatostatin and the immune and haematopoietic system: a review. *Eur J Clin Invest* 1994; **24**: 91–9.
19 Jenkins SA, Baxter JN, Day DW, *et al.* The effects of somatostatin and SMN 201-995 on experimentally-induced pancreatitis and endotoxinemia in rats and on monocyte activity in patients with cirrhosis and portal hypertension. *Klin Wochenschr* 1986; **64**: 100–6.
20 Kaplan O, Kaplan D, Casif E, *et al.* Effects of delayed administration of octreotide in acute experimental pancreatitis *J Surg Res* 1996, **62**: 109–117.
21 Friess H, Beger HG, Sulkowski U, *et al.* Randomised controlled multicentre study of the prevention of complications by octreotide in patients undergoing surgery for chronic pancreatitis. *Br J Surg* 1995; **82**: 1270–3.
22 Klar E, Rattner DW, Compton C, *et al.* Adverse effect of therapeutic vasoconstrictors in experimental acute pancreatitis. *Ann Surg* 1991; **214**: 168–74.
23 Wyncoll DL. The management of severe acute necrotising pancreatitis: an evidence-based review of the literature. *Intensive Care Med* 1999; **25**: 146–56.
24 Buchler M, Malfertheiner P, Uhl W, *et al.* Gabexate mesilate in human acute pancreatitis. *Gastroenterology* 1993; **104**: 1165–70.
25 Beger HG, Bittner R, Block S, Buchler M. Bacterial contamination of pancreatic necrosis: a prospective clinical study. *Gastroenterology* 1986; **91**: 433–8.
26 Pederzoli P, Bassi C, Vesentini S, Campedelli A. A randomised multicenter trial of antibiotic prophylaxis of septic complications in acute necrotizing pancreatitis with imipenem. *Surg Gynaecol Obstet* 1993, **176**: 480–3.
27 Sainio V, Kemppainen E, Puolakkainen P, *et al.* Early antibiotic treatment in acute necrotizing pancreatitis. *Lancet* 1995, **346**: 663–7.
28 Stoutenbeek C, van Saene H, Miranda D, *et al.* The effects of selective decontamination of the digestive tract on colonisation and infection rate in multiple

trauma patients. *Intensive Care Med* 1984; **10**: 185–92.

29 Lee TK, Medich DS, Melhem MF, Rowe MI, Schraut WH, Lee KK. Pathogenesis of pancreatic sepsis. *Am J Surg* 1993; **165**: 46–50.

30 Luiten EJT, Hop WCJ, Lange JF, Bruining HA. Controlled clinical trial of selective decontamination for the treatment of severe acute pancreatitis. *Ann Surg* 1995; **222**: 57–65.

31 D'Amoco R, Pifferi S, Leonetti C, *et al.* Effectiveness of antibiotic prophylaxis in critically ill adult patients: systematic review of randomised controlled trials. *BMJ* 1998; **316**: 1275–85.

32 Moore FA, Feliciano DV, Andrassy RJ, *et al.* Early enteral feeding, compared with parenteral, reduces postoperative septic complications – a meta-analysis. *Ann Surg* 1992; **216**: 62–9.

33 Heyland D, MacDonald S, Keefe L, Drover J. Total parenteral nutrition in the critically ill patient. A meta-analysis. *JAMA* 1998; **280**: 2013–19.

34 Pomposelli JJ, Bistrian BR. Is total parenteral nutrition immunosuppressive? *New Horiz* 1994; **2**: 224–9.

35 Sitzmann JV, Steinborn PA, Zinner MJ, Cameron JL. Total parenteral nutrition and alternate energy sub-strates in the treatment of severe acute pancreatitis. *Surg Gynecol Obstet* 1989; **168**: 311–17.

36 Sax HC, Warner BW, Talamini MA, *et al.* Early total parenteral nutrition in acute pancreatitis: Lack of beneficial effects. *Am J Surg* 1987; **153**: 117–24.

37 Pisters PWT, Ranson JHC. Nutritional support for acute pancreatitis. *Surg Gynecol Obstet* 1992; **175**: 275–84.

38 McClave SA, Greene LM, Snider HL, *et al.* Comparison of the safety of early enteral vs parenteral nutrition in mild acute pancreatitis. *J Parent Ent Nutr* 1997; **21**: 14–20.

39 Kalfarentzos F, Kehagias J, Mead N, *et al.* Enteral nutrition is superior to parenteral nutrition in severe acute pancreatitis: results of a randomised prospective trial. *Br J Surg* 1997; **84**: 1665–9.

40 Windsor AC, Kanwar S, Li AG, *et al.* Compared with parenteral nutrition, enteral feeding attenuates the acute phase response and improves disease severity in acute pancreatitis. *Gut* 1998; **42**: 431–5.

41 Boulanger BR, Brennemann FD, Rizoli SB, Nayman R. Insertion of a transpyloric feeding tube during laparotomy in the critically injured: rationale and plea for routine use. *Injury* 1995; **26**: 177–80.

36

Hepatic failure

F Hawker

ACUTE LIVER FAILURE

In acute liver failure (ALF) massive necrosis of hepatocytes leads to severely impaired liver function with hepatic encephalopathy, coagulopathy and jaundice.[1-5] It is usually the consequence of viral infection, hepatotoxic drugs, and toxins or other rarer causes and presents unique diagnostic and management challenges. Acute liver failure can be divided into three subgroups with differing aetiologies, clinical patterns and outcomes[6]:

- *hyperacute*, when the onset of encephalopathy is within 7 days of the development of jaundice;
- *acute*, when encephalopathy develops 8–28 days after the onset of jaundice;
- *subacute*, when encephalopathy develops 4–26 weeks after the onset of jaundice.

Patients with hyperacute liver failure are more likely to have paracetamol hepatoxicity or acute hepatitis A or B. There is a high incidence of cerebral oedema but patients in this group are most likely to survive with medical management. On the other hand, patients with subacute liver failure have a lower incidence of cerebral oedema, develop renal failure more frequently and have a very poor prognosis without liver transplantation. In this group the cause is often presumed to be non-A to E hepatitis.

AETIOLOGY (Table 36.1)

VIRAL HEPATITIS

Acute viral hepatitis accounts for 40–70% of patients with ALF. The clinical characteristics of the hepatitis viruses are shown in Table 36.2.

(a) *Acute hepatitis A (HAV)* infection rarely leads to ALF (0.35% of infections[7]), but accounts for up to 10% of cases because infection is common. It is diagnosed by the presence of the IgM antibody to HAV. Patients with ALF caused by HAV infection have a relatively good prognosis and the survival is approximately 60% without liver transplantation.[8]

Table 36.1 Causes of acute liver failure

		Incidence (% of cases)
Viral hepatitis		40–70
Hepatitis A	(5–30)[a]	
Hepatitis B	(25–75)	
Hepatitis C	(<1)	
Hepatitis E	(0–20)	
Drug-induced hepatitis		15
Poisoning (including paracetamol)		5[b]
Miscellaneous		10
Unknown		20–30

[a] Percentage of all viral cases given in parentheses.
[b] Incidence of paracetamol-induced acute liver failure is much higher in the UK.

(b) *Acute hepatitis B (HBV)* has been the cause of 25–75% of instances of ALF from viral hepatitis. However, its incidence should decrease markedly now that immunization is widely available. The liver injury is immunologically mediated. The mortality rate is around 60–70% with medical treatment.[8] It is diagnosed by the presence of the IgM antibody (HBcAb) to hepatitis B core antigen, with or without hepatitis B surface antigen (HbsAg). Co-infection with hepatitis D virus (HDV) increases the risk and severity of ALF in patients with HBV infection.

(c) *Hepatitis C (HCV)* infection is commonly associated with chronic liver disease. It is detected by the presence of antibodies to HCV in serum. It very rarely results in ALF in Western countries, although the incidence is sigher in Japan and Taiwan.[9]

(d) *Hepatitis E (HEV)* is a virus responsible for outbreaks of enterically transmitted hepatitis, particularly in the Indian subcontinent, Asia and Africa, and causes 50% of instances of ALF in these areas. There is a high mortality rate among infected pregnant women. It can be diagnosed by detection of antibodies to HEV in serum. HEV infection is also responsible for sporadic instances

Table 36.2 Clinical characteristics of the hepatitis viruses

	Hepatitis A	Hepatitis B	Hepatitis C	Hepatitis D	Hepatitis E
Spread	Faecal–oral	Parental Sexual Perinatal	Parental ?Sexual Perinatal	Parental ?Sexual	Faecal–oral
Incubation period Mean Range	28 days 14–49 days	70–80 days 28–160 days	6–12 weeks 2–26 weeks	? 28–140 days	42 days 14–63 days
Acute mortality	0.2%	0.2–1%	0.2%	2–20%	0.2%
Mortality from ALF	30–40%	50–60%	85%	(See HBV)	20% (pregnant women)
Chronicity	None	2–10%	>20%	2–70%	None
Antigens	HAVAg	HBsAg HBcAg HbeAg	HCVAg	HDVAg	HEVAg
Antibodies	Anti-HAV	Anti-HBs Anti-HBc Anti-Hbe	Anti-HCV	Anti-HDV	Anti-HEV

ALF = Acute liver failure.

of ALF in the Western world, particularly if the patient has recently travelled to endemic areas.

(e) *New hepatitis viruses* will doubtless be described. A major proportion of sporadic cases of ALF remain of uncertain cause, formerly called non-A non-B, non-NANB or non-A to E. It is possible that mutant hepatitis B viral strains, co- and superinfection with known hepatitis viruses and certain newly described agents may account for some of these.[9] Interestingly, there is a characteristic clinical picture with patients labelled as non-A to E hepatitis (slow onset, late encephalopathy, poor prognosis and female preponderance), suggesting a single causative agent.

(f) *Other viruses*, such as herpes simplex 1 and 2, varicella zoster virus, cytomegalovirus (CMV), Epstein–Barr virus and measles virus are all rare causes of ALF, particularly in the immunocompromised patient. Infections such as rift valley fever, dengue, yellow fever, lassa fever and the haemorrhagic fevers should be remembered in travellers returning from endemic areas.

ACUTE DRUG-INDUCED HEPATIC NECROSIS

Drug-induced hepatitis is responsible for approximately 15–25% of cases of ALF. In some patients there appears to be true hypersensitivity, and symptoms develop after a sensitization period of 1–5 weeks, recur promptly with readministration of the drug and may be accompanied by fever, rash and eosinophilia. In other patients, toxic drug metabolites are believed to be responsible. Many

drugs have been implicated; but isoniazid, phenytoin, salazopyrine, non-steroidal anti-inflammatory agents, antidepressants and allopurinol are reported frequently. Only approximately 12% of patients with drug-induced ALF survive without liver transplantation.[8]

Halothane hepatitis is the rare fulminant liver injury associated with administration of the volatile anaesthetic agent, halothane,[10] now rarely used. It is believed to be caused by an allergic reaction to a reactive intermediate of oxidative halothane metabolism.

HEPATIC NECROSIS FROM POISONING

(a) *Paracetamol poisoning* (see Chapter 78, *Management of acute poisoning*). Paracetamol poisoning is a more common cause of ALF in the UK than elsewhere in the world. Nausea and vomiting are usual early after overdose and these are followed by signs of liver failure 48–72 hours after paracetamol ingestion. Hepatotoxic effects are caused by a reactive metabolite that is normally efficiently detoxified by glutathione. Treatment is with *N*-acetylcysteine, which increases hepatic stores of glutathione because it is a source of cysteine. The recommended dosage schedule is 150 mg/kg in 5% dextrose over 15 minutes, followed by 50 mg/kg in 5% dextrose over 4 hours, followed by 100 mg/kg in 5% dextrose over 16 hours. Even late administration of *N*-acetylcysteine (up to 36 hours after ingestion) may improve outcome.[11,12] It has become evident that accidental overdosage with paracetamol in children[13] or therapeutic doses in the very young, and with starvation and chronic alcohol ingestion may also result in acute liver injury.

(b) *Mushroom poisoning.* Signs of hepatic necrosis can develop 2–3 days after ingestion of some mushrooms, of which *Amanita phalloides* is the most toxic.[14] There are severe associated gastrointestinal symptoms, resulting in dehydration and electrolyte imbalance. The liver injury is caused by amatoxins. The most useful treatment is forced diuresis, as large amounts of toxin are excreted in urine. Thioctic acid, silibinin and penicillin have been advocated as therapy, but have not been subjected to controlled trials.

(c) *Ecstasy (MDMA) and amphetamine intoxications.*[15] The social use of ecstasy (methylenedioxymethamphetamine) is becoming increasingly increasingly widespread. It is responsible for a growing proportion of cases of ALF in young people. The mechanism of the hepatotoxicity remains unclear but may involve a genetic predisposition, immune mechanisms and/or heatstroke. Patients with ALF should be transferred to a liver unit as liver transplantation may be necessary. Medical treatment should include control of hyperthermia.

(d) *Herbal hepatotoxicity.*[16] It is clear that herbal remedies can cause ALF as part of a wide spectrum of hepatotoxicity. Unfortunately, the incidence and clinical course are poorly characterized, because of the lack of clinical studies, multiple-herb products and the frequent failure to disclose herb use by patients and their families.

(e) *Others.* Acute yellow phosphorus, carbon tetrachloride, chloroform, trichloroethylene and xylene (in glue sniffers) are very rare causes of ALF.

MISCELLANEOUS CAUSES

Miscellaneous causes account for a small proportion of cases of ALF. These include fulminant Wilson's disease,[17] microvesicular steatosis (Reye's syndrome, acute fatty liver of pregnancy), hyperthermia, ischaemic liver necrosis, hepatic venous obstruction (Budd–Chiari syndrome), reactivation of chronic HBV infection, and complications of liver transplantation and hepatic resection surgery.

CLINICAL FEATURES

Patients may present a with history suggestive of a cause for ALF. However, in many cases no likely precipitating contact or incident can be identified. The disease typically evolves over several days, but deep coma can occur in hours or may develop over months with the subacute variant. Most patients become deeply jaundiced. The liver is usually small and impalpable. Signs of chronic liver disease, such as palmar erythema, spider naevi, splenomegaly and hypoalbuminaemia are usually absent at presentation, but ascites may develop in patients with subacute hepatic failure.

ENCEPHALOPATHY

Encephalopathy is a characteristic feature of ALF. It is classified, by severity, into four grades (Table 36.3). Cerebral oedema is present in over 80% of patients with grade IV encephalopathy, and is the major cause of death. Although documentation of the grade of encephalopathy is important, the clinical course can be followed more accurately by repeated clinical examination. One of the earliest signs of progression of encephalopathy is a generalized increase in muscle tone, which may progress to full decerebrate posturing. There is a parallel increase in briskness of the deep tendon reflexes, and an extensor plantar response and sustained clonus may be present as encephalopathy progresses. Lateralizing signs are virtually never present and suggest an alternate or additional diagnosis, such as intracerebral haemorrhage. Spontaneous hyperventilation is also common and can result in significant respiratory alkalosis. The pupils may become dilated in advanced encephalopathy, particularly in response to noxious stimuli, and may subsequently become sluggishly reactive. Despite the presence of cerebral oedema at this stage, papilloedema is unusual. If the pupils become dilated and unreactive to light, it is likely that brainstem coning has occurred. In this circumstance, the metabolic derangements preclude diagnosis of death by clinical tests, and death should be confirmed by demonstrating absence of cerebral blood flow by radiological or nuclear medicine techniques.

The precise cause of encephalopathy in ALF is unknown. It is generally attributed to accumulation of toxic substances in the circulation that can cause both coma and cerebral oedema. Substances arising from the gut, such as ammonia, mercaptans, fatty acids, phenols and γ-aminobutyric acid (GABA) have been implicated, as have endogenous benzodiazepines, glutamine and other neurotransmitters, such as octopamine. Although some of these substances may be important, alone or in combination, no useful specific treatment for hepatic encephalopathy or cerebral oedema has resulted from antagonizing their effects.

Table 36.3 Grades of encephalopathy

Grade	Features
I	Mild or episodic drowsiness, impaired intellect, concentration and psychomotor function, but rousable and coherent
II	Increased drowsiness with confusion and disorientation, rousable and conversant
III	Very drowsy, disorientated, responds to simple verbal commands, often agitated and aggressive
IV	Responds to painful stimuli at best, but may be unresponsive May be complicated by evidence of cerebral oedema

The cerebral blood flow in ALF is variable and changes with the progression of encephalopathy, so that it is high at some times and low at others.[20] Autoregulation of cerebral blood flow to pressure is lost.

BLEEDING DIATHESIS

The liver plays a central role in haemostasis, and ALF results in a complex coagulopathy.[21] All of the coagulation factors except factor VIII are synthesized in hepatocytes, and in ALF circulating concentrations of fibrinogen, prothrombin and factors V, VII, IX and X are reduced. The International Normalized Ratio (INR) for prothrombin or prothrombin time (PT) is prolonged, primarily because of reduced synthesis of factors of the extrinsic coagulation pathway. Prolongation of the INR is a useful prognostic indicator.

There is low-grade disseminated intravascular coagulation (DIC) in most patients, but a fulminant disorder is unusual. The principal causes are endotoxaemia and sepsis, although impaired synthesis of the naturally occurring inhibitors of coagulation (e.g antithrombin III and protein C) may contribute.

Quantitative and qualitative defects of platelet function occur. About two-thirds of patients have platelet counts $<100\,000 \times 10^6$ cells/l. Platelet aggregation is impaired but there is increased platelet adhesiveness.

Older studies report severe bleeding in 30% of patients with ALF, but this complication appears to have become less common in recent years. The deficiency of coagulation factors does not correlate directly with the risk of bleeding, and haemorrhage is most likely with thrombocytopenia and in the minority with frank DIC. The most common site of haemorrhage is the gastrointestinal tract. Other sites include the nasopharynx, respiratory tract, skin puncture sites or the retroperitoneal space. Spontaneous intracerebral haemorrhage is unusual.

CARDIOVASCULAR DISTURBANCES

Patients with ALF characteristically have high cardiac index (frequently greater than 5 l/min per m²) and low systemic vascular resistance[22]. A flow murmur is commonly present. The peripheral vasodilatation may result in hypotension, but this is usually responsive to appropriate volume loading. The mediators involved in the pathogenesis of this 'high output' state are not known with certainty, although nitric oxide may be involved. On the other hand, hypertension may occur in patients with advanced encephalopathy, and is probably an appropriate response to maintain cerebral perfusion pressure (CPP) in response to an elevated intracranial pressure.

RESPIRATORY FAILURE

The decreased level of consciousness may compromise the airway. Hyperventilation leading to respiratory alkalosis is a characteristic feature of hepatic encephalopathy. In the majority of patients who require endotracheal intubation and mechanical ventilation, the indication is airway management and treatment of cerebral oedema rather than hypoxaemia. If hypoxaemia occurs, it is most often the result of complications of decreased level of consciousness, such as bronchopneumonia, aspiration or atelectasis.

RENAL FAILURE

Renal failure occurs in approximately 75% of patients with grade IV encephalopathy resulting from paracetamol poisoning, largely due to drug nephrotoxicity. The incidence is lower with other aetiologies.[8] The usual form of renal failure associated with liver failure is the hepatorenal syndrome (HRS). The diagnosis of HRS is no longer dependent upon the presence of low urinary sodium or high urine:plasma osmolality ratio as agreed at a recent international forum[23,24] (Table 36.4). The acute form is termed type 1 HRS and is most frequently observed in ALF. In type 2 HRS there is a gradual decline in renal function over weeks or months. It is characterized by a progressive increase in the plasma creatinine concentration, oliguria, low urine sodium concentration (usually <10 mmol/l) and histologically normal kidneys. Acute tubular necrosis (ATN) may also occur as a result of hypotension, hypovolaemia or severe sepsis. It may be difficult to differentiate between these two syndromes, and often a diagnosis of HRS can only be made after correction of the predisposing causes for ATN.

In the past, associated renal failure requiring renal replacement therapy had a dismal prognosis. However,

Table 36.4 Criteria for diagnosis of the hepatorenal syndrome[24]

Major criteria
Chronic or acute liver disease with advanced hepatic failure and portal hypertension
Low GFR defined by serum creatinine >130 mmol/l or creatinine clearance <40 ml/min
Absence of shock, bacterial infection and recent treatment with nephrotoxic drugs
No sustained improvement of renal function after expansion with 1.5 l isotonic saline
Proteinuria <0.5 g/day, and no ultrasonographic evidence of renal tract disease
Additional criteria[a]
Urine volume <500 ml/day
Urine sodium <10 mmol/l
Urine osmolality > plasma osmolality
Urine red blood cell count <50 per high power field
Serum sodium <130 mmol/l

[a] The additional criteria relate to factors that are commonly present, but are NOT required for the diagnosis.

more recently survival has been shown to be 50% for renal failure associated with paracetamol-induced ALF and 30% with viral hepatitis A and B[8].

INFECTIVE COMPLICATIONS

Severe infection may complicate the course of ALF. Death from sepsis typically occurs after the first week and is most common in patients with subacute liver failure. Even when not the direct cause of death, sepsis causes worsening of liver function.[25,26]

Early infections are usually caused by Gram-positive and Gram-negative aerobes. The respiratory and urinary tracts are the most common sites. Spontaneous bacterial peritonitis is rare since ascites is an uncommon finding. Infections occurring after the first week of ICU treatment are often fungal.

Elevations of temperature and peripheral white blood cell count are not good indices of infection in patients with ALF. They are absent in 30% of patients with documented bacterial infection.

Rare complications of viral hepatitis include myocarditis, atypical pneumonia, aplastic anaemia, transverse myelitis and peripheral neuropathy.

METABOLIC DISTURBANCES

Hypoglycaemia is common, and results from impaired gluconeogenesis, reduced glycogen stores and increased circulating insulin concentrations. It should be considered whenever the mental state deteriorates, although the clinical signs may be masked in established encephalopathy. Both hypernatraemia and hyponatraemia may be present. The former is a consequence of treatment of cerebral oedema, with dehydration and a large salt load in blood products. Hyponatraemia appears to be dilutional. Hypokalaemia is present in approximately 50% of patients. It is closely related to the presence of metabolic alkalosis and may be both the cause and the result of this abnormality. Decreased plasma concentrations of magnesium, phosphate and zinc occur frequently.

It is a consequence of hepatic encephalopathy but the mechanism is unknown. Metabolic alkalosis occurs in 25–50% of patients. The predisposing factors are hypokalaemia and perhaps inability of the liver to synthesize urea. Gastric aspiration and vomiting do not seem to be important causes. Metabolic acidosis is common in patients with paracetamol poisoning, and it is the most reliable indicator of a poor prognosis in these patients; in others it is almost always associated with severe circulatory compromise.

IMPAIRED DRUG METABOLISM

Patients with ALF are particularly sensitive to the depressant effects of sedative and analgesic drugs. This is chiefly the result of impaired drug breakdown, but increased cerebral sensitivity and changes in plasma protein binding also contribute.

INVESTIGATIONS

Laboratory investigations. These should include serological investigations for hepatitis (hepatitis A, B, C and E, CMV, Epstein–Barr virus and herpes simplex) and a drug screen, specifically for paracetamol, to determine the cause of ALF. Plasma caeruloplasmin concentration and 24-hour urinary copper excretion exclude Wilson's disease.

Coagulation studies. The INR is a sensitive index of liver function and is an important determinant of prognosis and the need for liver transplantation. It should be measured every 6–12 hours.

Liver function tests. These should also be performed at least daily. A plasma bilirubin concentration of >300 μmol/l is a poor prognostic sign and is one of the criteria suggesting the need for transplantation. Plasma aminotransferase concentrations (alanine aminotransferase, ALT; aspartate aminotransferase, AST) show variable increases in ALF, and although peak levels are always high, plasma concentrations of these enzymes may be only mildly elevated by the time of ICU admission because of massive loss of hepatocytes. Plasma alkaline phosphatase (ALP) and γ-glutamyl transpeptidase (GGT) concentrations are usually normal. Plasma albumin and globulin concentrations are usually normal on presentation.

Other investigations. Blood glucose levels should be measured at least 4-hourly. Plasma electrolytes, urea and creatinine concentrations, arterial blood gases and full blood count should be measured at least twice daily, or more frequently if indicated. Specimens of sputum and urine should be cultured regularly, and blood taken for culture if there are signs of infection. Chest X-ray and 12-lead ECG should be performed daily.

Early studies suggested that signs of cerebral oedema on CT scan do not correlate well with the ICP until very late in the clinical course.[27] Although more recent studies claim that cerebral oedema can be quantified to an extent from the CT scan,[28] the risks of transporting patients with ALF are significant and the investigation is not indicated to estimate the ICP. It is useful, however, if intracerebral haemorrhage is suspected, particularly in the presence of an ICP monitoring device.

Liver biopsy may occasionally be necessary. If indicated, the transjugular route is preferred, because of a decreased risk of haemorrhagic complications.

MANAGEMENT

Patients with grade III and IV encephalopathy should be managed in an ICU. Because liver transplantation is indicated in many patients with ALF, early transfer to a liver transplant unit should be considered.

The mainstay of treatment in ALF is appropriate selection of transplant candidates and meticulous supportive care. The indications for liver transplantation are discussed further in Chapter 92, *Liver Transplantation*.

MONITORING

Oxygenation indices, ECG, haemodynamic variables and temperature should be measured continuously, and urine output measured hourly. Pulmonary artery catheterization may be required.

ICP monitoring is now well established in the management of patients with ALF and advanced encephalopathy. It allows early recognition and treatment of intracranial hypertension (also during liver transplantation). However, there is considerable potential for intracranial bleeding as a direct consequence of the monitoring device, in these coagulopathic patients. The incidence of fatal haemorrhage is as high as 5%. Fresh frozen plasma should be given prior to placement of the monitor, during which the patient should be anaesthetized to avoid elevations in ICP caused by pain and stimulation. An ICP over 25–30 mmHg (3.3–4.0 kPa) requires urgent treatment (see below). In the past, a cerebral perfusion pressure (CPP) of <50 mmHg (37.5 kPa) has been regarded as a contraindication to liver transplantation because of the likelihood of ischaemic cerebral injury. However, it is now clear that patients with CPP < 50 mmHg and ICP > 35 mmHg for 24–38 hours can survive with normal neurological function.[30] As with all forms of monitoring the risk–benefit ratio of ICP monitoring should be considered for each patient, as excellent results have been obtained without its use.[31] The applications of jugular bulb venous saturation monitoring in ALF are being explored.[20] Multimodality monitoring (ICP, cerebral function, cerebral blood flow using Doppler techniques and jugular oximetry) may well improve management in the future.

SUPPORTIVE CARE

- Mechanical ventilation at normocarbia is usually necessary in grade III and IV encephalopathy.
- An infusion of 10% dextrose will help avert hypoglycaemia.
- Lactulose (30 ml t.d.s. via the nasogastric tube) is widely used although there is no evidence that it will improve encephalopathy in ALF. Bowel distension associated with its use may complicate liver transplantation. Use of neomycin is not recommended because of its nephrotoxicity and ototoxicity.
- Normovolaemia should be maintained. Fluid overload may precipitate or worsen cerebral oedema, and hypovolaemia may result in hypotension, which may criti-

cally compromise the liver, other organs and CPP. If hypotension is not controlled with fluid replacement, inotrope or vasopressor infusions are indicated. The first aim of inotropic support is to main the CPP. *N*-acetylcysteine has been shown to improve tissue perfusion, oxygen extraction ratio and mean arterial pressure (MAP) in patients with ALF from various causes,[22] although a subsequent study does not confirm these findings.[32] Its effect on outcome has yet to be evaluated.

- Oliguria is managed initially with volume loading, but this must be balanced against the risk of worsening cerebral oedema. The prognosis is worse if renal failure develops, but many patients survive this complication. It is clearly a better result than brainstem coning. Low-dose dopamine has been used to increase urine output and promote diuresis, but as in other groups of patients no benefits are proven. If oliguric renal failure develops, early renal replacement therapy is indicated.
- Blood losses are replaced by blood transfusion, and platelet transfusions are indicated if the platelet count falls below $50\,000 \times 10^6$ cells/l.
- Infusions of clotting factors are indicated before invasive procedures or if there is overt bleeding. Because the INR is a major consideration in the decision to undertake transplantation, fresh frozen plasma is not given routinely unless a decision to proceed with transplantation has been made. Vitamin K should be administered daily.
- H_2-antagonists or omeprazole are given because of the high risk of gastrointestinal bleeding.
- Nutritional therapy is indicated, preferably by the enteral route. There is no evidence that protein restriction improves the outcome in ALF. Branched chain amino acid (BCAA) solutions have not been demonstrated to improve encephalopathy or overall mortality.
- Infective complications should be anticipated. Appropriate antibiotic therapy is instituted early. If empiric antibiotics are necessary, these should be effective against both Gram-positive and Gram-negative bacteria. Antifungal agents should be considered after a week of ICU care. Aminoglycosides should be avoided because of the increased risk of nephrotoxicity in patients with liver disease. Application of topical antifungal agents to the mouth and skin creases is a useful measure to reduce colonization, and is particularly important before liver transplantation.

MANAGEMENT OF CEREBRAL OEDEMA

Patients should be nursed with the head elevated to 20 degrees[33]; and venous return from the head must be unimpeded. Mannitol is the most effective treatment of cerebral oedema in ALF.[34] A dose of 0.5 g/kg is infused rapidly using a burette, but maximum reductions in ICP may not occur for 20 to 60 minutes. The dose can be repeated to control further episodes of intracranial hypertension, providing the serum osmolality remains <320 mosmol/kg. In patients with renal failure, mannitol should only be used in conjunction with renal replacement therapy, since fluid overload may exacerbate cerebral oedema. Furosemide (frusemide) may be useful adjunctive therapy to maintain the initial osmotic gradient established by mannitol.

Hyperventilation may be effective during an acute increase in ICP, but does not reduce the incidence or severity of cerebral oedema in the longer term.[35] It should not be used without jugular venous oximetry to prevent development of cerebral hypoxaemia.[20]

Barbiturate therapy (specifically thiopental by infusion) has been used to control ICP in patients with ALF,[36] but has not been subjected to a randomized controlled trial. Although reductions in ICP occur, the concomitant decrease in MAP resulting from cardiovascular depression can result in no change or a decrease in the CPP. This treatment may have a place in treating cerebral oedema refractory to mannitol therapy when liver transplantation is imminent, but only when ICP and therefore CPP is monitored.

Corticosteroids do not influence the incidence and severity of cerebral oedema.[37] The usefulness of benzodiazepine antagonists has not been established.

Moderate hypothermia to 32–33°C has been shown to be useful in the treatment of uncontrolled ICP in a small group of patients with ALF,[38] but further study is required to establish its place in management.

MEASURES TO IMPROVE LIVER FUNCTION

No drugs reverse the effects of hepatic failure. Drugs with cytoprotective properties, such as corticosteroids[37] and prostaglandin E_1 do not have beneficial effects.

There has been recent experimental interest in treatments that may stimulate hepatic regeneration. Insulin and glucagon therapy appears to have no benefit. However specific growth factors, such as hepatocyte growth factor (HGF)[39] may have therapeutic potential in the future.

ARTIFICIAL LIVER SUPPORT

Many patients with ALF have the capacity for hepatic regeneration but die from cerebral oedema before the liver recovers. For these patients, a period of successful artificial liver support could be life saving and also prevent the need for transplantation. Artificial liver support could also be used as a 'bridge to transplantation'.

Because of the many functions of the liver, involving detoxification, biotransformation and synthesis, the role of artificial liver support is complex.

Non-biological systems include the MARS system that incorporates a polysulphone membrane impregnated on both sides with albumin.[40] Clinical and biochemical improvements have been shown in patients with chronic liver disease using this system. The roles of high-flow haemofiltration,[41] plasma exchange and plasmapheresis[42] are being reinvestigated.

Hybrid hepatic support combines the use of biological tissue with the use of non-biological materials. In these systems, the patient's blood is perfused through a bioreactor containing hepatocytes supported in a matrix. The two systems that have been used clinically are the bioartificial liver developed by Rozga,[43] and the extracorporeal liver assist device developed by Sussman.[44] These methods of artificial liver support have shown some promise in clinical studies,[45,46] but benefits to survival have not yet been successfully demonstrated. Hepatocyte transplantation may play a role in bridging to transplantation,[47] but success is limited by the relatively small number of cells that may engraft.

LIVER TRANSPLANTATION

Liver transplantation for ALF is discussed in Chapter 92. It should be considered early in the course of all patients with ALF. The King's College Liver Unit criteria used to select patients for transplantation are shown Table 36.5.

PROGNOSIS

Overall, survival from ALF when all aetiologies are considered is approximately 20–25% with medical therapy alone, and 70% with liver transplantation. Adverse prognostic indicators are shown in Table 36.5. The aetiology

Table 36.5 Criteria adopted in King's College Hospital for liver transplantation in fulminant hepatic failure[8]

Paracetamol induced fulminant hepatic failure
  Ph <7.30 (irrespective of grade of encephalopathy) **OR**
  Prothrombin time >100 s and serum creatinine
  >300 µmol/l in patients with grade III or IV encephalopathy

Non-paracetamol-induced fulminant hepatic failure
  Prothrombin time >100 s (irrespective of grade of encephalopathy)[a] **OR**
  Any three of the following variables (irrespective of grade of encephalopathy):
    Age <10 or >40 years
    Aetiology – non-A, non-B hepatitis, halothane hepatitis, idiosyncratic drug reactions
    Duration of jaundice before encephalopathy >7 days
    Prothrombin time >50 s
    Serum bilirubin >300 µmol/l

---

[a] Prothrombin time 100 s is equivalent to an INR of 6; prothrombin time 50 s is equivalent to an INR of 3.5.

of ALF is particularly important. In general, the prognosis for spontaneous recovery is relatively good for HAV infection, paracetamol poisoning and acute fatty liver of pregnancy, intermediate for HBV infection, and poor for idiosyncratic drug reactions, fulminant Wilson's disease and when the aetiology is unknown (previously termed non-A, non-B hepatitis).[8]

CHRONIC LIVER FAILURE

Chronic liver failure is most often the result of:

- chronic infection with the hepatitis viruses B and C
- autoimmune diseases such as primary biliary cirrhosis, chronic active hepatitis and primary sclerosing cholangitis
- alcoholic liver disease
- cryptogenic cirrhosis.

The clinical signs include jaundice, ascites and encephalopathy, which may be present singly or in combination. Spider angiomata and palmar erythema are usually present. There is usually a high cardiac output, low resistance haemodynamic state,[48] and hypoxaemia caused by intrapulmonary shunting (the hepatopulmonary syndrome[49]) occurs in a proportion of patients. The hepatorenal syndrome (discussed above) also occurs in patients with chronic liver disease and is often a terminal complication.[50] Many of these clinical manifestations of chronic liver disease are the result of portal hypertension (Table 36.6). Laboratory tests show that the plasma albumin concentration is usually low and the INR or prothrombin time may be prolonged, reflecting a reduced capacity of the liver to synthesize proteins. Other liver function tests are often unremarkable.

Table 36.6 Complications of portal hypertension

Bleeding
Oesophageal varices
Portal hypertensive gastropathy
Ascites
Spontaneous bacterial peritonitis
Hypersplenism
Thrombocytopenia
Neutropenia
Portal-systemic shunting
Prolonged half-life of drugs metabolized by the liver
Systemic spread of gut-derived micro-organisms and endotoxin
Hypergammaglobulinaemia
Probable role in hepatic encephalopathy by allowing systemic spread of ammonia and gut-derived amines
?Role in circulatory manifestations of chronic liver disease
?Role in hepatorenal syndrome
?Role in hepatopulmonary syndrome

Acute episodes of decompensation may be caused by insults such as gastrointestinal bleeding, sepsis or dehydration. It is therefore important to recognize and treat these precipitants if possible. Unlike ALF, patients with chronic liver disease have minimal potential for hepatic regeneration, and ICU management has little to offer unless there is an acute reversible complication or if liver transplantation is feasible.

OESOPHAGEAL VARICES

Portal hypertension, oesophageal varices and the treatment of variceal bleeding are discussed elsewhere (Chapter 34). Variceal haemorrhage is a major cause of acute decompensation in chronic liver disease, and a common reason for admission to the ICU.

ASCITES[51,52]

Ascites is almost invariably present in patients with advanced chronic liver disease. Portal hypertension, hypoalbuminaemia, excessive hepatic lymph formation and abnormalities of sodium and water balance all contribute to its pathogenesis.

Ascites increases intra-abdominal pressure and may decrease cardiac output (through a decrease in venous return), embarrass pulmonary function (through elevation of the diaphragm) and may contribute to renal impairment. Although treatment of ascites traditionally includes salt and water restriction and diuretic therapy, these measures are usually unsuccessful or impractical in the critically ill patient. Paracentesis is the safest and most effective treatment of ascites in this setting. The total volume of ascites can be removed at a single paracentesis,[53] although blood pressure, urine output and CVP should be closely monitored. The procedure has been shown to have beneficial effects on pulmonary function, cardiac output and portal venous pressure. As ascites rapidly reaccumulates after paracentesis, colloid administration is usually required to prevent the consequent decrease in intravascular volume.

SEPSIS

Sepsis is a common cause of decompensation in patients with chronic liver disease. In some circumstances the site of infection will be known, but primary spontaneous bacterial peritonitis is common in patients with ascites and should be suspected if there are signs of sepsis, worsening encephalopathy or an unexplained general deterioration. The diagnosis is made by ascitic tap, and this procedure should be performed in all those sick enough to be admitted to the ICU. If the white cell count is $>250 \times 10^6$ cell/l, antibiotics should be commenced. The ascitic fluid should also be cultured. The infecting microorganism is usually a Gram-negative aerobe, often *Escherichia coli*. Intravenous albumin administration in addition to antibiotics has been shown to improve survival and reduce the incidence of renal impairment in cirrhotic patients with spontaneous bacterial peritonitis.[54]

ENCEPHALOPATHY

Hepatic encephalopathy (termed portal-systemic encephalopathy in patients with chronic liver disease) often develops or worsens after an episode of gastrointestinal bleeding, and may also be precipitated by sepsis, dehydration, protein loading and portal-systemic shunting procedures. It is treated with lactulose (30 ml, 3–4 times daily) instilled down the nasogastric tube, the gastric lumen of the balloon tamponade tube or rectally, and concurrently with treatment of the underlying cause. General management includes airway and ventilatory support and avoidance, where possible, of sedative drugs which may prolong the period of unconsciousness. Hepatic encephalopathy is very rarely associated with cerebral oedema in patients with chronic liver failure, and measures to control ICP are not necessary. It usually resolves with time if the precipitating cause can be controlled.

LIVER DYSFUNCTION IN THE ICU

Critically ill patients admitted to the ICU with primarily non-hepatic diseases frequently develop liver dysfunction.[55] There may be: (a) direct hepatocellular damage (hepatitis-like pattern) with a marked rise in plasma AST and ALT concentrations, a prolonged INR, and variable but usually minor elevation of the plasma bilirubin concentration; or (b) intrahepatic cholestasis, where there is elevation of the plasma bilirubin concentration, with relatively normal plasma concentrations of AST, ALT, ALP and GGT.

Multiple aetiological factors may be present, and hepatocellular damage and intrahepatic cholestasis may coexist. In patients with unexplained jaundice, ultrasonography of the liver should be performed to exclude extrahepatic bile duct obstruction.

ISCHAEMIC HEPATITIS

Ischaemic hepatitis is the most common cause of direct hepatocellular damage (AST >1000 IU/l) in the ICU and in the hospital in general.[56] It results from a critical reduction in liver blood flow in some patients with shock (particularly cardiogenic shock).[57] It is characterized biochemically by a marked elevation in the plasma concentrations of the aminotransferase enzymes and prolongation of the INR. It is often accompanied by other manifestations of shock such as renal failure and metabolic acidosis. The mortality rate is approximately 67%, but it is unclear whether the liver injury itself contributes to the poor prognosis or whether this is dependent on the severity of the underlying disease. The patient's low cardiac output state requires aggressive treatment.

VIRAL HEPATITIS

Exposure to viral hepatitis may very occasionally be the cause of abnormal liver function tests in the ICU patient. The clinical picture and management are as discussed above.

'ICU JAUNDICE'

This syndrome is associated with severe trauma and sepsis and develops approximately one week after the onset of critical illness. It is the 'classic' liver failure of the multiple organ failure syndrome, although conventional signs of liver failure are not present. Jaundice is the major clinical and biochemical finding, and other clinical signs reflect the underlying disease. The principle histological finding is intrahepatic cholestasis. The pathogenesis is thought to involve uncontrolled production of inflammatory cytokines by Kupffer cells primed by ischaemia and stimulated by endotoxin, perhaps derived from the gut. These cytokines act on adjacent hepatocytes to produce the classical metabolic changes of sepsis as well as the hyperbilirubinaemia. They may also be responsible for multiple organ dysfunction commonly seen in this setting. The treatment is that of the underlying disease.

DRUGS

Jaundice and liver dysfunction have been associated with many drugs. Drugs may impair metabolism of bilirubin or may be hepatotoxic (directly or due to metabolites). Hypersensitivity reactions may also cause hepatocellular dysfunction and, occasionally, massive liver cell necrosis. In such cases, there may be other allergic manifestations such as fever, arthralgia, urticaria and eosinophilia. Drugs may cause hepatocellular necrosis or intrahepatic cholestasis. Drug reactions should be considered in any patient with abnormal liver function tests.

TOTAL PARENTERAL NUTRITION (TPN)

Elevation of plasma AST, ALP and bilirubin concentration may occur with TPN, particularly if excessive calorie intake is prolonged. Histologically, there is fatty infiltration of the liver, associated with cholestasis and periportal inflammation. In general, the abnormalities reverse when enteral nutrition is established, although some infants have developed cirrhosis.

REFERENCES

1 Lee WM. Acute liver failure. *N Engl J Med* 1993; **329**: 1862–3.
2 Hawker F. *The Liver: Critical Care Management*. London: WB Saunders; 1993.
3 Bernal W, Wendon J. Acute liver failure: clinical features and management. *Eur J Gastro Enterol* 1999; 977–84.

4 Caraceni P, Van Thiel DH. Acute liver failure. *Lancet* 1995; **345**: 163–9.

5 Rahman T, Hodgson H. Clinical management of acute hepatic failure. *Intensive Care Med* 2001; **27**: 467–76.

6 O'Grady J, Schalm SW, Williams R. Acute liver failure: redefining the syndromes. *Lancet* 1993; **342**: 273–5.

7 Fagan EA, Williams R. Fulminant viral hepatitis. *Br Med Bull* 1990; **46**: 462–80.

8 O'Grady JG, Gimson AES, O'Brien CJ, *et al.* Controlled trials of charcoal hemoperfusion and prognostic factors in fulminant hepatic failure. *Gastroenterology* 1988; **94**: 1186–92.

9 Williams R, Riordan SMJ. Acute liver failure: Established and putative hepatitis viruses and therapeutic implications. *Gastroenterol Hepatol* 2000; **15**(Suppl): G17–25.

10 Ray DC, Drummond GB. Halothane hepatitis. *Br J Anaesthesia* 1991; **7**: 84–99.

11 Harrison PM, Keays R, Bray GP, *et al.* Improved outcome of paracetamol-induced fulminant hepatic failure by late administration of acetylcysteine. *Lancet* 1990; **335**: 1572–3.

12 Jones, AL. Mechanism of action and value of N-acetylcysteine in the treatment of early and late acetaminophen poisoning: a critical review. *J Toxicol Clin Toxicol* 1998; **36**: 277–85.

13 Miles FK, Kamath R, Dorney SFA, *et al.* Accidental paracetamol overdosing and fulminant hepatic failure in children. *Med J Aust* 1999; **171**: 472–5.

14 Pinson WC, Daya MR, Benner KG, *et al.* Liver transplantation for severe *Amanita phalloides* mushroom poisoning. *Am J Surg* 1990; **159**: 493–9.

15 Jones AL, Simpson KJ. Review article: mechanisms and management of hepatotoxicity in ecstasy (MDMA) and amphetamine intoxications. *Aliment Pharmacol Ther* 1999; **13**: 129–33.

16 Chitturi S, Farrell GC. Herbal hepatotoxicity: an expanding but poorly defined problem. *J Gastroenterol Hepatol* 2000; **15**: 1093–9.

17 Loudianos G, Gitlin JD. Wilson's disease. *Semin Liver Dis* 2000; **20**: 353–64.

18 Blei AT, Larsen FS. Pathophysiology of cerebral edema in fulminant hepatic failure. *J Hepatol* 1999; **31**: 771–6.

19 Albrecht J, Jones EA. Hepatic encephalopathy: molecular mechanisms underlying the clinical syndrome. *J Neurol Sci* 1999; **170**: 138–6.

20 Wendon J, Harrison P, Keays R, *et al.* Cerebral blood flow and metabolism in fulminant hepatic failure. *Hepatology* 1994; **19**: 1407–13.

21 Pereira SP, Langley PG, Williams R. The management of abnormalities of hemostasis in acute liver failure. *Semin Liver Dis* 1996; **16**: 403–14.

22 Harrison PM, Wendon JA, Gimson AES, Alexander GJM, Williams R. Improvement by acetylcysteine of haemodynamics and oxygen transport in fulminant hepatic failure. *N Engl J Med* 1991; **324**: 1852–7.

23 Moore K. Renal failure in acute liver failure. *Eur J Gastroenterol Hepatol* 1999; **11**: 967–75.

24 Arroyo V, Gines P, Gerbes AL, *et al.* Definition and diagnostic criteria of refractory ascites and hepatorenal syndrome in cirrhosis. *Hepatology* 1996; **23**: 164–76.

25 Rolando N, Harvey F, Brahm J, *et al.* Prospective study of bacterial infection in acute liver failure: an analysis of fifty patients. *Hepatology* 1990; **11**: 49–53.

26 Rolando N, Harvey F, Brahm J, *et al.* Fungal infection: a common, unrecognised complication of acute liver failure. *J Hepatol* 1991; **12**: 1–9.

27 Munoz S J, Robinson M, Northrup B, *et al.* Elevated intracranial pressure and computed tomography of the brain in fulminant hepatocellular failure. *Hepatology* 1991; **13**: 209–12.

28 Wijdicks EF, Plevak DJ, Rakela J, Wiesner RH. Clinical and radiologic features of cerebral edema in fulminant hepatic failure. *Mayo Clin Proc* 1995; **70**: 119–24.

29 Blei A T, Olafsson S, Webster S, Levy R. Complications of intracranial pressure monitoring in fulminant hepatic failure. *Lancet* 1993; **341**: 157–8.

30 Davies M, Mutimer D, Lowes J, *et al.* Recovery despite impaired cerebral perfusion in fulminant hepatic failure. *Lancet* 1994; **343**: 1329–30.

31 Sheil AGR, McCaughan GW, Isai H, *et al.* Acute and subacute fulminant hepatic failure: the role of liver transplantation. *Med J Aust* 1991; **154**: 724–8.

32 Walsh TS, Hopton P, Philips BJ, *et al.* The effect of N-acetylcysteine on oxygen transport and uptake in patients with fulminant hepatic failure. *Hepatology* 1998; **27**:1332-40.

33 Davenport A, Will EJ, Davison AM. Effect of posture on intracranial pressure and cerebral perfusion pressure in patients with fulminant hepatic failure and renal failure after acetaminophen self-poisoning. *Crit Care Med* 1990; **18**: 286–9.

34 Canalese J, Gimson A E S, Davis C, *et al.* Controlled trial of dexamethasone and mannitol for the cerebral oedema of fulminant hepatic failure. *Gut* 1982; **23**: 625–9.

35 Ede RJ, Gimson AES, Bihari D, Williams R. Controlled hyperventilation in the prevention of cerebral oedema in fulminant hepatic failure. *J Hepatol* 1986; **2**: 43–51.

36 Forbes A, Alexander GJM, O'Grady JG, *et al.* Thiopental infusion in the treatment of intracranial hypertension complicating fulminant hepatic failure. *Hepatology* 1989; **10**:306–10.

37 European Association for the Study of the Liver. Randomised trial of steroid therapy in acute liver failure. *Gut* 1979; **20**: 620–3.

38 Alan R, Damink SWM, Deutz NEP, *et al.* Moderate hypothermia for uncontrolled intracranial hypertension in acute liver failure. *Lancet* 1999; **354**: 1164–8.

39 Boros P, Miller CM. Hepatocyte growth factor: a multifunctional cytokine. *Lancet* 1995; **345**: 293–295.

40 Stange J, Mitzner S. A carrier-mediated transport of toxins in a hybrid membrane. Safety barrier between a patient's blood and a bioartificial liver. *Int J Artif Organs* 1996; **19**: 669–91.

41 Bernal W, Wong T, Wendon J. High volume continuous venous–venous haemofiltration in hyper-acute liver failure: a pilot study. *Crit Care* 1999; **3**: 106–10.

42 Kondrup J, Almdal T, Vilstrup H, Tygstrup N. High volume plasma exchange in fulminant hepatic failure. *Int J Artif Organs* 1992; **15**: 669–76.

43 Rozga J, Williams F, Ro MS, et al. Development of a bioartificial liver: properties and function of a hollow-fiber module inoculated with liver cells. *Hepatology* 1993; **17**: 258–65.

44 Sussman NL. Chong MG, Koussayer T, *et al.* Reversal of fulminant hepatic failure using an extracorporeal liver assist device. *Hepatology* 1992; **16**: 60–5.

45 Whatanabe FD, Mullon CJ, Hewitt WR, *et al.* Clinical experience with a bioartificial liver in the treatment of severe liver failure. A phase I clinical trial. *Ann Surg* 1997; **225**: 484–91.

46 Ellis AJ, Hughes RD, Wendon JA, *et al.* Pilot-controlled trial of the extracorporeal liver assist device in acute liver failure. *Hepatology* 1996; **24**: 1446–51.

47 Strom SC, Fisher RA, Thompson MT, *et al.* Hepatocyte transplantation as a bridge to orthotopic liver transplantation in terminal liver failure. *Transplantation* 1997; **63**: 559–69.

48 Groszmann RJ. Hyperdynamic circulation of liver disease 40 years later: pathophysiology and clinical consequences. *Hepatology* 1994; **20**: 1359–63.

49 Krowka MJ, Cortese DA. Hepatopulmonary syndrome: current concepts in diagnostic and therapeutic considerations. *Chest* 1994; **105**: 1528–37.

50 Arroyo V, Jimenez W. Complications of cirrhosis II. Renal and circulatory dysfunction. Lights and shadows in an important clinical problem. *J Hepatol* 2000; **32S**:157–70.

51 Runyon BA. Care of patients with ascites. N Engl J Med 1994; **330**:337–42.

52 Aiza I, Perez GO, Schiff ER. Management of ascites in patients with chronic liver disease. *Am J Gastroenterol* 1994; **89**: 1949–56.

53 Tito L, Gines P, Arroyo V, *et al.* Total paracentesis associated with intravenous albumin management of patients with cirrhosis and ascites. *Gastroenterology* 1990; **98**: 146–51.

54 Sort P, Navasa M, Arroyo V, *et al.* Effect of intravenous albumin on renal impairment and mortality in patients with cirrhosis and spontaneous bacterial peritonitis. *N Engl J Med* 1999; **341**: 403–9.

55 Hawker F. Liver dysfunction in critical illness. *Anaesth Intensive Care* 1991; **19**: 165–81.

56 Hickman PE, Potter JM. Mortality associated with ischaemic hepatitis. *Australian and New Zealand Journal of Medicine* 1990; **20**: 32–34.

57 Henrion J, Descamps O, Luwaert R, *et al.* Hypoxic hepatitis in patients with cardiac failure; incidence in a coronary care unit and measurement of hepatic blood flow. *J Hepatol* 1994; **21**: 696–703.

37

Abdominal surgical catastrophes

S J Streat

Intra-abdominal surgical catastrophes are common conditions in intensive care units1 and typically occur in elderly patients with comorbidity and reduced physiological reserve. They are often associated with sepsis, either primarily or secondarily, and with subsequent multiple organ failure. Overall mortality is high2 and there is usually a long period of intensive care in survivors. The long-term health outcomes of patients with these conditions may be poor, particularly if severe comorbidity and functional impairment were present before the catastrophe. These factors inevitably lead treating clinicians to consider carefully the costs and benefits3,4 of various treatment strategies during an illness which often has the character of a tragic saga. The clinical issues alone are complex and decision-making is often hampered by the lack of controlled trials of various strategic approaches.

These many difficulties create the potential for conflict to arise between intensivists and other involved clinicians who may have different perspectives on what constitute realistic goals and reasonable strategies, particularly for patients who are near the end of life.[5] It is in the care of these patients that the particular day-to-day work skills of the intensivist[6,7] ('seeing the big picture', providing meticulous bedside care, and negotiating and maintaining consensus, good communication and teamwork between various clinicians and the family) are tested to the limits. In this chapter, vascular catastrophes, intra-abdominal sepsis and a few serious abdominal complications are discussed.

VASCULAR CATASTROPHES

ABDOMINAL AORTIC ANEURYSM

Abdominal aortic aneurysm (AAA) is a disease of the elderly, which is up to six times more common in men than women.[8] Rupture of an abdominal aortic aneurysm is the most common vascular catastrophe seen in intensive care units and accounts for 2% of all deaths in men over 60 years of age.[9] The prevalence of AAA (defined as infrarenal aortic diameter of 30 mm or more) as detected by screening in men, rises from less than 1% at age 50 to

around 4% at aged 60, between 5 and 10% at age 70 and around 10% at age 80. Aortic diameter is the strongest predictor of the risk of rupture, which is below 1% per year with aortic diameter < 5 cm and about 17% per year with aortic diameter of 6 cm or more.[9] The risk of rupture is increased in women, current smokers and when hypertension is present. Aortic aneurysm expansion is around 0.3 cm per year for aneurysms smaller than 5 cm and around 0.5 cm per year for those larger than 5 cm and this rate might be reduced by a short course of macrolide or by stopping smoking.

Operative mortality for elective aneurysm repair is around 5% overall and somewhat higher in those with significant preoperative respiratory or renal dysfunction.[10] Operative mortality is increased to around 15% in urgently repaired (non-ruptured) aneurysms[11] and around 50% in ruptured aneurysms repaired as an emergency.[11] However, ruptured aneurysm may lead to death before hospital admission in around 30% of cases[12]; it is almost always lethal without surgery[13] and not all patients are offered surgery. Vascular surgeons are less selective (~10% non-operative) than general surgeons (~60% non-operative), without an increase in mortality in operated patients.[13]

These results have led to recommendations for population screening by ultrasound at age 65, continued surveillance for small aneurysms[15] and elective open operative repair in patients without severe comorbidity when aneurysm diameter exceeds 5 or 6 cm.[16] Some patients with severe comorbidity may be suitable for elective endovascular stenting with acceptable procedural mortality but anatomical contraindications and post-procedure endoleaks with persistent risk of rupture continue to seriously limit the applicability of this technique.

RUPTURE OF AN ABDOMINAL AORTIC (OR ILIAC ARTERY) ANEURYSM

The clinical features of rupture include the sudden onset of shock and back pain or abdominal pain or tenderness in a patient typically over the age of 70. Most ruptures are, initially at least, retroperitoneal with intraperitoneal rupture resulting in greater physiological disturbance and much higher subsequent operative mortality.[17] Many patients do not have shock when first seen and the correct clinical diagnosis is often not made by the first attending doctor.[18] Similarly, a pulsatile abdominal mass is commonly not detectable[17] and failure to find this should not lead to discounting the diagnosis. Although immediate bedside ultrasound may sometimes be able to confirm the clinical diagnosis without increasing delay, others have found that this investigation commonly delayed vascular surgical referral and subsequent operation without diagnostic benefit.[19] Although CT can readily make the diagnosis,[20] it carries a significant risk of sudden deterioration outside the operating room and probably has no place in determining the need for operation when a vascular surgeon remains uncertain of the diagnosis on clinical grounds alone.[20]

It may sometimes be inappropriate to proceed to operation (very severe comorbidity, poor quality of life) and this decision should be very carefully considered.[21] Lack of physiological reserve (often associated with advanced age) predicts high operative mortality and long periods of intensive care and hospitalization in survivors. Open repair remains the current treatment of choice but successful endovascular repair (sometimes with subsequent laparotomy for evacuation of haematoma) is now being reported.[22] A very small number of patients with aortic aneurysm have infection of the aneurysm, usually with staphylococcus or salmonella, which is often diagnosed at rupture.[23]

A period of postoperative intensive care is appropriate for most patients. During this time common physiological abnormalities (e.g. hypothermia, dilutional coagulopathy, minor bleeding, circulatory shock, renal tubular dysfunction) can be corrected and serious complications can be sought and, if possible, treated (e.g. major bleeding, renal failure, myocardial infarction, acute lung injury, peripheral ischaemia, stroke, pulmonary embolism, persistent ileus, mesenteric ischaemia, pancreatitis, acalculous cholecystitis, increased intra-abdominal pressure). In the absence of evidence of the efficacy of a particular approach, our own practice does not rely on invasive haemodynamic monitoring and includes rapid ventilator weaning and extubation with thoracic epidural anaesthesia[24] after abnormal coagulation has been corrected. We have abandoned abdominal decompression in these particular patients as we did not find it to be helpful.[25] Finally, an assessment of overall progress should be made after 24–48 hours. Severe or progressive multiple organ failure,[26] or major visceral or limb infarction should lead to a re-appraisal of the appropriateness of continuing intensive therapies. Persistent renal failure occurs more commonly after acute renal failure in this context than in other intensive care patients. Massive upper gastrointestinal haemorrhage (usually aortoduodenal) is a rare complication, usually resulting from infection of a previous aortic repair and less commonly from primary infection in an aortic aneurysm. Some of these patients can be rescued surgically.

ACUTE AORTIC OCCLUSION

This is an uncommon syndrome, usually caused by thrombotic occlusion (of a stenotic or aneursymal aorta) or by saddle embolism that presents with painful lower limb paraparesis or paraplegia and absent distal circulation. Minimizing delay to emergency re-vascularization is of the essence but mortality and multisystem morbidity remain high.[27]

MESENTERIC INFARCTION

This uncommon syndrome presents with an acute abdomen and may develop in critically ill patients. It is most commonly due to non-occlusive arterial ischaemia, arterial embolism or atherosclerotic arterial thrombosis, although venous occlusion and various low-flow or hypercoagulable states have also been reported.[28] A delay until operation is often reported and despite surgery (usually gut resection), mortality is high.

AORTIC DISSECTION

Aortic dissection is uncommon, occurring with an incidence of ~30 per million per year. The typical patient is elderly and has a history of hypertension,[29] but cases have been reported in young people after circumstances suggesting acute situational hypertension. Most aortic dissections originate in the ascending thoracic aorta and some of these will extend to involve the abdominal aorta or its branches. Spontaneous dissection of the abdominal aorta alone is rare. The most common presentation is with pain, the distribution of which can follow the site of dissection. Pericardial tamponade, haemothorax, myocardial infarction, stroke, paraplegia due to spinal cord ischaemia, anuria or an acute abdomen may be present. Mortality is high, but incidence may be falling as a result of early diagnosis and surgical treatment.

SPONTANEOUS RETROPERITONEAL HAEMORRHAGE

Excluding rupture of an aortic aneurysm, spontaneous retroperitoneal haemorrhage is uncommon. It is usually associated with vascular or malignant disease of the kidney or adrenal gland and less commonly with spontaneous rupture of the retroperitoneal veins or with anticoagulant therapy, including warfarin and heparin. We have also seen this complication in patients given low-molecular-weight heparin. The presentation is most often with acute abdominal pain, shock and a palpable abdominal or groin mass. CT scanning is useful when this diagnosis is suspected.[30] Correction of coagulopathy and interventional radiologic embolization may control some situations but surgery may be required in others, either to stop bleeding or to relieve associated intra-abdominal hypertension.

INTRA-ABDOMINAL SEPSIS

OVERVIEW

Intra-abdominal sepsis is very common in the ICU. In our own experience, the abdomen was the most common septic site in patients admitted with severe sepsis,[32] including peritonitis after chronic ambulatory peritoneal dialysis (CAPD), and accounted for 583 (35.9%) of the 1624 such admissions over the 17 years 1984–2000.[32] The incidence of sepsis in ICUs is reported to be increasing[33] and our experience is in keeping with this. The mortality of intensive care patients with severe intra-abdominal infections is variously reported between 25 and 80% but varies greatly dependent on the extent of comorbidity[33] and the severity of the acute illness.

The general principles treating severe sepsis are: (i) support oxygen transport as required; (ii) identify and, if at all possible, remove the septic source; and (iii) provide appropriate antimicrobial therapy. The place of adjunctive therapies is not yet established despite considerable research in this area and some recent promising reports. The issue of severe sepsis in general is covered in Chapter 59 of this volume.

In the critically ill patient with intra-abdominal sepsis, effective source control usually involves surgery, although occasionally interventional procedures may suffice. Laparotomy on clinical grounds and without delay is recommended for most patients presenting acutely with peritonitis. Diagnostic peritoneal aspiration or lavage, abdominal CT scanning or laparoscopy may have limited applicability in unusual circumstances that do not mandate immediate laparotomy.

Common syndromes include:

- faecal peritonitis
  – primarily, diverticular disease or colonic malignancy
  – secondarily, after prior anterior resection[34]
- perforated upper abdominal viscus (usually of a gastric or duodenal ulcer)
- biliary obstruction (sometimes with perforation)
- intestinal infarction without perforation (usually adhesive, less commonly ischaemic)
- appendicitis, which is more often perforated in older patients.

Less common syndromes include acalculous cholecystitis, toxic megacolon, perforation of a Fallopian tube abscess, spontaneous bacterial peritonitis (in nephrotic syndrome or end-stage liver disease) and CAPD-associated peritonitis (not all cases of which are non-surgical).

SURGICAL SOURCE CONTROL

Surgical source control should involve definitive control of the septic site at the first ('damage control') operation but definitive surgical therapy for the underlying disease may not always be feasible or desirable at this time. Initial surgery involves:

- removal of all peritoneal contamination (both macroscopically and by generous lavage)
- drainage of abscesses
- resection of devitalized tissue and
- defunctioning the gut to prevent ongoing contamination.

The abdomen may be left open if required for intra-abdominal hypertension or to facilitate repeat laparotomy. Temporary fascial closure with a variety of materials has been reported with apparently little to recommend one method over another. Although anastomotic healing is impaired by the presence of sepsis, some surgeons have recently reported successful primary anastomosis colonic (even left sided) after resection in the presence of sepsis.[35]

Failure of the sepsis syndrome to settle ('failure to thrive') after apparently definitive surgical source control should suggest ongoing contamination or ischaemia or the development of abscess. Repeat laparotomy on clinical grounds is recommended when postoperative progress is unsatisfactory early, whereas CT scanning followed by either directed laparotomy[36] or interventional radiologic drainage are more successful strategies for late abscess formation.

INTESTINAL-SOURCE PERITONITIS

Peritonitis secondary to contamination by intestinal contents usually results in mixed aerobic and anaerobic infection, and therefore recommended antibiotic regimens[32] involve either combination therapy with an aminoglycoside (or aztreonam) and metronidazole (or clindamycin) or, alternatively, monotherapy with a carbapenem. Similar antibiotic regimens are appropriate in sepsis following intestinal infarction without perforation. An agent active against *Staphylococcus aureus*[37] should be included in treatment for patients with peritonitis resulting from gastric or duodenal perforation.

BILIARY SEPSIS

Biliary ultrasound followed by endoscopic sphincteromy and stone removal is recommended for critically ill patients with cholangitis. Antibiotic regimens should cover enterococci and aerobic Gram-negative bacilli.

ACALCULOUS CHOLECYSTITIS

Acalculous cholecystitis is a rare but serious condition in ICUs. A small number of patients with the syndrome of acute cholecystitis will have acalculous cholecystitis, but these patients have low mortality and do not present to ICUs. Of greater concern are the perhaps half of all cases of acalculous cholecystitis that develop insidiously in intensive care patients who are already critically ill for another reason (e.g. recent trauma or surgery), and the condition can therefore go unrecognized until gangrene, perforation or abscess develops. The gallbladder histology in such patients usually includes prominent ischaemia and arteriosclerosis, and low cardiac output may predispose to the condition. An intensive care patient who develops new abdominal pain or clinical signs of sepsis should arouse a high index of suspicion. Although a variety of investigations including scintigraphy, CT scanning, ultrasound and laparoscopy have been used to help establish the diagnosis, none perform reliably[38] and many surgeons advocate a low threshold to exploratory laparotomy on clinical grounds where suspicion exists. Although percutaneous cholecystostomy has been used successfully, infarction or perforation of the gallbladder are commonly found at laparotomy and early cholecystectomy is advocated by others[39]. Reported mortality is commonly around 40% of patients.[38]

TOXIC MEGACOLON

Toxic megacolon[40] is now a rare indication for ICU admission. It is characterized by systemic toxicity accompanying a dilated, inflamed colon and is usually due to inflammatory bowel disease. Infection by *Clostridium difficile*, cytomegalovirus (in patients with HIV-disease or immunosuppression) or, rarely, other organisms may also precipitate toxic megacolon. The diagnosis should be considered in patients with diarrhoea and abdominal distension. Limited colonoscopy (despite the risk of perforation) and biopsy may both yield important microbiological information and help in the decision to operate. Supportive therapy in an intensive care unit is usually recommended and includes both antibiotics as for colonic perforation and steroids (equivalent of ~300 mg/day of hydrocortisone). Other immunosuppression has also been used. Frequent surgical re-assessment and abdominal X-rays are used to monitor progress. Intravenous nutrition may help to reduce the activity of Crohn's disease but does not reduce hospital stay or the need for surgery in ulcerative colitis. A period of several days of careful observation may be reasonable to assess the response to medical treatment but urgent surgery (subtotal colectomy with end-ileostomy) is indicated for perforation or for increasing colonic dilatation, bleeding, or systemic toxicity. Parenteral metronidazole may be effective in severe pseudomembranous colitis without megacolon (but early surgery is often recommended if megacolon develops).

RUPTURE OF A TUBO-OVARIAN ABSCESS

Rupture of a tubo-ovarian abscess is a rare cause of peritonitis presenting to intensive care units and is best treated with surgical extirpation. Antibiotic therapy should including activity against anaerobic organisms.

SPONTANEOUS BACTERIAL PERITONITIS

Spontaneous bacterial peritonitis (SBP) is most often caused by a monomicrobial infection, usually with *Escherichia coli*, *Klebsiella pneumoniae*, pneumococci or enterococci and rarely with anaerobes.[32] The development of SBP in patients with end-stage liver disease is a grave prognostic sign – hepatic decompensation and multiple organ failure commonly develop, and the median survival in such patients (without liver transplantation) is less than six months.[41] Early albumin supplementation has been shown to reduce both renal failure and mortality in SBP associated with end-stage liver disease.[42] Treatment with a broad-spectrum β-lactam antibiotic should be followed by secondary oral antibiotic prophylaxis.

CAPD-ASSOCIATED PERITONITIS

Peritonitis is not uncommon in CAPD patients but is rarely a cause of ICU admission. The development of (extra-renal) organ failure is an ominous sign and usually reflects delay in effective treatment, abscess formation, the presence of unusual organisms including a variety of fungi or an unrecognized gastrointestinal septic source.[43]

TERTIARY PERITONITIS

Tertiary peritonitis occurs occasionally in severely ill patients with prior laparotomy. It is seldom associated with intestinal contamination of the peritoneum and is usually monomicrobial, commonly due to *S. epidermidis*, enterococci, Enterobacter, Pseudomonas or *Candida albicans*[32]. Empiric treatment should initially include amoxycillin, gentamicin and metronidazole until culture results are available. When infection is due to *Candida* spp., other antimicrobial agents should be discontinued, any foreign bodies removed if possible, and treatment with amphotericin B given for at least 4 weeks.[44]

COMPLICATIONS

INTRA-ABDOMINAL HYPERTENSION: THE ABDOMINAL COMPARTMENT SYNDROME

This uncommon syndrome is now increasingly recognized in critically ill patients, particularly after surgery for trauma or sepsis, and delayed fascial closure is increasingly recommended in at-risk patients.[45] Intra-abdominal pressure (IAP) can be conveniently and easily measured via intravesical pressure,[25] is normally less than 10 mmHg (1.3 kPa) and is increased in patients with increased body mass index. Physiological impairment (including cardiorespiratory, renal, splanchnic, and neurological) can occur with acute increases in IAP to levels above 12 mmHg but the precise indications for decompression are unclear. In the absence of evidence from randomized controlled trials, expert opinion suggests that an acute increase of IAP to above 20–25 mmHg,[46] particularly if associated with severe cardiorespiratory impairment or impending renal failure,[25] warrants consideration of urgent decompression and temporary fascial closure. Despite abdominal decompression, mortality for such patients remains high (~50%).[25]

THE OPEN ABDOMEN AND STAGED ABDOMINAL REPAIR

The use of synthetic materials to provide temporary fascial closure has facilitated the care of the patient with an open abdomen and allowed repeat laparotomy and staged abdominal repair to proceed in a timely and unhurried manner. Our own practice[25] has been to use polypropylene mesh alone for this purpose if the period of open abdomen is likely to be short (less than a week) and the mesh can be removed before significant adhesion occurs. Two or more drains on moderate suction are laid over the mesh and then covered with a clear plastic adhesive dressing to provide a sterile waterproof seal and allow continual removal of ascites. If a longer period is required with an open abdomen then a non-adherent plastic material should be used, either under or instead of the mesh to prevent adherence and minimize the risk of gut perforation and fistula during removal of the material and fascial closure. The management of fistulation in the open abdomen remains problematic, as proximal surgical defunctioning is often technically impossible and control of wound contamination is not ideal with soft-catheter intubation of the small bowel via the fistulous tract.

ENTEROCUTANEOUS FISTULAS: INTESTINAL, BILIARY AND PANCREATIC

These are rare complications in intensive care practice, but they usually present formidable problems in such patients because of their common associations with serious gastrointestinal comorbidity (e.g. inflammatory bowel disease, intestinal malignancy, pancreatitis) and concurrent severe sepsis. In addition, complex fistulation with multiple collections, fistulation through an open abdomen, inability to proximally defunction or distal obstruction are commonly present. A standard approach to fistula management should apply,[47] including attention to drainage of sepsis, control of the fistula by drainage or, if necessary, by proximally defunctioning, protection of the skin from the deleterious effects of the fistula fluid, nutritional support and replacement of fluid and electrolyte losses. Somatostatin analogues have been shown to reduce high-output small bowel fistula losses and are commonly recommended, as are H_2-blockers,[47]

in fistulas of intestinal or pancreatic origin. However, their efficacy in achieving closure is less clear.[48] Parenteral nutrition is usually recommended for proximal small bowel fistulas but more distal intestinal, biliary or pancreatic fistulas can probably be safely treated with a trial of enteral nutrition. Recently, treatment with an anti-TNF antibody has been shown to be effective in chronic enterocutaneous fistulas in (non-ICU) patients with Crohn's disease.[49] Persistent high-output fistula should lead to investigation of possible causes,[47] including complete disruption of the gut lumen, distal obstruction or persistent intra-abdominal sepsis. Definitive operative treatment for fistulas that do not close should await clinical recovery and, if possible, nutritional repletion.

COLONIC PSEUDO-OBSTRUCTION

Colonic pseudo-obstruction (Ogilvie's syndrome) is a severe form of colonic ileus and is not uncommon in critically ill patients. There is a small risk of spontaneous perforation with high resultant mortality and the syndrome may also contribute to ventilatory difficulty, intra-abdominal hypertension and failure of enteral feeding. Conventional conservative treatment includes nasogastric drainage, i.v. fluid replacement and avoidance of opioids and anticholinergic agents. Treatment with neostigmine has been found to be highly effective[50] but caution is recommended as symptomatic bradycardia can occur.

REFERENCES

1 Streat SJ, Plank LD, Hill GL. Overview of modern management of patients with critical injury and severe sepsis. *World J Surg* 2000 Jun; **24**(6): 655–63.
2 McLauchlan GJ, Anderson ID, Grant IS, Fearon KC. Outcome of patients with abdominal sepsis treated in an intensive care unit. *Br J Surg* 1995 Apr; **82**(4): 524–9.
3 Sznajder M, Aegerter P, Launois R *et al*. A cost-effectiveness analysis of stays in intensive care units. *Intensive Care Med* 2001 Jan; **27**(1): 146–53.
4 Heyland DK, Konopad E, Noseworthy TW *et al*. Is it 'worthwhile' to continue treating patients with a prolonged stay (> 14 days) in the ICU? An economic evaluation. *Chest* 1998 Jul; **114**(1): 192–8.
5 Rabow MW, Hardie GE, Fair JM, McPhee SJ. End-of-life care content in 50 textbooks from multiple specialties. *JAMA*. 2000 Feb 9; **283**(6): 771–8.
6 Fisher MM. Critical care. A specialty without frontiers. *Crit Care Clin* 1997 Apr; **13**(2): 235–43.
7 Curtis JR, Patrick DL, Shannon SE *et al*. The family conference as a focus to improve communication about end-of-life care in the intensive care unit: opportunities for improvement. *Crit Care Med* 2001 Feb; **29**(2 Suppl): N26–33.
8 Vardulaki KA, Walker NM, Day NE *et al*. Quantifying the risks of hypertension, age, sex and smoking in patients with abdominal aortic aneurysm. *Br J Surg* 2000 Feb; **87**(2): 195–200.

9 Law M. Screening for abdominal aortic aneurysms. *Br Med Bull* 1998; **54**(4): 903–13.

10 Brady AR, Fowkes FG, Greenhalgh RM *et al.* Risk factors for postoperative death following elective surgical repair of abdominal aortic aneurysm: results from the UK Small Aneurysm Trial. On behalf of the UK Small Aneurysm Trial participants. *Br J Surg* 2000 Jun; **87**(6): 742–9.

11 Sayers RD, Thompson MM, Nasim A *et al.* Surgical management of 671 abdominal aortic aneurysms: a 13 year review from a single centre. *Eur J Vasc Endovasc Surg* 1997 Mar; **13**(3): 322–7.

12 Johansson G, Swedenborg J. Ruptured abdominal aortic aneurysms: a study of incidence and mortality. *Br J Surg* 1986 Feb; **73**(2): 101–3.

13 Basnyat PS, Biffin AH, Moseley LG *et al.* Mortality from ruptured abdominal aortic aneurysm in Wales. *Br J Surg* 1999 Jun; **86**(6): 765–70.

14 Scott RA, Vardulaki KA, Walker NM *et al.* The long-term benefits of a single scan for abdominal aortic aneurysm (AAA) at age 65. *Eur J Vasc Endovasc Surg* 2001 Jun; **21**(6): 535–40.

15 The UK Small Aneurysm Trial Participants. Mortality results for randomised controlled trial of early elective surgery or ultrasonographic surveillance for small abdominal aortic aneurysms. *Lancet* 1998 Nov 21; **352**(9141): 1649–55.

16 Scott RA, Ashton HA, Lamparelli MJ *et al.* A 14-year experience with 6 cm as a criterion for surgical treatment of abdominal aortic aneurysm. *Br J Surg* 1999 Oct; **86**(10): 1317–21.

17 Aburahma AF, Woodruff BA, Stuart SP *et al.* Early diagnosis and survival of ruptured abdominal aortic aneurysms. *Am J Emerg Med* 1991 Mar; **9**(2): 118–21.

18 Rose J, Civil I, Koelmeyer T *et al.* Ruptured abdominal aortic aneurysms: clinical presentation in Auckland 1993–1997. *Aust NZ J Surg* 2001 Jun; **71**(6): 341–4.

19 Acheson AG, Graham AN, Weir C, Lee B. Prospective study on factors delaying surgery in ruptured abdominal aortic aneurysms. *J R Coll Surg Edinb* 1998 Jun; **43**(3): 182–4.

20 Rosen A, Korobkin M, Silverman PM *et al.* CT diagnosis of ruptured abdominal aortic aneurysm. *Am J Roentgenol.* 1984 Aug; **143**(2): 265–8.

21 Prance SE, Wilson YG, Cosgrove CM *et al.* Ruptured abdominal aortic aneurysms: selecting patients for surgery. *Eur J Vasc Endovasc Surg* 1999 Feb; **17**(2): 129–32.

22 Greenberg RK, Srivastava SD, Ouriel K, *et al.* An endoluminal method of hemorrhage control and repair of ruptured abdominal aortic aneurysms. *J Endovasc Ther* 2000 Feb; **7**(1):1–7.

23 Muller BT, Wegener OR, Grabitz K *et al.* Mycotic aneurysms of the thoracic and abdominal aorta and iliac arteries: experience with anatomic and extra-anatomic repair in 33 cases. *J Vasc Surg* 2001 Jan; **33**(1): 106–13.

24 Rodgers A, Walker N, Schug S, *et al.* Reduction of postoperative mortality and morbidity with epidural or spinal anaesthesia: results from overview of randomised trials. *BMJ* 2000 Dec 16; **321**(7275): 1493–7.

25 Torrie J, Hill AA, Streat S. Staged abdominal repair in critical illness. *Anaesth Intensive Care* 1996 Jun; **24**(3): 368–74.

26 Meesters RC, van der Graaf Y, Vos A, Eikelboom BC. Ruptured aortic aneurysm: early postoperative prediction of mortality using an organ system failure score. *Br J Surg* 1994 Apr; **81**(4): 512–16.

27 Surowiec SM, Isiklar H, Sreeram S *et al.* Acute occlusion of the abdominal aorta. *Am J Surg* 1998 Aug; **176**(2): 193–7.

28 Newman TS, Magnuson TH, Ahrendt SA *et al.* The changing face of mesenteric infarction. *Am Surg* 1998 Jul; **64**(7): 611–16.

29 Meszaros I, Morocz J, Szlavi J *et al.* Epidemiology and clinicopathology of aortic dissection. *Chest* 2000 May; **117**(5): 1271–8.

30 Nazarian LN, Lev-Toaff AS, Spettell CM, Wechsler RJ. CT assessment of abdominal hemorrhage in coagulopathic patients: impact on clinical management. *Abdom Imaging* 1999 May–Jun; **24**(3): 246–9.

31 Bone RC, Balk RA, Cerra FB, *et al.* Definitions for sepsis and organ failure and guidelines for the use of innovative therapies in sepsis. The ACCP/SCCM Consensus Conference Committee. American College of Chest Physicians/Society of Critical Care Medicine. *Chest* 1992 Jun; **101**(6): 1644–55.

32 Thomas MG, Streat SJ. Infections in intensive care patients. In: Finch R, Greenwood D *et al.* (eds) *Antibiotic and Chemotherapy.* London: Harcourt Brace; p 2001 : pp. 564–576.

33 Angus DC, Linde-Zwirble WT, Lidicker J, Clermont G, Carcillo J, Pinsky MR. Epidemiology of severe sepsis in the United States: analysis of incidence, outcome, and associated costs of care. *Crit Care Med* 2001 Jul; **29**(7): 1303–10.

34 Hill GL. The leaking anterior resection and the management of SIRS, MODs and CHAOS. *Aust NZ J Surg* 2000 Feb; **70**(2): 90–4.

35 Umbach TW, Dorazio RA. Primary resection and anastomosis for perforated left colon lesions. *Am Surg* 1999 Oct; **65**(10): 931–3.

36 Bunt TJ. Non-directed relaparotomy for intra-abdominal sepsis. A futile procedure. *Am Surg* 1986 Jun; **52**(6): 294–8.

37 Brook I, Frazier EH. Microbiology of subphrenic abscesses: a 14-year experience. *Am Surg* 1999 Nov; **65**(11): 1049–53.

38 Kalliafas S, Ziegler DW, Flancbaum L, Choban PS. Acute acalculous cholecystitis: incidence, risk factors, diagnosis, and outcome. *Am Surg* 1998 May; **64**(5): 471–5.

39 Shapiro MJ, Luchtefeld WB, Kurzweil S *et al.* Acute acalculous cholecystitis in the critically ill. *Am Surg* 1994 May; **60**(5): 335–9.

40 Sheth SG, LaMont JT. Toxic megacolon. *Lancet* 1998 Feb 14; **351**(9101): 509–13.

41 Franca AV, De Souza JB, Silva CM, Soares EC. Long-term prognosis of cirrhosis after spontaneous bacterial peritonitis treated with ceftriaxone. *J Clin Gastroenterol* 2001 Oct; **33**(4): 295–8.

42 Sort P, Navasa M, Arroyo V *et al*. Effect of intravenous albumin on renal impairment and mortality in patients with cirrhosis and spontaneous bacterial peritonitis. *N Engl J Med* 1999 Aug 5; **341**(6): 403–9.

43 Carmeci C, Muldowney W, Mazbar SA, Bloom R. Emergency laparotomy in patients on continuous ambulatory peritoneal dialysis. *Am Surg* 2001 Jul; **67**(7): 615–18.

44 British Society for Antimicrobial Chemotherapy Working Party. Management of deep Candida infection in surgical and intensive care unit patients. *Intensive Care Med* 1994 Aug; **20**(7): 522–8.

45 Offner PJ, de Souza AL, Moore EE, *et al*. Avoidance of abdominal compartment syndrome in damage-control laparotomy after trauma. *Arch Surg* 2001 Jun; **136**(6): 676–81.

46 Joynt GM, Ramsay SJ, Buckley TA. Intra-abdominal hypertension – implications for the intensive care physician. *Ann Acad Med Singapore* 2001 May; **30**(3): 310–19.

47 Hill GL. Disorders of nutrition and metabolism in clinical surgery – understanding and management. Churchill Livingstone, Edinburgh 1992.

48 Li-Ling J, Irving M. Somatostatin and octreotide in the prevention of postoperative pancreatic complications and the treatment of enterocutaneous pancreatic fistulas: a systematic review of randomized controlled trials. *Br J Surg* 2001 Feb; **88**(2): 190–9.

49 Present DH, Rutgeerts P, Targan S, *et al*. Infliximab for the treatment of fistulas in patients with Crohn's disease. *N Engl J Med* 1999 May 6; **340**(18): 1398–405.

50 Ponec RJ, Saunders MD, Kimmey MB. Neostigmine for the treatment of acute colonic pseudo-obstruction. *N Engl J Med* 1999 Jul 15; **341**(3): 137–41.

Part Six

Acute Renal Failure

38.

Acute renal failure

R Bellomo

Acute renal failure (ARF) remains one of the major therapeutic challenges for the critical care physician. ARF describes a syndrome characterized by a rapid (hours to days) decrease in the kidney's ability to eliminate waste products. Such loss of excretory function is clinically manifested by the accumulation of end products of nitrogen metabolism (urea and creatinine) which are routinely measured in ICU patients. Other typical clinical manifestations include decreased urine output (not always present), accumulation of non-volatile acids and an increased potassium concentration.

Depending on the criteria used to define its presence, ARF has been reported to occur in 15–20% of ICU patients.[1] Acute renal injury (albuminuria, loss of small tubular proteins, inability to excrete a water load or a sodium load or amino acid load) is almost ubiquitous in critically ill patients. There is some evidence, however, that, when dialysis becomes necessary, mortality is increased.[2,3] The incidence of such severe ARF has been recently reported at approximately 11 cases per 100 000 people per year in the state of Victoria, Australia.[4]

The term 'acute tubular necrosis' (ATN) comes from old biopsy data, and from animal models that poorly reflect current clinical situations. In these patients, tubular 'necrosis' is patchy and mostly isolated to the thick ascending loop of Henle, and cells found in the urinary 'tubular casts' of such patients are viable on staining studies, partly invalidating the term 'necrosis'.

ASSESSMENT OF RENAL FUNCTION

Renal function is complex (control of calcium and phosphate, acid–base balance, water balance, erythropoiesis, etc.). In the clinical context, monitoring of renal function is commonly reduced to assessment of glomerular filtration rate (GFR) by the measurement of urea and creatinine in blood. These waste products are insensitive markers of GFR and are heavily modified by nutrition, muscle injury, the use of steroids, or the presence of gastrointestinal blood. They become abnormal only when more than 50% of GFR is lost; they do not reflect dynamic changes in GFR and are grossly modified by aggressive fluid resuscitation. However, the use of creatinine clearance (2 or 4 hour collections) or of calculated clearance by means of formulae increases accuracy but rarely, if ever, changes clinical management. The use of more sophisticated radionuclide-based tests is cumbersome in the ICU and only useful for research purposes.

DIAGNOSIS AND CLINICAL CLASSIFICATION

The most practically useful approach to the aetiological diagnosis of ARF is to divide its causes according to the probable source of renal injury: pre-renal, renal (parenchymal) and post-renal.

PRE-RENAL RENAL FAILURE

This form of ARF is by far the most common in ICUs. The term indicates that the kidney malfunctions predominantly because of systemic factors, which diminish renal blood flow and decrease GFR, or alter intraglomerular haemodynamics and thereby also decrease GFR. Renal blood flow can be diminished because of decreased cardiac output, hypotension or raised intra-abdominal pressure. Raised intra-abdominal pressure can be suspected on clinical grounds and confirmed by measuring bladder pressure with a urinary catheter. Decompression should be considered once the intra-abdominal pressure exceeds 25–30 mmHg (3.3–4.0 kPa) above the pubis. If the systemic cause of renal failure is rapidly removed or corrected, renal function improves and relatively rapidly returns to near normal levels. However, if intervention is delayed or unsuccessful, renal injury becomes established and several days or weeks are then necessary for recovery.

Several tests have been used to help clinicians identify the development of such 'established' ARF. These tests are included below for the sake of completeness (Table 38.1). The clinical utility of these tests in ICU patients who receive vasopressors, massive fluid resuscitation and, increasingly, loop diuretic infusions is

Table 38.1 Laboratory tests used to help diagnose 'established' acute renal failure (ARF)

Test	Pre-renal ARF	Established ARF
Urine microscopy	Normal	Casts
Specific gravity	High: >1.020	Fixed: 1.010–1.020
Urine sodium	Low: <20 mmol/l	High: >40 mmol/l
U/P creatinine ratio	High: >40	Low: <10
P urea/creatinine ratio	> Normal	Normal

U = urine; P = plasma.

untested and questionable. Furthermore, it is important to observe that pre-renal ARF and established ARF are part of a continuum, and their separation has limited clinical implications. The treatment is the same: treatment of the cause while promptly resuscitating the patient using invasive haemodynamic monitoring to guide therapy.

PARENCHYMAL RENAL FAILURE

This term is used to define a syndrome where the principal source of damage is within the kidney and where typical structural changes can be seen on microscopy. Disorders that affect the glomerulus or the tubule can be responsible (Table 38.2). Among these, nephrotoxins are particularly important, especially in hospitalized patients.[4] The most common nephrotoxic drugs affecting ICU patients are listed in Table 38.3.

Table 38.2 Causes of parenchymal acute renal failure

Glomerulonephritis
Vasculitis
Interstitial nephritis
Malignant hypertension
Pyelonephritis
Bilateral cortical necrosis
Amyloidosis
Malignancy
Nephrotoxins

Table 38.3 Drugs that may cause acute renal failure in the ICU

Radiocontrast agents
Aminoglycosides
Amphotericin
Non-steroidal anti-inflammatory drugs
β-lactam antibiotics (interstitial nephropathy)
Sulphonamides
Ayclovir
Methotrexate
Cisplatin
Cyclosporin A
FK-506 (Tacrolimus)

Many cases of drug-induced ARF rapidly improve upon removal of the offending agent. Accordingly, a careful history of drug administration is *mandatory* in all patients with ARF. In some cases of parenchymal ARF, a correct working diagnosis can be obtained from history, physical examination, radiological and laboratory investigations. In such patients, one can proceed to a therapeutic trial without the need to resort to renal biopsy. However, prior to aggressive immuno-suppressive therapy, renal biopsy is recommended to allow histological confirmation of the aetiology of ARF. Renal biopsy in ventilated patients under ultrasound guidance does not carry additional risks compared to standard conditions.

More than a third of patients who develop ARF in ICUs have chronic renal dysfunction[4] due to factors such as age-related changes, long-standing hypertension, diabetes or atheromatous disease of the renal vessels. It may be manifest by a raised serum creatinine. However, this is not always the case. Often, what may seem to the clinician to be a relatively trivial insult, which does not fully explain the onset of ARF in a normal patient, is sufficient to unmask lack of renal functional reserve in another.

HEPATORENAL SYNDROME

This condition is a form of ARF that occurs in the setting of severe liver dysfunction in the absence of other known causes of ARF. Typically, it presents as progressive oliguria with a very low urinary sodium concentration (<10 mmol/l). Its pathogenesis is not well understood but appears to involve severe renal vasoconstriction. However, in patients with severe liver disease other causes of ARF are much more common. They include sepsis, paracentesis-induced hypovolaemia, raised intra-abdominal pressure due to tense ascites, diuretic-induced hypovolaemia, lactulose-induced hypovolaemia, alcoholic cardiomyopathy, and any combination of these. The avoidance of hypovolaemia by albumin administration in patients with spontaneous bacterial peritonitis has been shown to decrease the incidence of renal failure in a recent randomized controlled trial.[5] These causes must be looked for and promptly treated. Recent uncontrolled studies suggest that vasopressin derivatives (omnipressin) may improve GFR in this condition.[6] The use of such agents remains controversial.

RHABDOMYOLYSIS-ASSOCIATED ARF

This condition accounts for close to 5–10% of cases of ARF in the ICU,[4] depending on the setting. Its pathogenesis involves pre-renal, renal and post-renal factors. It is now typically seen following major trauma, drug overdose with narcotics, vascular embolism, and in response to a variety of agents which can induce major muscle injury. The principles of treatment are based on retrospective data, small series and multivariate logistic regression analysis, because no randomized controlled trials have been conducted. They include prompt and aggressive fluid resuscitation, elimination of causative agents, correction of compartment syndromes, the alkalinization of urine (pH >6.5) and the maintenance of polyuria (>300 ml/h). The role of mannitol is controversial.

POST-RENAL RENAL FAILURE

Obstruction to urine outflow is the most common cause of functional renal impairment in the community,[7] but is uncommon in the ICU. Typical causes of obstructive ARF include bladder neck obstruction from an enlarged prostate, ureteric obstruction from pelvic tumors or retroperitoneal fibrosis, papillary necrosis or large calculi. The clinical presentation of obstruction may be acute or acute-on-chronic in patients with long-standing renal calculi. It may not always be associated with oliguria. If obstruction is suspected, ultrasonography can be easily performed at the bedside. However, not all cases of acute obstruction have an abnormal ultrasound and, in many cases, obstruction occurs in conjunction with other renal insults (e.g. staghorn calculi and severe sepsis of renal origin). Assessment of the role of each factor and overall management should be conducted in conjunction with a urologist.

PATHOGENESIS OF ACUTE RENAL FAILURE

The pathogenesis of obstructive ARF involves several humoral responses as well as mechanical factors. The pathogenesis of parenchymal renal failure is typically immunological. It varies from vasculitis to interstitial nephropathy and involves an extraordinary complexity of immunological mechanisms. The pathogenesis of pre-renal ARF is of greater direct relevance to the intensivist. Several mechanisms appear to play a major role in the development of renal injury:

- ischaemia of outer medulla with activation of the tubulo-glomerular feedback[8]
- tubular obstruction from casts of exfoliated cells[9]
- interstitial oedema secondary to back diffusion of fluid[9]
- humorally mediated afferent arteriolar renal vasoconstriction[10]

- inflammatory response to cell injury and local release of mediators[11]
- disruption of normal cellular adhesion to the basement membrane[12]
- radical oxygen species-induced apoptosis[13]
- phospholipase A_2 induced cell membrane injury[14]
- mitogen-activated protein kinases-induced renal injury[15]

In septic patients with hyperdynamic circulations, there may be adequate global blood flow to the kidney but intrarenal shunting away from the medulla causing medullary ischaemia, or efferent arteriolar vasodilatation causing decreased intraglomerular pressure and thus decreased GFR.

THE CLINICAL PICTURE

The most common clinical picture is that of a patient who has sustained a major systemic insult. When the patient arrives in the ICU resuscitation is well under way or surgery may have just been completed. Despite such efforts, the patient is already anuric or profoundly oliguric, the serum creatinine is rising and a metabolic acidosis is developing. Potassium and phosphate levels may be rapidly rising as well. Accompanying multiple organ dysfunction (mechanical ventilation and need for vasoactive drugs) is common. Fluid resuscitation is typically undertaken in the ICU under the guidance of invasive hemodynamic monitoring. Vasoactive drugs are often used to restore mean arterial pressure (MAP) to 'acceptable' levels, typically >70–75 mmHg (9.3–10.0 kPa). The patient may improve over time and urine output may return with or without the assistance of diuretic agents. If urine output does not return, however, renal replacement therapy needs to be considered.

If the cause of ARF has been removed and the patient has become physiologically stable, slow recovery occurs (from 4 to 5 days to 3 or 4 weeks). In some cases, urine output can be above normal for several days. If the cause of ARF has not been adequately remedied, the patient remains gravely ill, the kidneys do not recover and death from multiorgan failure occurs.

PREVENTING ACUTE RENAL FAILURE

The fundamental principle of ARF prevention is to treat its cause. If pre-renal factors contribute, these must be identified, and haemodynamic resuscitation quickly instituted.

RESUSCITATION

Intravascular volume must be maintained or rapidly restored, and this is often best done using invasive hemodynamic monitoring (central venous catheter, arterial cannula, and pulmonary artery catheter in some cases). Oxygenation must be maintained. An adequate hemoglobin concentration (at least >70 g/l) must be maintained or immediately restored. Once intravascular volume has been restored, some patients remain hypotensive, with a MAP <75 mmHg (10.0 kPa). In these patients, autoregulation of renal blood flow may be lost. Restoration of MAP to near normal levels is likely to increase GFR.[16-18] Such elevations in MAP require the addition of vasopressor drugs.[16-18] In patients with hypertension or renovascular disease, a MAP of 75–80 mmHg may still be inadequate. The nephroprotective role of additional fluid therapy in a patient with a normal or increased cardiac output and blood pressure is questionable. Despite these measures renal failure may still develop if cardiac output is inadequate. This may require a variety of interventions from the use of inotropic drugs to the application of ventricular assist devices.

NEPHROPROTECTIVE DRUGS

Following haemodynamic resuscitation and removal of nephrotoxins, it is unclear whether the use of additional pharmacological measures is of further benefit to the kidneys.

'Renal dose' or 'low-dose' dopamine

Evidence of the efficacy or safety of its administration in critically ill patients is lacking. However, this agent is a tubular diuretic and occasionally increases urine output. This may be incorrectly interpreted as an increase in GFR. Furthermore, a recent large phase III trial in critically ill patients showed low-dose dopamine to be as effective as placebo in the prevention of renal dysfunction.[19] In a patient with a low cardiac output, however, the administration of β-dose dopamine (as would dobutamine or milrinone) may increase cardiac output, renal blood flow and GFR.

Mannitol

A biological rationale exists for its use, as is the case for dopamine. Animal experiments offer some encouraging findings. However, no controlled human data exist to support its clinical use. The effect of mannitol as a renal protective agent remains questionable.[20]

Loop diuretics

These agents may protect the loop of Henle from ischaemia by decreasing its transport-related workload. Animal data are encouraging, as are *ex-vivo* experiments. There are no double-blind randomized controlled studies of suitable size to prove that these agents reduce the incidence of renal failure. However, several studies support the view that loop diuretics may decrease the need for dialysis in patients with developing ARF.[21] They appear to achieve this by inducing polyuria, which results

in the prevention or easier control of volume overload, acidosis and hyperkalemia, the three major triggers for renal replacement therapy in the ICU. Because avoiding dialysis simplifies treatment and reduces cost of care, loop diuretics may be useful in patients with renal dysfunction especially in the form of continuous infusion. Other agents such as theophylline, urodilatin, and anaritide (a synthetic atrial natriuretic factor) have also been proposed. Studies so far, however, have either been experimental, too small or have shown no beneficial effect.[23,24]

Radiocontrast nephropathy

In patients receiving radiocontrast a randomized controlled trial (RCT) suggested that saline infusion to maintain intra-vascular fluid expansion is superior to the addition of mannitol or furosemide.[20] A more recent RCT of similar patients demonstrated a beneficial effect of *N*-acetylcysteine treatment before and after radiocontrast administration.[25] Since these preventive interventions have minimal toxicity, they should be considered whenever a patient is scheduled for the administration of intravenous radiocontrast.

DIAGNOSTIC INVESTIGATIONS

An aetiological diagnosis of ARF must always be established. Such diagnosis may be obvious on clinical grounds. However, in many patients, it is best to consider all possibilities and exclude common treatable causes by simple investigations. Such investigations include the examination of urinary sediment and exclusion of a urinary tract infection (most if not all patients), the exclusion of obstruction when appropriate (some patients) and the careful exclusion of nephrotoxins (all patients).

In specific situations, other investigations are necessary to establish the diagnosis, such as creatine kinase and free myoglobin for possible rhabdomyolysis. A chest radiograph, a blood film, the measurement of non-specific inflammatory markers, and the measurement of specific antibodies (anti-GBM, anti-neutrophil cytoplasm, anti-DNA, anti-smooth muscle, etc.) are extremely useful screening tests to help support the diagnosis of vasculitis or of certain types of collagen disease or glomerulonephritis. If thrombotic-thrombocytopenic purpura is suspected, the additional measurement of lactic dehydrogenase, haptoglobin, unconjugated bilirubin and free hemoglobin are needed. In some patients, specific findings (cryoglobulins, Bence–Jones proteins) are almost diagnostic. In a few rare patients, the clinical picture, laboratory investigations, and radiological investigations are not sufficient to make a causative diagnosis with sufficient certainty. In such patients a renal biopsy becomes necessary.

MANAGEMENT OF ESTABLISHED ACUTE RENAL FAILURE

The principles of management of established ARF are the treatment or removal of its cause and the maintenance of physiological homeostasis while recovery takes place. Complications such as encephalopathy, pericarditis, myopathy, neuropathy, electrolyte disturbances or other major electrolyte, fluid or metabolic derangement should never occur in a modern ICU. Their prevention may include several measures, which vary in complexity from fluid restriction to the initiation of extra-corporeal renal replacement therapy.

Nutritional support must be started early and must contain adequate calories (30–35 kcal/kg per day) as a mixture of carbohydrates and lipids. Adequate protein (about 1–2 g/kg per day)[26] must be administered. There is no evidence that specific renal nutritional solutions are useful. Vitamins and trace elements should be administered at least according to their recommended daily allowance. The role of newer immunonutritional solution remains controversial. The enteral route is preferred to the use of parenteral nutrition.

Hyperkalaemia (serum $K^+ > 6$ mmol/l) must be promptly treated either with insulin and dextrose administration, the infusion of bicarbonate if acidosis is present, the administration of nebulized salbutamol, or all of the above together (also see Ch. 84). Spurious causes of hyperkalaemia secondary to haemolysis, thrombocytosis and a very high white cell count should be excluded. Laboratories are increasingly measuring plasma potassium which is not altered by platelet or white cell count; however, the normal range of plasma potassium is lower than serum, and care must be taken to reflect this difference. If the 'true' serum potassium is > 7 mmol/l or electrocardiographic signs of hyperkalaemia appear, calcium gluconate (10 ml of 10% solution i.v.) should also be administered. The above measures are temporizing actions, while renal replacement therapy is being set up. The presence of hyperkalaemia is a major indication for the immediate institution of renal replacement therapy.

Metabolic acidosis is almost always present but rarely requires treatment *per se*. Anaemia requires correction to maintain a haemoglobin > 70 g/l. More aggressive transfusion needs individual patient assessment.[27] Drug therapy must be adjusted to take into account the effect of the decreased clearances associated with loss of renal function. Stress ulcer prophylaxis is advisable and should be based on H_2-receptor antagonists or proton pump inhibitors in selected cases. Assiduous attention should be paid to the prevention of infection.

Fluid overload can be prevented by the use of loop diuretics in polyuric patients. However, if the patient is oliguric, the only way to avoid fluid overload is to institute renal replacement therapy at an early stage (see Ch. 39). Marked azotaemia ([urea] > 40 mmol/l or [creatinine] > 400 μmol/l) is undesirable and should probably be treated with renal replacement therapy unless recovery is imminent or already under way and a return toward normal values is expected within 24 hours.[28] It is recognized, however, that no RCTs exist to define the ideal time for intervention with artificial renal support.

PROGNOSIS

The mortality of critically ill patients with ARF remains high (40–80% depending on case-mix). It is frequently stated that patients die *with* renal failure rather than *of* renal failure. However, growing evidence suggests that better uraemic control and more intensive artificial renal support may improve survival by perhaps 30%.[29,30] Such evidence supports a careful and pro-active approach to the treatment of patients with ARF, which is based on the prevention of uncontrolled uremia and the maintenance of low urea levels throughout the patient's illness.

REFERENCES

1 Chew SL, Lins RL, Daelemans R, De Broe ME. Outcome in acute renal failure. *Nephrol Dial Transplant* 1993; **8**: 101–7.

2 Liano F, Garcia-Martin F, Gallego A, *et al.* Easy and early prognosis in acute tubular necrosis: a forward analysis of 228 cases. *Nephron* 1989; **51**: 307–13.

3. Vincent J-L. Incidence of acute renal failure in the Intensive Care Unit. *Contrib Nephrol* 2001; **132**: 1–6.

4 Cole L, Bellomo R, Silvester W, Reeves JH. A prospective, multicenter study of the epidemiology, management and outcome of severe acute renal failure in a 'closed' ICU system. *Am J Respir Crit Care Med* 2000; **162**: 191–6.

5 Sort P, Navasa M, Arroyo V, *et al.* Effect of intravenous albumin on renal impairment and mortality in patients with cirrhosis and spontaneous bacterial peritonitis. *N Engl J Med* 1999; **341**: 403–9.

6 Guevara M, Gines P, Fernandez-Esparrach G, *et al.* Reversibility of hepatorenal syndrome by prolonged administration of ornipressin and plasma volume expansion. *Hepatology* 1998; **27**: 35–41.

7 Feest TG, Round A, Hamad S. Incidence of severe acute renal failure in adults: results of a community-based study. *BMJ* 1993; **306**: 481–3.

8 Brezis M, Rosen SN, Silva P, Epstein FH. Selective vulnerability of the medullary thick ascending limb to anoxia in the isolated perfused rat kidney. *J Clin Invest* 1984; **73**: 182–90.

9 Burke TJ, Cronin RE, Duchin KL, *et al.* Ischemia and tubule obstruction during acute renal failure in dogs: mannitol in protection. *Am J Physiol* 1980; **238**: F305–14.

10 Tomita K, Ujiie K, Nakanishi T, *et al.* Plasma endothelin levels in patients in acute renal failure. *N Engl J Med* 1989; **321**: 1127–31.

11 Linas SL, Shanley PF, Whittenburg D, *et al*. Neutrophils accentuate ischemia– reperfusion injury in isolated perfused rat kidneys. *Am J Physiol* 1988; **255**: F728–35.

12 Schwartz JH, Shih T, Menza SA, Lieberthal W. ATP depletion increases tyrosine phoshorylation of beta-catenin and plakoglobin in renal tubular cells. *J Am Soc Nephrol* 1999; **264**: F1–8.

13 Bonventre JV. Mechanisms of ischemic acute renal failure. Kidney Int 1993; **43**: 1160–78.

14 Portilla D, Mandel LJ, Bar-Sagi D, Millington DS. Anoxia induces phospholipase A_2 activation in rabbit renal proximal tubules. *Am J Physiol* 1992; **262**: F354–60.

15 Di Mari JF, Davis R, Safirstein RL. MAPK activation determines renal epithelial cell survival during oxidative injury. *Am J Physiol* 1999; **277**: F195–203.

16 Bellomo R, Kellum JA, Wisniewski SR, Pinsky MR. Effects of norepinephrine on the renal vasculature in normal and endotoxemic dogs. *Am J Respir Crit Care Med* 1999; **159**: 1186–92.

17 Redl-Wenzel EM, Armbruster C, Edelman G, *et al*. The effects of norepinephrine on hemodynamics and renal function in severe septic shock. *Intensive Care Med* 1993; **19**: 151–4.

18 Bersten AD, Holt AW. Vasoactive drugs and the importance of renal perfusion pressure. *New Horiz* 1995; **3**: 650–61.

19 ANZICS Clinical Trials Group. Low-dose dopamine in patients with early renal dysfunction: a placebo-controlled randomised trial. *Lancet* 2000; **356**: 2139–3.

20 Solomon R, Werner C, Mann D, *et al*. Effects of saline, mannitol, and furosemide to prevent acute decreases in renal function induced by radiocontrast agents. *N Engl J Med* 1994; **331**: 1416–20.

21 Majumdar S, Kjellstrand CM. Why do we use diuretics in acute renal failure? *Seminars in Dialysis* 1996; **9**: 454–9.

22. Rudy DW, Voelker JR, Greene PK, *et al*. Loop diuretics for chronic renal insufficiency: a continuous infusion is more efficacious then bolus therapy. *Ann Intern Med* 1991; **115**: 360–6.

23 Conger JD. Interventions in clinical acute renal failure: what are the data? *Am J Kid Dis* 1995; **26**: 565–76.

24 Chertow GM, Lazarus JM, Paganini EP, *et al*. Predictors of mortality and the provision of dialysis in patients with acute tubular necrosis: The Auriculin Anaritide Acute Renal Failure Study Group. *J Am Soc Nephrol* 1998; **9**: 692–8.

25 Tepel M, van der Giet M, Schwarzfeld C, *et al*. Prevention of radiographic-contrast-agent-induced reductions in renal function by acetylcysteine. *N Engl J Med* 2000; **343**: 180–4.

26 Kierdorf HP. The nutritional management of acute renal failure in the intensive care unit. *New Horiz* 1995; **3**: 699–707.

27 Hebert P, Wells G, Blajchman MA, *et al*. A multicenter randomized controlled clinical trial of transfusion requirements in critical care. *N Engl J Med* 1999; **340**: 409–417.

28 Gettings LG, Reynolds HN, Scalea T. Outcome in post-traumatic acute renal failure when continuous renal replacement therapy is applied early vs. late. *Intensive Care Med* 1999; **25**: 805–13.

29 Paganini EP. Dialysis is not dialysis is not dialysis! Acute dialysis is different and needs help! *Am J Kidney Dis* 1998; **32**: 832–3.

30 Ronco C, Bellomo R, Homel P, *et al*. Effects of different doses in continuous veno-venous haemofiltration on outcomes of acute renal failure: a prospective randomized trial. *Lancet* 2000; **355**: 26–30.

39

Renal replacement therapy

R Bellomo

When acute renal failure (ARF) is severe, resolution can take several days or weeks. During this time, the kidneys cannot maintain homeostasis of fluid, potassium, metabolic acid and waste products. Life-threatening complications inevitably develop in these patients. Extracorporeal techniques of blood purification must therefore be applied to prevent such complications. These techniques, broadly named renal replacement therapy (RRT), include continuous haemofiltration, intermittent haemodialysis and peritoneal dialysis. Each has its technical variations, but they all rely on the principle of removing unwanted solutes and water through a semipermeable membrane, which is either biological (peritoneum) or artificial (haemodialysis or haemofiltration membranes), and offer advantages, disadvantages and limitations.

PRINCIPLES

The principles of RRT have been extensively studied and described.[1–3] This chapter summarizes some aspects that are particularly relevant to the critical care physician.

WATER REMOVAL

The removal of unwanted solvent (water) is therapeutically as important as the removal of unwanted solute (acids, uraemic toxins, potassium, etc.). During RRT, water is removed through a process called ultrafiltration, which is essentially the same as that performed by the glomerulus. It requires a driving pressure to move fluid across a semipermeable membrane, because such fluid would normally be kept within the circulation due to oncotic pressure. This pressure is achieved by: (i) generating a transmembrane pressure (as in haemofiltration or during intermittent haemodialysis) that is greater than oncotic pressure; (ii) increasing osmolarity of the dialysate (as in peritoneal dialysis).

SOLUTE REMOVAL

The removal of unwanted solute can be achieved by:

1 creating an electrochemical gradient across the membrane by using a flow past system with toxin-free dialysate (diffusion), as in intermittent haemodialysis (IHD) and peritoneal dialysis (PD);
2 creating a 'solvent drag' driven by transmembrane pressure, where solute moves together with solvent (convection) across a porous membrane, is discarded and then replaced with toxin-free replacement fluid, as in haemofiltration (HF).

The rate of diffusion of a given solute depends on its molecular weight, the porosity of the membrane, the blood flow rate, the dialysate flow rate, its binding to proteins, and its concentration gradient across the membrane. If standard, low-flux, cellulose-based membranes are used, middle molecules of >500 daltons cannot be removed. If synthetic high-flux membranes are used with a cut-off at 20–30 kilodaltons (kDa), larger molecules can be removed, and with these membranes convection can be about 20–30% superior to diffusion in achieving the clearance of middle molecules. During PD, larger molecules (albumin) can also be removed because of the porosity of the peritoneal membrane. However, because blood flow rate across the peritoneal membrane is limited, clearances are also limited.

INDICATIONS FOR RENAL REPLACEMENT THERAPY

In the critically ill patient, RRT should be initiated early, prior to the development of complications. Fear of early dialysis stems from the adverse effects of conventional IHD with cuprophane membranes, especially haemodynamic instability, and from the risks and limitations of continuous or intermittent PD.[4,5] However, continuous renal replacement therapy (CRRT),[6,7] or prolonged IHD[8] minimize these effects. The criteria for the initiation of RRT in patients with chronic renal failure may be inappropriate in the critically ill.[9,10] A set of modern criteria for the initiation of RRT in the ICU is presented in Table 39.1.

Table 39.1 Modern criteria for the initiation of renal replacement therapy (RRT) in the ICU[a]

- Oliguria (urine output: <200 ml/12 h)
- Anuria (urine output: 0–50 ml/12 h)
- [Urea] >35 mmol/l
- [Creatinine] >400 μmol/l
- [K+] >6.5 mmol/L or rapidly rising[b]
- Pulmonary oedema unresponsive to diuretics
- Uncompensated metabolic acidosis (pH <7.1)
- [Na+] <110 and >160 mmol/l
- Temperature >40°C
- Uraemic complications (encephalopathy/myopathy/neuropathy/pericarditis)
- Overdose with a dialyzable toxin (e.g. lithium)

[a] If one criterion is present, RRT should be considered. If two criteria are simultaneously present, RRT is strongly recommended.
[b] Be aware of differences between plasma vs. serum measurement in your laboratory.

With either IHD or CRRT there are limited data on what is 'adequate' intensity of dialysis. However, this should include maintenance of homeostasis at all levels,[10] and better uraemic control may translate into better survival.[11,12] An appropriate target urea is 15–25 mmol/l, with a protein intake around 1.5 g/kg per day. This can be easily achieved using CRRT at urea clearances of 35–45 litres per day, depending on patient size and catabolic rate. If IHD is used, daily treatment becomes desirable, as shown by a recent randomized controlled trial in which daily dialysis decreased mortality and accelerated renal recovery in medical critically ill patients.[13]

MODE OF RENAL REPLACEMENT THERAPY

There is a great deal of controversy as to which mode of RRT is 'best' in the ICU, due to the lack of randomized controlled trials comparing different techniques. Trials of sufficient statistical power are difficult to conduct and may never be performed. In their absence, techniques of RRT may be judged on the basis of the following criteria:

- haemodynamic side-effects
- ability to control fluid status
- biocompatibility
- risk of infection
- uraemic control
- avoidance of cerebral oedema
- ability to allow full nutritional support
- ability to control acidosis
- absence of specific side-effects
- cost

CRRT and slow low-efficiency extended dialysis (SLED) offer many advantages over PD and conventional IHD (3–4 h/day, 3–4 times a week),[13] and while CRRT is almost exclusively used in some centres,[14] only 10–20% of American ICU patients receive CRRT.[15]

CONTINUOUS RENAL REPLACEMENT THERAPY (CRRT)

First described in 1977, CRRT has undergone several technical modifications. Initially, it was performed as an arteriovenous therapy (continuous arteriovenous haemo-filtration, CAVH) where blood flow through the haemo-filter was driven by the patient's blood pressure. However, clearances were low and countercurrent dialysate flow was soon added to double or triple solute clearances (continuous arteriovenous haemodialysis/diafiltration, CAVHD or CAVHDF), with or without spontaneous ultrafiltration. The need to cannulate an artery, however, is associated with 15–20% morbidity. Accordingly, double-lumen catheters and peristaltic blood pumps have come into use (continuous veno-venous haemofiltration, CVVH) with or without control of ultrafiltration rate. Ultrafiltration rates of 2 l/h yield urea clearances of >30 ml/min. Diagrams illustrating typical haemofiltration circuits are presented in Figs 39.1 and 39.2.

In a veno-venous system, dialysate can also be delivered countercurrent to blood flow (continuous veno-

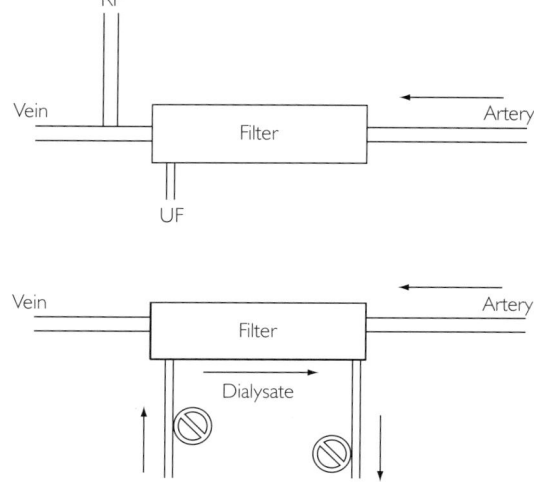

Fig. 39.1 Diagrams illustrating two standard arteriovenous circuit designs. The top circuit represents continuous arteriovenous haemofiltration (CAVH) with spontaneous generation of ultrafiltrate (UF) and post-filter administration of replacement fluid (RF). The bottom circuit represents continuous arteriovenous haemodialysis (CVVHD) with countercurrent dialysate flow. Dialysate is pump controlled, so that spent dialysate outflow is just 100–200 ml/h (as needed to maintain overall fluid balance) above dialysate inflow.

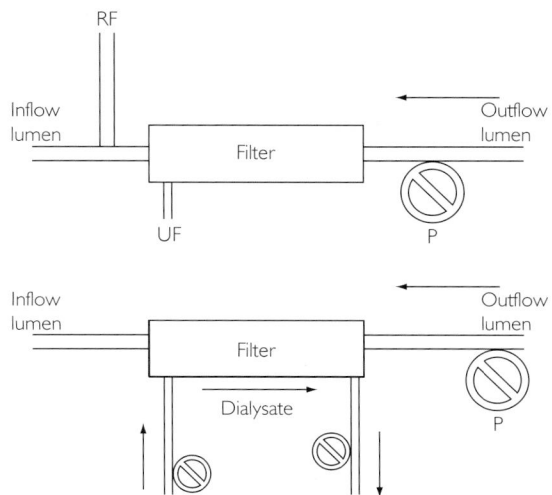

Fig. 39.2 Diagrams illustrating two standard veno-venous circuit designs with flow out of the double lumen catheter driven by a pump (P) from the outflow lumen of the catheter to the inflow lumen. The top circuit represents continuous veno-venous haemofiltration (CVVH) with spontaneous generation of ultrafiltrate (UF) and post-filter administration of replacement fluid (RF). The bottom circuit represents continuous veno-venous haemodialysis (CVVHD) with countercurrent dialysate flow. Dialysate is pump controlled so that spent dialysate outflow is just 100–200 ml/h (as needed to maintain overall fluid balance) above dialysate inflow.

venous haemodialysis/haemodiafiltration) to achieve either almost pure diffusive clearance or a mixture of diffusive and convective clearance.

No matter what technique is used, the following outcomes are predictable:

- continuous control of fluid status
- haemodynamic stability
- control of acid–base status
- ability to provide protein rich nutrition while achieving uraemic control
- control of electrolyte balance, including phosphate and calcium balance
- prevention of swings in intra-cerebral water
- minimal risk of infection
- high level of biocompatibility.

However, CRRT mandates the presence of specifically trained nursing and medical staff 24 hours a day. Small ICUs often cannot provide such level of support. If CRRT is used only 5–10 times a year, the cost of training may be unjustified and expertise may be hard to maintain. Furthermore, depending on the organization of patient care, CRRT may be more expensive that IHD. Finally, the issues of continuous circuit anticoagulation and the potential risk of bleeding have been a major concern.

ANTICOAGULATION DURING CRRT

The flow of blood through an extracorporeal circuit causes activation of the coagulation cascade and promotes clotting of the filter and circuit itself. In order to delay such clotting and achieve acceptable operational lives (approximately 24 hours) for the circuit, anticoagulants are frequently used.[16] However, circuit anticoagulation increases risk of bleeding. Therefore, the risks and benefits of more or less intense anticoagulation and alternative stategies (Table 39.2) must be considered.

In the vast majority of patients, low-dose heparin (<500 IU/h) is sufficient to achieve adequate filter life. It is easy and cheap to administer, and has almost no effect on the patient's coagulation tests. In some patients, a higher dose is necessary. In others (e.g. with pulmonary embolism or myocardial ischaemia), full heparinization may actually be concomitantly indicated. Regional citrate anticoagulation is very effective but requires a special dialysate or replacement fluid. Regional heparin/protamine anticoagulation is also somewhat complex, but may be useful if frequent filter clotting occurs and further anticoagulation of the patient is considered dangerous. Low-molecular-weight heparin is also easy to give but more expensive. Its dose must be adjusted for the loss of renal function. Heparinoids and prostacyclin may be useful if the patient has developed heparin-induced thrombocytopenia and thrombosis. Serine proteinase inhibitors are not available outside Japan. Finally, in perhaps 10–20% of patients, anticoagulation is best avoided because of endogenous coagulopathy or recent surgery. In such patients, mean filter lives >24 hours can be achieved provided that blood flow is kept at about 200 ml/min and vascular access is reliable.[17,18]

Many circuits clot for mechanical reasons: inadequate access; unreliable blood flow from the double-lumen catheter depending on patient position; kinking of the catheter. Responding to frequent filter clotting by simply increasing anticoagulation without making the correct aetiological diagnosis (checking catheter flow and position, taking a history surrounding the episode of clotting, identifying the site of clotting) is often futile and

Table 39.2 Strategies for circuit anticoagulation during continuous renal replacement therapy

- No anticoagulation
- Low-dose pre-filter heparin (<500 IU/h)
- Medium-dose pre-filter heparin (500–1000 IU/h)
- Full heparinization
- Regional anticoagulation (pre-filter heparin and post-filter protamine usually at a 100 IU : 1 mg ratio)
- Regional citrate anticoagulation (pre-filter citrate and post-filter calcium – special calcium-free dialysate needed)
- Low-molecular-weight heparin
- Prostacyclin
- Heparinoids
- Serine proteinase inhibitors (nafamostat mesylate)

exposes the patient to unnecessary risk. Particular attention needs to be paid to the adequacy/ease of flow through the double-lumen catheter. Smaller (11.5 Fr) catheters in the subclavian position are a particular problem. Larger catheters (13.5 Fr) in the femoral position appear to function more reliably.

CRRT TECHNOLOGY

The increasing use of veno-venous CRRT has led to the development of a field of CRRT technology, which offers different kinds of machines to facilitate its performance.[19] Some understanding of these devices is important to the successful implementation of CRRT in any ICU. The simplest technical approach is to allow ultrafiltration to occur spontaneously, measure it and replace it as indicated. In such a system, hourly measurement of effluent is necessary, and the only requirement is that of a blood pump to deliver blood to the filter and of a volumetric pump to administer replacement fluid at the appropriate rate. Such a system is inherently unsafe and labour intensive. However, a volumetric pump can easily regulate effluent flow. Thus, one can have a simple blood pump with safety features (air bubble trap and pressure alarms), and use widely available volumetric pumps to control replacement or dialysate flow and effluent flow. Such adaptive technology is inexpensive, but is not user-friendly. Also, volumetric pumps have an inherent inaccuracy of about 5%, which, in a system exchanging up to 50 l/day, can cause problems.[19] Various manufacturers have now produced custom-made machines for haemofiltration. These machines are safer and have much more sophisticated pump control systems, alarms and graphic displays. They are much more user-friendly, especially with the set-up procedure.

The choice of membrane is also a matter of controversy. Several biosynthetic membranes on the market have excellent biocompatibility (AN69, polyamide, polysulfone, cellulose triacetate). but no controlled studies have been undertaken to show that one of them confers a clinical advantage over the others. The AN69 is the most commonly used CRRT membrane in Australia. The issue of membrane size is also controversial, as no controlled studies have compared different membrane surface sizes. For the AN69 membrane, there is no increase in price up to a size of 1.2 m², thus there is no reason to use smaller membranes in adults. If high-volume haemofiltration is planned, the membrane surface needs to be in the 1.6–2 m² range.

INTERMITTENT HAEMODIALYSIS

Vascular access is typically by double lumen catheter, as in continuous haemofiltration. The circuit is also the same, with veno-venous blood flow driven by a peristaltic pump. Countercurrent dialysate flow is used as in CVVHD. The major differences are that standard IHD uses high dialysate flows (300–400 ml/min), generates

dialysate by using purified water, and concentrate and is applied for short periods of time (3–4 hours), usually every second day.

These differences have important implications. First, volume has to be removed over a short period of time and this may be poorly tolerated by critically ill patients, with a resulting high incidence of hypotension.[20] Repeated hypotensive episodes may delay renal recovery.[4] Second, solute removal is episodic. This translates into inferior uraemic control,[21] and acid–base control. Limited fluid and uraemic control imposes unnecessary limitations on nutritional support.[22] Furthermore, rapid solute shifts increase brain water content and raise intracranial pressure.[23] Finally, much controversy has surrounded the issue of membrane bioincompatibility. Standard low-flux dialysing membranes made of cuprophane are known to trigger the activation of several inflammatory pathways, when compared to high-flux synthetic membranes (also used for continuous haemofiltration). It is possible that such pro-inflammatory effect contributes to further renal damage and delays recovery or even affects mortality. Two studies have offered support to this hypothesis.[20,24] However, others have failed to confirm any advantage of using biocompatible membranes in all cases of ARF,[25] and the matter remains unresolved.[26] Given the minimal difference in cost between biocompatible and bioincompatible low-flux membranes, biocompatible membranes (polysulfone) are preferred.

The limitations of applying 'standard' IHD to the treatment of ARF[9] has led to the development of new approaches (so-called 'hybrid techniques') such as SLED, and intermittent extended haemofiltration.[13] These techniques seek to adapt IHD to the clinical circumstance[27] and thereby increase its tolerance and its clearances.

PERITONEAL DIALYSIS

This technique is now uncommonly used in the treatment of adult ARF in developed countries.[15] However, it may be an adequate technique in developing countries or in children because alternatives are considered too expensive, too invasive, or are not available. Typically, access is by the insertion of an intra-peritoneal catheter. Glucose-rich dialysate is then inserted into the peritoneal cavity and acts as the 'dialysate'. After a given 'dwell time', it is removed and discarded with the extra fluid and toxins that have moved from the blood vessels of the peritoneum to the dialysate fluid. Machines are also available which deliver and remove dialysate at higher flows, providing intermittent treatment or higher solute clearances.

Several major shortcomings make PD relatively unsuited to the treatment of adult ARF:

- limited and sometimes inadequate solute clearance
- high risk of peritonitis

- unpredictable hyperglycaemia
- fluid leaks
- protein loss
- interference with diaphragm function

There have not been any reports of the sole use of PD for the treatment of adult patients with ARF in the last 15 years.

OTHER BLOOD PURIFICATION TECHNIQUES

HAEMOPERFUSION

During haemoperfusion, blood is circulated through a circuit similar to one used for CVVH. However, a charcoal cartridge is perfused with blood instead of a dialysis membrane. In some cases an ion exchange resin (Amberlite) has been used. Charcoal microcapsules effectively remove molecules of 300–500 daltons in size, including some lipid soluble and protein bound substances. Heparinization is necessary to prevent clotting. Attention must also be paid to changes in intravascular volume at the start of therapy, because of the large priming volume of the cartridge (260 ml). Glucose absorption is significant and monitoring of blood glucose is necessary to avoid hypoglycaemia. Also thrombocytopenia is common, and can be marked. The role of charcoal haemoperfusion is controversial, as no controlled trials have ever shown it to confer clinically significant advantages. It may be useful, however, in patients with life-threatening theophylline overdose because it remove the agent effectively.

PLASMAPHERESIS OR PLASMA EXCHANGE

With this technique, plasma is removed from the patient and exchanged with fresh frozen plasma (FFP) and a mixture of colloid and crystalloid solutions. This technique can also be performed in an ICU familiar with CRRT techniques. A plasmafilter (a filter that allows the passage of molecules up to 500 kDa) instead of a haemofilter is inserted in the CVVH circuit, and the filtrate (plasma) discarded. Plasmapheresis can also be performed with special machines using the principles of centrifugation. The differences, if any, between centrifugation and filtration technology are unclear. Replacement (post-filter) will occur as in CVVH using, for example, a 50/50 combination of FFP and albumin. Plasmapheresis has been shown to be effective treatment for thrombotic thrombocytopenic purpura (TTP) and for several diseases mediated by abnormal antibodies (Guillain–Barré syndrome, cryoglobulinaemia, myasthenia gravis, Goodpasture's syndrome, etc.), in which antibody removal appears desirable. Its role in the treatment of sepsis remains uncertain.[28]

BLOOD PURIFICATION TECHNOLOGY OUTSIDE OF ARF

There is growing interest in the possibility that blood purification may provide a clinically significant benefit in patients with severe sepsis/septic shock by removing circulating 'mediators'. A variety of techniques including plasmapheresis, high-volume haemofiltration, very-high volume haemofiltration, and coupled plasma filtration adsorption[28-33] are being studied in animals and in phase I/II studies in humans. Initial experiments support the need to continue exploring this therapeutic option.[31] However, no suitably powered randomized controlled trials have yet been reported. Also, blood purification technology, in combination with bioreactors containing either human or porcine liver cells, is under active investigations as a form of artificial liver support for patients with fulminant liver failure or for patients with acute on chronic liver failure.[34,35] Such complex technology is beginning to show some promising results.[35]

DRUG PRESCRIPTION DURING DIALYTIC THERAPY

Acute renal failure and RRT profoundly affect drug clearance. A comprehensive description of changes in drug dosage according to the technique of RRT, residual creatinine clearance, and other determinants of pharmacodynamics is beyond the scope of this chapter and can be found in specialist texts.[36] The following table (Table 39.3) provides general guidelines for the prescription of drugs that are commonly used in the ICU.

SUMMARY

The area of renal replacement therapy has undergone remarkable changes over the last 5 years and is continuing to evolve rapidly. Technology is being improved to facilitate clinical application and new areas of research are developing. CRRT is now firmly established throughout the world as perhaps the most commonly used form of RRT. Conventional dialysis, however, which was slowly losing ground is reappearing in the form of extended, slow-efficiency treatment, especially in the USA. In the meantime, the use of novel membranes, of sorbents and of different intensities of treatment are being explored in the area of sepsis management and liver support. The intensivist needs to keep abreast of this rapid evolution if patients are to be offered the best of care.

Table 39.3 Drug dosage during dialytic therapy[a]

DRUG	CRRT	IHD
Aminoglycosides	Normal dose q. 36 h	50% normal dose q. 48 h-2/3 re-dose after IHD
Cefotaxime or Ceftazidime	1g q. 8–12 h	1g q.12–24 h after IHD
Imipenem	500 mg q.8 h	250 mg q.8 h and after IHD
Meropenem	500 mg q. 8 h	250 mg q. 8 h and after IHD
Metronidazole	500 mg q. 8 h	250 mg q. 8 h and after IHD
Co-trimoxazole	Normal dose q. 18 h	Normal dose q. 24 h after IHD
Amoxycillin	500 mg q. 8 h	500 mg daily and after IHD
Vancomycin	1 g q. 24 h	1 g q. 96–120 h
Piperacillin	3–4 g q. 6 h	3–4 g q. 8 h and after IHD
Ticarcillin	1–2 g q. 8 h	1–2 g q. 12 h and after IHD
Ciprofloxacin	200 mg q. 12 h	200 mg q. 24 h and after IHD
Fluconazole	200 mg q. 24 h	200 mg q. 48 h and after IHD
Acyclovir	3.5 mg/kg q. 24 h	2.5 mg/kg/d and after IHD
Gancyclovir	5 mg/kg/day	5 mg/kg/48 h and after IHD
Amphotericin B	Normal dose	Normal dose
Liposomal amphotericin	Normal dose	Normal dose
Ceftriaxone	Normal dose	Normal dose
Erythomycin	Normal dose	Normal dose
Milrinone	Titrate to effect	Titrate to effect
Amrinone	Titrate to effect	Titrate to effect
Catecholamines	Titrate to effect	Titrate to effect
Ampicillin	500 mg q. 8 hourly	500 mg daily and after IHD

[a] The above values represent approximations and should be used as a general guide only. Critically ill patients have markedly abnormal volumes of distribution for these agents which will affect dosage. CRRT is conducted at variable levels of intensity in different units also requiring adjustment. The values reported here relate to CVVH at 2 l/h of ultrafiltration. Vancomycin is poorly removed by CVVHD. IHD may also differ from unit to unit. The values reported here relate to standard IHD with low-flux membranes for 3–4 hours every second day. For abbreviations: see text.

REFERENCES

1 Sargent J, Gotch F. Principles and biophysics of dialysis. In: Maher J (ed.) *Replacement of Renal Function by Dialysis*. Dordrecht: Kluwer Academic Publishers; 1989: pp 87–102.

2 Henderson L. Biophysics of ultrafiltration and hemofiltration. In: Maher J (ed). *Replacement of Renal Function by Dialysis*. Dordrecht: Kluwer Academic Publishers; 1989: pp 300–2.

3 Nolph KD. Peritoneal dialysis. In: Brenner BM, Rector FC (eds) *The Kidney*, 1st edn., Philadelphia, PA: WB Saunders; 1986: pp 1791–45.

4 Conger JD. Does hemodialysis delay recovery from acute renal failure? *Seminars Dial* 1990; **3**: 146–5.

5 Howdieshell TR, Blalock WE, Bowen PA, *et al.* Management of post-traumatic acute renal failure with peritoneal dialysis. *Am Surg* 1992; **58**: 378–82.

6 Bellomo R, Boyce N. Continuous venovenous hemodiafiltration compared with conventional dialysis in critically ill patients with acute renal failure. *ASAIO J* 1993; **39**: M794–7.

7 Gettings LG, Reynolds HN, Scalea T. Outcome in post-traumatic acute renal failure when continuous renal replacement therapy is applied early vs. late. *Intensive Care Med* 1999; **25**: 805–81.

8 Chatoth DK, Shaver MJ, Marshall MR, Golper TA. Daily 12-hour sustained low-efficiency hemodialysis (SLED) for the treatment of critically ill patients with

acute renal failure: initial experience. *Blood Purif* 1999; **17**: Abstr 16.

9 Paganini EP. Dialysis is not dialysis is not dialysis! Acute dialysis is different and needs help! *Am J Kidney Dis* 1998; **32**: 832–3.

10 Bellomo R, Ronco C. Adequacy of dialysis in the acute renal failure of the critically ill: the case for continuous therapies. *Int J Artif Organs* 1996; **19**: 129–42.

11 Kanagasundaram NS, Paganini EP. Critical care dialysis – a Gordian knot (but is untying the right approach?). *Nephrol Dial Transplant* 1999; **14**: 2590–4.

12 Ronco C, Bellomo R, Homel P, *et al*. Effects of different doses in continuous veno-venous haemofiltration on outcomes of acute renal failure: a prospective randomized trial. *Lancet* 2000; **355**: 26–30.

13 Schiffl H. Lang SM, Fischer R. Daily hemodialysis and the outcome of acute renal failure. *N Engl J Med* 2002; **346**: 305–10.

14 Cole L, Bellomo R, Silvester W, Reeves JH. A prospective, multicenter study of the epidemiology, management and outcome of severe acute renal failure in a 'closed' ICU system. *Am J Respir Crit Care Med* 2000; **162**: 191–6.

15 Mehta R, Letteri JM. Current status of renal replacement therapy for acute renal failure. *Am J Nephrol* 1999; **19**: 377–82.

16 Mehta R, Dobos GJ, Ward DM. Anticoagulation procedures in continuous renal replacement. *Seminars Dial* 1992; **5**: 61–8.

17 Tan HK, Baldwin I, Bellomo R. Hemofiltration without anticoagulation in high-risk patients. *Intensive Care Med* 2000; **26**: 1652–7.

18 Bellomo R, Teede H, Boyce N. Anticoagulant regimens in acute continuous hemodiafiltration: a comparative study. *Intensive Care Med* 1993; **19**: 329–32.

19 Ronco C, Brendolan A, Bellomo R. Current technology for continuous renal replacement therapies. In: Ronco C, Bellomo R (eds) *Critical Care Nephrology*. Dordrecht: Kluwer Academic Publishers; 1998: pp 1327–34.

20 Hakim RM, Wingard R, Parker RA. Effect of dialysis membrane in the treatment of patients with acute renal failure. *N Engl J Med* 1994; **331**: 1338–42.

21 Macias WL, Clark WR. Azotemia control by extracorporeal therapy in patients with acute renal failure. *New Horiz* 1995; **3**: 688–93.

22 Kierdorf HP. The nutritional management of acute renal failure in the intensive care unit. *New Horiz* 1995; 3: 699–707.

23 Davenport A. The management of renal failure in patients at risk of cerebral edema/hypoxia. *New Horiz* 1995; **3**: 717–24.

24 Schiffl H, Lang SM, Konig A, *et al*. Biocompatible membranes in acute renal failure: prospective case controlled study. *Lancet* 1994; **344**: 570–2.

25 Jorres A, Gahl GM, Dobis C, *et al*. Hemodialysis-membrane biocompatibility and mortality of patients with dialysis-dependent acute renal failure: a prospective randomized multicentre trial. *Lancet* 1999; **354**: 1337–41.

26 Vanholder R, Lemaire N. Does biocompatibility of dialysis membranes affect recovery of renal function and survival? Lancet 1999; **354**: 1316–18.

27 Lameire N, Van Biesen W, Vanholder R. Dialysing the patient with acute renal failure in the ICU: the emperor's clothes. *Nephrol Dial Transplant* 1999; **14**: 2570–3.

28 Reeves JH, Butt WW, Shann F, *et al*. Continuous plasmafiltration in sepsis syndrome. *Crit Care Med* 1999; **27**: 2096–104.

29 Bellomo R. Continuous hemofiltration as blood purification in sepsis. *New Horiz* 1995; **3**: 732–7.

30 Tetta C, Mariano F, Ronco C, Bellomo R. Removal and generation of inflammatory mediators during continuous renal replacement therapies. In: Ronco C, Bellomo R (eds). *Critical Care Nephrology*, Dordrecht: Kluwer Academic Publishers; 1998: pp 1239–48.

31 Bellomo R, Baldwin I, Ronco C. Extracorporeal blood purification therapy for sepsis and systemic inflammation: its biological rationale. *Contrib Nephrol* 2001; **132**: 367–74.

32 Bellomo R, Baldwin I, Ronco C. High-volume hemofiltration. *Contrib Nephrol* 2001; **132**: 375–82.

33 Brendolan A, Bellomo R, Tetta C, *et al*. Coupled plasma filtration adsorption in the treatment of septic shock. *Contrib Nephrol* 2001; **132**: 383–91.

34 Rahman TM, Hodgson HJ. Liver support systems in acute hepatic failure. *Aliment Pharmacol Ther* 1999; **13**: 1255–72.

35 Mitzner SR, Stange J, Klammt S, *et al*. Extracorporeal detoxification using the molecular adsorbent recirculating system for critically ill patients with liver failure. *J Am Soc Nephrol* 2001; **12**: S75–82.

36 Buckmaster J, Davies AR. Guidelines for drug dosing during continuous renal replacement therapies. In: Ronco C, Bellomo R (eds) *Critical Care Nephrology*. Dordrecht: Kluwer Academic Publishers; 1998: pp 1327–34.

Part Seven

Neurologic Disorders

40

Disorders of consciousness

B Venkatesh

NEUROANATOMY AND PHYSIOLOGY OF WAKEFULNESS

A normal level of consciousness depends on the integrity of and the interaction between the cerebral hemispheres and the rostral reticular activating system (RAS) located in the upper brainstem. The RAS is a diffuse projection but the areas of RAS particularly pertinent to the maintenance of consciousness are located between the rostral pons and the diencephalon. As the anatomical areas subserving consciousness cover a large part of the brain, consciousness is not focally represented in the cerebral hemispheres and is in many ways related to the mass of functioning cortex. Altered consciousness may result from anatomical lesions in the hemispheres, either unilaterally or bilaterally, through compression of the upper brainstem or through lesions in the brain stem.[1] Metabolic processes either disrupting energy substrate delivery or altering neuronal excitability can alter consciousness. Disorders of consciousness are characterized either by an alteration in the level or content of consciousness (Table 40.1).

The last three conditions described in that table are a frequent source of confusion and require further discussion (Table 40.2).

These neurological states are seen more frequently in modern-day clinical practice, partly because of the advances in therapy of severe brain injury and intensive care which have led to the survival of many patients who would have otherwise died.

DIFFERENTIAL DIAGNOSIS OF COMA

Although the aetiology of coma is invariably multifactorial, the differential diagnosis of coma can be broadly grouped into three classes:

1 diseases that produce focal or lateralizing signs;
2 coma without focal or lateralizing signs, but with signs of meningeal irritation;

Table 40.1 Disorders of consciousness

Consciousness	An awake individual demonstrates full awareness of self and environment
Confusion	Inability to think with customary speed and clarity, associated with inattentiveness, reduced awareness and disorientation
Delirium	Confusion with agitation and hallucination
Stupor	Unresponsiveness with arousal only by deep and repeated stimuli
Coma	Unarousable unresponsiveness
Locked in syndrome	Total paralysis below third cranial nerve nuclei; normal or impaired mental function
Persistent vegetative state	Prolonged coma > 1 month, some preservation of brainstem and motor reflexes
Akinetic mutism	Prolonged coma with apparent alertness and flaccid motor tone

3 coma without focal or lateralizing signs or signs of meningeal irritation.

These are considered in greater detail in Table 40.3.

CLINICAL EXAMINATION OF THE COMATOSE PATIENT

The neurological examination of the comatose patient is of crucial importance to assess the depth of coma and locate the site of lesion. Although the detailed neurological examination that can be carried out in a conscious patient is not possible in a comatose individual, useful information can be obtained by performing a thorough general examination and a neurological examination, particularly evaluating the level of consciousness, brainstem signs and motor responses in coma.

Table 40.2 Coma like syndromes and related states

Syndrome	Features	Site of lesion	Comments
Locked-in syndrome (30) (de-efferented state)	Alert and aware, vertical eye movements present, and able to blink. Quadriplegic, lower cranial nerve palsies, no speech, facial or pharyngeal movements	Bilateral anterior pontine lesion which transects all descending motor pathways, but spares ascending sensory and RAS systems	Similar state seen with severe polyneuropathies, myasthenia gravis and neuromuscular blocking agents
Persistent vegetative state (PVS) (31) (32) (apallic syndrome, neo-cortical death)	Previously comatose, who now appear to be awake. Spontaneous limb movements, eye movements and yawning seen. However patient inattentive, no speech, no awareness of environment and total inability to respond to commands	Extensive damage to both cerebral hemispheres with relative preservation of the brainstem	PVS lasting for longer than 2 weeks implies a poor prognosis
Akinetic mutism (33) (coma vigile)	Partially or fully awake patient, immobile and silent	Lesion in bilateral frontal lobes or hydrocephalus or third ventricular masses	Abulia is the term applied to milder forms of akinetic mutism
Catatonia	Awake patients, sometimes a fixed posture, muteness with decreased motor activity	Usually of psychiatric origin	May be mimicked by frontal lobe disease and drugs

GENERAL EXAMINATION

General examination of the patient may point to the aetiology of coma. Some common clinical examples are described below.

- Skin changes
  - carbon monoxide poisoning (cherry red discolouration of skin)
  - alcoholic liver disease (telangiectasia, clubbing)
  - hypothyroidism (puffy facies)
  - hypopituitarism (sallow complexion).
- Skin lesions/rashes
  - cutaneous petechiae or ecchymoses meningococcemia
  - rickettsial infection or endocarditis
  - needle puncture marks (substance abuse)
  - bullous skin lesions (barbiturate overdose)
  - excessively dry skin (diabetic ketoacidosis or anticholinergic overdose)
  - periorbital haematomas (raccoon eyes), suggest anterior basal skull fracture (look for associated CSF rhinorrhoea). Other signs of a basal skull fracture include Battle's sign and CBF otorrhoea.
- Other physical signs
  - nuchal rigidity (meningoencephalitis and subarachnoid haemorrhage)
  - hepatomegaly or stigmata of chronic liver disease (hepatic encephalopathy)
  - bilateral enlarged kidneys (polycystic kidney disease) suggests subarachnoid haemorrhage as potential aetiology of coma.

- breath odour, from alcohol or other poisons (e.g. organophosphates). Ketones in the breath is an unreliable sign; hepatic and uraemic foetor are rare.

LEVEL OF CONSCIOUSNESS

This is assessed by the Glasgow Coma Scale (GCS),[2] which takes into account patient's response to command and physical stimuli and enables grading and outcome prognostication of head injury. (Table 40.4)

This scale has now been extended for all causes of impaired consciousness and coma. Important considerations are:

1 The GCS should always be determined prior to administration of sedative drugs or endotracheal intubation.
2 The GCS should also be defined with regard to patient's vital signs, namely, blood pressure, heart rate and temperature.
3 The GCS must be interpreted in light of previous or concomitant drug therapy.
4 The presence of alcohol in the breath or in the serum should always be documented.
5 Because of the considerable inter-observer variation in scoring, it is important to define the responses in descriptive terms rather than emphasising the numerical score associated with each response.

PUPILLARY RESPONSES IN COMA[3]

The presence of normal pupils (2–5 mm, equal in size and demonstrating both direct and consensual light reflexes)

Table 40.3 Differential diagnosis of coma

Category	Specific disorder	Features in history and examination	Investigations	Comments
Coma with focal signs	Trauma – extradural, subdural and parenchymal haemorrhage, concussions	History of trauma, findings of fracture base of skull, scalp haematoma, other associated body injuries	Usually an abnormal CT	Exclude coexisting drug or alcohol ingestion
	Vascular – Intracerebral haemorrhage	Sudden onset, history of headaches or hypertension, neck stiffness may be present	Abnormal CT scan	Consider causes of secondary hypertension in young hypertensives
	Vascular – thromboembolic	Sudden onset, atrial fibrillation, vascular bruits, endocarditis	An abnormal CT after a few days	Consider echocardiography to diagnose cardiac sources of emboli
	Brain abscess	Subacute onset, look for ENT and dental sources of infection .	Abnormal CT and CSF	Consider infective endocarditis and suppurative lung disease as sources of sepsis
Coma without focal signs, but with meningeal irritation	Infection Meningitis, encephalitis	Onset of illness over a few hours to days, neck stiffness, rash of meningococcemia	Abnormal CSF	Consider underlying immunosuppressive states
	Subarachnoid haemorrhage	Onset usually sudden, subhyaloid haemorrhages on fundoscopy	Abnormal CT and CSF	Consider polycystic kidney disease in subarachnoid haemorrhage
Coma without focal signs and no meningeal irritation	Metabolic causes Hyponatraemia Hypoglycaemia Hypoxia Hypercapnia Hypo and hyperthermia Hyper and hypoosmolar states	History might point to the cause of metabolic disturbance, asterixis a feature of hypercapnia induced coma	Abnormal blood results	Rapid correction of hyponatraemia and osmolality should be avoided
	Endocrine causes Myxoedema Adrenal insufficiency Hypopituitarism	Puffy facies, may be hypothermic	Abnormal electrolyte profile, hypoglycaemia	Multiple disorders may be present in the same patient
	Seizure disorders	History typical	Abnormal EEG, check anticonvulsant levels	CT scan to exclude an underlying space occupying lesion
	Organ failure Hepatic Renal	History of jaundice, chronic alcohol ingestion, stigmata of liver disease, asterixis	Abnormal hepatic and renal functions	Presence of A-V fistula may be a pointer to chronic renal failure

Table 40.3 Differential diagnosis of coma *continued*

Category	Specific disorder	Features in history and examination	Investigations	Comments
	Toxic/drug Sedatives Narcotics Alcohol Psychotropic Carbon monoxide Poisons	History, may be hypothermic at presentation except in psychotropic drug overdose	Metabolic screen is usually normal	Rapid improvement in conscious states with antidotes
	Behavioural Sleep deprivation Pseudocoma	No typical features	No specific diagnostic tests	Diagnosis of exclusion

Table 40.4   Glasgow Coma Scale

Eye Opening	Points
Spontaneous	4
To speech	3
To pain	2
Nil	1
Best verbal response	
Oriented	5
Confused	4
Inappropriate	3
Incomprehensible	2
Nil	1
Intubated	T
Best motor response	
Obeys commands	6
Localises to pain	5
Withdraws to pain	4
Abnormal flexion	3
Extensor response	2
Nil	1

confirms the integrity of the pupillary pathway (retina, optic nerve, optic chiasma and tracts, midbrain and 3rd cranial nerve nuclei and nerves). The size of the pupil is a balance between the opposing influences of both sympathetic (causing dilatation) and parasympathetic (causing constriction) systems. Pupillary abnormalities have localizing and diagnostic value in clinical neurology (Table 40 5). When the pupils are miosed, the light reaction is difficult to appreciate and may require a magnifying glass.

OPHTHALMOSCOPY IN COMA

The pupils should *never* be dilated pharmacologically without prior documentation of the pupillary size and the light reflex. The presence of papilloedema suggests the presence of intracranial hypertension, but is frequently absent when the lesion is acute. Subhyaloid and vitreous haemorrhages are seen in patients with subarachnoid haemorrhage.[4]

EYE MOVEMENTS IN COMA[5]

Horizontal eye movements to the contralateral side are initiated in the ipsilateral frontal lobe and closely co-ordinated with the corresponding centre in the contralateral pons. To facilitate conjugate eye movements, yoking of the 3rd, 4th and 6th cranial nerve nuclei is achieved by the medial longitudinal fasciculus.

To look to the left, the movement originates in the right frontal lobe and is co-ordinated by the left pontine region and vice versa. In contrast to horizontal gaze, vertical eye movements are under bilateral control of the cortex and upper midbrain.

Table 40.5   Pupillary abnormalities in coma

Abnormality	Cause	Neuroanatomical basis
Miosis (<2 mm in size)		
Unilateral	Horner's syndrome	Sympathetic paralysis
	Local pathology	Trauma to sympathetics
Bilateral	Pontine lesions	
	Thalamic haemorrhage	Sympathetic paralysis
	Metabolic encephalopathy	
	Drug ingestion	
	Organophosphate	*Cholinesterase inhibition*
	Barbiturate	
	Narcotics	Central effect
Mydriasis (>5 mm in size)		
Unilateral fixed pupil	Midbrain lesion	3rd nerve damage
	Uncal herniation	Stretch of 3rd nerve against the petroclinoid ligament
Bilateral fixed pupils	Massive midbrain haemorrhage	Bilateral 3rd nerve damage
	Hypoxic cerebral injury	Mesencephalic damage
	Drugs	
	Atropine	Paralysis of parasympathetics
	Tricyclics	Prevent local reuptake of catecholamines by nerve endings
	Sympathomimetics	Stimulation of sympathetics

The position and movements of the eyes are observed at rest. The presence of full and conjugate eye movements in response to oculocephalic and oculovestibular stimuli demonstrates the functional integrity of a large segment of the brainstem. Corneal reflexes are preserved until late in coma. Upward rolling of the eyes after corneal stimulation (Bell's phenomenon) implies intact midbrain and pontine function.

The presence of spontaneous roving eye movements excludes brainstem pathology as a cause of coma. Ocular bobbing, an intermittent downward jerking eye movement, is seen in pontine lesions due to loss of horizontal gaze and unopposed midbrain controlled vertical gaze activity.[6]

In a paralytic frontal lobe pathology, the eyes will deviate towards the side of the lesion, while in pontine pathologies, the eyes will deviate away from the side of the lesion. Skew deviation (vertical separation of the ocular axes) occurs with pontine and cerebellar disorders.[7]

LIMB MOVEMENTS AND POSTURAL CHANGES IN COMA

- Restlessness, crossing of legs and spontaneous coughing, yawning, swallowing and localizing movements suggest only a mild depression of the conscious state.
- Choreoathetotic or ballistic movements suggest a basal ganglion lesion.
- Myoclonic movements indicate a metabolic disorder usually of post-anoxic origin.
- Asterixis is seen with metabolic encephalopathies.
- Hiccup is a non-specific sign and does not have any localizing value.
- Decerebrate rigidity is characterized by stiff extension of the limbs, internal rotation of the arms and plantar flexion of the ankles. With severe rigidity, opisthotonos and jaw clenching may be observed. These movements may be unilateral or bilateral, and spontaneous or in response to a noxious stimulus.

While animal studies suggest that the lesion is usually in the midbrain or caudal diencephalon (leading to exaggeration of antigravity reflexes), in humans such posturing may be seen in a variety of disease states: (i) midbrain lesion; (ii) metabolic disorders, such as hypoglycaemia, anoxia, hepatic coma, or drug intoxication.

Decorticate posturing is characterized by flexion of elbows and wrists and extension of the lower limbs. The lesion is usually above the midbrain in the cerebral white matter.

RESPIRATORY SYSTEM[8]

Abnormal respiratory rate and patterns have been described in coma, but their precise localizing value is uncertain. As a general rule, at lighter levels of impaired consciousness tachypnoea predominates, while respiratory depression increases with the depth of coma. Some

Table 40.6 Disorders of respiratory rate and pattern in coma

Abnormality	Significance
Bradypnoea	Drug induced coma, hypothyroid coma
Tachypnoea	Central neurogenic hyperventilation (Mid brain lesion), Metabolic encephalopathy
Cheyne Stokes respiration	Deep cerebral lesions, metabolic encephalopathy
(Hyperpnoea alternating regularly with apnoea)	
Apneustic breathing (an inspiratory pause)	Pontine lesions
Ataxic breathing	Medullary lesions
(Ataxic breathing normally progresses to agonal gasps and terminal apnoea)	

of the commonly observed respiratory abnormalities are summarized in Table 40.6. Respiratory failure in comatose patients may result from hypoventilation, aspiration pneumonia and neurogenic pulmonary oedema, a syndrome seen in acute brain injury mediated by the sympathetic nervous system.

BODY TEMPERATURE IN COMA

The presence of altered core body temperature is a useful aid in the diagnosis of coma. Hypothermia (<35°C) is frequently observed with alcohol or barbiturate intoxication, sepsis with shock, drowning, hypoglycaemia, myxoedema coma and exposure to cold. Severe hyperthermia may be seen in pontine haemorrhage, intracranial infections, heat stroke and anticholinergic drug toxicity.

RECOGNITION OF BRAIN HERNIATION[9,10]

When patients with impaired levels of consciousness deteriorate, it is important to consider brain herniation as a possible cause of worsening. Brain herniation results from the downward displacement of the upper brainstem (central herniation) with or without involvement of the uncus (lateral herniation). The clinical signs of a central herniation are progressive obtundation, Cheyne–Stokes respiration, small pupils followed by extensor posturing and medium sized fixed dilated pupils. Uncal herniation differs from central herniation in that pupillary dilatation occurs early in the process because of 3rd cranial nerve compression.

The traditional Cushing's response of hypertension and bradycardia is not always a feature of herniation and any heart rhythm may be present.

DIFFERENTIATING TRUE COMA FROM PSEUDOCOMA

In patients feigning coma, the pattern of clinical 'abnormalities' do not fit any specific neurological syndromes. Patients may resist passive eye opening and may not demonstrate spontaneous roving eye movements. By contrast, they move the eyes concomitantly with head rotation, and with cold caloric testing they may wake up or demonstrate preservation of the fast component of nystagmus. They also demonstrate avoidance of 'self injury'.

MANAGEMENT OF THE COMATOSE PATIENT

EMERGENCY THERAPEUTIC MEASURES

Irrespective of the aetiology of coma, certain emergency therapeutic measures apply to the care of all patients. These take precedence over any diagnostic investigation.

- Ensure adequate airway and oxygenation.
- Secure intravenous access and maintain circulation.
- Administer 50% dextrose after drawing a sample of blood for serum glucose levels. Although there are theoretical concerns about augmentation of brain lactic acid production[11,12] in anoxic coma, the relatively good prognosis for hypoglycaemic coma when treated expeditiously far outweighs any potential risks of glucose administration.
- Thiamine must always be administered in conjunction with dextrose to prevent precipitation of Wernicke's encephalopathy.
- Consideration should be given to administering naloxone, when there is a suspicion of narcotic overdose with impending respiratory arrest.
- If hypertension, bradycardia and fixed dilated pupils are present at the time of the initial presentation, suggestive of marked intracranial hypertension and tentorial herniation, 20% mannitol at a dose 0.25–0.5 gm/kg body weight should be administered. Consideration should be given to the emergency placement of an external ventricular drain.
- Treat suspected meningitis with antibiotics, even if CSF results are not available. A combination of penicillin and ceftriaxone is usually recommended for a community acquired bacterial meningitis.
- Control of seizures must be achieved as outlined in the Chapter 41 on *Status Epilepticus*.
- Treat extreme body temperatures.

INVESTIGATIONS

The order of investigation depends on the clinical circumstances. In the majority of cases, history and examination will provide enough information to be able to perform specific cause related investigation. In general, the investigations can be grouped as follows:

ROUTINE INVESTIGATIONS

Measurements of serum glucose, electrolytes, arterial blood gases, liver and renal function tests, osmolality, and blood count and blood film are part of the routine investigations. When drug overdose is suspected a toxicology screen for alcohol, paracetamol, salicylates, benodiazepines and tricyclic antidepressants should be performed. A sample of serum should be stored for later analysis for uncommon drug ingestions.

NEUROIMAGING
Computerized Tomography (CT) Scanning

The most commonly used radiological investigation for evaluation of the comatose patient is CT scanning of the brain. This is useful for diagnosing CNS trauma, subarachnoid haemorrhage (SAH) and intracerebral haemorrhage, haemorrhagic and non-haemorrhagic strokes, cerebral oedema, hydrocephalus and the presence of space occupying lesion (SOL). (Please see Figs 40.1–40.10). Frequently, a CT scan is performed prior to a lumbar puncture to exclude rather than confirm the presence of severe cerebral oedema or a SOL. Other advantages include: lower cost; easy availability; short examination time; and safety in the presence of pacemakers, surgical clips and other ferromagnetic substances. The advent of helical CT whereby multiple images are possible has

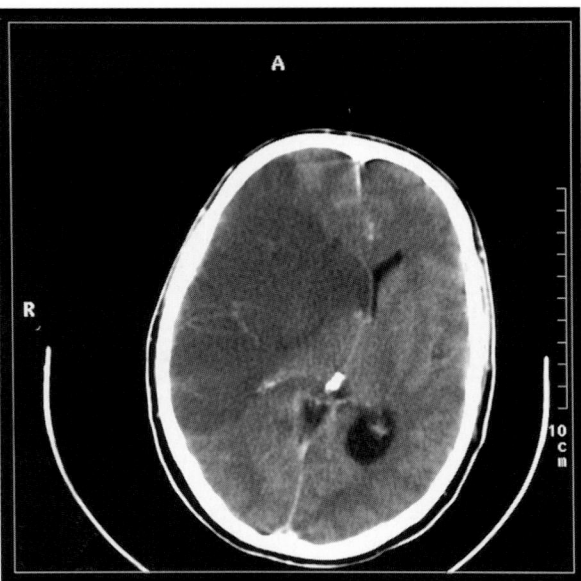

Fig. 40.1   Right middle cerebral artery infarct. There is anterior and posterior sparing. Loss of right latereal ventricle. Moderate mass effect with midline shift.

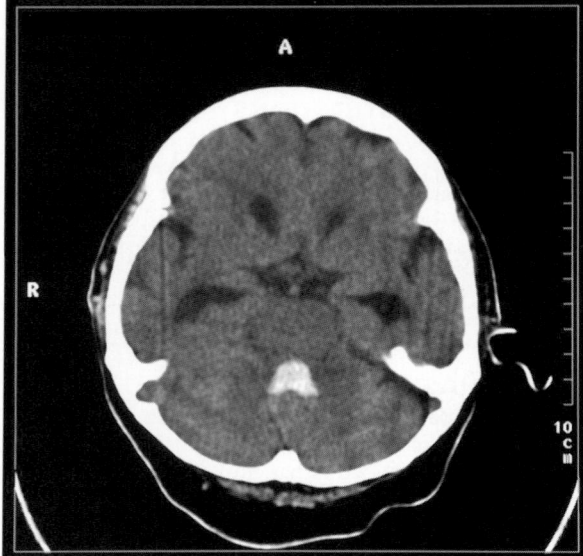

Fig. 40.2a Blood in the fourth ventricle.

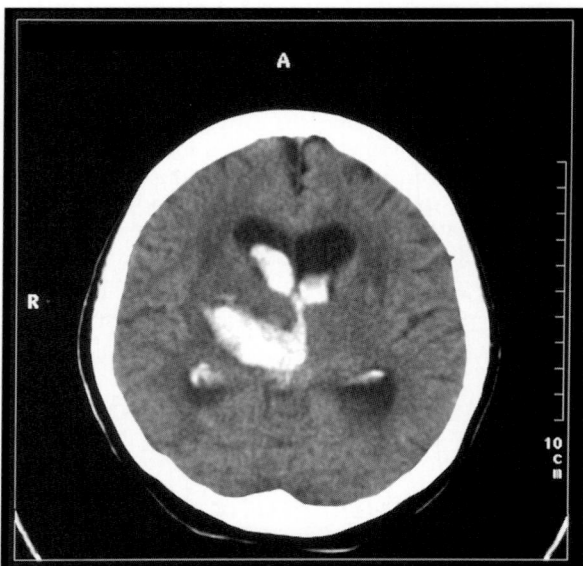

Fig. 40.2c Blood in both ventricles and intraparenchymal blood.

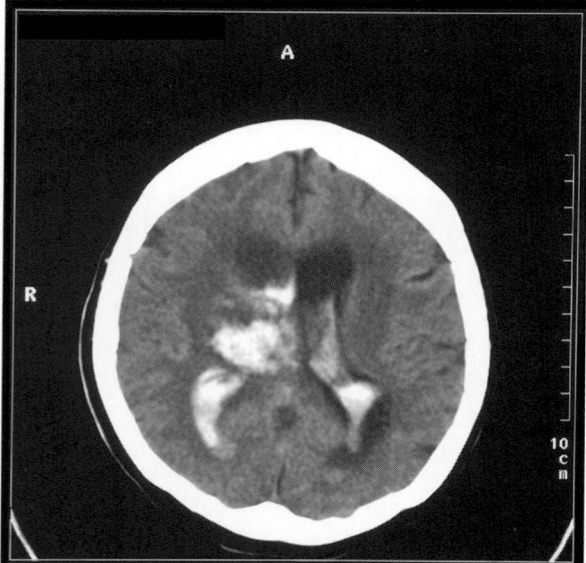

Fig. 40.2b Blood in both lateral ventricles

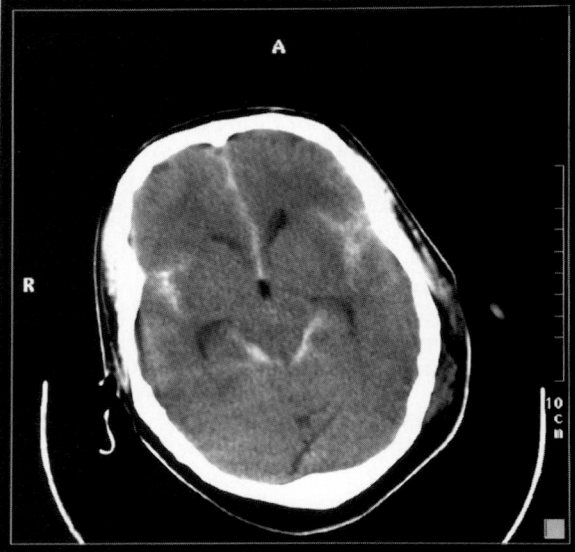

Fig. 40.3 Subarachnoid haemmorrhage: blood in the sylvian fissure and in basal cisterns.

reduced scanning times and is suitable for the uncooperative patient. The limitations of a CT scan include:

- the need to transfer the patient to a site where resuscitation and monitoring facilities are limited;
- the need to sedate and possibly endotracheally intubate patients who are agitated;

- its low sensitivity to demonstrate an abnormality in the acute phase of a stroke;
- its low sensitivity for detecting brainstem lesions;
- the need to administer i.v. contrast agents.

The two major side effects of i.v. contrast are anaphylaxis (with an approximate death rate of 1 in 40 000) and

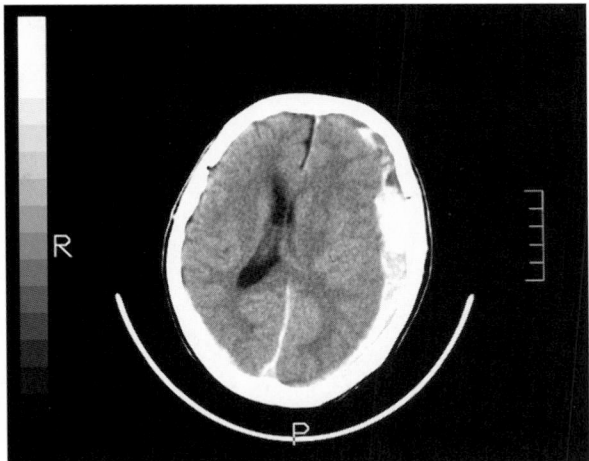

Fig. 40.4 Acute left subdural. Rescentric within the skull with high attenuation. Loss of ventricle.

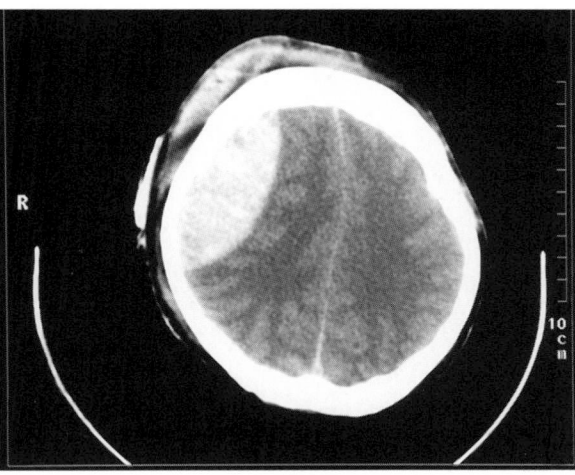

Fig. 40.6 Right extradural. Note the convex angle the acute extradural makes with the skull and the soft tissue swelling extracranially.

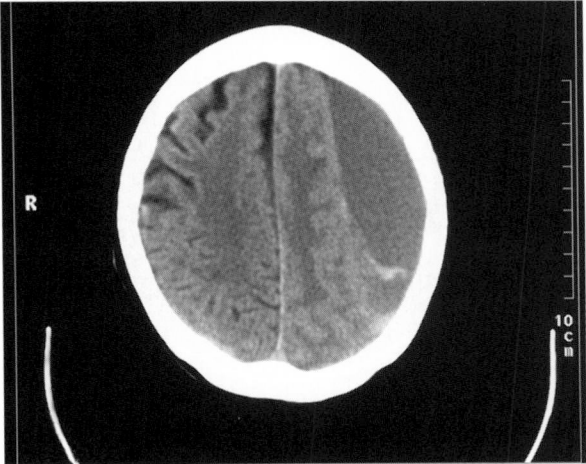

Fig. 40.5 Chronic left subdural. Isodens fluid filling space. The white area may suggest a recent acute bleed.

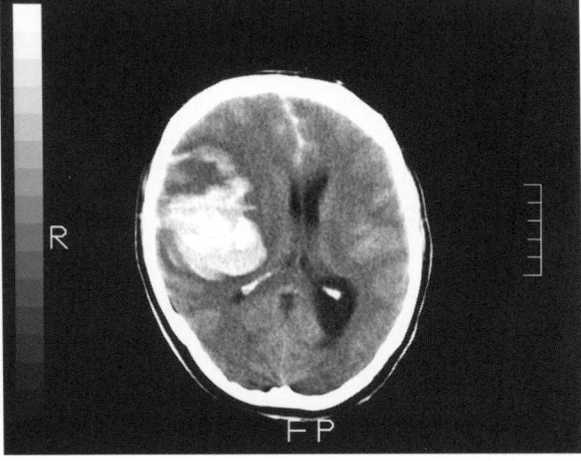

Fig. 40.7 Right fronto parietal bleed. Note oedema, loss of lateral ventricle and minor midline shift.

renal failure. The risk of nephrotoxicity may be minimized by the administration of acetylcysteine before and after the procedure.[13]

Magnetic Resonance Imaging (MRI) (Figs 40.11 and 40.12)

MRI scans provide superior contrast and resolution of the grey and white matter as compared to CT scans, thus facilitating easy identification of the deep nuclear structures within the brain. Brainstem and posterior fossa structures are better visualized. The other advantage of MRI is the use of non-ionizing energy. The use of

gadolinium, a paramagnetic contrast agent, permits sharp definition of lesions. MRI coupled with angiography (MRA) may enable diagnosis of vascular lesions. The limitations of MRI are:

- the need for special equipment;
- long imaging times;
- the need to transfer the patient to a site where resuscitation and monitoring facilities are limited;
- the need to sedate and possibly endotracheally intubate patients who are agitated;
- risk of dislodgement of metal clips on blood vessels and resetting of pacemakers.

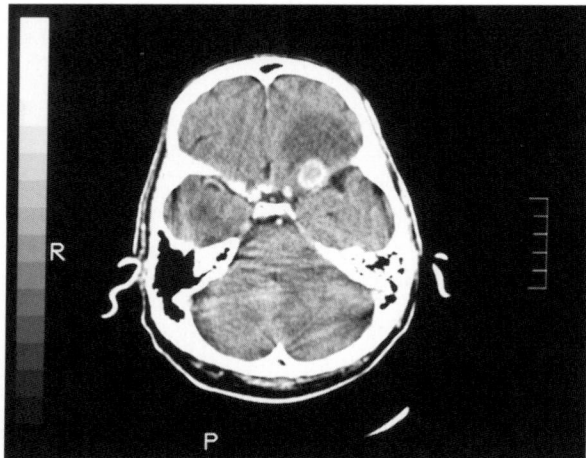

Fig. 40.8a   Left frontal lesion

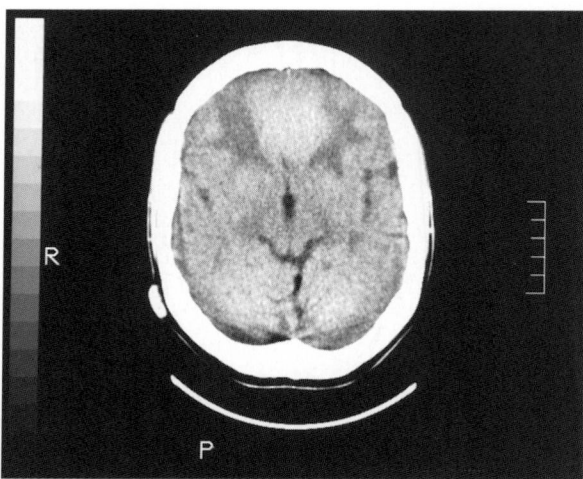

Fig. 40.9a   Frontal meningioma pre contrast.

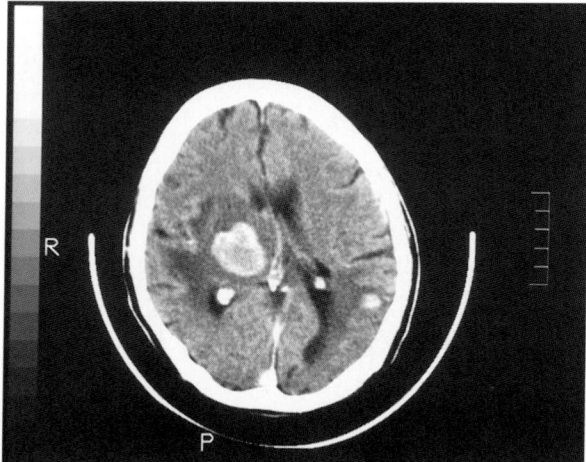

Fig. 40.8b   Right thalamic lesion with large zone of oedema around it.

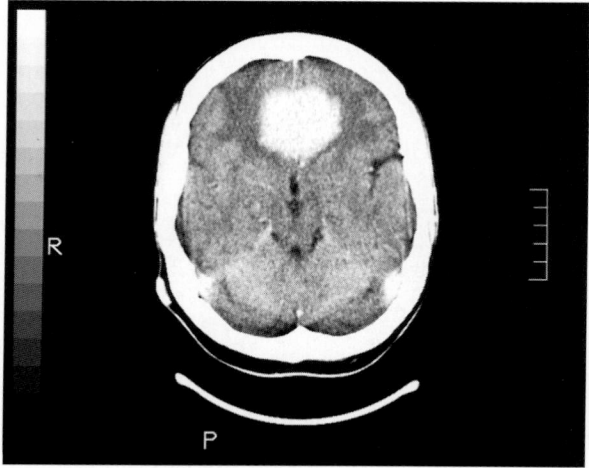

Fig. 40.9b   Frontal meningioma post contrast.

PET and SPECT Scans

Newer nuclear medicine scan techniques such as SPECT (single photon emission with computerized tomography) and PET (positron emission tomography) are useful for the assessment of cerebral blood flow and oxygenation and in the prognostication of neurotrauma, but have little role to play in the management of acute disorders of consciousness. In PET scans, positron emitting isotopes such as ^{11}C, ^{18}F, and [15]O are incorporated into biologically active compounds such as deoxyglucose or fluorodeoxyglucose which are metabolized in the body. By determining the concentration of the various tracers in the brain and constructing tomographic images, cerebral blood flow and metabolism can be measured.

SPECT scans use iodine-containing isotopes incorporated into biologically active compounds and, like PET scans, their cranial distribution is determined after a dose of tracer. Information on cerebral blood flow and metabolism can be obtained from SPECT scans. The advantage of a PET scan is that it does not require a cyclotron for the generation of isotopes. Despite their many advantages, both these technologies continue to be research tools and are not routinely available in many medical centres.

LUMBAR PUNCTURE (LP)[14]

Cerebrospinal fluid is most commonly obtained by means of a lumbar puncture (LP). This should be performed after ensuring that raised intracranial pressure has

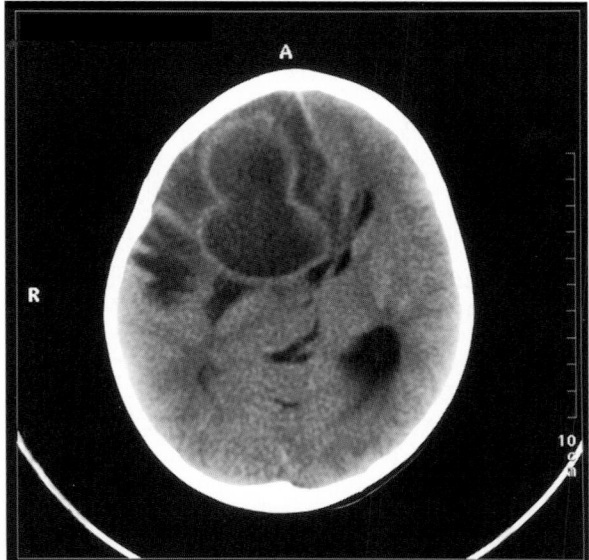

Fig. 40.10a   Large abscess in the right frontal lobe with ring enhancement when contrast is given, 10a pre contrast 10b post contrast.

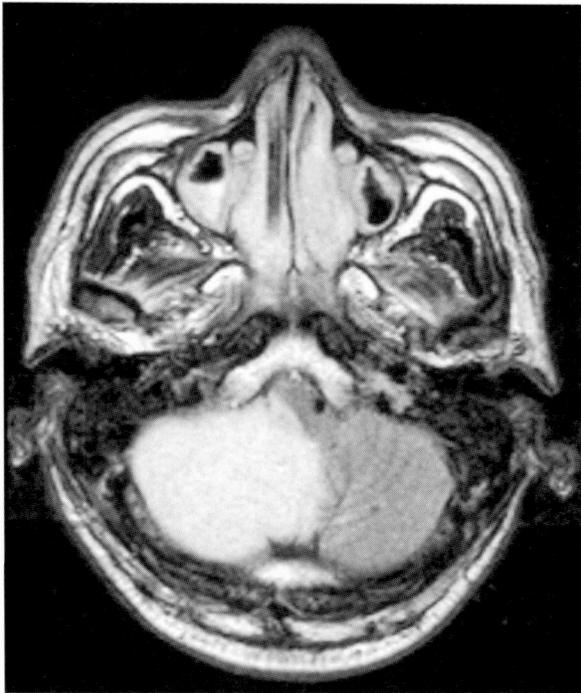

Fig. 40.11   MRI, large cerebellar infarct.

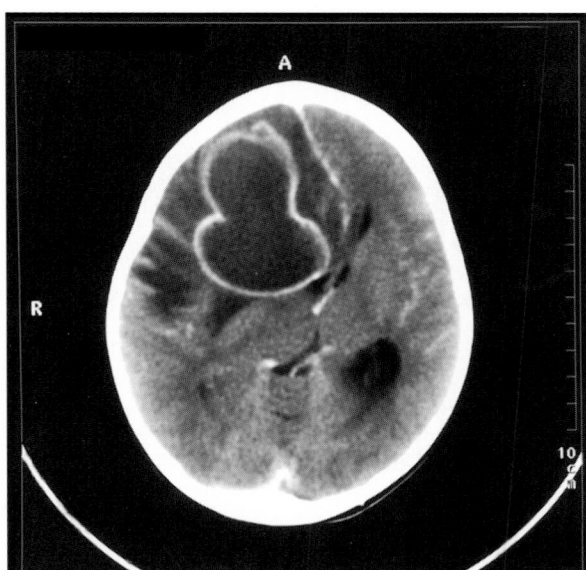

Fig. 40.10b   Post contrast.

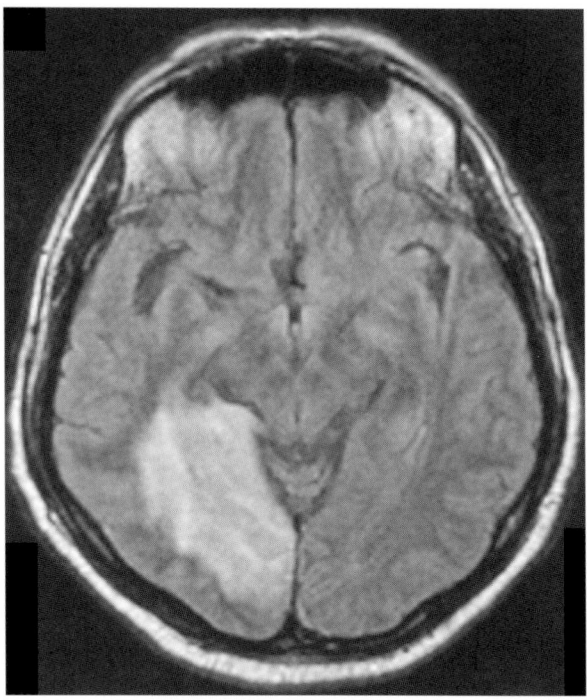

Fig. 40.12   MRI, Posterior cerebral bleed.

been excluded clinically or radiologically. The major use of a lumbar puncture is to diagnose an intracranial infection and to detect abnormal cytology in cases of suspected malignant meningeal infiltration. The advent of CT scans has diminished the role of LP in the diagnosis of SAH. Some of the commonly reported complications after lumbar puncture include, post-puncture headache (12–39%) and traumatic tap (15–20%). Brain herniation is a rare potential complication seen with conditions associated with raised intracranial pressure due to a space-occupying lesion.

ENCEPHALOGRAPHY (EEG) IN COMA[15,16]

Continuous EEG monitoring in the ICU has been reported to be useful in the identification of acute cerebral ischaemia and non-convulsive seizures. The usefulness of EEG in coma is summarized below:

- Identification of non-convulsive status epilepticus.
- Diagnosis of hepatic encephalopathy
  - presence of paroxysmal triphasic waves.
- Assessing severity of hypoxic encephalopathy
  - presence of theta activity
  - diffuse slowing
  - burst suppression (seen with more severe forms)
  - alpha coma (seen with more severe forms).

EVOKED POTENTIALS

Visual, brainstem and somatosensory evoked potentials test the integrity of neuroanatomical pathways within the brain and the spinal cord. They may be used in the diagnosis of blindness in comatose patients and in the assessment of 'locked-in' states. Data suggest that they have better prognostic value than clinical judgement in patients with anoxic coma.[17]

CARE OF THE COMATOSE PATIENT

Airway. Assessment of airway adequacy takes precedence over any diagnostic investigation in comatose patients.

Assess the patient's response to command and physical stimulation, and whether a gag reflex is present. Securing the airway will depend on the level of consciousness. Simple manoeuvres such as jaw thrust, chin lift, use of oropharyngeal airways are helpful but in the comatose patient endotracheal intubation is mandatory. All of these patients are at risk of pulmonary aspiration. There must be a low threshold for establishing a definitive airway.

As a general rule, patients presenting with medical causes of coma may be nursed on their side (coma position, if the airway is adequate. However, all traumatized patients should be assumed to have a potential cervical spine injury and must be nursed with the cervical spine in the neutral position and/or with a rigid collar until an injury is excluded by definitive radiological views. All patients with disordered consciousness must receive supplemental oxygen.

Ventilation. It is important to ensure optimal gas exchange and avoid hypoxia and hypercapnia. Generally, a Pa_{O_2} of >80 mmHg (9 kPa) and Pco_2 of 35–40 mmHg

(5 kPa) are acceptable. If either spontaneous ventilatory efforts or respiratory function is inadequate to achieve these levels of arterial blood gases, mechanical ventilatory support may be necessary.

Circulation. Adequacy of circulation should be assessed. The goals of circulatory therapy in coma include prompt restoration of appropriate mean arterial blood pressure, correction of dehydration and hypovolaemia and urgent attention to life-threatening causes of shock.

Specific treatment. This will depend on the underlying aetiology of the coma and is discussed in the relevant chapters. Avoidance of secondary insults (hypoperfusion and inadequate oxygen delivery) is of paramount importance in the management of these patients.[18]

Nursing care. Meticulous eye and mouth care, regular changes in limb position, limb physiotherapy, bronchial toilet and psychological support are mandatory. Nosocomial infections and iatrogenic complications are associated with an increased mortality and morbidity in these patients and must be promptly diagnosed and treated.

Other therapy. Stress ulcer and deep vein thrombosis prophylaxis should be instituted. Early establishment of enteral feeding via a nasoenteric tube is preferable. It is important to exclude a basal skull fracture is before insertion of a nasoenteric tube.

ANOXIC COMA/ENCEPHALOPATHY

Cardiac arrest is the third leading cause of coma resulting in ICU admission after trauma and drug overdose. The symptomatology and clinical outcome of patients with anoxic brain damage depend on the severity and duration of oxygen deprivation to the brain. A number of criteria have been developed to prognosticate outcome in anoxic coma. Although a number of laboratory and imaging criteria contribute to the prognostic assessment, clinical signs still have major prognostic impact. The important clinical predictors of outcome are listed in Table 40.7. However, there are data to suggest that electrophysiological studies using evoked potential have far greater prognostic accuracy as compared to clinical assessment.[19]

THE CONFUSED/ENCEPHALOPATHIC PATIENT IN THE ICU

Encephalopathy is a term used to describe the alteration in the level or content of consciousness due to a process extrinsic to the brain. Metabolic encephalopathy, particularly of septic aetiology, is the most common cause of altered mental status in the ICU setting.[20] A number

Table 40.7   Clinical predictors of unfavourable prognosis in anoxic coma[17,34,35]

Clinical predictor	Unfavourable prognosis
Duration of anoxia	8–10 min
(Time interval between collapse and initiation of CPR)	
Duration of CPR	>30 min
(Time interval between initiation of CPR and ROSC)	
Duration of postanoxic coma	>72 hours
Pupillary reaction	Absent on day 3
Motor response to pain	Absent on day 3
(Absent = a motor response worse than withdrawal)	
Roving spontaneous eye movements	Absent on day 1

of processes can lead to metabolic encephalopathy (Table 40.8).

A number of features in the history and examination help to differentiate metabolic from structural causes of altered conscious states (Table 40.9).

Owing to their increased frequency in and exclusiveness to the critical care setting, two types of encephalopathy will be considered in detail: septic encephalopathy and ICU syndrome.

SEPTIC ENCEPHALOPATHY

This condition has been reported to occur in 8–80% of patients with sepsis.[21] Criteria for diagnosis include:

- impaired mental function;
- evidence of an extracranial infection ;
- absence of other obvious aetiologies for the altered conscious state.

Although the precise mechanism of damage to the brain has not been delineated, the pathogenesis of the encephalopathy is thought to be multifactorial:

- alteration in cerebral blood flow induced by mediators of inflammation;
- generation of free radicals by activated leukocytes, resulting in erythrocyte sludging in the microcirculation;
- breakdown of the blood–brain barrier resulting in cerebral oedema;
- reduced brain oxygen consumption induced by endotoxin and cytokines;

Table 40.8   Aetiology of metabolic/toxic encephalopathy[36–38]

Hepatic failure
Renal failure
Respiratory failure
Sepsis
Electrolyte abnormalities: Hyponatraemia, hypernatraemia, hypercalcaemia
Hypoglycaemia and Hyperglycaemia
Acute pancreatitis
Endocrine – Addisonian crisis, myxoedema coma, thyroid storm
Drug withdrawal – Benzodiazepine, opiates
Hyperthermia
Toxins: Alcohols, glycols, tricyclic antidepressants
ICU syndrome
D-Lactic Acidosis

Table 40.9   Distinguishing features of structural and metabolic encephalopathy[38]

Feature	Structural	Metabolic
State of consciousness	Usually fixed level of depressed conscious state, may deteriorate progressively	Milder alteration of conscious state, waxing and waning of altered sensorium
Fundoscospy	May be abnormal	Usually normal
Pupils	May be abnormal, either in size or response to light	Usually preserved light response (although pupil shape and reactivity affected in certain overdoses-see above)
Eye movements	May be affected	Usually preserved
Motor findings	Asymmetrical involvement	Abnormalities usually symmetrical
Involuntary movements	Not common	Asterixis, tremor, myoclonus frequently seen

Plum, F sustained impairment of conciousness. In: Bennett CPF (ed.) Cecil's Texbook of Medicine. Philadelphia, PA: WB Saunders; 1996; 1970-8.

- neuronal degeneration;
- increases in aromatic amino acids resulting in altered neurotransmitter function and increased GABA-mediated neurotransmission, leading to general inhibition of the CNS.

Hypotension may contribute to the encephalopathy. The asterixis, tremor and myoclonus – features of other metabolic encephalopathies – are uncommon in sepsis. The mortality of patients with septic encephalopathy is higher than in those with sepsis without encephalopathy.[22,23] Therapy is largely directed at the underlying septic process.

ICU ENCEPHALOPATHY OR ICU SYNDROME[24,25]

This is a term used to describe behavioural disorders that develops in patients 5–7 days after admission to intensive care. Clinically, this may present as agitation, restlessness and frank delirium. This is attributed to sleep deprivation,[26,27] distortion of perception with loss of day-night cycles, immobilization and a noisy environment. These coupled with administration of multiple sedatives and neurological consequences of the underlying disease can precipitate psychotic behaviour in the ICU. It is important to bear in mind that *this is a diagnosis of exclusion and that all other reversible causes are looked for* before this diagnostic label is applied.

Abnormal behaviour can increase patient morbidity (self-extubation, ripping of catheters, soft tissue damage, etc). It is important to identify the underlying cause of the abnormal behaviour to institute appropriate therapy. Management of this condition may require the use of restraints, sedation and major tranquilizers. Improvement of sleep quality (minimizing interruption of nocturnal sleep, adjusting lighting in the ICU), reducing patient boredom by the use of television and music and better communication with the patient may reduce the incidence and severity of this syndrome.

PROGNOSIS IN COMA

Drug induced comas usually have a good prognosis unless hypoxia and hypotension have resulted in severe secondary insults. Coma following head injury has a statistically better outcome as compared to non-traumatic coma (coma occurring during the course of a medical illness). In non-traumatic coma lasting for 6 hours or greater, only 15% of the patients make a meaningful recovery that enables return to their pre-morbid state of health.[29] The prognosis following anoxic coma has been described in a separate section above (p. 480). Within the non-traumatic coma category, coma resulting from infection, metabolic causes and multiple organ dysfunction syndrome have better outcome as compared to anoxic coma.[29]

REFERENCES

1 Ropper A, Martin J. Coma and other disorders of consciousness. In: Isselbacher K (ed.) *Harrison's Principles of Internal Medicine*. Maidenhead and New York: McGraw Hill; 1994: pp. 146–52.

2 Teasdale G, Jennett B. Assessment of coma and impaired consciousness. A practical scale. *Lancet* 1974; **2**(7872): 81–4.

3 Adams R, Victor M, Ropper A. Coma and Related Disorders of Consciousness. In: *Principles of Neurology*. New York: McGraw Hill; 1997. pp. 344–66.

4 Keane JR. Retinal hemorrhages. Its significance in 100 patients with acute encephalopathy of unknown cause. *Arch Neurol* 1979; **36**: 691–4.

5 Keane J. Eye movements in coma. In: Jakbiec AA (ed.). *Principles and Practice of Ophthalmology*. Philadelphia, PA: WB Saunders; 2000. pp. 4075–83.

6 Fisher C. Ocular bobbing. *Arch Neurol* 1964; *11*: 543.

7 Keane JR. Ocular skew deviation. Analysis of 100 cases. *Arch Neurol* 1975; **32**: 185–90.

8 North JB, Jennett S. Abnormal breathing patterns associated with acute brain damage. *Arch Neurol* 1974; **31**: 338–44.

9 Kernohan J, Woltman H. Incisura of the crus due to contralateral brain tumour. *Arch Neurol Psych* 1929; **21**: 274.

10 McNealy D, Plum F. Brainstem dysfunction with supratentorial mass lesions. *Arch Neurol* 1962; **7**: 10.

11 De Salles AA, Muizelaar JP, Young HF. Hyperglycemia, cerebrospinal fluid lactic acidosis, and cerebral blood flow in severely head-injured patients. *Neurosurgery* 1987; **21**: 45–50.

12 Penney DG. Hyperglycemia exacerbates brain damage in acute severe carbon monoxide poisoning. *Med Hypotheses* 1988; **27**: 241–4.

13 Tepel M, van der Giet M, Schwarzfeld C, *et al.* Prevention of radiographic-contrast-agent-induced reductions in renal function by acetylcysteine. *N Engl J Med* 2000; **343**: 180–4.

14 Venkatesh B, Scott P, Ziegenfuss M. Cerebrospinal fluid in critical illness. *Crit Care Resusc* 2000; **2**: 43–55.

15 Bauer G. Coma and brain death. In: Niedermeyer E, Da Silva F. (eds) *Electroencephalography: Basic Principles, Clinical Applications and Related Fields*: Baltimore, Williams and Wilkins; 1999, 459–475.

16 Nuwer MR. Continuous EEG monitoring in the intensive care unit. *Electroencephalogr Clin Neurophysiol Suppl* 1999; **50**: 150–5.

17 Zandbergen EG, de Haan RJ, Stoutenbeek CP, *et al.* Systematic review of early prediction of poor outcome in anoxic-ischaemic coma. *Lancet* 1998; **352**(9143): 1808–12.

18 Chesnut RM, Marshall LF, Klauber MR, *et al.* The role of secondary brain injury in determining outcome from severe head injury. *J Trauma* 1993; **34**: 216–22.

19 Madl C, Kramer L, Domanovits H, *et al.* Improved outcome prediction in unconscious cardiac arrest survivors with sensory evoked potentials compared with clinical assessment. *Crit Care Med* 2000; **28**(3): 721–6.

20 Bleck TP, Smith MC, Pierre-Louis SJ, *et al.* Neurologic complications of critical medical illnesses. *Crit Care Med* 1993; **21**: 98–103.

21 Papadopoulos MC, Davies DC, Moss RF, *et al.* Pathophysiology of septic encephalopathy: a review. *Crit Care Med* 2000; **28**: 3019–24.

22 Young GB, Bolton CF, Austin TW, *et al.* The encephalopathy associated with septic illness. *Clin Invest Med* 1990; **13**: 297–304.

23 Sprung CL, Peduzzi PN, Shatney CH, *et al.* Impact of encephalopathy on mortality in the sepsis syndrome. The Veterans Administration Systemic Sepsis Cooperative Study Group. *Crit Care Med* 1990; **18**: 801–6.

24 McGuire BE, Basten CJ, Ryan CJ, Gallagher J. Intensive care unit syndrome: a dangerous misnomer. *Arch Intern Med* 2000; **160**: 906–9.

25 Weber RJ, Oszko MA, Bolender BJ, Grysiak DL. The intensive care unit syndrome: causes, treatment, and prevention. *Drug Intell Clin Pharm* 1985; **19**: 13–20.

26 Krachman SL, D'Alonzo GE, Criner GJ. Sleep in the intensive care unit. *Chest* 1995; **107**: 1713–20.

27 Shilo L, Dagan Y, Smorjik Y, *et al.* Patients in the intensive care unit suffer from severe lack of sleep associated with loss of normal melatonin secretion pattern. *Am J Med Sci* 1999; **317**: 278–81.

28 Plum F, Levy DE. Outcome from severe neurological illness; should it influence medical decisions? *Ciba Found Symp* 1979; No. 69: 267–77.

29 Levy DE, Bates D, Caronna JJ, *et al.* Prognosis in nontraumatic coma. *Ann Intern Med* 1981; **94**: 293–301.

30 Nordgren RE, Markesbery WR, Fukuda K, Reeves AG. Seven cases of cerebromedullospinal disconnection: the 'locked-in' syndrome. *Neurology* 1971; **21**: 1140–8.

31 Multi Society Task Force on PVS. Medical aspects of the persistent vegetative state (1). *N Engl J Med* 1994; **330**: 1499–1508.

32 Jennett B, Plum F. Persistent vegetative state after brain damage. A syndrome in search of a name. *Lancet* 1972; **1**(7753): 734–7.

33 Cairns H, Oldfield R, Pennybacker K. Akinetic mutism with an epidermoid cyst of the third ventricle. *Brain* 1941; **64**: 273.

34 Berek K, Jeschow M, Aichner F. The prognostication of cerebral hypoxia after out-of-hospital cardiac arrest in adults. *Eur Neurol* 1997; **37**(3): 135–45.

35 Levy DE, Caronna JJ, Singer BH, *et al.* Predicting outcome from hypoxic-ischemic coma. *JAMA* 1985; **253**: 1420–6.

36 Surtees R, Leonard JV. Acute metabolic encephalopathy: a review of causes, mechanisms and treatment. *J Inherit Metab Dis* 1989; **12**(Suppl 1): 42–54.

37 Uribarri J, Oh MS, Carroll HJ. D-Lactic acidosis. A review of clinical presentation, biochemical features, and pathophysiologic mechanisms. *Medicine (Baltimore)* 1998; **77**: 73–82.

38 Plum F. Sustained impairment of consciousness. In: Bennett CPF (ed.) *Cecil's Textbook of Medicine.* Philadelphia:PA: W.B. Saunders; 1996: pp. 1970–8.

41

Status epilepticus
H Opdam

Status epilepticus (SE) is a medical emergency requiring prompt intervention to prevent the development of irreversible brain damage. It is generally defined as more than 30 minutes duration of either a single seizure, or intermittent seizures with no regaining of consciousness between seizures.[1]

A definition that allows an earlier diagnosis of SE, such as after 5 minutes of continuous seizure activity, or after two or more discrete seizures with no intervening recovery of consciousness, may be more useful. This is based on the generally accepted need to rapidly initiate treatment for SE (before 30 minutes have elapsed), and the observation that isolated convulsive seizures in adults rarely last more than a few minutes.[2]

Refractory SE refers to seizures that fail to respond to appropriate first-line drug treatment such as benzodiazepines, phenytoin and phenobarbitone.

SE is commonly separated into three categories:

- *Generalized convulsive SE.* Seizures are primary or secondarily generalized and the patient has generalized tonic and/or clonic convulsive movements with loss of consciousness.
- *Non-convulsive SE.* There is altered consciousness without convulsive movements. This category includes absence SE and complex partial SE.
- *Simple partial SE.* Persistent focal seizures with no alteration of consciousness.

The incidence of SE is U-shaped, being greatest under 1 year and over 60 years of age.[3,4]

PATHOPHYSIOLOGY[5]

Ongoing or recurrent seizures result from either excessive excitation causing seizure activity to persist or the failure of normal seizure terminating mechanisms. The major inhibitory mechanisms in the brain include γ-aminobutyric acid$_A$ (GABA$_A$) receptor-mediated inhibition and possibly neuropeptide Y.[5,6]

The pathophysiological effects of seizures on the brain are thought to result from both direct excitotoxic neuronal injury and secondary injury due to systemic complications such as hypotension, hypoxia and hyperthermia. High concentrations of excitatory amino acids such as glutamate, result in excessive intracellular calcium through the opening of NMDA (*N*-methyl-D-aspartate) receptor-mediated calcium channels and other mechanisms, inducing a cascade of intracellular neurochemical events that damage or kill the cell.[5]

AETIOLOGY

Status epilepticus may occur *de novo* (approximately 60% of presentations) or less commonly in a previously diagnosed epileptic.[3,4] The aetiologies of SE, in decreasing order of frequency as they occur in adults, are given in Table 41.1.[3]

For SE that has its onset in the ICU, the following should be considered as possible causes[7]:

- drug withdrawal (narcotics, benzodiazepines, omission of anticonvulsant medications)
- metabolic disturbance (hyponatraemia, hypocalcaemia, uraemia, hyperglycaemia, hypoglycaemia)

Table 41.1   Causes of status epilepticus in adults

Low anti-epileptic drug levels (poor compliance, recent dose reduction or discontinuation)
Temporally remote causes (previous CNS injury, e.g. stroke, trauma, tumour, meningitis, and no acute precipitant)
Stroke – vascular occlusion or haemorrhage
Hypoxia/anoxia
Metabolic disturbances (electrolyte abnormalities, uraemia, hyperglycaemia, hypoglycaemia)
Alcohol – withdrawal or intoxication
Tumour – primary or metastatic CNS tumours
Systemic infection
Idiopathic
CNS infection – meningitis, encephalitis
Head trauma
Drug toxicity (tricyclic antidepressants, phenothiazines, theophylline, isoniazid, cocaine, amphetamine)

- drug toxicity (theophylline, pethidine, antibiotics e.g penicillins, imipenem in renal failure, cyclosporine)
- stroke – vascular occlusion or haemorrhage.

GENERALIZED CONVULSIVE STATUS EPILEPTICUS (GCSE)

GCSE is the most common and most dangerous type of SE and accounts for approximately 75%.[3] It encompasses a broad spectrum of clinical presentations, from overt generalized tonic-clonic seizures to subtle convulsive movements in a profoundly comatose patient.[8,9]

Clinical
Typically, early in the evolution of seizures, patients are unresponsive with obvious tonic (sustained contractions) and/or clonic (rhythmic jerking) movements (overt GCSE). Motor manifestations may be symmetrical or asymmetrical.

With time, the clinical manifestations may become subtle, and patients have only small amplitude twitching movements of the face, hands, or feet or nystagmoid jerking of the eyes (late or subtle GCSE).[8]

Later still, some patients will have no observable repetitive motor activity, and the detection of ongoing seizures requires electroencephalography (EEG) (electrical GCSE). Some classify these later phases of GCSE, in which there are few or no clinical manifestations of SE despite ongoing electrical seizure activity on the EEG, as a form of non-convulsive SE.[10] Such patients are still at risk of CNS injury and require prompt treatment.

EEG changes
Just as there is a progression from overt to increasingly subtle motor manifestations of GCSE, there is also a predictable sequence of EEG changes during untreated GCSE. Initially, discrete electrographic seizures merge to a waxing and waning pattern of seizure activity, followed by continuous monomorphic discharges, which become interspersed with increasing periods of electrographic silence and, eventually, periodic epileptiform discharges on a relatively flat background.[9] The presence of any of these EEG patterns should suggest the diagnosis of GSCE.

Endocrine and metabolic effects
Early in GCSE there is a marked increase in plasma catecholamines, producing systemic physiologic changes that resolve if SE is stopped early (Table 41.2). However, if seizures continue, many of these early physiologic changes reverse and the resultant hypotension and hypoglycaemia may exacerbate neurological injury.[11]

Hyperthermia is due to both muscle activity and central sympathetic drive, and thus may still occur when motor activity is prevented by paralysing agents. In early SE, both cerebral metabolic activity and CBF are increased. However, in late SE, although cerebral metabolic activity

Table 41.2 Physiological changes of generalized convulsive status epilepticus[11,12]

Hypoxia
Respiratory acidosis
Lactic acidosis
Hyperpyrexia
Hypertension (early)
Hypotension (late)
Hyperglycaemia (early)
Hypoglycaemia (late)
Tachycardia
Cardiac arrhythmias
Blood leukocytosis
CSF pleocytosis, increased CSF protein
Intracranial hypertension
Neurogenic pulmonary oedema
Aspiration pneumonitis
Rhabdomyolysis

Table 41.3 Features suggestive of pseudoseizures

Lack of stereotyped seizures, with behavioural manifestations varying from event to event
Lack of sustained convulsive activity – 'on-off' appearance
Clonic movements that have a different rate on each side, or vary in rate.
Poor response to treatment, refractory status epilepticus
Abolition of motor movements with reassurance or suggestion
Gaze aversion and resistance to examination during seizure
Absence of pupillary dilatation
Normal tendon reflexes and plantar responses immediately after convulsion
Lack of metabolic consequences despite some hours of apparent fitting

remains high, CBF may fall due to hypotension and loss of cerebral autoregulation, leading to cerebral ischaemia.

An important differential diagnosis of generalized convulsive epilepsy is pseudoseizures.[13] Clinical features suggestive of pseudoseizures are listed in Table 41.3. Distinction between the two may be extremely difficult, and can only be made with complete certainty using EEG monitoring.[14] Serum prolactin concentrations are often increased following a single true fit, and can be used to distinguish a single fit from a pseudoseizure, but concentrations are not usually raised in status epilepticus.[15] Pseudostatus, misdiagnosed as true SE, is often refractory to initial therapy and can lead to patients receiving general anaesthesia and mechanical ventilation.

NON-CONVULSIVE STATUS EPILEPTICUS (NCSE)[16,17]

This may account for approximately 20% of SE, though its incidence is probably underestimated because of failure to recognize and diagnose the condition.[18]

Considerable debate exists regarding the precise criteria for diagnosing NCSE, and published reports often describe diverse cohorts of patients. NCSE is generally divided into absence status epilepticus (bilateral synchronous EEG seizure activity) and complex partial status epilepticus (focal EEG seizure activity), though differentiating the two types may not always be possible.[16,17,19]

The diagnosis of NCSE generally requires the presence of:

1 At least a 30 minute period of behavioural change from baseline
2 EEG evidence of epileptic activity
3 A response (clinical and EEG) to anti-epileptic drugs.

A wide variation in clinical features and conscious state is possible, from mild confusion to coma (Table 41.4).

NCSE is often mistaken for other conditions, resulting in a delay in diagnosis and treatment. A high index of suspicion must therefore be present to trigger investigation with an EEG.[17]

The differential diagnosis of NCSE is:

- metabolic encephalopathy
- drug intoxication
- cerebrovascular disease, cerebral vasculitis
- psychiatric syndromes (dissociative reactions, acute psychosis)
- post-ictal confusion

ABSENCE STATUS EPILEPTICUS (ASE)

There are two forms of ASE, typical and atypical.

Typical ASE is characterized by altered behaviour or loss of responsiveness associated with generalized 3 Hz spikes and slow-wave EEG activity. It is most commonly seen in children and adolescents with idiopathic generalized epilepsy who are otherwise normal. Although recurrent attacks may occur, no deaths or long-term morbidity have been reported.

Atypical ASE is a heterogeneous syndrome, associated with generalized spike-waves on the EEG at frequencies of < 3 Hz.[9] It occurs in patients with mental retardation and epilepsy with multiple seizure types, or with other forms of diffuse cerebral dysfunction. The

Table 41.4 Common clinical features of non-convulsive status epilepticus

Fluctuating confusional states, partial responsiveness
Agitation, lethargy, or aggressive behaviour
Decreased speech, mutism, verbal perseveration
Confusion or delirium
Blank staring, blinking, chewing, or picking
Subtle myoclonic movements of the eyes, face or limbs
Bizarre behaviour
Inappropriate laughing, crying, or singing

prognosis is usually poor and is related to the underlying condition.

Coma is almost never caused by ASE and patients rarely require admission to the ICU.

COMPLEX PARTIAL STATUS EPILEPTICUS (CPSE)

There is considerable disagreement as to whether the clinical and electrographic seizure activity observed in patients with CPSE causes brain injury. Some case series suggest that the seizures are relatively benign,[20] whereas others suggest that CPSE can result in direct neurological injury.[21] Most morbidity appears attributable to the underlying illness rather than to the CPSE itself.[22] None the less, prompt treatment is generally recommended.[16,22]

Diagnosis of this condition may be difficult due to its variable presentation and CPSE should be considered in the differential diagnosis of any unresponsive or confused patient.

The EEG may also not clearly suggest the diagnosis, lacking the organized discharges of GCSE or ASE, but instead have a waxing and waning rhythmic activity in one or several cerebral regions. A diagnostic trial of an intravenous benzodiazepine may be necessary to diagnose CPSE.[23]

SIMPLE PARTIAL STATUS EPILEPTICUS

In simple partial SE, there is no impairment of consciousness, and the clinical features reflect the focal ictal discharges confined to one area of the cortex. The condition is uncommon and outcome is dependent on the underlying cause.[24]

EPILEPTIFORM ENCEPHALOPATHIES[16]

Some other less well-established and more controversial variants of SE deserve mention. These include comatose patients in whom there are epileptiform patterns on the EEG. Some of these cases may be late or subtle GCSE. However, these clinical and electrographic features often occur without prior clinical convulsions. In such situations it is unclear whether the abnormal discharges seen on the EEG are responsible for, or contribute to, the altered consciousness and abnormal movements, or are merely a reflection of a severe cerebral insult.

Myoclonic SE that follows an anoxic insult falls into this category. Patients have incessant, at times asynchronous, rhythmic jerks that may involve the entire body. This clinical appearance after an anoxic insult is associated with an extremely poor outcome.[25,26]

Table 41.5   Investigations in status epilepticus

Initial studies
Blood glucose, electrolytes (sodium, potassium, calcium,
    magnesium), urea
Oximetry SpO_2 or arterial blood gases
Anticonvulsant drug levels
Full blood count
Urinalysis

Further investigations after stabilization
Liver function tests, lactate, creatine kinase
Toxicology screen
Lumbar puncture
Electroencephalogram (EEG)
Brain imaging with CT or MRI

INVESTIGATIONS

Not all of the investigations listed in Table 41.5 need to be performed in every patient. The selection of tests depends on both the patient's history and presentation.

CT scan. Most patients with SE should have a CT scan of the brain performed at some point. This is true for all adults with new onset seizures, but not for children. In children, the indications for imaging include seizures that begin after head trauma, focal seizures, focal neurological signs, or focal EEG abnormalities. Many patients with established epilepsy who have already been thoroughly evaluated do not require another brain imaging procedure after an episode of SE. However, if there is reason to suspect a new problem, and when the need for imaging is not urgent, magnetic resonance imaging (MRI) may be preferable because it occasionally reveals abnormalities not visualized on CT scans.

Lumbar puncture. In any patient, especially in young children with fever and SE, CNS infection and lumbar puncture (LP) should be considered. Contraindications to LP include intracranial hypertension, suspected mass lesion and hydrocephalus. In adults, unless the suspicion of CNS infection is high, brain imaging should be performed before an LP. Even in suspected meningitis, lumbar puncture should be delayed for 30 minutes after a fit, because of the accompanying transient rise in intracranial pressure.[27] If meningitis is suspected but an LP cannot be performed expediently, antibiotics should be administered immediately rather than delayed. Note that whereas approximately 20% of patients have a modest CSF pleocytosis after SE (white cell counts rarely greater than $30 \times 10^6/l$), so-called benign postictal pleocytosis, meningitis is an uncommon cause of SE in adults.[3,12] Patients with CSF pleocytosis should be treated for suspected meningitis until the diagnosis is excluded by culture or other means.[1]

MANAGEMENT

GENERALIZED CONVULSIVE STATUS EPILEPTICUS (GCSE)

An accurate history should be obtained, with particular emphasis on eye-witness accounts of the onset and nature of the seizures, and a full physical examination performed. However, neither should delay initial emergency management. There is evidence in both humans and animals that the longer SE goes untreated, the harder it is to control with drugs.[28,29]

Management of SE involves termination and prevention of recurrence of seizures, treating precipitating causes and underlying conditions, and management of complications.

Few controlled data are available to support the use of any particular agents. A recent randomized, double-blind clinical trial for treatment for GCSE found that lorazepam, phenobarbitone or diazepam followed by phenytoin are all acceptable as initial treatment, but that phenytoin alone was not as effective as lorazepam.[30]

Various protocols for SE management have been suggested.[1,2,23,31] One approach is outlined in Box 41.1.

ABSENCE STATUS EPILEPTICUS (ASE)

These patients do not usually require admission to the ICU. Treatment should not be unduly delayed, for although ASE does not appear to present the same degree of risk of neurological injury as GCSE or CPSE, distinguishing ASE from CPSE can be difficult.[16,17] Intravenous benzodiazepines are the usual first-line drugs. Intravenous sodium valproate has also been used successfully in ASE.[32] An EEG should be obtained before and after therapy. Once seizures are controlled, treatment with long-term sodium valproate or ethosuximide should be started to prevent recurrence. However, in patients who have a treatable precipitating cause and no prior history of epilepsy, long-term maintenance therapy may not be necessary.

COMPLEX PARTIAL STATUS EPILEPTICUS

CPSE includes a heterogenous group of patients who are likely to vary in their response to and outcome from treatment. Most recommend prompt initiation of treatment, which is generally the same as for GCSE.[16,22] The potential side-effects of aggressive treatment (hypotension and respiratory depression) need to be balanced against the potential neurologic morbidity of CPSE.[16,17] Also, in elderly patients, it is questionable as to whether admission to ICU and treatment with benzodiazepines improves outcome.[33]

Box 41.1   *Protocol for management of generalized convulsions*

1. Assess A, B, C, GCS
2. Give O_2 and consider need for intubation/ventilation
3. Monitor blood pressure (BP), ECG, pulse oximetry
4. Obtain i.v. access and draw blood for investigations
5. If patient hypoglycaemic, or if blood glucose estimation is not available, give glucose:
   adults, give thiamine 100 mg i.v., and glucose 50 ml of 50% i.v.
   children, give 2 ml/kg of 25% glucose i.v.
6. Seizure control.
   A. Give benzodiazepine*, for example:
      diazepam 0.2 mg/kg i.v. at 5 mg/min up to total dose of 20 mg;
      lorazepam 0.1 mg/kg i.v. at 2 mg/min up to total dose of 10 mg;
      clonazepam 0.01–0.02 mg/kg i.v. at 0.5 mg/min up to total dose of 4 mg.
   If diazepam stops the seizures, phenytoin should be given next to prevent recurrence.
   Repeat dose every 2–5 min if required. Note: risk of respiratory depression with cumulative doses.
   B. If seizures persist, give phenytoin:
      phenytoin 15–20 mg/kg (adults ≤50 mg/min; children ≤1 mg/kg/min) or fosphenytoin 15–20 phenytoin equivalents (PE) mg/kg
      i.v. (adults ≤150 mg/min; children ≤3 mg/kg per min).
      If seizures persist, give extra doses of 5 mg/kg i.v, to a maximum dose of 30 mg/kg.
      Monitor blood pressure and the ECG during infusion. If hypotension or arrhythmias develop, stop or slow the rate of the
      infusion.
   C. If seizures persist, consider phenobarbitone.
      phenobarbitone 20 mg/kg i.v at 100 mg/min.
   Be prepared for tracheal intubation and ventilatory support as the risk of apnoea is high.
   D. If seizures persist (refractory status), intubate and ventilate patient. Give either
      thiopental: slow bolus 3–5 mg/kg i.v., followed by infusion 1–5 mg/kg per h; or
      propofol: slow bolus 1–2 mg/kg i.v., followed by infusion 2–5 mg/kg per h;[†] or
      midazolam: slow bolus 0.1–0.2 mg/kg, followed by infusion 0.03–0.6 mg/kg per h.
   Titrate doses based on clinical and electrographic evidence of seizures and/or burst suppression.
   Monitor BP and maintain normotension by reducing infusion rate and/or giving fluids/pressor agents.
   E. Insert nasogastric tube and administer usual anticonvulsant medications if patient receiving treatment for pre-existing epilepsy.
   F. Beware of ongoing unrecognized seizures.
   Use EEG monitoring until seizures are controlled and then for 1–2 hours after seizures stop. Continue to monitor the EEG
   continuously, or for periods of more than 30 minutes every 2 hours, during the maintenance phase.
   Avoid muscle relaxants (use continuous EEG if giving repeated doses of muscle relaxants).
   G. Discontinue midazolam or thiopental, or start reducing propofol, approximately 12 hours after resolution of seizures. Use con-
      tinuous EEG monitoring and observe for further clinical and/or electrographic seizure activity. If seizures recur, reinstate the
      infusion and repeat this step at 12–24 hour intervals or longer if the patient's seizures remain refractory.
   In addition:
   Look for and treat cause and precipitant[††]
   Look for and treat complications: hypotension, hyperthermia, rhabdomyolysis

*If i.v. access is not obtainable, consider rectal diazepam, buccal/sublingual or intranasal or i.m. midazolam, i.m. fosphenytoin.
[†]Higher infusion rates for prolonged periods require caution.
[††]In refractory SE, consider giving pyridoxine for children <18 months or if isoniazid toxicity is suspected in adults.

For patients who have medically intractable localization-related epilepsy, surgical intervention should be considered.

DRUGS FOR STATUS EPILEPTICUS

BENZODIAZEPINES

Benzodiazepines are fast-acting anti-seizure drugs and are therefore preferred as initial therapy. They act mainly by enhancing the neuroinhibitory effects of γ-aminobutyric acid$_A$ (GABA$_A$).

Diazepam is a highly lipid soluble drug with rapid CNS penetration, but with a short duration of action. It can be administered intravenously or by the rectal route. Rectal administration can be achieved using a specially formulated rectal gel, which is effective in both children and adults. Alternatively, the intravenous preparation can be diluted with an equal amount of saline and flushed into the rectum. Rectal administration should be considered when vascular access is delayed and may be particularly useful in the prehospital setting.

Lorazepam is less lipid-soluble than diazepam and, after intravenous injection, brain and CSF levels rise at a slower rate than those of diazepam.[34] However, a double-blind, randomized comparison of intravenous diazepam and lorazepam in patients with SE found both drugs to be equally fast-acting and efficacious.[35] Despite their equivalence as initial therapies, lorazepam has a longer duration of anti-seizure effect than diazepam, and has a lower incidence of seizure recurrence when used alone.[1]

Midazolam has a short duration of action that may allow earlier assessment of the patient's post-ictal neurologic condition than longer acting benzodiazepines. Midazolam administered by bolus and infusion may terminate seizures when other agents have failed. It may also have fewer side effects than alternative agents available for the treatment of refractory SE.[36,37]

For the initial therapy of SE, midazolam may also be given via the buccal/sublingual route, having similar efficacy as rectal diazepam.[38] Intranasal administration is also possible.[39] These routes offer advantages in terms of convenience and acceptability over the rectal and intramuscular routes. Whereas intramuscular administration of diazepam and lorazepam is not recommended owing to their slow absorption, intramuscular midazolam is rapidly absorbed; in one study it was equally efficacious as intravenous diazepam in treating motor seizures in children.[40] These alternative routes of administration may be particularly useful in the out-of-hospital setting and when intravenous access is difficult.

Clonazepam has a longer duration of action than diazepam and is given by intravenous bolus. Early reports suggested that it has better efficacy and fewer side effects than diazepam, though there are no published comparisons.[41]

PHENYTOIN

Phenytoin is useful for maintaining a prolonged anti-seizure effect after rapid termination of seizures with a benzodiazepine, or when benzodiazepines fail. When used alone as initial therapy phenytoin is not as efficacious as benzodiazepines for terminating seizures.[30]

The recommended intravenous loading dose is 20 mg/kg. The common practice of giving a standard loading dose of 1000 mg of phenytoin may provide inadequate therapy for some adults.

When phenytoin is infused at the maximal adult recommended rate of 50 mg/min, hypotension occurs in up to 50% of patients and cardiac rhythm disturbance occurs in 2%.[42] These adverse effects are more common in older patients and those with cardiac disease and are due to the phenytoin itself as well as the propylene glycol diluent. Blood pressure and the ECG should be monitored during infusion of phenytoin and the infusion slowed or stopped if cardiovascular complications occur.

The intramuscular administration of phenytoin is not recommended as absorption is erratic and it can cause local tissue reactions.

Fosphenytoin, a new water-soluble prodrug of phenytoin, is converted to phenytoin by endogenous phosphatases.[43] Doses of fosphenytoin are expressed as phenytoin equivalents (PE). Fosphenytoin can be administered at rates of up to 150 PE mg/min, since it is not formulated with propylene glycol. Therapeutic serum concentrations of fosphenytoin are attained within 10 minutes when fosphenytoin is administered at maximal infusion rates.[31] However, this may not necessarily result in more rapid CNS penetration and onset of action.[44]

Systemic side-effects are similar for phenytoin and fosphenytoin, although reactions at the infusion site are less common with fosphenytoin.[43]

Fosphenytoin can also be administered intramuscularly, though absorption is slower than intravenous administration, and this route should only be used when intravenous access is not possible.[31]

SODIUM VALPROATE

Valproate is now available in an intravenous form, and there are reports of intravenous valproate being used to treat both GCSE and NCSE in adults and children.[32,45] The recommended infusion rate is 20 mg/min, though rates of up to 200 mg/min have been well tolerated.[45] The exact role of valproate in the management of SE remains to be established in trials assessing its efficacy as a primary or secondary agent.

BARBITURATES

Phenobarbitone is a potent anticonvulsant with a long duration of action and is usually administered in SE by a short intravenous infusion. It may be used as a first, second or third line agent. Intubation, ventilatory and resuscitative facilities must be available with its use.

Thiopental is an intravenous anaesthetic agent used for refractory SE. A dose of 3–5 mg/kg is usually given for intubation, followed by repeated doses of 0.5–1 mg/kg until seizures are controlled. Following bolus intravenous administration, the drug is rapidly redistributed into peripheral fat stores and an infusion of 1–5 mg/kg per h is required for ongoing suppression of seizures. Once lipid stores are saturated the duration of action is prolonged and recovery may take hours to days. Prolonged therapy requires the use of EEG monitoring to ensure that seizures remain suppressed and to use the minimal dose that achieves the usual target of burst suppression. Side-effects include hypotension, myocardial depression and immunosuppression with increased risk of infection.

PROPOFOL

Propofol (2,6-diisopropylphenol) is an anaesthetic agent that has become increasingly popular for the treatment of refractory SE, despite anecdotal reports that suggest it may occasionally induce seizures.[46] It is administered as an intravenous bolus followed by infusion and intubation and ventilation are required.

Compared with high-dose barbiturates (pentobarbital) in adult patients with refractory SE, propofol has been found to more quickly control seizures.[47] However, seizures tend to recur with sudden discontinuation of propofol, necessitating recommencement of the infusion and a more gradual tapering of the dose, such that both drugs ultimately may result in similar duration of ventilation and ICU stay.[47]

Propofol has also been used successfully for SE in children. However, there have been reports of prolonged infusions at high dose (>5 mg/kg per h) being associated with severe hypotension, myocardial failure, hypoxia, metabolic acidosis and rhabdomyolysis in children and more recently in adults and, as such, its use requires caution.[48–50]

PARALDEHYDE

Paraldehyde is usually given rectally or by deep intramuscular injection as a second or third-line drug for controlling SE. Intravenous infusion is problematic as the drug reacts with plastic and tends to precipitate. Reported adverse effects include right heart failure, pulmonary oedema and pulmonary haemorrhage, as well as nerve damage and sterile abscesses following intramuscular injection. Despite its problems, it continues to be used by experienced units when intravenous administration is difficult, or where conventional drugs are contraindicated or have proved ineffective.[51]

NEUROMUSCULAR BLOCKING AGENTS

Paralysis is indicated if uncontrolled fitting causes respiratory embarrassment or severe lactic acidosis. Neuromuscular blockade should only be used if continuous EEG monitoring is available, as the clinical expression of seizure activity is abolished.

OTHER AGENTS OF POTENTIAL USE IN REFRACTORY SE

Ketamine may be a useful adjuvant in the treatment of refractory SE.[52] Lignocaine administered by bolus and infusion may also be useful in refractory SE in neonates, children and adults.[53] Isoflurane has been seen to rapidly control seizures in refractory SE, but seizures tend to recur upon its cessation.[54]

INTENSIVE CARE MONITORING

Monitoring using ECG, intra-arterial and central venous catheters, capnography and pulse oximetry should be

Table 41.6 Indications for EEG monitoring[10]

Refractory SE, to aid the titration of anticonvulsant drugs (minimizing dose and toxicity) and ensure suppression of seizure activity†
Patients receiving neuromuscular blockade†
Patients who continue to have a poor conscious state after apparent cessation of seizures
Suspected non-convulsive status epilepticus in a patient with an altered conscious state

† Continuous or regular intermittent EEG monitoring recommended

considered in patients with, or at risk of, cardiorespiratory compromise. Indications for EEG monitoring are listed in Table 41.6. Cerebral function monitors are useful in titrating doses of anaesthetic agents to burst suppression, but may not have sufficient sensitivity to detect seizure activity at other times. Intracranial pressure monitoring should be considered if elevated intracranial pressure is suspected.

OUTCOME[26]

The prognosis of patients with SE is related to the aetiology, age, duration of seizures and time to provision of adequate treatment. Overall mortality is approximately 20% and increases with age. Paediatric patients have a mortality of 3%, adults 26% and adults over 60 years of age have a mortality of 38%.[3] The underlying aetiology is probably the most important factor influencing outcome.[26,55,56] SE in young patients that is precipitated by low anti-epileptic drug levels or systemic infection has a very low mortality.[26] SE in the setting of acute cerebrovascular disease has a mortality of 35% and that associated with anoxic injury is usually fatal.[25,26,57] The duration of status and delay in diagnosis and treatment influences the ease with which seizures can be controlled and the risk of residual neurological deficits and mortality.[19,56]

Neurological sequelae that may follow SE include intellectual impairment, focal neurological deficits and the development of epilepsy.[55]

After resolution of SE, the EEG can provide prognostic information, with a burst suppression pattern, electrographic ictal discharges and periodic lateralizing epileptiform discharges in the 24 hours after SE being associated with a poor prognosis.[58] A normal EEG post-resolution of SE predicts a good outcome, whereas epileptiform EEG abnormalities may indicate a risk of further seizures and influence the decision to institute long-term anti-epileptic drug therapy.[1]

Neurone-specific enolase (NSE) is a well studied marker of brain injury and high serum levels have been found in GCSE and NCSE, particularly CPSE.[59] Elevated levels may reflect either the severity of brain

Table 41.7 Causes of status epilepticus in children

Febrile
Remote (e.g. brain malformations, cerebral palsy, previous
    trauma or meningitis)
Low anti-epileptic drug levels
Idiopathic
CNS infection – meningitis, encephalitis
Stroke – vascular occlusion or haemorrhage
Metabolic abnormalities
Hypoxia/anoxia
Drug toxicity
Progressive neurologic conditions
Head trauma
Tumour – primary or metastatic CNS tumours

injury resulting from SE, the underlying brain pathology or both. Increases in serum NSE have been correlated with the duration and outcome of GCSE.[59]

STATUS EPILEPTICUS IN CHILDREN[23,60]

The majority of paediatric cases of status epilepticus occur in young children, with more than 40% occurring in those below two years of age.[61]

More than 90% of cases are convulsive and the majority are generalized.[60]

The distribution of causes is highly age dependent, with febrile SE and that due to acute neurological disease (e.g. CNS infection) being more common in children under 2 years. Idiopathic and remote symptomatic causes are more common in older children.[61] The most frequent aetiologies of SE in children are listed in Table 41.7.

Treatment of SE in children is essentially the same as in adults.[60] The outcome is generally good and is related to the aetiology. Neurological sequelae in children with idiopathic or febrile SE are rare. The risk of subsequent seizures in a child with idiopathic or febrile SE is no greater than a child who presents with a brief fit.[60,62] Recurrent SE and seizures occur primarily in neurologically abnormal children, particularly those with remote symptomatic causes or progressive neurological disease.[61]

REFERENCES

1 Treatment of convulsive status epilepticus. Recommendations of the Epilepsy Foundation of America's Working Group on Status Epilepticus. *JAMA* 1993; **270**: 854–9.
2 Lowenstein DH, Alldredge BK. Status epilepticus. *N Engl J Med* 1998; **338**: 970–6.
3 DeLorenzo RJ, Hauser WA, Towne, *et al.* A prospective, population-based epidemiologic study of status epilepticus in Richmond, Virginia. *Neurology* 1996; **46**: 1029–35.
4 Hesdorffer DC, Logroscino G, Cascino G *et al.* Incidence of status epilepticus in Rochester, Minnesota, 1965–1984. *Neurology* 1998; **50**: 735–41.

5 Wasterlain CG, Fujikawa DG, Penix L, Sankar R. Pathophysiological mechanisms of brain damage from status epilepticus. *Epilepsia* 1993; **34**(Suppl 1): S37–53.
6 Kapur J. Status epilepticus and seizures. *Curr Opin Critical Care* 1998; **4**: 83–88.
7 Wijdicks EF, Sharbrough FW. New-onset seizures in critically ill patients. *Neurology* 1993; **43**: 1042–4.
8 Treiman DM. Generalized convulsive status epilepticus in the adult. *Epilepsia* 1993; **34**(Suppl 1): S2–11.
9 Treiman DM. Electroclinical features of status epilepticus. *J Clin Neurophysiol* 1995; **12**: 343–62.
10 DeLorenzo RJ, Waterhouse EJ, Towne AR, *et al.* Persistent nonconvulsive status epilepticus after the control of convulsive status epilepticus. *Epilepsia* 1998; **39**: 833–40.
11 Walton NY. Systemic effects of generalized convulsive status epilepticus. *Epilepsia* 1993; **34**(Suppl 1): S54–8.
12 Simon RP. Physiologic consequences of status epilepticus. *Epilepsia* 1985; **26**(Suppl 1): S58–66.
13 Howell SJ, Owen L, Chadwick DW. Pseudostatus epilepticus. *Q J Med* 1989; **71**(266): 507–19.
14 Betts T. Pseudoseizures: seizures that are not epilepsy. *Lancet* 1990; **336**(8708): 163–4.
15 Bauer J. Epilepsy and prolactin in adults: a clinical review. *Epilepsy Res* 1996; **24**: 1–7.
16 Krumholz A. Epidemiology and evidence for morbidity of nonconvulsive status epilepticus. *J Clin Neurophysiol* 1999; **16**: 314–22. [Discussion 353]
17 Kaplan PW. Assessing the outcomes in patients with nonconvulsive status epilepticus: nonconvulsive status epilepticus is underdiagnosed, potentially overtreated, and confounded by comorbidity. *J Clin Neurophysiol* 1999; **16**: 341–52. [Discussion 353]
18 Towne AR, Waterhouse EJ, Boggs JG, *et al.* Prevalence of nonconvulsive status epilepticus in comatose patients. *Neurology* 2000; **54**: 340–5.
19 Young GB, Jordan KG, Doig GS. An assessment of nonconvulsive seizures in the intensive care unit using continuous EEG monitoring: an investigation of variables associated with mortality. *Neurology* 1996; **47**: 83–9.
20 Cockerell OC, Walker MC, Sander JW, Shorvon SD. Complex partial status epilepticus: a recurrent problem. *J Neurol Neurosurg Psychiatry* 1994; **57**: 835–7.
21 Krumholz A, Sung GY, Fisher RS, *et al.* Complex partial status epilepticus accompanied by serious morbidity and mortality. *Neurology* 1995; **45**: 1499–504.
22 Drislane FW. Evidence against permanent neurologic damage from nonconvulsive status epilepticus. *J Clin Neurophysiol* 1999; **16**: 323–31. [Discussion 353]
23 Weise KL, Bleck TP. Status epilepticus in children and adults. *Crit Care Clin* 1997; **13**: 629–46.
24 Scholtes FB, Renier WO, Meinardi H. Simple partial status epilepticus: causes, treatment, and outcome in 47 patients. *J Neurol Neurosurg Psychiatry* 1996; **61**: 90–2.
25 Wijdicks EF, Parisi JE, Sharbrough FW. Prognostic value of myoclonus status in comatose survivors of cardiac arrest. *Ann Neurol* 1994; **35**: 239–43.

26 Logroscino G, Hesdorffer DC, Cascino G, *et al.* Short-term mortality after a first episode of status epilepticus. *Epilepsia* 1997; **38**: 1344–9.

27 Mellor DH. The place of computed tomography and lumbar puncture in suspected bacterial meningitis. *Arch Dis Child* 1992; **67**: 1417–19.

28 Lowenstein DH, Alldredge BK. Status epilepticus at an urban public hospital in the 1980s. *Neurology* 1993; **43**: 483–8.

29 Walton NY, Treiman DM. Response of status epilepticus induced by lithium and pilocarpine to treatment with diazepam. *Exp Neurol* 1988; **101**: 267–75.

30 Treiman DM, Meyers PD, Walton NY, *et al.* A comparison of four treatments for generalized convulsive status epilepticus. Veterans Affairs Status Epilepticus Cooperative Study Group. *N Engl J Med* 1998; **339**: 792–8.

31 Lukovits TG, Smith MC. Update on status epilepticus. *Curr Opin Critical Care* 1999; **5**: 107–111.

32 Uberall MA, Trollmann R, Wunsiedler U, Wenzel D. Intravenous valproate in pediatric epilepsy patients with refractory status epilepticus. *Neurology* 2000; **54**: 2188–9.

33 Litt B, Wityk RJ, Hertz SH, *et al.* Nonconvulsive status epilepticus in the critically ill elderly. *Epilepsia* 1998; **39**: 1194–202.

34 Arendt RM, Greenblatt DJ, deJong RH, *et al.* In vitro correlates of benzodiazepine cerebrospinal fluid uptake, pharmacodynamic action and peripheral distribution. *J Pharmacol Exp Ther* 1983; **227**: 98–106.

35 Leppik IE, Derivan AT, Homan RW, *et al.* Double-blind study of lorazepam and diazepam in status epilepticus. *JAMA* 1983; **249**: 1452–4.

36 Rivera R, Segnini M, Baltodano A, Perez V. Midazolam in the treatment of status epilepticus in children. *Crit Care Med* 1993; **21**: 991–4.

37 Igartua J, Silver P, Maytal J, Sagy M. Midazolam coma for refractory status epilepticus in children. *Crit Care Med* 1999; **27**: 1982–5.

38 Scott RC, Besag FM, Neville BG. Buccal midazolam and rectal diazepam for treatment of prolonged seizures in childhood and adolescence: a randomised trial. *Lancet* 1999; 353(9153): 623–6.

39 Kendall JL, Reynolds M, Goldberg R. Intranasal midazolam in patients with status epilepticus. *Ann Emerg Med* 1997; **29**: 415–17.

40 Chamberlain JM, Altieri MA, Futterman C, *et al.* A prospective, randomized study comparing intramuscular midazolam with intravenous diazepam for the treatment of seizures in children. *Pediatr Emerg Care* 1997; **13**: 92–4.

41 Gastaut H, Courjon J, Poire R, Weber M. Treatment of status epilepticus with a new benzodiazepine more active than diazepam. *Epilepsia* 1971; **12**: 197–214.

42 Cranford RE, Leppik IE, Patrick B, *et al.* Intravenous phenytoin: clinical and pharmacokinetic aspects. *Neurology* 1978; **28**: 874–80.

43 Browne TR. Fosphenytoin (Cerebyx). *Clin Neuropharmacol* 1997; **20**: 1–12.

44 Walton NY, Uthman BM, El Yafi K, *et al.* Phenytoin penetration into brain after administration of phenytoin or fosphenytoin. *Epilepsia* 1999; **40**: 153–6.

45 Lowe MR, DeToledo JC, Vilavizza N, *et al.* Efficacy, safety, and tolerability of fast IV loading of valproate in patients with seizures and status epilepticus. *Epilepsia* 1998; **39**:S235. [Abstr]

46 Brown LA, Levin GM. Role of propofol in refractory status epilepticus. *Ann Pharmacother* 1998; **32**: 1053–9.

47 Stecker MM, Kramer TH, Raps EC, *et al.* Treatment of refractory status epilepticus with propofol: clinical and pharmacokinetic findings. *Epilepsia* 1998; **39**: 18–26.

48 Parke TJ, Stevens JE, Rice AS, *et al.* Metabolic acidosis and fatal myocardial failure after propofol infusion in children: five case reports. *BMJ* 1992; **305**: 613–16.

49 Hanna JP, Ramundo ML. Rhabdomyolysis and hypoxia associated with prolonged propofol infusion in children. *Neurology* 1998; **50**: 301–3.

50 Cremer OL, Moons KG, Bouman EA, *et al.* Long-term propofol infusion and cardiac failure in adult head-injured patients. *Lancet* 2001; **357**: 117–18.

51 Shorvon S. *Status Epilepticus: its Clinical Features and Treatment in Children and Adults.* Cambridge, UK: Cambridge University Press; 1994.

52 Sheth RD, Gidal BE. Refractory status epilepticus: response to ketamine. *Neurology* 1998; **51**: 1765–6.

53 Walker IA, Slovis CM. Lidocaine in the treatment of status epilepticus. *Acad Emerg Med* 1997; **4**: 918–22.

54 Kofke WA, Young RS, Davis P, *et al.* Isoflurane for refractory status epilepticus: a clinical series. *Anesthesiology* 1989; **71**: 653–9.

55 Cascino GD, Hesdorffer D, Logroscino G, Hauser WA. Morbidity of nonfebrile status epilepticus in Rochester, Minnesota, 1965–1984. *Epilepsia* 1998; **39**: 829–32.

56 Maytal J, Shinnar S, Moshe SL, Alvarez LA. Low morbidity and mortality of status epilepticus in children. *Pediatrics* 1989; **83**: 323–31.

57 Waterhouse EJ, Vaughan JK, Barnes TY, *et al.* Synergistic effect of status epilepticus and ischemic brain injury on mortality. *Epilepsy Res* 1998; **29**: 175–83.

58 Jaitly R, Sgro JA, Towne AR, *et al.* Prognostic value of EEG monitoring after status epilepticus: a prospective adult study. *J Clin Neurophysiol* 1997; **14**: 326–34.

59 DeGiorgio CM, Heck CN, Rabinowicz AL, *et al.* Serum neuron-specific enolase in the major subtypes of status epilepticus. *Neurology* 1999; **52**: 746–9.

60 Wolf SM, Ochoa JG, Conway EE. Seizure management in pediatric patients for the nineties. *Pediatr Ann* 1998; **27**: 653–64.

61 Shinnar S, Pellock JM, Moshe SL, *et al.* In whom does status epilepticus occur: age-related differences in children. *Epilepsia* 1997; **38**: 907–14.

62 Maytal J, Shinnar S. Febrile status epilepticus. *Pediatrics* 1990; **86**: 611–16.

42

Acute cerebrovascular complications
B Riley

Cerebrovascular disease is common and its acute manifestations, known as stroke, produce considerable morbidity and mortality. Stroke is defined as an acute focal neurological deficit caused by cerebrovascular disease, which lasts for more than 24 hours or causes death before 24 hours. Transient ischaemic attack (TIA) also causes focal neurology, but this resolves within 24 hours. In the UK, stroke is responsible for 12% of all deaths and is the most common cause of physical disability in adults. The incidence in most developed countries is about 1–2/1000 population per year.[1] The main causes of stroke are cerebral infarction as a consequence of thromboembolism and spontaneous intracranial haemorrhage (either intracerebral or subarachnoid haemorrhage), causing about 85% and 15% of strokes, respectively. The main risk factors are increasing age, hypertension, ischaemic heart disease, atrial fibrillation, smoking, obesity, some oral contraceptives and raised cholesterol or haematocrit. The manifestations of stroke are:

- Cerebral infarction
- thrombosis
- embolism
- Spontaneous intracranial haemorrhage
- intracerebral haemorrhage
- subarachnoid haemorrhage

CEREBRAL INFARCTION

Infarction of cerebral tissue occurs as a result of inadequate perfusion from occlusion of cerebral blood vessels in association with inadequate collateral circulation. It may occur due to cerebral thrombosis or embolism.

AETIOLOGY AND PATHOLOGY

CEREBRAL THROMBOSIS

Atherosclerosis is the major cause of major arterial occlusion and most often produces symptoms if it occurs at the bifurcation of the carotid artery or the carotid syphon. Progressive plaque formation causes narrowing and forms a nidus for platelet aggregation and thrombus formation. Ulceration and rupture of the plaque exposes its thrombogenic lipid core activating the clotting cascade. Hypertension and diabetes mellitus are common causes of smaller arterial thrombosis. Rarer causes of thrombosis include any disease resulting in vasculitis, vertebral or carotid artery dissection (either spontaneous or post-traumatic) or carotid occlusion by strangulation or systemic hypotension after cardiac arrest. Cerebral venous thrombosis, responsible for less than 1% of strokes, may occur in hypercoagulable states such as dehydration, polycythaemia, thrombocythaemia, some oral contraceptive pills, protein C or S deficiency or antithrombin III deficiency, or vessel occlusion by tumour or abscess.

CEREBRAL EMBOLISM

Embolism commonly occurs from thrombus or platelet aggregations overlying arterial atherosclerotic plaques, but 30% of cerebral emboli will arise from thrombus in the left atrium or ventricle of the heart. This is very likely in the presence of atrial fibrillation, left-sided valvular disease, recent myocardial infarction, chronic atrial enlargement or ventricular aneurysm. The presence of a patent foramen ovale or septal defects allows paradoxical embolism to occur. Iatrogenic air embolism may occur during cardiopulmonary bypass, cardiac catheterization or cerebral angiography. It may also occur as a complication of attempted coil embolization of cerebral aneurysms after subarachnoid haemorrhage.

CLINICAL PRESENTATION

In cerebral thrombosis, there is initially no loss of consciousness or headache and the initial neurological deficit develops over several hours. Cerebral embolism may be characterized by sudden onset and rapid development of complete neurological deficit. No single clinical sign or symptom can reliably distinguish a thrombotic from embolic event. Where infarction occurs in a limited arterial territory the clinical signs are often characteristic. The commonest site involves the middle cerebral artery, which classically produces acute contra-lateral brachiofacial hemiparesis with sensory or motor deficits, depending on the precise area of infarction.

- Infarction of the middle cerebral territory leads to a dense contralateral hemiplegia, contralateral facial paralysis, contralateral hemianopia and ipsilateral eye deviation.
- Dominant left hemisphere lesions result in language difficulties from aphasia, dysphasia, dysgraphia and dyscalculia.
- Non-dominant right hemispheric lesions cause the patient to neglect the left side, and may not communicate with anyone approaching from that side.

Other cognitive effects of stroke include memory impairment, anxiety, depression, emotional lability, aprosody and spatial impairment. Bilateral brainstem infarction after basilar artery thrombosis may produce deep coma and tetraparesis. Pontine stroke may produce the 'locked in' syndrome. The precise clinical presentation depends on the size of the infarcted area and its position in the brain.

INVESTIGATIONS

A full history and examination from the patient are required, and the results of this will produce a differential diagnosis that will require specific investigations. The aim is to make the diagnosis, establish the nature, size and position of the pathology, so that correct treatment can be administered to compensate for the effects of the primary injury and prevent extension of the lesion or complications occurring.

Blood tests. Haemoglobin, white cell count and platelets are determined to look for polycythaemia, infection or thrombocythaemia. A raised erythrocyte sedimentation rate or C-reactive protein level may indicate vasculitis, infection or carcinoma, warranting further appropriate investigations.

Coagulation screen should be taken together with serum cholesterol, triglyceride and syphilis serology. Specific investigation for thrombophilia due to protein C, protein S, Leiden factor V and antithrombin III abnormalities should be undertaken in patients with venous thrombosis or patients with otherwise unexplained cerebral infarction or TIA.

Electrocardiography. This may demonstrate atrial fibrillation or other arrhythmia, or recent myocardial infarct.

Echocardiography. Either transthoracic or transoesophageal echocardiography (TOE) may demonstrate mural or atrial appendage thrombus as a source of embolism. TOE is more effective in detecting patent foramen ovale, aortic arteriosclerosis or dissection.

CT or MRI scanning. These techniques are used to distinguish infarction from haemorrhage. Tumour, abscess or subdural haematoma may also produce the symptoms and signs of stroke. Ideally, the scans should be undertaken as soon as possible to exclude conditions that are treatable by neurosurgery. Early scanning is vital if interventional treatment such as thrombolysis, anticoagulation, anti-platelet therapy or surgery is planned.

The CT scan may be normal or show only minor loss of grey/white matter differentiation in first 24 hours after ischaemic stroke but haemorrhage is seen as areas of increased attenuation within minutes. After a couple of weeks the CT appearances of an infarct or haemorrhage become very similar and it may be impossible to distinguish them if CT is delayed beyond this time. Multi-modal MRI, a combination of diffusion and perfusion-weighted MRI and MR angiography, is much more sensitive in demonstrating small areas of ischaemia and targeting those patients most suitable for thrombolysis.[5] Other imaging techniques are appropriate to identify the source of stroke in specific areas. Any patient with a stroke or TIA in the internal carotid artery territory should have Duplex–Doppler ultrasonography which may demonstrate stenosis, occlusion or dissection of the internal carotid. Where trauma is an aetiological factor then plain radiographs of skull and cervical spine may be indicated. (See Figs 40.1 and 40.12).

MANAGEMENT

Ideally, treatment for stroke patients should be co-ordinated within a Stroke Unit, as there is a 28% reduction in mortality and disability at 3 months compared to patients treated on general medical wards.[6] In general only those patients with a compromised airway due to depressed level of consciousness or life-threatening cardiorespiratory disturbances require admission to medical or neurosurgical ICUs. In either case, attention to basic resuscitation involving stabilization of airway, breathing and circulation are self-evident.

AIRWAY AND BREATHING

Patients with Glasgow coma scores of 8 or less or those with absent gag will require intubation to preserve their airway and prevention of aspiration. Where this requirement is likely to be prolonged, early tracheostomy should be considered. Adequate oxygenation and ventilation should be confirmed by arterial blood gas analysis, and supplemental oxygen prescribed if there is any evidence of hypoxia. If hypercarbia occurs then ventilatory support to achieve normocarbia is necessary to prevent exacerbation of cerebral oedema. Ventilatory support in such cases has been shown to result in improved prognosis.[7]

CIRCULATORY SUPPORT

A large number of stroke patients will have raised blood pressure on admission presumably as an attempt by the vasomotor centre to improve cerebral perfusion. Hypertensive patients may have impaired autoregulation and regional cerebral perfusion may be very dependent on blood pressure.[8] The patient's clinical condition and neurological status should determine treatment rather than an arbitrary level of blood pressure. Control of even very high blood pressure (220/120 mmHg; 29.3/16.0 kPa) is not without risk and may result in progression of ischaemic stroke, so reduction should be monitored closely.[9] It would seem reasonable on physiological grounds to avoid drugs that cause cerebral vasodilatation in that they may aggravate cerebral oedema, although there is no hard evidence for this. Animal experiments have suggested that haemodilution could improve blood flow by reducing whole blood viscosity but a recent multicentre study has failed to identify any clinical benefit.[10] Cardiac output should be maintained and any underlying cardiac pathology such as failure, infarction and atrial fibrillation treated appropriately.

METABOLIC SUPPORT

Both hypo- and hyperglycaemia have been shown to worsen prognosis after acute stroke, therefore blood sugar levels should be maintained in the normal range.[11] In the long term, nutritional support must not be neglected and early enteral feeding instituted by percutaneous gastrostomy if necessary.

ANTICOAGULATION

In theory, the use of anticoagulation reduces the propagation of thrombus and should prevent further embolism. In practice, the reduction in risk of further thromboembolic stroke is offset by a similar number of patients dying from cerebral or systemic haemorrhage as a result of anticoagulation.[12,13] Anticoagulation can only be recommended in individuals where there is a high risk of recurrence, such as in those patients with prosthetic heart valves, atrial fibrillation with thrombus or those with thrombophilic disorders. A CT scan must be obtained prior to commencing therapy to exclude haemorrhage, and careful monitoring used. In patients with large infarcts there is always the risk of haemorrhage into the infarct and early heparinization is best avoided.

THROMBOLYSIS

Systemic thrombolysis with streptokinase carries a very high risk of cerebral haemorrhage and should not be used.[14] There is some evidence that intravenous recombinant tissue plasminogen activator (alteplase) has a better safety/efficacy profile. The National Institute of Neurological Disorders and Stroke (NINDS) trial showed a significant improvement in those patients given alteplase rather than placebo within 3 hours of acute stroke.[15] This benefit was not found to be statistically significant in two European trials[16,17] and the ATLANTIS trial showed no significant benefit at 90 days in the alteplase group together with an increased risk of intracranial haemorrhage.[18] Currently, thrombolysis cannot be recommended for acute ischaemic stroke in

routine clinical practice and further trials are required to identify those patients most likely to benefit.[19]

CEREBRAL PROTECTION

Various agents such as free-radical scavengers, calcium antagonists, magnesium, AMPA antagonists, glutamate antagonists, γ-aminobutyric acid antagonists, etc. have been used in attempts to limit the deleterious effects of the biochemical changes that occur intracellularly following ischaemia. No agent has been shown to be effective in placebo controlled phase III trials.

DECOMPRESSIVE CRANIOTOMY

This is an option in young patients with large middle cerebral artery territory infarcts in the non-dominant hemisphere. Untreated, these normally have a mortality of 80% and it is suggested that this procedure can reduce mortality to around 30% but with residual neurological deficit. This procedure is limited to specialist centres.[20] Other forms of surgical intervention proven to be effective are drainage of secondary hydrocephalus, evacuation of haemorrhage into infarcted areas resulting in new compressive symptoms, especially in the posterior fossa.

COMPLICATIONS

Local complications include cerebral oedema, haemorrhage into infarcted areas or secondary hydrocephalus. General complications include bronchopneumonia, aspiration pneumonia, deep vein thrombosis, urinary tract infections, pressure sores, contractures and depression. A team approach of specialist nursing, physiotherapists, occupational and speech and language therapists is best able to avoid these complications.

SPONTANEOUS INTRACRANIAL HAEMORRHAGE

Spontaneous intracranial haemorrhage producing stroke may occur from either, intracerebral haemorrhage (10%) or, subarachnoid haemorrhage (5%).

INTRACEREBRAL HAEMORRHAGE

The incidence of intracerebral haemorrhage is about 9/100 000 of the population, mostly in the age range of 40–70 years with an equal incidence in males and females.

AETIOLOGY AND PATHOLOGY

The commonest cause is the effect of chronic systemic hypertension. This results in degeneration of the walls of vessels or microaneurysms by the process of lipohyalinosis, which then suddenly rupture. This may also occur in malignant tumour neo-vasculature, vasculitis, mycotic aneurysms, amyloidosis, sarcoidosis, malignant hypertension, primary haemorrhagic disorders or over-anticoagulation. Occasionally, cerebral aneurysms or arteriovenous malformations (AVMs) may cause intra-cerebral haemorrhage without subarachnoid haemor-rhage. The rupture of microaneurysms tends to occur at the bifurcation of small perforating arteries. Common sites of haemorrhage are the putamen (55%), cerebral cortex (15%), thalamus (10%), pons (10%) and cerebel-lum (10%). Haemorrhage is usually due to rupture of a single vessel, and the size of the haemorrhage is influ-enced by the anatomical resistance of the site into which it occurs. The effect of the haemorrhage is determined by the area of brain tissue that it destroys. Cortical haemorrhages tend to be larger than pontine bleeds but the latter are much more destructive.

CLINICAL PRESENTATION

Usually, there are no prodromal symptoms and a sudden onset of focal neurology or depressed level of conscious-ness occurs. Headache and neck stiffness will occur in conscious patients if there is subarachnoid extension by haemorrhage into the ventricles. As with ischaemic stroke, focal neurology is determined by which area of the brain is involved. The only way to differentiate absolutely between ischaemic, intracerebral or subarach-noid haemorrhage is by appropriate imaging. The symp-toms relate to tissue destruction, compression and raised intracranial pressure which, if progressive will result in brain stem ischaemia and death.

INVESTIGATIONS

The general investigations are essentially those listed previously for ischaemic stroke, since in the early stages it is difficult to distinguish between the two. In addi-tion, CT and/or MRI should be performed at the ear-liest opportunity. Lumbar puncture may be performed to exclude infection if mycotic aneurysm is suspected, but only after CT has excluded raised intracranial pres-sure or non-communicating hydrocephalus. Digital subtraction angiography will enable localization of the source of the haemorrhage and will facilitate any surgical intervention for aneurysm or AVM. (See Figs 40.7, 42.1 and 42.2).

MANAGEMENT

The general management principles are identical to those for ischaemic stroke. There is, of course, no place for anti-coagulation or thrombolysis, and reversal of any coagula-tion defect either primary or secondary to therapeutic anticoagulation must be undertaken as a matter of urgency. A full coagulation screen must be performed and the administration of vitamin K, fresh frozen plasma, cryopre-cipitate, etc. directed by the results. Operative decompres-sion of the haematoma should be undertaken only in neurosurgical centres and safe transfer must be assured if this is considered. The administration of mannitol prior to transfer should be discussed with the Neurosurgical Unit. There is no place for steroids, and hyperventilation to $PaCO_2$ of 30 mmHg (4kPa) or less to control raised intra-

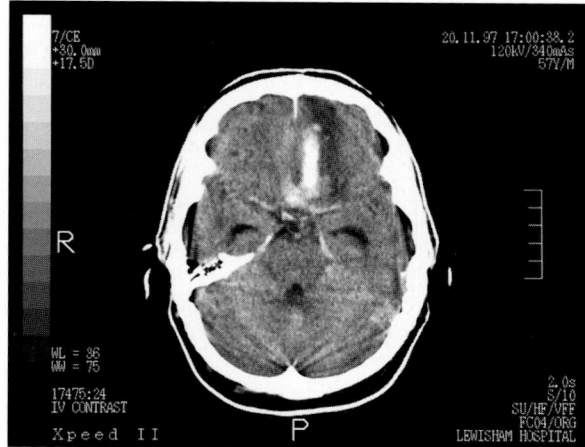

Fig. 42.1 Left frontal intraparenchmal bleed. With local oedema.

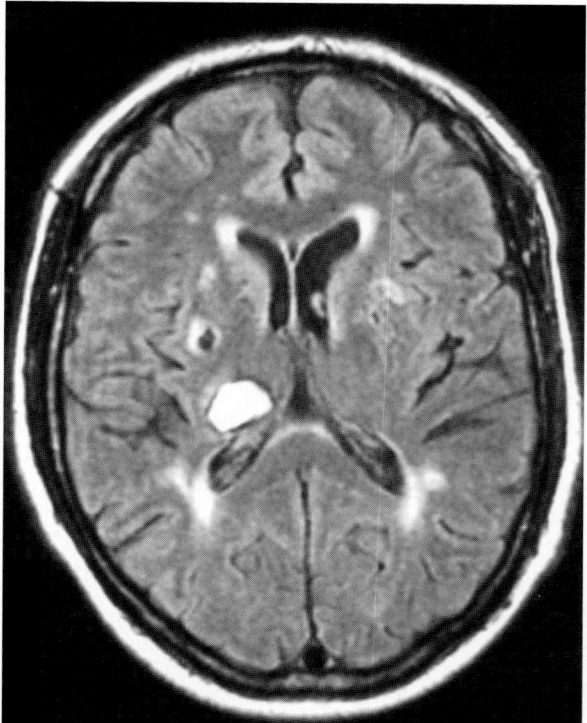

Fig. 42.2 MRI. Thalamic Bleed.

cranial pressure will have detrimental effects on cerebral blood flow in other areas of the brain. Ideally clot evacua-tion within 6 hours maximum should be the goal. Not all intracerebral haematomata are amenable to surgery, and the CT scans should be reviewed by the Neurosurgical Unit, preferably by digital image link, prior to patient transfer.

SUBARACHNOID HAEMORRHAGE

Subarachnoid haemorrhage (SAH) refers to bleeding which occurs principally into the subarachnoid space and not into the brain parenchyma. The incidence of SAH is around 6/100 000, the apparent decrease, compared with earlier studies, is due to more frequent use of CT scanning which allows exclusion of other types of haemorrhage. Risk factors are the same as for stroke, but SAH patients are usually younger, peaking in the sixth decade, with a female to male ratio of 1.6:1. Black people have twice the risk for SAH as whites. Between 5 and 20% of patients with SAH have a positive family history, with first degree relatives having a 3–7-fold risk while second degree relatives have the same degree of risk as the general population. Specific inheritable disorders are rare and account for only a minority of all patients with SAH.[21] The only modifiable risk factors for SAH are smoking, heavy drinking and hypertension which increase the risk odds ratio by 2 or 3.[22] Overall mortality is 50% of which 15% die before reaching hospital with up to 30% of survivors having residual deficit producing dependency.

AETIOLOGY AND PATHOLOGY

The majority of cases of SAH are caused by ruptured saccular (berry) aneurysms (85%), the remainder being caused by non-aneurysmal perimesencephalic haemorrhage (10%) and rarer causes such as arterial dissection, cerebral or dural AVMs, mycotic aneurysm, pituitary apoplexy, vascular lesions at the top of the spinal cord and cocaine abuse. Saccular aneurysms are not congenital, almost never occur in neonates and young children and develop during later life. It is not known why some adults develop aneurysms at arterial bifurcations in the Circle of Willis and some do not. It was thought that there was a congenital weakness in the tunica media, but gaps in the arterial muscle wall are equally as common in patients with or without aneurysms and once the aneurysm is formed, the weakness is found in the wall of the sac and not at its neck.[23] The association with smoking, hypertension and heavy drinking would suggest that degenerative processes are involved. Sudden hypertension plays a role in causing rupture as shown by SAH in patients taking crack cocaine or rarely with sulfenidil.

CLINICAL PRESENTATION

Classically, there is a 'thunderclap' headache developing in seconds, with half of patients describing its onset as instantaneous. This is followed by a period of depressed consciousness for less than an hour in 50% of patients with focal neurology in about 30% of patients.[24] About a fifth of patients recall similar headaches and these may have been due to 'warning leaks'. The degree of depression of consciousness depends upon the site and extent of the haemorrhage. Meningism – neck stiffness, photophobia, vomiting and a positive Kernig's sign – is common in those patients with higher Glasgow coma scores. The clinical severity of SAH is often described by a grade, the

Table 42.1 Clinical neurological classification of subarachnoid haemorrhage

Grade	Signs
I	Conscious patient with or without meningism
II	Drowsy patient with no significant neurological deficit
III	Drowsy patient with neurological deficit – probably intracerebral clot
IV	Deteriorating patient with major neurological deficit (because of large intracerebral clot)
V	Moribund patient with extensor rigidity and failing vital centres

WFNS grade	GCS	Motor deficit
I	15	Absent
II	14–13	Absent
III	14–13	Present
IV	12–7	Present or absent
V	3–6	Present or absent

most widely used being that described by the World Federation of Neurological Surgeons (WFNS)[2], which is summarized in Table 42.1.

This grading, together with the extent of the haemorrhage and the age of the patient, gives some indication of the prognosis, in that the worse the grade the bigger the bleed, and the older the patient the less likely a good prognosis.

COMPLICATIONS

The clinical status of the patient may be complicated by factors other than the physical effect of initial bleed, and factors such as acute hydrocephalus, early re-bleeding, cerebral vasospasm, parenchymal haematoma, seizures and medical complications must be considered.

Acute hydrocephalus. This may occur within the first 24 hours post-ictus and is often characterized by a 1 point drop in the Glasgow Coma Scale, sluggish pupillary responses and bilateral downward deviation of the eyes ('sunset eyes'). If these signs occur, CT scan should be repeated and if hydrocephalus is confirmed, or there is large amount of intraventricular blood, then a ventricular drain may be inserted. This is not without risk as it may provoke more bleeding and introduce infection. Only observational studies exist and these are contradictory so no firm recommendation can be made.

Re-bleeding. This may occur within the first few hours after admission and 15% of patients may deteriorate from their admission status.[26] They may require urgent intubation and resuscitation but not all re-bleeds are unsurvivable and such deterioration should be treated. The chance of re-bleeding is dependent on the site of the aneurysm, presence of clot, degree of vasospasm, age and sex of the patient. A preliminary report of the Co-operative

Aneurysm Study gave the re-bleeding rate in the first 2 weeks after the initial SAH was reported as 19% cumulative and then approximately 1.5% per day for the next 13 days in 1983.[27]

Cerebral vasospasm. This is the term used to describe narrowing of the cerebral blood vessels in response SAH seen on angiography. It occurs in up to 70% of patients, but not all of these patients will have symptoms.[28] Use of transcranial Doppler (TCD) to estimate middle cerebral artery blood velocity has shown that a velocity of more than 120 cm/s correlates with angiographic evidence of vasospasm. This technology allows diagnosis in the ICU and provides a means of monitoring the success of treatment to reduce vasospasm, which is undertaken to reduce the severity of delayed neurological deficit secondary to vasospasm. The problem is that not all patients who have angiographic vasospasm or high Doppler velocities have symptoms. If there is evidence of a depressed level of consciousness in the absence of re-bleeding, hydrocephalus or metabolic disturbances, but there is evidence of vasospasm on TCD or angiogram, then it would seem appropriate to initiate treatment to reduce the vasospasm.

Parenchymal haematoma. This may occur in up to 30% of SAH following aneurysm rupture and has a much worse prognosis than SAH alone.[29] If there is mass effect with compressive symptoms then evacuation of haematoma and simultaneous clipping of the aneurysm may improve outcome.

Medical complications. During the placebo-controlled study of nicardipine in WFNS grade I and II SAH patients, there was a 40% incidence of at least one life-threatening medical complication in the placebo group.[30] The mortality due to medical complications was almost the same as that due to the combined effects of the initial bleed, re-bleeds and vasospasm. The types of medical complication seen are shown in Table 42.2.

INVESTIGATIONS

The general investigations for stroke should be performed and early CT imaging is mandatory. Blood

Table 42.2 Types of medical complication seen in patients with subarachnoid haemorrhage

Medical complication	Incidence
Arrhythmias	35%
Liver dysfunction	24%
Neurogenic pulmonary oedema	23%
Pneumonia	22%
ARDS and atelectasis	20%
Renal dysfunction	5%

ARDS = acute respiratory distress syndrome.

appears characteristically hyperdense on CT and the pattern of haemorrhage may enable localization of the arterial territory involved. Very rarely, a false positive diagnosis may be made if there is severe generalized oedema resulting in venous congestion in the subarachnoid space. Small amounts of blood may not be detected and the incidence of false negative reports is around 2%.[31] It may be difficult to distinguish between post-traumatic SAH and primary aneurysmal SAH, which precipitates a fall in the level of consciousness that provokes an accident or fall.[32] MR scanning is particularly effective for localizing the bleed after 48 hours when extravasated blood is denatured, and provides a good signal on MRI.[33]

Lumbar puncture is still necessary in those patients where the suspicion of SAH is high despite a negative CT, or there is a need to exclude infection. There must be no raised intracranial pressure and at least 6 hours should have passed to give time for the blood in the CSF to lyse, enabling xanthochromia to develop.

Angiography via arterial catheterization is still the most commonly used investigation for localizing the aneurysm or other vascular abnormality prior to surgery. It is generally performed on patients who remain, or become, conscious after SAH. It is not without risk and aneurysms may rupture during the procedure and a meta-analysis has shown a complication rate of 1.8%.[34] Other methods under investigation include CT angiography and MR angiography, and it is likely that these techniques may replace catheter angiography for diagnosis, although intra-arterial catheterization would still be needed for endovascular therapy.[35,36]

Intracranial pressure monitoring is of limited use in SAH patients except in those where hydrocephalus or parenchymal haematoma is present and early detection of pressure increases may be the trigger for drainage or decompressive surgery.

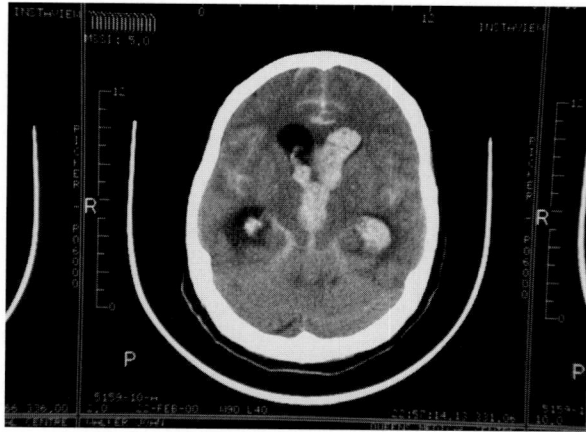

Fig. 42.3 Spontaneous subarachnoid haemorrhage and secondary hydrocephalus.

Transcranial Doppler studies may be useful in detecting vasospasm or those patients in whom autoregulation is impaired.[37] The technique is dependent on there being a 'window' of thin temporal bone allowing isonation of the Doppler signal along the middle cerebral artery. It is very user-dependent and 15% of patients do not have an adequate bone window (See Figs 40.3 and 41.3).

MANAGEMENT

GENERAL CARE

The initial management of SAH is influenced by the grading, medical comorbidity or complications, and the timing or need for surgery. Patients with decreased Glasgow coma scoring may need early intubation and ventilation, simply for airway protection, whereas those with less severe symptoms require regular neurological observation, analgesia for headache, and bed rest prior to investigation and surgery. Other management options are:

- stress ulcer prophylaxis
- deep vein thrombosis prophylaxis using compression stockings or boots
- seizures control with phenytoin or barbiturates.

If the patent is sedated and ventilated, the use of an analysing cerebral function monitor should be considered to detect subclinical fitting.

Hyponatraemia is a common finding and adequate fluid therapy with normal saline is required with electrolyte levels maintained in the normal range.

BLOOD PRESSURE CONTROL

Elevation of blood pressure is commonly seen after SAH and there are no precise data on what constitutes an unacceptably high pressure that is likely to cause re-bleeding. Equally, there are no precise data on a minimum level of pressure below which infarction is likely to occur, since this will depend on the patient's normal pressure, degree of cerebral oedema and the presence or absence of intact autoregulation. One observational study has demonstrated reduced re-bleeding but higher rates of infarction in newly treated compared with untreated post-SAH hypertensive patients.[38] If blood pressure exceeds 200 mmHg (26.6 kPa) systolic or 100 mmHg (13.3 kPa) diastolic, then empirically it would seem wise to reduce this pressure in SAH patients who have unclipped aneurysms. β-adrenergic blockers or calcium antagonists are the most widely used agents, since drugs producing cerebral vasodilation may increase intracranial pressure.

VASOSPASM

Angiographic demonstration of vasospasm may be seen in about 70% of SAH patients but only about 30% develop cerebral symptoms related to vasospasm. Transcranial Doppler derived flow velocities in the middle cerebral arteries of more than 120cm/s are accurate in predicting ischaemia.[37] Symptoms tend to occur between 4 and 14 days post-bleed, which is the period when cerebral blood flow is decreased after SAH.

One method of pre-empting vasospasm is the prescription of oral nimodipine at 60 mg given 4-hourly for 21 days, which has been shown to achieve a reduction in the risk of ischaemic stroke of 34%.[39] Intravenous nimodipine should be used in the patients who are not absorbing, but it must be titrated against blood pressure to avoid hypotension. Other calcium antagonists, notably nicardipine and the experimental drug AT877, reduce vasospasm but do not improve outcome.

Low cerebral blood flow is known to worsen outcome and this resulted in the development of prophylactic hypertensive hypervolaemic haemodilution, so called 'Triple-H Therapy'.[40] As originally described, the therapy involved the use of fluid loading to achieve haemodilution and vasopressor therapy to increase cerebral blood flow, and was combined with surgery within 24 hours if possible. The therapy was continued for 21 days and all patients remained neurologically stable or improved as a result, apparently, of the absence of vasospasm. Very few centres use the strict protocol as originally described, but fluid loading rather than fluid restriction is the norm and inotropes or vasopressors are used subsequently if neurological function decreases. Despite its widespread use, there remains no prospective randomized trial that demonstrates its utility.

The use of intravascular catheters to deliver papaverine into vasospastic vessels remains experimental. Where symptoms develop it is important to exclude other causes such as re-bleeding, hydrocephalus or metabolic disorder.

SURGERY

Clipping of the aneurysm is the surgical treatment of choice with wrapping, proximal ligation or bypass grafting being used if the aneurysm is inaccessible to Yasargil clipping. The timing of surgery remains debatable. Early surgery, within 3 days of the bleed, has the advantage of fewer deaths occurring from re-bleeding but is technically difficult due to the friability of associated tissues. Delayed surgery, around 10–12 days post-bleed, gives better operating conditions but allows some patients to suffer a re-bleed. There is no type 1 evidence but an observational study suggested that there is no difference in outcome after early or late operation.[41]

ENDOVASCULAR COILING

The development of detachable micro-coils made of platinum by Gugliemi in 1990 has resulted in endovascular embolization of aneurysms or AVMs by interventional radiology.[42] A micro-catheter is passed from the femoral artery to the cerebral aneurysm and the coils positioned sequentially in the lumen of saccular aneurysms to occlude it. Rupture of the aneurysm or adjacent vessel occlusion, causing ischaemia, are the most frequent complications.[43] A small randomized study of surgery versus coiling found no difference in outcome at 3 months but a much larger trial is in progress.[44] Interim analysis suggests a survival advantage in the coiling group.

NEUROPROTECTIVE THERAPY

There has been a great deal of research on the cellular and biochemical responses to brain injury and several drugs have been investigated to try and reduce mortality in SAH. The 21-amino steroid tirilizad, nicaraven and ebselen, all free-radical scavengers, have been the most widely investigated. None has been shown to consistently improve outcome in all types of patient with SAH.

THERAPY OF MEDICAL COMPLICATIONS

This is obviously specific to the type of complication. Pneumonia may require continuous positive airways pressure or ventilatory support together with directed anti-microbial therapy; acute respiratory distress syndrome requires lung protective/recruitment ventilatory strategies; and renal failure necessitates an appropriate means of renal replacement therapy. Arrhythmias require correction of trigger factors such as hypovolaemia and electrolyte or acid–base disturbances prior to the appropriate anti-arrhythmic drug or DC cardioversion. Neurogenic pulmonary oedema may be associated with severe cardiogenic shock, which may require inotropic support or even temporary intra-aortic balloon counter-pulsation. The cardiogenic shock is reversible and patients can make a good recovery despite the need for aggressive support.[45]

PROGNOSIS IN ACUTE CEREBROVASCULAR DISEASE

Mortality after stroke averages 30% within a month, with more patients dying after subarachnoid haemorrhage or intracerebral haemorrhage than after cerebral infarction, although survival to 1 year is slightly better in the haemorrhagic group. In all types of stroke about 30% of survivors remain disabled to the point of being dependent on others. Risk of stroke increases with age, so that it rises from 3/100 000 in the third and fourth decades to 300/100 000 in the eighth and ninth decades.[2] Thus stroke is often accompanied by significant age-related medical comorbidity. This may in the past have been partially responsible for a relatively non-aggressive approach to the treatment of stroke patients. So that the gloomy prognosis of stroke becomes a self-fulfilling prophecy. It has been suggested that by regarding stroke as a medical emergency, a 'brain attack' analogous to 'heart attack', and ensuring early intensive care support, outcome may be improved.[3,4]

REFERENCES

1 Wolfe CDA. The impact of stroke. *Br Med Bull* 2000; **56**: 275–6.
2 Bonita R. Epidemiology of stroke. *Lancet* 1992; **339**: 342–4.
3 Treib J, Grauer MT, Woessner R, Morgenthaler M. Treatment of stroke on an intensive stroke unit: a novel concept. *Intensive Care Med* 2000; **26**: 1598–11.
4 Wolfe C, Rudd A, Dennis M, *et al*. Taking acute stroke care seriously. *BMJ* 2001; **323**: 5–6.
5 Jansen O, Schellinger P, Fiebach J, *et al*. Early recanalisation in acute ischaemic stroke scar tissue at risk defined by MRI. *Lancet* 1999; **353**: 2036–7.
6 Stroke Trialists Collaboration. Collective systematic review of the Randomised Trials of Organised Inpatient (Stroke Unit) Care after stroke. *BMJ* 1997; **314**: 1151–9.
7 Steiner T, Mendoza G, De Gorgia M, *et al*. Prognosis of stroke patients requiring mechanical ventilation in a neurological critical care unit. *Stroke* 1997; **28**: 711–15.
8 Fujii K, Satoshima S, Okada Y, *et al*. Cerebral blood flow and metabolism in normotensive and hypotensive patients with transient neurological deficits. *Stroke* 1990; **21**: 283–90.
9 Treib J, Haa BA, Stoll M, Grauer MT. Monitoring and management of antihypertensive therapy induced deterioration in acute ischaemia stroke. *Am J Hypertens* 1996; **9**: 513–14.
10 Aichner FT, Fazehar F, Bainin M, *et al*. Hypervolaemic hemodilution in acute ischaemic stroke. The Multicenter Austrian Hemodilution Stroke Trial (MAHST). *Stroke* 1998; **29**: 743–9.
11 Jorgensen HS, Nakayam H, Raaschon HO, *et al*. Effect of blood pressure and diabetes on stroke in progression. *Lancet* 1994; **344**: 156–9.
12 International Stroke Trial Collaborative Group. The International Stroke Trial (IST): a randomised trial of aspirin, subcutaneous heparin, both or neither among 19 435 patients with acute ischaemic stroke. *Lancet* 1997; **349**: 1564–5.
13 The Publications Committee for the Trial ORG 10172 in Acute Stroke Treatment (TOAST). Low molecular weight heparinoid ORG 10172 (Danaparoid) and outcome after acute ischaemic stroke. *JAMA* 1998; **279**: 1265–72.
14 Multicentre Acute Stroke Trial – Europe Study Group. Thrombolytic therapy with streptokinase in acute ischaemic stroke. *N Engl J Med* 1996; **335**: 145–50.
15 National Institute of Neurological Disorders and Stroke rt-PA Stroke Study Group. Tissue plasminogen activator for acute ischaemic stroke. *N Engl J Med* 1996; **333**: 1–7.
16 Hacke W, Kaste M, Fieschi C, *et al*. Intravenous thrombolysis with recombinant tissue plasminogen activator for acute hemispheric stroke. The European Co-operative Acute Stroke Study (ECASS) *JAMA* 1995; **274**: 1017–25.
17 Hacke W, Kaste M, Fieschi C, *et al*. for the Second European–Australasian Acute Stroke Study Investigators.

Randomised double blind placebo-controlled trial of thrombolytic therapy with intravenous alteplase in acute ischaemic stroke (ECASS II). *Lancet* 1998; **352:** 1245–51.

18 Clark WM, Wissman S, Albers GW, *et al.* Recombinant tissue type plasminogen activator (alteplase) for ischaemic stroke 3 to 5 hours after symptom onset. The ATLANTIS study: a randomised controlled trial. Alteplase thrombolysis for acute non-interventional therapy in ischaemic stroke. *JAMA* 1999; **282:** 2019–26.

19 Wardlow JM, del Zoppo G, Yamaguchi T. Thrombolysis for acute ischaemic stroke. [Cochrane Review] In: *The Cochrane Library*, Issue 3. Oxford: Update Software; 2001.

20 Siddique MS, Mendelow AD. Surgical treatment of intracerebral haemorrhage. *Br Med Bull* 2000; **56:** 444–56.

21 Van Gijn J, Rinkel GJE. Subarachnoid haemorrhage: diagnosis, causes and management. *Brain* 2001; **124:** 249–8.

22 Teunissen LL, Rinkel GJE, Algra A, *et al.* Risk factors for subarachnoid haemorrhage – a systematic review. *Stroke* 1996; **27:** 544–9.

23 Stehbens WE. Etiology of intracranial berry aneurysms. *J Neurosurg* 1989; **70:** 823–31.

24 Linn FH, Rinkel GJ, Algra A, van Gijn J. Headache characteristics in subarachnoid haemorrhage and benign thunderclap headache. *J Neurol Neurosurg Psychiatry* 1998; **65:** 791–3.

25 Drake CG, Hunt WE, Kassell NF, *et al.* Report of the World Federation of Neurological Surgeons Committee on a universal subarachnoid haemorrhage grading scale. *J Neurosurg* 1996; **84:** 985–6.

26 Fujii Y, Takeuchi S, Sasaki O, *et al.* Ultra-early rebleeding in spontaneous subarachnoid haemorrhage. *J Neurosurg* 1996; **84:** 35–42.

27 Kassell NF, Torner JC. Aneurysmal rebleeding: a preliminary report from the Cooperative Aneurysm Study. *Neurosurgery* 1983; **13:** 479–81.

28 Weir B, MacDonald L. Cerebral vasospasm. *Clin Neurosurg* 1992; **40:** 40–5.

29 Hauerberg J, Eskesen V, Rosenova J. The prognostic significance of intracerebral haematoma as shown on CT scanning after subarachnoid haemorrhage. *Br J Neurosurg* 1994; **8:** 333–9.

30 Solenski NJ, Haley EC, Kassell NF, *et al.* Medical complications of aneurysmal subarachnoid haemorrhage: a report of the multicenter cooperative aneurysm study. *Crit Care Med* 1995; **25:** 1007–17.

31 Van der Wee N, Rinkel GJ, Hasan D, *et al.* Detection of subarachnoid haemorrhage on early CT: is lumbar puncture still needed after a negative scan? *J Neurol Neurosurg Psychiatry* 1995; **58:** 357–9.

32 Vos PE, Zwienenberg M, O'Hannion KL, *et al.* Subarachnoid haemorrhage following rupture of an ophthalamic artery aneurysm presenting as traumatic brain injury. *Clin Neurol Neurosurg* 2000; **102:** 29–32.

33 Noguchi K, Ogawa T, Seto H, *et al.* Sub-acute and chronic subarachnoid haemorrhage: diagnosis with fluid attenuated inversion – recovery MR imaging. *Radiology* 1997; **203:** 257–62.

34 Cloft HJ, Joseph GJ, Dion JE. Risk of cerebral angiography in patients with subarachnoid haemorrhage, cerebral aneurysm and arteriovenous malformation: a meta-analysis. *Stroke* 1999; **30:** 317–20.

35 Wardlaw JM, White PM. The detection and management of unruptured intracranial aneurysms. *Brain* 2000; **123:** 205–21.

36 Hashimoto H, Iida J, Hironaka Y, *et al.* Use of spiral CT angiography in patients with subarachnoid haemorrhage in whom subtraction angiography did not reveal cerebral aneurysms. *J Neurosurg* 2000; **92:** 278–83.

37 Vora YY, Suarez-Almazor M, Steinke DE, *et al.* Role of transcranial doppler in the diagnosis of cerebral vasospasm after subarachnoid haemorrhage. *Neurosurgery* 1999; **44:** 1237–47.

38 Wijdicks EF, Vermeulen M, Murray GD, *et al.* The effects of treating hypertension following aneurysmal subarachnoid haemorrhage. *Clin Neurol Neurosurg* 1990; **92:** 111–17.

39 Pickard JD, Murray GD, Illingworth R, *et al.* Effect of oral nimodipine on cerebral infarction and outcome after subarachnoid haemorrhage: British Aneurysm Nimodipine Trial (BRANT). *Br Med J* 1989; **298:** 636–42.

40 Origatano TC, Wascher TM, Reichman OU, *et al.* Sustained increased cerebral blood flow with prophylactic hypertensive hemodilution ('triple-H' therapy) after subarachnoid haemorrhage. *Neurosurgery* 1990; **27:** 729–40.

41 Kassell NF, Torner JC, Jane JA, *et al.* The International Cooperative Study on the Timing of Aneurysm Surgery. Part 2: surgical results. *J Neurosurg* 1990; **73:** 18–36.

42 Guglielmi G, Vinuela F, Duckwriter G, *et al.* Endovascular treatment of posterior circulation aneurysms by electrothrombosis using electrically detachable coils. *J Neurosurg* 1992; **77:** 515–24.

43 Brilstra EH, Hop JW, van der Graaf Y, *et al.* Treatment of intracranial aneurysms by embolisation with coils: a systematic review. *Stroke* 1999; **30:** 470–6.

44 Vannine R, Koivisto T, Saari T, *et al.* Ruptured intracranial aneurysms: acute endovascular treatment with electrically detachable coils; a prospective randomised study. *Radiology* 1999; **211:** 325–36.

45 Parr MJ, Finfer SR, Morgan MK. Reversible cardiogenic shock complicating subarachnoid haemorrhage. *BMJ* 1996; **313:** 681–3.

43

Cerebral protection

M Hayes

The concept of cerebral or neural protection has taken on many forms, from prophylaxis in stroke prevention to resuscitation in the treatment of ongoing ischaemia or recent infarction. A complete review is beyond the scope of this chapter, but current understanding of cerebral protection is beneficial to intensivists in treating cerebral insults.

NORMAL BRAIN PHYSIOLOGY

The brain is an energetic tissue, utilizing approximately 3–5 ml O_2/min per 100 g tissue (45–75 ml O_2/min per 1500 g brain) and 5 mg glucose/min per 100 g tissue (75 mg glucose/min per 1500 g brain). It has little ability to store precursors of metabolism and thus depends on a constant supply of nutrients from the blood. At a cerebral blood flow (CBF) of 50 ml/min per 100 g tissue (750 ml/min per 1500 g brain) and a normal oxygen content of 20 ml O_2/100 ml blood, the brain receives approximately 150 ml O_2/min per 1500 g brain, or 2–3 times the amount needed for normal brain activity. The brain extracts 35–50% of the oxygen delivered to fuel metabolism. Similarly, assuming the same CBF of 50 ml/min per 100 g tissue and a blood glucose concentration of 5.5 mmol/l (100 mg/100 ml blood), then there is 50 mg/min per 100 g tissue (750 mg/min per 1500 g brain) delivery of glucose. Glucose extraction by the brain, as 5 mg/min per 100 g brain tissue, is minimal compared with oxygen.

Cerebral injury has many aetiologies, but the mechanisms of injury are thought to be few. The most common by far is caused by the lack of essential nutrients, oxygen and glucose. This can occur separately with preserved blood flow (i.e. hypoxia or hypoglycaemia), or more often together, because of reduced/absent perfusion (i.e. ischaemia or infarction). Reduced supply of these energy precursors is a major contributor in the mechanism of brain injury, regardless of the aetiology.

NATURAL PROTECTIVE MECHANISMS

The importance of the brain to the whole being is highlighted by the mechanisms in place to protect the cerebral elements from ischaemia.

COLLATERAL BLOOD SUPPLY

An elaborate vascular architecture is designed to ensure adequate CBF. Circulation to the head is divided into anterior (carotid arteries) and posterior (vertebral arteries) systems, each providing bilateral supply. Carotid arteries divide before entering the skull to form the external carotid branches (feeding the face and scalp) and the internal branches supplying the anterior cerebrum (frontal, parietal and temporal lobes) and anterior diencephalon (basal ganglia and hypothalamus). Vertebral arteries join once inside the cranium to form the basilar artery, which runs the length of the posterior fossa, supplying the brainstem, cerebellum and posterior portion of the cerebrum (occipital lobes) and diencephalon (thalamus). Adequacy of arterial blood supply is ensured by connections between these two circulations, called collaterals. The circle of Willis (Fig. 43.1), which joins the large branches of the anterior and posterior circulations at the base of the brain, is the major component of this collateral network in humans. Between these arterial distributions are watershed zones fed by leptomeningeal connections. In addition, persistent fetal arteries can infrequently provide collateral routes between the anterior and posterior arterial systems in the brain.

CEREBRAL BLOOD FLOW (CBF)

CEREBRAL PERFUSION PRESSURE

The amount of blood delivered to the brain is highly regulated and is determined by several factors. CBF is determined in part by the perfusion pressure across the

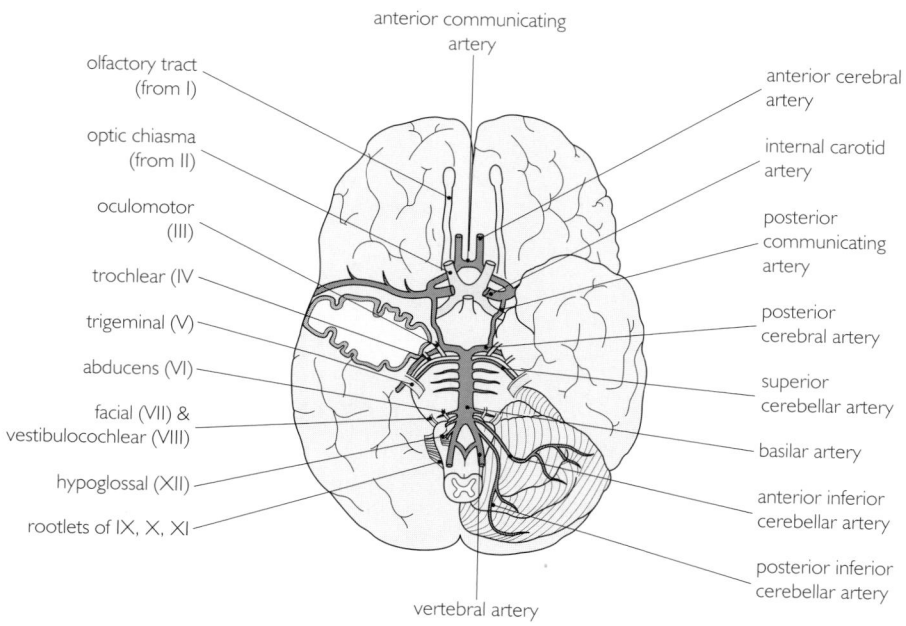

Fig. 43.1 Circle of Willis

brain, called cerebral perfusion pressure (CPP). CPP, in fact, is the difference between the arterial pressure in the feeding arteries as they enter the subarachnoid space and the pressure in the draining veins before they enter the major dural sinuses. Because these pressures are difficult to measure, CPP is derived from the difference between the systemic mean arterial pressure (MAP) and the intracranial pressure (ICP), which is an estimate of tissue pressure.

The cerebral vessels change diameter inversely with changing perfusion pressure: as CPP rises, the vessels constrict and as CPP falls the vessels dilate, such that blood flow is kept constant over a wide range of CPP (Fig. 43.2a). This pressure autoregulation is thought to be controlled by local myogenic responses of the vessel wall to changes in intra-arterial pressure. At pressures above and below this range of 6.7–20 kPa (50–150 mmHg), cerebral perfusion becomes pressure-passive and increases or decreases in direct proportion to changes in CPP. The autoregulatory range varies with age, being shifted to the left in newborns and to the right in those with chronic hypertension. The latter is important to remember to avoid overtreating systolic blood pressure in such patients and thus incur the risk of cerebral ischaemia at the lower limits of autoregulation. Alternatively, cerebral perfusion above normal can be caused by acute hypertension overcoming the upper limits of autoregulation. This may lead to cerebral oedema secondary to increased hydrostatic pressures (hypertensive encephalopathy) and potentially lead to seizures or cerebral haemorrhage.

Pao_2 AND $Paco_2$ EFFECTS

A second group of factors control CBF through an influence on the local metabolic milieu. Prominent in this mechanism are oxygen and carbon dioxide. Arterial content or partial pressure of oxygen in the normal or hyperoxic ranges causes very little change in CBF. Perhaps this represents a demand for another nutrient (i.e. glucose) or a need to remove waste products (i.e. carbon dioxide or metabolic acid). With the onset of hypoxaemia (Pao_2 60 mmHg or 8 kPa), there is a prompt increase in CBF proportional to the decrease in blood oxygen content, in order to maintain oxygen delivery constant (Fig. 43.2b).

There is also a direct relationship between CBF and $Paco_2$, such that cerebral perfusion increases with increasing $Paco_2$ (Fig. 43.2b). This probably represents the need of the brain to maintain homeostatic pH by removing metabolic breakdown products more efficiently by increased blood flow. Unlike the response to oxygen, the CBF response to changes in $Paco_2$ is dramatic in the physiological range, such that for every 0.13 kPa (1.0 mmHg) change in $Paco_2$ there is a 1–2 ml/min per 100 g tissue change in CBF. Therefore, an increase in $Paco_2$ to 10.6 kPa (80 mmHg) will increase CBF to approximately 100 ml/min per 100 g and a decrease in $Paco_2$ to 2.7 kPa (20 mmHg) will decrease CBF to 25 ml/min per 100 g. Thus:

- doubling of $Paco_2$ doubles CBF and
- halving $Paco_2$ halves CBF within this range.

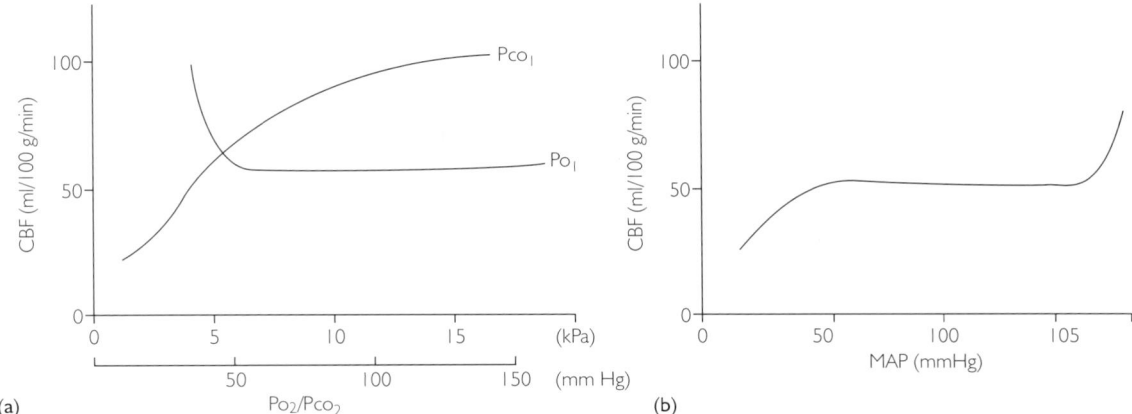

Fig. 43.2 (a) The relationship between the partial pressure of oxygen and carbon dioxide and cerebral blood flow. (b) The relationship between mean arterial pressure and cerebral blood flow under normal circumstances illustrating the range of autoregulation.

Understanding this basic physiology will make treatment logical (see below), as increases in CBF often lead to increases in cerebral blood volume, which in turn can increase ICP – a common cause of cerebral ischaemia.

AETIOLOGY

Vascular insufficiency or disruption, trauma, tumour, infection/inflammation, and metabolic and nutritional derangement can all cause damage. Whatever the cause, the mechanism of injury is usually hypoxic and/or ischaemic injury.

- Hypoxia is lack of oxygen.
- Ischaemia is lack of flow.

Therefore, it is possible to have high flow but no oxygen or, alternatively, no flow but plenty of oxygen. At the cellular level the consequence is the same.

The protective mechanisms afforded by the ability to increase CBF many-fold in response to hypoxaemia and the generous oversupply of nutrients under normal conditions allows for sufficient blood flow, with maintenance of oxygen delivery and supply of other nutrients in many cases. Limitation in the ability to alter CBF, whether through cerebrovascular disease restricting perfusion or intracranial masses, oedema and increased ICP exerting excess local pressure, and thereby altering flow, will cause hypoxic/ischaemic injury. Systemic problems such as severe or prolonged hypoxaemia will eventually disturb systemic circulatory homeostasis, leading to hypotension and eventual ischaemia. Thus hypoxic and ischaemic injury may be considered synonymous, although there may be aetiological differences between them. A more important distinction is to be made between global and focal hypoxic/ischaemic insults.

GLOBAL HYPOXIC/ISCHAEMIC INSULTS

Hypoxic and low/no-flow states are caused by hypoxaemia and cardiovascular insufficiency or arrest, respectively. These are usually sudden, short and severe. If there is to be recovery, prompt return of oxygen delivery and spontaneous circulation are necessary. The recovery may be variable, depending on the severity and duration of the insult and the selective vulnerability of certain cell types. After 4–6 minutes of complete global ischaemia, there are signs of permanent histological damage in selective neuronal populations and the beginnings of neurological deficits in survivors. Outcome worsens significantly after 15 minutes of global ischemia.[1]

FOCAL HYPOXIC/ISCHAEMIC INSULTS

Focal hypoxic/ischaemic insults often occur suddenly but are usually of more prolonged duration. They may be less severe if the surrounding brain is preserved by collateral blood supply. Even if perfusion does not return to the area in jeopardy, patient survival initially is not a concern, because a subtotal area of the brain is affected.

The area of the focal ischaemic area supplied by end-arteries will result in cell death unless reperfusion is established rapidly. The periphery of an infarcted area is the ischaemic penumbra. Here, CBF is greater than at the infarcted core, but less than in the normal tissue around it. Animal studies suggest that the time course for infarction and irreversible damage to brain from a focal hypoxic/ischaemic event is around 30–60 minutes. The focus of therapeutic intervention is the penumbral area, after a focal infarction, on the basis that if blood flow can be normalized in this region, or pharmacological agents can be delivered despite the reduced blood flow, there is a potential for recovery. Conversely, failure to maintain this area will result in a coalescing of the penumbra into the infarcted area, as the ischaemic stimulus continues.

It is likely that the ongoing ischaemic penumbral area of a focal insult and transient whole brain ischaemia (e.g. during early cardiac arrest, low flow cardiopulmonary resuscitation (CPR) or elevated ICP states) are subject to similar pathophysiological processes. As pretreatment is usually impossible, prevention and treatment of the secondary insults is the focus in neuroprotection and tissue salvage strategies.

BRAIN ISCHAEMIC AND INFARCTION PROCESSES

Changes in normal physiology begin to occur when blood flow is reduced.

- At CBF below 50 ml/min per 100 g neurological function is impaired and there is slowing of the electroencephalogram (EEG).
- A CBF of 15–25 ml/min per 100 g results in loss of electrical activity.
- A CBF between 10 and 15 ml/min per 100 g can maintain ATP levels sufficiently to support ionic pump function for a time, despite the lack of electrical activity and normal neurological function.
- At a CBF of 10 ml/min per 100 g membrane failure occurs, due to a critical loss of ATP, which causes ionic imbalance between the cell and the extracellular milieu. If prolonged or worsened, CBF at this level will lead to permanent neurological impairment as a result of cell death.

EFFECTS OF ISCHAEMIA

Ischaemia results in reduced available oxygen and glucose to support aerobic production of ATP. Levels of ATP are depleted within 2–3 min of complete ischaemia (animal studies). There is little brain storage of either glucose or oxygen, and ATP production during ischemia relies on anaerobic glycolysis for as long as stores last. This results in continued ATP use but suboptimal production of ATP to fuel aerobic metabolism, so a lactic acidosis develops. Loss of ATP causes failure of membrane ionic pump function, leading to an efflux of potassium and an influx of sodium, calcium and chloride ions. This begins a cascade of events resulting in eventual cell death.

The potassium leakage probably causes cell depolarization, with voltage-sensitive ion channel opening and release of excitatory amino acid (EAA) neurotransmitters. EAA neurotransmitters will begin a wave of further depolarization that affects neighbouring cells and parts of the brain removed from the initial injury. These depolarizations (agonist-operated) will allow influx of sodium and chloride through activation of kainate (K) and quisqualate (Q) receptors and influx of calcium by activation of the N-methyl-D-aspartate (NMDA) receptors. Influx of sodium (and chloride) is followed by water, leading to intracellular oedema. Calcium influx or release from intracellular stores can lead to further release of excitatory transmitters. It also leads to conversion of phosphorylases, with uncoupling of oxidative phosphorylation in the mitochondria, activation of proteases, with degradation of cystosolic protein and stimulation of lipases. These lipases liberate arachidonic acid and other free fatty acids that cause tissue damage via production of oxygen radicals and prostaglandins.

Other effects occur at the nuclear level, interfering with DNA and RNA production and hence inhibiting protein production. This may explain why cellular and clinical recovery is partial even with restoration of ionic equilibrium and near normal ATP levels after successful reperfusion.

EXTRACELLULAR EFFECTS

Leukocytes are thought to be major contributors to reperfusion injury in that:

- they may plug up small capillaries under conditions of low blood flow and prevent reflow in certain areas, thus hindering restoration of perfusion;
- they may enhance production of oxygen radicals and begin a cascade of inflammatory mediators, which may potentiate cell destruction in injured tissue.

The injury frequently results in tissue oedema. This may affect the core lesion by narrowing blood vessels and worsening chances of reperfusion and can alter function in neighbouring tissue by mechanical compression of tissue or its blood supply. The alteration in volume is of extreme importance in the adult brain because the cranial vault is non-distensible, preventing accommodation to an expanding lesion. This will impede CBF both locally and globally.

Hypoxic/ischaemic insults are rarely predictable, so that the process is usually well established when clinicians intervene. It is, therefore, highly likely that the injury will be only partially remediable.

MANAGEMENT

The first approach to neurological injury is to establish adequate vital function. Assessment of the airway and respiration are the first priority, closely followed by optimization of the circulation.

In cases of head trauma, but also other intracranial injury, it is very important to prevent secondary brain injury. Reviews of intensive care practice have resulted in recommendations for treatment in this group of patients.[2] These involve:

- institution of monitoring
- early treatment of hypotension, hypoxia, hyperthermia and intracranial hypertension
- maintenance of cerebral perfusion pressure.

Following stroke, it is also important to optimize homeostasis and address any hypertension, hyperglycaemia, hyperthermia and intracranial hypertension, as these are independent factors of a poor prognosis.[3]

Hypertension. There is no definitive evidence of how to treat hypertension. Most experts recommend leaving it alone unless the level is particularly high. It has, however, been suggested that hypertension should be treated if thrombolytics are to be administered, since trials of these agents have lowered blood pressure prior to treatment.[4]

Hyperglycaemia. This has also been associated with an increased mortality and reduced functional outcome after stroke.[5] Insulin, as well as having a glucose lowering effect, has been shown to be directly neuroprotective.[6] No large trials have tested the effect of relatively aggressive normalization of glucose levels with insulin.

Hyperthermia increases cerebral metabolism, thereby increasing oxygen requirements, CBF and intracranial pressure. A raised temperature should, therefore, be treated aggressively and any evidence of infection identified early and treated with appropriate antibiotics.

REVASCULARIZATION

For global ischaemia following cardiac arrest, the theoretical principles are to re-establish systemic blood pressure and to consider the no-reflow phenomenon in certain areas of the brain. Current research is addressing attempts to increase blood pressure during cardiopulmonary resuscitation and to open up capillaries that may have collapsed during the arrest period.

For focal cerebral ischaemia:

- start treatment as early as possible
- increase local CBF (fibrinolysis)
- effect ischaemic cascade blockade (neuroprotection).

The speed at which ischaemic neuronal degeneration proceeds after the onset of perfusion failure mandates that interventional therapy must begin immediately after discovery of the patient. Unfortunately, thrombolytic agents will never be administered out of hospital unless a portable reliable imaging modality is made available. The results from the National Institute of Neurological Disorders and Stroke (NINDS) study of recombinant tissue plasminogen activator (rtPA) for acute ischaemic stroke suggest efficacy if intravenous thrombolytic therapy is initiated within the first 3 hours of stroke symptoms.[7] Clearly, this may be difficult to achieve and, taking into account the potential risks of this therapy, the search continues for an ideal neuroprotective agent which would complement thrombolytic therapy. This area is currently very contentious with differing opinions on the actual places of thrombolytics, if at all, see chapter on acute cerebrovascular. Hopefully a definitive view on their place will emerge in the near future.

HAEMODILUTION

Decreasing haematocrit and viscosity by haemodilution has the potential for facilitating blood and oxygen delivery to areas that have narrowed arterial supply. This benefit has been shown in animal models of ischaemia but in clinical trials of stroke, results are not impressive. Three major studies have shown no benefit of normovolaemic[8,9] and hypervolaemic haemodilution,[10] mainly because of complications of volume therapy in patients with an associated risk of heart disease.

Blood substitutes derived from human haemoglobin can have a neuroprotective effect, improving tissue oxygenation and perfusion in the ischaemic territory. Based on the results obtained in animal models with DCL Hb, a phase II clinical trial was performed. In this trial, unfortunately, the treated group had more adverse events and mortality than the control group; consequently clinical development of this drug was discontinued.[11] Hypervolaemic haemodilution and deliberate hypertension with augmentation of cardiac output using vasopressors and inotropic agents are currently being used in many centres for the treatment of delayed ischaemic deficits after subarachnoid haemorrhage related to vasospasm. This therapy can be administered safely with intensive monitoring, but benefits are anecdotal, as it has not been tested with concurrent controls.[12] If nothing else, this therapeutic approach has changed the long-held belief that dehydration is best for patients with central nervous system disease.

INTRACRANIAL PRESSURE

Raised ICP can cause global ischaemia. To maintain adequate cerebral perfusion, treatment should be targetted at both, ensuring an adequate perfusion pressure and a reduction in ICP. MAP should be raised to a level at or above the usual pressure for that patient, within the zone of pressure autoregulation. Knowledge of his/her normal blood pressure is important. If the majority of the vasculature is autoregulating, raising the blood pressure may decrease vascular diameter and reduce blood volume within the cranium. If the cause of the raised ICP cannot be corrected (e.g. blood clot or brain tumour), then the focus should be to prevent secondary injury around the lesion. An increased ICP can cause further ischaemia, so a reduction of ICP should facilitate adequate perfusion to areas at risk. Treating ICP requires knowledge of the three compartments (blood, brain and CSF) within the intracranial vault. Whenever possible, the offending compartment should be treated primarily (e.g. tumour removal, blood evacuation and drainage of hydrocephalus). If this is not advisable, reducing the relative volumes of other compartments may improve compliance overall and reduce the ICP.

MONITORING OF ICP (Fig. 43.3)

Fluid-coupled catheters. Intraventricular catheterization is probably the most accurate method of measuring ICP. A

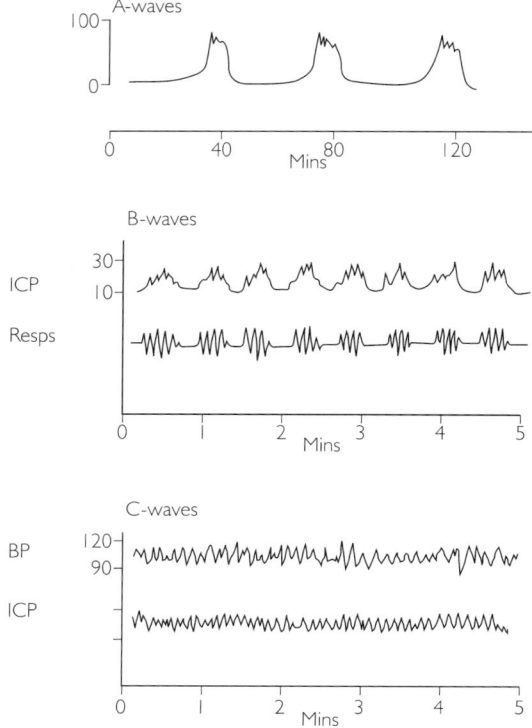

Fig. 43.3 ICP waveforms. A-waves are plateau waves of 50–100mmHg, sustained for 5–15 minutes. Associated with raised ICP and compromised CBF. B-waves are small changes in pressure every 0.5–2 minutes, often associated with breathing patterns and possibly due to local variations in the partial pressure of oxygen and carbon dioxide. C-waves are low amplitude oscillations with a frequency of about 5 per minute. Associated with variation in vasomotor tone.

catheter can be used as a therapeutic device to drain CSF when intracranial hypertension is present, or for culture. Air, blood or debris, collapse of the ventricles can all adversely affect measurement.

All externally transduced ICP systems require an atmospheric pressure reference that should be zero-balanced to account for variations in patient head position. Two anatomical reference points used are the external auditory meatus, or the Lundberg point, 1.5 cm below the uppermost part of the head regardless of position.

Fluid-coupled surface devices. These are easy to place and usually provide a reliable ICP wave-form and pressure reading. They may become unreliable with a damper trace when the dural perforations become plugged with blood or debris, or if brain swelling obliterates communication with the CSF space. Debris can be flushed from the open bolt surface with 0.2 ml of preservative-free (non-bacteriostatic) saline solution and this may restore

accurate ICP readings. It is unusual to cause any sustained ICP elevation with this technique.

The SA bolt measures the local ICP at the surface of the hemisphere, so it can be inaccurate if there is a pressure gradient between the left and right supratentorial compartments. These gradients can occur between the left and right hemispheres or the supratentorial and infratentorial compartments, but are usually transient; they should be considered if there is a discrepancy between the apparent ICP and the patient's clinical condition. Clarification should be sought by computed tomographic (CT) scanning if there is doubt about whether to intervene with treatment of the elevated ICP.

Solid-state devices. These are air-referenced and do not require repositioning of the external transducer element. As there is no fluid coupling for pressure transduction, the problems of wave-form damping and artefacts from poor coupling are avoided. The transducer cannot be calibrated to zero once it has been inserted.

The Camino system accuracy is reliable in the subdural space, the brain parenchyma and the ventricles but there may be disparities with other systems. Parenchymal fibreoptic pressures may consistently exceed intraventricular catheter pressures by nearly 1.3 kPa (10 mmHg).

Baseline drift is a problem after a few days use (± 0.8 kPa; 6 mmHg) and may necessitate transducer replacement.

COMPLICATIONS OF ICP MONITORING
Infection

The risk of meningitis or ventriculitis associated with the intravascular catheter (IVC) appears to be related to the duration of catheter insertion, and increases significantly after 5 days. Irrigation of the catheter or drainage system, and intraventricular blood increase the risk. The role of prophylactic antibiotics during external CSF drainage is still unclear but monitoring of the CSF for infection would seem sensible.

The infection risk from SA bolts is extremely low (consistently below 5%), and infections are nearly always superficial and rarely involve the brain or meninges. Again, the risk is higher if the device is opened and flushed to improve the wave-form. Prophylactic antibiotics for SA bolts are not recommended.

There are few reports on complications associated with solid-state devices.

Placing the device

Placing an IVC can cause brain parenchymal damage with parenchymal or subdural haemorrhage. Bleeding probably occurs, because during placement it is possible to tear unseen pial vessels. Deeper vital structures such as the thalamus, hypothalamus or midbrain can be damaged.

SA bolts are rarely associated with brain injury, but cortical laceration or puncture can occur if the needle used to puncture the dura is passed too deeply. Epidural or subdural haemorrhage can also occur at the SA bolt site, but this usually happens when coagulation is disordered and the likelihood of epidural or subdural haemorrhage is increased.

Solid-state devices are the subject of few reports, but injury will relate to site of insertion. The risk should be higher with intraventricular or parenchymal insertion, and lower with subarachnoid or epidural insertion.

REGULATION OF ICP

Brain compartment
Reduction in the parenchymal compartment depends on removal of either free water or the lesion causing the raised ICP.

Free water must be moved across an intact blood–brain barrier. Mannitol increases plasma osmolarity and reduces brain oedema. In addition, it may have a beneficial effect on microcirculatory flow. It is also thought to have antioxidant effects, although these may not be clinically important. Hypertonic saline has been used not only for volume resuscitation (7.5%), but also for treatment of raised ICP refractory to mannitol (23.4%).[13–15]

Removal of tumour or blood clot, drainage of abscesses, extirpation of infarcted brain are all therapies aimed at improving compliance. Mounting evidence now suggests that there is a penumbra of functionally impaired but potentially reversible neuronal injury surrounding a haematoma. Indications for clot removal, however, are controversial.[16] A prospective, randomized study is presently underway to determine whether a policy of early surgical evacuation of the haematoma in patients with spontaneous supratentorial intracranial haemorrhage will improve outcome compared with a policy of initial conservative treatment. The rationale for removing part of the skull overlying the stroke in patients with or at risk of developing cerebral oedema and intracranial hypertension is simply to decompress the brain swelling and prevent herniation. Decompressive craniectomy has been assessed in experimental cerebral infarction and was effective in reducing death and neurological impairment whether performed 1 hour or 24 hours after induction of permanent middle cerebral artery occlusion.[17] An uncontrolled trial comparing patients with hemicraniectomy with historical controls found that mortality rates were reduced from 80 to 35% in the surgical group.[18] These non-randomized studies are clearly at risk of bias and properly controlled trials of craniectomy for malignant middle cerebral artery infarction are required.

Blood compartment
Although a small component of intracranial volume, the blood compartment is most compliant. Reduction in blood volume is useful in the treatment of raised ICP, especially in the acute setting. As explained above, hypoxia and hypercarbia can lead to hyperaemia and an increase in cerebral blood volume, potentially worsening ICP. Alternatively, induced hypocarbia leads to very rapid changes in blood flow and blood volume. Hyperventilation as a treatment for raised ICP in severe head injury is now the subject of much debate. Unfortunately, the reduction in cerebral blood volume may be accompanied by a fall in global CBF, which may result in ischaemia and a worsened outcome. It is recommended that a secondary treatment be instituted as soon as possible to allow slow withdrawal of hyperventilation.[19] If adaptation to hypocapnia has not occurred, hyperventilation can be reinstituted with the same effect. Finally, CBF and volume are reduced by lowering the need for blood supply and nutrients to the brain, through prevention and treatment of seizures and hyperthermia.

CSF compartment
CSF drainage can be used to reduce ICP; however, this is only possible if there is a ventricular catheter in place. Care is taken regarding the route and rate of CSF drainage to avoid herniation of a mass lesion, either towards the other side of the brain or through the tentorium. In recent years there has been a move towards the use of less invasive methods to measure intracranial pressure. However, the brain trauma foundation guidelines, for the management of severe head injury, provide some evidence supporting the increased use of CSF drainage for ICP control.[20]

HYPOTHERMIA

METABOLIC THERAPY

Injury to the central nervous system is temperature dependent. Fever can make an existing neurological dysfunction more apparent and may worsen an ongoing insult. Cooling the body and, in turn, the brain has been known for years to offer protection. Drowning victims who were cold have survived long periods of ischaemia. Therefore it is suggested that treatment of fever should be aggressive, using cooling blankets, cool water, cool intravenous fluids, fans and antipyretic medications. Induced hypothermia (28–30°C) is commonplace for coronary artery bypass surgery, and deep hypothermia (<20°C) has allowed prolonged circulatory arrest in order to repair high thoracic and giant cerebral aneurysms. Treatment with moderate, systemic hypothermia has been shown to reduce the rate of cerebral oedema and death after injury to the cerebral cortex in laboratory animals. In the absence, therefore, of any proven drug therapies for patients with severe head injuries, several centres began to cool patients almost routinely, despite the potential risks and the considerable effort required.

Unfortunately, a recent study, which hoped to obtain definitive evidence of the efficacy of hypothermia in head injuries, was halted after the enrolment of 392 patients because the treatment was ineffective.[21] They found that cooling patients to a target bladder temperature of 33°C within eight hours after injury, and maintaining hypothermia for 48 hours was not effective in improving the clinical outcome at 6 months. In fact, patients older than 45 years of age in the hypothermia group had a higher incidence of poor outcome. These results conflict with two earlier studies,[22,23] both of which demonstrated an improvement in outcome with cooling to 32°C. It is unclear why the recent study showed a different result; it may be related to different percentages of patients who had hypothermia on admission or differences in the protocols for re-warming.

No randomized, controlled trials of hypothermia in patients with stroke have been reported; however, experimental studies in animal models of permanent and transient ischaemic stroke have confirmed the hypothesis that inducing hypothermia reduces stroke lesion size.[24,25] An uncontrolled study of inducing moderate hypothermia in 25 cases of severe middle cerebral artery infarction found that lowering temperature reduced mortality from an expected value of 78% to 44%[26]. Randomized, controlled studies will need to be performed to confirm this benefit.

ANAESTHETIC AGENTS

Pharmacological reduction in cerebral metabolism with general anaesthetics has received much interest over the years. Suppression of EEG activity and an associated 50% reduction in the cerebral metabolic rate has been used in many animal models of global and focal ischaemia. Studies using barbiturates in many animal species have shown some convincing benefit, especially for focal ischaemia. However, only one clinical study has shown reduction in focal deficits, using the induction of barbiturate coma during coronary bypass surgery.[27] However, this study was criticized due to the small numbers of patients included, and so barbiturates are not commonly used in this situation or in situations of global ischaemia. Generally, barbiturates are now less commonly used in head injured patients but may have a role to play in those patients who have intractable intracranial hypertension.

Propofol is commonly used but does have some side-effects, which include hypotension, with a reduction in cerebral perfusion pressure and hyperlipidaemia when an infusion of 200 μg/kg per min is used to produce burst suppression.[28] This latter problem has been lessened by the introduction of a more concentrated formulation.

Midazolam has also been used for sedation. It reduces the cerebral metabolic rate for oxygen; CBF and volume; however, even in large doses it will not produce burst suppression or an isoelectric EEG.

Neuromuscular blockade is often used in head injured patients to prevent any coughing on the tracheal tube and subsequent rise in ICP. It is interesting that their use is not associated with better outcome despite the improvements in ICP control.

CALCIUM ANTAGONISTS

The influx of calcium from the extracellular space and from intracellular organelles, which is normally in minute quantities unbound within the cytosol, has been implicated as the common mediator of cell death from a variety of causes. Calcium antagonists were among the first neuroprotective agents studied to prevent cerebral ischaemia. Despite the effects seen in animal models, human studies in both global and focal ischaemia have been disappointing. The two largest clinical trials with intravenous nimodipine in acute ischaemic stroke had to be terminated early when it was shown that the neurological and functional outcome was significantly poorer in the active group compared with the placebo group.[29,30] A close relationship was found between a reduction in diastolic and mean blood pressure in the group treated with nimodipine and an unfavourable neurological outcome. Nimodipine has, however, become standard therapy in the prophylactic treatment of cerebral vasospasm after subarachnoid haemorrhage.[31–33] Benefits appear to be due to an effect on smaller penetrating vessels not seen by angiography, or a neuroprotective effect at the cellular level,[32] rather than cerebral vasodilatation as determined by angiography. Studies have also suggested that nimodipine may improve outcome in head injured patients with traumatic subarachnoid haemorrhage,[34,35] although this is controversial.[36]

STEROIDS

Glucocorticoids are thought to decrease cerebral oedema associated with breakdown of the blood–brain barrier (i.e. vasogenic oedema). Improvement in central nervous system function has been seen with brain tumours and abscesses.[37,38]

In the treatment of acute spinal cord injury, high dose methyl prednisolone for 24 hours has been shown to offer small but significant benefit provided treatment begins within eight hours of injury.[39,40]

Glucocorticoids are not effective for cytotoxic oedema, which is seen with ischaemic disease whether focal[41] or global[42] in aetiology. Patients with head injuries have in the past not been thought to benefit from steroids[43,44]; however, there has been renewed interest in the subject and a randomized, controlled study has recently commenced.

The 21-amino steroids form a group of drugs developed from methylprednisolone of which one is tirilazad. This is a free-radical scavenger that has been used in patients with ischaemic stroke, subarachnoid haemorrhage and head injury. It has shown no evidence of benefit in patients with focal cerebral ischaemia in one major trial which was terminated prematurely on the advice of the independent monitoring committee.[45] Nor has it shown any benefit on outcome in patients with head injury.

EXPERIMENTAL THERAPY

Laboratory studies have identified numerous potential therapeutic interventions that have clinical application for the treatment of head injury, many of which have progressed to clinical trials. Dizocilbine, the non-competitive glutamate antagonist acting at the NMDA receptor, never reached large scale clinical trials because of fears regarding hippocampal neurotoxicity. Other compounds tested have acted at presynaptic sites to reduce glutamate release or act at non-NMDA glutamate receptors. The results of all completed trials have been disappointing compared with the successes of these interventions in laboratory animals.

Thrombolysis has been effective following ischaemic stroke, within the first few hours after onset. Brain tissue can be salvaged and functional outcome can be improved. Unfortunately however this treatment is limited to relatively small numbers. Therefore the search continues for safe neuroprotective strategies which can be used alone or in combination with thrombolysis. The primary aim of cerebral protection is to interfere with the biochemical changes occurring in the penumbra area to block the ischaemic cascade in order to delay or prevent cell death. In experimental circumstances, treatment after the onset of ischaemia with free radical scavengers, glutamate antagonists, or anti-inflammatory strategies can limit the size of the infarct.

Several classes of cerebral protective agents have been investigated in phase III trials. Antagonists of excitatory amino acids, such as gavestinel, an antagonist of the glycine site of the NMDA receptor. It was administered up to 6 hours after an acute ischaemic stroke[46] but unfortunately there was no improvement in functional outcome at 6 months. At high doses, magnesium acts as an endogenous vasodilator of brain circulation and behaves pharmacologically as a non-competitive antagonist of NMDA receptors and of the voltage-dependent calcium channels. A phase III trial is currently ongoing (IMAGES) to assess the efficacy of the administration of magnesium within 12 hours after stroke. Other studies have looked at monoclonal antibodies, clomethiazole (a GABA agonist)[47] and a sodium channel and nitric oxide blocker (lubeluzole)[48,49] among others. Lubeluzole inhibits glutamate release in the penumbra area and decreases post ischaemic excitotoxicity. It also appears to inhibit glutamate-induced nitric oxide neurotoxicity.

Most of the completed trials have yielded disappointing efficacy results and some showed safety problems, including increased mortality or psychotic effects which resulted in their early termination. Despite this, it is believed that with the increased understanding of the mechanism of cell death and new targets for drug treatment, it is only a matter of time before an effective cerebral protective agent will become available.

REFERENCES

1 Bedell S, Delbanco T, Cook E, Epstein P. Survival after cardiopulmonary resuscitation in the hospital. *N Engl J Med* 1983; **309**: 569–76.
2 Maas AIR, Dearden M, Teassdale GM, *et al*. EBIC guidelines for management of severe head injury in adults. *Acta Neurochir* 1997; **139**: 286–94.
3 Bath PMW. Optimising homeostasis. *Br Med Bull* 2000; **56**: 422–35.
4 Brott T, Lu M, Kothari R, *et al*. Hypertension and its treatment in the NINDS rt-PA stroke trial. *Stroke* 1998; **29**: 1504–9.
5 Weir CJ, Murray GD, Dyker AG, Lees KR. Is hyperglycaemia an independent predictor of poor outcome after acute stroke? Results of a long term follow up study. *BMJ* 1997; **314**: 1303–6.
6 Strong AJ, Fairfield JE, Monteiro E, *et al*. Insulin protects cognitive function in experimental stroke. *J Neurol Neurosurg Psychiatry* 1990; **53**: 847–53.
7 The National Institute of Neurological Disorders and Stroke rt-PA Stroke Study Group. Tissue Plasminogen Activator for acute ischaemic stroke. *N Engl J Med* 1995; **333**: 1581–7.
8 Scandinavian Stroke Study Group. Multicenter trial of hemodilution in acute ischemic stroke. Results in the total patient population. *Stroke* 1987; **18**: 691–9.
9 Italian Acute Stroke Study Group. Haemodilution in acute stroke: results of the Italian haemodilution trial. *Lancet* 1988; **1**: 318–21.
10 The Hemodilution in Stroke Study Group. Hypervolemic hemodilution treatment of acute stroke. Results of a randomised multicenter trial using pentastarch. *Stroke* 1989; **20**: 317–23.
11 Saxena R, Wijnhoud AD, Carton H, *et al*. Controlled safety study of a haemoglobin-based oxygen carrier, DCL Hb, in acute ischaemic stroke. *Stroke* 1999; **30**: 993–6.
12 Solomon R, Fink M, Lennihan L. Early aneurysm surgery and prophylactic hypervolemic, hypertensive therapy for the treatment of aneurysmal subarachnoid hemorrhage. *Neurosurgery* 1988; **23**: 699–704.
13 Worthley LI, Cooper DJ, Jones N. Treatment of resistant intracranial hypertension with hypertonic saline. Report of two cases. *J Neurosurg* 1988; **68**: 478–81.
14 Henschen S, Busse MW, Zisowsky S, *et al*. Short term volume effects of a hypertonic saline bolus during neurosurgery. *Neurochirurgie* 1991; **34**: 163–5.
15 Fisher B, Thomas D, Peterson B. Hypertonic saline lowers raised intracranial pressure in children after head trauma. *J Neurosurg Anesthesiol* 1992; **1**: 4–10.
16 Siddique MS, Mendelow AD Surgical treatment of intracerebral haemorrhage. *Br Med Bull* 2000; **56**: 444–6.
17 Forsting M, Reith W, Shabitz W-R, *et al*. Decompressive craniectomy for cerebral infarction. An experimental study in rats. *Stroke* 1995; **26**: 259–64.

18 Rieke K, Schwab S, Horn M, *et al*. Decompressive surgery in space occupying hemispheric infarction: results of an open, prospective trial. *Crit Care Med* 1995; **23**: 1576–87.

19 Muizelaar JP, Marmarou A, Ward JD, *et al*. Adverse effects of prolonged hyperventilation in patients with severe head injury: a randomized clinical trial. *J Neurosurg* 1991; **75**: 731–9.

20 Bullock MR, Povilshock JT. Indications for intracranial pressure monitoring. *J Neurotrauma* 1996; **13**: 667–9.

21 Clifton GL, Miller ER, Choi SC, *et al*. Lack of effect of induction of hypothermia after acute brain injury. *N Engl J Med* 2001; **344**: 556–63.

22 Clifton GL, Allen S, Barrodale P, *et al*. A phase II study of moderate hypothermia in severe brain injury. *J Neurotrauma* 1993; **10**: 263–71.

23 Marion DW, Obrist WD, Carlier PM, *et al*. The use of moderate therapeutic hypothermia for patients with severe head injuries: a preliminary report. *J Neurosurg* 1993; **79**: 354–62.

24 Baker J, Onesti T, Solomon R. Reduction by delayed hypothermia of cerebral infarction following middle cerebral artery occlusion in the rat: a time-course study. *J Neurosurg* 1992; **77**: 438–44.

25 Ridenour TR, Warner DS, Todd MM, *et al*. Mild hypothermia reduces infarct size resulting from temporary but not focal ischaemia in rats. *Stroke* 1992; **23**: 733–8.

26 Schwab S, Schwarz S, Spranger M, *et al*. Moderate hypothermia in the treatment of patients with severe middle cerebral artery infarction. *Stroke* 1998; **29**: 2461–6.

27 Nussmeier NA, Arlund C, Slogoff S. Neuropsychiatric complications after cardiopulmonary bypass: cerebral protection by a barbiturate. *Anesthesiology* 1986; **64**: 165–70.

28 Menon DK. Cerebral protection in severe brain injury: physiological determinants of outcome and their optimisation. *Br Med Bull* 1999; **55**: 226–58.

29 Wahlgren NG, MacMahon DG, De Keyser J, *et al*. Intravenous Nimodipine West European Stroke Trial (INWEST) of nimodipine in the treatment of acute ischaemic stroke. *Cerebrovasc Dis* 1994; **4**: 204–10.

30 Bridgers S, Koch G, Munera C, *et al*. Intravenous nimodipine in acute stroke: Interim analysis of randomised trial. *Stroke* 1991; **22**: 29.

31 Allen GS, Ahn HS, Preziosi TJ, *et al*. Cerebral arterial spasm – a controlled trial of nimodipine in patients with subarachnoid hemorrhage. *N Engl J Med* 1983; **308**: 619–24.

32 Petruk KC, West M, Mohr G, *et al*. Nimodipine treatment in poor-grade aneurysm patients. Results of a mulicenter double-blind placebo-controlled trial. *J Neurosurg* 1988; **68**: 505–17.

33 Pickard JD, Murray GD, Illingworth R, *et al*. Effect of oral nimodipine on cerebral infarction and outcome after subarachnoid haemorrhage: British aneurysm nimodipine trial. *BMJ* 1989; **298**: 636–42.

34 Harders A, Kakarieka A, Braakman R, *et al*. Traumatic subarachnoid haemorrhage and its treatment with nimodipine. *J Neurosurg* 1996; **85**: 82–5.

35 European Study Group on Nimodipine in Severe Head Injury. A multicentre trial of the efficacy of nimodipine on outcome after severe head injury. *J Neurosurg* 1994; **80**: 797–804.

36 Murray GD, Teasdale GM, Schmitz H. Nimodipine in traumatic subarachnoid haemorrhage – a reanalysis of the HIT-I and HIT-II trials. *Acta Neurochir* 1996; **138**: 1163–7.

37 Reulen H. Vasogenic brain oedema. New aspects in its formation, resolution and therapy. *Br J Anaesth* 1976; **48**: 741–52.

38 French LA, Galicich JH. The use of steroids for control of cerebral oedema. *Clin Neurosurg* 1964; **10**: 212–23.

39 Bracken M, Shepard M, Collins W, *et al*. Methylprednisolone or naloxone treatment after acute spinal cord injury: one-year follow-up data. *J Neurosurg* 1992; **76**: 23–31.

40 Bracken MB, Shepard MJ, Collins W, *et al*. A randomized, controlled trial of methylprednisolone or naloxone in the treatment of acute spinal-cord injury. Results of the second national acute spinal cord injury study. *N Engl J Med* 1990; **322**: 1405–11.

41 Patten BM, Mendell J, Brunn B, *et al*. Double-blind study of the effects of dexamethasone on acute stroke. *Neurology (Minneapolis)* 1972; **22**: 377–83.

42 Jastremski M, Sutton Tyrrell K, Vaagenes P, *et al*. Glucocorticoid treatment does not improve neurological recovery following cardiac arrest. Brain Resuscitation Clinical Trial I Study Group. *J Am Med Assoc* 1989; **262**: 3427–30.

43 Braakman R, Schouten JHA, Blaauw-Van Dischoeck M, Minderhoud JM. Megadose steroid in severe head injury. *J Neurosurg* 1983; **58**: 326–30.

44 Cooper PR, Moody S, Clark WK, *et al*. Dexamethasone and severe head injury. A prospective double-blind study. *J Neurosurg* 1979; **51**: 307–16.

45 The RANTTAS Investigators. A randomised trial of tirilazad mesylate in patients with acute stroke (RANTTAS). *Stroke* 1996; **27**: 1453–8.

46 Sacco RL, DeRosa JT, Clarke Haley Jr E, *et al*. Glycine antagonist in neuroprotection for patients with acute stroke. GAIN Americas: A randomised controlled trial. *JAMA* 2001; **285**: 1729–8.

47 Wahlgren NG, for the CLASS study group. The clomethiazole acute stroke study (CLASS): results of a randomised controlled trial of clomethiazole versus placebo in 1360 acute stroke patients. *J Stroke* 1999; **230**: 21–8.

48 Grotta J, for the US and Canadian Lubelozole Ischaemic Stroke Study Group. Lubelozole treatment of acute ischaemic stroke. *Stroke* 1997; **28**: 2338–46.

49 Diener HC, for the European and Australian Lubelozole Ischaemic Stroke Study Group. Multinational randomised controlled trial of lubelozole in acute ischaemic stroke. *Cerebrovasc Dis* 1998; **8**: 172–81.

44.

Brain death

T E Oh

Today, ICUs can maintain cardiopulmonary function by artificial means and death cannot always be equated with cessation of spontaneous heartbeat. It has become necessary to reappraise death based on the integrity of the central nervous system.[1] The ability to certify death when there is irrecoverable cessation of brain function enables intensivists to withdraw treatment on ethical, humanitarian and utilitarian grounds. Relatives are relieved of unnecessary prolonged anxiety and false hopes, and the burden on expensive medical resources is reduced. A potential benefit for the community is a greater availability of physiologically sound organs for transplantation. Causes of brain death in adults are mostly traumatic brain injury and subarachnoid haemorrhage. In children, trauma, including physical abuse, is the main cause. Infections (e.g. encephalitis) are less common causes. Hypoxia may be the sole cause (e.g. cardiac arrest or drowning) or a complicating factor. Cerebral oedema may be a contributory or principal cause (e.g. secondary to hypoglycaemia).

DEFINITION OF DEATH

In Australia and many countries, for the purposes of organ removal for transplantation, the statutory definition of death is irreversible cessation of all brain function. In most jurisdictions, precise means to determine irreversible brain function are not specified by law, but have been drafted by medical bodies (see below). The role of intensivists is vital in diagnosing brain death and supporting organ donation. Brain death is associated with death of the brainstem and is a requisite for the donation of organs for transplantation.

PERSISTENT VEGETATIVE STATE

There is a clear difference between severe brain damage and brain death. Comatose patients with severe brain damage may recover (albeit with various degrees of disability) or remain in persistent coma (Fig. 44.1). Those

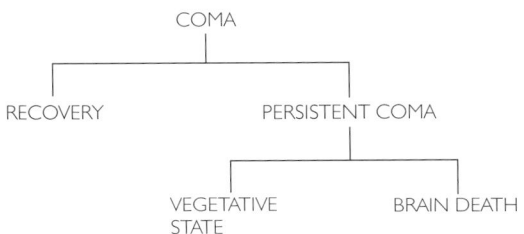

Fig. 44.1 The outcome of coma.

who remain in a persistent vegetative state (PVS) have lost cortical (higher brain) activity, but are able to breathe spontaneously. If properly cared for, PVS patients can live a considerable time. Patients with brain death due to permanent structural brain damage have irreversible loss of consciousness and the capacity to breathe.

ESTABLISHMENT OF BRAIN DEATH CRITERIA

The concept of accepting a clinical state of brain death as 'death' was proposed in 1968 by Harvard Medical School (the Harvard Criteria).[2] Two neurosurgeons introduced in 1971 the diagnostic importance of irreversible brainstem damage and emphasized that an EEG was not necessary for diagnosis (the Minnesota Criteria).[3] The Statement on brain death made in 1976 and 1979 by the UK Medical Royal Colleges and their Faculties[4,5] defined brain death as a complete, irreversible loss of brainstem function, and specified clinical criteria to certify brain death. In the USA, the Report to the President's Commission[6] confirmed in 1981 the need for the irreversible cessation of the brain and brainstem function to diagnose death. This Report recommended confirmatory tests to reduce the required time of observation. Current guidelines to certify brain death in Australasia, the UK and many countries are based on the UK Statement and the US Report.

ROLE OF THE BRAINSTEM

The brainstem maintains consciousness and the sleep–waking cycle. Pathways through the brainstem are required for cranial nerve reflexes and voluntary and coordinated trunk and limb movement. The pathways serving eye movements pass through both the mid-brain and pons. Spontaneous ventilation is dependent on medullary nuclei. As brain death occurs, the patient loses brainstem reflexes in a caudal direction, and complete brainstem destruction may take several hours. The medulla oblongata is the last part of the brainstem to cease functioning. Brain death will always result in cardiac asystole within days or weeks, despite continuation of mechanical ventilation and full life-support.[7] Myocardial function progressively deteriorates but the pathogenesis is unclear.

CLINICAL PROCEDURE TO DIAGNOSE BRAIN DEATH [8–11]

PRECONDITIONS

Certain preconditions and exclusions must be fulfilled before considering a diagnosis of brain death.

1 THE PATIENT'S CONDITION IS DUE TO IRREVERSIBLE STRUCTURAL BRAIN DAMAGE

The diagnosis of a disorder that can lead to brain death must be established. This is fairly straightforward in head injuries and cerebrovascular bleeds, but confirmation of the diagnosis may take longer in coma of hypoxic or other causes. A CT scan and full neurological examinations are essential.

2 THE PATIENT IS DEEPLY COMATOSE

(a) Effects of depressant drugs must be excluded. The drug history should be obtained or reviewed; if suspicion so indicates, a toxicology screen is obtained. Assays of drugs detected in blood or urine may be necessary. If a depressant drug is present, adequate time must be allowed for its effects to be excluded. This is especially important when pharmacological toxic effects were the cause of the coma and resultant hypoxic brain destruction. The observation period depends on the drug pharmacokinetics, dose used, half-life, and the patient's renal and hepatic status. This period could last four times the drug's half-life, or until the blood concentration decreases below its therapeutic range. Most commonly used drugs would be adequately cleared within 8–12 hours, but a longer observation period may be advisable if the clinician suspects the presence of an undetected drug.

(b) Hypothermia as a cause of coma must be excluded. Body temperature may be low because of depression of temperature regulation by drugs or brainstem damage. Core temperature should be at least 35°C (and achieved by active warming if necessary) before diagnostic tests are performed. A low reading thermometer should be used.

(c) Metabolic or endocrine disturbances that may cause or contribute to coma must be excluded. Possible factors should be carefully assessed. There must be no profound abnormality of serum urea and electrolytes, acid–base status, or blood glucose concentrations.

3 THE PATIENT IS APNOEIC

The patient must be on a ventilator with no spontaneous breathing efforts. Effects of muscle relaxants if used, must be excluded by demonstrating intact neuromuscular conductance with a peripheral nerve stimulator. Persistent effects of opioids and central depressants on respiration must also be excluded.

DIAGNOSTIC TESTS TO CONFIRM BRAIN DEATH [8–12]

These tests are intended to demonstrate the absence of brainstem reflexes in brain death. They should not be performed in the presence of seizures. Facial trauma or obstruction to both external ear canals may preclude adequate assessment (see below).

1 Motor responses within the cranial nerve distribution (e.g. grimacing) are absent when painful stimuli are applied to any somatic area, for example, pressing on the supraorbital nerve, temporomandibular joint, or finger nail bed. (Tests trigeminal V sensory supply to upper face and facial VII cranial nerves.) Tendon stretch reflexes and plantar reflexes are of spinal cord origin, and may persist in the presence of brainstem death.[3]

2 Both pupils are fixed in diameter and unresponsive to bright light (direct and consensual responses). Pupil size is irrelevant, although most will be dilated. (Tests oculomotor III cranial nerve.)

3 Corneal reflexes are absent in response to a firm touch on the cornea using a cotton wool swab. (Tests trigeminal V and facial VII cranial nerves.)

4 Vestibulo-ocular reflexes are absent (the caloric response). No eye movement occurs during or after a slow injection of 20 ml of ice-cold water into one, or preferably each, ear canal. Intact reflexes show movement towards the side of cold stimulus. Clear access to the tympanic membrane must be confirmed by direct inspection with an auroscope. (Tests vestibulo-cochlear VIII, occulomotor III and abducen VI cranial nerves.)

5 The gag and cough reflexes are absent in response to pharyngeal, laryngeal or tracheal stimulation. (Tests glossopharyngeal IX and vagus X cranial nerves.)

6 Spontaneous ventilation is absent. Testing for apnoea involves disconnection from the ventilator when $PaCO_2$ is near normal, ensuring that it reaches the threshold required to stimulate the medullary centre, and observing the patient for respiratory movements. Normally, a $PaCO_2$ of 50 mmHg (6.7 kPa) would be sufficient to stimulate the medullary centre, but a threshold of 60 mmHg (8 kPa) is recommended. Arterial blood gas analysis must be used to assess $PaCO_2$. A decrease in arterial pH to 7.30 will also confirm that respiratory stimulus is adequate.

Ventilation with 5% carbon dioxide in oxygen can be used to increase $PaCO_2$ and achieve some denitrogenation before ventilator disconnection. Alternatively, $PaCO_2$ is allowed to rise with apnoea, after first ventilating with 100% oxygen. Hypoxia is avoided during apnoea by diffusion oxygenation via a catheter delivering 4–6 l/min of oxygen into the trachea. The rate of rise of $PaCO_2$ during apnoea is about 3 mmHg/min (0.40 kPa), but is reduced in these patients who are mildly hypothermic and flaccid with a depressed metabolic rate. The threshold $PaCO_2$ in patients with chronic obstructive airways disease need to be increased accordingly, for example, 20 mmHg (2.67 Pa) above the patient's baseline value.

CONFIRMATORY TESTS

Some jurisdictions (but not in the UK, Australia or New Zealand) require tests to confirm the clinical criteria of brain death.[12] Confirmatory tests are required if conditions for clinical criteria cannot be met (Table 44.1). The following confirmatory tests have been used.

1 *Electroencephalography.* Recordings are obtained for over 30 minutes using at least 8 scalp electrodes to demonstrate absence of electrical activity. Artefacts from the high levels of sensitivity used are common, due to the ICU environment. The EEG does not adequately assess brainstem function but is used in selected patients such as young children (see below).
2 *Cerebral angiography.* Four-vessel angiography (injection of contrast medium into both vertebral and carotid arteries from the aortic arch) or three-vessel angiography (both carotid arteries and a basilar artery) will confirm absence of intracerebral filling at the level of vessel entry into the skull.

Table 44.1 Indications for confirmatory tests to diagnose brain death

No clear cause for coma exists
Possible drug or metabolic effect on coma
Cranial nerves cannot be adequately tested
Cervical vertebra or cord injury is present
Cardiorespiratory instability that precludes testing for apnoea

Ischaemia oedema, and death of brain tissue cause increased intracranial pressure and occlusion of blood flow. Isolated or minimal filling will necessitate a repeat examination. Cerebral angiography is invasive, cumbersome and time-consuming, involving patient transfer to the Radiology Suite.
3 *Magnetic resonance imaging.* Diffusion-weighted MRI can show structural changes secondary to brain death,[13] but its use is time-consuming and cumbersome.
4 *Transcranial Doppler ultrasonography.*[14–16] This is a relatively new and, being non-invasive, more easily applied test. The middle cerebral and vertebral arteries are examined and recordings are compared with extracranial vessel recordings. Occlusion of blood flow in brain death is manifested by (i) oscillating signals, (ii) systolic spikes and (iii) disappearance of flow signals. In brain death, systolic flow expands the arterial tree without any flow through the microcirculation. During diastole, the contractive forces of the arteries force flow in the reverse direction, thus giving rise to oscillating flow signals. Systolic spikes are signals in early systole with very short peak velocities due to reduced blood movement. Ventricular drains or skull openings may interfere with recordings.
5 *Radionuclide imaging.*[17] This is increasingly used in place of cerebral angiography. Imaging of radioactive-labelled substances that cross the blood–brain barrier, such as technetium-99m, can reliably show absence of brain perfusion in brain death ('hollow-skull' sign).
6 *Multimodality evoked potentials* can demonstrate successive loss of function of various afferent pathways of the brainstem. Their use to confirm brain death is advocated by some,[18] but this remains to be validated.

In the unusual situation of the brainstem being the primary site of injury with loss of all reflexes, but confirmatory tests reveal residual blood flow to the supratentorial part of the brain, brain death cannot be diagnosed.

OTHER CONSIDERATIONS

1 *Retesting.* Two full and separate examinations are usually required to demonstrate irreversibility. The first should be undertaken after at least 4 hours of observed coma and absent cough, gag, and muscle activity. The second examination should be carried out after an interval of at least 6 hours.[8,11] For victims of primary hypoxic brain damage and encephalitis, prolonged observation periods before both examinations are recommended.
2 *Assessors.* Protocols for diagnosing brain death may require examination by two doctors. Separate examinations are not always specified, but should be undertaken. Both doctors may be present at both examinations. Rather than being specifically neurosurgeons or neurologists, the doctors should have the

experience, expertise and authority to conduct the examinations. Neither doctor should be principally involved in organ removal or transplant.

3 *Certification of death.* Laws in many countries such as Australia specify that death must be certified by the two doctors who conducted the examinations. The time of death for certification purposes will be the time after the second confirmatory examination.

4 *Spontaneous movements* of the limbs, neck or body, and deep tendon, abdominal, and Babinski reflexes may be seen. These are generated by the spine and are compatible with, and do not invalidate, the diagnosis of brain death.

5 *Atropine* 0.6–1.0 mg i.v. has been used. An increase in heart rate denotes persistent medullary activity, but changes are often inconclusive. It is unreliable in a patient with autonomic neuropathy. Nil increase in heart rate indicates loss of vagal tone but does not unequivocally indicate circulatory arrest. It is not a requirement for assessing brain death.

6 *Oculocephalic reflex.* Absence of the oculocephalic reflex (denoted by the eyes remaining fixed when the head is briskly turned side-to-side (i.e 'doll's eye phenomenon') is not a requirement. Confirmation of the sign is often subjective.

7 *Misdiagnosis.* There has been no report of a patient who developed clinically detectable brain function after having fulfilled the criteria for brain death. There is no evidence to suggest errors in diagnosing brain death if the examination is properly conducted. None the less, some conditions may mimic brain death, such as severe hypothermia, drug intoxication, locked-in syndrome, and Guillain–Barré syndrome.[19] Strict adherence to the preconditions and assessment of brain death, and knowledge of the history of illness will eliminate these conditions to prevent errors.

8 *Policies and protocols* must be developed by hospitals for diagnosing brain death. These should include educational information, a list of designated assessing doctors, standard forms, and organ donation procedures.

BRAIN DEATH IN CHILDREN

Caution is recommended in applying the above brain death testing criteria in children under 5 years old, on the assumption that the young brain has a greater capacity for recovery after acute damage. In general, the same principles for adults are applied, but a longer observation period and a confirmatory test (EEG or cerebral blood flow study) are usually conducted. The following modifications have been recommended.[20]

● *Term newborns to 2 months.* A clinical examination and a radionuclide brain flow study be done.

● *2 months to 1 year.* Two examinations and EEGs, separated by 24 hours, need to be performed. The second examination and EEG can be omitted if absent cerebral blood flow is demonstrated by a radionuclide study.

● *Over 1 year.* Criteria are the same as those for older children and adults. An observation period of at least 12 hours is recommended, and longer for those with hypoxic/ischaemic coma.

REFERENCES

1 Pallis C. ABC of brainstem death. Reappraising death. *BMJ* 1982, **285**: 1409–12.

2 Ad Hoc Committee of the Harvard Medical School. A definition of irreversible coma. *JAMA* 1968; **205**: 85–8.

3 Mohandas A, Chou SN. Brain death – a clinical and pathological study. *J Neurosurg* 1971; **35**: 211–18.

4 Conference of Medical Royal Colleges and their Faculties in the UK. Diagnosis of brain death. *BMJ* 1976; **2**: 1187–8.

5 Conference of Medical Royal Colleges and their Faculties in the UK. Diagnosis of brain death. *BMJ* 1979; **i**: 3320.

6 Report of the Medical Consultants on the Diagnosis of Death to the President's Commission for the Study of Ethical Problems in Medicine and Biomedical and Behavioural Research. Guidelines for the determination of death. *JAMA* 1981; **246**: 2184–6.

7 Pallis C. Prognostic significance of a dead brainstem. *BMJ* 1983; **286**: 123–4.

8 Recommendations on Brain Death and Organ Donation, 2nd edn. Australian and New Zealand Intensive Care Society, Melbourne; 1998

9 Widjicks EFM. Current concepts: the diagnosis of brain death. *N Engl J Med* 2001; 344: 1215–21.

10 Canadian Neurocritical Care Group. Guidelines for the diagnosis of brain death. *Can J Neurol Sci* 1999; **26**: 64–66.

11 Pallis C. Diagnosis of brainstem death I and II. *BMJ* 1982; **285**: 1558–60, 1641–4.

12 Haupt WF, Rudolf J. European brain death codes: a comparison of national guidelines. *J Neurol* 2000; **246**: 432–7.

13 Lovblad KO, Bassetti C. Diffusion-weighted magnetic resonance imaging in brain death. *Stroke* 1999; **31**: 539–42.

14 Ducrocq X, Hassler W, Moritake K, *et al.* Consensus opinion on diagnosis of cerebral circulatory arrest using Doppler-sonography. *J Neurol Sci* 1998; **159**: 145–50.

15 Azevedo E, Teixeira J, Neves JC, Vaz R. Transcranial doppler and brain death. *Transplant Proc* 2000; **32**: 2579–81.

16 Hadani M, Bruk B, Ram Z, *et al.* Application of transcranial doppler for the diagnosis of brain death. *Intensive Care Med* 1999; **25**: 822–8.

17 Weckesser M, Schober O. Brain death revisited: Utility confirmed for nuclear medicine. *Eur J Nucl Med* 1999; **26**: 1387–91.

18 De Tourtchaninoff M, Hantson P, Mahieu P, Guerit JM. Brain death diagnosis in misleading conditions. *Q J Med* 1999; **92**: 407–14.

19 Vargas F, Hilbert O, Gruson D, *et al.* Fulminant Guillain–Barré syndrome mimicking cerebral death. *Intensive Care Med* 2000; **26**: 623–7

20 Task Force for the Determination of Brain Death in Children. Guidelines for the determination of brain death in children. *Arch Neurol* 1998; **44**: 587–8.

45

Meningitis and encephalomyelitis
A Kennedy

Infections of the cranial contents can be divided into those which affect the meninges (meningitis) and those which affect the brain parenchyma (encephalitis). Chronic, insidious or rare infections are beyond the scope of this chapter which will focus on acute bacterial and viral causes of meningitis and encephalomyelitis.

- *Meningitis*: defined as infection or inflammation of the meninges and subarachnoid space. The infection can be caused by viruses, bacteria, fungi or protozoa. Meningeal inflammation may be caused by subarachnoid haemorrhage, vaccination or be a manifestation of other multiorgan diseases, such as systemic lupus erythematosus, sarcoidosis, lymphoma or multiple meningeal metastases from a disseminated carcinoma.
- *Aseptic meningitis*: aseptic meningitis is a generic term for cases of meningitis in which bacteria cannot be isolated from the cerebrospinal fluid. The differential diagnosis in this situation includes: (1) viral meningitis; (2) partially treated bacterial meningitis; (3) TB meningitis; (4) fungal meningitis; (5) lymphoma; (6) sarcoidosis; and (7) other collagen vascular diseases. The most common causes of aseptic meningitis are due to viral infection most often due to an enterovirus or coxsackie infection.
- *Encephalitis*: encephalitis is an infection of the brain parenchyma.
- *Tuberculous meningitis*: causes a subacute lymphocytic meningitis. Patients may have a non-specific prodromal phase, including symptoms such as headache, vomiting and fever.
- *Subdural empyema*: subdural empyema is a suppurative process in the space between the pia and dura mata.
- *Brain abscess*: Brain abscess is a collection of pus within the brain tissue.

BACTERIAL MENINGITIS

GENERAL POINTS

Bacterial meningitis is an inflammatory response due to infection of the lepto meninges and subarachnoid space. This is characterized by the clinical syndrome of fever, headache, neck stiffness and cerebrospinal fluid pleocytosis.

The bacterial organisms are usually not confined to the brain and meninges and frequently cause systemic illness; for example, severe sepsis, shock, acute respiratory distress syndrome, and bleeding disorders such as disseminated intra-vascular coagulation.[1,2]

A variety of other pathogens cause meningeal inflammation, resulting in very similar clinical presentations. Bacterial infections must be treated urgently and appropriately to limit ongoing central nervous system damage. It is also important to treat the complications of meningitis such as seizures and raised intracranial pressure (ICP).

Where possible, spinal fluid examination following a lumbar puncture is required in order to confirm the diagnosis and establish the pathogenic organism responsible. A cerebrospinal fluid (CSF) examination may be contraindicated if there are signs of raised intracranial pressure, including:

- papilloedema
- focal neurological signs
- seizures

These features raise the possibility of an undiagnosed cerebral mass lesion which, in turn, could cause cerebral herniation should lumbar puncture be performed. A computed tomography (CT) brain scan is required prior to CSF examination in order to rule out this possibility. Even if the CT brain scan is normal, intracranial pressure may be raised. The importance of performing a safe CSF examination must be balanced against the need to commence immediate treatment in each individual patient.[3,4]

AETIOLOGY

The three main causes of meningitis are spread by droplet infection or exchange of saliva. Meningitis may occur when pathogenic organisms colonize the naso pharynx and reach the blood–brain barrier. Meningitis can occur as a result of infection in the middle ear, sinus or teeth leading to secondary meningeal infection. Most bacteria obtain entry into the central nervous system via the haematogenous route. As the organisms multiply, they release cell wall products and lipopolysaccharide, and generate a local inflammatory reaction which in itself also releases inflammatory mediators. The net result of the release of cytokines, tumour necrosis factor and other factors is associated with a significant inflammatory response. Vasculitis of central nervous system (CNS) vessels, thrombosis, cell damage and exudative material all contribute to vasogenic and cytotoxic oedema, altered blood flow and cerebral perfusion pressure. Later on infarction and raised intracranial pressure occur.[5]

The inflammatory events seen with infection are summarized in Fig. 45.1.

ORGANISMS

Acute bacterial meningitis can be caused by many species of bacteria, although three organisms are commonly reported, including:

- *Haemophilus influenzae*
- *Streptococcus pneumoniae*
- *Neisseria meningitidis* (which account for 70% of cases in the neonatal period)

Until the advent of the meningitis vaccination programme *H. influenzae* type B was the most common cause of bacterial meningitis. Recently *S. pneumoniae* and *N. meningitidis* are considered the main causes, although one study suggested that *Listeria monocytogenes* is the second most common isolate in adult population. The occurrence of pneumococcal strains which are resistant to penicillin has also influenced the epidemilogy of meningitis.[6]

NOSOCOMIAL INFECTIONS
Common systemic nosocomial pathogens such as *Escherichia coli*, *Pseudomonas* spp., *Klebsiella* and *Acinetobacter* spp. account for a high percentage of nosocomial infections of the meninges.

IMMUNOCOMPROMISED HOSTS
In the immunocompromised patient with meningitis (e.g. human immunodeficiency virus, HIV), fungal viral and cryptocococal meningitis should be considered.[7]

NEUROSURGERY AND TRAUMA
Infections following skull trauma are frequently caused by *Staphylococcus aureus* and *Staphylococcus epidermis*

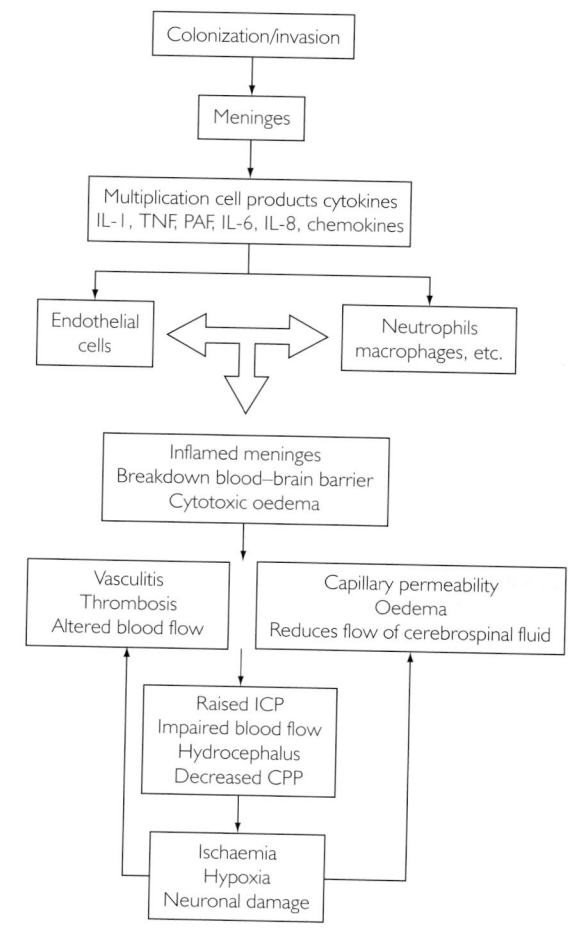

Fig. 45.1 Cascade of events in meningitis

which should be considered in those with shunts or other intra-cranial devices.

CLINICAL PRESENTATION

The history may reveal evidence of trauma or infection. Meningitis usually presents with an acute onset of:

- Fever
- Headache
- Neck stiffness
- Photophobia
- Altered conscious level
- Irritabilty
- Seizures (paediatric)

However, in the immunocompromised, elderly or infant patient, non-specific features such as a low-grade fever or mild behavioural change may be all that is apparent.

It is important to identify from the history reports about preceding trauma, upper respiratory tract infection or ear infection. Symptoms may develop over hours or days. Specific infections relate partly to an individual's age.

Neurological signs can be present with meningitis but signs such as nuchal rigidity, stiffness and a positive Kernigs sign (pain and hamstring spasm resulting from attempts to straighten, e.g. with the hip flexed), in addition to Brudzinski's sign (neck flexion produces flexion of lower limbs) should be noted. There may be focal neurological signs. Systemic signs may occur most often in meningococcal disease where a haemorrhagic, petechial or purpuric rash may be observed. Digital gangrene or skin necrosis may occur. Some patients are severely septic with acute respiratory distress syndrome and disseminated intravascular coagulation.

Approximately 25% of patients have a seizure during the course of the illness. Differential diagnosis may include subarachnoid haemorrhage, migraine, encephalitis and tumour.

INVESTIGATIONS

The patient with suspected bacterial meningitis requires immediate blood cultures and should be given empirical i.v. antibiotics if there is likely to be any delay in further assessment (Table 45.1).

CSF FINDINGS

The pressure may be raised (CT first)

- Polymorph leukocystosis
- Low CSF glucose relative to the plasma value
- Raised CSF protein concentration

An urgent gram stain and microbiological culture is mandatory. The gram stain is usually positive in approximately 50–60% of cases. A CSF examination shortly after empirical antibiotics does not necessarily decrease the diagnostic sensitivity of CSF culture. Polymerase chain reaction (PCR) techniques can be used to detect different organisms. A throat swab should be routinely taken.

Blood cultures comprise an important investigation in patients with meningitis, as spread is haematogenous, and a number of sets of cultures should be sent. It is advisable to routinely check a full blood count clotting profile and biochemistry including blood glucose level. A chest X-ray and blood gases should be performed to identify systemic involvement. Obviously, relevant areas such as infected sinuses or ears should be examined if there is an indication that they are implicated.

MANAGEMENT

Antibiotics should be started as early as possible (Table 45.2). The selection of antibiotics is influenced by the clinical situation in conjunction with known allergies or local patterns of antibiotic resistance and the CSF findings. Delays in administering antibiotics are a significant risk factor for a poor prognosis. In the absence of a known organism, empirical choice for antibiotics has been complicated by the development of resistance strains. Penicillin G, ampicillin and third generation

Table 45.1   Cerebrospinal fluid changes in meningitis

	Normal	Bacterial	Viral
Appearance	Clear	Turbid/purulent	Clear/turbid
White cell count	<5 per mm³ mononuclear	200–10 000 per mm³ predominantly polymorphonuclear	<500 per mm³ mainly lymphocytes
Protein	0.2–0.4 g/l	0.5–2.0 g/l	0.4–0.8 g/l
Glucose	Blood glucose	≤ Blood glucose	Blood glucose pressure is usually raised

Table 45.2   Empiric antibiotics for meningitis

Indication	Antibiotic	Dose
<50 years	Ceftriaxone or cefotaxime	2–4 g q. 24 h 2 g q. 4 h
>50 years or impaired cell immunity	Ceftriaxone	2–4 g q. 24 h
	or cefotaxime	2 g q. 4 h
	Cefotaxime + ampicillin or penicillin G	2 g q. 4 h or 3–4 MU q. 4 h
Drug resistant *Strep pneumoniae*	Ceftriaxone	2-4 g q. 8 h
	+ rifampicin	2 g q. 4 h
	or vancomycin	0.5 g q. 6 h
Neurosurgery shunts trauma	Ceftazidime	2 g q. 8 h
	+ nafcillin or	2 g q.4 h
	Vancomycin +	0.5 g q. 6 h
	aminoglycoside 2 mg l kg q. 8 h. (gentamicin 5–7 mg/kg stat)	

cephalosporins are typical first line agents. Until recently, ampicillin was appropriate for pneumococcal, meningococcal and listeria infections. The emergence of resistant strains influences local antibiotic practice. If there is a history of recent head injury, a broad spectrum cephalosporin may be indicated with vancomycin. Discussions with local microbiology services are recommended. If the CSF examination identifies the organism, then specific regimens can be prescribed (Table 45.3).

It is more difficult to select an appropriate empirical antibiotic in the immunocompromised patient. When the organism has been identified and sensitivity results are available, it may be necessary either to change the antibiotic or to rationalize those being given.[8,9]

In all cases, it is important to monitor the clinical response to therapy and, if necessary, antibiotics should be reviewed and appropriately altered once antibiotic sensitivities are known or a patient is not considered to be improving. A repeat CSF examination should be performed if there is concern about antibiotic sensitivity or selection. In those with penicillin resistant pneumococcal meningitis, a CSF examination 48 h after presentation is recommended to ensure bacteriological improvement. Antibiotics should be given for 10–14 days, although a shorter course may be adequate in some circumstances. Intrathecal antibiotics are not recommended.

STEROID ADMINISTRATION

A few large clinical trials have shown some benefits for steroid administration in paediatric meningitis. These studies confirm a benefit for those with *H. influenzae* type B infection and reduce the frequency of post meningitis deafness.

RECOMMENDATIONS

15 mg/kg i.v. 6-hourly for 4 days starting and correlating with antibiotics administration.

Indications for steroid therapy in meningitis in adults are less clear. There have been some reported benefits in pneumococcal patients but it is possible that steroids may influence the penetration of antibiotics in the CSF.

ANTICONVULSANTS

Focal or generalized seizures should be treated immediately with i.v. benzodiazepines to stop the seizures and the individual then subsequently loaded with i.v. phenytoin. The possibility of the following should be considered

- Raised intracranial pressure
- Cerebritis
- Cerebral abscess
- Septic venous thombosis

The development of seizures may be indicative of a poor prognosis.

ICP

Intracranial hypertension is a common complication of meningitis. Intracranial pressure monitoring may be required and standard measures such as hyperventilation, mannitol infusion or CSF drainage may be considered. Depending upon the particular circumstance, serial lumbar punctures or external ventricular drainage should be implemented.

GENERAL MANAGEMENT CONSIDERATIONS[10]

INTRAVENOUS FLUID THERAPY

Normal haemodynamics should be maintained. Currently, there is emphasis on maintaining the cerebral perfusion pressure at around 70 mmHg. Inappropriate antidiuretic hormone secretion may occur in meningitis.

RESPIRATORY

It is important to secure the airway and respiratory support may be required for those with severe shock or profound coma. Attention should be paid to management of the unconscious patient with appropriate mouth and eye care. Physiotherapy will be required in order to prevent the onset of pressure sores. Surgical evaluation may be needed for skin necrosis.[11,12]

PUBLIC HEALTH

Meningitis prophylaxis is commended for close (kissing contacts) associates and for those medical personnel with

Table 45.3 General recommendation for known organisms. Always check local sensitiviity as resistance patterns are variable

Organism	Antibiotic	2nd line or allergy
Strep pneumoniae (penicillin resistant)	Ceftriaxone + Vancomycin or Rifampicin	Vancomycin + rifampicin
Penicillin sensitive	Penicillin G	Ceftriaxone or chloramphenicol
β-haemolytic strep	Penicillin or ampicillin	Cefotaxime or chloramphenicol or vancomycin
Haemophilus influenzae	Ceftriaxone or cefotaxime	Chloramphenicol
Neisseria meningitidis	Penicillin G	Ceftriaxone or chloramphenicol
Listeria monocytogenes	Ampicillin + gentamicin	Trimethoprim = sulphamethoxazole
Enterobacteriaceae	Ceftriaxone + gentamicin	Quinolones
Pseudomonas aeruginosa	Ceftazidime + tobramycin	Quinolones

close contact. A 2-day course of oral rifampacin 600 mg 12 hourly is recommended. There should be procedures for alerting infectious disease team.

PROGNOSIS

Untreated bacterial meningitis is usually fatal. Appropriate therapy significantly reduces the mortality rate; however, recent studies still show that the overall mortality is approximately 18%. Mortality is slightly higher in those who have seizures and when there have been delays introducing treatment, or it the patient is elderly or very young[12,13] (Table 45.3).

VIRAL MENINGITIS

The majority of cases of viral meningitis are benign usually self-limiting conditions which are often caused by enterovirus or coxsackie infection. Some are caused by arboviruses. The same viruses that produce meningitis can also cause encephalitis. Herpes simplex virus type 1 usually produces encephalitis but rarely causes meningitis. Other viruses causing CNS infections include echoviruses, mumps, polio and HIV.

CLINICAL PRESENTATION

Patients usually present symptoms of meningeal irritation, fever, headache, neck stiffness, retrobulbar pain, photophobia, vertigo, nausea and vomiting which are less severe than those with bacterial meningitis. The presence of intellectual impairment, focal neurological symptoms or seizures suggest that the brain parenchyma is involved and, consequently, these are due to meningoencephalitis. True viral meningitis develops over hours to days but rarely lasts longer than 7–10 days. A variety of associated symptoms, such as nausea, vomiting and generalized malaise, may accompany this condition.[14]

INVESTIGATIONS

A CSF examination is important and usually shows:

- A mild to moderate lymphocytic pleocytosis
- A mildly elevated CSF protein concentration
- Normal glucose concentration.

Staining for microorganisms, including bacteria, mycobacterium tuberculosis and cryptococcal meningitis, may be necessary. Sites for culture include the mucous membranes, throat, skin and rectum.

MANAGEMENT

Acute viral meningitis is usually a self-limiting condition and only supportive therapy is required with analgesia and bedrest. Viral meningitis caused by Herpes Simplex Virus (HSV) 1 or II may require i.v. acyclovir. Acute HIV infection causing meningitis may respond to retroviral therapy.

ENCEPHALITIS

Encephalitis is a viral infection of the brain. HSV 1 is the most common cause of focal encephalitis, which usually affects the temporal and frontal lobes. There are a large number of arboviruses that cause epidemics of encephalitis. These are usually borne by arthropod vectors, such as mosquitoes and ticks, and therefore are considered as airborne viruses.[15]

CLINICAL PRESENTATION

The key clinical pointer of encephalitis is the presence of focal neurological symptoms indicating involvement of the brain parenchyma. Particularly, the presence of speech disturbance, seizures, altered cognition, disturbance of conscious level suggest this.

Diagnosis is difficult.

- Abnormalities on cranial imaging such as T2-weighted magnetic resonance imaging (MRI) may support this diagnosis (Fig. 45.2)
- Electroencephalogram (EEG) studies may show slow wave activity or epileptiform discharges in temporal lobe.
- PCR examination of the CSF examination may confirm the virus at a later date.

TREATMENT

Specific treatment for HSV encephalitis requires i.v. acyclovir at a dose of 30 mg/kg per day for 14 days. Left untreated, the mortality of HSV encephalitis is approximately 70% but there is still a 25% mortality in patients treated with optimal therapy. Patients can be left with significant disability in terms of cognitive dysfunction or seizures. Most patients with significant cerebral oedema receive empirical steroids, although there are no clinical trials to support this therapy. Acyclovir can cause renal impairment and the patient should be hydrated intravenously and renal function monitored.[16]

Cytomegalovirus (CMV) infection requires antiviral therapy with ganciclovir. CMV may cause a ganglionitis and polyradiculitis, which may suggest this diagnosis clinically in an immunocompromised patient.

Most CNS viruses cause neuronal damage but chronic Creuzfeldt–Jacob virus infection in oligodendrocyes causes the syndrome of progressive multifocal leukoencephalopathy (PML). This condition presents with a subacute onset of confusion, weakness and visual symptoms, usually in an immunosuppressed individual.

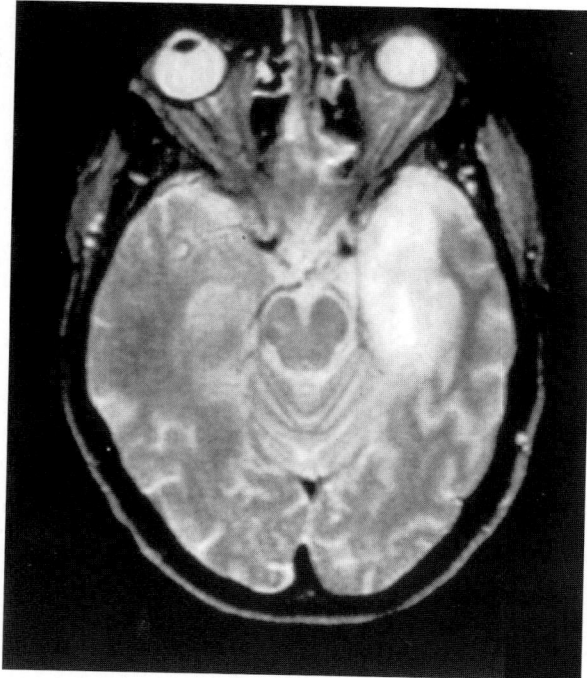

Fig. 45.2 Enhanced temporal lobe with Herpes encephalitis

The MRI scan is usually suggestive but CSF examination with PCR amplification of the Creuzfeldt–Jacob virus particles may be required. Currently, no specific therapy for PML exists. The survival of HIV patients with associated PML is poor, averaging 6 months in 90% of individuals.

Viral infection with HIV 1, measles and rubella can also cause chronic CNS infection leading to chronic encephalitides.

A number of systemic neurological conditions (e.g. lymphoma, Lyme disease, sarcoidosis and vasculides such as Behçets disease) may present with aseptic meningitis. It is therefore important to consider these systemic conditions in those presenting with viral meningitis or encephalitis.

TUBERCULOUS MENINGITIS

Tuberculous meningitis has a variable natural history with a range of different clinical presentations. This and the lack of specific and sensitive tests hinders the diagnosis of this condition. Approximately 10% of individuals with tuberculosis develop meningeal involvement. A variety of risk factors such as HIV, diabetes mellitus and the recent use of steroid use may increase the risk of tuberculous meningitis.[17]

CLINICAL FEATURES

Tuberculous meningitis has a very varied clinical presentation. Often, it is heralded by a non-specific prodromal phase, frequently but not necessarily including headache, vomiting and fever. Of one case series which included those admitted to an intensive care unit, only 65% had fever, 52% had focal neurology and 88% had signs of meningism. A variety of cranial nerve palsies can occur but other presentations include those seen with stroke, hydrocephalus and tuberculoma.

DIAGNOSIS

An investigation of the differential diagnosis of tuberculous meningitis is important. PCR amplification of mycobacterial DNA has not been fully evaluated in this technique which, in the case of TB meningitis, usually requires a lumbar puncture examination. Those who are immunosuppressed may have atypical CSF appearance including normal CSF examinations in occasional HIV individuals. Tuberculosis culture from CSF is required but may take up to 6 weeks before a positive culture result is available. Imaging studies may show a basal meningitis and hydrocephalus but these features are non-specific.[18]

Current advice suggests that the first 2 months of treatment should comprise quadruple therapy:

- Isoniazid oral/i.v. 10 mg/kg per day up to 300 mg. It is bactericidal and has good CNS penetration.
- Pyrazinamide oral/i.v. 25 mg/kg per day up to 2.5 g/day.
- Rifampicin high dosage as poor penetration, 10 mg/kg per day up to 600 mg.
- Ethambutol i.v. high dosage as it is highly protein bound and therefore has poor penetration.

Streptomycin is used rarely. The toxicity of the agents must be monitored in terms of renal and liver function and the effect on other organs such as the eye.

There is increasing multi drug resistant tuberculous meningitis, especially in the HIV positive population and so sensitivity is important. Some clinical trials suggest that steroids have a beneficial effect in some groups of patients.[19] Patients may require neurosurgical intervention for the treatment of hydrocephalus.

SUBDURAL EMPYEMA

This is a collection of pus between the dural and arachnoid space and usually is a consequence of middle ear or sinus disease. It may follow cranial osteomyelitis related to previous neurosurgery. Head trauma can also be responsible.

Individuals present acutely with headache, fever, neck stiffness, seizures and focal neurological symptoms. Meningeal signs and evidence of hemispheric dysfunction with sinusitis should suggest the diagnosis.

DIAGNOSIS

CT and MRI are both effective in demonstrating a fluid collection.

Surgical intervention, drainage and appropriate antibiotic regimes are required. Both Gram-positive, staphylococcus and streptococcus and Gram-negative organisms may be implicated. Initial broad spectrum cover should be narrowed to targeted treatment when the organism or organisms are known.

PROGNOSIS

This condition if left untreated is invariably fatal. With treatment mortality is in the order of 20% and neurological sequelae are common.

EPIDURAL INFECTION

Cranial and spinal epidural abscess is an infection between skull and dura often as a consequence of osteomyelitis, from an orbital infection or malignancy. There is a very low but occasional incidence following an epidural. It is similar to subdural empyema. The organism involved where a catheter or drain is implicated is often the same as that found at the skin; hence, *Staphylococcus aureus* is frequently responsible.

PRESENTATION

Commonly present on the back, which may be generalized to the area of the back involved. There may be local tenderness over the site associated with redness of the catheter insertion site. Fever is common. Initially mild neurological deficit may rapidly progress leading to para/quadrapareses.

Blood cultures may be positive and may indicate the organism.

DIAGNOSIS

CT and MRI are both effective in diagnosis.

Spinal decompression and drainage is urgently required. This usually a nosocomial infection and therefore resistant organisms are commonly found. Antibiotics should be specific for the organisms involved and may need to be continued for prolonged periods, often weeks, to eradicate the infection.

Where there have been neurogical symptoms and signs prior to surgery, residual deficit is common. In one series, the recovery rate for patients with paresis/plegia after lumbar epidural abscess was 50%, while no patients with paresis/plegia following a thoracic abscess recovered. The majority of long-term survivors had severe neurological deficits.

CEREBRAL VENOUS AND SAGITTAL SINUS THROMBOSIS

Venous and sinus thrombosis may occur in the context of infection; in particular meningitis, and epidural or subdural abscess. It may also be secondary to facial or dental infection. It may have no septic aetiology but can occur either as an isolated event or in association with prothrombotic problems such as diabetic ketoacidosis, MDMA abuse (ectsasy), oral contraceptives and hereditary prothrombotic conditions in pregnancy.[20]

Clinical signs at presentation include:

- Headache
- Focal neurological deficits in particular cranial nerves
- Seizures
- Papilloedema

The diagnostic sensitivity of CT, MRI and digital subtract angiography are 59%, 86% and 100%, respectively but MRI with magnetic resonance angiography reaches 96% (Fig. 45.3).

TREATMENT

- Treat the primary infection if present
- Anticoagulants are the mainstay of treatment.

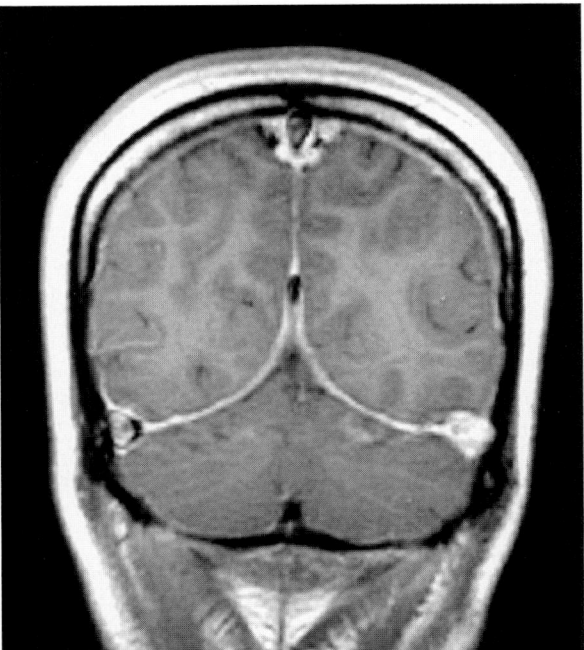

Fig. 45.3   Magnetic resonance imaging (MRI) of superior sagittal sinus thrombosis. Coronal T1-weighted post contrast MRI. Patient developed a sinus thrombosis following protracted labour and delivery

BRAIN ABSCESS

AETIOLOGY

Direct spread from bone or dura or may be via haemato-genous spread. Predisposition includes cranial trauma, neurosurgery, chronic ear or sinus disease, suppurative lung disease, congenital heart disease and recurrent sepsis. Immunological compromise may predispose to more exotic organisms but more common organisms include *Staphylococcus* spp. associated with trauma, and *Streptococcus*, *Bacteroides* and Gram-negative bacteria which are common with lung disease or recurrent sepsis.

PRESENTATION

Severe headache, vomiting, obtundation, seizures and focal neurological signs. Neck stiffness is often absent. Clinical sepsis may not be obvious.

DIAGNOSIS (Fig. 45.4)

- An obvious primary source of infection
- Evidence of raised ICP
- Focal cerebral or cerebellar signs.

INVESTIGATIONS

- Lumbar puncture is dangerous and contraindicated
- CT scan. Contrast will usually show enhancement.
- MRI

TREATMENT

Indications for surgery include large single lesions, relief of raised ICP and the need for tissue diagnosis.

Antibiotics are the mainstay of therapy. If the organism is known, then the treatment should be specific. In the absence of a definitive organism, penicillin plus chloram-phenicol (as for meningitis) and metronidazole 500 mg i.v. 8-hourly or 500 mg rectally 12-hourly should be empirical therapy. Cefotaxime 1–2 g i.v. 6–8-hourly and metronidazole 500 mg i.v. 8-hourly. If there is a recent history of trauma or neurosurgery, then a regimen that will cover staphylococcus should he used. Antibiotics should be continued for 3–6 weeks.

Supportive therapy limits morbidity, which is never-theless high. Mortality from cerebral abscesses is still 10–20%.[21]

LYME DISEASE

This is a tick borne multisystem disease with dermato-logical, cardiological, rheumatological and neurological effects caused by the spirochaete *Borrelia burgdorferi*.

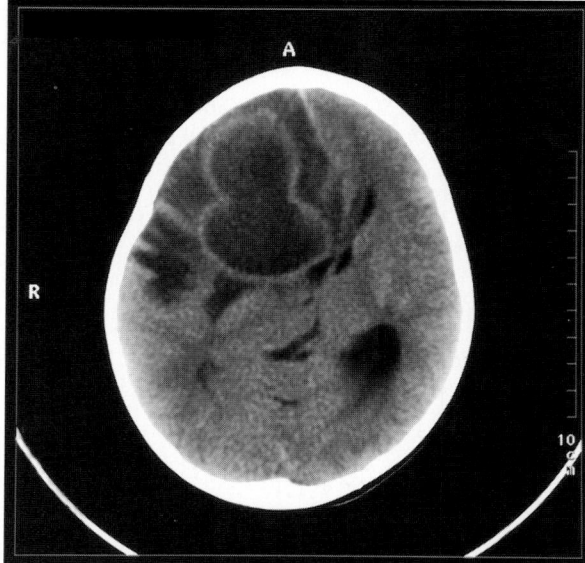

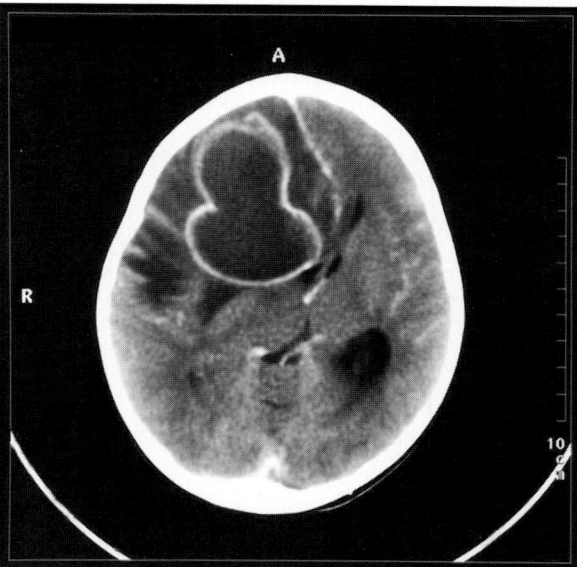

Fig. 45.4 Abscess: pre (a) and post (b) contrast

Usually presents as an acute febrile illness with gastro-intestinal upset, but it may present as an encephalitis or as a radiculitis. Facial palsy may occur. It may also present as a lymphocytic meningitis and may have been diag-nosed as a 'viral' meningitis in the past.

INVESTIGATIONS

CSF

White cell count is equivocal but may be raised. Protein is normal or marginally raised and sugar is normal or marginally low. Serology and ELISA may be difficult. PCR may be helpful. It may have characteristic MRI appearances. Vaccination is the only empirically demonstrated method to prevent Lyme disease.

TREATMENT

β-lactam antibacterials such as penicillin V, amoxicillin and cefuroxime are effective first-line treatment. The optimal duration of treatment is not known, but 10–21 days is recommended.[22,23]

OTHER DISEASES

There are several other diseases that may have an encephalopathic component. Cerebral malaria is dealt with elsewhere. Legionella may lead to subclinical or clinical neurological manifestations, ranging from headache to coma or encephalopathy usually seen in conjunction with pneumonia, in addition to possible renal impairment. Similarly, mycoplasma has been associated with an encephalitic picture characterized by impaired consciousness and seizures, and by normal or non-specific neuroradiological findings. Occasionally, symmetrical lesions in the putamen and its external surrounding areas have been seen.

Septic encephalopathy has been described as a common complication in the critically ill, presenting in a panoply of ways, from the agitated confused state seen in acute sepsis through to profound loss of consciousness. The aetiology is almost certainly multifactorial involving changes in cerebral blood flow, alteration in oxygen extraction, cerebral oedema, disruption of the blood–brain barrier, the presence and effects of diverse inflammatory mediators and abnormal neurotransmitter activity. Deranged liver and renal function contribute. It is a syndrome of exclusion based on observation and circumstantial evidence. The EEG is usually abnormal with decreased fast activity and an increase of slow wave activity, but the findings are not pathognomonic. There are no specific treatments. In general terms, outcome appears to correlate with the management of the underlying sepsis.[24]

REFERENCES

1 Isenberg H. Bacterial meningitis: signs and symptoms. *Antibiot Chemother* 1992; **45**: 79–95.
2 Spach DH, Jackson LA. Bacterial meningitis. *Neurol Clin* 1999; **17**: 711–35.
3 Roos KL. Acute bacterial meningitis. *Semin Neurol* 2000; **20**: 293–306.
4 Anderson M. Management of cerebral infection. *J Neurol Neurosurg Psychiatry* 1993; **56**: 1243–58.
5 Pfister HW, Fontana A, Tauber MG, *et al.* Mechanisms of brain injury in bacterial meningitis: workshop summary. *Clin Infect Dis* 1994; **19**: 463–79.
6 van Deuren M, Brandtzaeg P, van der Meer JW. Update on meningococcal disease with emphasis on pathogenesis and clinical management. *Clin Microbiol Rev* 2000; **13**: 144–66.
7 Gottfredsson M, Perfect JR. Fungal meningitis. *Semin Neurol* 2000; **20**: 307–22.
8 Vandecasteele SJ, Knockaert D, Verhaegen J, *et al.* The antibiotic and anti-inflammatory treatment of bacterial meningitis in adults: do we have to change our strategies in an era of increasing antibiotic resistance? *Acta Clin Belg* 2001; **56**: 225–33.
9 Tenover FC. Development and spread of bacterial resistance to antimicrobial agents; an overview. *Clin Infect Dis* 2001; **15**: S108–15.
10 Raser K, Deziel PJ. The danger of bacterial meningitis in the adult. 1. *JAAPA* 2001; **14**: 16–8, 21–4.
11 Hussein AS, Shafran SD. Acute bacterial meningitis in adults. A 12-year review. *Medicine (Baltimore)* 2000; **79**: 360–8.
12 Durand ML, Calderwood SB, Weber DJ, *et al.* Acute bacterial meningitis in adults. A review of 493 episodes. *N Engl J Med* 1993; **328**: 21–8.
13 Pfister HW, Feiden W, Einhaupl KM. Spectrum of complications during bacterial meningitis in adults. Results of a prospective clinical study. *Arch Neurol* 1993; **50**: 575–81.
14 Robert HA. Viral meningitis. *Semin Neurol* 2000; **20**: 277–92.
15 Schmutzhard E. Viral infections of the CNS with special emphasis on herpes simplex infections. *J Neurol* 2001; **248**: 469–77.
16 Gutierrez KM, Prober CG. Encephalitis. Identifying the specific cause is key to effective management. *Postgrad Med* 1998; **103**: 123–5, 129–30, 140–3.
17 Thwaites G, Chau TT, Mai NT, *et al.* Tuberculous meningitis. *J Neurol Neurosurg Psychiatry* 2000; **68**: 289–99.
18 Roos KL. Mycobacterium tuberculosis meningitis and other etiologies of the aseptic meningitis syndrome. *Semin Neurol* 2000; **20**: 329–35.
19 Prasad K, Volmink J, Menon GR. Steroids for treating tuberculous meningitis. *Cochrane Database Syst Rev* 2000; **3**: Cd002244.
20 de Bruijn SF, Stam J, Koopman MM, Vandenbroucke JP. Case-control study of risk of cerebral sinus thrombosis in oral contraceptive users and in carriers of hereditary prothrombotic conditions. The Cerebral Venous Sinus Thrombosis Study Group. *BMJ* 1998; **316**: 589–92.
21 Yildizhan A, Pasaoglu A, Ozkul MH, *et al.* Clinical analysis and results of operative treatment of 41 brain abscesses. *Neurosurg Rev* 1991; **14**: 279–82.
22 van Dam AP. Recent advances in the diagnosis of Lyme disease. *Expert Rev Mol Diagn* 2001; **1**: 413–27.
23 Glaser C, Lewis P, Wong S. Pet-, animal-, and vector-borne infections. *Pediatr Rev* 2000; **21**: 219–32.
24 Papadopoulos MC, Davies DC, Moss RF, *et al.* Pathophysiology of septic encephalopathy: a review. *Crit Care Med* 2000; **28**: 3019–24.

46

Tetanus

J Lipman

Tetanus is a preventable, often Third-World disease, frequently requiring expensive First-World technology to treat. It is an acute, often fatal disease caused by exotoxins produced by *Clostridium tetani,* and is characterized by generalized muscle rigidity, autonomic instability and sometimes convulsions.

EPIDEMIOLOGY

Recently, tetanus has become a disease of the elderly and debilitated in developed countries, as younger people are likely to have been immunized.[1] In the USA, its incidence decreased from 0.23 per 100 000 in 1955 to 0.04 per 100 000 in 1975, and remained stable thereafter.[1] The annual world mortality from tetanus is estimated to be 400 000–2 000 000. Tetanus claimed the lives of over 433 000 infants in 1991, and accounts for 5 deaths for every 1000 live births in Africa. It is geographically prevalent in rural areas with poor hygiene and medical services. Thus, tetanus remains a significant public health problem in the developing world, primarily because of poor access to immunization programmes. In addition, modern management requires ICU facilities, which are rarely available in the most severely afflicted populations.[2] Therefore, tetanus will continue to afflict developing populations in the foreseeable future.

PATHOGENESIS

Clostridium tetani is an obligate anaerobic, spore-bearing, Gram-positive bacillus. Spores exist ubiquitously in soil and in animal and human faeces. After gaining access to devitalized tissue, spores proliferate in the vegetative form, producing toxins, tetanospasmin and tetanolysin. Tetanospasmin is extremely potent; an estimated 240 g could kill the entire world population,[2] with 0.01 mg being lethal for an average man. Tetanolysin is of little clinical importance.

C. tetani is non-invasive. Hence, tetanus occurs only when the spores gain access to tissues to produce vegeta-

tive forms. The usual mode of entry is through a puncture wound or laceration, although tetanus may follow surgery, burns, gangrene, chronic ulcers, dog bites, injections such as with drug users, dental infection, abortion and childbirth. Tetanus neonatorum usually follows infection of the umbilical stump. The injury itself may be trivial, and in 20% of cases there is no history or evidence of a wound.[1] Germination of spores occurs in oxygen-poor media (e.g. in necrotic tissue), with foreign bodies, and with infections. *C. tetani* infection remains localized, but the exotoxin tetanospasmin is distributed widely via the blood stream, taken up into motor nerve endings, and transported into the nervous system. Here, it affects motor neurone end-plates in skeletal muscle (to decrease release of acetylcholine), the spinal cord (with dysfunction of polysynaptic reflexes) and the brain (with seizures, inhibition of cortical activity and autonomic dysfunction). Tetanus is not communicable from person to person.

The symptoms of tetanus appear only after tetanospasmin has diffused from the cell body through the extracellular space, and gained access to the presynaptic terminals of adjacent neurones.[1] Tetanospasmin spreads to all local neurones, but is preferentially bound by inhibitory interneurones, that is, glycinergic terminals in the spinal cord, and γ-aminobutyric acid (GABA) terminals in the brain.[2] Its principal effect is to block these inhibitory pathways. Hence stimuli to and from the central nervous system (CNS) are not 'damped down'.

ACTIVE IMMUNOPROPHYLAXIS[1,3]

Natural immunity to tetanus does not occur. Tetanus may both relapse and recur. Victims of tetanus must be *actively immunized.* Tetanus toxoid is a cheap and effective vaccine, which is thermally stable.[3] It is a non-toxic derivative of the toxin which, nevertheless, elicits and reacts with antitoxic antibody. By consensus, an antibody titre of 0.01 U/ml serum is protective.[4] None the less, tetanus has been reported in a few victims with much higher serum antibody titres.[1]

In adults, a full immunization course consists of three toxoid doses, given at an optimal interval of 6–12 weeks between the first and second doses, and 6–12 months between the second and third doses. A single dose will offer no immediate protection in the unimmunized, but a full course should never be repeated. Neonates have immunity from maternal antibodies. Children over 3 months should be actively immunized, and need four doses in total. Two or more doses to child-bearing females over 14 years will protect any child produced within the next 5 years. Pregnant females who are not immunized should thus be given two spaced-out doses 2 weeks to 2 months before delivery. Booster doses should be given routinely every 10 years.

Side-effects of tetanus toxoid are uncommon and not life-threatening. They are associated with excessive levels of antibody due to indiscriminate use.[5] Common reactions include urticaria, angio-oedema and diffuse, indurated swelling at the site of injection.

CLINICAL PRESENTATION[1,4,6]

The incubation period (i.e. time from injury to onset of symptoms) varies from 2 to 60 days. The period of onset (i.e. from first symptom to first spasm) similarly varies. Nearly all cases (90%), however, present within 15 days of infection.[6] The incubation period and the period of onset are of prognostic importance, with shorter times signifying more severe disease.

Presenting symptoms are pain and stiffness. Stiffness gives way to rigidity, and there is difficulty in mouth opening – trismus or lockjaw. Most (75%) of non-neonatal generalized tetanus present with trismus.[6] Rigidity becomes generalized, and facial muscles produce a characteristic clenched-teeth expression called risus sardonicus. The disease progresses in a descending fashion. Typical spasms, with flexion and adduction of the arms, extension of the legs and opisthotonos, are very painful, and may be so intense that fractures and tendon separations occur.[1] Spasms are caused by external stimuli, for example, noise and pressure. As the disease worsens, even minimal stimuli produce more intense and longer-lasting spasms. Spasms are life-threatening when they involve the larynx and/or diaphragm.

Neonatal tetanus presents most often on day 7 of life,[4] with a short (1 day) history of failure of the infant to feed. The neonate displays typical spasms that can be easily misdiagnosed as convulsions of another aetiology. In addition, because these infants vomit (as a result of the increased intra-abdominal pressure) and are dehydrated (because of their inability to swallow), meningitis and sepsis are often considered first.

Autonomic dysfunction occurs in severe cases,[6–8] and begins a few days after the muscle spasms (the toxin has further to diffuse to reach the lateral horns of the spinal cord.) There is increased basal sympathetic tone, mani-

festing as tachycardia and bladder and bowel dysfunction. Also, episodes of marked sympathetic overactivity involving both α and β-receptors occur. Vascular resistance, central venous pressure and, usually, cardiac output are increased, manifesting clinically as labile hypertension, pyrexia, sweating, and pallor and cyanosis of the digits.[7] These episodes are usually of short duration and may occur without any provocation. They are caused by reduced inhibition of postsynaptic sympathetic fibres in the intermediolateral cell column, as evidenced by very high circulating noradrenaline concentrations.[1,8] Other postualated causes of this variable sympathetic overactivity include loss of inhibition of the adrenal medulla with increased adrenaline secretion, direct inhibition by tetanospasmin of the release of endo-genous opiates, and increased release of thyroid hormone.[1,2]

The role of the parasympathetic nervous system is debatable. Episodes of bradycardia, low peripheral vascular resistance, low central venous pressure and profound hypotension are seen, and are frequently preterminal.[7] Sudden and repeated cardiac arrests occur, particularly in intravenous drug abusers.[8] These events have been attributed to total withdrawal of sympathetic tone, since it is unresponsive to atropine.[9] However, they may be caused by catecholamine-induced myocardial damage[8,10] or direct brainstem damage.[8] Whatever the mechanism, patients afflicted with the autonomic dysfunction of tetanus are at risk of sudden death.

Local tetanus is an uncommon, mild form of tetanus with a mortality of 1%. The signs and symptoms are confined to a limb or muscle, and may be the result of immunization. *Cephalic tetanus* is also rare: it results from head and neck injuries, eye infections and otitis media. The cranial nerves, especially the seventh are frequently involved, and the prognosis is poor. This form may progress to a more generalized form. Tetanus in heroin addicts seems to be severe, with a high mortality, but numbers are small.[8,11]

DIAGNOSIS

The diagnosis is clinical and often straightforward. There are no laboratory tests specific to tetanus. *C. tetani* is cultured from the wound only in a third of cases. The most common differential diagnosis is dystonic reaction to tricyclics. Other differential diagnoses include strychnine poisoning, local temporomandibular disease, local oral disease, convulsions, tetany, intra-cranial infections or haemorrhage and psychiatric disorders.

MANAGEMENT

Initial objectives of treatment are to neutralize circulating toxin (i.e. passive immunization) and prevent it from entering peripheral nerves (i.e. wound care), as well as eradicating the source of the toxin (i.e. extensive surgery, hygiene, wound care and antibiotics). Treatment then aims to minimize the effect of toxin already bound in the nervous system, and to provide general supportive care.

PASSIVE IMMUNIZATION[1,12]

Human antitetanus toxin has now largely replaced antitetanus serum (ATS) of horse origin, as it is less antigenic. Antitetanus toxin will at best neutralize only circulating toxin, but does not affect toxins already fixed in the CNS, that is it does not ameliorate symptoms already present. Although never prospectively tested, present recommendations for human antitetanus toxin in tetanus are 3000–6000 units i.v. It has been suggested that unimmunized patients or those whose immunization status is unknown should be given human rich antiserum on presentation with contaminated wounds. No controlled study has shown this to be more effective than wound toilet and penicillin administration.

Intrathecal administration of antitetanus toxin is still controversial. A large meta-analysis reported it to be ineffective.[13] Moreover, suitable intrathecal preparations are not widely available. Side-effects of human antitetanus toxin include fever, shivering and chest or back pains. Cardiovascular parameters need to be monitored, and the infusion may need to be stopped temporarily if significant tachycardia and hypotension present.[1,5,12] If human antiserum is not available, equine ATS can be used after testing and desensitization.[1]

ERADICATION OF THE ORGANISM

WOUND CARE

Once human antitetanus toxin has been given, the infected site should be thoroughly cleaned and all necrotic tissue extensively debrided.

ANTIBIOTICS

Tetanus spores are destroyed by antibiotics. The vegetative form (bacillus) is sensitive to antibiotics *in vitro*. However, *in vivo* efficacy depends on the antibiotic concentration at the wound site, and large doses may be required. Recommended antibiotic regimens include:

1 Metronidazole 500 mg i.v. 8-hourly for 10 days: The drug has a spectrum of activity against anaerobes, is able to penetrate necrotic tissue, and has been shown to be more effective than penicillin in this situation.[14]
2 Penicillin G 1–3 Mu i.v. 6-hourly intervals for 10 days: penicillin is a GABA antagonist in the CNS,[15] and may aggravate the spasms. Nevertheless, it is still often used in this situation.
3 Erythromycin has been used, but should not be used routinely.

SUPPRESSION OF EFFECTS OF TETANOSPASMIN

CONTROLLING MUSCLE SPASMS

In the early stages of tetanus, the patient is most at risk from laryngeal and other respiratory muscle spasm. Therefore, if muscle spasms are present, the airway should be urgently secured by endotracheal intubation or tracheostomy. If respiratory muscles are affected, mechanical ventilation is instituted. In severe tetanus, spasms usually preclude effective ventilation, and muscle relaxants may be required. Pancuronium bromide may cause tachycardia and hypertension by stimulating noradrenaline release from sympathetic nerve endings,[16] but has been used safely in tetanus.[17] Heavy sedation alone may prevent muscle spasms and improve autonomic dysfunction (see below).

MANAGEMENT OF AUTONOMIC DYSFUNCTION

Autonomic dysfunction manifests in increased basal sympathetic activity[18] and episodic massive outpourings of catecholamines.[18-20] During these episodes, noradrenaline and adrenaline may be up to ten times basal levels.[18,19] The clinical picture is variable.[20] Hypertension, tachycardia and sweating do not always occur concurrently.

Traditionally, a combination of α and β-adrenergic blockers has been used to treat sympathetic overactivity. Phenoxybenzamine, phentolamine, bethanidine and chlorpromazine have been used as α-receptor blockers. Ganglion blockers and nitroprusside have occasionally been used. Propranolol and labetalol have had limited success.[21-23] However, unopposed β-adrenergic blockade cannot be advised. Deaths from acute congestive cardiac failure have resulted.[21,22] Removal of β-mediated vasodilatation in limb muscle causes a rise in systemic vascular resistance, and β-blocked myocardium may not be able to maintain adequate cardiac output. Also, with β-blockade, hypotension follows when sympathetic overactivity abates. Esmolol, a very short-acting β-adrenergic blocker given i.v., has been reported to be useful.[24] However, although sympathetic crises can be controlled by esmolol, catecholamine levels remain raised.[20] This raises concern, because excessive catecholamine secretion is associated with myocardial damage.[10]

From the above, it appears more logical to decrease catecholamine output. This can be done with sedatives. Benzodiazepines and morphine are successfully used.[19] Morphine and diazepam act centrally to minimize the effects of tetanospasmin. Morphine probably acts by replacing deficient endogenous opioids.[1] Benzodiazepines increase the affinity and efficacy of GABA.[1] Very large doses of these agents, for example, diazepam 3400 mg/day[19] and morphine 235 mg/day,[25] may be required, and are well-tolerated.

Magnesium has been used as an adjunct to sedation.[19,26] Magnesium sulphate infusions to keep serum concentrations between 2.5 and 4.0 mmol/l have decreased systemic vascular resistance and pulse rate, with a small decrease in cardiac output.[19,26] In animal studies, magnesium inhibits release of adrenaline and noradrenaline, and reduces the sensitivity of receptors to these neurotransmitters. Magnesium also has a marked neuromuscular blocking effect, and may reduce the intensity of muscle spasms. However, magnesium sulphate must be used with sedatives,[19] and calcium supplements may be needed when it is infused. Anecdotally, clonidine, a central α_2 stimulant, has successfully produced sedation with control of autonomic dysfunction.[27] It seems sensible to attempt to make use of the central nervous system effects of an α_2-adrenergic agonist, namely sedation and vasodilatation.[28] In this regard dexmedetomidine may be even better than clonidine.[28] Intrathecal baclofen has produced similar beneficial results in a series of cases, but significant respiratory depression occurred in a third of patients.[29] When given intrathecally, baclofen can diminish spasms and spasticity, allowing for a reduction in sedative and paralysis requirements.[30]

SUPPORTIVE TREATMENT

Steps should be taken to prevent contractures, nosocomial pneumonias and deep vein thrombosis. The patient (including the mother if a neonate is afflicted) must be actively immunized. Where possible, supportive psychotherapy should be offered to both patient and family.

COMPLICATIONS[1,4,6,10,31]

Muscle spasms disappear after 1–3 weeks, but residual stiffness may persist. Although most survivors recover completely by 6 weeks, cardiovascular complications, including cardiac failure, arrhythmias, pulmonary oedema and hypertensive crises can be fatal. No obvious cause of death can be found at autopsy in up to 20% of deaths. Other complications include those associated with factors shown in Table 46.1

OUTCOME

Recovery from tetanus is thought to be complete. However, in 25 non-neonatal patients followed for up to 11 years,[32] 15 were reported to have one or more abnormal neurological features, such as intellectual or emotional changes, fits and myoclonic jerks, sleep disturbance, and decreased libido. Of the 10 apparently normal survivors, 6 had electroencephalogram changes. Some of these symptoms resolved within 2 years.

Table 46.1 Factors contributing to death in tetanus

Hypoxia
Complications of mechanical ventilation
Myoglobinuria and its attendant problems
Sepsis, particularly pneumonia
Fluid and electrolyte problems (including inappropriate antidiuretic hormone secretion)
Deep vein thrombosis and embolic phenomena
Bed sores
Bony fractures

Mortality figures depend on the availability of intensive care. In neonates, the mortality from African countries with no ICU facilities can be up to 80% of cases, but falls to about 10% when artificial ventilation is used. In the USA, mortality in non-neonates relates directly to age, with rates from 0% in patients under 30 years rising to 50% in those 60 years or older. An average of 10% mortality would seem to be reasonable for most ICUs. However, as this disease is easily and completely preventable, loss of life is unacceptable.

REFERENCES

1 Bleck TP. Tetanus: pathophysiology, management and prophylaxis. *Dis Mon* 1991; **37**(9): 556–603.
2 Ackerman AD. Immunology and infections in the pediatric intensive care unit. Part B: Infectious diseases of particular importance to the pediatric intensivist. In: Rogers MC (ed.) *Textbook of Pediatric Intensive Care*, vol 26. Baltimore: Williams and Wilkins; 1987: pp. 866–75.
3 Editorial. Prevention of neonatal tetanus. *Lancet* 1983; **1**: 1253–4.
4 Stoll BJ. Tetanus. *Pediatr Clin N Am* 1979; **26**: 415–31.
5 Editorial. Reactions to tetanus toxoid. *BMJ* 1974; **1**: 48.
6 Alfery DD, Rauscher LA. Tetanus: a review. *Crit Care Med* 1979; 7: 176–81.
7 Kerr JH, Corbett JL, Prys-Roberts C, *et al.* Involvement of the sympathetic nervous system in tetanus. *Lancet* 1968; **2**: 236–41.
8 Tsueda K, Oliver PB, Richter RW. Cardiovascular manifestations of tetanus. *Anesthesiology* 1974; **40**: 588–92.
9 Kerr J. Current topics in tetanus. *Intensive Care Med* 1979; **5**: 105–10.
10 Rose AG. Catecholamine-induced myocardial damage associated with phaeochromocytomas and tetanus. *S Afr Med J* 1974; **48**: 1285–9.
11 Sun KO, Chan YW, Cheung RT, *et al.* Management of tetanus: a review of 18 cases. *J Roy Soc Med* 1994; **87**: 135–7.
12 Annotation. Antitoxin in treatment of tetanus. *Lancet* 1976; **1**: 944.
13 Abrutyn E, Berlin JA. Intrathecal therapy in tetanus: a meta-analysis. *JAMA* 1991; **266**: 2262–7.

14 Ahmadsyah I, Salim A. Treatment of tetanus: An open study to compare the efficacy of procaine penicillin and metronidazole. *BMJ* 1985; **291**: 648–50.

15 Clarke G, Hill RG. Effects of a focal penicillin lesion on responses of rabbit cortical neurones to putative neurotransmitters. *Br J Pharmacol* 1972; **44**: 435–41.

16 Barnes PK, Brindle Smith G, White WD, Tennant R. Comparison of the effects of Org NC 45 and pancuronium bromide on heart rate and arterial pressure in anaesthetized man. *Br J Anaesth* 1982; **54**: 435–9.

17 Spelman D, Newton-John H. Continuous pancuronium infusion in severe tetanus. *Med J Aust* 1980; **1**: 676.

18 Domenighetti GM, Savary G, Stricker H. Hyperadrenergic syndrome in severe tetanus: extreme rise in catecholamines responsive to labetalol. *BMJ* 1984; **288**: 1483–4.

19 Lipman J, James MFM, Erskine J, *et al.* Autonomic dysfunction in severe tetanus: magnesium sulphate as an adjunct to deep sedation. *Crit Care Med* 1987; **15**: 987–8.

20 Beards SC, Lipman J, Bothma P, Joynt GM. Esmolol in a case of severe tetanus: adequate haemodynamic control despite markedly elevated catecholamine levels. *S Afr J Surg* 1994; **32**: 33–5.

21 Buchanan N, Smit L, Cane RD, De Andrade M. Sympathetic overactivity in tetanus: Fatality associated with propanolol. *BMJ* 1978; **2**: 254–5.

22 Wesley AG, Hariparsad D, Pather M, Rocke DA. Labetalol in tetanus. *Anaesthesia* 1983; **38**: 243–9.

23 Edmondson RS, Flowers MW. Intensive care in tetanus: management, complications and mortality in 100 cases. *BMJ* 1979; **1**: 1401–4.

24 King WW, Cave DR. Use of esmolol to control autonomic instability of tetanus. *Am J Med* 1991; **91**: 425–8.

25 Rocke DA, Wesley AG, Pather M, *et al.* Morphine in tetanus – the management of sympathetic nervous system overactivity. *S Afr Med J* 1986; **70**: 666–8.

26 James MFM, Manson EDM. The use of magnesium sulphate infusions in the management of very severe tetanus. *Intensive Care Med* 1985; **11**: 5–12.

27 Sutton DN, Tremlett MR, Woodcock TE, Nielsen MS. Management of autonomic dysfunction in severe tetanus: the use of magnesium sulphate and clonidine. *Intensive Care Med* 1990; **16**: 75–80.

28 Kamibayashi T, Maze M. Clinical uses of alpha2-adrenergic agonists. *Anesthesiology* 2000; **93**: 1345–1349.

29 Saissy JM, Demaziere J, Vitris M, *et al.* Treatment of severe tetanus by intrathecal injections of baclofen without artificial ventilation. *Intensive Care Med* 1992; **18**: 241–4.

30 Boots RJ, Lipman J, O'Callaghan J, *et al.* The treatment of tetanus with intrathecal baclofen. *Anaesth Intens Care* 2000; **28**: 438–42.

31 Potgieter PD. Inappropriate ADH secretion in tetanus. *Crit Care Med* 1983; **11**: 417–18.

32 Illis LS, Taylor FM. Neurological and electroencephalographic sequelae of tetanus. *Lancet* 1971; **1**: 826–30.

47

Neuromuscular diseases in intensive care

G Skowronski

A number of disorders producing generalized neuromuscular weakness can require admission to the ICU, or complicate the course of ICU patients. These may involve:

- Spinal anterior horn cells – motor neurone disease, poliomyelitis.
- Peripheral nerve conduction – Guillain–Barré syndrome (GBS) and related disorders.
- The neuromuscular junction – myasthenia gravis, botulism.
- Muscle contraction – critical illness myopathy, periodic paralysis.

GUILLAIN–BARRÉ SYNDROME AND RELATED DISORDERS

In 1834 James Wardrop reported a case of ascending sensory loss and weakness in a 35-year-old man, leading to almost complete quadriparesis over 10 days, and complete recovery over several months.[1] In 1859, Landry described an acute ascending paralysis occurring in 10 patients, 2 of whom died. Guillain, Barré and Strohl[2] in 1916 reported two cases of motor weakness, paraesthesiae and muscle tenderness in association with increased protein in the cerebrospinal fluid. (Lumbar puncture for cerebrospinal fluid (CSF) examination was first described only in the 1890s.)

Many variants of this syndrome have since been reported, and this has resulted in confusion in nomenclature. The lack of specific diagnostic criteria has also been a problem. Clinical, electrical and laboratory criteria for the predominant variant – acute inflammatory demyelinating poly-radiculopathy (AIDP) – are now well described,[3] though 10–15% of cases do not fit these criteria, and GBS is best regarded as a heterogeneous group of immunologically mediated disorders of peripheral nerve function.

INCIDENCE

Since the incidence of poliomyelitis has markedly declined due to mass immunization programmes, GBS has become the major cause of rapid-onset flaccid paralysis in previously healthy people, with an incidence of approximately 1.7 per 100 000.[4] Epidemics have occurred in large populations exposed to viral illness or immunization.[5] Immunosuppression and concurrent autoimmune disease may also be predisposing factors.[6,7] The disorder is slightly commoner in males, and up to four times commoner in the elderly. No consistent seasonal or racial predilection has been demonstrated.[4]

AETIOLOGY

Most recent evidence supports the proposition that GBS is caused by immunologically mediated nerve injury.[8] Cell-mediated immunity, in particular, probably plays a significant role, and inflammatory cell infiltrates are often seen in association with demyelination, which is generally regarded as the primary pathologic process. Antibodies to a number of nervous system components have been demonstrated in GBS patients, but none is of clear diagnostic or pathogenic importance.

Although the precise mechanism of sensitization is not known, clinical associations suggest that antecedent viral infections or immunizations are commonly involved. Infective agents implicated include influenza A, parainfluenza, varicella-zoster, Epstein–Barr virus, chickenpox, mumps, human immunodeficiency virus (HIV),[9] measles virus and *Mycoplasma*. *Campylobacter jejuni* gastroenteritis now appears to be the most common predisposing infection and may be associated with a more severe clinical course; 26–41% of GBS patients show evidence of recent *C. jejuni* infection.[10] Cytomegalovirus infection accounts for a further 10–22% of cases.[11] Immunizations against viral infections, tuberculosis, tetanus, and typhoid have all preceded the development of GBS. Most of these associations are anecdotal and of doubtful aetiological significance, but about 65% of patients present within a few weeks of minor respiratory (43%) or gastrointestinal (21%) illness.

PATHOGENESIS

The peripheral nerves of patients who have died of GBS show infiltration of the endoneurium by mononuclear cells, in a predominantly perivenular distribution. The inflammatory process may be distributed throughout the length of the nerves, but with more marked focal changes in the nerve roots, spinal nerves and major plexuses. Electron micrographs show macrophages actively stripping myelin from the bodies of Schwann cells and axons. In some cases, Wallerian degeneration of axons is also seen, and failure of regeneration in these cases may correspond with a poor clinical outcome.

The underlying immune response is complex and poorly understood, but serum from GBS patients produces myelin damage *in vitro* when complement is present.[13] Although antibodies to various glycolipids have been demonstrated in GBS, these are generally in low titre and can occasionally be seen in controls. Patients with recent *C. jejuni* infection have a high incidence of antibodies to the ganglioside GM_1. The basis of the effectiveness of plasma exchange and immunoglobulin therapy is likely to be blocking of demyelinating antibodies by several mechanisms.[14]

CLINICAL PRESENTATION

The majority of patients describe a minor illness in the 8 weeks prior to presentation, with a peak incidence 2 weeks beforehand. Approximately half the patients initially experience paraesthesiae, typically beginning in the hands and feet. One-quarter complain of motor weakness, and the remainder have both.[15] Motor weakness proceeds to flaccid paralysis, which becomes the predominant complaint. Objective loss of power and reduction or loss of tendon reflexes usually commence distally and ascend, but a more haphazard spread may occur. Cranial nerves are involved in 45% of cases, most commonly the facial nerve, followed by the glossopharyngeal and vagus nerves. One third of patients require ventilatory support.

In the Miller–Fisher syndrome, a variant of GBS,[16] cranial nerve abnormalities predominate, with ataxia, areflexia and ophthalmoplegia as the predominant features. This is strongly associated with recent *C. jejuni* infection.

Another subgroup of patients presents with a primarily axonal neuropathy – acute motor-sensory axonal neuropathy (AMSAN). In these cases, motor and sensory axons appear to be the primary targets of immune attack, rather than myelin. These patients have a more fulminant and severe course, and there is again a strong association with *C. jejuni* infection.[17]

Sensory loss is generally mild, with paraesthesiae or loss of vibration and proprioception, but occasionally sensory loss, pain or hyperaesthesia can be prominent features. Autonomic dysfunction is common, and a major contributor to morbidity and mortality in ventilator-dependent cases.[18] Orthostatic or persistent hypotension, paroxysmal hypertension, and bradycardia are all described, as are fatal ventricular tachyarrhythmias. Adynamic ileus, urinary retention and abnormalities of sweating are also commonly seen.

DIFFERENTIAL DIAGNOSIS

Most of the important alternative diagnoses are listed as exclusion criteria in Table 47.1. In patients with prolonged illness, the possibility of chronic inflammatory demyelinating polyradiculopathy (CIDP) should be considered.[19] In this condition, which is usually distinguished from GBS, preceding viral infection is uncommon, the onset is more insidious and the course is one of slow worsening or stepwise relapses. Corticosteroids and plasma exchange are possibly effective in this disorder, but adequate studies of immunosuppressive drugs have not been carried out.

An intermediate *subacute* polyradiculopathy (SIDP) as well as a recurrent form of GBS are also described, and all of these variants may be part of the spectrum of a single condition. However, a purely motor axonal neuropathy (acute motor-axonal neuropathy, AMAN), which causes seasonal childhood epidemics mimicking classical GBS in China and elsewhere,[20] appears to be a distinct entity. Once again, this is strongly associated with *C. jejuni* infection.

INVESTIGATIONS

In over 90% of patients, cerebrospinal fluid (CSF) protein is increased (>0.4 g/l), within a week of onset of symptoms. The level does not correlate with the clinical findings. A pleocytosis with lymphocytes and monocytes in the CSF may be seen in a small proportion of

Table 47.1 Diagnostic criteria for typical Guillain–Barré syndrome[3]

Features required for diagnosis
Progressive weakness in both arms and both legs
Areflexia

Features strongly supportive of the diagnosis
Progression over days to 4 weeks
Relative symmetry of symptoms
Mild sensory symptoms or signs
Cranial nerve involvement, especially bilateral weakness of facial muscles
Recovery beginning 2–4 weeks after progression ceases
Autonomic dysfunction
Absence of fever at onset
High concentration of protein in cerebrospinal fluid protein with fewer than 10×10^6 cells/l
Typical electrodiagnostic features

Features excluding diagnosis
Diagnosis of botulism, myasthenia, poliomyelitis or toxic neuropathy
Abnormal porphyrin metabolism
Recent diphtheria
History or evidence of lead intoxication
Purely sensory syndrome, without weakness

patients, especially later in the disease. Nerve conduction studies may demonstrate reduced conduction velocity and prolonged distal latencies.[21] Severely reduced distal motor amplitude and a predominantly axonal pattern are associated with more severe disease and a guarded prognosis.

MANAGEMENT

The management of the patient with severe and protracted GBS provides a major challenge, as the prognosis is generally excellent if complications can be treated early or avoided. These complications may be life-threatening, affect any of the major organ systems or result in permanent disability, and can be prevented only by meticulous attention to detail.

SPECIFIC THERAPY

Plasma exchange (plasmapheresis) is of value in GBS. Two large controlled trials showed a reduction in patients requiring mechanical ventilation, reduced duration of mechanical ventilation for those who required it, reduced time to motor recovery and time to walking without assistance.[22,23] Mortality, however, was not altered. Plasma exchange was most effective when carried out within 7 days of onset of symptoms. The plasma exchange schedules consisted of three to five exchanges of 1–2 plasma volumes each, over 1–2 weeks. Adverse events are common, and some relate to the disease itself.[24] Fresh frozen plasma is reported to have more side-effects than albumin as the replacement fluid.

Immunoglobulin therapy was as effective as plasmapheresis[25] and previous concerns of higher recurrence rates may be unfounded. Because of its ease of use, many authorities now advocate immunoglobulin as the treatment of choice. A dose of 0.4 g/kg body weight intravenously, daily for 5 days, was used in the most recent trials.

About 10% of patients relapse after initial treatment with either plasmapheresis or immunoglobulin; most respond well to a further course.

Available studies suggest that low or high dose corticosteroids are of no value.[26] However, there has been a suggestion of a beneficial interaction between steroids and immunoglobulin. This awaits further study.

SUPPORTIVE CARE

RESPIRATORY SYSTEM

In the spontaneously breathing patient, chest physiotherapy and careful monitoring of respiratory function are of paramount importance. Regular measurement of vital capacity is probably the best way to predict respiratory failure, and is more reliable than arterial blood gases.[27] The latter nevertheless remain a useful guide. Any patient with a vital capacity of less than 15 ml/kg

or 30% of the predicted level, or a rising $Pa\text{CO}_2$ is likely to require mechanical ventilation.

Bulbar involvement should be carefully sought, as there is a significant risk of aspiration of upper airway secretions, gastric contents or ingested food. The cough reflex may be inadequate, and airway protection by tracheal intubation or tracheostomy is then required. Oral feeding should be stopped in any patient in whom bulbar involvement is suspected.

Mechanical ventilation is mandatory if coughing is inadequate, pulmonary collapse or consolidation develop, arterial blood gases are significantly abnormal, vital capacity is less than predicted tidal volume (approximately 10 ml/kg), or the patient is dyspnoeic, tachypnoeic or appears exhausted. Mechanical ventilation, if necessary, will probably be required for several weeks (although there is wide variation), and early tracheostomy should be considered.

CARDIOVASCULAR SYSTEM

Cardiac rhythm and blood pressure should be monitored. Induction of anaesthesia appears particularly likely to induce serious arrhythmias. Use of suxamethonium may contribute significantly to this,[28] and, as with many other neuromuscular disorders, should be avoided. Cardiovascular instability may also be exacerbated by a number of other drugs (Table 47.2). These, likewise, should be avoided or used with great care.

Mild hypotension and bradycardia may require no treatment, particularly if renal and cerebral function are maintained. However, blood volume expansion or inotropic drugs may be required in some cases. Hypertension is often transient, but occasionally requires

Table 47.2 Drugs associated with cardiovascular instability in Guillain–Barré syndrome[a]

Exaggerated hypotensive response
Phentolamine
Nitroglycerin
Hexamethonium
Edrophonium
Thiopentone
Morphine
Furosemide
Exaggerated hypertensive response
Phenylephrine
Ephedrine
Dopamine
Isoprenaline
Arrhythmias
Suxamethonium
Cardiac arrest
General anaesthesia

[a] Modified from: Dalos et al.,[77] with permission.

appropriate drug therapy. Hypoxia, hypercarbia, pain and visceral distension should be excluded as causes.

FLUIDS, ELECTROLYTES AND NUTRITION

Paralytic ileus is not uncommon, especially immediately following the institution of mechanical ventilation, and a period of parenteral nutrition may be required. However, wherever possible, nasoenteric feeding should be instituted because of its significantly greater safety. Energy and fluid requirements are considerably reduced in these patients.

SEDATION AND ANALGESIA

In non-ventilated patients, sedation should be avoided because of the potential for worsening respiratory and upper airway function. In ventilated patients, sedation becomes less necessary as the patient becomes accustomed to the ventilator, but night sedation may help to preserve diurnal rhythms. Limb pain, particularly with passive movement, is very common and often quite severe. Quinine, minor and non-steroidal analgesics and antidepressant drugs may all be tried, but the pain can be difficult to control and opioids are often required. Methadone, transdermal fentanyl and tramadol have all been advocated.

GENERAL AND NURSING CARE

A comprehensive programme of physiotherapy should be implemented by nurses and physiotherapists, with careful attention to pressure area care, the maintenance of joint mobility and pulmonary function. Opportunistic infection should be actively sought with culture of urine and respiratory secretions at least twice weekly. Sites of vascular access should be inspected frequently, and changed whenever necessary. It may be possible to manage stable long-term patients without venous access. Care should be taken to prevent corneal ulceration and faecal impaction.

Prophylaxis against venous thromboembolism should be given, and enterally administered low-dose warfarin may be preferable to twice-daily heparin injections in long-stay patients. Psychological problems, especially depression, are common, and some patients are helped by antidepressant drugs. Good communication and rapport between the patient and staff, involvement of allied health practitioners, the provision of television, radio and reading aids, and, where possible, occasional trips out of the ICU, are all of great value.

PROGNOSIS

The nadir of the disease is reached within 2–4 weeks, and gradual resolution follows over weeks to months. Of those who survive the acute illness, 70% are fully recovered within one year, and a further 20% are left with only minor limitation. Poor prognostic features include age over 60 years, rapid progression to quadri-

paresis in less than 7 days, the need for mechanical ventilation (except for children),[29] and a preceding diarrhoeal illness.[30] Even in patients ventilated for more than 2 months, gradual improvement may continue for 18 months to 2 years.[31] These severely affected patients require a protracted period of rehabilitation.

Death in up to 25% of GBS patients has been reported in those requiring intensive care.[32] Many of these deaths were due to potentially avoidable problems such as respiratory arrest, ventilator malfunction and intercurrent sepsis, and considerably better results have been achieved. A more representative estimate of the overall mortality is 5–8%.[33]

WEAKNESS SYNDROMES COMPLICATING CRITICAL ILLNESS[34,35]

A number of neuromuscular disorders specifically associated with critical illness have been described over the last 30 years, and remain poorly understood. These include neuropathies, myopathies and combinations of both. Variations in nomenclature, the lack of a satisfactory classification or diagnostic test, and confusion with other disorders, such as GBS, have further complicated this area. There is also considerable overlap among the various subtypes. Sepsis, neuromuscular blocking drugs (NMBA), disuse atrophy, asthma, corticosteroids and the multiple organ dysfunction syndrome (MODS) have all been implicated. Although the two major subgroups are outlined below, a number of rarer variants have also been described. No specific therapies are available, but most patients improve after a period of supportive care.

Critical illness polyneuropathy. This acute, diffuse, mainly motor neuropathy is probably the commonest of these disorders. It usually presents in the recovery phase of a severe systemic illness with persistent quadriparetic weakness, hyporeflexia and difficulty in weaning from respiratory support. There appears to be a specific association with severe sepsis and MODS. Histological and electrophysiological features are consistent with axonal degeneration. The mortality in this group is high, presumably reflecting that of the underlying condition. However, among those who survive the acute illness, the outlook for recovery of function appears quite good, with 70% recovering completely over an average of 4–5 months.[36]

Critical illness myopathy. This disorder is linked with asthma and with the use of corticosteroids, NMBA and, less convincingly, aminoglycosides and β-adrenergic agonists. Reflexes are preserved except in severe cases, as is sensation. Elevated blood creatine phosphokinase (CPK) concentrations are often seen. A few patients have a more severe, fulminant form with very high CPK levels, frank rhabdomyolysis and, rarely, renal failure. Electrophysiological findings are somewhat variable, though muscle necrosis is usually apparent on histology.

Although steroidal muscle relaxants (pancuronium or vecuronium)[37] have been particularly implicated, the disorder has also been seen with other types of NMBA. On the basis of two small case series, the outlook for functional recovery appears good.

DIFFERENTIAL DIAGNOSIS

The influence of drugs, metabolic abnormalities and hyperthermia should always be excluded when unexplained neuromuscular weakness appears in an intensive care patient. The possibility of a coincident illness such as the Eaton–Lambert syndrome, myasthenia gravis, vasculitis or GBS must also be carefully considered. Severe catabolism and disuse atrophy are common in many of these patients and can themselves result in significant weakness.

MYASTHENIA GRAVIS

Myasthenia gravis (MG) is an autoimmune disorder caused by antibodies directed against acetylcholine (ACh) receptors in skeletal muscle. Despite its relative rarity, it is the most studied and best understood clinical disorder of neuroreceptor function, and arguably the best understood organ-specific autoimmune disease. It is characterized clinically by weakness or exaggerated fatigability on sustained effort. Intensive care is most commonly required because of severe involvement of the bulbar or respiratory muscles, which may be the result of a spontaneous exacerbation of the disease, a complication of drug therapy, intercurrent illness or surgery, or following surgical thymectomy – the treatment of choice for most patients.

INCIDENCE

The incidence of MG is approximately 1 in 20 000 in the USA. There is no racial or geographic predilection. Although MG can occur at any age, it is very rare in the first 2 years of life, and the peak incidence is in young adult females. Overall, females are affected about twice as often as males. This sexual predilection decreases with increasing age, and there is a smaller, second incidence peak in elderly males.[38]

AETIOLOGY AND PATHOPHYSIOLOGY

In 75% of cases, there is histological evidence of thymic abnormality. Thymic hyperplasia is present in the majority of patients, but approximately 10% have a thymoma. The latter appears more common in the older age group. The precise role of the thymus is uncertain, but ACh receptors are present in the myoid cells of the normal thymus, and there is evidence that anti-ACh receptor antibody production is mediated by both B and T lymphocytes of thymic origin. Other organ-specific autoimmune disorders, most commonly thyroid disease,[39] but also rheumatoid arthritis, lupus erythematosus and pernicious anaemia, are significantly associated with MG, and autoantibodies to other organs may be seen in MG patients without evidence of disease.

Children born to mothers with MG demonstrate transient weakness ('neonatal MG') in about 15% of cases. A number of congenital myasthenic syndromes exist, in which symptoms develop in infancy without evidence of autoantibody production.[40] A familial tendency is more common in this group, and structural changes at the neuromuscular junction have been demonstrated.

The stimulus to autoantibody production is not known, but these can be detected in about 90% of patients with generalized myasthenia. They may interfere with neuromuscular transmission by competitively blocking receptor sites, by initiating immune-mediated destruction of receptors, or by binding to portions of the receptor molecule which are not part of the ACh receptor site, but which, nevertheless, are important in allowing ACh to bind.

CLINICAL PRESENTATION

Ptosis and diplopia are the most common initial symptoms, and in 20% of cases, the disorder remains confined to the eye muscles (ocular MG).[41] Bulbar muscle weakness is common and may result in nasal regurgitation, dysarthria and dysphagia. Limb and trunk weakness can occur with varying distribution, and is usually asymmetrical. Some patients complain of fatigue rather than weakness, and may be misdiagnosed as having psychogenic symptoms. However, weakness can be elicited by sustained effort of an involved muscle group, for example, sustained upward gaze is often worse at the end of the day and improves with rest.

INVESTIGATIONS

Impairment of neuromuscular transmission may be confirmed by a positive edrophonium (Tensilon) test. Atropine 0.6 mg is given i.v. to prevent muscarinic side-effects, and this is followed by 1 mg edrophonium. If there is no obvious improvement within 1–2 min, a further 5 mg may be given. Some authors recommend the use of a saline placebo injection, and the presence of a second doctor as a 'blinded' observer. Resuscitation facilities should be available, as profound weakness may ensue, especially in patients already receiving anticholinesterase drugs. Intramuscular neostigmine, 1–2 mg, may produce a positive response in 5–10% of patients who do not respond to edrophonium.[42]

The presence of autoantibodies against ACh receptors is quite specific, but false positives occur in patients with penicillamine-treated rheumatoid disease, other autoimmune diseases and in some first-degree relatives of myasthenic patients.[43] Electromyography shows characteristic changes in 90% of patients with generalized MG, and also in many patients with ocular symptoms only.

A syndrome of myasthenic weakness occurs in association with malignancy and other autoimmune diseases (Eaton–Lambert syndrome). Although fatigability is present, the pelvic and thigh muscles are predominantly affected, whereas ocular and bulbar involvement are rare. Tendon reflexes are reduced or absent, and there are specific electromyographic changes.

MANAGEMENT

1 *Symptomatic treatment* is provided by anticholinesterase drugs which potentiate the action of ACh at receptor sites. Pyridostigmine (Mestinon) is the most commonly used, and is usually commenced at a dose of 60 mg orally 4 times daily. Considerable adjustment of dosage may be required.

2 *Thymectomy* produces the best results, and early thymectomy is now advocated as the treatment of choice in virtually all patients with more than mild disease, regardless of the presence of a thymoma.[44] Compared with medical therapy, thymectomy results in an earlier onset of remission, lower mortality and greater delay in the appearance of extrathymic recurrences.[45]

Preoperative optimization of neuromuscular function is essential, using anticholinesterase drugs, supplemented by plasma exchange if necessary. Though anticholinesterase requirements are usually reduced in the immediate postoperative period to about three-quarters of the preoperative dose, sustained improvement following thymectomy may not be seen for many months. A transcervical approach has been advocated, but doubts remain about the completeness of excision by this route. A thoracoscopic approach may achieve equivalent results with less short-term morbidity,[46] but the traditional sternotomy approach continues to be much more widely used.[47]

3 *Corticosteroids* are effective in approximately 70% of patients, and give best results when high doses (e.g. prednisolone 50–100 mg/day) are used initially, and then gradually reduced. However, transient exacerbation upon commencement of steroids is very common,[48] and severely affected patients are often hospitalized for the initiation of therapy with gradually increasing doses. Older patients are more likely to respond, but an average of 4 months' treatment is required to achieve clinical stability, and the majority will require continuing treatment indefinitely.[49]

4 *Azathioprine and cyclophosphamide* are both effective adjuncts to corticosteroid therapy. Overall, 80% of patients are helped, but improvement may be seen only after some months. A few patients may achieve complete remission.[50] Cyclosporine is also effective, and patients may show benefit more quickly than with azathioprine.[51]

5 *Plasma exchange* is effective in producing short-term clinical improvement.[52] It is mainly used in myasthenic crisis or to improve severely affected patients before thymectomy. Its use should be considered, particularly in patients with severe respiratory failure refractory to conventional therapy (see below).[53] Typically, five exchanges of 3–4 litres each are performed over a 2-week period, and this results in improvement within days. However, the benefits are short-lived, lasting only weeks.[54]

6 *γ-Globulin* given intravenously has similar effects to those of plasma exchange. A dose of 400 mg/kg per day is usually given for 5 successive days, and occasional patients derive long-term benefit.[55] Interestingly, γ-globulin has no consistent effect on ACh receptor antibody concentrations, and its mechanism of action is unknown.

MYASTHENIC AND CHOLINERGIC CRISIS

Patients with known MG may undergo life-threatening episodes of acute deterioration affecting bulbar and respiratory function. These may follow intercurrent infection, pregnancy or the administration of various drugs[56] (Table 47.3). Such episodes, known as myasthenic crises, usually resolve over several weeks, but occasionally last

Table 47.3   Drugs which may exacerbate myasthenia gravis

| *Antibiotics* |
| Streptomycin |
| Kanamycin |
| Tobramycin |
| Gentamicin |
| Polymyxin group |
| Tetracycline |
| *Antiarrhythmics* |
| Quinidine |
| Quinine |
| Procainamide |
| *Local anaesthetics* |
| Procaine |
| Lignocaine |
| *General anaesthetics* |
| Ether |
| *Muscle relaxants* |
| Curare |
| Suxamethonium |
| *Analgesics* |
| Morphine |
| Pethidine |

months. The incidence of myasthenic crisis increases markedly with age.[57]

These patients should be admitted directly to the ICU, as there is a significant risk of pulmonary aspiration due to bulbar involvement, bacterial pneumonia due to stasis, and acute respiratory failure or cardiorespiratory arrest. After stabilization and resuscitation, if necessary, an edrophonium (Tensilon) test should be performed. This will indicate whether the patient can be expected to respond to increased dosage of anticholinergic drugs.

If the condition is worsened by edrophonium, the patient is likely to be suffering from over administration of anticholinesterase drugs (i.e. cholinergic crisis). Abdominal cramps, diarrhoea, excessive pulmonary secretions, sweating, salivation and bradycardia may be present; the patient may improve if anticholinesterase drugs are reduced in dosage or withdrawn temporarily and restarted after 1–2 days. Frequent estimations of vital capacity and maximum inspiratory force should be made and recorded. Tracheal intubation and mechanical ventilation should be considered in patients with significant bulbar involvement or clinical evidence of worsening respiratory failure. As with other neuromuscular disorders, deterioration of blood gases may occur late, and is an unreliable sign of progressive respiratory failure.[58] Aggressive chest physiotherapy, urinary drainage and nasogastric feeding may be required. Hypokalaemia, hypocalcaemia and hypermagnesaemia should be avoided, as all may exacerbate muscle weakness.

If the patient's clinical status cannot be rapidly improved by the adjustment of anticholinesterase dosage and aggressive treatment of intercurrent illness, high-dose corticosteroids and plasma exchange should be commenced simultaneously, and may produce some benefit within as little as 24 hours.

PERIOPERATIVE MANAGEMENT

MG patients often require intensive care in relation to surgery for intercurrent illness or, more often, thymectomy. Unstable patients should be admitted to hospital some days in advance for stabilization. In severely affected patients, preoperative high-dose corticosteroids and/or plasma exchange may be used to improve the patient's fitness for surgery. It may be prudent to omit premedication, and an anaesthetic technique which avoids the use of non-depolarizing muscle relaxants is usually advocated, though vecuronium and atracurium are probably acceptable in reduced dosage.[60,61] Suxamethonium can be used safely in normal dosage.[62]

Up to one-third of patients require continuing mechanical ventilation postoperatively following thymectomy. Predictive factors include a long preoperative duration of myasthenia, coexistent chronic respiratory disease, high anticholinesterase requirements (e.g. pyri-

dostigmine >750 mg/day), and a preoperative vital capacity of less than 2.9 litres.[63] In those cases requiring mechanical ventilation, some authors advocate temporary cessation of anticholinesterase drugs to reduce respiratory secretions,[64] but in all other cases they should be continued, though dosage requirements must be reassessed carefully and repeatedly.

MOTOR NEURONE DISEASE (AMYOTROPHIC LATERAL SCLEROSIS, LOU GEHRIG'S DISEASE)[65]

Motor neurone disease refers to a large group of related disorders (Table 47.4), a few of which are clearly genetically determined, while most arise sporadically, are of completely unknown aetiology, and are generally untreatable. The most common variant is the sporadic form known as amyotrophic lateral sclerosis (ALS), a relentlessly progressive degenerative disease which most commonly affects males over 50 years of age.[66] In North America, the term ALS is often used more generically, essentially equivalent to the broader term motor neurone disease.

PATHOGENESIS

The disease affects both upper and lower motor neurones. The involvement of either can predominate early on, giving rise to several clinically recognizable subgroups (Table 47.4). The cerebral cortex as well as the anterior horns of the spinal cord are involved, with shrinkage, degenerative pigmentation and, eventually, disappearance of the affected cells accompanied by gliosis of the lateral columns ('lateral sclerosis'). As muscles are denervated, there is progressive atrophy of muscle fibres ('amyotrophy'), but, remarkably, sensory neurones as well as those concerned with autonomic function, co-ordination and higher cerebral function are all spared. The precise cause remains unknown. Postulated pathogenetic causes include oxygen free-radicals, viral or prion

Table 47.4 Degenerative motor neurone diseases[a]

Amyotrophic lateral sclerosis
Spinal muscular atrophy
Bulbar palsy
Primary lateral sclerosis
Pseudobulbar palsy
Heritable motor neurone diseases
Autosomal recessive spinal muscular atrophy
Familial amyotrophic lateral sclerosis
Other
Associated with other degenerative disorders

[a] Modified from Beal et al.,[78] with permission.

infection, excess excitatory neurotransmitters and growth factor, and immunological abnormalities.[67] The only established clinical risk factors are age and family history.

CLINICAL PRESENTATION[68]

The earliest symptoms are those of insidiously developing limb weakness, often asymmetrical, accompanied by obvious muscle wasting. This classically affects the small muscles of the hand and may be accompanied by fasciculation. As time passes, the disease becomes more generalized and more symmetrical, with a mixture of upper and lower motor neurone signs (i.e. spasticity and hyperreflexia in addition to gross wasting). Bulbar and respiratory muscles are affected but awareness and intellect are completely preserved. Death occurs in 50% of cases within 3–5 years, usually due to respiratory infection, aspiration or ventilatory failure from profound weakness. However, there is wide variability, and a few patients may survive for many years.

DIAGNOSIS

There are no specific investigations, and the diagnosis must be made on clinical grounds together with electromyogram (EMG) evidence of denervation in at least 3 limbs. Experienced neurologists correctly diagnose the condition with 95% accuracy.[69] The most important differential diagnosis is multifocal motor neuropathy. The distinction is of clinical importance, as the latter is amenable to treatment. Poliomyelitis can also result in a syndrome of progressive weakness, wasting and fasciculation, beginning many years after the initial illness (the post-polio syndrome), and leading occasionally to respiratory failure and death.[70]

MANAGEMENT

Treatment is essentially symptomatic and supportive. No benefit has been shown with antioxidants, growth factors and immunosuppressants. However, the centrally acting glutamate antagonist riluzole has been shown to slow slightly the progression of ALS.[71] Admission to an ICU is sometimes requested when these patients present with an acute deterioration or intercurrent illness. The intensivist may be asked to assist with ambulatory or home respiratory support for gradually worsening chronic respiratory failure. Such cases present major ethical as well as clinical problems, but the provision of assisted ventilation can result in an improved quality of life, and possibly prolonged survival for carefully selected individuals.[72] Respiratory support may be given by facemask, nasal mask or, rarely, by tracheostomy using simple, compact ventilators. Some patients require only intermittent support, particularly at night or during periods of acute deterioration due to intercurrent illness. Long-term respiratory support outside the ICU is a major undertaking, requiring specific equipment and extensive liaison with the patient, the family and numerous specialized support services.

RARE CAUSES OF ACUTE WEAKNESS IN THE ICU

PERIODIC PARALYSIS[73]

This term describes a group of rare primary disorders, mostly inherited as autosomal dominant traits, producing episodic weakness. They must be distinguished from other causes of intermittent weakness, including electrolyte abnormalities, MG and transient ischaemic attacks. In the inherited disorders, the underlying abnormality is a defect of skeletal muscle ion channels. Symptoms begin early in life (before age 25), and follow rest or sleep rather than exertion. Alertness during attacks is completely preserved, and muscle strength between attacks is normal. Treatment is usually successful in preventing both the attacks and the chronic weakness, which can develop after many years in untreated patients.

The *hypokalaemic* form of periodic paralysis is predominantly inherited, but can also arise sporadically in association with thyrotoxicosis. Involvement of bulbar or respiratory muscles occurs rarely, as can cardiac arrhythmias. The degree of hypokalaemia during attacks is mild, but patients rapidly respond to potassium administration. Effective prophylaxis is conferred by acetazolamide, but not by oral potassium.

The *hyperkalaemic* form is milder, almost always inherited and virtually never requires intensive care. During attacks the serum potassium may be modestly elevated or normal. Patients respond to carbohydrate administration, and thiazide diuretics or acetazolamide provide effective prophylaxis.

BOTULISM[74,75]

Botulism is a widespread but very uncommon potentially lethal disease caused by exotoxins produced by *Clostridium botulinum*, which is an anaerobic, spore-forming Gram-positive bacillus. The vast majority of botulism is food-borne and outbreaks occur largely in home-preserved vegetables (type A toxin), meat (type B) or fish (type E), but high-risk foods also include low-acid fruit and condiments. Signs and symptoms are caused by toxin produced *in vitro* and then ingested.

Wound botulism arises rarely, when wounds (typically open fractures) are contaminated by soil containing type A or B organisms. Intravenous drug abusers are an increasing source of this condition through infected injection sites.

Infantile botulism arises in infants under 6 months of age, and is due to the active production of toxin by organisms in the gut rather than the direct ingestion of toxin.

Hidden botulism describes the adult equivalent of infantile botulism, and is a rare complication of various gastrointestinal abnormalities.

Inadvertent botulism is the most recently described form, and occurs as a complication of the medical use of botulinum toxin.

Botulism has also been recognized for its potential as a biological weapon, which could be adopted by terrorist groups.

In most cases, exogenously produced exotoxin is absorbed (primarily in the upper small intestine), and carried by the blood stream to cholinergic nerves at the neuromuscular junction, postganglionic parasympathetic nerve endings and autonomic ganglia, to which it irreversibly binds. The toxin enters the nerve endings to interfere with ACh release.

Most patients become ill about 3 days after ingestion of toxin, with gastrointestinal symptoms (nausea, vomiting, abdominal pain, diarrhoea or constipation), dryness of the eyes and mouth, dysphagia and generalized weakness, which progresses in a symmetrical, descending fashion, with ventilatory failure in severe cases. Cranial nerve dysfunction is manifested by ptosis and diplopia, facial weakness and impaired upper airway reflexes.

The differential diagnosis includes food poisoning from other causes, MG and GBS. Botulism can be confirmed by the presence of toxin (either in the patient's serum or stool, or in contaminated food) in about two-thirds of cases.

Treatment is mainly supportive, with airway protection and mechanical ventilation when required. Clearance of toxin from the bowel with enemas and cathartics has been advocated. Guanidine hydrochloride, which enhances the release of ACh from nerve terminals, has been reported to improve muscle strength, especially in ocular muscles, and may be useful in milder cases.[76] Antibiotics have not been clearly shown to be useful. Equine antitoxins are available, but side effects are common and their efficacy is limited. Trials of a human antitoxin are currently in progress. In wound botulism, aggressive debridement is recommended.

Most patients begin to improve after a week or so, but mild weakness and constipation may persist for months.

REFERENCES

1 Wardrop J. Clinical observations on various diseases. *Lancet* 1834; **1**: 380.

2 Guillain G, Barré JA, Strohl A. Sur un syndrome de radiculo-nevrites avec hyperalbuminose du liquide cephalorachidren sans reaction cellulaire. Remarques sur les caracteres cliniques et graphiques des reflexes tendineaux. *Bull Soc Med Hop Paris* 1916; **40**: 1462.

3 Asbury AK, Aranson BG, Karp HR, MacFarlin DF. Criteria for diagnosis of Guillain–Barré syndrome. *Ann Neurol* 1998; **3**: 565–6.

4 Hahn AF. Guillain–Barré syndrome. *Lancet* 1998; **352**: 635–41.

5 Sliman NA. Outbreak of Guillain–Barré syndrome associated with water pollution. *BMJ* 1978; **1**: 751–2.

6 Lisak RP, Mitchell M, Zweiman B, *et al*. Guillain–Barré syndrome and Hodgkin's disease. Three cases with immunological studies. *Ann Neurol* 1977 **1**: 72–8.

7 Korn-Lubetzki I, Abramsky O. Acute chronic demyelinating inflammatory polyradiculoneuropathy: association with auto-immune diseases and lymphocyte response to human neuritogenic protein. *Arch Neurol* 1986; **43**: 604–8.

8 Giovannoni G, Hartnung H-P. The immunopathogenesis of multiple sclerosis and Guillain–Barré syndrome. *Curr Opin Neurol* 1996; **9**: 165–77.

9 Simpson DM, Olney RK. Peripheral neuropathies associated with human immunodeficiency virus infection. *Neurol Clin* 1992; **10**: 685–711.

10 Jacobs BS, van Doorn PA, Schmitz PIM, *et al*. *Campylobacter jejuni* infection and anti-GM$_1$ anti bodies in Guillain–Barré syndrome. *Ann Neurol* 1996; **40**: 181–7.

11 Visser LH, van der Meché FGA, Meulste J, *et al*. Cytomegalovirus infection and Guillain–Barré syndrome: the clinical, electrophysiological and prognostic features. *Neurology* 1996; **47**: 668–73.

12 Newton N, Janoti A. Guillain–Barré syndrome after vaccination with purified tetanus toxoid. *South Med J* 1987; **80**: 1053–4.

13 Sawant S, Clark MB, Koski CL. *In vitro* demyelination by serum antibody from patients with immune complexes. *Ann Neurol* 1991; **29**: 397–404.

14 Slater RA, Rostomi A. Treatment of Guillain–Barré syndrome with intravenous immunoglobulin. *Neurology* 1998; **51**(Suppl 5): S9–S15.

15 Loffel NB, Rossi LN, Mumethaler M, *et al*. Landry–Guillain–Barré syndrome: complications, prognosis and natural history in 123 cases. *J Neurol Sci* 1977; **33**: 71–9.

16 Fisher CM. Unusual variant of acute idiopathic polyneuritis (syndrome of ophthalmoplegia, ataxia and areflexia). *N Engl J Med* 1956; **255**: 57–65.

17 Powell HC, Myers RR. The axon in Guillain–Barré syndrome: immune target or innocent bystander? *Ann Neurol* 1996; **39**: 4–5.

18 Truax BT. Autonomic disturbances in the Guillain–Barré syndrome. *Semin Neurol* 1984; **4**: 462–8.

19 Hughes RA. The spectrum of acquired demyelinating polyradiculopathy. *Acta Neurol Belg* 1994; **94**: 128–32.

20 McKhann GM, Cornblath DR, Griffin JW, *et al*. Acute motor axonal neuropathy: a frequent cause of acute flaccid paralysis in China. *Ann Neurol* 1993; **33**: 333–42.

21 Olney RK, Aminoff MJ. Electrodiagnostic features of the Guillain–Barré syndrome: the relative sensitivities of different techniques. *Neurology* 1990; **40**: 471–5.

22 French cooperative group on plasma exchange in Guillain–Barré syndrome. Efficiency of plasma exchange in Guillain–Barré syndrome: role of replacement fluids. *Ann Neurol* 1987; **22**: 753–61.

23 The Guillain–Barré study group. Plasmapheresis and acute Guillain–Barré syndrome. *Neurology* 1985; **35**: 1096–104.

24 Bouget J, Chevret S, Chastang C, *et al.* Plasma exchange morbidity in Guillain–Barré syndrome: results from the French prospective, double-blind, randomized, multi-center study. *Crit Care Med* 1993; **21**: 651–8.

25 Plasma Exchange/Sandoglobulin Guillain–Barré Syndrome Trial Group. Randomised trial of plasma exchange, intravenous immunoglobulin and combined treatments in Guillain–Barré syndrome. *Lancet* 1997; **349**: 225–30.

26 Guillain–Barré syndrome steroid trial group. Double-blind trial of intravenous methylprednisolone in Guillain–Barré syndrome. *Lancet* 1993; **341**: 586–90.

27 Hund EF, Borel CO, Cornblath DR, *et al.* Intensive management and treatment of severe Guillain–Barré syndrome. *Crit Care Med* 1993; **21**: 433–66.

28 Fergusson RJ, Wright DJ, Willey RJ, *et al.* Suxamethonium is dangerous in polyneuropathy. *BMJ* 1981; **282**: 298–9.

29 Cole GF, Matthew DJ. Prognosis in severe Guillain–Barré syndrome. *Arch Dis Child* 1987; **62**: 288–91.

30 Rees JH, Soudain SE, Gregson NA, Hughes RAC. *Campylobacter jejuni* infection and Guillain–Barré syndrome. *N Engl J Med* 1995; **333**: 1374–9.

31 Ropper AH. Severe acute Guillain–Barré syndrome. *Neurology* 1986; **36**: 429–32.

32 Scott IA, Seeley G, Wright M, *et al.* Guillain–Barré syndrome: a retrospective review. *Aust NZ J Med* 1988; **18**: 149–55.

33 Ng KKP, Howard RS, Fish DR, *et al.* Management and outcome of severe Guillain–Barré syndrome. *QJM* 1995; **88**: 243–50.

34 Nates JL, Cooper DJ, Day B, Tuxen DV. Acute weakness syndromes in critically ill patients – a reappraisal. *Anaesth Intens Care* 1997; **25**: 502–13.

35 Sliwa JA. Acute weakness syndromes in the critically ill patient. *Arch Phys Med Rehabil* 2000; **81**: S45–52.

36 Op de Cool AAW, Verheul GAM. Leijten ACM, *et al.* Critical illness polyneuropathy after artificial respiration. *Clin Neurol Neurosurg* 1991; **93**: 27–33.

37 Margolis B, Kachikian D, Friedman Y *et al.* Prolonged reversible quadriparesis in mechanically ventilated patients who received long-term infusions of vecuronium. *Chest* 1991; **100**: 877–8.

38 Kurtze JF, Kurland LT. The epidemiology of neurologic disease. In: Joynt RJ (ed.) *Clinical Neurology*, vol 4. Philadelphia, PA: JB Lippincott; 1992: pp. 80–8.

39 Osserman KE, Tsairis P, Weiner LB. Myasthenia gravis and thyroid disease. Clinical and immunological correlation. *Mt Sinai J Med* 1967; **34**: 469–83.

40 Engel AG, Ohno K, Sine SM. Congenital myasthenic syndromes. *Arch Neurol* 1999; **56**: 163–7.

41 Sharp HR, Degrip A, Mitchell D, Heller A. Bulbar presentations of myasthenia gravis in the elderly patient. *J Laryngol Otol.* 2001; **115**: 1–3.

42 Osserman KE, Genkins G. Critical reappraisal of the use of edrophonium (Tensilon) chloride tests in myasthenia gravis and significance of clinical observation. *Ann NY Acad Sci* 1966; **135**: 312–26.

43 Vincent A, Newsom-Davis J. Acetylcholine receptor antibody as a diagnostic test for myasthenia gravis: results in 153 validated cases and 2967 diagnostic assays. *J Neurol Neurosurg Psychiatry* 1986; **48**: 1246–52.

44 Busch C, Machens A, Pichlmeier U, *et al.* Long-term outcome and quality of life after thymectomy for myasthenia gravis. *Ann Surg* 1996; **224**: 225–32.

45 Papatestas AE, Genkins G, Kornfeld P, *et al.* Effects of thymectomy in myasthenia gravis. *Ann Surg* 1987; **206**: 79–88.

46 Ruckert JC, Walter M, Muller JM. Pulmonary function after thoracoscopic thymectomy versus median sternotomy for myasthenia gravis. *Ann Thorac Surg* 2000; **70**: 1656–61.

47 Younger DS, Jaretzky A IIIrd, Penn AS, *et al.* Maximum thymectomy for myasthenia gravis. *Ann NY Acad Sci* 1987; **505**: 832–5.

48 Johns TR. Long-term corticosteroid treatment of myasthenia gravis. *Ann NY Acad Sci* 1987; **505**: 568–83.

49 Sghirlanzoni A, Peluchetti D, Mantegazza R, *et al.* Myasthenia gravis: pro-longed treatment with steroids. *Neurology* 1984; **34**: 170–4.

50 Niakan E, Harati Y, Rolak LA. Immunosuppressive drug therapy in myasthenia gravis. *Arch Neurol* 1986; **43**: 155–6.

51 Schalke BCG, Kappos L, Rohrbach E, *et al.* Cyclosporine A vs. azathioprine in the treatment of myasthenia gravis: final results of a randomised, controlled double-blind clinical trial. *Neurology* 1988; **38**(Suppl 1): 135. [Abstr]

52 Dau PC, Lindstrom JM, Cassel CK, *et al.* Plasmapheresis and immunosuppressive drug therapy in myasthenia gravis. *N Engl J Med* 1977; **297**: 1134–40.

53 Gracey DR, Howard FM, Divertie MB. Plasmapheresis in the treatment of ventilator-dependent myasthenia gravis patients. Report of four cases. *Chest* 1984; **85**: 739–43.

54 Drachman DB. Myasthenia gravis. *N Engl J Med* 1994; **330**: 1797–810.

55 Arsura E. Experience with intravenous immunoglobulin in myasthenia gravis. *Clin Immunol Immunopathol* 1989; **53**(suppl): S170–9.

56 Wittbrodt ET. Drugs and myasthenia gravis. *Arch Intern Med* 1997; **157**: 399–408.

57 Sellman MS, Mayer RF. Treatment of myasthenic crisis in late life. *South Med J* 1985; **78**: 1208–10.

58 Harrison BDW, Collins JV, Brown KGE, Clarke THJ. Respiratory failure in neuromuscular diseases. *Thorax* 1971; **26**: 579–84.

59 Berroschot J, Baumann I, Kalischewski P, *et al.* Therapy of myasthenic crisis. *Crit Care Med* 1997; **25**: 1228–35.

60 Bell CF, Florence AM, Hunter JM, *et al.* Atracurium in the myasthenic patient. *Anaesthesia* 1984; **39**: 691–8.

61 Eisenkraft JB, Sawkney RK, Papatestas AE. Vecuronium in the myasthenic patient. *Anaesthesia* 1986; **41**: 666–7.

62 Wainwright AP, Broderick PM. Suxamethonium in myasthenia gravis. *Anaesthesia* 1987; **42**: 950–7.

63 Eisenkraft JB, Papatestas AE, Kahn CH, *et al.* Predicting the need for postoperative mechanical ventilation in myasthenia gravis. *Anaesthesiology* 1986; **65**: 79–82.

64 Gracey DR, Divertie MB, Howard FM, Payne WS. Postoperative respiratory care after transternal thymectomy in myasthenia gravis. *Chest* 1984; **86**: 67–71.

65 Rowland LP, Shneider NA. Amyotrophic lateral sclerosis. *N Engl J Med* 2001; **344**: 1688–700.

66 Williams DB, Windebank AJ. Motor neuron disease (amyotrophic lateral sclerosis). *Mayo Clin Proc* 1991; **66**: 54–82.

67 Jerusalem F, Pohl Ch, Karitzky J, Ries F. ALS. *Neurology* 1996; **47**(Suppl 4): S218–20.

68 Dengler R. Current treatment pathways in ALS: A European perspective. *Neurology* 1999; **53** (Suppl): S4–S10.

69 Rowland LP. Diagnosis of amyotrophic lateral sclerosis. *J Neurol Sci* 1998; **160**(Suppl 1): S6–S24.

70 Fisher DA. Poliomyelitis: late respiratory complications and management. *Orthopedics* 1985; **8**: 891–894.

71 Bensimon G, Lacomblez L, Meininger V for the ALS/Riluzole Study Group. A controlled trial of riluzole in amyotrophic lateral sclerosis. *N Engl J Med* 1994; **330**: 585–91.

72 Edwards PR, Howard P. Methods and prognosis of non-invasive ventilation in neuromuscular disease. *Monaldi Arch Chest Dis* 1993; **48**: 176–82.

73 Gutman L. Periodic paralyses. *Neurol Clin* 2000; **18**: 195–202.

74 Cherington M. Clinical spectrum of botulism. *Muscle Nerve* 1998; **21**: 701–10.

75 Shapiro RL, Hatheway C, Swerdlow DL. Botulism in the United States: a clinical and epidemiologic review. *Ann Intern Med* 1998; **129**: 221–8.

76 Puggiari M, Cherington M. Botulism and guanidine. Ten years later. *J Am Med Assoc* 1978; **240**: 2276–7.

Part Eight

Endocrine Disorders

48.

Diabetic emergencies
R Keays

Diabetes mellitus is due to an absolute or relative deficiency of insulin. The sustained effect of poor glycaemic control results in a wide array of end-organ damage as a consequence of small and large vessel pathology. Mortality and morbidity are related to the progress of this damage, but often there are acute metabolic deteriorations that can be life threatening. Diabetic ketoacidosis (DKA) and hyperosmolar hyperglycaemic state (HHS) are two of the most common acute complications of diabetes, both accompanied by hyperglycaemia. The pathophysiologic changes that occur in both disease states represent an extreme example of the super-fasted state. Coma may also result from severe hypoglycaemia due to over-treatment – usually with insulin.

DIABETES MELLITUS

TYPE I

Insulin dependant diabetes mellitus (IDDM) has a peak incidence in the young, rising from 9 months to 14 years and declining thereafter. It varies across race and regions, being highest in northern Europe and the USA and lowest in Asia and Australasia.[1] In 25% of patients the presentation is with ketoacidosis especially in those under 5 years of age.[2] Usually, the fasting plasma glucose is >7.8 mmol/l and glucose and ketones may be present in the urine. In the asymptomatic patient with an equivocal fasting plasma glucose an impaired glucose tolerance test may be demonstrated.

TYPE II

Non-insulin dependant diabetes mellitus (NIDDM) is prevalent in the elderly, but can occur at any age. Truncal obesity is a risk factor and there is ethnic variation in susceptibility. Diagnosis is often delayed and may be incidental from blood or urine sugar screening.[3] It may present with classical symptoms, as a diabetic emergency, or with complications such as organ damage or vascular disease. It is aetiologically diverse

and shows clustering in families, although only maturity-onset diabetes of the young (MODY) shows autosomal dominant inheritance.

PATHOGENESIS

Normal carbohydrate metabolism depends upon the presence of insulin (Figure 48.1) however, different tissues handle glucose in different ways. For example, red blood cells lack mitochondria and therefore pyruvate dehydrogenase and the enzymes involved in β-oxidation whereas liver parenchymal cells are able to perform the full range of glucose disposal (Figure 48.2). Both DKA and HHS result from a reduction in the effect of insulin with a concomitant rise in the counterregulatory hormones such as glucagon, catecholamines, cortisol and growth hormone. Hyperglycaemia occurs as a consequence of three processes: increased gluconeogenesis, increased glycogenolysis and reduced peripheral glucose utilization. The increase in glucose production occurs in both the liver and the kidneys as there is a high availability of gluconeogenic precursors such as amino acids (protein turnover shifts from balanced synthesis and degradation to reduced synthesis and increased degradation). Lactate and glycerol also become available due to an increase in skeletal muscle glycogenolysis, and an increase in adipose tissue lipolysis, respectively. Lastly, there is an increase in gluconeogenic enzyme activity enhanced further by stress hormones. While hepatic gluconeogenesis is the main mechanism for producing hyperglycaemia a significant proportion can be produced by the kidneys.[4] What is unclear is the temporal relationship of these changes, although an increase in both catecholamines and the glucagon/insulin ratio are early features.[5]

Decreased insulin and increased epinephrine levels activate adipose tissue lipase, causing a breakdown of triglycerides into glycerol and free fatty acids (FFAs). Once again glucagon is implicated as hepatic oxidation of FFAs to ketone bodies is stimulated predominantly by its inhibitory effect on acetyl-CoA carboxylase. The resultant reduced synthesis of malonyl-CoA causes a disinhibition of acyl-carnitine synthesis and subsequent

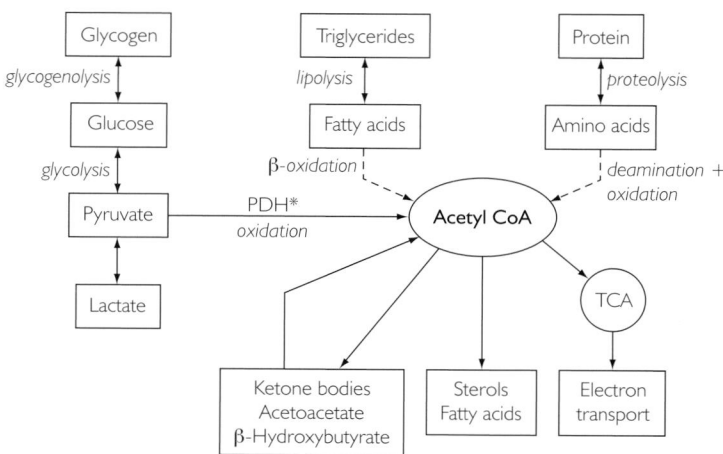

Fig. 48.1 Sources and fate of acetyl CoA. *Pyruvate conversion by pyruvate dehydrogenase (PDH) is essentially irreversible therefore no net conversion of fatty acids to carbohydrates can occur.

promotion of fatty acid transport into mitochondria where ketone body formation occurs. Both cortisol and growth hormone are capable of increasing FFA and ketone levels, and once again the exact contribution of insulin deficiency or stress hormone increase to ketogenesis is undetermined.

As HHS does not share the ketogenic features of DKA it is interesting to examine how these two conditions differ. Reduced levels of FFAs, glucagon, cortisol and growth hormone have been demonstrated in HHS relative to DKA although this is by no means a consistent observation. However, the presence of higher levels of C-peptide in HHS (with lower levels of growth hormone) relative to DKA suggests there is just enough insulin present in HHS to prevent lipolysis but not enough to promote peripheral glucose utilization.[6]

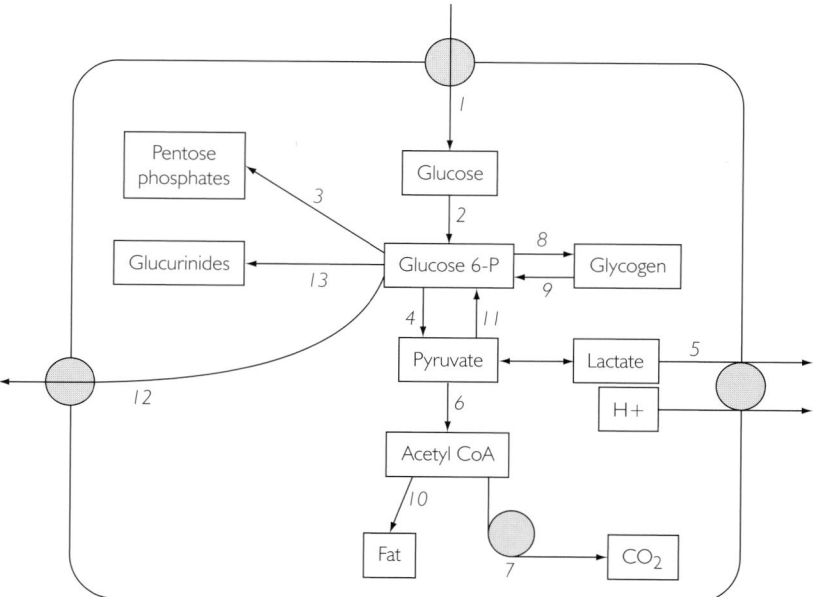

Fig. 48.2 Glucose metabolism within hepatocyte. (*1*) Glucose transport GLUT-1, (*2*) hexokinase phosphorylation, (*3*) pentose phosphate pathway (hexose monophosphate shunt), (*4*) glycolysis, (*5*) lactate transport out of cell, (*6*) pyruvate decarboxylation, (*7*) TCA cycle, (*8*) glycogenesis, (*9*) glycogenolysis, (*10*) lipogenesis, (*11*) gluconeogenesis, (*12*) G-6-P hydrolysis and release of glucose, (*13*) glucuronidation.

Hyperosmolarity, which is a prominent feature of HHS is caused by the prolonged effect of an osmotic diuresis with impaired ability to take adequate fluids. It has been shown that even when well, patients who have suffered from HHS have impaired thirst reflexes. However, the hyperosmolarity seen in about one-third of patients with DKA results from a shorter osmotic diuresis, and to variable fluid intake due to nausea and vomiting – which is often ascribed to the brainstem effects of ketones.

CLINICAL PRESENTATION

DKA and HHS represent the two extremes of presentation due to the absolute or relative deficiency of insulin. However, up to one third of cases can present with mixed features.[7] DKA develops over a shorter time period whereas HHS appears more insidiously (see Table 48.1). Polyuria, polydipsia and weight loss are experienced for a variable period prior to admission and, in patients with DKA, nausea and vomiting is also a common symptom. Abdominal pain is commonly seen in children and occasionally in adults and may mimic an acute abdomen. Dehydration presents with loss of skin turgor, dry mucous membranes, tachycardia and hypotension. Mental obtundation occurs more frequently in HHS than DKA as more patients, by definition, are hyperosmolar. The presence of stupor or coma in patients who are not hyperosmolar requires consideration of other potential causes for altered mental status.[8] However, loss of consciousness is not a common presentation with DKA or HHS (<20%). Most hospitalizations are caused by infection (29%) or non-compliance with medication (17%) in previously diagnosed diabetics, however, in some patients it is the first presentation with undiagnosed diabetes (17%).[9] Given that there is a high likelihood of concurrent infection most patients have a normal or low temperature and most patients also have a leukocytosis, whether there is infection present or not.

DIABETIC KETOACIDOSIS

Tends to occur more often in patients with Type I diabetes and the predominant feature is ketoacidosis. Rapid, deep breathing due to the acidosis (Kussmaul breathing) may be present as may the breath odour that is characteristic of ketones, which is somewhat like nail polish remover. A history of insulin therapy omission is common and patients using continuous insulin delivery devices are particularly at risk due to the use of short-acting insulin which provides no insulin reserve if the pump fails. Diagnostic criteria include pH <7.3, HCO_3^- <15 mmol/l and blood glucose >14 mmol/l. Increasing acidaemia, ketonaemia and deteriorating conscious level indicate an increasing severity. Blood glucose *per se* is not a good determinant of severity and euglycaemic keto-

Table 48.1 Comparison of diabetic ketoacidosis (DKA) and hyperosmolar hyperglycaemic state (HHS)

	DKA	HHS
Presentation		
Prodromal illness	Days	Weeks
Coma	++	+++
Blood glucose	++	+++
Ketones	+++	0 or +
Acidaemia	+++	0 or +
Anion gap	++	0 or +
Osmolality	++	+++
Typical deficits		
Total water (litres)	6	9
Water (ml/kg)	100	100–200
Na^+ (mEq/kg)	7–10	5–13
Cl^- (mEq/kg)	3–5	5–15
K^+ (mEq/kg)	3–5	4–6
PO_4^{3-} (mEq/kg)	5–7	3–7
Mg^{2+} (mEq/kg)	1–2	1–2
Ca^{2+} (mEq/kg)	1–2	1–2

acidosis is possible, depending on the hepatic glycogen stores *prior* to the onset of DKA – a patient who has not been eating well in the recent past may well have a minimally elevated blood glucose. A high amylase is frequently seen and may be extra-pancreatic in origin. It should be interpreted cautiously as a sign of pancreatitis.

HYPEROSMOLAR HYPERGLYCAEMIC SYNDROME

This is more often seen in patients with Type II diabetes and the dominant feature is hyperosmolarity (>320 mOsm/kg). HHS is typically observed in elderly patients with non-insulin-dependent diabetes mellitus, although it may rarely be a complication in younger patients with insulin-dependent diabetes, or those without diabetes following severe burns,[10] parenteral hyperalimentation, peritoneal dialysis, or haemodialysis. Patients receiving certain drugs including diuretics, corticosteroids, β-blockers, phenytoin, and diazoxide are at increased risk of developing this syndrome. HHS may be caused by lithium induced diabetes insipidus.[11] Not only may mental obtundation occur but occasionally focal neurological features or seizures are present.

MANAGEMENT

ICU admission is indicated in the management of DKA, HHS, and mixed cases in the presence of cardiovascular instability, inability to protect the airway, altered sensoria, and the presence of acute abdominal signs or symptoms suggestive of acute gastric dilatation.

INITIAL ASSESSMENT

These conditions are medical emergencies and a prompt and thorough history and physical examination should be obtained with special attention paid to airway patency, conscious level, cardiovascular and renal status, possible sources of infection and state of hydration. Some assessment of the severity of DKA is also aided by the degree of acidosis.

FLUID REQUIREMENTS

Dehydration and sodium depletion develop as a result of the osmotic diuresis that accompanies hyperglycaemia in both DKA and HHS. In DKA there is an additional keto-anion excretion which is approximately half that of glucose. This obligates cation (sodium, potassium and ammonium) excretion and contributes to the electrolyte losses. Despite the dual osmotic load of glucose and ketones in DKA, dehydration is often worse in HHS due to the more prolonged onset. Insulin itself also promotes salt, water and phosphate reabsorption in the kidney and its lack can contribute further to these losses. The total osmolar load on the kidney in DKA can be as much as 2000 mOsm/day.[12] Fluid resuscitation is initially directed to repleting the intravascular volume and colloids achieve this more rapidly than crystalloids. There is individual variation as to how much fluid will be required and simple vital signs, such as heart rate, blood pressure and peripheral perfusion should guide the resuscitation. Fluid challenges with assessment of response may be less likely to avoid the problems of fluid overload. The usual urinary sodium concentration is 60–70 mmol/l, which is roughly similar to half-normal saline and this is the logical fluid to use for rehydration.[13] This avoids too great a sodium load and is less likely to produce a hyperchloraemic acidosis which, if rhabdomyolysis occurs, will further acidify the urine and promote precipitation of myoglobin in the renal tubule. As insulin therapy is commenced extracellular water is driven into the intracellular compartment exacerbating hypovolaemia.

Inappropriate fluid replacement can lead to problems. Studies of DKA and cerebral oedema are limited but there is some evidence that over aggressive replacement of water losses can precipitate cerebral and other forms of oedema. Water losses do not need to be corrected rapidly and hyperosmolality should not be corrected more rapidly than 3 mOsm/kg H_2O/h. Inappropriate resuscitation fluid can also lead to further overshoot in plasma sodium levels and a further increase in plasma osmolarity which has been associated with pontine myelinolysis.[14]

General guidelines are given in Figure 48.3 but it must be remembered that each case needs individual tailoring of treatment. It is mostly agreed that the first litre should be isotonic saline, even in patients with marked hypertonicity. This should be given over the first hour. If there is any evidence of cardiovascular compromise due to hypovolaemia plasma expansion with colloids should also be given as a matter of urgency. For the next 2 h, 0.45% saline can be given if the serum sodium is normal or high. If the corrected sodium is low then 0.9% saline should be continued. When the blood glucose falls to 15 mmol/l or below then a combination of 5% dextrose solution (100–250 ml/h) with some further saline containing solution should be commenced. Assuming cardiovascular stability, the aim should be to correct the

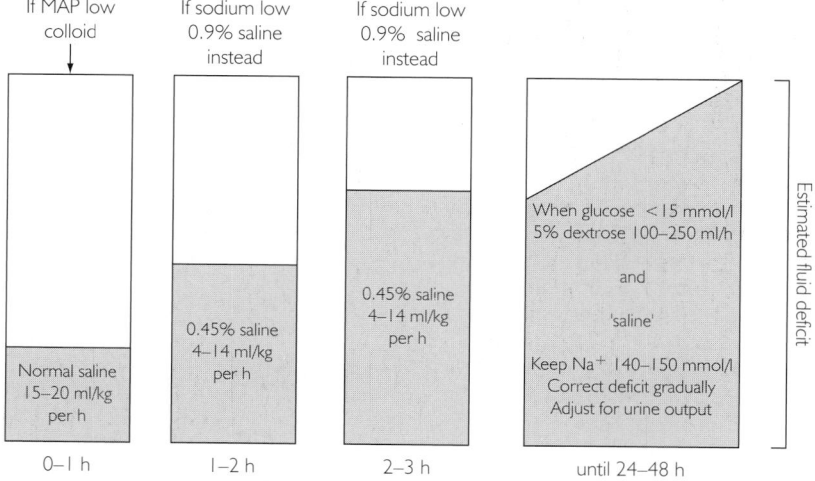

Fig. 48.3   Fluid regimen in hyperglycaemic emergencies. No major differences between diabetic ketoacidosis (DKA) and hyperosmolar hyperglycaemic state (HHS), except glucose supplement needs to be given at an earlier stage of correction in HHS when the blood glucose is 15 mmol/l or less. MAP, Mean arterial pressure.

remaining fluid deficit gradually over the next 24–48 h, while also taking account of on-going urinary losses.

INSULIN THERAPY

It is now clear that an intial bolus dose of 0.15 U/kg followed by low dose (0.1 U/kg per h) insulin infusions and gradual correction of hyperglycaemia in DKA results in a reduced mortality.[15] This is because there are less therapy-induced episodes of hypoglycaemia and hypokalaemia. Intravenous rather than subcutaneous or intramuscular delivery is preferable as glucose decrement is the same whatever route is chosen but intravenous insulin reduces ketone body production faster. It is mandatory to use the intravenous route where hypovolaemic shock is present. Appropriate rehydration also acts to reduce blood glucose levels by increased glomerular filtration and a reduction in counterregulatory hormone levels. Inadequate glucose decrement may indicate inadequate fluid resuscitation. Severe insulin resistance, which occurs in 10% of cases, will necessitate the use of higher doses.

ELECTROLYTE THERAPY

POTASSIUM

Hyperosmolarity causes a shift of potassium from within cells to the extracellular space and this potassium is lost as a result of the osmotic diuresis. Renal losses are augmented by secondary hyperaldosteronism and ketoanion excretion as potassium salts. Typical total body deficits are shown in Table 48.1. Serum potassium levels may initially be high and potassium replacement should not commence until this has fallen to <5.5 mmol/l. Potassium can be replaced as a combination of the chloride and phosphate salt as this can avoid hyperchloraemia and hypophosphataemia. Occasionally the potassium level will be low (<3.3 mmol/l), representing profound potassium depletion (600–800 mmol), and replacement should commence immediately, and before insulin therapy is initiated. If the patient is in between these two levels then 20–40 mmol of potassium may be given in the first hour – this should not generally be exceeded. Further decisions regarding potassium replacement need to be adjusted with respect to serum levels and the urine output, but usually 20–30 mmol/h is required. ECG monitoring has been recommended where potassium replacement is needed in patients who present with hypokalaemia or cardiac rhythms other than sinus tachycardia.[6]

PHOSPHATE

A total body phosphate deficit of greater than 1 mmol/kg is typical. Once again, the shift is from the intracellular compartment with subsequent urinary loss, however, serum levels are typically normal or increased.

Insulin causes an intracellular shift of phosphate and, although hypophosphataemia rarely results in adverse complications, muscle weakness, haemolytic anaemia and impaired cardiac systolic performance can occur. Routine phosphate replacement has not been shown to be beneficial in DKA[16] but correction of severely low levels (<0.4 mmol/l) may be necessary. Excessive phosphate replacement leads to hypocalcaemia, and serum calcium should be monitored.

MAGNESIUM

A chronic magnesium deficiency may be present in type I or II diabetes and may be exacerbated by renal impairment. The benefits of magnesium replacement have not been demonstrated in diabetic emergencies, but the principles of magnesium supplementation are similar to other critical care situations.

CORRECTION OF ACIDOSIS

This occurs more slowly than the correction of blood glucose but the use of bicarbonate in DKA remains controversial. Sodium bicarbonate is associated with side-effects that may overshadow any potential benefits. These include increased CO_2 production, CSF acidosis, hypokalaemia, rebound alkalosis, volume overload and altered tissue oxygenation. At pH >7.0 insulin will block lipolysis and ketoacid production, however, when the pH is between 6.9 and 7.1 it remains uncertain whether bicarbonate is beneficial or otherwise. Below pH 6.9 most authorities would recommend the use of bicarbonate to correct the pH partially to the threshold. The threshold for correction is debatable (between pH 6.9–7.15) but life-threatening hyperkalaemia is an undisputed indication for bicarbonate therapy.

Sometimes there is a persistent acidosis without ketosis. Regeneration of bicarbonate in DKA once insulin activity has been restored occurs via two mechanisms: renal and hepatic. The latter requires a metabolizable substrate, typically ketones, which are lost to the body especially if the diuresis is substantial. The former is slow and hyperchloraemia may persist, particularly if a high chloride containing fluid such as normal saline is used.[17]

UNDERLYING CAUSE

Attention must also focus on any underlying precipitant. The two major factors involved are inadequate insulin treatment and infection causing a change in insulin responsiveness. The latter must be actively looked for in the management of these patients.

MONITORING

The following monitoring parameters are also undertaken as investigations on presentation:

- Blood glucose concentration; initially every hour, then less frequently.
- Blood urea and creatinine concentrations; on admission and then at least daily. Creatinine assays that rely on a colorimetric method may be interfered with by the presence of acetoacetate, giving a falsely elevated value.
- Serum electrolytes:
  (a) *Serum sodium*: on admission and at least daily. It represents the relative water and electrolyte losses and cannot be used to infer a state of hydration. It may be normal (50% of cases), raised or lowered. Each 3.0 mmol/l rise in blood glucose will decrease serum sodium by 1 mmol/l, so hypernatraemia represents a profound loss of water. This formula is often used to calculate the 'corrected sodium' (see also Ch. 84).
  (b) *Serum potassium*: initially every hour, then less frequently (every 2–4 h). DKA patients have a K+-deficit of 3–5 mmol/kg. However, serum concentrations are usually normal or raised because of a shift from the intracellular to the extracellular compartment due to acidaemia, insulin deficiency and hypertonicity. Hypokalaemia on admission represents severe potassium depletion (>600–800 mmol) and requires potassium administration before starting insulin therapy.
  (c) *Serum chloride*: as often as needed to calculate the anion gap, which decreases to normal as DKA is treated. It also allows differentiation of the different causes of acidosis (see Ch. 82).
  (d) *Serum phosphate*: on admission and every 1–2 days. Routine replacement is not of any benefit. Despite evidence that hypophosphataemia leads to a decrease in 2,3-diphosphoglycerate levels, subsequent correction has no impact on the oxyhaemoglobin dissociation curve and dangerous hypocalcaemia may result.[16]
  (e) *Serum magnesium*: on admission and every 1–2 days. Chronic hypomagnesaemia may be present and may contribute to insulin resistance, carbohydrate intolerance and hypertension. Severe uncontrolled diabetes also results in magnesium depletion. However, the benefits of replacement therapy have not been demonstrated but may be necessary if arrythmias are present.
- Serum ketones (if available): on admission. This test relies on the nitroprusside reaction and, because it does not measure β-hydroxybutyrate (which is the main ketoacid in DKA), it consequently underestimates the degree of ketoacidosis.
- Urinary glucose and ketones: 4-hourly. Ketonuria may persist up to 2 days after the correction of acidosis due to the presence of acetone, which is not an acid anion and is highly lipid-soluble.
- Arterial blood gases: frequently as indicated.
- Serum osmolality and anion gap: initially and as indicated. Serum osmolality can be measured with an osmometer or estimated from the equation:

Osmolality (normal 285–300 mosmol/l) = $2(Na^+ + K^+)$ + glucose + urea

All values in mmol/l. The anion gap is calculated by the equation:

Anion gap (normal 10–17 mmol) = $(Na^+ + K^+) - (Cl^- + HCO_3^-)$

All values in mmol/l.

- Serum lactate: if acidosis is severe and anion gap is large.
- Full blood count and coagulation studies: daily and as indicated. Leukocytosis with left shift may occur in the absence of sepsis.
- Chest X-ray.
- Blood cultures, urine and sputum microscopy and culture and culture of relevant specimens as indicated.
- Pulse oximetry continuously.
- Electrocardiogram – 12 lead recording and continuous monitoring.
- Invasive haemodynamic monitoring as indicated.
- Neurological status and observations: including Glasgow coma scale and computed tomography scans as indicated for persistent coma or worsening neurological state.
- Other investigations as indicated (e.g. liver function tests, serum amylase, cardiac enzymes and creatinine clearance).

COMPLICATIONS

EARLY

The commonest early complications are hypoglycaemia due to over-treatment with insulin, hypokalaemia due to inadequate replacement and hyperglycaemia due to interruption of insulin. A hyperchloraemic acidosis can develop in about 10% of patients with DKA. It can be exaggerated by excessive saline use and is not usually clinically significant except in cases of acute renal failure or extreme oliguria.

Cerebral oedema is a rare but extremely serious complication of DKA occurring predominantly in children (0.7–1%). It does also occur in young adults and may be associated with rapid deterioration in conscious level with or without seizures. If progressive signs of brain stem herniation are present the mortality is high with only 7–14% likely to make a complete recovery. The risks of brain herniation are related to the degree of acidosis and the volume of initial fluid resuscitation. The mechanism for oedema formation is unknown but is most likely due to intracellular shift of water when plasma osmolality declines too rapidly.[18] It has been recommended that plasma osmolality is reduced slowly and that glucose must be added to the hydrating fluids when the plasma glucose has fallen to 15 mmol/l in DKA and possibly before this in HHS. Fatal cases of cerebral oedema have been reported in HHS as well, and treatment is aimed at maintaining plasma osmolality with intravenous mannitol.

Some degree of brain dysfunction is apparent even in those patients who are not comatose but who have severe DKA as measured by sensory evoked potentials. This reverts to normal with correction of the ketoacidosis.[19]

Hypoxia and non-cardiogenic pulmonary oedema can also occur and the increase in lung water and resultant reduced lung compliance is attributed to the reduction in colloid oncotic pressure. Myocardial infarction can also occur – particularly in the elderly.

INTERMEDIATE

A reversible critical illness motor syndrome has been described in HHS leading to prolonged stupor, and reversible tetraplegia.[20] Deep venous thrombosis and pulmonary embolism occur more frequently in DKA and is a significant cause of mortality in HHS.[21,22] Prophylaxis with subcutaneous heparin is advisable.

LATE

Various movement disorders can rarely persist after recovery from HHS[23]. The effects of hypoglycaemia can result in an array of late neurological complications from amnesia to optic atrophy.

PROGNOSIS

In a series of 610 patients with DKA or HHS the overall mortality was 6.2%. HHS is a more serious disease and has an associated mortality 2–3 times higher than DKA, nevertheless DKA is approximately six times commoner. Although HHS tends to occur in the older age groups, age *per se* is not a poor prognostic indicator whereas mortality is age related in DKA. A retrospective analysis of causes of death in this group of patients revealed that pneumonia was the commonest cause of death (37%), followed by myocardial infarction (21%) with mesenteric or iliac thrombosis accounting for 16% of deaths.[24] Rhabdomyolysis has been reported in both DKA and HHS and, when present, increases the mortality.[25] Pregnant women with type I diabetes are more likely to have worse outcome from DKA than non-pregnant diabetic women who develop DKA. The presence of hypothermia is also a poor prognostic sign.

Survival depends upon establishing a high index of suspicion and making a rapid diagnosis.[26]

HYPOGLYCAEMIC COMA

This results from overtreatment with insulin and is the commonest cause of diabetic coma. Clinically, there is confusion, agitation progressing to coma and fitting. Tremor, tachycardia and sweating may be blunted by diabetic autonomic neuropathy. It may be precipitated in known type I diabetic patients (up to 10% of patients per year) by changing therapy or insulin periods, missed meals, exercise and overdose of insulin or oral hypoglycaemic agents, particularly long-acting sulphonylureas. Alcoholic ketoacidosis is a syndrome of hypoglycaemia, ketoacidosis and dehydration associated with starvation, vomiting, upper abdominal pain and neurological changes including seizures and coma. Hypoglycaemia may complicate other disease states (e.g liver and renal failure, or adrenocortical insufficiency).

Severe hypoglycaemia (blood glucose <2 mmol/l) is a medical emergency. Brain metabolism uses half the glucose produced by the liver and neuronal stores of glycogen are depleted in 2 min, after which the brain is susceptible to damage. Urgent glucose infusion (50 ml of 50% glucose) is required and leads to rapid resolution of coma. Intramuscular glucagon is an alternative especially suited to out of hospital circumstances but achieves a slower result when compared with intravenous glucose.[27] Hypoglycaemia due to long-acting insulins or oral hypoglycaemic agents will require on-going glucose infusion.

REFERENCES

1 Karvonen M, Tuomilehto J, Libman I, LaPorte R. A review of the recent epidemiological data on the worldwide incidence of type 1 (insulin-dependent) diabetes mellitus. World Health Organization DIAMOND Project Group. *Diabetologia* 1993; **36**: 883–92.

2 Pinkey JH, Bingley PJ, Sawtell PA, *et al.* Presentation and progress of childhood diabetes mellitus: a prospective population-based study. The Bart's-Oxford Study Group. Diabetologia 1994; **37**: 70–4.

3 Harris MI. Undiagnosed NIDDM: clinical and public health issues. *Diabetes Care* 1993; **16**: 642–52.

4 Meyer C, Stumvoll M, Nadkarni V, *et al.* Abnormal renal and hepatic glucose metabolism in type 2 diabetes mellitus. *J Clin Invest* 1998; **102**: 619–24.

5 Schade DS, Eaton RP. The temporal relationship between endogenously secreted stress hormones and metabolic decompensation in diabetic man. *J Clin Endocrinol Metab* 1980; **50**: 131–6.

6 Kitabchi AE, Umpierrez GE, Murphy MB, *et al.* Management of hyperglycemic crises in patients with diabetes. *Diabetes Care* 2001; **24**: 131–53.

7 Magee MF, Bhatt BA. Management of decompensated diabetes. Diabetic ketoacidosis and hyperglycemic hyperosmolar syndrome. *Crit Care Clin* 2001; **17**: 75–106.

8 Umpierrez GE, Khajavi M, Kitabchi AE. Review: diabetic ketoacidosis and hyperglycemic hyperosmolar nonketotic syndrome. *Am J Med Sci* 1996; **311**: 225–33.

9 Wachtel TJ, Tetu-Mouradjian LM, Goldman DL, *et al.* Hyperosmolarity and acidosis in diabetes mellitus: a

three-year experience in Rhode Island. *J Gen Intern Med* 1991; **6**: 495–502.

10 Inglis A, Hinnie J, Kinsella J. A metabolic complication of severe burns. *Burns* 1995; **21**: 212–4.

11 Hyperosmolar coma due to lithium-induced diabetes insipidus. *Lancet* 1995; **346**(8972): 413–7.

12 DeFronzo RA, Goldberg M, Agus ZS. The effects of glucose and insulin on renal electrolyte transport. *J Clin Invest* 1976; **58**: 83–90.

13 Hillman K. Fluid resuscitation in diabetic emergencies – a reappraisal. *Intensive Care Med* 1987; **13**: 4–8.

14 McComb RD, Pfeiffer RF, Casey JH, *et al.* Lateral pontine and extrapontine myelinolysis associated with hypernatremia and hyperglycemia. *Clin Neuropathol* 1989; **8**: 284–8.

15 Wagner A, Risse A, Brill HL, *et al.* Therapy of severe diabetic ketoacidosis. Zero-mortality under very-low-dose insulin application. *Diabetes Care* 1999; **22**: 674–7.

16 Fisher JN, Kitabchi AE. A randomized study of phosphate therapy in the treatment of diabetic ketoacidosis. *J Clin Endocrinol Metab* 1983; **57**: 177–80.

17 Matz R. Severe diabetic ketoacidosis. *Diabet Med* 2000; **17**: 329.

18 Hyperglycemic crises in patients with diabetes mellitus. *Diabetes Care* 2001; **24**: 154–61.

19 Eisenhuber E, Madl C, Kramer L, *et al.* Detection of subclinical brain dysfunction by sensory evoked potentials in patients with severe diabetic ketoacidosis. *Intensive Care Med* 1997; **23**: 587–9.

20 Kennedy DD, Fletcher SN, Ghosh IR, *et al.* Reversible tetraplegia due to polyneuropathy in a diabetic patient with hyperosmolar non-ketotic coma. *Intensive Care Med* 1999; **25**: 1437–9.

21 Ceriello A. Coagulation activation in diabetes mellitus: the role of hyperglycaemia and therapeutic prospects. *Diabetologia* 1993; **36**: 1119–25.

22 Whelton MJ, Walde D, Havard CW. Hyperosmolar non-ketotic diabetic coma: with particular reference to vascular complications. *Br Med J* 1971; **1**(740): 85–6.

23 Lin JJ, Chang MK, Hemiballism-hemichorea and non-ketotic hyperglycaemia. *J Neurol Neurosurg Psychiatry* 1994; **57**: 748–50.

24 Hamblin PS, Topliss DJ, Chosich N, *et al.* Deaths associated with diabetic ketoacidosis and hyperosmolar coma, 1973–1988. *MJA* 1989; **151**: 439–444.

25 Wang LM, Tsai ST, Ho LT, *et al.* Rhabdomyolysis in diabetic emergencies. *Diabetes Res Clin Pract* 1994; **26**: 209–14.

26 Small M, Alzaid A, MacCuish AC. Diabetic hyperosmolar non-ketotic decompensation. *Q J Med* 1988; **66**: 251–7.

27 Patrick AW, Collier A, Hepburn DA, *et al.* Comparison of intramuscular glucagon and intravenous dextrose in the treatment of hypoglycaemic coma in an accident and emergency department. *Arch Emerg Med* 1990; **7**: 73–7.

49.

Diabetes insipidus
A E Vedig

Diabetes insipidus (DI) is a syndrome characterized by polyuria, excessive thirst and polydipsia. *Central* or *neurogenic* DI results from an inappropriately low amount of antidiuretic hormone (ADH) being released into the circulation in response to an osmotic stimulus. Persistent severe central DI occurs rarely, as does the syndrome of DI, which is precipitated by excessive intake of water caused by abnormalities of thirst mechanisms or psychological function (*dipsogenic* or *psychogenic* DI). Transient, usually incomplete, central DI is noticed frequently by intensivists in patients with severe head injuries. *Nephrogenic* DI, caused by deficient action of ADH, occurs very uncommonly in its classical form, but may be recognized frequently, often as an acquired, less severe form, in patients on lithium therapy. A vasopressin-resistant, transient pregnancy-related disorder of water metabolism is recognized where the polyuria is responsive to vasopressin analogues.

BASIC PHYSIOLOGY[1-6]

Water balance and body fluid tonicities are maintained by the double-negative system of feedback involving thirst, ADH secretion and its renal effects. The basic mechanisms of stimulating and decreasing thirst are not as well-understood, but involve neuroendocrine reflexes, mediation by ADH and angiotensin II, osmotic mechanisms and pharyngeal distension. Thirst is stimulated by plasma osmolalities in excess of 290 mosmol/kg. Intravascular volume depletion simulates intense thirst. Cold fluids held in the oropharynx inhibit ADH release. Ageing and drugs affect these processes.

Normally, plasma osmolality is maintained in a very narrow range, ±1% for an individual, with a population range of 275–295 mosmol/kg. As plasma osmolality increases from 280 mosmol/kg, there is a steady increase in ADH secretion. Small changes (1% increase or decrease) in plasma osmolality influence ADH secretion. Stress, disease states, many drugs and the ageing process can influence the hypothalamic osmostat and the ADH-secretory response to an osmotic change (Table 49.1).

Table 49.1 Factors influencing antidiuretic hormone (ADH) secretion or action

ADH secretion is *increased* by:
  Hyperosmolality
  Hypotension
  Stress, emotional stimuli
  Trauma, surgery, pain
  Exercise, increased temperature
  Positive-pressure ventilation
  Cholinergic and β-adrenergic drugs
  Nicotine, angiotensin II, barbiturates
  Chlorpropamide
ADH action is *potentiated* by:
  Chlorpropamide
  Carbamazepine
  Clofibrate
  Thiazide diuretics
  Prostaglandin synthetase inhibitors
ADH secretion is *inhibited* by:
  Causes of central diabetes insipidus
  Diphenylhydantoin
  Opioid antagonists
ADH action is *antagonized* by:
  Hypokalaemia
  Hypercalcaemia
  Prostaglandin E_2
  Drugs (e.g. demeclocycline, lithium carbonate,
    amphotericin B)
  Excess vasopressinase

Hormonal release is also mediated by peripheral stretch receptors (in atria, great veins, arterial vasoreceptors and lungs). Hypotension or depletion of effective blood volume will stimulate the release of very large amounts of ADH, overriding any osmotic stimulus.

ADH (8-arginine vasopressin), a nonapeptide, is synthesized in neurones of the hypothalamus, predominantly in the paired supraoptic and paraventricular nuclei. It has structural and some functional similarities to oxytocin. ADH is transported intra-axonally to the pituitary gland (neurohypophysis). Here, the hormone is stored in granules bound to the carrier protein neurophysin. Some neurones containing ADH terminate in the median eminence, where adrenocorticotrophic hormone release may be stimulated. The half-life in blood is 10–15 min, with metabolism undertaken by hepatic and renal peptidases. Seven to 10% of active hormone is excreted in the urine. Plasma concentrations range from 1–5 μg/ml (antidiuretic action) to greater than 40 μg/ml with 20% blood volume depletion. Nausea is also a potent stimulus for ADH secretion.

ACTIONS OF ADH

ANTIDIURESIS

Antidiuresis results from ADH action on V_2 receptors in the distal renal tubule, mainly in the collecting duct. The V_2 agonist action stimulates adenylcyclase generation of 3,5 cyclic adenosine monophosphate (AMP) within the tubular cytoplasm, which allows a protein kinase to open microtubular passages for water ingress from the renal filtrate. The final pathway involves the creation of a highly selective water channel protein (aquaporin-2, one of many aquaporins). Up to 12% of glomerular filtrate may be reabsorbed. This regulation of free water excretion maintains osmotic and volume homeostasis. Severe DI may result in the excretion of very large amounts of dilute urine (e.g. 20 l/day). Stimulation of V_2 receptors also results in tachycardia, facial flushing, decreased blood pressure and increased plasma renin concentration.

ADH stimulates renal prostaglandin E_2 synthesis, which in turn modulates the antidiuresis by inhibiting ADH-induced cyclic AMP generation. Prostaglandin E_1, hypokalaemia, hypercalcaemia and drugs such as demeclocycline and lithium, antagonize the ADH effect on adenyl cyclase.

VASOCONSTRICTION[7–11]

Vasoconstriction results from V_{1a} receptor stimulation, which occurs when higher concentrations of ADH exist. This is clinically significant in hypotensive states, where high concentrations of ADH contribute to the maintenance of blood pressure. The skin and mesenteric and coronary vessels are particularly sensitive to this vasoconstriction. This action is not antagonized by α-adrenergic blocking agents or by vascular denervation. Intravenous infusions of ADH have been used to diminish bleeding from oesophageal varices. More recently, ADH deficiency and pressor hypersensitivity of blood pressure effect has been recognized in unstable brain dead organ donors, patients with septic shock, postcardiac surgery and following cardiac arrest. Other V_{1a} effects include glycogenolysis, stimulation of renal prostaglandin synthesis and inhibition of renal renin secretion.

COAGULATION[12–16]

Coagulation effects are extrarenal V_2 receptor-mediated. Prostacyclin generation is stimulated; tissue-type plasmino-

gen activator activity, factor VIII-related antigen activity, factor VIII coagulant activity and von Willebrand's factor multimers all increase. ADH and its analogues, in pharmacological doses, induce coagulant activity in healthy individuals, as well as disease states (e.g. haemophilia, renal and hepatic disease) and after cardiac surgery. Desmopressin is the treatment of choice in most patients with type 1 and 2 von Willebrand's disease.

OTHER ACTIONS

ADH via V_{1a} receptors affects learning, memory and water permeability of the brain. V_{1b} receptors are found in the pituitary. Activation results in secretion of corticotrophin.

CENTRAL DIABETES INSIPIDUS[1–3,17–20]

AETIOLOGY

Causes of persistent central DI invariably involve destruction of the hypothalamus or pituitary gland, and sometimes produce defects in thirst mechanisms. Permanent, complete or incomplete central DI may follow severe head injury and, rarely, quite minor trauma. Transient complete or incomplete central DI occurs quite commonly with severe head injuries and particularly brain death. Fatal central diabetes mellitus and insipidus resulting from untreated hyponatraemia has been described.

Pituitary apoplexy continues to be described after hypovolaemic and septic shock. The enlarged pituitary that occurs with pregnancy may be more vulnerable to vasospasm. Obvious polyuria is unusual; the first sign may be inability to lactate. Transient central DI can follow infectious meningitis, chemical meningitis, electrical burns and is associated with amiodarone therapy. Transient DI has also been described with penetrating thoracic trauma and coronary artery bypass surgery. Some causes (e.g. lithium and sarcoidosis) may have variable components of central and nephrogenic DI and thirst disorder.

The nature and level of interruption of the neurohypophyseal tract will influence the time course and severity of central DI. Almost complete lesions, at or above the median eminence, or lesser lesions of the neural stalk, will probably result in a permanent state of DI. However, localized cerebral oedema and lower lesions are more likely associated with milder or temporary deficiency in ADH secretion.

PATHOPHYSIOLOGY[1–6]

The syndrome of DI results from a failure of appropriate ADH secretion or action, in response to the physiological stimulus of water deficiency, which is characterized by relative plasma hyperosmolality. If the ADH deficiency is complete, over 20 l/day of very dilute urine may be passed. Frequently, the ADH deficiency is relative, with a reduction in the slope and sensitivity of the ADH response to a change in plasma tonicity, resulting in lesser amounts of hypotonic urine output (3–6 l/day). Nocturia may be the major symptom. Even if the ADH limb of the regulatory feedback is completely lost, the excess thirst mechanism ensures that plasma osmolality stabilizes at a level only slightly above normal, no matter how severe the polyuria. Hyperosmolaemia and hypernatraemia are associated with a defect in thirst or water intake. If the thirst mechanism or water intake is very impaired in severe ADH deficiency, plasma will become hyperosmotic and grossly depleted in volume. Extra fluid losses such as vomiting and diarrhoea will complicate management. Death may result from the hypernatraemia and cardiovascular collapse.

The pathophysiological responses to worsening deficiency of ADH secretion vary between blunted ADH secretion with mild hyperosmolality, to absent secretion and effector response to hypovolaemia.

Antidiuresis to a number of physiological or pathological events or drug therapy (Table 49.1) may occur if any ADH secretory response exists.

Central DI is less severe in the presence of simultaneous failure of the anterior pituitary. A deficiency of adrenocorticotrophic hormone and cortisol results in a lower metabolic rate, renal solute load and glomerular filtration rate, and inhibition of free water excretion. Corticosteroid replacement therapy may exacerbate DI. The converse situation, of relative ADH excess, is the syndrome of inappropriate antidiuretic hormone (SIADH) (see Ch. 83).

CLINICAL PRESENTATION AND DIAGNOSIS[1–3,17–22]

The usual clinical manifestations of DI are sudden onset of polyuria (sometimes the major complaint is nocturia), resultant thirst and excessive intake of (usually) cold drinks. Lack of thirst, inability to drink, inadequate water replacement or excessive saline administration may result in signs of hypovolaemia and hypernatraemia (e.g. lethargy, confusion, delirium and coma; convulsions are uncommon).

Urine volumes over 4–6 l/day or 3 ml/kg for 4–6 consecutive hours in neurosurgical patients suggests DI. In severe forms, urine is very hypotonic (urine osmolality 50–200 mosmol/kg) but, in incomplete forms, particularly if hypovolaemia is present, urine osmolality may rise well above plasma osmolality (up to 700 mosmol/kg). The essential feature is that urine osmolality is inappropriately low compared to the plasma osmolality

Following neurosurgery on the hypothalamus and pituitary, four patterns of urine output have been observed:

1 Temporary polyuria, which may last several days.
2 The classic triphasic pattern, which consists of transient polyuria, an interphase of essentially normal urine output which may last a week, and then permanent polyuria.
3 An immediate and permanent polyuria, without an interphase.
4 A variation of the triphasic pattern where there is a diminution of urine output during the interphase, but it does not return to normal and is followed by worsening polyuria which becomes permanent.

Early polyuria is not due to decreased concentrations of circulating ADH, but may be related to the release of the biologically inactive precursor neurophysin I. It is hypothesized that this may lead to renal refractoriness to effects of ADH.

Additional signs relating to an underlying disease state (e.g. neoplasia, sarcoid and intracranial haemorrhage) may be evident, as may signs of anterior hypopituitarism (particularly after hypophyseal radiotherapy or transsphenoidal operative procedures). Central DI must be distinguished from other causes of polyuria (Table 49.2). Solute diuresis can be recognized and quantified by specific measurements (e.g. glucose in plasma and urine) or measurement of total daily urine osmolality (e.g. salts and urea) or measurement and calculation of plasma or urine osmolar gaps (e.g. mannitol and i.v. contrast agents).

Other causes of polyuria, such as primary defects in thirst or psychogenic polydipsia, will present very rarely to the intensivist, but endogenous or exogenous fluid overload may occur much more frequently. Plasma osmolality generally remains low in fluid overload after water deprivation, as opposed to becoming hyperosmolar with incomplete central DI. Recovery from fluid overload in association with SIADH has a similar pattern of plasma and urine osmolality changes. However, unrecognized excess exogenous solute administration may complicate the diagnosis.

A predictor of the development of the triphasic pattern of ADH deficit and osmoreceptor impairment is the absence or impairment of thirst in hypernatraemic patients (especially after hypothalamic surgery).

Nephrogenic DI is recognized by a failure to concentrate urine even after ADH administration. Where acquired partial nephrogenic DI exists, together with incomplete central DI in patients with an altered conscious state, the precise diagnosis is irrelevant to the central aim of maintaining plasma volume and osmolality within appropriate limits.

INVESTIGATIONS[1–3,23–28]

RANDOM PLASMA AND URINE OSMOLALITY (WITH LIBERAL WATER INTAKE OR INPUT)

Subjects with DI have higher plasma osmolalities, but there is considerable overlap with the normal range, and this determination is not diagnostic in individual patients. Urine osmolality is low (often 50–100 mosmol/kg) but the degree varies inversely with the severity of the

Table 49.2 Major polyuric syndromes

EXCESS WATER LOAD
Exogenous
  Iatrogenic
  Thirst disorders
  Hypothalamic disease
  Drugs: thioridazine, chlorpromazine, anticholinergics
  Psychogenic polydipsia
Endogenous
  Recovery from unrecognized overload
SOLUTE (OSMOTIC) DIURESIS
Exogenous or endogenous solute load
  Glucose, urea
  Mannitol, i.v. contrast media
  Sodium chloride
Abnormal solute handling
  Chronic renal disease
  Diuretics
RENAL TUBULAR UNRESPONSIVENESS TO ADH
Nephrogenic DI
  Congenital and familial
Acquired nephrogenic DI
  Drug-induced:
  Lithium, foscarnet, clozapine, demeclocycline,
    methoxyflurane, gentamicin, rifampicin, frusemide
  Chronic electrolyte disturbances
    Hypercalcaemia (hyperparathyroidism)
    Hypokalaemia (primary hyperaldosteronism)
  Renal disease
  Postobstructive, pyelonephritis
  Post acute tubular necrosis
  Post renal transplant
  Systemic disorders
  Amyloid, multiple myeloma, Sjögren's syndrome, polycystic
    disease, sickle-cell disease
  Pregnancy
    Excess vasopressinase
    Acquired nephrogenic
CENTRAL DI
Neoplastic, infective or infiltrative lesions of hypothalamus or
  pituitary
  Primary and secondary neoplasms
  Granulomatous diseases
  Tuberculosis, mycoses, toxoplasmosis, encephalitis, basal
    meningitis
Pituitary or hypothalamic surgery or ablative radiotherapy
Head injuries
Vascular lesions
  Postpartum necrosis
  Aneurysm, haemorrhage
  Hyperviscosity syndrome
Idiopathic
  Familial (usually autosomal dominant)

Table 49.3 Normal plasma/urine osmolality relationship

Plasma osmolality (mosmol/kg)	Urine osmolality (mosmol/kg)
>288	>125
>290	>200
>292	>400
>294	>600

nations of serum sodium, potassium glucose and urea: osmolarity = $1.86 \times (Na^+, K^+)$ + glucose + urea (where all values are in mmol/l).

A diagnosis of DI may usually be made when there is an elevated plasma osmolality due to increased sodium, and an inappropriately low urine osmolality (see below). Often, there is no need for a dehydration test, and desmopressin (DDAVP) may be given to examine the renal response.

BLOOD CHEMISTRY
Blood glucose, 24-h urinary osmolality and electrolytes, blood and urine electrolytes, urea and creatinine are useful for determining solute load and renal function.

PLASMA AND URINE OSMOLALITY RELATIONSHIPS, AND WATER DEPRIVATION
If required, comparison of simultaneously determined plasma and urine osmolality during dehydration may be conducted at any time. Fluid replacement regimens are simply ceased (or restricted for limited time if laboratory reports take too long). The rate of change of plasma osmolality is proportional to the degree of continuing polyuria. In normal subjects, there is a relationship between increasing plasma osmolality and increasing urine osmolality. Provided solute diuresis has been excluded and assuming blood urea and glucose are normal, failure to concentrate urine adequately suggests either central or nephrogenic DI. The normal plasma/urine osmolality relationship is shown in (Table 49.3).

Where there is an elevated urea (e.g. renal failure), a corrected osmolality may be calculated substituting a urea measurement of 8 mmol/l. Allowances can be made with hyperglycaemia, but corrections are less helpful. The hypothalamic-pituitary axis responds to tonicity changes rather than strictly osmolality. During pregnancy, there is a resetting of the osmostat, resulting in generally lower plasma sodium concentrations and plasma osmolality for a corresponding urine osmolality.

The degree of failure to concentrate urine and an examination of the relationship may indicate the type of DI and its severity. Excess water load states usually manifest a hypotonic urine (e.g. osmolality <150 mosmol/kg) with persistently low plasma osmolality (e.g. <288 mosmol/kg). Following demonstration of failure to concentrate urine adequately in response to water deprivation, renal response to exogenous ADH should be examined.

polyuria. Solute diuresis may be suspected if urine osmolality is measured between 250 and 320 mosmol/kg, and particularly if an abnormal plasma or urine osmolar gap exists. Plasma osmolality may be calculated from determi-

ADH TEST

If dehydration exists, as indicated by elevated plasma osmolality, and there is inadequate urine concentration, then ADH (as 10 μg DDAVP nasally, or 1 μg s.c. or i.v.) should be given. A rise in urine osmolality of 50% following ADH is almost always sufficient to differentiate central from nephrogenic diabetes insipidus if severe DI is present. Unfortunately, if urine is able to be concentrated greater than 300 mosmol/kg with dehydration, then ADH administration in supraphysiological amounts does not reliably differentiate between chronic severe excess water loads, chronic incomplete central DI or partial nephrogenic DI.

ADH ASSAY

Reliable, simple and highly sensitive radioimmunoassays are commercially available. Plasma and/or urine ADH can be measured before and during dehydration tests, and results analysed together with plasma and urine osmolality changes. Nomograms are available to compare these relationships. Basal plasma ADH is normal or high in the presence of polyuria associated with nephrogenic DI. Basal concentrations are low and remain clearly subnormal with central DI. ADH concentrations rise appropriately in response to hyperosmolaemia with thirst disorders and psychogenic polydipsia.

Careful studies using reliable and sensitive ADH assays have cast doubt on the diagnostic veracity of the classical dehydration and ADH administration test. It has been found that the maximum concentrating capacity of the kidney in all types of DI is decreased equally in proportion to the polyuria. Furthermore, for partial nephrogenic DI, incomplete central DI and primary polydipsia, the relationships between urine osmolality and plasma ADH differ only at submaximal concentrations of plasma ADH. It is possible that these relationships may not be precise with acute DI because of the release of inactive precursors.

ADH TRIAL

If the diagnosis is unclear after clinical assessment and the above investigations, then a carefully conducted clinical trial is indicated for both diagnostic and therapeutic purposes. DDAVP (1–2 μg s.c. 12-hourly) is administered for several days. If thirst and polydipsia are abolished without excessive fluid retention, then the patient probably has incomplete central DI. Administration of larger amounts of ADH may decrease polyuria in partial nephrogenic DI.

HYPERTONIC SALINE

Infusions of hypertonic saline, according to a specific protocol, may be used to evaluate the set-point of the osmoreceptor mechanism.

SPECIFIC INVESTIGATIONS

Special investigations, including magnetic resonance imaging (MRI) and assessment of anterior pituitary function, may be required for suspected lesions of the hypothalamus and pituitary gland. MRI studies demonstrate the anatomy and provide insights into the underlying pathology. T1-weighted imaging may differentiate primary polydipsia from central DI. The presence of a hyperintense signal is consistent with a diagnosis of primary polydipsia, whereas it is absent with central DI.

MANAGEMENT[1–3,7–16,26,29–32]

Management problems in intensive care unit (ICU) are usually focused on the polyuria and hypovolaemia, associated with varying states of plasma osmolality. Priorities in diagnosis and treatment have to be balanced carefully. Water restriction and administration of ADH may be required. Rapid return to normal plasma osmolality is not always the major objective, particularly where an increase in cerebral volume is undesirable.

Provided there is cardiovascular stability, mild polyuria (e.g. 3 ml/kg per h) is often best observed with frequent determinations of plasma and urine osmolality, unless hyperosmolaemia occurs. Even if a provisional diagnosis of incomplete central DI is made, at this level of urine output, it is often advantageous simply to replace output with an appropriate solution or allow the patient to drink rather than initiate specific drug therapy. If the polyuria is persistent (>24 h) or severe (>7 ml/kg per h for 4–6 h), drug therapy should be considered as specific replacement therapy or as part of a diagnostic and therapeutic trial. Resuscitation may be necessary in dehydrated patients in shock. The priority is almost always restoration of circulatory stability rather than reversal of hyperosmolaemia. If parasellar pathology is suspected, then one should assume anterior pituitary deficiency and routinely use stress-dose steroids even though polyuria may be worsened with steroid use.

Routine management will require accurate fluid balance with daily patient weighing (usually impractical in the ICU), and at least twice daily plasma and urine osmolality and electrolytes in the acute phase. Water is lost far in excess of electrolytes, so i.v. replacement fluid as 5% dextrose is generally satisfactory. Large volumes of 5% dextrose may cause hyperglycaemia and further exacerbate polyuria, particularly if corticosteroids are being administered. Large sodium inputs are unnecessary and may confuse the diagnosis. Dextrose 4% with 0.18% saline is often a convenient way of supplying daily sodium requirements. Potassium requirements are generally small. Disturbances of thirst, whether due to primary polydipsia or habit, can complicate management. Hormone therapy other than ADH will be required in panhypopituitarism.

ADH THERAPY

ADH replacement is the most effective means of reducing the polyuria, nocturia and polydipsia of central DI. Significant regeneration of ADH secretion may occur even months postoperatively, allowing a decrease in

ADH supplementation. The volume of i.v. replacement must be decreased with the onset of ADH action or water overload will result.

SHORT-ACTING AGENTS: AQUEOUS VASOPRESSIN (ARGININE)

In the ICU, it is generally given i.v. by continuous infusion and occasionally in ultra-low doses (e.g. 1–2 IU/24 h) Although vasopressin is a V_1 and V_2 agonist, small i.v. doses are not associated with undesirable V_1 effects (e.g. coronary vasoconstriction, abdominal and uterine cramps). There is particular utility in the use of aqueous vasopressin in the setting of organ donation in haemodynamically unstable donors. Its use is not just to counter the effects of polyuria but rather because of the pressor sensitivity exhibited. Doses of 0.04–0.1 U/h are effective in reversing polyuria and in reducing catecholamine requirements. There is no detrimental effect on transplant kidneys.

LONG-ACTING AGENTS

DDAVP, 1-deamino-8-O-arginine-vasopressin (desmopressin), is an analogue of arginine vasopressin with specific V_2 agonist effects. It has generally been given intranasally in doses of 0.1–0.4 ml (10–40 μg) in adults, but may be administered parenterally (1–4 μg) and as a continuous infusion. Dosing is less flexible with metered-dose inhalers (minimum dose 10 μg), but is preferred by many patients. The duration of action of 12–24 h, when given intranasally, is due to slow absorption, resistance to enzymatic breakdown and an enhanced effect on the kidney. In individuals, the duration of effect is relatively constant, although there is inconsistency between patients. Larger doses are sometimes required in the very early phase of central DI, possibly due to receptor blockade by biologically active precursors of ADH released by the acutely damaged hypothalamic–pituitary tract.

Although DDAVP is a polypeptide, it has been successfully administered sublingually (0.4 μg/kg) and orally, when about 10–20 times the intranasal dose is required (100–400 pg t.d.s. in adults). In young children aged below 6 months, an initial dose of 5–10 p.g orally 2–3 times a day is recommended. A newer oral formulation of desmopressin acetate is available.

There are problems with nasal absorption, storage and compliance, particularly in children. Use during pregnancy appears to be safe although antibodies to vasopressin have occasionally occurred in patients treated with arginine and lysine vasopressin, causing secondary resistance. In these patients the antidiuretic response to DDAVP is normal. There is no detrimental effect on organs transplanted except in experimental pancreas transplants.

NON-HORMONAL THERAPY (NOT FOR EMERGENCY MANAGEMENT)

These agents either increase renal sensitivity to ADH or potentiate ADH release, and are only considered in partial central DI. Usually, these patients do not require antidiuretic therapy or may be managed with small doses of DDAVP.

Thiazide Diuretics

These have a paradoxical action in decreasing diuresis. Treatment, including salt restriction, causes contraction of circulatory volume, decreased glomerular filtration rate, and enhanced proximal tubular sodium chloride reabsorption such that less chloride is available for reabsorption in the diluting segment.

Chlorpropamide

This oral hypoglycaemic agent enhances the release and potentiates the renal action of residual ADH in incomplete DI. It may also restore thirst perception. Dosage is 200–500 mg daily. Hypoglycaemia still occurs despite frequent meals. Its latency of action is 3 days.

Carbamazepine (Tegretol)

This anticonvulsant is thought to stimulate ADH release, but is not used in the long term because of toxicity at the dose required (400–600 mg daily).

NEPHROGENIC DIABETES INSIPIDUS[1–6,29,30,33–43]

CONGENITAL NEPHROGENIC DI

The more common (90%) congenital form is X-linked, affecting males from birth. A less common autosomal-recessive or autosomal dominant mode of inherited nephrogenic DI also occurs. These forms are rare and unlikely to present undiagnosed to an intensivist. Most of these patients are V_2 receptor deficient in the kidneys and often lack V_2 receptors extrarenally. Mutations have been identified in the aquaparin-2 gene. Hypercalcaemia, hypokalaemia and drugs (e.g. lithium, methoxyflurane and amphotericin) are likely to exacerbate the disorder and should be avoided. ADH and its analogues are ineffective in this disorder. However, thiazide diuretics and salt restriction decrease the diuresis. Additional benefit is obtained with prostaglandin synthetase inhibitors (e.g. indomethacin and tolmetin sodium), especially in children where severe salt restriction is difficult. A newer approach involves a combination of thiazide, indomethacin and DDAVP.

ACQUIRED NEPHROGENIC DI

Acquired nephrogenic DI occurs commonly. Drug induced DI is always of the nephrogenic type. Nephrogenic DI occurs in 10% of patients receiving long-term lithium therapy, even when plasma lithium concentrations are kept within the normal range. Lithium causes relative unresponsiveness to exogenous ADH.

Larger doses of ADH will increase renal concentrating ability. Lithium decreases renal cyclic AMP production, which may, in turn, be increased by non-steroidal anti-inflammatory drugs. Unfortunately, amelioration of lithium-induced nephrogenic DI by indomethacin may produce its own complications of increasing plasma lithium concentrations and potentiating toxicity. Amiloride, rather than thiazides, has been advocated for lithium-induced DI. Lithium-induced nephrogenic DI may be persistent and occasionally permanent. Chronic renal failure may predispose to persistence of the DI.

Nephrogenic DI has long been recognized as a side-effect of amphotericin B. Resolution of the DI has been described shortly after commencing therapy with its liposomal counterpart. Other drugs causing nephrogenic DI include foscarnet, clozapine and antibiotics. A case of massive vasopressin resistant polyuria has been discribed with dexamethasone.

Demeclocycline, which inhibits cyclic-AMP accumulation and action, may be used deliberately in doses 600–1200 mg/day in the management of SIADH.

TRANSIENT DIABETES INSIPIDUS OF PREGNANCY[44–48]

A vasopressin-resistant DI of pregnancy is recognized. This is a transient condition caused by excessive placental-generated vasopressinase, an aminopeptide that metabolizes ADH. There is a brisk response with DDAVP, which is not metabolized by vasopressinase. Associated acute fatty liver and liver failure have been described. Transient nephrogenic DI of pregnancy unresponsive to DDAVP has also been recognized. The normal pregnancy-induced elevation in vasopressinase may unmask partial central or nephrogenic DI. Vasopressinase concentrations decrease rapidly after delivery.

REFERENCES

1 Robertson GL. Diabetes insipidus. *Endocrinol Metab Clin North Am* 1995; **24**: 549–72.
2 Robinson AG, Verbalis JG. Diabetes insipidus. *Curr Ther Endocrinol Metab* 1997; **6**: 1–7.
3 Hendy GN, Bichet DG. Diabetes insipidus. *Baillières Clin Endocrinol Metab* 1995; **9**: 509–24.
4 King LS, Agre P. Pathophysiology of the aquaporin water channels. *Annu Rev Physiol* 1996; **58**: 619–48.
5 Agre P, King LS, Yasui M, *et al*. Aquaporin water channels – from atomic structure to clinical medicine. *J Physiol* 2002; **542**: 3–16.
6 Nielsen S, Frokiaer J, Marples D, *et al*. Aquaporins in the kidney: from molecules to medicine. *Physiol Rev* 2002; **82**: 205–44.
7 Guesde R, Barrou B, Leblanc I, *et al*. Administration of desmopressin in brain-dead donors and renal function in kidney recipients. *Lancet* 1998; **352**: 1178–81.
8 Chen JM, Cullinane S, Spanier TB, *et al*. Vasopressin deficiency and pressor hypersensitivity in hemodynami-cally unstable organ donors. *Circulation* 1999; **100**: 244.
9 Landry DW, Levin HR, Gallant EM, *et al*. Vasopressin deficiency contributes to the vasodilation of septic shock. *Circulation* 1997; **95**: 1122–5.
10 Wenzel V, Lindner KH. Arginine vasopressin during cardiopulmonary resuscitation: laboratory evidence, clinical experience and recommendations, and a view to the future. *Crit Care Med* 2002; **30**: S157–61.
11 Morales DL, Gregg D, Helman DN, *et al*. Arginine vasopressin in the treatment of 50 patients with post-cardiotomy vasodilatory shock. *Ann Thorac Surg* 2000; **69**: 102–6.
12 Mannucci PM, Canciani MT, Rota L, *et al*. Response of factor VIII/von Willebrand factor to dDAVP in healthy subjects and patients with haemophilia A and von Willerbrand's disease. *Br J Haematol* 1981; **47**: 283–93.
13 Mannucci PM. Hemostatic drugs. *N Engl J Med* 1998; **339**: 245–53.
14 Mannucci PM. Desmopressin (DDAVP) in the treatment of bleeding disorders: the first twenty years. *Haemophilia* 2000; **6**: 60–7.
15 Federici AB, Mannucci PM. Advances in the genetics and treatment of von Willebrand disease. *Curr Opin Pediatr* 2002; **14**: 23–33.
16 DeLoughery TG. Management of bleeding with uremia and liver disease. *Curr Opin Hematol* 1999; **6**: 329–33.
17 Wang LC, Cohen ME, Duffner PK. Etiologies of central diabetes insipidus in children. *Pediatr Neurol* 1994; **11**: 273–7.
18 Maghnie M, Cosi G, Genovese E, *et al*. Central diabetes insipidus in children and young adults. *N Engl J Med* 2000; **343**: 998–1007.
19 Outwater KM, Rockoff MA. Diabetes insipidus accompanying brain death in children. *Neurology* 1984; **34**: 1243–6.
20 Fraser CL, Arieff AI. Fatal central diabetes mellitus and insipidus resulting from untreated hyponatraemia: a new syndrome. *Ann Intern Med* 1990; **112**: 113–9.
21 Robertson GL. Differential diagnosis of polyuria. *Annu Rev Med* 1988; **39**: 425–42.
22 Delhaye F, Vincent JL, Fery F *et al*. Extreme polyuria: decompensated diabetes mellitus and/or diabetes insipidus? *Intens Care Med* 1995; **21**: 515–21.
23 Sakurai H, Kanai A, Nomura K, *et al*. A simple and highly sensitive radio-immunoassay for 8-arginine vasopressin in human plasma using a reversed-phase C18 silica column. *J Tokyo Wom Med Coll* 1986; **56**: 394–403.
24 Robertson GL. The use of vasopressin assays in physiology and pathophysiology. *Semin Nephrol* 1994; **14**: 368–83.
25 Diederich S, Eckmanns T, Exner P, *et al*. Differential diagnosis of polyuric/polydipsic syndromes with the aid of urinary vasopressin measurement in adults. *Clin Endocrinol (Oxf)* 2001; **54**: 665–71.
26 Baylis PH, Cheetham T. Diabetes insipidus. *Arch Dis Child* 1998; **79**: 84–9.

27 Elster AD. Imaging of the sella: anatomy and pathology. *Semin Ultrasound CT MR* 1993; **14**: 182–94.

28 Moses AM, Clayton B, Hochhauser L. The use of T1-weighted magnetic resonance imaging to differentiate between primary polydipsia and central diabetes insipidus. *Am J Neuroradiol* 1992; **13**: 1273–7.

29 Singer I, Oster JR, Fishman LM. The management of diabetes insipidus in adults. *Arch Intern Med* 1997; **157**: 1293–301.

30 Seckl JR, Dunger DB. Diabetes insipidus. Current treatment recommendations. *Drugs* 1992; **44**: 216–24.

31 Ray JG. DDAVP use during pregnancy: an analysis of its safety for mother and child. *Obstet Gynecol Surv* 1998; **53**: 450–5.

32 Keck T, Banafsche R, Werner J, *et al.* Desmopressin impairs microcirculation in donor pancreas and early graft function after experimental pancreas transplantation. *Transplantation* 2001; **72**: 202–9.

33 Knoers N, Monnens LAH. Nephrogenic diabetes insipidus: clinical symptoms, pathogenesis, genetics and treatment. *Paediatr Nephrol* 1992; **6**: 476–82.

34 Bichet DG. Nephrogenic diabetes insipidus. *Am J Med* 1998; **105**: 431–42.

35 Deen PM, Marr N, Kamsteeg EJ, *et al.* Nephrogenic diabetes insipidus. *Curr Opin Nephrol Hypertens* 2000; **9**: 591–5.

36 Morello JP, Bichet DG. Nephrogenic diabetes insipidus. *Annu Rev Physiol* 2001; **63**: 607–30.

37 Bendz H, Aurell M. Drug-induced diabetes insipidus: incidence, prevention and management. *Drug Saf* 1999; **21**: 449–56.

38 Lam SS, Kjellstrand C. Emergency treatment of lithium-induced diabetes insipidus with nonsteroidal anti-inflammatory drugs. *Ren Fail* 1997; **19**: 183–8.

39 Grindlinger GA, Boylan MJ. Amelioration by indomethacin of lithium-induced polyuria. *Crit Care Med* 1987; **15**: 538–9.

40 Batlle DC, von Riotte AB, Graviria M, *et al.* Amelioration of polyuria by amiloride in patients receiving long-term lithium therapy. *N Engl J Med* 1985; **312**: 408–14.

41 Guirguis AF, Taylor HC. Nephrogenic diabetes insipidus persisting 57 months after cessation of lithium carbonate therapy: report of a case and review of the literature. *Endocr Pract* 2000; **6**: 324–8.

42 Markowitz GS, Radhakrishnan J, Kambham N, *et al.* Lithium nephrotoxicity: a progressive combined glomerular and tubulointerstitial nephropathy. *Am Soc Nephrol* 2000; **11**: 1439–48.

43 Toftegaard M, Knudsen F. Massive vasopressin-resistant polyuria induced by dexamethasone. *Intensive Care Med* 1995; **21**: 238–40.

44 Barron WM, Cohen LH, Ulland LA, *et al.* Transient vasopressin-resistant diabetes insipidus of pregnancy. *N Engl J Med* 1984; **310**: 442–4.

45 Lindheimer MD, Davison JM. Osmoregulation, the secretion of arginine vasopressin and its metabolism during pregnancy. *Eur J Endocrinol* 1995; **132**: 133–43.

46 Robinson AG, Amco JA. 'Non Sweet' diabetes of pregnancy. *N Engl J Med* 1991; **324**: 556–8.

47 Usta IM, Barton JR, Amon EA, *et al.* Acute fatty liver of pregnancy: an experience in the diagnosis and management of fourteen cases. *Am J Obstet Gynecol* 1994; **171**: 1342–7.

48 Iwasaki Y, Oiso Y, Kondo K, *et al.* Aggravation of subclinical diabetes insipidus during pregnancy. *N Engl J Med* 1991; **324**: 522–6.

50.

Thyroid emergencies

A E Vedig

Thyroid disease is common in Western countries. Myxoedema coma and thyroid crisis are rare, but have a high mortality without specific treatment. Abnormal thyroid hormone concentrations commonly occur in critically ill patients.

BASIC PHYSIOLOGY AND PATHOPHYSIOLOGY[1–5]

The thyroid gland actively uptakes and concentrates iodide, which is oxidized and organified to produce tetraiodothyronine (T_4) and triiodothyronine (T_3). When iodine deficiency exists, the gland increases the efficiency of uptake, whereas excess iodine inhibits synthesis and release of the thyroid hormones. Both T_4 and T_3 are extensively bound to plasma proteins (thyroxine-binding globulin, thyroxine-binding pre-albumin and albumin) with small amounts (T_4, approximately 0.03%; T_3, approximately 0.3%) circulating free. The total concentrations of T_4 and T_3 are affected by protein binding. T_4 is produced only by the thyroid gland. T_3 is secreted by the thyroid, but most arises from α-deiodination of T_4 in peripheral tissues (particularly the liver and kidney), which also yields an inactive metabolite, reverse T_3 (rT_3), also by α-deiodination. Peripheral deiodination of T_4 is decreased in pathological states and by some pharmaceutical agents (Table 50.1). The half-life of T_4 in the circulation is 7 days; the half-life of T_3 is approximately 24 h. Free hormone (FT_3) enters cells and attaches to specific intracellular receptors (TR). The brain, heart, liver and kidney have high concentrations of TR. T_3 has a much greater effect than T_4 on metabolic state, which correlates more closely to concentrations of free hormones rather than total hormones in plasma. The rate of synthesis of a variety of proteins is affected through messenger RNA. Thyroid hormones increase sodium-potassium ATPase activity, stimulate β-adrenergic receptors, increase cycling of fatty acids and generally increase cell respiration and energy expenditure.

Syndromes with distinctive clinical features of generalized thyroid hormone resistance are recognized. Abnormal function of thyroid receptors results in a euthyroid or hypothyroid state with elevated circulating FT_3 and FT_4.

There are two distinct mechanisms of regulation of thyroid function. First, thyroid hormones regulate, in a classic negative feedback manner, the secretion of thyroid-stimulating hormone (TSH) from the anterior pituitary. The level of circulating FT_4 and FT_3 and intrapituitary-generated T_3 from T_4 influences TSH secretion, as does thyrotrophin-releasing hormone (TRH), which sets the threshold of feedback. In turn, TRH is also influenced by circulating thyroid hormones and higher centres in the brain. Dopamine and somatostatin are physiological inhibitors of TRH secretion, as are glucocorticoids. Cytokines and tumor necrosis factor also inhibit TSH secretion.

Autoregulation is the second mechanism of regulating thyroid hormones by maintaining the pool of organic iodine within the thyroid gland. A negative feedback exists between the size of the organic pool of iodine, the sensitivity of the thyroid gland to TSH, and the activity of the iodide transport mechanism in the gland. When autoregulation is unable to sustain normal secretion of thyroid hormone, increased activation of the hypothalamic–pituitary axis occurs. Large amounts of iodine inhibit thyroid hormone synthesis (Wolff-Chaikoff effect), but normal auto-regulation permits 'escape'. Failure of escape leads to continued inhibition of hormone synthesis with consequent TSH-induced goitre and enhanced iodide transport, which further inhibits hormone synthesis, often resulting in hypothyroidism. Neonatal and damaged glands (e.g. Hashimoto's disease, radioiodine-treated Grave's disease and patients treated with lithium and phenazone) are susceptible to failure of escape. If there is

Table 50.1 States associated with decreased deiodination of T_4 to T_3

Systemic illness
Fasting
Malnutrition
Postoperative state
Trauma
Drugs: propylthiouracil, glucocorticoids, propranolol, amiodarone
Radiographic contrast agents (ipodate, ipanoate)

a basic failure in autoregulation, then iodide excess, rather than inhibiting synthesis of thyroid hormones, will lead to sustained hypersecretion (Jod–Basedow disease).

Laboratory tests usually available include FT_4 and FT_3 concentrations in blood, and sensitive and ultra-sensitive TSH measurements.

THYROID FUNCTION WITH NON-THYROIDAL ILLNESS[6–9]

The euthyroid sick syndrome is used to describe clinically euthyroid patients with severe non-thyroidal illness (NTI) who have low T_3, normal or low T_4, elevated rT_3, and a TSH that is normal or low, but occasionally increased in the recovery phase of an illness (Table 50.2). A normal TSH suggests a euthyroid state, but the TSH level is probably inappropriately low for the circulating thyroid hormone concentrations, although synthesis of T_3 tissue receptors is increased which in effect maintains a 'euthyroid' state. Starvation, stress, effects of cytokines and drugs (dopamine, steroids and opioids) reduce thyrotropin secretion and effect. Although rT_3 is unmeasurable with hypothyroid sick patients and is usually elevated with euthyroid sick syndrome, levels are not diagnostically reliable.

Conditions such as hepatic cirrhosis and chronic renal failure may elevate TSH. As the underlying illness improves, a TSH concentration that has been low or normal may rise and be transiently elevated. Specific variants of thyroid function abnormality have been described with severe NTI. Low T_4 and/or T_3 and TSH correlate with the severity of illness and mortality in many non-thyroidal disorders.

Rarely, euthyroid hyperthyroxinaemia occurs in sick patients. This condition is characterized by elevated FT_4 and high, normal or low FT_3. The diagnosis may be difficult in an elderly patient with severe NTI where apathetic hyperthyroidism is a consideration. TSH concentrations are normal, reduced or increased. The mechanism is sometimes associated with drugs that inhibit peripheral T_4 conversion to T_3 (e.g. amiodarone, propranolol and contrast agents), hyperemesis, acute psychiatric illness and hyponatraemia. Failure to recognize these clinical entities may result in inappropriate therapy.

Table 50.2 Changes in thyroid hormone concentrations

	FT_4	T_3	TSH
Euthyroid	N	N	N
Hyperthyroid	↑	↑	↓
Hypothyroid	↓	↓N	↑
Non-thyroid illness	↑N↓	↓	N↓

FT_4, Free tetraiodothyronine; T_3, triiodothyronine; TSH, thyroid-stimulating hormone; N = normal; ↑ = increased; ↓ = decreased.

In general, patients who have low thyroid hormone concentrations in blood in the setting of NTI do not benefit from treatment with thyroid hormones.

THYROID CRISIS (THYROID STORM)[10–17]

Thyroid crisis is the life-threatening clinical extreme of hyperthyroidism. It is more common in women than in men, and has a mortality rate of 10–20% with treatment. The onset is usually abrupt, and precipitating factors may be identified in about 50% of cases.

FT_3 or FT_4, although usually high in crisis, does not correlate well with the severity of the condition. The essential feature of crisis is that it is a condition of decompensation, where target organs lose their ability to modulate their response to excess T_3 or T_4. Pathogenesis is obscure and, curiously, many of the precipitating conditions are normally associated with inhibition of T_4 to T_3 conversion. TSH is undetectable.

PRECIPITATING FACTORS[10–19]

The majority of patients presenting in crisis have unrecognized or poorly-controlled Grave's disease. Intercurrent illness, particularly infection, trauma, operative procedures, uncontrolled diabetes mellitus, labour and eclampsia, are the most commonly described provoking factors. Crisis is now uncommon as a complication of thyroid surgery, but has been reported following excessive palpation of the thyroid gland, incomplete preparation and inadequate dosage of β-adrenergic antagonists perioperatively. Uncommon factors include the use of radioiodine in unprepared patients, and drugs such as iodides in patients with impaired autoregulation (Jod–Basedow phenomenon), haloperidol or massive overdose of thyroid hormone preparations. Overdoses of less than 10 mg usually cause few problems, but massive doses may precipitate a thyrotoxic crisis within days.

Amiodarone may cause two forms of hyperthyroidism. Type 1 is caused by iodine excess typically in patients with nodular goitres. Type 2 is mediated by an inflammatory process in the thyroid gland releasing T_4 and T_3.

CLINICAL PRESENTATION[10–17,20–23]

Exaggerated manifestations of hyperthyroidism (Table 50.3) are usually present. Hyperpyrexia, tachycardia with atrial fibrillation (AF), delirium, agitation or coma, vomiting, diarrhoea and muscle weakness are the main features. Rarely, apathetic hyperthyroidism (usually occurring in the elderly) may present in crisis with the features of profound exhaustion, tachycardia, hyporeflexia, severe myopathy, marked weight loss and hypotension. The usual differential diagnosis is sepsis, but the presentation may be confused with other hyperthermic syndromes, delerium tremens, opioid withdrawal, adrenergic or cholinergic overdose. Clinical presentation may be complicated by the precipitating factors and coexistent disease.

FEVER
Fever may be extreme (>41°C) and is generally regarded as essential to the diagnosis. Pyrexia is not usually present in uncomplicated thyrotoxicosis. The skin is usually moist and warm.

CARDIOVASCULAR FEATURES
Cardiovascular features are very common, even in patients with the apathetic presentation. Sinus tachycardia (often >160 beats/min), heart failure, AF and ventricular arrhythmias are common. Mitral valve prolapse occurs frequently in patients with treated or active hyperthyroidism. Cardiomegaly and electrocardiogram (ECG) changes of left ventricular hypertrophy may be seen. Decreasing pulse rate and systemic blood pressure with the development of shock are poor prognostic features.

NEUROLOGICAL AND MUSCULAR DISTURBANCES
These are very common. A clinical picture of tremor and increasing restlessness progressing to delirium, coma and death is characteristic of untreated cases. Profound muscular weakness may occur, particularly with apathetic thyrotoxic crisis. Other syndromes of muscle weakness have been described, including descriptions of an upper motor neurone abnormality with asymmetrical reflexes, and sudden-onset episodic thyrotoxic periodic paralysis. Rhabdomyolysis can also occur.

GASTROINTESTINAL DISTURBANCES
Vomiting, nausea and diarrhoea may be present and complicate management, particularly due to the poor bioavailability of orally administered drugs. Severe abdominal pain may suggest an underlying abdominal emergency. Jaundice is sometimes present and is a poor prognostic sign.

HYPERCALCAEMIA
Hypercalcaemia is relatively common (15%) in severe thyrotoxicosis, but rarely an independent emergency. Hypo-

kalaemia and leukocytosis occur frequently, and hypomagnesaemia may be severe, particularly with apathetic thyrotoxicosis.

MANAGEMENT[10–17]
Management includes diagnosis and specific management of the precipitating event, supportive measures, reducing the synthesis, release, peripheral conversion and peripheral effects of thyroid hormones, and searching for the cause of hyperthyroidism. The diagnosis of thyroid crisis is clinical and management must be aggressive. A protocol that includes rapid access to required drugs must be formulated in advance. Blood should be collected for thyroid hormone and TSH assays before commencing therapy. Responses to treatment can be monitored by observation of clinical signs (e.g. pulse, temperature and agitation) and T_3 concentrations.

β-ADRENERGIC BLOCKADE[10–17,24–28]
β-Adrenergic blockade antagonizes the effect of thyroid hormones and the hypersensitivity to the action of catecholamines. Propranolol is the drug of choice, as it also inhibits the peripheral conversion of T_4 to T_3. Tachycardia, fever, hyperkinesis and tremor respond promptly. Other beneficial effects include improvement in proximal myopathy, periodic thyrotoxic paralysis, bulbar palsy and thyrotoxic hypercalcaemia. Blockade is achieved with i.v. increments of 0.5 mg, with continuous cardiovascular monitoring, usually to a total of 10 mg. Further amounts are given 4–6-hourly. Unfortunately parenteral propranolol is not now generally available. The usual oral doses of propranolol are 20–120 mg 6-hourly, but because of the markedly increased clearance, very large doses (>720 mg) may be required to achieve β-blockade.

β[1]-Selective antagonists do not inhibit T_4 to T_3 conversion as effectively as propranolol, but may be favoured in the presence of complicating factors (e.g. reactive airways and heart failure). Use of β[1]-blockers should be combined with other therapy, since the basic metabolic abnormalities are not inhibited. β-blockers may precipitate cardiogenic shock if significant cardiomyopathy or heart failure is already evident.

Esmolol 250–500 μg/kg i.v. loading dose followed by an infusion of 50–100 μg/kg per min may be titrated to a desired effect. Because of its ultrashort action, undesirable side-effects will be short-lived.

Reserpine and guanethidine, although largely superseded by the β-adrenergic blockers, may be life-saving, and should be considered in propranolol resistant hyperthyroidism and if propranolol is contraindicated. Onset of action is slow, and adverse effects include central nervous system depression and diarrhoea. The parenteral formulation of reserpine is no longer manufactured.

Diltiazem reduces pulse rate as effectively as propranolol and could be considered as an alternative to β-blockers in thyroid crisis.

Table 50.3 Clinical manifestations of hyperthyroidism

Nervousness, insomnia, tremor, hyperkinesis, muscle weakness, hyperactive reflexes
Heat intolerance, hot and moist skin, increased sweating, acropachy, onycholysis
Bowel hyperactivity, increased appetite, weight loss
Eye symptoms, stare, lid retraction, lid lag, ophthalmopathy (if Grave's disease)
Dyspnoea, fatigue, tachycardia, atrial fibrillation, congestive cardiac failure, mitral valve prolapse
Goitre, dysphagia, thyroid bruit (if Grave's disease)

CORTICOSTEROIDS

Corticosteroids are usually administered during a crisis, because a relative deficiency may be present, and gluco-corticoids inhibit the peripheral conversion of T_4 to T_3. Hydrocortisone 100 mg i.v. 6-hourly or dexamethasone 5 mg i.v. 12-hourly together with iodides, can produce a rapid reduction in the degree of thyroxtoxicosis. Steroids are the most effective treatment for amiodarone induced type-2 thyrotoxicosis.

THIOAMIDES
Propylthiouracil

Propylthiouracil is given orally or administered as a slurry via a nasogastric tube. Unfortunately, gastrointestinal absorption is impaired or unreliable in thyroid crisis, but no parenteral preparation of this thioamide is available. It has a rapid onset of action, and exerts its effects by blocking the iodination of tyrosine and partial inhibition of the peripheral conversion of T_4 to T_3. A loading dose of 100 mg may be given, followed by 100 mg 2-hourly.

Methimazole

Methimazole may be less rapidly absorbed, but is longer acting. It does not inhibit peripheral conversion of T_4. Equipotent doses are one-tenth of propylthiouracil. A dose of 100 mg may be given orally, followed by 20 mg 8-hourly.

Carbimazole

Carbimazole is metabolized to methimazole (relative potency 0.62:1.0). Transient leukopenia is common (20%) with antithyroid drugs, but agranulocytosis is rare.

IODINE

When given in large doses, iodine inhibits the synthesis and release of thyroid hormones. Its administration is generally delayed for at least 1 h after thioamides. Oral iodine/iodide preparations include Lugol's iodine (130 mg total iodine/ml), potassium iodide or sodium iodide. Intravenous preparations are not always available, but can be easily prepared. Sodium iodide, 1 g i.v., can be given 12-hourly as either a continuous infusion or a bolus over a few minutes. Equivalent doses of other available preparations are given orally or via a nasogastric tube. Iodine-containing contrast media (Ipodate 1 g orally twice daily for the first day and then 1 g daily for a maximum of 2 weeks) may specifically ameliorate the cardiac effects of thyroxine. In addition they are the most potent blockers of T_4 to T_3 conversion. These agents are probably the drugs of choice rather than simple iodides.

LITHIUM CARBONATE

Lithium carbonate is an alternative in patients who are allergic to iodine. It has a similar, but much weaker action in blocking thyroid hormone release and synthesis. Doses of 500–1500 mg daily have been used.

Frequent drug level monitoring is required to maintain lithium concentrations of 0.7–1.4 mmol/l.

DIGOXIN

Digoxin is indicated following the correction of hypo-kalaemia when AF or heart failure is present. Larger doses than usual will be required because of pharmaco-kinetic and pharmacodynamic changes associated with the hyperthyroid state. Adequate slowing of ventricular responses is not usually achieved with digoxin alone. β-Adrenergic blockers, verapamil, or even reserpine may be considered. Thyrotoxic patients are very sensitive to warfarin and the risk benefit of anticoagulation for AF is not favourable.

AMIODARONE

Amiodarone may be useful when given parenterally to control acute arrhythmias, and has been shown to inhibit peripheral deiodination of T_4 to T_3. It has been used by itself and in combination with thioamides to treat thyro-toxicosis. Acute antithyroid hormone effects on the heart are also described.

SUPPORTIVE MEASURES[10–17,29–32]

Supportive measures include identification and treatment of the precipitating cause. This is complicated by the non-specific symptoms and signs of severe hyper-thyroidism. These patients are grossly hypermetabolic and may require large amounts of fluids, electrolytes and glucose. Careful monitoring is required. Vitamins, par-ticularly thiamine, are usually given. Usual measures are used for the treatment of hyperpyrexia, except that sali-cylates are avoided. They displace thyroid hormones from their binding proteins. Frusemide is also a competi-tor for binding proteins and causes abrupt increases in FT_3 and FT_4 concentrations, and should be similarly avoided. Ethacrynic acid is a suggested alternative. The markedly increased metabolism and clearance of drugs may complicate management. Specimens should be taken for microbiological purposes and consideration should be given to empiric antibiotics.

Plasma exchange and charcoal haemoperfusion have been successfully used in refractory cases following 24–48 h of aggressive conventional therapy. However, lack of efficacy has also been reported.

Dantrolene has been used with symptomatic improve-ment, when thyrotoxic crisis mimicked malignant hyper-thermia, and in the treatment of recognized thyrotoxic crisis.

MYXOEDEMA COMA[10,17,33–38]

Overt hypothyroidism is present in 0.5–0.8% of the pop-ulation. While hypothyroidism may occur in either sex or at any age, myxoedema coma occurs typically during winter in elderly (60 years and older) females. Myxoedema coma represents the terminal stage of decompensated hypothyroidism, and has a high mortality, even if recognized. Most patients present in an earlier stage with neither coma nor obvious myxoedema. Instead, the cardinal manifestation is a deterioration of the patient's mental status. Patients presenting with decompensated hypothyroidism or coma usually have long-standing unrecognized thyroid hypofunction, most commonly caused by autoimmune thyroiditis, radioiodine therapy or thyroidectomy.

Drugs (e.g. phenytoin, frusemide, non-steroidal anti-inflammatory drugs, glucocorticoids and dopamine) can affect thyroid hormone concentrations, such that hypothyroidism is falsely suggested. Diagnosis of hypothyroidism in patients with critical illness should be made with caution. Thyroid hormone replacement in hypothyroxinaemic sick patients simply to achieve normal levels of circulatory hormone is not recommended. True hypothyroidism may be produced by antithyroid drugs, iodine, lithium and amiodarone. Amiodarone, because of its high iodine content, inhibits thyroid hormone synthesis and secretion. T_3 levels decrease by 20–30% in normal patients. Although T_4 and TSH increase initially and then decline, most of the 5–25% of patients on amiodarone who become hypothyroid have pre-existing thyroid disease.

Thyroid hormone concentrations will indicate whether the hypothyroidism is probably due to intrinsic thyroid disease (primary and most common), a failure of secretion of TSH (secondary) or hypothalamic dysfunction (tertiary).

PRECIPITATING FACTORS[4,10,17,33–41]

Coma is often precipitated by hypothermia, sometimes consequent to central nervous system depressant drugs (that inhibit thermogenesis or interfere with neurovascular adaptation to reduced thermogenesis), infections (pneumonia or urosepsis), trauma, cardiac failure or cerebrovascular accident, or drugs with antithyroid actions, including amiodarone or failure to reinstate thyroid replacement therapy during hospitalization. There is usually a long history of pre-existing hypothyroidism.

CLINICAL PRESENTATION[10,17,33–38,42–43]

The diagnosis of myxoedema coma is dependent on recognizing the triad of altered mental state, hypothermia, and clinical features of hypothyroidism (Table 50.4). When the typical features of hypothyroidism are present, diagnosis is straightforward. Difficulties arise when the features are atypical, the onset is relatively rapid, or when complicated by precipitating factors. Myxoedemic coma and coma in association with the euthyroid sick syndrome may be difficult to differentiate.

Table 50.4 Clinical manifestations of hypothyroidism

Cold intolerance, decreased energy, muscular weakness, bradykinesia, dementia, delayed tendon reflexes
Dry, yellowish skin, hoarse voice, coarse facial features, lateral eyebrow thinning, periorbital oedema, brittle hair
Constipation, weight gain, pleural and pericardial effusions, ischaemic heart disease, anaemia

COMA

This is due to the combination of hypothermia, hypercarbia, hypoxia, cerebral oedema and other metabolic derangements. All patients have deterioration of their mental state. Its onset may be quite abrupt. Tendon reflexes are usually symmetrical, but show a slow relaxation phase. Major seizures precede coma in about 25% of patients. Myopathy may be present. Creatine phosphokinase is frequently elevated.

HYPOTHERMIA

This may be profound, particularly when ambient temperatures are low. A low reading thermometer is required. Patient's temperatures are usually less than 35.5°C but some patient's temperatures may be normal.

HYPOVENTILATION

This occurs very frequently. Quantitation and monitoring of hypoxaemia and hypercarbia require blood-gas analysis. Multifactorial contributions to the respiratory failure include decreased ventilatory responsiveness to hypoxia and carbon dioxide, respiratory muscle fatigue, obesity, myxoedematous thickening of the vocal cords and sensitivity to the depressant effects of drugs.

HYPOTENSION

This is common and usually accompanied by an inappropriate sinus bradycardia. Baroreceptor dysfunction and reduction in plasma volume contribute. Tissue hypoxia is compounded by shock and anaemia. Myocardial myxoedematous infiltrates occur, but while pericardial effusions are frequently present, cardiac tamponade is uncommon. A small heart suggests adrenal insufficiency secondary to either pituitary hypothyroidism or coincidental primary adrenal failure. Lactic acidosis is frequent and may be severe. Increased creatine kinase MB, may be due to hypothermia rather than myocardial infarction. The ECG may show a slow-rate, low-voltage trace, with prolongation of QT interval and T-wave flattening or inversion.

HYPOGLYCAEMIA

This is often present and requires rapid recognition and treatment.

HYPONATRAEMIA

Together with low serum osmolality and increased total body water and sodium associated with oedema, this will be evident if hypothyroidism is long-standing and severe. Increased antidiuretic hormone concentrations and altered renal clearance of free water contribute to fluid accumulation. Despite excess total body sodium and water, plasma volume is usually depleted by 10–20% of predicted. Azotaemia and hypophosphataemia are common.

HYPOFUNCTION OF GUT AND BLADDER

Together with paralytic ileus, megacolon and urinary retention, these are frequent accompaniments.

MANAGEMENT[10,17,33–38]

Management of myxoedema coma includes careful assessment, treating precipitating factors and complications, and appropriate administration of thyroid hormone. Treatment should begin once the clinical diagnosis is made without awaiting laboratory confirmation. Rapid availability of appropriate formulations of thyroid hormone is very important. Blood should be collected for thyroid function tests and plasma cortisol determination before thyroid hormone is administered.

THYROID HORMONES[10,17,33–38,44–49]

The emphasis in severe and long-standing hypothyroidism is on initial low doses, with gradual escalation of hormone replacement. This may take months and never reach normal requirements, if complicated by ischaemic heart disease. More rapid replacement has been associated with sudden death due to arrhythmias or myocardial infarction, because of the imbalance in myocardial oxygen supply and demand. Angina improves in the majority of patients treated with thyroid hormone but intervention with angiography, angioplasty or cardiac surgery may be required. Oral T_4 (of variable, but approximately 50% bioavailability) is usually commenced at 50–100 μg/day with 25 μg increments, although 12.5–25 μg/day is an appropriate initial dose if ischaemic heart disease is present. There may be advantages in the use of T_3 orally (10 μg/day with 5 μg increments). It has good oral bioavailability and there is rapid cessation of hormone action if arrhythmias occur or angina worsens.

The optimum regimen for thyroid hormone replacement in myxoedema coma is unknown. Intestinal absorption of thyroid hormones, particularly T_4, is very variable with severe hypothyroidism, and the peripheral conversion of T_4 to T_3 is decreased. Larger dose proponents suggest that loading doses are necessary in myxoedema coma to saturate binding protein, and restore hormone levels to a low-normal euthyroid state. If T_4 is to be used, it must initially be given i.v. The large dose regimen involves a bolus of 400–500 μg (300 μg/m^2) followed by 50 μg i.v. daily. Changeover to orally administered T_4 may occur when gastrointestinal function resumes. Although a safer, smoother response is claimed for the use of T_4 (because of a gradual increase in the T_4 to T_3 conversion), this response is slow. Improvements in body temperature, heart rate and mental state barely begin within 24 h. Doses of T_4 (300 μg/m^2) have been given to euthyroid sick patients without detectable adverse effects. Alternatively, it is argued that large doses are not essential for recovery and may be harmful. An initial dose of 200–300 μg of thyroxine i.v. may be quite adequate.

Intravenous infusions of T_3, either continuously (20 μg/day) or very slow boluses repeated 8-hourly, may be preferred. The solubility and stability of T_3 in solution can be maintained if albumin 2% is added to the normal saline diluent, and minimum-volume polyvinyl chloride extension tubes are used. The advantage of more rapid onset and cessation of action may be achieved with infusions of T_3, or even repeated smaller doses (5 μg) via nasogastric tube, without obtaining dangerously high plasma concentrations.

The degree of hypothyroidism (as indicated by thyroid hormone concentrations) is not directly related to the severity of illness (e.g. degree of hypothermia or metabolic acidosis). Hence, initial doses of thyroid hormones should not necessarily relate to illness severity.

CORTICOSTEROIDS

Corticosteroids are usually administered, as patients with myxoedema coma may have impaired glucocorticoid response to stress, or even frank coexistent adrenal insufficiency (Schmidt's syndrome). Hydrocortisone, at least 200–300 mg/day, should be administered until normal adrenocortical function is demonstrated.

SUPPORTIVE MEASURES[10,17,33–38,50–51]

These patients have reduced ventilatory response to hypoxia and hypercarbia, and are very sensitive to central nervous system depressants. Endotracheal intubation and ventilation will often be required for airway protection and symptomatic management of hypercarbia. An additional benefit of intubation is the provision of warm humidification to treat hypothermia. Delayed gastric emptying and the anatomical abnormalities of the upper airway require specific care with intubation.

Shock is managed in accordance with usual principles, except that thyroid hormone and corticosteroids must be given. Intravascular fluid depletion is common despite oedema. There is resistance to inotropic agents, due to a reduction in β-adrenergic receptor expression. α-Adrenergic activity appears to remain intact. Hyponatraemia usually responds to water restriction. Rarely, rapid onset, severe hyponatraemia (less than 110 mmol/l) in association with coma and convulsions will require hypertonic saline. Sodium bicarbonate (8.4%) should be considered if severe metabolic acidosis coexists.

Intravenous glucose, 25 g statum, is given for hypoglycaemia. Hypertonic (20–50%) glucose may be infused via a central vein commensurate with glucose and water restriction requirements.

Mild hypothermia (e.g. 34–36°C) requires little more than prevention of further heat loss, treating hypoglycaemia, and warming of inspired gases. Moderate to severe hypothermia (<32°C) requires specific active management to bring core temperatures to greater than 34°C. Provided there is adequate monitoring of body temperature gradients and appropriate responses to haemodynamic and metabolic changes to prevent rewarming shock and acidosis, there is little to support the often repeated traditional warning against active warming.

Precipitating events and complications (e.g. septicaemia and pneumonia) will require specific therapy. Impaired bioavailability and clearance of drugs complicate therapy (e.g. sensitivity to digoxin, but resistance to anticoagulants).

REFERENCES

1 Woeber KA. Iodine and thyroid disease. *Med Clin North Am* 1991; **75**: 169–78.
2 Dayan CM. Interpretation of thyroid function tests. *Lancet* 2001; **357**: 619–24.
3 McDermott MT, Ridgway EC. Thyroid hormone resistance syndromes. *Am J Med* 1993; **94**: 424–32.
4 Klein I, Ojamaa K. Thyroid hormone and the cardiovascular system. *N Engl J Med* 2001; **344**: 501–9.
5 Jordan RM. Myxedema coma: pathophysiology, therapy, and factors affecting prognosis. *Med Clin North Am* 1995; **79**: 185–94.
6 McIver B, Gorman CA. Euthyroid sick syndrome: an overview. *Thyroid* 1997; **7**: 125–32.
7 Umpierrez GE. Euthyroid sick syndrome. *South Med J* 2002; **95**: 506–13.
8 Burmeister LA. Reverse T$_3$ does not reliably differentiate hypothyroid sick syndrome from euthyroid sick syndrome. *Thyroid* 1995; **5**: 435–41.
9 Papanicolaou DA. Euthyroid sick syndrome and the role of cytokines. *Rev Endocr Metab Disord* 2000; **1**: 43–8.
10 Smallridge RC. Metabolic and anatomic thyroid emergencies: a review. *Crit Care Med* 1992; **20**: 276–91.
11 Burch HB, Wartofsky L. Life-threatening thyrotoxicosis. Thyroid storm. *Endocrinol Metab Clin North Am* 1993; **22**: 263–77.
12 Tietgens ST, Leinung MC. Thyroid storm. *Med Clin North Am* 1995; **79**: 169–84.
13 Pronovost PH, Parris KH. Perioperative management of thyroid disease. Prevention of complications related to hyperthyroidism and hypothyroidism. *Postgrad Med* 1995; **98**: 83–6, 96–8.
14 Rennie D. Thyroid storm. *JAMA* 1997; **277**: 1238–43.
15 Dillmann WH. Thyroid storm. *Curr Ther Endocrinol Metab* 1997; **6**: 81–5.
16 Lazarus JH. Hyperthyroidism. *Lancet* 1997; **349**: 339–43.
17 Ringel MD. Management of hypothyroidism and hyperthyroidism in the intensive care unit. *Crit Care Clin* 2001; **17**: 59–74.
18 Nystrom E, Lindstedt G, Lundberg PA. Minor signs and symptoms of toxicity in a young woman in spite of massive thyroxine ingestion. *Acta Med Scand* 1980; **207**: 135–6.
19 Ratnaike S, Campbell DG, Melick RA. Thyroxine overdose. *Aust NZ J Med* 1986; **16**: 514.
20 Jiang YZ, Hutchinson KA, Bartelloni P, *et al.* Thyroid storm presenting as multiple organ dysfunction syndrome. *Chest* 2000; **118**: 877–9.
21 Choudhary AM, Roberts I. Thyroid storm presenting with liver failure. *J Clin Gastroenterol* 1999; **29**: 318–21.
22 Homma M, Shimizu S, Ogata M, *et al.* Hypoglycemic coma masquerading thyrotoxic storm. *Intern Med* 1999; **38**: 871–4.
23 Ghobrial MW, Ruby EB. Coma and thyroid storm in apathetic thyrotoxicosis. *South Med J* 2002; **95**: 552–4.
24 Ko GTC, Chow C-C, Sanderson JE, *et al.* Should β-blocking agents be used in thyrotoxic heart disease? *Med J Aust* 1995; **162**: 426–7.
25 Stockigt JR. Hyperthyroidism and the heart: clinical dilemmas. *Med J Aust* 1995; **162**: 398.
26 Isley WL, Dahl S, Gibbs H. Use of esmolol in managing a thyrotoxic patient needing emergency surgery. *Am J Med* 1990; **89**: 122–3.
27 Thorne AC, Bedford RF. Esmolol for perioperative management of thyrotoxic goitre. *Anesthesiology* 1989; **71**: 291–4.
28 Roti E, Montermini M, Roti S. The effect of diltiazem, a calcium-channel blocking drug, on cardiac rate and rhythm in hyperthyroid patients. *Arch Int Med* 1988; **148**: 1919–21.
29 Lim CF, Curtis AJ, Barlow JW. Assessment of loop diuretics as inhibitors of thyroid hormone binding in serum. *Proc Endocrinol Soc Aust* 1989; **32**: 143.
30 Henderson A, Hickman P, Ward G, *et al.* Lack of efficacy of plasmapheresis in a patient overdosed with thyroxine. *Anaesth Intens Care* 1994; **22**: 463–4.
31 Samaras K, Marel GM. Failure of plasmapheresis, corticosteriods and thionamides to ameliorate a case of protracted amiodarone-induced thyroiditis. *Clin Endocrinol (Oxf)* 1996; **45**: 365–8.
32 Ebert RJ. Dantrolene and thyroid crisis. *Anaesthesia* 1994; **49**: 924.
33 Nicoloff JT, LoPresti JS. Myxedema coma. A form of decompensated hypothyroidism. *Endocrinol Metab Clin North Am* 1993; **22**: 279–90.
34 Jordan RM. Myxedema coma. Pathophysiology, therapy, and factors affecting prognosis. *Med Clin North Am* 1995; **79**: 185–94.
35 Tsitouras PD. Myxedema coma. *Clin Geriatr Med* 1995; **11**: 251–8.
36 Pittman CS, Zayed AA. Myxedema coma. *Curr Ther Endocrinol Metab* 1997; **6**: 98–101.
37 Mathes DD. Treatment of myxedema coma for emergency surgery. *Anesth Analg* 1998; **86**: 450–1.
38 Wall CR. Myxedema coma: diagnosis and treatment. *Am Fam Physician* 2000; **62**: 2485–90.
39 Yamamoto T, Fukuyama J, Fujiyoshi A. Factors associated with mortality of myxedema coma: report of eight cases and literature survey. *Thyroid* 1999; **9**: 1167–74.

40 Mazonson PD, Williams ML, Cantley LK, *et al.* Myxedema coma during long-term amiodarone therapy. *Am J Med* 1984; **77:** 751–4.

41 Waldman SA, Park D. Myxedema coma associated with lithium therapy. *Am J Med* 1989; **87:** 355–6.

42 Hickman PE, Silvester W, Musk AA, *et al.* Cardiac enzyme changes in myxedema coma. *Clin Chem* 1987; **33:** 622–4.

43 Nee PA, Scane AC, Lavelle PH, *et al.* Hypothermic myxedema coma erroneously diagnosed as myocardial infarction because of increased creatine kinase MB. *Clin Chem* 1987; **33:** 1083–4.

44 Ladenson PW, Goldenheim PD, Ridgway EC. Rapid pituitary and peripheral tissue responses to intravenous L-triiodothyronine in hypothyroidism. *J Clin Endocrinol Metab* 1983; **56:** 1252–9.

45 Chernow B, Burman KD, Johnson DL. T_3 may be a better agent that T_4 in the critically ill hypothyroid patient: evaluation of transport across the blood–brain barrier in a primate model. *Crit Care Med* 1983; **11:** 99–104.

46 McCulloch W, Price P, Hinds CJ, *et al.* Effects of low dose oral triiodothyronine in myxoedema coma. *Intensive Care Med* 1985; **11:** 259–62.

47 Odgers CL, Phillips PJ, Shanks G. Intravenous liothyronine sodium (T_3) for myxoedema coma – pharmaceutical considerations. *Aust J Hosp Pharm* 1984; **14:** 181–8.

48 Arlot S, Debussche X, Lalau JD, *et al.* Myxoedema coma: response of thyroid hormones with oral and intravenous high-dose L-thyroxine treatment. *Intensive Care Med* 1991; **17:** 16–8.

49 Toft AD. Thyroxine therapy. *N Engl J Med* 1994; **331:** 174–80.

50 Frank DH, Robson MC. Accidental hypothermia treated without mortality. *Surg Gynecol Obstet* 1980; **151:** 379–81.

51 Fitzgerald FT, Jessop C. Accidental hypothermia: a report of 23 cases and review of literature. *Adv Intern Med* 1982; **27:** 127–50.

51

Adrenocortical insufficiency

A E Vedig

Adrenocortical insufficiency may present as an insidious, occult disorder, unmasked by conditions of stress, or as a catastrophic syndrome that may result in death. In the critically ill patient, occult 'relative' adrenal insufficiency is common, with the usual clinical presentation being hyperdynamic vasopressor-dependent shock. Empirical treatment is often required before the diagnosis is confirmed by investigations.

PHYSIOLOGY AND PATHOPHYSIOLOGY[1-9]

The adrenal cortex synthesizes and secretes three major types of hormones: glucocorticoid (cortisol), mineralocorticoids (aldosterone and 11 deoxycorticosterone) and adrenal androgens. The major pathogenic effects of disease result from cortisol and aldosterone deficiency.

Anatomically, the adrenal gland is unique in that the arteries and veins do not run in parallel. There is a very rich autonomic innervation and vascular supply. Venous drainage is limited to one or two veins which have an eccentric muscular arrangement, making the gland sensitive to stress states and coagulopathy. Histologically, the adrenal cortex is divided into three major zones: zona fasciculata, zona glomerulosa and zona reticularis.

CORTISOL

Cortisol is secreted by the zona fasciculata which is the thickest intermediate layer of the adrenal gland. This hormone affects intermediary metabolism via a type II glucocorticoid receptor. It regulates protein, carbohydrate, lipid and nucleic acid metabolism, resulting in increased gluconeogenesis and enhanced catabolism and lipolysis. Anti-inflammatory activity is related to the inhibition of neutrophil and macrophage migration, resulting in a microvascular stabilizing effect. Free water clearance is facilitated, and there is a permissive effect on peripheral vascular responses to endogenous vasoconstrictors.

There is normal diurnal output of cortisol with a lower level in the morning (08.00 h to 09.00 h, <140 nmol/l) and higher levels after midnight (110–520 nmol/l). Total output of cortisol is 40–80 μmol/day (i.e. 15–30 mg/day). Stress, in particular, sepsis and respiratory failure, results in levels in excess of 1500–2000 nmol/l. The half-life of cortisol is 60–90 min.

Cortisol secretion is directly controlled by adrenocorticotropic hormone (ACTH) which is, in turn, regulated by corticotrophin-releasing hormone (CRH). Release of these hypothalamic-pituitary hormones is influenced by circulating levels of cortisol or cortisol-like steroids, stress, antidiuretic hormone (ADH), oxytocin, angiotensin II, leptin, sleep–wake cycles and circulating levels of interleukin-1. ACTH is derived from a precursor molecule pro-opiomelanocortin (POMC). β-Lipotropin and several other POMC derivatives have melanocyte-stimulating activity.

Leptin, an adipose-produced hormone has recently been found to have previously unsuspected roles in the hypothalamus (H), anterior pituitary (P), HP-adrenal, HP-thyroid and HP-gonadal axes. Leptin has an inverse diurnal rhythm compared with cortisol, and while cortisol stimulates leptin expression, it only has a modulating effect. Cytokines and endotoxins stimulate leptin which itself inhibits activation of the HP axis. Leptin is important in energy homeostasis and weight balance.

ALDOSTERONE

The zona glomerulosa is the thin outermost layer of the adrenal gland, which secretes aldosterone. The hormone increases sodium conservation and potassium loss by the kidney, sweat glands and gastrointestinal tract. These actions are mediated by the type 1 glucocorticoid receptor. It is a major regulator of extracellular fluid volume. Fluid and electrolyte abnormalities of primary adrenal gland insufficiency are mostly due to aldosterone deficiency. Most glucocorticoid drugs have some mineralocorticoid like activity.

Prolonged administration of glucocorticoids results in adrenal atrophy and hyposecretion of endogenous glucocorticoid and androgens, although aldosterone responsiveness to sodium depletion is maintained. Aldosterone secretion is controlled by the renin–angiotensin system, in particular angiotensin II activity, serum potassium concentration and ACTH (which plays a minor role). Aldosterone output normally is 200–500 nmol/day (70–100 μg/day) but with shock, severe sodium restriction or heart failure output may increase to 1100–1400 nmol/day (400–500 mg/day).

ANDROGENS

The zona reticularis is the inner layer which secretes androgens. Deficiency produces a decrease in body hair in adult female patients, while male patients notice little or no change because of gonadal testosterone production. Androgen deficiency in females may contribute to anaemia and osteoporosis

PRIMARY ADRENOCORTICAL INSUFFICIENCY (ADDISON'S DISEASE)[10–14]

This is a rare disorder that occurs equally in males or females at any age. Most of the adrenal gland (90%) is destroyed if symptoms are present. More than 80% of cases are idiopathic, of whom 50% have anti-adrenal antibodies present. Other immune disorders are commonly associated with adrenocortical insufficiency. Specific polyglandular autoimmune syndromes and other associated neurological disorders are rare. Tuberculosis accounts for a lesser proportion than previously, but is more likely (50%) if adrenal calcification is present. Cryptococcosis, other fungi and cytomegalovirus (CMV) infections occur rarely, except in patients with AIDS. CMV adrenalitis is a common abnormality present in autopsy specimens of patients with AIDS, although clinically less than 50% have overt adrenal insufficiency. Individual patients with known CMV infection have a higher rate of adrenal infarction.

Destruction of the gland may occur with metastic neoplasms, and rarely with granulomatous or amyloid infiltration, irradiation or haemochromatosis. Other causes include haemorrhage, congenital adrenal hyperplasia and drugs such as ketoconazole, fluconazole and those used to treat hyperadrenalism (e.g. metyrapone). More recently, thrombosis and infarction of the adrenal glands have been recognized in patients with the antiphospholipid (anticardiolipin) syndrome, who may present in the intensive care unit with thromboembolic disease. Physical destruction of the adrenal glands will result in varying degrees of glucocorticoid, mineralocorticoid and androgen deficiency. Specific diseases and drugs may result in a preponderance of glucocorticoid or mineralocorticoid insufficiency.

SECONDARY ADRENOCORTICAL INSUFFICIENCY[10–16]

This condition may be due to ACTH deficiency from pituitary and hypothalamic disease, or to hypothalamic–pituitary–adrenal (HPA) gland suppression by exogenously administered corticosteroid. Adrenocortical insufficiency associated with corticosteroid therapy occurs frequently. The type of steroid, dose, route and duration influence the likelihood of HPA suppression. Prednisolone (or other equivalent) in excess of 7.5 mg/day for longer than 2–3 weeks may suppress the HPA and, with continued use, result in adrenal atrophy. Suppression may continue for months after the cessation of therapy, during which time acute deficiency may occur if the patient is stressed. Suppression may occur with topically applied, inhaled and depot-type preparations. Neither the dose and duration of corticosteroid therapy, nor basal cortisol levels can reliably predict the functional reserve.

Pituitary dysfunction as a cause of secondary adrenocortical insufficiency occurs rarely, and may be due to neoplasms, infections, haemorrhage (Sheehan's syndrome), infarction (pituitary apoplexy), radiation and granulomatous infiltration. Pituitary apoplexy is usually acute in presentation and may require immediate hormone replacement whereas Sheehan's syndrome is less fulminant in presentation. Aldosterone secretion continues normally (as it is not controlled predominantly by ACTH), but severe fluid losses may reveal a subnormal aldosterone secretory capacity. Isolated mineralocorticoid deficiency due to reduced renin activity is uncommon although hyperreninaemic hypoaldosteronism occurs frequently in critically ill patients. If panhypopituitarism exists, hypogonadism, growth retardation and hypothyroidism may be present. Secondary hormonal deficiencies (e.g. hypothyroidism) may further complicate glucocorticoid metabolism.

CLINICAL PRESENTATION OF DEFICIENCY STATES[10–15]

There may be few symptoms and presentation insidious. The only physical sign apparent in Addison's disease may be hyperpigmentation of skin which is exposed to light, friction or pressure. Gingival, scar, nipple, freckle, tongue and genital pigmentation may also be present, secondary to the combined effects of β-lipotropin and melanocyte-stimulating hormone. Clinical features common to primary and secondary adrenocortical deficiency include asthenia, muscle weakness, malaise, fever, anorexia, abdominal pain (which may be severe), vomiting, alternating diarrhoea and constipation, and weight loss. Postural and supine hypotension also occur, as do salt craving, myalgias, arthralgias, vitiligo, flexural contractures, alteration in personality, mental confusion and psychosis. There is increased sensitivity to central nervous system depressant drugs, including opioids.

Signs of reactive or fasting hypoglycaemia may be present (more common in pituitary insufficiency). In advanced disease, there may be hyponatraemia and/or hyperkalaemia, which may lead to a form of life-threatening ascending neuromyopathy. Hypercalcaemia is rarely present. A small heart may be demonstrated radiographically. Haemodynamic measurements may reveal increased cardiac output and low systemic vascular resistance. Eosinophilia, relative lymphocytosis and normocytic anaemia also occur. About one-quarter of critically ill patients with eosinophilia greater than 3% have depressed adrenal function. Although cortisol has a permissive role in haemosynthesis, androgen deficiency is responsible for the anaemia. Since the features of adrenocortical deficiency are non-specific and common in other severe debilitating disease, it is important to maintain a high index of suspicion.

Secondary insufficiency is more difficult to diagnose than primary insufficiency. Hyperpigmentation is absent. Major findings, in order of prevalence, are hypoglycaemia, weight loss, hypotension, anaemia, weakness and fatigue, hair loss, nausea, vomiting and hyponatraemia. Stiffman syndrome and delirium and fever are also described.

ACUTE ADRENOCORTICAL INSUFFICIENCY (ADDISONIAN CRISIS)[10–15,17]

AETIOLOGY

Acute adrenal insufficiency may present as an intensification of chronic hypoadrenalism, where there is insufficient hormonal resource to meet the stress requirements of trauma, infection and surgery. Sudden cessation or too rapid reduction of chronic exogenous steroids may precipitate an acute crisis. Unrecognized, inappropriately low-level therapy with corticosteroid drugs may result from drug interactions which increase steroid metabolism (e.g. with rifampicin, barbiturates and phenytoin). Also, drugs such as ketoconazole that inhibit steroid synthesis when given in the setting of stress (it also binds to the glucocorticoid receptor) may precipitate a crisis in patients with congenital adrenal hyperplasia or decreased adrenocortical reserve.

Sudden destruction of glands due to haemorrhage although unusual, may occur with severe sepsis, anticoagulant therapy (particularly heparin-induced thrombocytopenia), burns, surgery or trauma. The classical Waterhouse–Friederichsen syndrome was associated with meningococcaemia, but may occur with either Gram-positive or Gram-negative septicaemia. Chest, abdominal or investigation trauma has caused an Addisonian crisis secondary to haemorrhage. Surgical removal of a single gland, postpartum pituitary infarction (Sheehan's syndrome) and pituitary apoplexy may cause acute adrenal insufficiency.

Infusions of the anaesthetic agents etomidate and alfathesin (althesin) probably contributed in early reports to the adrenocortical insufficiency ascribed to critically ill patients.

CLINICAL PRESENTATION[10–15]

Patients present usually in a shocked state with a history of worsening prodromal symptoms of hypoadrenalism. Malaise, weakness, tiredness, anorexia, nausea, vomiting, mental disturbance, fever and severe abdominal pain are common presenting complaints. Precipitating events such as surgery or septicaemia may be elicited. Sudden flank or epigastric pain suggest adrenal haemorrhage. Anticoagulant-induced haemorrhage is more common in the middle-aged to elderly and thrombocytopenic patients. The shock presentation may be confused with sepsis (high cardiac output and low systemic vascular resistance) or hypovolaemia which is not so obvious with secondary insufficiency. Severe dehydration, hypotension and peripheral circulatory failure are evident terminally, and are refractory to treatment without steroid administration. The diagnosis of Addisonian crisis should be suspected in all shocked patients if they remain refractory to usual treatment and when the cause of their condition is not apparent, especially if associated hypoglycaemia and eosinophilia exist.

INVESTIGATIONS[18–23]

Those which assist diagnosis and management include the following:

BIOCHEMICAL AND HAEMATOLOGICAL TESTS

Hyponatraemia and hyperkalaemia ($Na^+ : K^+$ ratio of <25 : 1) are very suggestive of Addison's disease. Hypoglycaemia is common. Serum calcium may be elevated, although the ionized calcium is usually normal (but may rarely be increased). Metabolic and respiratory acidosis may be present, as may evidence of renal tubular acidosis (type IV) and dehydration. High urinary sodium excretion (>40 mmol/l) may occur despite hypovolaemia. Moderate neutropenia with relative eosinophilia and lymphocytosis may be seen. Antibodies to adrenal gland and other organs may be detected. C-reactive protein, and procalcitonin are normal in Addisonian crisis.

ELECTROCARDIOGRAM

Low voltage and slow conduction are present in severe hypoadrenalism. Hyperkalaemic changes may be present.

IMAGING

Chest X-rays may show evidence of old tuberculosis. The heart is small in chronic insufficiency. Heart enlargement suggests concomitant hypothyroidism. Ultrasound, computed tomography, MRI imaging may reveal pituitary or adrenal calcification, haemorrhage or neoplastic infiltration.

PLASMA HORMONES
Basal cortisol levels
These are sometimes <100 nmol/l (ACTH >200 ng/l). Levels <500 nml/l with marked stress suggest insufficiency.

Short ACTH test (0.25 mg synacthen)
This traditionally involves administration of 0.25 mg i.v. (or i.m.) synacthen. Plasma cortisol (plus sometimes renin, aldosterone and pituitary hormones) are measured at 30 and 60 min. A rise of 250 nmol/l or 2–3 times basal level, and levels more than 550 nmol/l should be achieved if there is 'normal' adrenal responsiveness. Basal levels >200 nmol/l are usual.

If hydrocortisone has been given inadvertently the short ACTH test may be repeated in 24 h. Stimulated plasma adosterone levels <14 000 pmol/l indicate insufficiency, as do basal plasma ACTH levels of >200 ng/l.

Low-dose ACTH test (LDACTH)
Baseline and 30 min plasma cortisols are taken after 1 μg i.v. ACTH is administered. A normal response is a plasma cortisol of >550 nmol/l. Sensitivity of the LDACTH test increases to 100% with a plasma cortisol cut-off value at 600 nmol/l.

TSH, thyroxine
Patients with Addison's disease may have low or normal thyroxine levels with elevated TSH. These normalize with hydrocortisone administration.

MANAGEMENT[10–15,24–28]

Treatment must be immediate, and should be initiated prior to confirmation of the diagnosis. Precipitating factors, if not apparent, should be sought and treated appropriately (e.g. sepsis and thrombocytopenia).

CORTICOSTEROIDS[24–28]
Acute management
If adrenal crisis is suspected, corticosteroids must be given without delay; results of plasma cortisol assays will not readily be available. The short or ultra-short synacthen test should be undertaken together with treatment, provided that there is no undue delay in corticosteroid administration. Blood is taken at baseline and at 30 min for cortisol concentrations, and other hormone and electrolyte measurement. Dexamethasone 10 mg i.v. is given, together with ACTH 0.25 mg i.v. (Synacthen, Cortrosyn) or 1 μg ACTH i.v. dexamethasone begins replacement therapy rapidly without interfering with the cortisol assay.

Corticosteroid treatment is continued as hydrocortisone 100 mg i.v. 6–8-hourly. On day 2, 100 mg hydrocortisone is given 8-hourly i.m. or i.v., then 12-hourly,

and changed to an oral maintenance regimen. Hydrocortisone has sufficient mineralocorticoid activity in higher doses (>120 mg/day) to allow omission of mineralocorticoid replacement.

Maintenance
When the crisis has been successfully treated, appropriate investigations help formulate a corticosteroid maintenance regimen, which will involve giving cortisol or its equivalent twice daily (on waking and at 18.00 h) to mimic circadian rhythm. Oral fludrocortisone 50–100 mg daily or every other day provides mineralocorticoid support if required. Concomitant phenytoin may cause adverse effects. The choice of corticosteroid and dosage will depend on the degrees of insufficiency of the two essential hormones. Although adrenal insufficiency is usually permanent when the glands have been destroyed by haemorrhage and infarction, recovery is possible.

Prevention
Recent studies have shown that cortisol production is lower than previously throught being only 5.7 mg/m^2 of body surface area. This is equivalent to 10–12 mg of oral hydrocortisone because of different potency and bioavailability. Major surgery may result in only 200–300 mg of cortisol secretion in the first 24 h. Steroid supplementation is not necessary to the level of previous recommendations which were 100 mg i.v. hydrocortisone just prior to surgery and then 100 mg i.v. 8-hourly for 1–3 days depending on whether major surgery occurred.

Patients with established disease of the adrenal cortex or HPA
These patients are not able to increase their cortisol response to stress and should routinely receive supplemental steroids for surgery or severe illness. The dose should be at least 100–150 mg of hydrocortisone daily.

If these lower dose recommendations are adopted these patients must be observed with continued care and awareness of the possibility of a beneficial affect of increased doses of steroids. Over treatment may contribute to hyperglycaemia and poorer wound healing.

MONITORING AND GENERAL SUPPORTIVE MEASURES

These include oxygen therapy, and assessment and management of metabolic and respiratory acidosis. Opioid and sedative drugs should be avoided. Frequent electrolyte (particularly potassium) and glucose determinations will be required. Continuous electrocardiogram and frequent arterial and central venous pressure measurements, and attention to fluid balance are essential. Repeated urinary electrolytes may be helpful. More invasive haemodynamic monitoring and inotropic drugs may be required in managing the precipitating event, or if shock remains unresponsive to appropriate fluid replacement.

INTRAVENOUS FLUIDS

Normal saline is infused rapidly, without awaiting monitoring catheter placement. The infusion rate could be 1 l or more in the first 30 mm. Subsequent infusion may be in the order of 1 l/h, but is determined by the response to initial infusion and monitoring of clinical signs. The volume deficit in acute adrenal crisis is seldom greater than 10% of total body water. Dextrose should be given at the same time as the saline infusion, as 5% dextrose in normal saline, or separately. Hypertonic dextrose can be given via a central line to treat hypoglycaemia. About 50 g of dextrose may be required in the first 1–2 h.

CORTICOSTEROID THERAPY[29–32]

Apart from substitution therapy in adrenocortical deficiency, the use of corticosteroids is largely empirical and palliative by virtue of the anti-inflammatory effects. A single dose (even a large one) or a few days of therapy is unlikely to produce harm, unless specific contraindications exist. In the long term, the likelihood of disabling and potentially lethal effects increases in proportion to the extent that the dose exceeds substitution therapy. Sudden cessation may precipitate an Addisonian crisis, or unmask an underlying disease. This may occur even with topically or rectally applied, inhaled and locally injected glucocorticoids. Alternate-day dosing with the shorter-acting steroids minimizes HPA suppression, but in acute situations, at least daily dosing must be used. Selection and dosing regimens are based on anti-inflammatory potency, mineralocorticoid activity and duration of action (Table 51.1). The pharmacodynamic effects of the corticosteroid drugs are more relevant than plasma half-lives when considering dosing schedules.

HYPOALDOSTERONISM[33,34–42]

INHERITED HYPOALDOSTERONISM[33]

Inherited hypoaldosteronism (congenital adrenal hyperplasia) is most commonly due to 21-hydroxylase defi-ciency. This autosomal recessive disorder occurs in 1 in 10 000–15 000 births. Infants present with hyponatraemia and hyperkalaemia, which can progress to shock and death. Girls usually have masculinized genitalia. Mineralocorticoids and glucocorticoids control the salt wasting. Aldosterone synthase deficiency occurs less commonly, as does pseudohypoaldosteronism.

ACQUIRED HYPOALDOSTERONISM

In the presence of normal glucocorticoid synthesis, acquired hypoaldosteronism may occur during prolonged heparin or heparinoid therapy and following operative removal of aldosterone-secreting adenomas, and is common with critical illness. Patients are unable to increase aldosterone secretion appropriately in response to sodium restriction or hypovolaemia. Unexplained hyperkalaemia is the commonest presenting feature. Once transcellular shifts of potassium have been excluded, hypoaldosteronism must be considered in patients with hyperkalaemia.

HYPORENINAEMIC HYPOALDOSTERONISM[34,35]

This is most frequently seen in adults with diabetes mellitus and mild renal failure, where the hyperkalaemia and metabolic acidosis are disproportionate to the degree of kidney impairment. Renin production is low, as is the aldosterone level in relationship to the degree of hyperkalaemia. Other associated diseases are gout, pyelonephritis, nephrosclerosis and amyloid.

HYPERRENINAEMIC HYPOALDOSTERONISM[36–42]

Hyperreninaemic hypoaldosteronism is common with prolonged, severe illness. Plasma renin activity and angiotensin II levels are elevated. The pathogenesis is unknown, but may result from prolonged stimulation of the adrenal cortex by ACTH, resulting in a shift from mineralocorticoid to glucocorticoid production. The aldosterone precursor 18-hydroxycorticosterone is

Table 51.1   Suggested glucocorticoid replacement regimen

Indication	Hydrocortisone dose (or equivalent)	Timing
Low dose maintenance (e.g. 5 mg prednisolone/day)	Consider omitting	
Minor stress (e.g. hernia repair)	25 mg i.v. stat	Taper over 1–2 days
Moderate stress (e.g. abdominal hysterectomy)	50–75 mg i.v. stat	Taper over 1–2 days
Major stress (e.g cardiac surgery)	100–150 mg i.v. per day	Maintenance for 1–3 days then taper over 1–2 days
Critically ill patients	50–100 mg i.v. 6–8-hourly	Maintenance for 3–7 days and then gradual taper

The contents of the table represent a consensus view from limited data.

frequently elevated, hypotension is common, and an increased mortality is associated. Although mild hyponatraemia is often seen, normokalaemia is usual. In the stressed critically ill patient, the high cortisol concentrations may inhibit the development of hyperkalaemia. Disorders associated with hyperreninaemic hypoaldosteronism include heparin therapy (low molecular weight heparin less so), diabetes mellitus, AIDS and secondary carcinoma of the adrenal gland. Hyperkalaemia is well-recognized in association with prolonged heparin therapy (unfractionated and low molecular weight heparin) and seems more common in less severely ill patients.

Both hyporeninaemic and hyperreninaemic hypoaldosteronism respond to mineralocorticoids. Hydrocortisone administration results in marked improvement in cardiovascular status, with dramatic reduction in inotropic requirement in hypotensive critically ill patients. Basal and ACTH-stimulated plasma cortisol levels are frequently very high. The patients with renal insufficiency often respond to a reduction in sodium intake and to administration of frusemide, which increases the stimulus for aldosterone secretion, improving the hyperkalaemia and metabolic acidosis.

HPA INSUFFICIENCY IN THE CRITICALLY ILL[42-54]

Adrenal insufficiency is common in critically ill patients (20%). It is part of a more complex HPA axis abnormality induced by sepsis, hypovolaemia, continued stress and drug therapies. Basal plasma cortisol concentrations, both low (<200 nmol/l) and high, have been associated with poor prognosis. In general, high levels of basal cortisol are found in patients with higher Acute Physiology, Age and Chronic Health Evaluation (APACHE) and Sepsis Related Organ Failure Assessment (SOFA) scores which are independently linked to poorer prognoses. Patients with respiratory failure or sepsis may have basal cortisol levels of >1200 nmol/l. Patients with a ruptured aortic aneurysm had average concentrations of 745 nmol/l, as do other critically and postoperative patients. There is no consensus on what constitutes a 'normal' cortisol concentration in critically ill patients. Normal values greater than 200–250 nmol/l for basal cortisol concentrations or as high as 550 nmol/l have been proposed. Responses to the rapid ACTH test (usually 250 μg i.v.) are perhaps more useful. Patients unable to respond with increases above baseline by 250 nmol/l appear to have poorer outcomes whereas patients with 'adequate' high baseline cortisols may only achieve small increments presumable due to an already maximally stimulated HPA axis. The more recently introduced low dose ACTH test using 1 μg i.v. may be a more sensitive tool for diagnosing adrenal insufficiency. High doses of ACTH may produce false negatives in patients with secondary adrenal insufficiency. Presently, there are no generally agreed guidelines for hormone concentrations in the diagnosis of adrenal insufficiency. Certainly, patients who have normal responses to 250 μg ACTH are demonstrated adrenally insufficient if subjected to insulin induced hypoglycaemia and metapyrone testing.

Leptin an adipocyte-produced hormone is important in energy homeostasis, being influential in the balance of fat stores and energy expenditure. It is found in the anterior pituitary, participates in the expression of CRH in the hypothalamus and interacts in a previously unsuspected neuroendocrine role in the HPA axis, HP-thyroid and HP-gonadal axis. While leptin expression is stimulated by glucocorticoids, cytokines and endotoxins, leptin itself inhibits activation of the HPA. Glucocorticoids have a modulatory effect on normal leptin output rather than a direct feedback role, even though there is a inverse diurnal rhythm of cortisol and leptin. In the critically ill, particularly when the illness is prolonged, leptins may play a major role and help explain some of the apparent inconsistencies of hormonal relationships and outcomes.

Occult 'relative' adrenal insufficiency in critical illness often presents with the clinical picture of vasopressor dependence in hyperdynamic shock. Relative eosinophilia (>3%) may also provide a clue. Stress doses of hydrocortisone show beneficial effects in the ability to withdraw vasopressors, wean patients from mechanical ventilation and improve survival. The mechanisms of these physiological responses and their relationships to aspects of hypoaldosteronism are not clear. In patients with suspected 'relative' adrenal insufficiency a therapeutic trial with hydrocortisone should be commenced pending results of diagnostic testing.

Table 51.2 Corticosteroids and synthetic analogues

Drug	Equivalent dose (mg)	Sodium-retaining activity	Plasma half-life (h)	Duration of action (h)
Cortisone	25	1	1.5	8–12
Hydrocortisone (cortisol)	20	1	+1.5	8–12
Prednisone, prednisolone	5	0.8	>3	>24
Methylprednisolone	4	0.5	>3	>24
Dexamethasone	0.75	0	>3	>36

REFERENCES

1 Chrousos GP. The hypothalamic-pituitary-adrenal axis and immune mediated inflamation. *N Engl J Med* 1995; **332**: 1351–62.

2 Tsigos C, Chrousos GP. Physiology of the hypothalamic-pituitary-adrenal axis in health and dysregulation in psychiatric and autoimmune disorders. *Endocrinol Metab Clin North Am* 1994; **23**: 451–66.

3 White PC. Disorders of aldosterone biosynthesis and action. *N Engl J Med* 1994; **331**: 250–8.

4 Chrousos GP. Regulation and dysregulation of the hypothalamic-pituitary-adrenal axis. The corticotropin-releasing hormone perspective. *Endocrinol Metab Clin North Am* 1992; **21**: 833–58.

5 Turnbull AV, Rivier CL. Regulation of the hypothalamic-pituitary-adrenal axis by cytokines: actions and mechanisms of action. *Physiol Rev* 1999; **79**: 1–71.

6 Gaillard RC, Spinedi E, Chautard T, Pralong FP. Cytokines, leptin, and the hypothalamo-pituitary-adrenal axis. *Ann NY Acad Sci* 2000; **917**: 647–57.

7 Leal-Cerro A, Soto A, Martinez MA *et al.* Influence of cortisol status on leptin secretion. *Pituitary* 2001; **4**: 111–6.

8 Pralong FP, Gaillard RC. Neuroendocrine effects of leptin. *Pituitary* 2001; **4**: 25–32.

9 Lloyd RV, Jin L, Tsumanuma I, *et al.* Leptin and leptin receptor in anterior pituitary function. *Pituitary* 2001; **4**: 33–47.

10 Vallotton MB. Endocrine emergencies. Disorders of the adrenal cortex. *Baillières Clin Endocrinol Metab* 1992; **6**: 41–56.

11 Werbel SS, Ober KP. Acute adrenal insufficiency. *Endocrinol Metab Clin North Am* 1993; **22**: 303–28.

12 Malchoff CD, Carey RM. Adrenal insufficiency. *Curr Ther Endocrinol Metab* 1997; **6**: 142–7.

13 Oelkers W. Adrenal insufficiency. *N Engl J Med* 1996; **335**: 1206–12.

14 Ten S, New M, Maclaren N. Clinical review 130: Addison's disease 2001. *J Clin Endocrinol Metab* 2001; **86**: 2909–22.

15 Rolih CA, Ober KP. Pituitary apoplexy. *Endocrinol Metab Clin North Am* 1993; **22**: 291–302.

16 Schlaghecke R, Kornely E, Santen RT, Ridderskamp P. The effect of long-term glucocorticoid therapy on pituitary-adrenal responses to exogenous corticotropin-releasing hormone. *N Engl J Med* 1992; **326**: 226–30.

17 Satta MA, Corsello SM, Della Casa S, *et al.* Adrenal insufficiency as the first clinical manifestation of the primary antiphospholipid antibody syndrome. *Clin Endocrinol* 2000; **52**: 123–6.

18 Oelkers W. The role of high- and low-dose corticotropin tests in the diagnosis of secondary adrenal insufficiency. *Eur J Endocrinol* 1998; **139**: 567–70.

19 Thaler LM, Blevins LS Jr. The low dose (1-microg) adrenocorticotropin stimulation test in the evaluation of patients with suspected central adrenal insufficiency. *J Clin Endocrinol Metab* 1998; **83**: 2726–9.

20 Rose SR, Lustig RH, Burstein S, *et al.* Diagnosis of ACTH deficiency. Comparison of overnight metyrapone test to either low-dose or high-dose ACTH test. *Horm Res* 1999; **52**: 73–9.

21 Tordjman K, Jaffe A, Trostanetsky Y, *et al.* Low-dose (1 microgram) adrenocorticotrophin (ACTH) stimulation as a screening test for impaired hypothalamo-pituitary-adrenal axis function: sensitivity, specificity and accuracy in comparison with the high-dose (250 microgram) test. *Clin Endocrinol* 2000; **52**: 633–40.

22 Beishuizen A, van Lijf JH, Lekkerkerker JF, Vermes I. The low dose (1microg) ACTH stimulation test for assessment of the hypothalamo-pituitary-adrenal axis. *Neth J Med* 2000; **56**: 91–9.

23 Suliman AM, Smith TP, Labib M, *et al.* The low-dose ACTH test does not provide a useful assessment of the hypothalamic-pituitary-adrenal axis in secondary adrenal insufficiency. *Clin Endocrinol* 2002; **56**: 533–9.

24 Salem M, Tainsh RE Jr, Bromberg J, *et al.* Perioperative glucocorticoid coverage. A reassessment 42 years after emergence of a problem. *Ann Surg* 1994; **219**: 416–25.

25 Lamberts SW, Bruining HA, de Jong FH. Corticosteriod therapy in severe illness. *N Engl J Med* 1997; **337**: 1285–92.

26 Nicholson G, Burrin JM, Hall GM. Peri-operative steroid supplementation. *Anaesthesia* 1998; **53**: 1091–104.

27 Oelkers W, Diederich S, Bahr V. Therapeutic strategies in adrenal insufficiency. *Ann Endocrinol* 2001; **62**: 212–6.

28 Coursin DB, Wood KE. Corticosteriod supplementation for adrenal insufficiency. *JAMA* 2002; **287**: 236–40.

29 Begg EJ, Atkinson HC, Gianarakis N. The pharmacokinetics of corticosteriod agents. *Med J Aust* 1987; **146**: 37–41.

30 Sweetman SC. *Martindale, The Complete Drug Reference*, 33rd edn. London: Pharmaceutical Press; 2002: pp. 1039–81.

31 Baxter JD. The effects of glucocorticoid therapy. *Hosp Pract* 1992; **27**: 111–23.

32 Buchman AL. Side Effects of corticosteroid therapy. *J Clin Gastroenterol* 2001; **33**: 289–94.

33 Merke DP, Bornstein SR, Avila NA, Chrousos GP. NIH conference. Future directions in the study and management of congenital adrenal hyperplasia due to 21-hydroxylase deficiency. *Ann Intern Med* 2002; **136**: 320–34.

34 Uribarri J, Oh MS, Carroll HJ. Hyperkalemia in diabetes mellitus. *J Diabet Complications* 1990; **4**: 3–7.

35 Williams ME. Endocrine crises. Hyperkalemia. *Crit Care Clin* 1991; **7**: 155–74.

36 Zipser RD, Davenport MW, Martin KL, *et al.* Hyperreninemic hypoaldosteronism in the critically ill: a new entity. *J Clin Endocrinol Metab* 1981; **53**: 867–3.

37 Davenport MW, Zipser RD. Association of hypotension with hyperreninemic hypoaldosteronism in the critically ill patient. *Arch Intern Med* 1983; **143**: 735–7.

38 Findling JW, Waters VO, Raff H. The dissociation of renin and aldosterone during critical illness. *J Clin Endocrinol Metab* 1987; **64**: 592–5.

39 O'Kelly R, Magee F, McKenna TJ. Routine heparin therapy inhibits adrenal aldosterone production. *J Clin Endocrinol Metab* 1983; **56**: 108–12.

40 Levesque H, Verdier S, Cailleux N, *et al.* Low molecular weight heparins and hypoaldosteronism. *BMJ* 1990; **300**: 1437–8.

41 Oster JR, Singer I, Fishman LM. Heparin-induced aldosterone suppression and hyperkalemia. *Am J Med* 1995; **98**: 575–86.

42 Bick RL, Frenkel EP. Clinical aspects of heparin-induced thrombocytopenia and thrombosis and other side effects of heparin therapy. *Clin Appl Thromb Hemost* 1999; **5** (suppl. 1): S715.

43 Rivers EP, Blake HC, Dereczyk B, *et al.* Adrenal dsyfunction in hemodynamically unstable patients in the emergency department. *Acad Emerg Med* 1999; **6**: 626–30.

44 Ligtenberg JJ, van der Werf TS, Tulleken JE, *et al.* Diagnosis of relative adrenal insufficiency in critically ill patients. *Lancet* 1999; **354**: 774–5.

45 Briegel J. Hydrocortisone and the reduction of vasopressor in septic shock: therapy or only chart cosmetics? *Intensive Care Med* 2000; **26**: 1723–6.

46 Woolf PD. Adrenal tea leaves: is the adrenal response to sepsis discernible? *Crit Care Med* 2001; **29**: 450–1.

47 Zaloga GP, Marik P. Hypothalamic-pituitary-adrenal insufficiency. *Crit Care Clin* 2001; **17**: 25–41.

48 Shenker Y, Skatrud JB. Adrenal insufficiency in critically ill patients. *Am J Respir Crit Care Med* 2001; **163**: 1520–3.

49 Ihle BU. Adrenocortical response and cortisone replacement in systemic inflammatory response syndrome. *Anaesth Intens Care* 2001; **29**: 155–62.

50 Beishuizen A, Thijs LG. Relative adrenal failure in intensive care: an identifiable problem requiring treatment? *Best Pract Res Clin Endocrinol Metab* 2001; **15**: 513–31.

51 Rivers EP, Gaspari M, Saad GA, *et al.* Adrenal insufficiency in high-risk surgical ICU patients. *Chest* 2001; **119**: 889–96.

52 Annane D. Corticosteroids for septic shock. *Crit Care Med* 2001; **29** (suppl. 7): S117–20.

53 Zaloga GP. Sepsis-induced adrenal deficiency syndrome. *Crit Care Med* 2001; **29**: 688–90.

54 Loisa P, Rinne T, Kaukinen S. Adrenocortical function and multiple organ failure in severe sepsis. *Acta Anaesthesiol Scand* 2002; **46**: 145–51.

Acute calcium disorders

B Venkatesh

Calcium is an important cation and the principal electrolyte of the body. A total of 1 to 2 kg is present in the average adult of which 99% is found in the bone. Of the remaining 1%, nine-tenths are present in the cells and only a tenth in the extracellular fluid. In the plasma, 50% of the calcium is ionized, 40% bound to plasma proteins mainly to albumin and the remaining 10% is chelated to anions such as citrate, bicarbonate, lactate, sulphate, phosphate and ketones.[1] The chelated fraction is usually of little clinical importance, but may become relevant in conditions where some of these anionic concentrations might be elevated, such as renal failure. While most calcium inside the cell is in the form of insoluble complexes, the concentration of intracellular ionized calcium is about 0.1 μmol/l, creating a gradient of 10 000:1 between plasma and ICF levels of ionized calcium.[2] A schematic illustration of calcium distribution within the various body compartments is shown in Figure 52.1.

Table 52.1 Functions of calcium[1,14]

Excitation–contraction coupling in cardiac, skeletal and smooth muscle
Cardiac action potentials and pacemaker activity
Release of neurotransmitters
Coagulation of blood
Bone formation and metabolism
Hormone release
Ciliary motility
Catecholamine responsiveness at the receptor site[7]

Because ionized calcium is the biologically active component of ECF calcium with respect to physiological functions (Table 52.1), and is the reference variable for endocrine regulation of calcium homeostasis, its measurement is recognized as being one of prime importance in the management of disorders of calcium homeostasis.

REGULATION OF CALCIUM HOMEOSTASIS

HORMONAL REGULATION OF CALCIUM HOMEOSTASIS

The concentration of ionized calcium in the plasma is subject to tight hormonal control[1,3]; particularly parathyroid hormone (PTH). In response to ionized hypocalcaemia, PTH secretion is stimulated, which in turns serves to restore serum calcium levels back to normal by increasing osteoclastic activity in bone, renal reabsorption of calcium, and stimulating renal synthesis of 1,25 OH-D3 (calcitriol – the active metabolite of Vit.D) which increases gut absorption of calcium.

Calcitriol production is stimulated by hypocalcaemia and vice versa. Calcitriol increases serum calcium largely by promoting gut reabsorption, and to a lesser extent renal reabsorption, of calcium.

Calcitonin, a peptide hormone, produced by the thyroid, has been shown to reduce serum calcium levels in animals by increasing renal clearance of

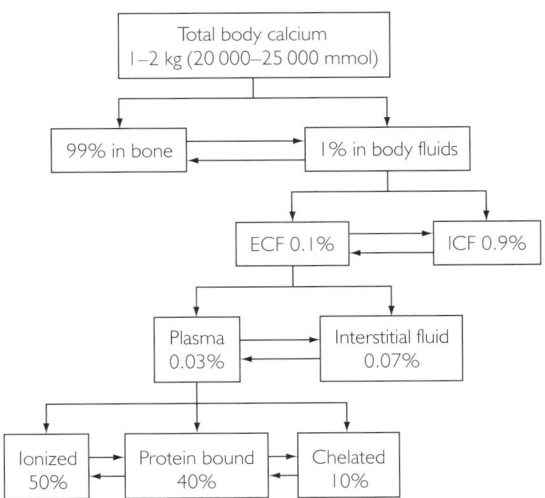

Fig. 52.1   Distribution of body calcium.

calcium and inhibiting bone resorption. Its role in humans is less clear. Despite wide variations in calcitonin concentrations in disease states, for example total lack of in patients who have undergone total thyroidectomy or excess plasma levels as seen in patients with medullary carcinoma of the thyroid gland, no significant changes in calcium and phosphate metabolism are seen. Calcitonin is useful as a pharmacological agent in the management of hypercalcaemia.

METABOLIC FACTORS INFLUENCING CALCIUM HOMEOSTASIS

Alterations in serum protein, pH, serum phosphate and magnesium alter serum calcium concentrations. Correction is made for hypoalbuminaemia by adding 0.2 mmol/l to the measured serum calcium concentration for every 10 g/l decrease in serum albumin concentration below normal (40 g/l). The corresponding correction factor for globulins is: 0.04 mmol/l of serum calcium for every 10 g/l rise in serum globulin.

Changes in pH alter protein binding of calcium. An increase in pH by 0.1 pH units results in a decrease in ionized calcium by approximately 0.1 mmol/l.[4]

Calcium and phosphate are closely linked by the following reaction in the extracellular fluid.

$$HPO_4^{2-} + Ca^{2+} \rightarrow CaHPO_4.$$

Increases in serum phosphate shift the reaction to the right. When the calcium phosphate solubility product exceeds the critical value of 5 mmol/l, calcium deposition occurs in the tissues, resulting in a fall in serum calcium concentration and a secondary increase in PTH secretion. Reductions in phosphate concentration lead to corresponding changes in the opposite direction.

As magnesium is required for PTH secretion and end organ responsiveness, alterations in serum magnesium have an impact on serum calcium concentration.

Turnover of calcium in bone is predominantly under control of PTH and calcitriol, although prostaglandins

Table 52.2 Daily calcium balance (Adapted from ScheinKestel and Oh[36]

		mg/day
Gastrointestinal tract	Diet	600–1200
	Absorbed	200–400
	Secreted	150–800
Renal	Filtered	11 000
	Reabsorbed (97% in the proximal convoluted tubule)	10 800
	Urinary calcium	200
Bone	Turnover	600–800

and some of the cytokines play a role. Bone resorption is mediated by osteoclasts, while osteoblasts are involved in bone formation. The daily calcium balance is summarized in Table 52.2

MEASUREMENT OF SERUM CALCIUM

Most hospital laboratories measure total serum or plasma calcium. The normal plasma concentration is 2.2–2.6 mmol/l. However, the ionized form (1.1–1.3 mmol/l) is the active fraction and its measurement is not routine in many laboratories although most state of the art blood gas analysers can measure serum ionized calcium concentrations. Estimation of ionized calcium from total serum calcium concentration using mathematical algorithms is unreliable in critically ill patients.[5–7] Heparin forms complexes with calcium and decreases ionized calcium.[8] A heparin concentration of <15 U/ml of whole blood is therefore recommended for the measurement of ionized calcium.[9] Anaerobic collection of the specimen is also recommended as CO_2 loss from the specimen may result in alkalosis and reduction in ionized calcium concentration. Calcium levels are also reduced by a concomitant lactic acidosis owing to chelation by lactate ion.[10] Free fatty acids (FFAs) increase calcium binding to albumin and may form a portion of the calcium binding site.[11] Increases in FFAs may be seen in relation to stress, use of steroids, catecholamines and heparin. The impact of pH on calcium measurements has been described above. The normal reference levels of serum calcium are reduced in pregnancy.

HYPERCALCAEMIA IN CRITICALLY ILL PATIENTS

The frequency of hypercalcaemia in critically ill patients is not well established, although it is not as common as hypocalcaemia. Depending on the patient population, the reported incidence ranges from 3–5% to as high as 32%.[12,13] Admission to the ICU with a primary diagnosis of a hypercalcaemic crisis is uncommon. Although a number of aetiologies have been described (Table 52.3), in the critically ill patient, it is usually due to malignancy related hypercalcaemia, renal failure or posthypocalcaemic hypocalcaemia.[14] False positive increases in serum calcium concentra-tion resulting from haemoconcentration due to poor blood sampling technique must be excluded prior to undertaking a diagnostic work up for hypercalcaemia. Ionized calcium levels are not affected by haemoconcentration.[15]

From a pathophysiological standpoint, hypercalcaemia may be due to an elevation in PTH, in which case the homeostatic regulatory and feedback mechanisms are preserved and this is termed *equilibrium hypercalcaemia*. Alternatively, it could be a non-parathyroid mediated hypercalcaemia with associated breakdown of homeostatic mechanisms and this situation is termed *dysequilibrium hypercalcaemia*.

MECHANISMS OF HYPERCALCAEMIA

Malignancy related hypercalcaemia might arise from bony metastases or humoral hypercalcaemia of malignancy. In the latter (seen with bronchogenic carcinoma and hypernephroma), tumour osteolysis of bone resulting from the release of PTH like substances (these cross react with PTH in the radioimmunoassay, but are not identical to PTH), calcitriol, osteoclast activating factor and prostaglandins is thought to be the major underlying mechanism. Aggravating factors include dehydration, immobilization and renal failure.

Post-hypocalcaemic hypercalcaemia is a transient phenomenon seen in patients following a period of hypocalcaemia.[14] This has been attributed to a parathyroid hyperplasia which then develops during the period of hypocalcaemia which results in a rebound hypercalcaemia.

Immobilization hypercalcaemia results from an alteration in balance between bone formation and resorption.[16–19] This leads to loss of bone minerals and, hypercalcaemia. In patients with normal bone turnover, immobilization rarely causes significant hypercalcaemia. However, in patients with rapid turnover of bone (children, adolescents during the growth spurt, patients with multiple fractures, hyperparathyroidism, Paget's disease, spinal injuries causing paraplegia and quadriplegia, long-standing stroke and Guillain–Barré syndrome), immobilisation might lead to hypercalcaemia.

Intravascular volume depletion reduces renal calcium excretion by a combination of reduced glomerular filtration and increased tubular reabsorption of calcium. Hypercalcaemia further compounds this problem by causing a concentrating defect in the renal tubules creating polyuria, further exacerbating the hypovolaemia.

Extrarenal production of calcitriol by lymphocytes in granulomata is thought to be the predominant mechanism of hypercalcaemia in granulomatous diseases.[20]

Only 10–20% of patients with adrenal insufficiency develop hypercalcaemia.[21,22] The aetiology of this is thought to be multifactorial: intravascular volume depletion, haemoconcentration of plasma proteins and the loss of anti-vitamin D effects of glucocorticoids.

MANIFESTATIONS OF HYPERCALCAEMIA

The clinical manifestations of hypercalcaemia (commonly encountered when total serum calcium exceeds

Table 52.3 Causes of hypercalcaemia

Common causes of hypercalcaemia in the critically ill patient
Complication of malignancy
  Bony metastases
  Humoral hypercalcaemia of malignancy
Posthypocalcaemic hypercalcaemia
  Recovery from pancreatitis[14]
  Recovery from acute renal failure following
  rhabdomyolysis[31–35]
Primary hyperparathyroidism
Adrenal insufficiency[21,22]
Prolonged immobilization[16–19]
Disorders of magnesium metabolism
Use of TPN[36]
Hypovolaemia
Iatrogenic calcium administration

Less common causes of hypercalcaemia in the critically ill patient
Granulomatous diseases – sarcoidosis, tuberculosis, berylliosis
Vit A & D intoxication
Multiple myeloma
Endocrine
  Thyrotoxicosis
  Acromegaly
  Phaeochromocytoma
Lithium – chronic therapy

Table 52.4 Clinical manifestations of hypercalcaemia (Modified from ScheinKestel and Oh[36])

Cardiovascular
  Hypertension
  Arrhythmias
  Digitalis sensitivity
  Catecholamine resistance
Urinary system
  Nephrocalcinosis
  Nephrolithiasis
  Tubular dysfunction
  Renal failure
Gastrointestinal
  Anorexia/nausea/vomiting
  Constipation
  Peptic ulcer
  Pancreatitis
Neuromuscular
  Weakness
Neuropsychiatric
  Depression
  Disorientation
  Psychosis
  Coma
  Seizures

Ectopic calcification is usually seen with chronic hypercalcaemia.

3 mmol/l) are outlined in Table 52.4. *Hypercalcaemic crisis* is defined as severe hypercalcaemia (total serum Ca >3.5 mmol/l) associated with acute symptoms and signs.

INVESTIGATIONS

The basic work up should include serum calcium, phosphate, alkaline phosphatase, PTH assay, renal function assessment and a skeletal survey.

THERAPY OF HYPERCALCAEMIA AND HYPERCALCAEMIC CRISIS

Mild asymptomatic hypercalcaemia does not require emergent treatment. Therapy is usually directed at the underlying cause.

The management of hypercalcaemic crisis consists of two principal components:

- increasing urinary excretion of calcium
- reducing bone resorption.

INCREASING URINARY EXCRETION OF CALCIUM

As almost all patients with hypercalcaemia are volume depleted, the initial therapy consists of rehydration with normal saline, followed by diuresis with frusemide. Rehydration with normal saline improves intravascular volume, reduces serum calcium by extracellular dilution, and saliuresis promotes calcium loss in the urine. Volume expansion should be titrated to clinical endpoints and CVP monitoring. A urine output of 4–5 l should be aimed for in these patients to promote calciuresis. In many patients, these measures would achieve a reduction in serum calcium by about 0.4–0.5 mmol/l. Hypokalaemia, hypomagnesaemia and calcium stone formation in the urine are potential side effects of this mode of treatment.

In patients with established renal failure in whom forced diuresis cannot be instituted, dialysis against a dialysate with zero or low calcium concentrations should be the treatment of choice.

REDUCTION OF BONE RESORPTION

Measures to increase urinary excretion of calcium should be followed up with administration of agents minimizing bone resorption. A number of agents are available and these are listed in Table 52.5.

The efficacy of biphosphonates, combined with a relative lack of side effects make them the agents of choice for the treatment of malignancy related hypercalcaemia. Disodium EDTA at a dose of 15–50 mg/kg i.v. rapidly lowers serum calcium. However, its propensity to rapidly reduce serum calcium coupled with its nephrotoxic effects limits its usefulness to life threatening hypercalcaemia. Other therapeutic modalities include the use of NSAIDs and parathyroidectomy. These, however, have a limited role in the management of acute hypercalcaemia.

ADJUNCTIVE MEASURES IN THE MANAGEMENT OF HYPERCALCAEMIA

Monitoring of vital signs and serial measurements of electrolytes are mandatory during therapy of hypercalcaemia. The dosage of digoxin may need to be adjusted as its effects can be potentiated by hypercalcaemia.

HYPOCALCAEMIA

Hypocalcaemia is in critically ill patients, has an estimated incidence of around 70–90%.[5] The frequency of ionized hypocalaemia, however, is far more varied, ranging from 15–70%.[5,23,24] *Spurious hypocalcaemia* is seen with poor storage of specimens prior to analysis resulting in CO_2 loss from the specimen, use of either EDTA or large doses of heparin as anticoagulants in the syringe.

AETIOLOGIES

The aetiology of ionized hypocalcaemia based on the predominant pathophysiological mechanism is listed in Table 52.6. Although a long list of causes exists for hypocalcaemia, calcium chelation and hypoparathyroidism constitute the common mechanisms of ionized hypocalcaemia in intensive care. Frequently, hypocalcaemia is accompanied by a number of other biochemical abnormalities, thus a pattern recognition approach towards the cause of hypocalcaemia will point to its aetiology and save a considerable amount of investigations for the patient. Common diagnostic patterns are listed below in Table 52.7. While alkalosis is frequently associated with ionized hypocalcaemia, the presence of a metabolic acidosis in the face of a low serum ionized calcium narrows the differential diagnosis even further (Table 52.8):

CLINICAL MANIFESTATIONS OF HYPOCALCAEMIA

Mild degrees of hypocalcaemia are usually asymptomatic. Ionized calcium levels less than 0.8 mmol/l may cause neuromuscular irritability and result in clinical symptoms. The clinical manifestations of hypocalcaemia are summarized in Table 52.9. The manifestations listed in the Table 52.9 are by no means a comprehensive list of all the clinical features but

Table 52.5 Therapeutic agents for reducing bone resorption (Modified from Polts JT Jr. et al[38])

Therapy	Indications	Dose	Onset time/duration	Limitations	Mechanism of action	Comments
Bi-phosponates Etidronate (1st generation)	Malignancy related hypercalcaemia	5 mg/kg per day	1–2 days, lasts 5–7 days	Hyperphosphataemia, short duration of action	Inhibits osteoclast activity, may have some effect on osteoblasts	High potency group. Pamidronate lowers Ca levels more rapidly than etidronate
Pamidronate (2nd generation)		90 mg as an infusion every 4 weeks	1–2 days, lasts 10–14 days	Hypophosphataemia, fever and hypomagnesaemia		
Calcitonin	Hypercalcaemia, Paget's disease	Initial i.v. dose 3–4 U/kg followed by 4 U/kg SC 12-hourly	Hours, lasts 2–3 days	Nausea, abdominal pain, flushing, tachyphylaxis, limited efficacy	Inhibits osteoclast activity, reduces renal tubular reabsorption of calcium	Tachyphylaxis minimized by concomitant steroid therapy
Glucocorticoids	Vit D toxicity, myeloma, lymphoma, granulomata	IV hydro-cortisone 200–400 mg/day	Days, lasts days to weeks	Glucocorticoid side-effects	Inhibits inflammatory cell production of calcitriol, reduce gut absorption of calcium	Improve the efficacy of calcitonin
Gallium nitrate	Malignancy related hypercalcaemia	100–200 mg/m² per day for 5–7 days	5 to 6 days, lasts 7 to 10 days	Nephrotoxic	Inhibits bone resorption and alters bone crystal structure	Lack of familiarity and data on long term efficacy limit its use
Plicamycin	Malignancy related hypercalcaemia	25 µg/kg i.v.	Rapid onset, lasts for a few days	Hepatotoxic, nephrotoxic and thrombocytopenia	Inhibits cellular RNA synthesis	Side effect profile limits the use of this drug
Intravenous phosphates	Limited clinical role	10–15 mmol as an infusion repeated at regular intervals	Hours, lasts 24–48 h after cessation	Ectopic calcification, severe hypocalcaemia	Ectopic calcification, reduce gut absorption, inhibition of bone resorption	Use superseded by the other modalities described.

include the ones most commonly seen in the critical care setting.

When eliciting tetany, Trousseau's sign (carpopedal spasm) is more specific for hypocalcaemia than Chvostek's sign (facial twitch in response to facial nerve stimulus – present in 10–30% of the normal population). ECG changes do not correlate well with the degree of hypocalcaemia. The symptoms of hypocalcaemia are exacerbated by a coexisting hypokalaemia and a hypomagnesaemia.

The laboratory work up should include serum calcium, phosphorus, magnesium and alkaline phosphatase, PTH and Vit D assays and renal function assessment.

Table 52.6 Aetiology of ionized hypocalcaemia

Calcium chelation
    Alkalosis (increased binding of calcium by albumin)
    Citrate toxicity (calcium chelation)
    Hyperphosphataemia (calcium chelation, ectopic calcification, reduced Vit D3 activity)
    Pancreatitis (calcium soap formation, reduced parathyroid secretion)
    Tumour lysis syndrome (hyperphosphataemia)
    Rhabdomyolysis (hyperphosphataemia and reduced levels of calcitriol)
Hypoparathyroidism
    Hypo- and hypermagnesaemia
    Sepsis (decrease PTH secretion, calcitriol resistance, intracellular shift of calcium)
    Burns (decrease in PTH secretion)
    Neck surgery (removal of parathyroid gland, calcitonin release during thyroid surgery and hungry bone syndrome post parathyroidectomy)
Hypovitaminosis D
    Inadequate intake
    Malabsorption
    Liver disease (impaired 25-hydroxylation of cholecalciferol)
    Renal failure (impaired 1-hydroxylation of cholecalciferol, hyperphosphataemia)
Reduced bone turnover
    Osteoporosis
    Elderly
    Cachexia
Drug induced
    Phenytoin (accelerated metabolism of Vit D3)
    Diphosphonates (see 'hypercalcaemia')
    EDTA (calcium chelation)
    Ethylene glycol (formation of calcium oxalate crystals in the urine)
    Cis-platinum (renal tubular damage leading to hypermagnesuria)
    Protamine
    Gentamicin (hypermagnesuria leads to hypomagnesaemia and hypocalcaemia)

APPROACH TO THE TREATMENT OF ASYMPTOMATIC AND SYMPTOMATIC HYPOCALCAEMIA

ARGUMENTS FOR AND AGAINST CORRECTION OF ASYMPTOMATIC HYPOCALCAEMIA

It is not clear if asymptomatic hypocalcaemia needs correction. Based on a higher mortality and increased length of stay in intensive care,[25–27] it is advocated that ionized hypocalcaemia be corrected routinely irrespective of the level. However, arguments exist against the routine correction of asymptomatic ionized hypocalcaemia. Increases in cytosolic calcium lead to disruption of intracellular processes, activation of proteases and can lead to ischaemia and reperfusion injury.[28] There are also data suggesting that ionized calcium is an important participant in the pathogenesis of coronary and cerebral vasospasm.[29] In rodent models of endotoxic shock, there are also data demonstrating an increased mortality when these rats were administered intravenous calcium.[30] Most clinicians agree that an ionized calcium level of <0.8 mmol/l needs correction even if asymptomatic.

Table 52.8 Hypocalcaemia with metabolic acidosis

Acute renal failure
Tumour lysis
Rhabdomyolysis
Pancreatitis
Ethylene glycol poisoning
Hydrofluoric acid intoxication

Table 52.7 Pattern recognition in the diagnosis of common causes of hypocalcaemia (Modified fron ScheinKestel and Oh[36])

Aetiology of hypocalcaemia	Clinical/biochemical patterns
Low serum albumin	Reduced total calcium, normal ionized calcium
Alkalosis	Normal total calcium, reduced ionized calcium
Hypomagnesaemia	Reduced ionized calcium and hypokalaemia
Pancreatitis	Hypocalcaemia, elevated serum lipase and glucose
Renal failure	Elevated blood urea nitrogen, elevated phosphate
Rhabdomyolysis	Hypocalcaemia, elevated phosphate, CK and urinary myoglobin
Tumour lysis syndrome	Hypocalcaemia, elevated phosphate, potassium and urate

Table 52.9 Clinical manifestations of hypocalcaemia

Central nervous system
Circumoral and peripheral paraesthesia
Muscle cramps
Tetany
Seizures
Extrapyramidal manifestations: tremor, ataxia, dystonia
Proximal myopathy
Depression, anxiety, psychosis
Cardiovascular
Arrhythmias
Hypotension, inotrope unresponsiveness
Prolonged QT intervals, T-wave inversion
Loss of digitalis effect
Respiratory
Apnoea
Laryngospasm
Bronchospasm

Table 52.10 Commonly used i.v. calcium preparations

Preparation	Dosage	Elemental calcium
Calcium gluconate	10 ml	93 mg (2.3 mmol)
Calcium chloride	10 ml	272 mg (6.8 mmol)

Table 52.11 Indications for calcium administration

Absolute
Symptomatic hypocalcaemia
Ionized Ca <0.8 mmol/l
Hyperkalaemia
Ca channel blocker overdose
Relative
Betablocker overdose
Hypermagnesaemia
Hypocalcaemia in the face of high inotrope requirement
Massive blood transfusion post cardiopulmonary bypass to augment cardiac contractility

MANAGEMENT OF ACUTE SYMPTOMATIC HYPOCALCAEMIA

Acute symptomatic hypocalcaemia is a medical emergency that requires immediate therapy. In addition to treatment of underlying cause and support of airway, breathing and circulation, the definitive treatment includes administration of intravenous calcium. Intravenous calcium is available as a calcium salt of chloride or gluconate. The main difference between the two formulations is the amount of elemental calcium available at equivalent volumes of drug (Table 52.10). Intravenous calcium can be administered as a bolus or as an infusion. Rapid administration of calcium may cause nausea, flushing, headache and arrhythmias. Digitalis toxicity may be precipitated. Extravasation of calcium may lead to tissue irritation, particularly with the chloride salt. Following an initial bolus, an infusion may be commenced at a rate of 1–2 mg/kg per h of elemental calcium to maintain target levels of ionized calcium. With correction of the underlying disorder and restoration of calcium to normal levels, the infusion can be tapered and stopped. Adequacy of calcium therapy can be monitored clinically and by performing serial determinations of ionized calcium. Failure of ionized calcium to increase after commencement of i.v. calcium may indicate an underlying magnesium deficiency. This can be corrected by administration of 10 mmol of intravenous magnesium over 20 min. Administration of calcium in the setting of hyperphosphataemia may result in calcium precipitation in the tissues. Calcium salts should not be administered with bicarbonate since the two precipitate. The other indications for calcium administration are listed in Table 52.11. Other therapy for hypocalcaemia consists of oral calcium supplements and calcitriol administration, although these are usually used in the management of chronic hypocalcaemia.

REFERENCES

1 Bourdeau J, Attie M. Calcium metabolism. In: Narins R (ed.) *Clinical Disorders of Fluid and Electrolyte Metabolism*, 5th edn. New York: McGraw-Hill; 1994: pp. 243–50.

2 Zaloga GP. Hypocalcemia in critically ill patients. *Crit Care Med* 1992; **20**: 251–62.

3 Holick M, Krane S, Potts J. Calcium, phosphorus and bone metabolism: Calcium-regulating hormones. In: Fauci AS (ed.) *Principles of Internal Medicine*: New York: McGraw Hill; 1998.

4 Watchko J, Bifano EM, Bergstrom WH. Effect of hyperventilation on total calcium, ionized calcium, and serum phosphorus in neonates. *Crit Care Med* 1984; **12**: 1055–6.

5 Zaloga GP, Chernow B, Cook D *et al*. Assessment of calcium homeostasis in the critically ill surgical patient. The diagnostic pitfalls of the McLean–Hastings nomogram. *Ann Surg* 1985; **202**: 587–94.

6 Vincent JL, Jankowski S. Why should ionized calcium be determined in acutely ill patients? *Acta Anaesthesiol Scand* 1995; **107(Suppl)**: 281–6.

7 Toffaletti J. Physiology and regulation. Ionized calcium, magnesium and lactate measurements in critical care settings. *Am J Clin Pathol* 1995; **104(Suppl 1)**: S88–94.

8 Landt M, Hortin GL, Smith CH *et al*. Interference in ionized calcium measurements by heparin salts. *Clin Chem* 1994; **40**: 565–70.

9 Sachs C, Rabouine P, Chaneac M *et al*. In vitro evaluation of a heparinized blood sampler for ionized calcium measurement. *Ann Clin Biochem* 1991; **28**: 240–4.

10 Toffaletti J, Abrams B. Effects of in vivo and in vitro production of lactic acid on ionized, protein-bound, and complex-bound calcium in blood. *Clin Chem* 1989; **35**: 935–8.

11 Zaloga GP, Willey S, Tomasic P, Chernow B. Free fatty acids alter calcium binding: a cause for misinterpreta-

tion of serum calcium values and hypocalcemia in critical illness. *J Clin Endocrinol Metab* 1987; **64**: 1010–4.

12 Forster J, Querusio L, Burchard KW, Gann DS. Hypercalcemia in critically ill surgical patients. *Ann Surg* 1985; **202**: 512–8.

13 Lind L, Ljunghall S. Critical care hypercalcemia – a hyperparathyroid state. *Exp Clin Endocrinol* 1992; **100**: 148–51.

14 Zaloga GP. Calcium homeostasis in the critically ill patient. *Magnesium* 1989; **8**: 190–200.

15 McMullan AD, Burns J, Paterson CR. Venepuncture for calcium assays: should we still avoid the tourniquet? *Postgrad Med J* 1990; **66**: 547–8.

16 Massagli TL, Cardenas DD. Immobilization hypercalcemia treatment with pamidronate disodium after spinal cord injury. *Arch Phys Med Rehabil* 1999; **80**: 998–1000.

17 Sato Y, Fujimatsu Y, Kikuyama M, *et al.* Influence of immobilization on bone mass and bone metabolism in hemiplegic elderly patients with a long-standing stroke. *J Neurol Sci* 1998; **156**: 205–10.

18 Kedlaya D, Brandstater ME, Lee JK. Immobilization hypercalcemia in incomplete paraplegia: successful treatment with pamidronate. *Arch Phys Med Rehabil* 1998; **79**: 222–5.

19 Evans RA, Lawrence PJ, Thanakrishnan G, *et al.* Immobilization hypercalcaemia due to low bone formation and responding to intravenous sodium sulphate. *Postgrad Med J* 1986; **62**: 395–8.

20 Sharma OP. Hypercalcemia in granulomatous disorders: a clinical review. *Curr Opin Pulm Med* 2000; **6**: 442–7.

21 Miell J, Wassif W, McGregor A, *et al.* Life-threatening hypercalcaemia in association with Addisonian crisis. *Postgrad Med J* 1991; **67**: 770–2.

22 Vasikaran SD, Tallis GA, Braund WJ. Secondary hypoadrenalism presenting with hypercalcaemia. *Clin Endocrinol* (Oxford) 1994; **41**: 261–4.

23 Zaloga GP, Chernow B. The multifactorial basis for hypocalcemia during sepsis. Studies of the parathyroid hormone–vitamin D axis. *Ann Intern Med* 1987; **107**: 36–41.

24 Desai TK, Carlson RW, Geheb MA. Prevalence and clinical implications of hypocalcemia in acutely ill patients in a medical intensive care setting. *Am J Med* 1988; **84**: 209–14.

25 Chernow B, Zaloga G, McFadden E, *et al.* Hypocalcemia in critically ill patients. *Crit Care Med* 1982; **10**: 848–51.

26 Desai TK, Carlson RW, Thill-Baharozian M, Geheb MA. A direct relationship between ionized calcium and arterial pressure among patients in an intensive care unit. *Crit Care Med* 1988; **16**: 578–82.

27 Broner CW, Stidham GL, Westenkirchner DF, Tolley EA. Hypermagnesemia and hypocalcemia as predictors of high mortality in critically ill pediatric patients. *Crit Care Med* 1990; **18**: 921–8.

28 Cheung JY, Bonventre JV, Malis CD, Leaf A. Calcium and ischemic injury. *N Engl J Med* 1986; **314**: 1670–6.

29 Lemmer JH Jr., Kirsh MM. Coronary artery spasm following coronary artery surgery. *Ann Thorac Surg* 1988; **46**: 108–15.

30 Zaloga GP, Sager A, Black KW, Prielipp R. Low dose calcium administration increases mortality during septic peritonitis in rats. *Circ Shock* 1992; **37**: 226–9.

31 Meneghini LF, Oster JR, Camacho JR, *et al.* Hypercalcemia in association with acute renal failure and rhabdomyolysis. Case report and literature review. *Miner Electrolyte Metab* 1993; **19**: 1–16.

32 Akmal M, Bishop JE, Telfer N, *et al.* Hypocalcemia and hypercalcemia in patients with rhabdomyolysis with and without acute renal failure. *J Clin Endocrinol Metab* 1986; **63**: 137–42.

33 Leonard CD, Eichner ER. Acute renal failure and transient hypercalcemia in idiopathic rhabdomyolysis. *JAMA* 1970; **211**: 1539–40.

34 Prince RL, Hutchison BG, Bhagat CI. Hypercalcemia during resolution of acute renal failure associated with rhabdomyolysis: evidence for suppression of parathyroid hormone and calcitriol. *Aust N Z J Med* 1986; **16**: 506–8.

35 Sperling LS, Tumlin JA. Case report: delayed hypercalcemia after rhabdomyolysis-induced acute renal failure. *Am J Med Sci* 1996; **311**: 186–8.

36 Izsak EM, Shike M, Roulet M, Jeejeebhoy KN. Pancreatitis in association with hypercalcemia in patients receiving total parenteral nutrition. *Gastroenterology* 1980; **79**: 555–8.

37 ScheinKestel CD, Oh TE. Acute calcium disorders, In Oh TE (ed) *Intensive Care Manual 4th edn.* Oxford: Butterworth-Heinemann; 1997: pp. 475–483.

38 Polts JT. Diseases of the parathyroid gland and other hyper- and hypocalcemic disorders, In Isselbacher KJ et al (ed) *Harrison's Principles of Internal Medicine 13th edn.* New York: McGraw-Hill: 1994: pp. 2151–2171.

Part Nine

Obstetric Emergencies

53

Pre-eclampsia and eclampsia

W D Ngan Kee and T Gin

Pre-eclampsia is a syndrome specific to pregnancy that is diagnosed clinically when hypertension and proteinuria occur after 20 weeks gestation (Table 53.1). It occasionally presents earlier in cases of hydatidiform mole. Diagnostic criteria vary internationally,[1,2] and in Australia, proteinuria is not considered mandatory in the presence of other clinical signs.[1] Pre-eclampsia may be superimposed upon pre-existing chronic hypertension, which can make diagnosis difficult.[2] Eclampsia in a pre-eclamptic woman describes the occurrence of seizures not attributable to other causes.

Pre-eclampsia complicates 2–10% of pregnancies, and is a leading cause of maternal deaths.[2,3] Maternal mortality from pre-eclampsia/eclampsia is 1.5 per 100 000 live births in the USA,[4] but it is much greater in developing countries. The incidence of eclampsia is 2–6 per 10 000 deliveries with a maternal mortality in the UK of 1.8% and fetal/neonatal mortality of around 7%.[5]

Factors associated with increased maternal risk include:[4,6,7]

- onset at ≤ 32 weeks gestation
- greater maternal age and parity
- pre-existing medical complications
- Afro-Caribbean descent
- nausea and vomiting and epigastric pain
- abnormal laboratory tests including raised liver enzymes, increased serum creatinine and increased serum uric acid.

Table 53.1 Basic diagnostic criteria for pre-eclampsia

Hypertension
Systolic arterial pressure ≥ 140 mmHg   **OR**
Diastolic arterial pressure* ≥ 90 mmHg
and
Proteinuria
≥ 300 mg protein in a 24 h collection

*Korotkoff phase V.
A rise in blood pressure above baseline and oedema are now not usually included.
A positive dipstick test for proteinuria should be confirmed by 24 h urine collection.

Patients are referred to an ICU mainly for poorly controlled hypertension or convulsions, pulmonary oedema, refractory oliguria, coagulopathy, haemorrhage and for postoperative care. Providing complications are avoided, the disease normally resolves completely after delivery.

AETIOLOGY

The aetiology of pre-eclampsia is unknown. There is a genetic predisposition and it is more likely in women with chronic hypertension, diabetes, multiple gestation and hydatidiform mole.[8] Pre-eclampsia is twice as common in primigravid compared with multiparous women although the risk in multiparous women increases if there is a change of paternity.[9]

PATHOGENESIS

Many theories have been suggested for the pathogenesis of pre-eclampsia.[8,10] A commonly accepted hypothesis is that absolute or relative placental ischaemia acts as a precipitating factor that leads to diffuse systemic vascular endothelial activation or damage. The nature of the placental hypoperfusion is incompletely understood but is thought to involve inadequate endovascular invasion of fetal trophoblast into the spiral arteries[8] which may be the result of immune maladaptation.[10] The link between placental triggering and the systemic response is unknown, but has been theorized to involve oxidative stress,[8] a generalized intravascular inflammatory reaction and circulating cytotoxic factors.[11] The result is an increase in sensitivity to vasoactive substances, a decrease in endothelial synthesis of vasodilator substances such as PGI_2 and nitric oxide, platelet activation with increased thromboxane A_2 release and activation of the coagulation cascade, and an increase in capillary permeability. This causes widespread vasoconstriction, fluid extravasation, proteinuria, decreased intravascular volume, haemoconcentration and decreased organ perfusion.

CLINICAL PRESENTATION

Pre-eclampsia is a clinical syndrome with a spectrum of presentations. Although hypertension is the most common diagnostic sign, some women present with convulsions, abdominal pain, or general malaise.[9] Several of the non-hypertensive complications may be life-threatening without a marked increase in blood pressure. Manifestations of pre-eclampsia that increase certainty of diagnosis and usually indicate severe disease are listed in Table 53.2.[1,2] Rarely, cocaine intoxication and phaeochromocytoma may be confused with pre-eclampsia.

The haemodynamic changes of pre-eclampsia traditionally have been described as hypertension, increased systemic vascular resistance, decreased intravascular volume and decreased cardiac output. However, in some patients an increase in cardiac output has been observed.[12] Serial investigation has shown that some patients initially have a hyperdynamic high output/low resistance state but subsequently there is a crossover to a low output/high resistance state which coincides with the onset of clinical symptoms.[13] Pulmonary oedema may occur because of iatrogenic fluid overload, decreased left ventricular function, increased capillary permeability, and narrowing of the colloid osmotic-pulmonary capillary wedge pressure gradient. This is more likely to occur after delivery, particularly in patients who are older or multiparous or have pre-existing chronic hypertension. Sudden ventricular tachycardia may occur during hypertensive crises.

Neurological complications include eclamptic convulsions, cerebral oedema, raised intracranial pressure and stroke, but these are decreasing in incidence.[3]

Table 53.2 Clinical features of severe pre-eclampsia

Blood pressure	Systolic arterial pressure ≥ 160 mmHg Diastolic arterial pressure ≥ 110 mmHg
Renal	Proteinuria ≥ 2 g / 24 h Oliguria < 500 ml / 24 h Serum creatinine ≥ 0.09 mmol/l
Hepatic	Epigastric or right upper quadrant pain Elevated bilirubin and/or transaminases
Neurological	Persistent headaches Visual disturbances Convulsions (eclampsia)
Haematological	Thrombocytopenia Deranged coagulation tests Haemolysis
Cardiac/respiratory	Pulmonary oedema Cyanosis

Renal changes include reduced glomerular filtration rate and renal plasma flow, which are associated with the characteristic lesion of glomeruloendotheliosis. Hyperuricaemia is associated with increased prenatal risk, particularly if serum uric acid concentration rises rapidly, and is an indication to consider termination of pregnancy.[14]

The most common haemostatic abnormality is thrombocytopenia, which may be associated with decreased platelet function. Associated coagulopathy abnormalities may occur but are unlikely unless the platelet count is $<100\,000 \times 10^9/l$.[15,16]

The leading causes of maternal death in pre-eclampsia/eclampsia are intracranial haemorrhage, pulmonary oedema and hepatic complications.[3,4] In recent decades, deaths from cerebral causes have decreased and pulmonary oedema has become relatively more important.[3] Fetal morbidity results from placental insufficiency or acute maternal deterioration, and there is an increased risk of abruptio placentae.

MANAGEMENT

The principles of management include:

(a) maintenance of placental perfusion with timely termination of pregnancy;
(b) control of blood pressure;
(c) prevention of seizures; and
(d) prevention and management of complications.

The definitive treatment of pre-eclampsia is delivery of the fetus and placenta. In milder cases, the disease may be controlled while allowing fetal maturation and cervical ripening. Expectant management for severe cases in mid-trimester has been advocated,[17] but the maternal risks of this have not been fully quantified.[18] Transfer of the mother to a tertiary centre before delivery should be considered if a Level III neonatal unit is not available. (See Ch. 1 *Design and Organization of Intensive Care Units.*) Admission into an ICU before delivery may be appropriate in severe cases, or when the labour ward lacks the expertise or equipment for intensive monitoring. After delivery, severe cases should preferably be managed in an ICU for 24–72 h.

GENERAL MEASURES

Before delivery, patients should be kept in the lateral or semi-lateral position and the fetal heart rate should be monitored. Regular oral or intravenous ranitidine will decrease gastric acidity and volume. Prophylactic steroids should be considered for fetal lung maturity if gestation is less than 34 weeks and early delivery is anticipated. Routine monitoring should include frequent clinical assessment, blood pressure, ECG and fluid balance. Pulse oximetry aids the detection of incipient pulmonary oedema.[19] Central venous pressure (CVP) monitoring, preferably via an antecubital vein, and/or pulmonary artery catheterization may assist in fluid balance (see below). Full blood count, coagulation screen, electrolytes, uric acid, renal function, liver function, and urinalysis should be performed serially to monitor disease progression.

ANTIHYPERTENSIVE THERAPY

The aim of antihypertensive therapy is to prevent maternal complications (intracerebral haemorrhage, cardiac failure, and abruptio placentae) while maintaining placental blood flow. Acute treatment is indicated when blood pressure is greater than 160–170 mmHg (21.2–22.6 kPa) systolic or 105–110 mmHg (14.0–14.6 kPa) diastolic. Initially, systolic blood pressure should be reduced by about 20–30 mmHg (2.7–4.0 kPa) and diastolic by 10–15 mmHg (1.3–2.0 kPa) while monitoring the fetus.[1] Concomitant plasma expansion reduces the risk of sudden hypotension when vasodilators are used.[1] Recommended antihypertensive drugs for acute treatment are summarized in Table 53.3 and described below.[1,2] The most commonly used drugs are hydralazine, labetalol and nifedipine.

HYDRALAZINE

Hydralazine is a direct arteriolar vasodilator with a long history of use in pre-eclampsia. However, recent evidence suggests that hydralazine is associated with more maternal and perinatal adverse effects compared with labetalol and nifedipine.[18] It has a relatively slow onset of action of 10–20 min and a duration of action of 6–8 h. Infusions of hydralazine can be difficult to titrate and may result in hypotension and fetal distress. This may also occur when hydralazine is given without intravenous volume expansion. Adverse effects include headache, tachycardia, tremor, nausea, and rare cases of neonatal thrombocytopenia.

LABETALOL

Labetalol is a non-selective β-adrenergic receptor blocker with some α_1-blocking effect. When given intravenously, it rapidly reduces blood pressure without decreasing uteroplacental blood flow,[20] and does not cause reflex tachycardia, headache or nausea. Although labetalol crosses the placenta, neonatal bradycardia and hypoglycaemia are rarely seen. Duration of action is variable. It should not be given to patients with asthma or myocardial dysfunction.

NIFEDIPINE

Nifedipine is a calcium-channel blocker that directly relaxes arterial smooth muscle. In pre-eclamptic patients with severe hypertension it causes a steady decrease in blood pressure and systemic vascular resistance within 30 min with a concomitant increase in maternal cardiac index and heart rate.[21] Although there have been concerns about the use of nifedipine capsules for management of acute hypertension, others have considered it safe in pre-eclampsia. Nifedipine can be given orally or sublingually although severe hypotension and fetal distress has been reported after sublingual administration. Sudden hypotension and potentiation of neuromuscular block has been reported in patients receiving magnesium sulphate. Nifedipine causes relaxation of uterine muscle which may increase the risk of postpartum haemorrhage. Mild side-effects include headache, flushing, and nausea.

OTHER AGENTS

Sodium nitroprusside can be used to rapidly reduce blood pressure in emergencies.[2] Direct arterial pressure monitoring should be used and care should be taken in patients with depleted intravascular volume. Fetal cyanide poisoning may occur if used for >4 hours.[2] **Nitroglycerin** infusion may be useful in cases complicated by pulmonary oedema. **Methyldopa** is often used for mild cases but its slow onset time makes it unsuitable for acute treatment. **Diazoxide** can be given by repeated small boluses of 30 mg i.v. but its use has been questioned because of the risk of profound hypotension.[22] **Ketanserin** has limited efficacy.[22] **β-blockers** other than labetalol may cause decreased uteroplacental perfusion, fetal bradycardia, and decreased fetal tolerance to hypoxia **Angiotensin converting enzyme inhibitors** have been associated with neonatal abnormalities, renal failure and intra-uterine death and should not be used before delivery.[1,2] **Diuretics** should

Table 53.3 Drugs used for acute management of hypertension in pre-eclampsia

Drug	Dosage guide
Hydralazine	*Bolus* 5 mg i.v. followed by 5–10 mg every 20 min to maximum of 40 mg as required
Labetalol	*Bolus* 20 mg i.v. followed by 40 mg after 10 min then 80 mg every 10 min for 2 further doses to a maximum of 220 mg as required *Infusion* 1–2 mg/min, reducing to 0.5 mg/min or less after blood pressure is controlled
Nifedipine	*Orally or sublingually* 10 mg, repeated after 30 min as required.
Sodium nitroprusside	*Infusion* 0.25 µg/kg per min, increased to maximum of 5 µg/kg per min. Limit duration of infusion to <4 h.

be avoided since most pre-eclamptic patients have reduced plasma volume.

ANTICONVULSANT THERAPY

Anticonvulsants are used in conjunction with blood pressure management to terminate or prevent convulsions.

MAGNESIUM SULPHATE

The drug of choice to prevent convulsions in pre-eclampsia and eclampsia is magnesium sulphate,[23–26] although it may not be effective in all cases. In eclampsia, there is good evidence supporting the use of magnesium to prevent recurrent convulsions.[24] In pre-eclampsia, the relative benefits and risks of magnesium to prevent initial convulsions are still under investigation. It is the authors' opinion that it should be started in severe cases. The mechanism of action of magnesium is unknown. Although abnormal electroencephalograms are frequent in pre-eclampsia and eclampsia, they are not altered by magnesium sulphate. By antagonism of calcium at membrane channels or intracellular sites, magnesium may reduce systemic and cerebral vasospasm. It amplifies release of prostacyclin by vascular endothelium, and this may inhibit platelet aggregation and vasoconstriction. Doppler ultrasonography suggests that magnesium vasodilates smaller diameter intracranial blood vessels, and some of its effects may be from relieving cerebral ischaemia. Part of the anticonvulsant activity of magnesium may be mediated by blockade or suppression of N-methyl-D-aspartate (NMDA) receptors. Magnesium has tocolytic effects and mild general vasodilator and antihypertensive actions and increases renal and uterine blood flow.

Guidelines for administration of magnesium sulphate are summarized in Table 53.4. It can be given intravenously or intramuscularly. Although intravenous dosing regimens vary, in the USA a loading dose of 6 g followed by an infusion of 2 g/h has been recommended. Suggested target serum concentration for severe pre-eclampsia is 2–3.5 mmol/l (4–7 mEq/l or 4.8–8.4 mg/dl). Monitoring of levels is usually not necessary if deep tendon reflexes are checked regularly as toxicity is unlikely when reflexes are present (the upper limb should be used during epidural analgesia).

Table 53.4 Dosage regimens for magnesium sulphate

Intravenous regimen	Loading dose: 4–6 g over 20 min
	Maintenance: 1–3 g/h
Intramuscular regimen	4 g every 4 hours

Reduce dose and monitor serum concentrations in oliguria or renal failure.
(1 g magnesium sulphate = 98 mg = 4.06 mmol = 8.12 mEq elemental magnesium).

Magnesium is rapidly excreted by the kidney. The half-life in patients with normal renal function is 4 h and 90% of the dose is excreted by 24 h after the infusion.[27] Renal function should be checked when magnesium is used and the dose should be reduced and serum concentrations measured when there is renal impairment or oliguria.

Magnesium toxicity is associated with muscle weakness and may lead to respiratory paralysis (>7.5 mmol/l). Increased conduction time with increased PR and QT intervals and QRS duration can lead to sinoatrial and atrioventricular block (>7.5 mmol/l) and cardiac arrest in diastole (>12.5 mmol/l). Magnesium toxicity can be treated with small intravenous doses of calcium. Other reported adverse effects of magnesium include death from overdose, increased bleeding, slowed cervical dilatation and increased risk of pulmonary oedema. Magnesium crosses the placenta and can cause neonatal flaccidity and respiratory depression. If repeated seizures occur despite therapeutic levels of magnesium, conventional anticonvulsants should be considered and other causes of convulsions excluded.

OTHER ANTICONVULSANTS

Phenytoin and **diazepam** are inferior to magnesium for preventing convulsions,[25,26] but they may be considered in cases refractory to magnesium. Phenytoin is given as an initial intravenous loading dose of 10 mg/kg, followed 2 h later by 5 mg/kg. Doses are diluted in normal saline and given no faster than 50 mg/min. Electrocardiogram and arterial pressure should be monitored. Maintenance doses of 200 mg p.o. or i.v. are started 12 h after the second bolus and given 8-hourly. Adverse effects include pain on injection, nystagmus, ataxia and lethargy at high plasma concentrations, and cardiotoxicity if given rapidly. Intravenous infusion of diazepam has been used for prevention of recurrent convulsions.[24,28] An infusion of 40 mg diazepam in 500 ml normal saline is titrated to keep patients sedated but rousable.[28] Potential adverse effects include oversedation, fetal heart rate changes, and neonatal respiratory depression, hypotonia, poor sucking and decreased body temperature.[28]

ECLAMPSIA

The priorities in the management of eclamptic seizures are airway protection, oxygenation, and termination and prevention of seizures. Delivery of the fetus should be considered after maternal stabilization. Eclampsia may occur without marked hypertension or without proteinuria.[5,29] Patients should be placed in the left lateral position and given oxygen. Seizures can be terminated by diazepam at 5–10 mg i.v. Alternatively, magnesium at 4 g i.v. can be given no faster than 1 g/min; further boluses to a maximum of 8 g total are given for repeated seizures. After termination of seizures, maintenance magnesium should be started if the patient is not already receiving magnesium. If seizures are not controlled, thiopentone and suxamethonium should be given and the airway secured. Recurrent convulsions or prolonged unconsciousness may indicate additional cerebral pathology (e.g. cerebral oedema, intracerebral haemorrhage, venous thrombosis) and a CT scan should be done. Intensive neurological management, aimed at controlling intracranial pressure and optimizing cerebral perfusion, has significantly reduced mortality in unconscious eclamptic patients.

FLUID BALANCE

Fluid management in pre-eclampsia is controversial. Pre-eclamptic patients usually have reduced circulating intravascular volume and oliguria is common in patients with pre-eclampsia. Therefore, fluid loading with crystalloid or colloid solution has been advocated to improve urine output, decrease arterial pressure, decrease systemic vascular resistance and increase cardiac output.[30] However, because pulmonary oedema is now a leading cause of mortality and morbidity,[3] this practice is questionable.

Initial maintenance fluid should consist of crystalloid at 75–125 ml/h i.v., aiming for urine output >0.5 ml/kg per h, averaged over 3–4 h. When there is oliguria or other signs of poor perfusion, repeated fluid challenge with 250–500 ml crystalloid or 100–200 ml colloid may be given, while monitoring with a pulse oximeter and examining for fluid overload.

Urinalysis is useful; sodium <20 mmol/l, osmolality >500 mosm/kg or fractional excretion of sodium of <1 support a pre-renal cause for oliguria. Low-dose dopamine infusion (1–5 μg/kg per min) was shown to improve urine output without detrimental haemodynamic effects.[31]

Invasive monitoring may be helpful in management of persistent oliguria. However, there is considerable controversy over the reliability of CVP and pulmonary capillary wedge pressure (PCWP) which have poor correlation, especially when CVP is greater than 6 mmHg (0.8 kPa).[32] Optimal CVP and PCWP values are unknown but the measured response to fluid challenge may be informative and useful. Pulmonary artery catheterization may be useful to differentiate patients with predominantly high systemic vascular resistance from those with high cardiac output. However, because insertion may be difficult and hazardous in patients who are oedematous and coagulopathic they should only be used for clear indications (e.g. refractory hypertension, pulmonary oedema, and refractory oliguria).[32] Pulmonary oedema is unlikely with a CVP less than 6 mmHg, but when it occurs, should be managed with oxygen therapy, positive end-expiratory pressure with or without ventilation, inotropes, vasodilators, morphine or diuretics as indicated. Renal failure in pre-eclampsia is now uncommon.

Some patients with persistent oliguria and a rising serum creatinine concentration may require a period of continuous renal replacement therapy but the majority of cases recover. However, the risk of irreversible renal damage is greater when there is associated abruptio placentae, disseminated intravascular coagulation (DIC), hypotensive shock, or sepsis.[9,33]

POSTPARTUM CARE

Patients are frequently referred to an ICU for postpartum care, particularly after caesarean delivery. About 40% of patients who develop eclampsia have the first seizure after the delivery.[5] The risk of pulmonary oedema is greatest after delivery and most maternal deaths occur then.[3,34] After delivery, there is often an initial improvement with a relapse in the first 24 h. Magnesium should be continued for 24–48 h. Antihypertensive drugs may be reduced according to the blood pressure. Some patients may require a change to oral medication which may need to be continued for several weeks. Psychological support is important, especially if there has been an adverse neonatal outcome. Full recovery from the organ dysfunction of pre-eclampsia is normally expected within six weeks.

HELLP SYNDROME AND HEPATIC COMPLICATIONS

HELLP syndrome is a form of severe pre-eclampsia characterized by the triad of *h*aemolysis (microangiopathic haemolytic anaemia), *e*levated *l*iver enzymes and *l*ow *p*latelets, which is of particularly high risk to the mother and fetus.[33,35] Onset may be insidious and not all patients have hypertension or proteinuria. Common presenting symptoms include epigastric or right upper quadrant pain, nausea, malaise, or features typical of severe pre-eclampsia. Important differential diagnoses include idiopathic thrombocytopenic purpura, systemic lupus erythematosis, thrombotic thrombocytopenic purpura, haemolytic uraemic syndrome and acute fatty liver of pregnancy.[35] Typically, HELLP syndrome presents at early gestational ages and is more common in white and multiparous women.[35] In about 30% of cases, it first manifests itself in the postpartum period and many of these patients will have had no evidence of pre-eclampsia before delivery.[33] After delivery, patients usually show a continuing deterioration in platelet count and liver enzymes with a peak in severity 24–48 h after delivery followed by gradual resolution and complete recovery if complications are avoided. Frequent complications of HELLP syndrome include DIC, abruptio placentae, acute renal failure, pulmonary oedema, severe ascites and pleural effusion.[33] Usual treatment of HELLP syndrome is stabilization and delivery. However, in some cases expectant management has improved neonatal and maternal outcome. Use of plasmapheresis and corticosterioids (dexamethasone 10 mg i.v. every 12 h) have been shown to accelerate recovery but their use is not fully established.[35]

Life-threatening complications occasionally occur in severe pre-eclampsia and HELLP syndrome.[36] Oedema, inflammatory infiltrates, obstructed sinusoidal blood flow or intrahepatic and subcapsular haemorrhage can cause liver swelling and rupture. If suspected, patients should have a CT scan or bedside ultrasound examination.[37] Hepatic rupture is a surgical emergency. Hepatic haemorrhage without rupture has been managed conservatively.

ANAESTHESIA AND ANALGESIA

Platelet count and coagulation tests should be checked before regional anaesthesia. Epidural analgesia in labour reduces fluctuations in arterial pressure and improves placental blood flow.[38] For caesarean section, the use of epidural and spinal anaesthesia[39] avoids the risks of aspiration, difficult intubation from airway oedema, exaggerated hypertensive response to intubation, and magnesium-induced sensitivity to muscle relaxants associated with general anaesthesia. If general anaesthesia is required, smaller size endotracheal tubes may be required. The following regimens have been reported to attenuate the hypertensive response to intubation: labetalol (up to 1 mg/kg), fentanyl (2.5 μg/kg), alfentanil (10 μg/kg), magnesium sulphate (40 mg/kg) or a combination of alfentanil (7.5 μg/ml) with magnesium sulphate (30 mg/kg). Occasionally, awake intubation under topical anaesthesia may be necessary when there is airway obstruction.

REFERENCES

1 Brown MA, Hague WM, Higgins J, *et al*. The detection, investigation and management of hypertension in pregnancy: executive summary. *Aust NZ J Obstet Gynaecol* 2000; **40**: 133–8.
2 Report of the National High Blood Pressure Education Program Working Group on High Blood Pressure in Pregnancy. *Am J Obstet Gynecol* 2000; **183**: S1–S22.
3 Department of Health. *Why mothers die. Report on Confidential Inquiries into Maternal Deaths in the United Kingdom 1994–96*. London: Stationery Office; 1999.
4 MacKay AP, Berg CJ, Atrash HK. Pregnancy-related mortality from preeclampsia and eclampsia. *Obstet Gynecol* 2001; **97**: 533–8.
5 Douglas KA, Redman CW. Eclampsia in the United Kingdom. *BMJ* 1994; **309**: 1395–400.
6 Mattar F, Sibai BM. Eclampsia. VIII. Risk factors for maternal morbidity. *Am J Obstet Gynecol* 2000; **182**: 307–12.

7 Martin JN Jr, May WL, Magann EF, Terrone DA, Rinehart BK, Blake PG. Early risk assessment of severe preeclampsia: admission battery of symptoms and laboratory tests to predict likelihood of subsequent significant maternal morbidity. *Am J Obstet Gynecol* 1999; **180**: 1407–14.
8 Roberts JM, Cooper DW. Pathogenesis and genetics of pre-eclampsia. *Lancet* 2001; **357**: 53–6.
9 Walker JJ. Pre-eclampsia. *Lancet* 2000; **356**: 1260–5.
10 Dekker GA, Sibai BM. Etiology and pathogenesis of preeclampsia: current concepts. *Am J Obstet Gynecol* 1998; **179**: 1359–75.
11 Roberts JM, Taylor RN, Musci TJ, *et al*. Preeclampsia: an endothelial cell disorder. *Am J Obstet Gynecol* 1989; **161**: 1200–4.
12 Cotton DB, Lee W, Huhta JC, Dorman KF. Hemodynamic profile of severe pregnancy-induced hypertension. *Am J Obstet Gynecol* 1988; **158**: 523–9.
13 Bosio PM, McKenna PJ, Conroy R, O'Herlihy C. Maternal central hemodynamics in hypertensive disorders of pregnancy. *Obstet Gynecol* 1999; **94**: 978–84.
14 Sagen N, Haram K, Nilsen ST. Serum urate as a predictor of fetal outcome in severe pre-eclampsia. *Acta Obstet Gynecol Scand* 1984; **63**: 71–5.
15 Leduc L, Wheeler JM, Kirshon B, *et al*. Coagulation profile in severe preeclampsia. *Obstet Gynecol* 1992; **79**: 14–18.
16 Sharma SK, Philip J, Whitten CW, *et al*. Assessment of changes in coagulation in parturients with preeclampsia using thromboelastography. *Anesthesiology* 1999; **90**: 385–90.
17 Visser W, Wallenburg HC. Maternal and perinatal outcome of temporizing management in 254 consecutive patients with severe pre-eclampsia remote from term. *Eur J Obstet Gynecol Reprod Biol* 1995; **63**: 147–54.
18 Magee LA, Ornstein MP, von Dadelszen P. Fortnightly review: management of hypertension in pregnancy. *BMJ* 1999; **318**: 1332–6.
19 Walker JJ. Care of the patient with severe pregnancy induced hypertension. *Eur J Obstet Gynecol Reprod Biol* 1996; **65**: 127–35.
20 Jouppila P, Kirkinen P, Koivula A, Ylikorkala O. Labetalol does not alter the placental and fetal blood flow or maternal prostanoids in pre-eclampsia. *Br J Obstet Gynaecol* 1986; **93**: 543–7.
21 Visser W, Wallenburg HC. A comparison between the haemodynamic effects of oral nifedipine and intravenous dihydralazine in patients with severe pre-eclampsia. *J Hypertens* 1995; **13**: 791–5.
22 Duley L, Henderson-Smart DJ. Drugs for rapid treatment of very high blood pressure during pregnancy (Cochrane Review). In: *The Cochrane Library*. Oxford: Update Software; 2001.
23 Lucas MJ, Leveno KJ, Cunningham FG. A comparison of magnesium sulfate with phenytoin for the prevention of eclampsia. *N Engl J Med* 1995; **333**: 201–5.
24 Collaborative Eclampsia Trial. Which anticonvulsant for women with eclampsia? Evidence from the

Collaborative Eclampsia Trial. *Lancet* 1995; **345**: 1455–63.

25 Duley L, Henderson-Smart D. Magnesium sulphate versus diazepam for eclampsia (Cochrane Review). In: *The Cochrane Library*. Oxford: Update Software; 2001.

26 Duley L, Henderson-Smart D. Magnesium sulphate versus phenytoin for eclampsia (Cochrane Review). In: *The Cochrane Library*. Oxford: Update Software; 2001.

27 Lu JF, Nightingale CH. Magnesium sulfate in eclampsia and pre-eclampsia: pharmacokinetic principles. *Clin Pharmacokinet* 2000; **38**: 305–14.

28 Crowther C. Magnesium sulphate versus diazepam in the management of eclampsia: a randomized controlled trial. *Br J Obstet Gynaecol* 1990; **97**: 110–17.

29 Sibai BM, McCubbin JH, Anderson GD, *et al.* Eclampsia. I. Observations from 67 recent cases. *Obstet Gynecol* 1981; **58**: 609–13.

30 Sehgal NN, Hitt JR. Plasma volume expansion in the treatment of pre-eclampsia. *Am J Obstet Gynecol* 1980; **138**: 165–8.

31 Mantel GD, Makin JD. Low dose dopamine in postpartum pre-eclamptic women with oliguria: a double-blind, placebo controlled, randomised trial. *Br J Obstet Gynaecol* 1997; **104**: 1180–3.

32 Clark SL, Cotton DB. Clinical indications for pulmonary artery catheterization in the patient with severe preeclampsia. *Am J Obstet Gynecol* 1988; **158**: 453–8.

33 Sibai BM, Ramadan MK, Usta I, *et al.* Maternal morbidity and mortality in 442 pregnancies with hemolysis, elevated liver enzymes, and low platelets (HELLP syndrome). *Am J Obstet Gynecol* 1993; **169**: 1000–6.

34 Sibai BM, Mabie BC, Harvey CJ, *et al.* Pulmonary edema in severe preeclampsia-eclampsia: analysis of thirty-seven consecutive cases. *Am J Obstet Gynecol* 1987; **156**: 1174–9.

35 Saphier CJ, Repke JT. Hemolysis, elevated liver enzymes, and low platelets (HELLP) syndrome: a review of diagnosis and management. *Semin Perinatol* 1998; **22**: 118–33.

36 Neerhof MG, Zelman W, Sullivan T. Hepatic rupture in pregnancy. *Obstet Gynecol Surv* 1989; **44**: 407–9.

37 Barton JR, Sibai BM. Hepatic imaging in HELLP syndrome (hemolysis, elevated liver enzymes, and low platelet count). *Am J Obstet Gynecol* 1996; **174**: 1820–5.

38 Jouppila P, Jouppila R, Hollmen A, *et al.* Lumbar epidural analgesia to improve intervillous blood flow during labor in severe preeclampsia. *Obstet Gynecol* 1982; **59**: 158–61.

39 Hood DD, Curry R. Spinal versus epidural anesthesia for cesarean section in severely preeclamptic patients: a retrospective survey. *Anesthesiology* 1999; **90**: 1276–82.

54

General obstetric emergencies in the ICU

T Gin and W D Ngan Kee

The ICU will receive obstetric patients who present with the usual range of medical and surgical emergencies, and also provide supportive care for patients who suffer specific obstetric complications. However, the proportion of obstetric patients in most ICUs is low, and this may lead to relative inexperience in management and teamwork between the intensivist and obstetrician. Scoring systems have not been validated in obstetric patients and, although there have been conflicting reports about their applicability, recent data suggest a low mortality for obstetric patients in general.[1,2]

Two important points to recognize in treating emergencies in obstetric patients are that: (i) physiological changes in pregnancy may modify the presentation of the problem, the normal physiological variables used to guide treatment and also the response to treat-ment; (ii) both mother and fetus are affected by the pathology and subsequent treatment.

Physiology. During pregnancy, the normal ranges for physiological variables change,[3] so that therapy is guided by different endpoints (Table 54.1).

- After 20 weeks' gestation, aortocaval compression by the gravid uterus can decrease uterine perfusion and venous return to the heart. This is best prevented by using the full left lateral position, but a left lateral tilt or manual displacement of the uterus may be more practicable.
- Oedematous tissues, delayed gastric emptying and increased oxygen consumption complicate tracheal intubation.
- Patients should be given prophylaxis for thrombo-embolism, typically with low-molecular-weight heparin (LMWH) and elastic compression stockings.
- The majority of physiological changes revert to normal several days after delivery.
- Perineal and breast nursing care should not be neglected.

Mechanical ventilation can be more problematic in the pregnant patient.[4] Although the changes in anatomy and lung compliance present no difficulty to the mechanics of ventilation, some of the recommended strategies for managing adult respiratory distress syndrome (ARDS) may be more difficult to implement.

- Permissive hypercapnia may cause fetal respiratory acidosis that will reduce the ability of fetal haemo-globin to bind oxygen.
- Low tidal volumes make it difficult to maintain the increased ventilation of pregnancy, and higher tidal volumes and alveolar plateau pressures up to 35 cmH$_2$O (0.34 kPa) may be necessary.
- There are no data on the prone position.
- Unlike in other obstetric-related diseases, delivery of the fetus does not appear to result in marked improvement of maternal respiratory failure.

Haemodynamic support should generally start with good hydration. The uterine vascular bed is considered

Table 54.1 Changes in physiological variables during late pregnancy

Systolic arterial pressure	−5 mmHg
Mean arterial pressure	−15 mmHg
Diastolic arterial pressure	−15 mmHg
Central venous pressure	No change
Pulmonary capillary wedge pressure	No change
Heart rate	+15%
Stroke volume	+30%
Cardiac output	+45%
Systemic vascular resistance	−15%
Tidal volume	+40%
Respiratory rate	+10%
Minute volume	+50%
Oxygen consumption	+20%
pH	No change
PaO$_2$	+10 mmHg
PaCO$_2$	−10 mmHg
HCO$_3^-$	−4 mmol/l
Total blood volume	+40%
Haematocrit	−0.06
Plasma albumin	−5 g/l
Oncotic pressure	−3 mmHg

maximally dilated but still responsive to stimuli that cause vasoconstriction, such as circulating catecholamines.[5] Ephedrine has traditionally been the vasoconstrictor used in obstetrics because it was thought to preserve uterine blood flow better than pure α-agonists. However, α-agonists such as phenylephrine are proving superior from both a maternal and fetal perspective in treating hypotension during caesarean delivery.[6] There is no evidence favouring any particular inotrope.

Mother and fetus. The mother's welfare usually takes precedence over fetal concerns, especially as fetal survival is dependent on optimal maternal management. However, the possibility of fetal viability also creates ethical dilemmas. It is important to monitor the fetus because of the problems associated with premature labour, placental transfer of drugs and maintenance of placental perfusion and oxygenation. An obstetric opinion should be sought as soon as possible regarding cardiotocography, ultrasound examination and timing of delivery. Nutrition is also very important for the fetus and adequate maternal feeding should be started as soon as possible.

CARDIOPULMONARY RESUSCITATION

Cardiac arrest is rare in pregnancy and estimated to occur once in every 30 000 deliveries.

At more advanced gestation, one must consider potential fetal viability and recognize that the aetiology of cardiac arrest may include particular obstetric complications, such as amniotic fluid embolism or drug toxicity from magnesium sulphate and local anaesthetics.

Normally, external cardiac massage produces only 30% of cardiac output and this is reduced further if there is vena caval compression. After about 20 weeks' gestation it becomes increasingly necessary to relieve aortocaval compression during basic life support (BLS). Left lateral tilt decreases the efficiency of closed chest compression, but a wedge providing an angle of 27° gives significant relief of vena caval obstruction while allowing 80% of the maximal force for chest compression.[7] During BLS, aortocaval compression may be minimized by manually displacing the uterus using a wedge, or positioning the pregnant patient's back on the rescuer's thighs. During advanced life support (ALS), drugs are given and defibrillation performed according to the normal protocol. Although sodium bicarbonate is not a drug of choice and may cause fetal acidosis, it has been suggested that the pH should eventually be kept above 7.3 to prevent uteroplacental vasoconstriction.[8]

Case reports at advanced gestation indicate that both maternal and fetal survival from cardiac arrest may depend on prompt caesarean delivery to relieve the effects of aortocaval compression. The International Liaison Committee on Resuscitation (ILCOR) advisory statement suggests that if there is no immediate response to ALS, perimortem caesarean delivery should be considered. The decision must be made quickly because the infant should be delivered within five minutes of the arrest.[9]

TRAUMA

Trauma occurs in approximately 6–7% of all pregnancies but only requires hospital admission in 0.3–0.4% of pregnancies. Even though only about 1% of trauma admissions are pregnant,[10] trauma is the leading non-obstetric cause of maternal mortality.[11,12] Head injuries and haemorrhagic shock account for most maternal deaths, while placental abruption and maternal death are the most frequent causes of fetal death. Case series show that different patterns of injury in different centres (motor vehicle accidents with or without seat belts) can cause wide variation in mortality rates.[13]

Initial resuscitation should follow the normal plan of attention to airway, breathing and circulation.[14,15] oxygen 100% should be given and cricoid pressure applied during tracheal intubation. Blood volume is increased during pregnancy and hypotension may not be evident until 35% or more of total blood volume is lost. Uterine blood flow is not autoregulated and may be decreased despite normal maternal haemodynamics, so that slight overhydration is preferred to underhydration. Femoral and lower limb venous catheters may not be appropriate because of pelvic injury. Treatment of hypotension always includes positioning or manual uterine displacement to avoid aortocaval compression. Drug treatment of modest hypotension can be started with ephedrine, but more potent vasopressors should be used if necessary.

Cardiotocographic monitoring is considered essential, but there is wide variation in practice and in the recommended duration of monitoring.

Necessary radiological investigations should be performed as indicated because radiation hazard to the fetus is very unlikely except in the first trimester where exposure to more than 5 cGy is cause for concern. A chest X-ray delivers less than 0.5 cGy to the lungs and very little to the shielded abdomen. However, the radiation dose with a pelvic film is 1 cGy, while an abdominal pelvic CT is about 5–10 cGy.

Assessment of trauma should note the increased significance of pelvic fractures for uterine injury and retroperitoneal haemorrhage.

- Ultrasound is the investigation of choice.
- Diagnostic peritoneal lavage should be performed through a surgical incision above the fundus.
- Chest drains are placed slightly higher than normal, in the third or fourth intercostal space.
- It is important to exclude herniation of abdominal contents through a ruptured diaphragm.

Fetal monitoring includes external cardiotocography, ultrasound and the Kleihauer–Betke test for transplacental haemorrhage.[16,17] Rh immune globulin at 300 μg given within 72 hours of injury should be considered for all Rh D-negative women. Premature labour and placental abruption may not be diagnosed unless regular monitoring is continued for at least six hours and even 24 hours if indicated.[18]

BURNS

Serious burns during pregnancy are seen more commonly in the developing world. Although the women are usually young and healthy, pregnancy is already a hypermetabolic state and the fetus is at great risk from many complications.[19]

- Severe burns and sepsis are associated with high levels of prostaglandins that may cause preterm labour.
- Replacement of fluid loss from burns must keep in mind the normally increased circulating volume of pregnancy.
- Inhalational injuries with hypoxia and carbon monoxide are especially detrimental to the fetus.
- Infection is responsible for many of the maternal and fetal deaths but prophylactic antibiotic policies are controversial.

Patients of advanced gestation should not be kept supine and nutritional support for the fetus is necessary early. Topical povodine–iodine solution should be avoided because the iodine may be absorbed and affect fetal thyroid function. Premature delivery may have to be considered, especially with extensive burns.

SEVERE OBSTETRIC HAEMORRHAGE

Antepartum haemorrhage is mostly from placenta praevia or placental abruption and both are ultimately managed by delivery.

In placenta praevia, the placenta implants in advance of the presenting part and classically presents as painless bleeding during the second or third trimester. Placenta praevia is relatively common (1 in 200 pregnancies) but severe haemorrhage is relatively rare.

In placental abruption, a normally implanted placenta separates from the uterine wall. The incidence of placental abruption is low (0.5–2%) but perinatal mortality may be as high as 50%. Several litres of blood may be concealed in the uterus as a retroplacental clot. Bleeding may continue after delivery for a variety of reasons, including disseminated intravascular coagulation, uterine atony, placenta accreta, and lacerations to cervix or vagina.

Peripartum haemorrhage contributes to 15% of maternal deaths, but if one includes ectopic pregnancy, 25% of maternal deaths are a result of haemorrhage. It seems obvious that the treatment of massive haemorrhage requires sufficient intravenous access and the logistic capability to quickly replace circulating volume with warmed fluids, blood and clotting factors. Unfortunately, many deaths have occurred because blood loss was often underestimated and volume replacement delayed.[20] In an emergency, the aorta can be compressed against the vertebral column by a fist pressed on the abdomen above the umbilicus. The control of haemorrhage allows time for resuscitation and more definitive surgical treatment.

Causes of postpartum haemorrhage are placenta accreta, cervical or vaginal lacerations and uterine atony.

MANAGEMENT

Uterine atony is managed initially with bimanual compression, uterine massage and intravenous oxytocin given intravenously by bolus (5 units) or infusion (20 units). Ergonovine (0.2 mg) may also be given intramuscularly, but for persistent atony the preferred drug is 15-methyl-prostaglandin $F_{2\alpha}$ (0.25 mg) given intramuscularly or intramyometrially every 15–30 min up to 2 mg.

Disseminated intravascular coagulation develops in 10–30% of cases, partly because tissue thromboplastin is released during abruption. Thus, blood should be sent for measurement of fibrinogen and fibrin degradation products and blood component therapy, and cryoprecipitate given as appropriate.

If bleeding persists, specific invasive procedures to be considered are angiographic arterial embolization, surgical ligation of the uterine, ovarian or internal iliac arteries or hysterectomy.

SEPTIC SHOCK[21,22]

Septic shock is a rare complication of maternal infection that may be seen following chorioamnionitis, postpartum endometritis, urinary tract infections, pyelonephritis and septic abortion. There are very few case series from which to make definitive conclusions.[23] Mortality varied from 20–28% and locating the source of infection was often difficult and delayed.

Gram-negative coliforms are the frequent causative organisms but streptococci and bacteroides may also be present. The physiological changes of pregnancy may influence the course and presentation of septic shock. Animal studies suggest that pregnancy increases the susceptibility to endotoxin, and that metabolic acidosis and cardiovascular collapse occur earlier.

Management of septic shock follows normal guidelines with eradication of the infectious source, although the normal range for haemodynamic variables may be different. Suggested antibiotic combinations are ampicillin, gentamicin and clindamycin, or imipenem, cilastatin and vancomycin.[24] Tetracyclines and quinolones should not be used in pregnancy.

VENOUS THROMBOSIS

Pulmonary thromboembolism is a common cause of maternal death, accounting for 15–25% of maternal mortality. Pregnancy is associated with a fivefold increase in thromboembolism because of:

- venous stasis
- hypercoagulable state
- vascular injury associated with delivery.

Patients with acquired and hereditary thrombophilias have an even greater risk.[25]

Accurate diagnosis of venous thromboembolism is crucial because of the long-term implications for therapy. Symptoms of dyspnoea or pain in the leg or chest require accurate diagnosis, especially in the immediate postpartum period. Real time or duplex ultrasonography is the first choice for diagnosis, but venography, perfusion lung scanning and pulmonary angiography should not be avoided, if indicated.

There are many recent reviews summarizing the various consensus guidelines for anticoagulant therapy during pregnancy.[26,27] LMWH has gradually replaced unfractionated heparin for the prophylaxis and treatment of deep venous thrombosis and pulmonary embolism in pregnancy as a result of low incidence of side-effects, ease of administration and the reduced need for monitoring.

Pregnant patients with suspected or proven deep vein thrombosis or pulmonary embolus should be given full anticoagulant therapy that is continued throughout pregnancy. Warfarin should not be used before delivery so heparin is continued until labour begins and restarted in the postpartum patient for at least 6–12 weeks.

With massive pulmonary embolus, surgical treatment or thrombolysis must be considered. Thrombolysis was thought to be relatively contraindicated during pregnancy because of the risk of maternal and fetal haemorrhagic complications. No controlled trials are feasible and outcome data must be extracted from case reports. A review in 1995 of the world's literature found 172 cases of pregnant women with thromboembolism that was treated with thrombolytic agents, mostly streptokinase.[28] The maternal mortality rate was 1.2%; haemorrhagic complications were reported in 8% and there were 10 pregnancy losses. These risks appear to be comparable to that obtained with surgical intervention in pregnant patients, and are actually lower than reported risks for surgery, thrombolysis or transvenous filters in non pregnant patients. Although heparin remains the treatment of choice, thrombolysis appears to be a viable option except during the immediate postpartum period.

AMNIOTIC FLUID EMBOLISM

Amniotic fluid embolism (AFE) is the cause of 5–10% of maternal deaths. The incidence of AFE varies between 1 in 20 000 and 1 in 80 000 deliveries, although there must be undetected and unsuspected cases where minimal amounts of amniotic fluid produce few symptoms. Between 25 and 50% of patients with suspected or proven AFE die within the first hour and the overall maternal mortality may be as high as 86% in symptomatic patients with a perinatal and neonatal mortality up to 40%.[29,30]

AFE was thought to be associated with vigorous labour and the use of oxytocics, but it may occur in any parturient. The exact pathogenic factors for the syndrome of AFE remain unclear.[31,32] Amniotic fluid is thought to enter the maternal circulation through endocervical or uterine lacerations, or uterine veins at the site of placental separation. Placental abruption may be a significant factor in the development of AFE. Amniotic fluid normally contains prostaglandins, leukotrienes, endothelin and fetal debris which can cause complement activation, pulmonary vasoconstriction, and physical blockage of pulmonary capillaries with resultant damage and release of further mediators. By these mechanisms, AFE has more in common with anaphylaxis and septic shock than other embolic diseases.

The initial diagnosis of AFE is made on clinical grounds and is often one of exclusion. Classically, patients may present with severe dyspnoea, cyanosis, sudden cardiovascular collapse, coma or convulsions during labour but AFE may occur earlier during pregnancy, during delivery or in the early puerperium. Some patients may present with bleeding and most patients eventually develop a coagulopathy.

Differential diagnoses include:

- thromboembolism
- air embolism
- aspiration pneumonitis
- eclamptic convulsions and coma
- local anaesthetic toxicity
- placental abruption
- haemorrhagic shock
- anaphylaxis
- intracranial haemorrhage
- acute heart failure.

Animal studies indicate that AFE causes a biphasic haemodynamic response. The early phase probably lasts less than half an hour and is characterized by severe hypoxia and right heart failure as a result of pulmonary hypertension from vasoconstriction or vessel damage. Half of the patients may die within the first hour.

Patients who survive this first phase develop left ventricular failure with return of normal right ventricular function. Left ventricular failure may be a result of the initial hypoxia or the depressant effects of mediators. Disseminated intravascular coagulation (DIC) is present in almost all patients but the mechanism is unknown. It could be caused by a specific activator of factor X, tissue factor or other substances, such as trophoblasts, in the amniotic fluid. Traditionally, AFE is confirmed by detection of squamous cells and fetal debris in the pulmonary circulation either at autopsy or in blood samples from a pulmonary artery catheter,[33] but squamous cells are a contaminant that can be found in other parturients and even non pregnant patients.

No specific therapy is available. Immediate cardiopulmonary resuscitation and 100% oxygen are necessary. Assessment of central venous pressure may be misleading, and early pulmonary artery catheterization has been advocated in a series reporting 100% survival in five patients by treating left ventricular failure aggressively.[34] The differential diagnoses must be evaluated quickly because urgent delivery of the fetus by caesarean section may improve resuscitation and prevent further AFE. Patients who survive the first few hours will continue to require supportive treatment for their acute lung injury. Blood component therapy is given as necessary to manage the coagulopathy. Cryoprecipitate has sometimes provided significant improvement in patient oxygenation.

Survivors of AFE regain normal cardiorespiratory function but may have neurological sequelae. There are two case reports of subsequent pregnancies, both with uncomplicated deliveries.[35]

ACID ASPIRATION (MENDELSON'S SYNDROME)

Obstetric patients are at increased risk of acid aspiration because of decreased gastric emptying, increased gastric acidity and volume and increased intra-abdominal pressure. Tracheal intubation is a particularly hazardous event because anatomic changes can make intubation difficult. Despite the notoriety of acid aspiration in obstetric patients, it is not known if pregnant patients' lungs are more susceptible to injury. Aspiration of acidic material will cause acute lung injury, the severity being related to the amount, content and acidity of the aspirate.

The initial presentation is hypoxaemia and bronchospasm. The chest X-ray may appear normal. Chemical pneumonitis and increased permeability pulmonary oedema develop over several hours.

Treatment includes standard respiratory support. Rigid bronchoscopy may be required to remove large food particles. Bronchoalveolar lavage and steroids are not useful and antibiotics should only be given for proven infection.

COCAINE TOXICITY[36]

Cocaine abuse during pregnancy has become a significant problem in the USA where maternal cocaine use may be as high as 5% in some populations. Cocaine causes:

- maternal hypertension
- tachycardia and increased cardiac output but decreases uterine blood flow
- increases uterine contractility.

Patients commonly present with placental abruption and fetal distress, while acute toxicity may also mimic pre-eclampsia by presenting with cerebral haemorrhage or convulsions.

For the treatment of hypertension, the drug of choice is controversial. Although hydralazine is often used in obstetrics to treat maternal hypertension, labetalol is preferable and widely used. However, concerns about using β-blockers may also be relevant to labetalol, and calcium-channel antagonists and nitroglycerine have also been advocated.

TOCOLYTIC THERAPY AND PULMONARY OEDEMA[37]

Pulmonary oedema is an uncommon (1 in 400 pregnancies) but serious complication of tocolytic therapy with β-adrenergic agonists. The underlying mechanism for pulmonary oedema is unclear but is probably due to fluid overload and increased hydrostatic pressure rather than increased pulmonary capillary permeability or left ventricular dysfunction. The initial management of pulmonary oedema is discontinuation of the β-adrenergic agonist and oxygen therapy, with further monitoring, diuretics and respiratory support as necessary.

OVARIAN HYPERSTIMULATION SYNDROME[38]

Ovarian hyperstimulation syndrome (OHSS) remains a significant but unpredictable and incompletely understood complication of ovarian stimulation. The syndrome is typically associated with:

- exogenous human chorionic gonadotrophin (hCG) regimens, used to induce ovulation in assisted reproduction techniques;
- increased capillary permeability, leading progressively to hypovolaemia with haemoconcentration, oedema and accumulation of fluid in the abdomen and pleural spaces.

The pathophysiology of OHSS has not been fully determined. A likely mediator is vascular endothelial growth factor, but many interacting cytokines and endocrine factors may be involved.

OHSS is most severe at several days to a week after a stimulated cycle, but early signs and symptoms can often be seen during the stimulatory phase. Fertility clinics will have their own protocols to try and minimize the incidence of OHSS and to detect its early stages. In general, symptoms resolve spontaneously over 2 weeks, in parallel with the decline in hCG from the last doses given. However, a successful pregnancy implantation will increase endogenous hCG and may temporarily worsen OHSS. Although subclinical OHSS may be found in most patients, only a small percentage require ward admission for careful fluid management to restore circulating volume, prevention of thrombosis with heparin, and treatment of ascites by paracentesis as necessary. Severe OHSS may cause renal failure, respiratory failure or thromboembolism, which requires supportive intensive care therapy. Invasive monitoring is essential for fluid management.

REFERENCES

1 Afessa B, Green B, Delke I, Koch K. Systemic inflammatory response syndrome, organ failure and outcome in critically ill obstetric patients treated in an ICU. *Chest* 2001; **120**: 1271–7.

2 Hazelgrove JF, Price C, Pappachan VJ, Smith GB. Multicenter study of obstetric admissions to 14 intensive care units in southern England. *Crit Care Med* 2001; **29**: 770–5.

3 Chamberlain G, Broughton-Pipkin F. *Clinical Physiology in Obstetrics*, 3rd edn. Oxford: Blackwell Science; 1998.

4 Campbell LA, Klocke RA. Implications for the pregnant patient. *Am J Respir Crit Care Med* 2001; **163**: 1051–4.

5 Greiss FC Jr. A clinical concept of uterine blood flow during pregnancy. *Obstet Gynecol* 1967; **30**: 595–604.

6 Lee A, Ngan Kee WD, Gin T. A quantitative systematic review of randomized controlled trials of ephedrine versus phenylephrine for the management of hypotension during spinal anesthesia for cesarean section. Anesth Analg 2002; **94**: 920–6.

7 Rees GAD, Willis BA. Resuscitation in late pregnancy. *Anaesthesia* 1988; **43**: 347–9.

8 Mauer DK, Gervais HW, Dick WF, *et al.* Cardiopulmonary resuscitation (CPR) during pregnancy. *Eur J Anaesthesiol* 1993; **10**: 437–40.

9 Kloeck W, Cummins RO, Chamberlain D, *et al.* Special resuscitation situations. An advisory statement from the international liaison committee on resuscitation. *Circulation* 1997; **95**: 2196–210.

10 Rogers FB, Rozycki GS, Osler TM, *et al.* A multi-institutional study of factors associated with fetal death in injured pregnant patients. *Arch Surg* 1999; **134**: 1274–7

11 Esposito TJ. Trauma during pregnancy. *Emerg Med Clin North Am* 1994; **12**: 167–99.

12 Kuhlmann RS, Cruikshank DP. Maternal trauma during pregnancy. *Clin Obstet Gynecol* 1994; **37**: 274–93.

13 Shah KH, Simons RK, Holbrook T, *et al.* Trauma in pregnancy: maternal and fetal outcomes. *J Trauma* 1998; **45**: 83–6.

14 Neufeld JDG. Trauma in pregnancy, what if ...? *Emerg Med Clin North Am* 1993; **11**: 207–24.

15 American College of Obstetricians and Gynecologists. *Trauma During Pregnancy.* ACOG Technical Bulletin Number 161. *Int J Gynecol Obstet* 1993; **40**: 165–70.

16 Pearlman MD, Tintinalli JE. Evaluation and treatment of the gravida and fetus following trauma during pregnancy. *Obstet Gynecol Clin North Am* 1991; **18**: 371–81.

17 Towery R, English TP, Wisner D. Evaluation of pregnant women after blunt injury. *J Trauma* 1993; **35**: 731–6.

18 Curet MJ, Schermer CR, Demarest GB, *et al.* Predictors of outcome in trauma during pregnancy: identification of patients who can be monitored for less than 6 hours. *J Trauma* 2000; **49**: 18–25

19 Polko LE, McMahon MJ. Burns in pregnancy. *Obstet Gynecol Surv* 1998; **53**: 50–6.

20 Hibbard BM, Anderson MM, Drife JO, *et al.* Report on Confidential Enquiries into Maternal Deaths in the United Kingdom 1988–1990. London: Her Majesty's Stationery Office; 1994.

21 Gonik B. Septic shock in obstetrics. *Clin Perinatol* 1986; **13**: 741–54.

22 Segal S, Carp H. Chestnut DH. Fever and infection. In: Chestnut DH (ed.) *Obstetric Anesthesia, Principles and Practice*, 2nd edn. St Louis, MO: Mosby; 1999: pp. 711–24.

23 Mabie WC, Barton JR, Sibai B. Septic shock in pregnancy. *Obstet Gynecol* 1997; **90**: 553–61.

24 American College of Obstetricians and Gynecologists. *Septic Shock.* ACOG Technical Bulletin No 204; April 1995.

25 Greer IA. Thrombosis in pregnancy: maternal and fetal issues. *Lancet* 1999; **353**: 1258–6.

26 Barbour LA. Current concepts of anticoagulant therapy in pregnancy. *Obstet Gynecol Clin North Am* 1997; **24**: 499–521.

27 Andres RL, Miles A. Venous thromboembolism and pregnancy. *Obstet Gynecol Clin North Am* 2001; **28**: 613–30.

28 Turrentine MA, Braems G, Ramirez MM. Use of thrombolytics for the treatment of thromboembolic disease during pregnancy. *Obstet Gynecol Surv* 1995; **50**: 534–41.

29 Morgan M. Amniotic fluid embolism. *Anaesthesia* 1979; **34**: 20–32.

30 Clark SL, Hankins GDV, Dudley DA, *et al.* Amniotic fluid embolism: analysis of the national registry. *Am J Obstet Gynecol* 1995; **172**: 1158–69.

31 Locksmith GJ. Amniotic fluid embolism. *Obstet Gynecol Clin North Am* 1999; **26**: 435–44.

32 Davies S. Amniotic fluid embolus: a review of the literature. *Can J Anaesth* 2001; **48**: 88–98.

33 Masson RG. Amniotic fluid embolism. *Clin Chest Med* 1992; **13**: 657–65.

34 Clark SL, Cotton DB, Gonik B, *et al*. Central hemodynamic alterations in amniotic fluid embolism. *Am J Obstet Gynecol* 1988; **158**: 1124–6.

35 Clark SL. Successful pregnancy outcomes after amniotic fluid embolism. *Am J Obstet Gynecol* 1992; **167**: 512–3.

36 Hughes SC, Kissin C. Anaesthesia and the drug-addicted mother. In: Hughes SC, Levinson G, Rosen MA (eds.) *Shnider and Levinson's Anesthesia for Obstetrics*, 4th edn. Philadelphia, PA: Lippincott, Williams and Wilkins; 2002: pp. 599–612.

37 Lamont RF. The pathophysiology of pulmonary oedema with the use of beta-agonists. *Br J Obstet Gynaecol* 2000; **107**: 439–44.

38 Whelan JG IIIrd, Vlahos NF. The ovarian hyperstimulation syndrome. *Fertil Steril* 2000; **73**: 883–96.

55

Severe pre-existing disease in pregnancy

S M Yentis

The two main sources of information about the spectrum of pre-existing conditions that result in severe morbidity in pregnancy are national or local registries/databases and published case series of admissions to intensive care, high-dependency units or obstetric units. Information about mortality comes from registries of maternal death such as the Reports on Confidential Enquiries into Maternal Deaths in the UK, or from individual case series. Differences in definitions and resources make it difficult to draw precise conclusions, but data from these various sources (e.g. within a unified system such as the UK) suggest that there is a discrepancy between those conditions which cause admission to the ICU and those which result in maternal death (Table 55.1). Reasons for this discrepancy might be because:

- some fatal disorders are rapidly fatal, with the mother dying before she reaches the ICU (e.g. severe pulmonary embolism)
- some conditions may be managed in non-ICU medical wards or specialized units (e.g. cardiac or neurological disease)

Table 55.1 Pooled results from four UK series of maternity patients admitted to ICU[1-4] (excluding deaths) and the two latest Reports on Confidential Enquiries into Maternal Deaths in the UK (1994–1996[5] and 1997–1999),[6] showing the most common causes of ICU admission and death respectively in women with pre-existing disease

Most common causes of admission to ICU (excluding deaths) in women with pre-existing disease, in descending order	Most common causes of death in women with pre-existing disease, in descending order
Connective tissue disease	Cardiac disease
Haematological disease	Neurological disease
Cardiac disease	Psychiatric disease
Drug addiction	Respiratory disease
Psychiatric disease	Haematological disease
Respiratory disease	Connective tissue disease
Neurological disease	Diabetes
	Drug addiction

- late deaths may not be recorded as being pregnancy related and thus not included in ICU series
- problems with small numbers, non-representative series and/or poor standardization of terms.

With increasingly successful medical care during childhood and early adulthood, the number of women with severe disease who survive to child-bearing age has increased. Part of such women's wishes to live a normal life includes the desire to have children, and this places increasing demands on obstetric, anaesthetic and ICU services, as well as on the women's physiological reserves.

It is important that women with severe disease are appropriately counselled before pregnancy since the risks to both them and their fetuses may be considerable. This early counselling should ideally include anaesthetic input.

CARDIAC DISEASE

There are more maternal deaths in the UK from cardiac disease than from pre-eclampsia and haemorrhage combined.[5,6] Over the last 20–30 years, there has been a shift away from acquired cardiac disease (mainly rheumatic heart disease) towards congenital heart disease, especially as modern techniques of cardiac surgery in early life enable girls to reach maturity with conditions that in previous years would have resulted in early death. Mortality varies from less than 1% in uncomplicated conditions to over 40% in Eisenmenger's syndrome, even with modern methods of medical management.[7]

PHYSIOLOGY AND PATHOPHYSIOLOGY

The physiological changes of pregnancy are discussed in Chapter 54 on *Pre-eclampsia*. The changes most relevant to cardiac disease are:

- susceptibility to aortocaval compression
- reduction in systemic vascular resistance

- increases in blood volume and cardiac output by up to 40–50% by the 20th week of gestation, with a potential further increase in cardiac output (up to 50%) during labour.

In patients with cardiac function already impaired, such as those with cardiomyopathy or valvular stenoses, inability to meet this challenge may result in cardiac failure. If there is a right-to-left shunt, the fall in systemic vascular resistance encourages blood to bypass the lungs; this, together with the increasing demands of the fetus and the reduced maternal pulmonary reserve, may lead to severe exacerbation of hypoxaemia.

GENERAL ANTEPARTUM AND PERIPARTUM MANAGEMENT

Antepartum management consists mainly of regular assessments and measures to reduce cardiac workload, for example, by reducing activity and treating arrhythmias/cardiac failure.

Electrocardiography, chest X-rays and echocardiography are the most useful investigations. Echocardiography is particularly helpful for measurement of valve areas, since flow across stenosed valves can be expected to increase as cardiac output increases in pregnancy. Pulse oximetry is a simple, non-invasive tool for monitoring the degree of right-to-left shunt.

An obstetric and anaesthetic plan should be prepared and the intensivists informed of the anticipated delivery date. Antithromboembolic prophylaxis should be considered since cardiac patients are more at-risk even without prolonged bed rest. Low-molecular-weight heparins are increasingly used, although both heparin and warfarin have been used for patients with prosthetic heart valves.[8] The requirements for heparin increase in pregnancy, so greater doses than normal should be used.

The principles of peripartum management are vaginal delivery unless caesarean section is indicated for obstetric indications. Elective caesarean section has been advocated in the past as a matter of course but the stresses of surgery are now generally felt to exceed those of a well-controlled vaginal delivery. Low-dose epidural regimens using weak solutions of local anaesthetic (e.g. 0.1% bupivacaine or less) with opioids such as fentanyl have been found to be effective and cardiostable.[9] Combined spinal–epidural anaesthesia using similar low doses are also suitable. In patients with marked exercise intolerance, outlet forceps or ventouse delivery is usually recommended to limit pushing and the duration of the second stage. If caesarean section is required, both regional and general anaesthesia have their advocates,[10,11] but either is acceptable as long as due care is taken.

Peripartum complications such as bleeding, pulmonary oedema, arrhythmias and sudden increases in pulmonary vascular resistance or drops in systemic vascular resistance, may be tolerated badly by patients with limited reserves.

Oxytocin analogue (Syntocinon) has marked cardiovascular effects[12] which although tolerable in normal patients, may cause a calamitous drop in systemic vascular resistance with hypotension, tachycardia and worsening of shunt in susceptible patients. If Syntocinon is required it should be diluted and given very slowly (e.g. 5 U over 10–20 minutes). This may be a problem as such patients may be especially sensitive to acute blood loss. In patients with fixed cardiac outputs and no pulmonary hypertension, ergometrine may be preferable. Exacerbation of right-to-left shunt are manifested by worsening hypoxaemia, which may be improved by vasoconstrictors such as phenylephrine – the chronotropic and inotropic effects of ephedrine are often undesirable in patients with cardiac disease.

Monitoring ranges from simple non-invasive methods to peripheral arterial, central venous and pulmonary arterial cannulation, depending on the severity of the underlying disease.[13] Arterial cannulation is usually straightforward but central venous cannulation is often difficult because of the increased maternal body weight and fluid retention, and the inability to lie flat, let alone head-down. The antecubital fossa should be considered as a route for cannulation first. Scrupulous attention must be paid to avoiding intravascular air in patients with right-to-left shunts.

The principles of haemodynamic support are generally the same as in non-pregnant patients, remembering that pregnant women have a propensity to acute lung injury if overloaded with fluid. The physiological changes of pregnancy, especially tachycardia and increased cardiac output, should be remembered. The risk from aortocaval compression is often forgotten and this must be reinforced at all times, with the woman placed in the lateral or supine wedged position. If a pregnant woman requires intensive care before the baby is born, there may be a conflict between the maternal need for vasopressors and the adverse effects of these drugs on uteroplacental blood flow. Similarly, attempts to prolong pregnancy with steroids and β_2-adrenergic agonists such as terbutaline or salbutamol may cause adverse cardiovascular effects (primarily, pulmonary oedema) in the mother.

Common peripartum complications are summarized in Table 55.2.

Table 55.2 Common peripartum problems in patients with pre-existing cardiac disease

- Arrhythmias
- Cardiac failure/pulmonary oedema
- Pulmonary embolism
- Susceptibility to the effects of haemorrhage
- Susceptibility to the effects of infection
- Severe iatrogenic reductions in systemic vascular resistance, e.g. regional anaesthesia, intravenous bolus of oxytocin

POSTPARTUM COMPLICATIONS

Women may continue to be at risk from bleeding, arrhythmias and cardiac failure postpartum. Specific problems need to be considered:

- If oxytocin has been withheld, postpartum haemorrhage may become a problem.
- Pulmonary embolism is a particular risk in the postpartum period, and the risks and benefits of anticoagulant therapy must be weighed up in each individual case.
- Patients with Eisenmenger's syndrome typically die on or around the 10th postpartum day of pulmonary haemorrhage, embolism or both.[14]
- Endocarditis should be prevented with appropriate antibacterial drugs (typically amoxycillin and gentamicin, or vancomycin if allergic to penicillin). The threat of endocarditis should always be considered.
- There is susceptibility to chest infection and its effects (and those of wound or other infection) may be devastating; thus a high index of suspicion and aggressive early management is required.

RESPIRATORY DISEASE

The most common respiratory causes of morbidity and mortality in pregnancy are pneumonia, asthma, and cystic fibrosis; thus the latter two conditions are the most common pre-existing respiratory diseases that cause mothers to present to ICUs.[5,6,15,16]

Asthma is very common but rarely causes serious morbidity in its own right although there is a higher risk of maternal and neonatal morbidity.[17]

Cystic fibrosis is relatively rare but is more likely to be associated with poor outcomes.[18] Recent studies suggest that pregnancy itself does not increase mortality in women with mild cystic fibrosis and that the risk factors are the same as in non-pregnant patients (prepregnancy forced expiratory volume in one second [FEV_1] <50–60% of predicted; colonization with *Burkholderia cepacia*; and pancreatic insufficiency).[19,20] Overall mortality has been reported as 5% within two years of pregnancy, 10–20% within five years of pregnancy and 21% within 10 years.[19,20]

Psychological support is an important consideration. The decision to have a child, with the risk of passing on the cystic fibrosis gene and the adverse effect that pregnancy might have on the mother, is one that imposes a great deal of stress on the mother, her partner and their relatives.

PHYSIOLOGY AND PATHOPHYSIOLOGY

If respiratory function is already impaired, the physiological effects of pregnancy add an extra burden on the respiratory system that may precipitate respiratory failure:

- reduced functional residual capacity
- splinting of the diaphragm
- increased oxygen demand
- the stimulus to hyperventilate.

In cystic fibrosis, an additional stress is the increased nutritional demand in a patient who may already be malnourished because of malabsorption. In addition, chronic hypoxaemia may lead to chronic pulmonary vasoconstriction, cor pulmonale and pulmonary hypertension.

GENERAL MANAGEMENT AND COMPLICATIONS

Antepartum management comprises regular assessment and adjustment of medical treatment when required. Patients may be taking a variety of drugs including steroids. This is particularly relevant in asthma, in whom there is a trend nowadays towards aggressive treatment of acute exacerbations of asthma, with early use of steroids. Although prednisolone is about 90% metabolized by the placenta, large doses have been associated with neonatal adrenal suppression.

Regional analgesia is indicated in patients with moderate or severe functional limitation, in order to reduce the demands of labour. If caesarean section is required, regional anaesthesia is thought to reduce the risk of postoperative pulmonary complications, although objective evidence is lacking. Care is required: if regional anaesthesia extends too high, ventilation and the ability to cough may be impaired.

In cystic fibrosis, the principles of intensive care are generally the same as in non-pregnant patients. Assessment of patients with respiratory disease requires knowledge of the physiological changes induced by pregnancy and parameters such as blood gases need to be considered in that context. An arterial partial pressure of carbon dioxide 45 mmHg (6 kPa) represents a much greater deviation from the normal value in pregnancy. The mainstay of supportive treatment is regular physiotherapy and antibiotic therapy. It is important to know whether the patient has been previously colonized with unusual and/or resistant organisms, for example, *B. cepacia*. The biggest single hazard for the mother is an acute infective exacerbation in the middle/third trimester provoking incipient respiratory failure. Infection has to be treated both early and aggressively. Exhaustion and respiratory failure has been managed with non-invasive ventilatory techniques with some success.

Problems with intermittent positive pressure ventilation during an acute exacerbation in severe disease appear to relate to widely disparate compliance in different lung areas. This produces $\dot{V}/\dot{Q}$ mismatch with a large effective physiological dead space. The key to management is control and clearance of the underlying infection but this can be very difficult.

The beneficial effect of delivery on maternal oxygenation is usually immediate, although pain following caesarean section may limit deep inspiration and encourage basal atelectasis. Fatigue can also be a problem. Just because the baby has been delivered, scrupulous respiratory support cannot be forgone.

NEUROLOGICAL DISEASE

Epilepsy has been highlighted as an important cause of maternal death in recent Reports on Confidential Enquiries into Maternal Deaths in the UK.[5,6] Many of these deaths are thought to be related to poor control of epilepsy, secondary to altered pharmacodynamics and pharmacokinetics of anticonvulsant drugs in pregnancy. A convulsion while in the bath was thought to have occurred in a large proportion of deaths.[5,6] In terms of pre-existing neurological disease leading to admission to the ICU during or shortly after pregnancy, no single condition stands out, although those potentially affecting respiratory function (e.g. myasthenia gravis, multiple sclerosis; high spinal cord lesions) might be expected to cause particular problems.

GENERAL MANAGEMENT

Until recently, regional analgesia and anaesthesia was traditionally avoided in most neurological disease, for fear of exacerbating the condition, or being blamed for an exacerbation should it occur. Nowadays, most authorities actively encourage regional analgesia for labour since it reduces the physiological demand and thus the risk of respiratory insufficiency or excess fatigue. Similarly, regional anaesthesia for caesarean section avoids the problems of excessive postoperative sedation and how or whether to use neuromuscular blocking drugs – including suxamethonium. Initial fears about an increased relapse rate of multiple sclerosis following regional anaesthesia have fortunately not been borne out by large prospective series.[21]

If there is raised intracranial pressure, the use of regional techniques is more controversial. On the one hand, labour and vaginal delivery without effective analgesia can result in marked increases in intracranial pressure; on the other, accidental dural puncture can be disastrous. Even if successfully placed, rapid epidural injection may be associated with increases in intracranial pressure.[22] This risk still exists with epidural analgesic techniques continued into the postoperative period.

Management of conditions in which there are spinal abnormalities are also controversial. Spina bifida and other lesions have been successfully managed using regional techniques, although in each case a careful balance between risk and benefit must be assessed. These patients are unlikely to present to intensivists unless they are associated with respiratory impairment.

Table 55.3 Guide to converting oral to systemic medication in mothers with myasthenia gravis. Approximate conversion doses are given

Drug	Oral dose	Intramuscular dose	Intravenous dose
Neostigmine	15 mg	0.7–1.0 mg	0.5 mg
Pyridostigmine	60 mg	3–4 mg	2 mg

Myasthenia gravis poses a particular problem because of the need for regular medication throughout labour and after delivery. Gastric emptying may be decreased during labour, especially if systemic opioids are given although this effect can also occur (albeit to a lesser extent) with boluses of epidural opioids. It is therefore important to consider alternative routes of administering the mother's drug therapy if opioids are given in this way. A useful guide is offered in Table 55.3. Epidural analgesia can be very helpful in limiting maternal fatigue during and after labour. The mother needs watching carefully for signs of increasing weakness up to 7–10 days postpartum.

PSYCHIATRIC DISEASE (INCLUDING DRUG ADDICTION)

Psychiatric disease features consistently in surveys of maternal morbidity and mortality, for example through parasuicide or suicide, violence or the complications of drug addiction. Psychiatric patients may be more vulnerable to becoming pregnant, and pregnant women more vulnerable to suffering from psychiatric disease either during or after pregnancy.

Abuse of drugs poses similar problems to those in the non-pregnant population, with the additional effect of fetal addiction and retarded growth. In particular, cocaine is commonly abused in parts of the developed world and has been implicated in causing placental abruption and maternal convulsions, hypertension and tachycardia, with increased morbidity and mortality for both mother and fetus.[23] Unplanned operative intervention for delivery is more likely, which may contribute to an increased requirement for intensive care. The combination of substance abuse and HIV infection poses a particular challenge in the obstetric patient.

Management in terms of intensive care is usually similar to that in non-pregnant patients, with special attention to the effects of maternal drugs on the fetus (if antepartum), for example those taken in overdose or those used for sedation, as antidotes, etc.

HAEMATOLOGICAL, CONNECTIVE TISSUE AND METABOLIC DISEASE

Several haematological conditions may predispose to critical illness in pregnancy, sickle-cell disease being one of the most common.[1-4] Patients with coagulopathy are clearly at increased risk of haemorrhage but, in general, ICU management of patients with haematological disease is as for non-pregnant patients. It is important that all staff appreciate that significant amounts of blood may be lost into the uterus or vagina without it being visible externally.

Connective tissue disease rarely presents to the intensivist unless there is widespread and severe systemic involvement. Cardiac and pulmonary manifestations are the usual culprits, which may be exacerbated by pregnancy because of the increased demands. Such patients are also at risk of obstetric complications such as bleeding (including postpartum).

Diabetes mellitus is the most important pre-existing metabolic disease in pregnancy. It is well known to increase both maternal and fetal morbidity but usually features in the ICU as a contributory factor to other conditions, for example, sepsis. Anecdotal reports suggest that diabetic coma presenting in pregnancy may be particularly difficult to treat and stability of blood glucose may only be achieved after delivery of the fetus.

REFERENCES

1 Umo-Etuk J, Lumley J, Holdcroft A. Critically ill parturient women and admission to intensive care: a 5-year review. *Int J Obstet Anesth* 1996; **5**: 79–84.

2 Wheatley E, Farkas A, Watson D. Obstetric admissions to an intensive therapy unit. *Int J Obstet Anesth* 1996; **5**: 221–4.

3 Margarson M, Dob D, Yentis SM. A retrospective survey of obsetric admissions to the Intensive Care Unit. *Int J Obstet Anesth* 1998; 7: 205–6.

4 Donnelly JA, Smith EA, Runcie CJ. Transfer of the critically ill obstetric patient. *Int J Obstet Anesth* 1995; **4**: 145–9.

5 Why mothers die. Report on Confidential Enquiries into Maternal Deaths in the United Kingdom 1994–96. London: Stationery Office; 1998.

6 Report on Confidential Enquiries into Maternal Deaths, 1997–99. London: Stationery Office; 2001.

7 Yentis SM, Steer P, Plaat F. Eisenmenger's syndrome in pregnancy: maternal and fetal mortality in the 1990s. *Br J Obstet Gynaecol* 1998; **105**: 921–2.

8 Chan WS, Anand S, Ginsberg JS. Anticoagulation of pregnant women with mechanical heart valves. A systematic review of the literature. *Arch Int Med* 2000; **160**: 191–6.

9 Suntharalingam G, Dob D, Yentis SM. Obstetric epidural analgesia in aortic stenosis: a low-dose technique for labour and instrumental delivery. *Int J Obstet Anesth* 2001; **10**: 129–34.

10 Brighouse D. Anaesthesia for Caesarean section in patients with aortic stenosis: the case for regional anaesthesia. *Anaesthesia* 1998; **53**: 107–9.

11 Whitfield A, Holdcroft A. Anaesthesia for Caesarean section in patients with aortic stenosis: the case for general anaesthesia. *Anaesthesia* 1998; **53**: 109–12.

12 Weis FR, Markello R, Mo B, Bochiechio P. Cardiovascular effects of oxytocin. *Obstet Gynecol* 1975; **46**: 211–14.

13 Nolan TE, Wakefield ML, Devoe LD. Invasive hemodynamic monitoring in obstetrics. A critical review of its indications, benefits, complications and alternatives. *Chest* 1992; **101**: 1429–33.

14 Stoddart P, O'Sullivan G. Eisenmenger's syndrome in pregnancy: a case report and review of the literature. *Int J Obstet Anesth* 1993; **2**: 159–68.

15 Bouvier-Colle MH, Varnoux N, Salanave B, *et al.* Case-control study of risk factors for obstetric patients' admission to intensive care units. *Eur J Obstet Gynecol Reprod Biol* 1997; **74**: 173–7.

16 Kilpatrick SJ, Matthay MA. Obstetric patients requiring critical care. A five-year review. *Chest* 1992; **101**: 1407–12.

17 Liu S, Wen SW, Demissie K, *et al.* Maternal asthma and pregnancy outcomes: a retrospective cohort study. *Am J Obstet Gynecol* 2001; **184**: 90–6.

18 Bose D, Fauvel NP, Yentis SM. Caesarean section in a parturient with respiratory failure caused by cystic fibrosis. *Anaesthesia* 1997; **52**: 578–81.

19 Edenborough FP, Stableforth DE, Webb AK, *et al.* Outcome of pregnancy in women with cystic fibrosis. *Thorax* 1995; **50**: 170–4.

20 Gilljam M, Antoniou M, Shin J, *et al.* Pregnancy in cystic fibrosis. Fetal and maternal outcome. *Chest* 2000; **118**: 85–91.

21 Confavreux C, Hutchinson M, Hours MM, *et al.* Rate of pregnancy-related relapse in multiple sclerosis. *N Engl J Med* 1998; **339**: 285–91.

22 Hilt H, Gramm HJ, Link J. Changes in intracranial pressure associated with extradural anaesthesia. *Br J Anaesth* 1986; **58**: 676–80.

23 Stackhouse RA, Hughes SC. Drug abuse and HIV disease in the obstetric patient: clinical issues in obstetric anaesthesia. *Curr Anaesth Crit Care* 2000; **11**: 97–103.

Part Ten

Infections and Immune Disorders

56.

Anaphylaxis

M M Fisher

Anaphylaxis is the symptom complex accompanying the acute reaction to a chemical recognized as hostile. Usually the patient has been previously sensitized (immediate hypersensitivity or type 1 hypersensitivity). The term anaphylactoid reaction is used to describe reactions clinically indistinguishable from anaphylaxis, in which the mechanism is non-immunological, or has not been determined. In conventional usage, the term 'anaphylaxis' implies severity, and anaphylactoid reactions are more common and less severe than anaphylactic reactions. Both conditions can be incorporated under the title 'clinical anaphylaxis'. The symptom complex may be produced by direct drug effects, physical factors or exercise, and a causative agent cannot always be determined. The mediators involved are the same as those in other acute inflammatory responses such as sepsis, but the rate of release is more rapid and of shorter duration.

AETIOLOGY

Clinical anaphylaxis in hospital commonly follows injection of drugs, blood products, plasma substitutes, contrast media, or exposure to latex products. Outside hospital drugs, ingestion of foods or food additives (especially peanut products) or insect stings are the common causes.

Neuget *et al.*[1] estimated 1400–1500 deaths per year in the USA and between 3.3 and 40.9 million patients at risk. They estimated radiocontrast media and penicillin to be the greatest cause of death with food and stings the next groups. In contrast a post mortem study of 56 deaths in the United Kingdom[2] attributed 19 deaths to venoms, 16 to foods and 19 to drugs and radiocontrast media.

In anaphylaxis, sensitization occurs following exposure to an allergenic substance, which either alone, or by combination with a protein or hapten, stimulates the synthesis of immunoglobulin E (IgE). Some IgE binds to the surface of mast cells and basophils. Later, re-exposure to antigen produces an antigen-cell surface IgE antibody interaction where two IgE molecules are bridged. This results in mast cell degranulation and the release of histamine and other mediators, including interleukin, prostaglandins, and platelet-activating factor. Histamine is responsible for the early signs and symptoms, but is rapidly cleared from plasma. The overall effects of the mediators are to produce vasodilatation, smooth muscle contraction, increased glandular secretion and increased capillary permeability. The mediators act both locally and upon distant target organs.

Anaphylactoid reactions have trigger mechanisms other than direct histamine release. Some intravenous drugs and X-ray contrast media may activate the complement system. Plasma protein and human serum albumin reactions may be induced by either albumin aggregates or stabilizing agent-modified albumin molecules. Other reactions, including those to dextrans and gelatin preparations, may be activated by non IgE antibody already present in the plasma or osmotic factors (dextrose, mannitol).

The direct histamine-releasing effects of some drugs may produce reactions due to the effect of histamine alone, and such reactions are related to volume, rate and amount of infusion. Recent work suggests that the site of release of histamine may be important in its clinical effects. Drugs such as morphine release histamine from skin alone,[3] and are unlikely to produce symptoms such as asthma, whereas drugs which produce release from lung mast cells (e.g. atracurium, vecuronium and propofol) may be more likely to produce bronchospasm.[4] Direct histamine release is usually a transient phenomenon, but in some patients severe manifestations may occur, particularly with Haemaccel and vancomycin.

Anaphylactic reactions are usually seen in fit patients. It is likely that the adrenal response to stress 'pretreats' sick patients, and blocks the release and effects of anaphylactic mediators. The exception to this appears to be patients with asthma, in whom reactions to the additives in steroid and aminophylline preparations may occur, and this may be related to the reduced catecholamine response in asthma.[5] Patients on β-blockers and with epidural blockade may be more likely to develop adverse responses due to histamine release, and this may also be related to reduced catecholamine responsiveness. Reactions occurring in these groups are more difficult to treat.

CLINICAL PRESENTATION

The latent period between exposure and development of symptoms is variable, but usually occurs within 5 min if the provoking agent is given parenterally. Reactions may be transient or protracted (lasting days), and may vary in severity from mild to fatal. Recurrent anaphylaxis is described. Cutaneous, cardiovascular, respiratory or gastrointestinal manifestations may occur singly or in combination. The incidence of clinical features is shown in Table 56.1.

Cutaneous features include erythematous flush, generalized or localized urticaria, angioneurotic oedema, conjunctival injection, pallor and cyanosis. Awake patients may experience an aura, warning of an impending reaction. Cardiovascular system involvement occurs most commonly and may occur as a sole clinical manifestation. It is characterized by initial bradycardia then sinus tachycardia, hypotension and the development of shock. Respiratory manifestations include rhinitis, bronchospasm and laryngeal obstruction. Gastrointestinal symptoms of nausea, vomiting, abdominal cramps and diarrhoea may be present. Other features include apprehension, metallic taste, choking sensation, coughing, paraesthesiae, arthralgia, convulsions, clotting abnormalities and loss of consciousness. Pulmonary oedema is a rare sign.

Anaphylaxis is rare in the ICU, probably because of the protective effects of the adrenal response to stress. Recently, use of the mast cell tryptase assay (see below) has detected anaphylaxis as an unsuspected cause of shock in intensive care.

PATHOPHYSIOLOGY OF CARDIOVASCULAR CHANGES

The traditional concept of the cardiovascular changes in clinical anaphylaxis is that of an initial vasodilatation, followed by capillary leak of plasma which produces endogenous hypovolaemia, reduced venous return and lowered cardiac output.

Whether or not cardiac function is impaired has been controversial. Although most anaphylactic mediators adversely affect myocardial function *in vitro*, most case reports of anaphylaxis in which invasive cardiovascular monitoring has been used suggest minimal impairment of cardiac function. Patients with normal cardiac function before the reaction rarely show evidence of cardiac failure or arrhythmias other than supraventricular tachycardia, but the incidence of serious arrhythmias and cardiac failure increases in those with prior cardiac disease.[6] Two reactions in patients with no previous cardiac disease where the major manifestation was prolonged global myocardial dysfunction and the use of a balloon counterpulsator was life-saving have been reported.[7]

TREATMENT

There are no randomized controlled trials of treatment in anaphylaxis and the unexpected onset, rapid course, and usual rapid response to treatment preclude performing such trials. Treatment recommendations are based on historical practice, case reports, series of cases, and animal models.

OXYGEN

Oxygen is given by facemask. Endotracheal intubation may be required to facilitate ventilation, especially if angioedema or laryngeal oedema is present. Oedema of the upper airway is more common when anaphylaxis is due to foods than to drugs.[2] Mechanical ventilation is indicated for severe bronchospasm, apnoea or cardiac arrest.

Table 56.1 Clinical features of anaphylaxis in 700 patients.

	Number	Sole feature	Worst feature
Cardiovascular collapse	612	75	548
Bronchospasm	268	34	127
Transient	104		
Asthmatics	98		
Cutaneous			
Rash	103		
Erythema	310		
Urticaria	59		
More than one	38		
Angioedema	167	9	22
Generalized oedema	43		
Pulmonary oedema	18	1	3
Gastrointestinal	39		

EPINEPHRINE

Epinephrine is universally recommended as the drug of choice for severe reactions. In the community epinephrine may be given intramuscularly in a dose of 0.3–1.0 mg early in anaphylaxis. Intramuscular epinephrine produces higher levels earlier in stable allergic patients than subcutaneous epinephrine.[8] In severe shock or in patients in whom muscle blood flow is thought to be compromised by shock, intravenous injection of 3–5 ml of 1:10 000 epinephrine is given. A second dose is necessary in 35%[9] and an infusion in 10%.

Epinephrine, by increasing intracellular levels of cyclic adenosine monophosphate (cAMP) in leukocytes and mast cells, inhibits further release of histamine. It has beneficial effects on myocardial contractility, peripheral vascular tone and bronchial smooth muscle. A common management error is not to institute external cardiac massage (ECM) as the arrhythmia is 'benign'. If the patient is pulseless, ECM should be instituted irrespective of rhythm, although there is no data to support its efficacy.

There has been controversy regarding the best route of administration of epinephrine outside hospital. Both case reports and patients self injecting show efficacy for intramuscular epinephrine when given early. Intravenous epinephrine may cause arrythmias and myocardial infarction particularly in unmonitored patients. Recent recommendations endorse the use of intramuscular epinephrine.[10]

OTHER SYMPATHOMIMETIC DRUGS

Other sympathomimetic drugs may reverse the symptoms, but appear (albeit in the absence of any randomized trials) to be less effective than adrenaline.

NOREPINEPHRINE

Norepinephrine by infusion may be life saving in the absence of a response to fluid loading and epinephrine.

COLLOIDS

Plasma expanders are given rapidly to correct the hypovolaemia consequent to acute vasodilatation and leakage of fluid from the intravascular space.[11] The author favours plasma protein solution, dextran 70 or gelatin preparations rather than crystalloids, as they remain in the vascular compartment earlier and for longer. There is, however, no data showing improved outcomes from colloid over crystalloid and there are many patients resuscitated successfully with either crystalloid or colloid alone. Greater volumes of crystalloid are necessary and on occasions very large volumes of fluid may be required and central venous pressure (CVP) monitoring and measurement of haematocrit are helpful.

BRONCHOSPASM

Nebulized salbutamol should be given for severe asthma. Aminophylline 5–6 mg/kg i.v. may be given over 30 min, if bronchospasm is unresponsive to epinephrine alone. Aminophylline increases intracellular cAMP by phosphodiesterase inhibition, and its effect on inhibiting histamine and interleukin release is theoretically additive to that of epinephrine. Adverse responses have not been observed in our series but a recent comprehensive review[12] suggested safer agents with proven efficacy should be preferred. Volatile anaesthesia, ketamine and magnesium sulphate may produce improvement in some patients with severe asthma.

CORTICOSTEROIDS

Steroids have no proven benefit, particularly early, and should be reserved for refractory bronchospasm. Conversely, steroids are often given and there is likewise no evidence of harm.

ANTIHISTAMINES

Antihistamines are the treatment of choice in localized non severe reactions. In severe reactions they are only indicated in protracted cases or in those with angioneurotic oedema which may recur. The data on antihistamines are not conclusive, but in protracted anaphylaxis, improvement is often reported with H_2 blockers.

DIAGNOSIS

The most important advance in the diagnosis of anaphylaxis has been the introduction of an assay for mast cell tryptase. The mast cell enzyme is elevated 1 h after a reaction begins, and the elevation may persist for up to 4 h. It can also be used to diagnose anaphylaxis from post mortem specimens.[13,14] The assay is highly specific and sensitive for anaphylaxis, although elevated levels are found with direct histamine release, and at post mortem in some patients with myocardial infarction.

FOLLOW-UP

Following successful acute management, the drug or agent responsible should be determined by *in vitro* or *in vivo* testing if possible. Hyposensitization should be considered for food, pollen and bee-sting allergy. A medic-alert bracelet should be worn and the patient given a letter stating the nature of the reaction to the particular causative agent.

If re-exposure to the allergen is likely at home, patients or their relatives should be instructed in the use of epinephrine, salbutamol inhalation and antihistamines. Clinical anaphylaxis may be modified by pretreatment with disodium cromoglycate, corticosteroids, antihistamines, salbutamol and isoprenaline.

In patients with recurrent anaphylaxis in whom no cause can be found corticosteroids on alternate days reduce the incidence and severity of attacks.

REFERENCES

1 Neugut AL, Ghatak AT, Miller RL. Anaphylaxis in the United States: an investigation into its epidemiology. *Arch Int Med.* 2001; **161**: 15–21.

2 Pumphrey RS, Roberts IS. Postmortem findings after fatal anaphylactic reactions. *J Clin Path* 2000; **53**: 273–6.

3 Tharp MD, Kagey-Sobotka A, Fox CC, *et al.* Functional heterogeneity of human mast cells from different anatomic sites: in vitro responses to morphine sulphate. *J Allergy Clin Immunol* 1987; **79**: 646–53.

4 Stellato C, de Paulis A, Cirillo R, *et al.* Heterogeneity of human mast cells and basophils in response to muscle relaxants. *Anesthesiology* 1991; **74**: 1078–86.

5 Ind PW, Causon RC, Brown MJ, Barnes PJ. Circulating catecholamines in acute asthma. *Br Med J* 1985; **290**: 267–9.

6 Fisher MM. Clinical observations on the pathophysiology and treatment of anaphylactic cardiovascular collapse. *Anaesth Intens Care* 1986; **14**: 17–21.

7 Raper RF, Fisher MM. Profound reversible myocardial depression following human anaphylaxis. *Lancet* 1988; **8582**: 386–8.

8 Simons FE, Roberts JR, Gu X, Simons KJ. Epinephrine absorption in children with a history of anaphylaxis. *J All Clin Immunol* 1988; **101**: 33–7.

9 Korenblat P, Lundie MJ, Dankner RE, Day JH. A retrospective study of epinephrine administration for anaphylaxis: how many doses are needed. *Allergy Asthma Proceedings* 1988; **20**: 83–6.

10 Project team of the Resuscitation Council UK. Emergency medical treatment of anaphylactic reactions. *Resuscitation* 1999; **41**: 93–9.

11 Fisher MM. Blood volume replacement in acute anaphylactic cardiovascular collapse related to anaesthesia. *Br J Anaesth* 1977; **49**: 1023–6.

12 Ernst ME, Graber MA. Methylxanthine use in anaphylaxis: what does the evidence tell us? *Annals Pharmacotherapy* 1999; **33**: 1001–4.

13 Yunginger JW, Nelson DR, Squilace DL. Laboratory investigation of deaths due to anaphylaxis. *J Forensic Sci* 1991; **36**: 857–65.

14 Fisher MM, Baldo BA. The diagnosis of fatal anaphylactic reactions during anaesthesia: employment of immunoassays for mast cell tryptase and drug-reaction IgE antibodies. *Anaesth Intens Care* 1993; **21**: 353–7.

57

Host defence failure and immunodeficiency

S Wesselingh and M A H French

There is a coordinated immunological response to infection involving both cellular and humoral components. The outcome of an infection will be determined by the balance between the body's ability to eliminate invading micro-organisms and the micro-organism's virulence. Humans have diverse host defence mechanisms to protect the different anatomical compartments of the body from a great variety of micro-organisms (see Table 57.1). There are many ways in which the immune system can be defective, leading to an increased propensity to infections. The immune response also needs to be controlled to avoid inappropriate and excessive activation, which may damage the host. A certain degree of host damage is inevitable during the response to infection, particularly if there is systemic activation resulting in disseminated intravascular coagulation (DIC) and an excessive inflammatory response.

HOST DEFENCE MECHANISMS

INNATE IMMUNE RESPONSES

The immune system is capable of reacting to micro-organisms without having been previously exposed to antigens from those micro-organisms. This innate immune system consists of plasma proteins, including alternative pathway components of the complement system and mannose binding lectin (MBL), a subset of lymphocytes with cytotoxic activity (natural killer or NK cells), and some macrophage functions. Innate immune responses provide a first line of defence against many pathogenic micro-organisms.

ACUTE PHASE REACTION

The acute phase reaction is a response of the haematopoietic and hepatic systems, involving at least 20 plasma proteins and the cellular components of the blood. The reaction occurs within hours of acute physical stress or infection. The functions of many of these acute-phase proteins remains unclear, but teleologically, they should be assumed to be beneficial to the patient. The falls in haemoglobin, serum iron and albumin are all

Table 57.1 Host defence mechanisms

Physical barriers
    Skin and mucosal surfaces
    Cilia
Fever
Lysozyme
Lactoferrin
Acute-phase proteins, e.g. C-reactive protein
Fibronectin
Mannose binding lectin
Immune system, including secondary mediators
Other mediators of inflammation
    Kinins
    Vasoactive amines
    Coagulation system

normal in the acute-phase reaction. Most of the proteins are inflammatory mediators or inhibitors of transport proteins. Fibrinogen, the bulk protein of the coagulation system, is one of the plasma proteins to show the greatest rise in the acute-phase reaction, and is responsible for the elevation in the erythrocyte sedimentation rate. The fall in albumin is due to redistribution and decreased synthesis and generally does not require supplementation.

THE ADAPTIVE IMMUNE SYSTEM

Adaptive immune responses are characterized by specificity, memory, amplification and diversity. The specificity of an immune response against a particular antigenic component of a micro-organism, and the memory which results in a prompt response on subsequent exposures, is determined by lymphocytes and antigen receptors on their surface. Amplification and diversity of immune responses is regulated by cytokines, which are secreted by lymphocytes and other cells, and through the effects of various lymphocyte surface molecules, including adhesion molecules and activation proteins. Cytokines which have immunoregulatory actions include the interleukins (of which there are at least 20), tumour necrosis factor (TNF), lymphotoxins and interferon-gamma (IFN-γ).

ANTIGEN PRESENTATION

The most important events in the initiation of an immune response are the processing and presentation of fragments of the micro-organism in a form which makes the fragments antigenic to lymphocytes. Major histocompatibility complex (MHC) class I (human leukocyte antigen (HLA)-A, B, C) and class II (HLA-DR, DP, DQ) molecules are the major cell-surface antigen presentation molecules. These molecules also determine the nature of the subsequent response against the antigen. Class I MHC molecules are present on most nucleated cells, and present processed endogenous peptides (such as fragments of viruses) to the antigen receptor (T-cell receptor; TcR) of T-cells expressing CD8 molecules. Class II MHC molecules present antigenic fragments of micro-organisms which are exogenous to cells and have been taken into the cell by phagocytosis, in the case of macrophages and monocytes, or by binding to antigen-specific surface immunoglobulins (the B-cell antigen receptor), in the case of B-cells. Antigens presented on class II MHC molecules bind to TcRs on CD4+ T-cells.

T-CELLS AND B-CELLS

CD8+ T-cells have a cytotoxic effect on cells expressing class I MHC-associated viral antigens, resulting in the death of the cell and inhibition of viral replication. Antigen-induced stimulation of CD4+ T-cells results in activation of the T-cell and the expression of cell-surface molecules and secretion of cytokines with immunoregulatory effects. These immunoregulatory molecules augment the functions of many other cells, including B-cells, T-cells and macrophages (T-cell help). A response to an antigen directed by CD4+ T-cells may also elicit macrophage activation and killing of the micro-organism expressing that antigen. Activation of macrophages by CD4+ T-cells is critically dependent on the production of IFN-γ.

The activation and proliferation of T-cells occurs under the influence of cytokines and other regulatory molecules, including T-cell membrane activation molecules such as the ligand of the B-cell membrane molecule CD40 (CD40L). Proliferating B-cells differentiate into plasma cells, which secrete immunoglobulins with antibody activity against the initiating antigen. Nine isotypes of immunoglobulin can be produced, each of which has a different function.

IMMUNOGLOBULINS

Immunoglobulin M (IgM) is a large pentameric molecule, which is particularly effective as a bacterial agglutinator and activator of the complement system, and has its major effect within the circulation. IgA1 and IgA2 are produced at secretory surfaces, such as the mucosa of the gut and respiratory tract, and also in the breast, where IgA is a major constituent of the colostrum and provides secretory antibody to the gut of the neonate. IgE antibodies are also produced at mucosal surfaces where they form an important part of the immune response against parasitic infections. Antibodies of the IgG1 and IgG3 subclass are particularly effective at activating the complement system and binding to Fc receptors on phagocytic cells. IgG2 antibodies are mainly active against polysaccharide antigens, such as those present in bacterial cell walls. The functions of IgG4 antibodies are unclear.

SECONDARY ANTIBODY FUNCTION

The elimination of a micro-organism by antibodies usually requires the activation of a secondary effector mechanism, of which there are several. The complement system consists of plasma proteins, which are sequentially activated by either antigen–antibody complexes through the classical pathway, or directly by components of micro-organisms through the alternative pathway. Activation of the complement system results in the generation of biologically active molecules, such as C3b, which is an important opsonin, and the activation of the membrane attack complex (MAC), which lyses bacterial cell walls. Like C3b, antibodies of the IgM, IgG1 and IgG3 isotype are also important opsonins. These molecules, when bound to the surface of a micro-organism, facilitate their opsonization and phagocytosis. These effects of complement and antibody are mediated through complement receptors (CRs) and receptors for the Fc portion of the immunoglobulin molecules (Fc receptors) on the phagocytic cell surface. The most important phagocytic cells are neutrophils and macrophages.

Th1/Th2 RESPONSES

The type of immune response produced against a micro-organism varies according to the nature of the infecting organism. Thus, virus-infected cells elicit a cytotoxic CD8+ T-cell response; intracellular pathogens such as mycobacteria and protozoa elicit a CD4+ T-cell response, which results in macrophage activation; encapsulated bacteria elicit an opsonizing antibody response; and some bacteria such as *Neisseria* spp. elicit a complement-activating antibody response, which lyses the cell wall of the bacterium. The nature of the immune response is regulated by cytokines, which provide T-cell help (Th) in the course of an immune responses. Thus, interleukin(IL)-2, IL-12 and IFN-γ production induces a predominantly cellular immune response (Th1), whereas the production of IL-4, IL-6 and IL-10 induces a predominantly antibody-mediated immune response (Th2).

IMMUNE DEFECTS UNDERLYING IMMUNODEFICIENCY SYNDROMES

Defects of the immune system that give rise to an immunodeficiency syndrome are generally of four types: antibody deficiency, cellular immunodeficiency, complement deficiency and phagocyte defects. Combined defects of antibody- and cell-mediated immune responses are referred to as combined immunodeficiency. In addition, patients with asplenism, and multi-organ failure will have degrees of immunodeficiency and will also be discussed.

ANTIBODY DEFICIENCY

A deficient systemic antibody response most commonly results in a lack of opsonizing antibody, and a propensity to infections with encapsulated bacteria such as pneumococci as well as *Haemophilus influenzae*. Recurrent respiratory tract infections including sinusitis are therefore the most common complication of this type of immune defect. Much less commonly, patients may develop chronic echovirus infections of the nervous system and infections with some mycoplasmas.

Deficient secretory antibody responses are common in patients with IgA deficiency, but most affected individuals are able to produce compensatory secretory IgM or IgG antibody responses and do not suffer from infections.

CELLULAR IMMUNODEFICIENCY

Impairment of cell-mediated immune responses leads to an increased propensity to infection with micro-organisms which are normally controlled by cellular immunity (Table 57.2). In general, these micro-organisms are intracellular pathogens, which cause persistent (latent) infections that reactivate when the cellular immune response against them becomes ineffective.

Table 57.2 Common micro-organisms causing disease in patients with cellular immunodeficiency

Protozoa	Toxoplasma gondii
	Cryptosporidia
Mycobacteria	Mycobacterium tuberculosis
	Non-tuberculous (atypical) mycobacteria
Bacteria	Salmonella spp.
	Shigella spp.
	Listeria monocytogenes
	Pneumocystis carinii
Fungi and yeasts	Candida spp. (mucosal infections)
	Cryptococci
	Aspergillus spp.
	Dermatophytes
	Pityrosporon spp.
Viruses	Herpes viruses
	Cytomegalovirus
	Varicella-zoster
	Herpes simplex
	Epstein–Barr virus
	Molluscum contagiosum virus
	JC virus (progressive multifocal leukoencephalopathy)

COMPLEMENT DEFICIENCY

Complement-mediated lysis of bacterial cell walls is a critical mechanism in the immune response against certain bacteria, especially *Neisseria* spp. and related bacteria such as *Moraxella* spp and *Acinetobacter* spp. Deficiency of complement components, particularly MAC components (C5–C9), may therefore result in infection with these bacteria. C3b is an important opsonin and C3 deficiency will often impair phagocytosis of bacteria. Deficiency of classical pathway components may also result in impaired antibody responses.

PHAGOCYTE DEFECTS

Depletion or functional impairment of phagocytes results in an increased propensity to bacterial and fungal infections, particularly infection with *Staphylococcus aureus*, gram-negative enteric bacteria, *Candida* spp and *Aspergillus* spp. Fungal and yeast infections are often systemic in patients with severe neutropenia, indicating the importance of phagocytes in the systemic immune response against these micro-organisms.

Phagocytosis of a bacterium or fungus by a neutrophil leukocyte or macrophage is dependent on chemotactic attraction of phagocytes to the site of infection, their adhesion to endothelial cells via adhesion molecules such as integrins, binding to opsonins on the microorganism, ingestion and intracellular killing. Intracellular killing involves both oxidative and non-oxidative mechanisms. Primary or acquired defects of phagocytes may result in localized pyogenic infections or pneumonia. However, in the neutropenic patient, localized infections may show little inflammatory reaction and overwhelming systemic infections are common.

IMMUNODEFICIENCY DISEASES

Immunodeficiency diseases are classified as primary or acquired. Primary immunodeficiency diseases are the result of a developmental anomaly or a genetically-determined defect of the immune system. Genetically determined defects are usually of two types:

1 The consequence of an absent or non-functional gene product, which is critical for the normal development or function of a component of the immune system.
2 Aberrant regulation of lymphocyte differentiation, which is probably determined by the products of several genes and possibly by environmental factors.

Immunodeficiency diseases caused by the latter type of defect usually present later in life than congenital immunodeficiency caused by a non-functioning gene product.

Acquired immunodeficiency syndromes are more common than primary immunodeficiency syndromes and may present at any time after early childhood. Most result from an immune defect that is a consequence of a disease process (disease-related immunodeficiency) or therapy for a disease, such as immunosuppressant therapy (therapy-related immunodeficiency).

Diagnosis of an immunodeficiency syndrome in a patient with an abnormal propensity to infections is dependent on the demonstration of an immune defect, as indicated in Table 57.3.

ANTIBODY DEFICIENCY

PRIMARY ANTIBODY DEFICIENCY SYNDROMES

Failure of B-cell production or the presence of immature B-cells due to a defect of differentiation are the cause of most primary antibody deficiency syndromes.[1] B-cells are absent from blood and secondary lymphoid tissues in patients with X-linked agammaglobulinaemia (XLA) because mutations of the Btk gene on the X-chromosome result in the absence of a B-cell tyrosine kinase necessary for the maturation of pre-B-cells to B-cells in the bone marrow. In the hyper-IgM immunodeficiency syndrome, B-cells are able to differentiate into plasma cells secreting IgM, but not IgG or IgA. The X-linked form of this condition results from mutations in the gene of CD40L, which is critical in delivering a T-cell signal to differentiating B-cells.

Common variable immunodeficiency (CVID) and IgA deficiency appear to be the consequence of an immunoregulatory defect which results in impaired B-cell differentiation. Hypogammaglobulinaemia and systemic antibody deficiency are characteristic of CVID, whereas most individuals with IgA deficiency are asymptomatic. Those IgA-deficient patients who suffer from recurrent infections often have a defect of systemic antibody responses, which commonly manifests as deficiency of an IgG subclass and/or impairment of antibody responses to polysaccharide antigens.[2]

The immunoregulatory defect underlying CVID and IgA deficiency sometimes results in an increased propensity to autoimmunity, which can include the production of anti-IgA antibodies. These antibodies may be the cause of anaphylactoid reactions to blood products.

ACQUIRED ANTIBODY DEFICIENCY SYNDROMES
Disease-related

B-cell chronic lymphocytic leukaemia or lymphoma and myeloma are commonly associated with reduced synthesis of normal immunoglobulins, which may result in antibody deficiency and bacterial infections.[3] A thymoma is also

Table 57.3 Tests of immunocompetence

Antibody-mediated immunity
 Serum immunoglobulins, including IgG subclasses
 Systemic antibody responses (after vaccination if necessary)
  Polysaccharide antigens, e.g. pneumococcal
  Protein antigen, e.g. tetanus toxoid
 Blood B-cell (CD19+, CD20+) numbers
Cell-mediated immunity
 Delayed-type hypersensitivity (DTH) skin test responses
  Multitest CMI method
  Mantoux method
 Blood T-cell (CD3+) and T-cell subset (CD4+ or CD8+) numbers
Phagocyte function
 Blood neutrophil numbers
 Tests of oxidative killing mechanisms, e.g. NBT test
 Leukocyte expression of CR3 (a CD18 integrin)
 Neutrophil migration assays
 Bacteria or *Candida* killing assays
Complement system
 Immunochemical quantitation of individual components
 Functional assays of the classical pathway (CH50) or alternative pathway (AH50)

IgG, immunoglobulin G; DTH, delayed-type hypersensitivity; CMI, cell-mediated immunity; NBT, nitroblue tetrazolium.

sometimes associated with hypogammaglobulinaemia, and should always be considered in a patient presenting with primary hypogammaglobulinaemia after the age of 40.[4]

Impaired production of antibodies against polysaccharide antigens contributes to the susceptibility which postsplenectomy patients have to infection with encapsulated bacteria, such as pneumococci and meningococci.[5]

Therapy-related

Drugs occasionally affect B-cell differentiation and cause immunoglobulin deficiency, particularly IgA deficiency. The most common offender is phenytoin. Most patients do not have antibody deficiency severe enough to cause infections. Intensive plasmapheresis may also cause severe immunoglobulin deficiency if immunoglobulin replacement is not used.

TREATMENT OF ANTIBODY DEFICIENCY DISEASE

Infections can be prevented by regular infusions of intravenous immunoglobulin (IVIG) in patients with primary or acquired antibody deficiency. The usual dose is 300–500 mg/kg given monthly. Acute infections should be treated with appropriate antibiotics. The use of IVIG as an adjunct in the management of sepsis, particularly pneumococcal infections, has been suggested. In the absence of documented antibody deficiency there is no evidence to support this practice.

CELLULAR IMMUNODEFICIENCY

PRIMARY CELLULAR IMMUNODEFICIENCY SYNDROMES

Complete or partial absence of the thymus gland resulting in depletion of T-cells from blood and lymphoid tissue is the characteristic immunological abnormality in children with the Di George syndrome.[6] Infections of the type listed in Table 57.2 occur from birth onwards. A less severe defect of cellular immunity is present in patients with chronic mucocutaneous candidiasis.[7] This syndrome is the result of several poorly defined immune defects, which result in an abnormal propensity to mucocutaneous infections with *Candida* spp. and other fungi.

ACQUIRED CELLULAR IMMUNODEFICIENCY SYNDROMES

Acquired defects of cellular immunity are by far the most common cause of cellular immunodeficiency.

Disease Related

Cellular immunodeficiency resulting from infection of the immune system by human immunodeficiency viruses (HIVs) 1 and 2 is common (see Chapter 58). Less commonly, Hodgkin's disease, T-cell lymphomas and sarcoidosis may also be complicated by opportunistic infections occurring as a consequence of cellular immunodeficiency. A thymoma may be associated with a chronic mucocutaneous candidiasis syndrome which, like thymoma and hypogammaglobulinaemia, occurs later in life.[4]

Therapy Related

Suppression of cellular immune responses is an intended effect of many immunosuppressant drugs used to treat allograft rejection, graft-versus-host disease (GVHD), autoimmune diseases and vasculitis. Opportunistic infections are a complication of this type of immunodeficiency, and may cause severe morbidity and death.

TREATMENT OF CELLULAR IMMUNODEFICIENCY DISEASES

Since most infections complicating cellular immunodeficiency are reactivated latent infections, an important aspect of management is prevention of infection by the use of prophylactic antimicrobial drugs, as exemplified by HIV-induced immunodeficiency.[8] In circumstances of acquired cellular immunodeficiency it is essential to take into account the degree and duration of immunodeficiency. It is possible to predict the likelihood of infection and the likely pathogens by determining the degree of cellular immunodeficiency. This allows for appropriate decisions to be made regarding investigations, treatment and prophylaxis.

Acquired cellular immunodeficiency may be corrected, at least temporarily, by removing its cause (e.g. by suppressing HIV infection or ceasing immunosuppressive therapy). Thymus transplantation may be effective in children with thymus aplasia.

COMPLEMENT DEFICIENCY

Deficiency of complement components is an uncommon but often overlooked cause of recurrent bacterial infections.

PRIMARY COMPLEMENT DEFICIENCY

Congenital deficiency of C3 is extremely rare and usually causes a propensity to severe pyogenic infections. Deficiency of MAC components (C5–9) is more common, and should be considered in patients with meningococcal infections, particularly when the infections are recurrent.[9] Deficiency of classical pathway components (C1, C2, C4) may also result in an increased propensity to infection with meningococci and some other bacteria, but most affected individuals do not experience recurrent infections.

ACQUIRED COMPLEMENT DEFICIENCY
Disease Related

Disease processes, which cause persistent activation of the complement system, may cause depletion of complement components, particularly classical pathway components. This can result in infections with *Neisseria* spp. or related bacteria, and sometimes overwhelming septicaemia when the complement deficiency is severe. Systemic lupus erythematous, myeloma and chronic atrioventricular shunt infections are the commonest causes.

MANAGEMENT OF PATIENTS WITH COMPLEMENT DEFICIENCY

An awareness of the possibility of complement deficiency is the most important aspect of management. If a complement deficiency is identified, appropriate prophylaxis can be implemented.

PHAGOCYTE DEFECTS

PRIMARY PHAGOCYTE DEFECTS

Congenital neutropenias are rare. Defects of phagocyte function usually affect chemotaxis, adhesion or intracellular killing, either alone or in combination. The best characterized defect of phagocyte adherence results from a congenital absence of the β-subunit of CD18 integrins in patients with leukocyte adhesion deficiency syndrome Type 1.[10] Defects of intracellular killing are usually caused by a deficiency of an enzyme critical for the functioning of killing mechanisms. In chronic granulomatous disease (CGD), deficiency of a phagosome enzyme (NADPH oxidase) results in ineffective oxidative killing mechanisms.[11] CGD usually presents in childhood but may present in adults, even as late as the seventh decade.[12] It should be considered in patients with recurrent abscesses or suppurative lymphadenitis, and in patients with pneumonia caused by *Staphylococcus aureus* or *Aspergillus* spp. infection.

ACQUIRED PHAGOCYTE DEFECTS
Disease Associations

Severe neutropenia may be complicated by bacterial or fungal infections. There are many causes of neutropenia, including autoimmune neutropenia, drug therapy and haematological diseases such as cyclic neutropenia, myelodysplastic syndromes and aplastic anaemia.

Therapy Related
Cytotoxic chemotherapy, used to treat various malignancies, commonly causes neutropenia, which is often complicated by severe bacterial and fungal infections.

TREATMENT OF PHAGOCYTE DEFECTS
Acquired neutropenia may be corrected by removing the underlying cause and/or use of granulocyte colony stimulating factor (G-CSF). Febrile neutropenia requires investigation for the source of sepsis and empirical antibiotics. If fever persists antifungals should be added. IFN-γ therapy may be effective in patients with CGD.

COMBINED IMMUNODEFICIENCY SYNDROMES

Several immunodeficiency syndromes result from a combination of immune defects. Some combinations of congenital immune defects are so severe that death is a common occurrence, unless the defect can be corrected. Such conditions are classified as severe combined immune deficiency (SCID) syndromes. Patients heavily treated with immunosuppressive therapy, e.g. heart-lung transplants, or bone marrow transplant patients may develop an acquired combined immunodeficiency syndrome.

PRIMARY COMBINED IMMUNODEFICIENCY DISEASES
There are many primary combined immunodeficiency syndromes, which present in early childhood.[13] Some are still classified descriptively, but the molecular defects have now been demonstrated for many of them. For example, defective expression of MHC class II molecules, adenosine deaminase (ADA) deficiency, and deficiency of the common γ-chain (γc) of the receptor for several interleukins (IL-2, 4, 7, 9, 15, 21) all result in a deficiency and/or functional impairment of B-cells, T-cells and sometimes NK cells. Deficiency of the interleukin receptor γc- chain results from mutations of its gene on the X-chromosome and is the underlying defect of X-linked SCID.

ACQUIRED COMBINED IMMUNODEFICIENCY DISEASES
Bone Marrow Transplantation

Combined immune defects can result in severe infections in patients who have received a bone marrow transplantation.[14] Following transplantation, the recipient's immune system is reconstituted with donor cells. A degree of immunocompetence is passively transferred from the donor to recipient by antigen-specific lymphocytes, but as this and any residual immunocompetence of the recipient declines, an immunodeficient state exists until the donor immune system is established. Consequently, both antibody-mediated and cell-mediated immunity are deficient in the first 3–4 months after transplantation and may remain deficient for a longer period of time in patients with graft versus host disease (GVHD). This combined immune defect is often compounded by neutropenia and/or the effects of corticosteroid or immunosuppressant therapy for GVHD. Defective antibody responses may persist for 1–2 years after transplantation, particularly antibody responses against polysaccharide antigens.

Critically Ill Patients
Many patients who are critically ill as a result of surgery, trauma, thermal injury or overwhelming sepsis also have acquired immune defects.[15] These defects include abnormalities of cellular immunity, immunoglobulin deficiency and impaired neutrophil function. They appear to be associated with an increased propensity to infections and arise from abnormalities that are complex and multifactorial. Impairment of cell-mediated immune responses usually manifests as decreased T-cell proliferation and impaired delayed-type hypersensitivity responses, and probably results from a combination of factors, including the effects of anaesthetic drugs, blood transfusion, negative nitrogen balance and serum suppressor factors, including cytokines such as TNF. Phagocyte defects are mostly due to impairment of neutrophil chemotaxis by serum factors, and impaired intracellular killing. Deficiency of serum immunoglobulins also occurs, especially IgG deficiency, and may be associated with antibody deficiency. Serum leakage is a factor in patients with thermal injuries, and reduced synthesis and increased catabolism of immunoglobulins occur in many critically ill patients.

TREATMENT OF COMBINED IMMUNODEFICIENCY DISEASES
Bone marrow transplantation is the treatment of choice for many types of primary SCID, though enzyme replacement therapy can be effective in ADA deficiency and gene replacement therapy has been used to treat X-linked SCID. Antibody replacement with IVIG therapy and prophylaxis for opportunistic infections are also important in primary SCID.

The correction of immune defects in critically ill patients has been intensely investigated, but no effective treatment regimen has been defined. General measures such as adequate nutrition, achieving a positive nitrogen balance and excision of thermally injured tissue are effective. Biological response modifiers, cytokine and mediator inhibitors, and IVIG therapy have all been evaluated. The number of acute infections, particularly pneumonia, can be reduced by the use of IVIG therapy, but patient survival is not increased.

Use of G-CSF

G-CSF levels are increased during critical illnesses and correlate with the severity of illness. Administration of G-CSF has been shown to be safe in intensive care patients with no apparent increases in acute respiratory distress syndrome or multiple organ dysfunction. However there is no current evidence that the administration of G-CSF improves outcome and until further evidence is presented G-CSF is not indicated in the treatment of critically ill ICU patients.

ASPLENISM

The spleen is an important part of the immune system's response to serious infections. In those people in whom the spleen is removed or does not function, best practice guidelines recommend lifelong education, vaccination and appropriate use of antibiotics. The risk of severe life-threatening infection related to splenectomy alone is in the order of 1 in 500 per annum with 50% mortality. The most common organisms identified with overwhelming post-splenectomy infection (OPSI) include encapsulated bacteria, such as pneumococcus, *Haemophilus influenzae*, and meningococcus for which vaccines are available. Other bacteria, which are sometimes important, include Group A Streptocccus, *Capnocytophagia canimorsus* following dog bites, Salmonella, Enterococcus and bacteroides.

Pneumococcus, *Haemophilus influenzae*, and meningococcus vaccines including regular boosters and annual influenza vaccine are recommended. This is consistent with US guidelines and broadly with UK guidelines, which make the last bacterial vaccine optional. Second, chemoprophylaxis with penicillin for at least 2 years after splenectomy, if the patient is not allergic, is indicated.

MICROBIOLOGICAL INVESTIGATION OF THE IMMUNODEFICIENT PATIENT

Advances in molecular biology have had significant impacts on the microbiological investigation of immunodeficient patients. The major advance in diagnostics has been the development of the polymerase chain reaction (PCR) and the application of this to the detection of small amounts of nucleic acid in body fluids. This has enabled the development of quick and very sensitive diagnostic assays. Following diagnosis, we now also have the capacity to monitor and optimise therapy.

SUMMARY: APPROACH TO THE IMMUNODEFICIENT PATIENT

1 Determine (a) type of immunodeficiency, (b) degree of immunodeficiency and (c) duration of immunodeficiency.

2 Predict (a) the likelihood of infection and (b) the type of infection.
3 Commence (a) empirical and (b) prophylactic therapy.
4 Targeted diagnostic tests.

REFERENCES

1 Buckley RH. Primary immunodeficiency diseases due to defects in lymphocytes. *N Engl J Med*. 2000; **343**: 1313–24.
2 French MAH, Denis K, Dawkins RL, Peter JB. Infection susceptibility in IgA deficiency: correlation with low polysaccharide antibodies and deficiency of IgG2 and/or IgG4. *Clin Exp Immunol* 1995; **100**: 47–53.
3 Tsiodras S, Samonis G, Keating MJ, Kontoyiannis DP. Infection and immunity in chronic lymphocytic leukemia. *Mayo Clin Proc* 2000; **75**: 1039–54.
4 Tarr PE, Sneller MC, Mechanic LJ, *et al*. Infections in patients with immunodeficiency with thymoma (Good syndrome). Report of 5 cases and review of the literature. *Medicine* (Baltimore) 2001; **80**: 123–33.
5 Di Padova F Durig, Wadstrom J, Harder F. Role of spleen in immune response to polyvalent pneumococcal vaccine. *BMJ* 1993; **287**: 1829–33.
6 Hong R. The DiGeorge anomaly. *Clin Rev Allergy Immunol* 2001; **20**: 43–60.
7 Kirkpatrick CH. Chronic mucocutaneous candidiasis. *Pediatr Infect Dis J* 2001; **20**: 197–206.
8 Kovacs JA, Masur H. Prophylaxis against opportunistic infections in patients with human immunodeficiency virus infection. *N Engl J Med* 2000; **342**: 1416–29.
9 Fijen CA, Kuijper EJ, te Bulte MT, *et al*. Assessment of complement deficiency in patients with meningococcal disease in The Netherlands. *Clin Infect Dis* 1999; **28**: 98–105.
10 Sullivan KE. Defects in adhesion molecules. *Clin Rev Allergy Immunol* 2000; **19**: 109–25.
11 Winkelstein JA, Marino MC, Johnston RB Jr, *et al*. Chronic granulomatous disease. Report on a national registry of 368 patients. *Medicine* (Baltimore). 2000; **79**: 155–69.
12 Schapiro BL, Newburger PE, Klempner MS, Dinauer MC. Chronic granulomatous disease presenting in a 69 year old man. *N Engl J Med* 1991; **325**: 1786–90.
13 Buckley RH. Advances in the understanding and treatment of human severe combined immunodeficiency. *Immunol Res* 2001; **22**: 237–51.
14 Ninin E, Milpied N, Moreau P, *et al*. Longitudinal study of bacterial, viral, and fungal infections in adult recipients of bone marrow transplants. *Clin Infect Dis* 2001; **33**: 41–7.
15 Napolitano LM, Faist E, Wichmann MW, Coimbra R. Immune dysfunction in trauma. *Surg Clin North Am* 1999; **79**: 1385–416.

58

HIV and acquired immunodeficency syndrome

S Wesselingh and M A H French

AETIOLOGY

Human immunodeficiency viruses (HIVs) 1 and 2 are retroviruses of the Lentivirus group. Like other lentiviruses, they exhibit tropism for cells of the immune system and cause immunological disorders, particularly immunodeficiency. Infection of immune cells in the nervous system may also cause neurological disease. Entry of HIV into cells of the immune system is via cell surface receptors. The major receptor is the CD4 molecule, but some chemokine receptors play an important role as co-receptors. Inside the cell, the viral RNA is reverse transcribed into DNA by a viral reverse transcriptase enzyme, and the DNA is incorporated into the DNA of the host cell as proviral DNA. The proviral DNA remains there until the cell is activated, when it is transcribed into RNA, which provides the template for assembly of new HIVs under the control of viral enzymes such as proteases. Budding of new virus from the cell is followed by infection of new cells and a repeat of the replication cycle.

PATHOPHYSIOLOGY

ACUTE HIV INFECTION

Initial infection by HIV-1 is associated with an acute HIV infection syndrome (also known as a seroconversion illness or primary HIV infection) in 50–70% of patients. This syndrome is similar to infectious mononucleosis, being characterized by fever, lymphadenopathy, headache, photophobia, fatigue and myalgia. However, mucocutaneous lesions, neurological disease and even transient immunodeficiency may also occur which, when present, differentiates it from infectious mononucleosis. It may take a number of weeks for HIV antibody (detected by enzyme linked immunosorbent assay [ELISA]) to become positive during acute seroconversion, however

the level of plasma HIV RNA is very high. The diagnostic test of choice during this period is the measurement of HIV viral load utilizing HIV RNA RT/PCR (reverse transcription of HIV RNA and amplification by polymerase chain reaction). HIV RNA peaks at a median of 10 days.[1]

CHRONIC HIV INFECTION

The viraemia associated with acute HIV infection is controlled by a cellular and antibody-mediated immune response, which results in resolution of symptoms. However, even though the great majority of people become asymptomatic, HIV replication continues to take place. This results in activation of the immune system, depletion of CD4+ T-cells and immunodeficiency, especially cellular immunodeficiency. These abnormalities develop at different rates in different individuals. In untreated patients the median time to develop the acquired immunodeficiency syndrome (AIDS) after acquiring HIV infection is 9 years, and about 5% of HIV-infected individuals have no abnormalities even after 15 years.

Early in the course of chronic HIV infection, virus is present in lymphoid tissues where it is bound to follicular dendritic cells. There is a persistent immune response against the HIV but, as this fails, viral replication increases and the viral load becomes larger and other cells become infected, including macrophages, microglial cells of the nervous system and CD4+ T-cells.

Chronic HIV infection may cause weight loss, fevers and diarrhoea, though such symptoms are more likely to be caused by an opportunistic infection in immunodeficient patients. Effects of worsening HIV infection are an immunodeficiency syndrome, which results in the development of opportunistic infections, tumours, and neurological disease. Neurological disease is a consequence of HIV infection of macrophages and microglial cells in the central and peripheral nervous system.

DIAGNOSIS

A diagnosis of HIV infection can usually be made by demonstrating anti-HIV antibodies in the patient's serum. However, the serological diagnosis of HIV infection can sometimes be problematic. A small minority of individuals who are not infected by HIV have serum antibodies which are reactive with some HIV proteins, and give false-positive results with some ELISAs. Many laboratories use two different types of ELISA to identify such sera. To ensure that HIV infection is not incorrectly diagnosed, an antibody test should only be considered positive if antibody is also detected according to defined criteria, using a confirmatory antibody test such as a Western blot immunoassay.[2] Anti-HIV antibodies may be absent from the serum of patients with acute HIV infection. They are usually detectable by 2–6 weeks after infection, and almost always detectable by 12 weeks. After this time, absence of HIV antibodies excludes HIV infection in all but the most advanced cases of AIDS, or in a patient with an antibody deficiency syndrome

MONITORING

VIROLOGICAL MONITORING

It could be argued that HIV has been one of the major driving forces in the development of modern virology.

HIV viral load monitoring has enabled the clinician for the first time to predict outcome, and monitor therapy during a viral infection.

HIV VIRAL LOAD MEASUREMENT

The major advance in viral diagnostics has been the development of the polymerase chain reaction (PCR) and the application of this to the detection and quantification of viral nucleic acid in body fluids. Measurement of the blood 'HIV load' can be done by quantitating HIV RNA in plasma. Knowledge of the HIV load is useful in prognostication and essential when making decisions to commence and optimize therapy[3] (see Figure 58.1).

GENOTYPING HIV TO DETECT DRUG RESISTANCE

Drug susceptibility testing of HIV from a clinical specimen is performed in order to detect mutations in the genome of the HIV that predict failure of individual antiviral therapeutic agents. The predominant genotype from an individual's plasma or cerebrospinal fluid sample is determined by sequencing of the reverse transcriptase and protease genes of complementary DNA (cDNA) obtained following RT/PCR. This information is used to assist the clinician and patient in the choice of an antiretroviral drug combination with the best chance of successful suppression of HIV replication, especially where resistance is suspected i.e. in a failing regimen.[4]

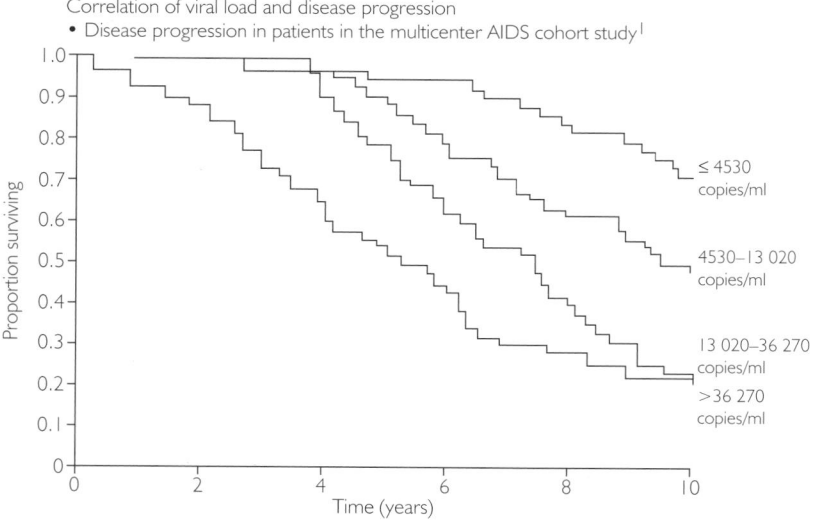

Correlation of viral load and disease progression
• Disease progression in patients in the multicenter AIDS cohort study[1]

1. Mellors JW, 3rd conference on rectroviruses and opportunistic infections, January 1996. Abstract number 522.

Fig. 58.1   Correlation of viral load with disease progression (from Mellors, JW, et al.[3] Copyright, American Association for the Advancement of Science, reproduced with permission).

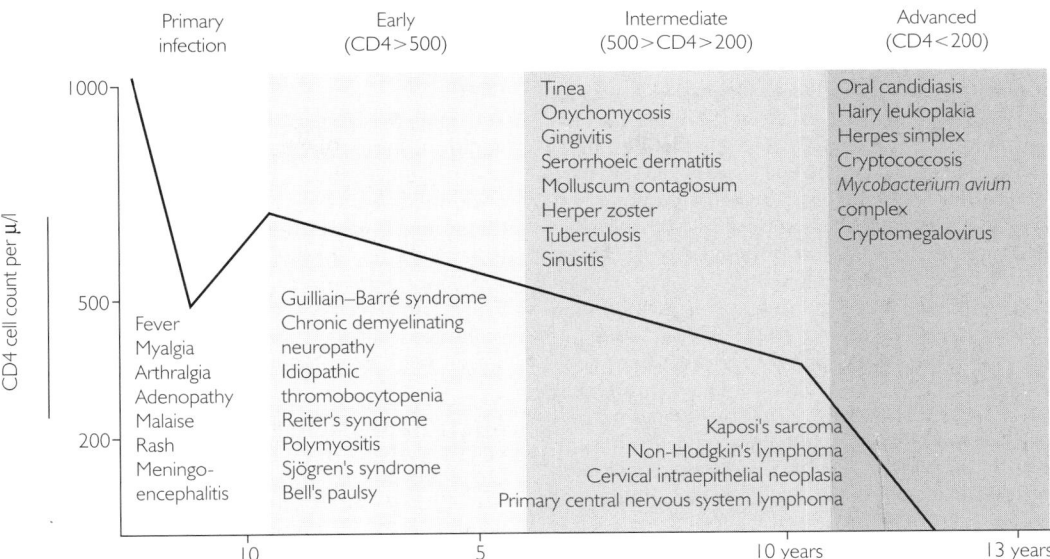

Fig. 58.2 Chronological framework for understanding HIV disease and its management. (From Stewart, G. 'Managing HIV', *The Medical Journal of Australia* 1997; **5**, reproduced with permission.)

IMMUNE MONITORING

Immunodeficiency and neurological disease caused by HIV infection usually develop gradually over months to years. It is important to monitor their severity to determine when to commence therapy, and when the patient is susceptible to various disease manifestations.

The blood CD4+ T-cell count or percentage is the best indicator of the severity of HIV-induced immunodeficiency and, therefore, of the patient's susceptibility to opportunistic infections. Measurement of the blood CD4+ T-cell count or percentage is therefore critical in determining if the symptoms of an HIV-infected patient are likely to be caused by an opportunistic infection, and if so, what type of infection (see Figure 58.2 and text below).[5]

MANAGEMENT OF THE HIV-INFECTED PATIENT

The impact of combination antiretroviral therapy on the morbidity and mortality associated with HIV infection has been dramatic. The HIV Outpatient Study demonstrated a stepwise reduction in opportunistic infections and mortality with increasing intensity of antiretroviral therapy.[6] In Australia, a comparison of cohorts before and after the introduction of combination antiretroviral therapy documented the effectiveness of these agents in reducing the risk of progression to the Acquired Immune Deficiency Syndrome (AIDS) and death.[7] This reflects similar epidemiological studies conducted in

Switzerland,[8] France[9] and the USA.[10] A 70–80% reduction in mortality over 5 years has been the norm. AIDS defining illnesses in Australia now occur predominantly in those without a past diagnosis of HIV infection.

Two classes of antiretroviral drugs are currently in use: reverse transcriptase inhibitors and protease inhibitors. Reverse transcriptase inhibitors are of three types. Nucleoside analogues and nucleotide analogues act by substituting for natural nucleosides during HIV replication, thereby inhibiting DNA chain elongation and the effects of the reverse transcriptase enzyme. Non-nucleoside reverse transcriptase inhibitors (NNRTIs) inhibit the reverse transcriptase enzyme by a different mechanism (Table 58.1).

All antiretroviral drugs have a limited duration of efficacy if used alone because the HIV eventually develops resistance to them. The use of drug combinations is much more effective than single drugs, partly because drug resistance develops more slowly. Adherence to combination regimens has therefore become a significant and difficult issue.

DRUG TOXICITY

With decreased rates of HIV morbidity and mortality, attention has now become focused on the toxicities of treatments. Adverse effects of antiretroviral drugs are common, and are a cause of significant morbidity and even mortality.

Recently, nucleoside analogue reverse transcriptase inhibitors (NRTIs) have been implicated in the development of syndromes that include fatigue, fat wasting, lactic acidosis and peripheral neuropathy. It has been suggested that these symptoms may be due to an inhibition of mitochondrial DNA (mtDNA) synthesis.[11,12] Pancreatitis has occurred uncommonly with ddI (5–7%) and d4T (1–2%).

The most common adverse effect of NNRTIs is a skin rash. This occurs in up to 25% of subjects started on nevirapine and can range from a mild rash to Steven–Johnson syndrome. Combination antiretroviral therapy is associated with a syndrome characterized by redistribution of fat (lipodystrophy) and fat atrophy (lipoatrophy). The biological mechanism responsible for the development of this syndrome is still unclear[13] although protease inhibitors in association with d4T have been implicated.

The use of antiretroviral therapy is also associated with hepatotoxicity in about 10% of patients.[14] Co-infection with hepatitis C virus is one risk factor for hepatotoxicity and at least some cases are probably a type of immune restoration disease.[15] Restoration of immune responses against pathogens also appears to be a cause of other types of inflammatory disease after the use of combination antiretroviral therapy.[16,17]

HIV INDUCED IMMUNODEFICIENCY

Patients who are not treated with antiretroviral therapy or whose antiretroviral therapy is ineffective, for whatever reason, often become immunodeficient. Both CD4+ T-cell depletion and the effects of other immune defects lead to the development of an immunodeficiency syndrome. This syndrome is characterized by impaired cellular immunity and an increased propensity to opportunistic infections. In addition, some patients have impaired antibody responses and phagocyte function, which results in infections with encapsulated bacteria and systemic fungal infections. As mentioned previously, during chronic HIV infection there is a strong relationship between the degree of immunodeficiency and susceptibility to opportunistic infections. The CD4+ T-cell count (or percentage) predicts the likely pathogens and is a guide to the need for prophylactic antimicrobials (see Figure 58.2).

MILD IMMUNODEFICIENCY (CD4 T-CELL COUNT >200/μl, 20%)

Infectious complications of cellular immunodeficiency may occur when there is relatively mild impairment of cellular immune responses (CD4+ T-cell counts of 200–500/μl). Mucocutaneous infections occur most commonly (see Table 58.2) but infections with bacteria such as *Campylobacter jejuni*, *Salmonella* spp., or *Shigella* spp. are a cause of diarrhoea, and occasionally bacteraemia. Bacteraemic pneumococcal disease is also more common in this group. Most of these infections are not restricted to patients with HIV infection, and are therefore not considered to be AIDS-defining opportunistic infections. However, when they present atypically, are severe or are recurrent, they may be the first indication of underlying HIV-induced immunodeficiency. In contrast to the other infections, oral hairy leukoplakia (due to EBV infection of epithelial cells) is almost always indicative of HIV infection.

MODERATE IMMUNODEFICIENCY (CD4 T-CELL COUNT 50–200/μl, 10–20%)

Cellular immunodeficiency which is severe enough to result in an increased propensity to systemic opportunistic infections is usually associated with a CD4 T-cell

Table 58.1 Antiretroviral drugs used to treat human immunodeficiency virus (HIV) infection

Reverse transcriptase inhibitors
Nucleoside analogues
Abacavir (ABV)
Didanosine (ddI)
Lamivudine (3TC)
Stavudine (d4T)
Zalcitabine (ddC)
Zidovudine (AZT)
Combivir (AZT + 3TC)*
Trizivir (AZT + 3TC + ABV)*
Nucleotide analogues
Tenofovir
Non-nucleoside reverse transcriptase inhibitors
Delavirdine
Efavirenz
Nevirapine
Protease inhibitors
Amprenavir
Indinavir
Lopinivir (+Ritonavir)**
Nelfinavir
Ritonavir
Saquinavir

*Combination tablets
**Low dose Ritonavir is co-formulated with Lopinavir to increase serum levels of Lopinavir

Table 58.2 Mucocutaneous opportunistic infections in patients with human immunodeficiency virus (HIV) induced immunodeficiency

Herpes zoster (varicella-zoster virus infection)
Mucosal candidiasis
Oral hairy leukoplakia (Epstein–Barr virus infection)
Seborrhoeic dermatitis (*Pityrosporon* spp. yeast infection)
Molluscum contagiosum (poxvirus infection)
Genital and cutaneous warts (human papillomavirus infection)
Fungal infections of the skin and nails
Recurrent mucocutaneous herpes simplex virus infections
Folliculitis (*Staphylococcus aureus, Pityrosporon* spp.)

count of $<200/\mu$l. Such infections are considered to be indicative of the presence of AIDS. Infection with many different micro-organisms may occur including infection with unusual micro-organisms. Only the most common are described here.

PNEUMOCYSTIS CARINII PNEUMONITIS

Infection of the lungs by *Pneumocystis carinii* causes an interstitial pneumonitis. Patients with this condition usually have a history of subacute progressive dyspnoea, cough, fever and weight loss. Examination often reveals basal pulmonary crackles. The chest X-ray usually shows interstitial infiltrates but is occasionally normal. Other findings which would support a diagnosis of *Pneumocystis carinii* pneumonitis (PCP) are hypoxaemia, an increased serum lactate dehydrogenase (LDH) concentration, diffuse uptake of radio-labelled gallium into the lungs on a gallium scan, ground glass pulmonary opacities on a computerized tomographic (CT) scan of the lungs, and detection of Pneumocystis by smear or DNA by PCR in induced sputum specimens. A definitive diagnosis can be made by demonstrating Pneumocystis cysts in an induced sputum specimen, bronchoalveolar lavage fluid or a transbronchial biopsy.[18]

PCP is treated with co-trimoxazole (trimethoprim-sulphamethoxazole), given orally or intravenously (i.v.) depending on disease severity. However, many patients develop a hypersensitivity reaction to co-trimoxazole which is usually mild and transient but if systemic and severe alternative medications, including oral dapsone and trimethoprim or i.v. pentamidine, can be used with equal efficacy. Steroid therapy should also be used if the PaO_2 is <70 mmHg (9.3 kPa)[19] with an FiO_2 of 0.21.

Pneumocystis infection can be prevented by prophylactic medications, which should be offered to all patients with a CD4 T-cell count of $<200/\mu$l. The most effective drug is co-trimoxazole. Alternatives for patients who are sensitive to co-trimoxazole include dapsone (with or without pyrimethamine), or inhaled pentamidine.[20]

OESOPHAGEAL CANDIDIASIS

Candida infection of the oesophageal mucosa presents with odynophagia and dysphagia. The occurrence of such symptoms in association with oral candidiasis is usually sufficient to make a presumptive diagnosis of oesophageal candidiasis and to start treatment. Endoscopy is required for a definitive diagnosis. Treatment is usually with an azole, such as fluconazole. However, in patients with severe immunodeficiency, resistance to azoles is not uncommon and treatment with i.v. amphotericin may be required.

CRYPTOCOCCAL MENINGITIS

Meningitis is the most common manifestation of infection with *Cryptococcus neoformans* in patients with AIDS. It usually presents with headache and fever, but sometimes confusion or behavioural abnormalities are the pre-dominant abnormalities. Neck stiffness is often minimal or absent. Cerebrospinal fluid examination may reveal little evidence of inflammation, particularly in the most severe cases, but cryptococcal antigen is virtually always present in both serum and CSF and cultures for crypto-cocci are positive.[21] Most patients also have cryptococcal antigen in their serum. Intravenous amphotericin is the treatment of choice, and must be followed by permanent suppressive therapy (or until immune reconstitution with ART; antiretroviral therapy) with oral fluconazole to prevent relapses.[22]

TOXOPLASMA ENCEPHALITIS

Reactivation of *Toxoplasma gondii* infection most commonly presents as a focal encephalitis. This may cause headaches, fever, focal neurological deficits, convulsions and even coma. One or more brain lesions may be present. They usually produce ring-enhancing lesions with surrounding oedema on a brain CT scan, and can occur in many sites, with a predilection for the basal ganglia. Serological evidence of previous Toxoplasma infection is present in virtually all patients, and absence of serum Toxoplasma antibody is strongly against the diagnosis. Treatment is with i.v. sulphadiazine or clindamycin and oral pyrimethamine. Hypersensitivity reactions to sulphadiazine and clindamycin are common, and an alternative drug regimen may be necessary. A brain CT scan should be repeated after 2–3 weeks of therapy, and an alternative diagnosis considered if there has been no resolution of the lesions. Cerebral lymphoma can produce very similar lesions to Toxoplasma encephalitis. A brain biopsy is often necessary to make the diagnosis.[23]

SEVERE IMMUNODEFICIENCY (CD4 T-CELLS $<50/\mu$l, 10%)

CYTOMEGALOVIRUS INFECTION

Cytomegalovirus (CMV) infection most often occurs in patients with very severe immunodeficiency (CD4 T-cell count $<50/\mu$l). The most common site for reactivation of CMV infection is the retina. CMV retinitis usually presents with unilateral blurred vision, visual field loss or 'floaters'. Diagnosis is by fundoscopy and confirmation by an ophthalmologist should be undertaken. Treatment is with i.v. ganciclovir or foscarnet, followed by suppressive therapy to prevent relapses, which should be continued indefinitely unless there is immune reconstitution following the use of combination ART.

CMV infection less commonly presents with disease of other organs, particularly the oesophagus, bile ducts or colon. Biopsy of affected tissue is necessary to make a definitive diagnosis. High or increasing CMV viral load in blood provides support for a diagnosis of CMV infection. In addition, CMV load can be utilized to monitor the response to therapy and early identification of resistance.

CRYPTOSPORIDIOSIS

Infection of the gastrointestinal tract by *Cryptosporidium parvum* causes a severe and intractable secretory diarrhoea, which is often associated with a malabsorption syndrome. It can also cause cholangitis. Diagnosis is by demonstrating *Cryptosporidium* oocysts in faeces and/or a rectal or duodenal biopsy. There is no satisfactory treatment, but paromomycin is of use in some patients. Response is common following successful ART.

MYCOBACTERIUM AVIUM COMPLEX INFECTION

Infection with *Mycobacterium avium* complex (MAC) is usually disseminated and affects blood leukocytes, liver, spleen and lymph nodes, and the gastrointestinal tract. This infection often results in weight loss, fatigue, fevers, anaemia and diarrhoea. The diagnosis is usually made by culturing MAC from blood, but sometimes stool microscopy and culture or biopsy of affected tissues are necessary. Treatment with multiple drug therapy is often successful. Commonly used drugs are clarithromycin, rifabutin and ethambutol. Suppressive therapy should be continued indefinitely, unless there is immune reconstitution following the use of combination ART.[24] An unusual painful necrotizing lymphadenopathy following initiation of ARV therapy has been identified as MAC immunerestoration disease.[16]

Certain neoplasms are a characteristic complication of cellular immunodeficiency, including HIV-induced immunodeficiency. Uncontrolled replication of an additional virus resulting from the immunodeficiency is probably involved in the pathogenesis of all of these neoplasms.

Kaposi's sarcoma (KS) is an angioproliferative tumour, which originates from vascular endothelium. There is much evidence implicating Human herpesvirus-8 (HHV-8) in the pathogenesis of KS. It usually presents as skin lesions, which have a reddish-brown colour. They vary in extent from one or two small papules to numerous bulbous lesions. The mucosal surface of the gastrointestinal tract, lymph nodes, and, rarely, internal organs may also be involved. A clinical diagnosis of KS can be confirmed by biopsy of a lesion. KS may present at any degree of immunodeficiency but occurs most often, and is more severe, in patients with moderate to severe immunodeficiency. New antimitotic agents plus ART have resulted in KS essentially disappearing as a clinical problem in treated individuals.

Lymphomas are also a complication of HIV-induced immunodeficiency. The great majority are B-cell lymphomas (non-Hodgkins), and reactivation of Epstein–Barr virus infection is implicated in the pathogenesis of many cases. Primary cerebral lymphoma or extracerebral lymphoma, which often has extranodal involvement, are common in patients with severe immunodeficiency. These lymphomas are usually high-grade with poor prognosis (stage 3/4, CD4 <100, median survival 44 weeks).[25]

Cervical intraepithelial neoplasia (CIN) is more common in women with HIV infection. This is presumably because human papillomavirus (HPV) infection is more likely to be present in women with HIV infection, and the cellular immunodeficiency permits HPV replication. As a consequence, the incidence of cervical carcinoma appears to be increased in HIV-infected women. Anal neoplasia is also increased in males.

In addition to the opportunistic infections of the nervous system discussed above, HIV infection of macrophages and microglial cells in the nervous system often results in neurological disease by incompletely understood mechanisms. Encephalopathy, myelopathy or peripheral neuropathy are all possible. In a small number of patients, the neurological disease is more problematical than the immunodeficiency. The encephalopathy usually develops insidiously in individuals with advanced immunodeficiency and eventually results in cognitive, motor and behavioural abnormalities. Myelopathy, which is now rare, results in an ataxic spastic paraparesis.[26]

Investigation of HIV patients with space occupying cerebral lesions requires analysis of serology, cerebrospinal fluid and neuro-imaging investigations. Analysis of CSF includes PCR for EBV (indicative of lymphoma), HSV, CMV VZV (viral encephalitis), JC virus (indicative of PML), toxoplasmosis and MTB.[27]

HIV/AIDS AND ADMISSION TO THE INTENSIVE CARE UNIT

HIV infection remains an incurable condition albeit chronically controllable with ART. However, the prognosis has improved significantly over the past 10 years with mathematical models indicating a median survival of 30 years. The admission of a patient with AIDS to an intensive care unit (ICU) is therefore often indicated.[28,29]

The most common indications are:

- Respiratory failure complicating PCP or other infective pulmonary conditions.
- Coma or convulsions complicating opportunistic infections or tumours of the brain.
- Non-HIV-related conditions, such as a self-poisoning and post-operative management.
- Drug toxicity, particularly related to antiretrovirals and drug–drug interactions.

Respiratory failure complicating PCP has been the most common reason for admitting an HIV-infected patient to an ICU. Survival following ventilation for PCP was poor in the early 1980s, but improved with treatment advances. In recent years, survival has worsened again in some cohorts, particularly for patients with a CD4 T-cell count of $<50/\mu$l and for those who develop pneumothorax as a result of barotrauma. The poor outcome in recent years may reflect the fact that patients are living longer because of improved therapy, and are hence often more immunodeficient when PCP develops. A first episode of PCP, a CD4 T-cell count of >50/μl and no previous antiretroviral therapy are all favourable factors for survival. Furthermore, ventilation may be avoided by the use of continuous positive airways pressure (CPAP) or bilevel positive airways pressure (BIPAP), thereby reducing the risks of a pneumothorax, airway obstruction and nosocomial infection. Prolonged illness antidating ICU admission, low serum albumin and few options for antiretroviral therapy should be considered when assessing predictors of survival.

Drug–drug interactions are of particular importance especially when ART includes protease inhibitors or efaverenz (metabolized via P450 hepatic enzyme system. Web based guidelines are very useful (www.HIV-druginteractions.org) when prescribing antimicobials, antiemetics and lipid lowering drugs.

NEEDLE-STICK INJURIES AND POST EXPOSURE PROPHYLAXIS

Patients with unrecognized HIV infection or AIDS may also be admitted to an ICU with the first manifestation of HIV disease. It is therefore important for all ICU staff to practise stringent infection control procedures at all times.

HIV transmission from needlesticks occurs at a rate of approximately 0.3%, and from mucosal exposure at a rate of approximately 0.009%. There have been no reported seroconversions after skin exposure. In addition, there have been no documented seroconversions in surgeons and no seroconversions due to suture needle exposure. The major risk factors for infection after a needlestick injury are (a) deep injury, (b) visible blood on device, (c) needle placement in a vein or artery, and (d) a source patient with late stage HIV/AIDS (high viral load).

There is evidence that antiretroviral prophylaxis is associated with a reduction in transmission rates. On the basis of this, antiretroviral prophylaxis guidelines have been published.[30] A protocol for dealing with blood and body fluid exposure should therefore be developed for every health-care institution.

REFERENCES

1 Tindall B, Cooper DA. Primary HIV infection: host responses and intervention strategies. *AIDS* 1991; **5**: 1–14.
2 Robertson P, Dwyer D. Western blot assay. In Lee N (ed.) *Clinical Microbiology Update* 1993; No 35. Sydney: University of New South Wales, pp. 9–16.
3 Mellors JW, Rinaldo CR, Gupta P, *et al.* Prognosis in HIV-1 infection predicted by the quantity of virus in plasma. *Science* 1996; **272**: 1167–70.
4 Durant J, Clevenbergh P, Halfon P, *et al.* Drug resistance genotyping in HIV-1 therapy: the VIRADAPT randomised controlled trial. *Lancet* 1999; **353**: 2195–9.
5 Mellors JW, Munoz A, Giogi JV, *et al.* Plasma viral load and CD4+ lymphocytes as prognostic markers of HIV-1 infection. *Ann Internal Med.* 1997; **126**: 946–54.
6 Palella FJ, Delaney KM, Moorman AC, *et al.* Declining morbidity and mortality among patients with advanced human immunodeficiency virus infection. *N Engl J Med* 1998; **338**: 853–60.
7 Correll PK, Law MG, McDonald AM, *et al.* HIV disease progression in Australia at the time of combination antiretroviral therapies. *MJA* 1998; **169**: 469–72.
8 Egger M, Hirschel B, Francioli P, *et al.* Impact of new antiretroviral combination therapies in HIV infected patients in Switzerland: prospective multicentre study: HIV Cohort Study. *BMJ* 1997; **315**: 1194–9.
9 Mouton Y, Alfandari S, Valette M, *et al.* Impact of protease inhibitors on AIDS defining events and hospitalizations in 10 French AIDS reference centres. *AIDS* 1997; **11**: F101–5.
10 Torres RA, Barr M. Impact of combination therapy for HIV infection in inpatient census. *N Engl J Med* 1997; **336**: 1531–2.
11 Brinkman K, Smeitink JA, Romijn JA, Reiss P. Mitochondrial toxicity induced by nucleoside-analogue reverse-transcriptase inhibitors is a key factor in the pathogenesis of antiretroviral-therapy-related lipodystrophy. *Lancet* 1999; **354**: 1112–5.
12 Carr A, Miller J, Law M, Cooper DA. A syndrome of liopatrophy, lactic acidaemia and liver dysfunction associated with HIV nucleoside analogue therapy: contribution to protease inhibitor-related lipodystrophy syndrome. *AIDS* 2000; **14**: F25–32.
13 Carr A, Cooper DA. Adverse effects of antiretroviral therapy. *Lancet* 2000; **356**(9239): 1423–30.
14 Monforte Ade A, Bugarini R, Pezzotti P, *et al.* The ICONA (Italian Cohort of Naive for Antiretrovirals) Study Group. Low frequency of severe hepatotoxicity and association with HCV coinfection in HIV-positive patients treated with HAART. *J Acquir Immune Defic Syndr* 2001; **28**: 114–23.
15 John M, Flexman J, French MA. Hepatitis C virus-associated hepatitis following treatment of HIV-infected patients with HIV protease inhibitors: an immune restoration disease? *AIDS* 1998; **12**: 2289–93.
16 French MA, Lenzo N, John M, *et al.* Immune restoration disease after the treatment of immunodeficient HIV-infected patients with highly active antiretroviral therapy. *HIV Medicine* 2000; **1**: 107–15.
17 DeSimone JA, Pomerantz RJ, Babinchak TJ. Inflammatory reactions in HIV-1-infected persons after initiation of highly active antiretroviral therapy. *Ann Intern Med* 2000; **133**: 447–54.
18 Frame P, Wilkin A. *Pneumocystis carinii* pneumonia. In: Crowe S, Hoy J, Mills J (eds) *Management of the HIV-Infected Patient*. London: Martin Dunitz; 2002: pp. 421–42.
19 Consensus statement on the use of corticosteroids as adjunctive therapy for *Pneumocystis* pneumonia in the

acquired immunodeficiency syndrome. The National Institutes of Health University of California expert panel for corticosteroids as adjunctive therapy for *Pneumocystis* pneumonia. *N Engl J Med* 1990; **323**: 500–504.

20 Kovacs JA, Masur H. Prophylaxis against opportunistic infections in patients with human immunodeficiency virus infection. *N Engl J Med* 2000; **342**: 1416–29.

21 Dismukes WE. Cryptococcal meningitis in patients with AIDS. *J Infect Dis* 1998; **157**: 624–8.

22 Powderly WG, Sagg MS, Cloud GA, *et al.* A controlled trial of fluconazole or amphotericin B to prevent relapse of cryptococcal meningitis in patients with the acquired immunodeficiency syndrome. *N Engl J Med*. 1992; **326**: 793–8.

23 Porter SB, Sande M. Toxoplasmosis of the central nervous system in the acquired immunodeficiency syndrome. *N Engl J Med*. 1992; **327**: 1643–8.

24 Aberg A J, Yajko DM, Jacobson MA. Eradication of AIDS-related disseminated *Mycobacterium avium* complex infection after twelve months of antimycobacterial therapy combined with highly active antiretroviral therapy. *J Inf Dis* 1998; **178**: 1446–9.

25 Straus DJ, Huang J, Testa MA, *et al.* Prognostic factors in the treatment of human immunodeficiency virus-associated non-Hodgkin's lymphoma: analysis of AIDS Clinical Trials Group Protocol 142-low-dose versus standard-dose m-BACOD plus granulocyte-macrophage colony-stimulating factor. *J Clin Oncol* 1998; **16**: 3601–6.

26 McArthur JC, Sacktor N, Selnes O. Human immunodeficiency virus-associated dementia. *Semin Neurol* 1999; **19**: 129–50.

27 Antinori A, Ammassari A, De Luca A, *et al.* Diagnosis of AIDS-related focal brain lesions: a decision-making analysis based on clinical and neuroradiologic characteristics combined with polymerase chain reaction assays in CSF. *Neurology* 1997; **48**: 687–94.

28 Nickas G, Wachter RM. Outcomes of intensive care for patients with human immunodeficiency virus infection. *Arch Intern Med*. 2000; **169**: 541–47.

29 JK Gill, L Greene, R Miller, *et al.* ICU admission in patients infected with the human immunodeficiency virus – a multicentre survey. *Anaesthesia* 1999; **4**: 727–32.

30 Post Exposure Prophylaxis (PEP) for Health Care Workers. *MMWR* 2001; 50(RR-1).

59

Severe sepsis
G M Clarke

Sepsis has traditionally implied infection accompanied by systemic inflammatory manifestations, such as fever, tachycardia and elevated white blood cell count. However, the systemic changes are indistinguishable from those of non-infective inflammatory conditions (e.g. pancreatitis, acute hepatic failure, immunological reactions and gross trauma, including burns). Consequently, much confusion arose when terms, such as sepsis and septic syndrome were applied to these latter conditions. This led to a consensus conference of the American College of Chest Physicians and Society of Critical Care Medicine to define terms related to infection and the systemic response (Table 59.1; Figure 59.1).[1] Thus, sepsis is the systemic inflammatory response to infection. It is the commonest contributor to death in the ICU.[2]

AETIOLOGY AND EPIDEMIOLOGY

Sepsis may be caused by Gram-negative and Gram-positive bacteria, fungi, protozoa, *Rickettsia*, viruses and spirochaetes. In the ICU, common infective Gram-negative organisms include *Escherichia coli*, *Pseudomonas*, *Klebsiella*, *Proteus*, *Enterobacter* and *Bacteroides*; Gram-positive organisms include staphylococci, streptococci and *Clostridium*. Systemic infection with fungi, especially *Candida*, is a risk in immunodeficient patients receiving broad spectrum antibiotics.

Nosocomial infection rates in ICU patients are 5–10 times higher than among general ward patients. Organisms posing serious resistance problems in the ICU setting include methicillin-resistant staphylococci,

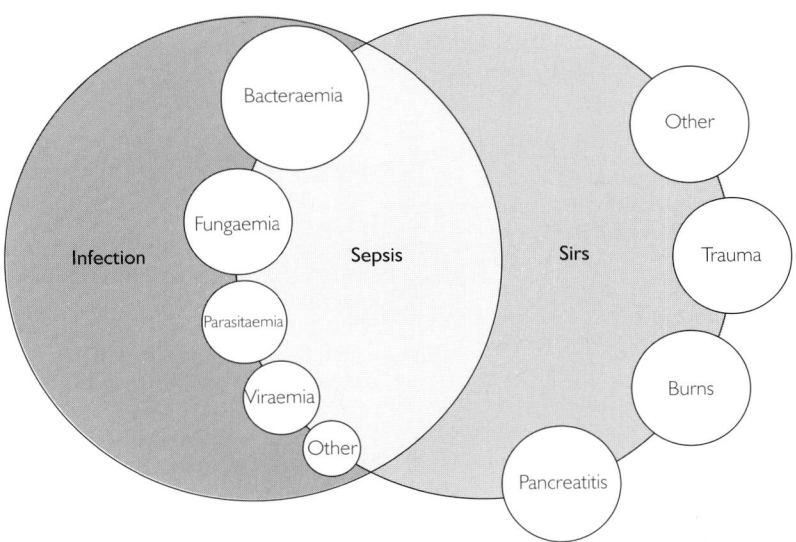

Fig. 59.1   Inter-relationship of systemic inflammatory response syndrome (SIRS), sepsis and infection. (From American College of Chest Physicians/Society of Critical Care Medicine,[2] with permission.)

Table 59.1 Definitions of sepsis[2]

Infection
Microbial phenomenon characterized by an inflammatory response to the presence of microorganisms or the invasion of normally sterile host tissue by those organisms

Bacteraemia
The presence of viable bacteria in the blood

Systemic inflammatory response syndrome
The systemic inflammatory response to a variety of severe clinical insults. The response is manifested by two or more of the following conditions:
    Temperature >38°C or <36°C
    Heart rate >90 beats/min
    Respiratory rate >20 breaths/min or $Paco_2$ <4.3 kPa (<32 Torr)
    White blood cell count >12 000 cells/mm³, <4000 cells/mm³, or <10% immature (band) forms

Sepsis
The systemic response to infection. This systemic response is manifested by two or more of the following conditions as a result of infection:
    Temperature >38°C or <36°C
    Heart rate >90 beats/min
    Respiratory rate >20 breaths/min or $Paco_2$ <4.3 kPa (<32 Torr)
    White blood cell count >12 000 cells/mm³, <4000 cells/mm³, or <10% immature (band) forms

Severe sepsis
Sepsis associated with organ dysfunction, hypoperfusion or hypotension. Hypoperfusion and perfusion abnormalities may include, but are not limited to, lactic acidosis, oliguria or an acute alteration in mental status

Septic shock
Sepsis with hypotension, despite adequate fluid resuscitation, along with the presence of perfusion abnormalities that may include, but are not limited to, lactic acidosis, oliguria or an acute alteration in mental status. Patients who are on inotropic or vasopressor agents may not be hypotensive at the time when perfusion abnormalities are measured

Hypotension
A systolic blood pressure of <90 mmHg or a reduction of >40 mmHg from baseline in the absence of other causes for hypotension

Multiple organ dysfunction syndrome
Presence of altered organ function in an acutely ill patient such that homeostasis cannot be maintained without intervention.

certain Enterobacteriaceae, *Pseudomonas aeruginosa*, *P. cepacia*, *Stenotrophomonas maltophilia*, *Acinetobacter*, *Candida* species and more recently, vancomycin resistant enterococci.

Many infections acquired in the ICU are endogenous and follow colonization of the alimentary tract by organisms usually insignificant in healthy individuals (e.g. *E. coli*, *Klebsiella*, *Proteus* and *Pseudomonas*). The EPIC study demonstrated a rise in Gram-positive infections, particularly *Staphylococcus aureus* and coagulase negative Staphylococci.[3] The latter organisms are normal skin commensals. Coagulase negative Staphylococci in particular, play a significant role in catheter related sepsis.

PATHOGENESIS

The host response, rather than the infecting organism, predominantly determines the severity of infection. Nonetheless, attributes of the infecting organism which include pathogenicity, virulence and inoculum size influence whether or not infection occurs. Also impor-tant are the status of the host's local and general defence mechanisms. Both are often impaired in the acutely ill or injured patient (Ch. 58).

INITIATORS OF THE SYSTEMIC INFLAMMATORY RESPONSE IN INFECTION[4,5]

Innate immunity (Table 59.2) with its germ line-encoded receptors for the recognition of microbial pathogens represents a phylogenetically ancient defence against micro-organisms. It is now generally assumed that severe sepsis usually results from over-stimulation of the innate rather than the adaptive immune system. Sepsis begins with the recognition of microbial products by phagocytic leukocytes and other immune cells. Toll-like receptors, an evolutionary conserved family of receptors on the surface of immune cells, mediate the subsequent cellular activation resulting in massive cytokine release. Some examples are given below.

For Gram-negative infection, endotoxin (LPS) triggers the systemic inflammatory response. LPS binds to a specific lipopolysaccharide binding protein (LBP) in the plasma. The LPS–LBP complex binds to receptor CD14 of macrophages and other immune cells. This receptor presents LPS to a Toll-like receptor (TLR4) which is a transmembrane protein having an extracellular domain and a cytoplasmic domain. Once LPS is presented to this signal transducing receptor (TLR4), macrophage activation occurs. This results in the production and release of an array of potent inflammatory cytokines such as tumour necrosis factor (TNF), interleukin-1 (IL-1), IL-6 and IL-8. Complex interaction of these cytokines and possibly LPS with other cells, leads to the release of adhesion molecules, metabolites of arachidonic acid pathways (leukotrienes, thromboxane and prostaglandins), and products of leukocytes, platelets and vessel walls (elastase, nitric oxide, platelet activating factor, toxic oxygen radicals). Also activated are the coagulation, complement and kinin systems.

Gram positive organisms can trigger sepsis and septic shock by the whole organism or cell wall components which include peptidoglycans, teichoic acids and lipoteichoic acid presenting to CD14 receptors and then to Toll-like receptors (TLR2). Massive cellular cytokine release follows. The complex end result is as described above.

Certain staphylococci and streptococci can trigger septic shock through the production of superantigens (staphylococcal toxic shock syndrome toxin-1, streptococcal pyrogenic exotoxin). Superantigens can induce T-cell proliferation without regard for antigenic specificity of T-cells.

SYSTEMIC INFLAMMATORY RESPONSE SYNDROME ONCE ESTABLISHED

The host response results in a multilayer highly complex array of mediators and proteolytic cascades with associated positive and negative feedback loops. Some mediators are pro-inflammatory, others anti-inflammatory (Table 59.3). It has been argued that if the former predominate systemic inflammatory response syndrome (SIRS) is evident and if the latter predominate anergy may be seen.[6]

POLYMORPHISM

Genetic variability (polymorphism) in the population is apparent in the variability of cytokine production in response to severe infection or injury. TNF B_2 homozygous individuals with severe sepsis had higher circulating TNF levels and higher mortality than heterozygous TNF B_1/TNF B_2 patients.[7]

CARDIOVASCULAR PATHOPHYSIOLOGY

Sepsis has early and often profound effects on the cardiovascular system. Though individual studies often implicate a particular mediator for a particular effect, it is likely that many factors and pathways have compounding effects.

Table 59.2 Innate and acquired immune systems

Innate	Acquired (adaptive)
Polymorphonuclear leukocyte	Complex, involving T and B cells and characterized by:
Natural antibodies, opsonins	memory
Macrophages	specificity
Dendritic cells	diversity
Natural killer cells (NKC)	
Complement system (alternative pathway)	
Coagulation system	

Table 59.3 Inflammatory mediators

Pro-inflammatory mediators and pathways	Anti-inflammatory mediators
Cytokines – TNF, IL-1, 6, 8, IFN-γ	Interleukin 4, 10, 11, 13
Contact system/coagulation pathways	Transforming growth factor β
Macrophages, monocytes, neutrophils	Colony stimulating factor
Endothelial cells, platelets	Soluble TNF receptors
Platelet activating factor	IL-1 receptor antagonist
Oxygen free radicals	Natural anticoagulants
Proteases	
Nitric oxide	

DECREASED SYSTEMIC VASCULAR RESISTANCE

Severe sepsis is commonly associated with a decreased systemic vascular resistance index (SVRI), which results in hypotension despite a normal or increased cardiac index (CI).[2] This is believed to be due principally to NO production in endothelial and vascular smooth muscle cells, via NO synthase, an enzyme that can be induced by endotoxin and certain cytokines (e.g. IFN-γ, TNF and some interleukins). Other mediators implicated include histamine, β-endorphins, decreased C3 complement, C3 proactivator and decreased prekallikrein. Arterial resistance vessels also become hyporesponsive to catecholamines and this appears to correlate with the severity of sepsis. This may in part be secondary to adrenocortical functional impairment.[8] Most non-survivors of severe sepsis show persistent vasodilatation with refractory hypotension prior to death.

INCREASED PULMONARY VASCULAR RESISTANCE

Pulmonary vascular resistance (PVR) may be normal initially, but frequently rises at a later stage of sepsis. The mechanisms of increased PVR are ill understood; PVR may still be increased in the absence of hypoxaemia or acidosis. Postulated causative factors include microthrombi, vasoactive amines, endotoxin, angiotensin, platelet activating factor (PAF), thromboxane A_2 and endothelin-1. Increased PVR has been associated with increased mortality.[9]

INCREASED VENOUS CAPACITANCE

Increased venous capacitance, due to decreased venous tone (probably due to increased NO production), results in relative hypovolaemia.

INCREASED CAPILLARY PERMEABILITY, THE ENDOTHELIUM AND COAGULATION

Permeability of both systemic and pulmonary capillary beds may increase rapidly, so that fluid is lost from the circulation. Clearance of radio-iodinated serum albumin has been shown to increase from a normal of 5–10%/h to 20–35%/h in severe sepsis. Although capillary leak is probably multifactorial, the expression of adherence molecules by the endothelium and subsequent endothelial-leukocyte interaction is thought to play an important role. NO may play an attenuating role.

Tissue factor (TF) can be rapidly induced on mononuclear cells and on vascular endothelium during infection and after stimulation with endotoxin or TNF. Activation of the coagulation cascade via the extrinsic TF/VIIa-dependent pathway is common in severe sepsis.[10] Concomitant derangements include depression of inhibitory mechanisms of coagulation (decreased antithrombin III and activated protein C) and inhibition of the fibrinolytic system by high circulating levels of plasminogen activator inhibitor-1.

The natural anticoagulation inhibitors antithrombin III, protein C and tissue factor pathway inhibitor (TFPI) play anticoagulant, anti-inflammatory and profibrinolytic roles in severe sepsis. Levels of anti-thrombin III are decreased in sepsis due to increased consumption, decreased hepatic synthesis and degradation by elastase released by activated neutrophils. Protein C is activated by a complex of thrombin with the endothelial cell surface protein thrombomodulin. Activated protein C (aPC) activity is facilitated by protein S. Impairment of the protein C system in sepsis is the result of increased consumption of protein S and protein C, and decreased activation of protein C by down regulation of thrombomodulin on endothelial cells.

Thrombin is capable of stimulating multiple inflammatory pathways. Like thrombin, factor VIIa and Xa can activate cells to release cytokines.[11] Though still debated, it is thought that disseminated intravascular coagulation (DIC) contributes to diffuse endovascular injury, multiple organ dysfunction and possible death.

HYPOVOLAEMIA

This major abnormality in severe sepsis is due to several factors: increased venous capacitance, increased capillary permeability (with loss of fluid to the interstitial space) and decreased systemic vascular resistance. Other factors may include increased permeability of cell membranes to sodium ion inducing fluid shifts to the intracellular space, decreased fluid intake and inappropriate polyuria.

SEPTIC CARDIOMYOPATHY

Myocardial dysfunction in severe sepsis is common and is associated with increased mortality. Despite this the majority of patients with septic shock who have been volume loaded have normal or increased cardiac output. Sepsis is characterized by biventricular systolic (decreased ejection fraction) and diastolic dysfunction (abnormal ventricular compliance) with increase in both end diastolic and end systolic volumes.[12] Such changes are seen within 24 h of the onset of sepsis. Ventricular function recovers in those surviving sepsis.[13,14] Survivors tend to develop more cardiac dilatation and have grossly reduced ejection fractions.[12] Non-survivors had normal initial ejection fractions and ventricular size that did not change during this study. A more abnormal echocardiographic pattern of left ventricular relaxation has been seen in non-survivors than survivors.

Decreased coronary blood flow is not the usual cause of myocardial dysfunction in severe sepsis as coronary sinus catheter studies showed normal coronary blood flow and increased myocardial lactate uptake. TNFα and interleukin-1β combination have been implicated as depressant to the myocardium in sepsis. Myocardial depression analogous to septic cardiomyopathy has been seen in non-infectious SIRS.[15] This suggests mediators common to infectious and non-infectious SIRS are the cause of the myocardial dysfunction.

OXYGEN TRANSPORT, CONSUMPTION AND THE MICROCIRCULATION

An increased blood lactate in severe sepsis and septic shock suggests inadequate oxygen delivery or utilization in the tissues. This need not always be the case. Other possible explanations exist. Hypermetabolism, increased transport of glucose into cells, increased glycolysis, gluconeogenesis and glycogenolysis are all characteristic of severe sepsis.[16] Glycolysis in excess of that needed for oxidative metabolism leads to some pyruvate being converted to lactate. In the absence of tissue hypoxia, however, though both lactate and pyruvate are increased, the lactate-pyruvate (L/P) ratio remains normal. Normal L/P ratios have been reported in septic patients with hyperlactataemia[17] and do not indicate inadequate oxygen availability to tissues. Decreased lactate clearance may also occur in severe sepsis.

In sepsis decreased oxygen extraction (i.e. increased mixed venous oxygen saturation with decreased A-VO$_2$ difference) is a common finding. This may result from peripheral arterio-venous shunts (due to maldistribution of blood flow secondary to impaired vasoregulation[18] and interstitial oedema), and/or cellular metabolism defects limiting the cells ability to utilize oxygen.

The concept of pathological supply dependency of oxygen uptake (VO$_2$) on oxygen delivery (DO$_2$) in sepsis has been challenged. Supply dependency of VO$_2$ was not demonstrated in sepsis when VO$_2$ was measured directly.

RELEVANCE OF GLOBAL TO REGIONAL BLOOD FLOW AND OXYGEN EXTRACTION

Regional changes in perfusion and oxygen extraction cannot be predicted from whole body changes in cardiac output in septic shock. During the acute phase of septic shock, whole body oxygen extraction may fall yet splanchnic blood flow, oxygen extraction and VO$_2$ can all rise.[19]

CLINICAL PRESENTATION

Sepsis, severe sepsis and septic shock (Table 59.1) are stages in a spectrum of pathophysiological disturbances in the infected patient. Sepsis is common and can present many faces. Many septic patients are referred to the ICU with such labels as cardiogenic shock, pulmonary embolism, hypovolaemic shock, profound hypothermia and haemolytic-uraemic syndrome. Conversely, there are many causes of systemic inflammatory response syndrome (SIRS) and multiple organ dysfunction syndrome (MODS) other than sepsis. However, as sepsis requires specific therapy, the patient with signs consistent with sepsis should be considered as being infected until proven otherwise.

The classic picture of severe sepsis is that of a hypermetabolic patient with a high temperature, flushed appearance, tachycardia, tachypnoea, a hyperdynamic vasodilated circulation with bounding pulses, low diastolic blood pressure and in some patients a 'pistol shot' sound audible over the femoral arteries. Oliguria is commonly present and the patient may be agitated, confused or drowsy. Leukocytosis is usually present and the urea may be disproportionately elevated with respect to the plasma creatinine suggesting rampant protein catabolism.

However, not all cases present such findings. Body temperature may be normal, increased or decreased. Though leukocytosis and increased numbers of immature band forms are common, leukopenia may be seen. Classically the erythrocyte sedimentation rate (ESR), C-reactive protein (CRP) and procalcitonin levels are all raised. Elevated blood lactate is common as is hyperglycaemia, though hypoglycaemia may be seen in those with liver dysfunction. Evidence of other organ failure (kidney, liver, gut, myocardial, and coagulopathy) may be evident. Other signs and symptoms may relate to the original site of infection. Hypotension, vasoconstriction and peripheral cyanosis ('cold shock') may be seen in septic patients who are hypovolaemic and/or have pre-existing myocardial dysfunction, or have been referred late and without any prior resuscitation.

MANAGEMENT

Septic shock has a high mortality rate. Efforts should be made to diagnose and treat sepsis before shock occurs. Once severe sepsis and septic shock are evident then an emergency situation exists. Management principles then include:

- combined initial assessment and resuscitation paying specific attention to the airway, oxygenation, ventilation and the circulation (ABC)
- when life threatening situations have been dealt with, making a more detailed secondary assessment aimed at establishing a diagnosis and initiating specific treatment.

GENERAL MEASURES

Initial general measures are set out in Table 59.4. Invasive procedures must not take precedence over basic common sense resuscitation though it is useful to have a central line (preferably multilumen), urethral catheter and arterial line *in situ* fairly early in the proceedings. Oxygen should be given by mask as hypoxaemia is

Table 59.4 Basic general measures – septic shock

Administer oxygen, ventilatory support if necessary Volume loading ± ionotropic/vasoactive drugs guided by monitoring	
Basic bedside monitoring:	pulse rate, pulse oximetry, ECG, systemic arterial pressure (SAP) central venous pressure (CVP) temperature, urine output chest X-ray (CXR)
Basic laboratory monitoring:	arterial blood gas (ABG) blood lactate plasma electrolytes/creatinine blood sugar (BSL), haemoglobin platelet and white blood cell count INR (consider APTT, fibrinogen level) liver function tests

common. If inadequate, consider CPAP or non-invasive ventilation by mask or invasive ventilatory assistance.

CORRECTION OF HYPOVOLAEMIA

Initial volume loading is a cornerstone of therapy in septic shock. It is guided by monitoring pulse rate, blood pressure, jugular venous pressure (or CVP) and by auscultation of the lung bases for crepitations. Crystalloid or colloid may be used though it will take more of the former than the latter[20] when aiming for a MAP 65–80 mmHg by increasing the CVP to the range of 8–12 mmHg (10–15 cmH$_2$O). Though in the past the haemoglobin was usually maintained at 100 g/l or higher, recent evidence indicates levels down to 70 g/l are usually safe except possibly in patients with severe ischaemic heart disease.[21,22] If the patient does not respond adequately to oxygenation and volume loading, then consider insertion of a Swan-Ganz catheter and undertaking advanced haemodynamic monitoring (Table 59.5). 'Practice parameters for haemodynamic support of sepsis in adult patients with sepsis' have been published by a task force of the American College of Critical Care Medicine.[23] Controversy in this area persists.

USE OF VASOACTIVE AND/OR INOTROPIC DRUG INFUSIONS

Having corrected hypovolaemia, if hypotension persists then further action may be required to deal with a very

Table 59.5 Advanced haemodynamic monitoring

Pulmonary artery pressure (PAP)
Pulmonary capillary wedge pressure (PCWP)
Cardiac output (CO)
Derived indices
Cardiac index (CI)
Systemic vascular resistance index (SVRI)
Oxygen delivery (DO$_2$)

low SVR and/or the effects of septic cardiomyopathy. Haemodynamic ranges (rather than absolute values) recommended here are: MAP 65–80 mmHg, CVP 8–12 mmHg (10–15 cmH$_2$O), PCWP 10–12 mmHg and CI 3.0–4.0 l/min per m^2. PCWP of 10–12 mmHg is reported as being associated with peak left ventricular stroke work and CI in septic patients.[24] These ranges are for guidance only as the individual patient and clinical situation (including comorbidities such as acute lung injury, ischaemic heart disease, other organ dysfunction) ultimately set the limit on what can be safely achieved. Indeed, in some patients these ranges are not achievable, in others a satisfactory outcome may result with figures outside of the ranges quoted.

Attaining a reasonable MAP is important as autoregulation may be lost in severe sepsis/septic shock such that perfusion of vital organs becomes pressure dependent. Also arterial pressure and SVRI correlate directly with survival in septic shock.[13,14] Norepinephrine raises SVRI, MAP, regional blood flow, oxygen extraction and urine output[19,25,26] and is the usual agent of first choice in this situation. The dose range is enormous: from 0 μg/min to over 100 μg/min. Epinephrine may have undesirable effects on the splanchnic circulation.[27]

If norepinephrine maintains an adequate MAP but CI remains low, then a separate infusion of dobutamine may lead to improvement.[28] Dobutamine has been shown to improve splanchnic blood flow in norepinephrine treated patients with septic shock.[27]

Hyporesponsiveness of vessels to catecholamines is a feature of septic shock and may in part be due to a relative deficiency of cortisol[8] (see the section 'Adjunctive therapies').

It is important that haemodynamic intervention should avoid:

- the use of inotropes/vasoconstrictors before hypovolaemia has been corrected
- overdriving the heart with excessive catecholamines which are cardiotoxic, arrhythmogenic and in some cases decrease gut blood flow and oxygen requirements
- using agents inappropriately, for example, dobutamine alone when a patient has a profoundly low SVRI or using vasoconstriction agents alone causing excessive elevation of SVRI in a patient with poor left ventricular function
- prolonged norepinephrine infusion masking the redevelopment of hypovolaemia by its effect of maintaining central filling pressures through venoconstriction.

Afterload reduction to improve right ventricular function is a consideration in pulmonary hypertension as the latter is associated with a high mortality.[9] Vasodilators such as hydralazine, sodium nitroprusside and prostacyclin lower PVRI and also SVRI, and are therefore prone to cause hypotension and increase pulmonary shunt. NO, by inhalation, is a selective pulmonary vasodilator,[29] which

Table 59.6 Specific measures – septic shock

Culture blood
Gram stain, microscopy and culture of specimens from
suspected infected sites
Test for specific antigens/serology as indicated
Administer antibiotics
Institute drainage/debridement
Other measures as indicated:
  prophylaxis for stress ulceration
  oral/nasogastric amphotericin for anticandida gut colonization
  deep vein thrombosis prophylaxis

may decrease both shunt and PAP without causing systemic hypotension. Its use is still experimental.

SPECIFIC MEASURES

Cultures of blood and from suspected sites of infection are preferably taken before antibiotics are given. Such specimens should be taken as a matter of urgency as antibiotic therapy should not be delayed. In suspected meningitis, if coagulopathy is suspected or proven, then antibiotics should be given immediately and lumbar puncture not undertaken (Table 59.6).

ANTIBIOTICS

Where the offending organism is unknown, then antibiotics are initially given on a best guess basis based on:

- the possible site of infection
- whether the infection was acquired outside or within the hospital
- the age of the patient
- any history of hypersensitivity
- renal function
- whether previous antibiotics have been given.

The regimen may need to be changed once the organism and sensitivities are known (see Ch. 63).

SURGICAL DRAINAGE

Surgical debridement or drainage of the infection source is vital. If intra-abdominal abscesses are left undrained, mortality approaches 100%. Locating sources of infection can prove difficult and frustrating. Drainable sites of infection which may be missed include the abdomen, pleural cavities, and paranasal sinuses. The presence of nasotracheal and nasogastric tubes, head injuries and facial fractures, as well as the supine 'nursed horizontal' position, all predispose to poor sinus drainage and infection.

In suspected intra-abdominal sepsis, plain abdominal X-rays, ultrasonography, computed tomography (CT) scan, gallium 67 citrate scan and indium 111-labelled leukocytes may be helpful, but may also be misleading. The choice of investigation is guided by availability, expertise and the clinical situation. If intra-abdominal

sepsis is strongly suspected, exploratory laparotomy should be undertaken. Direct percutaneous drainage may be attempted in selected cases, when a definite abscess is located by ultrasonography or CT scan.

Severe diffuse peritonitis has a high mortality, and aggressive forms of therapy have been tried. However, radical peritoneal debridement or postoperative continuous peritoneal lavage offers no benefit. Repeated laparotomies confer poor results especially when performed more than 48 h after the initial operation.[30] Electively staged laparotomies and open management of the abdomen (possibly with use of a mesh zipper) are also proposed. Advantages claimed for open management include maximal drainage, ease of repeated debridement and lowered intra-abdominal pressure.[31] This method should be reserved for severe cases; mortality remains high and its superiority remains unestablished.[32]

OTHER MEASURES

Prophylaxis against stress ulceration should be undertaken. Candidal overgrowth in the gastrointestinal tract is likely in patients on broad spectrum antibiotics, and can pass from the gastrointestinal tract to cause fungaemia in man.[33] Candida prophylaxis should be considered in high-risk patients. Prophylaxis against deep vein thrombosis should also be undertaken.

COMPLICATIONS OF SEPSIS

Local complications related to the initial site of infection may be evident. Severe sepsis and septic shock are common causes of multiple organ dysfunction or failure (see Ch. 13). Common findings are metabolic failure (lactic acidosis, hyper/hypoglycaemia), rampant hypercatabolism with gross muscle wasting and coagulopathy. Severe gastrointestinal bleeding is a life threatening complication of sepsis. Critical illness myopathy and/or neuropathy may occur.

ADJUNCTIVE AND EXPERIMENTAL THERAPY

CORTICOSTEROIDS

Though Schumer's trial of 1974 utilizing high dose steroids suggested benefit in septic shock, this was not confirmed in subsequent large double blind studies.[34] The subject of steroids in septic shock has re-surfaced though this time the focus is on the value of relatively low doses ('stress doses') of hydrocortisone. These have been either 200–300 mg hydrocortisone/d in divided doses or 100 mg i.v. stat followed by an i.v. infusion of 10 mg/h. Such regimens have been shown to reduce the duration of vasopressor support and improve the clinical condition of the patient.[35,36] The cessation time for vaso-pressor infusion was shorter in patients with impaired adenocortical function than in patients with normal responses to corticotropin.[36] However, hydrocortisone also reverses shock in patients with an appropriate response to corticotropin.[35]

THERAPIES MODULATING COAGULATION

Of the therapies listed below, much interest is currently focused on the effects of replacement of natural antico-agulants (aPC, AT-III and TFPI). They have anticoagu-lant, anti-inflammatory and profibrinolytic properties. APC and AT-III become depleted in severe sepsis.

ACTIVATED PROTEIN C
A randomized, double blind, placebo controlled, multi-centre trial conducted with recombinant human activated protein C (aPC) involved 840 patients in the placebo group and 850 patients in the treatment group. Mortality rate was 30.8% in the placebo group and 24.7% in the recombinant aPC (drotrecogin) group. The absolute reduction in the risk of death was 6.1% ($P = 0.005$). The incidence of serious bleeding was higher in the drotreco-gin group (3.5% vs 2.0%; $P = 0.06$). Thus, drotrecogin significantly reduced mortality.[37]

ANTITHROMBIN III
Three randomized, double blind trials each containing between 34 to 42 patients and a fourth with 120 patients,[38] failed to demonstrate statistically significant differences in mortality between treatment and placebo arms. However, DIC and existing organ failure resolved more quickly, while less organ failure developed in patients receiving antithrombin III (AT-III) in some of the trials. Publication of the results of a large phase III trial (~200 patients) is awaited.

TISSUE FACTOR PATHWAY INHIBITOR
Tissue factor pathway inhibitor (TFPI) is a protein made by endothelial cells and is active against tissue factor VIIa (TF/VIIa) complex. Plasma levels of TFPI in sepsis are generally normal or high. It has been suggested any supple-mentary therapy should achieve supranormal levels. TFPI in animal studies has inhibited DIC or reduced mortality. A phase II study in 210 patients with severe sepsis showed a trend toward reduction in mortality in the rTFPI treated group.[39] An international phase III study has commenced.

HEPARIN
The use of heparin to treat DIC in sepsis has not been shown to improve survival.[40] Heparin potentially has a detrimental effect on the inflammatory response by com-peting with cell surface heparin sulphate proteoglycans for AT-III binding, by decreasing the activation of protein C due to decreased thrombin production, or by displacing TFPI from the endothelium.[41]

ENHANCING FIBRINOLYSIS
This could be achieved by inhibition of plasminogen activator inhibitor-I, but no such therapy currently exists. An alternative strategy of administering recombinant tissue plasminogen activator to patients with purpura fulminans has been undertaken.[42] No controlled trials have been published.

DISAPPOINTING RESULTS OF IMMUNOMODULATING TRIALS

A number of immunomodulating therapies designed to reduce or ameliorate the damaging inflammatory response of severe sepsis and septic shock have produced disappointing results. This is despite initially encourag-ing results from phase II clinical trials. Larger studies have been unable to demonstrate a reduced mortality resulting from a variety of interventions.[43] Reasons for this include agents studied being ineffective, too much emphasis on mortality as an outcome, compensatory mechanisms negating the effect of the intervention, incorrect dose and timing, and population studies being too heterogeneous.

ANTI-ENDOTOXIN THERAPY
Non-specific immunoglobin was used in early studies though later specific human antibodies to *E. coli* J5 and murine E5 and humanized HA-1A antibodies were explored. Early encouraging studies were followed by larger clinical trials failing to show benefit.[43,44]

ANTI-TNF TRIALS
The North American Sepsis Trial (NORASEPT) and a subsequent International Sepsis Trial (Intersept) examined a murine IgG1 monoclonal antibody in the treatment of sepsis and septic shock. Though incon-clusive, there were encouraging features. A larger NORASEPT II study enrolled 1879 patients with septic shock. No improvement in survival or increased rate of shock reversal was seen in the treatment group receiving 7.5 mg/kg of the murine monoclonal anti-TNF-α antibody. The use of anti-TNF receptor fusion proteins (P75 or P55) to detoxify TNF have also been tried. The first study showed increased mortality in the treatment group receiving the higher dose (1.5 mg/kg) of P75 anti-TNF agent. The next study looked at three different dose levels of P55 TNF recep-tor fusion protein in septic patients. No benefit was seen at any dose level in patients with refractory septic shock. The above studies were reviewed by Abraham.[43] A third phase III study[45] was undertaken in 1342 patients with severe sepsis with and without early septic shock. The P55 TNF receptor fusion protein used was not identical to that in the previous study. No improve-ment in day 28 mortality or organ failure scores were found in treated patients.

INTERLEUKIN-1 RECEPTOR ANTAGONIST IL-1ra

Two large phase III trials did not demonstrate benefit of IL-1ra administration to septic patients.[46] It also has no effect on cardiac function in septic patients.

ANTI-PLATELET ACTIVATING FACTOR

Three phase III clinical trials of platelet activating factor receptor antagonist have been published, the last in 2000.[47] Overall these trials showed insignificant beneficial treatment effect.

BRADYKININ ANTAGONIST

A randomized, double blind, placebo controlled multi-centre trial in 504 patients with SIRS and documented evidence of infection plus either hypotension or dysfunction of two organs, evaluated deltiband, a novel bradykinin antagonist. There was no significant effect on risk-adjusted 28-day survival.[48]

ANTI-PROSTAGLANDINS

A randomized, double blind, placebo controlled trial of intravenous ibuprofen (10 mg/kg [maximum dose 800 mg], given every 6 h for eight doses) in 455 septic patients with acute failure of at least one organ system, did not demonstrate improved survival, nor prevent the development of shock or acute respiratory distress syndrome (ARDS).[49]

KETOCONAZOLE

The antifungal agent ketoconazole is a thromboxane synthetase inhibitor. Three clinical studies suggested ketoconazole may prevent ARDS developing in critically ill patients. A multicentre randomized controlled trial, including 234 patients with ALI on ARDS did not find ketoconazole beneficial in the early treatment of ALI on ARDS.[50]

ANTIOXIDANTS

Of three prospective, randomized, double blind, placebo controlled trials of N-acetylcysteine (NAC) (a sulfhydryl group donor and oxygen radical scavenger), the first in patients with septic shock showed depression in cardiac performance (CI, left ventricular stroke work index, MAP) in the NAC treated patients.[51] A second trial of NAC in ameliorating development or progression of multiple organ failure, suggested initiation of NAC therapy >24 h after hospital admission may be harmful. Mortality was 61% in the NAC group vs 32% in controls; $P = 0.05$.[52] A third study involving 60 septic shock patients showed improved liver blood flow index and liver function as determined by MEGX in the NAC group. This was associated with an increase in CI (which conflicts with the findings of the first study). ICU length of stay and mortality rate was the same in the two groups.[53]

VASOPRESSIN

Arginine vasopressin has been shown to elevate blood pressure in septic shock patients who were requiring norepinephrine, epinephrine (or both) to maintain an adequate blood pressure.[54] Vasopressin levels have been reported to be inappropriately low in vasodilatory septic shock.[55] In this small study it was shown to significantly increase blood pressure, systemic vascular resistance and to decrease cardiac output. A small double blind, placebo controlled clinical trial (treatment $n = 5$, placebo $n = 5$) assessed the role of low dose vasopresssin infused at 0.04 U/min as a pressor in patients with septic shock requiring conventional vasopressors. At 24 hours all vasopressin receiving patients had survived and conventional vasopressors virtually ceased. Two patients in the placebo group had died of refractory hypotension during this time period.[56] Use of vasopressin in septic shock is experimental. It may adversely affect coronary and splanchnic blood flow. It raises blood pressure by its vasoconstrictive effects and may cause adverse falls in cardiac output if used alone. Note that vasopressin is not a vasopressor in normal subjects nor is hypertension a feature of the syndrome of inappropriate antidiuretic hormone.

PENTOXIFYLLINE

This phosphodiesterase inhibitor has immunomodulatory and cardiovascular effects. It blocks chemotaxis and activation of neutrophils. It significantly decreases plasma TNF and IL-6 levels in septic premature infants and it reduced mortality.[57] In a study of 51 patients with severe sepsis, it beneficially influenced cardiopulmonary function.[58] Improved haemodynamics in septic patients had previously been reported. Large well constructed trials are needed.

INHIBITING NITRIC OXIDE PRODUCTION OR ITS EFFECTS

Though vasoplegia and myocardial depression in sepsis may in part be due to nitric oxide (NO), this substance has important roles in neurotransmission, regulation of vascular tone, platelet inhibition, leukocyte adhesion and has antibacterial and antitumour effects. NO synthase inhibitors have been used to treat hypotension in sepsis. Methylene blue which inhibits the effects of NO on guanylate cyclase, increased MAP with no fall in cardiac output or oxygen consumption in one clinical trial.[59] A phase III multicentre, randomized, placebo controlled, double blind study of the nitric oxide synthase inhibitor 546 C88 to see if this agent increased 28 day survival after a treatment period of up to 14 days, was ceased early. There was increased mortality in the NO synthase inhibitor group with increased adverse cardiovascular events: decreased cardiac output, pulmonary hypertension, systemic hypertension and heart failure.[60]

NALOXONE

Endogenous opioid peptides derived from β-lipotropin are released in septic shock and other stress states. A meta-analysis of therapy of shock found naloxone increased blood pressure. It concluded that its clinical usefulness in treating shock was still to be determined.[61]

GRANULOCYTE COLONY STIMULATING FACTOR

Granulocyte colony stimulating factor (G-CSF) has had extensive use in the treatment of neutropenia in patients with malignancy. In a randomized controlled trial, G-CSF was used as an adjunct to antibiotics for the treatment of community acquired pneumonia. Time to reduction of morbidity, mortality and length of hospital stay were unaffected.[62] G-CSF (Filgrastim) was found to be safe in intubated ICU patients, with no excess risk of development of ARDS or MOD.[63]

GROWTH HORMONE

Two prospective, multicentre, double blind, randomized, placebo controlled trials in parallel showed intensive care patients receiving growth hormone had more than double the mortality of those that did not receive it (P <0.001 for both studies). Morbidity was also increased in the treatment group. Multiple organ failure, septic shock or uncontrolled infection were the main causes of death in both treatment groups.[64]

HAEMOFILTRATION

The role of this modality in modifying SIRS is controversial (see Ch. 39). Adjuncts to haemofiltration have been the use of polymyxin B binding columns to remove endotoxin, and cytokine and other inflammatory mediator adsorption by resin in an animal model of endotoxaemia has been studied. Encouraging results are reported, but more work is needed.

PROGNOSIS

Mortality increases with increasing severity score (e.g. APACHE II), number of dysfunctional/failed organs and duration of such failure.[65,66] Several factors influence the prognosis in bacteraemia and fungaemia in adults[67,68]: source of infection, where acquired, blood pressure, organism isolated, body temperature, age and predisposing factors. Survival is improved by appropriate use of antibiotics and surgical drainage (where applicable).[68] The ability to maintain an increased CI, DO_2 and VO_2 is associated with better prognosis.[13,69] Pulmonary hypertension is an adverse factor.[9] Peripheral vascular failure may be a major haemodynamic determinant of mortality, as survivors of septic shock are more able to augment SVRI.[70] A high blood lactate is a marker of a poor prognosis.

REFERENCES

1 American College of Chest Physicians/Society of Critical Care Medicine Consensus Conference. Definitions for sepsis and organ failure and guidelines for the use of innovative therapies in sepsis. *Crit Care Med* 1992; **20**: 864–74.

2 Parillo JE, Parker MM, Natanson C, *et al.* Septic shock: advances in the understanding of pathogenesis, cardiovascular dysfunction, and therapy. *Ann Intern Med* 1990; **113**: 227–42.

3 Vincent J-L, Bihari DJ, Suter PM, *et al.* The prevalence of nosocomial infection in intensive care units in Europe. *JAMA* 1995; **274**: 639–44.

4 Glauser MP. Pathophysiological basis of sepsis: considerations for future strategies of intervention. *Crit Care Med* 2000; **28**(**Suppl**): S4–8.

5 Modlin RL, Brightbill HD, Godowski PJ. The toll of innate immunity on microbial pathogens. *N Engl J Med* 1999; **340**: 1834–5.

6 Bone RC. Sir Isaac Newton, sepsis, SIRS and CARS. *Crit Care Med* 1996; **24**: 1125–8.

7 Stuber F, Petersen M, Bokelmann F, Schade U. A genomic polymorphism within the tumor necrosis factor locus influences plasma tumor necrosis factor-α concentrations and outcome of patients with severe sepsis. *Crit Care Med* 1996; **24**: 381–4.

8 Briegel J. Hydrocortisone and the reduction of vasopressors in septic shock: therapy or only chart cosmetics? Editorial *Intensive Care Med* 2000; **26**: 1723–6.

9 Sibbald WJ, Paterson NAM, Holiday RL *et al.* Pulmonary hypertension in sepsis. Measurement by pulmonary arterial diastolic-pulmonary wedge pressure gradient and the influence of passive and active factors. *Chest* 1978; **73**: 583–91.

10 de Jonge E, Levi M, van der Poll T. Coagulation abnormalities in sepsis: relation with inflammatory responses. *Curr Opin Crit Care* 2000; **6**: 317–22.

11 Esmon CT. Are natural anticoagulants candidates for modulating the inflammatory response to endotoxin? *Blood* 2000; **95**: 1113–6.

12 Parker MM, Shelhamer JH, Bacharach SL, *et al.* Profound but reversible myocardial depression in patients with septic shock. *Ann Intern Med* 1984; **100**: 483–90.

13 Parker MM, Shelhamer JH, Natanson C, *et al.* Serial cardiovascular variables in survivors and non-survivors of septic shock: heart rate as an early predictor of prognosis. *Crit Care Med* 1987; **15**: 923–9.

14 Metrangolo L, Fiorillo M, Friedman G, *et al.* Early hemodynamic course of septic shock. *Crit Care Med* 1995; **23**: 1971–5.

15 Muller-Werdan U, Werdan K. Septic cardiomyopathy. *Curr Opin Crit Care* 1999; **5**: 415–21.

16 Mizock BA. Alterations in carbohydrate metabolism during stress: a review of the literature. *Am J Med* 1995; **98**: 75–84.

17 Gammaitoni C, Nasraway SA. Normal lactate/pyruvate ratio during overwhelming polymicrobial bacteremia and multiple organ failure. *Anesthesiology* 1994; **80**: 213–6.

18 Ince C, Sinaasappel M. Microcirculatory oxygenation and shunting in sepsis and shock. *Crit Care Med* 1999; **27**: 1369–77.

19 Ruokonen E, Takala J, Kari A *et al*. Regional blood flow and oxygen transport in septic shock. *Crit Care Med* 1993; **21**: 1296–303.

20 Marik PE, Varon J. The hemodynamic derangements in sepsis. *Chest* 1998; **114**: 854–60.

21 Hebert PC, Wells G, Blajchman MA, *et al*. A multi-center, randomised, controlled clinical trial of transfusion requirements in critical care. *N Engl J Med* 1999; **340**: 409–17.

22 Hebert PC, Yetisir E, Martin C, *et al*. Is a low transfusion threshold safe in critically ill patients with cardiovascular diseases? *Crit Care Med* 2001; **29**: 227–34.

23 Task Force of the American College of Critical Care Medicine, Society of Critical Care Medicine. Practice parameters for hemodynamic support of sepsis in adult patients in sepsis. *Crit Care Med* 1999; **27**: 639–60.

24 Packman MI, Racklow EC. Optimum left heart filling pressure during fluid resuscitation of patients with hypovolemic and septic shock. *Crit Care Med* 1983; **11**: 165–9.

25 Marik P, Mohedin M. The contrasting effects of dopamine and norepinephrine on systemic and splanchnic oxygen utilization in hyperdynamic sepsis. *J Am Med Assoc* 1994; **272**: 1354–7.

26 Schreuder WO, Schneider AJ, Groeneveld AB, Thijs LG. Effect of dopamine vs norepinephrine on hemodynamics in septic shock. Emphasis on right ventricular performance. *Chest* 1989; **95**: 1282–8.

27 Duranteau J, Sitbon P, Teboul JL, *et al*. Effects of epinephrine, norepinephrine, or the combination of norepinephrine and dobutamine on gastric mucosa in septic shock. *Crit Care Med* 1999; **27**: 893–900.

28 Martin C, Viviand C, Arnaud S *et al*. Effects of norepinephrine plus dobutamine or norepinephrine alone on left ventricular performance of septic shock patients. *Crit Care Med* 1999; **27**: 1708–13.

29 Rossaint R, Falke KJ, Lopez F *et al*. Inhaled nitric oxide for the adult respiratory distress syndrome. *N Engl J Med* 1993; **328**: 399–405.

30 Koperna T, Schulz F. Relaparotomy in peritonitis: prognosis and treatment of patients with persisting intra-abdominal infection. *World J Surg* 2000; **24**: 32–7.

31 Schein M, Saadia R, Decker GGA. The open management of the septic abdomen. *Surg Gynecol Obstet* 1986; **163**: 587–92.

32 Saadia MS, Freinkel Z, Decker G. Aggressive treatment of severe diffuse peritonitis: a prospective study. *Br J Surg* 1988; **75**: 173–6.

33 Krause W, Matheis H, Wulf K. Fungaemia and funguria after oral administration of Candida albicans. *Lancet* 1969; **i**: 598–9.

34 Lefering R, Neugebauer EA. Steroid controversy in sepsis and septic shock: a meta-analysis. *Crit Care Med* 1995; **23**: 1294–303.

35 Bollaert PE, Charpentier C, Levy B *et al*. Reversal of late septic shock with supraphysiologic doses of hydrocortisone. *Crit Care Med* 1998; **26**: 645–50.

36 Oppert M, Reinicke A, Graf K-J *et al*. Plasma cortisol levels before and during 'low dose' hydrocortisone therapy and their relationship to hemodynamic improvement in patients with septic shock. *Intensive Care Med* 2000; **26**: 1747–55.

37 Bernard GR, Vincent J-L, Laterre P-F, *et al*. for the PROWESS Study Group. Efficacy and safety of recombinant human activated protein C for severe sepsis. *N Engl J Med* 2001; **344**: 699–709.

38 Baudo F, Caimi TM, de Cataldo E, *et al*. Antithrombin III replacement therapy in patients with sepsis and/or surgical complications: a controlled, double blind, randomised, multicenter study. *Intensive Care Med* 1998; **24**: 336–42.

39 Abraham E. Tissue factor inhibition and clinical trial results of tissue factor pathway inhibitor in sepsis. *Crit Care Med* 2000; **28**(Suppl): S31–3.

40 Mant MJ, King EG. Severe, acute disseminated intravascular coagulation. *Am J Med* 1979; **67**: 557–63.

41 Esmon CT. Are natural anticoagulants candidates for modulating the inflammatory response to endotoxin? *Blood* 2000; **95**: 1113–6.

42 Aiuto LT, Barone SR, Cohen PS, *et al*. Recombinant tissue plasminogen activator restores perfusion in meningococcal purpura fulminans. *Crit Care Med* 1997; **25**: 1079–82.

43 Abraham E. Why immunomodulatory therapies have not worked in sepsis. *Intensive Care Med* 1999; **25**: 556–66.

44 Angus DC, Birmingham MC, Balk RA, *et al*. E5 murine monoclonal antiendotoxin antibody in Gram-negative sepsis: a randomised controlled trial. *JAMA* 2000; **283**: 1723–30.

45 Abraham E, Laterre P-F, Garbino, *et al*. for the Lenercept Study Group. Lenercept (p55 tumor necrosis factor receptor fusion protein) in severe sepsis and early septic shock: a randomised, double blind, placebo controlled, multicenter phase III trial with 1342 patients. *Crit Care Med* 2001; **29**: 503–10.

46 Opal SM, Fisher CJ, Pribble JP, *et al*. for the Interleukin-1 Receptor Antagonist Sepsis Investigator Group. The confirmatory interleukin-1 receptor antagonist trial in severe sepsis: a phase III randomised, double blind, placebo controlled, multicenter trial. *Crit Care Med* 1997; **25**: 1115–24.

47 Suputtamongkol Y, Intaranongpai S, Smith MD, *et al*. A double blind, placebo controlled study of an infusion of lexipafant (platelet activating factor receptor antagonist) in patients with severe sepsis. *Antimicrobial Agents and Chemotherapy* 2000; **44**: 693–6.

48 Fein AM, Bernard GR, Criner GJ, *et al*. Treatment of severe systemic inflammatory response syndrome and sepsis with a novel bradykinin antagonist, deltiband (CP-0127). Results of a randomised, double blind, placebo controlled trial. CP-0127 SIRS and Sepsis Study Group. *JAMA* 1997; **277**: 482–7.

49 Bernard GR, Wheeler AP, Russell JA, *et al*. The effects of ibuprofen on the physiology and survival of patients with sepsis. The Ibuprofen in Sepsis Study Group. *N Engl J Med* 1997; **336**: 912–8.

50 The ARDS Network. Ketoconazole for early treatment of acute lung injury and acute respiratory distress syndrome. *JAMA* 2000, **283**: 1995–2002.

51 Peake SL, Moran JL, Leppard PI. N-acetyl-L-cysteine depresses cardiac performance in patients with septic shock. *Crit Care Med* 1996; **24**: 1302–10.

52 Molnar Z, Shearer E, Lowe D. N-acetylcysteine treatment to prevent the progression of multisystem organ failure: a prospective, randomised, placebo controlled study. *Crit Care Med* 1999; **27**: 1100–4.

53 Rank N, Michel C, Haertel C, *et al*. N-acetylcysteine increases liver blood flow and improves liver function in septic shock patients: results of a prospective, randomised, double blind study. *Crit Care Med* 2000; **28**: 3799–807.

54 Landry DW, Levin HR, Gallant EM, *et al*. Vasopressin pressor hypersensitivity in vasodilatory septic shock. *Crit Care Med* 1997; **25**: 1279–82.

55 Landry DW, Levin HR, Gallant EM, *et al*. Vasopressin deficiency contributes to the vasodilation of septic shock. *Circulation* 1997; **95**: 1122–5.

56 Malay MB, Ashton RC Jr, Landry DW, *et al*. Low dose vasopressin in the treatment of vasodilatory septic shock. *J Trauma Inj Infect Crit Care* 1999; **47**: 699–703.

57 Lauterbach R, Pawlik D, Kowalczyl D, *et al*. Effect of immunomodulating agent pentoxifylline, in the treatment of sepsis in prematurely delivered infants: a placebo controlled, double blind trial. *Crit Care Med* 1999; **27**: 807–14.

58 Stauback K, Schroder J, Stuber F, *et al*. Effect of pentoxifylline in severe sepsis: results of a randomised, double blind, placebo controlled study. *Arch Surg* 1998; **133**: 94–100.

59 Preiser JC, Lejeune P, Roman A, *et al*. Methylene blue administration in septic shock: a clinical trial. *Crit Care Med* 1995; **23**: 259–64.

60 Grover R, Lopez A, Lorente J, *et al*. Multi-center, randomised, placebo controlled, double blind study of the nitric oxide synthase inhibitor 546C88: effect on survival in patients with septic shock. Abstract. *Crit Care Med* 1999; **27**; A33.

61 Boeuf B, Gauvin F, Guerguercon A, *et al*. Therapy of shock with naloxone: a meta-analysis. *Crit Care Med* 1998; **26**: 1910–6.

62 Nelson S, Balknep S, Carlson R, *et al*. A randomised controlled trial of filgrastim as an adjunct to antibiotics for treatment of hospitalised patients with community acquired pneumonia. *J Infect Dis* 1998; **178**: 1075–80.

63 Pettila V, Takkunen O, Varpula T, *et al*. Safety of granulocyte colony stimulating factor (filgrastim) in intubated patients in the intensive care unit: interim analysis of a prospective, placebo controlled, double blind study. *Crit Care Med* 2000; **28**: 3620–5.

64 Takala J, Ruokenon E, Webster N, *et al*. Increased mortality associated with growth hormone treatment in critically ill adults. *N Engl J Med* 1999; **341**: 785–92.

65 Knaus WA, Draper EA, Wagner DP, Zimmerman JE. Prognosis in acute organ system failure. *Ann Surg* 1985; **202**: 685–93.

66 Chang RWS, Jacobs S, Lee B. Predicting outcome among intensive care unit patients using computerised trend analysis of daily APACHE II scores corrected for organ system failure. *Intensive Care Med* 1988; **114**: 558–66.

67 An expert report of the European Society of Intensive Care Medicine. The problem of sepsis. *Intensive Care Med* 1994; **20**: 300–4.

68 Weinstein MP, Murphy JR, Reller LB, Lichtenstein KA. The clinical significance of positive blood cultures: comprehensive analysis of 500 episodes of bacteremia and fungemia in adults. Clinical observations, with special reference to factors influencing prognosis. *Rev Infect Dis* 1983; **5**: 54–70.

69 Rhodes A, Lamb FJ, Malagon I, *et al*. A prospective study of the use of a dobutamine stress test to identify outcome in patients with sepsis, severe sepsis, or septic shock. *Crit Care Med* 1999; **27**: 2361–6.

70 Groeneveld ABJ, Nauta JJP, Thijs LG. Peripheral vascular resistance in septic shock: its relation to outcome. *Intensive Care Med* 1988; **14**: 141–7.

60

Nosocomial infection

N Soni

Nosocomial or 'hospital-acquired infections' are a major problem in hospitals and in particular in the critically ill. ICUs represent 2–10% of hospital beds, but are responsible for 25% of all nosocomial blood stream and pulmonary infections. Nosocomial infection is, at least in theory, a preventable cause of morbidity and mortality (Table 60.1).

EPIDEMIOLOGY

The incidence of nosocomial infection is determined by a range of factors. The prevalence will vary between institutions (3–12%), as well as between in-hospital settings. A recent study demonstrated a range of 0–23% between ophthalmology and ICU patients.[1] The EPIC snap shot study found an ICU infection rate of 20.6%.[2]

Within a hospital population, urinary tract infection is the most frequent, followed by lower respiratory tract, with surgical wound infection and blood cultures less than 10% each. However, in the ICU, respiratory infections are more common, as are surgical wound and blood stream infections (8–12%), while urinary tract infections are relatively rare.

The impact of nosocomial infection is impressive with both prolonged length of stay, and an attributable morbidity and mortality.[3] Blood stream infections result in 14 attributable extra hospital days, surgical wound infections 12 days, and nosocomial pneumonia 13 days.[4] The mortality rates directly due to these infections are hard to separate from the mortality attributed to the presenting severity of illness, which in its own right may have predisposed to infection. However, it is clear that nosocomial infection is associated with increased mortality, and huge financial and resource costs.

THE MECHANISMS INVOLVED IN NOSOCOMIAL INFECTION

A range of factors come together to enable nosocomial infection to occur (Table 60.2).

Table 60.1 Principles of diagnosis of nosocomial infections

Diagnosis of infection usually requires the combination of both clinical findings and the results of diagnostic tests.

Clinical diagnosis of infection from direct observation at surgery, endoscopy or other diagnostic procedure is an acceptable criterion for an infection.

It must be hospital acquired. There must be no evidence that the infection was present or incubating at the time of hospital admission. Infection acquired in hospital, but only evident after hospital discharge also fulfils the criteria

Usually no specific time during or after hospitalization is given to determine whether an infection is nosocomial or community-acquired. Each infection is examined for evidence that links it to hospitalization (this is a matter of controversy).

HOST

The vulnerability of a potential host will be determined by several factors:

1 The acute illness or problem that required ICU admission.
2 The chronic health status and underlying disease. Conditions, such as diabetes, predispose to infective problems.
3 The status of their immunocompetence, which may involve medications, such as steroids.
4 The integrity of natural defences, such as the skin and mucous membranes. This may be disrupted by burns, surgery or by breakdown of tissues such as with pressure sores. The presence of invasive devices (e.g. endotracheal tube, intravenous devices) provides a conduit past the natural defences.
5 Antibiotics given to the patient which may encourage emergence of particular strains or resistant organisms.

ENVIRONMENT

Local environmental pressures play their part, such as antibiotic use and abuse. Pseudomembranous colitis from Clostridium difficile toxin is an example, although cross infection may also occur. Epidemiological patterns,

Table 60.2   Risk factors for nosocomial infection

Patient
   Severity of illness
   Underlying diseases
   Nutritional state
   Immunosuppression
   Open wounds
   Invasive devices
   Multiple procedures
   Prolonged stay
   Ventilation
   Multiple or prolonged antibiotics
Environment
   Changes in procedures or protocols
   Multiple changes in staff; new staff
   Poor aseptic practice – poor hand washing
   Patient to patient. Busy, crowded unit, staff shortages
The Organism
   Resistance
   Resilience in terms of survival
   Formation of slime or ability to adhere
   Pathogenicity
   Prevalence

such as the prevalence of *Enterococcus faecalis* as a common pathogen in the surgical population may be linked to widespread cephalosporin usage. Much of the multi-resistance problem probably originates from antibiotic pressures.[5] Transmission is by various means but the most common is by hands.[6]

ORGANISM

The host usually lives in synergistic or symbiotic tranquillity with a huge range of organisms (Table 60.3). Antibiotics may suppress many of the normal organisms and allow emergence and overgrowth of a usually insignificant organism. A classic example of an intrinsic organism causing problems with overgrowth might be the prevalence of symptomatic candidiasis in the presence of broad spectrum antibiotics. Extrinsic organisms are those that may be introduced from the environment, from other patients or from staff. These may be organisms which are thriving in that environment because of local pressures (e.g. antibiotics), or from poor hygiene. On admission, patients will be carrying a range of organisms that may cause problems, but during their stay they are likely to acquire a new ecology some of which is from their surroundings.

The individual characteristics of the organism are important, and include the ease with which they survive or thrive in the local environment, the ease of transmission and the individual pathogenicity. This clearly interacts with the vulnerability of the host as some usually innocuous organisms, such as candida or Serratia marcescens will only

cause problems in vulnerable hosts while others, such as some strains of Staph aureus, Acinetobacter or Clostridium difficile can be more virulent.

THE ORGANISMS

There is a wide range of organisms that can cause nosocomial infection (Table 60.6). It must be emphasized that each hospital and each ICU will have its own local ecology and that awareness of the organisms in the local environment is important. Regional, national and international surveys give indication of general trends but this does not supplant local knowledge.

The organisms with highest profile in nosocomial infection alter over time. Historically, gram positive infections in the 1950s and 1960s gave way to gram negative infections in the 1970s. The emergence of multiresistant gram positive organisms is currently the predominant problem, but already super resistant organisms, such as Stenotrophomonas and Acinetobacter are emerging as major contenders.

In ICU, where there is the combination of sick patients and widespread use of potent antibiotics, the environment will in effect tend to select multi resistant organisms that may dominate colonization patterns.

The organisms causing nosocomial infection may be endogenous or exogenous. In the critically ill there are striking changes in the patterns of colonization. Multiple factors, including the use of antibiotics, may alter the endogenous flora allowing predominance of organisms normally suppressed and thereby a change in ecology on the skin, in the oro/nasopharynx and in the gut. Exogenous organisms from the local environment are able to colonize the patient from whence they can either invade or be introduced by invasive procedures, by devices or simply through areas of injury.

Table 60.3   Common commensals that may cause infection in a vulnerable host

Site	Common commensal organisms
Skin	Staph. epidermidis, streptococci, corynebacterium (diphtheroids) candida
Throat	Strep. viridans, diphtheroids
Mouth	Strep viridans, Moraxella cattharalis, actinomyces, spirochaetes
Respiratory tract	Strep. viridans, Moraxella, diphtheroids, micrococci
Vagina	Lactobacilli, diphtheroids, streptococci, yeast
Intestines	Bacteroides, anaerobic streptococci, Clostridium perfringens, Escherichia coli, Klebsiella, proteus, enterococci.

MULTI-RESISTANT ORGANISMS

Many of the organisms that cause nosocomial infection are characterized by multi-resistance. There are several mechanisms involved in resistance and in its spread. Enzymes, such as the β-lactamases, render a large array of antibiotics useless. Class 1 β-lactamase is effective against some β-lactam containing antibiotics but extended spectrum β-lactamases (ESBL), which incorporate enzymes, such as TEM-24, will produce cross resistance to multiple classes of antibiotics including fluoroquinolones and aminoglycosides. Resistance may be produced by a combination of mechanisms such as in Pseudomonas aeruginosa where the resistance is due to a combination of derepression of protein efflux systems, cephalosporinases and derepression of AmpC enzyme.

Resistance is acquired in a variety of ways. Mutation of any gene occurs at a rate of one cell in 10^7 and if this cell is then presented with antibiotics that it can survive it will become a dominant cell reproducing at a rate of 10^9 overnight. An example of this might be the development of AmpC β-lactamase in enterobacter, when patients are treated with third generation cephalosporins. Similarly, the loss of porin OprD in *Pseudomonas aeruginosa* in the presence of imipenem.

Spread or resistance may be very rapid once the genes are encoded. The enzyme production may be encoded chromosomally within the organism, or may be transferred between bacteria by plasmids Transposons transfer genes between plasmids. This potentially allows rapid transmission of resistance between species. Examples of this include:

1 SHV-1 plasmid β-lactamase from klebsiella
2 plasmid AmpC β-lactamases from citrobacter
3 aminoglycoside-modifying enzymes from aminoglycoside producing streptomycetes.

Table 60.5 Principles for the diagnosis of nosocomial pneumonia

Crackles on auscultation or dullness to percussion on physical examinaion of the chest and any of the following:
New onset of purulent sputum
Organism isolated from blood cultures
Isolation of pathogen from specimen obtained by transtracheal aspirate, bronchial brushing or biopsy
Chest radiography examination shows ne or progressive infiltration, consolidation, cavitation or pleural effusion
Isolation of virus or detection of virus antigen in respiratory secretions
Diagnostic single antibody titre (IgM) or fourfold increase in paired serum samples (IgG) for pathogen
Histopathological evidence of pneumonia

IgM = Immunoglobulin M.

Table 60.4 The influence of ESBL on resistance in Klebsiella[7]

Antibiotics	ESBL negative (% resistant)	ESBL positive (% resistant)
Gentamicin	8	76
Amikacin	3	52
Ciprofloxacin	3	31
All the above	0	5

(From Livermore and Yuan).[7]

The phenomenon of induction is also seen. This is the process whereby the presence of an antibiotic appears to 'induce' or speed up the production of the relevant enzyme so that the organism rapidly becomes resistant.

Alternatively, the production of a resilient and resistant bacteria may allow it to dominate the local ecology where antibiotics are in use, antibiotic pressure. It may then be spread by vectors and thrive in other similar environments. Staphylococcal resistance to methicillin occurs due to an altered penicillin binding protein, which has low affinity for all beta-lactam agents. It is linked to a MecA gene. This gene does not develop readily, with the spread of methicillin resistant organisms through vector transmission, not *de novo* production of resistance[7] (Table 60.4).

SOME COMMON ORGANISMS

See Table 60.6 for organisms responsible for the majority of nosocomial infections.

E. COLI

One of the first organisms to become multi-resistant. The spread of its resistance is a model of how the problem develops in different environments. Currently in Europe, about 4% of E. Coli is resistant to ceftazidime but in Turkey, this figure is 26%. The trend towards an

Table 60.6 Organisms responsible for the majority of nosocomial infections

Methicillin resistant Staphylococcus aureus (MRSA)
Coagulase negative Staph. (CNS)
Enterococcus spp. (faecalis, faecium)
Pseudomonas aeruginosa
Acinetobacter baumanii
Stenotrophomonas maltophilia
Enterobacter spp
Klebsiella spp.
E. coli
Serratia marcescens
Proteus spp.
Candida spp. (albicans, glabrata, krusei)

Other organisms may be a problem in the severely immunocompromised, such as those with acquired immunodeficiency, AIDS (see Ch. 59).

increase in resistance seems to correspond with the use of quinolones.[8]

ENTEROBACTER SPECIES, CLOACAE AND AEROGENES

Part of the normal intestinal flora. They tend to develop ESBL relatively easily making them multi-resistant to a wide range of antibiotics including ceftazidime. The prevalence of resistance in many Western ICUs is running at about 35% and rising. This organism has been implicated in cross colonization in ICU and the relevant enzymes including TEM-24 impart cross-resistance to multiple classes of antibiotics.

KLEBSIELLA

Klebsiella has become increasingly resistant with the acquisition of extended spectrum beta-lactamases (ESBL) and can be multi-resistant. The incidence is incredibly variable between countries.

PSEUDOMONAS

Versatile opportunistic pathogens common in the critically ill. They may colonize patients with chronic lung disease. Resistance is able to develop in a range of ways and produces a very broad spectrum of resistance making it potentially very difficult to treat.

STENOTROPHOMONAS MALTOPHILIA

An increasingly common and troublesome environmental organism. Often resistant to β-lactam antibiotics, quinolones and to aminoglycosides. It also produces a carbapenamase, which makes it resistant to carbapenems.

ACINETOBACTER BAUMANII

Acinetobacter baumanii is an increasing and major problem. It survives even in dry environments and despite its name spreads and cross infects readily (*a-cineto* without movement). They are multi-resistant and while they were sensitive to carbapenems they are increasingly resistant even to these agents, presumably through gene exchange.

COAGULASE NEGATIVE STAPHYLOCOCCI

Coagulase negative staphylococci (CNS) are low virulence organisms, but are increasingly causing nosocomial infection. Frequently methicillin resistant, they are also resistant to multiple classes of antibiotics, but usually sensitive to glycopeptides. As glycopeptide resistance patterns alter newer agents, such as quinupristin, dalfopristin and linezolid will have a role.

STAPHYLOCOCCUS AUREUS

This is a virulent pathogen causing a wide range of infections. Methicillin resistance started in the early 1960s, and although rates between countries and ICUs vary considerably, there has been an inexorable rise in its prevalence in most countries. It is easily identified. It

both colonizes and infects, but is relatively easily treated with glycopeptides. More recent reports of occasional glycopeptide resistant organisms is therefore a major source of concern. It has been a model of the failure of some infection control methods.

ENTEROCOCCUS FAECALIS AND FAECIUM

These organisms emerged with increased third generation cephalosporin use. E. faecalis is more commonly isolated and may still be sensitive to ampicillin but more than 30% or more are resistant to aminoglycosides. This contrasts with E. faecium, which has a resistance rate of 7% to vancomycin (and rising), 53% to ampicillin and 30% to aminoglycosides. Glycopeptide resistance is increasing and vancomycin resistant enterococcus (VRE), unheard of 3 years ago, is now being regularly identified.

TUBERCULOSIS

Not normally seen as a nosocomial infection, this has the potential to become a nosocomial problem. As numbers increase and infected patients are not recognized on admission, there is the possibility of rapid spread to both other patients and staff. In particular multi-resistant TB is on the increase. At present there are occasional outbreaks but these could easily increase.

CANDIDA SEPSIS

Almost always a nosocomial problem. Probably related to overgrowth secondary to antibiotic pressures. The prevalence of species is defined by each unit but C. albicans is most common. There is some evidence to suggest that the widespread use of azoles may have influenced the relative increase in C. glabrata and C. krusei species. The sudden appearance of an unusual species, such as C. krusei on more than one patient, may well indicate cross infection. Definitive diagnosis is by blood culture but presumptive diagnosis is suggested by the triad of clinical infection, a high-risk patient and candida at more than two sites. Antifungal treatment should depend on the sensitivity of the species involved.

In the next decade, three organisms will dominate nosocomial infection and one, MRSA, will provide a historical perspective. The organisms are Stenotrophomonas and Acinetobacter, which are rapidly becoming more common and less easy to treat. The third relates to the rising incidence of tuberculosis, which is already providing infection control challenges in the critically ill (see Figure 60.1).

COLONIZATION AND INFECTION

Many of these organisms colonize and cause infection, but differentiating these is difficult and identifying the responsible organism even more challenging. The presence of an organism in the critically ill does not necessarily mean it is responsible for an infection. As a consequence, treatment is often based on probability or the weight of evidence, rather than certainty.

MRSA colonizes very readily and causes infection in a significant proportion of cases but is often easily identified and treated. VRE is still relatively uncommon. It does colonize although the incidence of overt infection appears low, at present although difficult to treat when it occurs. Acinetobacter colonizes and infects very readily, and is difficult to treat.[9]

SITES OF INFECTION

The main sites of nosocomial infection are the chest, wounds and intravenous lines. Urinary tract infection often quoted as common, seems to be seen rarely in the critically ill.

NOSOCOMIAL PNEUMONIA

Nosocomial pneumonia[10] is a common problem in the critically ill, particularly in ventilated patients with an incidence of 15–30%.[3,11]

AETIOLOGY

There are several possible mechanisms, including aspiration from the nasopharynx, local spread or haematogenous spread of infection. Some 45% of healthy adults aspirate in their sleep. In the sick the nasopharynx colonizes rapidly with a wide range of organisms, usually gram negatives, and aspiration is encouraged by the unconscious state, the presence of a nasogastric tube or by endotracheal intubation. Pneumonia will develop in up to 25% of colonized patients, compared with a 3% incidence in non-colonized patients. It may also be related to the colonization of the upper GI tract, which may in turn colonize the nasopharynx.

Factors that are likely to encourage colonization of the pharyngeal areas with organisms include antibiotics and nasogastric tubes. Also implicated are alterations in the host defences in the pharynx, changes in the local pH, the amount of surface mucin, and impairment of other local immune defence mechanisms

Patient factors predisposing to nosocomial pneumonia include acute severity of illness; chronic illness, especially chronic lung disease; diabetes; immunosuppression; advanced age; recent surgery to thorax or abdomen; intubation; and bronchoscopy. Environmental factors include broad spectrum and prolonged use of antibiotics; potential pathogens in the vicinity; bacterial properties such as ability to adhere to surfaces; cross infection; 24-hour ventilator tubing changes; and foreign bodies such as nasogastric tubes. Intubated and ventilated patients have a higher rate of nosocomial infection than patients receiving non-invasive ventilation. However, this may be due to different patient populations with different underlying problems and background morbidity.[12] Neutralization of gastric acid is also controversial. Meta-analyses seemed to show that the use of H_2-antagonists were associated with a marked increase in nosocomial pneumonia, implicating bacterial colonization of the upper GI tract as a potent source of pneumonia. However, recent data have not confirmed this.[13–15]

DIAGNOSIS

The general criteria for diagnosis[10,16] are general signs of infection; clinical signs of a chest infection; purulent sputum; radiological evidence, such as new pulmonary infiltrates; and positive cultures, from sputum or blood. These produce a non-specific diagnosis. Expectorated sputum is difficult to assess, but should contain <25 polymorphs and >10 squamous epithelial cells per low-power field. In ICU it is more usual to provide samples from the endotracheal tube and to then use quantitative techniques. This can achieved with protected brush specimens (PBS) bronchoalveolar lavage (BAL) and protected BAL. These are difficult and time consuming and it appears that non- bronchoscopic techniques such as blind tracheal aspirates through the endotracheal tube are both practical and reasonably effective from a clinical if not a research viewpoint.

THE ORGANISMS

Aerobic gram negatives predominate including Pseudomonas aeruginosa, Enterobacter sp., Klebsiella, E. coli, Serratia marcescens and Proteus; which between them account for about 70% of infections. Staphylococci, in particular MRSA, account for a small, but significant number of nosocomial pneumonias. Early onset VAP, between 48 hours to 5 days, may be due to community pathogens, such as methicillin-sensitive *Staphylococcus aureus*, *Streptococcus pneumoniae*, and *Haemophilus influenzae* as well as gram-negative enteric bacilli (GNEB). This has been described as early endogenous infection. In contrast

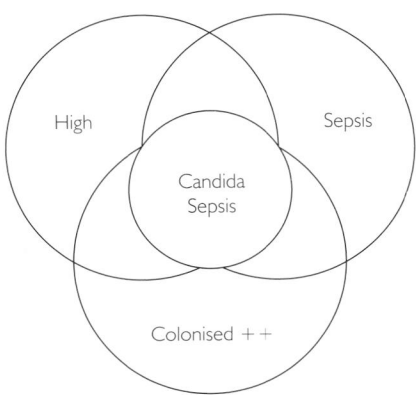

Fig. 60.1 Diagnostic triad of candida sepsis.

later onset, after 5–7 days, involves more resistant species such as MRSA, *Pseudomonas aeruginosa*, *Acinetobacter baumannii* and *Stenotrophomonas maltophilia*.[16,17] This has been called secondary endogenous and exogenous infection.

PREVENTION

Prevention is by methods that reduce aspiration, reduce cross infection and reduce contamination of respiratory devices. Several recommended methods are:

1. hand washing
2. limiting antibiotic use
3. changing ventilator circuits at longer intervals – 1 week.
4. orotracheal, rather than nasotracheal intubation
5. removing nasogastric tube
6. Semi-recumbent position; reduces aspiration
7. avoiding muscle relaxants
8. avoiding reintubation
9. Using non-invasive ventilation, where possible.

Other more controversial methods include:

1. antibiotic prophylaxis after intubation
2. continuous suctioning of subglottic secretions
3. early enteral nutrition: benefits of the colonization of the GI tract might be offset by problems with naso-gastric tubes and nasopharyngeal colonization
4. the use of heat moisture exchangers
5. closed suctioning: with some limited evidence it reduces VAP.[18]

TREATMENT

Inappropriate antibiotics, as with some empiric regimens, leads to an increased mortality. As the spectrum of resistance grows it is highly likely that it will be increasingly difficult to apply empiric treatment, especially with late onset VAP. Surveillance of current colonization, awareness of an individual ICU's ecology and targeted treatment will replace empiric regimens. At present, combination therapy is recommended, but there is little evidence to support it over monotherapy.[19–22]

The attributable mortality with nosocomial pneumonia is difficult to determine because the patients requiring ventilation have a high intrinsic mortality. Rates of 30% have been quoted, with pneumonia, probably accounts for 60% of deaths from nosocomial infections. In addition, nosocomial pneumonia increases length of stay by 12–23 days.[23]

WOUND INFECTION

Wound infections are common and represent 20% of all nosocomial infection. The organisms involved may be those introduced at the time or from later contamination.

RISK FACTORS[24]

1. the procedure itself and the level of contamination prior to or during surgery. In clean elective surgery the incidence should be less than 10%, but where contamination may occur (e.g. bowel surgery) it may be as high as 15%. In contaminated procedures, the rate rises to around 20%, and where infection already exists it may be 40% or higher.
2. the surgeons technical ability[25]
3. host factors, see Table 60.2.
4. the use of antibiotic prophylaxis
5. duration of stay in ICU.

THE ORGANISMS

The organisms are frequently determined by the type of surgery and procedure. Skin commensals are common, such as staphylococci or streptococci and are usually early infections. These are characterized by fever, pain and redness around the site. With streptococcal infection this may be quite confluent. Gram negative organisms may also cause infection. Drainage is important.

PREVENTION

Clean theatres, good operating technique and thorough asepsis both in the theatre and post operatively are important.

ANTIBIOTIC PROPHYLAXIS

This is a difficult and contentious area. The unnecessary use of broad spectrum antibiotics should be avoided, but there are some areas of surgery where prophylaxis has a proven place. If there is no risk of infection with a clean procedure there is no place for antibiotics. If there is contamination either seen or likely to occur, the use of antibiotics is to provide cover for the spillage. There may be other circumstances where the patient is particularly vulnerable to bacteraemia, such as with valve disease or where the consequences of infection would be disastrous. Effective prophylaxis requires an antibiotic(s):

1. which cover the most likely organisms
2. given prior to contamination
3. at peak dosage at time of contamination.

A single dose should suffice, although a second dose is recommended if the procedure extends beyond 3 hours. Prolonged administration:

1. increases the chance of antibiotic resistance
2. unnecessarily exposes the patient to adverse effects from the drugs
3. encourages colonization with resistant organisms
4. ensures that if a late infection occurs it will be with an organism resistant to the prophylaxis.

In many circumstances the evidence supporting prophylaxis is minimal, and frequently the antibiotics used are inappropriate to the perceived risk. Local factors including the local ecology will determine specific requirements. With grafts, mesh or prostheses the morbidity from infection are so great as to justify using prophylaxis even if the evidence is marginal (Table 60.7).

LINE SEPSIS[26,27]

The use of intravascular devices in hospital practice is ubiquitous. There is both a significant morbidity, resulting in prolongation of hospital stay, and an attributable mortality associated with their use due to infection.

PERIPHERAL LINES

The use of peripheral lines is commonly associated with phlebitis, which may be chemical but is frequently a precursor of infection. Usually peripheral lines should only be *in situ* for less than 72 hours.

ARTERIAL LINES

Curiously, arterial lines seem to become colonized and infected less frequently than other peripheral devices. Nevertheless they do become colonized and should be regularly changed. Complications include infected radial aneurysms or thrombosis.

PULMONARY ARTERY CATHETERS

The introducers are a potential source of infection, as is the part of the catheter in the introducer. They are frequently left *in situ* when they should have been removed earlier.[28]

CENTRAL VENOUS CATHETERS

Colonization of catheters is common and it is likely that this is a precursor of infection. Colonization rates are in the order of 5–40%, determined in part by the risk factors involved (see below). Infection rates are approximately 10% of the colonized catheters.[29]

DEFINITIONS

1 Colonized catheter: growth of >15 colony forming units (semi quantitative) or 10^3 (quantitative) from a proximal or distal catheter segment in the absence of accompanying clinical symptoms and signs.
2 Catheter related blood stream infection (CRS or CR-BSI): Isolation of the same organism from the catheter segment (see above) as from a peripheral blood culture in a patient with signs of infection and in the absence of another source. In the absence of laboratory confirmation of infection then defervescence of infection after removal of the catheter may be taken as circumstantial evidence.

Extrinsic mechanisms associated with developing catheter sepsis include infection from the skin and insertion site; contamination from the hub and then internally spread; and contamination of drugs or fluids administered through the catheter. Bacteraemia seeding to catheter is an intrinsic mechanism.

Table 60.7 Surgical prophylaxis

Type of surgery	
Abdominal wall	Insertion of mesh. Staphylococcal or streptococcal cover. In the groin, gram negative cover might be needed.
Cardiac	Protection of valves and grafts. Staphylococci may be resistant.
Vascular	Protection of grafts. Staph. are a major consideration. If the groin is involved, it may require gram negative cover.
Orthopaedic	Prostheses. Staphylococci are an increasing problem.
Biliary upper GI	Usually gram negative and anaerobic cover, with an awareness of resistant enterococci.
Colorectal	Protection against faecal flora. Cephalosporins and metronidazole have been popular but predispose to developing enterococci such as E. faecalis or faecium, which may be multi-resistant.
Gynaecological	Conventionally broad spectrum involving cephalosporins or currently, augmentin. Metronidazole is also favoured.
Urological	Protection from instrumentation of the urinary tract, gram negative cover. Awareness of any existing infection.

The actual mechanics by which the organisms colonize the catheter is important. Some organisms, such as CNS produce a polysaccharide film of 'slime' that develops on the catheter while the host's proteins such as fibronectin may also provide a matrix in which the organism can adhere and which may provide a protective barrier against both white cells and antibiotics. Polyvinyl chloride or polythene are more prone to this film developing than some other materials such as silicone (Table 60.8).

Organisms

The organisms involved in catheter sepsis are many and varied. There is a 25% incidence of coagulase negative staphylococci, which are increasingly recognized as

Table 60.8 Risk factors for catheter infection

Host risk factors
Site: subclavian is a lower risk than internal jugular and femoral
Catheter material: antibacterial catheters may reduce infection, antiseptic catheters reduce colonization
Number of lumens: multilumen catheters increase the infection risk[30]
Number of administrations through the lines
Dressing type frequency of changes
Skin preparation
Experience of technique of personnel
Occurrence of bacteraemia
Tunnelling: often used for long-term access but the data is contentious[31]

pathogens. Staph aureus and MRSA are prevalent. There may be seeding resulting in vertebral osteomyelitis and a variably reported incidence of endocarditis. Enterococci are increasingly seen. Occasionally fungi are found and may again be associated with seeding to the eyes or heart.

Treatment of Catheter Infection

The most important aspect of treatment[32] is a high index of suspicion that leads to removal of the device if infection is present either locally or systemically. Although fever and bacteraemia are likely to resolve rapidly after removal of the line, appropriate antibiotics are indicated. The recommended duration of treatment[32] varies: 5–7 days for CNS, 10–14 days for S. aurues, gram negative organisms and fungi, and 4–6 weeks if there is evidence of endocarditis, infected thrombus, osteomyelitis, or clinical line sepsis is still present after 3 days. Lines removed should be cultured. If an infection is present it is best to avoid replacing the CVC if possible for a few days. In situations where it is uncertain if the line is implicated in infection some advocate replacing a new line over a wire. If the removed catheter is subsequently shown to be infected, then it must be removed.

The situation is slightly different with Broviac or Hickman catheters. Occasionally the administration of antibiotics through the catheter will eradicate the infection and save the line. Unfortunately, it is not always successful with the risk of failure to be balanced against the value of the line. Some medical catastrophes have been the consequence of persisting with infected Hickman lines.

Prevention

Important issues include adequate hand-washing; adequate skin disinfection; insertion under aseptic conditions; intravenous team to insert and manage lines; anchoring of lines to prevent excessive movement; closed systems with limited interruptions to the lines; application of sterile dressings to the insertion site; and daily inspection of catheter site. Replacement of intravenous administration sets at 72 hours is optimal.[33] Stopcocks may be essential, but are portals of infection. Local antiseptics are advocated for site care, but there is little difference between gauze and transparent dressings, although efforts to reduce local humidity at the site may be important.

Techniques of unproven benefit include antiseptic cream at insertion site; routine changes of dressings at frequent intervals; occlusive antimicrobial dressings; in-line filters; tunnelling of central venous catheters; and routine flushing of long-term central venous catheters.

METHODS OF INFECTION CONTROL

Each hospital has an infection control team that can employ techniques to reduce infection (Table 60.9).

Table 60.9 Roles of infection control teams

Surveillance and investigation of infection outbreaks
Education of staff
Review of antibiotic utilization
Review of antibiotic resistance patterns
Review of infection control procedures and policies

The most important aspects of preventing nosocomial infection and facilitating infection control are simple hygiene, such as hand washing and being aware that the problem exists. There are several ways in which the issue of nosocomial infection can be addressed. These include surveillance, screening, isolation, eradication and strategic planning.

SURVEILLANCE

Routine cultures of both patients and environment provides information on the organisms currently prevalent, and is a useful tool in guiding management when infection occurs. It also provides information on cross infection rates. Using 'typing' techniques, individual organisms can be tracked, which is of particular importance in following outbreaks.

SCREENING

This tries to prevent multi-resistance by identifying patients carrying high-risk organisms. In the critically ill, to be effective it requires isolating the patient until cultures are available. It is clearly of benefit with rare or very threatening infection, such as the haemorrhagic fevers but cumbersome and ineffectual with an organism as prevalent as MRSA. Future problems with Acinetobacter may need re-evaluation of its role.

ISOLATION

Although physical barriers undoubtedly reduce cross-contamination, isolation may be hazardous as it often indicates lower intensity care. The relative risks need to be addressed.

ERADICATION

This requires the use of potent antibiotics ± antiseptics to eliminate the organism, which may be colonizing rather than infecting. It exposes potent therapeutic agents and facilitates the development of resistance or the emergence of more resistant strains. It is therefore a hazardous undertaking in strategic terms.

STRATEGIC PLANNING

There are two elements. One is enforcing hygienic practice, which is simple cheap and very effective. The other is looking towards means of reducing both nosocomial infection and the emergence of resistance. This is essentially the planned use of antibiotics.

Currently the same agents are used in agriculture, the community and in hospital, which provides vast potential for the emergence of resistance. In human practice the widespread use of potent agents in the community will impinge on hospitals. In hospitals focussed antibiotic use in one area will be undermined by generalized use in another. There should be controls across the boundaries of these areas of use.

On an individual basis the approach to management must change. In the past, empiric treatment on the basis of likely organisms led to the use of very broad spectrum antibiotics. It is already clear that in an individual who has been in hospital for any period of time using any antibiotic is likely to miss some resistant strains. Narrow spectrum targeted treatment will cease to be an option and will become a necessity. Prolonged broad spectrum antibiotic management aimed at dealing with any eventuality will be replaced by short duration specific and effective regimens.

SELECTIVE DECONTAMINATION OF THE DIGESTIVE TRACT (SDD)

There has been considerable interest in the role of colonization of the upper GI tract in the genesis of nosocomial infection. The theory is that if bacterial overgrowth of the gastrointestinal tract leads to nosocomial infection then eradication of gut flora should reduce infection rates. To achieve this oral non-absorbable antibiotics, such as polymyxin, tobramycin, gentamicin, neomycin, and nystatin and are applied to the oropharynx and administered through nasogastric tubes. Parenteral antibiotics have been added to some regimens.

Over the last decade, there have been major claims made for the efficacy of this approach; however, it has also been challenged.[33–36] There has been anxiety about the emergence of resistance, although at least one paper refutes this.[37] More recent studies in paediatric burns and in liver transplantation have been equivocal or poor.[38,39] It remains a controversial area.

REFERENCES

1 Sax H, Ruef C, Widmer AF. Qualitats standard fur Spitalhygiene an mittleren und grossen Spitalern der Schweiz: ein Konzeptvorschlag. *Schweiz Med Wochenschr* 1999; **129**: 276–84.

2 Vincent JL, Bihari DJ, Suter PM, *et al*. The prevalence of nosocomial infection in intensive care units in Europe. Results of the European Prevalence of Infection in Intensive Care (EPIC) Study. EPIC International Advisory Committee. *JAMA* 1995; **274**: 639–44.

3 Girou E, Stephan F, Novara A, *et al*. Risk factors and outcome of nosocomial infections: results of a matched case-control study of ICU patients. *Am J Respir Crit Care Med* 1998; **157**: 1151–8.

4 Pittet D. [Nosocomial pneumonia: incidence, morbidity and mortality in the intubated-ventilated patient]. *Schweiz Med Wochenschr* 1994; **124**: 227–35.

5 Edgeworth JD, Treacher DF, Eykyn SJ. A 25-year study of nosocomial bacteremia in an adult intensive care unit. *Crit Care Med* 1999; **27**: 1421–8.

6 Pittet D, Hugonnet S, Harbarth S, *et al*. Effectiveness of a hospital-wide programme to improve compliance with hand hygiene. Infection Control Programme. *Lancet* 2000; **356**(9238): 1307–12.

7 Livermore DM, Yuan M. Antibiotic resistance and production of extended-spectrum beta-lactamases amongst Klebsiella spp. from intensive care units in Europe. *J Antimicrob Chemother* 1996; **38**: 409–24.

8 Hanberger H, Diekema D, Fluit A, *et al*. Surveillance of antibiotic resistance in European ICUs. *J Hosp Infect* 2001; **48**: 161–76.

9 Theaker C, Ormond Walshe S, Azadian B, Soni N. MRSA in the critically ill. *J Hosp Infect* 2001; **48**: 98–102.

10 Guidelines for prevention of nosocomial pneumonia. Centers for Disease Control and Prevention. *MMWR Morb Mortal Wkly Rep* 1997; **46**(Rr-1): 1–79.

11 Richards MJ, Edwards JR, Culver DH, Gaynes RP. Nosocomial infections in combined medical-surgical intensive care units in the United States. *Infect Control Hosp Epidemiol* 2000; **21**: 510–5.

12 Girou E, Schortgen F, Delclaux C, *et al*. Association of noninvasive ventilation with nosocomial infections and survival in critically ill patients. *JAMA* 2000; **284**: 2361–7.

13 Cook D, Heyland D, Griffith L, *et al*. Risk factors for clinically important upper gastrointestinal bleeding in patients requiring mechanical ventilation. Canadian Critical Care Trials Group. *Crit Care Med* 1999; **27**: 2812–7.

14 Cook DJ, Reeve BK, Guyatt GH, *et al*. Stress ulcer prophylaxis in critically ill patients. Resolving discordant meta-analyses. *JAMA* 1996; **275**: 308–14.

15 Cook DJ, Reeve BK, Scholes LC. Histamine-2-receptor antagonists and antacids in the critically ill population: stress ulceration versus nosocomial pneumonia. *Infect Control Hosp Epidemiol* 1994; **15**: 437–42.

16 Hospital-acquired pneumonia in adults: diagnosis, assessment of severity, initial antimicrobial therapy, and preventive strategies. A consensus statement, American Thoracic Society, November 1995. *Am J Respir Crit Care Med* 1996; **153**: 1711–25.

17 Silvestri L, Monti Bragadin C, Milanese M, *et al*. Are most ICU infections really nosocomial? A prospective observational cohort study in mechanically ventilated patients. *J Hosp Infect* 1999; **42**: 125–33.

18 Combes P, Fauvage B, Oleyer C. Nosocomial pneumonia in mechanically ventilated patients, a prospective randomised evaluation of the Stericath closed suctioning system. *Intensive Care Med* 2000; **26**: 878–82.

19 Cometta A, Baumgartner JD, Lew D, *et al*. Prospective randomized comparison of imipenem monotherapy with imipenem plus netilmicin for treat-

ment of severe infections in nonneutropenic patients. *Antimicrob Agents Chemother* 1994; **38**: 1309–13.

20 Rello J, Paiva JA, Baraibar J, *et al*. International conference for the development of consensus on the diagnosis and treatment of ventilator-associated pneumonia. *Chest* 2001; **120**: 955–70.

21 Rello J, Sa-Borges M, Correa H, *et al*. Variations in etiology of ventilator-associated pneumonia across four treatment sites: implications for antimicrobial prescribing practices. *Am J Respir Crit Care Med* 1999; **160**: 608–13.

22 Costa SF, Newbaer M, Santos CR, *et al*. Nosocomial pneumonia: importance of recognition of aetiological agents to define an appropriate initial empirical therapy. *Int J Antimicrob Agents* 2001; **17**: 147–50.

23 Pittet D, Tarara D, Wenzel RP. Nosocomial bloodstream infection in critically ill patients. Excess length of stay, extra costs, and attributable mortality. *JAMA* 1994; **271**: 1598–601.

24 Pittet D, Ducel G. Infectious risk factors related to operating rooms. *Infect Control Hosp Epidemiol* 1994; **15**: 456–62.

25 Holzheimer RG, Haupt W, Thiede A, Schwarzkopf A. The challenge of postoperative infections: does the surgeon make a difference? *Infect Control Hosp Epidemiol* 1997; **18**: 449–56.

26 Pearson ML. Guideline for prevention of intravascular device-related infections. Hospital Infection Control Practices Advisory Committee. *Infect Control Hosp Epidemiol* 1996; **17**: 438–73.

27 Chatzinikolaou I, Raad II. Intravascular catheter-related infections: a preventable challenge in the critically ill. *Semin Respir Infect* 2000; **15**: 264–71.

28 Maki DG, Stolz SS, Wheeler S, Mermel LA. A prospective, randomized trial of gauze and two polyurethane dressings for site care of pulmonary artery catheters: implications for catheter management. *Crit Care Med* 1994; **22**: 1729–37.

29 Hannan M, Juste RN, Umasanker S, *et al*. Antiseptic-bonded central venous catheters and bacterial colonization. *Anaesthesia* 1999; **54**: 868–72.

30 Yeung C, May J, Hughes R. Infection rate for single lumen v triple lumen subclavian catheters. *Infect Control Hosp Epidemiol* 1988; **9**: 154–8.

31 Andrivet P, Bacquer A, Ngoc CV, *et al*. Lack of clinical benefit from subcutaneous tunnel insertion of central venous catheters in immunocompromised patients. *Clin Infect Dis* 1994; **18**: 199–206.

32 Mermel LA, Farr BM, Sherertz RJ, *et al*. Guidelines for the management of intravascular catheter-related infections. *Infect Control Hosp Epidemiol* 2001; **22**: 222–42.

33 Raad I, Hanna HA, Awad A, *et al*. Optimal frequency of changing intravenous administration sets: is it safe to prolong use beyond 72 hours? *Infect Control Hosp Epidemiol* 2001; **22**: 136–9.

34 Rommes JH, Zandstra DF, van Saene HK. [Selective decontamination of the digestive tract reduces mortality in intensive care patients]. *Ned Tijdschr Geneeskd* 1999; **143**: 602–6.

35 Silvestri L, Mannucci F, van Saene HK. Selective decontamination of the digestive tract: a life saver. *J Hosp Infect* 2000; **45**: 185–90.

36 van Nieuwenhoven CA, Bergmans DC, Bonten MJ. Ventilator-associated pneumonia: risk factors and patient mortality. *Hosp Med* 1999; **60**: 558–63.

37 Zandstra DF, Van Saene HK. Selective decontamination of the digestive as infection prevention in the critically ill. Does it lead to resistance? *Minerva Anestesiol* 2001; **67**: 292–7.

38 van Enckevort PJ, Zwaveling JH, Bottema JT, *et al*. Cost effectiveness of selective decontamination of the digestive tract in liver transplant patients. *Pharmacoeconomics* 2001; **19**: 523–30.

39 Barret JP, Jeschke MG, Herndon DN. Selective decontamination of the digestive tract in severely burned pediatric patients. *Burns* 2001; **27**: 439–45.

61

Severe soft-tissue infections

H Sax and D Pittet

The skin is the largest organ and acts as an excellent barrier against infection. It consists of the epidermis and dermis, and resides on fibrous connective tissue, the superficial and deep fasciae (Figure 61.1). The fascial cleft, with nerves, arteries, veins, lymphatic and adipose tissue, lies between these fascial planes. Normal skin flora includes *Corynebacterium* spp., coagulase-negative staphylococci, *Micrococcus* spp., *Lactobacillus* and rarely *Staphylococcus aureus*. Colonization by gram-negative bacteria occurs in hospital patients, and there are more *S. aureus* in the altered flora.

These colonizing microorganisms seldom cause skin and soft-tissue infections but serious infections can occur if:

- there is a break in the skin because of traumatic lesion or maceration
- soft tissues are ischaemic and non-viable
- colonizing bacteria are particularly virulent
- the patient is immunocompromised (Figure 61.2).[1–8]

Conditions predisposing to infection include diabetes mellitus, cirrhosis, malnutrition, major trauma, advanced age, renal failure, steroid use, collagen vascular disease and malignancies.[1–9] Differentiation between soft-tissue infection can be difficult, and one unified management approach to severe forms is appropriate.[10,11]

Soft-tissue infections are usually caused by bacterial entry through skin lesions or perforation of adjacent intestinal structures. Skin lesions can on occasion be the manifestations of systemic infection; examples of this are bacteraemia by meningococci, staphylococci, *Pseudomonas aeruginosa*, *Candida* spp., and bacterial endocarditis.[3] These will not be addressed here.

CLASSIFICATION

The bacteriology and subtypes of severe soft-tissue infections have not changed significantly over the last century.[12–14] The classification of soft-tissue infections can be confusing partly because individual organisms can cause different clinical syndromes. Consequently, there are a

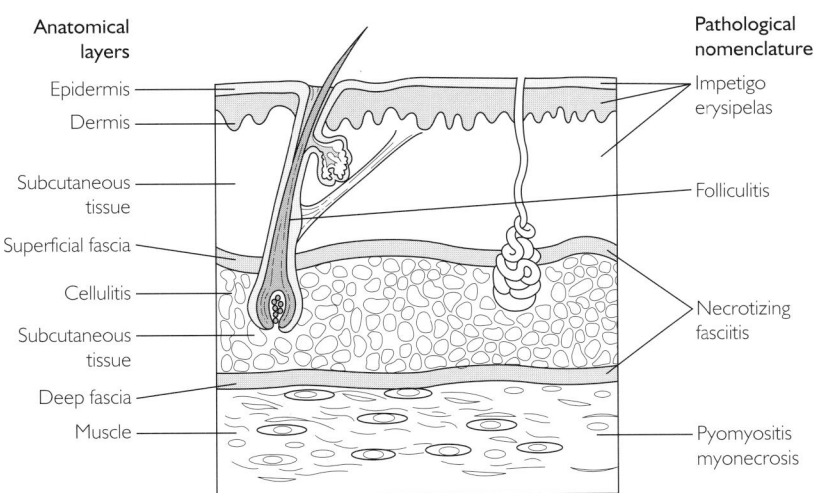

Fig. 61.1 Anatomy of skin and nomenclature of skin and deep tissue infections.

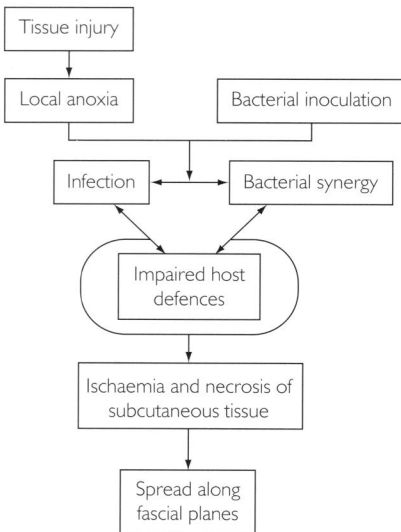

Fig. 61.2 Pathogenesis of severe soft-tissue infections.

wealth of terms often referring to the same diseases (e.g. Meleney's gangrene, haemolytic streptococcal gangrene and progressive bacterial synergistic gangrene).[12] Classification by the anatomical structure involved is more logical but it has to be borne in mind that some conditions involve several soft-tissue levels and that some cases may evolve from a minor entity to a more severe form with more diffuse anatomical involvement (Figure 61.1).

IMPETIGO

Impetigo,[1–3] more common in children, is a superficial skin infection caused by group A streptococci, *Staphylococcus aureus* or both. Mild infections can be managed with topical antibiotics; more serious infections need a first-generation cephalosporin. A penicillinase-resistant penicillin is mostly chosen in severe empirical conditions (e.g. dicloxacillin).[15] Increasing resistance in streptococci and staphylococci might prohibit the use of erythromycin which has been the alternative in the penicillin-allergic patient.

FOLLICULITIS

This is an infection arising in hair follicles and apocrine glands.[2,3] *S. aureus* is the usual causative organism. Topical antibiotic treatment is usually all that is required. When confluent, folliculitis can evolve to furunculosis and may need surgical drainage as sole effective therapy.

If accompanied by cellulitis and/or sepsis antibiotics are added (see cellulitis). Repeated folliculitis raises the possibility of chronic granulomatous disease, an inherited immunodeficiency syndrome based on granulocyte malfunction.[16] Affected individuals are at risk for severe soft-tissue infections, sometimes with rare pathogens such as *Aspergilllus* spp.

ERYSIPELAS[1,2]

This superficial dermal infection is caused largely by group A streptococci, and also by other streptococci and *S. aureus*. The prominent lymphatic blockade results in a painful, bright, red patch with a raised sharp border, which clearly demarcates the infection from normal surrounding skin. Fever and chills often precede the skin eruption. Predisposing conditions include ulcers, venous stasis, diabetes, alcoholism and paraparesis. Treatment is a first-generation cephalosporin or a penicillinase-resistant penicillin. If mobilization is premature, signs recur and treatment failure may falsely be suspected.

CELLULITIS

Cellulitis[1–3,5–8] is an acute spreading infection of the skin extending below the superficial fascia, usually to involve only the upper part of the subcutaneous tissue. It can occur at any body site, but is most frequent in the lower extremities and in the face. There is less lymphatic involvement so the borders of the infection are often not well-defined, and differentiation between cellulitis and erysipelas is sometimes difficult. Fever, malaise and rigors are common. It is more common in patients with tissue oedema. Cellulitis is most commonly due to *Streptococcus pyogenes* but other Gram-positive and negative organisms can also cause this condition.

Typically, *S. pyogenes* cellulitis may appear hours after surgical intervention with fast progression of the erythematic zone over a large surface and can be accompanied by bacteraemia and sepsis. Many of these organisms may produce gas, hence crepitus is sometimes present (Table 61.1).

Table 61.1 Infective causes of soft-tissue crepitus

Cellulitis	Usually anaerobic organisms, clostridial and non-clostridial
Bursitis	Gram-negative organisms
Necrotizing fasciitis	Usually type I (mixed infections, Gram-negative organisms)
Myonecrosis	Clostridial organisms
Infected vascular gangrene	Any organism

Other forms of cellulitis present with necrosis (gangrene). These include anaerobic infections with *Clostridium* spp. or non-clostridial anaerobes sometimes mixed with Gram-negative pathogens that are facultative anaerobes. This latter condition may be hard to distinguish from deeper forms of infection such as necrotizing fasciitis and myositis, and may be crepitant. Immediate assessment by MRI and surgical exploration determines fascial and muscular involvement and allows for adequate debridement. Potent empirical therapy must include all possible pathogens because of the impossibility of deducing bacterial aetiology and depth from the initial clinical presentation. For antimicrobial therapy, see under necrotizing fasciitis below.

Periocular cellulitis is a medical emergency. It needs immediate clinical and then radiological assessment to decide if the retrobulbar space is involved. Clinical signs for the latter include visual disturbance because of optical nerve involvement. Definite diagnosis can only be established by CT. External facial cellulitis may involve the venous system draining into the *sinus venosus* and, thus, lead to thrombosis.

A severe and fulminant form of cellulitis can be caused by marine bacteria of the *Vibrio* spp., mostly with a history of contact with sea-water or raw fish.[17]

TREATMENT

Appropriate microbiological tests are undertaken prior to starting antibiotics. Any skin abrasion or sites of drains are swabbed for Gram stain and culture. Needle aspiration, skin biopsy and blood cultures produce only a 25% positive yield.[1] Treatment involves site elevation and cloxacillin 2 g i.v. 4-hourly or a first-generation cephalosporin (e.g. cefazolin 2.0 g i.v. 6-hourly). If there is a possibility of methicillin-resistant *S. aureus*, vancomycin 1.0 g i.v. 12-hourly is indicated instead. In severe cases addition of clindamycin 600 mg i.v. 6-hourly is beneficial because of its antitoxic effect and enhanced intracellular activity.[18] If Gram-negative rods are suspected or identified (e.g. an immunocompromised patient or involvement of intestinal tract lesions), a third-generation cephalosporin should be considered. In a patient with prolonged hospitalization or in penetrating foot infections a cephalosporin with anti-pseudomonas activity is preferred. If *Vibrio* spp. is suspected or isolated, doxycycline 100 mg bid may be added, since in murine sepsis, activity of tetracyclines against *V. vulnificus* is better than third-generation cephalosporins.[19] In the absence of controlled studies, some authors recommend ceftazidime[20] in addition to tetracyclines because of the high mortality of 50%.[17]

Pyoderma gangrenosum has a similar appearance, but completely different aetiology and therapeutic management. It is a rare idiopathic, inflammatory, ulcerative disease of undetermined cause that is more frequent in patients with ulcerative colitis and rheumatoid arthritis

and presents as deep ulcers with undermined borders usually on lower extremities or abdomen. It is often triggered by surgical intervention and only secondarily colonized with skin flora. Treatment is conservative and includes steroid medication.[21]

NECROTIZING FASCIITIS

Necrotizing fasciitis[1–3,5–11,22–26] is a deeper infection of the skin with extensive undermining of surrounding tissues. Interest in this fulminant infection has recently increased.[12,22,27] The World Health Organization reports only 160 cases since 1989, but the incidence in the USA is about 100 cases annually and recently there has been an increased incidence of group A streptococcal fasciitis in Europe.[12,22]

It usually occurs on the extremities, perineum and abdominal wall. Involvement of male genitalia is known as Fournier's gangrene.[13] Two types are described, depending on causative organisms.[25] Type I are mixed infections usually caused by enteric bowel organisms or *Vibrio* spp. Type II infections are caused by group A streptococci (occasionally with *S. aureus*). Secondary infections with zygomycetes may occur.[24,26] There is no difference in the clinical course, morbidity, and mortality between the two types of infections.

CLINICAL PRESENTATION

A history of minor trauma is common, and necrotizing fasciitis can complicate surgery and varicella infections.[22,28] Predisposing factors include cirrhosis, diabetes and other immunocompromised states. Necrotizing fasciitis begins as an area of cellulitis that typically fails to improve on antibiotics and quickly spreads. Pathophysiological sequelae of sepsis result in microthrombi and impaired perfusion leading to gangrene. Pain is a predominant feature frequently out of keeping with other presenting symptoms and signs. Sometimes no external sign is apparent and increasing pain may even be the only initial symptom. Fever, rigors and shock are common.[22] Half of the cases of necrotizing fasciitis present together with a streptococcal toxic shock syndrome.[15] Manifestations of the systemic inflammatory response syndrome are evident and multiple organ dysfunction develops in most cases. Bullae may form, and late lesions may resemble deep burns that are pain free, because of the necrosis of nerve fibres. Reduced skin surface sensitivity and elevated creatine phosphokinase may suggest fascial involvement. Crepitus may be present (Table 61.1). The normally adherent fascia may be easily peeled off the underlying muscle bed.

Retroperitoneal necrotizing fasciitis is particularly vicious, with a high mortality due partly to the difficulty in diagnosis.[29] Abdominal or perineal trauma or sepsis is always the predisposing event. Diagnosis can only be made at laparotomy for the presenting acute abdomen. Broad-spectrum antibiotic therapy and aggressive surgery (repeated debridement of all necrotic tissue) with planned 'relook' laparotomies is strongly suggested.

Necrotizing fasciitis concerning the face, eyelid or lip are rather of the type II whereas that of the neck more often of type I, associated with a 4-fold mortality compared to the facial form.[30]

MANAGEMENT

Because of rapid progression, early diagnosis and treatment are crucial for the prognosis. Two major diagnostic tools are appropriate. An experienced surgeon should be involved as early as possible with surgical incision, probing of fascial consistency and histological diagnosis on a frozen section specimen of doubtful fascia intraoperatively.[31] The other mainstay of diagnosis is magnetic resonance imaging.

A complete microbiological investigation is of utmost importance. This includes sampling for culture by needle aspiration of any crepitant area and blood cultures. Treatment with antibiotics alone is usually inadequate. Immediate extensive surgical removal of necrotic and damaged tissues is essential.[10,11,22–24,26] Planned surgery at 24-h intervals to debride spreading necrotic tissue is necessary, until the necrotic process stops. If extremities are involved, amputation may be life-saving.

Initial antibiotic therapy includes a first-generation cephalosporin or a penicillinase-resistant penicillin plus gentamicin or a third-generation cephalosporin. Clindamycin 600 mg i.v. 6-hourly is added because of toxin inhibition and anaerobic activity.[18] If fungi (e.g. Mucormycosis) are isolated, amphotericin B 0.5 mg/kg per day i.v. should be given for at least 2 weeks.[24,26] As in cellulitis, *Vibrio* spp. may respond better to tetracyclines.[19]

Supportive care, especially organ support, is also fundamental treatment, and is discussed in other chapters. Hyperbaric oxygen therapy has no proven benefit, and is likely to delay surgical intervention. Mortality from necrotizing fasciitis is high, and survival appears improved when surgery is undertaken early.

Table 61.2 Pathogens and presumptive antibiotic therapy in severe soft-tissue infections*

Disease	Suspected pathogens	Antibiotic therapy	Remarks
Impetigo	S. aureus, group A streptococci	First generation cephalosporin, erythromycin, penicillin, dicloxacillin.	
Folliculitis	S. aureus, Candida spp., Pseudomonas aeruginosa, Pityrosporum ovale		Local therapy usually sufficient, antibiotic treatment only with cellulitis.
Erysipelas	Group A streptococci (occasionally, group B, C, G), S. aureus	Penicillin (if no underlying disease and possible to observe), 1st-generation cephalosporin, flucloxacillin.	Enterobacteriaceae in diabetes: 3rd-generation cephalosporin or carbapenem.
Cellulitis	Group A streptococci, S. aureus; rarely, various other organisms	Flucloxacillin, 1st-generation cephalosporin, erythromycin (for severe penicillin allergy).	Resistance in S. pyogenes and S. aureus against erythromycin exists.
Necrotizing fasciitis	Type I: Anaerobic species (Bacteroides, peptostreptococcus spp.), together with facultative anaerobes non-A streptococci, enterobacteriaceae (E. coli, Enterobacter, Klebsiella, etc.) Type II: group A streptococci alone or with S. aureus	Carbapenem, 3rd-generation cephalosporin plus clindamycin.	Surgical debridement absolutely essential. Empirical therapy must cover for all pathogens.
Pyomyositis	S. aureus, group A streptococci (rarely), Gram-negative bacilli (very rarely), anaerobic bacteria other than Clostridium	Flucloxacillin, or 1st generation cephalosporin plus clindamycin.	Surgical drainage absolutely essential. Cave compartment syndrome. Change to penicillin, if streptococcal origin.
Myonecrosis	Clostridium perfringens, C. septicum	High dose penicillin plus clindamycin 3 × 600 mg i.v.	Surgical exploration and debridement crucial with open wound healing; hyperbaric oxygen debated.

*Once causative pathogen(s) has(ve) been identified, antibiotic choice can be modified and spectrum narrowed.

PYOMYOSITIS AND MYONECROSIS

Muscles are remarkably resistant to infection, so bacterial infections are rare. Infections of muscles are termed myonecrosis when *Clostridium* spp. is the causative organism, and pyomyositis when infection is from other bacteria.[1,2,4–8,10,11,23,24,32,33] Often, more than one bacterial species is isolated from infected muscles. In such conditions, bacteria act synergistically, and often produce various toxins (Figure 61.2).[4,34] As infection is likely to be mixed, differentiation of pyomyositis and myonecrosis is bacteriological, and important only for antibiotic choices.

PYOMYOSITIS

Pyomyositis is more common in the tropics. The causative organism in over 90% of cases is *S. aureus*, with others being *S. pyogenes*, *E. coli* and *S. pneumoniae*. Pyomyositis often follows blunt trauma to torso, thigh or buttock muscles. Spontaneous staphylococcal muscle abscesses may occasionally occur.[2] Initial presentation is with aching muscles, which feel indurated on examination. If untreated, the muscles become erythematous and boggy, and are eventually destroyed. Spontaneous drainage of debris and pus does not occur. Instead, there is contiguous spread to surrounding tissues and metastatic spread to the chest (e.g. empyemas) and heart (e.g. endocarditis and pericarditis).

Investigations include needle biopsy (for Gram stain of the aspirate), ultrasound (for localized muscle oedema) and, more recently, magnetic resonance imaging.[2] Large increases in serum creatine phosphokinase may be indicative of the degree of muscle involvement.[33] Antibiotic therapy with a penicillinase-resistant penicillin or a first-generation cephalosporin adding metronidazole, may be successful in the early stages. More often, though, the condition is not recognized early because of diagnostic difficulties, and extensive surgical drainage is mandatory for a favourable outcome.[33] Even after disfiguring muscle destruction, functional prognosis is good.

MYONECROSIS

The bacterial infection of muscles by clostridial organisms (usually *Clostridium perfringens* or *C. septicum*) has been called gas gangrene as crepitus may occur. However, other causes of skin crepitus are just as common (Table 61.1). Predisposing causes are contaminated wounds (e.g. in trauma and septic abortions) and surgery in immunocompromised patients.

Onset is often abrupt, with involved areas being very painful and swollen. The patient presents with signs of severe sepsis. If a wound is present, there is usually a profuse serosanguinous discharge of sweet odour. Later, the skin becomes red, yellow, green or black. Bullae and crepitus may form.

A Gram stain revealing Gram-positive rods of *Clostridium* is diagnostic. Treatment of myonecrosis involves prompt, extensive surgical debridement of all infected tissue and antibiotics (i.e. penicillin plus clindamycin).[2] At surgery, the muscle is pale or brick-coloured and does not bleed. Hyperbaric oxygen has its proponents[35,36] and may be beneficial in conjunction with good supportive care. However, there is no prospective evidence to support use of hyperbaric oxygen.[37]

SPECIAL AREAS OF SOFT-TISSUE INFECTIONS

NECK INFECTIONS

Since the advent of antibiotics, oropharyngeal infections are no longer major causes of neck infections.[38–40] Dental infection and regional trauma are now more common causes. Neck infections include Ludwig's angina, retropharyngeal abscesses, parapharyngeal abscesses and necrotizing cervical fasciitis. Ludwig's angina is a submandibular space infection. There is deep and tender swelling of the submandibular and submaxillary area, with swelling of the floor of the mouth and elevation of the tongue.

Causative organisms are the usual mouth commensals, Gram-negative rods and *S. aureus*. Pain and odynophagia are almost always the presenting symptoms. Local swelling is usually present. Trismus and dental pathology are common. Systemic inflammatory signs occur in about two-thirds of patients.

Neck X-rays usually demonstrate some abnormality. Computerized tomography or magnetic resonance imaging will define anatomy and may help to decide on a course of conservative, expectant therapy.[40] Oesophagoscopy should be performed on all retropharyngeal abscesses, as foreign-body ingestion is a possible predisposing event.

Airway control must take top priority in any neck swelling. Antibiotics, in doses similar to necrotizing fasciitis, should incorporate cover for Gram-positive cocci and Gram-negative rods. Penicillin or clindamycin plus gentamicin, or a third-generation cephalosporin plus metronidazole are suitable. Some abscesses may be treated conservatively, especially those in children.[40] However, early surgical drainage remains the mainstay of management for large neck abscesses that impinge on airway patency, or deep infections that pursue a fulminant course.

Retrotonsillar abscess may evolve to Lemierre's syndrome, an infection with anaerobic bacteria, mostly *Fusobacterium necrophorum* that gain access to the jugular vein and lead to metastatic infections in the liver, lung, and brain. Because of possible involvement of anaerobes that produce β-lactamase, penicillin should be replaced by a beta-lactamase-resisting β-lactam antibiotic (e.g. amoxycillin-clavulanic acid).[41]

REFERENCES

1 Conly J. Soft tissue infections. In: Hall JB, Schmidt GA and Wood LDH (eds) *Principals of Critical Care.* New York: McGraw-Hill; 1992: pp. 1325–34.

2 Canoso JJ, Barza M. Soft tissue infections. *Rheum Dis Clin North Am* 1993; **19**: 293–309.

3 Swartz MN. Cellulitis and subcutaneous tissue infections. In: Mandell GL, Bennett JE and Dolin R (eds) *Principles and Practice on Infectious Diseases.* New York: Churchill Livingstone; 2000: pp. 1037–57.

4 Swartz MN. Myositis. In: Mandell GL, Bennett JE and Dolin R (eds) *Principles and Practice on Infectious Diseases.* New York: Churchill Livingstone; 2000: pp. 1058–65.

5 Ahrenholz DH. Necrotizing fasciitis and other soft tissue infections. In: Rippe JM, Irwin RS, Alpert JS and Fink MP (eds) *Intensive Care Medicine.* Boston: Little Brown; 1991: pp. 1334–42.

6 Cha JY, Releford BJ, Jr., Marcarelli P. Necrotizing fasciitis: a classification of necrotizing soft tissue infections. *J Foot Ankle Surg* 1994; **33**: 148–55.

7 Sutherland ME, Meyer AA. Necrotizing soft-tissue infections. *Surg Clin North Am* 1994; **74**: 591–607.

8 Ahrenholz DH. Necrotizing soft-tissue infections. *Surg Clin North Am* 1988; **68**: 199–214.

9 Ward RG, Walsh MS. Necrotizing fasciitis: 10 years' experience in a district general hospital. *Br J Surg* 1991; **78**: 488–9.

10 Kaiser RE, Cerra FB. Progressive necrotizing surgical infections – a unified approach. *J Trauma* 1981; **21**: 349–55.

11 Freischlag JA, Ajalat G, Busuttil RW. Treatment of necrotizing soft tissue infections. The need for a new approach. *Am J Surg* 1985; **149**: 751–5.

12 Loudon I. Necrotising fasciitis, hospital gangrene, and phagedena. *Lancet* 1994; **344**: 1416–9.

13 Fournier AJ. Clinical study of fulminating gangrene of the penis. *Sem Med* 1884; **4**: 69.

14 Meleney FL. Hemolytic streptococcus gangrene. *Arch Surg* 1924; **9**: 317–9.

15 Bisno AL, Stevens DL. Streptococcal infections of skin and soft tissues. *N Engl J Med* 1996; **334**: 240.

16 Lekstrom-Himes JA, Gallin JI. Immunodeficiency diseases caused by defects in phagocytes. *N Engl J Med* 2000; **343**: 1703–14.

17 Morris JG, Jr, Black RE. Cholera and other vibrioses in the United States. *N Engl J Med* 1985; **312**: 343–50.

18 Russell NE, Pachorek RE. Clindamycin in the treatment of streptococcal and staphylococcal toxic shock syndromes. *Ann Pharmacother* 2000; **34**: 936–9.

19 Bowdre JH, Hull JH, Cocchetto DM. Antibiotic efficacy against *Vibrio vulnificus* in the mouse: superiority of tetracycline. *J Pharmacol Exp Ther* 1983; **225**: 595–8.

20 Chuang YC, Yuan CY, Liu CY, *et al. Vibrio vulnificus* infection in Taiwan: report of 28 cases and review of clinical manifestations and treatment. *Clin Infect Dis* 1992; **15**: 271–6.

21 Bennett ML, Jackson JM, Jorizzo JL, *et al.* Pyoderma gangrenosum. A comparison of typical and atypical forms with an emphasis on time to remission. Case review of 86 patients from 2 institutions. *Medicine* (Baltimore) 2000; **79**: 37–46.

22 Chelsom J, Halstensen A, Haga T, *et al.* Necrotising fasciitis due to group A streptococci in western Norway: incidence and clinical features. *Lancet* 1994; **344**: 1111–5.

23 Baxter CR. Surgical management of soft tissue infections. *Surg Clin North Am* 1972; **52**: 1483–99.

24 Patino JF, Castro D. Necrotizing lesions of soft tissues: a review. *World J Surg* 1991; **15**: 235–9.

25 Giuliano A, Lewis F, Jr., Hadley K, *et al.* Bacteriology of necrotizing fasciitis. *Am J Surg* 1977; **134**: 52–7.

26 Patino JF, Castro D, Valencia A, Morales P. Necrotizing soft tissue lesions after a volcanic cataclysm. *World J Surg* 1991; **15**: 240–7.

27 Burge TS, Watson JD. Necrotising fasciitis. *Brit Med J* 1994; **308**: 1453–4.

28 Falcone PA, Pricolo VE, Edstrom LE. Necrotizing fasciitis as a complication of chickenpox. *Clin Pediatr* (Philadelphia) 1988; **27**: 339–43.

29 Mokoena T, Luvuno FM, Marivate M. Surgical management of retroperitoneal necrotising fasciitis by planned repeat laparotomy and debridement. *S Afr J Surg* 1993; **31**: 65–70.

30 Banerjee AR, Murty GE, Moir AA. Cervical necrotizing fasciitis: a distinct clinicopathological entity? *J Laryngol Otol* 1996; **110**: 81–6.

31 Stamenkovic I, Lew PD. Early recognition of potentially fatal necrotizing fasciitis: Use of frozen-section biopsy. *N Engl J Med* 1984; **310**: 1689–93.

32 Stone HH, Matin JD. Synergistic necrotizing cellulitis. *Ann Surg* 1972; **175**: 702–10.

33 Hird B, Byne K. Gangrenous streptococcal myositis: case report. *J Trauma* 1994; **36**: 589–91.

34 Kingston D, Seal DV. Current hypotheses on synergistic microbial gangrene. *Br J Surg* 1990; **77**: 260–4.

35 Thom S. A role for hyperbaric oxygen in clostridial myonecrosis. *Clin Infect Dis* 1993; **17**: 238.

36 Brown DR, Davis NL, Lepawsky M, *et al.* A multicenter review of the treatment of major truncal necrotizing infections with and without hyperbaric oxygen therapy. *Am J Surg* 1994; **167**: 485–9.

37 Heimbach D. Use of hyperbaric oxygen. *Clin Infect Dis* 1993; **17**: 239–40.

38 Sethi DS, Stanley RE. Deep neck abscesses—changing trends. *J Laryngol Otol* 1994; **108**: 138–43.

39 Linder HH. The anatomy of the fasciae of the face and neck with particular reference to the spread and treatment of intraoral infections (Ludwigs's) that have progressed into adjacent fascial spaces. *Ann Surg* 1986; **204**: 705–14.

40 Broughton RA. Nonsurgical management of deep neck infections in children. *Pediatr Infect Dis J* 1992; **11**: 14–8.

41 Sinave CP, Hardy GJ, Fardy PW. The Lemierre syndrome: suppurative thrombophlebitis of the internal jugular vein secondary to oropharyngeal infection. *Medicine (Baltimore)* 1989; **68**: 85–94.

62.

Principles of antibiotic use

J Lipman

The intensive care unit is always the area of any hospital associated with the greatest use of antibiotics. Resistance (and fungal overgrowth) is a direct consequence of usage, and every course of inappropriate antibiotics should be eliminated to help reduce the burden of resistance. Antibiotic cycling[1] has been suggested as a new strategy to help limit resistance, but it is probably better to have portions of the ICU population receive different classes of antibiotics at the same time.[1] Also, inadequate doses of even the 'correct' antibiotic may lead to survival of initially susceptible organisms. For the optimal use of antibiotics not only should antibiotic pharmacokinetics be understood, but there should be clear and rational principles on which each specific antibiotic prescription in the ICU is based.

GENERAL PRINCIPLES[2–6]

All appropriate microbiological specimens, including blood cultures, should be obtained before commencing antibiotic therapy. An immediate Gram-stain may indicate the appropriate antibiotic to use, otherwise a 'best guess' choice is made, which is dependent on the clinical situation. This important and common clinical phenomenon involves trying to predict the infecting organism(s).

Blood cultures should be taken from a venepuncture site, after adequate skin antisepsis, and not from an intravenous or arterial catheter. Two sets of 20 ml (for adults) should be taken, the timing of which is less important.[7] Depending on which system is used, 10 ml should be placed into two different blood culture bottles.

The decision for empiric therapy, that is, cover for the most 'likely' organisms causing any specific infection, must include various factors. These include (i) the site of the infecting organism (respiratory tract pathogens differ from those of abdominal infections); (ii) community vs hospital acquired infection; (iii) recent previous antibiotic prescription; (iv) ward vs ICU acquired infection; and (v) knowledge of the organisms commonly grown in patients in any specific area. This latter point is where ward/unit surveillance becomes important.[8,9]

A narrow spectrum antibiotic should be used whenever practicable. For example, cephalosporins should not generally be used first against *Staphylococcus aureus*, *Streptococcus pyogenes*, and *Streptococcus pneumoniae*. However, it would not be unreasonable under certain circumstances (e.g. for empirical choice for nosocomial sepsis) to start off with broad-spectrum antibiotics, perhaps a combination, until culture results are back. Inappropriate and/or delayed correct antibiotic use in the ICU has been shown to adversely impact on morbidity and mortality.[10]

Monotherapy with a single agent effective against the expected organisms aims to decrease the risk of drug antagonism, reaction or toxicity. Monotherapy often costs less than multiple antibiotic usage. However, prolonged use of a single broad-spectrum antibiotic may lead to resistant organisms[11,12] (see below).

The clinical response to treatment already given should always be considered when bacteriological results suggest a change in antibiotics.

In consultation with infectious disease specialists, additional tests such as antibiotic minimum inhibitory concentration (MIC), antibiotic assay, serum bactericidal activity, and synergy tests of antibiotic combinations may be useful in serious infections (e.g. endocarditis and infections in immunocompromised patients). Sensitivity tests should be interpreted carefully. *In vitro* sensitivity does not equate with clinical effectiveness; *in vitro* resistance generally predicts clinical ineffectiveness.

Consultations with the laboratory staff and infectious diseases/clinical microbiology specialists may be particularly useful in serious infections (e.g. meningococcal sepsis, methicillin-resistant Staphylococci, and multi-resistant Enterobacteriaceae).

The pharmacodynamics, pharmacokinetics (e.g. penetration into relevant tissues) as well as the spectrum of activity of the antibiotic must be considered. Antibiotic pharmacokinetic principles should determine the dosage and frequency of antibiotic regimens (see below).

Adequate drug doses should be given. The intravenous route is preferable in critically ill patients, but other routes should be considered when appropriate (e.g. rectal metronidazole).[13]

Serum levels of potentially toxic antibiotics should be monitored, especially if hepatic or renal dysfunction is present. Certain antibiotics, such as quinolones and carbapenems should not be recommended for routine use. They are best held in reserve for organisms resistant to commonly used agents.

Prophylactic use of antibiotics should be limited to certain situations, should cover organisms that potentially can cause infections in that specific group of patients (e.g. organisms causing skin and soft tissue infections differ from those implicated in intra-abdominal infections) and should be given at the appropriate timing (see below).

General signs of infection are signs of systemic inflammation. Although bacterial infection is likely, non-bacterial infection and non-infective causes should also be considered. High procalcitonin and C-reactive protein levels may be discriminatory for infection,[14] as are IL-6 levels although these are difficult to measure.

Antibiotic guidelines are only one aspect of infection control.[15] Hand washing and/or antiseptic hand sprays,[16,17] identification and elimination of reservoirs of infection, blocking transmission of infection, barrier nursing, interrupting progression from colonization to infection, and eliminating risk factors such as invasive devices are also important.

COMMON ERRORS WHEN USING ANTIBIOTICS

- Administration of antibiotics before microbiological specimens are obtained.
- Inadequate quantity and quality of blood cultures.
- Extended use of antibiotics after eradication of infection.
- Antibiotic 'surfing' (i.e. switching from one combination to another) when a patient is not improving, without delving into the cause of persistent inflammatory response.
- Inadequate and/or incorrect dosing of antibiotics.
- Failure to adequately predict 'resident' microbial flora and therefore inability to correctly choose empiric antibiotics for nosocomial infections (i.e. no adequate surveillance data).
- Failure to recognize toxic effects of antibiotics, particularly when polypharmacy is used.
- Use of combination therapy, irrespective of infection.

SPECIFIC ISSUES

PHARMACOKINETIC PRINCIPLES

The goal of antimicrobial prescription is to achieve effective active drug concentrations (a combination of dose and duration) at the site of infection while avoiding, or at least minimizing, toxicity. The various antibiotic classes have different 'kill characteristics' and therefore should be dosed differently.[18]

β-LACTAMS (ALL PENICILLINS AND CEPHALOSPORINS, MONOBACTAMS)

Studies of β-lactam[18,19] antibiotics on Gram-negative bacilli show a bactericidal activity that is relatively slow, time-dependent and maximal at relatively low concentrations. Bacterial killing is almost entirely related to the time that levels in tissue and plasma exceed a certain threshold. The maximum time plasma β-lactams levels should be allowed to fall below minimum inhibitory concentration (MIC) is 40% of the dosing interval. β-lactam antibiotics lack a significant post-antibiotic effect (PAE) particularly against Gram-negative organisms, and it is not necessary to achieve very high peak plasma concentrations. PAE is the continued suppression of bacterial growth, despite zero serum concentration of antibiotic. It is suggested that concentrations of any β-lactam should be maintained at about 4–5 times MIC for long periods, as maximum killing of bacteria *in vitro* occurs at this level. If antibiotic concentrations fall below this threshold in the *in vitro* models, bacterial growth is immediately resumed. Consequently, it is important for the efficacy of β-lactams that the dosing regime maintains adequate plasma levels for as long as possible during the dosing interval. It is not surprising then, that dosing regimes of β-lactam antibiotics are being re-evaluated, and aim to keep plasma levels above certain thresholds of MICs of Gram-negative organisms for longer periods of the dosing interval.[20]

AMINOGLYCOSIDES

The β-lactams contrast with the kill characteristic of the aminoglycosides,[18,21] which is concentration dependent. Experimentally, a high peak concentration of an aminoglycoside antibiotic provides a better, faster killing effect on standard bacterial inocula. All aminoglycosides exhibit a significant PAE. The duration of this effect is variable, but the higher the previous peak, the longer the PAE. This phenomenon allows drug concentration to fall significantly below MIC of the pathogen without allowing regrowth of bacteria and hence not compromising antibacterial efficacy. The phenomenon of PAE is much more prevalent in aminoglycosides than other antibiotics and more pronounced with Gram-negative bacilli than with other bacteria. These principles allow for single daily doses of aminoglycosides. Combining various meta-analyses involving thousands of patients, once daily administration was found to be more efficacious with reduced toxicity, higher peak/MIC ratios, further prolonged PAE and reduced administration costs. With renal dysfunction[22] the dose should be altered according to creatinine clearance (Table 62.1).

Table 62.1 Dose modification of gentamicin

Creatinine clearance	Gentamicin dose
≥60 ml/min	5–7 mg/kg daily
59–40 ml/min	5–7 mg/kg at an interval of 36 h
39–20 ml/min	5–7 mg/kg at an interval of 48 h

QUINOLONES[18,23,24]

Ciprofloxacin, in contrast, has a combination of both the above (concentration-dependent and time-dependent effects) as well as some PAE. Although one suggested 'target' parameter for a good clinical bactericidal effect is a high peak, the most validated parameter is the area under the inhibitor curve (AUIC), that is AUC/MIC, with values >125 associated with better clinical outcomes. There is general concern about the emergence of resistance related to inappropriately low doses of ciprofloxacin particularly of enterococci, *Pseudomonas* spp. and methicillin resistant Staphylococci.

GLYCOPEPTIDES AND CARBAPENEMS

Vancomycin induces a PAE and a post-antibiotic sub-MIC effect. These combined effects suggest that bacterial regrowth will not occur for prolonged periods following a fall in drug concentrations to levels below the MIC. Theoretically the carbapenems[18] should demonstrate characteristics similar to other β-lactam antibiotics. However, there are significant differences, specifically they exhibit some PAE effects.

GENERAL ISSUES

Aminoglycosides and glycopeptides distribute well into fluids of the extravascular, extracellular space, and less well into tissues. This has two important implications. First, these agents should not be first line agents for, nor monotherapy for, solid organ infections (lung, kidney, liver). Second, in situations where extravascular fluid shifts are significant, such as abdominal sepsis or severe burns, the volume of distribution of these drugs are significantly affected. Hence, for any serum level required, a larger dose may have to be administered. The volume of distribution of the quinolones (very large) suggest penetration is excellent into most tissues and these drugs are good for solid organ infections. Similarly β-lactams as a group (including carbapenems) all have good tissue penetration.

ANTIBIOTIC PROPHYLAXIS[2,4,5,25]

INDICATIONS

When surgery involves incision through an area of colonization or normal commensal flora and a resultant potential infection has morbidity or mortality.

When a procedure (e.g. catheterization, instrumentation, intubation, dental work) potentially produces a bacteraemia in the presence of an immuncompromised patient or when the potential bacteraemia occurs in the presence of an abnormal heart valve or a prosthesis.

BASIC PRINCIPLES OF CHOICE OF PROPHYLACTIC REGIMEN

The organisms colonizing the area through which the incision is made should be covered (Gram-positives if skin is breached, Gram-negatives and anaerobes if bowel is opened).

A similar case should be made for colonizing organisms through the area breached by catheterization or instrumentation (Gram-negatives for bladder catheterization, Gram-positives and anaerobes for dental procedures).

If prevalence of a resistant organism in a specific area is high (e.g. MRSA in burns units) then those organisms should be covered by the prophylactic regimen.

TIMING AND DURATION OF PROPHYLAXIS

Optimal blood levels of antibiotic(s) are needed when the occurrence of the potential bacteraemia occurs, that is for surgery optimal timing of the antibiotic should be at, or just prior to, induction of anaesthesia and skin incision.[25]

For prolonged procedures, where bacteraemias are still a potential occurrence, a second dose of antibiotic(s) may be considered.

There is no extra benefit of post-operative antibiotic prophylaxis.

ANTIBIOTIC DOSES

Doses suggested below are intravenous, for a 70 kg adult with normal renal function. All these drugs accumulate with renal dysfunction and modified doses should be used accordingly.

- Doses for β-lactams vary with each different drug *but* recent emphasis supports lower boluses with more frequent administration, i.e. 4-hourly vs 8-hourly or b.d. vs daily.
- Aminoglycosides: Tobramycin and gentamicin 7 mg/kg as a loading dose on the first day, followed by 5 mg/kg per day. Amikacin 20 mg/kg as the loading dose followed by 15 mg/kg per day. These doses are the same for adults and children, neonates excluded.
- Quinolones: Ciprofloxacin *at least* 400 mg b.d. (up to t.d.s.). Intravenous gatifloxacin may soon become widely available and useful.
- Glycopeptide: Vancomycin 2 g/d either as continuous infusion or in divided doses (40 mg/kg per day for children).

- Carbapenems: Meropenem or imipenem 2–3 g/d in three or four divided doses.

SURVEILLANCE

Some type of simple laboratory-oriented surveillance, which primarily collects data and resistance patterns of microbiological isolates is important. There are a few international projects,[9] but each unit should have access to their own such data, as there is increasing prevalence of resistant organisms in intensive care units. This is complicated even further by different units having differing resistance patterns.[8] Empiric antibiotic therapy must take these factors into account. Some form of surveillance that provides units with their own microbiological data, updateable quarterly or bi-annually, is therefore beneficial in helping choose empiric and prophylactic regimens that are applicable to any specific unit.[8]

MULTI-RESISTANT ORGANISMS

Without good, efficient and effective infection control policies in all areas treating critically ill patients, the spread of multi-resistant organisms would be rampant and the control thereof, useless.[15,26] Part of these policies should involve attention to good hand hygiene and the use of antiseptic soaps and alcohol-based hand rubs.[15–17] Hands are still the most documented and incriminated mode of transmission of infection. In this regard, a decrement in nursing numbers has also been incriminated in outbreaks of infections, possibly due to the time it takes to adequately wash between procedures.[15–17,26]

- Multi-resistant streptococci and vancomycin resistant enterococci (VRE) although not common in all countries, are an increasing world-wide problem.
- The prevalence of MRSA is wider, with many ICUs having this organism almost endemic.
- New agents are available for treatment of resistant Gram-positive infections.[27]
- Antibiotic resistance is agent specific. Often resistance is claimed to be against third generation cephalosporins, but this is largely to ceftazidime[11] (particularly the extended spectrum β-lactamases of *Klebsiella pneumoniae*, *E. coli* and some Enterobacteriaceae).
- Worrying Gram-negative organisms are *Klebsiella pneumoniae*, *Psuedomonas aeruginosa*, *Acinetobacter baumanii* spp. *and Stenotrophomonas maltophilia* (the latter specifically for which trimethaprim may need to be used). A common feature of these organisms is intrinsic resistance to multiple antibiotics.
- Since the carbapenems, there are no new agents for multi-resistant Gram-negative organisms. Sulbactam and polymixin B or colistin have been used for these problem organisms.[28,29]

MONO VS COMBINATION THERAPY[30]

Much of the work in this area was performed before the clinical introduction of the carbapenems, penicillin/ β-lactamase combinations and fourth generation cephalosporins. There is no clear evidence supporting the claim that combination antimicrobial therapy prevents emergence of resistance. However, combination therapy is often suggested for endocarditis and some Pseudomonal infections. When combination therapy is used, preference should be given to the combination therapy of two different classes of antibiotics and then classes that act synergistically. The combination of two β-lactam antibiotics should not be used. Also there is some evidence that in neutropenic patients combination therapy results in a better cure rate.

REFERENCES

1 Kollef MH. Is there a role for antibiotic cycling in the intensive care unit? *Crit Care Med* 2001; **29**(**suppl 4**): N135–42.
2 Reese RE, Douglas RG Jnr (eds) *A Practical Approach to Infectious Diseases*. Boston/Toronto: Little, Brown and Co; 1986.
3 Lundberg GD. Making use of the microbiology laboratory. 1. Use of the laboratory. *JAMA* 1982; **247**: 857–9.
4 Sanford JP. *Guide to Antimicrobial Therapy*. West Bethesda, Maryland: Antimicrobial Therapy Inc; 1993.
5 Mandell GL, Douglas RG, Bennett JE. *Principles and Practice of Infectious Diseases*, 4th edn. New York: Churchill Livingstone; 1994.
6 Neu HC. Antimicrobial agents: Role in the prevention and control of nosocomial infections. In: Wentzel RP (ed.) *Prevention and Control of Nosocomial Infections*, 2nd edn. Baltimore: Williams & Williams, Ch. 18.
7 Weinstein MP. Current blood culture methods and systems: clinical concepts, technology, and interpretation of results. *Clin Infect Dis* 1996; **23**: 40–6.
8 Namias N, Samiian L, Nino D *et al.* Incidence and susceptibility of pathogenic bacteria vary between intensive care units within a single hospital: implications for empiric antibiotic strategies. *J Trauma* 2000; **49**: 638–45.
9 Marchese A, Schito GC. Role of global surveillance in combating bacterial resistance. *Drugs* 2001; **61**: 167–73.
10 Kollef MH. Inadequate antimicrobial treatment: an important determinant of outcome for hospitalized patients. *Clin Infect Dis* 2000; **31**(**suppl 4**): S131–8.
11 Cunha BA. Antibiotic resistance. *Med Clin North Am* 2000; **84**: 1407–29.
12 Jenkins SG. Mechanisms of bacterial antibiotic resistance. *New Horiz* 1996; **4**: 321–32.
13 Baker EM, Aitchison JM, Crindland JS, Baker LW. Rectal administration of metronidazole in severely ill patients. *Brit Med J* 1983; **287**: 311–4.
14 Vincent J-L. Procalcitonin. THE marker of sepsis? *Crit Care Med* 2000; **28**: 1226–8.

15 Pittet D, Hugonnet S, Harbarth S *et al*. Effectiveness of a hospital-wide programme to improve compliance with hand hygiene. Infection Control Programme. *Lancet* 2000; **356**: 1307–12.

16 Boyce JM. Using alcohol for hand antisepsis: dispelling old myths. *Infect Control Hosp Epidemiol* 2000; **21**: 438–41.

17 Pittet D. Improving compliance with hand hygiene in hospitals. *Infect Control Hosp Epidemiol* 2000; **21**: 381–6.

18 Craig WA. Pharmacokinetic/pharmacodynamic parameters: rationale for antibacterial dosing of mice and men. *Clin Infect Dis* 1998; **26**: 1–10.

19 Turnidge JD. The pharmacodynamics of beta-lactams. *Clin Infect Dis* 1998; **27**: 10–22.

20 Lipman J, Wallis S, Rickard C. Low cefepime levels in critically ill septic patients: Pharmacokinetic modeling indicates improved troughs with revised dosing. *Antimicrob Agents Chemother* 1999; **43**: 2559–61.

21 Freeman CD, Nicolau DP, Belliveau PP, Nightingale CH. Once-daily dosing of aminoglycosides: review and recommendations for clinical practice. *J Antimicrob Chemother* 1997; **39**: 677–86.

22 Nicolau DP, Freeman CD, Belliveau PP, *et al*. Experience with a once daily aminoglycoside program administered to 2,184 adult patients. *Antimicrob Agents Chemother* 1995; **39**: 650–5.

23 Turnidge J. Pharmacokinetics and pharmacodynamics of fluoroquinolones. *Drugs* 1999; **58**(**suppl 2**): 29–36.

24 Schentag JJ. Clinical pharmacology of the fluoroquinolones: studies in human dynamic/kinetic models. *Clin Infect Dis* 2000; **31**(**suppl 2**): S40–4.

25 Classen DC, Evans RS, Pestotnik SL, *et al*. The timing of prophylactic administration of antibiotics and the risk of surgical-wound infection. *N Engl J Med* 1992; **326**: 281–6.

26 Fridkin SK. Increasing prevalence of antimicrobial resistance in intensive care units. *Crit Care Med* 2001; **29**(**suppl 4**): N64–8.

27 Lundstrom TS, Sobel JD. Antibiotics for gram-positive bacterial infections. Vancomycin, teicoplanin, quinupristin/dalfopristin, and linezolid. *Infect Dis Clin North Am* 2000; **14**: 463–74.

28 Evans ME, Feola DJ, Rapp RP. Polymyxin B sulfate and colistin: old antibiotics for emerging multi-resistant gram-negative bacteria. *Ann Pharmacother* 1999; **33**: 960–7.

29 Rodriguez-Hernandez MJ, Cuberos L, Pichardo C *et al*. Sulbactam efficacy in experimental models caused by susceptible and intermediate *Acinetobacter baumannii* strains. *J Antimicrob Chemother* 2001; **47**: 479–82.

30 Bouza E, Munoz P. Monotherapy versus combination therapy for bacterial infections. *Med Clin North Am* 2000; **84**: 1357–89.

63

Tropical diseases
R Sivakumar and M Pelly

Once an exotic and esoteric topic, modern travel and the quest for unusual holidays has the potential to bring tropical diseases to every ICU. This chapter covers some diseases, which are common in the tropical belt that are of global concern.

MALARIA

EPIDEMIOLOGY AND PATHOGENESIS

It is estimated that four species of *Plasmodium* (*vivax*, *malariae*, *ovale* and *falciparum*) cause 300 to 500 million infections per year. Most of the 1–3 million deaths per year are caused by *Plasmodium falciparum* and most of them are in children under 5 years in sub-Saharan Africa, but it is also found elsewhere such as Southeast Asia. It is transmitted from human to human by the bite of infected female Anopheles mosquitoes. In *vivax* and *ovale* infections, development to dormant forms can occur in liver, which may lead to relapse.

CLINICAL FEATURES

UNCOMPLICATED MALARIA

Classic symptoms of fever, aches, and headache are usually present, but not always. Other features, such as diarrhoea, vomiting, cough, and/or abdominal pain, may confuse the unwary. Unusual presentations are more common in children and may be missed. Classical rigors or fevers occurring on specific days (tertian or quartan) are usually absent in early *falciparum* infection. Clinical signs may be unhelpful although hepatospenomegaly may be present fairly early.

SEVERE MALARIA
Risk Factors for Severe Malaria

- children under 5 years in endemic regions
- adults and children in non-endemic areas
- non-immune travellers to endemic areas.

Definition
The diagnosis of severe malaria requires the presence of one or more of the following with no other confirmed cause occurring in a patient with asexual *Plasmodium falciparum* parasitaemia[1]:

- impaired conscious state
- multiple convulsions
- respiratory distress
- pulmonary oedema
- circulatory collapse
- abnormal bleeding
- jaundice
- haemoglobinuria
- severe anaemia.

The incubation period is 7 days (range 9–14 days), but this may be prolonged. Anaemia, jaundice, renal dysfunction, haemostatic abnormalities, thrombocytopenia, pulmonary oedema, shock, hypoglycaemia, and severe metabolic acidosis are common in severe malaria. Several of the above may coexist or may develop in rapid succession. Cough, convulsions, and hypoglycaemia are more common in children. Jaundice is common but hepatic failure is uncommon. The acidosis of malaria is multifactorial and probably very similar to other forms of sepsis involving tissue hypoxia, liver dysfunction, and impaired renal handling of bicarbonate.

The cytokines IL-6, IL-10, and TNF-α, and the IL-6:IL-10 ratio are elevated in severe malaria, but this is less marked in cerebral malaria, possibly reflecting more localized infection.

Pregnancy increases the risk of development of severe malaria. During pregnancy both maternal and fetal morbidity and mortality are increased.

The differential diagnosis of severe malaria includes:

- meningitis, typhoid fever, septicaemia
- severe influenza, dengue and other arboviral infections
- haemorrhagic fevers
- hepatitis, leptospirosis
- rickettsial diseases, e.g. scrub typhus
- relapsing fever (borrelia recurrentis)
- febrile convulsions in children.

Poor prognostic indicators include age under 3 years, cerebral malaria, circulatory collapse, and organ dysfunction. Laboratory evidence of poor prognosis includes hyperparasitaemia (>250 000/μl or >5%), peripheral schizontaemia, severe anaemia (PCV <15% or Hb <5 g/dl), blood urea >10 mmol/l (60 mg/dl) and serum creatinine >265 μmol/l (>3.0 mg/dl), venous lactate (>5 mmol/l), CSF lactate (>6 mmol/l) and low CSF glucose, very high concentration of TNF-α.

CEREBRAL MALARIA

Cerebral malaria may be the most common non-traumatic encephalopathy world-wide. The term is restricted to an altered conscious state due to malaria, which cannot be attributed to convulsions, sedatives, hypoglycaemia or to a nonmalarial cause. It is distinguished from the post-ictal state if unconsciousness persists for more than 30 min after a convulsion. Clinical, histopathological and laboratory studies have suggested two potential mechanisms:

- mechanical hypothesis: cytoadherence of parasitized erythrocytes
- cytotoxic hypothesis: neuronal injury by malarial toxin and excessive cytokine production, e.g. TNF-α.

In one study, jugular bulb venous oxygen saturation remained within the normal range in comatose patients, which would argue against a haemodynamic mechanism for altered consciousness during cerebral malaria.
  Clinical findings include:

- convulsions
- raised intracranial pressure
- hypoglycaemia
- acidosis
- abnormalities of tone and posture (the commonest being symmetrical pyramidal signs)
- retinopathy: retinal haemorrhages, cotton wool spots, papilloedema, retinal whitening and retinal vessel abnormalities which are all more common in children.

DIAGNOSIS

Microscopy of thick and thin films remains the gold standard both for diagnosis and for following the efficacy of treatment. In the non-immune patient there is a close association between parasite levels and complications; however severe complications can occur in patients with low counts.
  Rapid tests based on *P. falciparum* antigen histidine-rich protein 2 have a useful role especially in screening returning travellers with suspected malaria, but do not replace or remove the need for film examination. Parasight *F*-test (Becton Dickinson Advanced Diagnostics) has a sensitivity of 93.3% and a specificity of 98.3%.[2]

TREATMENT OF MALARIA[1] (Table 64.1)

BENIGN MALARIA

Chloroquine sensitive infections with *P. vivax, ovale, malariae* and *falciparum* malaria should be treated with this drug, but alternatives are quinine, mefloquine, halofantrine and artemisinin or its derivatives.

SEVERE MALARIA

In patients with features of severe malaria, if only a benign species alone is identified in the film, a mixed infection with *falciparum* should be assumed. If the clinical suspicion is high, a therapeutic trial is justified even if the film is negative. Severe malaria is in effect severe septic shock and the principles of management are the same. Initial doses of antimalarial drugs should not be reduced in renal failure. These patients are at risk of acute lung injury but do need adequate fluid resuscitation. Convulsions must be actively treated.

EXCHANGE BLOOD TRANSFUSION

Exchange blood transfuion (EBT) should be considered in the following situations if pathogen free compatible blood is available[5]:

Table 63.1 Anti-malarial drug treatment

Chloroquine sensitive malaria:
  Chloroquine: 10 mg base/kg i.v. over 8 h, followed by 15 mg/kg over the next 24 h.
or
  Chloroquine: 1 mg base/kg per hour i.v. for 30 h.
Chloroquine-resistant malaria or sensitivity unknown
  Quinine reduces the parasite burden by 50% in ~24 h, while artemisinin derivatives act about twice as fast.[3] A recent review suggests that artemisinin drugs are no worse than quinine in preventing death in severe or complicated malaria, and no artemisinin derivative appears better than another.[4] A loading dose of Quinine dihydrochloride salt 20 mg/kg in 10 ml isotonic fluid/kg i.v. over 4 h. Then 8 hours after the start of the loading dose, 10 mg/kg over 4 h every 8 hours, calculated from the beginning of the previous infusion until the patient can swallow, then quinine tablets 10 mg/kg (max 600 mg) every 8–12 h to complete 7 days of treatment, or a single dose of 25 mg/kg sulfadoxine and 1.25 mg/kg pyrimethamine (max 1500 mg sulfadoxine–75 mg pyrimethamine).
or
  Artesunate 2.4 mg/kg i.v. followed by 1.2 mg/kg at 12 h and 24 h, then 1.2 mg/kg daily for 6 days. If the patient is able to swallow, the daily dose can be given orally.
or
  Artemether: 3.2 mg/kg i.m., followed by 1.6 mg/kg daily for 6 days. If the patient is able to swallow, the dose can be given orally. If parenteral administration is not possible, artemisinin or artesunate suppositories may be given.

- Parasitaemia >30% even in the absence of clinical complications
- Parasitaemia >10% in the presence of severe disease especially cerebral malaria, acute renal failure, ARDS, jaundice and severe anaemia and/or poor prognostic factors (e.g. elderly patient, late stage parasites [schizonts] in the peripheral blood)
- Parasitaemia >10% and failure to respond to optimal chemotherapy after 12–24 h.

PROGNOSIS

Data are largely derived from endemic areas. Presentation with convulsions, acidosis or hypoglycaemia is associated with a poorer outcome. In patients requiring intensive care, one study has quoted a mortality of 12.5%. Cerebral malaria may have a high mortality in some endemic areas, 20–30%, but has a mortality of 2–6% in returned travellers, and these are usually related to late diagnosis. The prognosis of cerebral malaria frequently is determined by the management of other complications such as renal failure and acidosis but neurological sequelae are increasingly recognized.

TUBERCULOSIS

EPIDEMIOLOGY

Tuberculosis continues to be a devastating disease worldwide, and is increasing world-wide, with an estimated 8 million new cases and 2.6–2.9 million deaths annually. Medical conditions which predispose to tuberculosis include HIV infection, silicosis, diabetes, chronic renal failure/haemodialysis, malnutrition, solid organ transplantation, gastrectomy, jejunoileal bypass, injection and inhalational drug abuse, alcoholism, chronic pulmonary disease, and prolonged steroid use. Social factors such as institutional living conditions (nursing homes, homeless shelters, prisons), urban dwelling and poverty are also associated with an increased risk of tuberculosis.

PATHOGENESIS

Tuberculosis is usually caused by *Mycobacterium tuberculosis* and four others (*M. bovis*, *M africanum*, *M. microti* and *M. canetti*) grouped in Mycobacterium complex. The genus Mycobacterium consists of more than 80 different species all of which appear similar on acid-fast staining. Multiresistant TB is now a problem and should always be considered.

Inhalation of tubercle bacilli leads to one of the four possible outcomes: immediate clearance of the organism, primary or progressive primary disease, chronic or latent infection and reactivation disease. Latent infection refers to the presence of tuberculous infection (positive tuberculin reaction) without the disease.

The majority of primary TB infections are asymptomatic, while clinical pneumonia occurs in 5–10% of adults with a higher incidence in children and those HIV infected. *M. tuberculosis* microfoci that have remained dormant after primary infection may undergo reactivation resulting in secondary TB, often referred to as reactivation disease. This is responsible for 90% of TB in patients not infected with HIV.

CLINICAL SPECTRUM

The manifestations of TB are protean and TB should be considered in the differential diagnosis of all patients with fever of unknown origin, night sweats, or unexplained weight loss. Besides the lungs, it can also involve CNS, peritoneum, pericardium, gastrointestinal and genitourinary tract, bone and joints, lymph nodes and skin. Occasionally it can be disseminated in the form of miliary tuberculosis (Table 63.2).

PULMONARY TUBERCULOSIS

Typically, reactivation disease starts in the apex of one or both of lungs leading on to chronic inflammation and fibrosis. Pulmonary TB is often asymptomatic initially though cough, dyspnoea and haemoptysis are useful clues. Hilar lymphadenopathy is the most common pulmonary presentation in children. It may occasionally present very late as extensive disease in both lungs with severe lung injury including cavitation and development of pneumothoraces.

Diagnosis

Sputum, induced sputum, bronchial washings or transbronchial biopsy of infiltrates should be performed to isolate the organism. Computed tomography (CT) is more sensitive than chest radiography for detection of infiltrates, cavities, lymphadenopathy, miliary disease, bronchiectasis, bronchial stenosis, bronchopleural fistula, and pleural effusion.

TUBERCULOUS PLEURAL EFFUSION

Pleural TB may result in pleural effusion or pleural empyema, with or without bronchopleural fistula. Thoracentesis and pleural biopsy should be performed. Positive

Table 63.2 *Tuberculous emergencies*

Massive haemoptysis
Tuberculous meningitis
Pericardial tamponade
Small intestinal obstruction
Respiratory failure
Status epilepticus due to tuberculomas

cultures are found in less than 25% of cases. Pleural biopsy shows granulomatous inflammation in approximately 60% of patients. However, when culture of three biopsy specimens is combined with histologic examination, the diagnosis can be made in up to 90% of cases. Pleuroscopy-guided biopsies increase the yield in pleural sampling.

The pleural fluid should be examined for total protein and glucose content, WBC count and differential, and pH. Raised adenosine deaminase levels have been found to be useful in the diagnosis,[6] with levels more than 70 U/l in pleural fluid strongly favouring tuberculous aetiology and levels less than 40 U/l strongly negating it. Raised γ-interferon has also found to be useful.

TUBERCULOUS MENINGITIS

Tuberculous meningitis (TBM)[7] remains the most serious manifestation of TB, and the most relevant to the intensive care physician. Tuberculous meningitis results from haematogenous spread. There is thick gelatinous exudate around the sylvian fissures, basal cisterns, brainstem and cerebellum.

The majority of patients with TBM had recent contact with TB, followed by a prodrome of vague ill-health lasting 2–8 weeks. Later, signs and symptoms of meningeal irritation appear. Cranial nerve palsies occur in 20–25% of patients and papilloedema may be present. Choroidal tubercles are rare, but almost pathognomonic. Visual loss due to optic nerve involvement may occasionally be the presenting feature. There may be focal neurological deficit such as hemiplegia, extrapyramidal movements and seizures. As the disease progresses, cerebral dysfunction sets in and the mortality approaches 50%.

Diagnosis

A diagnostic algorithm has been suggested, but it is unlikely to provide sufficient assurance to confidently exclude other diagnosis.[8] The key is a high degree of clinical suspicion, especially in the critically ill. In one study, TBM was considered a diagnosis in only 36% of cases and only 6% received immediate treatment.[9] Definitive diagnosis of TBM depends upon the detection of the organism in CSF, either by smear examination or by bacterial culture. The yield of positive diagnosis from smear is variable, but generally low. Culture of the CSF for the organisms is not invariably positive. Raised adenosine deaminase level is not specific.

PCR on CSF samples has a reported sensitivity between 33–90% and a comparable specificity (88–100%) to culture. Computed tomography (CT) or magnetic resonance imaging (MRI) of the brain is sensitive but not specific, and may reveal thickening and intense enhancement of meninges, especially in basilar regions. Hydrocephalus or tuberculomas may also be present. Infarcts due to either vasculitis or mechanical strangulation of the vessels by the surrounding exudates are detected in up to 40% using CT scan. The radiological differential diagnosis includes cryptococcal meningitis, CMV encephalitis, sarcoidosis, meningeal metastases and lymphoma.

TB DIAGNOSIS

Once considered, isolate the patient, and sample all potential sites as dictated by their clinical state. Histologic examination for granulamatous infection is useful in bronchial tissue, pleural, peritoneal and skeletal tissues. Peritoneal biopsies are best obtained via laparoscopy.

Newer culture media have reduced the time for culture to 2 weeks. New innovations include nucleic acid amplification (NAA) techniques, which can be applied to clinical specimens within hours. They use either transcription mediated amplification (enhanced amplified Mycobacterium tuberculosis direct (E-MTD) test, Gen-Probe Inc., San Diego) or Polymerase chain reaction (PCR) based amplication (COBAS AMPLICOR Mycobacterium tuberculosis test, Roche Diagnostics) of specific target sequences of nucleic acids that can then be detected through the use of a nucleic acid probe.[10–12] Several in-house PCR assays have also been used.

- A positive NAA test in smear positive patients can differentiate *M. tuberculosis* from nontuberculous mycobacteria (NTM) and treatment can be started.
- The interpretation of smear positive but negative NAA test is controversial.
- In smear negative and NAA positive patients, if clinical suspicion is high, treatment should be started particularly in critically ill patients.
- If clinical suspicion is high, negative smear and NAA cannot exclude TB.
- NAA results may remain positive for months. This method should be used only for initial diagnosis and not follow-up evaluations of patients who are receiving anti-mycobacterial drugs.[13]

At present, amplification techniques for *M. tuberculosis* cannot replace the conventional diagnostic approach. Serodiagnosis of tuberculosis still remains a poor confirmatory tool, but may be useful in disease exclusion in areas of low incidence. Drug susceptibility tests should be performed on initial isolates from all patients in order to identify an effective antituberculous regimen and may have to repeated if the patient remains culture positive after 3 months.

TREATMENT OF TUBERCULOSIS

Local guidelines are of paramount importance and advice should be sought. The commonest regimen used is isoniazid (5 mg/kg), and rifampicin (10 mg/kg) for 6 months, with the addition of pyrazinamide (15–30 mg/kg) for the first 2 months. In the critically ill, absorption of these drugs may be a major problem. Ethambutol (5–25 mg/kg) is added in areas where the resistance to INH is high. Prothionamide is preferable as a fourth drug in tuberculous meningitis. Isoniazid, rifampicin and ethambutol are safe in pregnancy but pyrazinamide should be avoided. Steroids are generally recommended in severe tuberculous meningitis and pericardial tuberculosis.

DRUG RESISTANT TUBERCULOSIS

This is an increasing problem. Multidrug resistant tuberculosis means resistance to two or more of the first line anti-tuberculous drugs, usually INH and rifampicin, which can be primary (no prior anti-tuberculous therapy) or secondary (development of resistance during or after chemotherapy).

Diagnosis depends upon collecting adequate specimens for culturing prior to the initiation of anti-tuberculous therapy. With the improvements in the culture methods, and the availability of nucleic acid amplification, rapid identification of antibiotic resistance is possible.[14] When resistance is present to two or more first line agents, parenteral aminoglycosides (e.g. streptomycin, or amikacin) and a quinolone (e.g. ciprofloxacin or ofloxacin) are generally added.

TYPHOID FEVER

Typhoid fever is caused by *S. typhi* and less commonly by paratyphi B, A then C. Even non-typhoidal salmonellae have occasionally been isolated.[15] Typhoid fever, common in South and South East Asia, is almost exclusively caused by faecal-oral spread. In the developed world, cases are either seen in international travellers or occasionally caused by infected food.

CLINICAL FEATURES

The incubation period is 5–21 days. It presents non-specifically with fever, chills, abdominal pain and constitutional symptoms. Constipation may be more frequent than diarrhoea. Hepatosplenomegaly, erythematous macular rash (30%), and relative bradycardia, which although non-specific can be a useful clue.[16]

Complications include shock, ileal perforation, gastrointestinal haemorrhage, jaundice and encephalopathy,[17] neuropsychiatric manifestations, septic arthritis, pericarditis, and obstetric complications.

DIAGNOSIS

Anaemia, leukopenia or leukocytosis, and deranged liver function are common.

Blood cultures are positive in up to 80% of cases and are the investigation of choice. Though culturing urine, stool, rose spots and duodenal contents are useful, bone marrow culture is most sensitive and remains positive up to 5 days after commencement of antibiotics.[18] Serodiagnosis using the Widal agglutination test has limited clinical value.

TREATMENT

Multidrug resistant strains are common in the Indian subcontinent, Southeast Asia and Africa. There may be resistance to chloramphenicol, ampicillin and trimethoprim and sulphamethoxazole. This has led to the usage of fluoroquinolones (ciprofloxacin or ofloxacin for 7–10 days) and third generation cephalosporins for 7–14 days, as the empiral treatment in enteric fever, pending sensitivity results. Shorter courses have also been found to be effective. There is some concern in using fluoroquinolones in children, as they have been shown to cause cartilage toxicity in immature animals but this appears largely unfounded in clinical trials.[19,20]

Resistance to ciprofloxacin is being increasingly reported and should be taken into account in a seriously ill patient. Azithromycin has also been found to be useful.[21]

Dexamethasone was found to reduce mortality in severe typhoid fever patients who are delirious, obtunded, stuporous, comatose, or in shock.[22] In the absence of current evidence, steroids should be seriously considered in confirmed severe typhoid fever. Ileal perforation, which may occur late, classically in the third week of febrile illness, requires prompt surgical intervention and the segmental resection has been recommended as the procedure of choice.[23]

CHOLERA

It is caused by enterotoxin-producing *Vibrio cholerae*. The incubation period varies from 12 h to several days. The clinical case:infection ratio is about 1:10. It starts abruptly with painless watery diarrhoea associated with vomiting and painful muscle cramps.

Stool examination shows neither leukocytes nor erythrocytes. Dark field microscopy examination may reveal rapidly motile comma-shaped bacilli in fresh stool. Rapid (<5 min) commercial assays detecting O antigen in stool samples are as sensitive and specific as stool culture. Aggressive rehydration is the mainstay of treatment. Adjunctive antimicrobial therapy with tetracycline, trimethoprim/sulphamethoxazole, furazolidone or erythromycin are effective in shortening the duration of diarrhoea.

DENGUE FEVER

EPIDEMIOLOGY

It is estimated that 100 million dengue virus infections occur each year throughout the world.[24] The causative agent is a flavivirus with four distinct serogroups which is transmitted by the bite of Aedes mosquitoes. Two patterns of transmission have been recognized; epidemic due to isolated introduction of dengue to a region (usually due to a single serotype), and hyperendemic, which refers to the continuous circulation of multiple dengue virus serotypes.

PATHOGENESIS OF DENGUE INFECTION

Following a mosquito bite, viraemia begins after a few days and usually lasts up to 7 days. Infection with one of the four serotypes (primary infection) provides life-long immunity against that serotype, but not against the other serotypes (secondary infection). Epidemiological studies have suggested that the risk of severe disease (DHF/DSS) is significantly higher in secondary infection than primary infection.

CLINICAL FEATURES

The clinical presentation varies from mild febrile illness to severe haemorrhagic fever; however, most infections are asymptomatic. Dengue fever (DF) has an incubation period of 3–14 days; has associated chills, fever (as high as 40°C), arthralgia, myalgia, and retro-orbital pain on ocular movement. Injected conjunctivae, maculopapular rash, and hepatosplenomegaly are commonly found, and haemorrhagic manifestations can occur in DF and should not be confused with dengue haemorrhagic fever (DHF).

Dengue haemorrhagic fever occurs primarily in children <10 years. The key diagnostic criteria for DHF are:

- plasma leakage syndrome leading to haemoconcentration (20% or greater rise in haematocrit), pleural effusion or ascites
- thrombocytopenia (<100 000) associated with a bleeding tendency
- hepatomegaly and or abnormal liver function tests.

The mechanism underlying the profound capillary leak in DHF, but not DF, is poorly understood.

DIAGNOSIS

Dengue should be suspected in all febrile patients who live in, or have returned from, endemic areas in the preceding 2 weeks. Leukopenia, thrombocytopenia with a positive tourniquet test, and raised AST are frequently seen.[25] IgM immunoassay allows rapid confirmation of the diagnosis. If it is negative, particularly in the first 6 days of the illness, the diagnosis should not be ruled out. Acute and convalescent sera should be analysed by Haemagglutination assay or IgG immunoassay looking for a four-fold rise in titre. Virus isolation and reverse transcriptase PCR are available but are usually not used in the clinical setting.

TREATMENT

In addition to full supportive therapy for shock, a single dose of steroids have been used in DHF, but this has not been shown to alter mortality, bleeding severity or complications.[26]

VIRAL HAEMORRHAGIC FEVERS (VHF)

Arboviruses (arthropod-borne viruses) cause three syndromes (i) aseptic meningitis-encephalitis, (ii) arthralgia-arthritis, and (iii) haemorrhagic disease. Frequently, the disease will be a minor non-specific febrile illness, or most commonly asymptomatic infection. The mode of transmission is usually through ticks, mosquitoes and rodents. At least four of the haemorrhagic fevers (Lassa fever, Ebola virus, Marburg virus and Congo-Crimean haemorrhagic fever virus) are capable of person-to-person transmission through close contact with infected blood and other body secretions. Epidemiological studies of VHF in humans indicate that although possible, the airborne route does not readily transmit infection from person to person.

CLINICAL FEATURES

The patient will have either been in an endemic area or been in contact with someone from an endemic area. VHF cases generally have an abrupt onset after a short incubation period of <10 days, but this can be delayed up to 21 days.[27] They present as acute febrile illnesses with a prodrome that often includes severe headache, dizziness, flushing, conjunctival injection, myalgia, lumbar pain, and prostration. Gastrointestinal symptoms with nausea, vomiting, abdominal pain, and diarrhea may occur.

Leukopenia or leukocytosis, thrombocytopenia, and elevated serum aminotransferases may be evident early in the disease, and a petechial rash may appear on days 3–10. Coagulation profiles and fibrinogen degradation products and D-dimer values become progressively more abnormal, and overt haemorrhagic features of the disease (ecchymoses, epistaxis, gingival bleeding, maelena, haematuria,) may supervene from day 5 onward; sometimes even earlier. Multiple organ system failure supervenes and death may ensue. Clinical improvement becomes apparent toward the end of the second week of illness in patients who survive.

DIAGNOSIS

A high index of suspicion is needed and VHF should be suspected in the following circumstances:

- In unexplained fever in patients who have visited areas where VHF are endemic within 3 weeks of becoming ill. A history of camping in the bush, sleeping on the ground or in rural farms, tick bites or contact with sick animals increases the likelihood of VHF.
- Febrile medical and nursing staff in the endemic areas and laboratory workers who handle VHF viruses.
- Febrile contacts.

The diagnosis may be made by isolating from blood or body fluids, positive IgM antibody or by showing a four-fold rise in antibody titre. Detection of characteristic virions by electron microscopy establishes the diagnosis of Marburg and Ebola viruses. If needed for infection control, electron microscopy of tissues (especially liver) at autopsy is confirmatory.

TREATMENT

Therapy is essentially supportive for a severe shock state. Haemorrhage is managed by replacement of blood, platelets, and clotting factors as indicated. Ribavirin, a synthetic nucleoside analogue, is useful in treating Lassa fever and Congo-Crimean haemorrhagic fever. Ribavirin may reduce mortality by tenfold if treatment is begun within 6 days of onset. A 30 mg/kg i.v. loading dose is followed by 15 mg/kg q.i.d. for 4 days and then 7.5 mg/kg t.d.s. for another 6 days.

PRECAUTIONS

In most countries, these diseases must be notified immediately. In addition to universal blood and body fluid precautions, airborne isolation, including use of goggles, high-efficiency masks, a negative pressure room with no air circulation, and positive pressure filtered air respirators have all been recommended. Surveillance of contacts allows early detection. To prevent further mosquito transmission, patients should be isolated in well-screened rooms sprayed with residual insecticides.

REFERENCES

1 WHO. *Management of Severe Malaria. A Practical Handbook*, 2nd edn. Geneva: WHO; 2000.
2 Cropley IM, Lockwood DNJ, Mack D, *et al.* Rapid diagnosis of falciparum malaria by using the Parasight F test in travellers returning to the United Kingdom: prospective study. *Brit Med J* 2000; **321**: 484–5.
3 Hien TT, White NJ. Quinghausu. *Lancet* 1993; **341**: 603–8.
4 McIntosh HM, Olliaro P. Artemisinin derivatives for treating severe malaria. *Cochrane Database Syst Rev* 2000; **2**: CD000527.
5 WHO. Severe falciparum malaria. *Trans R Soc Trop Med Hyg* 2000: **94(suppl 1)**.
6 Riantawan P, Chaowalit P, Wongsangiem M, Rojanaraweewong P. Diagnostic value of pleural fluid adenosine deaminase in tuberculous pleuritis with reference to HIV coinfection and a Bayesian analysis. *Chest* 1999; **116**: 97–103.
7 Thwaites G, Chau TTH, Mai NTH, *et al.* Tuberculous meningitis. *J Neurol Neurosurg Psychiatry* 2000; **68**: 289–99.
8 Kumar R, Sing SN, Kohli N. A diagnostic rule for tuberculous meningitis. *Arch Dis Child* 1999; **81**: 221–4.
9 Kent SJ, Crowe SM, Yung A, *et al.* Tuberculous meningitis: a 30 year review. *Clin Infect Dis* 1993; **17**: 987–94.
10 American Thoracic Society. Rapid diagnostic tests for tuberculosis: what is the appropriate use? *Am J Respir Crit Care Med* 1997; **155**: 1804–14.
11 MMWR. Update: nucleic acid amplification tests for tuberculosis. *MMWR* 2000: **49**(26); 593–4.
12 American Thoracic Society. Diagnostic standards and classification of tuberculosis in adults and children. *Am J Respir Crit Care Med* 2000; **161**: 1376–95.
13 Shah S, Miller A, Mastellone A, *et al.* Rapid diagnosis of tuberculosis in various biopsy and body fluid specimens by the AMPLICOR Mycobacterium tuberculosis polymerase chain reaction test. *Chest* 1998; **113**: 1190–4.
14 Williams DL, Spring L, Gillis TP, *et al.* Evaluation of polymerase chain reaction based universal hetero-duplex assay for direct detection of rifampicin susceptibility of Mycobacterium tuberculosis from sputum specimens. *Clin Infect Dis* 1998; **26**: 446–50.
15 Obeogbulam SI, Oguike JU, Gugnani HC. Microbiological studies on cases diagnosed as typhoid/enteric fever in Nigeria. *J Commun Dis* 1997; **27**: 97–100.
16 Ostergaard L, Huniche B, Anderson PL. Relative bradycardia in infectious diseases. *J Infect* 1996; **33**: 185–91.
17 Kamath PS, Jalihal A, Chakraborty A. Differentiation of typhoid fever from fulminant hepatic failure in patients presenting with jaundice and encephalopathy. *Mayo Clin Proc* 2000; **75**: 462–6.
18 Gasem MH, Dolmans WM, Isbandri BB, *et al.* Culture of *Salmonella typhi* and paratyphi in blood and bone marrow in suspected typhoid fever. *Trop Geogr Med* 1995; **47**: 164–7.
19 Bethell DB, Hien TT, Phi LT, *et al.* The effects on growth of single short courses of fluoroquinolones. *Arch Dis Child* 1996; **74**: 44–6.
20 Doherty CP, Saha SK, Cutting WA. Typhoid fever, ciprofloxacin and growth in young children. *Ann Trop Paediatr* 2000; **20**: 297–303.
21 Frenck RW Jr, Nakhla I, Sultan Y. Azithromycin versus ceftriaxone for the treatment of uncomplicated typhoid fever in children. *Clin Infect Dis* 2000; **31**: 1134–8.
22 Hoffman SL, Punjabi NH, Kumala S, *et al.* Reduction of mortality in chloramphenicol-treated severe typhoid fever by high-dose dexamethasone. *N Engl J Med* 1984; **310**: 82–8.
23 Ameh EA, Dogo PM, Attah MM, *et al.* Comparison of three operations for typhoid perforation. *Br J Surg* 1997; **84**: 558–9.
24 Gubler DJ. Dengue and dengue hemorrhagic fever. *Clin Microbiol Rev* 1998; **11**: 480–96.
25 Kalayanarooj S, Vaughn D.W, Nimmannitya S, *et al.* Early clinical and laboratory indicators of acute dengue illness. *J Infect Dis* 1997; **176**: 313–21.
26 Tassniyom S, Vasanawathana S, Chirawatkul A, *et al.* Failure of methylprednisolone in established dengue shock syndrome: A placebo-controlled double blind study. *Pediatrics* 1993; **92**: 111–5.
27 Richards GA, Murphy S, Jobson R, *et al.* Unexpected Ebola virus in a tertiary setting: Clinical and epidemiologic aspects. *Crit Care Med* 2000; **28**: 240–4.

Part Eleven

Severe and Multiple Trauma

64.

Severe and multiple trauma

J A Judson

Trauma can be defined as physical injury from mechanical energy. It is usually categorized as blunt or penetrating. In Western countries, severe blunt trauma is common, caused by road crashes, falls and, less frequently, blows and assault. Severe penetrating trauma, usually from stabbings and gunshots, is less common except in larger cities of the USA,[1,2] South Africa and war zones. Blunt trauma is often more difficult to treat than penetrating trauma. Assessment is more difficult, because injuries are frequently internal, multiple and not obvious initially. The risk of missing serious injuries can only be lessened by a systematic approach and repeated assessments.[3–5]

ASSESSMENT AND PRIORITIES

TRIAGE

An important first step is triage – sorting patients with acute life-threatening injuries and complications from those whose lives are not in danger. The severity of total body injury is related to the number of separate injuries present, and to the severity of individual injuries. Assessment can be made either at the scene of injury or on arrival at hospital. As in any emergency, assessment, diagnosis and treatment need to be concurrent. There is limited time for detailed histories, examinations, investigations or well-considered diagnoses before starting emergency care. Most patients with severe injury can be distinguished early by the following:

- *Depressed consciousness* in the trauma patient can be related to brain injury, hypoxaemia, shock, alcohol or other ingested drugs, or precipitating neurological or cardiac events. Frequently, a combination of factors is present, and the precise extent of physical brain injury is not known initially. Initial treatment in any case is determined by the level of consciousness rather than its exact cause.
- *Breathing difficulties* are common in patients with trauma to the head, face, neck and chest. If rapid or distressed breathing is present, airway obstruction,

laryngeal injury, pulmonary aspiration and lung or chest wall injury (especially pneumothorax and lung contusion) must be considered.
- *Shock* is almost always hypovolaemic from blood loss, but other types of shock occasionally occur in trauma (see below).

PRIORITIES

A trauma patient often has multiple problems requiring attention. Determining priorities is not always easy. In general, the priorities are to:

- *Support life*: the patient is kept alive with resuscitative techniques, while the various injuries and complications are attended to
- *Locate and control bleeding*, which may be varied (see below)
- *Prevent brainstem compression* and spinal cord damage
- Diagnose and treat all other injuries and complications.

BASIC TREATMENT PRINCIPLES

A systematic approach to managing severe and multiple trauma is important. Effective programmes developed by the American College of Surgeons are now well established.[6] A number of basic treatment principles apply to all severe trauma patients.

EMERGENCY ASSESSMENT (PRIMARY SURVEY)

The following must be recognized and treated before anything else:

- *A – Airway obstruction*: suggested by noisy (or silent) breathing, with paradoxical chest movements and breathing distress, and inadequate airway protection from impaired gag reflexes in patients with depressed consciousness.

- B – *Breathing difficulty*: suggested by tachypnoea, abnormal pattern of breathing, cyanosis or mental confusion.
- C – *Circulatory shock*: manifested by cold peripheries with delayed capillary refill, rapid weak pulse or low blood pressure (see below).

OXYGEN AND VENTILATORY THERAPY

High-flow oxygen by mask is given to all trauma patients. However, patients with severe trauma frequently require ventilatory support. A restless unco-operative patient should be intubated under a rapid sequence induction to facilitate resuscitation.

BLOOD CROSS-MATCH AND TESTS

Six units of red cells should be cross-matched urgently, but it is impossible to predict the amount of blood that will be required. Blood is concurrently sent for baseline haematological and biochemical tests, including blood ethanol level. Blood ethanol is clinically useful in assessing individual patients with depressed consciousness, quite apart from epidemiologic and preventive medicine,[7] and legal considerations.

FLUID RESUSCITATION

Resuscitation fluids are given (see below). If necessary, two or three large 14 or 16-gauge i.v. cannulas are inserted in upper limb, external jugular or femoral veins.

ANALGESIA

Analgesia is easily overlooked. Opioid agents should he titrated i.v., and not given i.m. or subcutaneously. Large doses may he needed.

URINE OUTPUT

A urinary catheter is inserted unless a ruptured urethra is suspected (because of blood at the urinary meatus, severe fractured pelvis or abnormal prostate position on rectal examination), in which case a suprapubic catheter is indicated. Urine output monitoring is an important guide to resuscitation.

OTHER INJURIES

All injuries should be evaluated.

CLINICAL EVALUATION OF INJURIES (SECONDARY SURVEY)

Injuries are easily missed in an emergency, especially when one injury is obvious. A secondary, and even a ter-tiary, survey should be performed.[5] The back and the front of the patient should be examined. Special attention is paid to regions with external lacerations, contusions and abrasions. All body regions are examined systematically.

HEAD

Neurological observations are made. The ears and nose are inspected for cerebrospinal fluid and blood, and the scalp is examined thoroughly.

FACE

Bleeding into the airway should be excluded, and the face and jaws tested for abnormal mobility.

SPINE

A cervical spine fracture or dislocation is assumed in all patients with depressed consciousness until proved otherwise. Signs of spinal cord injury should be sought (e.g. warm dilated peripheries from loss of vasomotor tone, diaphragmatic breathing, paralysis, priapism and loss of anal tone). The thoracic and lumbar spine should be inspected and palpated.

THORAX

Fractured ribs in themselves are not usually life-threatening but haemothorax, pneumothorax, lung contusion and chest wall instability (flail chest) will require attention if present. Less common but very serious injuries can occur to the heart and great vessels (see Ch. 67).

ABDOMEN

The spleen, liver and mesenteries are often damaged. Retroperitoneal haemorrhage is common. Injuries to the pancreas, duodenum and other hollow viscera are less frequent, and may be missed until signs of peri-tonitis occur. Renal injury with retroperitoneal haemorrhage is suggested by haematuria and loin pain (see Ch. 69).

PELVIS

Pelvic fractures may be difficult to detect clinically, especially in the unconscious patient. Blood loss may be massive, particularly with posterior fractures involving sacroiliac dislocation. Ruptured bladder and ruptured urethra may occur with anterior fractures.

EXTREMITIES

A litre or more of blood may be lost into a fractured femur. Long bone fractures are more serious when they are open, comminuted or displaced, or if associated with nerve or arterial damage.

EXTERNAL

Contusions may be extensive and serious, especially in falls from heights, and may be overlooked if the victim's back is not examined. Road crash victims may sustain serious burns or abrasions.

SHOCK IN THE TRAUMA PATIENT

The earliest, most constant and reliable signs of shock are seen in the peripheral circulation. A patient with cold, pale peripheries has shock until proved otherwise. Tachycardia is not always present and hypotension is a late sign of shock. The commonest form of shock in trauma is hypovolaemic shock.

HYPOVOLAEMIC SHOCK

If the neck veins are empty, hypovolaemic shock should be inferred. Possible sites of blood loss causing shock are:

- *External loss,* which is obvious clinically from blood-soaked clothing and pooled blood.
- *Major fractures,* which are obvious clinically by deformity, swelling, crepitus, pain and tenderness (e.g. femurs) or seen on a plain X-ray (e.g. pelvis).
- *Pleural cavity,* detected on urgent chest X-ray. Intrapleural drains will reveal the amount and rate of blood loss.
- *Peritoneal cavity,* detected by laparotomy, diagnostic peritoneal lavage, computed tomography (CT) scan or ultrasound. Clinical examination of the abdomen can be misleading when the patient is intoxicated, has depressed consciousness or has multiple injuries. A single clinical examination is of limited value: changes over time are more important.
- *Retroperitoneum,* detected at laparotomy or by CT scan, or inferred when all the above are negative, especially in the presence of pelvic or lumbar spine fracture.

CARDIOGENIC SHOCK

If the trauma patient with shock has distended neck veins, possible causes are tension pneumothorax, concurrent myocardial infarction, cardiac tamponade or myocardial contusion.

NEUROLOGIC SHOCK

Patients with paraplegia or tetraplegia from spinal cord injury may have low blood pressure with warm dilated peripheries accompanied by lax anal tone and by priapism in the male (see Ch. 70). This is a diagnosis of exclusion and all causes of hypovolaemic shock (see above) must be sought.

SEPTIC SHOCK

Occasionally, patients with pulmonary aspiration may develop septic shock. This is unlikely to confuse the initial trauma assessment soon after injury, but may require consideration some hours or a day or two later.

DIAGNOSTIC PERITONEAL LAVAGE

Diagnostic peritoneal lavage is indicated to diagnose intra-abdominal bleeding

- In shocked patients who are not proceeding straight to laparotomy
- In patients without shock when repeated clinical examination of the abdomen for 6 h is not possible because of sedation or anaesthesia

Caution is needed with pregnancy, previous abdominal surgery or massive pelvic injury. Isotonic saline 1 l (or 10 ml/kg) is instilled into the peritoneal cavity, after drainage of the stomach and bladder. The presence of more than 10 ml frank blood on catheter aspiration necessitates immediate laparotomy; otherwise a lavage fluid specimen should be examined for red and white cell counts and amylase concentration. A red cell count over 100 000 per mm^3, white cell count over 500 per mm^3, or an increased amylase concentration suggests bleeding or viscus injury, and laparotomy should be undertaken immediately. These absolute figures are debatable and lower values are accepted in penetrating trauma.[6,8] Peritoneal lavages inevitably result in some false-positive laparotomies. However, in severe trauma, morbidity of a non-therapeutic laparotomy (i.e. no definitive surgery) is small compared with the dire consequences of missing significant intra-abdominal injury.[9]

CT ABDOMEN

Abdominal CT is not indicated in shock, but can be useful in the stable patient. Improved availability of CT scanning, and technologic advances with reduced scanning times and better definition, is increasingly favouring CT abdomen over diagnostic peritoneal leavage (DPL) in stable patients, if it can be performed quickly and safely, with gastric and i.v. contrast, and interpreted by radio-logists experienced in trauma. Visualization of abdomi-nal and pelvic organs and haemorrhage is excellent,[10,11] but results can be misleading and disastrous with poor technique.[4]

ABDOMINAL ULTRASOUND

Technologic advances in ultrasound scanning, and the increasing availability of FAST scanning (Focussed Assessment by Sonography for Trauma) in emergency departments make this modality attractive in trauma, and it is becoming increasingly used. However:

- It is operator-dependent
- It may have an unacceptably high false negative rate
- There is a small but important false positive rate for intra-abdominal bleeding[12]
- It is unable to diagnose ruptured bowel.
- It is not good for bleeding in the pelvis

Its main usefulness is probably in the unstable patient when it is positive, to indicate the need for laparotomy without the necessity to proceed to DPL.[13] FAST scans performed by enthusiastic amateurs in emergency departments without a treatment algorithm can be misleading and therefore worse than useless.

FLUID RESUSCITATION

FLUIDS

Almost all patients who are hypotensive or noticeably vaso-constricted will need blood transfusion. However, as cross-matched blood is not immediately available, other fluids are used first. Uncross-matched group O Rh-negative blood is occasionally indicated in the exsanguinating patient, but in general transfusion of large quantities of blood is wasteful while bleeding is uncontrolled. The place of hypertonic fluids in trauma resuscitation is unresolved.

Isotonic saline or a balanced salt solution should be the first fluids infused. Shocked patients may need 2–3 l in the first few minutes. One litre bags or bottles and giving sets with in-line pumps should be used on all i.v. lines. If fluid resuscitation is likely to be extensive, warmed fluids and rapid infusion devices should be used. A colloid plasma expander can be the second fluid used. By 20–30 min cross-matched red cells should be available. Platelets and fresh frozen plasma are reserved for documented or suspected coagulopathy (i.e. dilutional coagulopathy from fluids deficient in haemostatic factors, and disseminated intravascular coagulopathy (DIC) from prolonged shock).

All resuscitation fluids have a high sodium concentration, similar to that of extracellular fluid. Glucose 5% and glucose–saline solutions are not effective resuscitation fluids. Few trauma patients actually require them in the first day.

LIMITED FLUID RESUSCITATION

In penetrating trauma, there is some evidence that extensive fluid resuscitation prior to haemostasis may be detrimental, presumably because of higher blood pressure, displacement of blood clot and dilution of coagulation factors.[14]

In blunt trauma, there is no such evidence. Furthermore, it is not appropriate to generalize the evidence from penetrating trauma to blunt trauma because these two types of trauma are quite different. In penetrating trauma, the bleeding is often from single arteries without extensive tissue injury, and complete haemostasis can often be easily achieved.

In contrast, in blunt trauma, the bleeding is often venous as well as arterial, with capillary oozing into the soft tissues which may continue for hours. It can often not be controlled, or can be only partly controlled, by operative surgery, interventional radiology or reduction and fixation of fractures. Accordingly, fluid resuscitation in the face of continuing blood loss is an important part of the treatment of circulatory shock in blunt trauma (see section on Inadequate Resuscitation). Nevertheless, fluid resuscitation is not an alternative to haemostasis and must not be used as an excuse for delaying haemostasis in blunt trauma.

Furthermore head injury is often present in blunt trauma, which frequently involves several body regions.

Hypotension is disastrous to an already injured brain, and must not be prolonged by deliberate under-resuscitation (see section on Head Trauma – Emergency Treatment).[15–17]

URINE OUTPUT

Hourly urine output is a useful guide to resuscitation from shock. Minimal acceptable urine output is 0.5 ml/kg per h, but 1–2 ml/kg per h is more adequate. Frusemide has no place in initial resuscitation. Apart from adequate resuscitation, diuresis can be due to ethanol, mannitol, dopamine, nephrogenic or neurogenic diabetes insipidus, or non-oliguric renal failure. Polyuria may mask early recognition of acute renal failure.

INADEQUATE RESUSCITATION

Patients in shock have depleted interstitial fluid as well as circulating blood volume, and need trauma resuscitation fluid volumes greater than the actual volume of blood lost. With blunt injury, volume losses often continue for 24–48 h. Prolonged shock from delayed and inadequate resuscitation leads to renal failure, acute respiratory distress syndrome (ARDS), sepsis, DIC and multiple organ dysfunction.[18,19]

PULMONARY OEDEMA

Pulmonary oedema during resuscitation may be related to fluid overload, direct lung trauma, aspiration of gastric contents, pulmonary responses to non-thoracic trauma and reactions to resuscitation fluids. They can all cause leaky capillaries and produce non-cardiogenic pulmonary oedema.

RADIOLOGY FOR TRAUMA PATIENTS

Patients with depressed consciousness, breathing difficulties or unstable circulation, should be X-rayed in the emergency department, and not sent to a radiology department remote from skilled resuscitation facilities. Conversely, extensive imaging examinations of shocked patients in the emergency department are unacceptable. Only three examinations should be requested in the emergency department.

CHEST

This is the only X-ray ever justified in an unresuscitated patient. A supine film is usually sufficient. An erect film is better for showing intrapleural air or fluid, ruptured diaphragm, free abdominal gas and for defining an abnormal mediastinum, but is often impractical in shock or suspected spinal injury. It can be done later if feasible.

An obvious pneumothorax does not require a chest X-ray before insertion of an intercostal drain.

LATERAL CERVICAL SPINE

This should be performed in all patients with head injury or multiple injuries, as cervical spine fractures are often missed. With head or facial injuries, a cervical fracture should be assumed initially and a cervical collar applied. A lateral cervical spine X-ray can be taken after the patient has been resuscitated. In the comatose patient, adequate examination requires anteroposterior and odontoid views, and possibly a CT scan.[4]

PELVIS

Unexplained blood loss can be due to a missed pelvic fracture. A dislocated hip can be missed in multiple injuries. Pelvic X-ray is not needed in awake patients with no pelvic abnormalities.

OTHER RADIOLOGICAL INVESTIGATIONS

Other X-rays should be performed after adequate resuscitation in the radiology department, operating room or intensive care unit (ICU):

- *Skull*: plain skull X-rays do not guide immediate treatment. A CT scan of the brain is a more useful urgent investigation.
- *Extremities*: X-rays of the extremities to assess bony injuries are not urgent unless there is vascular injury. Therefore, these films should not be taken in the emergency department for diagnosis, unless the patient is going directly to the operating room for fracture fixation.
- *Spine*: X-rays of thoracic or lumbosacral spine are seldom indicated in the emergency department.
- *Abdomen*: a plain abdominal X-ray is of limited value in the initial evaluation of trauma.
- *CT abdomen*: this can be valuable to evaluate a patient who is haemodynamically stable.
- *CT head*: this is vital in the treatment of severe head injuries.
- *Aortography*: if aortic rupture is suspected, aortography is currently the definitive diagnostic test although, when available, helical CT scanning of the thorax with contrast can be diagnostic and is less invasive. As the incidence of positive aortography is low (10–20%),[20] the priority given to this investigation depends on the other injuries which are present (see Ch. 68).
- *CT thorax*: this is of limited value in the trauma patient. Visualization of thoracic structures is excellent but it seldom discovers important undiagnosed injuries which affect patient treatment.[21] In general, it is only useful in the patient without thoracic cage injury where it may rule out mediastinal haematoma (and therefore, by implication, trauma to the great vessels). It cannot diagnose aortic injury unless helical CT scanning with contrast is used.

- *Urethrography and cystography* are used when urethral and bladder injury are suspected.
- *Interventional radiology*: percutaneous transcatheter embolization is therapeutic rather than diagnostic. It can provide life-saving haemostasis in massive retroperitoneal haemorrhage associated with pelvic fracture.[22] The logistics of managing such haemodynamically unstable patients in the radiology department are formidable.

THE EXSANGUINATING PATIENT

With exsanguination secondary to penetrating thoracic injury, there is a place for Emergency Room thoracotomy, but this approach has little place in blunt trauma.[23] The exsanguinating blunt trauma patient needs rapid intubation, volume resuscitation, bilateral intrapleural drains or thoracostomies, chest and pelvic X-ray, and a rapid trip to the operating room if it seems likely that the bleeding is in the thorax or abdomen.

HEAD TRAUMA (see Ch. 66)

Head injuries are common, but those requiring urgent cranial operations are less so. The head injury may initially be the most obvious in multiple injuries, but may not be the most important. Conversely, a severe head injury may seem unimportant initially. Head injury is a major determinant of outcome in critically injured patients.

EMERGENCY TREATMENT

Resuscitation measures, as in the Emergency assessment (primary survey) section above are undertaken. Victims with one or both dilated unreactive pupils, or a rapidly deteriorating level of consciousness not due to hypoxia or shock, should be given mannitol 1 g/kg i.v. to relieve brainstem compression, until definitive diagnosis and treatment can be arranged. Mannitol should be given only if the patient has been adequately volume resuscitated as it may add to hypovolaemia. There is currently much interest in hypertonic saline, particularly in head trauma, and concentrated salt may eventually turn out to be a better agent than mannitol in this setting because it does not produce hypovolaemia.[24,25]

Shocked trauma patients with or without head injuries require the same resuscitation fluids. Treatment of shock and maintenance of cerebral perfusion are vital, as hypotension is disastrous to an already damaged brain.[15–17] Contrary to common belief, sodium-containing fluids are not inherently dangerous in head trauma. However, after adequate resuscitation, further sodium administration is usually not indicated. Excessive (free) water is potentially dangerous, as it can lead to hypo-osmolar brain swelling.[26]

NEUROLOGICAL EVALUATION

Factors such as hypoxaemia, shock, alcohol, analgesics, anaesthetic agents, muscle relaxants and other drugs depress consciousness and confound neurological signs. Clinical neurological evaluation includes the Glasgow coma score (GCS),[27,28] and a search for lateralizing signs.

CT scanning is indicated in all patients who will not obey verbal commands, especially if they are rendered neurologically inaccessible by sedative and relaxant agents. Lateralizing motor or pupillary signs with a deteriorating level of consciousness are indications for immediate CT scanning (or, if unavailable, emergency burr holes). In an unstable patient, a laparotomy for intra-abdominal haemorrhage should take priority over a head CT scan.[29]

SEVERITY AND MORBIDITY OF TRAUMA

Severity of injury is measured by the abbreviated injury scale (AIS), updated several times over the years,[30–32] which divides the body into six regions – head and neck, face, thorax, abdomen, pelvis and extremities, and external. Specific injuries in each body region are coded on a scale of 1 (minor), 2 (moderate), 3 (serious, not life-threatening), 4 (severe, life-threatening, survival probable), 5 (critical, survival uncertain) and 6 (unsurvivable). The AIS was designed for motor vehicle injuries, but has been validated for blunt and penetrating trauma. It can provide a basis for research, education, audit and allocation of resources.

Severity of trauma is related not just to the severity of individual injuries, but also to the combined effects of multiple injuries. Multiple injuries are graded by the injury severity score (ISS), which is an empirical system based on the AIS grades for the three worst body regions.[33,34] ISS gives a score between 0 and 75 for total body injury; 16 or more indicates major trauma. Death with an ISS below 24 should be rare. Above an ISS of 25, there is a stepwise increase in mortality, with very high rates over 50.[35,36]

AIS and ISS study mostly the anatomy of injury. Other factors influence trauma mortality and morbidity, including age, pre-existing health, degree of physiological derangement, standard of pre-hospital and early hospital care and complications. Degree of physiological derangement can be measured by the revised trauma score,[37] which is computed from the coded values of GCS, systolic blood pressure and respiratory rate, usually at admission to the emergency department. The TRISS severity index is based on the revised trauma score, ISS, and patient age.[38] It correlates well with outcome, and has been used to compile survival norms for blunt and penetrating trauma.[35,36] Physiological scoring systems such as APACHE do not work well for trauma patients (see Ch. 2).[39,40] Preinjury illness (comorbidity) has a profound effect on trauma outcome.[41]

Shock influences trauma mortality and morbidity. The 'Golden Hour' is a catchy concept based on the observation that the longer the patient is in shock, the higher is the probability of an immediate or delayed complications. However, the specific time frame of an hour has no real validity. Complications of shock include renal failure, acute respiratory distress syndrome, sepsis, liver failure and multiorgan dysfunction.[18,19,42] Acute oliguric renal failure on the first day after trauma is now rare, but non-oliguric renal failure is often seen 2–4 days later, caused by the shock and delayed or inadequate resuscitation. It is often heralded by polyuria, which is misinterpreted as a sign of adequate resuscitation.

EPIDEMIOLOGY OF INJURIES

Only a minority of victims of severe trauma reach hospital alive.[1,43,44] Of trauma deaths, the time interval between injury and death has three peaks.[1] The majority of deaths are immediate (within minutes) at the scene of injury. Some deaths are early (within hours) in the emergency department or the operating room, while some are late (after days or weeks) and occur in the ICU or ward. Those in the ICU are mostly from severe head injury

Table 64.1 Percentage of ICU trauma patients with grades of injury in different body regions

	AIS ≥4	AIS = 3	AIS <2	AIS = 0
Head and neck	63	8	11	17
Face	2	11	9	78
Thorax	10	17	6	67
Abdomen	16	5	1	78
Extremities	1	34	10	55
External	0	<1	67	33

Data on 2877 adult trauma patients (excluding burns) in the DCCM, Auckland Hospital, 1988–2000. Abbreviated injury scale (AIS-80) codes[31]: 0 = no injury; 1 = minor; 2 = moderate; 3 = serious; not life-threatening; 4 = severe; life-threatening, survival probable; 5 = critical; survival uncertain; 6 = unsurvivable. In tertiary referral centres, these figures will vary with the mix of local and referred patients.[47]

within a few days and, less commonly, multiorgan dysfunction later.

Of trauma admissions to hospital, only a minority have severe or multiple trauma.[45] In order of frequency, life-threatening injuries involve the head, abdomen, and chest (Table 64.1), and are often multiple. The hospital services which this small number of severely injured patients use out of proportion to their numbers are major surgery, intensive care, radiography and CT scanning.[45] Major trauma outcome studies in the USA,[35] the UK[36] and Australia[46] offer valuable epidemiological data. The USA study found that the mortality of direct admissions is strongly related to serious head injury.

ORGANIZATION OF TRAUMA CARE

Many of the problems of trauma care are organizational. Problems faced by health authorities are the provision of advanced care at the scene of injury, rapid transportation to hospital, policies on which hospitals should receive trauma patients, systems for rapid evaluation and decision-making in hospitals, and rapid, safe patient transfer between hospitals. If survival from major trauma is to be maximized, prehospital and hospital care must be co-ordinated.

Regionalization of trauma care has become an accepted concept.[2,48] Trauma centres are designated hospitals which meet certain requirements. Main prerequisites are in-house experienced surgeons, anaesthetists and neurosurgeons, and a minimum number of patients seen annually for staff expertise. Regionalization involves the concept of ambulances bypassing non-designated hospitals.[2] Helicopters are used increasingly to speed patient transportation.[49] Trauma teams are teams of surgeons and intensivists or anaesthetists who immediately attend the trauma victim on arrival at hospital.[2–4,42,42]

Trauma registries and databases are important tools in organizing and improving trauma care. The UK major trauma outcome study[36] showed that the doctors in charge of resuscitation were often junior, delays in performing urgent operations were common, and the number of preventable deaths was significant. A hospital may not see enough trauma patients to justify a trauma team or supply adequate experience for its staff, and may not have all the facilities required by trauma patients. Transfer to a trauma hospital may be desirable, but geography and limited transport facilities may make such transfers hazardous.

In Western countries, trauma is a leading cause of death and disability under the age of 38 years.[35] Reduction of mortality and morbidity depends on public education, new legislations, on-site advanced care, rapid evacuation (see Ch. 3), hospital trauma expertise and co-ordination of services.[50,51]

REFERENCES

1 Trunkey DD. Trauma. *Sci Am* 1983; **249**: 20–7.

2 Trunkey DD. Overview of trauma. *Surg Clin North Am* 1982; **62**: 3–7.

3 Trunkey DD. Initial treatment of patients with extensive trauma. *N Engl J Med* 1991; **324**: 1159–263.

4 Enderson BL, Maull KI. Missed injuries: the trauma surgeon's nemesis. *Surg Clin North Am* 1991; **71**: 399–418.

5 Janjua KJ, Sugrue M, Deane SA. Prospective evaluation of early missed injuries and the role of tertiary trauma survey. *J Trauma* 1998; **44**: 1000–6.

6 Committee on Trauma, American College of Surgeons. *Advanced Trauma Life Support (ATLS) Program for Physicians*, 5th edn. Chicago: American College of Surgeons; 1993.

7 Soderstrom CA, Cowley RA. A national alcohol and trauma center survey: missed opportunities, failures of responsibility. *Arch Surg* 1987; **122**: 1067–71.

8 Day AC. Rankin N, Charlesworth P. Diagnostic peritoneal lavage: integration with clinical information to improve diagnostic performance. *J Trauma* 1992; **32**: 52–7.

9 Weigelt JA, Kingman RG. Complications of negative laparotomy for trauma. *Am J Surg* 1988; **156**: 544–7.

10 Trunkey DD, Federle MP. Computed tomography in perspective (editorial). *J Trauma* 1986; **26**: 660–1.

11 Padbani HR, Watson CJE, Clements L, *et al*. Computed tomography in abdominal trauma: an audit of usage and image quality. *Br J Radiol* 1992; **65**: 397–402.

12 Shackford SR, Rogers FB, Osler TM, *et al*. Focused abdominal sonogram for trauma: the learning curve of nonradiologist clinicians in detecting hemoperitoneum. *J Trauma* 1999; **46**: 553–64.

13 Branney SW, Moore EE, Cantrill SV, *et al*. Ultrasound based key clinical pathway reduces the use of hospital resources for the evaluation of blunt abdominal trauma. *J Trauma* 1997; **42**: 1086–90.

14 Bickell WH, Wall MJ, Pepe PE, *et al*. Immediate versus delayed fluid resuscitation for hypotensive patients with penetrating torso injuries. *N Engl J Med* 1994; **331**: 1105–9.

15 Chestnut RM, Marshall LF, Klauber MR, *et al*. The role of secondary brain injury in determining outcome from severe head injury. *J Trauma* 1993; **34**: 216–92.

16 Wilden JN. Rapid resuscitation in severe head injury. *Lancet* 1993; **342**: 1378.

17 Brain Trauma Foundation. Guidelines for the management of severe traumatic brain injury. http://www.braintrauma.org/

18 Cowley RA, Trump BF. Editors' summary: Organ dysfunction in shock. In: Cowley RA, Trump BF (eds). *Pathophysiology of Shock. Anoxia, and Ischaemia*. Baltimore, MD: Williams & Wilkins; 1982: pp. 281–4.

19 Faist E, Baue AE, Dittmer H, Heberer G. Multiple organ failure in polytrauma patients. *J Trauma* 1983; **23**: 775–87.

20 Lee RB, Stahlmann GC, Sharp KW. Treatment priorities in patients with traumatic rupture of the thoracic aorta. *Am Surg* 1992; **58**: 37–43.

21 Paul A, Blostein PA, Hodgman CG. Computed tomography of the chest in blunt thoracic trauma:

results of a prospective study. *J Trauma* 1997; **43**: 13–8.

22 Panetta T, Selafari SJA, Goldstein AS, *et al.* Percutaneous transcatheter embolisation for massive bleeding from pelvic fractures. *J Trauma* 1985; **26**: 1021–9.

23 Boyd M, Vanek VW, Bourguet CC. Emergency room resuscitative thoracotomy: when is it indicated? *J Trauma* 1992; **33**: 714–21.

24 Suarez JI, Qureshi AI, Bhardwaj A, *et al.* Treatment of refractory intracranial hypertension with 23.4% saline. *Crit Care Med* 1998; **26**: 1118–22.

25 Prough DS, Zornow MH. Mannitol: an old friend on the skids? *Crit Care Med* 1998; **26**: 997–8.

26 Fishman RA. Effects of isotonic intravenous solutions on normal and increased intracranial pressure. *Arch Neural Psychiatry* 1953; **70**: 350–60.

27 Teasdale G, Jennett B. Assessment of coma and impaired consciousness: a practical scale. *Lancet* 1974; **2**: 81–4.

28 Jennett B, Teasdale G. Aspects of coma after severe head injury. *Lancet* 1977; **1**: 878–81.

29 Thomason M, Messick J, Rutledge R, *et al.* Head CT scanning versus urgent exploration in the hypotensive blunt trauma patient. *J Trauma* 1993; **34**: 40–5.

30 American Medical Association committee on medical aspects of automotive safety. Rating the severity of tissue damage: I – the abbreviated scale. *JAMA* 1971; **215**: 277–80.

31 Committee on Injury Scaling. *The Abbreviated Injury Scale – 1980 Revision*. Morton Grove, IL: American Association for Automotive Medicine; 1980.

32 Committee on Injury Scaling. *The Abbreviated Injury Scale – 1995 Revision*. Des Plaines, IL: American Association for Automotive Medicine; 1995.

33 Baker SP, O'Neill B, Haddon W, Long WB. The injury severity score: a method for describing patients with multiple injuries and evaluating emergency care. *J Trauma* 1974; **14**: 187–96.

34 Baker SP, O'Neill B. The injury severity score: an update. *J Trauma* 1976; **16**: 882–5.

35 Champion HR, Copes WS, Sacco WJ, *et al.* The major trauma outcome study: establishing national norms for trauma care. *J Trauma* 1990; **30**: 1356–65.

36 Yates DW, Woodford M, Hollis S. Preliminary analysis of the care of injured patients in 33 British hospitals: first report of the United Kingdom major trauma outcome study. *BMJ* 1992; **305**: 737–40.

37 Champion HR, Sacco WJ, Copes WS, *et al.* A revision of the trauma score. *J Trauma* 1989; **29**: 623–9.

38 Boyd CR, Tolson MA, Copes WS. Evaluating trauma care: the TRISS method. *J Trauma* 1987; **27**: 370–8.

39 McAnena OJ, Moore FA, Moore EE, *et al.* Invalidation of the APACHE II scoring system for patients with acute trauma. *J Trauma* 1992; **33**: 504–7.

40 Roumen RMH, Redl H, Schlag G, *et al.* Scoring systems and blood lactate concentrations in relation to the development of adult respiratory distress syndrome and multiple organ failure in severely traumatized patients. *J Trauma* 1993; **35**: 349–55.

41 Sacco WJ, Copes WS, Bain LW, *et al.* Effect of pre-injury illness on trauma patient survival outcome. *J Trauma* 1993; **35**: 538–43.

42 Cowley RA, Dunham CM (eds). *Shock Trauma/Critical Care Manual*. Baltimore, MD: University Park Press; 1982.

43 Baker CC, Oppenheimer L, Stephens B, *et al.* Epidemiology of trauma deaths. *Am J Surg* 1980; **140**: 144–50.

44 Smeeton WMI, Judson JA, Synek BJ, *et al.* Deaths from trauma in Auckland: a one year study. *NZ Med J* 1987; **100**: 337–40.

45 Streat SJ, Donaldson ML, Judson JA. Trauma in Auckland: an overview. *NZ Med J* 1987; **100**: 441–4.

46 Cameron P, Dziukas L, Hadj A, *et al.* Major trauma in Australia: a regional analysis. *J Trauma* 1995; **39**: 545–52.

47 Gardiner JP, Judson JA, Smith GS, *et al.* A decade of ICU trauma admissions in Auckland, New Zealand. *NZ Med J* 2000; **113**: 326–7.

48 Eggold R. Trauma care regionalisation: a necessity. *J Trauma* 1983; **23**: 260–2.

49 Freeark RJ. The trauma center: its hospitals, head injuries, helicopters, and heroes (1982 AAST presidential address). *J Trauma* 1983; **23**: 173–8.

50 Judson JA. Trauma management: modern concepts (editorial). *NZ Med J* 1985; **98**: 8–9.

51 Trunkey DD. On the nature of things that go bang in the night. *Surgery* 1982; **92**: 123.

65

Severe head injury

J A Myburgh

Despite improvements in resuscitation and vital organ support, the management of patients with traumatic brain injury in the intensive care unit (ICU) presents a challenge to all members of the critical care team. As head injury is associated with a high mortality and morbidity, the benefits of intensive treatment and care may not become apparent until months or years later during rehabilitation after injury.

EPIDEMIOLOGY

Traumatic brain injury has been termed a 'silent global epidemic'.[1,2] It accounts for up to 30% of all trauma related deaths and is the leading cause of death in young males in developed countries. The impact of mechanization in developing countries has resulted in a sharp increase in the incidence and mortality from vehicular trauma.[3]

In addition to this distressingly high mortality, the cost of survivors in these societies in emotional, social and financial terms is substantial, as the effects of the original injury may persist for many years.

AETIOLOGY

Vehicular trauma, industrial accidents, falls and assaults account for the majority of head injury, with marked variations in patterns of injury across the world.[4] For example, in Australasia and Western Europe, the incidence of head injury caused by vehicular trauma is decreasing owing to the success of preventive strategies such as restraint devices, speed control and stricter drink–driving legislation. This trend is reversed in developing countries.[5]

In the United States and South Africa, the incidence of penetrating head injury due to firearm injuries is increasing with associated increased mortality.

DEMOGRAPHICS

The numbers of patients with traumatic brain injury presenting to hospitals vary widely in accordance with hospital admission policies and capabilities. Typical figures of all-cause head injury admissions in developed countries range from 200 to 300 per 100 000 patients.

Age and gender specific data typically show two peaks: one in the second and third decades, with a male to female ratio of 2:1; the latter in the seventh to nine decades, with a more equivalent gender ratio.

PATTERNS OF INJURY

Traumatic brain injury represents a range of injury from mild head injury that may fully recover to severe injury associated with high mortality or high levels of disability. Injury may be either blunt or penetrating, with the latter associated with a higher mortality.

Although the majority of head injuries (70–80%) are minor, a significant proportion of these patients may have poor functional outcomes due to secondary insults, missed injuries and comorbidities. Of the 20–30% who constitute moderate to severe head injury, approximately 10% of these are dead on admission, while the remainder will usually require admission to the ICU for management in the first 7–10 days.

PATHOPHYSIOLOGY

Brain injury is a heterogeneous pathophysiological process. It encompasses a spectrum of injury that includes the degree of brain damage at the time of injury (primary injury) in addition to insults that occur during the post-injury phase (secondary injury). These processes are depicted in Fig. 65.1.

Both primary and secondary injuries are associated with the development of intracranial inflammation and disruption to cerebrovascular autoregulation. An understanding of these processes is essential in order to quantify the severity of injury, direct appropriate management strategies and to interpret information from clinical monitoring systems.

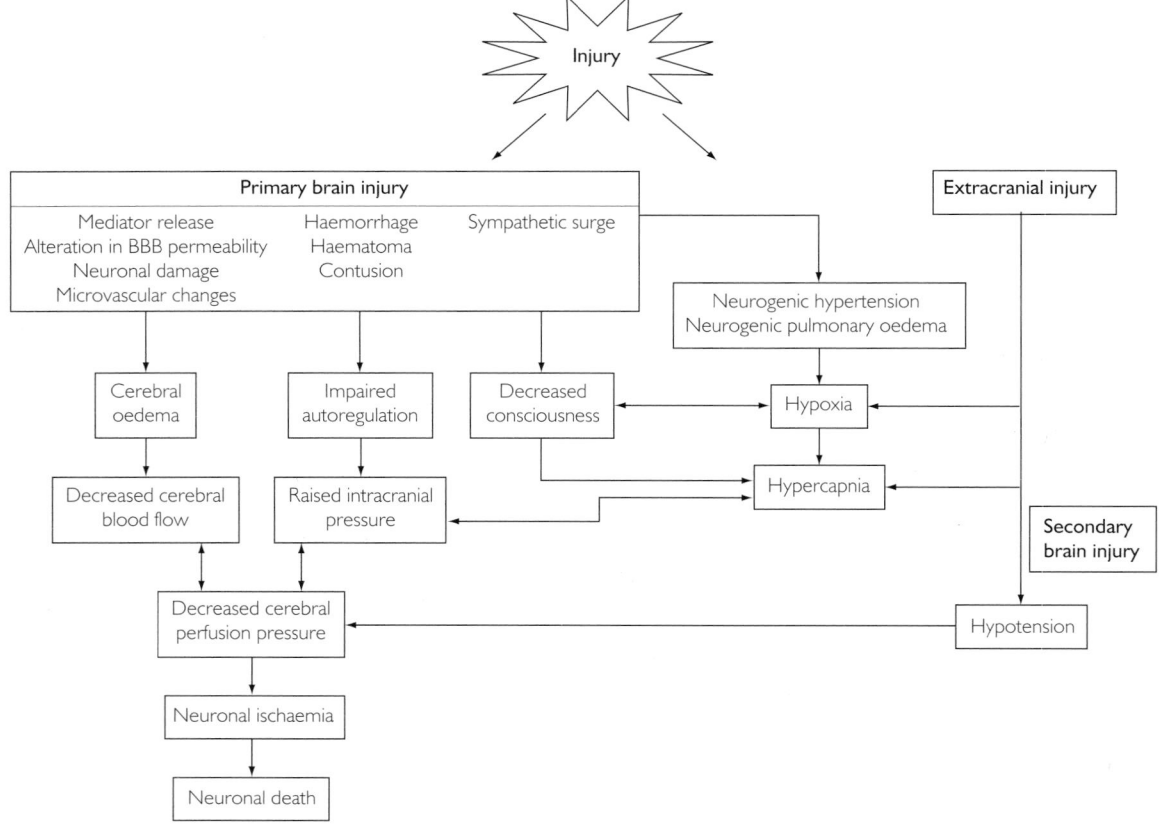

Fig. 65.1 Pathophysiology of traumatic brain injury.

PRIMARY BRAIN INJURY

The severity of primary injury is determined by the degree of neuronal damage or death at the time of impact. This is a major determinant of outcome from traumatic brain injury and, with the exception of surgically evacuable mass lesions, is usually irreversible.

Primary brain injuries include all types of injury to the brain parenchyma and vasculature. Primary injuries that are associated with adverse outcome include traumatic subarachnoid haemorrhage and non-evacuable mass lesions, particularly in critical parts of the brain such as the posterior fossa.

SECONDARY BRAIN INJURY

Secondary brain insults are characterized by a reduction in cerebral substrate utilization, particularly oxygen (Table 65.1). Of these insults, hypotension (defined as a systolic blood pressure of <90 mmHg; 12.0 kPa), hypoxia (oxygen saturation <90% or PaO_2 <50 mmHg; 6.7 kPa), hypoglycaemia, hyperpyrexia (temperature

Table 65.1 Secondary brain insults following traumatic brain injury that are associated with increased morbidity and mortality

Systemic	Intracranial
Hypoxia	Seizure
Hypotension	Delayed haematoma
Hypocapnia	Subarachnoid haemorrhage
Hypercapnia	Vasospasm
Hyperthermia	Hydrocephalus
Hypoglycaemia	Neuroinfection
Hyperglycaemia	
Hyponatraemia	
Hypernatraemia	
Hyperosmolality	
Infection	

>39°C) and prolonged hypocapnia ($PaCO_2$ <30 mmHg; 4.0 kPa) have been shown to independently worsen survival following traumatic brain injury.[6]

Secondary insults may occur during initial resuscitation, transport both between and within hospitals, surgery, and subsequently in the ICU.[7] Inadequate substrate delivery and utilization may initiate or propagate pathophysiologic processes, which may fatally damage neurones already rendered susceptible by the primary injury. Consequently, a vicious circle of secondary brain damage may develop with adverse outcomes.

INTRACRANIAL INFLAMMATION

As the brain is enclosed within the rigid skull and dura, small increases in intracranial volume result in sharp increases in intracranial pressure (Monro–Kelly doctrine). Consequently, the brain is a poorly compliant organ that has a limited capacity to accommodate pathological increases in intracranial pressure.

Traumatic brain injury invokes an intense inflammatory response characterized by the release of cytokines, free radicals, excitatory amino acids and other mediators.[8] The consequence of this response is disruption and alteration in the permeability of the blood–brain barrier, glial swelling and alterations in regional and global cerebral blood flow. The extent of this inflammatory process is an important determinant of intracranial pressure that may persist for some time following injury. Furthermore, alteration in blood–brain permeability may render the cerebral circulation susceptible to the effects of drugs that normally do not cross such as osmotic diuretics and catecholamines.

CEREBRAL BLOOD FLOW AND AUTOREGULATION

Normally, cerebral blood flow is maintained at a constant rate in the presence of changing perfusion pressures by myogenic and metabolic autoregulation. These homeostatic mechanisms, particularly myogenic autoregulation, are impaired following head injury due to neuronal damage and intracranial inflammation.[9-12] Distinct patterns of cerebral blood flow have been described following head injury that have direct clinical relevance with regard to management.[12] (See Fig. 65.2.)

THE HYPOPERFUSION PHASE

Cerebral blood flow is reduced by extrinsic and intrinsic mechanisms in the first 72 hours following injury, with resultant global and regional ischaemia.[12,13] Because myogenic autoregulation is markedly impaired during this period, cerebral blood flow in the hypoperfusion phase is directly dependent on systemic blood pressure. Resultant neuronal ischaemia may lead to 'cytotoxic' cerebral oedema and increased intracranial pressure.

In order to defend cerebral perfusion, systemic blood pressure must be assiduously maintained during this phase so that cerebral perfusion pressure (defined as the difference between mean arterial pressure and intracranial pressure) is maintained ≥70 mmHg (9.3 kPa).

THE HYPERAEMIC PHASE

Following the hypoperfusion phase, autoregulatory mechanisms may start to recover with improved cerebral blood flow. This hyperaemic phase may persist for up to 7–10 days post-injury and occurs in 25–30% patients.

During this phase, the combination of hyperaemia, intracranial inflammation and altered blood–brain permeability may result in 'vasogenic' cerebral oedema. In this context, medical therapies directed at maintaining

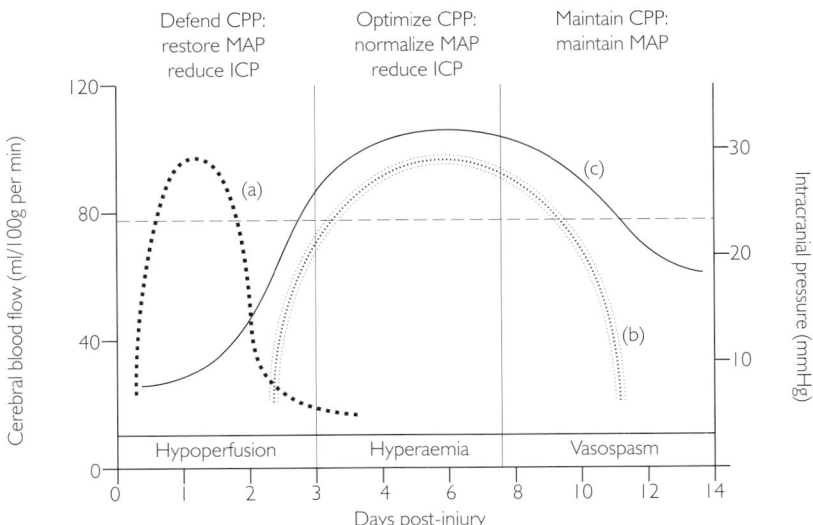

Fig. 65.2 Conceptual changes in cerebral blood flow and intra cranial pressure (ICP) over time following traumatic brain injury: (a) cytotoxic oedema; (b) vasogenic oedema; (c) cerebral blood flow. CPP = cerebral perfusion pressure; MAP = mean arterial pressure.

adequate cerebral perfusion pressure[14] may result in increased intracranial pressure.

As there is restoration or increased cerebral blood flow during this phase, a range of cerebral perfusion pressure is acceptable (50–70 mmHg; 6.7–9.3 kPa).[12]

THE VASOSPASTIC PHASE

In a small cohort of patients (10–15%), particularly those with severe primary and secondary injuries or those with significant traumatic subarachnoid haemorrhage, a vasospastic phase characterized by typical cerebral blood flow patterns may persist. This phase represents a complex of cerebral hypoperfusion due to arterial vasospasm, post-traumatic hypometabolism and impaired autoregulation.[12]

RESUSCITATION

INITIAL ASSESSMENT

The resuscitation of head injured patients should follow the principles outlined in the Advanced Trauma Life Support (ATLS®) guidelines for the early management of severe trauma.[15]

The initial emphasis is directed at assessing and controlling the airway, ensuring adequate oxygenation and ventilation, establishing adequate intravenous access and correcting haemodynamic inadequacy. Neurological assessment and brain specific treatment should only follow once cardiorespiratory stability has occurred. Given the direct association between hypotension and hypoxia in traumatic brain injury, this is an absolute priority.

With respect to the head injured patients, the following principles in the initial assessment apply.[16,17]

AIRWAY

All patients with severe head injury (traumatic coma), marked agitation or significant extracranial trauma require early oral endotracheal intubation. Depending on the skill of the operator and available facilities, this should be performed using a rapid sequence induction with cricoid pressure and in-line immobilization of the cervical spine.

All head injured patients should be assumed to have a potential cervical spine injury, and should be immobilized in a rigid collar until that possibility is definitively excluded.

BREATHING (=VENTILATION)

Patients should be ventilated in 100% oxygen using 5–7 ml/kg tidal volumes until blood gas analysis is available.

Oxygenation should be maintained at at least 100 mmHg (13.3 kPa) and the ventilator adjusted to achieve a normal arterial carbon dioxide tension (35–40 mmHg; 4.5–5.0 kPa).

Non-depolarizing muscle relaxants and narcotics such as fentanyl may facilitate ventilation in the immediate post-intubation period in combative patients.

Empirical hyperventilation during initial resuscitation is not indicated until adequate oxygenation, haemodynamic stability and urgent computerized tomography has been achieved.[18]

CIRCULATION (= CONTROL OF SHOCK)

Prompt restoration of circulating blood volume and restoration of a euvolaemic state is critical.[19,20] There is no evidence to recommend crystalloid or colloid volume resuscitation – either will suffice. Hypertonic saline may have a role as a small-volume, resuscitation fluid that is useful in expanding intravascular volume, with additional beneficial effects on cerebral blood flow and reduction of cerebral oedema.

Early arterial monitoring for accurate measurement of mean arterial pressure and central venous catheter placement for providing a guide to volume replacement and administration of blood and drugs is essential. The placement of these lines must not delay volume resuscitation.

Inotropes, such as epinephrine or norepinephrine, or vasopressors such as phenylephrine or metaraminol may be used to defend blood pressure once correction of hypovolaemia is underway or achieved.[22–24] This may be necessary if sedatives or narcotics are required.

The use of military anti-shock trousers (MAST suit) in traumatic brain injury is not recommended.[25]

DISABILITY (= NEUROLOGICAL ASSESSMENT)

Assessment of neurological function following injury is important to quantify the severity of neurotrauma and to provide prognostic information. The level of function may be influenced by associated injuries, hypoxia, hypotension and/or drug or alcohol intoxication. Similarly, the mechanism of injury is important, as high velocity injuries are associated with a greater degree of neuronal damage. It is important to review ambulance and emergency personnel and records in order to obtain the most accurate information.

Level of consciousness

The ATLS® recommends an initial assessment during initial resuscitation based on the response to stimulation: Awake, Verbal, Pain, Unresponsive (AVPU). This provides a rapid and practical grading of function with severe head injuries defined as those who respond to pain only, or who are unresponsive.

The Glasgow Coma Score (GCS) has an established place in the management of traumatic brain injury and is the most widely accepted and understood scale.[26] While originally described as a prognostic index, it provides an overall assessment of neurological function, derived from three parameters: eye opening, verbal response and motor response (Table 65.2).

Table 65.2 The Glasgow Coma Score.[25] The best response following non-surgical resuscitation is scored.

Best eyes open score		Best verbal response		Best motor response	
Spontaneously	4	Orientated, adequate	5	Obeys spoken command	6
On spoken command	3	Disorientated, confused	4	Localized pain	5
To pain	2	Inappropriate words	3	Flexion withdrawal	4
No response	1	Incomprehensible	2	Abnormal flexion	3
		No response	1	Extension	2
				No response	1
		Intubated patients:			
		Appears able to converse	5		
		Questionable ability to converse	3		
		Unresponsive	1		

The best responses in the GCS components should be recorded following cardiorespiratory resuscitation and prior to surgical intervention in order to provide prognostic information. In general, a GCS of 14–15 indicates a mild injury, 9–13 a moderate injury, and 3–8 is classified as severe. In the severely injured, such as intubated patients or those with ocular or facial trauma, the motor response is the most useful.

Pupillary responses

Pupil size and reactivity are important when consciousness is impaired. While not part of the GCS, pupillary function should always be assessed and recorded at the same time as the GCS, particularly prior to the administration of narcotics, sedatives or muscle relaxants.

In the absence of traumatic mydriasis, abnormalities of the pupil size and reactivity may indicate compression of the third cranial nerve, suggesting raised intracranial pressure or impending herniation, particularly when associated with lateralizing motor signs and depressed consciousness.

Papilloedema is uncommon in the acute phase of head injuries.

Motor function

In addition to the motor response of the GCS, decerebrate or decorticate posturing, hemiparesis or lateralizing signs, paraparesis and quadriparesis (given the high association with spinal injuries with traumatic brain injury) should be documented concurrently with the GCS and pupillary responses.

SECONDARY SURVEY

Once the initial assessment is complete and resuscitation underway, a thorough secondary survey adopting a 'top-to-toe' approach is mandatory. This is outlined in the ATLS® approach to the traumatized patient.

The principles outlined in the initial assessment form the basis for prioritizing interventions in the secondary survey in traumatic brain injury. Extracranial causes of hypoxia such as pulmonary contusion, haemo/

pneumothorax must be excluded and promptly treated. Haemorrhage – both externally from fractures or lacerations or internally such as major vascular disruption or visceral injuries – must be aggressively treated until circulatory stability is achieved. There is no place for 'permissive hypotension' in head injured patients, as has been advocated in selected cases of penetrating trauma.

Target mean arterial pressure should be estimated in the context of the patient's premorbid blood pressure. Higher pressures may be necessary in hypertensive or elderly patients. The early use of inotropes such as norepinephrine or epinephrine may be necessary to achieve this.

An approach of 'damage control surgery' is now advocated in head injured patients to minimize secondary insults. In the initial 24–48 hours following injury, only life or limb threatening injuries should be addressed, following which patients are transferred to the ICU for stabilization and monitoring. Thereafter, semi-urgent surgery such as fixation of closed fractures or delayed plastic repairs may be done.[27] Patients with severe head injury undergoing prolonged emergency surgery should ideally have intracranial pressure monitoring placed as soon as possible.

Routine X-rays of the chest, pelvis and cervical spine and baseline blood tests (including blood alcohol level in appropriate cases) are part of the secondary survey.

BRAIN SPECIFIC RESUSCITATION

The place of interventions and therapies specifically directed at reducing intracranial pressure has been extensively reviewed in evidence-based guidelines for the management of severe head injury. While there is little evidence for the role of therapies such as empirical hyperventilation and osmotherapy during resuscitation, they continue to be widely used in clinical practice.

HYPERVENTILATION

Ventilation induced reductions in $Pa\text{CO}_2$ result in marked reductions in cerebral blood flow and consequently in intracranial pressure. However, as cerebral blood flow may be reduced during the initial period following injury, further reductions in cerebral perfusion will result if hyperventilation is used during this phase (Fig. 65.2).

Hyperventilation is associated with reductions in cerebral oxygenation, particularly in areas of neuronal damage, potentially exacerbating cerebral hypoxia. The combination of induced cerebral oligaemia and hypoxia in the damaged brain therefore offsets the theoretical benefit of reducing intracranial pressure. Consequently, empirical hyperventilation is not indicated during initial resuscitation when cerebral blood flow is compromised.[28]

However, hyperventilation remains the most potent non-surgical clinical tool of reducing intracranial pressure. In the resuscitated head injured patient with unequivocal clinical signs of raised intracranial pressure or impending tentorial herniation (pupillary dilatation, lateralizing signs or a witnessed neurological deterioration), hyperventilation is an option. Reductions of $PaCO_2$ to levels ≤30 mmHg (4.0 kPa) may be therefore considered prior to urgent imaging or surgery for evacuation of a mass lesion.[18]

OSMOTHERAPY

Osmotically active agents, such as mannitol, are widely used in the treatment of traumatic brain injury. Theoretically, mannitol is administered to increase plasma osmolality in order to cause net efflux of fluid from areas of damaged, oedematous brain, with resultant reduction in intracranial pressure. An intact blood–brain barrier is necessary for this to occur. Following intravenous administration of mannitol, an immediate plasma expanding effect that reduces haematocrit and viscosity ensues, which temporarily increases cerebral blood flow. Subsequent reductions in intracranial pressure probably result from restoration in cerebral perfusion pressure and rheological changes in cerebral blood flow, rather than specific cerebral dehydration.[29]

Osmotherapy is associated with a number of potentially adverse effects. Mannitol exerts an osmotic effect over a narrow range of plasma osmolality (290–330 mosmol/l), above which theoretically beneficial effects may be negated. Mannitol will induce an osmolal gap between measured and calculated osmolality, so that regular measurements of serum osmolality are necessary to monitor the amount administered. This gap may be further increased by alcohol, which is frequently present in the acute period. Mannitol will enter the brain where the blood–brain barrier is damaged, thereby potentially increasing cerebral oedema by increasing brain osmolality. Mannitol is a potent osmotic diuretic that may compromise haemodynamic stability by inducing an inappropriate diuresis in a hypovolaemic patient. Consequently, systemic hypotension may ensue, which may cause further cerebral ischaemia or subsequent organ dysfunction such as acute renal failure. This effect may be exacerbated by the concomitant administration of catecholamines in order to defend systemic blood pressure.

Given the high risk with minimal benefit during resuscitation, the routine use of mannitol is not recommended in the absence of raised intracranial pressure and in patients where cerebral blood flow is compromised.[30]

Similarly to hyperventilation, mannitol is considered as an option only in resuscitated patients with unequivocal signs of raised intracranial pressure prior to imaging or evacuation of a mass lesion. Although doses are frequently quoted as 0.25–1.0 g/kg, lower doses are equally as effective as higher doses in terms of improving cerebral perfusion and are associated with a lower incidence of side-effects.[31]

Hypertonic saline (3% solution) exerts similar osmotic plasma expanding effects to mannitol. These solutions do not exert an osmolal gap, so that serum sodium reflects serum osmolality, allowing easier titration. These solutions have been advocated as 'small volume resuscitation fluids' that may be very effective in restoring systemic and cerebral perfusion in the acute phase following injury. In addition to reducing intracranial pressure, these solutions would appear to be superior to mannitol for resuscitation.[21,32]

EMERGENCY SURGICAL DECOMPRESSSION ('BURR HOLES')

The advent of better equipped in-field resuscitation, medical retrieval, imaging and innovations such as tele-radiology and telemedicine has largely superseded the need to perform urgent burr hole surgery in head injured patients. In most instances, patients are resuscitated, stabilized and imaged with computerized tomography (CT) scanning prior to any surgical intervention. This may involve transfer to a specialized trauma centre. CT scanning provides accurate information and directs the surgeon to a mass lesion that needs evacuation under optimal circumstances.

In remote communities without immediate access to CT scanning, surgical evacuation may be life-saving in patients with a clear history of an expanding mass lesion such as an extradural or subdural haematoma. These include patients with low velocity injuries to the temporal region and an associated skull fracture that have clinical signs of intracranial herniation or a witnessed deterioration.

IMAGING

X-RAYS

All head injured patients receive the routine 'trauma series' of X-rays; namely, chest, pelvis and cervical spine (lateral, antero-posterior and peg views). These should be reviewed by a radiologist and areas of concern, particularly in the upper and lower regions of the cervical spine, should be clarified with further investigations such as CT scan.

Skull X-rays have essentially been superseded by CT scanning and their routine use in the emergency evaluation of head-injured patients has been questioned.

CT SCAN

CT scanning is the most informative radiological technique in the evaluation of the acute head injury and is now standard after head injury in virtually all patients. CT scanning invariably requires moving the patient to a radiological suite. This must only be done once initial assessment and resuscitation are complete and the patient is stable enough to be transported by appropriately trained and equipped personnel.

The following patients should undergo CT head scan following traumatic brain injury:

- All patients with a history of loss of consciousness or traumatic coma.
- Combative patients where clinical assessment is masked by associated alcohol, drugs, or extracranial injuries. These patients may require endotracheal intubation, sedation and ventilation to facilitate completion of CT scanning.

Technological advances in imaging now enable quick, high resolution digital images of the brain parenchyma and bony compartments. The most important role of CT scanning is prompt detection of mass lesion such as extradural or subdural haematomas. Thereafter, the degree of brain injury may be quantified by radiological criteria (Table 65.3; Plates 65.4a and 65.4b).[33,34] These criteria are important for:

1 providing an index of injury severity
2 providing criteria for intracranial pressure monitoring

Table 65.3 Classification of CT scan appearance following traumatic brain injury.[32] Examples are shown in Fig. 65.3a

Category	Definition
Diffuse injury (DI) I	No visible intracranial pathology seen on CT scan
DI II (diffuse injury)	Cisterns are present with midline shift 0–5 mm and/or Lesion densities present No high or mixed density >25 mm May include bony fragments and foreign bodies
DI III (swelling)	Cisterns are compressed or absent with midline shift 0–5 mm NO high or mixed density >25 mm
DI IV (shift)	Midline shift >5 mm NO high or mixed density >25 mm
Evacuated mass lesion	Any lesion surgically evacuated
Non-evacuated mass lesion	High or mixed density lesion >25 mm, not surgically evacuated

3 comparing the progression of injuries with subsequent scans
4 providing an index for prognosis.

These criteria should be recorded following each CT scan, particularly when patients are transferred to secondary or tertiary centres. Examples of typical injuries appear in Plates 65.4a and 65.4b.

The presence of traumatic subarachnoid haemorrhage should be recorded. This is an important index of severity of injury and is relevant for prognostication.[35]

CEREBRAL ANGIOGRAPHY

Cerebral angiography should be considered when a vascular injury such as carotid artery dissection is suspected in head injured patients. This may be indicated by a large isodense lesion on CT scan or when the patient's clinical condition is not consistent with the CT findings, for example, a dense hemiparesis in the absence of a mass lesion.

In the absence of a CT scanner, cerebral angiography may be used in the diagnosis of intracranial haematoma, although this is now rare.

MAGNETIC RESONANCE IMAGING

Magnetic resonance imaging (MRI) provides accurate detail of parenchymal damage, specifically small collections and non-haemorrhagic contusions. However, the information provided is not significantly better than that obtained from CT scanning to warrant routine use of MRI in the acute phase of injury. In addition, the placement and monitoring of an acute traumatized patient in an MRI scanner poses an additional risk that does not justify its use in this situation.

MRI may have an important role in prognostication at a later stage in management, particularly in mild and moderate head injury.

INTER-HOSPITAL TRANSFER

All severely head injured patients should be managed in a specialized neurotrauma centre in close collaboration with intensivists and neurosurgeons.[36] This may involve intra- or inter-hospital transportation. This is a potentially hazardous exercise that may adversely affect outcome by causing secondary insults. Consequently, appropriately skilled and equipped personnel should only do this once resuscitation, stabilization and initial imaging is completed.

A full primary and secondary survey and review of all documentation and investigation is required following transfer to a secondary or tertiary centre.

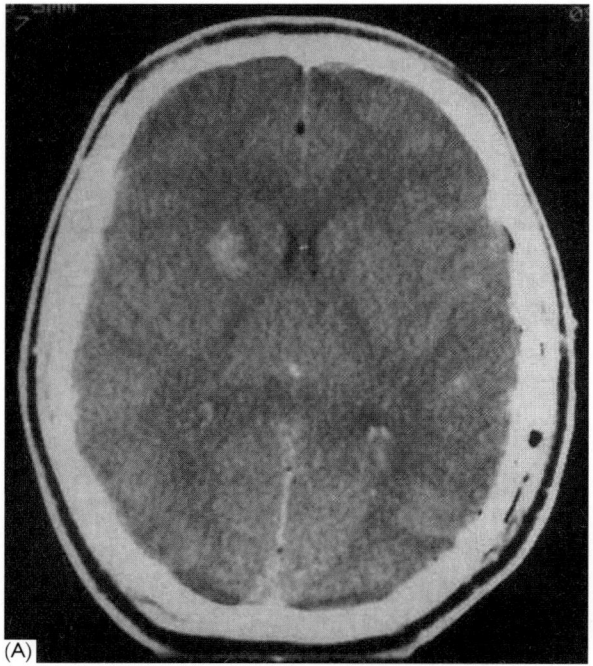

(A)

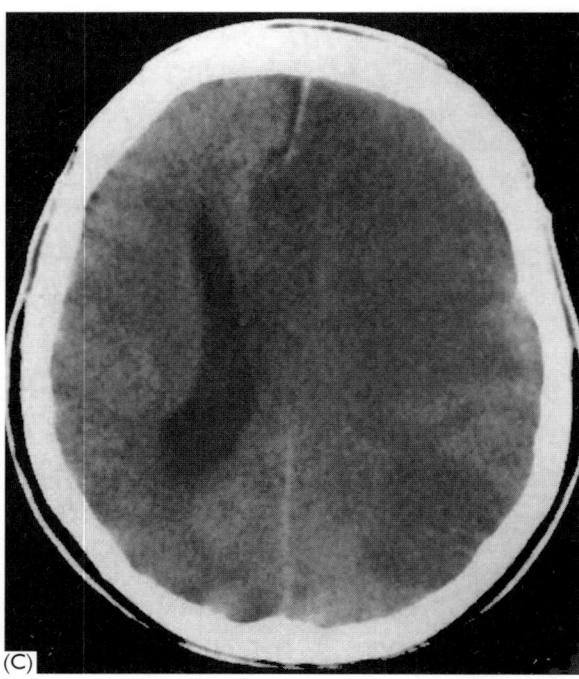

(C)

Plate 65.4a Computerized tomographic classification of Diffuse Axonal Injury (Table 65.3).[32] Panel (A) Diffuse injury II; (B) Diffuse injury III; (C) Diffuse injury IV.

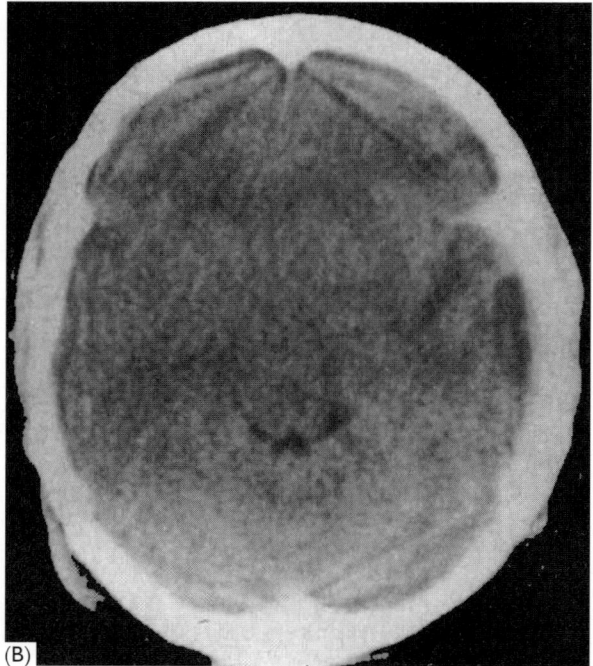

(B)

countries have demonstrated wide differences in practices with regard to monitoring, management strategies and ethical philosophies.[37–40] Most practices are determined by local preferences and experience, case-mix and resources.

The Brain Trauma Foundation of the American Association of Neurological Surgeons[41] and the European Brain Injury Consortium[42] have published evidence-based management guidelines for the management of severe brain injury. These publications provide very few standards by which to direct therapy, and the majority of issues addressed are presented either as management guidelines or options.[43]

Although management of head injury in the ICU will be considered in two sections – supportive therapy and brain specific therapy – these occur simultaneously. The principles of management focus on the integration of all monitoring information in the context of the underlying injury, so that secondary brain injury is prevented.

INTENSIVE CARE MANAGEMENT

There is no standard or uniform method of managing traumatic brain injury in the ICU. Surveys in several

SUPPORTIVE THERAPY

Following initial resuscitation, good intensive care management forms the basis of head injury management and is regarded as a continuum of care. This takes priority

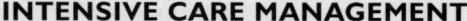

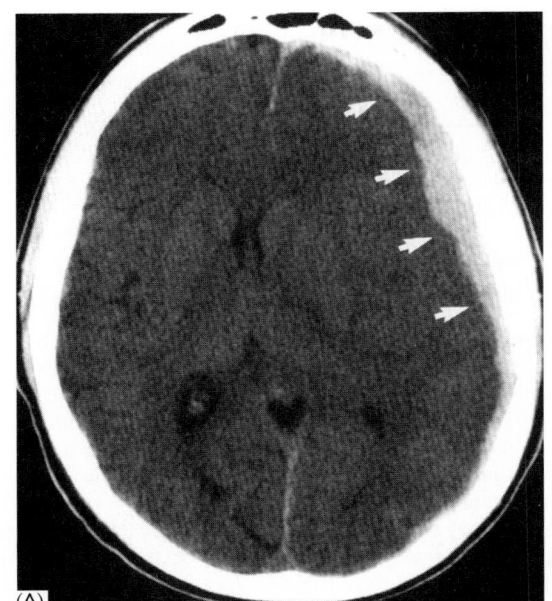

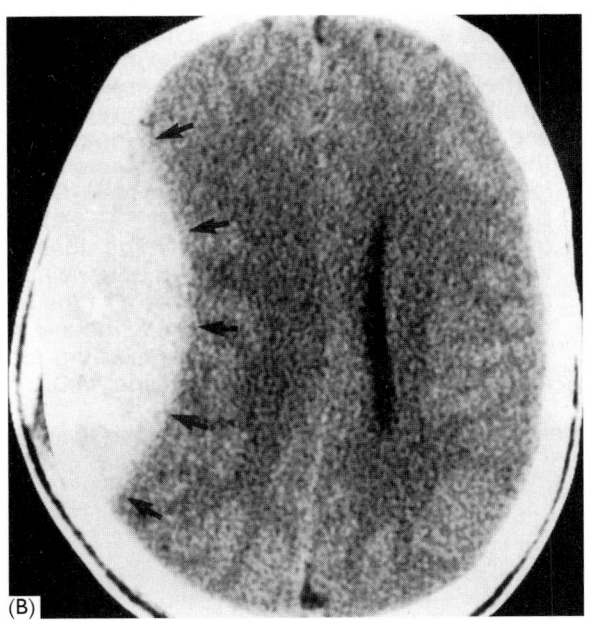

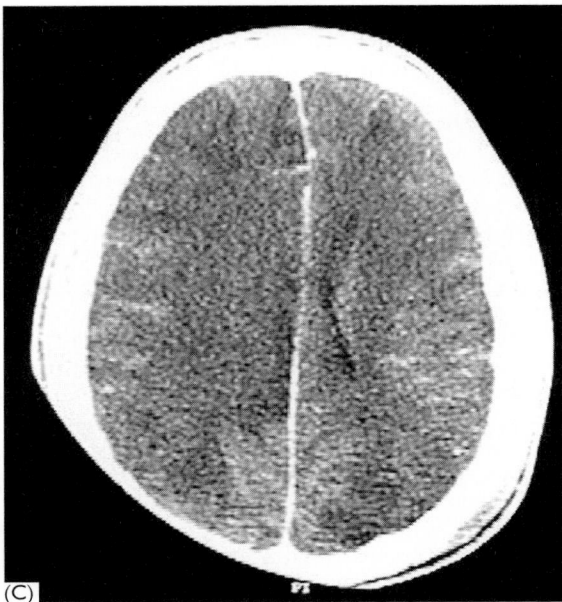

Plate 65.4b Intracranial haemorrhages. Panel (A) acute subdural haematoma; (B) acute extradural haematoma; (C) acute traumatic subarachnoid haemorrhage.

over brain specific therapies, which, to date, remain inconclusive in their efficacy.

HAEMODYNAMIC MANAGEMENT
Monitoring

Accurate measurement of systemic blood is essential and should be measured via an arterial catheter referenced to the aortic root. A large artery such as the femoral artery should be considered in haemodynamically unstable patients, as radial or dorsalis pedis arterial catheters may underestimate true systemic pressure in shocked patients. Given the importance of maintaining adequate systemic pressures, non-invasive measurement of blood pressure is not recommended during the acute phase of monitoring.[19]

Therapy should be titrated to mean arterial pressure in accordance with the patient's premorbid blood pressure; that is, in older patients, higher mean arterial pressure (e.g. 80 mmHg; 10.6 kPa) may be necessary.

Volume status should be assessed using central venous pressure monitoring, and hourly urine output.

Pulmonary artery catheterization for the measurement of cardiac output and pulmonary artery pressures is rarely indicated in head injured patients, unless there is associated cardiac dysfunction.

Fluid management

The attainment of a euvolaemic state is essential throughout intensive care management. This is determined by standard measurements such as serum sodium and osmolality, urea and creatinine, pulse rate, right atrial and mean arterial pressure and urine output.

Resuscitative fluids depend on local preferences, as there is no evidence to recommend crystalloids over colloids.

Optimal rheology for the cerebral circulation requires a haematocrit of approximately 30%: patients should be transfused if actively bleeding or to maintain a haemoglobin between 8.5 and 10 g/l.

Maintenance fluids should be directed at maintaining a normal osmolality. As a general principle, glucose-containing solutions are not recommended; however, these may be required (i.e. as 5% dextrose in water) if patients become hyperosmolar (>320 mosmol/l).

Inotropic therapy

Inotropes such as epinephrine, norepinephrine, or dopamine are frequently used to augment mean arterial pressure to attain an adequate cerebral perfusion pressure. These should only be commenced once volume resuscitation is actively underway or complete. The early use of inotropes is increasingly advocated during resuscitation as an important strategy during the hypoperfusion phase.[22,44]

There are no conclusive trials to recommend one inotrope over another or combination of inotropes. Epinephrine, norepinephrine and dopamine are equally effective in augmenting cerebral perfusion pressure. The degree to which these agents directly effect the cerebral circulation following head injury is unknown, although there is some evidence suggesting that dopamine has a direct effect.[45]

Epinephrine is widely used as an initial intropic agent in doses titrated to achieve a desired mean or cerebral perfusion pressure. While effective, it may be associated with metabolic side-effects such as hyperlactataemia and hyperglycaemia, which may complicate metabolic management. For this reason, norepinephrine is currently regarded by many as the initial agent of choice.[24]

Other agents that have a predominantly vasoconstrictor action such as phenylephrine or metaraminol have been advocated.[23]

Doses may range widely and high doses may be required to attain a desired cerebral perfusion pressure, particularly if cerebral perfusion pressures are targeted for >72 hours. It is important to prescribe inotropes in the context of the underlying injury. Lower cerebral perfusion pressure targets (i.e. 50–70 mmHg; 6.7–9.3 kPa), and therefore lower doses of inotropes, may be necessary if patients develop cerebral hyperaemia. Titration of inotropes may require an index of cerebral blood flow, such as jugular venous saturation monitoring, during this phase (see below).

Neurogenic hypertension

Neurogenic hypertension is common in the latter phases following injury (>5 days) and is usually centrally mediated. It may be associated with ECG changes and/or supraventricular arrhythmias. It is usually self-limiting and correlates with the severity of injury. Treatment depends on the severity of the problem: β-blockers or centrally acting agents such as clonidine are usually effective; vasodilators are relatively contraindicated.

RESPIRATORY THERAPY
Monitoring

Continuous measurement of arterial oxygen saturation is essential.

Continuous measurement of end-tidal carbon dioxide is frequently performed, although the reliability is questionable and should be checked with intermittent arterial blood gases.

Monitoring of ventilatory parameters should be consistent with standard approaches and includes measurement of tidal volumes, respiratory rates, inspiratory and expiratory airway pressures.

Ventilation

The majority of patients with severe head injury will require mechanical ventilation to ensure adequate oxygenation and to maintain an arterial carbon dioxide tension between 36 and 40 mmHg (4.8 and 5.3 kPa).

Strategies such as permissive hypercapnia, that are advocated for selected patients with acute lung injury or acute respiratory distress syndrome, do not have a role in head injured patients owing to the requirement to maintain normocapnia.

Positive end-expired pressure (PEEP) is recommended at low levels (5–10 cmH_2O; 0.49–0.98 kPa) to maintain functional residual capacity and oxygenation. Higher levels may compromise blood pressure, particularly in hypovolaemic patients, and should be used with caution. High levels of PEEP (>15 cmH_2O; 1.47 kPa) may compromise cerebral venous return and increase intracranial pressure, although this is uncommon.[46]

Weaning from ventilation should commence once intracranial pathology has stabilized – resolution of cerebral oedema on CT scan, control of intracranial hypertension and adequate cerebral perfusion pressures.

Trials of extubation should be carefully considered, so that subsequent hypoxic episodes do not occur, as these are potent secondary insults.

Patients with slow recovery of adequate consciousness should be considered for early tracheostomy, either percutaneously or surgically.

Neurogenic pulmonary oedema

This is a dramatic clinical syndrome that occurs in most patients with severe head injury and correlates with severity of injury. The underlying pathophysiological process is complex, but is primarily related to centrally mediated sympathetic nervous system overactivity. It is characterized by sudden onset of clinical pulmonary oedema, hypoxia, low filling pressures, poor lung compliance and bilateral lung infiltrates usually within 2–8 hours after injury.[47,48]

The process is usually self-limiting and treatment is primarily supportive, aiming at ensuring adequate oxygenation and ventilation. This usually requires endotracheal intubation and mechanical ventilation with the administration of PEEP. Ablation of sympathetic overactivity is effectively done with adequate sedation; β-blockade is usually unnecessary. Diuretics are effective but must be titrated against the volume status of the patient so that cerebral perfusion pressure is not compromised.[49]

The development of pulmonary oedema in patients with cardiac disease should be regarded as cardiogenic until proven otherwise.

Nosocomial pneumonia

Head injured patients who require prolonged ventilation are at increased risk of nosocomial pneumonia. This is associated with secondary brain injury and an increased mortality.[50] Risk factors include barbiturate and hypothermia therapy.

SEDATION, ANALGESIA AND MUSCLE RELAXANTS

There are no standards for sedation and analgesia in head injured patients – protocols will depend on local preferences and resources. The level of sedation and analgesia required for head injured patients depends on the degree of traumatic coma, haemodynamic stability, intracranial pressure and systemic effects of the head injury itself.

During the resuscitation phase, where cerebral hypoperfusion is common, sedation should be titrated to cause the least effect on systemic blood pressure. During this period, short acting narcotics such as fentanyl are useful, particularly if patients have associated extracranial injuries. These agents are relatively cardiostable and have the additional benefit of tempering systemic sympathetic surges that frequently occur after injury. As narcotics affect pupillary responses, these must be documented before administration, and CT scan should be performed soon afterwards to define baseline intracranial pathology. Short-term muscle relaxants such as vecuronium, are useful during this phase to control combative patients following intubation, ventilation and sedation.

During the intensive care phase, the requirements for sedation are different. Sedation should be titrated to have the patient sedated as lightly as possible to allow clinical assessment of neurological function and to facilitate mechanical ventilation. The level of sedation will depend on haemodynamic stability and the degree of intracranial pressure. Infusions of narcotic and benzodiazepines (e.g. morphine and midazolam) are useful in providing moderate to deep levels of sedation and are effective in controlling surges of intracranial pressure. However, these agents may accumulate resulting in a delay in return of consciousness or if used for prolonged periods, may be associated with an emergence delirium state.[51]

The use of propofol as a sole sedating agent has become popular.[52] It provides deep levels of sedation, which are effective in controlling systemic sympathetic swings and rises in intracranial pressure. It is rapidly reversible on cessation allowing prompt assessment of neurological status and does not accumulate. In addition, pupillary responses are not directly affected. Propofol should be used with caution in haemodynamically unstable patients, as it is a potent negative inotrope. The prolonged use of propofol is associated with tachyphylaxis and significant caloric loading from the lipid vector. Concerns have been raised about myocardial depression and sudden cardiac death, particularly if large doses are administered.[53]

The routine use of muscle relaxants is not recommended either to facilitate sedation or to control raised intracranial pressure. The prolonged use of these agents is associated with adverse outcome in traumatic brain injury.[54] Prolonged use of non-depolarizing muscle relaxants is associated with polyneuromyopathies.

BODY POSITION

Patients should be nursed at 30–45° head elevation to facilitate ventilation, improve oxygenation, and reduce the risk of aspiration. The head should be kept in a neutral position.[55]

PHYSIOTHERAPY

Physiotherapy has an important role to play in the removal of lung secretions, prevention of contractures and venous thrombosis. Patients with raised intracranial pressure may require boluses of sedation before chest physiotherapy to prevent acute rises in intracranial pressure.

METABOLIC MANAGEMENT

Routine measurement of biochemistry is essential with the aim of keeping all parameters within normal limits. The syndrome of inappropriate antidiuretic hormone secretion (SIADH) and diabetes insipidus may occur following head injury.

Hyperglycaemia is common following severe head injury and is usually centrally mediated and transient. Blood sugar levels should be maintained within normal limits with insulin infusions. Hypoglycaemia is a recognized secondary insult and must be avoided.

Core temperature should be routinely monitored, as hyperthermia has been identified as a cause of secondary injury. However, the real incidence of hyperpyrexic secondary brain damage may be underestimated, as a temperature gradient of 1–2°C between core and brain temperature has been demonstrated, and efforts should be directed at maintaining core temperature at 37.5°C.[56]

NUTRITION

The caloric needs of head injured patients must be addressed as soon as possible following resuscitation. Early enteral feeding is recommended.[57,58]

Placement of a nasogastric and/or enteral feeding tubes in head injured patients is usually via the oral route until an anterior cranial fossa (fractured cribriform plate) is excluded. Thereafter, postpyloric tubes, either via the oral, nasal or percutaneous routes are recommended, as gastroparesis is common following head injury.

STRESS ULCER PROPHYLAXIS

The incidence of gastric erosions and 'stress ulceration' has markedly decreased with better resuscitation and early enteral feeding. Head injured patients are at no more risk than other critically ill patients for developing stress ulceration. H_2-antagonists, such as ranitidine, should be used in ventilated patients until enteral feeding is established, after which they may be ceased.

Patients with a previous history of peptic ulceration should remain on antacid therapy for the duration of their ICU stay.

THROMBOPROPHYLAXIS

Head injured patients, particularly those requiring prolonged ventilation and sedation, or with extracranial injuries, are at increased risk for developing thromboembolism. The use of anticoagulants such as fractionated or low-molecular-weight heparins is contraindicated in patients with intracranial haemorrhage. Consequently, the role of thromboprophylaxis in head injury is difficult and there are no standards for their use.[59] As a general rule, anticoagulants should not be used in head injured patients with any evidence of destructive intracranial pathology or haemorrhage, until there is resolution of these processes on CT scan.

Non-pharmacological methods of thromboprophylaxis such as elastic stockings or pneumatic calf compressors are unproven, but provide a reasonable alternative.[60] Frequent surveillance using Doppler ultrasound of the iliofemoral veins in high risk patients, such as those with pelvic fractures, should be performed.

Patients who develop deep vein thromboses and cannot be given anticoagulation treatment should be considered for inferior vena caval filters.[61] The use of anticoagulants in a head injured patient with proven pulmonary embolism will depend on the relative risk to the patient's life.

ANTIBIOTICS

These should be used sparingly and in accordance with accepted microbiological principles. Prophylactic antibiotics should only be prescribed to cover insertion of intracranial pressure monitors and not recommended for basal skull fractures.[62] Frequent cultures of leaking or draining cerebrospinal fluid should be taken and infection treated specifically.

BRAIN SPECIFIC MONITORING

The most accurate assessment of brain function following traumatic brain injury is a full clinical neurological examination in the absence of drugs or sedatives. However, this is invariably not possible for the majority of head injured patients managed in the ICU.

Ideally, neuromonitoring should provide accurate and integrated information about intracranial pressure/volume relationships (elastance), patterns and adequacy of cerebral perfusion and an assessment of cerebral function. No such monitor exists, although each of these parameters may be monitored in various ways with variable levels of accuracy and clinical utility.

CLINICAL ASSESSMENT

Regular assessments of GCS, pupillary signs and motor responses should be made and recorded on the ICU flow chart. Concomitant sedation may influence the level of consciousness and this should be recorded. Initially, these assessments are recorded hourly, but this may change as patients become more stable.

A witnessed deterioration in GCS, especially the motor response, or the development of new lateralizing signs should be regarded as life-threatening intracranial hypertension or tentorial herniation until proven otherwise.

INTRACRANIAL ELASTANCE
Intracranial pressure monitoring

The recognition that raised intracranial pressure is associated with adverse outcome led to the measurement of this parameter in order to quantify the degree of injury and to assess the response to treatments directed at reducing intracranial pressure.[63]

The Brain Trauma Foundation guidelines recommend intracranial pressure monitoring in patients with traumatic coma (severe head injury: GCS ≤ 8 following non-surgical resuscitation) with either[64]:

- Abnormal CT scan:
  - Diffuse injury II–IV (Table 65.3) or
  - High or mixed density lesions >25 mm.
- Normal CT scan with two or more of the following features:
  - age >40 years
  - unilateral or bilateral motor posturing
  - significant extracranial trauma with systolic hypotension (<90 mmHg; 12.0 kPa)

Coagulopathy is a contraindication to intracranial pressure monitoring

Measurement of intracranial pressure[65] with an intraventricular catheter is the most accurate and clinically useful method. It has the advantages of zero calibration, cerebrospinal fluid drainage for raised intracranial pressure and allows dynamic testing of pressure volume relationships. Disadvantages include technical difficulty with insertion, particularly in patients with cerebral oedema and compression of the lateral ventricles and an increased incidence of infection.

Solid state systems such as fibreoptic (e.g. Camino®) or strain-gauge tipped catheters (e.g. Codman®) may be placed intraparenchymally or intraventricularly. These systems transduce intracranial pressure to provide high fidelity waveforms. They are small calibre, requiring a small craniotomy (burr hole) for insertion, but may be inserted at the bedside. Disadvantages include inability to perform zero calibration after insertion and baseline drift that may be clinically significant after 5 days.[66]

Fluid-filled, subdural catheters have been used for many years. However, these are no longer recommended due to the development of more accurate solid state systems. Subdural pressures do not accurately reflect global intracranial pressure, particularly in the presence of a craniectomy. Pressure readings may also be affected by local clot formation within the catheter.

Measurements are used to calculate cerebral perfusion pressure: mean arterial pressure minus intracranial pressure. For this calculation, both measurements should be referenced to the external auditory meatus (equivalent to the circle of Willis).

Intracranial pressure monitoring should be continued until the patient can be assessed clinically, intracranial pressure has stabilized to <25 cmH$_2$O 2.45 kPa and cerebral oedema has resolved on CT scan. This occurs in the majority of patients within 7 days. Patients with refractory intracranial hypertension may require monitoring for longer periods, although this may be complicated by drift (with solid state systems), infection (with intraventricular catheters) or occlusion (subdural catheters). In this situation, intracranial pressure monitors may need to be replaced or removed and patients assessed by serial CT scan or clinically.

Pressure/volume relationships

Determination of the change in intracranial pressure following a small increment in intracranial volume may provide information about the degree of elastance of the injured brain within the cranial vault.

The pressure volume index (PVI) is defined as the response in intracranial pressure after the injection of ml of fluid into an intraventricular catheter over 1 second. A change of >3 mmHg/ml (0.4 kPa/ml) is regarded as an index of reduced intracranial elastance, which may provide a criterion for surgical decompression in patients with progressive intracranial hypertension.

The PVI test has not assumed widespread use due to the risk of repeated intraventricular injection and associated risk of infection. Secondary waves of raised intracranial pressure may follow from a PVI test.[67]

CEREBRAL BLOOD FLOW

Currently, there is no method of routinely measuring cerebral blood flow at the bedside. Technological advances such as mapping with labelled xenon under CT, laser Doppler flowmetry[68] and thermal diffusion flow measurement provide useful imaging of regional and cerebral blood flow. However, these techniques are intermittent, labour intensive and limited to research based units.

A number of qualitative measurement techniques are available that provide an indirect assessment of cerebral blood flow which may be useful, particularly when used in conjunction with other modalities such as intracranial pressure monitoring and CT scanning. Interpretation of these measurements must be taken within the clinical context, particularly the time course of the underlying injury (Fig. 65.2).

Jugular bulb oximetry

Measurement of oxygen saturation in the jugular bulb by the retrograde placement of a fibreoptic catheter provides an indirect assessment of cerebral perfusion.[69,70] The principles of jugular bulb oximetry are shown in Fig. 65.3. Essentially, jugular venous saturation is inversely proportional to the cerebral blood flow for a given metabolic rate.[71] Adequate signal quality and calibration of saturations from the fibreoptic catheter are essential for accuracy.

Changes in jugular venous saturation usually occur independently of changes in intracranial pressure. Low jugular venous saturations (<55%) are indicative of cerebral hypoperfusion. The occurrence and duration of episodes of jugular venous desaturation is associated with adverse outcome.[72,73] These episodes are most common during the hypoperfusion phase and are usually associated with systemic or cerebral hypoperfusion or hypocapnia.[74]

Conversely, high levels of jugular venous saturation (>85%) may be indicative of cerebral hyperaemia or inadequate neuronal metabolism. Prolonged episodes of high jugular venous saturations are associated with adverse outcomes.[75] These episodes usually occur during the hyperaemic phase or during the evolution of brain death.

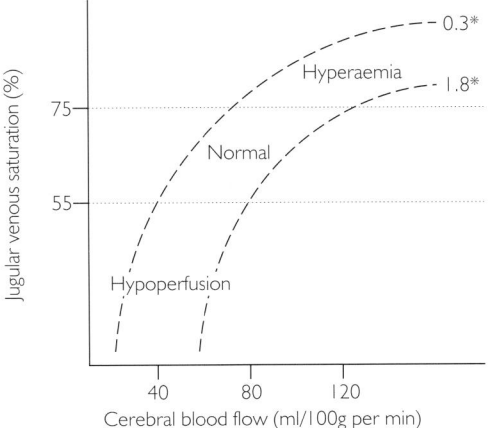

Fig. 65.3 Relationship between jugular venous saturation and cerebral blood flow over a range of cerebral metabolic rates (*) for oxygen.[70] Jugular venous saturation <55% is suggestive of cerebral hypoperfusion, while a level >80% is suggestive of hyperaemia.

There are insufficient data to provide evidence-based indications for the routine use of jugular bulb oximetry (SjO_2).

The following criteria may be considered as indications in selected patients.

1 Defence of cerebral perfusion pressure by maintaining SjO_2 >55%:
    (a) Haemodynamic instability, for example, during urgent extracranial surgery within 72 hours following injury.
    (b) Haemodynamic stability, but requiring high dose of catecholamines to achieve CPP of >70 mmHg (9.3 kPa); for example, 72 hours after injury, lower cerebral perfusion pressures may be tolerated provided SjO_2 is >55%.
2 Quantification of hyperaemia (defined as SjO_2 >85%) in patients with raised intracranial pressure >72 hours after injury.
3 Assessment and titration of adjunctive therapies in patients with severe intracranial hypertension by maintaining SjO_2 at 55–85%, for example, barbiturate coma, hyperventilation or hypothermia.

Cerebral lactate fluxes
Other applications of jugular bulb catheters include calculation of cerebral lactate fluxes from intermittent blood samples.[76] Arterio-jugular lactate difference (AJDL) of −0.4 mmol/l or a lactate oxygen index (AJDL/arteriojugular oxygen saturation difference) of >0.08 is suggestive of cerebral ischaemia or infarction.[77] These indices have limited clinical utility as titratable endpoints.

Near infrared spectroscopy
This is a non-invasive method of measuring regional cerebral oxygen saturations using a scalp oximeter similar to pulse oximetry. The accuracy and reliability of these monitors has been questioned due to the influence of extracranial signals.[78] Currently, they are not recommended for routine clinical use and do not provide a non-invasive alternative to jugular venous oximetry.

Transcranial Doppler
Transcranial Doppler ultrasonography with a 2 MHz pulsed Doppler probe allows non-invasive, intermittent or continuous assessment of the velocity of blood flow through large cerebral vessels. Insonation through a naturally occurring acoustic window such as the transtemporal approach allows insonation of the anterior, middle and posterior cerebral arteries, terminal internal carotid artery and anterior and posterior communicating arteries.[79]

Measured indices of flow include systolic, mean and diastolic flow velocities. Distinct patterns associated with normal, hyperaemic, vasospastic and absent flow are recognized. Derived indices such as the Gosling pulsatility index (systolic/diastolic difference divided by the mean velocity) and Lindegaard ratio (between middle cerebral artery to extracranial internal carotid artery) may assist in differentiating these flow patterns.[80,81]

Despite increasing use of transcranial Doppler to diagnose post-traumatic hyperaemia and vasospasm, there is insufficient data to provide evidence-based indications for the routine use of transcranial Doppler.

Continuous measurements and trends of transcranial Doppler provide a better assessment of flow/velocity patterns than intermittent or daily measurements. The technique is operator dependent and there may be significant variations in velocity patterns during the course of the injury. Consequently, interpretation of intermittent measurements should be made in conjunction with other variables such as CT scan appearance, intracranial pressure and where applicable jugular venous saturation.

CEREBRAL FUNCTION AND METABOLISM
Electroencephalography

Electroencephalography has been used for many years to assess seizure activity that may be masked by sedatives or muscle relaxants and to provide an objective estimate of the degree of electrical neuronal depression with barbiturate therapy. While seizures may not be clinically apparent in a proportion of patients, and may constitute an important secondary insult, the accuracy and reliability of electroencephalography in ICUs is questionable due to outside electrical interference from monitors and ventilators.[82]

The development of bispectral index as a measurement of depth of anaesthesia has led to the suggestion that this may be an alternative to the use of electroencephalography with barbiturate or sedative therapy in traumatic brain injury. Bispectral index has not been validated in this context and cannot be recommended as a titration endpoint.

Other forms of electroencephalography such as processed electroencephalography and integrated cerebral function monitors have a limited role in head injured patients, due to the amount of data generated and the need for skilled personnel to acquire and interpret the data.

Evoked potentials
Measurement of evoked potentials, assessing the integrity of sensor and motor pathways, may provide diagnostic and prognostic information, but because of the complexity of the technique is not recommended for general use.[83] The reliance of one variable, such as evoked potentials, to predict outcome from traumatic brain injury is not recommended.

Neuronal function
Research developments in microprobe technology have resulted in specific electrodes that may be placed into the brain parenchyma to measure brain oxygen, pH and

carbon dioxide tensions. These may be individual electrodes or combined with other sensors such as pressure monitors to form multimodal tissue monitors.[84]

Cerebral microdialysis is a technique that measures brain extracellular fluid metabolites. Dialysate is obtained through a microdialysis catheter inserted through the same burr hole as an intracranial pressure monitor to measure concentration and fluxes of markers of intracranial inflammation (e.g. lactate, pyruvate and purines).[85]

While these systems provide highly specific information about the biochemical milieu of focal areas of brain tissue, their clinical utility is limited to research centres.

BRAIN INJURY SURVEILLANCE

Serial assessment of the anatomical injury is an essential part of monitoring head injury. This is done by serial CT scanning at frequent intervals depending on the neurological status of the patient.

Any patient who develops an unexplained neurological deterioration or significant validated deviation of monitored parameters should have a CT scan so that new or delayed intracranial mass lesions are identified.

CT scans should be assessed and scored according to the classification outlined in Table 65.3. The progression or resolution of axonal injury, cerebral oedema, contusion and haemorrhages should be recorded. Other parameters such as intracranial pressure and jugular venous saturation should be interpreted in accordance with the CT scan appearance.

However, as CT scanning requires transport of the patient to a radiology suite, this should only be done by experienced personnel when the patient is stable.

BRAIN SPECIFIC THERAPY

Treatment options directed at ameliorating brain injury are limited. Despite intensive research into defining the pathobiological processes in primary injury, studies analysing therapies designed to modulate intracranial inflammation have not been successful. These include aminosteroids, calcium-channel blockade and N-methyl-D-aspartic acid antagonists.[86]

Brain specific, or targeted therapy is directed at maintaining cerebral perfusion pressure and minimizing intracranial pressure. While there is inherent relationship between these two principles, priorities are different depending on the time course of underlying injury. This is important as strategies directed at one may have adverse effects in the other (Fig. 65.2).

DEFENCE OF CEREBRAL PERFUSION PRESSURE

The pathophysiological principles outlined are important in defining strategies to optimize cerebral perfusion pressure following injury. While the Brain Trauma Foundation guidelines recommend a cerebral perfusion pressure of 70 mmHg (9.3 kPa), this figure may not be applicable over the entire time course after injury.[87]

This requires a change from a 'set and forget' philosophy to one of 'titration against time' in order to prescribe desirable therapeutic targets.

Hypoperfusion phase (0–72 hours)

Cerebral hypoperfusion is present in the majority of patients with severe head injury (GCS ≤ 8). During this phase, augmentation of cerebral perfusion pressure is paramount and should be done by maintaining adequate haemodynamic function.[20,88]

The principles outlined above on 'Haemodynamic management' become the mainstay of defence of cerebral perfusion pressure. This phase should be regarded as an extension of resuscitation and supportive treatment. During this period, a cerebral perfusion pressure of at least 70 mmHg (9.3 kPa) is recommended. In addition to reduced cerebral blood flow, intracranial pressure may be increased by mass lesions or 'cytotoxic' cerebral oedema. The latter will usually respond to restoration of cerebral perfusion pressure.

During this phase, medical therapies directed at raised intracranial pressure such as osmotherapy or hyperventilation should only be used if cerebral perfusion pressure is maintained at an appropriate level and the patient is adequately monitored.

Assessment of adequacy of the response to augmentation of cerebral perfusion pressure is made by intracranial pressure trends, CT scan appearance and where possible, neurological assessment. If patients appear to have stabilized, sedation may be reduced with the aim of extubation.

Hyperaemic phase (3–7 days)

Approximately 25–30% of patients will develop clinical signs of cerebral hyperaemia, characterized by raised intracranial pressure, persistent cerebral oedema on CT scan and/or high jugular venous saturations.[12,89,90] This may be due to vasogenic cerebral oedema caused by intracranial inflammation or by catecholamine infusions used to augment cerebral perfusion pressure.[14]

The diagnosis of catecholamine induced cerebral hyperaemia is difficult. This should be suspected in patients who require progressively increasing doses of catecholamines (e.g. >40 μg/min of epinephrine or norepinephrine) to attain a prescribed cerebral perfusion pressure of 70 mmHg (9.3 kPa). This phenomenon is due to tachyphyllaxis to prolonged catecholamine infusions and may be responsible for iatrogenically increasing intracranial pressure.

If CT appearance is unchanged, cerebral perfusion pressure targets may be lowered in order to use lower doses of inotropes. This exercise may be facilitated by jugular venous saturation monitoring or transcranial Doppler to provide an index of adequate cerebral blood flow for the lower cerebral perfusion pressure.

If patients continue to have raised intracranial pressure, strategies directed at reducing intracranial pressure should be considered.

REDUCTION OF INTRACRANIAL PRESSURE

In the absence of intracranial mass lesions, raised intracranial pressure is usually an indicator of severity of the underlying injury and represents exhausted intracranial elastance. The most effective methods of reducing raised intracranial pressure are surgical or mechanical, such as removal of mass lesions, drainage of cerebrospinal fluid and decompressive craniectomy.

A number of medical strategies directed at reducing intracranial pressure have been used for many years. Despite widespread use and firmly held beliefs, there is little evidence to support the use of routine use of these therapies.[91,92]

Intracranial pressure should be maintained at <25 cmH$_2$O (2.45 kPa).[93] Trends of intracranial pressure are equally as important and should be assessed within the context of cerebral perfusion pressure and the methods used to defend it.

Surgical evacuation of mass lesions

The prompt detection and evacuation of mass lesions causing raised intracranial pressure is the most effective method of relieving intracranial hypertension. Although the majority of these lesions will be present immediately after injury and will be treated during the resuscitative phase, approximately 10% patients will develop delayed intracranial haematomas. These are detected by sudden unexplained rises in intracranial pressure or by CT scan surveillance.

Close liaison with neurosurgeons is essential.

Cerebrospinal fluid drainage

Drainage of cerebrospinal fluid through an intraventricular catheter is an effective method of reducing intracranial pressure. If present, these catheters should be placed 5–10 cm above the head and opened for drainage every 1–4 hours.

Decompressive craniectomy

Wide, bilateral fronto-parietal craniectomies are increasingly being advocated to reduce intracranial pressure in patients with refractory intracranial hypertension. While there are numerous case series demonstrating dramatic improvements, there are no conclusive outcome based trials on which to base firm recommendations.[94,95]

Recent experience in paediatric patients is encouraging and the role of pre-emptive decompressive craniectomy in high risk patients is yet to be determined.[96]

Osmotherapy

The rationale and role of osmotherapy using mannitol or hypertonic solution is addressed on p. 694. The same principles during resuscitation apply during intensive care management.

Mannitol or hypertonic saline should only be used in patients with validated intracranial hypertension who are euvolaemic, haemodynamically stable, with a serum osmolality <320 mosmol/l.

There is no evidence that osmotherapy or induced dehydration improves outcome or is more effective in cytotoxic than vasogenic cerebral oedema.[30]

Hyperventilation

The role of hyperventilation during intensive care management is limited to the indications outlined on p. 693.

The routine, prolonged use of hyperventilation in head injured patients is associated with a worse outcome than patients ventilated to normocapnia.[97] This is probably due to reductions of cerebral blood flow and secondary brain ischaemia. The use of 'optimized hyperventilation' in selected patients with proven cerebral hyperaemia is a strategy that has a theoretical basis,[98] but efficacy is yet to be determined.

Current evidence-based guidelines do not recommend the use of routine hyperventilation.[18]

Hypothermia

Induced hypothermia has been used for many years to reduce cerebral metabolism and thereby raise intracranial pressure. A sound theoretical benefit exists in experimental models where hypothermia is induced immediately following injury with prompt reduction in raised intracranial pressure.[100] However, these benefits have not translated into improved outcomes in a number of clinical trials.[101]

Induced hypothermia (to temperatures of 30–33°C) is associated with prolonged ventilation, increased susceptibility to nosocomial infection, and may be associated with increased morbidity and mortality in head injured patients.

Currently, hypothermia is regarded as a 'second tier' option in patients with refractory intracranial hypertension, but on current evidence, cannot be recommended.

Barbiturate coma

The role of barbiturates in traumatic brain injury is similar to hypothermia. Despite strong experimental evidence that barbiturates reduce cerebral metabolism and reduce intracranial pressure, no definitive studies have shown a benefit in clinical trials. Barbiturates have invariably been used in patients with refractory intracranial hypertension where a positive outcome was unlikely, making interpretation of these trials difficult.[102]

Titration of barbiturate coma to burst suppression on the electroencephalograph is suggested as a reasonable endpoint. However, this is often difficult to obtain and measure.

Barbiturates may cause hypotension and reduce cerebral blood flow, potentially exacerbating secondary insults in patients with cerebral oligaemia. Prolonged use of barbiturates will delay awakening and predispose the patient to nosocomial infection.

Barbiturates are a 'second tier' option in patients with refractory intracranial hypertension and not recommended on current evidence.

Steroids

Steroids have been advocated for many years to ameliorate intracranial inflammation, thereby reducing intracranial pressure. To date, no definitive studies have shown a positive benefit and may be associated with an increased risk of infection.

On current evidence, steroids have no place in the management of traumatic brain injury.

Cerebral blood volume regulation

Following resuscitation and stabilization, a strategy reducing cerebral perfusion pressure to >50 mmHg (6.7 kPa) using β-blockade, clonidine and dihydroergotamine may be effective in minimizing secondary cerebral hyperaemia and vasogenic oedema. This strategy requires a measurement of cerebral blood flow to demonstrate adequate cerebral perfusion.[105,106] This interesting approach will require further evaluation.

CEREBRAL VASOSPASM

Post-traumatic cerebral vasospasm occurs in approximately 10–15% patients. It is associated with a high morbidity and mortality.[107] It is frequently present in patients with traumatic subarachnoid haemorrhage and is marker of severity of injury.

Cerebral angiography and transcranial Doppler are frequently used to diagnose vasospasm, although false positives and negative exist with both techniques and the true incidence of clinically significant vasospasm is uncertain.[108]

Treatment options remain limited. Calcium antagonists, such as nimodipine, have not been shown to be effective in traumatic subarachnoid haemorrhage.[109,110] Strategies that have been used in aneurysmal subarachnoid haemorrhage such as 'triple H' therapy (induced hypertension, hypervolaemia and haemodilution) or chemical angioplasty have not been evaluated in traumatic subarachnoid haemorrhage and are not recommended.

SEIZURE PROPHYLAXIS

Seizures are infrequent after traumatic brain injury and usually present at the time of injury. These should be treated with anticonvulsants (e.g. diazepam, midazolam) when they occur. Subsequent prophylaxis with phenytoin is recommended only in patients with destructive parenchymal lesions on CT scan and continued for 10 days following injury.[111] Short-term seizure prophylaxis does not prevent late onset posttraumatic epilepsy.[112]

OUTCOME AND PROGNOSIS

Patient factors that determine outcome from traumatic brain injury include severity of primary and secondary injuries, low GCS on presentation,[113] advanced age (>60 years)[114] and comorbidities. Prediction of outcome is difficult and must be made with circumspection

Table 65.4 The extended Glasgow Outcome Score.[112] This should be assessed at 6 and 12 months post-injury.

Score	Classification	Essential features
1	Death	
2	Persistent vegetative state	Eyes open, sleep–wake cycles. No speech, communication or response to external stimuli.
3	Severe disability	Lower grade: usually dependent in activities of daily living and institutionalized. May be living at home with a large degree of family and nursing support. Upper grade: may be largely self-caring, but unable to work, even in a sheltered environment, or travel independently.
4	Moderate disability	Lower grade: able to travel independently, work in a sheltered environment or at lesser level than pre-injury. Upper grade: able to work in a reduced capacity, may have deficits in speech, memory and personality change.
5	Good recovery	Lower grade: able to participate in social activities outside the home, but to a less extent than pre-injury. Upper grade: resumption of normal life, minor neurological or psychological deficits may persist.

as significant functional improvements, particularly in young patients, may occur over time.

There are patients in whom the prognosis is clearly very poor or hopeless. A proportion of these patients will become brain dead and may be considered for organ donation. This is discussed elsewhere. In other patients, it may be appropriate to withdraw active treatment. This increasingly complex process requires time, careful consideration and consensus with all members of the health care and relatives.

Outcome from traumatic brain injury is difficult to quantify. While mortality is an easy endpoint to measure, functional outcome is an equally important measurement. The extended Glasgow Outcome Scale (Table 65.4) is a blunt tool that is widely used to assess outcome from head injury. This takes the form of structured interviews of the patient or their caregiver and should be performed at 6 and 12 months post-injury.[115]

The future challenge facing intensive care management of traumatic brain injury is to determine whether standards of practice and innovations improve mortality and functional survival. There is a responsibility to ensure that accurate outcome data is collected both at institution and regional levels. This will define the epidemiology and provide the basis for future studies.[116]

REFERENCES

1 Goldstein M. Traumatic brain injury: a silent epidemic. *Ann Neurol* 1990; **27**: 327.

2 Feinstein A, Rapoport M. Mild traumatic brain injury: the silent epidemic. *Can J Public Health* 2000; **91**: 325–6, 332.

3 Jennett B. Epidemiology of head injury. *J Neurol Neurosurg Psychiatry* 1996; **60**: 362–9.

4 Alaranta H, Koskinen S, Leppanen L, *et al.* Nationwide epidemiology of hospitalized patients with first-time traumatic brain injury with special reference to prevention. *Wien Med Wochenschr* 2000; **150**: 444–8.

5 Brown DS, Nell V. Epidemiology of traumatic brain injury in Johannesburg. I. Methodological issues in a developing country context. *Soc Sci Med* 1991; **33**: 283–7.

6 Chesnut RM, Marshall LF, Klauber MR, *et al.* The role of secondary brain injury in determining outcome from severe head injury. *J Trauma* 1993; **34**: 216–22.

7 Chesnut RM, Marshall SB, Piek J, *et al.* Early and late systemic hypotension as a frequent and fundamental source of cerebral ischemia following severe brain injury in the Traumatic Coma Data Bank. *Acta Neurochir Suppl (Wien)* 1993; **59**: 121–5.

8 McKeating EG, Andrews PJ. Cytokines and adhesion molecules in acute brain injury. *Br J Anaesth* 1998; **80**: 77–84.

9 Bouma GJ, Muizelaar JP. Cerebral blood flow, cerebral blood volume, and cerebrovascular reactivity after severe head injury. *J Neurotrauma* 1992; **9** (Suppl 1): S333–48.

10 Bouma GJ, Muizelaar JP. Cerebral blood flow in severe clinical head injury. *New Horiz* 1995; **3**: 384–94.

11 Golding EM, Robertson CS, Bryan RM Jr. The consequences of traumatic brain injury on cerebral blood flow and autoregulation: a review. *Clin Exp Hypertens* 1999; **21**: 299–332.

12 Martin NA, Patwardhan RV, Alexander MJ, *et al.* Characterization of cerebral hemodynamic phases following severe head trauma: hypoperfusion, hyperemia, and vasospasm. *J Neurosurg* 1997; **87**: 9–19.

13 Bouma GJ, Muizelaar JP, Choi SC, *et al.* Cerebral circulation and metabolism after severe traumatic brain injury: the elusive role of ischemia. *J Neurosurg* 1991; **75**: 685–93.

14 Dunn-Meynell AA, Hassanain M, Levin BE. Norepinephrine and traumatic brain injury: a possible role in post-traumatic edema. *Brain Res* 1998; **800**: 245–52.

15 American College of Surgeons Committee on Trauma. Advanced Trauma Life Support for Doctors. 1997. Chicago IL.

16 The Brain Trauma Foundation. The American Association of Neurological Surgeons. The Joint Section on Neurotrauma and Critical Care. Initial management. *J Neurotrauma* 2000; **17**: 463–70.

17 The Brain Trauma Foundation. The American Association of Neurological Surgeons. The Joint Section on Neurotrauma and Critical Care. Resuscitation of blood pressure and oxygenation. *J Neurotrauma* 2000; **17**: 471–8.

18 The Brain Trauma Foundation. The American Association of Neurological Surgeons. The Joint Section on Neurotrauma and Critical Care. Hyperventilation. *J Neurotrauma* 2000; **17**: 513–20.

19 The Brain Trauma Foundation. The American Association of Neurological Surgeons. The Joint Section on Neurotrauma and Critical Care. Hypotension. *J Neurotrauma* 2000; **17**: 591–5.

20 Chesnut RM. Avoidance of hypotension: conditio sine qua non of successful severe head-injury management. *J Trauma* 1997; **42**: S4–9.

21 Qureshi AI, Suarez JI. Use of hypertonic saline solutions in treatment of cerebral edema and intracranial hypertension. *Crit Care Med* 2000; **28**: 3301–13.

22 Scalea TM, Maltz S, Yelon J, *et al.* Resuscitation of multiple trauma and head injury: role of crystalloid fluids and inotropes. *Crit Care Med* 1994; **22**: 1610–15.

23 Alspaugh DM, Sartorelli K, Shackford SR, *et al.* Prehospital resuscitation with phenylephrine in uncontrolled hemorrhagic shock and brain injury. *J Trauma* 2000; **48**: 851–63.

24 Ract C, Vigue B. Comparison of the cerebral effects of dopamine and norepinephrine in severely head-injured patients. *Intensive Care Med* 2001; **27**: 101–6.

25 Palafox BA, Johnson MN, McEwen DK, *et al.* ICP changes following application of the MAST suit. *J Trauma* 1981; **21**: 55–9.

26 Teasdale G, Jennett B. Assessment of coma and impaired consciousness. A practical scale. *Lancet* 1974; **2**: 81–4.

27 Townsend RN, Lheureau T, Protech J, *et al.* Timing fracture repair in patients with severe brain injury (Glasgow Coma Scale score <9). *J Trauma* 1998; **44**: 977–82.

28 Schierhout G, Roberts I. Hyperventilation therapy for acute traumatic brain injury. *Cochrane Database Syst Rev* 2000CD000565.

29 Schierhout G, Roberts I. Mannitol for acute traumatic brain injury. *Cochrane Database Syst Rev* 2000CD001049.

30 The Brain Trauma Foundation. The American Association of Neurological Surgeons. The Joint Section on Neurotrauma and Critical Care. Mannitol. *J Neurotrauma* 2000; **17**: 521–6.

31 Myburgh JA, Lewis SB. Mannitol for resuscitation in acute head injury: effects on cerebral perfusion and osmolality. *Critical Care and Resuscitation* 2000; **2**: 344–53.

32 Doyle JA, Davis DP, Hoyt DB. The use of hypertonic saline in the treatment of traumatic brain injury. *J Trauma* 2001; **50**: 367–83.

33 Marshall LF, Marshall SB, Klauber MR, et al. The diagnosis of head injury requires a classification based on computed axial tomography. *J Neurotrauma* 1992; **9**(Suppl 1): S287–2.

34 The Brain Trauma Foundation. The American Association of Neurological Surgeons. The Joint Section on Neurotrauma and Critical Care. Computed tomography scan features. *J Neurotrauma* 2000; **17**: 597–627.

35 Kakarieka A, Braakman R, Schakel EH. Clinical significance of the finding of subarachnoid blood on CT scan after head injury. *Acta Neurochir (Wien)* 1994; **129**: 1–5.

36 The Brain Trauma Foundation. The American Association of Neurological Surgeons. The Joint Section on Neurotrauma and Critical Care. Trauma systems. *J Neurotrauma* 2000; **17**: 457–62.

37 Fearnside MR, Cook RJ, McDougall P, *et al.* The Westmead Head Injury Project outcome in severe head injury. A comparative analysis of pre-hospital, clinical and CT variables. *Br J Neurosurg* 1993; **7**: 267–79.

38 Ghajar J, Hariri RJ, Narayan RK, *et al.* Survey of critical care management of comatose, head-injured patients in the United States. *Crit Care Med* 1995; **23**: 560–7.

39 Matta B, Menon D. Severe head injury in the United Kingdom and Ireland: a survey of practice and implications for management. *Crit Care Med* 1996; **24**: 1743–8.

40 Murray GD, Teasdale GM, Braakman R, *et al.* The European Brain Injury Consortium survey of head injuries. *Acta Neurochir (Wien)* 1999; **141**: 223–36.

41 The Brain Trauma Foundation. The American Association of Neurological Surgeons. The Joint Section on Neurotrauma and Critical Care. Management and prognosis of severe traumatic brain injury. *J Neurotrauma* 2000; **17**: 449–604.

42 Maas AI, Dearden M, Teasdale GM, *et al.* EBIC-guidelines for management of severe head injury in adults. European Brain Injury Consortium. *Acta Neurochir (Wien)* 1997; **139**: 286–94.

43 Chesnut RM. Guidelines for the management of severe head injury: what we know and what we think we know. *J Trauma* 1997; **42**: S19–22.

44 DeWitt DS, Prough DS. Should pressors be used to augment cerebral blood flow after traumatic brain injury? *Crit Care Med* 2000; **28**: 3933–4.

45 Myburgh JA, Upton RN, Grant C, *et al.* A comparison of the effects of norepinephrine, epinephrine, and dopamine on cerebral blood flow and oxygen utilisation. *Acta Neurochir Suppl (Wien)* 1998; **71**: 19–21.

46 Cooper KR, Boswell PA, Choi SC. Safe use of PEEP in patients with severe head injury. *J Neurosurg* 1985; **63**: 552–5.

47 Chen HI. Hemodynamic mechanisms of neurogenic pulmonary edema. *Biol Signals* 1995; **4**: 186–192.

48 Rogers FB, Shackford SR, Trevisani GT, *et al.* Neurogenic pulmonary edema in fatal and nonfatal head injuries. *J Trauma* 1995; **39**: 860–6.

49 McManis P, Lee C, Morgan M, *et al.* Neurogenic pulmonary oedema. *Aust NZ J Med* 2000; **30**: 514.

50 Ewig S, Torres A, El Ebiary M, *et al.* Bacterial colonization patterns in mechanically ventilated patients with traumatic and medical head injury. Incidence, risk factors, and association with ventilator-associated pneumonia. *Am J Respir Crit Care Med* 1999; **159**: 188–98.

51 McCollam JS, O'Neil MG, Norcross ED, *et al.* Continuous infusions of lorazepam, midazolam, and propofol for sedation of the critically ill surgery trauma patient: a prospective, randomized comparison. *Crit Care Med* 1999; **27**: 2454–8.

52 Kelly DF, Goodale DB, Williams J, *et al.* Propofol in the treatment of moderate and severe head injury: a randomized, prospective double-blinded pilot trial. *J Neurosurg* 1999; **90**: 1042–52.

53 Cremer OL, Moons KGM, Bouman ACB, *et al.* Long-term propofol infusion and cardiac failure in adult head-injured patients. *Lancet* 2001; **357**: 117–18.

54 Hsiang JK, Chesnut RM, Crisp CB, *et al.* Early, routine paralysis for intracranial pressure control in severe head injury: is it necessary? *Crit Care Med* 1994; **22**: 1471–6.

55 Winkelman C. Effect of backrest position on intracranial and cerebral perfusion pressures in traumatically brain-injured adults. *Am J Crit Care* 2000; **9**: 373–80.

56 Rumana CS, Gopinath SP, Uzura M, *et al.* Brain temperature exceeds systemic temperature in head-injured patients. *Crit Care Med* 1998; **26**: 562–7.

57 The Brain Trauma Foundation. The American Association of Neurological Surgeons. The Joint Section on Neurotrauma and Critical Care. Nutrition. *J Neurotrauma* 2000; **17**: 539–48.

58 Yanagawa T, Bunn F, Roberts I, *et al*. Nutritional support for head-injured patients. *Cochrane Database Syst Rev* 2000CD001530.

59 Hammond FM, Meighen MJ. Venous thromboembolism in the patient with acute traumatic brain injury: screening, diagnosis, prophylaxis, and treatment issues. *J Head Trauma Rehabil* 1998; **13**: 36–50.

60 Spain DA, Bergamini TM, Hoffmann JF, *et al*. Comparison of sequential compression devices and foot pumps for prophylaxis of deep venous thrombosis in high-risk trauma patients. *Am Surg* 1998; **64**: 522–5.

61 Langan EM IIIrd, Miller RS, Casey WJ IIIrd, *et al*. Prophylactic inferior vena cava filters in trauma patients at high risk: follow-up examination and risk/benefit assessment. *J Vasc Surg* 1999; **30**: 484–8.

62 Jacobs DG, Westerband A. Antibiotic prophylaxis for intracranial pressure monitors. *J Natl Med Assoc* 1998; **90**: 417–23.

63 Lane PL, Skoretz TG, Doig G, *et al*. Intracranial pressure monitoring and outcomes after traumatic brain injury. *Can J Surg* 2000; **43**: 442–8.

64 The Brain Trauma Foundation. The American Association of Neurological Surgeons. The Joint Section on Neurotrauma and Critical Care. Indications for intracranial pressure monitoring. *J Neurotrauma* 2000; **17**: 479–92.

65 The Brain Trauma Foundation. The American Association of Neurological Surgeons. The Joint Section on Neurotrauma and Critical Care. Recommendations for intracranial pressure monitoring technology. *J Neurotrauma* 2000; **17**: 497–506.

66 Signorini DF, Shad A, Piper IR, *et al*. A clinical evaluation of the Codman MicroSensor for intracranial pressure monitoring. *Br J Neurosurg* 1998; **12**: 223–7.

67 Bouma GJ, Muizelaar JP, Bandoh K *et al*. Blood pressure and intracranial pressure–volume dynamics in severe head injury: relationship with cerebral blood flow. *J Neurosurg* 1992; **77**: 15–19.

68 Lam JM, Hsiang JN, Poon WS. Monitoring of autoregulation using laser Doppler flowmetry in patients with head injury. *J Neurosurg* 1997; **86**: 438–45.

69 De Deyne C. Jugular bulb oximetry: the link between cerebral and systemic management of severe head injury. *Intensive Care Med* 1999; **25**: 430–1.

70 Macmillan CS, Andrews PJ. Cerebrovenous oxygen saturation monitoring: practical considerations and clinical relevance. *Intensive Care Med* 2000; **26**: 1028–36.

71 Robertson CS, Cormio M. Cerebral metabolic management. *New Horiz* 1995; **3**: 410–22.

72 Gopinath SP, Robertson CS, Contant CF *et al*. Jugular venous desaturation and outcome after head injury. *J Neurol Neurosurg Psychiatry* 1994; **57**: 717–23.

73 Robertson CS, Valadka AB, Hannay HJ *et al*. Prevention of secondary ischemic insults after severe head injury. *Crit Care Med* 1999; **27**: 2086–95.

74 Lewis SB, Myburgh JA, Reilly PL. Detection of cerebral venous desaturation by continuous jugular bulb oximetry following acute neurotrauma [see comments]. *Anaesth Intensive Care* 1995; **23**: 307–14.

75 Macmillan CS, Andrews PJ, Easton VJ. Increased jugular bulb saturation is associated with poor outcome in traumatic brain injury. *J Neurol Neurosurg Psychiatry* 2001; **70**: 101–4.

76 Murr R, Stummer W, Schurer L, *et al*. Cerebral lactate production in relation to intracranial pressure, cranial computed tomography findings, and outcome in patients with severe head injury. *Acta Neurochir (Wien)* 1996; **138**: 928–36.

77 Cruz J, Hoffstad OJ, Jaggi JL. Cerebral lactate–oxygen index in acute brain injury with acute anemia: assessment of false versus true ischemia. *Crit Care Med* 1994; **22**: 1465–70.

78 Lewis SB, Myburgh JA, Thornton EL, *et al*. Cerebral oxygenation monitoring by near-infrared spectroscopy is not clinically useful in patients with severe closed-head injury: a comparison with jugular venous bulb oximetry [see comments]. *Crit Care Med* 1996; **24**: 1334–8.

79 Castillo MA. Monitoring neurologic patients in intensive care. *Curr Opin Crit Care* 2001; **7**: 49–60.

80 Lewis SB, Wong ML, Bannan PE, *et al*. Transcranial Doppler identification of changing autoregulatory thresholds after autoregulatory impairment. *Neurosurgery* 2001; **48**: 369–75.

81 Vajramani GV, Chandramouli BA, Jayakumar PN, *et al*. Evaluation of posttraumatic vasospasm, hyperaemia, and autoregulation by transcranial colour-coded duplex sonography. *Br J Neurosurg* 1999; **13**: 468–73.

82 Procaccio F, Polo A, Lanteri P, *et al*. Electrophysiologic monitoring in neurointensive care. *Curr Opin Crit Care* 2001; **7**: 74–80.

83 Carter BG, Butt W. Review of the use of somatosensory evoked potentials in the prediction of outcome after severe brain injury. *Crit Care Med* 2001; **29**: 178–86.

84 Meixensberger J, Jager A, Dings J, *et al*. Multimodal hemodynamic neuromonitoring – quality and consequences for therapy of severely head injured patients. *Acta Neurochir Suppl (Wien)* 1998; **71**: 260–2.

85 Peerdeman SM, Girbes AR, Vandertop WP. Cerebral microdialysis as a new tool for neurometabolic monitoring. *Intensive Care Med* 2000; **26**: 662–9.

86 Maas AI, Steyerberg EW, Murray GD, *et al*. Why have recent trials of neuroprotective agents in head injury failed to show convincing efficacy? A pragmatic analysis and theoretical considerations. *Neurosurgery* 1999; **44**: 1286–98.

87 The Brain Trauma Foundation. The American Association of Neurological Surgeons. The Joint Section on Neurotrauma and Critical Care. Guide-

lines for cerebral perfusion pressure. *J Neurotrauma* 2000; **17**: 497–506.

88 DeWitt DS, Prough DS. Ameliorating cerebral hypoperfusion after traumatic brain injury. *Crit Care Med* 1999; **27**: 2592–3.

89 Kelly DF, Kordestani RK, Martin NA, *et al.* Hyperemia following traumatic brain injury: relationship to intracranial hypertension and outcome. *J Neurosurg* 1996; **85**: 762–71.

90 Marmarou A, Fatouros PP, Barzo P, *et al.* Contribution of edema and cerebral blood volume to traumatic brain swelling in head-injured patients. *J Neurosurg* 2000; **93**: 183–93.

91 Allen CH, Ward JD. An evidence-based approach to management of increased intracranial pressure. *Crit Care Clin* 1998; **14**: 485–95.

92 The Brain Trauma Foundation. The American Association of Neurological Surgeons. The Joint Section on Neurotrauma and Critical Care. Critical pathway for the treatment of established intracranial hypertension. *J Neurotrauma* 2000; **17**: 537–8.

93 The Brain Trauma Foundation. The American Association of Neurological Surgeons. The Joint Section on Neurotrauma and Critical Care. Intracranial pressure treatment threshold. *J Neurotrauma* 2000; **17**: 493–5.

94 Guerra WK, Gaab MR, Dietz H, *et al.* Surgical decompression for traumatic brain swelling: indications and results. *J Neurosurg* 1999; **90**: 187–96.

95 Munch E, Horn P, Schurer L, *et al.* Management of severe traumatic brain injury by decompressive craniectomy. *Neurosurgery* 2000; **47**: 315–22.

96 Taylor A, Butt W, Rosenfeld J, *et al.* A randomized trial of very early decompressive craniectomy in children with traumatic brain injury and sustained intracranial hypertension. *Childs Nerv Syst* 2001; **17**: 154–62.

97 Muizelaar JP, Marmarou A, Ward JD, *et al.* Adverse effects of prolonged hyperventilation in patients with severe head injury: a randomized clinical trial. *J Neurosurg* 1991; **75**: 731–9.

98 Cruz J. The first decade of continuous monitoring of jugular bulb oxyhemoglobin saturation: management strategies and clinical outcome. *Crit Care Med* 1998; **26**: 344–51.

99 Chesnut RM. Hyperventilation in traumatic brain injury: friend or foe? [Editorial; comment] [See comments] *Crit Care Med* 1997; **25**: 1275–8.

100 Clifton G. Hypothermia and severe brain injury. *J Neurosurg* 2000; **93**: 718–19.

101 Clifton GL, Miller ER, Choi SC, *et al.* Lack of effect of induction of hypothermia after acute brain injury. *N Engl J Med* 2001; **344**: 556–63.

102 Roberts I. Barbiturates for acute traumatic brain injury. *Cochrane Database Syst Rev* 2000CD000033.

103 The Brain Trauma Foundation. The American Association of Neurological Surgeons. The Joint Section on Neurotrauma and Critical Care. Use of barbiturates in the control of intracranial hypertension. *J Neurotrauma* 2000; **17**: 527–30.

104 The Brain Trauma Foundation. The American Association of Neurological Surgeons. The Joint Section on Neurotrauma and Critical Care. Steroids. *J Neurotrauma* 2000; **17**: 531–6.

105 Asgeirsson B, Grande PO, Nordstrom CH. A new therapy of post-trauma brain oedema based on haemodynamic principles for brain volume regulation. *Intensive Care Med* 1994; **20**: 260–7.

106 Grande PO, Asgeirsson B, Nordstrom CH. Physiologic principles for volume regulation of a tissue enclosed in a rigid shell with application to the injured brain. *J Trauma* 1997; **42**: S23–31.

107 Kakarieka A. Review on traumatic subarachnoid hemorrhage. *Neurol Res* 1997; **19**: 230–2.

108 Martin NA, Doberstein C, Zane C, *et al.* Post-traumatic cerebral arterial spasm: transcranial Doppler ultrasound, cerebral blood flow, and angiographic findings. *J Neurosurg* 1992; **77**: 575–83.

109 Langham J, Goldfrad C, Teasdale G, *et al.* Calcium channel blockers for acute traumatic brain injury. *Cochrane Database Syst Rev* 2000CD000565.

110 A multicenter trial of the efficacy of nimodipine on outcome after severe head injury. The European Study Group on Nimodipine in Severe Head Injury. *J Neurosurg* 1994; **80**: 797–804.

111 Temkin NR, Dikmen SS, Wilensky AJ, *et al.* A randomized, double-blind study of phenytoin for the prevention of post-traumatic seizures. *N Engl J Med* 1990; **323**: 497–502.

112 The Brain Trauma Foundation. The American Association of Neurological Surgeons. The Joint Section on Neurotrauma and Critical Care. Role of antiseizure prophylaxis following head injury. *J Neurotrauma* 2000; **17**: 549–54.

113 The Brain Trauma Foundation. The American Association of Neurological Surgeons. The Joint Section on Neurotrauma and Critical Care. Glasgow Coma Scale Score. *J Neurotrauma* 2000; **17**: 563–72.

114 The Brain Trauma Foundation. The American Association of Neurological Surgeons. The Joint Section on Neurotrauma and Critical Care. Age. *J Neurotrauma* 2000; **17**: 573–82.

115 Pettigrew LE, Wilson JT, Teasdale GM. Assessing disability after head injury: improved use of the Glasgow Outcome Scale. *J Neurosurg* 1998; **89**: 939–43.

116 Wilson JT, Pettigrew LE, Teasdale GM. Structured interviews for the Glasgow Outcome Scale and the extended Glasgow Outcome Scale: guidelines for their use. *J Neurotrauma* 1998; **15**: 573–85.

66

Maxillofacial and upper airway injuries

C Edibam

MAXILLOFACIAL INJURIES

Life threatening haemorrhage and airway obstruction are common complications accompanying severe blunt or penetrating maxillofacial and neck injury. Injuries may be isolated or part of multisystem trauma. Up to 20% of people with facial injury will have life-threatening associated injuries: 15% with closed head injury, 3.5% with airway obstruction and 1.5% with pulmonary contusion and/or aspiration.[1-3] Urgent skilled airway management and awareness of other commonly associated injuries to the brain, cervical spine, thorax and oesophagus are paramount in preventing adverse outcomes. Here, the basic anatomy, pathology, complications and common pitfalls in the emergency management of maxillofacial, upper airway and non-bony neck trauma are outlined.

EPIDEMIOLOGY

Maxillofacial trauma occurs most frequently in the 20–25 years age group, decreasing in frequency either side of this age group. It is three- to five-fold more likely to occur in males than in females. Blunt injury is by far the commonest mechanism, accounting for nearly 97% of all maxillofacial injuries.[4] Motor vehicle accidents (MVA) account for nearly three quarters of blunt injuries, with falls, physical assault, contact sports and industrial accidents accounting for the remainder. Legislative changes and preventative measures involving drink driving, seatbelt and airbag use have seen a reduction in the incidence of MVA related maxillofacial injury.[5,6] In multiple trauma patients with an Injury Severity Score >12, maxillofacial injury occurs in up to 17%, with a corresponding mortality rate of 13%.[4]

ANATOMICAL ASPECTS

Fractures, haemorrhage, soft tissue damage and oedema are the commonest manifestations of blunt facial trauma. The severity of facial injury is directly related to the velocity of force applied.[7] Common fractures of facial bones are maxilla (23%), orbital region (22%), zygoma (16%), nasal bones (15%), mandible (13%), teeth (8%), alveolar ridge (2%) and temporomandibular joint (TMJ) 1%.[4]

MANDIBULAR FRACTURES

The mandible is a unique horseshoe shaped bone that is tubular and weakest where the cortices are thinnest; most fractures occur at vulnerable points, regardless of the point of impact.[8] Common sites are the ramus (condylar neck and angle of the mandible) and body at the level of the first or second molar. Multiple fractures are common (64%),[8] with body of mandible fractures often being accompanied by fractures of the opposite angle or neck due to transmitted forces. Mandibular fragments are often distracted due to the action of the lower jaw muscles. Respiratory obstruction may occur after bilateral mandibular angle or body fractures due to the posterior displacement of the tongue – the 'Andy Gump' fracture.[9,10]

MIDFACIAL FRACTURES

The bones of the middle third of the face are relatively thin and poorly reinforced. Fracture dislocations occur through the bones and suture lines and the facial skeleton acts as a compressible energy-absorbing mass that gives on impact. The series of compartments (nasal cavity, paranasal sinuses and orbits) within the bony framework collapses progressively, absorbing energy and protecting the brain, spinal cord and other vital structures.[11] Multiple complex facial fractures usually result and isolated facial bone fractures are rare. Le Fort described three great lines of weakness in the facial skeleton and thus derived the Le Fort classification of fractures[12] (Fig. 66.1).

Le Fort fractures are perpendicular to the three main vertical buttresses of the facial skeleton – the nasomaxillary, zygomaticomaxillary and pterygomaxillary 'pillars'. Le Fort fractures rarely occur in their pure form with mixed patterns prevailing (e.g. right hemifacial Le Fort I and left hemifacial Le Fort II). Airway obstruction from posterior movement of the soft palate against the tongue and the posterior pharyngeal wall may occur. Oral secretions, blood, bone

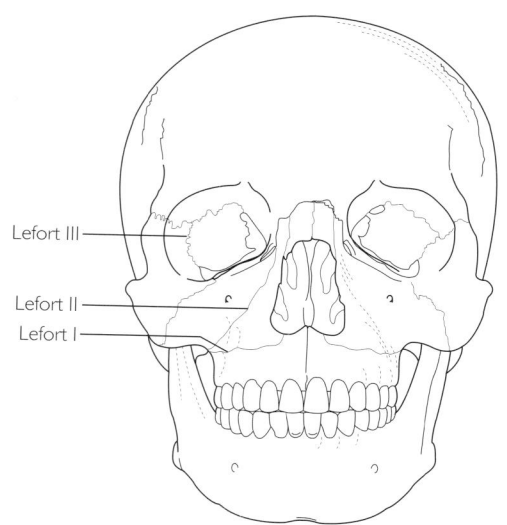

Fig. 66.1 LeFort classification of facial fractures

and tooth debris and pharyngeal wall haematomas may worsen airway compromise.

LE FORT I (ALSO KNOWN AS GUERIN'S FRACTURE)

This fracture involves only the maxilla at the level of the nasal fossa. It follows a horizontal plane at the level of the nose. The fracture separates the palate from the remainder of the facial skeleton (i.e. palate facial disjunction) and is usually caused by direct low-maxillary blows or by a lateral blow to the maxilla.

LE FORT II

This is the most common midface fracture.[13] The maxilla, nasal bones and medial aspect of the orbit are involved, which results in a freely mobile pyramidal shaped portion of the maxilla (i.e. pyramidal disjunction). The fracture line extends from the lower nasal bridge through the medial wall of the orbit, and crosses the zygomaticomaxillary process. It is caused by direct blows to the mid-alveolar area, or by lateral impacts and inferior blows to the mandible when the mouth is closed.

LE FORT III

This is known as cranio-facial disjunction because the fracture line runs parallel to the base of the skull, separating the midfacial skeleton from the cranium. The fracture extends through the upper nasal bridge and most of the orbit and across the zygomatic arch. It involves the ethmoid bone, and thus may transect the cribriform plate at the base of the skull.[13,14] These fractures result from superiorly directed blows to the nasal bones.[13]

TEMPOROMANDIBULAR JOINT

Mechanical TMJ impairment may result from condylar or zygomatic arch fractures and can prevent jaw opening even after muscle relaxants have been administered.[15]

ZYGOMATIC, ORBITAL AND NASAL FRACTURES

Zygomatic fractures are uncommon, but its attachment to the maxilla, frontal and temporal bones are vulnerable and may be disrupted. When the zygoma is displaced, disruption of the lateral wall and floor of the orbit may ensue. Orbital injury is commonly associated with midface trauma. The severity of injury in the orbital region varies from oedema and ecchymosis of the periosteal soft tissue to subconjunctival haemorrhage and loss of visual acuity or ocular rupture. Blinding injuries reported with facial fractures occur in 3–12% and most are secondary to globe perforation rather than optic nerve injury.[16] Orbital blow-out fractures occur when pressure is directly applied to the eye, and is hydraulically transmitted via the globe to the interior bony structures. The weaker inferior wall usually fractures, causing enophthalmos, diplopia, impaired eye movement and infraorbital hypoaesthesia. Nasal fractures are common, with epistaxis and septal haematoma being the prime concerns.

SOFT TISSUE INJURIES

Abrasions, contusions, lacerations to the tongue, palate, pharynx, cheek, eyelids, nasolacrimal duct, ear, parotid, gland and facial nerve can occur. Oedema evolving over 24–48 h can be massive and cause gross distortion of soft tissue structures. Patency of an initially unobstructed airway may become compromised during this period.

HAEMORRHAGE

Haemorrhage following blunt maxillofacial injury is extremely common but life threatening bleeding is fortunately rare. The reported incidence is between 1–10%.[1,17–19]

Most severe haemorrhage is associated with midfacial fractures although soft tissue lacerations alone can cause significant blood loss. The degree of haemorrhage may be concealed if the patient is swallowing blood and this will also predispose to aspiration.[20]

The source of bleeding in facial trauma is complex, as the vascular supply is derived from both the internal and external carotid arteries, with anastomoses occurring between them as well as between both halves of the face. In facial injuries, the internal maxillary artery, involving the intraosseous branches, is the main source of bleeding because the artery passes within the common Le Fort fracture borders.[16] The comminuted nature of maxillary fractures makes the detection of an exact site of vessel damage nearly impossible.[16] Branches of the internal carotid artery such as the lacrimal and zygomatic branches as well as the anterior and posterior ethmoidal arteries may contribute to bleeding.

ASSOCIATED INJURIES

More than half of all patients with maxillofacial injuries will have other injuries.

BASILAR SKULL FRACTURE

The anterior cranial fossa is often involved in craniofacial injuries. Fractures involving the frontal bone, frontal sinus, nasoethmoid complex, or fronto-orbital complex result in bone defects in the skull base and can cause dural tears with resultant leakage of cerebrospinal fluid (CSF). CSF fistulae occur in 10–30% of basilar skull fractures.[21] The clinical finding of CSF rhinorrhoea is not diagnostic for anterior cranial fossa lesions because this represents only the site of exiting CSF. The origin may be from a temporal bone fracture as CSF from the middle ear discharges into the nose via the Eustachian tube. A middle cranial fossa defect can produce rhinorrhoea through the sphenoid sinus. The vast majority of fistulae present within 1 week of injury. Meningitis in patients with midface fractures is uncommon despite the fact approximately 36% of patients sustaining Le Fort fractures with anterior cranial fossa fractures have CSF leaks.[22,23]

Pulsating exophthalmos and the presence of an orbital bruit may lead to the diagnosis of a carotido-cavernous fistula, which may develop following fractures involving the skull base and orbit.

HEAD AND CERVICAL SPINE INJURY

The incidence of head injury in those with maxillofacial trauma has been variably reported to be between 15% for severe head injury, increasing to 80% if all grades of head injuries are included.[1,4,24] Cervical spine injury has been reported in up to 11% of patients. The association between maxillofacial and cervical spine injury depends on the mechanism of injury. Falls and motor vehicle accident victims are more likely to have cervical injury than sporting or personal assault victims.[25] Cervical spine fracture occurs with mandibular injury in 3%[16] and is attributed to forces exerted directly or indirectly from the facial skeleton to the neck. C1/C2 and C5–C7 are at particular risk.

OTHER INJURIES

Thoracic (9–40%), abdominal (5–40%), limb fractures (30%) are other common co-existent injuries.[24,26] Carotid artery injury (dissection) following mandibular injury has been reported and should be considered in cases with neurological deficit or impaired conscious level with no obvious head injury.[27]

ASSESSMENT OF INJURY

The obvious priorities are airway management and control of haemorrhage and identifying other life-threat-

ening injuries. These are discussed later in detail. Once the patient is stable, formal assessment of the facial injuries can proceed.

HISTORY

Evaluation of facial fractures begins with a history of the injury. The mechanism of injury is important in order to assess the likelihood of other injuries.

EXAMINATION

Physical examination includes inspection of the deformity, presence of enophthalmos, asymmetry, dental malocclusion, nasal septal deviation or haematoma, CSF rhinorrhoea and the extent of jaw opening. Other signs associated with basal skull fracture should also be noted (haemotympanum, Battle's sign, Raccoon eyes). Tenderness and mobility on bimanual palpation of the alveolar process and the infraorbital rim or frontozygomatic suture indicates the presence of a complex midfacial fracture. Naso-orbito-ethmoid instability can also be established by bimanual palpation. Visual acuity (in the conscious patient), corneal integrity and pupillary reflexes as well as eye movements (failure of upward movements in orbital blowout fracture) should be assessed early and thoroughly. Facial nerve function should also be assessed if possible. The presence of a bruit over the orbit may indicate a carotido-cavernous fistula.

INVESTIGATION

Radiographic studies include a posterior–anterior, lateral oblique, stereo Water's view, stereo Caldwell's view and Panorex views. However, the use of computed tomography (CT) scan, especially with the three-dimensional reconstructive ability, is now the preferred and most accurate method of imaging. In addition to bony distortion, fluid in the paranasal sinuses, optic nerve integrity and soft tissue distortion, the brain, upper cervical spine and other body areas can be visualized concurrently. Other investigations such as colour Doppler ultrasound studies and/or angiography of the great vessels in the neck may be required in cases of possible carotid dissection or carotido-cavernous fistulae. Nasal discharge should be tested for glucose or a 'target test' can be performed on blotting paper to determine the presence of a CSF fistula.[23]

AIRWAY MANAGEMENT

Airway management in maxillofacial injury is potentially complex due to multiple concurrent compromising factors (Table 66.1).

IMMEDIATE PRIORITIES

- Assess and monitor for signs of airway obstruction
- Clear airway, assist respiration
- Definitive airway intervention

Table 66.1 Airway problems in maxillofacial trauma

General problems	Management
Haemorrhage/debris	Suction, volume replacement
Impaired laryngoscopy	Head down
Aspiration risk from blood swallowing	Definitive control of haemorrhage (see text)
Clot inhalation /obstruction	
Teeth, bone fragments	
Oedema soft tissue haematomas	Monitor airway closely
Increases over 48 hours	Head up 30°
Mask fit can be poor	Maintain spontaneous ventilation during airway manipulation; laryngeal mask ventilation
Specific problems	
Bilateral mandibular body/angle fractures	Anterior traction on tongue or jaw, towel clip or suture through tongue and elevate
Posterior displacement of tongue	
TMJ impairment	
Mandibular condyle, zygomatic arch	Nasotracheal intubation (blind/fibreoptic) or surgical airway may be required (see text)
Mouth opening limited	
Midfacial fracture	
Mask seal poor	Anterior traction on mobile segment.
Soft palate collapses against pharynx	
Basilar skull	
Nasotracheal intubation contraindicated	Avoid nasal intubation
Pneumocephalus from mask ventilation	
Cervical spine injury	Orotracheal intubation with in-line stabilization; fibreoptic intubation; surgical airway.

As swelling and oedema are progressive in the initial hours after injury, even an unobstructed airway may become compromised. Careful close monitoring in an intensive care unit (ICU) or high dependency unit (HDU) is essential. Maintaining the head-up position and the use of humidified oxygen may lessen the likelihood of later airway compromise. Sudden obstruction may occur with clot dislodgement and inhalation. Signs of partial obstruction include noisy breathing, stridor, intercostal, supraclavicular recession and restlessness.

Occasionally, patients may assume positions that lessen airway obstruction (e.g. sitting forward or even prone).[28] Simple measures such as suction and clearing the airway and insertion of an oropharyngeal airway may suffice.

In midfacial injuries, anterior digital traction on the mobile mid-segment may relieve obstruction.

In bilateral mandibular fractures of the angle or body, a towel clip or suture through the tongue may allow anterior traction on the unsupported tongue and relieve obstruction.

Bag and mask ventilation may be difficult due to distorted anatomy, and this should be borne in mind when a decision to intubate is made. Failure of these simple manoeuvres necessitates definitive airway management

TECHNIQUES (Fig. 66.2)

Facilities to perform a surgical airway must be available prior to elective intubation. The chosen technique for securing the airway depends on the presence of airway obstruction and the likelihood of difficult direct laryngoscopy (extent of jaw opening, gross anatomical distortion and swelling, operator experience).

In a combative patient, or if urgent intubation is necessary, then a rapid sequence induction can be used if laryngoscopic difficulty is not anticipated. If direct laryngoscopy is likely to be difficult or impossible, then spontaneous respiration must be maintained and intubation carried out under local anaesthesia. Analgesia can be achieved with a combination of sprayed or nebulized lignocaine (4%) to the posterior pharynx as well as a trans-cricoid injection of 2–4 ml lignocaine (2%). Adjunctive superior laryngeal and glossopharyngeal nerve blocks can be used.[29,30] The orotracheal route for intubation is the route of choice in the presence of basal skull fracture. If cervical spine injury is present or suspected, in-line stabilization is mandatory. A variety of intubation techniques can be used [e.g. direct laryngoscopy, fibreoptic guided laryngoscopy (oral/nasal), use of a light wand stylet, blind nasal and retrograde intubation techniques].[31,32] The operator should use the technique that he/she is most comfortable with. Excessive bleeding may render fibreoptic techniques useless. Failure to intubate in the presence of airway obstruction necessitates emergency cricothyroidotomy. Tracheostomy may be required in those likely to need prolonged ventilatory support (e.g. multiple facial fractures combined with a head injury) and

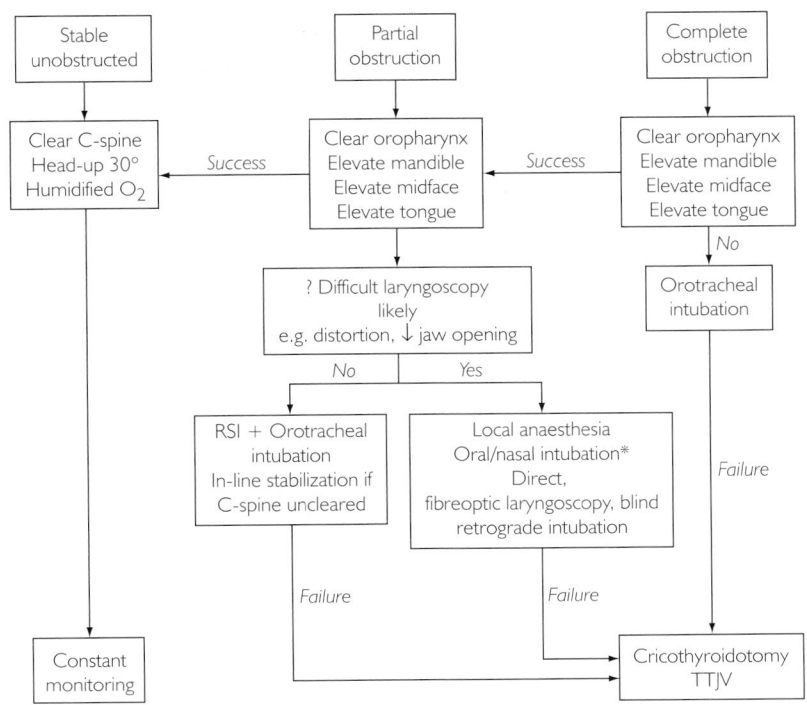

Fig. 66.2   An airway management algorithm for maxillofacial trauma. C-spine, cervical spine; TTJV, transtracheal jet ventilation; RSI, rapid sequence induction. *Nasotracheal route contra-indicated in basilar skull fracture

is best performed as a semi-elective procedure in the operating room.[16]

MANAGEMENT OF HAEMORRHAGE

Topical vasoconstrictors may not be effective with ongoing nasal haemorrhage. Anterior nasopharyngeal packs are sometimes effective at reducing blood loss. Foley catheters passed into the posterior nasopharynx with the balloons filled with air may stem blood loss, especially if anterior traction is applied.[20] Plastic or maxillofacial surgical opinion should be sought regarding operative reduction and stabilization of fractures and direct ligation of bleeding vessels if haemorrhage is persistent. External carotid ligation and angiographic embolization can be used as a last resort.

DEFINITIVE MANAGEMENT

Definitive surgery is generally delayed 4–10 days to allow swelling to subside. The timing of surgery may be further delayed if a severe head injury co-exists. Early surgery may be warranted if orbital injury with optic nerve compromise is present.

The use of high dose steroids in optic nerve compression is controversial and good data does not exist regard-

ing its efficacy[16]. Irrigation and debridement of open wounds, closure of facial lacerations and removal of foreign bodies must be undertaken as soon as is practicable, preferably within 24 h. The use of prophylactic antibiotics in the presence of basilar skull fracture and CSF leak is controversial and local protocols should be followed.[21] Appropriate tetanus prophylaxis must be given. Persistent CSF leaks (>2 weeks) or those complicated by meningitis, pneumocephalus are repaired surgically.[21] The use of modern internal fixation techniques have reduced the need for intermaxillary fixation following elective facial fracture repair, with only unstable comminuted fractures requiring this form of fixation. Submental intubation during fracture repair is now being used as an alternative to tracheostomy.[33]

INJURIES TO THE LARYNX AND TRACHEA

Direct trauma to the airway is rare, accounting for less than 1% of traumatic injury seen in most major centres.[15,34] The bony protection afforded to the airway by the sternum and mandible and death from asphyxia at the accident scene account for the rarity of the injury. Laryngotracheal injury can be classified as blunt or penetrating. Failure to recognize these injuries, their complications and specific pitfalls in airway management can lead to death.[35,36]

MECHANISM OF INJURY

BLUNT INJURY

Common causes include motor vehicle accidents where the extended neck impacts with the steering wheel or dashboard. The 'clothes line injury' occurs when a cyclist or horse rider collides with a cable or wire causing direct injury to the upper airway. Assaults and strangulation account for the remainder of blunt injuries. Direct blows are more likely to injure the cartilages of the larynx while flexion/extension injuries are most commonly associated with tracheal tears and laryngotracheal transection.[35] The larynx above the cricoid cartilage is injured in 35%, manifesting as oedema, contusions, haematomas, lacerations, avulsion and fracture dislocation, most commonly of the thyroid and arytenoid cartilages.

The cricoid cartilage itself is injured in 15%, which may cause recurrent laryngeal nerve dysfunction.[34] The cervical trachea is injured in 45%.[36] Tracheal transection most often occurs at the junction between the cricoid cartilage and trachea.[37] Oedema fluid and air dissecting within submucosal layers of the larynx and trachea may cause airway obstruction. Air in the soft tissues can cause epiglottic emphysema and narrowing of the supra glottic airway.[38] Straining, talking and coughing may worsen the oedema.

PENETRATING INJURY

Penetrating injuries usually result from stab and gunshot wounds. The anterior triangle of the neck is the most common site of entry. The cervical trachea is most commonly involved in stab wounds. The larynx is injured in about one-third of those with upper airway injuries.[36]

ASSOCIATED INJURIES

Common associations with blunt laryngotracheal injury include cervical spine, head injury and multisystem trauma. Of those with penetrating neck trauma, major vascular injuries (carotid, jugular, subclavian, vertebral arteries) occurs in 25–50%, pharyngeal or oesophageal injury in 30%, neural injury (spinal cord, brachial plexus) in 12% and apical thoracic injury in 10%.[7]

ASSESSMENT OF INJURY

Definitive investigation and management depend on the airway status and presence of associated injury. The degree of injury is not readily assessable on the basis of any one clinical symptom or sign (Table 66.2) and delayed diagnosis is common. Plain radiography (chest X-ray, cervical spine) is performed in all cases. CT scanning demonstrates fractures of cartilages, haematomas and other injuries, and is used in stable patients with laryngeal tenderness, endolaryngeal oedema and small haema-

tomas. When obvious signs of injury are not present and there is a satisfactory airway, fibreoptic laryngotracheoscopy under local anaesthesia can demonstrate vocal cord dysfunction, integrity of the cartilaginous framework and laryngeal mucosa. Rigid laryngoscopy can be used when adequate visualization is not achieved with the former. Pharyngo-oesophagoscopy, contrast studies, open exploration and angiography may be required to exclude aerodigestive tract and major vascular injuries.

AIRWAY MANAGEMENT

Major complications from airway manipulation can occur after laryngotracheal trauma. Blind intubation can lead to complete airway obstruction due to creation of false passages and mucosal disruption.[15] Cricoid pressure can lead to laryngotracheal separation and is contraindicated. Positive pressure ventilation can rapidly worsen air leaks and, wherever possible, the patient should maintain spontaneous respiration until a tube has been placed distal to the site of injury. Cricothyroidotomy is not recommended as it may compound laryngeal injury. Gaping airway wounds can be intubated under direct vision pending subsequent surgery.[36] The optimal mode of intubation is thus tracheostomy under local anaesthesia (Fig. 66.3). Excessive movement of the cervical spine during airway manipulation should be avoided in cases of blunt trauma.

Table 66.2 Clinical features in laryngotracheal injury

Symptoms
  Respiratory distress
  Hoarseness
  Dysphonia
  Cough
  Stridor, noisy breathing
  Dysphagia
Signs
  Abnormal laryngeal contour
  Subcutaneous emphysema
  Cervical ecchymosis
  Haemoptysis
Investigations
  Plain radiography
    Air in soft tissues
    Pneumomediastinum
    Pneumothorax
    Cervical spine fracture
  Computed tomography scan
    Cartilage and soft tissue injury
    Altered airway patency
  Laryngoscopy
    Vocal paralysis
    Mucosal or cartilage disruption
    Haematoma
    Laceration

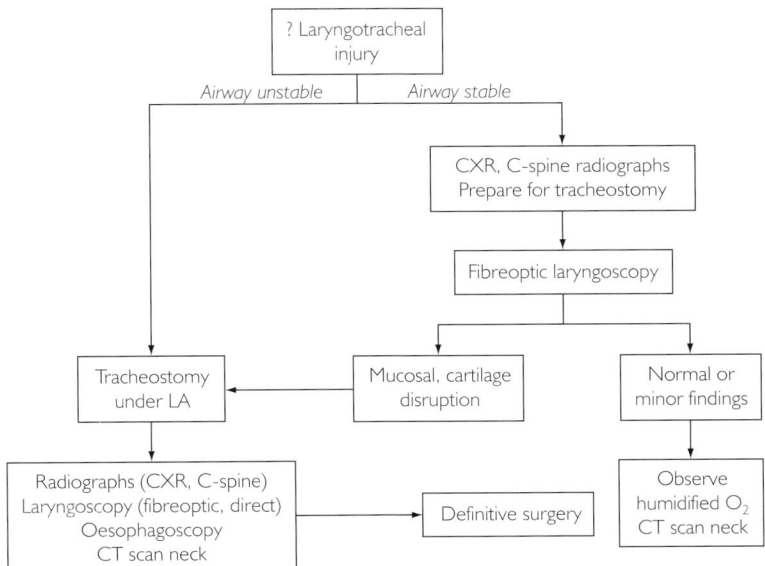

Fig. 66.3 Airway assessment and management algorithm for laryngotracheal trauma. CXR, chest X-ray; C-spine, cervical spine; CT, computed tomography; LA, local anaesthesia

REFERENCES

1 Gwyn PP, Carraway JH, Horton CE. Facial fractures: associated injuries and complications. *Plast Reconstr Surg* 1971; **47**: 225–30.
2 Tung T, Tseng WS, Chen CT, *et al*. Acute life threatening injuries in facial trauma patients: a review of 1025 patients. *J Trauma* 2000; **49**: 420–4.
3 Luce EA, Tubb TD, Moore AM. Review of 1000 major facial fractures and associated injuries. *Plast Reconstr Surg* 1979; **63**: 26–30.
4 Hogg NJ, Stewart TC, Armstrong JE, Girotti MJ. Epidemiology of maxillofacial injuries at trauma hospitals in Ontario, Canada, between 1992 and 1997. *J Trauma* 2000; **49**: 425–32.
5 Telfer MR, Jones GM, Shepherd JP. Trends in the aetiology of maxillofacial fractures in the United Kingdom (1977–1997). *Br J Oral Maxillofac Surg* 1991; **29**: 250–5.
6 Hussain KW, Wijetunge DB, Grubnic S, Jackson IT. A comprehensive analysis of craniofacial trauma. *J Trauma* 1994; **36**: 34–7.
7 Miller RH, Duplechain JK. Penetrating wounds of the neck. *Otolaryngologic Clin North Am* 1991; **24**: 15–29.
8 Halazonetis JA. The weak regions of the mandible. *Br J Oral Surg* 1968; **6**: 37–48.
9 Bavitz JB, Collicott PE. Bilateral mandibular fractures contributing to airway obstruction. *Int J Oral Maxillofac Surg* 1995; **24**: 273–5.
10 Seshul MB, Sinn DP, Gerlock AJ Jr. The Andy Gump fracture of the mandible: a cause of respiratory obstruction or distress. *J Trauma* 1978; **18**: 611–2.
11 Wenig BL. Management of panfacial fractures. *Otolaryn Clin North Am* 1991; **24**: 93–101.
12 Le Fort R. Experimental study of fractures of the upper jaw. *Rev Chir Paris* 1901; **23**: 208–27, 360–79 [reprinted in *Plast Reconstr Surg* 1972; **50**: 497–506].
13 Manson PN, Hoopes JE, Su CT. Structural pillars of the facial skeleton: an approach to the management of Le Fort fractures. *Plast Reconstr Surg* 1980; **66**: 54–61.
14 Cruise CW, Blevins PK, Luce EA. Naso-ethmoidal-orbital fractures. *J Trauma* 1980; **20**: 551–6.
15 Crosby R. The difficult airway 2. *Anesthesiol Clin North Am* 1997; **13**: 495–749.
16 Ardekian L, Rosen D, Peled M, *et al*. Life-threatening complications and irreversible damage following maxillofacial trauma. *Injury* 1998; **29**: 253–6.
17 Ardekian L, Samet N, Shoshani Y. Life threatening bleeding following maxillofacial trauma. *J Cranio-Maxillofac Surg* 1993; **21**: 336–40.
18 Thaller SR, Beal SL. Maxilofacial trauma: a potentially fatal injury. *Ann Plastic Surg* 1991; **27**: 281–90.
19 Buchanan RT, Holtmann B. Severe epistaxis in facial fractures. *Plast Reconstr Surg* 1983; **71**: 768–90.
20 Murakami WT, Davidson TM, Marshall LF. Fatal epistaxis and craniofacial trauma. *J Trauma* 1983; **23**: 57–61.
21 Marentette LJ, Valentino J. Traumatic anterior fossa cerebrospinal fluid fistulae and craniofacial considerations. *Otolaryn Clin North Am* 1991; **24**: 151–63.
22 Maxwell JA, Goldware SI. Use of adhesive in surgical treatment of cerebrospinal fluid leaks. *J Neurosurg* 1973; **39**: 322–36.
23 Laun A. Traumatic cerebrospinal fluid fistulae in the anterior and middle cranial fossae. *Acta Neurochir* 1982; **84**: 215–222.

24 Adams C, Januszkiewicz J, Judson J. Changing patterns of severe craniomaxillofacial trauma in Auckland over eight years. *Aust NZ J Surg* 2000; **70**: 401–4.

25 Davidson JSD, Birdsell BD. Cervical spine injury in patients with skeletal trauma. *J Trauma* 1989; **29**: 1276–8.

26 Schultz RC, Oldham RJ. An overview of facial injuries. *Surg Clin North Am* 1977; **57**: 987–1010.

27 Marciani RD, Israel S. Diagnosis of blunt carotid artery injuries in patients with facial trauma. *Oral Surg Oral Med Oral Pathol Oral Radiol Endod* 1997; **83**: 5–9.

28 Neal MR, Groves J, Gell IR. Awake fibreoptic intubation in the semi-prone position following facial trauma. *Anaesthesia* 1996; **51**: 1053–4.

29 Webb AR, Fernando SS, Dalton HR, *et al.* Local anaesthesia for fibreoptic bronchoscopy: transcricoid injection or the spray as you go technique. *Thorax* 1990; **45**: 474–7.

30 Gotta AW, Sullivan CA. Superior laryngeal nerve block: an aid to intubating the patient with a fractured mandible. *J Trauma* 1984; **24**: 83–5.

31 King H, Huntington C, Wooten D. Translaryngeal guided intubation in an uncooperative patient with maxillofacial injury: a case report. *J Trauma* 1994; **36**: 885–6.

32 Verdile VP, Chang JL, Bedger R. Nasotracheal intubation using a flexible lighted stylet. *Ann Emerg Med* 1990; **19**: 506–10.

33 Chandu A, Smith ACH, Gebert R. Submental intubation: an alternative to short-term tracheostomy. *Anaesth Intens Care* 2000; **28**: 193–5.

34 Gussack GS, Jurkovich GJ, Luterman F. Laryngotracheal trauma: a protocol approach to a rare injury. *Laryngoscope* 1986; **96**: 660–5.

35 Mathison DJ, Grillo H. Laryngotracheal trauma. *Ann Thorac Surg* 1987; **43**: 254–63.

36 Cicala RS, Kudsk KA, Butts A, *et al.* Initial evaluation and management of upper airway injuries in trauma patients. *J Clin Anesth* 1991; **3**: 91–8.

37 Trone TH, Schaefer SD, Carder HM. Blunt and penetrating laryngeal trauma: a 13 year review. *Otolaryngol Head Neck Surg* 1980; **88**: 257–61.

38 Sacco JJ, Halliday DW. Submucosa epiglottic emphysema complicating bronchial rupture. *Anesthesiology* 1987; **66**: 555–7.

67.

Chest injuries
G M Clarke

The commonest form of chest trauma in Australia is closed chest injury secondary to road traffic accident. Associated extrathoracic injuries, which themselves may be life threatening, are often present. Initial management is directed toward detection and correction of life threatening disorders. Swift assessment and resuscitation are carried out simultaneously. A team approach is necessary, with the team leader having clear management priorities. In almost every case, respiratory and circulatory resuscitation take precedence.

A secondary assessment is made after the initial assessment. During this time, detailed radiological and other imaging investigations are undertaken. The chest X-ray is an integral part of initial assessment and should be obtained as soon as possible. The 12-lead electrocardiogram (ECG) is an excellent filter for detecting myocardial injury in blunt chest trauma.[1]

IMMEDIATE MANAGEMENT

Obvious external bleeding is controlled and circulatory resuscitation initiated. Blood is sampled for cross-match, biochemistry and haematological tests. At the same time, respiratory and general measures (Table 67.1) are undertaken.

OXYGENATION

A clear airway must be assured. Oxygen is administered by face mask and ventilation assessed. Immediate endo-

Table 67.1 Immediate management of chest trauma

Assure patent airway, oxygenation and ventilation
Exclude or treat:
   Pneumothorax
   Haemothorax
   Cardiac tamponade
Assess for extrathoracic injuries
Decompress stomach
Provide pain relief
Reconsider endotracheal intubation, ventilation

tracheal intubation and controlled ventilation are indicated in compromised airways, severe head injury and gross hypoventilation and/or hypoxaemia unrelated to pneumothorax. Emergency cricothyroidotomy or tracheostomy is only rarely required when an upper respiratory tract obstruction cannot be bypassed by translaryngeal intubation.

PNEUMOTHORAX AND HAEMOTHORAX

Any pneumothorax and significant haemothorax is treated. Controlled ventilation in the presence of tension pneumothorax is potentially fatal. A 12 or 14-Fr i.v. cannula may be inserted percutaneously to relieve tension pneumothorax in dire emergencies. Usually, however, there is time to insert a wide bore intercostal catheter (ICC) under sterile conditions. An ICC directed superiorly through the second anterior intercostal space, 4 cm lateral to the sternal edge in adults, will adequately drain a non-loculated pneumothorax. Insertion through the mid-axillary line at the level of the nipple or above is recommended if a more lateral position is required. This site is preferred if a haemothorax is to be drained, with the tube directed posteriorly. Pneumothoraces are expected to be situated anteriorly in the supine patient and are hence more likely to be seen at the lung base. Radiological clues are basal hyperlucency, distinct visualization of diaphragm which may be depressed, distinct cardiac border and deepened costophrenic angle.

When inserting a chest tube, trocars are not recommended (to avoid penetration into lung or other organ). After sterile preparation and widespread infiltration with 1% lignocaine, the skin is incised and a pair of blunt forceps is used to dissect down to the pleura, which is then gently ruptured (Fig. 67.1). A gloved finger through this tract ascertains that lung is not adherent to chest wall, and the ICC is inserted. The ICC is attached to an underwater seal drain, with suction applied if necessary. It is unusual to require more than 20 cmH$_2$O suction pressure, although the system should have the capacity for 40–60 cmH$_2$O suction, with an airflow volume of 15–20 l/min.[2,3]

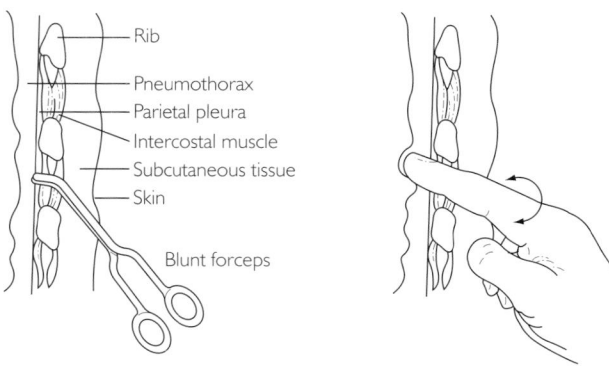

Fig. 67.1 Inserting an intercostal drain. Dissection is performed by blunt forceps. A gloved finger ascertains separation of lung from chest wall

CARDIAC TAMPONADE

Cardiac tamponade is suspected in any patient with thoracic trauma who has low blood pressure and raised venous pressure. Differential diagnoses include tension pneumothorax (most likely) and severe heart failure (usually due to gross myocardial contusion, or prolonged and inadequately treated shock). If readily available, transthoracic echocardiography (TTE) or transoesophageal echocardiography (TOE) can rapidly confirm or exclude tamponade. TTE performed in the emergency department (ED) by surgeons or ED specialists, is the diagnostic test of choice.[4,5] Table 67.2 shows the good results of surgeon performed ultrasound in rapid detection of pericardial effusion and haemothorax. Computed tomography (CT) scan will also reveal pericardial effusion, but is unsuitable for the unstable patient. In urgent situations the clinical diagnosis should be acted upon.

Emergency treatment of cardiac tamponade is aspiration of the pericardial sac, preferably under ECG control. The patient is positioned supine 35° head up. ECG limb leads are attached, and the chest lead is connected to the metal hub of the 16-Fr aspirating needle by a sterile wire. The needle with its plastic cannula is advanced towards the left shoulder at a 35° angle to the skin, from a point 2 cm below the apex of an angle formed between the xiphoid process and the left seventh costal cartilage (Fig. 67.2). Aspiration is made as the needle is slowly advanced. Remarkable improvement may follow the removal of as little as 30 ml of blood. Contact with the myocardium is denoted by ST elevation on the ECG, or ectopic beats. When a positive tap is obtained, the plastic cannula is left *in situ* for continued drainage. Alternatively, a pigtail catheter

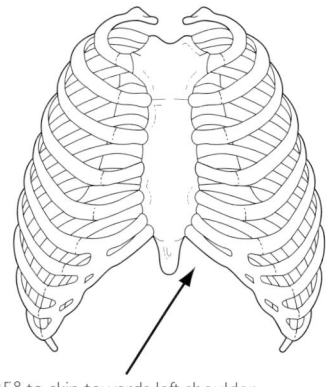

35° to skin towards left shoulder

Fig. 67.2 Approach to drain a pericardial effusion

(e.g. Pericardiocentesis set C-PCS-RPH-1 William A Cook, Australia) may be placed into the pericardial sac using a guidewire. Subsequent thoracotomy and full exploration will usually be necessary.

Many centres proceed to prompt thoracotomy with pericardial decompression, bypassing attempts at aspiration.[7,8] The surgical approach for penetrating chest wounds has been described.[9]

EXTRATHORACIC INJURIES

Extrathoracic trauma (i.e. head, neck, abdominal injuries and significant concealed blood loss) must be excluded. This initial rapid assessment should be made before potent analgesics are administered.

Table 67.2 Ultrasound diagnosis of pericardial effusion/haemothorax

	Sensitivity	Specificity
Ultrasound for pericardial effusion[5]	100%	96.9%
Ultrasound versus chest X-ray for haemothorax[6]	97.5 vs 92.5%	99.7 vs 99.7%

GASTRIC DECOMPRESSION

Gastric distension with attendant risks of regurgitation, vomiting and aspiration is extremely common, especially in patients with associated head injury. The stomach should be decompressed by a nasogastric tube (or orogastric tube in suspected base of skull fractures). If urgent endotracheal intubation is necessary, a rapid sequence intubation (with cricoid pressure) is recommended.

PAIN RELIEF

Pain relief is obtained at this early stage with i.v. opioids. This will frequently relieve respiratory distress in patients with fractures of the ribs and/or sternum.

RECONSIDERATION OF MECHANICAL VENTILATORY SUPPORT

After the initial management, mechanical ventilatory support should be reconsidered (Table 67.3). Ventilation should also be considered for patients with borderline respiratory distress associated with:

- Gross obesity
- Significant pre-existing lung disease
- Severe pulmonary contusion or aspiration
- Severe abdominal injuries requiring surgery

SPECIFIC THORACIC INJURIES

Specific thoracic injuries should be systematically excluded. Imaging techniques play an important role. Choice of investigation is influenced by clinical findings including the degree of haemodynamic and respiratory instability, which determines whether a patient can be moved to an imaging facility. Local availability of equipment, and the expertise of clinicians and imaging specialists are important.

RUPTURED AORTA

The majority of traumatic ruptures of the aorta occur at the isthmus situated at the junction of the mobile arch and fixed descending aorta, immediately beyond the origin of the left subclavian artery. Rupture at this site is attributed to forward movement of the mobile arch

Table 67.3 Major indications for endotracheal intubation and ventilation

Dangerous hypoxaemia and/or hypercarbia
Significant head injury
Gross flail segment and contusion and respiratory distress

against the tethered descending aorta in a deceleration situation (e.g. motor vehicle accident). In about 10% of cases, rupture is in the ascending aorta or near the origin of the other great vessels. These tears are usually due to direct trauma.

Vascular injury in blunt chest trauma may be suspected on clinical or chest X-ray findings, or on the history of how the patient was injured. Clinical findings may be unequal upper limb pulses or acute coarctation syndrome (such clinical findings are uncommon).

A widened mediastinum always arouses suspicion of a ruptured aorta.[10] In one series, mediastinal width greater than 8 cm at the level of the aortic arch was present in all 10 patients with ruptured thoracic aorta.[11] Diagnosis is enhanced by one or more of the following radiological features:

- Left haemothorax
- Depressed left main bronchus
- Blurred outline of the arch or descending aorta
- Fractured first rib or left apical haematoma
- Displacement of the mid-oesophagus to the right (easily detectable with a nasogastric tube *in situ*)

Other suspicious radiological features include loss of the aorticopulmonary window, anterior or lateral deviation of the trachea, loss of the paraspinal 'stripe', thoracic spine fracture and calcium layering in the aortic arch. Despite suggestive findings in some cases, the chest X-ray alone is of limited utility in the diagnosis of blunt traumatic aortic laceration.[12] Strongly suggestive history includes: motor vehicle, motor cycle or pedestrian versus car crash at greater than 40–45 mph (64–72 kph), significant deceleration in motor vehicle crash, severe broad side collision, death of another victim in the crash, all indicating that further investigation should be considered.[1] Although, in most centres, aortography remains the gold standard investigation,[13] the selective advantages of contrast enhanced CT, TOE and angiography in differing situations is increasingly recognized.[14] Table 67.4 outlines the advantages, disadvantages and accuracy of commonly used imaging techniques.[15–20] TOE can be undertaken in haemodynamically unstable patients without moving to an imaging facility. It provides excellent images of the distal aortic arch and descending aorta, especially the isthmus.[20–24] Although of similar sensitivity as helical CT in diagnosing subadventitial disruption, TOE is more sensitive in diagnosing intimal and medial layer aortic injuries.[14] Disadvantages of TOE are that it is operator dependent and visualization of the ascending aorta and branches coming off the arch may be less than ideal. Fig. 67.3 shows an investigational flow chart suitable for centres where helical CT and multiplane TOE are readily available.

Traditionally management of traumatic aortic injury has been prompt surgery. Over the past 10–15 years, significant variations have included non-operative or delayed definitive management,[25] use of endovascular stents for repair[26] and use of centrifugal pumps during

Table 67.4 Comparison of imaging techniques with special reference to aortic and great arterial injury

	Advantages	Disadvantages	Sensitivity %	Specificity %	Accuracy %
Chest X-ray	Readily available. Essential screen for thoracic injuries	Low positive predictive value 10–15%	90–95[11,15]	5–10[11,15]	
Helical CT	Accurate Detects intramural lesion	Moving the unstable patient Concurrent CT imaging of other body areas	100[16], 100[17], 100[18]	81.7[16], 83[17], 99.7[18]	86[17], 99.7[18]
TEE	No need to move unstable patient Rapid assessment Aortic isthmus Cardiac lesions Detects intramural lesion, intimal tears	Distal aortic arch and branches poorly seen Need for sedation, possible ET intubation Problem if facial, larynx, pharyngeal, oesophageal injury	93[19], 100[20]	98[19], 98[20]	98[19]
Angiography	Image entire aorta and branches.	Takes time and more staff, expertise May miss intramural lesion and small tears	94.4[16], 92[17]	96.3[16], 99[17]	97[17]

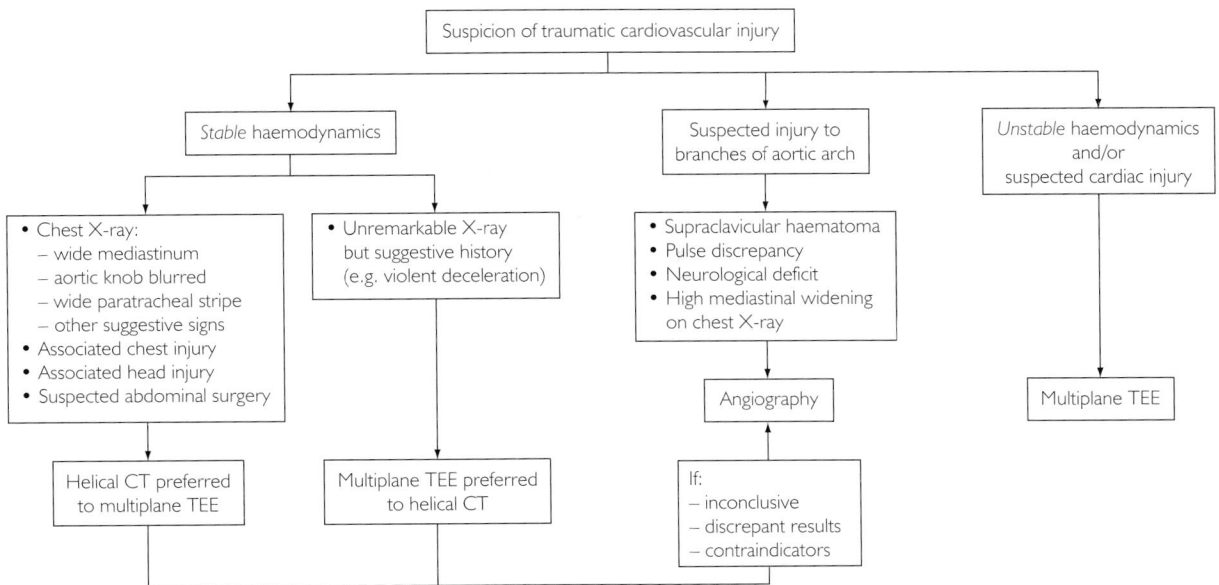

Fig. 67.3   Investigational flow chart for traumatic cardiovascular injury (adapted from Vignon *et al.*[14])

operative repair.[27] Patients with multiple associated injuries, particularly brain and lungs, are a subset who benefit most from deferred repair.[1] Similarly, those with injuries limited to intimal and medial layers of the aorta may be managed medically. Such management is similar to that for descending thoracic aortic dissection with β-blockers and vasodilators, maintaining a mean arterial pressure of 60–70 mmHg. The use of centrifugal pumps during operative repair may decrease the incidence of paraplegia.[1]

RUPTURED DIAPHRAGM AND DIAPHRAGMATIC PARESIS

The usual cause of a ruptured diaphragm is gross abdominal compression, and the incidence may have risen since seat belts were made compulsory.[28] Rupture of the left diaphragm is more common.[29] A haemopneumothorax is commonly misdiagnosed when the dilated stomach gives a horizontal air–fluid interface on the erect chest X-ray. Misdiagnosis is less likely if a nasogastric tube is *in situ*, when the distal end is noted to be in an abnormal position. A ruptured diaphragm as an isolated injury is often surprisingly well tolerated by the patient. Nevertheless, with a left diaphragmatic rupture, there is significant risk of gut strangulation, and surgical repair should follow basic resuscitation.

Rupture of the right diaphragm is more difficult to diagnose because of the liver. The radiographic appearance is similar to a paralysed right diaphragm. In the absence of right sided rib fractures, a small haemothorax with a high right diaphragm is suggestive evidence. Magnetic resonance imaging provides coronal and sagittal imaging, and

direct visualization of the diaphragm. It has been recommended to diagnose ruptured diaphragm if CT is non-diagnostic.[30] Video thoracoscopy is another diagnostic approach. Repair of ruptured diaphragm via an abdominal approach is recommended, as more than 75% of such cases have associated intra-abdominal injury.[31]

Unilateral and bilateral phrenic nerve palsy are occasionally seen after blunt chest trauma. The bilateral form results in classical paradoxical abdominal to chest wall movement, orthopnoea, reduced vital capacity and difficulty in weaning from ventilation.[32] Diaphragmatic dysfunction may also occur following upper abdominal surgery. This is possibly due to reflex inhibition of diaphragmatic activity.[33] Any respiratory dysfunction secondary to diaphragmatic paresis will be greatly magnified by the presence of other chest wall or lung injury.

DISRUPTION OF MAJOR AIRWAYS

Although signs and symptoms may vary according to the level of the rupture, the clinical picture is frequently that of respiratory distress, subcutaneous emphysema and haemoptysis.[34] A pneumothorax, which may be under tension, is invariably present with ruptured bronchus. Mediastinal emphysema is commonly seen on the chest X-ray. With tracheal injuries, immediate management involves endotracheal intubation (with the cuff positioned distal to the tear) to prevent aspiration and ablate the air leak. Any pneumothorax must be drained. Suction to the intercostal catheter may be necessary.

When initial priorities are achieved, bronchoscopy and early primary repair are undertaken. A double-lumen tube may be necessary for operative repair and if air leak is significant. If a neck wound is large, an endotracheal tube can be passed via the neck and tracheal wound in emergency situations. Difficult intubation may be accomplished by a flexible bronchoscope. Once the airway is secure, general anaesthesia and other interventions may be undertaken.[35]

MASSIVE HAEMOTHORAX

Disruption of intercostal and/or internal mammary arteries is a common cause.[36] The condition is usually fatal if caused by massive bleeding from the aorta or major pulmonary arteries. Immediate management involves insertion of a wide bore ICC and adequate resuscitation. Continued significant blood loss is an indication for early thoracotomy,[36] a recent study recommending this be undertaken if chest drain blood loss exceeds 1500 ml within 24 hours.[37] Inadequate drainage of a haemothorax may require a thoracotomy and decortication at a later date, but this is rarely necessary.[38]

PULMONARY CONTUSION

The classical view of pulmonary contusion is that bruised lung is not confined within anatomical segments, and becomes more oedematous over the next 48 h. However, CT evaluation has revealed that such pulmonary infiltration and consolidation is, in fact, a pulmonary laceration surrounded by intra-alveolar haemorrhage ('blood pneumonia') without significant interstitial injury.[39] Such lacerations have been classified into four types according to CT pattern, mechanism of injury, location of rib fracture or surgical findings.[40] When pulmonary contusion is associated with a severe flail segment and respiratory distress, assisted ventilation is required (which is usually short-term).[41] Laceration involving the lung surface may be treated using video-assisted thoracoscopy.[42] This technology has also been used to diagnose and treat diaphragmatic injuries and to evacuate clotted haemothoraces.[1]

MYOCARDIAL CONTUSION

Myocardial contusion is common in blunt chest trauma and may result in arrhythmias, conduction disturbances, and cardiac failure. Such complications should be managed as in myocardial infarction. A standard 12-lead ECG may show a variety of abnormalities, ranging from non-specific T wave changes to pathological Q waves. TOE may show cardiac wall motion abnormalities.[12] Abnormalities can also be demonstrated by myocardial nuclear scanning (not normally undertaken in the acutely injured patient). Serious damage to virtually every cardiac structure has been reported.[43] Cardiac injuries (e.g. rupture of the ventricular free wall, interventricular septum and valvular apparatus) and disruption of major coronary arteries are usually associated with penetrating injuries, but have also been reported in non-penetrating chest trauma.[44] Again, TOE may aid in diagnosis. Creatine-kinase myocardial-type enzymes and troponin I are frequently elevated in cases of suspected myocardial contusion. Sternal fractures (more common in females, the elderly and in those wearing seat belts) are associated with a low incidence of cardiac contusion and arrhythmias.[45,46]

SYSTEMIC AIR EMBOLISM

This is more frequent in penetrating injuries and is immediately life threatening. It is probably under-diagnosed, as it is unlikely to be proven at conventional autopsy.[47] Air embolism is usually caused by a bronchopulmonary vein fistula. It is suspected in the chest injured patient if:

- Focal neurological signs exist in the absence of head injury
- Circulatory collapse immediately follows controlled ventilation in the absence of tension pneumothorax
- Froth is obtained when arterial blood is sampled from a collapsed patient
- Cranial CT reveals negative density streaks reproducing casts of cerebral arteries

When suspected, the FiO_2 should be increased to 1.0 and ventilation pressures and volumes reduced to a minimum. Hyperbaric oxygen therapy, though indicated, is unlikely to be practical. Mattox[48] recommends urgent thoracotomy, to clamp the ascending aorta, remove air source (e.g. by clamping the pulmonary hilum) and aspirate free air from the left ventricle and ascending aorta. Spontaneous ventilation is preferred in any patient at risk of systemic air embolism,[49] especially those with penetrating lung wounds. If assisted ventilation is necessary, it has been recommended lung isolation devices be considered (double lumen tube or bronchial blocker) and/or high frequency ventilation.[49]

OESOPHAGEAL PERFORATION

Although usually due to penetrating injury, it can occur rarely with closed chest trauma. The patient may complain of retrosternal pain and difficulty in swallowing, and exhibit haematemesis and cervical emphysema. A chest X-ray may show mediastinal emphysema, widened mediastinum, pneumothorax, hydrothorax or hydro-pneumothorax. If suspected, a gastrografin swallow and/or endoscopy is performed. Treatment is immediate surgical repair.

SIGNIFICANCE OF FLAIL CHEST

A flail segment is no longer the dominant issue in chest injuries, but its significance should not be overlooked. The concept of pendulluft (to-and-fro movement of air between the flail and less affected sides of the thorax) has been shown to be incorrect.[50] With flail chest, overall ventilation may be reduced, but it is distributed to both lungs, because the mediastinal shift equalizes the pleural pressures. Nevertheless, there is poor expansion in contused, low compliant lung areas, impairment of coughing and seriously reduced ventilation in gross cases. Moreover, the greater the flail segment, the less the negative intrapleural pressure that can be generated for inspiration. Gross mediastinal shifts may impair systemic circulation.

PAIN CONTROL

Adequate pain relief is extremely important. It is the major determinant of whether deep breathing and efficient coughing are possible, thereby avoiding endotracheal intubation in non-severe injuries. Choice of pain relief may vary during the course of management. Options include:

- i.v. opioids by frequent, intermittent small doses, or by continuous infusion.
- Entonox inhalation during physiotherapy.
- Intercostal nerve block
  (a) multiple individual nerve blocks (repeated as necessary)
  (b) single large volume (e.g. 20 ml 0.5% bupivacaine) into one intercostal space (unilaterally or bilaterally), spreading to block nerves above and below the site injected[51]
  (c) intrapleural bupivacaine (0.25–0.5%) via unilateral or bilateral ICCs (epidural catheters have been used), using intermittent injections or continuous infusion[52]
- Epidural anaesthesia.
- Epidural or spinal opioids.
- Non-steroidal anti-inflammatory agents (in fully resuscitated patients with normal renal function).

RESPIRATORY SUPPORT

While several basic approaches to managing the chest injured patient have emerged (Table 67.5), the ultimate strategy is determined by the severity of chest injury, associated injuries and effectiveness of pain relief. All these factors influence respiratory dysfunction.

CONSERVATIVE THERAPY

Conservative treatment involves oxygen by mask, adequate pain relief and physiotherapy. It is the treatment in mild injury (i.e. isolated thoracic injury with fractured ribs, but without significant flail or disturbed blood gases). Similarly, it may be employed in moderate chest injury (i.e. significant flail but with adequate blood gases and the ability to cough). Prophylactic ventilation in these two groups is deemed inappropriate, with possible disadvantages of barotrauma, infection, tracheostomy complications and prolongation of hospitalization.[53,54]

Table 67.5   Respiratory support of the chest injured patient

Conservative
Non-invasive respiratory assistance (via face mask)
    Continuous positive-airways pressure (CPAP)
    Pressure support ventilation (PSV)
    Bi-level positive airway pressure (BiPAP)
Invasive respiratory assistance (via a tracheal tube)
    CPAP
    PSV ± positive end-expiratory pressure (PEEP)
    intermittent mandatory ventilation ± PEEP ± PSV
    pressure control ventilation ± PEEP
    volume control ventilation ± PEEP
    high frequency ventilation (major air leaks)
    independent lung ventilation ± PEEP
Surgical stabilization ± other measures

NON-INVASIVE RESPIRATORY ASSISTANCE

Even with moderately severe, isolated chest injuries, endotracheal intubation can be avoided, provided adequate analgesia is assured, and the patient can tolerate a close fitting face mask for non-invasive respiratory assistance. A preset airway pressure and the face mask lessen the risk of barotrauma. Patient tolerance for these non-invasive methods is variable. In a trial where 69 patients were randomly allocated to continuous positive-airways pressure (CPAP) by mask combined with regional analgesia, or endotracheal intubation and mechanical ventilation plus positive end-expiratory pressure, clinical outcomes were superior in the CPAP group. With CPAP there was significantly shorter duration of active treatment, shorter intensive care unit (ICU) stay and less infection.[55]

INVASIVE RESPIRATORY ASSISTANCE

This is necessary in severe chest injuries and if head injury is associated. Tracheal intubation is achieved by oral or nasal routes or a tracheostomy. Tracheostomy offers advantages over translaryngeal intubation in the conscious patient

- Decreased discomfort
- Reduced need for sedation
- Less resistance to breathing

Percutaneous tracheostomy may be undertaken in the ICU. Early use of intermittent mandatory ventilation is claimed to result in a shorter duration of assisted ventilation.[56] Currently, most centres use pressure control and pressure support ventilation to promote early weaning and reduce the incidence of barotrauma. Pressure ventilatory modes also provide some compensation for air leaks. Continuous positive airway pressure alone has not been fully evaluated, although it is used extensively during weaning. In patients with flail segments, inappropriate conservative therapy or poor ventilatory support may result in increased residual chest deformity. Independent lung ventilation may be used to treat a unilateral pulmonary contusion and/or flail.[57]

SURGICAL STABILIZATION

Interest is periodically revived in surgical stabilization of the chest wall. Advantages claimed are a shorter period of assisted ventilation or a shorter hospital stay.[58,59] Internal surgical stabilization undoubtedly reduces deformity, and a stable chest wall will help a patient to cope with an underlying lung problem. However, except for a fractured sternum, rupture of the diaphragm, and in the course of an otherwise necessary thoracotomy, the case for surgical repair has yet to be established.[60]

COMPLICATIONS

Following resuscitation and initial management, complications may follow and require treatment.

SPUTUM RETENTION

Sputum retention can precipitate or worsen respiratory distress and lead to pulmonary collapse. Infection is then more likely. Minimizing sputum retention in the spontaneously breathing patient includes adequate analgesia without marked respiratory depression. In the intubated/ventilated patient, efficient humidification and endobronchial toilet are essential. Frequent position changes are important. If clearing secretions remains difficult despite adequate pain relief, a minitracheostomy (e.g. 5.4 mm outer diameter tube via a percutaneous cricothyroidectomy) may avoid conventional endotracheal intubation or tracheostomy.

BRONCHOSPASM

Bronchospasm is managed conventionally. Its occurrence suggests the possibility of aspiration.

BAROTRAUMA

Barotrauma is more common in the mechanically ventilated patient. It may also occur in the spontaneously breathing patient with chest injuries several days after admission, especially if respiratory distress is present. Surgical emphysema, mediastinal emphysema, pneumothorax, pulmonary interstitial emphysema and pneumoperitoneum can all occur.

In patients with surgical and/or mediastinal emphysema, some authorities recommend insertion of ICCs if anaesthesia or mechanical ventilation is planned, even though pneumothorax is not evident on chest X-ray. CT scan is very sensitive to confirm or exclude pneumothorax, and may be used to avoid ICC tube insertion.

ACUTE RESPIRATORY FAILURE

Acute respiratory failure is common. When the acute lung injury (or acute respiratory distress syndrome, ARDS) occurs early after trauma, possible causes include pulmonary contusion, aspiration, prolonged shock or delayed resuscitation, and massive mediator release following multitrauma and fat embolism. When ARDS develops many days after injury, infection, which may originate from a site remote from the lungs, is a more likely cause.

INFECTION

Infection remains a major cause of death in chest injuries. The source of such infection is invariably endogenous, mainly from bacteria colonizing the patient's oropharynx and alimentary tract. Some authorities recommend parenteral antibiotic prophylaxis (e.g. cefotaxime) active against community bacteria (e.g. *Streptococcus pneumoniae, Haemophilus influenzae, Branhamella catarrhalis, Staphylococcus aureus,* or *Escherichia coli*) from the time of admission for four days. At the same time, oral and intragastric non-absorbable combinations of polymyxin E, tobramycin and amphotericin B are administered, to prevent colonization and infection by *Enterobacter, Pseudomonas* and fungi such as *Candida*.[61] However, the value of this strategy continues to attract analysis and discussion.[62,63]

The importance of hand washing between attending patients and meticulous attention to sterile techniques in respiratory care and management of invasive catheters cannot be over-emphasized. Early enteral feeding may decrease translocation of bacteria and toxins from the gut and thus reduce the incidence of sepsis.[64]

THROMBOEMBOLISM

Preventative measures include frequent movement, leg stockings, avoidance of pressure on limbs, and low dose subcutaneous heparin (5000 units b.d. or t.d.s.), or low molecular weight heparin in appropriate dose.

INADEQUATE NUTRITION

Gastric atony and stasis are common. In many cases adequate enteral nutrition is possible by appropriate posturing (e.g. on right side during feeding). Metoclopramide or cisapride may be used to promote gastric emptying. Nasojejunal feeding is usually successful when these measures fail. Parenteral nutrition is sometimes necessary.

STRESS ULCERATION

Ranitidine 50 mg i.v. t.d.s. or 150 mg orally b.d. is commonly used for prophylaxis. Early resuscitation is considered to be an important factor in reducing the incidence of this complication, as is early introduction of enteral feeding.

COAGULOPATHIES

Prompt resuscitation, control of haemorrhage, and possibly use of blood filters for massive blood transfusion help in this regard.

PROGNOSIS

Reported mortality rates in chest injured patients vary greatly, reflecting severity of the chest injury and associ-

Table 67.6   Chest related death in blunt chest trauma[67]

Chest injury	Chest related death	Odds ratio
Three fractured ribs unilateral	17.3%	1.01
Three fractured ribs bilaterally	40.9%	3.43
Lung contusion unilateral	25.2%	1.82
Contusion bilateral and haemothorax	53.5%	5.1

ated extrathoracic injuries. In one Australian series[65] of 1119 patients with chest and other injuries, the overall mortality rate was 5.3%. The three commonest causes of death were respiratory tract sepsis (35.6%), severe head injury (33.9%) and exsanguination (18.6%). Mortality was 37.5% for patients over 60 years who had respiratory failure, and 22.8% for all age groups requiring mechanical ventilation. Trunkey reported a 16% mortality in patients with isolated pulmonary contusion. When combined with a significant flail chest, the mortality rose to 42%.[66] The results of a more recent retrospective study of 1495 patients with thoracic trauma and multiple associated injuries are shown in Table 67.6.[67]

REFERENCES

1 Feliciano DV, Rozycki GS. Advances in the diagnosis and treatment of thoracic trauma. *Surg Clin North Am* 1999; **79**: 1417–29.

2 Symbas PN. Chest drainage tubes. *Surg Clin North Am* 1989; **69**: 41–6.

3 Munnel ER, Thomas EK. Current concepts in thoracic drainage systems. *Ann Thoracic Surg* 1975; **19**: 261–8.

4 Rozycki GS, Ballard RB, Feliciano DV *et al.* Surgeon performed ultrasound for the assessment of truncal injuries: lessons learned from 1540 patients. *Ann Surg* 1998; **228**: 557–67.

5 Rozycki GS, Feliciano DV, Ochsner MG, *et al.* The role of ultrasound in patients with possible penetrating cardiac wounds; a prospective, multicentre study. *J Trauma* 1999; **46**: 543–52.

6 Sisley AC, Rozycki GS, Ballard RB, *et al.* Rapid detection of traumatic effusion using surgeon performed ultrasonography. *J Trauma* 1998; **44**: 291–7.

7 Bodai BI, Smith JP, Blaisdell FW. The role of emergency thoracotomy in blunt trauma. *J Trauma* 1982; **22**: 487–90.

8 Baker CC, Thomas AN, Trunkey DD. The role of emergency room thoracotomy in trauma. *J Trauma* 1980; **20**: 848–55.

9 Mitchell ME, Muakkassa FF, Poole GV, *et al.* Surgical approach of choice for penetrating cardiac wounds. *J Trauma* 1993; **34**: 17–20.

10 Turney SZ, Attar S, Ayella R, *et al.* Traumatic rupture of the aorta. A five year experience. *J Thorac Cardiovasc Surg* 1976; **72**: 727–32.

11 Kram HB, Wohlmuth DA, Appel PL, Shoemaker WC. Clinical and radiological indications for aortography in blunt chest trauma. *J Vasc Surg* 1987; **6**: 168–75.

12 Cook AD, Klein JS, Rogers FB, *et al.* Chest radiographs of limited utility in the diagnosis of blunt traumatic aortic laceration. *J Trauma* 2001; **50**: 843–7.

13 Fabian TC, Richardson JD, Croce MA, *et al.* Prospective study of blunt aortic injury: multicentre trial of the American Association for the Surgery of Trauma. *J Trauma* 1997; **42**: 374–83.

14 Vignon P, Boncoeur M-P, Francois B, *et al.* Comparison of multiplane transoesophageal echocardiography and contrast enhanced helical CT in the diagnosis of blunt cardiovascular injuries. *Anesthesiology* 2001; **94**: 615–22.

15 Woodring JH. The normal mediastinum in blunt traumatic rupture of the thoracic aorta and brachiocephalic arteries. *J Emerg Med* 1990; **8**: 467–76.

16 Gavant ML, Menke PG, Fabian T, *et al.* Blunt traumatic aortic rupture: detection with helical CT of the chest. *Radiology* 1995; **197**: 125–33.

17 Fabian TC, Davis KA, Gavant ML, *et al.* Prospective study of blunt aortic injury: helical CT is diagnostic and antihypertensive therapy reduces rupture. *Ann Surg* 1998; **227**: 666–77.

18 Mirvis SE, Shanmuganathan K, Buell J, *et al.* Use of spiral computed tomography for the assessment of blunt trauma patients with potential aortic injury. *J Trauma* 1998; **45**: 922–30.

19 Chirillo F, Totis O, Cavarzerani A *et al.* Usefulness of transthoracic and transoesophageal echocardiography in recognition and management of cardiovascular injuries after blunt chest trauma. *Heart* 1996; **75**: 301–6.

20 Smith MD, Cassidy JM, Souther S, *et al.* Transesophageal echocardiography in the diagnosis of traumatic rupture of the aorta. *N Engl J Med* 1995; **332**: 356–62.

21 Riou B, Goarin JP, Saada M. Assessment of severe blunt chest trauma. In: Vincent J-L (ed). *Yearbook of Intensive Care and Emergency Medicine*. Springer-Verlag, Berlin, Heidelberg, New York; 1993: pp. 611–8.

22 Brathwaite CE, Cilley JM, O'Connor WH, *et al.* The pivotal role of transesophageal echocardiography in the management of traumatic thoracic aortic rupture with associated intra-abdominal haemorrhage. *Chest* 1994; **105**: 1899–901.

23 Books SW, Young JC, Cmolik B, *et al.* The use of transesophageal echocardiography in the evaluation of chest trauma. *J Trauma* 1992; **32**: 761–5.

24 Goarin JP, Le Bret F, Riou B, *et al.* Early diagnosis of traumatic aortic rupture by transesophageal echocardiography. *Chest* 1993; **103**: 618–9.

25 Pate JW, Gavant ML, Weiman DS, *et al.* Traumatic rupture of the aortic isthmus: program of selective management. *World J Surg* 1999; **23**: 59–63.

26 Fujikawa T, Yukioka T, Ishimaru S, *et al.* Endovascular stent grafting for the treatment of blunt thoracic aortic injury. *J Trauma* 2001; **50**: 223–9.

27 Oliver JF Jr, Maher TD, Liebler GA, *et al.* Use of the BioMedicus centrifugal pump in traumatic tears of the thoracic aorta. *Ann Thorac Surg* 1984; **38**: 586–92.

28 Ryan P, Ragazzon R. Abdominal injuries in survivors of road trauma before and since seat belt legislation in Victoria. *Aust NZ J Surg* 1979; **49**: 200–2.

29 Aronoff RJ, Reynolds, J, Thal ER. Evaluation of diaphragmatic injuries. *Am J Surg* 1982; **144**: 671–4.

30 Mirvis SE, Keramati B, Anderson JC. MR imaging of traumatic diaphragmatic rupture. *J Comput Assist Tomogr* 1988; **12**: 147–9.

31 Strug B, Noon GP, Beall AC Jr. Traumatic diaphragmatic hernia. *Ann Thorac Surg* 1974; **17**: 444–9.

32 Sandham JD, Shaw DT, Guenter CA. Acute supine respiratory failure due to bilateral diaphragmatic paralysis. *Chest* 1977; **72**: 96–8.

33 Ford GT, Whitelaw WA. Rosenal TW, *et al.* Diaphragm function after upper abdominal surgery in humans. *Am Rev Resp Dis* 1983; **127**: 431–6.

34 Lewis FR. Thoracic trauma. *Surg Clin North Am* 1982; **62**: 97–104.

35 Pate JW. Tracheobronchial and oesophageal injuries. *Surg Clin North Am* 1989; **69**: 111–23.

36 Kish G, Kozloff L, Joseph WL, Adkins PC. Indications for early thoracotomy in the management of chest trauma. *Ann Thorac Surg* 1976; **22**: 23–8.

37 Karmy-Jones R, Jurkovich GJ, Nathens AB, *et al.* Timing of urgent thoracotomy for haemorrhage after trauma. *Arch Surg* 2001; **136**: 513–8.

38 Wilson JM, Boren CH Jr, Peterson SR, Thomas AN. Traumatic hemothorax: is decortication necessary? *J Thorac Cardiovasc Surg* 1979; **77**: 489–94.

39 Wagner RB, Jamieson PM. Pulmonary contusion. *Surg Clin North Am* 1989; **69**: 31–40.

40 Wagner RB, Crawford WO Jr, Schimpf PP. Classification of parenchymal injuries of the lung. *Radiology* 1988; **167**: 77–82.

41 Richardson JD, Adams L, Flint LM. Selective management of flail chest and pulmonary contusion. *Ann Surg* 1982; **196**: 481–6.

42 Kaseda S, Aoki T, Hangai N, *et al.* A case of deep laceration of the lung treated with video-assisted thoracic surgical lobectomy: case report. *J Trauma* 1997; **43**: 856–8.

43 Bancewicz J, Yates D. Blunt injury to the heart. *Br Med J* 1983; **286**: 497.

44 Madoff IM, Desforges G. Cardiac injuries due to nonpenetrating thoracic trauma. *Ann Thorac Surg* 1972; **14**: 504–11.

45 Hills MW, Delprado AM, Deane SA. Sternal fractures: associated injuries and management. *J Trauma* 1993; **35**: 55–60.

46 Brookes JG, Dunn RJ, Roger IR. Sternal fractures: a retrospective analysis of 272 cases. *J Trauma* 1993; **35**: 46–54.

47 Thomas AN, Stephen BG. Air embolism: a cause of morbidity and death after penetrating chest trauma. *J Trauma* 1974; **14**: 633–8.

48 Mattox K. Indicators for thoracotomy: deciding to operate. *Surg Clin North Am* 1989; **69**: 47–58.

49 Ho AM, Ling E. Systemic air embolism after lung trauma. *Anesthesiology* 1999; **90**: 564–75.

50 Maloney JV, Schmutzer KJ, Raschke E. Paradoxical respiration and 'Pendulluft'. *J Thorac Cardiovasc Surg* 1961; **41**: 291–8.

51 O'Kelly E, Garry B. Continuous pain relief for multiple fractured ribs. *Br J Anaesth* 1981; **53**: 989–91.

52 Rocco A, Reiestad F, Gudman J, McKay W. Intrapleural administration of local anesthetics for pain relief in patients with multiple rib fractures. *Regional Anesth* 1987; **12**: 10–4.

53 Shackford SR, Smith DE, Zarins CK, *et al.* The management of flail chest. A comparison of ventilatory and non-ventilatory treatment. *Am J Surg* 1976; **132**: 759–62.

54 Trinkle JK, Richardson JD, Franz JL, *et al.* Management of flail chest without mechanical ventilation. *Ann Thorac Surg* 1975; **19**: 355–63.

55 Bolliger CT, Van Eeden SF. Treatment of multiple rib fractures. Randomised controlled trial comparing ventilatory and non-ventilatory management. *Chest* 1990; **97**: 943–8.

56 Cullen P, Modell JH, Kirby RR, *et al.* Treatment of flail chest. Use of intermittent mandatory ventilation and positive end expiratory pressure. *Arch Surg* 1975; **110**: 1099–103.

57 Hillman KM, Barber JD. Asynchronous independent lung ventilation (AILV). *Crit Care Med* 1980; **8**: 390–5.

58 Paris F, Tarazona V, Blasco E, *et al.* Surgical stabilization of traumatic flail chest. *Thorax* 1975; **30**: 521–7.

59 Moore BP. Operative stabilisation of non-penetrating chest injuries. *J Thorac Cardiovasc Surg* 1975; **70**: 619–30.

60 Editorial. Management of the stove-in chest with paradoxical movement. *Br Med J* 1977; **1**: 1242.

61 Van Saene HKF, Stoutenbeek CHP, Miranda DR, *et al.* Symposium paper: recent advances in the control of infection in patients with thoracic injury. *Injury* 1986; **17**: 332–5.

62 Cook D. Selective digestive decontamination: a critical appraisal. In: Vincent J-L (ed). *Yearbook of Intensive Care and Emergency Medicine.* Springer-Verlag, Berlin, Heidelberg, New York; 1993: 281–6.

63 Ramsay G, van Saeme RH. Selective decontamination in intensive care and surgical practice: where are we? *World J Surg* 1998; **22**: 164–70.

64 Alexander JW. Prevention of bacterial translocation with early enteral feeding — a feasible approach? In: Faist E, Meakins J, Schildberg FW (eds). *Host Defense Dysfunction in Trauma, Shock and Sepsis.* Berlin: Springer-Verlag; 1992; pp. 903–9.

65 James OF, Moore PG. Causes of death after blunt chest injury. *Aust NZ J Surg* 1983; **53**: 37–42.

66 Trunkey DD. Torso trauma. *Curr Probl Surg* 1987; **24**: 209–65.

67 Pape HC, Remmers D, Rice J, *et al*. Appraisal of early evaluation of blunt chest trauma: development of a standardised scoring system for initial clinical decision making. *J Trauma* 2000; **49**: 496–504.

68

Spinal injuries
G Gutteridge

There are few injuries that have a more devastating impact on both the patient and their family than spinal cord injuries (SCI). The physical, psychological and functional sequelae of permanent disability are immense. In addition, the economic cost to the individual and to society, with the loss of productivity and costs of hospitalization, rehabilitation and ongoing care, are enormous.

AETIOLOGY

The incidence of SCI in Australia is 15–20 new cases per million population per year (excluding deaths before reaching hospital), and appears to be decreasing.[1] In comparison, the incidence in the USA is 30–50 cases per million per year,[2] for which 75% are male, usually in the 15–35 years age group.

Traumatic SCI is due mainly to motor car and motor bike accidents (50%), falls (15–20%) and sporting injuries (10–15%, with about two-thirds of these due to diving). Alcohol ingestion is frequently an associated factor. Physical violence especially due to gunshot injury is responsible for 15–20% SCI in the USA.[2] Ischaemic SCI is occasionally due to aortic injury or cross clamping. Pre-existing spinal pathology predisposes to SCI, including osteoarthritis, spinal canal stenosis, ankylosing spondylitis, rheumatoid arthritis and congenital abnormalities.

With major trauma, the incidence of cervical spine injury (CSI) is 1.5–3%, with 50% of these being unstable.[3]

PATHOGENESIS

SPINAL INJURY

CERVICAL SPINE

Injury to the cervical spine has been classified several ways[4–6] relating to the mechanism of injury using the two-column concept. Differences appear to be due to the fact that compression of the anterior column is associated with distraction of the posterior column, and vice-versa.

Injuries may be grouped according to the predominant mechanism of injury (Table 68.1) with characteristic radiologic patterns and diagnostic utility.

THORACOLUMBAR SPINE

The classification of Denis[7] using the three-column concept of the spine has been widely adopted. Major injuries are classified in Table 68.2.

SPINAL CORD INJURY

Trauma to the spinal cord results in immediate primary and delayed secondary injury processes.

PRIMARY INJURY

Direct mechanical injury may produce focal compression, laceration or traction injury to the cord. Actual transection is unusual. Ischaemic injury may result from interference to the segmental spinal arterial supply.

Table 68.1 Cervical spine injuries

Hyperflexion
Hyperflexion and rotation
Hyperextension
Hyperextension and rotation
Vertical compression or burst injury
Lateral flexion
Direct shearing
Penetrating
Other

Table 68.2 Major thoracolumbar spine injuries

Compression fractures
Burst fractures
Seat belt type injuries
Fracture dislocations

SECONDARY INJURY

An understanding of secondary injury mechanisms has come from experimental SCI in animals.[8] Local hypoperfusion and ischaemia begin at the site of injury, extending progressively over hours from the site of injury in both directions. There is loss of spinal cord autoregulation, complicated by arterial hypotension with high SCI. Apart from ischaemia, other mechanisms may contribute to the secondary injury. These include the release of free radicals, eicosanoids, calcium, excitotoxic neurotransmitters (e.g. glutamate), proteases and phospholipases.

Petechial haemorrhages and oedema begin in the grey matter and progress over hours. There is cellular chromatolysis and vacuolation and, ultimately, neuronal necrosis. In the white matter, vasogenic oedema, axonal degeneration and demyelination follow. Infiltration of polymorphs occurs in the haemorrhagic areas. Late coagulative necrosis and cavitation subsequently take place.

CLINICAL PRESENTATION

Spinal and spinal cord injuries should be suspected after severe trauma or head injuries, if there are motor or sensory symptoms or signs, or the patient reports neck or back pain.

NEUROLOGICAL ASSESSMENT

A detailed neurological examination is essential, including motor function, sensory function (spinothalamic and dorsal column) and reflexes, as well as anal motor function, sensation and reflexes. The vital capacity should be measured. This neurological examination provides the most useful information with respect to assessment of the SCI and to prognosis. However, it may be difficult to conduct on presentation due to head or other injuries, pain, alcohol or the administration of analgesic or other drugs.

In an alert patient, SCI may be obvious with limb paralysis or weakness, numbness and absence of reflexes.

With a complete SCI, there is muscle paralysis, with somatic and visceral sensory loss below a discrete segmental level. Spinal shock is usually present, with the additional features of muscle flaccidity, absence of tendon reflexes, vaso- and venodilation, loss of bladder function and paralytic ileus. This term refers to a form of neurogenic 'shock' with temporary loss of somatic and autonomic reflex activity below the neurological level of injury. It usually lasts for 1–3 weeks before the recovery of distal reflex activity in the isolated cord segment.

TERMINOLOGY

The terminology for SCI has now been standardized.[9]

- *Tetraplegia* (preferred to quadriplegia) refers to impairment or loss of motor and/or sensory function in the cervical segments of the spinal cord due to damage of the neural elements within the spinal canal
- *Paraplegia* refers to impairment or loss in the thoracic, lumbar or sacral segments of the cord, as well as conus and cauda equina injuries within the spinal canal
- *Neurological level* is reported as the most caudal cord segment with normal motor and sensory function on both sides. As differences often exist, it is preferred to describe the individual motor and sensory levels on each side (as the most caudal segment with normal motor and sensory function respectively)
- *Skeletal level* refers to the level with the greatest vertebral damage on X-ray
- *Complete* injury refers to the absence of motor and sensory function in the lowest sacral segment.[10] If partial preservation of motor and sensory function is found below the neurological level, and includes the lowest sacral segment (with anal sensation and voluntary external anal sphincter contraction), the injury is defined as *incomplete*

INCOMPLETE SCI

Incomplete SCI tend to occur in characteristic syndromes.[11]

- The *central cord syndrome* is the most common, usually resulting from hyperextension injury to the neck, often in the elderly with a narrow spinal canal. There is disproportionate paralysis in the arms compared to the legs, and variable sensory loss
- The *anterior cord syndrome* has extensive bilateral paralysis with loss of pain and temperature sensation, but preservation of sensory function in the posterior white columns
- The *Brown–Sequard syndrome* is due to damage to one side of the spinal cord with loss of ipsilateral motor and proprioceptive function, as well as contralateral pain and temperature sensation. It usually results from penetrating injury
- The *conus medullaris syndrome* is due to T12/L1 injury with damage to lumbar and sacral cord segments producing extensive paralysis in the legs of both upper and lower motor neurone type
- The *cauda equina syndrome* results from skeletal injuries below L1 with damage to the lumbosacral nerve roots, resulting in lower motor neuron paralysis, and bladder and bowel areflexia
- Spinal cord injury without radiological abnormality (SCIWORA) occurs mainly in children, but is now very uncommon with magnetic resonance imaging (MRI)

UNCONSCIOUS OR UNCO-OPERATIVE PATIENTS

The neurological examination may be difficult if the patient is unconscious or unco-operative. In this case, a

Table 68.3 Signs of SCI in unconscious or unco-operative patients

Response to pain above, but not below a suspected level
Flaccid areflexia in the arms, and/or legs
Elbow flexion with the inability to extend suggestive of
   cervical SCI
Paradoxical pattern of breathing with indrawing of upper chest
   on inspiration (in the absence of upper respiratory tract
   obstruction or chest injury)
Inappropriate vasodilatation (in association with hypothermia,
   or in the legs but not the arms with thoracolumbar SCI)
Unexplained bradycardia, hypotension
Priapism
Loss of anal tone and reflexes

number of signs may be helpful in drawing attention to a SCI (Table 68.3). Confirmation of SCI may be established by MRI or somato-sensory evoked potentials.

SPINE

Alert patients will report neck or back pain and tenderness with spinal injuries. A palpable gap may be felt between the spinous processes of thoracolumbar vertebrae. However, a spinal injury is readily overlooked in association with head or other major injuries, or alcohol ingestion.[12]

ASSOCIATED INJURIES

CERVICAL SPINE INJURY/TETRAPLEGIA

Head injuries are commonly associated. Some 4–6% of patients with head injuries have a CSI, with two-thirds of these being unstable.[13] Patients with head injuries should be assumed to have a CSI until proved otherwise. Of patients with a cervical SCI, 25% have some degree of head injury, with 2–3% having a severe injury.

THORACOLUMBAR SPINE INJURY/PARAPLEGIA

Chest injuries are often present and are difficult to assess with the inability to take an erect chest X-ray, and the presence of a mediastinal haematoma associated with the vertebral injury. Contrast enhanced helical computed tomography (CT) of the chest may be used to exclude an aortic injury and to assess other chest injuries.[14]

Abdominal injuries are difficult to diagnose if there is a SCI. However, they should be suspected if there is excessive hypotension, referred shoulder pain, or free gas or fluid seen on X-ray of the spine or chest. Abdominal CT, diagnostic peritoneal lavage or ultrasound may be used to delineate these injuries.[15]

IMAGING

PLAIN X-RAYS (Fig. 68.1)

Plain X-rays remain the primary screening method for suspected spinal injuries (Table 68.4). However, the absence of a detectable abnormality does not exclude a spinal injury. Lesions may not be seen if the views are inadequate or of poor technical quality, or the observer is inexperienced. Even without these limitations, plain X-rays of the neck frequently miss fractures and subluxations,[16,17] and a high index of suspicion should be maintained. Adequate views of the entire cervical spine from the base of the skull down to and including the C7–T1 junction should always be obtained. Abnormalities of the prevertebral soft tissues are often present and indicative of subtle injuries.[5]

With the cervical spine the three-view trauma series is standard in most hospitals. This consists of a lateral, antero–posterior (AP) and odontoid (open mouth) views. A five-view series with supine oblique views has been recommended as improving the diagnostic yield,[18] but other studies show no difference in the detection rate.[19] If no injury is seen, flexion/extension X-rays may be undertaken to exclude cervical spine instability due to ligamentous injury.[13,20] Lateral and AP views are standard screening views for the thoracolumbar spine.

Although familiarity with common injuries is desirable, in view of the severe consequences of a missed spinal injury, 'clearance' of the spine must only be undertaken by a suitably experienced specialist after adequate imaging.

CT SCANNING

The sensitivity of CT is much greater than plain X-rays in the detection of spinal injuries.[16,17] Indications for CT scanning include:

- Inadequate plain X-rays
- High clinical suspicion of injury despite normal plain X-rays
- Suspicious plain X-ray findings
- Further investigation of fracture, subluxation or dislocation seen on plain X-rays. Additional fractures are frequently found in the same or adjacent vertebrae
- Evaluation of the spinal canal

Sagittal and coronal reconstructions should be routinely obtained. CT scanning of the spine should be co-ordinated with CT of other regions if needed. CT myelography has now been replaced by MRI, but may be indicated if MRI is not available or is contraindicated.

MRI (Fig. 68.2)

MRI allows visualization of soft tissues including ligaments, intervertebral discs and the spinal cord itself

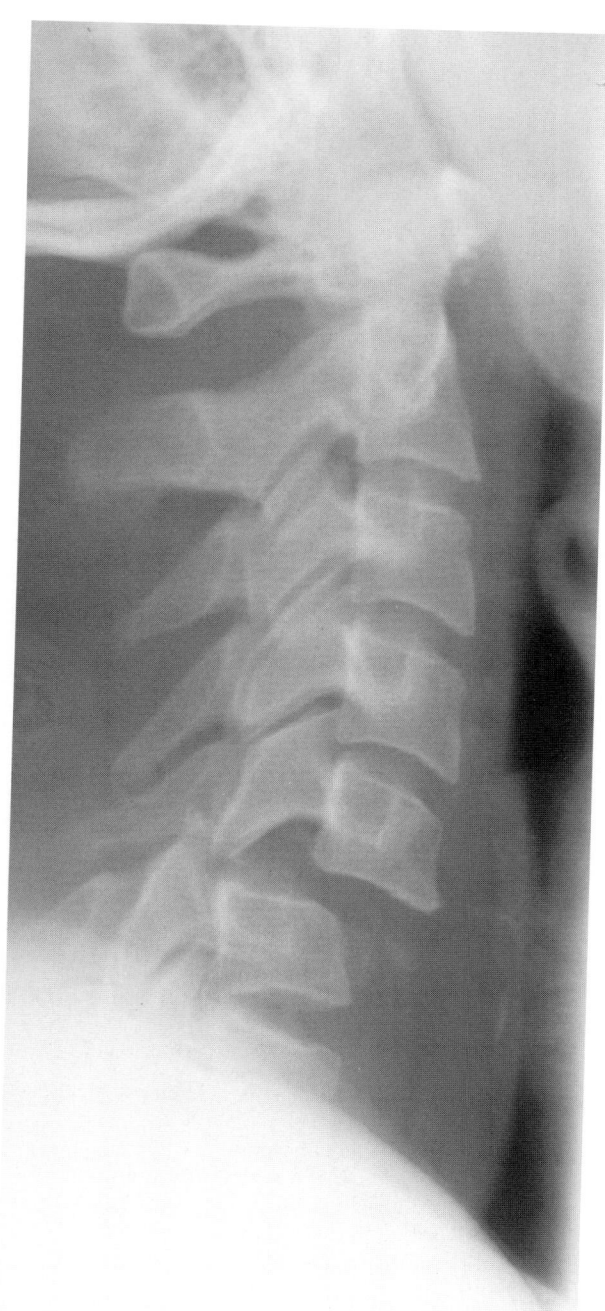

Fig. 68.1 Plain lateral X-ray of the cervical spine showing a C5/6 dislocation

Table 68.4 Basic examination of plain X-rays of cervical spine

Must include occipital condyles to C7–T1 junction.
Lateral is the most important view and will show most injuries.
Check for:

Alignment:	
Vertebral bodies	Anterior, posterior spinal lines
	Lateral alignment
Spinous processes	Spinolaminar line
	Posterior cervical line
Pedicles in AP view	
Laminae in oblique views	
Bony changes:	
Bony integrity, density, contour	
Vertebral body height	Anterior, posterior, lateral
Pedicles, laminae	
Spines, transverse processes	
Atlas, dens	
Spaces:	
Intervertebral disc spaces	
Interspinous spaces	
Predental (atlas-dens) space	
Facet joints	
Atlanto-axial, atlanto-occipital joints	
Soft tissues:	
Prevertebral soft tissue shadow	

evaluation of the neurological deficit, assessment of prognosis and in the planning of surgical management of SCI. It is also useful if the neurological deficit does not correlate with the bony injury seen on X-ray or CT.

MANAGEMENT

The main principles in the early management of a spinal injury relate to the prevention of secondary injury and the provision of optimum conditions for neurological recovery. Emphasis should be on resuscitation measures and immobilization, together with good protocols for clearance of the spine.

PREHOSPITAL MANAGEMENT

It should be assumed that all severe trauma patients have a spinal injury until proven otherwise. If a SCI is obvious, basic trauma assessment and resuscitation principles still apply.

RESPIRATION AND CIRCULATION

An adequate airway must be established by clearance of foreign material, jaw thrust and an oro- or nasopharyngeal airway if necessary. Adequate ventilation must be ensured with the provision of supplementary oxygen by

where it may show the site, extent and nature of the SCI.[5,21] However, it involves a prolonged study with physical isolation of the patient in a difficult environment. Nevertheless, it provides important information in

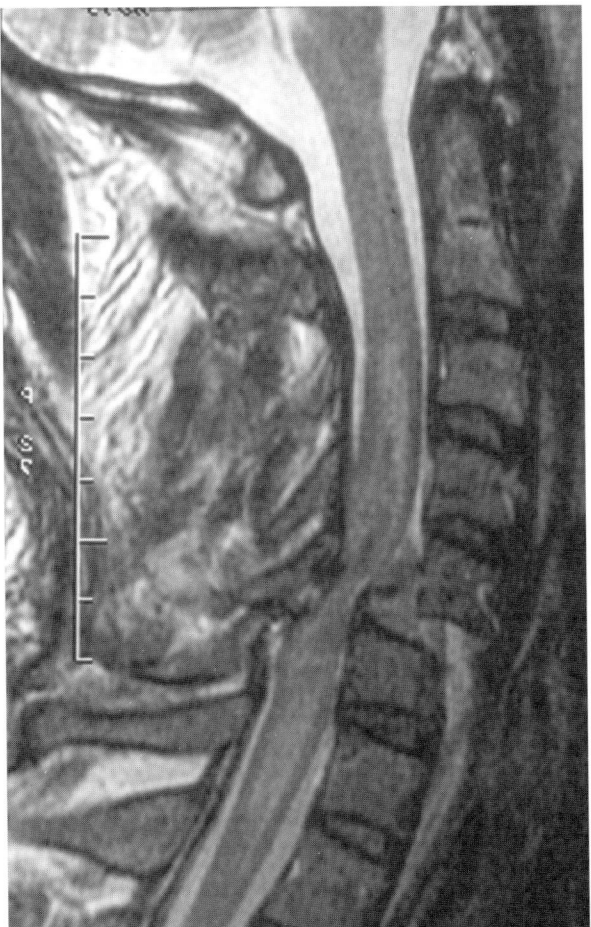

Fig. 68.2 T2 weighted MRI of the same patient as in Fig. 68.1 showing severe spinal cord damage

facemask. Immediate endotracheal intubation and artificial ventilation may be required.

Hypotension may be due to a high SCI and will need some plasma volume expansion to correct relative hypovolaemia. Excessive volume expansion should be avoided. Hypovolaemia may also be due to other injuries.

IMMOBILIZATION

If a CSI is suspected, the patient may have to be extricated from the scene of the accident. Manual stabilization of the head in a neutral position is used with four people lifting and one controlling the head and neck. The neck is immobilized in a rigid, hard collar that should be applied without neck movement. The patient is placed on a rigid spine board, supine with occipital padding. Sandbags should be placed on either side of the head, and the head secured with the application of broad tape across the forehead. With a

suspected thoracolumbar spinal injury (TLSI), the patient is again lifted as a single unit or log rolled as necessary.

HYPOTHERMIA

Prevention of hypothermia in the field is important with SCI.

EMERGENCY MANAGEMENT

The initial management of spinal injuries follows the usual trauma triage principles with a primary survey, resuscitation and a careful secondary survey. The measures previously mentioned for establishing an adequate airway, and for providing adequate ventilation and circulation, should be continued to minimize any further spinal cord insult.[22]

After stabilization, definitive X-rays and CT are undertaken whilst maintaining spinal immobilization. The prevention of hypothermia is a continuing issue in both the emergency and radiology departments. Morphine analgesia is likely to be required for pain at the spinal fracture site and/or other injury.

With SCI, a nasogastric tube should be inserted to prevent aspiration of gastric content and bowel distension from the associated ileus. A urinary catheter should also be inserted to monitor the urine output and prevent overdistension of the bladder. Attention to the skin, taking care to prevent pressure areas, is important. High dose corticosteroids should be started if within 8 h from the time of SCI (see pharmacological treatment). If stable, early transport to a definitive care facility such as a multidisciplinary SCI referral centre is recommended. This approach has been shown to result in fewer complications and a reduced hospital length of stay.[23]

HOSPITAL/INTENSIVE CARE UNIT (ICU) MANAGEMENT

RESPIRATORY

Respiratory Dysfunction

Respiratory dysfunction is a major cause of morbidity after SCI, especially in tetraplegics.[24]

Tetraplegia

The diaphragm is innervated by the C3–5 segments. With a C5 SCI, the diaphragm is intact but about 50% still need short-term mechanical ventilation (MV). With a C4 SCI, there is partial loss of diaphragmatic innervation, and nearly all need short-term MV. With a C3 SCI, most of the diaphragmatic innervation is lost, and all need initial MV with about 50% requiring permanent MV.[24] Intercostal muscle paralysis leads to a paradoxical pattern of breathing, and abdominal muscle paralysis produces an inability to cough.

The vital capacity (VC) is markedly reduced and is usually 1.0–1.5 l on presentation. In C5–6 complete SCI, the VC is decreased to 31% of predicted during the first week, and with C4 lesions to 24%.[25] It often undergoes a further decrease due to atelectasis, and sometimes from ascent of the neurological level. However, there is usually a significant increase in VC by 3–5 weeks after injury, reaching values of 44–51% of predicted by 3 months.[25] This is thought to be due mainly to the resolution of spinal shock with intercostal muscle tone preventing indrawing of the chest wall. The VC is dependent on posture and surprisingly is greatest in the supine position.[26] Hypoxaemia is very common in the early phase.

Paraplegia

The diaphragm is intact, but there is paralysis of the intercostal and abdominal muscles dependent on the neurological level of the SCI. The VC is reduced but is usually adequate, and there is variable impairment of the cough mechanism.

Respiratory Management

The aims of respiratory management are to prevent the development of respiratory complications and failure. Humidified oxygen should be provided by facemask. A regimen of 2-hourly postural change is instituted on a turning bed, or with log rolling, to prevent atelectasis. An intensive physiotherapy regimen is started with 4-hourly deep breathing, non-invasive ventilatory support by mouthpiece and bronchodilators if necessary. Assisted coughing (where the physiotherapist pushes on the abdomen synchronous with glottic closure as the patient attempts to cough) may be used to clear sputum. Serial evaluation of respiratory rate, oxygenation, vital capacity and chest X-ray is necessary.

Respiratory Complications

Respiratory complications are frequent and the major reason for SCI patients to be admitted to the ICU.[27] They are dependent on the level of the SCI, associated injuries and the presence of underlying respiratory disease. Respiratory complications are the leading cause of death after SCI with most attributed to pneumonia.[28]

These complications consist of atelectasis, sputum retention, pneumonia, aspiration, adult respiratory distress syndrome and acute respiratory failure (ARF). Indications for intubation and MV include an inability to clear secretions, progressive atelectasis or pneumonia, or frank ARF. Intubation and MV should also be undertaken for associated head or chest injuries, or if the VC falls below 12–15 ml/kg.

Endotracheal Intubation with CSI

The options are awake blind or fibreoptic nasotracheal intubation, or orotracheal intubation under general anaesthesia. No particular approach has been shown to be superior, and either is acceptable depending on individual circumstances. Factors determining the choice include the urgency of the situation, the skill and training of medical staff, the availability of equipment, the conscious state of the patient and the associated injuries.[3,29,30]

Awake nasotracheal intubation allows continuous neurological assessment, but should only be attempted with an alert co-operative patient. It is contraindicated if urgent intubation is required, or if there is coagulopathy, nasal obstruction or basal skull fracture. Blind intubation often requires multiple attempts, and has a significant complication and failure rate. Fibreoptic intubation, with appropriate topical anaesthesia, is a more acceptable technique.

Orotracheal intubation under anaesthesia is a safe technique, despite the greater potential for neck movement, and there is no evidence to suggest that neurological outcome is worse.[31] Preparation should be made for a rapid sequence induction and a difficult intubation. The anterior part of the collar is removed to allow adequate mouth opening, manual stabilization of the head is performed without traction, and cricoid pressure is applied; i.v. atropine is given, followed by the induction agent and muscle relaxant. Suxamethonium should be avoided between 10 days and 7 months after SCI to prevent severe hyperkalaemia.[32] Rocuronium is then the preferred relaxant.

Tracheostomy

Once intubated, tracheostomy is usually necessary. It improves comfort and communication, and facilitates weaning from MV and discharge from the ICU. Percutaneous tracheostomy may be used after internal fixation of the cervical spine, but often the neck can not be extended into the optimal position. Surgical tracheostomy is preferred and is ideally performed in the ICU.

Weaning from MV

With high tetraplegics, weaning can be very prolonged, difficult and is frequently complicated by recurrent atelectasis. Weaning is usually started after resolution of any pulmonary pathology and having a VC of at least 10 ml/kg. No method of weaning has been shown to be superior. Weaning is most conveniently begun by conversion to pressure support ventilation, ideally with flow triggering. Incremental reduction in the pressure support level is carried out as tolerated, before conversion to a T-piece. Alternatively, T-piece trials may be used from the outset but need much more psychological support to prevent patient anxiety and loss of confidence. Nearly all C4 or lower tetraplegics, and about 50% of C3 tetraplegics, can be weaned from MV given time.[24]

C1–3 tetraplegics who cannot be weaned are usually managed with permanent MV via a home ventilator. Some of these patients may be suitable for electrophrenic ventilation.[33]

CARDIOVASCULAR
Cardiovascular Dysfunction
With tetraplegia, there is loss of supra-spinal sympathetic control of the heart and peripheral vasculature with unopposed vagal activity. In the early phase of spinal shock, there is also loss of autonomic reflex activity in the isolated cord segment. These changes lead to sinus bradycardia and arterial hypotension associated with systemic vaso- and venodilation. Similar problems are seen in paraplegia, especially with SCI above T6. Patients are sensitive to further hypotension with postural change, blood or fluid loss and intermittent positive-pressure ventilation.

Cardiovascular Management
Monitoring should include electrocardiogram, arterial blood pressure, subclavian or femoral central venous pressure (CVP), and urine output. Some plasma volume expansion is necessary to correct a degree of relative hypovolaemia. Ideally normotension will be restored; however, mean arterial pressures of 60–70 mmHg are tolerated if the urine output is adequate (>0.5 ml/kg per h). Sometimes, a pressor agent such as dopamine is needed to elevate the heart rate and systemic vascular resistance in order to establish an adequate blood pressure. It is important to prevent severe hypotension that may produce additional ischaemic SCI.[8]

Cardiovascular Complications
Venous Thromboembolism
Venous thromboembolism has a 40% incidence without prophylaxis, with pulmonary embolism accounting for up to 15% deaths in the first year after SCI. Consensus guidelines[34] for prevention consist of compression stockings or external pneumatic compression device for 2 weeks, plus adjusted dose unfractionated heparin (to a high normal activated partial thromboplastin time) or enoxaparin 30 mg twice daily, starting within 72 h and continued for 8–12 weeks depending on risk factors. If high risk and anticoagulation fails or is contraindicated, a vena cava filter should be inserted.

Bradycardia, Asystole
Due to disruption of sympathetic pathways and unopposed vagal activity, these problems are extremely common after high SCI. With severe cervical SCI, the incidence of persistent bradycardia was 100% and transient marked bradycardia (heart rate <45 per min) 71%, with cardiac arrest occurring in 16% patients. These arrhythmias peaked in the first week and resolved 2–6 weeks after injury.[35] Tracheal suction in the presence of hypoxia appears to be a cause of cardiac arrest preventable with atropine.[36]

Acute Pulmonary Oedema
This is now less common, but does occur with misguided attempts to correct hypotension with excessive volume expansion, in the absence of CVP monitoring.

Autonomic Hyperreflexia
This is not a problem in the early phase. It begins within 6 months of SCI after recovery from spinal shock, and is usually only significant with SCI above the T6 level.[37] In response to an afferent stimulus below the neurological level, there is excessive paroxysmal autonomic reflex activity. The stimulus is often bladder or bowel distension, but may be cutaneous stimulation or surgery. The massive sympathetic efferent response causes intense vasoconstriction which produces severe hypertension, with the risk of seizures and cerebral haemorrhage. Baroreceptor mediated bradycardia may occur with reflex vasodilatation above the neurological level in paraplegics. Treatment consists of preventing or removing the stimulus, placing the patient in an upright posture and, if necessary, short-acting i.v. antihypertensive drugs such as nitroprusside.

NEUROLOGICAL
Drug treatment strategies are aimed to reduce secondary injury mechanisms, and to allow recovery of damaged neurones. Encouraging results have been achieved with animal experiments but only minimal improvement in human SCI using corticosteroids. In the NACSIS 2 trial,[38] methylprednisolone if started within 8 h of SCI (30 mg/kg bolus followed by 5.4 mg/kg per h for 23 h) resulted in mildly improved motor and sensory scores at 6 months and 1 year. A further trial (NACSIS 3)[39] showed some improvement in motor score and functional outcome if methylprednisolone started within 3–8 h of SCI was given for 48 h rather than 24 h. However, this was associated with more sepsis and pneumonia. The administration of methylprednisolone has been widely, but not universally, accepted. Criticism of these studies has followed from reanalysis of the NACSIS data[40,41] and systematic review of all published studies.[42] In a small study, GM-1 ganglioside appeared to improve neurological outcome after SCI.[43] A multicentre trial is now in progress. In human studies, tirilazad, naloxone and nimodipine have shown no benefit.

Muscle spasticity is a late problem not seen in the acute phase in ICU. It develops after resolution of spinal shock.

SKELETAL
The principles of management include adequate reduction, maintenance of position, and immobilization until stability has been achieved. There are both conservative and surgical options to management of the injury to the spine.

Conservative measures for CSI include traction in head tongs or a halo, or the application of a halo-thoracic brace. For TLSI, postural realignment may be used. However, these techniques require prolonged periods of immobilization in bed. Mechanical turning beds facilitate this approach.

Surgical techniques utilize open reduction and internal fixation to provide sufficient stability to allow early mobilization. External supports such as a collar or brace may added. Surgery is now utilized more frequently in order to achieve early stability and pain control, earlier mobilization and rehabilitation with less muscle wasting, fewer hospital complications and earlier time for hospital discharge. It is probably best undertaken at the earliest opportunity that other injuries and complications allow. In a multicentre study in North America, surgery was performed on 65% of acute SCI with little agreement as to timing.[44] Although claims have been made for fewer complications, and earlier mobilization and hospital discharge, there is little evidence to support this. In addition, human studies provide very little support for the role of early 'decompressive' surgery to improve neurological recovery after SCI.[45]

Physiotherapy measures are needed to preserve a full range of movement in paralysed joints and to prevent contractures.

TEMPERATURE
With high SCI, the loss of sympathetic nerve function and an inability to shiver leads to poikilothermia. Regular temperature monitoring is needed together with an approach to prevent hypothermia.

GASTROINTESTINAL
A range of gastrointestinal problems are associated with SCI.[46] Paralytic ileus and acute gastric dilatation are frequent problems in the first few days. A nasogastric tube should be inserted immediately to protect against aspiration and respiratory impairment from abdominal distension. It may then be used for early enteral nutrition once these problems have resolved. Stress ulceration with gastrointestinal bleeding has an incidence of 3–5%.[38] Ranitidine should be used for prevention. Acute acalculous cholecystitis,[47] pancreatitis and the superior mesenteric artery syndrome are uncommon. Constipation and faecal impaction readily develop after a number of days. A preventative bowel regimen consisting of faecal softeners, suppositories and laxatives should be started early.

URINARY
After SCI, there is paralysis of the bladder detrusor and urinary retention with the risk of bladder overdistension. A urethral catheter should be inserted early and placed on continuous drainage. Bladder training techniques with intermittent catheterization are delayed until the patient is stable and has been discharged from the ICU. Bacterial colonization of the urine is accepted while catheterized.

SKIN
Pressure sores readily develop and may cause considerable morbidity, prolonged hospitalization and need extensive plastic surgery for closure. They must be prevented by meticulous attention to 2-hourly postural change, the use of pneumatic pressure mattresses or pillows, and to the protection of bony pressure points.

METABOLIC
Hyponatraemia is very common after SCI.[48] Immobility after SCI leads to calcium mobilization from bone, hypercalciuria and, occasionally, hypercalcaemia. Muscle wasting and negative nitrogen balance are marked.

PSYCHOLOGICAL
Prolonged supportive care is necessary for both patients and their families to deal with depression, and to help them accept and adapt to neurological disability. After intubation or tracheostomy, tetraplegics have great difficulty with communication, as they are unable to write or use an alphabet board. Lip reading is utilized until a speaking tracheostomy tube can be used, or one-way speaking valve can be attached to the tracheostomy tube.

OUTCOME

After the acute care phase, SCI patients undergo extensive periods of rehabilitation to maximize their functional ability before returning to the community.

NEUROLOGICAL RECOVERY

The prognosis for neurological recovery is best judged by neurological examination 72 h post SCI. Most complete tetraplegics regain one motor level and do not recover functional lower limb movement. More than 50% of incomplete tetraplegics become ambulatory.[49] Spinal cord haemorrhage seen on MRI indicates a very low probability of motor recovery.[21]

SURVIVAL

Hospital survival after SCI is more than 90%. Long-term survival studies have shown a higher mortality risk with a higher neurological level, complete SCI, older age and earlier year of injury.[50] Most deaths are due to respiratory disease, urinary complications or heart disease.

REFERENCES
1 Yeo JD. Prevention of spinal cord injuries in an Australian study. *Paraplegia* 1993; **31**: 759–63.
2 Lobosky JM. The epidemiology of spinal cord injury. In: Narayan RK, Wilberger JE, Povlishock JT (eds). *Neurotrauma*. New York: McGraw-Hill; 1996: pp. 1049–58.
3 Abrams KJ, Grande CM. Airway management of the trauma patient with cervical spine injury. *Curr Opin Anaesthesiol* 1994; 7: 184–90.
4 Holdsworth F. Fractures, dislocations and fracture-dislocations of the spine. *J Bone Joint Surg* 1970; **52A**: 1534–51.

5 Harris JH, Mirvis SE. *The Radiology of Acute Cervical Spine Trauma*, 3rd edn. Baltimore: Williams & Wilkins; 1996: pp. 213–244.

6 Allen BL, Ferguson RL, Lehmann TR, O'Brien RP. A mechanistic classification of closed, indirect fractures and dislocations of the lower cervical spine. *Spine* 1982; 7: 1–27.

7 Denis F. The three column spine and its significance in the classification of acute thoracolumbar spinal injuries. *Spine* 1983; 8: 817–31.

8 Tator CH, Fehlings MG. Review of the secondary injury theory of acute spinal cord trauma with emphasis on vascular mechanisms. *J Neurosurg* 1991; 75: 15–26.

9 Maynard FM, Bracken MB, Creasey G, *et al.* International standards for neurological and functional classification of spinal cord injury. *Spinal Cord* 1997; 35: 266–74.

10 Waters RL, Adkins RH, Yakura JS. Definition of complete spinal cord injury. *Paraplegia* 1991; 29: 573–81.

11 Tator CH. Classification of spinal cord injury based on neurological presentation. In: Narayan RK, Wilberger JE, Povlishock JT (eds). *Neurotrauma*. New York: McGraw-Hill; 1996: pp. 1059–73.

12 Meldon SW, Moettus LN. Thoracolumbar spine fractures: clinical presentation and the effect of altered sensorium and major injury. *J Trauma* 1995; 39: 1110–14.

13 Chesnut RM. Emergency management of spinal cord injury. In: Narayan RK, Wilberger JE, Povlishock JT (eds). *Neurotrauma*. New York: McGraw-Hill; 1996: pp. 1121–38.

14 Lang-Lazdunski L, Pons F, Jancovici R. Update on the emergency management of chest trauma. *Curr Opin Crit Care* 1999; 5: 488–99.

15 Schuster-Bruce M, Nolan J. Priorities in the management of blunt abdominal trauma. *Curr Opin Crit Care* 1999; 5: 500–10.

16 Woodring JH, Lee C. Limitations of cervical radiography in the evaluation of acute cervical trauma. *J Trauma* 1993; 34: 32–9.

17 Acheson MB, Livingston RR, Richardson ML, Stimac GK. High resolution CT scanning in the evaluation of cervical spine fractures: comparison with plain film examinations. *AJR* 1987; 148: 1179–85.

18 Turetsky DB, Vines FS, Clayman DA, Northup HM. Technique and use of supine oblique views in acute cervical spine trauma. *Ann Emerg Med* 1993; 22: 685–89.

19 Freemyer B, Knopp R, Piche J, *et al.* Comparison of five-view and three-view cervical spine series in the evaluation of patients with cervical trauma. *Ann Emerg Med* 1989; 18: 818–21.

20 Ajani AE, Cooper DJ, Scheinkestel CD, *et al.* Optimal assessment of cervical spine trauma in critically ill patients: a prospective evaluation. *Anaesth Intens Care* 1998; 26: 487–91.

21 Bondurant FJ, Cotler HB, Kulkarni MV, *et al.* Acute spinal cord injury. A study using physical examination and magnetic resonance imaging. *Spine* 1990; 15: 161–8.

22 Meguro K, Tator CH. Effect of multiple trauma on mortality and neurological recovery after spinal cord or cauda equina injury. *Neurol Med Chir* 1988; 28: 34–41.

23 DeVivo MJ, Kartus PL, Stover SL, Fine PR. Benefit of early admission to an organized spinal cord injury care system. *Paraplegia* 1998; 28: 545–55.

24 Mansel JK, Norman JR. Respiratory complications and management of spinal cord injuries. *Chest* 1990; 97: 1446–52.

25 Ledsome JR, Sharp JM. Pulmonary function in acute cervical cord injury *Am Rev Respir Dis* 1981; 124: 41–4.

26 Ali J, Qi W. Pulmonary function and posture in traumatic quadriplegia. *J Trauma* 1995; 39: 334–7.

27 Jackson AB, Groomes TE. The incidence of respiratory complications following spinal cord injury. *Arch Physical Med Rehabilit* 1994; 75: 270–5.

28 Carter RE. Respiratory aspects of spinal cord injury management. *Paraplegia* 1987; 25: 262–6.

29 Hastings RH, Marks JD. Airway management for trauma patients with potential cervical spine injuries. *Anesth Analg* 1991; 73: 471–82.

30 Wood PR, Lawler PG. Managing the airway in cervical spine injury. *Anaesthesia* 1992; 47: 792–7.

31 Shatney CH, Brunner RD, Nguyen TQ. The safety of orotracheal intubation in patients with unstable cervical spine fracture or high spinal cord injury. *Am J Surg* 1995; 170: 676–80.

32 Yentis SM. Suxamethonium and hyperkalaemia. *Anaesth Intens Care* 1990; 18: 92–101.

33 Carter RE. Experience with ventilator dependent patients. *Paraplegia* 1993; 31: 150–3.

34 Prevention of thromboembolism in spinal cord injury. *J Spinal Cord Med* 1997; 20: 259–83.

35 Lehmann KG, Lane JG, Piepmeier JM, Batsford WP. Cardiovascular abnormalities accompanying acute spinal cord injury in humans: incidence, time course and severity. *J Am Coll Cardiol* 1987; 10: 46–52.

36 Welply NC, Mathias CJ, Frankel HL. Circulatory reflexes in tetraplegics during artificial ventilation and general anaesthesia. *Paraplegia* 1975; 13: 172–82.

37 Colachis SC. Autonomic hyperreflexia with spinal cord injury. *J Am Paraplegia Society* 1992; 15: 171–86.

38 Bracken MB, Shepard MJ, Collins WF, *et al.* A randomized controlled trial of methylprednisolone or naloxone in the treatment of acute spinal cord injury. *N Eng J Med* 1990; 322: 1405–11.

39 Bracken MB, Shepard MJ, Holford TR, *et al.* Administration of methylprednisolone for 24 or 48 hours or tirilazad mesylate for 48 hours in the treatment of acute spinal cord injury. *JAMA* 1997; 277: 1597–604.

40 Hurlbert JR. Methylprednisolone for acute spinal cord injury: an inappropriate standard of care. *J Neurosurg (Spine 1)* 2000; 93: 1–7

41 Nesathurai S. Steroids and spinal cord injury: revisiting the NACSIS 2 and NACSIS 3 trials. *J Trauma* 1998; 45: 1088–93.

42 Short DJ, El Masry WS, Jones PW. High dose methylprednisolone in the management of acute spinal cord

injury – a systematic review from a clinical perspective. *Spinal Cord* 2000; **38**: 273–86.

43 Geisler FH, Dorsey FC, Coleman WP. Recovery of motor function after spinal cord injury – a randomized placebo-controlled trial with GM-1 ganglioside. *N Eng J Med* 1991; **324**: 1829–38.

44 Tator CH, Fehlings MG, Thorpe K, Taylor W. Current use and timing of spinal surgery for management of acute spinal cord injury in North America: results of a prospective multicenter study. *J Neurosurg (Spine 1)* 1999; **91**: 12–8.

45 Fehlings MG, Tator CH. An evidence-based review of decompressive surgery in acute spinal cord injury: rationale, indications and timing based on experimental and clinical studies. *J Neurosurg (Spine 1)* 1999; **91**: 1–11.

46 Gore RM, Mintzer RA, Calenoff L. Gastrointestinal complications of spinal cord injury. *Spine* 1981; **6**: 538–44.

47 Romero Ganuza FJ, La Band F, Montalvo R, Mazaira J. Acute acalculous cholecystitis in patients with acute traumatic spinal cord injury. *Spinal Cord* 1997; **35**: 124–8.

48 Peruzzi WT, Shapiro BA, Meyer PR, *et al.* Hyponatremia in acute spinal cord injury. *Crit Care Med* 1994; **22**: 252–8.

49 Kirshblum SC, O'Connor KC. Levels of spinal cord injury and predictors of neurological recovery. *Physical Med Rehabilit Clin North Am* 2000; **11**: 1–27.

50 Frankel HL, Coll JR, Charlifue SW, *et al.* Long term survival in spinal cord injury: a fifty year study. *Spinal Cord* 1998; **36**: 266–74.

69

Abdominal and pelvic injuries
C J McArthur

Although important abdominal injuries are present in only 16–27% of hospital trauma admissions,[1] abdominal and pelvic injuries can represent up to 60% of missed diagnoses in preventable trauma deaths.[2] Most abdominal and pelvic injuries are caused by blunt trauma; penetrating aetiologies account for 6–21% of cases, depending on the society concerned.[1,3] Important considerations with abdominal and pelvic injuries are:

- potential for severe haemorrhage
- difficulties in diagnosing visceral injury
- severity of associated injuries (e.g. chest and head)
- complications, especially sepsis

MECHANISMS OF INJURY

BLUNT INJURIES

Road crashes account for most abdominal and pelvic blunt injuries. Injuries may also result from falls, assaults and industrial accidents.[1] Associated injuries are frequent, involving the thorax (most common), head and extremities. Seat belts and airbags reduce mortality in motor vehicle crashes (mainly by limiting brain injury), but are associated with more lower body injuries. Abdominal and pelvic injuries are more likely with vehicular side-on collisions, and when crashes result in a deformed steering wheel.[4]

PENETRATING INJURIES

Stab and gunshot wounds account for most penetrating injuries to the abdomen.

STAB AND LACERATION WOUNDS

Entry sites do not accurately predict the nature of deeper injury. Penetration of the thoracic cavity should be suspected with upper abdominal wounds; conversely, lower chest wounds may involve abdominal structures. Selective management of haemodynamically stable patients using investigation algorithms that accurately predict intra-abdominal injury has superseded mandatory laparotomy.[5]

GUNSHOT WOUND (see Ch. 75)

Injuries depend on missile calibre, and its velocity and trajectory. Intra-abdominal, thoracic and multiple organ injuries and mortality are substantially greater than with stab wounds. Laparotomy should be performed in all cases when peritoneal violation cannot be excluded, as most patients have intra-abdominal injury.

INITIAL TREATMENT AND INVESTIGATIONS

RESUSCITATION

Ensuring adequacy of airway, ventilation and oxygenation are immediate priorities. However, circulatory resuscitation should not delay surgery for uncontrolled haemorrhage. End-points for replacement of blood volume are controversial.[6] If rapid surgical haemostasis is provided in penetrating trauma, delaying or limiting fluid resuscitation before surgery may improve outcome.[7] Pneumatic antishock garments provide no benefit.[6,8]

CLINICAL ASSESSMENT

A full clinical examination (including the back) by experienced clinicians is most important. The mechanism of injury may direct attention to particular anatomical areas.[4]

- contusions, external wounds and their relationship to underlying viscera are noted
- abdominal distension, tenderness and peritonism are sought
- the rectum is examined for prostatic position, anal tone, blood or other evidence of injury
- gastric aspirate and urine are inspected for blood. Auscultation for bowel sounds is not useful

Isolated penetrating injuries present few diagnostic problems, but the decision to explore the abdomen can be difficult. Blunt abdominal trauma is often part of multiple injuries, and is more difficult to diagnose clinically, except when abdominal signs are obvious.

Nevertheless, in conscious patients, serial assessments can accurately identify those with significant intra-abdominal pathology. In the presence of impaired consciousness, intellectual disability or spinal, chest or pelvic injury, clinical assessment is unreliable. Other more visually spectacular injuries may also divert attention from the abdomen.

Laparotomy is indicated on clinical grounds when there is:

- shock with signs of intra-abdominal haemorrhage (e.g. peritonism or increasing distension)
- in penetrating trauma, laparotomy is indicated for evisceration or peritonism without shock

In all other situations where clinical examination is inadequate, further investigations must be undertaken.[9]

PLAIN X-RAYS

A chest X-ray (preferably erect) is essential. It may demonstrate free intraperitoneal gas, herniation of abdominal contents through a ruptured diaphragm, or other abnormalities.

Plain films of the abdomen are of no benefit.

An anteroposterior pelvic X-ray is indicated for all victims of blunt trauma, except conscious patients with normal pelvis on examination.[10]

INVESTIGATIONS FOR OCCULT ABDOMINAL INJURY

PERITONEAL LAVAGE

Diagnostic peritoneal lavage (DPL)[11] is indicated in blunt trauma when there is haemodynamic instability or uncertain clinical findings, and in penetrating trauma when peritoneal breach is suspected.

Open and closed (percutaneous guide wire) methods are both satisfactory.[12]

DPL is unjustified when an indication for laparotomy already exists. It is relatively contraindicated in:

- pregnancy
- significant obesity
- previous abdominal surgery

If required in these situations (or with pelvic fractures), the supraumbilical open method should be considered. DPL undertaken early remains reliable in the presence of pelvic fractures.[13] DPL detects intra-peritoneal injury with up to 98% accuracy,[11] but its high sensitivity can result in a significant non-therapeutic laparotomy rate. Cell counts of lavage effluent are more accurate than qualitative methods but hollow viscus injury is difficult to detect. Generally accepted criteria for a positive DPL are shown in Table 69.1.

COMPUTED TOMOGRAPHY (CT)

CT requires a still patient, a high-resolution scanner and experienced interpretation to match the sensitivity of

Table 69.1 Criteria for positive diagnostic peritoneal lavage

Clinical
Initial aspiration of >10 ml frank blood
Egress of lavage fluid via chest tube or urinary catheter
Bile or vegetable material in lavage fluid

Laboratory

	Blunt injury	Penetrating injury
Red cells		
Definite	$>100 \times 10^9/l$	$>20 \times 10^9/l$
Indeterminate	$50–100 \times 10^9/l$	$5–20 \times 10^9/l$
White cells	$>0.5 \times 10^9/l$	$0.5 \times 10^9/l$
Amylase	>20 IU/l	>20 IU/l
Alkaline phosphatase	>10 IU/l	>10 IU/l

peritoneal lavage. The routine use of enteral contrast is controversial.[14] Cuts from the top of the diaphragm to the symphysis pubis are required. The safety of undertaking CT in acute trauma depends on the degree of cardiorespiratory stability relative to the speed of scanning and access to resuscitation support. CT is particularly useful to assess the retroperitoneum and pelvic fractures, and delineate the nature of abdominal injury (thus guiding nonoperative management of some solid organ injuries). However, it may not detect all hollow viscus trauma.[15] Magnetic resonance imaging offers no advantage over CT in evaluating acute abdominal trauma, and poses significant logistical problems.

ULTRASONOGRAPHY

Focused Abdominal Sonography for Trauma (FAST) can be performed rapidly in the resuscitation room without compromising ongoing treatment. It requires significant training to achieve acceptable accuracy,[16] and although highly specific, is less sensitive than DPL or CT in detecting injury from either blunt[17] or penetrating[18] trauma. FAST can also identify pericardial fluid, but does not reliably demonstrate the nature of organ injury.[17] The small but important false negative rate must be considered in determining its role in abdominal assessment algorithms.

CHOICE OF INVESTIGATION

- DPL is invasive, reasonably rapid and accurate in identifying intraperitoneal bleeding or contamination, but may miss diaphragmatic injuries and does not examine the retroperitoneum. Its primary role is in unstable patients with blunt trauma and stable patients with anterior stab wounds
- FAST is non-invasive, particularly rapid, and reasonably accurate when used by trained staff. It is an alternative to DPL but negative studies should be followed by another investigation[17,18]
- CT is non-invasive, time-consuming, accurate, and has a primary role in defining the location and magnitude of intra-abdominal injuries in stable patients with blunt trauma or penetrating trauma to the flank or back

- DPL and CT are complementary,[19] and should both be available. If CT is unavailable, DPL rather than FAST is indicated in the stable patient with blunt trauma in whom clinical examination is inadequate

LAPAROSCOPY

Diagnostic laparoscopy may be useful in the haemodynamically stable patient. It is good at visualizing the diaphragm and identifying a need for laparotomy, but may miss specific organ injuries, particularly of the bowel. Laparoscopy appears best suited for the evaluation of equivocal penetrating wounds.[20]

ANGIOGRAPHY

Selective angiography and embolization are valuable in detecting and treating the source of major haemorrhage from liver, pelvis and retroperitoneal structures.

LAPAROTOMY

Laparotomy can be regarded as both therapeutic and diagnostic. Intra-abdominal injury may be detected by means discussed above, but often only laparotomy can accurately diagnose specific injuries. In severe and multiple trauma, the morbidity of a negative laparotomy is insignificant compared to the dire consequences of not diagnosing and treating a serious injury.

Operative treatment of more severe injuries with difficult haemostasis can cause a lethal triad of hypothermia, acidosis and coagulopathy. A 'damage control' laparotomy[21] with control of haemorrhage and contamination, intraperitoneal packing, elective re-exploration and removal of packs 24–48 h later should be performed.

- Angiography should be considered and may be required for inaccessible arterial bleeding
- Temporary prosthetic closure is often required to avoid elevated intra-abdominal pressure
- Survival is better when the decision to terminate the initial procedure is made earlier

SPECIFIC INJURIES

SPLEEN

The spleen is the organ most frequently injured by blunt trauma. Injuries vary from a small subcapsular haematoma to hilar devascularization or shattered spleen, but are rarely fatal with good medical care.[22] Diagnosis may be delayed in mild trauma. When associated chest or neurological injuries are severe, minor splenic injury may not initially be detected unless further investigation is undertaken. Fractures of the lower left ribs are a common association. Minor trauma may cause splenic injury when the spleen is enlarged (e.g. from malaria, lymphomas and haemolytic anaemias).

Immediate splenectomy is indicated in patients with severe multiple injuries, splenic avulsion, fragmentation or rupture, extensive hilar injuries, failure of haemostasis, peritoneal contamination from gastrointestinal injury or rupture of diseased spleen.[22] However, overwhelming infection by encapsulated organisms, such as *Pneumococcus*, can occur early or late (even years) after splenectomy in 0–2% of individuals. It is a particular risk following splenectomy in children and young adults. Polyvalent pneumococcal vaccine (Pneumovax) should be administered following splenectomy.

A conservative non-operative approach is possible in observable stable younger patients, in whom associated abdominal injuries have been excluded.[22] CT grading systems may identify patients in whom expectant management will fail.[23]

Other treatment alternatives include operative procedures to conserve splenic tissue (e.g. topical haemostatic agents, suture repair, absorbable mesh, partial splenectomy and splenic artery ligation). Benefits of splenectomy with autotransplantation of splenic tissue are unproven.

LIVER

The liver is the second most commonly injured organ after blunt abdominal trauma, and has been the most frequently missed injury in deaths from trauma.[2] Diagnosis is made by laparotomy in unstable patients, or CT in stable patients. Injuries range from small subcapsular haematomas to major parenchymal disruption and laceration of hepatic veins or even hepatic avulsion.

CT assessment enables most patients to be managed without operation. Patients should be haemodynamically stable, have associated major abdominal injuries excluded, and be assessed repeatedly. Follow-up CT scans can show the resolution of injury, which typically takes 2–3 months.

If surgery is required, early determination of indications for damage control approach is important. Perihepatic packing gives best haemostasis. Angiography may identify and treat uncontrolled arterial bleeding. Early complications of liver injury relate to the effects of hypoperfusion or massive blood transfusion. Late complications are usually associated with sepsis.[24]

GASTROINTESTINAL TRACT (GIT)

Injury to the GIT is more common following penetrating than blunt trauma. The very high likelihood of bowel injury in abdominal gunshot wounds mandates laparotomy. Laparoscopy can be used to identify those with stab wounds for laparotomy, when peritoneal violation cannot be excluded. Posterior stab wounds may damage retroperitoneal structures. CT examination with contrast enema may identify colonic injury better than clinical assessment or DPL.[5]

Blunt abdominal injuries to stomach, duodenum, small intestine, colon and their mesenteries are difficult to evaluate. Physical signs may be absent initially.

FAST or DPL may provide a general indication for laparotomy, but are not accurate in diagnosing isolated bowel trauma (especially of the duodenum) because of its retroperitoneal location.

CT is a sensitive indicator of free intraperitoneal air, but signs of duodenal perforation or haematoma are subtle, even with enteral contrast. Consequently, duodenal injury is often missed. A high index of suspicion should be maintained in patients with persistent abdominal pain and tenderness.[25]

Bleeding from mesenteric vessels is often self-limiting and may not require surgical control. However, vessel damage can cause ischaemia and infarction, and may require resection of affected bowel. Uncomplicated blunt or penetrating bowel injury can usually be managed by primary repair and anastomosis rather than colostomy.[26] A faecal diversion procedure with delayed repair is indicated in significant peritoneal contamination.

PANCREAS

Blunt injuries to the pancreas require considerable force and are often associated with duodenal, liver and splenic trauma. CT is the most useful investigation. Acute hyperamylasaemia does not predict pancreatic or hollow viscus injury.[27]

Minor injuries require simple drainage and haemostasis. Severe injuries to the body and tail of the pancreas are best managed by distal pancreatectomy. Severe injuries involving the proximal pancreas and duodenum with intact ampulla and common bile duct can be treated by drainage and pyloric exclusion. Pancreaticoduodenectomy is required in only 10% of cases. Complications such as pancreatitis, fistula, abscess and pseudocyst are common.[28]

KIDNEY AND URINARY TRACT

Blunt injury to the urinary tract is more common than penetrating injury. Identification and treatment of other major injuries often take precedence. Gross haematuria should be investigated; CT is the examination of choice. Contrast should be given 5–20 min before scanning to identify urinary extravasation. Unless there is unexplained shock, microscopic haematuria does not require further investigation. Renovascular pedicle or ureteric injuries may not cause any haematuria. Most renal injuries resolve with expectant management. Lacerations involving the collecting system or injury to the renal pedicle usually require operative intervention, although restoration of renal function following long warm ischaemic times is unusual. If major renal injury is discovered at emergency laparotomy, intraoperative i.v. urography is prudent to ensure contralateral function and will identify urinary extravasation.[29]

Bladder rupture is commonly associated with pelvic fractures. Over 95% of patients have macroscopic haematuria. Retrograde cystography is the investigation of choice because CT is neither sensitive nor specific enough. Intraperitoneal bladder rupture requires operative repair and urinary drainage. Patients with sterile urine and extraperitoneal rupture can be managed with catheter drainage alone.[30]

Urethral trauma is caused by direct blunt injury, or occurs in association with pelvic injury. It should be suspected if there is blood at the urinary meatus, perineal injury or abnormal position of the prostate on rectal examination in the male. In the absence of these findings, cautious urethral catheterization is appropriate. Treatment of urethral trauma is suprapubic drainage and subsequent definitive repair.

DIAPHRAGM

Diaphragmatic injury occurs in fewer than 5% of cases of blunt injury, is left-sided in 80% of cases, and is commonly associated with injuries to abdominal organs. It should also be suspected in penetrating trauma below the fifth rib. Diagnosis can be difficult, especially in the presence of positive-pressure ventilation, and may become evident only after ventilatory support is discontinued.

- Chest X-rays are commonly abnormal but often with non-specific findings
- DPL is insensitive for isolated diaphragmatic injuries
- Laparoscopy and thoracoscopy provides good views of the diaphragm

Spontaneous healing does not occur, and all defects should be repaired. The risk of associated injuries in acute cases mandates an abdominal approach.[31]

BONY PELVIS AND PERINEUM

Pelvic fractures are primarily caused by vehicular trauma or falls. Associated injuries to the bladder, urethra and intra-abdominal organs are common. Injuries may be life-threatening initially from major haemorrhage, or later from sepsis. Significant morbidity can result from damage to pelvic nerves, urethra or the structural integrity of the pelvis. Pelvic injury is suggested by pain on movement, structural instability, gross haematuria or peri-pelvic ecchymosis. Rectal examination is mandatory to identify rectal injury and prostatic position.

Radiography can confirm bony injury, but CT is required to identify associated intra-abdominal injuries (in the haemodynamically stable) and can assist in planning operative stabilization.

FAST has a significant false-negative rate with major pelvic fractures.[32]

Patients with haemodynamic instability and pelvic fractures must have intra-abdominal haemorrhage excluded. Early open supraumbilical DPL or FAST are the investigations of choice. If grossly positive, laparotomy should precede external fixation or angiography. If DPL is positive by cell count alone or FAST negative, the risk of life-threatening intra-abdominal haemorrhage is relatively low, and achieving haemostasis for pelvic bleeding becomes the priority; CT and/or laparotomy should follow if the patient is still unstable.

- Emergency measures to improve tamponade by reducing pelvic volume (pelvic binding or C-clamp) and prompt angiography and selective embolization can significantly reduce mortality[33]
- External fixation of the pelvis can control venous and small arteriolar bleeding near fracture sites, and will also reduce the volume of an open pelvis
- Bleeding from large vessels such as the aorta, common and external iliac arteries, and common femoral artery requires surgical control

Pelvic fractures range from simple fractures of individual bones requiring bed rest alone to complex fractures. Early operative stabilization of complex pelvic fractures is preferred in the intensive care unit (ICU), as it facilitates respiratory care, pain control and early mobilization. Compound pelvic fractures involving the perineum, rectum or vagina require aggressive surgery (including diversion of the faecal stream) to avoid high mortality.

RETROPERITONEAL HAEMATOMA

Retroperitoneal haematoma is frequent following blunt trauma, and is commonly caused by injury to the lumbar spine, bony pelvis, bladder or kidney or, less commonly, to the pancreas, duodenum or major vascular structures. Diagnosis may be inferred by excluding other sites of major blood loss, or presumed by signs of underlying organ injury.

CT is the most useful investigation in the stable patient.

A central haematoma should be explored with proximal vascular control, because of the risk of pancreatic, duodenal or major vascular injury. A lateral or pelvic haematoma should not be explored, unless there is evidence of major arterial injury, intraperitoneal bladder rupture or colonic injury. Treatment of major renal injury remains controversial.[34]

TRAUMA IN PREGNANCY

Women injured during pregnancy pose problems of altered physiology, risk to the gravid uterus and fetus, and conflict of priorities between mother and fetus.

- High-flow oxygen must be given until maternal hypoxaemia, hypovolaemia and fetal distress have been excluded
- Reduced respiratory reserve demands earlier intervention

- Maternal compensation for blood loss is at the expense of uteroplacental blood flow
- Mothers should be positioned to avoid aortocaval compression
- i.v. access should be in the upper limbs
- Transfusions should be Rhesus compatible
- All Rhesus-negative mothers should receive immune globulin, because of the immunological risk of even minor fetomaternal haemorrhage[35]

Only X-rays that may significantly alter therapy should be taken (with appropriate shielding), especially if under 20 weeks' of gestation.

Ultrasound is the preferred investigation as it is safe and can accurately detect free intra-abdominal fluid, confirm gestation and fetal well-being, and identify placental abnormalities.

DPL is safe if performed by the open method above the fundus.

CT may miss injuries due to abdominal crowding.

Retroperitoneal haemorrhage is more common in pregnant patients. Placental abruption may conceal significant blood loss. Treatment may be expectant or by caesarean section, depending on the condition of the mother and fetus. Uterine rupture is unusual and will often require hysterectomy. Rarely, perimortem caesarean section may be indicated in a dead or dying mother, to attempt to save the fetus.[35]

Placental abruption, fetal distress and fetal loss are rare following blunt injury, but premature uterine contractions are common.

Continuous cardiotocography is the most sensitive test to detect obstetric complications, but is required for only 6 h unless abnormalities are noted. Kleihauer–Betke tests to identify fetomaternal haemorrhage are not predictive of fetal or maternal morbidity.

COMPLICATIONS

HAEMORRHAGE

Patients with haemorrhage from abdominal and pelvic injuries can suffer the same complications of shock and massive transfusion as any patient with severe haemorrhage. Dilutional coagulopathy is common following resuscitation with fluids deficient in haemostatic factors. Patients resuscitated with crystalloids, colloids and red cells often require platelet and fresh frozen plasma transfusions. Disseminated intravascular coagulation occurs infrequently in trauma, usually when shock has been prolonged.

SEPSIS

Intra-abdominal sepsis remains an important preventable cause of death after trauma. Predisposing factors include

- peritoneal contamination from GIT injury
- external wounds

- invasive procedures
- delayed diagnosis of hollow viscus injuries
- splenectomy
- devitalized tissue

Early diagnosis and effective lavage and drainage procedures may reduce the incidence of intra-abdominal sepsis.

Prophylactic antibiotics for 24 h are satisfactory for penetrating injuries. Intra-abdominal sepsis should be excluded if unexplained fever and/or neutrophil leukocytosis, or multiple organ failure develops. Septic shock may represent a second shock insult to the trauma patient, leading to multiorgan dysfunction.

GASTROINTESTINAL FAILURE

GIT failure in various forms, ranging from stress ulceration and delayed gastric emptying to paralytic ileus, is a frequent occurrence. Prophylaxis against stress ulceration may be indicated. Enteral nutrition is associated with a lower incidence of sepsis following trauma.[36] Feeding through a jejunostomy tube placed during surgery or radiologically in the ICU is usually feasible. Parenteral nutrition may be necessary in patients with severe bowel or retroperitoneal injuries.

RAISED INTRA-ABDOMINAL PRESSURE

Abdominal distension with raised intra-abdominal pressure may be seen in the critically injured, as a consequence of haemorrhage, bowel oedema, ileus or surgical packs. This can have severe adverse effects on respiratory, cardiovascular and renal function.[37] Alleviation is by abdominal decompression using interposed synthetic mesh[38] or by leaving the abdomen open, with or without visceral packing. The abdomen is subsequently closed by staged repair as the distension resolves.

REFERENCES

1 Cameron P, Dziukas L, Hadj A, *et al*. Patterns of injury from major trauma in Victoria. *Aust NZ J Surg* 1995; **65**: 848–52.
2 Anderson ID, Woodford M, de Dombal FT, Irving M. Retrospective study of 1000 deaths from trauma in England and Wales. *BMJ* 1988; **296**: 1305–8.
3 Champion HR, Copes WS, Sacco WJ, *et al*. The Major Trauma Outcome Study: establishing norms for trauma care. *J Trauma* 1990; **30**: 1356–65.
4 Yoganandan N, Pintar FA, Gennarelli TA, Maltese MR. Patterns of abdominal injuries in frontal and side impacts. Proceedings of the Annual Conference. *Assoc Advance Automot Med* 2000; **44**: 17–36.
5 Chiu WC, Shanmuganathan K, Mirvis SE, Scalea TM. Determining the need for laparotomy in penetrating torso trauma: a prospective study using triple contrast enhanced abdominopelvic computed tomography. *J Trauma* 2001; **51**: 860–8.
6 Roberts I, Evans P, Bunn F, *et al*. Is the normalisation of blood pressure in bleeding trauma patients harmful? *Lancet* 2001; **357**: 385–7.
7 Bickell WH, Wall MJ, Pepe PE, *et al*. Immediate versus delayed resuscitation for hypotensive patients with penetrating torso injuries. *N Engl J Med* 1994; **331**: 1105–9.
8 Mattox KL, Bickell WH, Pepe PE, *et al*. Prospective MAST study in 911 patients. *J Trauma* 1989; **29**: 1104–12.
9 Prall JA, Nichols JS, Brennan R, Moore EE. Early definitive abdominal evaluation in the triage of unconscious normotensive blunt trauma patients. *J Trauma* 1994; **37**: 792–7.
10 Koury HI, Peschiera JL, Welling RE. Selective use of pelvic roentgenograms in blunt trauma patients. *J Trauma* 1993; **34**: 236–7.
11 Nagy KK, Roberts RR, Joseph KT, *et al*. Experience with over 2500 diagnostic peritoneal lavages. *Injury* 2000; **31**: 479–82.
12 Hodgson NF, Stewart TC, Girotti MJ. Open or closed diagnostic peritoneal lavage for abdominal trauma? A meta-analysis. *J Trauma* 2000; **48**: 1091–5.
13 Mendez C, Gubler KD, Maier RV. Diagnostic accuracy of peritoneal lavage in patients with pelvic fractures. *Arch Surg* 1994; **129**: 477–82.
14 Tsang BD, Panacek EA, Brant WE, Wisner DH. Effect of oral contrast administration for abdominal computed tomography in the evaluation of acute blunt trauma. *Ann Emerg Med* 1997; **30**: 7–13.
15 Wolfman NT, Bechtold RE, Scharling ES, Meredith JW. Blunt upper abdominal trauma: evaluation by CT. *Am J Roentgenol* 1992; **158**: 493–501.
16 Gracias VH, Frankel HL, Gupta R, *et al*. Defining the learning curve for the Focussed Abdominal Sonogram for Trauma (FAST) examination: implications for credentialling. *Am Surg* 2001; **67**: 364–8.
17 Stengel D, Bauwens K, Sehouli J, *et al*. Systematic review and meta-analysis of emergency ultrasonography for blunt abdominal trauma. *Br J Surg* 2001; **88**: 901–12.
18 Boulanger BR, Kearney PA, Tsui B, Ochoa JB. The routine use of sonography in penetrating torso injury is beneficial. *J Trauma* 2001; **51**: 230–5.
19 Gonzalez RP, Ickler J, Gachassin P. Complementary roles of diagnostic peritoneal lavage in the evaluation of blunt abdominal trauma. *J Trauma* 2001; **51**: 1128–34.
20 Poole GV, Thomas KR, Hauser CJ. Laparoscopy in trauma. *Surg Clin North Am* 1996; **76**: 547–56.
21 Shapiro MB, Jenkins DH, Schwab CW, Rotondo MF. Damage control: collective review. *J Trauma* 2000; **49**: 969–78.
22 Wilson RH, Moorehead RJ. Management of splenic trauma. *Injury* 1992; **23**: 5–9.
23 Sanders MN, Civil I. Adult splenic injuries: treatment patterns and predictive indicators. *Aust NZ J Surg* 1999; **69**: 430–2.
24 Carrillo EH, Richardson JD. The current management of hepatic trauma. *Adv Surg* 2001; **35**: 39–59.

25 Hughes TM. The diagnosis of gastrointestinal tract injuries resulting from blunt trauma. *Aust NZ J Surg* 1999; **69**: 770–7.

26 Demetriades D, Murray JA, Chan L, *et al.* Penetrating colon injuries requiring resection: diversion or primary anastomosis? An AAST prospective multicenter study. *J Trauma* 2001; **50**: 765–75.

27 Boulanger BR, Milzman DP, Rosati C, Rodriguez A. The clinical significance of acute hyperamylasemia after blunt trauma. *Can J Surg* 1993; **36**: 63–9.

28 Boffard KD, Brooks AJ. Pancreatic trauma – injuries to the pancreas and pancreatic duct. *Eur J Surg* 2000; **166**: 4–12.

29 Santucci RA, McAninch JW. Diagnosis and management of renal trauma: past, present and future. *J Am Coll Surg* 2000; **191**: 443–51.

30 Bodner DR, Selzman AA, Spirnak JP. Evaluation and treatment of bladder rupture. *Semin Urol* 1995; **13**: 62–5.

31 Rosati C. Acute traumatic rupture of the diaphragm. *Chest Surg Clin North Am* 1998; **8**: 371–9.

32 Ballard RB, Rozycki GS, Newman PG, *et al.* An algorithm to reduce the incidence of false-negative examinations in patients at high risk for occult injury. Focussed assessment for the sonographic examination of the trauma patient. *J Am Coll Surg* 1999; **189**: 145–50.

33 Biffl WL, Smith WR, Moore EE, *et al.* Evolution of a multidisciplinary pathway for the management of unstable patients with pelvic fractures. *Ann Surg* 2001; **233**: 843–50.

34 Feliciano DV. Management of traumatic retroperitoneal haematoma. *Ann Surg* 1990; **211**: 109–23.

35 Esposito TJ. Trauma during pregnancy. *Emerg Med Clin North Am* 1994; **12**: 167–99.

36 Kudsk KA, Croce MA, Fabian TC, *et al.* Enteral versus parenteral feeding. Effects on septic morbidity after blunt and penetrating abdominal trauma. *Ann Surg* 1992; **215**: 503–13.

37 Saggi BH, Sugerman HJ, Ivatury RR, Bloomfield GL. Abdominal compartment syndrome. *J Trauma* 1998; **45**: 597–609.

38 Torrie J, Hill AA, Streat SJ. Staged abdominal repair in critical illness. *Anaesth Intens Care* 1996; **24**: 368–74.

Part Twelve

Environmental Injuries

70.

Submersion injuries
C Edibam

DEFINITIONS

The American Heart Association Guidelines for Resuscitation[1] suggest that the term 'Submersion victim' be used to describe a person who experiences some swimming related stress that is sufficient to require support in the field, plus transportation to an emergency facility for further observation and treatment. 'Drowning' refers to death within 24 h following a submersion event and the term 'Near drowning' should no longer be used.

EPIDEMIOLOGY

Drowning causes over 140 000 deaths world-wide, with 9000 reported from the USA,[2] 500 from Australia[3] and 700 from the UK.[4] The incidence of non-fatal submersion events has been estimated to be 2–20 times more common than drowning.[5] More than half of all submersion events occur in children less than 5 years, the majority being 1–2 years old.[6,7] Males predominate with peaks at 5 and 20 years of age. Private swimming pools and natural water bodies close to home present the greatest risk to young children.[7] Other sites include bathtubs, fish tanks, buckets, toilets and washing machines. Adolescent drowning tends to occur in rivers, lakes, canals and beaches.[8] Lack of adult supervision is almost always to blame for toddler accidents, however, child abuse must also be considered. Alcohol and drug intoxication is associated with up to 40% of adolescent drowning.[9] Other risk factors include epilepsy (18%), trauma (16%), and cardiopulmonary disease (14%).[10] Hyperventilation prior to underwater swimming suppresses the physiologic response to rising carbon dioxide tension, allowing hypoxia to ensue with consequent loss of consciousness and water breathing.[11]

PATHOPHYSIOLOGY

Voluntary apnoea and reflex responses occur upon submersion. The 'diving response' is characterized by apnoea, marked generalized vasoconstriction and bradycardia in response to cold-water stimulus of the ophthalmic division of the trigeminal nerve. Blood is then shunted preferentially to the brain and heart. In infants, the response may be marked,[12] but only 15% of fully clothed adults show a significant response. The diving reflex appears to play a powerful role in oxygen conservation in animals, but in humans its role is unknown but may be protective.[13]

At some point after submersion, involuntary inspiration occurs, which leads to aspiration of water and often vomitus. Laryngeal spasm may occur which may explain the approximate 15% incidence of 'dry drowning,' where little or no fluid is found in the lungs.[14,15] Gasping then occurs and water aspiration continues. Up to 22 ml/kg of water has been estimated to be the maximal survivable inhaled water volume.[16] This is followed by a phase of secondary apnoea and loss of consciousness.

Hypoxaemic death ensues if the person is not retrieved and resuscitated. Acute lung injury (ALI) (see Ch. 27, ARDS), often termed 'secondary drowning', occurs in up to 72% of symptomatic survivors.[17] Multiple organ dysfunction and cerebral damage may become evident in those that survive to hospital.

SALT VS FRESH WATER ASPIRATION

The differences between salt and fresh water drowning should be downplayed.[1] On the basis of animal studies, it was thought that hypertonic seawater aspiration should draw plasma volume into the pulmonary interstitial space leading to hypovolaemia, hypernatraemia and haemoconcentration. Similarly, aspiration of hypotonic fresh water should lead to the passage of large volumes into the bloodstream leading to hypervolaemia, dilutional hyponatraemia, haemolysis and haemoglobinuria. Modell and colleagues[18] showed that volumes of water normally aspirated rarely translate into clinically meaningful syndromes. Of 91 patients seen with severe submersion, no patient had serious electrolyte abnormalities or haemolysis. In another series, only 15% of retrieved but unresuscitable patients had any of the expected electrolyte changes.[16] Generally, most patients with ALI will be hypovolaemic by the time they have reached hospital.[11] No clinically detectable difference in the patterns of lung injury is seen between salt and fresh water drowning, and both types reduce pulmonary surfactant quantity and function.[19]

WATER CONTAMINANTS

The incidence of pneumonia complicating submersion injury exceeds 15%.[17] Rivers, lakes and coastal waters are greater reservoirs for microbes than well-kept swimming pools. In fresh water, gram-negative bacteria predominate along with anaerobes and Staphylococci spp., fungi, algal and protozoan species. Aeromonas spp. are ubiquitous water-borne bacteria and can be responsible for severe pneumonia.[20] Chemicals in polluted water (e.g. kerosene,[21] chlorine[22]) and particulate matter (e.g. sand[23]) can cause severe pulmonary dysfunction.

TEMPERATURE

Victims of submersion may develop primary or secondary hypothermia. If submersion occurs in icy water (<5°C), hypothermia may develop rapidly and provide some protection against hypoxia. Surface cooling is unlikely to produce adequate protective hypothermia before hypoxia ensues.[13] Most survivors of prolonged submersion almost always involve small children in icy water, and it has been postulated that protective core cooling occurs rapidly due to cold-water aspiration, ingestion and absorption, though the mechanisms remains controversial.[24] Of more importance, in cold-water submersion, are the detrimental 'cold-shock' responses.[25] These responses include a 'gasp' followed by uncontrollable hyperventilation and reduction in maximal breath hold times, vasoconstriction, tachycardia, hypertension and increased myocardial oxygen consumption. These responses may lead to motor dyscoordination and swimming failure as well as cardiac arrhythmias. Hence, even strong swimmers may drown quickly in icy waters.

MANAGEMEMENT

BASIC LIFE SUPPORT

Prompt retrieval from the water and immediate on-site resuscitation are essential for survival. Expired air resuscitation and external cardiac compression should be applied immediately after retrieval. If trauma is suspected, especially in diving and surfing accidents, head and spinal injuries should be assumed, and the cervical spine stabilized during airway manipulation and transport. The Heimlich manoeuvre is no longer recommended in the management of submersion injury, as the volume of aspirated water removed at the time of attempt is small and the risk of gastric aspiration is great.[1] When experienced personnel arrive, bag and mask ventilation and advanced cardiac life support is initiated.

INITIAL HOSPITAL MANAGEMENT

Resuscitation continues on arrival to hospital. Endotracheal intubation and mechanical ventilation is instituted if hypoxaemia is severe, despite high flow oxygen or assisted bag and mask respiration. Ventilatory failure, characterized clinically by increasing respiratory distress and rising carbon dioxide levels, and the presence of an impaired conscious level or severe agitation may also necessitate intubation. Insertion of a nasogastric tube to decompress the stomach should be performed if possible but may be difficult in a hypoxic agitated patient. Attempts to re-warm the patient are initiated as soon as possible.

ASSESSMENT

HISTORY

Attempts should be made to elucidate the time and the duration of submersion, the presence of polluted water and likely contaminants, delay in resuscitation attempts and the likelihood of alcohol ingestion, drug use, pre-existing medical conditions and co-existing trauma.

EXAMINATION

A thorough secondary survey is carried out, concentrating on cardiorespiratory examination. Particularly important are signs of respiratory distress, wheeze, crackles and peripheral circulatory insufficiency. Neurological status should also be assessed. Clinical deterioration in those with minor symptoms and signs can occur and the patient should be reassessed at frequent intervals.

INVESTIGATIONS

These depend upon the clinical circumstance, but could include:

- arterial blood gases/ lactate level
- plasma biochemistry/serum osmolality: electrolyte abnormalities are unlikely in sea or fresh water drowning. CK should be measured as rhabdomyolysis has been reported[26]
- haematology: tests for haemolysis, e.g. total haemoglobin (tHb), free Hb and myoglobin concentrations in the plasma and urine
- toxicological assays for drug and alcohol levels should be considered
- chest X-ray, 12 lead ECG
- microbiology: tracheal aspirates or sputum for gram stain, microscopy and culture

● trauma imaging: cervical and/or thoracic lumbar spine X-rays; CT head if traumatic brain injury is suspected or the patient is comatose. Imaging of other body areas is dependent upon the clinical likelihood of injury.

ADMISSION CRITERIA

Asymptomatic patients with no clinical findings on cardiorespiratory examination and a normal chest radiograph and blood gas are unlikely to develop ALI and pneumonia, and do not require hospital admission.[17,27] All other patients should be admitted to a high-dependency area or intensive care unit for continuous monitoring and re-warming.

RESPIRATORY SUPPORT

Severe agitation or coma mandates intubation and mechanical ventilation. However, adequate oxygenation can often be maintained with high flow oxygen or continuous positive airway pressure (CPAP) by tight fitting facemask. Superimposed ventilatory failure may be managed by adding positive inspiratory pressure to CPAP, but this usually signals severe respiratory dysfunction that requires intubation and mechanical ventilation. The principals of respiratory support are discussed in Chapters 25 (Mechanical Ventilation) and 27 (ARDS).

CARDIOVASCULAR SUPPORT

Patients with ALI are often hypovolaemic regardless of the type of water ingestion. Cautious volume expansion and the use of catecholamine infusion may improve cardiac output and blood pressure. Fluid replacement with isotonic fluids is aimed at restoring adequate end-organ perfusion without compromising respiratory function. The use of a central venous or Swan-Ganz catheter may be necessary to achieve these goals.

CEREBRAL PROTECTION

No specific cerebral protective measures have proven efficacy in post anoxic encephalopathy associated with drowning.[28] Maintenance of an adequate cerebral perfusion pressure (by maintaining mean arterial pressure >90 mmHg in adults, or >60–70 mmHg in children) is the most important goal of therapy. Prevention of cerebral venous and thus intracranial hypertension can be achieved by neutral neck positioning, avoiding occlusive endotracheal tube ties and head up positioning. Avoiding hypocapnia ($PaCO_2$ <30 mmHg), reducing cerebral metabolic rate with sedation, preventing hypoglycaemia and hyperthermia and the use of anticonvulsants in those with documented seizures are simple measures to prevent secondary cerebral injury.

Table 70.1 Predictors of death or severe neurological impairment after submersion

At site of immersion
 Immersion duration >10 min[30]
 Delay in commencement of CPR[7]
In the emergency department
 Asystole on arrival[31] or CPR duration >25 min
 Fixed dilated pupils[32] and Glasgow Coma Score <5[33]
 Fixed dilated pupils and arterial pH <7.0[34]
In the ICU
 No spontaneous, purposeful movements and abnormal
  brainstem function 24 h after immersion
 Abnormal CT scan within 36 h of submersion

OTHER THERAPIES

There is no role for prophylactic corticosteroid therapy in the prevention of acute lung injury after submersion.[11] Prophylactic antibiotic therapy is unproven and the decision to commence therapy is made on the degree of water contamination, need for mechanical ventilation and severity of respiratory failure.[17] Baseline microbiological studies should be sent prior to commencement of therapy.

PROGNOSIS

Mortality rate for those surviving more than 24 h was 24% in a recent large series,[17] with three-quarters succumbing in the early stages after injury. Moderate to severe brain damage is reported in 33% of survivors.[7] The outcome in children is similar with 30% having selective deficits and 3% with persistent vegetative state.[29] No difference in mortality between fresh and salt water submersion has been documented.[10] Lower core temperatures appear to be associated with a better prognosis, except if this occurs after rescue. However, hypothermia in warm water immersion and severe hypothermia (<30°C) in cold water immersion is indicative of prolonged immersion and poor outcome.[25] Table 70.1 lists some factors associated with death or severe neurological impairment. None of these predictors are infallible and survival with normal cerebral function has been noted despite the presence of some or all of these factors.[11]

REFERENCES

1 AHA Resuscitation Guidelines Submersion or Near-Drowning. *Circulation* 2000; **102(suppl I)**: I-233–6.
2 Spyker DA. Submersion injury: epidemiology, prevention and management. *Pediatr Clin North Am* 1985; **32**: 113–25.
3 Pearn J. Drowning in Australia: a national appraisal with particular reference to children. *Med J Aust* 1977; ii: 770–1.

4 Golden F St C, Rivers JF. The immersion accident. *Anaesthesia* 1975; **30**: 364–73.

5 Weinstein M, Kreiger BP. Near drowning: epidemiology, pathophysiology and initial treatment. *J Emerg Med* 1996; **14**: 461–7.

6 Centers for Disease Control. Fatal injuries to children – United States, 1986. *MMWR* 1990; **39**: 442–51.

7 Orlowski JP. Drowning, near drowning, and ice-water submersions. *Pediatr Clin North Am* 1987; **34**: 75–92.

8 Wintemute GJ. Childhood drowning and near drowning in the United States. *Am J Dis Child* 1990; **144**,663–9.

9 Wintemute GJ, Kraus JF, Teret SP, Wright M. Drowning in childhood and adolescence: a population based study. *Am J Public Health* 1987; **77**: 830–2.

10 Spilzman D. Near drowning and drowning classification. A proposal to stratify mortality based on the analysis of 1831 cases. *Chest* 1997; **112**: 660–5.

11 Modell JH. Drowning. *N Engl J Med* 1993; **328**: 253–6.

12 Daly M deB, Angell-James JE, Elsner R. Role of carotid-body chemoreceptors and their reflex interactions in bradycardia and cardiac arrest. *Lancet* 1979; **1**: 764–7.

13 Gooden BA. Why some people do not drown: hypothermia versus the diving response. *Med J Aust* 1992; **152**: 629–32.

14 Karch SB. Pathology of the lung in near drowning. *Am J Emerg Med* 1986; **4**: 1–15.

15 Kringsholm B, Filskov A, Kock K. Autopsied cases of drowning in Denmark 1987–1989. *Forensic Sci Int* 1991; **52**: 85–92.

16 Modell JH, Davis JH. Electrolyte changes in human drowning victims. *Anesthesiology* 1969; **30**: 414–20.

17 van Berkel M, Bierens JJL, Lie RLK, *et al.* Pulmonary oedema, pneumonia and mortality in submersion victims: a retrospective study in 125 patients. *Intensive Care Med* 1996; **22**: 101–7.

18 Modell JH, Graves SA, Ketover A. Clinical course of 91 consecutive drowning victims. *Chest* 1976; **70**: 231–8.

19 Sachdev R. Near drowning. *Crit Care Clin* 1999; **15**: 281–96.

20 Ender PT, Dolan MJ, Farmer JC, *et al.* Near-drowning associated Aeromonas pneumonia. *J Emerg Med* 1996; **14**: 737–41.

21 Segev D, Szold O, Fireman E *et al.* Kerosene-induced severe acute respiratory failure in near-drowning. Reports on four cases of the literature. *Crit Care Med* 1999; **27**: 1437–40.

22 DeNicola LK, Falk JL, Swanson ME, *et al.* Submersion injuries in children and adults. *Crit Care Clin* 1997; **13**: 477–502.

23 Dunagan D, Cox J, Chang M.C *et al.* Sand aspiration with near drowning. Radiographic and bronchoscopic findings. *Am J Respir Crit Care Med* 1997; **156**: 292–5.

24 Conn AW, Miyassaka K, Katayama M *et al.* A canine study of cold water drowning in fresh versus saltwater. *Crit Care Med* 1995; **23**: 2023–36.

25 Golden F St C, Tipton MJ, Scott RJ. Immersion and near drowning. *Br J Anaesth* 1997; **79**: 214–25.

26 Agar JW. Rhabdomyolysis and acute renal failure after near drowning in cold salt water. *Med J Aust* 1994; **161**: 686–7.

27 Causey AL, Tilelli JA, Swanson ME. Predicting discharge in uncomplicated drowning. *Am J Emerg Med* 2000; **18**: 9–11.

28 Bohn DJ, Biggard WJ, Smith CR *et al.* Influence of hypothermia, barbiturate therapy and intracranial pressure monitoring on morbidity and mortality after near drowning. *Crit Care Med* 1986; **14**: 529–34.

29 Pearn J. Medical aspects of drowning in children. *Ann Acad Med Singapore* 1992; **21**: 433–55.

30 Quan L, Kinder D. Pediatric submersions: prehospital predictors of outcome. *Pediatrics* 1992; **90**: 909–13.

31 Nagel FO, Kibel SM, Beatty DW. Childhood near drowning- factors associated with poor outcome. *S Afr Med J* 1990; **78**: 422–5.

32 Frates RC Jr. Analysis of predictive factors in the assessment of warm-water near drowning in children. *Am J Dis Child* 1981; **135**: 1006–8.

33 Dean JM, Kaufman ND. Prognostic factors in childhood near-drowning: the Glasgow coma scale. *Crit Care Med* 1981; **9**: 536–9.

34 Orlowski JP. Prognostic factors in pediatric cases of near drowning. *JACEP* 1979; **8**: 176–9.

71.

Burns

D P Mackie

The last half of the twentieth century has witnessed a sustained improvement in the survival of patients suffering thermal injury. Arguably, the single most important development has been the establishment of centralized burn care, which made possible advances in fluid resuscitation, life support techniques and the prevention of infection. With optimal care, children and young adults with burns of more than 80% of total body surface area (TBSA) now stand a reasonable chance of survival.[1]

Improvements in survival have gradually led to a shift of emphasis in burn care towards aspects of care, such as rehabilitation and quality of life. The complexity of care has led to the concept of the multi-disciplinary burn team, in which all aspects of care are co-ordinated in an integrated approach to clinical management.[1]

PATHOPHYSIOLOGY

LOCAL EFFECTS

Thermal injury produces complex local and systemic responses. The local inflammatory response results in local vasodilatation and an increase in vascular permeability. The changes are immediate and combine to produce extravasation of fluid and plasma protein at the site of injury. In extensive burns, oedema becomes generalized. The greatest rate of oedema formation occurs in the first few hours, but further extravasation occurs up to 24 h post burn.[2] The total amount of oedema formed depends on the type of injury and the extent of resuscitation. Without fluid replacement, hypovolaemic shock occurs, limiting the extent of extravasation. On the other hand, excessive fluid administration will produce excessive oedema. By 24 h post-burn oedema formation is largely complete and local vascular integrity restored.

The process of deepening of the burn wound beyond the area of heat necrosis following injury is associated with microvascular stasis. Events occurring within minutes and hours of injury, which contribute to stasis include microthrombus formation, neutrophil adherence, fibrin deposition and endothelial swelling. Diverse agents, including anti-oxidants and anti-inflammatory drugs, have been shown to attenuate this process in experimental settings, but none are yet established in clinical practice. Empirically, it is assumed that maintenance of good tissue oxygenation, avoidance of over-resuscitation and prevention of wound dehydration all contribute to wound healing by preventing undue extension of necrosis in the wound bed.

CIRCULATORY EFFECTS

Circulatory effects of burn injury become significant in burns of over 15% TBSA. Changes are rapid and the magnitude is roughly proportional to the extent of burn injury. Cardiac output is reduced immediately following injury. Secretion of epinephrine, norepinephrine, vasopressin and angiotensin cause an increase in systemic and pulmonary vascular resistance. There is good evidence for the presence of circulating myocardial depressant factors, but developing hypovolemia and reduced venous return may be equally important.[3,4]

Cardiac output recovers gradually during the second post-burn day (PBD), reaching supra-normal levels by post-burn day 3 as the hypermetabolic response to burn injury becomes manifest. Circulatory dynamics are complicated by resorption of oedema fluid and by continuing evaporative fluid loss from the wounds. Prolonged elevation of renin/angiotensin and ADH has been well documented and circulating blood volume may remain subnormal into the second week post burn.[5]

METABOLIC EFFECTS

The hypermetabolic state, which ensues from around the third PBD until the wounds are substantially healed, is currently regarded as a manifestation of the systemic inflammatory response syndrome. The state is partly sustained by evaporative and radiant heat loss through the wounds[6] and energy expenditure can be reduced by increasing the ambient temperature and by the use of occlusive dressings.[6,7] Other factors shown to influence the metabolic rate include hypovolemia, pain, fear, and anxiety.[8] There is also a suggestion that bacterial colonization may aggravate hypermetabolism.[9,10]

PHARMACOLOGICAL EFFECTS

The pharmacokinetics and pharmacodynamics of many drugs are markedly altered in burn patients. During the first 24 h, when the cardiac output is depressed; absorption and distribution of administered drugs are delayed. Thereafter, increased cardiac output leads to accelerated drug absorption and distribution, while oedema fluid acts as an ill-defined third space. At the same time, renal blood flow and creatinine clearance are increased, particularly in younger patients. Drugs excreted via this route, such as the quinolone and aminoglycoside antibiotics, may therefore fail to reach effective levels at conventional dosages.[11,12] On the other hand, toxic levels may ensue if renal failure supervenes. If possible, therefore, antibiotic administration should be guided by measurement of plasma concentrations.

Drugs bound to albumin, including some benzodiazepines, will show increased bio-availability, In addition, detoxification via oxidative pathways, such as cytochrome P-450, is depressed, lengthening the half-life of drugs such as diazepam.[13] Accumulation of benzodiazepine derivatives may be increased.

The pharmacodynamics of muscle relaxants are significantly altered, by an apparent increase in receptor numbers.[14] Patients become relatively insensitive to non-depolarizing agents, while administration of succinylcholine may give rise to excessive release of potassium, and cardiac arrest.

The burn wound is a significant route of drug absorption as well as drug loss. For example the topical sulfonamide agent, mafenide, may cause metabolic acidosis through inhibition of renal carbonic anhydrase; deafness has been reported following the topical use of gentamicin.

CLINICAL MANAGEMENT

FIRST AID

Immediate aid comprises stopping the burn process, followed by the removal of clothing and cooling the wound, preferably with cold, running water, for 10–20 min. This provides pain relief and may prevent deepening of the wound.[15] Hypothermia should be avoided. Oxygen should be given, if available, and patients with burns to head and neck should be kept in a semi-upright position. Burn injury can only be assessed properly in hospital conditions, and priority should be given to early evacuation of the victim.

GENERAL MANAGEMENT: 0–24 HOURS

On admission, a careful history should be taken of the circumstances of the injury, and to elucidate past medical history. The patient should be undressed, weighed, and carefully examined to exclude additional traumatic injury.

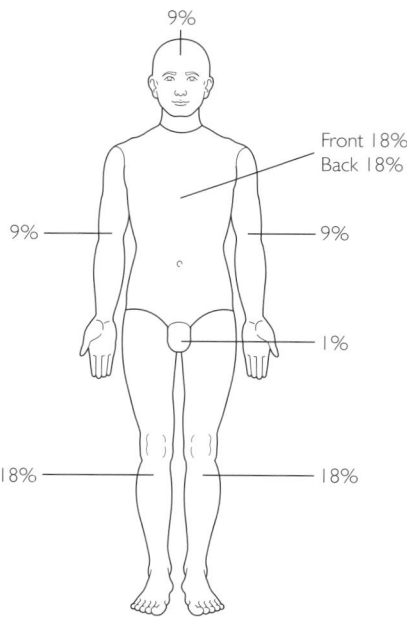

Fig. 71.1   Rule of nine to estimate body surface area burns in adults.

The extent and depth of injury is assessed with the aid of printed Lund and Browder charts, or by using the 'rule of nines' (Figure 71.1). The rule of nines is modified for children (Figure 71.2). A naso-gastric tube and urine catheter should be inserted in patients requiring resuscitation therapy. Escharotomies may be required for circular burns of the trunk and limbs.

FLUID THERAPY: 0–24 HOURS

Fluid therapy is required for injuries exceeding 15% of body surface area (10% in children and the elderly), preferably via a wide-bore peripheral i.v. cannula. The aim is to provide sufficient salt and water to preserve normal organ function, while minimizing oedema formation. Excessive fluid administration increases the risk of circulatory overload in the days following the resuscitation period. Potentially fatal complications of excessive fluid administration include the abdominal compartment syndrome in adults[16] and the occurrence of cerebral oedema in children.[17]

Various resuscitation formulae have been published in the past to guide initial fluid therapy. These formulae are entirely experience-based and many are of historical interest only, but all comprise a fluid intake of 2–4 ml/kg body weight per % burn in 24 h, and a sodium intake of approximately 0.5 mmol/kg per % burn.[18,19] These findings have led some to employ resuscitation regimens based on the administration of hypertonic sodium solutions, which require a smaller volume of fluid. However, the solute load may be excessive, requiring extra water administration in subsequent days, with an increased risk of fluid overload. The use of isotonic fluids is therefore preferred by those without widespread experience of burns resuscitation.

The most widely used resuscitation formula for adults is based on the Parkland Formula, which has been adopted by major training programmes, such as the Advanced Trauma Life Support and the Emergency Medicine for Severe Burns:

> 4 ml Ringer-Lactate solution × kg body weight × % TBSA burn in the first 24 h, of which half should to be given in the first 8 h *post burn*

The formula thus incorporates a faster rate of administration if initial treatment has been delayed.

Children require extra fluid to compensate for basal needs. For children under 30 kg, the resuscitation formula of Carvajal[20] is useful:

> Fluid requirement (ml): 0–24 h post burn = 2000 × TBSA + 5000 × TBSAB

where TBSA is the total body surface area (m²) and TBSAB is total body surface area burned (m²). Again half of the calculated amount is given in the first 8 h.

These formulae are to be regarded as guidelines only. The actual amount of fluid given depends on the clinical condition and the actual amount of fluid administered can vary widely from that predicted. Adequacy of resuscitation is monitored by vital signs, and a targeted urine output of 0.5–1 ml/kg per h. Other indicators include warm extremities and return of gut peristalsis. Fluid intake may be adjusted to maintain urine output at the desired range. Requirements are increased in the presence of inhalation injury, additional traumatic injury, and dehydration (e.g. fire-fighters).

Invasive monitoring is not essential in uncomplicated burns and the results may be misleading, as central pressures are often low. Thirst is common, but unrestricted oral fluids will increase oedema formation. Controlled quantities of nutritional liquids are recommended to protect gut integrity.[20,21]

Hypoalbuminaemia develops rapidly and may be extreme. The extent to which burn patients will tolerate hypoalbuminaemia is unknown and clinical studies into best practice are awaited. In our unit at present, albumin is given to maintain serum albumin above 15 g/l, com-

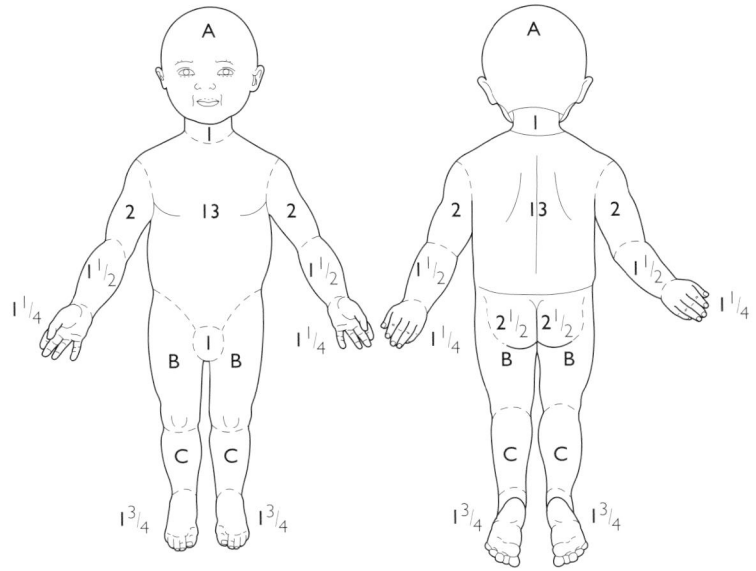

Age	< 1 year	1 year	5 years	10 years	15 years	Adult
Area A = ¹/₂ of head (%)	9.5	8.5	6.5	5.5	4.5	3.5
Area B = ¹/₂ of one thigh (%)	2.75	3.25	4.0	4.25	4.5	4.75
Area C = ¹/₂ of one leg (%)	2.5	2.5	2.75	3.0	3.25	3.5

Fig. 71.2   Surface area percentages by age.

mencing 12 h post burn when capillary integrity has been largely restored.

FLUID THERAPY AFTER 24 HOURS

During the second 24 h, enteral nutritional intake is increased, while the total rate of fluid administration is gradually reduced. At the end of the second day, fluid intake should allow for generous urine production, while compensating for evaporative losses through the wounds.

The actual fluid loss through wounds varies widely, and depends on the type of burn and topical wound treatment. A useful formula to obtain a rough estimate for fluid loss is:

(25+ % body surface burn) × m² body surface area = evaporative fluid loss (ml/h)

Electrolyte disturbance is common following burn injury and requires treatment. Hypernatraemia is often a sign of hypovolaemia, confirmed if urine sodium is low. The condition is perilous, especially in the first week post burn, as oligurea and renal failure may develop unexpectedly. The amount of free water given should be increased gradually, particularly in the elderly, to avoid fluid overload. Patients who are in fluid balance may require sodium supplementation to compensate for solute loss in wound exudates.

HAEMOGLOBINUREA/MYOGLOBINUREA

Tissue injury from deep burns, particularly electrical injury, causes the release of myoglobin and haemoglobin from damaged cells. Diagnosis is made on observing discoloration of the urine, from faint pink in mild cases to almost black. Fluid administration should be increased and mannitol (12.5 g/l resuscitation fluid) given to encourage diuresis. The addition of bicarbonate (25 mmol/l resuscitation fluid) will alkalinize the urine and increase the rate of pigment excretion.

PAIN THERAPY

During the first 24 h, pain management is best achieved by incremental doses of i.v. morphine. Thereafter, the pain suffered by burn patients may be divided into background pain, which is continuous, and procedural pain caused by interventions.[22] The recurring ordeal of dressing changes, physiotherapy exercises and surgical procedures generates apprehension and anxiety, which compound distress.

Regular pain therapy is required to counter background pain, topped up by extra analgesics prior to procedures. NSAIDs, slow-release oral morphine and continuous i.v. morphine, with incremental boluses can be titrated, alone or in combination, as required. Patient-controlled analgesia is effective, although modification of the control button may be necessary for those with bandaged hands. Ketamine in sub-anaesthetic doses is extremely useful for procedural pain in children. The influence of anxiety and depression on pain perception suggests additional avenues of therapy.[23]

Non-pharmacological interventions, such as hypnosis and other distraction techniques, are an effective adjunct in susceptible patients.[24] Above all, an attitude of reassurance and understanding by all carers is indispensable.

NUTRITION

The hypermetabolic response is roughly proportional to the extent of injury. In young adults and children with extensive burns, energy expenditure may be doubled. In addition, protein and substantial amounts of trace elements, such as zinc, copper and selenium are lost in wound exudate.[25]

There is no doubt that burn patients require additional calories and proteins, but traditional formulae for calculating requirements produce overestimates in the context of current burn care.[26] In the absence of direct metabolic measurements we currently use the empirical formula for minimal caloric intake:

Caloric requirement = REE + (REE × %TBSA burn/100)

where REE is the resting energy expenditure calculated from the Harris & Benedict equation.

Patients with extensive burns invariably require tube feeds, which are generally well tolerated. If gastric retention is problematic, a duodenum tube is usually effective. A high-protein proprietary feed is usually adequate, if supplemented by trace elements and vitamins. The role of arginine and glutamine supplements are reviewed in Ch. 85. Adequacy of feeding is best assessed by monitoring body weight.

WOUND HEALING

Treatment of extensive, full-thickness burn wounds by early excision and grafting has been firmly linked to survival.[27] Wound excision should be completed within the first week, before bacterial colonization and neovascular infiltration of the wound bed emerge. These operations are therefore urgent. Successfully grafted wounds will heal within 5 weeks, reducing the time available for bacterial infection to develop, and shortening the period of physiological disturbance. Wounds covered with widely meshed autografts lose large amounts of fluid, unless covered with a protective, such as allograft skin. Autograft donor sites are a further source of fluid loss.

For wounds treated conservatively, the main effort is devoted to the prevention of infection. Topical antimicrobial agents are commonly used, but may have potential side-effects (Table 71.1). These compounds change the appearance of the wound and should never be

Table 71.1 Commonly used topical anti-microbial agents

Agent	Comments
Silver sulfadiazine (SSD)	The most widely used agent with broad spectrum cover. Hypersensitivity (rarely) and transient leucopenia have been reported.
Cerium nitrate 0.5%	Often added to SSD, and forms a stable eschar. It is reported to bind 'burn toxins.'
Silver nitrate 0.5%	Applied as a soak, and is especially effective against pseudomonas. However, it may increase sodium loss, and potentially can cause methaemoglobinaemia.
Mafenide acetate 5–10%	Effective but short-lived antimicrobial, requiring repeated application. It has good penetration, and its side-effects (pain and metabolic acidosis) are less evident with 5% solution.
Chlorhexidine	Aqueous solution (0.2%) or 1% gel provides broad spectrum cover, but is rapidly inactivated, and may cause local pain, and rarely hypersensitivity.
Nitrofurazone	In polyethylene glycol (PEG) solution it is effective against *S. aureus*, but resistance develops early. Side-effects include hypersensitivity (common), hyperosmolarity, and renal failure due to PEG absorption has been reported.
Povidone iodine	In PEG solution provides broad spectrum cover, but is rapidly inactivated. It prevents wound maceration. Side-effects include occasional hypersensitivity, renal dysfunction due to excessive PEG, metabolic acidosis and rarely dysfunction.
Antibiotics	Have been used in solutions, creams, gels and sprays, but selection and development of resistant strains is inevitable, with a risk of systemic toxicity through absorption. Their usage is generally discouraged.

applied until expert wound inspection is complete. A number of bio-synthetic materials are currently available, which are designed to improve cosmetic and functional outcome. Despite the use of antiseptic dressings or biosynthetic coverings there is still a risk of microbial infection developing and unexplained signs of sepsis may necessitate urgent revision of the treated areas.

PREVENTION OF WOUND INFECTION

Bacterial infection is still the most common cause of death in burns. Depression of the immune system is well-documented.[28,29] At the same time, the burn wound presents a favourable medium for bacterial growth.

BACTERIOLOGICAL SURVEILLANCE

Routine bacteriological surveillance of burn patients (at least twice-weekly) is essential. The growth of pathogens from wound swabs may reflect growing resistance to topical wound therapy, indicating a need for change. When infection is suspected, the choice of an appropriate antibiotic will be governed by prior knowledge of the colonizing micro-organisms and their antibiograms. In addition, the effectiveness of prophylactic measures can only be assessed by regular monitoring of the microflora present within the burns unit.

PATIENT ISOLATION

In an effort to reduce wound colonization and contamination from cross-infection, barrier-nursing of patients with extensive injuries is mandatory. The importance of isolation measures has been stressed,[30] but a significant proportion of patients still become colonized by micro-organisms from endogenous reservoirs, which cannot be controlled by barrier nursing alone.[31-33]

THE GASTRO-INTESTINAL TRACT

Loss of gut integrity following burn injury has been well demonstrated.[34,35] In addition to reactive damage following reperfusion of the ischaemic gut, mediators derived from the burn wound itself may also be involved.[36] Clinical strategies aimed at protecting the gastro-intestinal tract include optimal fluid therapy during the first hours following injury to prevent mesenteric hypoperfusion, and the institution of early enteral nutrition, which can be safely commenced within a few hours of injury.[21] Diets enriched with specific amino acids, such as arginine and glutamine, may contribute to the maintenance of gut integrity.[37,38] Selective decontamination of the digestive tract has been advocated,[11,39] but the concept remains controversial.[40] Whatever the merits of each approach, all are secondary to the maintenance of effective hygienic policies in all aspects of patient care.

WOUND SEPSIS

Local effects include disruption of wound healing[41] and deepening of the injury.[42]

Systemic effects are often insidious. Prodromal signs are common and may include gastro-intestinal stasis, increasing positive fluid balance, glucose intolerance and increasing pyrexia. As sepsis progresses, clinical deterioration becomes manifest: tachypnoea, circulatory instability, thrombocytopenia and oliguria may herald the onset of multi-organ failure.

Antibiotic therapy, chosen on the basis of bacteriological surveillance data, should be given early, if possible. Fluid therapy in burn patients is complicated by evaporative fluid loss, which may increase if the wound surface degenerates. Supportive therapy for (multi-) organ failure should be implemented as indicated.

The causes of sepsis will persist until wound coverage is achieved and operative wound treatment should not be postponed. Although mortality is appreciable, experience has repeatedly shown that the prognosis is by no means hopeless.

INHALATION INJURY

The term inhalation injury includes three distinct types of injury which often, but not always, occur together.

HEAT INJURY TO THE UPPER AIRWAYS

Airway burns due to the inhalation of hot gases (steam excepted) rarely extend beyond the larynx. The development of mucosal and facial oedema can cause respiratory obstruction, particularly in children.

DIAGNOSIS

Facial burn, singed nasal hairs, visible burn to oropharynx, and hoarseness are typical features.

TREATMENT

If the condition is suspected, early endotracheal intubation is safest, before the procedure is rendered hazardous by oedema formation.

EFFECTS OF SMOKE ON THE RESPIRATORY SYSTEM

Many of the chemicals that are contained in smoke are highly reactive and produce immediate damage to the tracheo-bronchial tree. Detachment of epithelial cells and the development of tracheo-bronchial oedema cause airway narrowing and cast formation. Small airway closure leads to hypoxaemia and respiratory failure. Later, bronchorrhoea and mucosal sloughing may cause atelectasis and provide a focus for infection. In the absence of a cutaneous injury the clinical course is usually benign. However, the presence of an extensive skin burn increases the likelihood of ARDS; respiratory infection may follow.

DIAGNOSIS

History of exposure in a confined space, cough, breathlessness, wheeze, stridor, hypoxaemia, soot particles in pharynx. Diagnosis is confirmed by bronchoscopy, which may reveal soot in bronchial tree, mucosal injury, and tracheo-bronchial oedema.

TREATMENT

Mild cases may be treated by high-flow oxygen administration by mask. The mainstay of treatment in severe cases is intubation and ventilatory support with PEEP to maintain small-airway patency. Regular bronchial toilet is recommended to clear debris and to prevent respiratory infection.

Prolonged respiratory assistance may be necessary. The added respiratory requirements of the hypermetabolic state combined with inevitable loss of muscle mass frequently frustrate early weaning efforts.

INHALATION OF TOXIC GASES

Of the many toxic compounds[43] in smoke (Table 71.2), carbon monoxide (CO) deserves special mention. The affinity of CO for haemoglobin is 240 times that of oxygen. The loss of oxygen transport capacity is dependent on the concentration of inhaled CO and the duration of exposure. In addition, CO binds to cytochrome systems, inhibiting cellular oxidative processes. The half-life of COHb is 4 h when breathing air, compared with 45 min when breathing 100% oxygen.

DIAGNOSIS

Carbon monoxide poisoning should be suspected in all cases of exposure to combustion products in a closed space. The classical cherry red appearance of the CO victim is seldom evident; early signs may be mistaken for inebriation. Symptoms range from a throbbing headache in mild exposure (10–25% COHb) to weakness, dizziness, confusion and nausea (25–40% COHb), progressing to collapse, unconsciousness and convulsions (40–60% COHb). Death is increasingly likely at COHb concentrations of >60%. Patients exposed to high levels of CO may exhibit signs of cardiac instability. Signs of

Table 71.2 Common inhaled toxic gases

Gas	Source	Effect
Carbon monoxide	Organic matter	Tissue hypoxia, lipid peroxidation
Carbon dioxide	Organic matter	Narcosis tachycardia hypertension
Nitrogen dioxide	Wallpaper, wood	Bronchial irritation, dizziness, pulmonary oedema
Hydrogen chloride	Plastics	Severe mucosal irritation
Hydrogen cyanide	Wood, silk, nylons, polurethane	Headache, coma, acidosis
Benzene	Petrol, plastics	Mucosal irritation, coma
Ammonia	Nylon	Mucosal damage, extensive lung injury
Aldehyde	Wood, cotton, paper	Mucosal irritation

cerebral irritability may persist for days or weeks following apparent recovery.

TREATMENT
Administration of the highest concentration of oxygen available, as soon as possible after exposure. Loss of consciousness is an indication for oxygen delivery via an endotracheal tube. The use of hyperbaric oxygen, if immediately available, seems logical, but additional benefit has not been proven.

HYDROGEN CYANIDE TOXICITY
Hydrogen cyanide (HCN) toxicity frequently occurs in conjunction with CO inhalation. Inhaled concentrations of 200 ppm are rapidly fatal and HCN may account for many deaths at fire accident scenes.[44] Conventional treatment is as for CO intoxication. Removal by chelating agents, such as hydroxycobalamin or by the administration of sodium thiosulphate is also possible, but treatment would have to be immediate, based on a presumptive diagnosis, and is therefore not generally recommended.

FUTURE PROSPECTS

The outlook for young patients with extensive burn injuries, treated under optimal conditions, is now such that little further progress may be expected in terms of survival alone. Mortality among the elderly does, however, remain high. The major thrust of research is currently directed at improving functional and cosmetic outcome following burns. While the most visible efforts concern the development of techniques and materials to improve the quality of wound healing, advances in the field of intensive care are also relevant: strategies aimed at preventing ventilator-associated morbidity are equally applicable to burn patients, who often require prolonged ventilatory support; new insights into the inflammatory responses may improve the general condition of burn patients, increasing resistance to infection and improving tissue repair. There is growing interest in the psychological effects of thermal trauma, which includes new approaches to the management of pain and mental distress.

In the past, the establishment of burn centres has been largely opportunistic, often depending on the dedication of individual specialists. As the provision of medical services undergoes increasing scrutiny, the organization of burn care in many countries may be subject to reorganization. It is of the utmost importance that specialists involved in the field of burn care become actively engaged in this process, in order to guarantee continued quality of care for their population.

REFERENCES
1 Herndon DN, Muller MJ, Blakeney PE. Teamwork for total burn care: achievements, directions and hopes. In: Herndon DN (ed.) *Total Burn Care*. London: W.B. Saunders; 1996: pp. 1–4.
2 Demling RH, Mazess RB, Witt RM, *et al*. The study of burn wound edema using dichromatic absorptiometry. *J Trauma* 1978; **18**: 124–8.
3 Cioffi WG, De Meules JE, Gamelli RL. The effects of burn injury and fluid resuscitation on cardiac function in vitro. *J Trauma* 1986; **26**: 638–43.
4 Hilton JG, Marullo DS. Effects of thermal trauma on cardiac force of contraction. *Burns* 1986; **12**: 167–71.
5 Cioffi WG, Vaughan GM, Heironimus JD, *et al*. Disassociation of blood volume and flow in regulation of salt and water balance in burn patients. *Ann Surg* 1991; **214**: 213–9.
6 Wilmore DW, Mason AD, Johnson DW, *et al*. Effect of ambient temperature on heat production and heat loss in burn patients. *J Appl Physiol* 1975; **38**: 593–7.
7 Caldwell FT, Bowser GH, Crabtree JH. The effects of occlusive dressings on the energy expenditure of severely burned children. *Ann Surg* 1981; **193**: 579–91.
8 Arturson GS. Transport and demand of oxygen in severe burns. *J Trauma* 1977; **17**: 179–98.
9 Waymack JP. Antibiotics and the post-burn hypermetabolic response. *J Trauma* 1990; **30**: S30–5.
10 Mackie DP, van Hertum WAJ, Schumburg T, *et al*. Prevention of infection in burns: preliminary experience with selective decontamination of the digestive tract in patients with extensive injuries. *J Trauma* 1992; **32**: 570–5.
11 Loirat P, Rohan J, Bailet E *et al*. Increased glomerular filtration in patients with major burns and its effect on the pharmacokinetics of tobramycin. *N Engl J Med* 1978; **299**: 915–9.
12 Alexander D, Richard K, Morris S, *et al*. Application of newer antibiotic concepts in the use of ciprofloxacin for treatment of infections in the burn patient. *J Burn Care Rehab* 2001; **22**: S137.
13 Martyn JAJ, Greenblatt GS, Quinby WC. Diazepam kinetics following burn injury. *Anaesth Analgesia* 1983; **62**: 293–7.
14 Martyn JAJ, Goldhill DR, Goudsouzian NG. Clinical pharmacology of muscle relaxants in patients with burns. *J Clin Pharm* 1986; **26**: 680–5.
15 Davies JWL. Prompt cooling of the burned area: a review of the benefits and the effector mechanisms. *Burns* 1982; **9**: 1–6.
16 Ivy ME, Atweh NA, Palmer J, *et al*. Intra-abdominal hypertension and abdominal compartment syndrome in burn patients. *J Trauma* 2000; **49**: 387–91.
17 Prekop R, Bardosova G, Simko S, *et al*. Brain oedema in burned children. *Acta Chir Plast* 1984; **26**: 184–92.
18 Settle JAD. Principles of replacement fluid therapy. In: Settle JAD (ed.) *Principles and Practice of Burns Management*. London: Churchill Livingstone; 1996: pp. 217–22.
19 Carvajal HF. A physiologic approach to fluid therapy in severely burned children. *Surg Gyn Obstetrics* 1980; **150**: 379–84.
20 Klasen HJ, ten Duis HJ. Early oral feeding of patients with extensive burns. *Burns* 1987; **13**: 49–52.

21 Alexander JW, Gottschlich MM. Nutritional immuno-modulation in burn patients. *Crit Care Med* 1990; **18**: S149–53.

22 Choinière M, Melzak R, Rondeau J, *et al.* The pain of burns: characteristics and correlates. *J Trauma* 1989; **29**: 1531–9.

23 Taal LA, Faber AW, van Loey NEE, *et al.* The abbreviated burn-specific anxiety scale: a multi-centre study. *Burns* 1999; **25**: 493–7.

24 Miller AC, Hickman LC, Lemasters GK. A distraction technique for control of burn pain. *J Burn Care Rehabilitation* 1992; **13**: 576–80.

25 Berger MM, Cavadini C, Chiolero R, *et al.* Influence of large intakes of trace elements on recovery after burns. Nutrition 1994; **10**: 327–34.

26 Wolfe RR. Caloric requirements of the burned patients. *J Trauma* 1981; **21**: 712–4.

27 Muller MJ, Nicolai M, Wiggins R, *et al.* Modern treatment of a burn wound. In: Herndon DN (ed.) *Total Burn Care*. London: WB Saunders; 1996: pp. 136–47.

28 Abraham E. Physiologic stress and cellular ischemia: relationship to immunosuppression and susceptibility to sepsis. *Crit Care Med* 1991; **19**: 613–8.

29 Gibran NS, Heimbach DM. Mediators in thermal injury. *Seminars Nephrology*, 1993; **13**: 344–58.

30 McManus AT, Mason WF, McManus WF, *et al.* A decade of reduced Gram negative infections and mortality. *Abstracts, 5th European Burns Association Congress* 1992: M2.

31 Lowbury EJL, Babb JR, Ford PM. Protective isolation in a burns unit: the use of plastic isolators and air curtains. *J Hygiene* 1971; **69**: 529.

32 Burke JF, Quimby WC, Bondoc CC, *et al.* The contribution of a bacterially isolated environment to the prevention of infection in seriously burned patients. *Ann Surg* 1977; **186**: 377–87.

33 Lee JJ, Marvin JA, Heimbach DM, *et al.* Infection control in a burns centre. *J Burn Care Rehabilitation* 1990; **11**: 575–80.

34 Dobke MK, Simoni J, Ninnemann JL, *et al.* Endotoxemia after burn injury: effect of early excision on circulating endotoxin levels. *J Burn Care Rehab* 1989; **10**: 107–11.

35 Deitch EA. Intestinal permeability is increased in burn patients shortly after injury. *Surgery* 1990; **107**: 411–6.

36 Trop M, Schiffrin EJ, Carter EA. Effect of platelet activating factor on reticulo-endothelial system function. *Burns* 1991; **17**: 193–7.

37 Wilmore DW, Smith RJ, O'Dwyer ST, *et al.* The gut: a central organ after surgical stress. *Surgery* 1988; **104**: 917–23.

38 Burke DJ, Alverdy JC, Aoys E, *et al.* Glutamine-supplemented total parenteral nutrition improves gut immune function. *Arch Surg* 1989; **124**: 1396.

39 Manson WL, Klasen HJ, Sauer EW. Selective intestinal decontamination for prevention of wound colonization in severely burned patients: a retrospective analysis. *Burns* 1992; **18**: 98–102.

40 Deitch EA. Selective decontamination of the digestive tract: theory or therapy. *Crit Care Med* 1993; **21**: 1629–31.

41 Burke JF, Morris PJ, Bondoc CC. The effect of bacterial inflammation on wound healing. In Dunphy JE and van Winkle W (eds) *Repair and Regeneration*. New York: McGraw-Hill; 1969: pp. 19–31.

42 Order SE, Mason AD, Walker HL, *et al.* The pathogenesis of second and third degree burns and conversion to full thickness injury. *Surg Gyn Obst* 1965; **120**: 983–91.

43 Prien T, Traber DL. Toxic smoke compounds and inhalation injury – a review. *Burns* 1988; **14**: 451–60.

44 Purser DA, Grimshaw P, Berril KR. Intoxication by cyanide in fires: a study in monkeys using poly-acrylonitrile. *Arch Environmental Health* 1984; **39**: 394–400.

72.

Thermal disorders
A Hussein

Body temperature is normally very tightly controlled by a balance between heat production and heat loss, through a complex feedback mechanism involving the thermoregulatory centre in the hypothalamus. In the ICU, fever (pyrexia) is usually due to resetting of the thermoregulatory set-point at a higher level by activation of heat-conserving mechanisms, whereas hyperthermia is due to failure of effector mechanisms to maintain body temperature at the normal set-point.

Although the pathogenesis of hyperthermia varies between different aetiologies, the complications are similar:

- metabolic acidosis
- hyperkalaemia
- rhabdomyolysis
- renal failure
- disseminated intravascular coagulation
- liver failure
- death.

THERMOREGULATION

Control of body temperature, like most complex biological systems, is maintained by a complicated system of sensors and controls. The target set-point varies by $<1°C/d$ on a circadian basis, and by $<\frac{1}{2}°C$ monthly in women. However, at any given time the core temperature is within a few tenths of $1°C$ of the set-point.

The three major components of the thermoregulatory system are:

- afferent input
- central control
- effector responses.

Temperature is sensed by A-Δ fibres (most cold signals) and unmyelinated C fibres (most warm signals). These sensors are distributed throughout the body but the largest contribution is from the thermal core (deep abdominal and thoracic tissues, and neuraxis).

Signals from these sensors ascend via the spinothalamic tracts in the anterior spinal cord to the thermoregulatory centre located in the preoptic region of the hypothalamus near the floor of the third ventricle. This region contains heat-sensitive neurones but also receives neural input from other thermoreceptors. The preoptic region receives afferent information from peripheral thermoreceptors, determines the thermoregulatory set-point and co-ordinates appropriate responses.

Temperature is then regulated by a variety of central structures that compare integrated thermal inputs from skin, neuraxis and deep tissues with reference temperatures for each thermoregulatory response.

The most important effector response in humans against extreme environments is behavioural, and outweighs autonomic changes. At extremes of age, hypothalamic temperature regulation is impaired and less effective.

Humoral mediators from the circulation act to alter temperature primarily via the organum vasculosum of the lamina terminalis (OVLT), an area of fenestrated capillaries in the hypothalamus that permits cytokine access to neuronal receptors. Cytokines appear to be the endogenous pyrogens, with interleukin-6 (IL-6) and prostaglandin-E_2 (PGE_2) being a final common pathway. In addition to elevating body temperature, several cytokines also reduce the thermoregulatory set-point, and are known as endogenous cryogens.[1]

Patients in the ICU are likely to have disturbance of both heat production and heat loss. Heat is produced as a result of metabolic activity and energy expenditure. Inflammation or infection as part of an acute phase response results in an increase in body temperature and energy expenditure. Pyrexia in turn results in an increased metabolic rate, however, reducing activity with sedation and muscle relaxation reduces energy expenditure.

Regulation of heat loss, which is the predominant effector of thermoregulation, is usually disturbed in the ICU population. Patients are usually nursed seminaked, bed-bathed frequently, sedated and sometimes paralysed, and infused with drugs and fluids at ambient temperature. This effect is particularly pronounced during renal replacement therapy. Peripheral blood flow may be affected by vasopressors and the ability to shiver abolished by muscle relaxants. Behavioural defences may be compromised by sedative use. All of these effects play a variable part and, together with the method of temperature measurement, should be considered when evaluating fever in the ICU.

FEVER IN THE ICU

Fever is defined by a *regulated* hyperthermia, that is, it is a regulated elevation in the preoptic set-point temperature. Endogenous pyrogens as well as other mediators inhibit warm-sensitive neurones that normally facilitate heat loss and suppress heat production. This elevates the set-point temperature for all thermoregulatory responses and activates cold defences such as vasoconstriction and shivering, which decrease heat loss and increase metabolic heat production respectively. The set-point temperature returns to normal when pyrogen concentrations decrease, triggering heat loss by vasodilatation and sweating.[2]

Fever may reflect a wide variety of pathological processes including infection, inflammation, trauma, malignancy and connective tissue diseases (Table 72.1),

necessitating a systematic and comprehensive diagnostic approach.[3] It is often assumed that a patient presenting with a fever should be treated, regardless of the presence or absence of other symptoms. However, the evidence that anti-fever treatments lead to an improvement in morbidity or mortality, or even patient comfort, is lacking.[4]

The development of fever in response to infection may be a protective adaptive response, and appears to be a phylogenetically preserved evolutionary response because of its survival value.[5] In mammalian models, increasing body temperature results in enhanced resistance to infection. In humans, retrospective clinical trials have shown a positive correlation between maximum temperature on the day of bacteraemia and increased survival in patients with gram negative bacteraemia and spontaneous bacterial peritonitis.[6] Also, septic patients with hypothermia have a poorer outcome than those who develop fever, although this causality is less clear. Both local and systemic hyperthermia has been used to facilitate cancer treatment.

The protective effects of fever result from increased immune and cytokine functions.[7-10]

Temperature elevation has been shown to enhance:

- antibody production
- neutrophil and macrophage mobility and function

Table 72.1   Causes of fever in the ICU

System	Infectious aetiology	Non-infectious aetiology
Cardiovascular	Endocarditis	Myocardial infarction
	Catheter-related infection	Deep vein thrombosis
	Pacemaker infection	Pericarditis
Respiratory	Pneumonia	Atelectasis
	Empyema	Chemical pneumonitis
	Sinusitis	Pulmonary emboli
Alimentary	Abdominal abscess	Inflammatory bowel disease
	Biliary infection	Acalculous cholecystitis
	Peritonitis	Pancreatitis
	Diverticulitis	Ischaemic colitis
	Viral hepatitis	Non-viral hepatitis
	Antibiotic-related colitis	Gastrointestinal haemorrhage
Renal	Pyelonephritis	
	Urinary tract infection	
Central nervous	Meningitis	Cerebral haemorrhage/infarct
	Encephalitis	Seizures
Rheumatological	Septic arthritis	Connective tissue disease
	Osteomyelitis	Vasculitis
		Gout
Endocrine		Adrenocortical insufficiency
		Alcohol and drug withdrawal
		Hyperthyroidism
Skin/soft tissue	Cellulitis	Burns
	Decubitus ulcer	Intramuscular injections
	Wound infections	Haematoma
Other	Parotitis	Drug fever
	Pharyngitis	Transfusion reaction
	Otitis media	Neoplasms

- cytokine production
- T-lymphocyte activity
- and to reduce serum iron, which is required for bacterial growth.

In addition, elevated temperatures inhibit some pathogens, such as *Streptococcus pneumoniae*.[11]

Moderate fever is a common occurrence in ICU patients, but approximately half of these are non-infectious in origin.[12–14] The presence of fever frequently results in the performance of diagnostic tests and exposes the patient to unnecessary invasive procedures and inappropriate use of antibiotics.[15]

While very high fevers (>40°C) are dangerous, it is less clear whether moderate elevation of body temperature is detrimental and, indeed, may be protective.[4] Moreover, artificially lowering the temperature of a febrile patient may mask the signs of infection and make diagnosis and monitoring more difficult. Any decision to adopt anti-fever measures, physical or pharmacological, must take into consideration the variable response by this patient population. Anti-pyretics may be ineffective. The usual concern about external cooling measures inducing peripheral vasoconstriction, reducing heat loss and making the pyrexia worse by shivering and hypermetabolism, may not be observed in sedated ICU patients.[16] The most likely cause for this response is the drugs used to maintain sedation.[17,18]

Pyrexia is associated with a number of deleterious physiological effects. Cardiac output, oxygen consumption, carbon dioxide production and energy expenditure are all increased, particularly in the presence of shivering. Oxygen consumption is increased on average by 10%/°C.[2] These changes are poorly tolerated by patients with limited cardiorespiratory reserve, and this group of patients would probably derive benefit from cooling measures. Other patient groups that require special consideration include those with immunosuppression, prosthetic implants and acute brain injury. Recent trials of therapeutic moderate hypothermia and traumatic brain injury indicate that hypothermia is a complicated treatment that is likely to benefit only a subgroup of patients with head injury.[19–21]

HEAT STROKE

A diagnosis of heat stroke is suggested when hyperthermia is associated with neurological abnormalities after exposure to high ambient temperature and/or vigourous exercise. Rectal temperature is usually greater than 42°C. Two distinct forms are recognized, and the spectrum of injury includes milder forms of thermal injury often termed heat stress.

Exertional heat stroke is a consequence of prolonged, intense exercise in warm humid environments, often seen in athletes and military recruits. Classic heat stroke is

Table 72.2 Predisposing factors to heat stroke

Age	Elderly
Environmental	High ambient temperature and humidity
	Heat waves
	Poor ventilation
Behavioural	Lack of acclimatization
	Salt and water deprivation
	Obesity
Underlying conditions	Infection/fever
	Diabetes
	Malnutrition
	Alcoholism
	Hyperthyroidism
	Impaired sweat production
	Healed burns
	Ectodermal dysplasia
	Impaired sweating
	Cardiovascular disease
	Fatigue
	Potassium deficiency
Drugs	Anticholinergics
	Antiparkinsonians
	Antihistamines
	Butyrophenones
	Phenothiazines
	Tricyclics
	Diuretics
	Sympathomimetics

commonly seen in sedentary, elderly patients with underlying illnesses during heat waves. Factors predisposing to heat stroke are listed in Table 72.2. About 80% of heat stroke deaths occur in people aged 50 years and older, because of the diminished ability of the older body to compensate for increased core temperatures. Heat stroke is estimated to be the cause of approximately 1700 deaths each year in the USA.[22] During the 1987 Islamic pilgrimage to Mekkah, about 2000 cases were reported with 50% fatality.[23] A study of former heat stroke patients suggests that susceptible individuals have a poorer physiological response to heat stress in terms of core temperature, heart rate and sweat response.

There are two autonomic responses to heat stress: sweating and active precapillary vasodilatation. Sweating is extremely effective and can dissipate up to ten times the basal metabolic rate, provided that environmental conditions, such as ambient temperature, humidity and wind speed are optimal. The resemblance between heat illness and the effects of antimuscarinic drugs, which produce a central anticholinergic syndrome, is explained by the postganglionic, cholinergic sympathetic innervation of sweat glands. Vascular responses to heat stress include vasodilatation of peripheral vascular beds and vasoconstriction of splanchnic and renal beds. During severe heat stress, blood flow through the top millimetre of skin can be equal to the entire resting cardiac output.

PATHOGENESIS

The pathogenesis of multiple organ failure in heat stroke is complex. Although direct cellular damage from increased temperature constitutes the initiating insult,[24] the precise sequence of injury and responsible mediators are poorly understood. At the cellular level, thermal injury results in increased membrane permeability, which in turn stimulates membrane enzymes, such as Na^+K^+-ATPase to maintain membrane integrity. This ATP-consuming enzyme activity is also responsible for nerve impulse conduction, which is markedly curtailed when ATP is depleted. This results in tissue oedema, reduced oxygen extraction and neuronal injury. High temperatures ameliorate ATP synthesis leading to fatigue.

Recent evidence suggests that the pathways for tissue injury in heat stroke share many features with that of sepsis, endotoxaemia and systemic inflammation. Increased levels of circulating endotoxin and cytokines have been identified in patients with heat stroke.[25,26]

The use of anti-endotoxin antibodies in primate models of heat stroke suggests that endotoxin at least in part mediates the tissue injury associated with hyperthermia. There was also a significant correlation between plasma IL-6 concentration and the severity of heat stroke. Since this cytokine is known to modulate the hypothalamic set-point, the ramifications of such a response in an already hyperthermic patient are obvious.

Activation of coagulation factors,[27] and release of endothelin and adhesion molecules[28,29] from activated or injured endothelium has also been demonstrated in heat stroke. These recent observations lead to the speculation that certain mediators that are implicated in the pathogenesis of acute organ injury are also elevated in heat stress, but become intense when heat stroke develops and are not normalized upon cooling.

CLINICAL PRESENTATION

Heat stroke induces multiple organ failure and the clinical presentation reflects this. The first clinical signs may be neurological, and include restlessness, delirium, pupillary abnormalities, seizures and coma. Brain-stem reflexes may be lost in the presence of brainstem-evoked potentials. There may be focal pathology including cerebellar injury, which may remain permanent. Lumbar puncture may show increased protein, xanthochromia and lymphocytic pleocytosis.

The signs of distributive shock, with a hyperdynamic haemodynamic profile not dissimilar to that of sepsis, are present in a large number of patients. The marked hyperventilation results in respiratory alkalosis, and hypoxaemic respiratory failure may be due to cardiac failure or acute lung injury.

Dehydration follows excessive insensible losses, although sweating is generally absent in the terminal stages of classic heat stroke leaving a hot, dry skin. Hypovolaemia is a consequence of dehydration and fluid redistribution, and results in reduced organ perfusion. A severe metabolic (lactic) acidosis is present. The major biochemical abnormalities include hyperglycaemia, hypophosphataemia, and raised serum enzymes and acute phase proteins (Table 72.3). Haematological findings include leucocytosis, thrombocytopenia, and activation of coagulation and fibrinolysis.

Exertional heat stroke differs slightly in that additional findings include rhabdomyolysis and acute renal failure that is associated with hyperkalaemia, hyperphosphataemia and hypocalcaemia (Table 72.3).

MANAGEMENT

Heat stroke is a medical emergency. The principal therapeutic objectives are rapid cooling to below 40°C and support of vital organ systems. Heat is dissipated by:

- conduction (immersion in ice-cold water or packed ice)
- evaporation (repeated wetting of skin with tepid water and fanning the patient at room temperature and low humidity).

Table 72.3 Biochemical differences between classic and exertional heat stroke

	Classic heat stroke	**Exertional heat stoke**
Arterial gases	Mixed respiratory alkalosis	Severe metabolic acidosis
Serum electrolytes	Na^+, Mg^+, Ca^{2+}, Mg^{2+} are usually normal	Hyperkalaemia
		Hypocalcaemia
	Hypophosphataemia	Hyperphosphataemia
Blood glucose	Hyperglycaemia	Hypoglycaemia
Creatinine kinase	Moderately increased	Markedly increased
Hepatic enzymes	Markedly increased	Moderately increased
Acute phase proteins	Markedly increased	Moderately increased

Evaporation is considerably more effective. Pharmacological treatment with anti-pyretic agents, or dantrolene,[30] is ineffective. Prevention of vasoconstriction and shivering by overcooling is important because of the danger of subsequent rebound hyperthermia. Core and skin temperature monitoring is useful, but measurement of rectal temperature should be avoided because it lags considerably during cooling. Cooling can be stopped when core temperature reaches below 39°C. However, despite cooling, about 25% of patients experience failure of one or more organ systems.

Fluid and electrolyte imbalance, and acid-base disturbances must be corrected cautiously with appropriate fluids tailored to the individual and guided by measurements of filling pressure, serum electrolytes and haematocrit.

The mechanism of acute renal failure is multifactorial but rhabdomyolysis is the major component. Early institution of alkaline diuresis and mannitol may obviate the need for renal replacement therapy.

Oxygen therapy and controlled ventilation may be indicated, and anti-convulsants required. Prophylactic antibiotics and steroids are not recommended. Blood glucose must be controlled aggressively. Finally, any underlying illness should be sought and treated accordingly.

OUTCOME

The mortality from heat stroke has ranged from 5–50%, but in recent years this has fallen to around 12% due to early recognition and aggressive treatment. The incidence of permanent neurological deficit remains at 7–15%. Prognostic factors include:

- age
- severity
- neurological deficits
- serum concentrations of hepatic and muscle enzymes
- cooling time
- presence of lactic acidosis.

DRUG-INDUCED HYPERTHERMIAS

In contrast to fever, the thermoregulatory set-point during hyperthermia remains unchanged at normothermic levels, however body temperature increases in an uncontrolled fashion and overrides the ability of effector mechanisms to dissipate heat. Although a raised body temperature is not necessarily due to increased heat production but rather due to an imbalance between heat production and loss, most hyperthermias result as a consequence of net heat gain. Hyperthermia can result in dangerously high core temperatures by two mechanisms:

1 Excessive exogenous heat exposure
2 Excessive endogenous heat production.

Table 72.4 Causes of hyperthermia

Disorders of excessive heat production	Exertional hyperthermia
	Heat stroke (exertional)
	Malignant hyperthermia
	Neuroleptic malignant syndrome
	Lethal catatonia
	Thyrotoxicosis
	Phaeochromocytoma
	Salicylate intoxication
	Sympathomimetic drug abuse
	Delirium tremens
	Seizures
	Tetanus
Disorders of diminished heat dissipation	Heat stroke (classic)
	Dehydration
	Autonomic dysfunction
	Anticholinergic poisoning
	Neuroleptic malignant syndrome
Disorders of hypothalamic function	Cerebrovascular accidents
	Encephalitis
	Trauma
	Granulomatous diseases
	Neuroleptic malignant syndrome

The numerous causes of hyperthermia are listed in Table 72.4. This section will review the relatively common causes of drug-induced hyperthermias, including malignant hyperthermia, neuroleptic malignant syndrome, and the sympathomimetic and anticholinergic syndromes.

MALIGNANT HYPERTHERMIA

Malignant hyperthermia (MH) is a rare pharmacogenetic myopathy usually manifested when a susceptible individual is exposed to anaesthetic triggering agents. It is characterized by an intense hypermetabolic state and skeletal muscle rigidity upon exposure to volatile anaesthetics and depolarizing muscle relaxants. In extreme cases, body temperature may exceed 42°C and the arterial pH reach 6.8, and can be rapidly fatal. The incidence of an MH reaction during general anaesthesia varies between 1/60 000 when succinylcholine is used, and 1/250 000 when only volatile agents are used. It is more frequent in children (1/15 000), with more than 50% of cases before the age of 15 years.

PATHOGENESIS

Skeletal muscle is the principal tissue involved in a MH reaction. The primary defect is thought to be in the sarcolemma, and in particular the calcium release channel also termed the ryanodine receptor (RYR1). In MH, exposure of skeletal muscle to triggering agents depolarizes the muscle hypersensitively to release massive amounts of calcium ions from the sarcoplasmic reticulum (SR), thus vastly increasing its cytoplasmic concentration. It is believed that the altered kinetics of the RYR1 receptor is due to exaggerated release of calcium by small increases in cytoplasmic calcium concentration (calcium-induced calcium release), as well as a decrease in inhibitory effects of high calcium concentrations. ATP-dependent membrane pumps (Ca^{2+}-ATPase) attempt to return the calcium back to the SR resulting in a sustained glycolytic and aerobic metabolism. Recovery of calcium by the SR is often incomplete, causing prolonged excitation-contraction coupling and leading to muscle rigidity. Muscle contractures impede blood flow and perturb nutrient supply and waste removal from this hypermetabolic reaction. Eventually, oxidative phosphorylation is uncoupled, metabolism becomes anaerobic, and a severe lactic and respiratory acidosis develops. As muscle constitutes about 40% of body mass and is a major source of body heat, increased activity results in hyperthermia.

Membrane phospholipase A_2 is also activated by calcium leading to an increase in mitochondrial and sarcoplasmic permeability, with further loss of calcium regulation and release of intracellular contents (potassium [K^+], calcium [Ca^{2+}], creatinine kinase (CK), myoglobin) into the circulation.

CLINICAL PRESENTATION

The earliest sign of an impending MH crisis is an unexplained rise in end-tidal CO_2 and heart rate, and not necessarily an increase in body temperature. This classical crisis of acute fulminant MH with its multiplicity of marked metabolic and muscle anomalies, and sympathetic stimulation is unmistakable, but now rare. The pattern of presentation has altered since its first description in 1960, as anaesthetic techniques and succinylcholine use have changed.

The more gradual appearance of signs following exposure to triggering agents may be more difficult to diagnose, as the signs may be subtle, non-specific and have variable intensity, incidence and temporal association (Table 72.5).[31] Apart from the classical crisis, other forms of MH including smouldering, recurring, delayed and abortive forms may also occur. Clinical diagnosis is made on the basis of the pattern of features in Table 72.5. Other conditions that may mimic MH include inadequate levels of anaesthesia or analgesia, sepsis, ischaemia or anaphylaxis. Early diagnosis is important, as immediate treatment is associated with improved outcome. Masseter muscle spasm (MMS) has been associated with MH.[32] When MMS is the only presenting sign, the incidence of MH susceptibility is likely to be low. However, this incidence is increased if MMS is associated with other muscle or metabolic signs.

Halothane is the most potent of the contemporary volatile anaesthetic agents at inducing sustained contractures in isolated muscle strips from MH patients, and has formed the basis of diagnostic testing for MH for 30 years. There may be a difference amongst the volatile anaesthetics in their relative potency to trigger an MH reaction. Succinylcholine will cause an increase in the calcium concentration in the cytosol of normal muscle, and it appears that this release of calcium is exaggerated in MH muscle. Non-depolarizing muscle relaxants are generally accepted to be safe in MH. A list of safe and implicated drugs is shown in Table 72.6.

Table 72.5 Clinical features of malignant hyperthermia (adapted from Hopkins, 2000[31] with permission)*

Timing	Clinical signs	Changes in monitored variables	Biochemical changes
Acute	Sustained jaw rigidity after succinylcholine		
	Tachypnoea	Increased minute ventilation	
	Rapid exhaustion of soda lime	Rising end-tidal CO_2	Increased $PaCO_2$
	Hot soda lime canister		Decreased pH
	High pulse rate	Tachycardia	
	Irregular pulse	Ventricular ectopics	Increased [K^+]
		Peaked T waves on ECG	
Intermediate	Patient hot to touch	Rising core body temperature	
	Cyanosis	Falling SpO_2	Decreased PaO_2
	Dark blood in wound		
	Irregular pulse	Ventricular ectopics	Increased [K^+]
		Peaked T waves on ECG	
Late	Generalized muscle rigidity		
	Prolonged bleeding		
	Dark urine		Increased creatine kinase
	Oliguria		Myoglobinuria
	Irregular pulse	Ventricular ectopics	
		Peaked T waves on ECG	Increased [K^+]
	Death		

Table 72.6 Drug use in malignant hyperthermia

Contraindicated drugs	Safe drugs
Halothane	Nitrous oxide
Enflurane	Barbiturates
Isoflurane	Propofol
Desflurane	Etomidate
Sevoflurane	Ketamine
Succinylcholine	Opiates
Verapamil	Amide/ester local anaesthetics
Nifedipine	Noradrenaline
Diltiazem	Adrenaline
	Dopamine
	Dobutamine

Several neuromuscular and musculoskeletal abnormalities such as scoliosis, strabismus, muscular dystrophy and central core disease have been associated with MH susceptibility but definitive evidence for this association is lacking. Patients with neuroleptic malignant syndrome are not considered at risk of developing MH under general anaesthesia.

MH susceptibility has been diagnosed for the last 30 years on the basis of abnormal *in vitro* contractures to separate exposures to halothane and caffeine performed on freshly biopsied muscle strips. Recently, a ryanodine contracture test has been shown to be more specific and may be of additional value.

MOLECULAR GENETICS OF MALIGNANT HYPERTHERMIA

Malignant hyperthermia (MH) is a heterogenetic disorder that is autosomal dominant with variable penetration and expression. Recent advances in molecular genetics have supported the concept for a role of the RYR1 gene in the pathogenesis of MH. The RYR1 gene is found at position 13.1 on chromosome 19q and codes for the ryanodine receptor that regulates calcium transport across the calcium release channel. However, only 50% of MH families show genetic linkage to the RYR1 gene, and more than 17 mutations at this locus have been described so far. The mutation does not always segregate with *in vitro* contracture testing within a family. Furthermore, RYR1 linkage is not found in some MH families. Although all known mutations share the final common pathway of excessive calcium release from the SR, the genetic diversity of this disease precludes DNA-based diagnosis at present.

MANAGEMENT

Once a diagnosis of MH is suspected, and other diagnoses excluded, treatment should be based as follows:

- Stop all anaesthetic triggering drugs, increase fresh gas flow to purge the anaesthetic machine, and substitute a new breathing circuit. Valuable time should not be lost changing the machine and is no longer

recommended. Increase ventilation to 2–3 times the minute volume to aid removal of CO_2.

- Abandon surgery if possible, or continue using safe drugs (Table 72.6).
- Administer intravenous dantrolene, which is the only specific therapy, at an initial dose of 2.5 mg/kg and repeat at 5–10 min intervals until the drug reverses the metabolic derangements of MH (maximum dose 10 mg/kg). Dantrolene acts by inhibition of SR calcium release but without affecting uptake. It may be repeated at 1–2 mg/kg 4-hourly for 1–3 days and then given orally if still required.
- Arrhythmias not responsive to correction of acidosis and hyperkalaemia should be treated in the conventional manner. However, calcium antagonists are contraindicated as these drugs interact with high-dose dantrolene to cause severe hyperkalaemia and cardiovascular collapse.
- Cool the patient using simple measures such as tepid sponging, fanning and cool intravenous fluids in order to avoid vasoconstriction, which impedes heat loss. Occasionally, more aggressive cooling methods may be required.
- Frequent blood samples should be taken for analysis of blood gases, potassium, creatinine kinase, myoglobin and coagulation. Treat hyperkalaemia and acidosis early and aggressively.
- Measure urine output for impending signs of acute renal failure. Diuresis with mannitol or frusemide may be required in addition to fluids in order to prevent myoglobin precipitation in renal tubules. Mannitol doses should incorporate that contained in dantrolene preparations.
- Continue monitoring closely in the post acute phase according to signs and severity. Renal protection therapy and control of coagulopathy is desirable.
- Consider alternative diagnoses if there is no response to dantrolene, e.g. other myopathies, sepsis, thyrotoxic storm, phaeochromocytoma etc.
- After recovery, patients and relatives should be referred to a MH screening centre.

OUTCOME

The mortality rate from MH has declined from 70% in the 1960s to less than 10% world-wide. This vast improvement is attributed to increased awareness and understanding by anaesthetists, improved monitoring techniques especially capnography and pulse oximetry, and to the availability and early use of intravenous dantrolene. Late recognition of MH may result in a poor outcome despite treatment with dantrolene.

NEUROLEPTIC MALIGNANT SYNDROME

The neuroleptic malignant syndrome (NMS) is a relatively rare but potentially fatal idiosyncratic reaction to neuroleptic drugs that is not dose related. Many features of this syndrome remain controversial as several other medical conditions generate similar symptoms, but characteristic findings include:

- encephalopathy
- muscle rigidity
- hyperthermia
- autonomic dysfunction.

The incidence is estimated to vary between 0.07% to 2.2%. All ages are affected, but males are disproportionately represented in some studies.

PATHOGENESIS

The pathophysiology of NMS remains unclear. Two mechanisms, a neuroleptic-induced perturbation of central thermo- and neuro-regulatory mechanisms, and an abnormal reaction of skeletal muscle have been proposed.

Hypothalamic thermoregulation involves noradrenergic, serotonergic, cholinergic and central dopaminergic pathways. Neuroleptic blockade of dopamine receptors in the hypothalamus leads to disturbances in thermoregulation and heat dissipation. In addition, blockade of dopamine receptors in the basal ganglia is thought to cause muscle hypertonicity and contraction, leading to further heat production. Drugs linked to MNS appear to share the ability to antagonize dopamine receptors (primarily D_2 receptors) or to lower synaptic dopamine levels. Recent work suggests that glutaminergic excitatory amino acids may influence central dopamine activity and be more important in the development of NMS.

A common pathogenesis of NMS and MH has been suggested by virtue of similar clinical features (hyperthermia, rigidity, raised serum muscle enzymes), abnormal *in vitro* contracture tests and, interestingly, successful treatment with dantrolene in both. However, conflicting results have been reported regarding the prevalence of MH susceptibility among NMS patients. Neuroleptic agents induce muscle contracture *in vitro*, however, no difference was found in response to 4 neuroleptic drugs between muscle from NMS patients and normal individuals.[33]

Biochemical studies suggest the involvement of genetic factors in the pathogenesis of NMS but the molecular basis of this remains elusive. There does not appear to be an association between NMS and the mutations in the RYR1 gene associated with MH.

CLINICAL PRESENTATION

The presentation and course of NMS can be quite variable; it may take a relatively benign and self-limiting course, or it may be fulminant and fatal, although the latter is rare. NMS usually develops within 2–4 weeks of starting antipsychotic therapy but the majority of the cases develop within the first week. The main symptoms that indicate a high probability of NMS include:

- hyperthermia
- muscle rigidity

- elevated serum creatinine kinase
- autonomic instability.

A predictable progression of symptoms may be identified in many patients with NMS where mental status changes and rigidity precede hyperthermia and autonomic dysfunction.[34]

- temperature elevation can be mild or severe, but is rarely greater than 42°C as seen in heat stroke
- muscle rigidity is characterized by a 'lead pipe' increase in tone that may result in decreased chest wall compliance and hypoventilation
- extrapyramidal symptoms may also be present
- autonomic instability is demonstrated by labile hypertension (hypotension is rare), tachycardia and sweating
- altered consciousness is typically of the form of delirium and agitation that may progress to stupor and coma

Other clinical features of lesser frequency include dysarthria, dysphagia, chorea, mutism and seizures. Elevated serum creatinine kinase is now considered to be a major feature of NMS. Other non-specific laboratory abnormalities include leucocytosis, mildly elevated hepatic enzymes, and secondary electrolyte disturbances including hypocalcaemia, hypomagnesaemia and hypophosphataemia. Urine analysis often reveals proteinuria and myoglobinuria from rhabdomyolysis. The electroencephalograph (EEG) may show diffuse slowing. CT scans of the brain as well as examination of cerebrospinal fluid is usually normal in NMS.

All classes of neuroleptic medications have been implicated in NMS including butyrophenones, phenothiazines, thioxanthenes, benzamides, as well as newer drugs such as clozapine and resperidone. Haloperidol and fluphenazine are the most frequently reported agents. Other agents that block dopamine receptors or inhibit dopamine release have been associated with NMS including metoclopramide, reserpine and α-methylparatyrosine. Discontinuation of anti-parkinsonian drugs (leading to a relative decrease in dopamine levels), has also been associated with NMS.

Risk factors include organic brain disease, functional psychoses, dehydration and rapid loading of antipsychotics.

Complications include:

- acute renal failure from rhabdomyolysis
- respiratory failure from hypoventilation and aspiration pneumonia
- cardiovascular collapse
- irreversible neurological injury may result from extreme temperatures.

The differential diagnosis of NMS includes all disorders that can present with a combination of hyperthermia, rigidity and encephalopathy. These include CNS infections, cerebral masses, tetanus, heat stress, MH, catatonia and drug toxicities (lithium, atropine and monoamine oxidase inhibitors).

Neuroleptic-induced heat stroke is differentiated from NMS by its faster onset, absence of extrapyramidal signs and sweating (anticholinergic properties of neuroleptics), and a history of physical exertion and exposure to a hostile environment. Like NMS, lethal catatonia can present with hyperthermia, akinesia and muscle rigidity. The importance of distinguishing the catatonias from NMS lies in the differential treatment. Benzodiazepines are usually required for the former.

SEROTONERGIC SYNDROME

Drugs that enhance serotonergic neurotransmission or lead to a relative increase in synaptic levels of serotonin can result in a toxic state that resembles features of NMS. These drugs include selective serotonin reuptake inhibitors (SSRIs), monoamine oxidase inhibitors (MAOIs) and tricyclic antidepressants (TCAs), either alone or in combination. The serotonin syndrome is a toxic effect that appears to be due to hyperstimulation of 5-HT1A receptors in the brain and spinal cord. This is differentiated from NMS, which is an idiosyncratic response to antipsychotics and not serotonergic drugs.

Clinical features of the serotonergic syndrome include encephalopathy, hyperreflexia, nausea and vomiting, and autonomic instability. Sweating and mild increases in temperature are evident in 50% of cases. Rhabdomyolysis, hyperkalaemia, renal failure, DIC and seizures are all rare but reported findings. The serotonergic syndrome is usually self-limited, and resolves uneventfully once the offending drug has been withdrawn. However, rarely severe forms require more aggressive supportive therapy analogous to the treatment of NMS. Specific treatments, including the use of serotonin antagonists, have been proposed, however, these cannot be recommended at present due to lack of well-designed studies.

MANAGEMENT

Management of mild forms of NMS may only require early recognition, withdrawal of all neuroleptic, dopamine depleting or dopamine-antagonist medication and general supportive therapy. Cessation of all psychotropic drugs should be considered. Rarely, severe cases require aggressive treatment of fluid/electrolyte and acid-base balance as well as cardiorespiratory function. Because acute renal failure is the most frequent complication of NMS, therapy must be directed at renal protection from myoglobin injury. The hyperthermic patient should be cooled as described previously in this chapter. Haemodialysis may be required for renal failure, but is not useful for clearing neuroleptic drugs, as these are protein-bound and therefore too large to dialyse.

The benefit of adding specific pharmacotherapies in addition to supportive measures is unclear, but potential use cannot be excluded. Treatments with bromocriptine (a dopamine agonist) and dantrolene have led to a faster resolution of symptoms than with supportive therapy alone.[35] However, the place of dantrolene in the treatment of NMS is less well defined. Bromocriptine seems to be well tolerated by psychotic patients despite being a strong central dopamine agonist. The drug is effective within 24 h, with a reduction in rigidity followed by resolution of temperature and normalization of blood pressure. Similarly, amantadine, as well as a combination of levodopa-carbidopa, has also been reported to be effective. Anticholinergic drugs have little effect on muscle rigidity or hyperthermia. Non-specific adjuncts, such as the use of benzodiazepines, have been reported to be useful in agitated patients. Electroconvulsive (ECT) therapy may be of value in selected patients, for example, those with refractory NMS, those who remain catatonic, or those with ECT-responsive psychotic symptoms.

OUTCOME

A mortality of 22% prior to 1980 has been halved since 1984. This reduction has occurred largely due to early diagnosis, supportive therapy and advances in critical care medicine, rather than a consequence of therapy with either dantrolene, or dopamine agonists. Renal failure increases the mortality rate to approximately 50%, however, prognosis remains good in survivors.

SYMPATHOMIMETIC AND ANTICHOLINERGIC SYNDROMES

SYMPATHOMIMETIC POISONING

Mild to severe hyperthermia may be associated with all centrally acting sympathomimetics. These drugs produce their clinical effects by increasing synaptic concentrations of norepinephrine, dopamine and serotonin.

Cocaine predominantly blocks the presynaptic uptake of norepinephrine, although neurotransmission of dopamine and serotonin is also affected. Amphetamines and related drugs augment the release of norepinephrine, dopamine and serotonin from presynaptic nerve terminals and inhibit their uptake from the synapse. Some amphetamine metabolites also inhibit monoamine oxidase.

Central thermoregulatory disturbances from sympathomimetics may arise from complex interactions of these neurotransmitters in the brainstem and hypothalamus. The syndrome of hyperthermia associated with sympathomimetic poisoning bears similarity to that of heat stroke, MH, NMS and serotonin syndrome. This may reflect the final common pathway associated with the consequences of severe hyperthermia. Sympathomimetics such as MDMA ('ecstasy') have been shown to induce marked hyperthermia, through central mechanisms involving 5-HT$_2$ receptors, with subsequent rhabdomyolysis, disseminated intravascular coagulation and multi-organ failure.[36] Hyperkinetic muscle action, motor excitability and seizures may contribute to the rise in core temperature. Furthermore, elevated levels of both cocaine and amphetamine result in peripheral vasoconstriction thus impairing heat dissipation. Mortality appears to be related to the extent and duration of hyperthermia.

Therapy involves rapid cooling measures as outlined previously, together with support of failing organ systems. Benzodiazepines may relieve myotonic and hyperkinetic thermogenesis. However, patients who remain agitated and noncompliant should be paralysed and ventilated to permit institution of aggressive cooling measures. In moderately severe hyperthermia, dantrolene therapy has been described to improve outcome by enabling rapid muscle relaxation and control of temperature. However, the basis of its utility in this setting has not been established.

ANTICHOLINERGIC POISONING

The central and peripheral symptoms of anticholinergic syndrome result from the blockade of muscarinic acetylcholinergic receptors. Central toxicity results in:

- confusion
- tremor
- hallucinations
- myoclonus
- agitation

whereas peripheral signs of toxicity include

- dry mucous membranes
- mydriasis
- blurred vision
- tachycardia
- urinary retention.

Muscular hyperactivity from agitation, restlessness and convulsions in combination with impaired sweating may result in hyperthermia and rhabdomyolysis. Excessive temperatures can lead to multi-organ failure as described for other types of heat illness.

HYPOTHERMIA

Hypothermia is defined as a core body temperature below 35°C. In the UK, hypothermia accounts for 1% of winter admissions, particularly among the elderly population. The leading causes of hypothermia in the USA are exposure due to alcoholism, drug addiction, mental illness, or accidents involving immersion in cold water. The mortality rate from accidental hypothermia varies according to its severity, but averages 21% when core temperature is decreased to 28–32°C.[37] However, a core temperature of 32°C or less in trauma victims is associated with a mortality rate near 100%, and any hypothermia is considered a poor prognostic sign.[38,39]

Hypothermia is traditionally classified as:

- mild (temperature 32–35°C),

- moderate (temperature 28–32°C)
- severe (temperature below 28°C)

Significant hypothermia in terms of severity and duration results in multiple systemic derangements that ultimately lead to impaired tissue oxygenation. The major defence against cold stress is behavioural adaptation. However, autonomic thermoregulatory responses orchestrated by the hypothalamus are also activated to prevent heat loss and generate heat production. These include:

- peripheral vasoconstriction
- shivering
- increase in metabolism.

The four physical mechanisms of heat loss from the body surfaces are conduction, convection, radiation and evaporation.

Hypothermia may be induced deliberately for therapeutic purposes, for example, cardiovascular surgery or neuroprotection, or it may be accidental. Primary accidental hypothermia occurs when an otherwise healthy individual experiences overwhelming cold stress, for example, cold-water immersion. Secondary accidental hypothermia occurs despite mild environmental conditions and is due to illness or injury induced perturbations in thermoregulation and heat production, for example, drug intoxication or trauma.

The causes and predisposing conditions of hypothermia are listed in Table 72.7; however, the most frequent causes appear to be exposure, hypoglycaemia and the use of depressant drugs including alcohol. An impaired thermoregulatory system together with a reduced functional reserve makes the elderly more susceptible.

Administration of anaesthesia impairs the ability to maintain thermal homeostasis, decreases heat production and causes heat loss due to vasodilatation and exposure. General anaesthesia also alters the threshold for thermoregulatory vasoconstriction and shivering in the non-paralysed patient.[40]

PATHOGENESIS AND CLINICAL PRESENTATION

Hypothermia depresses all organ functions resulting in decreased cardiac function, shock, respiratory failure, confusion, muscle rigidity, renal failure and death. The cardiovascular response in hypothermia initially comprises an increase in heart rate, cardiac output and blood pressure in response to shivering and increased metabolic demand. Peripheral vasoconstriction is due to activation of the sympathetic nervous system as well as local cutaneous reflexes, resulting in shunting of peripheral blood to the central pool. With worsening hypothermia there is:

- progressive cardiovascular depression leading to a reduction in tissue perfusion

- cardiac output is halved at 28°C as a result of decreased heart rate and contractility
- conduction and pacemaker activity are reduced, and there is prolongation of PR, QRS, and QT intervals as well as non-specific ST-T wave changes. The characteristic J or Osborn wave may be seen when core temperature is below 33°C
- atrial fibrillation and heart block are also common below this temperature. Ventricular fibrillation can occur below 28°C and asystole when core temperature drops below 20°C. Fibrillation may occur earlier if the myocardium is diseased or stimulated, either mechanically or pharmacologically

An initial increase in respiratory rate during hypothermia is followed by progressive depression of rate, vital capacity and minute volume. The cough reflex is abolished, exposing the patient to an increased risk of aspiration pneumonia. Bronchial secretions, atelectasis and pulmonary oedema may develop. Apnoea may occur below 24°C. The oxyhaemoglobin dissociation curve is shifted to the left, resulting in reduced oxygen delivery to the tissues, but this is partially balanced by a right shift due to the underlying acidosis.

Shivering occurs in the early phase of hypothermia and is characterized by intense heat and energy production from the metabolism of stored fuels. Non-shivering thermogenesis is probably only of importance in children. Metabolic processes slow by approximately 6%/°C, and the metabolic rate is reduced by half at 28°C.[41] A mixed respiratory and metabolic acidosis results from hypoventilation and reduced tissue perfusion, leading to lactate accumulation from anaerobic metabolism. Hepatic function is depressed, affecting most enzymatic and detoxifying processes. There is a high risk of developing pancreatitis.

There is generalized cerebral depression as the metabolism of the brain declines with a fall in core temperature. This adaptation is neuroprotective and may improve the chances of survival even after prolonged hypothermic arrest. Cerebral blood flow falls as a consequence of reduced cardiac output and increased blood viscosity at a rate of 7%/°C drop in temperature.[42] Confusion can cause illogical behaviour, for example, aggression, and paradoxical undressing. Coma, pupillary dilatation, absence of tendon reflexes and rigidity are present below 28°C. Cerebral electrical activity ceases below 20°C.

Hypothermia causes an initial increase in catecholamine and cortisol release as a result of the stress response. There is a delayed increase in serum thyroxine levels. Below 30°C, pituitary and pancreatic functions, as well as catecholamine secretion, are blunted. Blood sugar concentration is increased as a result of increased glycogenolysis and insulin resistance.

Haemoconcentration develops as a consequence of hypovolaemia as well as fluid shifts between compartments. Hypothermia increases blood viscosity by 2%/°C. Splenic sequestration results in leucopenia and thrombocytopenia. Low temperature also interferes with the intrinsic coagulation cascade. In severe hypothermia, platelet dysfunction and disseminated intravascular coagulation is common.

Table 72.7 Causes and predisposing conditions of hypothermia

Age	Extremes of age
Environmental	Exposure to cold
	Immersion
	Poor living conditions
Drugs	Anaesthetic agents
	Phenothiazines
	Barbiturates
	Alcohol
Central nervous System disorders	Cerebrovascular accidents
	Trauma
	Spinal cord transections
	Brain tumours
	Wernicke's encephalopathy
	Alzheimer's and Parkinson's disease
	Mental illness
Endocrine dysfunction	Hypoglycaemia
	Diabetic ketoacidosis
	Hyperosmolar coma
	Panhypopituitarism
	Hypoadrenalism
	Hypothyroidism
Trauma	Major trauma
Debility	Severe cardiac, renal, hepatic impairment
	Malnutrition, sepsis
Skin disorders	Burns
	Exfoliative dermatitis

MANAGEMENT

Once the diagnosis of hypothermia has been made, further heat loss must be prevented and re-warming started with close monitoring to avoid complications. Individual management should be modified according to aetiology and severity of hypothermia, as well as the functional reserve of the patient. Severe hypothermia, especially in the immersion victim, can mimic death, with apnoea, cardiac standstill, coma, unreactive pupils, and a silent electrocardiogram and electroencephalogram. Successful resuscitation of such patients has been reported and death should not be assumed until resuscitation has failed in an adequately warmed patient (at least 35°C).[43]

General measures begin with removal of the patient from the cold environment as rapidly as possible. Rough handling must be avoided during transport as this may precipitate fatal arrhythmias in severe hypothermia. Also, transport in the upright position must be avoided because cerebral blood flow may be compromised due to orthostatic hypotension.

Recommendation for basic and advanced life support for hypothermic patients is according to the principles of Advanced Cardiorespiratory Life Support (ACLS). Aggressive re-warming should be continued during resuscitation until the core temperature is at least 35°C. A resuscitation protocol based on core temperature and cardiac monitoring may be used.[44] If core temperature is unknown or known to be above 28°C, cardiorespiratory resuscitation (CPR) should be instituted for apparent cardiac arrest. If the patient is known to be severely hypothermic (<28°C) but maintains sinus rhythm, chest compression may precipitate ventricular fibrillation (VF) and may be best withheld.

Vascular cannulation may be difficult in the presence of intense vasoconstriction and a central catheter is inevitably required, taking precautions to avoid myocardial stimulation.

For the same reasons, a pulmonary artery catheter should be deferred until normothermia has been re-established. Hypotension should be treated with aggressive warm fluid therapy. Lactated Ringers should be avoided because the liver may not be able to metabolize lactate to bicarbonate.

Atrial arrhythmias, bradycardia or atrioventricular block generally do not require treatment with anti-arrhythmic agents unless decompensated, and resolve on re-warming.

Electrical defibrillation may not be effective at body temperature below 30°C. Indeed, VF may resolve spontaneously upon re-warming.

Sodium bicarbonate should be avoided because of paradoxical intracellular acidosis, and severe alkalosis on re-warming may induce refractory VF and left shift of the oxyhaemoglobin dissociation curve, thereby reducing tissue oxygen uptake. Progressive cardiac depression during re-warming ('recovery shock', 'after-drop') may be due to further cooling of blood as it redistributes from the core to the relative colder periphery.[45]

The increased metabolic demand during re-warming requires oxygen therapy. Patients in coma or respiratory failure should be intubated and ventilated with warm gases. Drug administration during hypothermia may reach toxic levels after re-warming because of functionally prolonged half-lives, and therefore should be used sparingly. Insulin treatment should be delayed until the temperature is above 30°C. It should be administered in small doses because degradation is slow and accumulation may occur with rebound hypoglycaemia as the patient is warmed.

RE-WARMING

Various methods of re-warming have been employed depending upon the severity of the hypothermia

Table 72.8 Re-warming methods

Passive	Warm environment >30°C (rate 0.5–1.0°C/h) Insulating cover (warm blanket)
Active, external	Conduction methods Warmed pads, blanket Convective methods (rate at 2–3°C/h) Hot air blower (e.g. Bair Hugger) Radiant methods
Active, core	Humidified warm inspired gases (rate 0.5–1.5°C/h) Warmed intravenous fluids Body cavity lavage (rate 2–3°C/h) Gastric irrigation Pleural irrigation Peritoneal dialysis Extracorporeal methods Haemodialysis, continuous arterio-venous or veno-venous re-warming (rate 5°C/h) Cardiopulmonary bypass (rate up to 10°C/h)

(Table 72.8). Careful monitoring and supportive therapy are mandatory during re-warming.

Passive warming involves removing the patient from a cold environment and allowing to re-warm spontaneously in a warm room (30°C). It is best for patients with mild hypothermia who have no circulatory compromise. Re-warming is gradual at 0.5–1.0°C/h.

Patients with moderate or severe hypothermia should be treated with active re-warming, which consists of active external re-warming or active core re-warming. Patients with moderate hypothermia and no evidence of circulatory collapse can initially be treated with active external re-warming techniques. These include use of immersion, radiant heat, forced air and electric blankets. Convective (forced air) warming at 43°C has been shown to increase body temperature by 2–3°C/h and is extremely effective in both preventing and treating hypothermia, as well as preventing shivering in the postoperative period.[46,47]

Active core re-warming is best used for patients with moderate to severe hypothermia. Techniques include:

* airway re-warming
* gastrointestinal
* peritoneal or pleural cavity lavage
* extracorporeal re-warming
* cardiopulmonary bypass.

Active core re-warming methods are extremely rapid but invasive, and the inherent risks should be considered in the management.

In airway re-warming, inspired gas is heated and humidified up to 40°C, and delivered either through a facemask or endotracheal tube. It insulates the respiratory tract and stops heat and moisture loss through breathing. The rate of re-warming is about 0.5–1.5°C/h. Volume expansion with intravenous fluids warmed with heat exchangers or by microwave can also be used. However, this method is insufficient by itself as very large volumes would be required to achieve a significant rise in body temperature.

Peritoneal lavage with heated dialysate, and closed pleural irrigation using warm sterile saline (temperature 40–42°C) through large bore tubes may also be attempted.[48,49] These methods are equally effective in raising temperature (2–3°C/h), but impossible in patients with thoracoabdominal injuries.

Haemodialysis and continuous arterio-venous or veno-venous re-warming techniques are extremely effective in raising body temperature (5°C/h). The advantages of this technique include non-requirement of heparinization if heparin-bonded tubing is used, rapid reversal of hypothermia, decreased total fluid requirements, decreased organ failure, decreased length of ICU stay, and decreased early mortality.[50] Patients with severe cardiovascular dysfunction may not tolerate high arterio-venous fistula flows.

The best method for re-warming patients with severe hypothermia who have haemodynamic instability involves the use of cardiopulmonary bypass. Its advantages include the highest re-warming rate (up to 10°C/h), control of re-warming rate, oxygenation, fluid composition and haemodynamic support.[51] However, associated risks include heparinization, haemolysis and air embolism.

Afterdrop is a phenomenon seen with re-warming where tissues that have been vasoconstricted and very cold start to become perfused again. Blood returning from these areas may be cold and will result in a late reduction in core temperature. This may be seen when core temperature is approaching normal and after active measures have been stopped.

OUTCOME

Poor prognostic factors include aetiology and severity of hypothermia, advanced age, comorbid states and cardiorespiratory arrest. Hypothermia associated with trauma or sepsis carries a high mortality.

REFERENCES

1 Kluger MJ. Fever: role of pyrogens and cryogens. *Physiological Reviews* 1996; **71**: 93–127.
2 Lenhardt R, Kurz A, Sessler DI. Thermoregulation and hyperthermia. *Acta Anaesthesiologica Scandinavica Suppl* 1996; **40**: 34–38.
3 O'Grady WP, Barie PS, Bartlett JG, *et al.* Practice guidelines for evaluating new fever in critically ill adult patients. *Clin Infect Dis* 1998; **26**: 1042–59.
4 Gozolli V, Schottker P, Suter PM, *et al.* Is it worth treating fever in intensive care unit patients? *Arch Int Med* 2001; **161**: 121–3.
5 Kluger MJ, Kozak W, Conn CA, *et al.* The adaptive value of fever. *Infect Dis Clin North Am* 1996; **10**: 1–20.
6 Weinstein MR, Iannini PB, Stratton CW, *et al.* Spontaneous bacterial peritonitis: a review of 28 cases with emphasis on improved survival and factors influencing prognosis. *Am J Med* 1978; **64**: 592–8.
7 Azocar J, Yunis EJ, Essex M. Sensitivity of human natural killer cells to hyperthermia. *Lancet* 1982; **1**: 16–17.
8 Biggar W, Bohn DJ, Kent G, *et al.* Neutrophil migration *in vitro* and *in vivo* during hyperthermia. *Infect Immunol* 1984; **46**: 857–9.
9 Jampel HD, Duff GW, Gershon RK, et al. Fever and immunoregulation: III. Hyperthermia augments the primary *in vitro* humoral immune response. *J Exp Med* 1983; **157**: 1229–38.
10 van Oss CJ, Absolom DR, Moore LL, *et al.* Effect of temperature on chemotaxis, phagocyte engulfment, digestion and oxygen consumption of human polymorphonuclear leucocytes. *J Reticuloendothel Soc* 1980; **27**: 561–5.
11 Styrt B, Sugarman B. Antipyresis and fever. *Arch Intern Med* 1990; **150**: 1589–97.
12 Cunha BA, Shea KW. Fever in the intensive care unit. *Infect Dis Clin North Am* 1996; **10**: 185–209.
13 Circiumaru B, Baldock G, Cohen J. A prospective study of fever in the intensive care unit. *Intensive Care Med* 1999; **25**: 668–73.
14 Cunha BA. Intensive care, not intensive antibiotics. *Heart Lung* 1994; **23**: 361–2.
15 Marik PE. Fever in the ICU. *Chest* 2000; **117**: 855–69.
16 Poblette B, Romand JA, Pilchard C, et al. Metabolic effects of intravenous propacetamol, metamizol or external cooling in critically ill febrile sedated patients. *Brit J Anaesth* 1997; **78**: 123–7.
17 Kurz A, Go JC, Sessler DI. Alfentanil slightly increases the sweating threshold and markedly reduces the vasoconstrictor and shivering thresholds. *Anesthesiology* 1995; **83**: 293–9.
18 Kurz A, Sessler DI, Annadata R, *et al.* Midazolam minimally impairs thermoregulatory control. *Anesth Analg* 1995; **81**: 393–398.
19 Hindman BJ, Todd MM, Gelb AW, *et al.* Mild hypothermia as a protective therapy during intracranial aneurysm surgery: a randomized prospective pilot trial. *Neurosurgery* 1999; **44**: 23–33.
20 Marion DW, Penrod LE, Kelsey SF, *et al.* Treatment of traumatic brain injury with moderate hypothermia. *New Engl J Med* 1997; **336**: 540–6.
21 Bernard SA, Jones BM, Buist M. Experience with prolonged induced hypothermia in severe head injury. *Crit Care* 1999; **3**: 167–72.
22 Center for Disease Control. Heat related illness and deaths: United States, 1994–95. *MMWR* 1995; **44**: 465–8.
23 Ghaznawi HI, Ibrahim MA. Heat stroke and heat exhaustion in pilgrims performing the Haj (annual pilgrimage) in Saudi Arabia. *Ann Saudi Med* 1987; **7**: 323–6.
24 Sminia P, van der Zee J, Wondergem J, *et al.* Effect of hyperthermia on the central nervous system: a review. *Intl J Hyperthermia* 1994; **10**: 1–30.

25 Bouchama A, Parhar RS, El-Yazigi A, *et al.* Endotoxaemia and release of TNF and IL-1 in acute heat stroke. *J Appl Physiol* 1991; **70**: 2640–4.

26 Bouchama A, Al-Sedairy S, Siddiqui S, *et al.* Elevated pyrogenic cytokines in heat stroke. *Chest* 1993; **104**: 1498–2644.

27 Bouchama A, Bridley F, Hammami MM, *et al.* Activation of coagulation and fibrinolysis in heat stroke. *Thrombosis Haemostasis* 1996; **76**: 909–15.

28 Bouchama A, Hammami MM, Hay A, *et al.* Evidence for endothelial cell activation/injury in heatstroke. *Crit Care Med* 1996; **24**: 1173–8.

29 Hammami MM, Bouchama A. Levels of soluble L-selectin and E-selectin in heatstroke and heatstress. *Chest* 1998; **114**: 949–50.

30 Bouchama A, Cafege A, deVol EB, *et al.* Ineffectiveness of dantrolene sodium in the treatment of heatstroke. *Crit Care Med* 1991; **19**: 176–80.

31 Hopkins PM. Malignant hyperthermia: advances in clinical management and diagnosis. *Brit J Anaesth* 2000; **85**: 118–28.

32 Ramirez JA, Cheetham ED, Laurence AS. Succinylcholine, masseter spasm and later malignant hyperthermia. *Anaesthesia* 1998; **53**: 1111–16.

33 Reyford HG, Cordonnier C, Adnet P, *et al.* The *in vitro* exposure of muscle strips from patients with neuroleptic malignant syndrome cannot be correlated with the clinical features. *J Neurol Sci* 1990; **98**: 527.

34 Velamoor VR, Norman R, Caroff SN, *et al.* Progression of symptoms in neuroleptic malignant syndrome. *J Nerv Ment Dis* 1994; **182**: 168–73.

35 Rosenberg MR, Green M. Neuroleptic malignant syndrome: a review of response to therapy. *Arch Int Med* 1989; **149**: 1927–31.

36 McKenna DJ, Peroutka SJ. Neurochemistry and neurotoxicity of 3, 4 methylenediaoxymetamphetamine (MDMA, 'ecstasy'). *J of Neurochemistry* 1990; **54**: 14–22.

37 Danzl D, Pozos RS, Auerbach PS, *et al.* Multicentre hypothermia survey. *Ann Emerg Med* 1987; **16**: 1042–55.

38 Jurkovic GJ, Greiser WB, Luterman A, *et al.* Hypothermia in trauma victims: an ominous predictor of survival. *J Trauma* 1987; **27**: 1019.

39 Smith CE. Focus on: Perioperative hypothermia. Trauma and hypothermia. *Curr Anaesth and Crit Care* 2001; **12**: 87–95.

40 Sessler DI. Consequences and treatment of perioperative hypothermia. *Anesthesiology Clin North Am* 1994; **12**: 425–56.

41 Corneli HM. Accidental hypothermia. *J Pediatr* 1990; **120**: 671–79.

42 Morley-Forster PK. Unintentional hypothermia in the operating room. *Can Anaest Soc J* 1986; **33**: 516–27.

43 Larach MG. Accidental hypothermia. *Lancet* 1995; **345**: 493–8.

44 Zell SC, Kurtz KJ. Severe experimental hypothermia: a resuscitation protocol. *Ann Emer Med* 1985; **4**: 339–45.

45 Giesbrecht GG, Bristow GK. A second post cooling afterdrop: more evidence for a convective mechanism. *J Appl Physiol* 1992; **73**: 1253–8.

46 Smith CE, Yamat RA. Avoiding hypothermia in the trauma patient. *Curr Opin Anaesthesiol* 2000; **13**: 167–74.

47 Smith CE, Patel N. Hypothermia in adult trauma patients: anaesthetic considerations. Part II. Prevention and treatment. *Am J Anesthesiol* 1997; **24**: 29–36.

48 Otto KJ, Metzler MH. Re-warming from experimental hypothermia: comparison of heated aerosol inhalation, peritoneal lavage and pleural lavage. *Crit Care Med* 1988; **16**: 869–75.

49 Brunette DD, Biros M, Mlinek EJ, *et al.* Internal cardiac massage and mediastinal irrigation in hypothermic cardiac arrest. *Am J Emerg Med* 1992; **10**: 32–4.

50 Gentilello LM, Jurkovic GJ, Stark MS, *et al.* Is hypothermia in the victim of major trauma protective or harmful? *Ann Surg* 1997; **226**: 439–49.

51 Walpoth BH, Walpoth-Aslan BN, Mattle HP, *et al.* Outcome of survivors of accidental deep hypothermia and circulatory arrest treated with extracorporeal blood warming. *New Engl J Med* 1997; **337**: 1500–5.

73

Electrical safety and injuries

L A H Critchley

Patients suffering from the consequences of electrocution and associated burns occasionally require ICU management. Patients and staff in the ICU are at risk of electrocution from faulty electrical equipment. The necessity of direct patient contact with electrical equipment increases this risk, and when therapy involves an invasive contact close to the heart, microshock is an additional hazard. Faulty electrical equipment can also result in power failures, fires, and explosions. The use of mobile phones and related devices nearby patient equipment can lead to malfunctioning.

PHYSICAL CONCEPTS

Electricity is produced by the movement of negatively charged electrons. A potential difference or voltage, measured in volts (V), exists between two points if the number or density of electrons is greater at one point. When these points are connected by a conductor, the potential difference will cause electrons or an electric current (I), measured in amperes (A), to flow. Resistance (R), measured in ohms (Ω), opposes this flow of electrons. Resistance is low in a conductor, because electrons can move freely from atom to atom. However, resistance is high in an insulator as electrons are unable to move. Voltage, current and resistance are related by Ohm's Law:

$$V = I \times R$$

When an electric current flows through a resistance, it dissipates energy as heat. The heating effect per second, or power, is measured in Joules(J)/s or Watts(W):

$$Power = V \times I = I^2 \times R$$

When a current flows in one direction, such as produced by a battery, it is called a direct current. Electricity to homes, hospitals, and factories is supplied as an alternating current which flows back and forth at a frequency, i.e. cycles per second or hertz (Hz). Two configurations are commonly used. Australasia and the UK use 240 V at 50 Hz, and North America uses 120 V at 60 Hz.

A current flowing in a circuit produces magnetic fields, which induce currents to flow in neighbouring circuits. When this results in a current flowing between the two circuits, it is called capacitive and inductive coupling, respectively. With capacitive coupling, high frequency currents are most easily passed, and the size of the current is greatest when the circuits are close. Inductive coupling can result from the strong magnetic fields produced by heavy duty electrical equipment, such as transformers, electric motors, and magnetic resonance imaging machines. The most common problem associated with coupling is electrical interference or 'noise'. Monitoring equipment is designed to 'filter' out this noise. However, in certain circumstances, such as the use of high frequency surgical diathermy and magnetic resonance, sufficient amperage can be induced to cause microshock and burns.[1,2] Smaller electromagnetic fields emitted by hand-held devices, such as mobile phones can effect the programming of microprocessors. Cases of patient equipment malfunctions have been reported.[3]

Static electricity has no free flow of electrons. Insulated objects can become highly charged, usually by repeated rubbing. The charge is dissipated by electrons jumping onto another neighbouring object of a different potential. 'Jumping' electrons ionize and heat the air through which they pass, causing a spark which may ignite an inflammable liquid or gas. Lightning is a type of static electrical discharge. Direct currents of 12 000–200 000 A and voltages in the millions are involved; however, flow lasts only a fraction of a second.[4]

PHYSIOLOGICAL CONSIDERATIONS

For a current to flow through the body, the body must complete a circuit. Usually this involves the current flowing from its source to ground through the body. The pathophysiological effects depend on the size of the current, and this depends on the voltage and electrical resistance of the body, most of which occurs in the skin. Dry skin has a resistance in excess of 100 000 Ω.[5] However, skin resistance is markedly reduced (to ~1000 Ω)[6] if the skin is wet, or if a conductive jelly has been applied. Hence, from Ohm's law, dry skin in contact with 240 V mains supply will result in a 0.24 mA current flowing through the body, whereas moist or wet skin will result in a 240 mA current.

ELECTROCUTION

Most cases of electrocution occur in the workplace (about 60%) or at home (about 30%), where misuse of extension cables is the main culprit.[6] Pathophysiological processes involved in true electrical injuries are poorly understood. The extent of injury depends on (i) the amount of current that passes through the body, (ii) the duration of the current, and (iii) the tissues traversed by the current (Table 73.1).

The extent of injury is most directly related to amperage. However, usually only the voltage involved is known. In general, lower voltages cause less injury, although voltages as low as 50 V have caused fatalities. An electric current passing through the body produces these main effects.

TISSUE HEAT INJURY

Currents in excess of 1 A generate sufficient heat energy to cause burns to the skin and occult thermal injury to internal tissues and organs. Blood vessels and nervous tissue appear to be particularly susceptible.[6]

DEPOLARIZATION OF MUSCLE CELLS

An alternating current of 30–200 mA will cause ventricular fibrillation.[7] Currents in excess of 5 A cause sustained cardiac asystole, which is the principle used in defibrillation. Apart from ventricular fibrillation, other arrhyth-

Table 73.1 Origin and pathophysiological effects of different levels of electrical injury

Current (A)	Source	Effects on victim
10–100 μA	Earth leakage	Microshock (ventricular fibrillation)
300–400 μA	Faulty equipment	Tingling (harmless)
>1 mA	Faulty equipment	Pain (withdraw)
>10 mA	Faulty equipment	Tetany (cannot let go)
>100 mA	Faulty equipment	Macroshock (ventricular fibrillation)
>1 A	Faulty equipment	Burns and tissue damage
>1,000 A	High tension injury	Severe burns and loss of limbs
>12,000 A	Lightning	Coma, severe burns and loss of limbs

mias may occur. Myocardial damage is common and may result in ST and T-wave changes. Global left ventricular dysfunction may occur hours or days later, despite initial minimal ECG changes.[8,9] Myocardial infarction has been reported, and the diagnosis is often difficult, because of the elevated creatine phosphokinase concentrations (even MB isoenzymes) from the extensive muscle injury.[10,11]

Tetanic contractions of skeletal muscle occur with currents in excess of 15–20 mA. The threshold is particularly low with alternating currents at the household frequency of 50–60 Hz. Tetanic contraction will prevent voluntary release of the source of electrocution, and violent muscle contractions may cause fractures of long bones and spinal vertebrae.[6]

VASCULAR INJURIES

Blood vessels may become thrombosed and occluded as a result of the thermal injury. Compartment syndromes are seen secondary to tissue oedema, causing tissue ischaemia and necrosis. Effected limbs may even require amputation.[12]

NEUROLOGICAL INJURIES

Neurological injuries may be central or peripheral, and immediate or late in onset. Monoparesis may occur in effected limbs, and the median nerve is particularly vulnerable.[6,13] Electrocution to the head may result in unconsciousness, paralysis of the respiratory centre, and late complications such as epilepsy, encephalopathy, and Parkinsonism.[6,13] Spinal cord damage resulting in para- or tetraplegia can result from a current traversing both arms.[6,13] Autonomic dysfunction may also occur causing acute vasospasm or a late sympathetic dystrophy.[6]

RENAL FAILURE

Acute renal failure may result from the myoglobinuria and toxins produced by extensive muscle necrosis.[13]

OTHER INJURIES

Electrocution can cause the victim to fall or be thrown, and clothing to catch fire, resulting in associated injuries. High voltage injuries can rupture the ear drum.[14] Cataracts may later develop.[13]

MICROSHOCK

The above domestic/industrial electrocution is known as macroshock, when current flowing through the intact skin and body passes through the heart. In the ICU, potential microshock electrocution exists. Microshock occurs when there is a direct current path to the heart

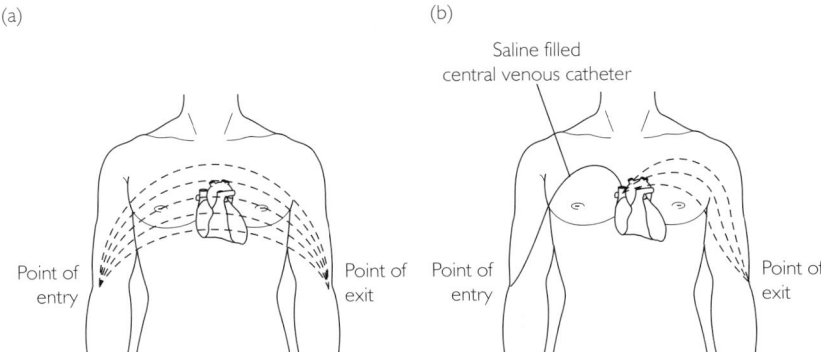

Fig. 73.1 Microshock. (a) low current density at the heart; (b) high current density at the heart if there is a conducting pathway, such as a saline-filled catheter.

muscle. The pathway may be provided by a saline-filled monitoring catheter, pulmonary artery catheter, or transvenous pacemaker wires. The current required to produce ventricular fibrillation in microshock is extremely small, in the order of 60 μA.[15] Currents of 1–2 mA are barely perceptible and produce tingling of the skin (Table 73.1). Hence a lethal microshock may be transmitted to a patient via a staff member who is unaware of the conducted current. Microshock can result from direct contact with faulty electrical equipment, or stray currents from capacitive coupling, or earth leakage. Such small currents are potentially lethal because a high current density is produced at the heart (Figure 73.1).

HIGH TENSION AND LIGHTNING INJURIES

High tension electricity (>1000 V) involves voltage much greater than domestic supply, usually many thousands of volts. Tissue damage is mainly due to the generation of heat, as high amperage currents are involved. Witnesses have described tissues actually exploding.[16]

Lightning injury is a type of high tension injury. It is rare and its incidence depends upon geographic location. Victims can be thrown several feet as a result of violent muscular contractions. Electrical arcing of the air causes intense heat, resulting in superficial burns and clothes igniting. Characteristic entrance and exit site burns are seen, which have a spider like appearance with redness and blistering. Victims are usually unconscious in the initial phase. However, many victims survive,[4] and good recovery has been reported despite initial hopeless neurological responsiveness (e.g. fixed dilated pupils).[17] Immediate death usually results from cardiorespiratory arrest; asystole is more common than ventricular fibrillation.[4]

MANAGEMENT OF ELECTRICAL INJURIES

Treatment of electrical injuries is mainly supportive. They include the following.

FIRST AID AND RESUSCITATION

It is imperative to make the immediate environment safe for rescuers. Power sources should be switched off and wet areas avoided where possible. Instinctive attempts to grab the electrocuted victim must be avoided until it is safe to do so. Cardiopulmonary resuscitation is carried out when indicated, and continued even if the prognosis seems hopeless. The neck and spine should be protected from possible fractures.

INVESTIGATIONS

Investigations are indicated to detect damaged organs. They include ECG, echocardiography, CT of the head, EEG, X-rays of the spine and long bones, haemoglobin, serum electrolytes, creatine kinase and urine myoglobin to assess muscle damage, and nerve conduction studies. Arteriograms may help in the decision to amputate a limb.[12]

HOSPITAL AND ICU MANAGEMENT

Management is directed towards treatment of burns, ischaemic and necrotic tissue, and injured organs. The principle of treating electrical burns is complete excision because of the risks of acute renal failure and sepsis. Fasciotomies and amputations may be necessary. Tetanus toxoid and antibiotics, especially penicillin, are given if indicated.

ELECTRICAL HAZARDS IN ICU

The ICU has the potential to inflict both macroshock and microshock injuries to staff and patients. Potential sources of these electrical hazards are:

MAJOR ELECTRICAL FAULTS

The casing and insulated wiring of electrical equipment protect against electric shock. Faulty wiring or components, and deterioration of internal insulation, can result in the casing becoming 'live'. Contact with live casing or wires can result in an electric current flowing through the victim to ground. The outcome largely depends on the resistance offered by the body to the current. If it is low, such as in a wet environment, sufficient current can flow to cause death.

MICROSHOCK CURRENTS

EARTH LEAKAGE CURRENTS

Within all pieces of electrical equipment, stray low amperage electrical currents exist that usually flow to earth, called earth leakage currents. They originate from current leaks across imperfect insulation of wires, capacitive and inductive coupling within the equipment, and coupling from electric and magnetic fields that exist in the working environment, such as the 50–60 Hz mains supply. Normally these currents are small and harmless, but they have the potential to cause microshock.

PACING WIRES AND CENTRAL VENOUS LINES

In certain circumstances, sufficient current to cause microshock can be passed by capacitive and inductive coupling to intracardiac pacing wires and central venous lines. Ventricular fibrillation has resulted from capacitive coupling with thermistor wires in a pulmonary artery catheter.[1]

DIFFERENT EARTH POTENTIALS

Inadequate or faulty earthing can result in separate earthing points being at different resting potentials. If contact is made between the two earthing points, sufficient current can flow to cause microshock.

STAFF–PATIENT CONTACT

Small currents capable of causing microshock can be transmitted unknowingly to a patient by a staff member who simultaneously touches faulty electrical equipment and the patient. If this current returns to earth via an intracardiac connection, a high current density will pass through the heart resulting in microshock.

INDUCTIVE CURRENTS

Inductive coupling from the strong magnetic fields produced by magnetic resonance imaging can cause over heating of wires and equipment. Severe burns have resulted from the use of pulse oximetry during magnetic resonance imaging, and specially designed wiring and probes are recommended.[2] Similar problems can exist with any intravascular device containing wires, such as a pulmonary artery catheter. More recently problems have arisen from the interference caused by personal computers, mobile phones and related devices with patient equipment. Many hospitals have banned the use of such devices in areas where patients are treated.

OTHER RELATED HAZARDS

Electrical equipment has the potential to cause other hazards such as thermal injury, fires, and power failures. Preliminary critical incident reports suggest that power failures are the most commonly encountered incidents involving electricity in the ICU. Power failures can be disastrous, as many patients' lives depend on electrically driven 'life support' equipment. As the intensivist frequently works outside the ICU, he should also be aware of potential electrical hazards outside ICU.

ELECTRICAL SAFETY STANDARDS

Most western countries have standards of electrical safety that apply to the use of medical equipment. For example, Australian Standards (AS 3003 and AS 3200) set minimum requirements for Australian hospitals. AS 2500 covers the safe use of electricity in patient care areas.[18] Britain and Europe follow the International Electrotechnical Commission Code[19,20] and the USA follows the National Electric Code 1993.[21] Hospitals should establish their own committees to ensure that adequate standards are applied. However, patient care areas differ in their safety requirements and commonly used classifications are listed below. The ICU should conform to (1b) and preferably (1c).

1. (a) *Unprotected areas*, where only routine electrical safety standards are applied.
   (b) *Body protected areas*, where the level of electrical safety is sufficient to minimize the risk of macroshock when the patient is in direct contact with electrical equipment and the skin impedance is reduced or bypassed.
   (c) *Cardiac protected areas*, where the level of electrical safety is sufficient to minimize the risk of direct microshock to the heart.
2. *Wet locations*, where spillage of water and physiological solutions, such as saline and blood, frequently occurs.

3 Until recently, standards existed for the safe use of inflammable anaesthetics agents.

MEASURES TO PROTECT STAFF AND PATIENTS[22,23]

EARTHING, FUSES AND CIRCUIT BREAKERS

Earthing reduces the risk of macroshock. The casing in most electrical equipment is connected to ground by a very low resistance wire. If a fault arises, the earth wire offers a low resistance path to ground. The high amperage current that results will blow the main fuse or circuit breaker, thus warning that a fault is present. Additional protection can be achieved by connecting all the earthing points in a patient care area together by a very low resistance wire. This reduces the risk of microshock occurring from earthing points at different potentials, and is commonly used in cardiac protected areas.

POWER SUPPLY ISOLATION

MAINS ISOLATION

The power supply is isolated from earth using a mains isolation transformer. If contact is made with live faulty circuitry, the risk of electric shock is reduced because stray currents no longer preferentially flow through patient or staff member to earth. Presence of stray earth leakage currents can be detected by using a line isolation monitor. This type of system is particularly useful in wet locations where the body may offer a very low resistance to earth.

INTERNAL ISOLATION

The mains power supply is isolated from the patient connection by using transformers and photoelectric diodes. The casing is still earthed to protect against faulty circuitry. This method of protection is commonly used in ICU equipment.

EARTH LEAKAGE CIRCUIT BREAKERS

These are devices that switch off the electrical supply if small currents are detected flowing to earth. They can be used to protect against microshock. A major disadvantage is that power supply to essential life supporting equipment is switched off.

EQUIPMENT CHECKS

The purchase of new equipment should be strictly controlled, and circuit diagrams should be provided. All new equipment should be checked for function and current leaks before use in the ICU. Preventative maintenance of equipment should be done regularly. Dated stickers should be used to show when the equipment was last checked. All faulty equipment must be removed from service, labelled appropriately, and recommissioned only after thorough checking.

RESERVE POWER SUPPLIES AND ALARMS

All essential equipment should have a reserve power supply (usually a battery), and alarms that warn of power failure. All hospitals should provide an emergency backup power supply in case of power cuts.

PERSONNEL EDUCATION

Staff should be taught correct ways to handle electrical equipment. Equipment with frayed wires should never be used, plugs should never be tugged, trolleys should never be wheeled over power cords, and two pieces of equipment should never be handled simultaneously. Staff should also respond appropriately to alarms.

REFERENCES

1 McNulty SE, Cooper M, Staudt S. Transmitted radiofrequency current through a flow directed pulmonary artery catheter. *Anesth Analg* 1994; **78**: 587–9.
2 Peden CJ, Menon DK, Hall AS *et al.* Magnetic resonance for the anaesthetist. *Anaesthesia* 1992; **47**: 508–17.
3 Hayes DL, Carrillo RG, Findlay GK *et al.* State of the science: pacemaker and defibrillator interference from wireless communication devices. *Pacing Clin Electrophysiol* 1996; **19**: 1407–9.
4 Apfelberg DB, Masters FW, Robinson DW. Pathophysiology and treatment of lightning injuries. *J Trauma* 1974; **14**: 453–60.
5 Bruner JMR. Hazards of electrical apparatus. *Anesthesiology* 1976; **28**: 396–424.
6 Fontneau NM, Mitchell A. Miscellaneous neurologic problems in the intensive care unit. In: Irwin RS, Cerra FB, Rippe JM (eds) *Intensive Care Medicine*, 4th edn. Philadelphia: Lippincott-Raven; 1999: 2127–35.
7 Loughman J, Watson AB. Electrical safety in hospitals and proposed standards. *Med J Aust* 1971; **2**: 349–55.
8 Lewin RF, Arditti A, Sclarovsky S. Non-invasive evaluation of cardiac injury. *Br Heart J* 1983; **49**: 190–2.
9 Jensen PJ, Thomsem PEB, Bagger JP *et al.* Electrical injury causing ventricular arrhythmias. *Br Heart J* 1987; **57**: 279–83.
10 Walton AS, Harper RW, Coggins GL. Myocardial infarction after electrocution. *Med J Aust* 1988; **148**: 365–7.
11 McBride JW, Labrosse KR, McCoy HG. Is serum creatine kinase–MB in electrical injured patients predictive of myocardial injury. *JAMA* 1986; **255**: 764–8.

12 Hunt JL, McManus WF, Haney WP, Pruitt BA. Vascular lesions in acute electric injuries. *J Trauma* 1974; **14**: 461–73.

13 Solem L, Fischer RP, Strate RG. The natural history of electrical injury. *J Trauma* 1977; **17**: 487–92.

14 Ogren FP, Edmunds AL. Neuro-otologic findings in the lightning-injured patient. *Semin Neurol* 1995; **15**: 256-62.

15 Watson AB, Wright JS, Loughman J. Electrical thresholds for ventricular fibrillation in man. *Med J Aust* 1973; **1**: 1179–82.

16 Burke JF, Quinby WC, Bondoc C *et al.* Patterns of high tension electric injury in children and adolescents and their management. *Am J Surg* 1977; **133**: 492–4.

17 Hanson GC, McIlwaith GR. Lightning injury: Two case histories and a review of management. *Br Med J* 1973; **4**: 271–4.

18 Australian Standard 2500. *Guide to the Safe Use of Electricity in Patient Care*, Standards Association of Australia: 1988.

19 CEI–IEC 601–1&2. *Medical Electrical Equipment*, Geneve: International Electrotechnical Commission; 1988: 2nd edn.

20 Herrmann D. A preview of IEC safety requirements for programmable electronic medical systems. *Med Dev Diag Indust* 1995; **17**: 106–11.

21 Early, MW, Murray, RH, Caloggero, JM. *National Electrical Code Handbook*. Quincy: National Fire Protection Association; 1993: 6th edn.

22 Litt L, Ehrenwerth J. Electrical safety in the operating room: Important old wine, disguised new bottles. *Anesth Analg* 1994; **78**: 417–9.

23 Ehrenwerth J. Electrical safety in and around the operating room. *ASA Refresher Course in Anesthesia.* Philidelphia: JB Lippincott; 1994: 123.

74.

Envenomation
J Tibballs

Envenomation by species of snakes, spiders, ticks, bees, ants, wasps, jellyfish, octopuses or cone shell snails may threaten life, while envenomation by others may cause serious illness.[1] Although this chapter focuses on Australia, the principles of management are widely applicable. Advice on management may be obtained from the Australian Venom Research Unit advisory service on their 24-hour telephone number: 03 9483 8204.

SNAKES

EPIDEMIOLOGY

Australia is habitat to a large number of venomous terrestrial and marine snakes (Families Elapidae and Hydrophiidae). The genera responsible for the majority of serious illness are Brown Snakes (*Pseudonaja*), Tiger Snakes (*Notechis*), Taipans (*Oxyuranus*), Black Snakes (*Pseudechis*) and Death Adders (*Acanthophis*).

The mean death rate in Australia from 1981 to 1999 was 2.6 per year[1] (~0.014/100 000) usually occurring only because of massive envenomation, snake bite in remote locations, rapid collapse, or due to delayed or inadequate antivenom therapy. However, as many as 2000 people are bitten each year and of these at least 300 require antivenom treatment. This morbidity and mortality is far less than that observed in surrounding countries. Death and critical illness is due to (i) progressive paralysis leading to respiratory failure, (ii) bleeding, or (iii) renal failure occurring as a complication of rhabdomyolysis, disseminated intravascular coagulation (DIC), haemorrhage, haemolysis or to their combinations. Rapid collapse within minutes after a snake bite is due to anaphylaxis to venom or possibly due to the myocardial effects of DIC causing hypotension.

Snake bite is often 'accidental' when a snake is trodden upon or suddenly disturbed. However, many bites occur when humans deliberately interfere with snakes or handle them. The herpetologist or snake collector is at special risk. Not only do they invariably sustain bites in the course of their work[2] or hobby, but they are also at risk of developing allergic reactions to venoms and to the antivenoms used in their treatment.

SNAKE VENOMS

Venoms are complex mixtures of toxins, usually proteins, which kill the snake's prey and aid its digestion. Many are phospholipases. The main toxins cause paralysis, coagulopathy, rhabdomyolysis and haemolysis (Table 74.1). Coagulopathy may be due to a procoagulant effect by prothrombin activators (Factor Xa-like enzymes), with consumption of clotting factors, or due to a direct anticoagulant effect.

Table 74.1 Main components of Australian snake venoms

Neurotoxins
Presynaptic and postsynaptic neuromuscular blockers present in all dangerous venomous snakes. May cause paralysis.
Postsynaptic blockers readily reversed by antivenom.
Presynaptic blockers are more difficult to reverse, particularly if treatment is delayed.
Some presynaptic blockers are also rhabdomyolysins.

Prothrombin activators
Present in many important species.
Cause disseminated intravascular coagulation with consumption of clotting factors including fibrinogen.
Intrinsic fibrin(ogen)lysis generates fibrin(ogen) degradation products.
Significant risk of haemorrhage.

Anticoagulants
Present in a relatively small number of dangerous species.
Prevent blood clotting without consumption of clotting factors.

Rhabdomyolysins
Some presynaptic neurotoxins also cause lysis of skeletal and cardiac muscle.
Apart from loss muscle of mass, may cause myoglobinuria and renal failure.

Haemolysins
Present in a few species.
Rarely a serious clinical effect.

SNAKE BITE AND ENVENOMATION

Although a bite is usually observed, envenomation is less common because no venom or a variable amount of venom is injected. Bites are relatively painless and may be unnoticed. This is in marked contrast to many overseas crotalid and viperid snakes, where massive local reaction and necrosis are often a major feature as a result of proteolytic enzymes. Paired fang marks are usually evident but sometimes only scratches or single puncture wounds are found. In general, Australian snake venoms do not cause extensive damage to local tissues. There is usually mild swelling and bruising, and continued bleeding from the bite-site may be a feature.

SYMPTOMS AND SIGNS OF ENVENOMATION

Not all possible symptoms and signs occur in a particular case and in some cases, one symptom or sign may predominate the clinical picture, and in other cases they may wax and wane (Table 74.2). These phenomena are explained by variations in toxin content of venoms of the same species in different geographical areas, and by variable absorption of different toxins.

The cause of transient hypotension soon after envenomation is obscure but it may be related to intravascular coagulation.[3,4] Prothrombin activators gain access to the circulation within a number of minutes after subcutaneous

Table 74.2 Progressive onset of major systemic symptoms and signs of untreated envenomation (in massive envenomation or in a child, a critical illness may develop in minutes rather than hours)

<1 h after bite
Headache
Nausea, vomiting, abdominal pain
Transient hypotension associated with confusion or loss of consciousness
Coagulopathy (laboratory testing)
Regional lymphadenitis
1–3 h after bite
Paresis/paralysis of cranial nerves, e.g. ptosis, double vision, external ophthalmoplegia, dysphonia, dysphagia, myopathic facies
Haemorrhage from mucosal surfaces and needle punctures
Tachycardia, hypotension
Tachypnoea, shallow tidal volume
>3 h after bite
Paresis/paralysis of truncal and limb muscles
Paresis/paralysis of respiratory muscles (respiratory failure)
Peripheral circulatory failure (shock), hypoxaemia, cyanosis
Rhabdomyolysis
Dark urine (due to myoglobinuria or haemoglobin)
Renal failure

injection. There is often tachycardia and relatively minor ECG abnormalities. Other causes of hypotension such as direct cardiac toxicity remain unproven. Hypotension may be secondary to myocardial hypoxaemia.

Tender or even painful regional lymph nodes are moderately common but are not *per se* an indication for antivenom therapy, since lymphadenitis also occurs with bites by mildly venomous snakes which do not cause serious systemic illness.

Occasionally intracranial haemorrhage occurs. In the case of untreated or massive envenomation, rhabdomyolysis may occur. This usually involves all skeletal musculature and sometimes cardiac muscle. The resultant myoglobinuria may cause renal failure. Direct nephrotoxicity has been suspected in a few cases of Brown Snake bites, but is as yet unproven.

A high intake of alcohol before snake-bite is common, and may make management quite difficult initially. Pre-existing treatment (e.g. warfarin therapy) or disease (e.g. gastro-intestinal tract ulceration) may complicate management of coagulopathy.

SNAKE BITE IN CHILDREN
Snake bite in young children presents additional problems. It is difficult to diagnose when a bite has not been observed. The symptoms of early envenomation may pass unsuspected and the signs, particularly cranial nerve effects, are difficult to elicit. Bite marks may be difficult to distinguish from the effects of everyday minor trauma. Lastly, the onset of syndrome of envenomation is likely to be more rapid than in adults and the severity of envenomation more severe because of the relatively higher ratio of venom to body mass. Presentation may be cardiorespiratory failure.

IDENTIFICATION OF THE SNAKE

Identification of the snake guides selection of the appropriate antivenom, and provides an insight into the expected syndrome. Administration of the wrong antivenom may endanger the victim's life because there may be very little cross reactivity. A venom detection kit (VDK) can be used to identify the snake venom. If the snake cannot be identified, a specific antivenom, or a combination of monovalent antivenoms or polyvalent antivenom should be administered on a geographical basis (see Tables 74.3 and 74.4).

IDENTIFICATION BY VENOM DETECTION KIT TEST

The venom detection kit (VDK) is an *in vitro* test for detection and identification of snake venom at the bite site, in urine, blood or other tissue in cases of snake bite in Australia and Papua New Guinea. A positive result will indicate the type of antivenom to be administered. It detects venom from a range of snake genera including Tiger, Brown, Black, Death Adder and Taipan. Individual species of snake cannot be identified by the test and several genera may yield a positive result in a specified well. It is an enzyme immunoassay using rabbit antibodies and chromogen and peroxide solutions. The incidences of false positive and false negative tests of the kit remain unknown, but are generally regarded as low. It is very sensitive, able to detect venom in concentrations as low as 10 ng/ml. It yields a visual qualitative result in test wells in approximately 25 min. On occasions, a positive test may be present, but the patient is asymptomatic. A decision to administer antivenom should be made on clinical grounds. A very high concentration of venom in a sample may overwhelm the test and yield a spuriously negative result (Hook effect). If that possibility exists, a diluted sample should be re-tested.

IDENTIFICATION BY PHYSICAL CHARACTERISTICS

This can be misleading. Non-herpetologists should consult an identification guide[1] with reference to scale patterns, to correctly identify a specimen if antivenom therapy is based on morphological characteristics alone.

IDENTIFICATION BY CLINICAL EFFECTS

The appearance of a bite site cannot be used to reliably identify the snake.

Table 74.3 Antivenom and *initial* dosages when snake identified

Snake	Antivenom	Dose (units)
Common Brown Snake	Brown Snake	4 000
Chappell Island Tiger Snake	Tiger Snake	12 000
Copperheads	Tiger Snake	3 000–6 000
Death Adders	Death Adder	6 000
Dugite	Brown snake	4 000
Gwardar	Brown Snake	4 000
Mulga (King Brown) Snake	Black Snake	18 000
Papuan Black Snake	Black Snake	18 000
Red-bellied Black Snake	Tiger Snake *or*	3 000
	Black Snake*	18 000
Rough-scaled (Clarence River) Snake	Tiger Snake	3 000
Sea-Snakes	Sea-Snake *or*	1 000
	Tiger Snake	3 000
Small-scaled (Fierce) Snake	Taipan	12 000
Taipans	Taipan	12 000
Tasmanian Tiger Snake	Tiger Snake	6 000
Tiger Snake	Tiger Snake	3 000

*Smaller protein mass Tiger Snake antivenom preferable. Antivenom units per ampoule: Brown Snake 1000; Tiger Snake 3000; Black Snake 18 000; Taipan 12 000; Death Adder 6000; Polyvalent 40 000.
Note: (1) if the victim on presentation is critically ill, 2–3 times these amounts should be given initially; (2) additional antivenom may be required in the course of management since absorption of venom may be delayed.

Table 74.4 Antivenom and *initial* dosages when identity of snake uncertain

State	Antivenom	Dose (units)
Tasmania	Tiger Snake	6 000
Victoria	Tiger Snake *and*	3 000
	Brown Snake	4 000
New South Wales and ACT; Queensland; South Australia; Western Australia; Northern Territory	Polyvalent	40 000
Papua New Guinea	Polyvalent	40 000

Note: (1) If the victim on presentation is critically ill, 2–3 times these amounts should be given initially; (2) additional antivenom may be required in the course of management since absorption of venom may be delayed.

The constellation of symptoms and signs may be used to a limited degree in identification. For example, within the common genera, paralysis associated with procoagulopathy may be caused by a Tiger Snake, Taipan, Brown Snake, Rough-scaled Snake, *Hoplocephalus* spp. or Red-bellied Black Snake, but if rhabdomyolysis also occurs, a bite by a Brown Snake is improbable. Paralysis associated with anticoagulation may be caused by a Black Snake (other than Red-bellied Black Snake), Copperhead or Death Adder but if rhabdomyolysis occurs, a bite by a Death Adder is improbable. Paralysis with neither coagulopathy nor rhabdomyolysis may be caused by a Death Adder bite.

This information is of limited practical importance. It is essential to administer antivenom at the first opportunity when indicated, rather than wait until the full syndrome becomes apparent to enable an 'educated clinical guess' in selection of the appropriate antivenom.

MANAGEMENT OF SNAKE ENVENOMATION

The essentials of management are:

- resuscitation: mechanical ventilation and restoration of blood pressure with intravenous fluids, inotropic and vasoactive agents as needed
- application of a pressure-immobilization bandage
- administration of antivenom
- performance of investigations.

From a practical point of view, one of three clinical situations arise after snake bite. A plan of management for each of these is summarized in Figure 74.1.

- Victim presents with a critical illness
- Victim is envenomated but not critically ill
- Victim bitten but does not appear envenomated

When the envenomated victim is not critically ill, more time is available to identify the snake by investigations and to administer specific monovalent antivenom. A pressure-immobilization bandage should be applied if not already in place, and not removed until antivenom has been administered.

When the victim has been bitten, but not apparently envenomated, admission to hospital is advisable with observation and examination at least hourly for at least 12 h in the case of a child but less time for an adult. The syndrome of envenomation may be very slow in onset over numerous hours with a symptom free initial period. A test of coagulation should always be performed. If a coagulopathy is present, specific monovalent antivenom should be administered after identification of the species or as indicated by a VDK test. If only a mild coagulopathy is present it may be acceptable to withhold antivenom in the hope of spontaneous resolution but coagulation should be checked at intervals and the victim

maintained under surveillance until coagulation is normal.

THE PRESSURE-IMMOBILIZATION TECHNIQUE OF FIRST AID

Since at least 95% of snake bites occur on the arms or legs,[1] Sutherland's pressure-immobilization technique[5] is applicable to the majority of cases. With this technique, a crepe (or crepe-like) bandage is applied from the fingers or toes up the limb as far as possible, encompassing the bite site. It should be as firm as required for a sprained ankle. Additional immobilization is applied to the entire limb by a rigid splint, in particular immobilizing the joints either side of the bite site.

Venom is usually deposited subcutaneously. The systemic spread of venom largely is dependent on its absorption by way of the lymphatics[6] or the small blood vessels. Application of a pressure less than arterial to the bitten area when combined with immobilization of the limb effectively delays the movement of venom to the central circulation.[5] Although it is a first aid technique designed for use in the field, it should be part of initial management in hospital since it halts further absorption of venom. There is some experimental[1] and anecdotal evidence[7] with Death Adder bites that the technique inactivates some venom at the bite site but prolonged application has not been subjected to a controlled study.

REMOVAL OF THE PRESSURE-IMMOBILIZATION BANDAGE

Removal may precipitate a sudden elevation in blood concentration of venom and collapse of the victim. On the other hand, first aid has not been proven to inactivate venom in humans. Its removal therefore should be dictated by the circumstance. When an asymptomatic snake-bite victim reaches hospital with the recommended first aid measures in place, these should not be disturbed until antivenom, appropriate staff and equipment have been assembled. If the victim is symptomatic and antivenom is indicated, the first aid measures should not be removed until after antivenom has been administered, and re-applied if the victim's condition deteriorates. A swab of the bite site may be obtained by removing the splint temporarily and then cutting a window in the bandage. Thereafter the bandage should be made good and the splint re-applied.

ANTIVENOM

CHOICE

CSL Ltd (Parkville, Australia) produces highly purified equine monovalent antivenoms against the venoms of the main terrestrial snakes including Tiger Snake, Brown Snake, Black Snake, Death Adder and Taipan. A polyvalent antivenom, a mixture of aliquots of all these is also

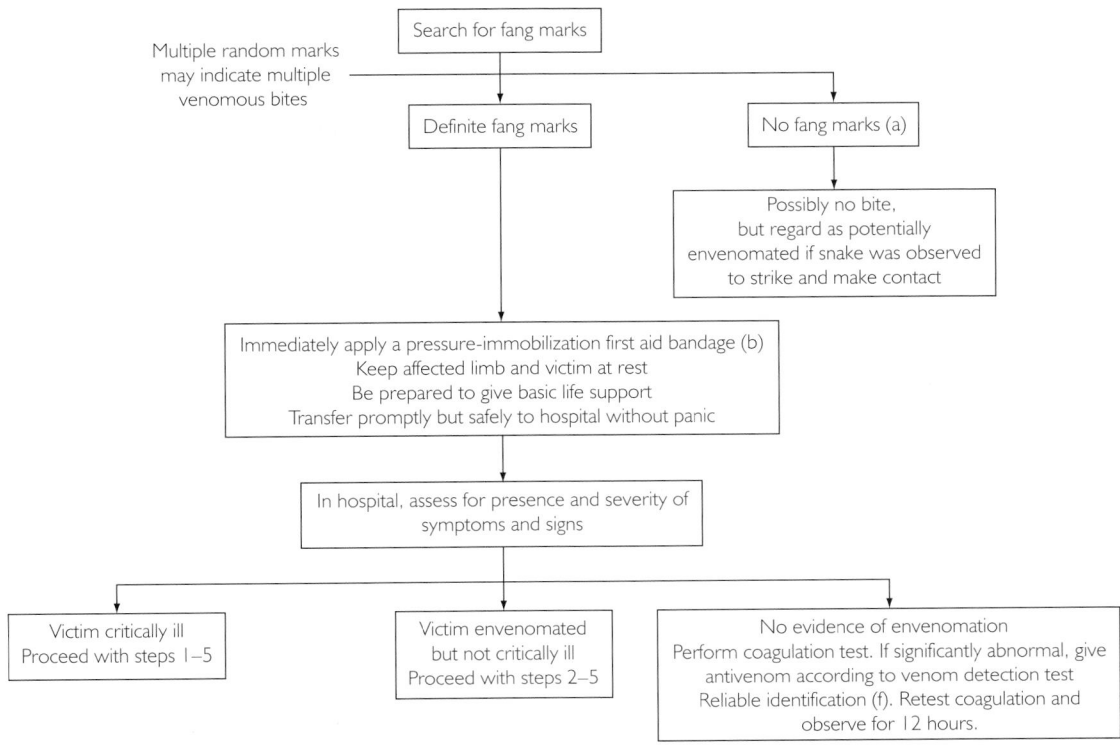

Multiple random marks may indicate multiple venomous bites

Search for fang marks

Definite fang marks

No fang marks (a)

Possibly no bite, but regard as potentially envenomated if snake was observed to strike and make contact

Immediately apply a pressure-immobilization first aid bandage (b)
Keep affected limb and victim at rest
Be prepared to give basic life support
Transfer promptly but safely to hospital without panic

In hospital, assess for presence and severity of symptoms and signs

Victim critically ill
Proceed with steps 1–5

Victim envenomated but not critically ill
Proceed with steps 2–5

No evidence of envenomation
Perform coagulation test. If significantly abnormal, give antivenom according to venom detection test
Reliable identification (f). Retest coagulation and observe for 12 hours.

1. Resuscitate (treat hypoxaemia and shock)
   Be prepared to intubate and mechanically ventilate. Admit to intensive care.
2. Apply pressure-immobilization bandage. Do not remove if already applied (b)
3. Give antivenom intravenously (c,d,e,f,g)
   - Give monovalent if species reliably known or appropriate antivenom indicated by venom detection test.
   - In critically ill victim, don't wait for venom detection test result or if species cannot be determined; give according to geographic location:
     Victoria – Brown and tiger snake
     Tasmania – tiger snake
     Other states and territories – polyvalent
   - Titrate antivenom against clinical and coagulation status (NOTE: Death Adders don't cause significant coagulopathy).
4. Perform investigations
   - Bite swab for venom detection. (First aid bandage may be cut to expose bite site, and then reinforced)
   - Blood for venom detection, coagulation, type and cross-match blood (if bleeding), fibrin degradation products, full blood examination, enzymes, electrolytes, urea, creatinine
   - Urine for venom detection, red blood cells, haemoglobin, myoglobin.
5. Examine frequently to detect slow onset of paralysis (h), coagulopathy, rhabdomyolysis and renal failure.

Dangers and mistakes in management

a. Fang marks not visible to naked eye.
b. Premature release of bandage may result in sudden systemic envenomation. Leave *in situ* until victim reaches full medical facilities. If clinically envenomated, remove only after antivenom given.
c. Erroneous identification of snake may cause wrong antivenom to be given. If in any doubt treat as unidentified.
d. Antivenom without premedication. Anaphylaxis is not rare and may not respond to treatment.
e. Insufficient antivenom. Titrate dose against clinical and coagulation status.
f. Blood and coagulation factors (fresh frozen plasma, cryoprecipitate) not preceded by antivenom will worsen coagulopathy.
g. Antivenom given without clinical or laboratory evidence of envenomation.
h. Delayed onset of paralysis may be missed. Victim must be examined at least hourly.

Fig. 74.1   Management of snake bite

available. A sea snake antivenom is produced from horses immunized with Beaked Sea Snake (*Enhydrina schistosa*) and Tiger Snake venom.

Antivenom should be administered according to the identity of the snake or if unknown or doubtful, according to the result of a venom detection kit (Table 74.3). If neither of these criteria can be fulfilled, and if the situation warrants immediate antivenom therapy, the geographical location may be used a guide, since the distribution of many species is limited (Table 74.4). Polyvalent antivenom should not be used when a monovalent antivenom could be used appropriately. For bites by uncommon snakes, when antivenom is indicated, polyvalent antivenom should be chosen or a monovalent antivenom as indicated by a VDK test.

DOSE

The initial doses of antivenom are given in Tables 74.3 and 74.4. The need for subsequent doses should be guided by the clinical response. After bites by species with coagulopathic effects the victim's coagulation status is a useful guide.

The dose of antivenom required varies. The amount of venom injected cannot be determined, and snakes may bite multiple times. Victims may present late after envenomation when toxins have already become bound to target tissues and cannot be easily neutralized. Some victims in this circumstance have required mechanical ventilation for many weeks despite large amounts of appropriate antivenom. A child requires more antivenom than an adult envenomated by the same amount of venom, and a victim in poor general health will likewise require more. Finally, antivenoms are manufactured against specific species and may have less neutralizing ability against different species of the same genus or against unrelated species or even when the antivenom chosen is nonetheless appropriate.

One ampoule of specific antivenom neutralizes *in vitro* the average yield on 'milking' – a process whereby venom is harvested by inducing the snake to bite through a latex membrane. If the amount of venom injected at a bite is greater than the average yield on milking, one ampoule of antivenom will not be adequate therapy. In severe cases of envenomation, a number of ampoules of antivenom will need to be administered. Absorption of venom from a bite site(s) is a continuing process.

ADMINISTRATION

The decision to administer antivenom must be based on clinical criteria of envenomation, not restricted to the result of a VDK test. A positive VDK test establishes the diagnosis of envenomation and the choice of antivenom but does not imply that antivenom should or should not be given.

However, if the victim is significantly envenomated, antivenom must be administered. There is no other effective treatment. Antivenom may be withheld if envenomation is so mild that spontaneous recovery may occur or the consequences of antivenom administration are likely to outweigh the benefit to be gained, for example, in a herpetologist known to have allergy to antivenom.

Snake antivenoms must be given by the intravenous route, or in dire circumstances if a vein cannot be cannulated, by the intraosseous route in a child. The large volume of fluid and slow absorption renders the intramuscular route useless in emergencies.

A test dose of antivenom to determine allergy should not be done. It is unreliable and a waste of precious time.

PREMEDICATION

Antivenom should be preceded by premedication with subcutaneous epinephrine approximately 0.25 mg for an adult and 0.005–0.01 mg/kg for a child about 5–10 min before commencement of infusion. In the moribund or critically ill victim, when it is essential to administer antivenom quickly, the epinephrine may be given intramuscularly or even intravenously in smaller doses. However, in general, epinephrine is not recommended by either of those routes because of the risk of intracerebral haemorrhage due to the combination of possible hypertension and coagulopathy. Although intracerebral haemorrhage has been recorded in the past in association with premedication, all such cases were accompanied by intravenous epinephrine, none with subcutaneous epinephrine. On the other hand, the incidence of adverse reactions (8–13%) to antivenom is sufficient to warrant premedication with epinephrine, which is the only medication proven effective in reducing the incidence of antivenom induced reactions and their severity.[8] It is not prudent to forgo premedication and elect to treat anaphylaxis if it occurs. Iatrogenic anaphylaxis has a high mortality despite vigourous and expert resuscitation.[9] If an adverse reaction to the first ampoule of antivenom has not occurred, subsequent ampoules do not need to be preceded by epinephrine. The reaction rate to polyvalent antivenom is higher than to monovalent antivenoms and should not be used when a monovalent antivenom or combinations will suffice.

The antihistamine, promethazine, is ineffective in this setting[10] and may cause obtundation and hypotension which may both exacerbate and confound a state of envenomation. It is not recommended. Other drugs such as steroids and aminophylline are also not useful in preventing anaphylaxis because their actions, apart from being unproven, are too slow in onset, but steroids are useful for preventing serum sickness.

INFUSION

The antivenom may be injected slowly into a running intravenous line or diluted in Hartmann's or other crystalloid solution in approximately 1 in 10 volumes in a burette and administered over 15–30 min if the situation is not critical. This measure reduces the risk of an anaphylactoid reaction resulting from its binding with complement. For small children if multiple ampoules are required the dilution may be less to prevent excessive fluid administration. In emergencies the antivenom may be infused quickly in high concentration.

ADVERSE REACTIONS

Antivenom infusion should always be administered in a location equipped and staffed by personnel capable of managing anaphylaxis. Management of anaphylaxis is discussed in detail in Chapter 57. Intramuscular epinephrine is the key treatment in a dose of approximately 0.25–1.00 mg for adults and 10 μg/kg for children. Antivenom therapy should be discontinued temporarily and re-started when the victim's condition is stable.

Lesser degrees of immediate adverse reaction restricted to headache, chest discomfort, fine rash, arthralgia, myalgia, nausea, abdominal pain, vomiting, and pyrexia may be managed by temporary cessation of infusion and administration of steroids and antihistamine before re-commencement.

A delayed hypersensitivity reaction, serum sickness, should be anticipated and patients warned of the symptoms and signs which usually appear several days to two weeks after antivenom administration. Severity may range from a faint rash and pyrexia to serious multi-system disease including lymphadenitis, polyarthralgia, urticaria, nephritis, neuropathy and vasculitis. The incidence of serum sickness appears to be greater with use of multiple doses of monovalent antivenom and with polyvalent antivenom. The treatment is a course of steroids, e.g. prednisolone 1 mg/kg per day, which may be required for several weeks.

INVESTIGATIONS AND MONITORING

Tests should be performed regularly, interpreted quickly and treated promptly to counter venom effects and its complications. Serial coagulation tests and tests of renal function are especially important. Absorption of venom from the bite site is a continuing process and management must anticipate unabsorbed venom. Apart from regular monitoring of vital signs and oxygenation, the following are specifically needed.

BITE SITE

A swab for venom testing should be done. It has the highest likelihood of detecting venom provided the site has not been washed. The site may be squeezed to yield venom if it has been washed.

URINE

Test the urine for venom that may be present when venom in blood has been bound by antivenom and is therefore undetectable. Urine should also be tested for

blood and protein. If the urine is pigmented a distinction should be made between haemoglobinuria and myoglobinuria – which is impossible with simple ward tests. Urine output should be recorded.

BLOOD

- Coagulation tests should include prothrombin time, activated thromboplastin time, serum fibrinogen and fibrin degradation products.
- A full blood examination and blood film for haemoglobin level, evidence of haemolysis and platelet count. A mild elevation in white cell count is expected.
- Electrolytes, urea, creatinine, and creatine phosphokinase (isoenzymes and troponin are useful) to monitor rhabdomyolysis and possible renal compromise.

ELECTROCARDIOGRAM

Sinus tachycardia, ventricular ectopy and ST segment and T-wave changes are not uncommon. These effects may be the result of venom toxins or from electrolyte disturbances caused by rhabdomyolysis or renal failure.

SECONDARY MANAGEMENT

COAGULATION FACTOR AND BLOOD TRANSFUSION

Although coagulopathy often resolves after several doses of antivenom it does not *per se* restore coagulation – it permits newly released or manufactured coagulation factors to act unopposed by venom. If coagulation is not restored after several doses of antivenom over several hours, it is prudent to administer fresh frozen plasma and to re-measure coagulation at intervals. Because regeneration of coagulation factors takes many hours, treatment of isolated coagulopathy entirely with antivenom while waiting for their regeneration exposes the patient to serious haemorrhage and implies overdosage with antivenom. Administration of coagulation factors should be preceded by antivenom to neutralize venom prothrombin activator. Platelets may be required. Whole blood is rarely needed.

INTRAVENOUS FLUIDS, RHABDOMYOLYSIS AND RENAL PROTECTION

After acute resuscitation, intravenous fluids in sufficient volume to maintain urine output at about 40 ml/kg per day in an adult and 1–2 ml/kg per hour in a child to prevent tubular necrosis as a consequence of rhabdomyolysis. Life-threatening hyperkalaemia and hypocalcaemia may develop with rhabdomyolysis. Haemofiltration or dialysis may be required.

HEPARIN

Although this anticoagulant has prevented the action of prothrombin activators in animal models of envenomation, it does not improve established disseminated intravascular coagulation.[11] It is not recommended. Emphasis instead should be on treating the cause by neutralizing venom with antivenom.

ANALGESIA AND SEDATION

Australian snake bite does not cause severe pain. However, sedation is required for the mechanically ventilated venom-paralysed victim and analgesia for rhabdomyolysis.

CARE OF THE BITE SITE

Usually no specific care is required. Occasionally the site may blister, bruise, ulcerate or necrose, particularly when first aid bandage has been in place for a considerable time or when the bite was from a member of the Black Snake genus, such as a Mulga Snake or Red-bellied Black Snake.

OTHER DRUGS

Antibiotics are not routinely required but should be considered as for any potentially contaminated wound. Sea snake bites may cause Gram-negative infections. Tetanus prophylaxis should be reviewed.

SEA-SNAKE BITE

Some sea-snake venoms cause widespread damage to skeletal muscle with consequent myoglobinuria, neuromuscular paralysis or direct renal damage. Many have not been researched. The principles of treatment are essentially the same as for envenomation by terrestrial snakes. The venoms of significant species are neutralized with CSL Ltd Beaked Sea-Snake (*Enhydrina schistosa*) antivenom. If that preparation is not available, Tiger Snake or polyvalent antivenom should be used. Sea-snake bites are uncommon in Australia and no deaths have been recorded.

UNCOMMON AND EXOTIC SNAKE BITE

Zoo personnel, herpetologists and amateur collectors who catch, maintain and breed species of uncommon Australian snakes or who import or breed exotic (overseas) snakes are at risk. There are no specific antivenoms to the venoms of uncommon Australian snakes, but neutralization is provided by polyvalent antivenom or by monovalent antivenom, as indicated by the Venom Detection Kit. Exotic snake antivenoms are maintained by Venom Supplies Ltd., Tanunda, South Australia (Tel: 08 8563 0001), Royal Melbourne Hospital (Tel: 03 9342 7000), Royal Adelaide Hospital (Tel: 08 8223 4000), Australian Reptile Park (Tel: 02 4340 1022) and by Taronga Zoo (Mosman, Tel: 02 9969 2777).

LONG-TERM EFFECTS OF SNAKE BITE

After appropriate treatment, recovery is expected but it may be slow, taking many weeks or months particularly from a critical illness or after delayed presentation with neurotoxicity and rhabdomyolysis. Isolated neurological or ophthalmic signs may persist. Long-term loss of taste or smell occurs occasionally.

SPIDERS

Although several thousand species of spiders exist in Australia, only Funnel-web Spiders (Genera *Atrax* and *Hadronyche*) and the Red-back Spider (*Latrodectus hasselti*) have caused death or significant systemic illness. All spiders have venom and a few, particularly the White-tailed Spider (*Lampona cylindrata*) and the Common Black House Spider (*Badumna insignis*) are capable of causing severe local injury.

FUNNEL-WEB SPIDERS

Several species of the genera *Atrax* and *Hadronyche* cause significant illness and are potentially lethal. *Atrax robustus* (Sydney Funnel-web Spider) is a large aggressive spider inhabiting an area within an approximate 160 km radius of Sydney. It has caused the deaths of more than a dozen people. The male spider is more dangerous than the female, in contrast to other species, and is inclined to roam after rainfall. In doing so, it may enter houses and seek shelter among clothes or bedding and give a painful bite when disturbed.

Bites do not always result in envenomation, but envenomation may be rapidly fatal. The early features of the envenomation syndrome include nausea, vomiting, profuse sweating, salivation and abdominal pain. Life-threatening features usually are heralded by the appearance of muscle fasciculation at the bite site, which quickly involves distant muscle groups. Hypertension, tachyarrhythmias, vasoconstriction, hypersalivation and bronchorrhoea occur. The victim may lapse into coma, develop central hypoventilation and have difficulty maintaining an airway free of secretions. Finally, respiratory failure, pulmonary oedema and severe hypotension culminate in death. The syndrome may develop within several hours but it may be more rapid. Several children have died within 90 min of envenomation, and one has died within 15 min. An active component in the venom is a polypeptide, which stimulates the release of acetylcholine at neuromuscular junctions and within the autonomic nervous system and the release of catecholamines.

Treatment consists of the application of a pressure-immobilization bandage, intravenous administration of antivenom and support of vital functions, which may include airway support and mechanical ventilation. No deaths or serious morbidity have been reported since the introduction of antivenom in 1981.

RED-BACK SPIDER

This spider is distributed throughout Australia and is found outdoors in household gardens in suburban and rural areas. Related species and similar effects of envenomation ('Latrodectism') occur in many parts of the world. Red-back spider bite is the most common cause for antivenom administration in Australia at 300–400/annum. The adult female is identified easily. Its body is about 1 cm in size and has a distinct red or orange dorsal stripe over its abdomen. When disturbed, it gives a pin prick like bite. The site becomes inflamed. During the following minutes to several hours, severe pain, exacerbated by movement, commences locally and may extend up the limb or radiate elsewhere. The pain may be accompanied by profuse sweating, headache, nausea, vomiting, abdominal pain, fever, hypertension, paraesthesias and rashes. In a small percentage of cases when treatment is delayed, progressive muscle paralysis may occur over many hours, requiring mechanical ventilation. Untreated, muscle weakness, spasm and arthralgia may persist for months after the bite. Death has not occurred since introduction of an antivenom in 1956. If the effects of a bite are minor and confined to the bite site, antivenom may be withheld but otherwise, antivenom should be given intramuscularly. The rate of anaphylaxis to antivenom is very low (<0.5%). A premedication with promethazine is recommended and epinephrine should be at hand. In contrast to a bite from a snake or Funnel-web spider, a bite from a Red-back spider is not immediately life threatening. There is no effective first aid, but application of a cold pack or iced-water may help relieve pain. Bites by *Steatoda* spp. (Cupboard spiders) may cause a similar syndrome and can be treated effectively with Red-back spider antivenom.

BOX JELLYFISH

This creature, *Chironex fleckeri*, is probably the most venomous in the world. It has caused at least 63 deaths in the waters off northern Australia.[12] It has a cuboid bell up to 30 cm in diameter. Numerous tentacles arise from the corners of the bell and trail several metres. It is semi-transparent and difficult to see by anyone wading or swimming in shallow water. The tentacles are lined with millions of nematocysts, which on contact with skin, discharge a threaded barb, which pierces subcutaneous tissue, including small blood vessels. Contact with the tentacles causes severe pain and envenomation from which death may occur within minutes. Death is probably due to both neurotoxic effects causing apnoea and direct cardiotoxicity, although the precise mode of action of the venom is unknown. In mechanically ventilated animals, fatal hypotension occurs rapidly on envenomation.[13] The skin which sustains the injury may heal with disfiguring scars.

First aid, which must be administered on the beach, consists of dousing the skin with acetic acid (vinegar) which inactivates undischarged nematocysts. Adherent tentacles can then be removed. Cardiopulmonary resuscitation may be required on the beach. An ovine antivenom is available but prevention is of paramount importance. Water must not be entered when this jellyfish is known to be close inshore. Wet suits, clothing and 'stinger suits' offer protection.

IRUKANDJI

Stings by the Irukandji, *Carukia barnesi*, and possibly by other jellyfish may cause a syndrome known as the Irukandji syndrome. The Irukandji is a small cubozoan jellyfish with a squarish bell up to several centimetres in diameter. Single tentacles trail from its corners. When submerged it is virtually impossible to see.

Its sting is mild and marked only by a small area of erythema. However, severe general symptoms which may follow include abdominal cramps, hypertension, back pain, nausea and vomiting, limb cramps, chest tightness and marked distress.[14] Occasionally, cardiogenic pulmonary oedema has ensued necessitating mechanical ventilation and inotropic therapy.[15] The mechanism is uncertain but experimental studies in animals have shown that Irukandji extracts cause a massive release of catecholamines[16] which may explain at least in part the cause of heart failure.

AUSTRALIAN PARALYSIS TICK

This tick (*Ixodes holocyclus*) injects a toxin that causes flaccid paralysis after some 3–5 days of feeding on humans. The onset of illness resembles that of Guillain–Barré syndrome. Prompt, careful and entire removal of tick(s) is necessary, followed by a period of observation to ensure that late onset paralysis does not occur. A tick antitoxin is available.

BEES, WASPS AND ANTS

Anaphylactic reactions to bee and wasp stings cause approximately the same number of deaths in Australia each year as does snake bite (i.e an average of 2.3 per annum[17]). The common European Honey Bee (*Apis mellifera*) is largely responsible. Jumper and Bull Ants (*Myrmecia* spp) may also cause anaphylaxis. Persons who develop reactions to bites should seek immunotherapy and carry injectable epinephrine.

BLUE-RINGED OCTOPUSES

Several species of *Hapalochlaena* inhabit the Australian coastline. When handled, these octopuses bite and inject tetrodotoxin – a neurotoxin found in many different species of marine animals. It causes flaccid paralysis. Approximately a dozen deaths are recorded. The required treatment is mechanical ventilation until spontaneous recovery occurs.

STINGING FISH

Numerous marine and fresh-water fish carry venom in glands attached to stinging spines. The most dangerous is the Stonefish (*Synanceia* spp.). When trodden upon, venom is injected. The immediate effect is extreme pain. Several deaths have been recorded, presumedly due to the known depressive effects of the toxins on cardiovascular and neuromuscular function, and myotoxicity. An antivenom is available. Local or regional nerve blockade may be required for pain relief. Other stinging fish, such as the freshwater Bullrout (*Notesthes robusta*) also cause excruciating pain when their spines are contacted. Immersion of the affected limb in warm-to-hot water provides pain relief.

VENOMOUS CONE SHELLS

From within their beautiful shells, many gastropod molluscs rapidly eject a venom-laden harpoon to almost instantaneously immobilize and kill prey. The numerous conotoxins, short proteins, stimulate or block neuronal and neuromuscular receptors, causing rapid death. A handful of human deaths have been recorded, when shells have been carelessly or unwittingly handled. There is no antivenom. Mechanical ventilation would be required until spontaneous recovery occurs.

REFERENCES

1 Sutherland SK, Tibballs J. *Australian Animal Toxins.* Melbourne: Oxford University Press; 2001.
2 Pearn JH, Covacevich J, Charles N, Richardson P. Snakebite in herpetologists. *Med J Aust* 1994, **161**: 706–8.
3 Tibballs J, Sutherland S, Kerr S. Studies on Australian snake venoms. Part I: the haemodynamic effects of Brown Snake (*Pseudonaja*) species in the dog. *Anaesth Intens Care* 1989, **17**: 466–9.
4 Tibballs J. The cardiovascular, coagulation and haematological effects of Tiger Snake (*Notechis scutatus*) venom. *Anaesth Intens Care* 1998, **26**: 529–35.
5 Sutherland SK, Coulter AR, Harris RD. Rationalization of first-aid measures for elapid snakebite. *Lancet* 1979, **1**: 183–6.
6 Howarth DM, Southee AE, Whyte IM. Lymphatic flow rates and first-aid in simulated peripheral snake or spider envenomation. *Med J Aust* 1994, **161**: 695–700.
7 Oakley J. Managing death adder bite with prolonged pressure bandaging. *6th Asia-Pacific Congress on Animal, Plant and Microbial Toxins and 11th Annual Scientific Meeting of the Australasian College of Tropical Medicine*, 8–12 July 2002. Cairns, Australia: pp. 29.
8 Premawardhena AP, de Silva CE, Fonseka M, *et al.* Low dose subcutaneous adrenaline to prevent acute adverse reactions to antivenom serum in people bitten by snakes: randomised, placebo controlled trial. *BMJ* 1999, **318**: 1041–3.
9 Pumphrey RS. Lessons for management of anaphylaxis from a study of fatal reactions. *Clin Exp Allergy* 2000, **30**: 1144–50.
10 Fan HW, Marcopito LF, Cardoso JL, *et al.* A Sequential randomised and double blind trial of promethazine prophylaxis against early anaphylactic reactions to antivenom for *Bothrops* snake bites. *BMJ* 1999, **318**: 1451–3.
11 Tibballs J, Sutherland SK. The efficacy of heparin in the treatment of Common Brown Snake (*Pseudonaja textilis*) envenomation. *Anaesth Intens Care* 1992, **20**: 33–7.
12 Williamson JA, Fenner PJ, Burnett JW, Rifkin JF. *Venomous and Poisonous Marine Animals.* Sydney: University of New South Wales Press; 1996.
13 Tibballs J, Williams D, Sutherland SK. The effects of antivenom and verapamil on the haemodynamic actions of *Chironex fleckeri* (Box jellyfish) venom. *Anaesth Intens Care* 1998, **26**: 40–5.
14 Little, M, Mulcahy RF. A year's experience of Irukandji envenomation in far north Queensland. *Med J Aust* 1998, **169**: 638–41.
15 Little M, Mulcahy RF, Wenck DJ. Life-threatening cardiac failure in a healthy young female with Irukandji syndrome. *Anaesth Intens Care* 2001, **29**: 178–80.
16 Tibballs J, Hawdon G, Winkel KD, *et al.* The in vivo cardiovascular effects of Irukandji (*Carukia barnesi*) venom. *XIIIth World Congress of the International Society of Toxinology.* 18–22nd September, Paris, 2000: P276.
17 Levick NR, Schmidt JO, Harrison J, *et al.* Review of bee and wasp sting injuries in Australia and the USA. In: Austin AD, Dowton M (eds) *Hymenoptera,* Melbourne: CSIRO Publishing; 2000.

75

Blast injury and gunshot wounds: pathophysiology and principles of management

S J Brett

Conflict, violent crime and terrorism continue to be a feature of twenty-first century life. Since the break-up of the Warsaw Pact, the Soviet Union and numerous recent conflicts, sophisticated military hardware is easily available to *ad hoc* militias, criminals and terrorist groups at modest cost. In addition, the detritus of conflict injures large numbers of innocent people on a daily basis. Thus all physicians with responsibility for the injured must have an appreciation of the pathology of injury due to explosive devices and gunshot wounds.

BLAST INJURY

PHYSICS OF EXPLOSIONS

An explosion is the almost instantaneous release of stored energy.[1] The energy may come from, for example, pressurized gas, a nuclear reaction or stored chemical energy. Thus specific 'explosives' are not necessarily required. Explosives are materials that contain stored chemical energy that may be released rapidly. High performance explosives release this energy by means of a chemical reaction which propagates through the explosive material faster than the speed of sound; thus the detonation velocity is of the order of 8 km/s compared with the speed of sound in air, 0.33 km/s.[1] This produces a supersonic shock front (blast wave) with a rapidly expanding cloud of gaseous reaction products, which cause damage to structures and people in the vicinity. In effect, there is an extremely rapid increase in atmospheric pressure, 'positive overpressure', the duration of which is dependent on the magnitude of the explosive charge. This dies away exponentially and is followed by a negative pressure phase produced by gases forced away from the centre of the blast leaving a vacuum. Blast winds may subsequently move paradoxically towards the explosion as pressures equalize.

The blast wave carries with it energized environmental debris and device fragments. These are propelled substantial distances. In air, the blast wave intensity dies away rapidly with distance (with an inverse cube relationship) while debris travels further with the capacity to damage and injure at much greater distances. This is reversed in an underwater blast. Water propagates the blast wave effectively but 'drag' reduces the range of debris and device fragments.

In addition to the kinetic energy released, heat and light energy are also produced and can contribute to damage and injury. For a deliberate explosion, such as that produced by a military or terrorist device, the precise characteristics depend upon a number of factors including the size and nature of the container, the environment, and the dispositions of buildings and rooms.

CLASSIFICATION OF BLAST INJURY

By convention, blast injuries are classified according to which feature of the explosion was involved in wound generation.[2,3] They can be outlined as follows.

PRIMARY INJURY

Primary injury caused by interaction of the blast wave and the body, particularly injuring the lungs, abdominal contents, the ears and contributing to traumatic amputation.

SECONDARY INJURY

Secondary injury produced by energized debris and weapon fragments – predominantly penetrating and soft tissue injuries.

TERTIARY INJURY

Tertiary injury caused by displacement of the victim by the mass movement of air – 'blast winds'; this group includes long bone fractures and head injury.

QUATERNARY INJURY

This is a miscellaneous group including crush injury from falling masonry (leading to renal failure) and flash burns.

Table 75.1 Types of explosive devices

Conventional munitions: e.g. grenades, aerial bombs, mortar bombs, rockets	All types of blast injury may occur, but penetrating injuries from multiple fragments predominate. Primary fragments are derived from the munition; preformed within the shell or from the casing when the munition explodes. Other materials (building debris, vehicle components) energized by the blast form secondary fragments.
Terrorist devices: typically contain a few kilograms of explosive	Although the reported incidence of primary blast injuries varies from 1%–76%, serious primary blast injury is uncommon and secondary and tertiary injuries predominate. Mortality is low (5%) unless the device is large, explodes in a confined space or there is structural collapse. Less than 50% of those presenting to hospital will require admission.
Antipersonnel landmines: common in developing countries. Indiscriminate in action	Patterns of injury: (a) Traumatic amputation of foot or leg, due to standing on a buried 'point detonating' mine. Mine fragments, grass, soil, parts of shoe and foot are blown upwards with substantial proximal tissue damage and contamination. (b) More random distribution of penetrating injuries caused by fragment mine triggered near victim by a trip-wire. (c) Severe upper limb and facial injuries due to handling of a mine.
Enhanced-blast munitions: e.g. fuel-air explosives	Designed to injure by primary blast effect rather than by fragmentation. Reportedly used by Soviet and American forces in Afghanistan.

EXPLOSIVE DEVICES

Conventional military anti-personnel devices (Table 75.1) rely on fragment generation to produce 'secondary' injuries. The device's casing is designed to produce fragments, and may contain preformed fragments or notched wire to increase the fragment load. An 81 mm mortar round contains a small quantity (~1 kg) of high explosive; the blast itself would only be lethal within 2–3 m, but the fragment cloud generated will seriously injure or kill within a radius of around 85 m. Improvised explosive devices (IED) built by terrorists contain material (bolts, nails etc.) to increase secondary injury. Larger devices, such as air-delivered free fall bombs, missiles or artillery shells contain sufficient explosive to produce secondary injury by throwing bricks, masonry debris, and glass substantial distances. In addition, the blast may collapse physical structures such as walls and buildings.

Anti-personnel mines are broadly of two types: buried mines, which detonate and disrupt the foot and lower leg, blasting debris from the ground, footwear and device fragments up fascial planes towards the knee; and above ground mines, which are initiated by trip- or command-wires or electronic sensors and produce a preformed fragment load and thus secondary injury, with a high incidence of ocular damage.

PRIMARY BLAST INJURY

A blast wave passing through an individual behaves like an acoustic wave, giving up energy at interfaces between materials of differing acoustic quality, causing damage. Air-containing organs – the lungs, the gut and the ears, are particularly vulnerable.[4,5] Massive pressure pulses, causing body wall distortion, can tear solid organs from their vascular supplies. Recent work suggests that traumatic amputation caused by shock wave induced stress concentrations fracture the long bones which are subsequently removed by flailing and blast wind effects.[6] This explains why amputations are generally not through joints.[7]

Primary blast injury (PBI) is unusual among survivors,[8] but very common in those killed immediately.[9] The blast wave dies away rapidly with distance, but device fragments and energized debris travel and injure at greater distances. If a casualty is close enough to sustain a primary injury, there will be overwhelming secondary and tertiary damage. The majority of survivors from an explosion will have sustained secondary or tertiary injuries.[8] Military and terrorist devices are specifically designed to maximize casualties by the use of fragments. Primary injury does sometimes occur and an understanding of mechanisms is useful in guiding management of such casualties. Survivors presenting with signs of one PBI (e.g. visceral perforation) must be assumed to have damage to other vulnerable regions and investigated accordingly. Casualties as close to the blast as other overwhelmingly injured fatalities must be investigated carefully for PBI. The absence of eardrum damage does not exclude PBI, as eardrum rupture depends on a number of factors, including the orientation of the head to the blast.

THE LUNG

Immediate effects of severe blast exposure may include apnoea and bradycardia.[5] The blast wave produces disruption of the alveolar-capillary barrier leading to intra-alveolar haemorrhage that may be massive. This occurs in regions of the chest subjected most directly to the incident blast wave (not by a pressure pulse travelling down the trachea). The wave may 'echo' around the pleural cavity, exhibiting interference effects and injuring other regions at points of stress wave concentration. Such regions include the juxta-mediastinal tissue and the diaphragmatic recesses. Pulmonary contusions are produced, with associated shunt and reduction in compliance. The surface of the lung may evolve bullae, which are mechanically weak and may rupture producing pneumothoraces. These may present early or late, perhaps triggered by mechanical ventilation. Damage to hilar structures may be produced by severe and long duration over-pressures; pulmonary artery and vein injuries are usually rapidly fatal. A variety of clinical features have been described and these are summarized in Table 75.2. Radiological features are outlined in Table 75.3.

Investigations obtained may depend on availability and prioritization if the casualty burden is high. Chest X-ray (CXR), blood gas analysis and pulse oximetry monitoring are useful. CXR will provide data concerning pneumothorax, pneumomediastinum, subcutaneous and interstitial emphysema and sub-diaphragmatic air from visceral perforation. The CXR is a poor modality for quantifying extent of contusion, for which computed tomography (CT) is better.[10,11] CT may be unavailable or overwhelmed with demand. In the majority of cases, CT will not provide management altering data. The priority is close clinical observation of conventional parameters to identify the drift toward respiratory failure.

The management of significant PBI is similar to that of any other pulmonary contusion with a number of corollaries from the pathology. PBI renders the lungs prone to development of pneumothorax, and importantly, significant air emboli may be created.[12] Historically CPAP and mechanical ventilation were regarded as so hazardous at to be treatments of last resort. This was due to fear of creating or exacerbating air embolism. Modern strategies based around modest gas exchange targets, with limited volume excursion and pressure change, has ameliorated these concerns.[13] A variety of non-conventional strategies including hyperbaric chambers, inhaled NO, high frequency jet ventilation and ECMO have been tried with varying success. The prognosis for pulmonary function in survivors is generally excellent.[14]

THE ABDOMEN

The hollow viscera are at risk of primary blast injury (particularly in cases of immersion blast). Isolated PBI to

Table 75.2   Clinical features of blast lung

Symptoms	Dyspnoea
	Cough – dry to productive with frothy sputum. Haemoptysis
	Chest pain or discomfort (typically retrosternal)
Signs	Cyanosis
	Torrential pulmonary haemorrhage
	Tachypnoea
	Reduced breath sounds, dullness to percussion
	Coarse crepitations, rhonchi
	Features of pneumothorax or haemopneumothorax. Subcutaneous emphysema
	Retrosternal crunch (pneumomediastinum)
	Retinal artery air emboli

Table 75.3   Radiological evidence of blast lung

Diffuse pulmonary opacities 'infiltrates'. (Typically these develop within a few hours, become maximal at 24–48 h and resolve over 7 days)
Pneumothorax/haemopneumothorax
Interstitial (peribronchial) emphysema
Subcutaneous emphysema
Pneumomediastinum
Pneumoperitoneum (usually secondary to perforation of an abdominal viscus, but tension pneumoperitoneum has been ascribed to blast lung)

the gut is unusual in air-blast, and generally occurs in the presence of severe secondary and tertiary injuries. At high overpressures, immediate rupture of the gut wall occurs with bleeding and spillage of intraluminal contents into the peritoneal cavity. More commonly and at lower overpressures, haemorrhage develops within the intestinal wall. These haemorrhages range in size from small petechiae to confluent haematomas. These lesions are characterized by varying degrees of vascular damage and some will progress to necrosis of the gut wall and late perforation.[15]

With large numbers of casualties, surgical triage is difficult. In a pig model[16] bowel contusions >15 mm diameter and colonic contusions >20 mm diameter were at higher risk and warranted resection; smaller lesions could be treated conservatively. Circumferential lesions and those on the antimesenteric border were also associated with greater evidence of microvascular damage and perforation risk. Subcapsular haematomas, lacerations of solid organs, testicular rupture and retroperitoneal haematomas have all been described. These result from high blast loads and are likely to present early with abdominal signs and cardiovascular instability. In some patients, the indications for exploratory laparotomy are obvious; in others primary blast injury to the abdomen represents a diagnostic challenge, since it may be clinically silent until complications are advanced.

THE EARS

Damage to the ears[17] includes sensorineural deafness, tympanic membrane rupture, injury to the ossicles and implantation cholesteatoma. These injuries are clearly not of major importance in the immediate management of the critically injured. Acute deafness may be very distressing to the victim, and impair assessment of conscious level. It may prevent gaining an accurate history of the circumstances of the blast, which might assist in assessing risk of PBI. The absence of PBI to the ear has a poor negative predictive value for PBI to the lungs and gut.

TRAUMATIC AMPUTATION

Common in mine injury, traumatic amputation is unusual in blast survivors. It is common in those who are killed immediately or die quickly.[9] The amputations do not generally occur through joints.[6] That situation is seen in ejecting fast jet pilots exposed to high wind speeds (1100 km/h). The common sites are the upper third of the tibia, and the upper or lower third of the femur. Computer modelling and evidence from isolated animal limb studies[7] demonstrate that the blast wave generates stress concentrations at particular points in long bones causing fractures before displacement occurs. Subsequently, blast wind induced displacement removes the limb. The implication of this is that any survivors with traumatic amputation must be regarded as at very high risk for PBI to the lungs and gut even if not manifested immediately.

The surgical strategy is initially one of extensive debridement leaving only viable tissue. The resulting wound is loosely packed and allowed to drain, with planned secondary inspection and soft tissue closure after a few days.[18] Bone stock is preserved with the intention that a myoplastic stump can be organized at a later date, but the surgeon must acknowledge that this *may* be the final stump.[19] The vascular damage which occurs under these circumstances is severe, and heroic efforts to revascularize partially amputated limbs may be counter productive; any venous anastomosis attempted is likely to be precarious, and may jeopardize survival due to prolonged shock.

SPECIAL CIRCUMSTANCES

Under certain circumstances a relatively high incidence of PBI may be encountered, for example if casualties are protected from fatal secondary injury by personal body armour or environmental structures. Alternatively, an explosion in a confining space may produce exacerbation of the overpressure experienced by an individual, by summation of incident blast energy and that reflected from rigid surfaces. Thus casualties at a distance from the explosion normally considered safe (for primary effects) for a 'free field' blast, might experience an enhanced blast effect and be at risk for PBI. This has been well described for terrorist bombs in buses.[20,21]

Conventional military devices exert their anti-personnel effects by secondary and tertiary action. Fuel-air weapons function by delivering a cloud of fuel vapour over or around a target which, once optimally mixed with air, is then detonated. These devices have a very low integral fragment load, but have an enhanced blast effect experienced throughout the fuel cloud that may cover a wide area; the thermal output is also substantial. Originally designed to assist in mine clearance, these weapons are ideal for attacking enemy troops in trenches or built up areas.[22,23] The development of these weapons was initially difficult but most of the technical problems have been overcome, and new generations have appeared. Such devices are reported to have been deployed in recent conflicts (Afghanistan, Chechnya), and are available in air-delivered, artillery, tank-mounted and shoulder-launched variants. Now fairly widely available, this class of enhanced blast effect weapon is likely to become an increasing threat. Individuals caught in the centre of the vapour cloud are unlikely to survive, but people at the margins can be predicted to have a high incidence of PBI, significant burns and injuries associated with collapse of buildings.

SECONDARY BLAST INJURY

Secondary injury can be due either to the effects of energized environmental debris or to material integral to the explosive device itself. Environmental debris may include glass fragments, or material from any vehicle used to deliver the device. Clearly a careful exposure and physical and radiological examination is required; bearing in mind that material penetrating one body cavity may travel some distance and produce damage in another. In the terrorist context material removed, and excised and amputated tissue must be retained for forensic examination.

Surgical strategy hinges around the identification and removal of large pieces of foreign material, or those associated with, or likely to cause neurovascular compromise.[24] Systematic removal of all minute fragments may cause more tissue destruction than might otherwise have occurred.[25,26]

Modern anti-personnel munitions (grenades, mortar rounds) are designed to incapacitate or kill by delivering high energy small fragments into the target. Such weapons have caused the majority of wounds to military personnel in recent conflicts.[27] Pre-formed fragments often have a mass of 0.1–0.2 g and an initial velocity of ~1500 m/s. Because of irregular shape

Table 75.4 Factors to be considered in the management of small fragment wounds

Risk factors for infection[29]	Criteria where non-operative management may be appropriate[25,30,31]
Prolonged time between wounding and presentation for treatment	Entry/exit wound <1 cm
	No evidence of permanent cavitation within the wound
Lack of prior wound cleansing	No neuro-vascular compromise
Wound size >1 cm	No compartment syndrome
Failure to comply with wound care instructions	Stable fracture pattern
Low to medium energy transfer fractures	No signs of infection
	Have been treated early with dressings and antibiotics

velocity falls rapidly, but penetration can still occur at substantial distances. Soldiers in field conditions wear clothes contaminated with soil (and *Clostridia* spp.), and the skin is covered with faecal organisms and pyogenic *Streptococci* and *Staphylococci* spp.[28] High energy fragments produce temporary cavities (see below) with negative intra-cavity pressure. Small fragments shred clothing and contaminated clothing fibres are driven or drawn in to the wound. Wounds characterized by cavitation will have contamination distributed throughout a greater volume of tissue than might have been anticipated, or exhibited by lower energy wounds. The benefit of the early administration of antibiotics to prevent or retard the development of infection is well established.

Many of these wounds are to the limbs and these are small and multiple. The orthodox operative doctrine was derived from experiences in World War I, where large fragments produced the majority of wounds. Newer weapons producing smaller wounds have caused a re-examination of this philosophy; selected wounds may be managed conservatively with cleansing, closed fracture management, antibiotics and observation, and criteria (Table 75.4) have been published.[29–31]

High-energy fragments can produce fractures, and can penetrate the body wall and injure the lungs or visceral structures. As the body wall is penetrated, the fragment energy is significantly reduced so that in survivors reaching hospital intra-cavity damage will tend to be localized.[24] Thus, mesenteric and gut perforations tend to be small and discrete. Small bowel wounds can generally be repaired primarily, but the management of large bowel wounds remains contro-versial. There is an increasing enthusiasm for primary resection and repair with or without proximal diversion.[32] The pursuit of small fragments, which have transited the colon in to the retroperitoneal tissues, may be counterproductive.[33]

TERTIARY BLAST INJURY

Head injuries, long bone, spinal and pelvic fractures and soft tissue injuries can all be caused by casualties being displaced by the blast winds. Furthermore limb flailing contributes to the pathogenesis of traumatic amputation. The management of such injuries follows conventional trauma doctrines.

QUATERNARY BLAST INJURY

This classification includes injuries not otherwise classified and includes superficial flash burns and crush injury from collapsing buildings.

MINES

It has been estimated that around 100 million anti-personnel mines are currently in the ground world-wide and a further 250 million are stockpiled. A mine explodes every 20 min, injuring or killing approximately 26 000 people per year, most commonly children and agricultural workers. Many of these people die before reaching medical assistance[34] (Table 75.5).

An anti-personnel mine is designed to incapacitate and maim rather than to kill, an exception being trip-

Table 75.5 Classification of anti-personnel mine injury[34]

	Activation	Injury pattern
Pattern 1	Mine stepped on	Severe lower limb, perineal and genital injuries
Pattern 2	Device explodes near victim: activated by other victim or an above ground mine	Less severe lower extremity injuries; injuries to head chest and abdomen common
Pattern 3	Handling injury	Severe facial and upper limb injury

or command-wire detonated above-ground mines (e.g. 'Claymore' mines). A small quantity of explosive is detonated by pressure and device fragments, soil, and footwear remnants are forced upwards. The shock wave is concentrated in the tibia, which fractures; the subsequent expansion of explosive products opens up tissue plains; causes substantial damage, contamination and often completes the traumatic amputation. Limbs not amputated at first instance often require surgical amputation due to overwhelming soft tissue damage. Damage to the contralateral limb is likely to be less severe, but meticulous attention must be paid to avoid complications leading to a second amputation. In addition, up to 5% of casualties suffer ocular injuries, and this figure is higher for handling injuries and above ground mines. Injuries to the perineum, the external genitalia and the rectum are all common. Many patients will require laparotomy for penetrating trauma.[34]

The wounds are heavily contaminated with soil organisms. The surgical strategy consists of:

- initial débridement – exposing and exploring all tissue plains
- removing devitalized tissue and foreign material
- subsequent delayed closure.

Primary closure of wounds,[35] and heroic limb salvage for limited posterior foot injuries[36] have been reported. Complication rates are likely to be high under all but the most ideal circumstances and the expertise and facilities required to attempt this approach safely are not available to the vast majority of those injured.

GUNSHOT WOUNDS

Small arms ammunition can be divided broadly into two types: rifle rounds, which are supersonic; and subsonic handgun or sub-machine gun rounds. This leads to a superficially attractive classification of gunshot wounds (GSW) into high or low velocity wounds. This has now been superseded with the realization that *energy transfer* is the important factor. The kinetic energy available is governed by the equation:

$$\text{Kinetic energy} = \tfrac{1}{2} \times \text{mass} \times \text{velocity}^2$$

High velocity rounds have inherently more energy available. The amount of energy transferred is governed by a variety of factors including; the resistance of the tissues penetrated, direct impact on to bone, and whether the round penetrated point first or was unstable in flight. Thus low velocity wounds caused by hand guns (or even shotguns) at close range may cause massive tissue destruction, and occasionally high velocity rounds may pass directly through a casualty causing very little damage.

PATHOLOGY AND MANAGEMENT OF GUNSHOT WOUNDS

The phenomenon of *temporary cavitation* is generally a feature of high velocity rounds.[37] The bullet penetrating a casualty is preceded by a shock wave which forces tissue away from its path producing a temporary cavity the diameter of which is many times that of the projectile itself (Figure 75.1). The cavity is instantly under negative pressure and thus draws environmental debris, clothing fragments and resident skin organisms in to the casualty, via the entry wound. In addition, the tissue forming the walls and margins of the cavity is damaged and devitalized, and forms a substrate for infection with the inoculating organisms. Shock wave and cavitation effects may be responsible for fractures not directly involved with the wound track.[38] Skeletal muscle is fairly elastic and tolerates cavitation reasonably well, whereas organs constrained by inelastic capsules or bony structures, such as the liver and brain, fair very badly.

Rounds may yaw and tumble prior to or after impact, and thus travel on an unpredictable path through the victim; this is a particular feature of bullets from high velocity smaller calibre rifles, known as assault rifles. Such injuries commonly involve more than one body cavity. Thus extensive radiological studies must be performed prior to surgical exploration if at all possible. Occasionally minute fragments of radio-opaque bullet debris may mark the path of the wound track.[39] The presence or absence and size of any exit wound are an imperfect guide to the magnitude of wound trauma.[37] The behaviour of bullets is unpredictable and attempting to predict this from knowledge of the weapon and firing distance may produce a misleading treatment plan.

The severity of fractures produced by direct impact on bone is governed largely be energy transfer. High-energy weapons such as military and hunting rifles produce fractures with a high degree of comminution, whereas the majority of ballistic fractures due to handguns are minimally fragmented.[40–42]

Gunshot wounds become infected quickly due to the effects outlined above. Military surgical doctrine is for extensive wide local excision and delayed primary closure of limb wounds (Figure 75.2). This strategy evolved from conflicts during which time of wounding to time of surgery intervals were long, and contamination with coliforms and soil organisms was likely. In civilian practice the wounding to treatment interval is usually short and a less mutilating surgical strategy can sometimes be adopted. Under certain circumstances, upper limb wounds can be treated on an outpatient basis, with suitable wound cleansing, immobilization and perhaps an antibiotic prescription.[30,43]

The majority of casualties surviving to hospital admission will require surgical exploration. The degree of debridement required will be governed by the operative findings and anatomy, rather than assumptions derived from knowledge of the weapon.

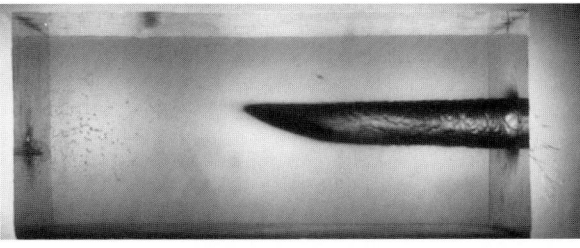

(a)

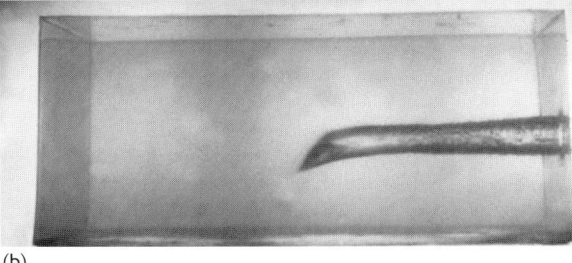

(b)

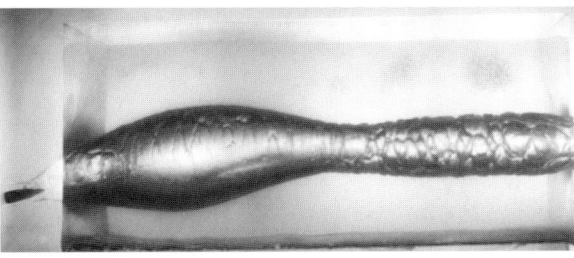

(c)

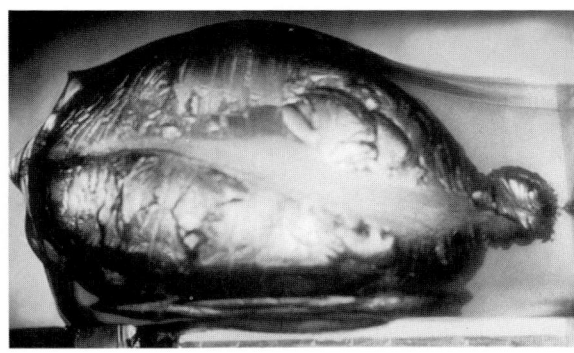

(d)

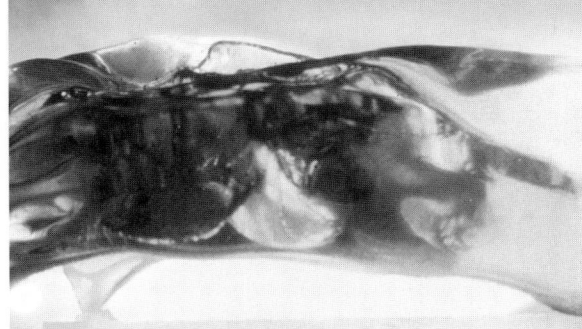

(e)

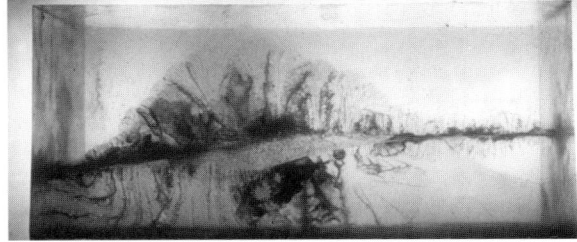

(f)

Fig. 75.1 High speed camera capturing (a) a rifle round penetrating a block of ballistic gelatin; the round is fired through simulated clothing. (b) The round yaws and tumbles shortly after penetration, (c) a temporary cavity forms, (d) oscillates and (e) collapses. (f) Cloth fragments that have been drawn in to the 'wound' are clearly visible.

ANTIBIOTIC CONSIDERATIONS

The combination of a wound, devitalized tissue and foreign material is ideal for the development of infection. Whether or not an infection develops depends on the quantity of bacteria and foreign material inoculated, and the time interval during which the bacteria can divide prior to wound irrigation, surgery or antibiotic administration.[44,45] Antibiotics can lengthen the safe period prior to establishment of infection if surgery is to be delayed.[46] The mainstay of treatment is surgery, but during conflict this may not be available immediately and thus early dressing and antibiotics have an important role. *Clostridia* spp. and beta-haemolytic *Streptococci* have caused the majority of infective complications of war wounds and thus simple benzyl penicillin has been the most valuable first line prophylactic and therapeutic agent; there is still strong evidence to support its continued use.[28,46] Ballistic fractures carry a significant risk of Staphylococcal osteomyelitis and require flucloxacillin. In civilian circumstances the bacterial inoculum is orders of magnitude less. Thus for simple limb gunshot wounds, if there is minimal inoculated material and the wound is attended to early, a far weaker argument for prophylactic use exists.

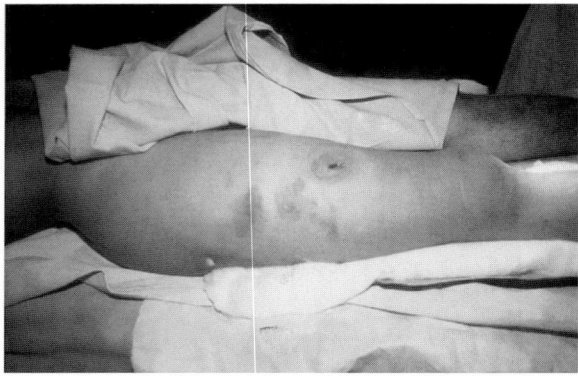

(a)

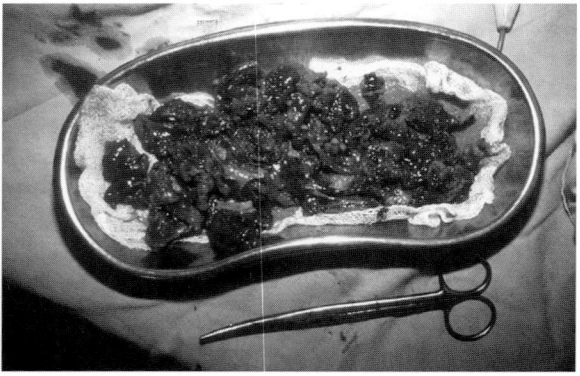

(c)

Fig. 75.2 (a) Rifle wound of the thigh with small entrance wound, (b) substantial damage to muscle visible at exploration, and (c) typical mass of devitalized, contaminated tissues removed. Both Figures 75.1 and 2, courtesy of Professor Jim Ryan, Leonard Cheshire Professor of Conflict Recovery, University College, London.

REFERENCES

1 Cullis IG. Blast waves and how they interact with structures. *J R Army Med Corps* 2001; **147**: 16–26.

2 Zuckerman S. Experimental study of blast injury to the lungs. *Lancet* 1940; **2**: 219–24.

3 Krohn PL, Whitteridge D, Zuckerman S. Physiological effects of blast. *Lancet* 1942; **1**: 252–8.

4 Horrocks CL. Blast injuries: biophysics, pathophysiology and management principles. *J R Army Med Corps* 2001; **147**: 28–40.

5 Guy RJ, Kirkman E, Watkins PE, Cooper GJ. Physiologic responses to primary blast. *J Trauma* 1998; **45**: 983–7.

6 Hull JB, Cooper GJ. Pattern and mechanism of traumatic amputation by explosive blast. *J Trauma* 1996; **40**: S198–S205.

7 Hull JB, Bowyer GW, Cooper GJ, Crane J. Pattern of injury in those dying from traumatic amputation caused by bomb blast. *Br J Surg* 1994; **81**: 1132–5.

8 Brismar B, Bergenwald L. The terrorist bomb explosion in Bologna, Italy, 1980: an analysis of the effects and injuries sustained. *J Trauma* 1982; **22**: 216–20.

9 Mellor SG, Cooper GJ. Analysis of 828 servicemen killed or injured by explosion in Northern Ireland 1970–84: the Hostile Action Casualty System. *Br J Surg* 1989; **76**: 1006–10.

10 Schild HH, Strunk H, Weber W, *et al.* Pulmonary contusion: CT vs plain radiograms. *J Comput Assist Tomogr* 1989; **13**: 417–20.

11 Wagner RB, Jamieson PM Pulmonary contusion. Evaluation and classification by computed tomography. *Surg Clin North Am* 1989; **69**: 31–40.

12 Keren A, Stessman J, Tzivoni D. Acute myocardial infarction caused by blast injury of the chest. *Br Heart J* 1981; **46**: 455–7.

13 Sorkine P, Szold O, Kluger Y, *et al.* Permissive hypercapnia ventilation in patients with severe pulmonary blast trauma. *J Trauma* 1998; **45**: 35–8.

14 Hirshberg B, Oppenheim-Eden A, Pizov R, *et al.* Recovery from blast lung injury: one-year follow-up. *Chest* 1999; **116**: 1683–8.

15 Cripps NPJ, Cooper GJ. Intestinal injury mechanisms after blunt abdominal impact. *Ann R Coll Surg Engl* 1997; **79**: 115–20.

16 Cripps NPJ, Cooper GJ. Risk of late perforation in intestinal contusions caused by explosive blast. *Br J Surg* 1997; **84**: 1298–303.

17 Kerr AG. Blast injury to the ear: a review. *Rev Environ Health* 1987; 7: 65–79.

18 Covey DC, Lurate RB, Hatton CT. Field hospital treatment of blast wounds of the musculoskeletal system during the Yugoslav civil war. *J Orthop Trauma* 2000; **14**: 278–86.

19 Coupland RM. Amputation for antipersonnel mine injuries of the leg: preservation of the tibial stump using a medial gastrocnemius myoplasty. *Ann R Coll Surg Engl* 1989; **71**: 405–8.

20 Katz E, Ofek B, Adler J, *et al.* Primary blast injury after a bomb explosion in a civilian bus. *Ann Surg* 1989; **209**: 484–8.

21 Pizov R, Oppenheim-Eden A, Matot I, *et al.* Blast lung injury from an explosion on a civilian bus. *Chest* 1999; **115**: 165–72.

22 Demonstration of fuel–air weapon, available at: http://www.nawcwpns.navy.mil/clmf/faeseq.html

23 Grau L, Smith T. A 'Crushing' Victory: Fuel-air explosives and Grozny 2000, available at: http://call.army.mil/fmso/fmsopubs/issues/fuelair/fuelair.htm

24 Hill PF, Edwards DP, Bowyer GW. Small fragment wounds: biophysics, pathophysiology and principles of management. *JR Army Med Corps* 2001; **147**: 41–51.

25 Coupland RM. Hand grenade injuries among civilians. *JAMA* 1993; **270**: 624–6.

26 Bowyer GW. Management of small fragment wounds: experience from the Afghan border. *J Trauma* 1996; **40**: S170–2.

27 Ryan JM, Cooper GJ, Haywood IR, Milner SM. Field surgery on a future conventional battlefield: strategy and wound management. *Ann R Coll Surg Engl* 1991; **73**: 13–20.

28 Mellor SG, Easmon CSF, Sanford JP. Wound contamination and antibiotics. In: Ryan JM, Rich NM, Dale RF, Morgans BT, Cooper GJ (eds) *Ballistic Trauma*. London: Edward Arnold; **1997**: pp. 61–71.

29 Ordog GJ, Sheppard GF, Wasserberger JS, *et al.* Infection in minor gunshot wounds. *J Trauma* 1993; **34**: 358–65.

30 Ordog GJ, Wasserberger J, Balasubramanium S, Shoemaker W. Civilian gunshot wounds – outpatient management. *J Trauma* 1994; **36**: 106–11.

31 Bowyer GW. Management of small fragment wounds in modern warfare: a return to Hunterian principles? *Ann R Coll Surg Engl* 1997; **79**: 175–82.

32 Gonzalez RP, Falimirski ME, Holevar MR. Further evaluation of colostomy in penetrating colon injury. *Am Surg* 2000; **66**: 342–6; discussion: 346–7.

33 Edwards DP, Brown D, Watkins PE. Should colon-penetrating small missiles be removed? An experimental study of retrocolic wound tracks. *J Invest Surg* 1999; **12**: 25–9.

34 Coupland RM, Korver A. Injuries from antipersonnel mines: the experience of the International Committee of the Red Cross. *BMJ* 1991; **303**(6816): 1509–12.

35 Atesalp AS, Erler K, Gur E, Solakoglu C. Below-knee amputations as a result of land-mine injuries: comparison of primary closure versus delayed primary closure. *J Trauma* 1999; **47**: 724–7.

36 Selmanpakoglu N, Guler M, Sengezer M, *et al.* Reconstruction of foot defects due to mine explosion using muscle flaps. *Microsurgery* 1998; **18**: 182–8.

37 Cooper GJ, Ryan JM. Interaction of penetrating missiles with tissues: some common misapprehensions and implications for wound management. *Br J Surg* 1990; **77**: 606–10.

38 Hill PF, Parker SJ, Clasper JC, Watkins PE. Contaminated fractures of the tibia: The results of immediate intramedullary nailing in an animal model. *Proceedings of the British Orthopaedic Society*: 1998; Oct 5–6: 28.

39 Ragsdale BD, Sohn SS. Comparison of the terminal ballistics of full metal jacket 7.62 mm M80 (NATO) and 5.56 mm M193 military bullets: a study in ordnance gelatin. *J Forensic Sci* 1988; **33**: 676–96.

40 Ragsdale BD, Josselson A. Experimental gunshot fractures. *J Trauma* 1988; **28**: S109–15.

41 Rose SC, Fujisaki CK, Moore EE. Incomplete fractures associated with penetrating trauma: etiology, appearance, and natural history. *J Trauma* 1988; **28**: 106–9.

42 Robens W, Kusswetter W. Fracture typing to human bone by assault missile trauma. *Acta Chir Scand Suppl* 1982; **508**: 223–7.

43 Knapp TP, Patzakis MJ, Lee J, *et al.* Comparison of intravenous and oral antibiotic therapy in the treatment of fractures caused by low-velocity gunshots. A prospective, randomized study of infection rates. *J Bone Joint Surg Am* 1996; **78**: 1167–71.

44 Zimmerli W, Waldvogel FA, Vaudaux P, Nydegger UE. Pathogenesis of foreign body infection: description and characteristics of an animal model. *J Infect Dis* 1982; **146**: 487–97.

45 Robson MC, Duke WF, Krizek TJ. Rapid bacterial screening in the treatment of civilian wounds. *J Surg Res* 1973; **14**: 426–30.

46 Tikka S. The contamination of missile wounds with special reference to early antimicrobial therapy. *Acta Chir Scand Suppl* 1982; **508**: 281–7.

76

Biochemical terrorism

M Pelly and M Grover

Biochemical terrorism is defined as the use of biological or chemical agents to intimidate, incapacitate, or eradicate crops, livestock, civilian and military personnel.[1] It is well suited for attack by poorer nations against the rich, and is known as a poor man's atom bomb, or asymmetric method of attack. The large scale use of mustard and nerve gases in the Iran/Iraq war,[2] the dissemination of nerve gas sarin on the Tokyo underground,[3] and the discovery by UN inspectors in Iraq of SCUD missiles, rockets and aerial bombs primed with Botulinum and aflatoxins[4,5] have highlighted the need for planning.

CHARACTERISTICS OF BIOLOGICAL WEAPONS

Intended target effects are due to either infection with disease-causing micro-organisms and other replicative entities, including viruses, fungi, and prions, or due to the toxins they elaborate. Their effects depend on the ability to multiply in the person, animal, or plant attacked.[6] Sequelae depend on host factors (state of nutrition, immunocompetence) and environment (sanitation, temperature, humidity, water quality, population density).[7] (See table 76.1.)

Table 76.1   Potential weapons

Biological diseases	Chemical agents
Bacillus anthracis (anthrax)	Blisters/vesicants
Clostridium botulinum toxin (botulism)	Distilled mustard (HD)
Yersinia pestis (plague)	Lewsite (L)
Variola major (smallpox)	Mustard gas (H)
Francisella tularensis (tularaemia)	Nitrogen mustard (HN-2)
Viral haemorrhagic fever	Phosgene oxime (CX)
Coxiella burnetii (Q fever)	Blood
Brucella melitensis (brucellosis)	Arsine (SA)
Burkholderia mallei (glanders)	Cyanogen chloride (CK)
Ricin toxin (*Ricinus communis* – castor beans)	Hydrogen chloride
Staphylococcus enterotoxin B	Hydrogen cyanide (AC)
Niaph virus	Choking/pulmonary damage
Hantaviruses	Chlorine (CL)
	Nitrogen oxide (NO)
	Phosgene (CG)
	Nerve
	Sarin (GF)
	Soman (GD)
	Tabun (GA)
	VX
	Incapacitating
	LSD
	Cannabinoids

CLASSIFICATION

Although classification of biological weapons can be taxonomy based, for example, bacterial/viral/fungal; it is also useful to examine particular features such as:

- Infectivity: proportion of persons exposed to a given dose who become infected. Reflects capability of agent to enter, survive and replicate.
- Virulence: Ratio of the number of clinical cases to the number of infected hosts. May differ for strains of the same pathogen.
- Lethality: Ability of agent to cause death in an infected population.
- Pathogenicity: Ratio of number of clinical cases to the number of exposed persons, reflects capability of agent to cause disease.
- Incubation period: Time elapsing between exposure to the agent and first signs and symptoms of disease.
- Contagiousness: Number of secondary cases following exposure to a primary case in relation to the total number exposed.
- Stability: Ability of an agent to survive the environment (see table 76.2).

ROUTES OF DISSEMINATION

Inhalational exposure using sprays or aerosols. Optimal particle size for alveolar deposition is 0.6–5 microns. Larger than this are filtered by the nose and smaller are exhaled. This can be achieved using aerosol generators mounted on stationary objects or primed onto trucks, cars, boats, cruise missiles and planes. Environmental factors such as wind velocity, cloud cover, rainfall and humidity effect the efficiency of dissemination.[7]

Cutaneous: via wounds and mucous membranes.

Ingestion via food and water. Hand to mouth contact is a suitable vehicle, for example the Rajneeshee cult successfully disseminated Salmonella via salads, infecting 750 people in 1984.

Table 76.2 Criteria for a successful biological weapon[6]

Assailant
Has methods to treat own forces and population
Target population
Non-immune
Little or no access to immunization or treatment
Bioweapon
Consistently produces disease/death
Highly contagious or infective in low doses
Short and predictable incubation period
Difficult to identify in target population
Suitable for mass production, storage, and weaponization
Stable during dissemination
Low persistence after delivery

Table 76.3 Epidemiological evidence of an attack

Increasing incidence of disease in a normally healthy population
Higher incidence in subgroups, e.g. outdoor workers/shared ventilation
Increasing numbers seeking help with similar symptoms
Rise in endemic disease at an uncharacteristic time
Large numbers of rapidly fatal cases
Any patient with an uncommon disease which has bioterrorist potential
Large numbers of dying animals or fish, and unusual swarms of insects

DETECTION OF A BIOTERRORIST EVENT

This may be obvious if large numbers of military personnel become ill with similar syndromes, but any release is likely to be a covert event (see table 76.3). Furthermore, genetic engineering may result in altered pathogenicity, incubation periods, clinical effects and response to treatment or immunization.

SPECIFIC AGENTS

ANTHRAX

Anthrax[8] is an acute infectious zoonosis caused by *Bacillus anthracis*, a Gram positive spore forming bacillus. The infective dose is 8000–50 000 spores and routes of transmission include inhalation, ingestion and skin contact. Person to person transmission does not occur for the pulmonary form but secondary cutaneous lesions may occur after direct exposure to vesicle secretions.

CLINICAL FEATURES
Pulmonary Exposure[9,10]

- Incubation period is 2–60 days.
- Prodrome with flu-like symptoms.
- Interim improvement followed by respiratory failure, cardiovascular collapse. Widened mediastinum on CXR, due to haemorrhagic mediastinitis and lymphadenopathy.
- Gram positive bacilli on blood cultures.

Cutaneous Exposure

- Incubation period is 1–7 days.
- Mostly head, hands, and forearms.
- Pruritis, erythema, oedema, and maculopapular lesions progress to depressed black eschars within 2–6 days. Eschars fall off without scarring.

Gastrointestinal Exposure

- Incubation period is 1–7 days.
- Usually follows ingestion of infected meat.

- Presents with abdominal pain, cramps, haematemesis, and bloody diarrhoea followed by toxaemia and cardiovascular collapse.
- Gram positive blood cultures.

Post Exposure Management[11]

- Universal precautions for medical personnel.
- Warning to laboratory and coroners personnel regarding pathology specimens.
- Contact infection control team.
- Minimal handling of fomites.
- Thorough decontamination with soap and water.
- Disinfection of surfaces with 0.5% hypochlorite solution.

TREATMENT

Most strains used for bioterrorism will produce β-lactamases; and cephalosporinases were produced by the latest cases in the USA. Appropriate antibiotics include:

- Ciprofloxacin: adults 500 mg b.d. for 8 weeks; children 20–30 mg/kg per day.
- Doxycycline: adults 100 mg b.d. for 8 weeks; children 5 mg/kg per day.
- In children and pregnant patients amoxycillin 40 mg/kg per day (max 500 mg t.d.s.) is appropriate if the organism is penicillin sensitive.

Immunization with anthrax vaccine consists of 3 doses at 0, 2, 4 weeks. Prophylaxis of contacts should continue for 8 weeks and include immunization if exposure is confirmed. Preventative immunization using an inactivated cell free vaccine is available but presently only administered to military personnel.

BOTULISM

Botulism[5] is caused by *Clostridium botulinum*, an anaerobic Gram positive bacillus that produces a neurotoxin. Seven forms of the toxin have been identified from A to G, but human botulism is due mainly to strains A, B, E. The neurotoxin contains a zinc protease that acts at the presynaptic terminal of the neuromuscular junction, to prevent the fusion of vesicles of acetylcholine with the presynaptic membrane, therefore preventing release of acetylcholine and causing a flaccid paralysis. The LD_{50} for type A is 0.001 μg/kg. Routes of exposure are either inhalation or ingestion, and there is an incubation period of 12–36 h. Person to person transmission does not occur.

Clinical features include a responsive patient withno fever. There is a symmetric descending flaccid paralysis in a proximal to distal pattern without a sensory deficit. Cranial neuropathies (mainly bulbar) lead to diplopia, dysphagia, dysphonia, and dysarthria. Respiratory dysfunction may occur due to upper airway obstruction or muscle paralysis. The diagnosis is clinical, and confirmation is with the mouse bioassay in which mice are pre-treated with antitoxin and exposed to the patient's serum. A pentavalent toxoid vaccine is available for prevention, but routine immunization is not recommended.

TREATMENT

Patients should be monitored with frequent assessment of gag, cough reflexes, inspiratory force, and vital capacity. Mechanical ventilation may be protracted, and may be punctuated by nosocomial infections requiring antibiotics. Aminoglycosides and clindamycin are contraindicated because of their ability to increase blockade.[12] Administration of the trivalent (A, B, E) antitoxin should not be delayed while awaiting confirmation of the diagnosis. This horse serum has <9% hypersensitivity reactions, and <2% incidence of anaphylaxis. Skin testing is advisable.[13] A heptavalent antitoxin is under investigation. Passive administration of neutralizing antibody minimizes further damage.[14] Treatment of children, pregnant women and immunocompromised patients should be no different, all have received equine antitoxin without short-term sequelae.

Prophylaxis of contacts involves close observation and at the first sign of illness, treatment with antitoxin, neutralising antibody and administration of the pentavalent toxoid vaccine.

SMALLPOX

Smallpox[15] is an acute viral illness caused by variola virus (orthopoxvirus). The last documented case was in Somalia in 1977. It is transmitted from person to person via the airborne route, and its release into a non-immune population would be catastrophic.[16] The infective dose is 10–100 virions, with an incubation period of 7–17 days.

CLINICAL FEATURES[17]

There is a flu-like prodrome with malaise, fever, and headache. There is also a synchronously evolving maculopapular rash forming pustules over the head and extremities, and the mouth and pharynx may also be affected. Multi-organ failure commonly complicates smallpox. Diagnosis is clinical with confirmation by identification of brick-shaped virions from vesicular fluid using electron microscopy.

PREVENTION

Routine vaccination with vaccinia virus stopped in 1972. The immune status of vaccinated individuals is unclear, but if a single dose vaccine was administered it is assumed the subject is non immune. A preventative vaccination program is not currently recommended.

TREATMENT

Vaccination within 4 days of exposure.[18] However, complications include:

- Post-vaccinial encephalitis
- Vaccinia gangrenosa
- Eczema vaccinatum
- Generalized vaccinia
- Inadvertant innoculation.

Five groups are considered high risk for these complications. These are pregnancy, HIV infection, chemotherapy, eczema, and immune disorders.[19] In these cases, vaccinia immune globulin should be given simultaneously. Other treatments include:

- supportive care with isolation
- antibiotics for secondary bacterial infections
- cidofovir, a nucleoside DNA polymerase inhibitor, is under investigation but needs to be given i.v. and causes renal toxicity.[20]

PLAGUE

Plague[21] is an acute bacterial disease caused by the Gram negative *Yersinia pestis*, from the enterobacter species.[22] Although usually transmitted by fleas causing bubonic and septicaemic plague, a bioterrorist event is likely to be airborne resulting in pneumonic plague. The infective dose is <100 organisms, and has an incubation period of 2–3 days. It is unlikely that spread would be person to person.

Plague presents with fever, haemoptysis, chest pain, and dyspnoea. Gram negative rods are found in mucopurulent sputum, and on Wright's, Giemsa or Wayson stain appear as bipolar rods with a safety pin appearance. The diagnosis can be confirmed on blood culture, and with fluorescent antibody testing. There is radiographic evidence of bronchopneumonia, and multi-organ failure soon develops. Until 72 h of antibiotic therapy have been completed, plague is communicable.

A formalin-killed vaccine exists but is ineffective and unavailable. Post exposure immunization has no benefit.

TREATMENT[21]

Once the diagnosis is considered, isolation and universal precautions should be instituted. Historically streptomycin (1 g b.d. i.m.) reduced mortality to 5%, and gentamicin (5 mg/kg per day) has also been used successfully. Tetracycline and doxycycline (100 mg b.d.), have been used, but in Madagascar 13% of strains were resistant to doxycycline. Animal studies have demonstrated efficacy of fluoroquinolones including ciprofloxacin (400 mg b.d.), ofloxacin and levofloxacin. No human trials exist so far. Chloramphenicol (25 mg/kg q.i.d.) is recommended for plague meningitis.

CHARACTERISTICS OF CHEMICAL AGENTS

The North Atlantic Treaty Organization definition of a chemical agent is a 'chemical substance which is intended for use in military operations to kill, seriously injure, or incapacitate people because of its physiological effects'.[2] In addition to physiological effects these agents promote psychological warfare.[23]

ROUTES OF DISSEMINATION

The principal hazard is inhalation of liquid, vapour, or droplets (0.6–5 microns). Delivery may be by artillery shells, missiles or aerial bombing. In the Tokyo subway attack in 1995, terrorists left plastic bags on the subway filled with Sarin after piercing them with umbrella tips. There were 3796 casualties and 12 deaths.[3]

Toxicity depends on the concentration and time of exposure, is measured in units of concentration and time (mg/min m³), known as the Haber product.[7] Most chemical agents are designed to penetrate the skin, respiratory epithelium and cornea, unlike biological agents. Penetration is promoted by thinner, more vascular, moister, hairy skin, and by high humidity, spills and aerosols.

SARIN

Sarin ($C_4H_{10}FO_2P$, isopropylmethylphosphofluoridate) is a colourless, and odourless liquid at room temperature. It is volatile and incompatible with metals or concrete, which lead to production of hydrogen gas. Hydrolysis of sarin forms acids. It is thermally stable <49°C, but clings to clothing and releases slowly for 30 min. Toxicity is through inhibition of the enzyme acetylcholinesterase (see table 76.4).

Table 76.4   Sarin toxicity

Mild	Rhinorrhitis
	Dyspnoea
	Meiosis
	Blurred vision
Moderate	Diaphoresis
	Drooling
	Bronchospasm
	Nausea, vomiting, cramps
	Weakness
	Twitching
	Headache
	Confusion
Severe	Involuntary defecation/urination
	Convulsions
	Respiratory arrest
	Coma, death

The route of exposure determines which clinical features appear first.[24] Post inhalation respiratory and eye symptoms appear, whereas post cutaneous exposure diaphoresis and muscle fasciculation occur. Immediate first aid is to remove the patient from the area of danger to a well-ventilated area before removal of clothing, and decontamination of the skin. This can be achieved using mists of water, or dilute sodium hypochlorite. Eyes are irrigated with water or normal saline.

Assessment follows airway, breathing and circulation. Patients with compromised airways, either due to direct effects or secondary to reduced level of consciousness, require intubation and positive pressure ventilation. Aggressive suctioning may be needed for the bronchial secretions.

TREATMENT

- Anticholinergics to antagonize the muscarinic effects, usually i.v. atropine in 2 mg doses, every 3–5 min, until the patient is atropinized. It may need to be continued for 24 h at 2 mg/h.[2]
- Oximes to reactivate the anticholinesterase enzyme at nicotinic sites, e.g. pralidoxime mesilate 30 mg/kg by slow i.v. injection, up to 2–4 g. This should be prompt, as dealkylation of the inhibited enzyme renders it resistant to reactivation.
- Prophylactic anticonvulsants to prevent seizures. Diazepam 5 mg by any route, has been shown to reduce morbidity in animal studies.

MUSTARD GAS

Mustard gas ($C_4H_8Cl_2S$, Bis-(2-Chloroethyl) sulphide) is a yellow oily liquid at room temperature. It has a faint garlic odour and evaporates to form a vapour that penetrates clothing. There is a low mortality, but tends to incapacitate. It is a bifunctional alkylating agent that is carcinogenic (oral cavity, larynx, bronchus), and irritates skin and mucosa. Mustard gas is also myelotoxic (pancytopenia) and teratogenic. Assessment is similar to Sarin.[25] (See Table 76.5.)

TREATMENT

Patients with large burns are resuscitated as any other burn injuries; however, fluid losses are transudates, so protein losses are less.[26] Pain control is important and frequently requires analgesics, such as morphine. Tense blisters are dressed with silver sulfadiazine. Mustard burns take at least 12 weeks to heal, but early excision and grafting does not reduce healing time.[27,28] Eye lesions usually heal in 2 weeks, and are aided by topical antibiotics and saline irrigation. Oxygen, antibiotics for secondary pneumonia, physiotherapy and ventilation are the mainstays of treatment for respiratory effects.

Table 76.5 Features of mustard gas toxicity

Eyes	Lacrimation, conjunctivitis, photophobia
Skin	Erythema, blistering, partial to full thickness burns
Respiratory tract	Rhinorrhoea, tracheobronchitis, bronchopneumonia
Systemic	Nausea, vomiting, diarrhoea, bradycardia, hypotension

REFERENCES

1 Spencer R, Wilcox M. Agents of biological warfare. *Rev Med Microbiol* 1993; **4**: 138–43.
2 Evison D, Hinsley D, Rice P. Chemical weapons. *BMJ* 2002; **324**: 332–5.
3 KB O. Aum Shinrikyo: once and future threat? *Emerg Infect Dis* 1999; **5**: 513–6.
4 Zilinskas R. Iraq's biological weapons: the past as future? *JAMA* 1997; **278**: 418–24.
5 Arnon SS, Schechter R, Inglesby TV, *et al.* Botulinum toxin as a biological weapon. Medical and Public Health Management. *JAMA* 2001; **285**: 1059–70.
6 Beeching NJ, Dance DA, Miller AR, Spencer RC. Biological warfare and bioterrorism. *BMJ* 2002; **324**: 336–9.
7 WHO. *Health Aspects of Chemical and Biological Weapons.* WHO; 2001: 2.
8 Inglesby TV, Henderson DA, Bartlett JG, *et al.* Anthrax as a biological weapon. Consensus statement. *JAMA* 1999; **281**: 1735–45.
9 Meselson M, Guillemin J, Hugh-Jones M, *et al.* The Sverdlovsk Anthrax outbreak of 1979. *Science* 1994; **266**: 1202–7.
10 Swartz M. Recognition and management of anthrax – an update. *N Engl J Med* 2001; **345**: 1621–6.
11 English JF. Overview of bioterrorism readiness plan: a template for health care facilities. *Am J Infect Control* 1999; **27**: 468–9.
12 Schulze J, Toepfer M, Schroff KC, *et al.* Clindamycin and nicotinic neuromuscular transmission. *Lancet* 1999; **354**: 1792–3.
13 Black R, Gunn R. Hypersensitivity reactions with botulinal antitoxin. *Am J Med* 1980; **69**: 567–70.
14 Amersdorfer P, Marks J. Phage Libraries for the generation of anti-botulinum scFv antibodies. *Methods Mol Biol* 2000; **145**: 219–40.
15 Breman J, Henderson D. Poxvirus dilemmas: monkeypox, smallpox and biological terrorism. *N Engl J Med* 1998; **339**: 556–59.
16 Gani R, Leach S. Transmission potential of smallpox in contemporary populations. *Nature* 2001; **414**: 748–51.
17 Henderson DA, Inglesby TV, Bartlett JG, *et al.* Smallpox as a biological weapon: medical and public health management. *JAMA* 1999; **281**: 2127–30.

18 Vaccinia vaccine: recommendations of the Immunization Practices Advisory Committee (ACIP). *MMWR Recomm Rep* 1991; **40**: 1–10.

19 Redfield RR, Wright DC, James WD, *et al.* Disseminated vaccinia in a military recruit with human immunodeficiency virus. *N Engl J Med* 1987; **316**: 673–76.

20 Lalezari JP, Stagg RJ, Kuppermann BD, *et al.* Intravenous cidofovir for peripheral cytomegalovirus retinitis in patients with AIDS: a randomised, controlled trial. *Ann Intern Med* 1997; **126**: 257–63.

21 Inglesby TV, Dennis DT, Henderson DA, *et al.* Plague as a biological weapon: medical and public health management. *JAMA* 2000; **285**: 2763–73.

22 Perry R, Fetherston J. *Yersinia pestis* – aetiologic agent of plague. *Clin Microbiol Rev* 1997; **10**: 35–66.

23 Wesseley S, Hyams K, Bartholomew R. Psychological implications of chemical and biological weapons. *BMJ* 2001; **323**: 878–9.

24 Tu A. Overview of sarin terrorist attacks on Japan. *American Chemical Society Symposium Series* 2000; **745**: 304–7.

25 Newman-Taylor A, Morris A. Experience with mustard gas casualties. *Lancet* 1991; **337**: 242.

26 Mellor S, Rice P, Cooper G. Vesicant burns. *Br J Plast Surg* 1991; **44**: 434–7.

27 Eldad A, Weinberg A, Breiterman S, *et al.* Early non-surgical removal of chemically injured tissue enhances wound healing in partial thickness burns. *Burns* 1998; **24**: 166–72.

28 Rice P, Brown RF, Lam DG, *et al.* Dermabrasion a novel concept in the surgical management of sulphur mustard injuries. *Burns* 2000; **26**: 34–40.

Part Thirteen

Pharmacological Considerations

77

Pharmacokinetics, pharmacodynamics and drug monitoring in critical illness

T G Short and G C Hood

Critically ill patients usually receive multiple drug therapy, including specific treatment for their condition (e.g. antibiotics), for the pathophysiological consequences of their condition (e.g. inotropes) and to control sedation (e.g. benzodiazepines, opioids). Factors to be considered include:

- The drugs are nearly always given i.v.
- Most have a narrow therapeutic index
- Critically ill patients have altered pharmacokinetics
- Multiple drug therapy may lead to unexpected interactions between drugs
- Interventions such as haemodialysis and plasmapheresis may profoundly alter drug disposition
- The individual response to drugs can also change quickly
- A detailed knowledge of pharmacological changes in the critically ill is required to administer drugs safely. However, information about changes in drug handling and drug response has been mostly derived from normal patients or those with stable single organ failure, and may be less relevant to critically ill patients with multiple organ dysfunction
- It is essential to monitor the effects of all drug treatment regularly
- Individualizing drug therapy has been shown to improve survival of critically ill patients

PHARMACOKINETICS

Pharmacokinetics is the study of the absorption, distribution, metabolism and elimination of drugs. Several mathematical models can be used to describe drug disposition, but common pharmacokinetic concepts include volume of distribution (V), clearance (Cl) and half-life ($t_{1/2}$). These can be used to design rational dosing regimens.[1]

VOLUME OF DISTRIBUTION

The *apparent* volume of distribution (V) of a drug is the volume into which an amount (A) of a drug appears to be dispersed, given the concentration (C) measured in the blood according to the formula $V = A/C$. Drug dispersion is not instantaneous, and hence more than one apparent volume of distribution can be calculated.

The apparent *initial* volume of distribution (V_1) is the volume into which drug appears to be dispersed immediately after i.v. injection.

The apparent volume of distribution at steady-state (V_{ss}) is the larger volume calculated after distribution of drug throughout the body has occurred, or when the rate of drug administration equals the rate of drug elimination.

The V_1 is useful for calculating the initial i.v. loading dose (D_L) to achieve a target concentration (C) (i.e. $D_L = V_1 \times C$), so long as high initial concentrations do not cause unwanted effects (e.g. theophylline).

The V_{ss} similarly allows calculation of the loading dose when the therapeutic index is high and it is desirable to achieve therapeutic concentrations quickly (e.g. penicillin). Volumes of distribution depend upon physicochemical characteristics of drugs and can be drastically altered by pathophysiological changes. The V_{ss} of many drugs has been calculated from relatively brief infusions. When prolonged infusions are used, such as of the sedative propofol in intensive care, the V_{ss} is often found to be much larger, contributing to the often slow recovery after discontinuation of the infusion.

CLEARANCE

Clearance is defined as the volume of blood completely cleared of drug per unit time, and can be calculated for specific organs or the total body. The liver is the main organ for drug metabolism. It has a different intrinsic clearance (metabolizing capacity) for different drugs. Depending on the drug, metabolism may be altered by:

- enzyme inhibition
- enzyme induction
- changes in hepatic blood flow
- protein binding

The rate of elimination of drugs is usually proportional to the amount of drug reaching the liver – a first order process. However, when the concentration of some drugs is relatively large (e.g. ethyl alcohol, phenytoin, high-dose barbiturates), the metabolic pathway becomes saturated, and drug is slowly eliminated at a fixed rate – a zero order process. A corollary is that small doses of a drug will cause marked sustained increases in plasma concentration during zero-order kinetics compared with administration during first order kinetics.

Total body clearance (C_{TB}) can be used to calculate the infusion rate (k_{01}) of a drug to maintain a given blood concentration, when steady-state conditions have been reached (C_{ss}) by the formula $k_{01} = C_{ss} \times C_{TB}$. Clearance is the most useful indicator of drug elimination. Clearance and volume of distribution determine the elimination half-life.

HALF-LIFE

Half-life is the time taken for the drug concentration in the blood to decrease by 50%.

After a bolus dose of drug or after stopping an infusion, drug concentrations decrease because of re-distribution and metabolism. The initial distribution half-life of a drug ($t_{1/2\alpha}$) describes the initial rapid decrease in blood concentration mainly caused by drug redistribution to tissue. The elimination half-life ($t_{1/2\beta}$) describes the slower decrease in blood concentration caused mainly by drug elimination. If the concentration-time curve is best fitted by a tri-exponential curve, a terminal elimination half-life ($t_{1/2\gamma}$) can be calculated to describe drug elimination when there is a slow return of drug from peripheral reservoirs. The relevance of these half-lives depends on the drug concentration required to have an observable effect relative to the concentration in the patient. Elimination half-life is of limited use if termination of drug effect is caused by redistribution (e.g. propofol). The plasma half-life will thus be less than the terminal elimination half-life. However, as the duration of infusion becomes sufficient to achieve steady-state, the half-life upon stopping the infusion will increase until it equals the terminal elimination half-life.[2] Half-life, none-the-less, determines the time required for an exponential process to approach an equilibrium or steady-state. For a given dose rate, whether given by boluses or infusion, four half-lives are required for 94% completion of

steady-state and five half-lives are required for 97% completion.

PROTEIN BINDING

For most drugs, it is the free (unbound) drug that exerts the drug's effect at its site of action. It is also the free fraction that can be distributed across membranes and be metabolized or eliminated. Most acidic drugs, including all antibiotics, bind to albumin, with binding being proportional to the log of the concentration of albumin. When albumin concentrations fall below 20 g/l, increases in free concentration are likely to be significant. Basic drugs, such as lignocaine, pethidine, phenytoin and propanolol, bind mainly to α_1 acid glyco-protein. During acute illness, α_1 acid glycoprotein concentrations increase, with increased drug binding.[3] Changes in protein binding were once considered important for drugs which are highly protein bound (>80%), because small changes in protein binding would result in large changes in the free concentration (e.g. warfarin displacement of phenytoin). However, the free drug is also available for distribution and metabolism in the body and even large changes in protein binding only have a small effect on free concentration in the blood.

PRACTICAL APPLICATIONS

A knowledge of pharmacokinetics enables use of appropriate dosing regimens. If a drug has limited toxicity in above therapeutic doses, a large loading dose can be given to achieve and maintain a therapeutic concentration quickly (e.g. penicillins). With a drug of narrow therapeutic index, a small loading dose (calculated using V_1) is better. Maintenance doses are then based on clearance and closely monitored response (e.g. aminophylline).

The immediate effect of changing the rate of drug infusion will depend on the half-life of the drug. For drugs with long half-lives (e.g. midazolam and morphine), an increase in dose requirements should be met by titrating small boluses to achieve the new state, and then increasing the infusion rate by an appropriate amount. Decreases in requirements should be met by switching off the infusion and then restarting at a lower rate after the new desired state has been reached. Simply increasing or decreasing the infusion rate for morphine, which has an elimination half-life of at least 3 h in healthy individuals, will require five half-lives or 15 h for the drug concentration to reach the new steady-state (Fig. 77.1). If severe illness causes the volume of distribution of a drug to be doubled, then its half-life will also be doubled. Severe illness may also decrease clearance of drug, halving clearance will cause a similar doubling of half-life. Should both effects occur together, half-life will be increased four-fold, having a significant effect on the duration of action of a drug.

Recently, use of continuous infusion of drugs to maintain an effective concentration in the central blood volume (V_1) have been used to partially overcome some of the disadvantages of lack of predictability of drug concentrations in the blood and transient effect following i.v. bolus dosing of drugs.

PHARMACODYNAMICS

Pharmacodynamics is the study of the effects of drug on the body. The relationship between drug dosage or concentration and drug effect is complex. Drug effects are caused by the presence of active drug at its sites of action. For most drugs, the logarithmic dose–response curve is sigmoid in shape (Fig. 77.2). This curve may be modified by drug interactions and patient tolerance.

BIOPHASE

Drugs do not usually work in the blood, but rather at sites in various organs (e.g. muscle relaxants at receptors in the neuromuscular junction, antibiotics in bronchial secretions in a patient with pneumonia). This site of action is known as the biophase. There is a delay between achieving an adequate concentration of drug in the blood and a therapeutic concentration in the biophase. This delay is the result of two factors, the amount of blood flow to the organ and the time taken for the drug to pass from the blood to the biophase. Intravenous drug therapy differs from enteral routes of administration in that very high drug concentrations are achieved in the blood and highly perfused organs, compared with organs that are poorly perfused (Table 77.1). Thus rapid administration of drugs with a narrow therapeutic index may cause transient toxicity at the main or

secondary site of action (e.g. rapid administration of vancomycin can cause severe hypotension due to histamine release). The concentration of drug in the biophase may bear a poor relationship to the concentration of drug in the plasma. For example, drugs such as morphine and midazolam are transported out of the brain by active transport, utilizing glycoprotein P. Absence or inhibition of glycoprotein P, in animal models, leads to increased sensitivity to these drugs. It is possible that alterations in glycoprotein P activity may account for some of the increased sensitivity seen to these drugs in acute illness.

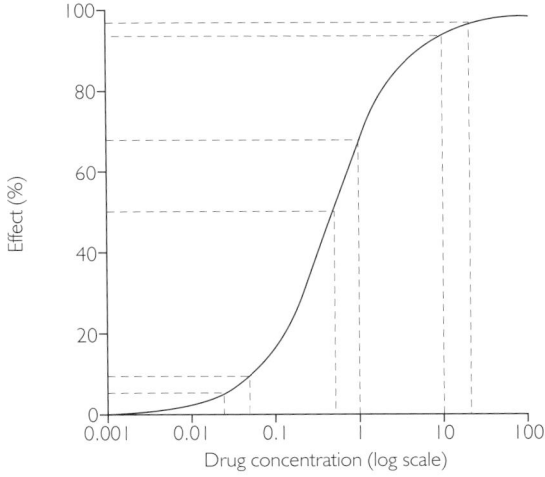

Fig. 77.2 A typical dose–response curve. In the middle part of the curve, a small change in drug concentration causes a large change in effect. At the extremes of the curve, large changes in concentration are required to observe much change in effect

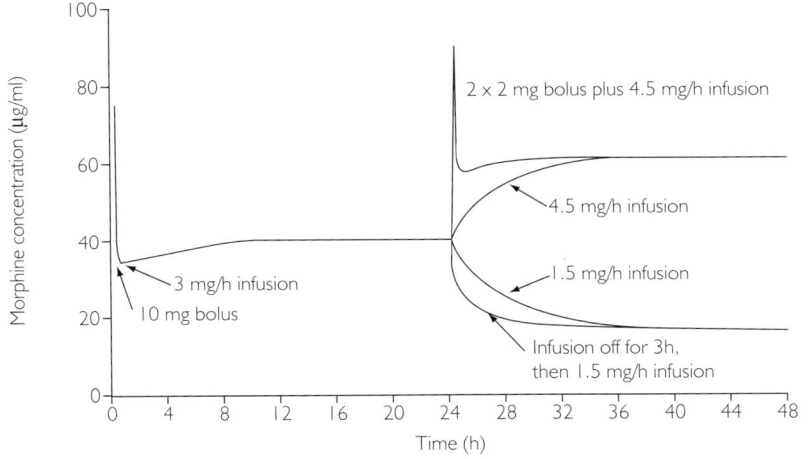

Fig. 77.1 Effect of methods of changing infusion rate on plasma concentration of morphine in a healthy patient

Table 77.1 Distribution of cardiac output in healthy and critically ill patients

Organ	% Body weight	% Cardiac output	Change in % of cardiac output in critical illness
Lungs	2	100	Nil
Heart	0.5	5	+++
Brain	2	14	+++
Kidneys	0.5	23	---
Liver/splanchnic	10	28	---
Endocrine/bone marrow	2	6	--
Skin	6	9	--
Muscle	50	16	--
Fat	15	5	--
Other	12	5	--

After i.v. injection in a healthy patient, initial organ concentrations depend on their blood flow and mass. In the critically ill, cardiac output may vary widely depending on therapy and distribution will depend on the amount of peripheral vasoconstriction (e.g. from hypovolaemia) or vasodilation (e.g. from systemic inflammatory response syndrome)

DOSE–RESPONSE

Drug effect is usually proportional to the logarithm of the free concentration of drug, and is described by a sigmoid shaped dose–response curve (Fig. 77.2). This relationship means that the dose of drug required to significantly increase or decrease its effects is highly dependent on drug concentration. In the middle part of the curve, small changes in dose (and thus concentration) will have large clinical effects; at the low or high ends of the curve, large changes in dose are required to obtain a change in clinical effect. The sigmoid shape of the curve results from the fact that for any drug there is a maximum observable therapeutic effect. Dose–response curves can be drawn for any aspect of drug pharmacology, and the ratio between the median toxic dose and the median effective dose is termed the therapeutic index. When this ratio is low, it is essential to titrate the drug, and observe or measure response carefully (e.g. aminoglycosides, theophylline). Drug effects also depend upon interactions with other drugs and concurrent disease. The effects of drugs with similar effects are not necessarily additive. The sedative effects of an opioid plus a benzodiazepine or propofol are up to 50% more than expected if the effects were simply additive.[4,5]

Many drugs have a wide dose range to achieve a given response. For example, for sedatives such as propofol and midazolam and opioids such as morphine, there is typically a ten-fold range in dose to achieve a given response (Fig. 77.3).[6,7] Typical dose recommendations ignore this variability. Combinations of drugs may also reduce the dose range required to achieve a given response, as is seen using the combination of fentanyl and midazolam for sedation (Fig. 77.3).

CHANGES IN CRITICAL ILLNESS

ROUTE OF ADMINISTRATION

The enteral route is usually best avoided because of alterations in gut motility, blood flow, pH, function and first past metabolism by the liver. Gastric emptying is impaired by many factors including:

● anticholinergics, antacids, phenothiazines and opioids
● inotropes, especially dopamine.
● traumatic brain injury
● diabetes mellitus

Subcutaneous and i.m. injection is also unpredictable because systemic transfer of drug is dependent on blood

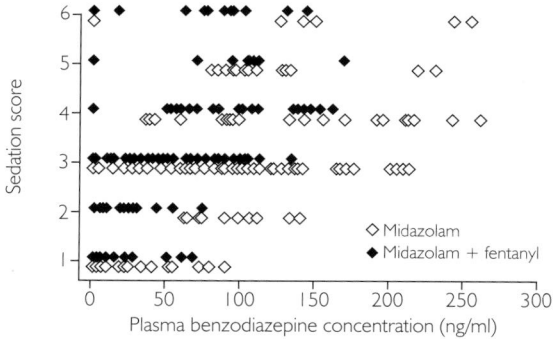

Fig. 77.3 Ramsay sedation score versus measured plasma midazolam concentrations for midazolam in the presence and absence of i.v. fentanyl target controlled infusion of 1.5 ng/ml, a concentration equivalent of an infusion of 1.7 μg/kg per h at steady-state[8]

flow at the site of injection, which in turn depends on posture, activity, site of injection and degree of vaso-constriction or vasodilatation at that site. Paradoxically systemic concentrations of drugs with high first-pass metabolism may be increased (e.g. propranolol).

Enteral feeding may reduce drug availability due to absorption of drug onto enteral feed components, naso-gastric tubing or by reduced absorption due to the pH of the feed.

The i.v. route is used for speed, convenience, reliabi-lity, titratability and lack of enteral formulations of some drugs. Intravenous apparatus including glass, plastics and rubber may absorb drugs, decreasing the dose delivered (e.g. insulin, heparin, isosorbide). When several drugs are delivered through the same i.v. line, chemical incompat-ibility may also occur. This may be a result of pH effects altering solubility, solvent effects (e.g. precipitation of the propylene glycol used to dissolve some preparations of diazepam when diluted excessively) and cation–anion interactions causing precipitation or formation of less active, yet soluble complexes (e.g. thiopentone or calcium in combination with most other drugs). Al-though precipitation can be detected by visual inspec-tion, lack of visual changes does not mean there has not been loss of potency (e.g. heparin and dopamine, insulin and total parenteral nutrition).[8,9]

When infusing drugs i.v., the method of administration can alter the amount of drug delivered dramatically. Simple infusions using a drip chamber to regulate flow are not adequate when infusing inotropes, and mechanical drop counters and peristaltic pumps may be erratic, espe-cially if drug is not adequately diluted and the flow rate is low. Syringe pumps are the most accurate, but may also be unreliable at low flow rates (1–2 ml/h). As siphoning from or flushing of i.v. lines can also result in drug over-dose, it is essential that anti-reflux valves are used when more than one infusion is running into a single i.v. site.

PHARMACOKINETIC AND PHARMACODYNAMIC CHANGES

Critically ill patients often have multiple organ dysfunc-tion, causing alterations in drug handling and effect in the body at all levels. The net effect of these multiple changes is difficult to predict. Frequently, the main effect is to increase interpatient variability in response, even if typical patient response is altered little. Intrapatient variability also occurs over surprisingly brief periods of time in response to changes in a patient's condition. Midazolam may fail to be metabolized in septic shock, and cardiogenic shock can cause rapid increases in lignocaine concentrations even after the infusion has been ceased.[10,11]

CIRCULATORY FAILURE

Circulatory failure causes a greater percentage of cardiac output to go to essential organs (e.g. heart and

brain) and decreased blood flow to peripheral tissues (Table 77.1). The net effects are:

- Increased blood concentrations in the heart and brain
- Decreased blood concentrations in the periphery
- Decreased renal blood flow and shunting of blood from cortical to juxtamedullary nephrons. Glomerular filtration rate and tubular excretion are decreased, decreasing extraction of drugs and metabolites
- Decreased liver blood flow. Hepatocellular function may be impaired, decreasing clearance of both highly extracted drugs due to failure of delivery to the liver, and of poorly extracted drugs due to failure of cellular metabolism[12]

Mechanical ventilation may cause further decreases in liver blood flow by increasing intrathoracic and therefore venous pressure.

The initial effect is a large decrease in V_1, and a decrease in V_{ss} and Cl of drugs. The effects are more profound on drugs that are usually rapidly distributed such as sedatives or lignocaine, where standard doses may cause central nervous system toxicity, than with slowly distributed drugs such as digoxin. Fluid and inotropic therapy may alter these effects over brief periods of time. With volume overload, there may be an increase in V_1 but with a more prolonged distribu-tion half-life. Acidaemia may exacerbate these changes by increasing the free concentration of highly bound drugs, but decrease the pharmacological response to some drugs by altering receptor affinity (e.g. cate-cholamines). Hypovolaemic shock causes increased sensitivity to central nervous system depressants even after restoration of circulating volume; this effect is probably secondary to as yet unidentified circulating factors.[13]

HEPATIC FAILURE

Hepatic failure may increase or decrease volume of dis-tribution and total body clearance and increases excre-tion half-life of hepatically metabolized drugs. Loading doses are often not greatly affected. Extrahepatic meta-bolism is considerable in anhepatic animal models. In the severely ill, there is usually a decrease in liver blood flow and therefore the rate at which drugs are delivered to the liver for metabolism. Flow-dependent drugs include lignocaine, morphine, midazolam.

Vasopressors do not usually decrease liver blood flow because of increases in cardiac output compensating for potential vasoconstriction.

Phase 1 reactions, which involve cytochrome P_{450}, are usually more affected than phase 2 reactions. There is a poor correlation between derangement of conventional tests of liver function and the degree of impairment of drug metabolism and the degree of impairment may vary widely over short periods of time. In the severely ill, metabolism of some drugs will almost cease, as indicated by a lack of formation of metabolites and very high plasma concentrations (e.g. midazolam).[10]

Hepatic failure tends to decrease the amount of drug bound because of accumulation of metabolites which compete for binding sites on protein. For example, elevated concentrations of bilirubin decrease protein binding of sulphonamides, tetracyclines, penicillins and cephalosporins. A decrease in protein binding will offset increases in volume of distribution when the drug is highly protein bound, such as most penicillins and erythromycin. For drugs with low protein binding, such as aminoglycosides, a decrease in protein binding will have little effect on free plasma concentrations.

RENAL FAILURE

Total body clearance Cl_{TB} is reduced by renal failure and volumes V_1 and V_{ss} will increase if there is significant fluid retention. Renal failure tends to decrease renal clearances and increase half-lives of drugs cleared by the kidneys. Drug doses may be decreased to as little as 10% of normal. In the case of drugs that are metabolized by the liver and metabolites excreted by the kidneys, there may be accumulation of active metabolites (e.g. morphine-6-glucuronide). Renal failure usually affects glomerular function more than tubular function, so excretion of aminoglycosides which depend more on glomerular filtration are affected more than excretion of penicillins which are dependent on tubular function.

Creatinine clearance is usually a poor guide to renal function in the critically ill because there may be alterations in the rate of formation of creatinine as well as its excretion by the kidneys. Algorithms for drug dose based on creatinine clearance may be similarly unreliable. Some assays of creatinine are also interfered with in jaundiced patients. Effects of disease may also not be as anticipated. For example, propranolol excretion is thought to be via metabolism in the liver but elimination is impaired in renal failure by an unknown mechanism. Accumulation of metabolic products may cause decreases in protein binding of drugs. For example, uraemia decreases binding of penicillins, sulphonamides and cephalosporins and in the case of phenytoin excretion is increased.

Renal replacement (dialytic) therapy drastically alters volumes and clearances of drugs. Effects vary with the mode of dialysis and the type of membrane in use and the drugs in question. For most modern membranes little information is available, but several reviews of what is known are available.[14,15]

SEPTIC INFLAMMATORY RESPONSE SYNDROME

In acute severe illness, such as sepsis, and multiple organ failure, there is an increase in capillary permeability and total body water secondary to the leaky capillaries. This usually increases volume of distribution of drugs, so that increased loading doses may be required to attain a satisfactory therapeutic concentration. Similar changes occur in patients with major burns and may be due to circulating leukotrienes. The volume of distribution may also change over short periods of time. When patients start to recover, serum concentrations may increase because of the decreasing volume of distribution of the drug (e.g. vancomycin[16]) as well as decrease because of resumption of normal metabolism and clearance (e.g. midazolam[10]). Circulatory, hepatic and renal failure may also add the characteristic changes already described, of decreased clearance or metabolism and accumulation of active metabolites.

CHANGES IN RECEPTORS IN ACUTE ILLNESS

Many drugs act at receptors and some receptors may change in the critically ill, affecting drug response. One cause of tolerance, which is a decreased drug effect for a given dose or plasma concentration, is altered receptor function.

Catecholamines show an increase in receptor numbers in response to a lack of agonist (up-regulation) and a decrease in receptor numbers in response to increased concentrations of agonist (down-regulation). Drug affinity for receptors is also pH dependent. Acidosis decreases the affinity of catecholamines for their receptors, and is a significant problem when there is a pH < 7.1. Hypothermia also decreases drug affinity for receptors.

Proliferation of extrajunctional acetylcholine receptors on muscle after acute injuries such as burns and denervation can lead to hyperkalaemia following the use of suxamethonium.

DRUG MONITORING

During critical illness there is substantial variation both between patients and within the same patient over time in factors affecting therapeutic drug concentrations. When a drug has a narrow therapeutic index, or there is a major risk of treatment failure if inadequate drug concentrations are achieved, it is essential to monitor drug effect. For some medicines, such as analgesics, sedatives and inotropes, this involves clinical and physiological observation. When clinical observation is not possible and drugs have a narrow therapeutic index, plasma concentrations are measured. Toxicity may relate to peak concentration (e.g. seizures and arrhythmias from theophyllines) or to mean concentration (e.g. ototoxicity from aminoglycosides). Some drugs for which there are accepted therapeutic and toxic concentrations are shown in Table 77.2.

Drug assays usually measure total plasma concentration. Plasma protein levels, protein binding and critical illness itself can modify the relationship between measured drug concentration and clinical effect. Regardless of measured concentration, evidence of clinical efficacy or toxicity must be monitored for constantly. Given these considerations the expense of therapeutic drug monitoring must be weighed against the risks of toxicity or treatment failure.

Use of pharmacokinetic software to modify drug therapy is increasingly widespread. Such systems vary from models using population-derived data to Bayesian feedback systems comparing measured drug levels with those predicted by a mathematical model of drug effect and modifying dosage recommendations accordingly. The Bayesian approach uses computerized algorithms that incorporate population-based pharmacokinetics (pharmacokinetics adjusted for patient characteristics such as weight, sex, age, serum creatinine) and measured drug levels (looking at the individual's pharmacokinetics), taking into account the variability of population parameters and serum level measurements. Generally, as long as the population model is carefully derived and is appropriate for the patient being treated, it performs better than a simple fixed dosing regimen.

Whilst adverse drug events may be reduced using such programmes they are still no substitute for good clinical judgement.[17]

SEDATIVES

Benzodiazepines (especially midazolam) with or without opioids are widely used for sedation in intensive care units (ICUs).

Whilst 'short acting' in the critically ill, midazolam's elimination half-life is increased as is that of its active metabolite 1-hydroxymidazolam, their metabolism changing in parallel with patient condition.[18] Midazolam (usually 96% protein-bound) increases its effect in renal failure despite increased clearance, due to reduced protein binding.[19] Tolerance theoretically develops over

time to benzodiazepines but is seldom a clinical issue. Clearance of concomitantly administered opioids also affects recovery time after sedation.

Propofol may be useful for selected patients and may be more predictable in its effects due to its more rapid elimination from the blood. In the critically ill, increases in propofol's large V, reductions in its clearance, with hypoalbuminaemia increasing its free fraction (propofol is 98% protein-bound), means that a reducing dosage strategy may be required for prolonged propofol infusion.

Propofol pharmacokinetics have been studied in patients without hepatic impairment receiving 2–4-day infusions of 1–3 mg/kg per h, a sedative dose. After cessation, due to its high clearance propofol concentrations halved by 10 min and thereafter gradually declined, usually leading to rapid awakening. Other concomitant medicines and disease can delay full awakening. Long terminal half-lives (12–50 h) at concentrations too low for clinical effect have been described, particularly after prolonged infusion.[6] Significant triglyceride and calorie load may be associated with long-term propofol infusion, and recently there has been a move to 2% solutions in this setting.

Thiopentone infusion for control of intracranial pressure carries risks of hypotension, impaired leukocyte function and infection. Dosage should be titrated to clinical effect on intracranial pressure and to an electroencephalogram (EEG) end-point of burst-suppression. Blood levels should be measured as clearance tends to increase over time. Thiopentone has a long elimination half-life of around 17.5 h and residual levels exist for prolonged periods, necessitating cerebral angiography for confirmation where brain death is suspected.[20]

Up to 40% of patients in ICU report some awareness whilst receiving muscle relaxants.[21] Subjective clinical assessment tools for assessing adequacy of sedation, such as the Ramsay Sedation Scale (Table 77.3), assign numeric value to clinical findings but have limited effectiveness due to inter-observer variability and cannot be

Table 77.2 Therapeutic drug monitoring in the critically ill

Drug	Therapeutic concentrations	Toxic effects and guidelines to dosage
Antiarrhythmics		
Digoxin	0.8–2.5 μg/ml	>5 μg/ml. Monitor ECG–dysrhythmia/conduction defects
Lignocaine	3–6 mg/ml	Increased toxicity congestive heart failure
Antibiotics		
Gentamicin	Peak 5–10 μg/ml, trough <2	Renal and ototoxicity. Once daily high dose. Check trough
Amikacin	Peak 8–16 μg/ml, trough <4	As above
Vancomycin	Peak 20–40 μg/ml, trough <10	
Anticonvulsants		
Phenytoin	10–20 mg/ml	Arrhythmias. Check free concentration if uraemia/ low albumin
Theophyllines		
Aminophylline	10–20 mg/l	>25 mg/l

Table 77.3 Ramsay Sedation Scale[23]

Level of sedation	Characteristics
Awake	
1	Anxious and/or agitated, baseline agitated state
2	Co-operative, oriented, and tranquil
3	Responsive to commands
Asleep	
4	Quiet, asleep, with brisk response to light glabellar tap or loud auditory stimulus
5	Sluggish response to light glabellar tap or loud auditory stimulus
6	Little or no response to stimuli

used during neuromuscular blockade.[22,23] Other measures of sedation effect open to interpretation include haemodynamic variables, respiratory rate and pattern, lacrimation and diaphoresis. There is increasing interest in EEG-based tools for monitoring and titrating sedation. Limitations include equipment size and complexity and data interpretation. The bispectral index, developed to monitor sedation during anaesthesia, shows more promise. The EEG is recorded as a numeric value between 0 and 100, calculated by computer, and has been shown to correlate with Ramsay score.

- 100 corresponds to awake
- 60 moderate to deep sedation
- less than 40 to deep hypnotic state[23–25]

OPIOIDS

Opioid doses need to be titrated and monitored as requirements vary up to ten-fold between patients and tolerance rapidly develops. Opioids for analgesia alone may be best delivered via patient controlled analgesia devices, with analgesia and side-effects monitored using various analogue or ordinal scales. Morphine and fentanyl are commonly used in ICU, pethidine less so because of its toxic metabolite norpethidine, which may accumulate with prolonged use.

Although morphine is primarily metabolized in the liver, liver failure seldom impacts on its metabolism.[26] Renal failure is more significant, leading to accumulation of both morphine and its active metabolite morphine-6-glucuronide, which has an elimination half-life of up to 38 h. Where fentanyl is used via infusion, the recovery time depends on the length of infusion, with elimination half-life being 6 h, it has no active metabolites.[4] Fentanyl is 84% protein bound and hepatically metabolized. Hepatic and renal failure have little effect on its pharmacokinetics, except for reduced protein binding.[27]

MUSCLE RELAXANTS

Prolonged paralysis and weakness may result from neuromuscular blockade in the ICU setting. Regular real-time monitoring of neuromuscular blockade via peripheral nerve stimulation during infusion aiming for maintenance of one to two twitches in train-of-four is simple, inexpensive and recommended.

The clearance and effect of common neuromuscular blocking agents is prolonged in hepatic and renal impairment, with the exception of atracurium. Other variations in neuromuscular blockade occur with drug interactions, electrolyte disturbance and neuromuscular disease. Vecuronium's principle metabolite, 3-desacetylvecuronium, contributes to prolonged paralysis after prolonged vecuronium infusion and has an elimination half-life of 116 min (cf vecuronium 36 min). Rocuronium requirements are lower when bolus administered rather than infused whereas the converse has been recorded for pancuronium.[28]

ANTI-ARRHYTHMICS

Lignocaine clearance and V_{ss} are reduced in cardiac and hepatic failure whilst active metabolites accumulate in renal failure. In critical illness increased α_1 acid glycoprotein binding may increase total lignocaine concentrations without affecting free concentrations. Concentrations should be measured daily and patients monitored for signs of toxicity including drowsiness and paraesthesiae.[29]

Digoxin maintenance doses should be reduced with renal impairment and concurrent use of amiodarone, erythromycin, quinidine or tetracyclines. Arrhythmias and cardiac conduction defects due to toxicity may be enhanced by hypokalaemia, hypocalcaemia and hypomagnesaemia. Regular monitoring of digoxin levels should be considered but in renal or hepatic failure a digoxin-like immunoreactive factor may interfere with the assay.[30] Toxicity is rare with concentrations $<2.5\ \mu g/l$ but common $>5\ \mu g/l$.

ANTIBIOTICS

β-Lactam antibiotics have slow bactericidal activity. Outcome for infections in which they are used is dependent upon the time for which tissue concentrations are maintained at levels four- to five-fold higher than minimum inhibitory concentration (MIC). Higher concentrations are not beneficial. Plasma concentrations in ICU patients can vary up to ten-fold due to increases in V and have been found to fall below MIC towards the end of an 8-h dosing interval. Data from animals and, more recently, neutropenic patients and critically ill children, suggest that bactericidal levels of ceftazidime in particular are better maintained with the same daily dose administered via continuous infusion rather than bolus injection.[31] No difference between effect for bolus vs infusion has been identified for penicillin. For susceptible Gram-negative infections, especially those not responding to treatment, consideration should be given to infusion rather than bolus therapy. Measuring MIC and C_{ss} plasma levels can help guide dosage although target tissue concentration determines efficacy. Continuous renal replacement therapy (CRRT) removes one-third to one-half the dosage for all β-lactam antibiotics, necessitating dose adjustment.[32–36]

Aminoglycosides and vancomycin have narrow therapeutic indices, with potential for nephrotoxocity and ototoxicity in overdose. They should be used with caution in renal impairment or avoided. Effective peak concentrations correlate with clinical response and induce post antibiotic inhibition of bacterial growth. With aminoglycosides, once daily dosing reduces toxicity and improves clinical outcome. Because the VD is increased in critically ill patients, an increased loading dose may be required (5–7 mg/kg for gentamicin) and conventional nomograms do not produce adequate concentrations.[37–40] Vancomycin nephrotoxicity is associated with trough levels of 20–30 μg/ml and ototoxicity with concentrations of 22–100 μg/ml. Nephrotoxicity is enhanced by concomitant aminoglycoside use. Concomitant use of medicines which increase cardiac output enhance vancomycin clearance and, conversely, lead to a reduction in these results in increased vancomycin trough levels.[41] Around 500 mg daily of vancomycin is removed by CRRT.[42] Peak and trough levels should be monitored.

Fluconazole and ganciclovir are also removed by CRRT, which may necessitate dose modification, although fluconazole elimination is generally reduced in critical illness. Burns patients have markedly increased V and reduced clearance for most antibiotics except imipenem.[43]

ANTICOAGULANTS

Heparin infusions should be titrated to effect of activated partial thromboplastin time (APTT) measured 6–12 hourly, aiming for 1.5–3 times normal APTT depending on diagnosis. Weight-based nomograms have been shown to take shorter times to reach C_{ss} than empiric therapy.[44] Acquired antithrombin III (AT III) deficiency is not uncommon in the critically ill and, where 'heparin-resistance' occurs as measured by APTT, AT III levels should be measured and, where deficient, corrected with AT III or plasma. Fixed-dose regimens of subcutaneous low molecular weight heparins, which have a greater anti-Xa effect, have

become increasingly popular for the treatment of deep vein thrombosis and pulmonary embolus. Reliable monitoring of their efficacy is not possible and their anticoagulant effect is not completely reversible in the event of bleeding, making their usefulness in the ICU setting limited if not contraindicated.

ANTICONVULSANTS

Phenytoin clearance varies widely in the critically ill. Concentrations are usually monitored, the therapeutic range being 10–20 mg/ml (40–80 μmol/l) but seizures may be well controlled outside this level. Low total concentrations may be misleading as reduced protein binding increases the unbound concentration. Enteral absorption is both delayed and impaired by enteral feed preparations, although the basis for this remains uncertain.[45] Hepatic metabolism is saturable, but may be increased by concurrent barbiturate therapy causing hepatic enzyme induction.[46] Toxic effects of other anticonvulsants, including valproic acid and phenobarbitone, can occur within their therapeutic ranges and levels are affected by many medicines affecting hepatic metabolism.

THEOPHYLLINES

Aminophylline has a long elimination half-life (8–9 h) and a narrow therapeutic index due to cardiac and neurotoxicity. Its hepatic metabolism varies depending upon age, gender, smoking, viral and bacterial illness, heart failure, hepatic cirrhosis and concurrent drugs including cimetidine and erythromycin. Hypoxia reduces both clearance and protein binding (normally 40–60%).[47] Plasma levels should be measured at least daily and maintained between 10–20 mg/l (55 and 110 μmol/l) although toxicity can occur within this range. Clinical efficacy is difficult to measure. Subtherapeutic levels can be corrected by top-up bolus whereas for excessive levels infusion should be stopped and recommenced later at lower dose.

REFERENCES

1 Hull CJ. *Pharmacokinetics for Anaesthesia*. Oxford: Butterworth Heinemann; 1991.

2 Hughes MA, Glass PSA, Jacobs JR. Context-sensitive half time in multicompartment pharmacokinetic models for intravenous drugs. *Anesthesiology* 1992; **76**: 334–41.

3 Craig WA, Welling PG. Protein binding of antimicrobials: clinical pharmacokinetic and therapeutic implications. *Clin Pharmacokinet* 1977; **2**: 252–68.

4 Short TG, Plummer JL, Chui PT. Interactions between propofol, alfentanil and midazolam. *Br J Anaesth* 1992; **69**: 162–7.

5 Smith C, McEwan AI, Jhaveri R, *et al.* The interaction of fentanyl on the Cp50 of propofol for loss of consciousness and skin incision. *Anesthesiology* 1994; **81**: 820–8.

6 Barr J, Egan TD, Sandoval NF, *et al.* Propofol dosing regimens for ICU sedation based upon an integrated pharmacokinetic-pharmacodynamic model. *Anesthesiology* 2001; **95**: 324–33.

7 Barr J, Zomorodi K, Bertaccini EJ, Shafer SL. A double-blind, randomized comparison of IV lorazepam versus midazolam for sedation of ICU patient via a pharmacologic model. *Anesthesiology* 2001; **95**: 286–98.

8 Rudy AC, Brater DC. Drug interactions. In: Chernow B (ed.) *The Pharmacologic Approach to the Critically Ill Patient*, 3rd edn. Philadelphia: Williams and Wilkins; 1994: pp. 18–40.

9 Florence AT, Attwood D. *Physicochemical Principals of Pharmacy*, 2nd edn. London: Baillière Tindall; 1988: pp. 271–303.

10 Shelly MP, Mendel L, Park GR. Failure of critically ill patients to metabolize midazolam. *Anaesthesia* 1987; **42**: 619–26.

11 Runciman WB, Myburgh JA, Upton RN. Pharmacokinetics and pharmacodynamics in the critically ill. In: Dobb GJ (ed.) *Clinical Anaesthesiology*. London: Baillière Tindall; 1990: pp. 271–303.

12 Wagner BKJ, Angaran DM, Fuhs DW. Therapeutic drug monitoring. In: Chernow B (ed.) *The Pharmacologic Approach to the Critically Ill Patient*, 3rd edn. Philadelphia: Williams and Wilkins; 1994: pp. 182–201.

13 Klockowski PM, Levy G. Kinetics of drug action in disease states. XXV. Effect of experimental hypovolaemia on the pharmacodynamics and pharmacokinetics of desmethyldiazepam. *J Pharmacol Exp Ther* 1988; **245**: 508–12.

14 Bugge JF. Pharmacokinetics and drug dosing adjustments during continuous venovenous hemofiltration or hemodiafiltration in critically ill patients. *Acta Anaesthesiol Scand* 2001; **45**: 929–34.

15 Bohler J, Donauer J, Keller F. Pharmacokinetic principles during continuous renal replacement therapy: drugs and dosage. *Kidney Int Suppl* 1999; **72**: S24–8.

16 Gous AGS, Dance M, Luyt D, *et al.* Vancomycin pharmacokinetics in critically ill septic infants. *Crit Care Med* 1994; **22**: A181.

17 Evans RS, Pestotnik SL, Classen DC, Burke JP. Evaluation of a computer-assisted antibiotic-dose monitor. *Ann Pharmacother* 1999; **33**: 1026–31.

18 Boulieu R, Lehmann B, Salord F, *et al.* Pharmacokinetics of midazolam and its main metabolite 1-hydroxymidazolam in intensive care patients. *Eur J Metab Pharmacokinet* 1998; **23**: 255–8.

19 Vinik HR, Reves JG, Greenblat DJ, *et al.* The pharmacokinetics of midazolam in chronic renal failure patients. *Anesthesiology* 1983; **59**: 390–4.

20 Russo H, Dubboin MP, Bressolle F, Urien S. Time-dependent pharmacokinetics of high dose thiopental infusion in intensive care patients. *Pharm Res* 1997; **14**: 1583–8.

21 Wagner BKJ, Zavotsky KE, Sweeney JB, *et al.* Patient recall of therapeutic paralysis in a surgical critical care unit. *Pharmacotherapy* 1998; **18**: 358–63.

22 Avramov MN, White PF. Methods for monitoring the level of sedation. *Crit Care Clin* 1995 **11**: 803–26.

23 Ramsay MA, Savage TM, Simpson BR, Goodwin R. Controlled sedation with alphaxalone-alphadolone. *Br Med J* 1974; **2**: 656–9.

24 Roscow C, Manberg PJ. Bispectral index monitoring. *Anesthesiol Clin North Am* 1998; **2**: 89–107.

25 Campbell ML, Bizek KS, Stewart R. Integrating technology with compassionate care: withdrawal of ventilation in a conscious patient with apnoea. *Am J Crit Care* 1998; **7**: 85–9.

26 Shelly MP, Cory EP, Park GR. Pharmacokinetics of morphine in two children before and after liver transplantation. *Br J Anaesth* 1986; **58**: 1218–23.

27 Haberer JP, Schoeffler P, Couderc E, Duvaldstin P. Fentanyl pharmacokinetics in anaesthetised patients with cirrhosis. *Br J Anaesth* 1982; **54**: 1267–70.

28 Sparr HJ, Wierda JM, Proost JH, *et al.* Pharmacodynamics and pharmacokinetics of rocuronium in intensive care patients. *Br J Anaesth* 1997; **78**: 267–73.

29 Park GR. Pharmacokinetics and pharmacodynamics in the critically ill patient. *Xenobiotica* 1993; **23**: 1195–1230.

30 Howarth DM, Sampson DC, Hawker FH, Young A. Digoxin like immunoreactive substances in the plasma of intensive care unit patients: relationship to organ dysfunction. *Anaesth Int Care* 1990; **18**: 45–52.

31 Lipman J, Gomersall CD, Gin T, *et al.* Continuous infusion ceftazidime in intensive care: a randomised control trial. *J Antimicrob Chemother* 1999; **43**: 309–311.

32 Bressolle F, Kinowski JM, de la Coussaye JE, *et al.* Clinical pharmacokinetics during continuous haemofiltration. *Clin Pharmacokinet* 1994; **26**: 457–71.

33 Reetze-Bonorden P, Bohler J, Keller E. Drug dosage in patients during continuous renal replacement therapy. Pharmacokinetic and therapeutic considerations. *Clin Pharmacokinet* 1993; **24**: 362–79.

34 Keller E, Bohler J, Busse-Grawitz A, *et al.* Single dose kinetics of piperacillin during continuous arteriovenous hemodialysis in intensive care patients. *Clin Nephrol* 1995; **43** (suppl. 1): S20–3.

35 Ververs TF, van Dijk A, Vinks SA, *et al.* Pharmacokinetics and dosing regimen of meropenem in critically ill patients receiving continuous venovenous hemofiltration. *Crit Care Med* 2000; **28**: 3412–6.

36 Giles LJ, Jennings AC, Thomson AH, *et al.* Pharmacokinetics of meropenem in intensive care patients receiving continuous veno-venous hemofiltration or hemodiafiltration. *Crit Care Med* 2000; **28**: 632–7.

37 van Dalen R, Vree TB. Pharmacokinetics of antibiotics in critically ill patients. *Int Care Med* 1990; **16**: S235–8.

38 Reed RL, Wu AH, Miller-Crotchett P, *et al.* Pharmacokinetic monitoring of nephrotoxic antibiotics in

surgical intensive care patients. *J Trauma* 1989; **29**: 1462–70.

39 Moore RD, Lietman PS, Smith CR. Clinical response to aminoglycoside therapy: importance of the ratio of peak concentration to minimal inhibitory concentration. *J Infect Dis* 1987; **155**: 93–9.

40 Marik PE, Havlik I, Monteagudo FSE, Lipman J. The pharmacokinetics of amikacin in critically ill adult and paediatric patients: comparison of once- versus twice-daily dosing regimens. *J Antimicrob Chemother* 1991; **27C**: 81–9.

41 Pea F, Porreca L, Baraldo M, Furlanut M. High vancomycin dosage regimens required by intensive care unit patients cotreated with drugs to improve haemodynamics following cardiac surgical procedures. *J Antimicrob Chemother* 2000; **45**: 329–35.

42 Boereboom FT, Ververs FF, Blankestijn PJ, *et al.* Vancomycin clearance during continous venovenous

haemofiltration in critically ill patients. *Intensive Care Med* 1999; **25**: 1100–4.

43 Boucher BA, Kuhl DA, Hickerson WL. Pharmacokinetics of systemically administered antibiotics in patients with thermal injury. *Clin Infect Dis* 1992; **14**: 458–63.

44 Brown G, Dodek P. An evaluation of empiric vs. nomogram-based dosing of heparin in an intensive care unit. *Crit Care Med* 1997; **25**: 1534–8.

45 Bauer LA. Interference of oral phenytoin absorption by continuous nasogastric feedings. *Neurology* 1982; **32**: 570–2.

46 Yoshida N, Oda Y, Nishi S, *et al.* Effect of barbiturate therapy on phenytoin pharmacokinetics. *Crit Care Med* 1993; **21**: 1514–22.

47 Richer M, Lam YWF. Hypoxia, arterial pH and theophylline deposition. *Clin Pharmacokinet* 1993; **25**: 283–99.

78

Management of acute poisoning
D L A Wyncoll

Acute poisoning remains one of the commonest medical emergencies, accounting for 10–20% of hospital medical admissions. Although, in the majority of cases, the drug ingestion is intentional, the mortality remains low. There are specific antidotes available for a small number of poisons and drugs; however, in most intoxications, basic supportive care is the main requirement and recovery will follow. This chapter is a hands-on guide to the general management of acute poisoning and drug intoxication. Larger reference books should be sourced, if specific detail is required.

Clinical toxicology remains an experience-based specialty; consequently, many recommendations are based on a small literature of case reports, rather than controlled clinical studies. In recent years, toxicological experts have produced position statements and clinical guidelines on certain aspects of care, and these will be referenced when possible.

GENERAL PRINCIPLES

The general principles of the management of poisoned patients are diagnosis, clinical examination and resuscitation, investigations, drug manipulation, specific measures and continued supportive care. In the more acute situations, these actions often have to be carried out simultaneously.

AIRWAY AND VENTILATION

In acute poisoned patients who are unconscious, dentures should be removed and the oropharynx cleared of food and vomit. Tracheal intubation and airway protection is almost always necessary when a patient tolerates insertion of an oropharyngeal airway. Inadequate spontaneous ventilation, determined clinically or by arterial blood gas (ABG) analysis, obviously requires ventilatory support. Venous access should be established, and circulatory assessment must be made. Basic observations, including blood pressure, pulse rate, peripheral perfusion and urine output, should be

recorded. There are very few tricks or traps as to the use of invasive monitoring and inotropic drugs, and the principles are similar to those covered elsewhere in this book.

CLINICAL EXAMINATION

A standard clinical examination should be carried out, looking particularly for needle marks or evidence of previous self-harm. The Glasgow Coma Scale, although designed for head injured patients, is frequently used. However, descriptive documentation of the degree of impaired consciousness is much more valuable. When patients are unconscious and no history is available, the diagnosis depends upon excluding other common causes of coma (Table 78.1) and consideration of any circumstantial evidence. Specific attention should be paid to the temperature, pupil size, respiratory and heart rate, as these may help to restrict the list of potential toxins (Table 78.2).

INVESTIGATIONS

Important initial investigations include:

- *Urinalysis*: with a sample kept for later analysis if required (rapid reaction dipsticks are available to screen for common drugs of abuse/recreational drugs).
- *Basic biochemistry*: many drugs are dependent on renal elimination. Significant renal insufficiency may alter management.

Table 78.1 Common causes of coma other than acute poisoning

Intracranial bleeds
   Subarachnoid haemorrhage
   Subdural/extradural haematomas
Meningitis or encephalitis
Diabetic comas
Uraemic encephalopathy

Table 78.2 Clinical effects of the common poisons

Skin	
Bullae	Barbiturates, tricyclics
Sweating	Salicylates, organophosphates, amphetamines, cocaine
Pupils	
Constricted	Opioids, organophosphates
Dilated	Hypoxia, hypothermia, tricyclics, phenothiazines, anticholinergics
Convulsions	Tricyclics, isoniazid, lithium, amphetamines, theophylline, carbon monoxide, phenothiazines, cocaine
Temperature	
Pyrexia	Anticholinergics, tricyclics, salicylates, amphetamine, cocaine
Hypothermia	Barbiturates, alcohol, opioids
Cardiac rhythm	
Bradycardia	Digoxin, β-blockers, organophosphates
Tachycardia	Salicylates, theophylline, anticholinergics
Arrhythmias	Digoxin, phenothiazines, tricyclics, anticholinergics

- *ABG analysis*: metabolic and/or respiratory acidosis are most common. Aspirin may initially cause a respiratory alkalosis. Metabolic alkaloses are unusual.
- *Anion gap* = $([Na^+] + [K^+]) - ([Cl^-] + [HCO_3^-])$: it is normally 10–14. Ethanol, methanol, ethylene glycol, metformin, cyanide, isoniazid or salicylates are the most frequent causes of a high anion gap metabolic acidosis in clinical toxicology.
- *Osmolal gap*: this is the difference between the laboratory measured osmolality (O_m) and the calculated osmolality (O_c). $O_c = 2(Na^+ + K^+)$ + urea + glucose. The osmolal gap is normally <10. Causes of a raised osmolal gap are ethanol, methanol and ethylene glycol.
- *Chest X-ray*: inhalation of gastric contents is not uncommon.
- *Drug levels*: these are rarely helpful except in specific poisonings. They include paracetamol, salicylates, iron, digoxin and lithium.

GUT DECONTAMINATION

EMESIS

Ipecacuanha-induced emesis is no longer recommended for two reasons.[1] First, it is ineffective at removing significant quantities of poisons from the stomach and, second, it limits the use of activated charcoal.

GASTRIC LAVAGE

Unless performed within 1 h of drug ingestion, it is no longer recommended.[2] If performed after this time, the amount of poison removed is insignificant and lavage may only propel unabsorbed poison into the small intestine.[3] Prior intubation is essential when laryngeal competence is absent or doubtful, especially because, in the majority of overdoses, pulmonary aspiration is more lethal than the ingested drug. To perform gastric lavage, the patient should be positioned head-down on the left side, and then a large-bore tube (36–40 Fr) with large side-holes is passed into the stomach. The tube is aspirated before lavage is started, then tepid water instilled and recovered completely before continuing. The lavage is repeated until the return is clear; stomach massage or gastroscopy may assist removal of coalesced drug masses. Sodium, water and heat balance are of major importance in children. Gastric lavage is contraindicated in ingestions of corrosives, caustics and acids; oesophageal or gastric perforation may occur. Inhalation of petrol, paraffin or white spirits can cause intense pneumonitis.

ACTIVATED CHARCOAL

Activated charcoal is now the first-line treatment for most acute poisonings.[4] Owing to its large surface area and porous structure, it is highly effective at adsorbing many toxins with few exceptions. Exceptions include elemental metals, pesticides, strong acids and alkalis, and cyanide. It should be given to all patients who present within 1 h of ingestion, although it is also acceptable to administer it after 1 h, if it follows an overdose of a substance that slows gastric emptying (e.g. opioids, tricyclic antidepressants). Repeated doses of charcoal can increase the elimination of some drugs by interrupting their entero-enteric and enterohepatic circulation. Indications for repeated dose activated charcoal are shown in Table 78.3.[5] Activated charcoal is given in 50 g doses for adults and 1 g/kg for children. It commonly causes vomiting; therefore consider giving an anti-emetic prior to administration. Repeated doses are given at 4-hourly intervals.

WHOLE BOWEL IRRIGATION

This is a newer method of gastric decontamination that is indicated for a limited number of poisons.[6] Whole bowel irrigation involves administration of non-absorbable polyethylene glycol solution to cause a liquid stool and

Table 78.3 Drug intoxications where multiple-dose activated charcoal may be beneficial

Carbamazepine
Theophylline
Digoxin
Quinine
Phenobarbitone
Dapsone
Sustained-release preparations

reduce drug absorption by physically forcing contents rapidly through the gastrointestinal tract. Polyethylene glycol preparations are still occasionally used in surgical units for 'bowel preparation' prior to surgery. Indications include large ingestions of iron or lithium, ingestion of drug-filled packets/condoms ('body packers'), and large ingestions of sustained-release or enteric-coated drugs (e.g. theophylline). At present, efficacy is based on case reports alone.

ENHANCING DRUG ELIMINATION

In the overwhelming majority of patients who present after an overdose, gut decontamination techniques and supportive care are all that is required. In a limited number of acute poisonings, it may be necessary to consider methods to enhance elimination.

FORCED ALKALINE DIURESIS (URINARY ALKALINIZATION)

Alkaline diuresis may be useful for serious poisonings with:

- Salicylates[7]
- Chlorpropamide
- Phenobarbitone

This technique is difficult to perform well and potentially hazardous. Essentially a diuresis is induced with an osmotic diuretic such as mannitol to produce a urine output of 2–3 ml/kg per h. Intravenous sodium bicarbonate (approximately 1.26%) is infused to maintain a neutral balance and to attempt to achieve a urine pH of approximately 7–8 and blood pH >7.45. Care must be taken to ensure the potassium does not fall rapidly.

EXTRACORPOREAL TECHNIQUES

Numerous extracorporeal techniques are potentially available to aid drug removal in the poisoned patient. These include plasmapheresis, haemodialysis, haemofiltration, haemodiafiltration and haemoperfusion. There are limited data on drug clearance by these techniques in the literature and it is not possible to extrapolate from one system to the other. At present, knowledge of the principles of the methods and the kinetics of the drug involved is relied upon.

Extracorporeal techniques should only be considered when there are clinical features or markers of severe toxicity, failure to respond to full supportive care coupled with poisoning by a drug that can potentially be removed. Impairment of the normal route of elimination of the compound may also influence the decision. Use of extracorporeal techniques is probably only worthwhile if total body clearance is increased by at least 30%. Haemoperfusion is rarely performed in most intensive care units and intermittent haemodialysis often confined to renal units. Consequently, the use of continuous haemofiltration with or without dialysis, using filtration rates of greater than 50–100 ml/kg per h, is likely to be equally effective when an extracorporeal technique is indicated.

CONTINUED SUPPORTIVE THERAPY

Self-poisoned patients do not always meet with the sympathies of the admitting medical team. Try to think of such patients as medical challenges rather than merely instances of self-inflicted illness. Apart from specific measures that are described subsequently, general care of the unconscious unstable patient should be continued. This includes monitoring of vital signs and provision of organ support when necessary. Attention should also be paid to fluid balance, correction of electrolytes, initiation of nutritional support and prompt treatment of nosocomial infection. Overall, in spite of the significant initial physiological disturbance, this group of patients usually has a good outcome.

SPECIFIC THERAPY OF SOME COMMON OR DIFFICULT OVERDOSES

This section emphasizes only those features that may aid clinical diagnosis or prognosis. Treatment suggestions are always intended to support those measures described under general principles. Some new and controversial therapies are mentioned.

AMPHETAMINES (INCLUDING ECSTASY)

CLINICAL FEATURES
Symptoms of mild overdose include sweating, dry mouth and anxiety. Although the majority of ecstasy patients are dehydrated, a proportion have hyponatraemia from drinking water to excess. More severe features include hypertonia, hyperreflexia, hallucinations and hypertension. Supraventricular dysrhythmias may follow with coma, convulsions and the risk of haemorrhagic stroke. A hyperthermic syndrome may develop with hyperpyrexia

leading to rhabdomyolysis, metabolic acidosis, acute renal failure, disseminated intravascular coagulation (DIC) and multiple organ failure.

TREATMENT

Activated charcoal should be considered up to 1 h post ingestion. Benzodiazepines are useful for agitated or psychotic patients and may have a central effect in reducing tachycardia, hypertension and hyperpyrexia. If benzodiazepines fail to control hypertension, other classes of antihypertensives should be started, such as alphablockers, labetalol or direct vasodilators. Hyperpyrexia should be treated in the standard manner including administration of cold fluids. Beyond this, there have been a few reports of the use of dantrolene.[8] In the future, specific centrally acting agents such as cyproheptadine and ketanserin may be available to reduce temperature.

BARBITURATES

CLINICAL FEATURES

The central nervous, cardiovascular and respiratory systems are depressed. Cardiovascular depression is due to vasomotor centre depression and a toxic effect on myocardium and peripheral vessels. Hypotension and relative hypovolaemia may be significant.

TREATMENT

Treatment is supportive, however, urinary alkalinization hastens elimination of phenobarbitone.

BENZODIAZEPINES

CLINICAL FEATURES

Overdose is common, but clinical features are not usually severe unless complicated by other drugs, pre-existing disease or the extremes of age.

TREATMENT

Flumazenil is a specific antagonist; however, its brief duration of action limits its use to diagnostic purposes. Moreover, flumazenil may cause other symptoms in patients who have ingested a cocktail of drugs (e.g. precipitation of fits in patients co-ingesting tricyclic antidepressants), consequently treatment remains supportive.

β-BLOCKERS

CLINICAL FEATURES

There is a wide variation in the individual response to β-blocker overdose. Those with cardiac disease are more at risk of complications. Hypotension and bradycardia predominate, and the degree of heart block can range from a prolonged PR interval through to complete heart block and asystole. Cardiogenic shock and pulmonary oedema are not uncommon.[9]

TREATMENT

Activated charcoal should be considered up to 1 h post ingestion and multiple-dose charcoal in patients who have ingested sustained-release preparations. The role of atropine is not clear, although it is commonly used in patients who have bradycardia and hypotension.[10] If symptomatic treatment fails then other options such as glucagon (up to 10 mg i.v.), an adrenaline infusion or cardiac pacing are indicated. Glucagon often comes as a dried powder with a phenol diluent. The powder should be dissolved in 5% dextrose, as the phenol diluent in large amounts is a myocardial depressant.

BUTYROPHENONES (INCLUDING HALOPERIDOL)

CLINICAL FEATURES

Drowsiness and extrapyramidal effects are most common. Rarely hypotension, QT prolongation, arrhythmias and convulsions develop.

TREATMENT

Activated charcoal should be considered up to 1 h post ingestion, otherwise treatment is supportive. Extrapyramidal symptoms can be treated with procyclidine or benztropine. If ventricular arrhythmias do occur, they are best treated with cardioversion; class 1a antiarrhythmics are theoretically detrimental.

CALCIUM CHANNEL BLOCKERS

CLINICAL FEATURES

The cardiac effects of these drugs predominate in overdose, particularly hypotension and atrioventricular block, although reflex tachycardia occurs with nifedipine. Hypotension occurs due to peripheral vasodilatation and negative inotropy. Severe toxicity may occur in patients who initially appear well, when sustained-release preparations have been ingested.[11]

TREATMENT

Activated charcoal should be considered up to 1 h post ingestion and multiple-dose charcoal in patients who have ingested sustained-release preparations. Treatment remains supportive; however, i.v. calcium chloride is often given in patients who remain hypotensive despite fluid administration.[12] Atropine is often used for bradycardia, and occasionally cardiac pacing may be necessary.

CANNABIS

CLINICAL FEATURES

Overdose is unusual following smoking of cannabis; however, high doses can produce an acute paranoid psychosis. Ataxia, nystagmus, tachycardia and confusion have been reported after ingestion in children. In adults, i.v. abuse of the crude extract may cause abdominal pain, fever, hypotension, pulmonary oedema and DIC.

TREATMENT

Treatment is supportive and most patients only have mild symptoms. Activated charcoal should be considered for children who have ingested cannabis.[13]

CARBAMAZEPINE

Absorption is slow and unpredictable; moreover, maximum serum concentrations may not be achieved until 72 h after ingestion. Carbamazepine undergoes enterohepatic recirculation and is metabolized to an active metabolite.

CLINICAL FEATURES

Nystagmus, ataxia, tremor and fits are common but, in severe overdose, fluctuating coma and severe tachycardia or bradycardia may occur. Plasma concentrations of carbamazepine and the active metabolite can be measured, but they do not correlate well with toxicity.

TREATMENT

Gastric lavage should be used if a patient presents within 1 h of a massive overdose. Multiple-dose activated charcoal is indicated in large ingestions or symptomatic patients, and may help elimination even if initiated several hours after the overdose.

CARBON MONOXIDE (CO)

Haldane first described symptoms of CO toxicity in 1919 and the mechanisms of toxicity remain unclear. Smokers may have up to 10% of their haemoglobin bound to CO (i.e. carboxyhaemoglobin, COHb) without deleterious effects. During CO poisoning, oxygen delivery to the heart and brain is increased. There is no marker that reliably detects CO poisoning. Whilst coma and/or COHb levels >40% always indicate serious poisoning, delayed deterioration can occur in their absence. Affinity of CO for haemoglobin is approximately 240 times that of oxygen.

CLINICAL FEATURES

Neurological signs vary from mild confusion through to seizures and coma. A history of loss of consciousness should always be sought and may be the only indicator of significant poisoning. ST segment changes may be present on electrocardiogram (ECG). In the absence of respiratory depression or aspiration, PaO_2 will be normal. It is essential that SaO_2 is measured directly by a co-oximeter, and not calculated. Cherry-pink skin is only seen in textbooks; cyanosis is far more common.

TREATMENT

After basic resuscitative measures, high flow oxygen (up to 100% if possible) should be administered and continued until the COHb level is less than 5%. This some-times takes up to 24 h. Hyperbaric oxygen, although often used, remains controversial. There have been two randomized, prospective and blinded studies comparing the use of oxygen at atmospheric and hyperbaric pressures.[14,15] The results are not entirely consistent but there is a suggestion of benefit for significant exposures if used early. The logistical difficulties of transporting unstable poisoned patients to hyperbaric centres should not be underestimated.

CHLOROQUINE

CLINICAL FEATURES

Hypotension, hypokalaemia, convulsions, ventricular arrhythmias and sudden cardiac arrest may result from severe poisoning.

TREATMENT

Activated charcoal should be considered up to 1 hour post ingestion. Vasopressors may be required until hypotension is reversed, together with diazepam for agitated patients. Hypokalaemia is common and may be protective in the early stage. It is self-correcting and, consequently, aggressive potassium replacement is not recommended.[16]

CLOZAPINE

CLINICAL FEATURES

Clinical effects in large overdose include tachycardia, hypotension, arrhythmias and coma.

TREATMENT

Treatment is supportive; however, extrapyramidal symptoms can be treated with procyclidine or benztropine.

COCAINE

CLINICAL FEATURES

Features of severe intoxication include hyperreflexia, drowsiness and convulsions.[17] Severe hypertension may cause subarachnoid or intracerebral haemorrhage, and coronary artery spasm may result in myocardial infarction or ventricular arrhythmias; fatalities generally occur early. Hyperthermia associated with rhabdomyolysis, acute renal failure and DIC may also occur.

TREATMENT

The toxic dose is variable and depends upon tolerance, presence of other drugs and route of administration, but ingestion of >1 g is potentially fatal. Blood pressure and ECG monitoring should be instituted early and activated charcoal administered within 1 h of ingestion. Benzodiazepines are useful for agitated or psychotic patients and may have a central effect in reducing tachycardia, hypertension and hyperpyrexia. If benzodiazepines fail to control hypertension, other classes of antihypertensives should be started, such as α-blockers, labetalol or direct vasodilators. The use of β-blockers is controversial and should be used with caution because of the risk of unopposed alpha-stimulation. Hyperthermia should be treated in the standard manner including administration of cold fluids, physical cooling measures and in the presence of convulsions, sedation, paralysis and ventilation.

CYANIDE

CLINICAL FEATURES

Severe toxicity is rapidly fatal; however, features include coma, respiratory depression, hypotension and metabolic acidosis. More moderate features include brief loss of consciousness, convulsions and vomiting. Rescuers must ensure that they do not become contaminated themselves.

TREATMENT

Inhaled amyl nitrate and 100% oxygen may well have been given at the scene, and it is present in 'cyanide antidote kits'. Following this, there are a number of options:

1 Patients with severe features need dicobalt edetate 300 mg i.v. over 1 min, followed by 50 ml dextrose 50% i.v., with a further 300 mg if there is no response.
2 Patients with moderate features should be given sodium thiosulphate 12.5 g i.v.
3 Hydroxocobalamin i.v. can also be given, but suitable preparations are not always available.
4 Patients with a metabolic acidosis should be given sodium bicarbonate.

DIGOXIN

CLINICAL FEATURES

Toxicity may result from ingestion of greater than 2–3 mg or, more commonly, from taking too high a daily dose and/or a reduction in renal elimination. Any cardiac arrhythmia may occur and adverse effects may be delayed for some hours. Severe poisoning can produce hyperkalaemia and hypotension.

TREATMENT

Activated charcoal should be considered up to 1 h post ingestion and multiple-dose charcoal may be effective by interrupting enterohepatic recirculation of the drug. A digoxin level may be helpful and hyper/hypokalaemia should be corrected. Hypomagnesaemia must also be excluded. Cardiac pacing may be necessary to control symptomatic bradyarrhythmias and amiodarone may be useful for tachyarrhythmias. DC shock should be avoided if possible, but when essential must be initiated at low energy levels (e.g. 20–50 J). Digoxin-specific antibodies are indicated in severe hyperkalaemia, resistant to basic treatment, bradycardia resistant to atropine, or ventricular arrhythmias.[18]

IRON

CLINICAL FEATURES

The corrosive action on gastric mucosa results in vomiting, pain, haematemesis and melaena and gastric perforation. Severe poisoning is reflected by plasma concentrations more than 90 μmol/l in children and 145 μmol/l in adults within 4 h of ingestion.

TREATMENT

Desferrioxamine mesylate (an iron chelator) 5 g is left in the stomach after lavage. Simultaneously, 2 g is injected i.m. and an infusion of 15 mg/kg per h (maximum 80 mg/kg) is commenced. Treatment is continued until serum concentration and clinical status are satisfactory.

ISONIAZID

CLINICAL FEATURES

Severe toxicity is characterized by coma, respiratory depression, hypotension and convulsions, and may result from doses >80 mg/kg. Protracted convulsions can cause rhabdomyolysis and acute renal failure.

TREATMENT

Gastric lavage followed by activated charcoal should be considered for large ingestions seen within 1 h. Convulsions should be controlled with diazepam and pyridoxine, which is a specific antidote for isoniazid poisoning. Pyridoxine should be given prophylactically for large ingestions as early as possible, since it may prevent the development of complications.

LITHIUM

CLINICAL FEATURES

Serum lithium levels >1.5 mmol/l are toxic, with the main feature being varied neurological symptoms and signs. Severe poisoning may result in permanent neurological damage and nephrogenic diabetes insipidus.

TREATMENT

Serum concentrations >3.5–4.0 mmol or patients with signs of severe toxicity generally require extracorporeal elimination techniques. Nevertheless, the majority of patients respond to general supportive measures.

METHANOL (INCLUDING ETHYLENE GLYCOL)

CLINICAL FEATURES

Methanol and ethylene glycol are essentially non-toxic. The metabolism of these products to their aldehydes and associated acids, following a latent period of 12–18 h, accounts for the metabolic acidosis, ocular toxicity and mortality that are occasionally seen. Mild features include dizziness, drowsiness and abdominal pain. When treatment is delayed, metabolic acidosis develops with drowsiness, coma and convulsions. The osmolal and the anion gap are increased.

TREATMENT

Activated charcoal does not adsorb alcohols. Metabolic acidosis should be treated with bicarbonate and serum electrolytes measured. Ethanol prevents formation of the toxic metabolites and is the most established treatment. 4-methylpyrazole has also been used and may be preferable in patients with impaired conscious levels.[19]

MONOAMINE-OXIDASE INHIBITORS (MAOIS)

CLINICAL FEATURES

MAOIs cause an accumulation of amine neurotransmitters and are readily absorbed from the gastrointestinal tract and metabolized in the liver. Overdose results in neuromuscular excitation (muscle spasm, rigidity and opisthotonus) and sympathetic overactivity (tremor, tachycardia, hyperthermia, hypertension with fixed and dilated pupils).

TREATMENT

Management is similar to that of intoxication with amphetamines and cocaine (see above).

NON-STEROIDAL ANTI-INFLAMMATORY DRUGS (NSAIDS)

CLINICAL FEATURES

Most overdoses with NSAIDS do not cause serious problems other than a bad attack of gastritis. Exceptions to this rule include mefenamic acid or large ingestions of ibuprofen where self-limiting convulsions and renal failure have been reported.[20]

TREATMENT

Activated charcoal can be given for large ingestions that are seen within 1 h of the overdose. Seizures should be treated with a benzodiazepine and an oral H_2 blocker may ease symptoms of gastrointestinal irritation.

OPIOIDS

CLINICAL FEATURES

Overdose is characterized by pinpoint pupils, drowsiness, shallow breathing and ultimately respiratory failure.

TREATMENT

Activated charcoal may be effective for oral ingestions, otherwise treatment is supportive. Naloxone 0.1–0.4 mg i.v. can be given by bolus and, if there is an inadequate response, repeat doses may be required. Intubation and mechanical ventilation are required if respiratory failure is not rapidly reversed by naloxone.

PARACETAMOL

In normal adults, doses >10 g may exceed the ability of hepatic glutathione to conjugate the toxic metabolite. Plasma concentrations >200 mg/l at 4 h or ≥50mg/l at 12 h (Fig. 78.1) are usually associated with hepatic damage. The treatment should begin at lower levels for those considered to be high risk (Table 78.4). While i.v. acetylcysteine administered more than 16 h after ingestion may not prevent severe liver damage, it should still be given since outcome from paracetamol-induced fulminant hepatic failure is improved.[21] Severe hepatic injury has a 10% mortality. The majority of patients recover within 1–2 weeks.

CLINICAL FEATURES

Nausea and vomiting may be the only features present in the first 24 h.

TREATMENT

- Gastric lavage, administration of activated charcoal, and assaying drug concentrations are performed as described in general principles.

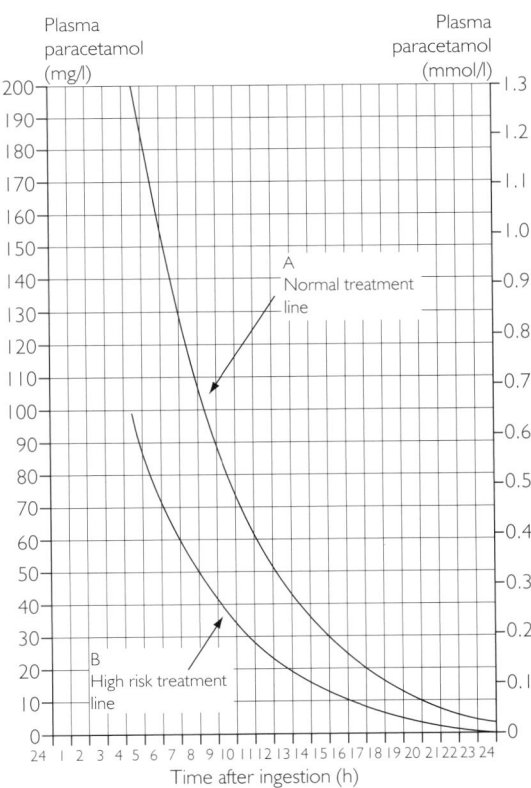

Fig. 78.1 Treatment lines following paracetamol overdose in relation to time after ingestion and plasma levels. (Figure from Paracetamol Information Centre, London and the Welsh National Poisons Unit Cardiff)

Table 78.4 Those at high risk of liver damage following paracetamol overdose

1	Regular alcohol consumption
2	Regular use of enzyme inducing drugs
	Phenytoin, carbamazepine, phenobarbitone, rifampicin
3	Conditions causing glutathione depletion
	HIV, eating disorders, malnutrition and cystic fibrosis

- *N*-acetylcysteine 150 mg/kg in 200 ml 5% dextrose is infused over 15 min, followed by 50 mg/kg in 500 ml 5% dextrose over 4 h and 100 mg/kg in 1 l 5% dextrose over 16 h (total dose 300 mg/kg in 20 h). Maximum protective effect is time-dependent. An ingestion-treatment interval of less than 10 h gives the best results.
- In fulminant hepatic failure, the last dose (100 mg/kg in 1 l 5% dextrose over 16 h) is repeated until the patient's INR is <2.
- Expert opinion should be sought early on from a regional centre if liver failure is progressive since liver transplantation may become necessary.

PARAQUAT

In adult humans the lethal dose is 3–6 g (i.e. 15–30 ml of 20% w/v liquid concentrate). The mortality rate in patients ingesting the liquid concentrate is 25–75%. The lung is the primary target organ, with the injury being enhanced by oxygen. Peak concentrations are achieved between 0.5 and 2.0 h.

CLINICAL FEATURES

Initial symptoms are gastrointestinal pain and vomiting with corrosive effects on the mouth, pharynx and oesophagus. Dyspnoea and pulmonary oedema follow within 24 h, progressing to irreversible fibrosis and death. Cardiac, renal and hepatic dysfunctions are common.

TREATMENT

Activated charcoal should be given if the patient presents within 1 h. Other than basic measures, such as antiemetics, analgesics and fluid replacement, the efficacy of specific treatment options is not established. A recent trial suggests that pulse therapy with cyclophosphamide 15 mg/kg and methyl prednisone 1 gm has been beneficial although this remains to be confirmed.[22] Palliative care is probably the best approach in patients with very high plasma levels.

PHENOTHIAZINES

CLINICAL FEATURES

Anticholinergic and cardiac effects are similar to tricyclic overdose.

TREATMENT

Treatment is supportive.

PHENYTOIN

CLINICAL FEATURES

Absorption is slow and unpredictable; moreover, maximum serum concentrations may not be achieved until 72 h after ingestion. After initial nausea and vomiting, neurological symptoms develop including drowsiness, dysarthria and ataxia, and may ultimately progress to seizures. Cardiovascular toxicity is rare unless the overdose has been given i.v.

TREATMENT

Most patients require nothing more than supportive measures.

SALICYLATES (ASPIRIN)

Moderate toxicity occurs with serum concentrations 500–750 mg/l (3600–5500 μmol/l), and severe toxicity with concentrations >750 mg/l. Serum concentrations alone do not determine prognosis. The elimination half-life increases significantly with increasing concentrations. Small reductions in pH produce large increases in non-ionized salicylate, which then penetrates tissues.

CLINICAL FEATURES

Tinnitus, deafness, diaphoresis, pyrexia, hypoglycaemia, haematemesis, hyperventilation and hypokalaemia may all occur. Coma, hyperpyrexia, pulmonary oedema and acidaemia are reported as more common in fatal cases, which present late.

TREATMENT

Multiple-dose activated charcoal may be effective but is not established. Vitamin K and glucose are used to correct hypoprothrombinaemia and hypoglycaemia. A forced alkaline diuresis (see above), will decrease the amount of non-ionized drug available to enter tissues, but is hazardous and should only be used for the most severely ill patients. Extracorporeal techniques are very effective in removing salicylates and correcting acid–base disturbance, although indications for their use are yet to be defined; however, they should be considered for severe cases.

SELECTIVE SEROTONIN REUPTAKE INHIBITORS (SSRIS) OR 5-HT DRUGS

Drugs include citalopram, fluoxetine, fluvoxamine, paroxetine and sertraline.

CLINICAL FEATURES

Drowsiness, tachycardia and mild hypertension are the commonest features.

TREATMENT

Activated charcoal should be considered up to 1 h post ingestion, otherwise treatment is supportive.[23]

THEOPHYLLINE

CLINICAL FEATURES

Acute theophylline poisoning is potentially very serious and severe poisoning carries a high mortality. Toxic effects such as agitation, tremor, nausea, vomiting and sinus tachycardia become evident at <30 mg/l (167 μmol/l). Concentrations >60 mg/l (333 μmol/l) in acute poisoning or >40 mg/l (222 μmol/l) in chronic usage frequently result in seizures, malignant ventricular arrhythmias, severe hypotension and death.[24] A key feature is hypokalaemia, which predisposes to arrhythmias and rhabdomyolysis. Measuring plasma theophylline levels confirms the ingestion and may help in deciding elimination methods; in the majority of poisoned patients, they do not aid management. Sustained-release preparations may result in delayed onset and prolonged toxicity.

TREATMENT

Gastric lavage is indicated for those who present early, but multiple-dose activated charcoal is highly effective. Electrolyte and acid–base disturbances should be corrected rapidly since this may be the only treatment required in many cases. Convulsions should be treated with benzodiazepines and cardiac arrhythmias with beta-blockers in non-asthmatic patients. Extracorporeal elimination techniques may be indicated for severe cases. Whole bowel irrigation may be of use for sustained-release preparation overdoses.

TRICYCLIC ANTIDEPRESSANTS (TCAS)

CLINICAL FEATURES

These drugs remain the leading cause of death from overdose in patients arriving at the emergency department alive and account for up to one-half of all overdose related adult intensive care admissions.[25] Features include anticholinergic effects such as warm dry skin, tachycardia, blurred vision, dilated pupils and urinary retention. Severe features include respiratory depression, reduced conscious level and cardiac arrhythmias, fits and hypotension. Arrhythmias may be predicted by a QRS duration >100 ms on the ECG; a QRS duration of >160 ms increases risk of seizures.[26] All forms of rhythm and conduction disturbance have been described, and are not necessarily predicted by the ECG.[27] Amoxapine typically causes features of severe poisoning in the absence of QRS widening. Cardiac toxicity is due mainly to quinidine-like actions, slowing phase 0 depolarization of the action potential. Other mechanisms include impaired automaticity, cholinergic blockade and inhibition of neuronal catecholamine uptake. Toxicity is worsened by acidaemia, hypotension and hyperthermia.

TREATMENT

After supportive care as outlined above, including multiple-dose activated charcoal, continuous cardiac monitoring is essential. Increasing arterial pH to ≥ 7.45 significantly reduces the available free drug and this may be the best way to avoid TCA toxicity. Mild hyperventilation and 8.4% sodium bicarbonate in 50 mmol aliquots achieves this strategy and may improve outcome.[28] Bicarbonate should probably be given in all cases of QRS prolongation (even in the absence of metabolic acidosis), malignant arrhythmias, hypotension or metabolic acidosis. If arrhythmias occur, avoid class 1a agents; lignocaine may be best. Benzodiazepines are the drug of choice for sedation, treatment of seizures and may prevent emergence delirium.

VALPROATE

CLINICAL FEATURES

Most overdoses follow a benign course, with nausea, mild drowsiness and confusion. Coma can occur in large ingestions with cerebral oedema.

TREATMENT

Valproate levels are of little value, except to confirm the ingestion. There is poor correlation between depth of coma and free or total valproate levels. Supportive management is all that is usually required. Rapid absorption occurs and therefore gastric lavage or activated charcoal is of little benefit.

VIGABATRIN

CLINICAL FEATURES

Often used for complex partial seizures as an adjunct when monotherapy has failed. Initial symptoms in overdose include vertigo and tremor, progressing to drowsiness and coma.[29]

TREATMENT

No specific care is required beyond general measures.

REFERENCES

1 American Academy of Clinical Toxicology; European Association of Poison Control Centres and Clinical Toxicologists. Position statement: ipecac syrup. *Clin Tox* 1997; **35**: 699–709.

2 American Academy of Clinical Toxicology; European Association of Poison Control Centres and Clinical Toxicologists. Position statement: gastric lavage. *Clin Tox* 1997; **35**: 711–9.

3 Saetta JP, March S, Gaunt ME, *et al*. Gastric emptying procedures in the self-poisoned patient: are we forcing gastric content beyond the pylorus? *J R Soc Med* 1991; **84**: 274–6.

4 American Academy of Clinical Toxicology; European Association of Poison Control Centres and Clinical

Toxicologists. Position statement: single-dose activated charcoal. *Clin Tox* 1997; **35**: 699–709.

5 American Academy of Clinical Toxicology; European Association of Poison Control Centres and Clinical Toxicologists. Position statement and practice guidelines on the use of multi-dose activated charcoal in the treatment of acute poisoning. *Clin Tox* 1999; **37**: 731–51.

6 American Academy of Clinical Toxicology; European Association of Poison Control Centres and Clinical Toxicologists. Position statement: whole bowel irrigation. *Clin Tox* 1997; **35**: 753–62.

7 Prescott LF, Balali-Mood M, Critchley JAJH, Johnstone AF. Diuresis or urinary alkalinisation for salicylate poisoning? *BMJ* 1982; **285**: 1383–6.

8 Singarajah C, Lavies NG. An overdose of ecstasy. A role for dantrolene. *Anaesthesia* 1992; **47**: 686–7.

9 Lip GY, Ferner RE. Poisoning with anti-hypertensive drugs: beta-adrenoceptor blocker drugs. *J Hum Hypertens* 1995; **9**: 213–21.

10 Taboulet P, Cariou A, Berdeaux A, Bismuth C. Pathophysiology and management of self-poisoning with beta-blockers. *J Toxicol Clin Toxicol* 1993; **31**: 531–51.

11 Lip GY, Ferner RE. Poisoning with anti-hypertensive drugs: calcium antagonists. *J Hum Hypertens* 1995; **9**: 155–61.

12 Kenny J. Treating overdose with calcium channel blockers. *BMJ* 1994; **308**: 992–3.

13 MacNab A, Anderson E, Susak K. Ingestion of cannabis: a cause of coma in children. *Pediatr Emerg Care* 1989; **5**: 238–9.

14 Scheinkestel CD, Biley M, Myles PS, *et al.* Hyperbaric or normobaric oxygen for acute carbon monoxide poisoning: a randomised controlled clinical trial. *Med J Aust* 1999; **170**: 203–10.

15. Weaver LK, Hopkins RO, Chan KJ, *et al.* Hyperbaric oxygen for Acute Carbon Monoxide poisoning. *N Engl J Med* 2002; **347**: 1057–67.

16 Jaeger A, Sauder P, Kopferschmitt J, Flesch F. Clinical features and management of poisoning due to antimalarial drugs. *Med Toxicol Adverse Drug Exp* 1987; **2**: 242–73.

17 Paul S, York D. Cocaine abuse: an expanding health-care problem for the 1990s. *Am J Crit Care* 1992; **1**: 109–13.

18 Taboulet P, Baud FJ, Bismuth C. Clinical features and management of digitalis poisoning – rationale for immunotherapy. *J Toxicol Clin Toxicol* 1993; **31**: 247–60.

19 Barceloux DG, Krenzelok EP, Olson K, Watson W. American Academy of Clinical Toxicology Practice Guidelines on the Treatment of Ethylene Glycol Poisoning. *J Toxicol Clin Toxicol* 1999; **37**: 537–60.

20 Smolinske SC, Hall AH, Vandenberg SA. Toxic effects of nonsteroidal anti-inflammatory drugs in overdose. *Drug Safety* 1990; **5**: 252–74.

21 Keays R, Harrison PM, Wendon JA, *et al.* Intravenous acetylcysteine in paracetamol induced fulminant hepatic failure: a prospective controlled study. *N Engl J Med* 1991; **303**: 1026–9.

22 Lin Am J, *Respir Crit Care Med* 1999; **159**: 357–360.

23 Borys DJ, Setzer SC, Ling LJ, *et al.* The effects of fluoxetine in the overdose patient. *J Toxicol Clin Toxicol* 1990; **28**: 331–40.

24 Shannon M. Predictors of major toxicity after theophylline overdose. *Ann Intern Med* 1993; **119**: 1161–7.

25 Newton EH, Shih RD, Hoffman RS. Cyclic antidepressant overdose: a review of current management strategies. *Am J Emerg Med* 1994; **12**: 376–9.

26 Boehert MT, Lovejoy FH. Value of the QRS duration versus the serum drug level in predicting seizures and ventricular arrhythmias after an acute overdose of tricyclic antidepressants. *N Engl J Med* 1985; **313**: 474–9.

27 Harrigan RA, Brady WJ. ECG abnormalities in tricyclic antidepressant ingestion. *Am J Emerg Med* 1999; **17**: 387–93.

28 Hoffman JR, Votey SR, Bayer M, Silver L. Effect of hypertonic sodium bicarbonate in the treatment of moderate-to-severe cyclic antidepressant overdose. *Am J Emerg Med* 1993; **11**: 336–41.

29 Jones AL, Proudfoot AT. Features and management of poisoning with modern drugs used to treat epilepsy. *Q J Med* 1998; **91**: 325–32.

79

Sedation, analgesia and muscle relaxation in the intensive care unit

P V van Heerden

Despite the widespread use of sedative and analgesic agents in the intensive care unit (ICU), the goals of sedation and analgesia are not well-established.[1] Indications for the use of sedative agents include:

- to enable the critically ill patient to tolerate invasive and uncomfortable monitoring and treatment procedures
- to reduce oxygen consumption[2] by reducing patient arousal and activity
- to promote amnesia for events in the ICU.[3]

Sedatives may also be used as specific treatment for conditions, such as epilepsy or tetanus. The delirious patient may require sedation to maintain safety of the patient and carers.

Combinations of opioids and benzodiazepines are commonly used to provide 'sedation' in the ICU. High doses of opioid analgesics may result in significant sedation in their own right and are synergistic with sedative agents such as benzodiazepines. The distinction between *sedation* and *analgesia* is therefore blurred, and makes the definition and attainment of clear sedation goals elusive.

Skilled use of analgesics in the modern ICU ensures that critically ill patients should no longer suffer pain. Pain management relies largely on the use of opioid analgesics, together with regional anaesthetic techniques.

SEDATION

Sedation of patients in the ICU is an integral part of what healthcare workers perceive to be *care and compassion* for the critically ill patient.

Sedative agents are used in an attempt to:

- allay anxiety over the patient's own illness, the welfare of relatives or the risk of death
- ensure adequate rest

- reduce the impact of unpleasant sensations, such as thirst
- reduce the distress of invasive treatment and monitoring, such as endotracheal intubation
- blunt awareness of the environment over which the patient has very little control and in which he/she may be unable to communicate.

Attention to such details as avoiding potentially distressing situations, where possible, allowing adequate access to caring visitors, maintenance of adequate communication with the patient and a positive outlook by the carers will satisfy many of these goals. Small comforts, such as ice chips by mouth, a comfortable mattress or relaxation audio tapes all help this process.

LEVEL OF SEDATION

The level of sedation required will vary, depending on the indication, e.g. heavy sedation may be necessary during the control of status epilepticus, while a much lower level of sedation will be required to tolerate endotracheal intubation. Modern modes of mechanical ventilation do not demand heavy sedation in order to be comfortably tolerated.[4] The aim of sedation should be clear to the treating team and the desired level of sedation should be determined and documented. Once sedation is instituted, the level of sedation should be regularly assessed. Protocol-based therapy reduces drug costs and enhances the quality of sedation and analgesia.[5] Failure to follow such a protocolized approach can result in significant problems, such as[6]:

- 'oversedation' with an increased risk of nosocomial pneumonia
- the need for more frequent neurological assessments including computed axial tomography (CT) scans
- prolonged stay in the ICU
- an increased incidence of psychological problems, such as post traumatic stress disorder and depression.

Table 79.1 Ramsay scale

Level	Response
Awake levels	
1	Patient anxious and agitated or restless or both
2	Patient co-operative, orientated and tranquil
3	Patient responds to commands only
Asleep levels	
4	Brisk response to a light glabellar tap or loud auditory stimulus
5	Sluggish response to a light glabellar tap or loud auditory stimulus
6	No response to a light glabellar tap or loud auditory stimulus

Level of sedation may be assessed by means of a number of measurement tools including:

- Scoring systems such as the Ramsay scale (see Table 79.1), which is a six point scale that ranges from anxious and agitated (level 1) to unresponsive (level 6), judged in response to a standardized stimulus (loud auditory stimulus or glabellar tap).[6] This scale has good interrator reliability and provides a numerical score, suitable for charting on the ICU observation chart and for descriptive purposes.
- Electroencephalography (EEG), which may be either 'raw' or 'processed' and is able to provide a measure of cerebral activity. This monitor is more suitable for assessing depth of anaesthesia and may be difficult to interpret in the encephalopathic patient. Newer easy to use devices using integrated EEG are now appearing but their efficacy and role in ICU have yet to be established.
- Visual analogue scales, which are more suited to the assessment of pain (see below), or for use as a research tool.
- Evoked potentials.[7]

Level of sedation may also be assessed by monitoring physiological parameters for signs of distress. A 'drug free' period every day, when sedative agents are completely withdrawn, is an excellent means of assessing level of sedation[8] – by taking note of the time for a patient to either *wake up* or rise to a predetermined level on the Ramsay Scale.

THE IDEAL SEDATIVE

There is no ideal sedative agent. Sedatives in the future may target specific aspects of sedation, such as hypnosis, anxiolysis or amnesia, without necessarily providing the whole spectrum of sedation for each patient. Currently the ideal sedative would address the following:

- hypnosis/sleep
- anxiolysis
- amnesia
- anticonvulsant
- be non-cumulative
- be independent of renal or hepatic metabolic pathways
- not produce respiratory or cardiovascular depression
- be of modest cost
- have a rapid onset and short offset time
- have no prolonged effects on memory
- have no long-term psychological effects.[9]

SEDATIVE AGENTS USED IN THE ICU

BENZODIAZEPINES

Benzodiazepines (BZAs), as a class, are probably the most widely used sedatives in ICUs. These agents provide hypnosis, amnesia and anxiolysis. They do not provide analgesia. BZAs are good anticonvulsant drugs and also provide for some muscle relaxation. They act via BZA receptors, which are closely associated with $GABA_A$ receptors, resulting in intracellular influx of chloride when activated. These drugs may be given by mouth (PO), per rectum (PR) or intravenously (i.v.). Most commonly in the ICU they are administered by intermittent or continuous i.v. infusion, e.g. midazolam in 1 mg/ml dilution, titrated to effect.

Dosage of these agents is by titration and may vary widely depending on factors such as:

- prior exposure to BZA (increased tolerance)
- age and physiological reserve
- volume status (hypovolaemic patients are more sensitive)
- renal and hepatic dysfunction
- co-administered drugs (whether BZA is combined with an opioid)
- history of alcohol consumption (increased tolerance).

Although some BZAs (e.g. midazolam) are reported to be short-acting, water-soluble agents, there is still potential for accumulation of both parent compound and active metabolites in patients with hepatic and renal dysfunction. This may result in prolonged sedation and increased length of mechanical ventilation and ICU stay. In the critically ill, there may be extensive derangement of the pharmacokinetic profiles of BZAs.[10,11] There is therefore some difficulty in predetermining suitable dosages of these agents. Typically, midazolam in doses of 0.02–0.2 mg/kg per hour may be suitable, with the level titrated to individual response. Longer acting agents, such as diazepam, may be given by intermittent i.v. injection, e.g diazepam 5–10 mg i.v., as necessary.

BZAs are often combined with opioids in a compound 'sedative' infusion. This allows lower doses of BZA to be used, while capitalizing on the opioid effects of respiratory and cough suppression, to facilitate mechanical ventilation.

Flumazenil, the specific BZA antagonist, may be used to reverse the effect of BZAs to reduce unwanted acute side-effects, such as severe hypotension or respiratory depression, or to allow acute neurological assessment of the sedated patient.

INTRAVENOUS ANAESTHETIC AGENTS
Propofol

The i.v. anaesthetic agent propofol (2,6-di-isopropylphenol) is frequently used for sedation in the ICU. It is fast-acting, very effective and with a rapid offset of action (due to its rapid metabolism to inactive metabolites in the liver). These features make it very suitable for use in patients requiring short-term sedation or for anaesthesia for procedures in the ICU. Although propofol has been shown to reduce time on mechanical ventilation compared with BZA (specifically midazolam) sedation, it has not been shown to reduce time in ICU.[12,13] Caution is required in hypovolaemic patients or those with impaired myocardial function as severe hypotension may result. Doses for ICU sedation are generally much lower than the 6–12 mg/kg per hour required for anaesthesia. The diluent in which propofol is delivered is lipid-rich and may have to be taken into account as a source of nutrition and indeed cause of hyperlipidaemia, depending on dosage and duration of therapy. Disodium edetate, present in the propofol solution, does not appear to be harmful in patients receiving long-term infusions of propofol.[14,15]

Thiopentone
Thiopentone is reserved for specific indications, such as management of intractable intracranial hypertension (to reduce cerebral metabolism) or for the treatment of status epilepticus. It is not commonly used as a general sedative agent. Its use is limited by its long duration of action and long terminal half-life when used for prolonged infusions.

Ketamine
Ketamine acts by blocking NMDA-receptors. It produces a sedative state known as 'dissociative anaesthesia', with the following characteristics:

- mild sedation
- amnesia
- analgesia
- reduced motor activity.

The lack of respiratory and cardiovascular depression at lower doses makes this a very safe drug for use in the ICU. Limitations to its use include hallucinations and delirium during the recovery/withdrawal phase. These may be ameliorated by BZA administration. Ketamine may be used specifically for sedation in severe asthmatics (for its bronchodilator effect),[16] in patients following head injury (for its effect at the NMDA receptor)[17] or in patients where analgesia is difficult (e.g. extensive burns).

Etomidate
Etomidate is no longer used for ICU sedation due to its adrenocortical suppressant (immunosuppressant) action.

MAJOR TRANQUILLIZERS
Butyrophenones (e.g. haloperidol) and phenothiazines (e.g. chlorpromazine) are very useful agents for the sedation of delirious patients in the ICU. They act via a range of receptors including dopaminergic (D_1 and D_2), α-adrenergic, histamine, serotonin and cholinergic receptors. Main actions include:

- reduced motor activity
- apathy and reduced initiative
- sedation and drowsiness
- reduced aggression
- antiemetic.

Unwanted effects with these drugs are common and include:

- extrapyramidal effects (dystonia and tardive dyskinesia)
- endocrine effects (e.g. lactation)
- anticholinergic effects (e.g. blurred vision, dry mouth, urinary retention, constipation)
- hypotension
- neuroleptic malignant syndrome.

The main advantage of major tranquillizers over large doses of minor tranquillizers is that they can be used to gain control in difficult situations (e.g. when delirious patients may be a risk to themselves or their carers), without a major risk of respiratory depression. These agents should not be used for long-term sedation, except where they are used for the specific treatment of psychosis. Typically haloperidol, diluted to a 1 mg/ml solution, may be given by repeated i.v. injection in doses of 5–20 mg/h until the delirious patient is approachable. Repeat dosages would then be titrated to allow easy arousal of the patient, with the patient otherwise calm. Haloperidol may also be given by mouth or by i.m. injection.

Olanzapine, a newer 'atypical' antipsychotic agent,[18] is also a useful agent for the sedation of delirious patients when given in oral doses of 5–20 mg/d. It has a much lower side-effect profile than the more 'typical' antipsychotics, especially with respect to motor side-effects.

VOLATILE ANAESTHETIC AGENTS
The widespread use of volatile anaesthetic agents for sedation in the ICU has been limited by:

- the cost of prolonged administration
- the more complex set-up required for the administration of these agents (vapourizer, scavenging apparatus etc.)

- specific side-effects (e.g. 'halothane' hepatitis, accumulation of fluoride ions and consequent renal dysfunction (enflurane and isoflurane) and inactivation of methionine synthase and bone marrow depression (nitrous oxide)).

Volatile agents are useful for short periods of anaesthesia during invasive procedures in the ICU. They may be used, with effect, for longer periods for sedation (up to a few days) in acute severe asthma, due to their bronchodilatory action. Short-term administrations of Entonox (50% nitrous oxide in oxygen) are still useful for analgesia and sedation during painful procedures (e.g. removal of intercostal catheters). This may be given by demand valve (controlled by the patient) or be administered by the medical staff.

OPIOIDS
Although opioids are used primarily for their analgesic action in the ICU (see below), they also produce a degree of sedation. They therefore complement the effect of other sedatives used in the ICU, with which they are often given in combination.

DEXMEDETOMIDINE
Dexmedetomidine is a highly selective novel α_2-agonist, which has been shown to provide safe analgesia and sedation in the ICU[19–21] when given as a single agent by i.v. infusion.

Dosages are: loading dose of 1 μg/kg over 10 min, followed by an infusion of 0.2–0.7 μg/kg per hour.

Infusions longer than 24 hours are currently not recommended. Side-effects may be predicted from the mechanism of action and include hypotension, bradycardia, hypoxaemia and atrial fibrillation. More established α_2-agonists, such as clonidine, may be used to enhance sedation and analgesia when BZA and opioids are used as the mainstay of sedation in the ICU.

ANALGESIA

Pain management is an important priority in the care of critically ill patients.

Many patients present to the ICU with painful conditions or undergo painful procedures during their ICU stay. Pain has a number of adverse consequences:

- it produces anxiety
- it contributes to lack of sleep
- it worsens delirium
- it enhances the stress response – increases circulating catecholamine levels and oxygen consumption
- it results in respiratory embarrassment due to atelectasis and sputum retention
- it leads to immobility and venous and gut stasis.

Pain management comprises a number of modalities in addition to analgesics and local and regional anaesthesia/analgesia such as:

- a caring and supportive medical team, whom the patient can trust
- warm and comfortable surroundings
- attention to pressure areas (e.g. regular turning)
- the use of warm packs
- the use of simple analgesics as appropriate
- bowel and bladder care
- adequate hydration and amelioration of thirst (e.g. moistening the mouth)
- early tracheostomy where indicated to reduce the discomfort of endotracheal intubation
- splinting and early fixation of fractures.

When drug therapy is required to alleviate pain, the following groups of drugs are commonly used:

- opioid analgesics
- simple analgesics
- non-steroidal anti inflammatory (NSAIDS) drugs
- novel agents, such as dexmedetomidine (see above) and tramadol
- local anaesthetic agents
- inhaled agents (see volatile anaesthetic agents above)
- ketamine (see above)
- 'multimodality' supplemental treatments such as acupuncture, acupressure, massage and transcutaneous electrical nerve stimulation (TENS).

OPIOIDS

Opioids remain the mainstay of analgesia in the ICU. This group of drugs encompasses:

- morphine and its analogues (e.g. morphine, diamorphine, codeine)
- semi-synthetic and synthetic agents
  - phenylpiperidine derivatives (e.g. pethidine, fentanyl)
  - methadone derivatives (e.g. methadone, dextropropoxyphene)
  - benzomorphan derivatives (e.g. pentazocine)
  - thebaine derivatives (e.g. buprenorphine).

The effects of opioids are mediated via the three main opioid receptor subtypes μ, κ and σ, which are G-protein coupled receptors and inhibit adenyl cyclase and include:

- analgesia (supraspinal, spinal and peripheral)
- sedation
- pupillary constriction
- respiratory depression and cough suppression
- euphoria or dysphoria
- reduced gastrointestinal motility
- physical dependence.

Opioids are titrated to effect by intermittent injection (usually i.v. in the ICU), or by continuous infusion, which may be nurse-controlled (nurse-controlled analgesia or NCA) or controlled by the patient (patient controlled analgesia or PCA). A suitable regimen is a 1 mg/ml dilution of morphine given by continuous i.v.

infusion, titrated to patient comfort. This is often combined with a BZA, such as midazolam to produce a 'sedative/analgesic' infusion for use in very ill patients on mechanical ventilation (see sedation above). Opioids are also administered via the subarachnoid, extradural, transdermal and intranasal routes.

The effect of analgesia in the clinical setting is judged by:

- patient response, if they are conscious, either verbally by describing the level of pain subjectively or by using a visual analogue score (Figure 79.1)[6]
- physiological markers of distress, e.g. tachycardia, hypertension, diaphoresis, restlessness.

These indicators should be assessed in the clinical context, i.e., is the pathophysiological process likely to be responsible for some, or considerable pain? Analgesia should be administered for a specific indication and to the desired effect. Many factors lead to a wide variation in the experience of pain including:

- personality traits
- the previous experience of pain
- fear
- interpretation of events/disorientation/depersonalization
- age
- degree of tissue damage
- chronic disease and debility.

In the critically ill, the use of opioids may be complicated by:

- wide inter-individual responses to similar dosages, mandating titration of the analgesic especially in debilitated and elderly patients
- severe hypotension following rapid administration, particularly in hypovolaemic patients. Fentanyl and sufentanil may offer advantages over morphine in terms of 'cardiostability'.
- prolonged duration of action, due to accumulation of parent compound and metabolites (e.g. morphine and its major metabolites morphine-3-glucuronide and morphine-6-glucuronide) in the elderly and in patients with renal and hepatic dysfunction. Use of drugs with shorter half-lives (such as alfentanil) or which are less dependent on hepatic and renal pathways for metabolism and excretion (such as remifentanil)[3,17] can reduce this problem.
- constipation, requiring careful attention to detail and the judicious use of prokinetic agents (e.g. metoclopramide, cisapride), to overcome gastric stasis and enable enteral feeding, or prurients to aid evacuation
- the development of tolerance requiring increasing doses to achieve the same effect
- withdrawal symptoms on cessation/reduction of opioid medication. The 'abstinance syndrome' is characterized by:
  - irritabilty
  - tremor

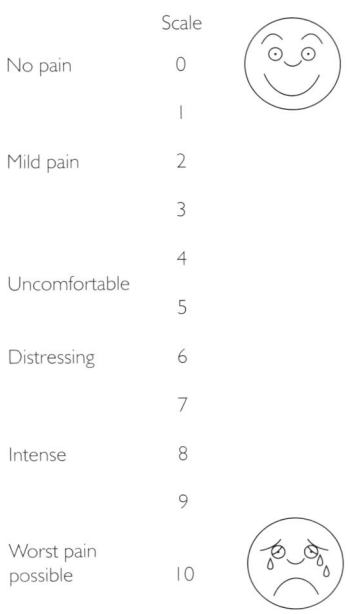

Fig. 79.1 Visual analogue score for the assessment of pain.[6]

  - aggression
  - fever
  - diaphoresis
  - piloerection
  - pupillary dilation
  - diarrhoea
  - insomnia.

Early recognition of these symptoms in not always simple in the ICU patient and may be mistaken for sepsis or delirium. Treatment is by reinstitution of and then slow withdrawal of the opioid, especially after prolonged periods of administration. Alternately, symptoms may be controlled with a combination of long-acting opioid (e.g. methadone), BZA and α_2 agonists (e.g. clonidine).

A knowledge of drug-related (as opposed to class-related) side-effects is important when using opioids other than morphine, e.g. the interaction between pethidine and the older monoamine oxidase inhibitors, the potential for seizures with high dose or prolonged use of pethidine, chest wall rigidity occasionally seen with high doses of fentanyl.

The specific opioid antagonist naloxone has little role to play in the ICU, except for the treatment of severe hypotension, unwanted sedation or respiratory depression following opioid usage. Rapid reversal of opioid effect for the purpose of neurological assessment may be another valid use of naloxone.

PHARMACOKINETIC CONSIDERATIONS

The pharmacokinetics[22,23] of analgesics and sedatives can be affected by such factors as:

- patient's fluid volume status
- capillary leak (changing volume of distribution)
- serum protein levels
- renal function
- hepatic function
- hepatic blood flow
- competition of combinations of drugs for carrier molecules, metabolic and excretory pathways.

All of these factors make the rational choice of an appropriate drug in the appropriate dose difficult in the critically ill patient.

Use of simple analgesics or NSAIDS to treat pain will reduce the amount of opioid required.

SIMPLE ANALGESICS

Paracetamol and other simple analgesics (e.g. salicylates) are particularly effective for:

- bone and joint pain
- soft tissue pain
- perioperative pain
- inflammatory conditions.

These drugs are given by mouth, via a nasogastric tube or per rectum to supplement analgesia in the critically ill (e.g. paracetamol 1–2 g 4–6-hourly). Use is limited by the need to use the enteral route and the risk of hepatic dysfunction if used in high dose or for prolonged periods.

NSAIDS

The commonly-used NSAIDs are carboxylic acids (e.g. indomethicin, ibuprofen, mefenamic acid) or enolic acids (e.g. piroxicam). NSAIDs are useful for supplemental analgesia in the ICU for the conditions listed for simple analgesics above. They are given by mouth, via a nasogastric tube, per rectum or by intramuscular injection (e.g. indomethacin 100 mg twice daily PR or ketorolac 10–15 mg 4–6-hourly IMI) for pain and pyrexia. Side-effects:

- renal dysfunction
- gastrointestinal haemorrhage
- increased bleeding tendency due to platelet inhibition.

The newer cyclooxygenase 2 specific inhibitors, such as valdecoxib and its injectable precursor parecoxib, have a much lower side effect profile than traditional NSAIDs.

TRAMADOL

Tramadol is a recent addition to the analgesic range. It acts via the μ receptor, as well as by inhibiting the uptake of serotonin and norepinephrine, with presynaptic stimulation of serotonin release, thereby enhancing the effects of the descending analgesia system.[24] It is useful for moderate to severe pain in the post-operative patient in

doses of 50–100 mg i.v., oral or i.m. 4–6-hourly to a maximum of 600 mg/day.

LOCAL ANAESTHETICS – REGIONAL ANAESTHESIA/ANALGESIA

The use of local anaesthetic techniques in the critically ill patient is limited by:

- pain often emanating from multiple sources, and therefore not amenable to a single regional technique
- the requirement for 'mandatory' sedation/analgesia in order for the patient to tolerate endotracheal intubation, making a regional technique for another source of pain (e.g. laparotomy wound) superfluous
- the need to treat pain over a prolonged period, mandating either repetition of the regional block (e.g. intercostal nerve blocks for pain from an upper abdominal incision, or femoral nerve blocks for a fractured femur) or the placement of an indwelling catheter (e.g. epidural catheter). Indwelling catheters also have a defined safe duration of insertion (usually 3–4 days), before they need to be removed and replaced.
- coagulopathy frequently seen in this group of patients
- co-morbidities (e.g. severe ischaemic heart disease) in the critically ill patient.

When a regional technique is considered viable (e.g. thoracic epidural for the treatment of pain due to fractured ribs), then the following need to be considered:

- the procedure should be carried out by adequately trained personnel (usually with an anaesthesia background)
- regional techniques may be very time-consuming, requiring additional staff to properly position the patient and assist the proceduralist
- regional techniques may carry serious complication risks (e.g. subarachnoid injection of local anaesthetic or epidural haematoma during placement of epidural catheters, with serious haemodynamic, neurological and respiratory consequences)
- good preparation is paramount:
  - informed consent from patient or legal surrogate
  - recent normal coagulation profile, or correction of abnormal profile
  - the knowledge and ability to deal with complications (e.g. sudden hypotension)
  - experience with the drugs being used (typically a mixture of local anaesthetic, such as bupivacaine 0.1%, and an opioid, such as fentanyl 2 μg/ml, are used for epidural infusion)
- adequate training of nursing staff to monitor the level of block, haemodynamic parameters and for possible complications.

Within the context above, the following blocks may be useful in individual patients:

- femoral nerve block for lower limb injuries (10 ml of 0.5% bupivacaine or 7.5 mg/ml ropivacaine injected intermittently 8–12-hourly into the region of the femoral nerve immediately inferior to the inguinal ligament)
- intercostal nerve blocks for thoracic and upper abdominal injuries or wounds (2–3 ml of 0.5% bupivacaine or 7.5 mg/ml ropivacaine injected into the region of appropriate intercostal nerves – usually at 3–4 sites unilaterally or bilaterally)
- brachial plexus or intravenous regional anaesthesia for isolated upper limb injuries or procedures (e.g. fracture manipulation)
- epidural analgesia for thoracic and abdominal pain
- intrapleural analgesia/anaesthesia, applied either via a catheter placed for this purpose or via intercostal drains previously placed for treatment of pneumothorax.

MUSCLE RELAXANTS

The routine use of muscle relaxants for prolonged periods is a rare occurrence in the ICU since the advent of mechanical ventilators that provide assisted modes of ventilation (as opposed to mandatory modes used previously). Spontaneous, assisted ventilation for almost all mechanically ventilated patients is now encouraged. Current indications for the use of muscle relaxants in the ICU include:

- to complement general anaesthesia for endotracheal intubation and initiation of mechanical ventilation or for short surgical procedures (e.g. tracheostomy)
- to facilitate the safe transport of patients and the acquisition of adequate radiographic images (e.g. CT or MRI)
- to facilitate mandatory mechanical ventilation when adequate sedation/analgesia alone is not adequate to achieve control e.g.:
  – to increase chest wall compliance (e.g. in the severe asthmatic or to facilitate venous drainage in the patient with severe intracranial hypertension)
  – to facilitate precise control of respiratory parameters, such as airway pressure or $PaCO_2$ (e.g. permissive hypercapnia in patients with ARDS or normocapnia in patients with impaired cerebral autoregulation)
  – to reduce $\dot{V}O_2$ in the severely hypoxaemic patient
- specific indications, such as treatment of muscle spasm in tetanus.

Before muscle relaxants are used, patients should already be (or about to be commenced) on mechanical ventilation, there should be the expertise and equipment available to deal with 'difficult intubation' or accidental extubation and patients should be sedated/anaesthetized to prevent the awareness of being paralysed while inadequately sedated. Muscle relaxants may be given by intermittent i.v. injection or by continuous i.v. infusion.

CHOICE OF MUSCLE RELAXANT

Depolarizing muscle relaxants are to be used with caution in the ICU patient who has:

- multiple injuries
- renal failure
- neurological problems (such as paraplegia)
- burns
- who has been immobilized for a prolonged period of time.

The risk of severe hyperkalaemia following administration of suxamethonium in these settings is high.

Non-depolarizing agents are the most commonly-used relaxants in the ICU. Their use may be complicated by:

- Accumulation of the parent compound or active metabolites in patients with hepatic or renal insufficiency. Atracurium or cisatracurium are useful agents in these patients due to their inactivation pathways being independent of the kidney and the liver. Accumulation of the epileptogenic metabolite laudanosine may be a problem with atracurium.
- Histamine release following usually rapid injection of certain of these agents (e.g. atracurium). Vecuronium has been shown to be very 'cardiostable'.
- Protective reflexes (e.g. cough, gag, blink) are abolished and the patient is not able to move and posture him/herself. This requires increased vigilance and attention from the attendants.
- Neurological assessment of the paralysed patient is not possible and requires strict attention to detail to ensure the patient is adequately sedated while paralysed.
- Prolonged duration of action may result from use of these drugs due to:
  – patient factors, such as electrolyte disturbances (e.g. hypokalaemia, hypophosphataemia)
  – drug factors, such as myopathy associated with the use of steroidal relaxants (e.g. pancuronium, vecuronium), especially when used in conjunction with corticosteroids or aminoglycoside antibiotics.

When muscle relaxants are to be used, they should be used for a clearly-defined indication, for as short a time as possible. In addition, the appropriate drug should be used and its use should be monitored regularly (e.g. train of four, post-tetanic count or double burst stimulation). Alternately, muscle relaxants may be withheld at least once a day, until the return of muscle activity. This drug-free period may be combined with a sedation-free period every day in stable patients to allow adequate neurological assessment.

REFERENCES

1 Piccolo R, Lipman J, Hon H, Burrows RC. Analgesia and sedation in the critically ill – a practical approach. *S Afr J Surg* 1999; **37**: 15–20.

2 Rhoney DH, Parker DJ. Use of sedative and analgesic agents in neurotrauma patients: effects on cerebral physiology. *Neurol Res* 2001; **23**: 237–59.

3 Mastronardi P, Cafiero T. Rational use of opioids. *Minerva Anestesiol* 2001; **67**: 332–7.

4 Lerch C, Park GR. Sedation and analgesia. *Br Med Bull* 1999; **55**: 76–95.

5 MacLaren R, Plamondon JM, Ramsay KB, *et al*. A prospective evaluation of empiric versus protocol-based sedation and analgesia. *Pharmacotherapy* 2000; **20**: 662–72.

6 Wiener-Kronish JP. Problems with sedation and analgesia in the ICU. *Pulm Pers* 2001; **18**: 1–3.

7 Habibi S, Coursin DB. Assessment of sedation, analgesia, and neuromuscular blockade in the perioperative period. *Int Anesthesiol Clin* 1996; **34**: 215–41.

8 Kress JP, Pohlman AS, O'Connor MF, Hall JB. Daily interruption of sedative infusions in critically ill patients undergoing mechanical ventilation. *New Engl J Med* 2000; **342**: 1471–7.

9 Wagner BK, O'Hara DA, Hammond JS. Drugs for amnesia in the ICU. *Am J Crit Care* 1997; **6**: 192–201.

10 Wagner BK, O'Hara DA. Pharmacokinetics and pharmacodynamics of sedatives and analgesics in treatment of agitated critically ill patients. *Clin Pharmacokinet* 1997; **33**: 426–53.

11 Watling SM, Dasta JF, Seidl EC. Sedatives, analgesics, and paralytics in the ICU. *Ann Pharmacother* 1997; **31**: 148–53.

12 Hall RI, Sandham D, Cardinal P, *et al*. Propofol vs midazolam for ICU sedation: a Canadian multicenter randomized trial. *Chest* 2001; **119**: 1151–9.

13 Walder B, Elia N, Henzi I, *et al*. A lack of evidence of superiority of propofol versus midazolam for sedation in mechanically ventilated critically ill patients: a qualitative and quantitative systemic review. *Anesth Analg* 2001; **92**: 975–83.

14 Herr DL, Kelly K, Hall JB, *et al*. Safety and efficacy of propofol with EDTA when used for sedation of surgical intensive care unit patients. *Intensive Care Med* 2000; **26(suppl 4)**: S452–62.

15 Abraham E, Papadakos PJ, Tharratt RS, *et al*. Effects of propofol containing EDTA on mineral metabolism in medical patients with pulmonary dysfunction. *Intensive Care Med* 2000; **26(suppl 4)**: S422–32.

16 Youssef-Ahmed MZ, Silver P, Nimkoff L, Sagy M. Continuous infusion of ketamine in mechanically ventilated children with refractory bronchospasm. *Intensive Care Med* 1996; **22**: 972–6.

17 Kolenda H, Gremmelt A, Rading S, *et al*. Ketamine for analgosedative therapy in intensive care treatment of head injured patients. *Acta Neurochir* (Wien) 1996; **138**: 1193–9.

18 Anonymous. Zyprexa. In: E-MIMS (ed.) *MIMS Abbreviated Prescribing Information, 1996–2001*. St Leonards, New South Wales: Vivendi Universal Publishing Company; 2001.

19 Venn RM, Hell J, Grounds RM. Respiratory effects of dexmedetomidine in the surgical patient requiring intensive care. *Crit Care* 2000; **4**: 302–8.

20 Hall JE, Uhrich TD, Barney JA *et al*. Sedative, amnestic, and analgesic properties of small-dose dexmedetomine infusions. *Anesth Analg* 2000; **90**: 699–705.

21 Venn RM, Bradshaw CJ, Spencer R, *et al*. Preliminary UK experience of dexmedetomidine, a novel agent for postoperative sedation in the intensive care unit. *Anaesthesia* 1999; **54**: 1136–42.

22 Scholz J, Steinfath M, Schulz M. Clinical pharmacokinetics of alfentanil, fentanyl, and sufentanil. An update. *Clin Pharmacokinet* 1996; **31**: 275–292.

23 Power BM, Forbes AM, van Heerden PV, Ilett KF. Pharmacokinetics of drugs used in critically ill adults. *Clin Pharmacokinet* 1998; **34**: 25–56.

24 Budd K, Langford R. Tramadol revisited. *Br J Anaesth* 1999; **82**: 493–5.

80

Inotropes and vasopressors

J A Myburgh

The pharmacological support of the failing circulation is a fundamental part of critical care. The principle aim of these drugs is to restore inadequate systemic and regional perfusion to physiological levels.

DEFINITIONS

Inotropic agents are defined as drugs that act on the heart by increasing the velocity and force of myocardial fibre shortening. The resultant increase in contractility results in increased cardiac output and blood pressure. Characteristics of the ideal inotrope are shown in Table 80.1.

Vasopressors are drugs that have a predominantly vasoconstrictive action on the peripheral vasculature, both arterial and venous. These drugs are primarily used to increase mean arterial pressure.

The distinction between these two groups of drugs is often confusing. Many of the commonly used agents, such as the catecholamines, have both inotropic and variable effects on the peripheral vasculature that include venoconstriction, arteriolar vasodilatation and constriction.

Vasoregulatory agents modulate the responsiveness of the peripheral vasculature to vasoactive drugs in pathological states, such as sepsis. These agents have an increasingly important role in intensive care and include vasopressin and corticosteroids.

THE FAILING CIRCULATION

PHYSIOLOGY

Traditionally, cardiac output is discussed in terms of factors that govern cardiac function. These include preload, afterload, heart rate and rhythm and contractility. Whilst this perspective is helpful in managing patients whose circulatory function is limited by cardiac disease, it is incomplete.

Cardiac output is controlled by the peripheral vasculature that is as energetic at returning blood to the

Table 80.1   The ideal inotrope

Increases contractility
   Increases mean arterial pressure
   Increases cardiac output
   Improves regional perfusion
No increase in myocardial oxygen consumption
   Avoidance of tachycardia
   Non-arrhythmogenic
   Maintenance of diastolic blood pressure
Does not develop tolerance
Titratable
   Rapid onset
   Rapid termination of action
Compatible with other drugs
Non-toxic
Cost effective

heart as the heart is at pumping blood to the periphery[1] (Figure 80.1).

Blood is pumped down a pressure gradient that is determined by the force of myocardial ejection (contractility) and impedance to ventricular ejection (afterload). The resultant mean arterial pressure is the major 'afferent' determinant of regional perfusion pressure. A total of 20% of the blood volume is contained in the arterial ('conducting') vessels. There is a marked drop in perfusion pressure and flow across the capillary beds to allow diffusion of substrates and oxygen. The difference between mean arterial pressure and the pressure in end capillaries ('efferent' perfusion pressure) determines regional, or organ specific, perfusion pressure.

Blood enters the venous system and is returned to the heart via a pressure gradient determined by mean systemic pressure and right atrial pressure.[1,2] The amount of blood returned to the heart determines the degree of ventricular filling prior to systole (preload), which subsequently determines stroke volume and cardiac output.

Under physiological conditions, the venous ('capacitance') system contains approximately 70% of the total blood volume which acts as a physiological reservoir ('unstressed' volume). Under conditions where circula-

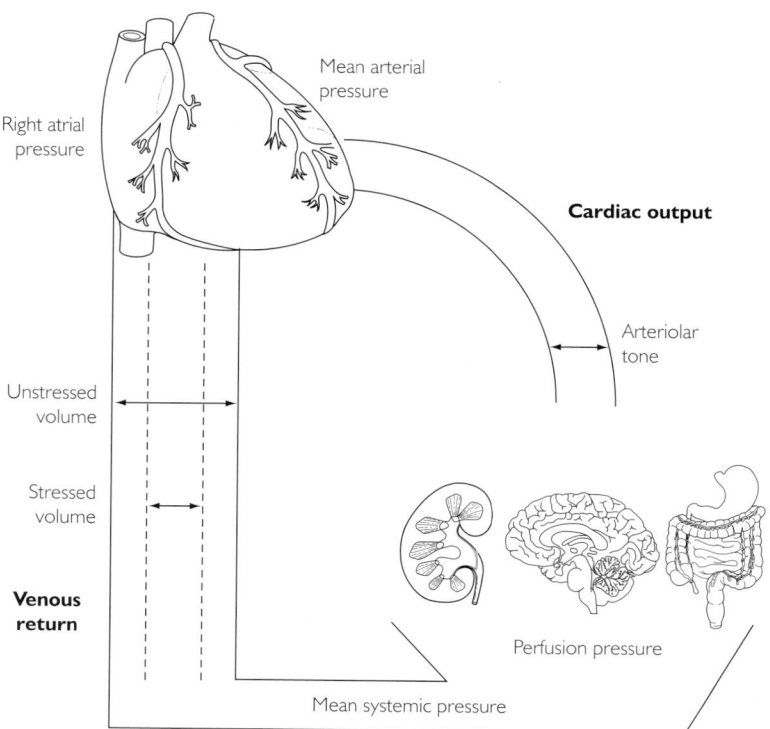

Fig. 80.1 Schematic relationship of the determinants of cardiac output and venous return.

tory demands increase, increased sympathetic tone will cause contraction of this reservoir. The resultant auto-transfusion ('stressed' volume) may increase venous return by approximately 30% and subsequently cardiac output.[1,3]

Both the arterial and venous systems are integrated under complex neurohormonal influences. These include the adrenergic, renin-angiotensin-aldosterone, vasopressinergic and glucocorticoid systems in addition to local mediators, such as nitric oxide, endothelin, endorphins and the eicosanoids.[4]

PATHOPHYSIOLOGY

Circulatory dysfunction or failure may be considered in terms of the major determinants of cardiac output, although there is marked interdependence between these factors.

HEART RATE FAILURE

Profound bradycardia will reduce both cardiac output and mean arterial pressure if sympathetic tone is compromised. Inotropes will increase both rate and speed of conduction, in addition to augmenting peripheral venous

return, thereby restoring cardiac output and mean arterial pressure.

Tachycardia is associated with decreased left coronary artery perfusion, due to reduction of diastolic time, during which coronary perfusion occurs. This may exacerbate myocardial ischaemia in patients with coronary artery disease, particularly if mean arterial pressure, specifically diastolic blood pressure, is compromised. Therefore, drugs that shorten diastolic time or compromise coronary perfusion should be used with caution in susceptible patients.

PRELOAD FAILURE

Loss of intravascular blood volume or extracellular fluid is the most common cause of inadequate ventricular preload. This is corrected with appropriate fluids to maintain a euvolaemic state. Correction of hypovolaemia is essential before drugs, such as inotropes or vasoactive agents are used.

There are other determinants of ventricular preload and venous return. Factors, such as loss of muscle pump, positive intrathoracic pressure, loss of atrial systole (atrial fibrillation) and ablation of sympathetic tone will also compromise preload by reducing venous return. Under these circumstances, volume replacement alone may be insufficient to maintain adequate preload and vasoactive agents may be required to increase venous return.

MYOCARDIAL FAILURE

Myocardial or 'pump' failure may be divided into disorders of systolic ejection (systolic dysfunction) and diastolic filling (diastolic dysfunction).

Systolic dysfunction occurs as a result of reduced effective myocardial contractility. This may be due to primary myocardial factors, such as ischaemia, infarction or cardiomyopathy. Myocardial depression of both right and left ventricular function may occur in severe sepsis or following prolonged infusions catecholamines. Increased impedance to ventricular ejection, such as hypertensive states or structural abnormalities such as aortic stenosis or hypertrophic obstructive cardiomyopathy may cause systolic dysfunction.

Diastolic dysfunction is characterized by reduced ventricular compliance or increased resistance to ventricular filling during diastole. It may be due to mechanical factors, such as structural abnormalities of the ventricle such as restrictive cardiomyopathy or due to impaired diastolic relaxation that occurs with myocardial ischaemia or severe sepsis. This results in elevated end diastolic pressure and pulmonary venous congestion. Episodic or 'flash' pulmonary oedema is a common clinical sign of diastolic dysfunction.[5] Tachycardias that shorten diastolic time may exacerbate diastolic failure. Diastolic dysfunction frequently accompanies systolic failure both in acute and chronic cardiac failure, particularly in elderly patients.[6]

In the presence of systolic dysfunction, adequate stroke volume may be maintained by an increase in left ventricular end-diastolic volume (Frank Starling relationship) provided diastolic function is optimal. However, if the loss of effective myocardial mass is critical, the ventricle will be unable to maintain an adequate stroke volume and cardiac output will fall.

In this situation, systolic dysfunction usually requires treatment with inotropic agents in order to augment stroke volume, thereby increasing cardiac output and mean arterial pressure.

VASOREGULATORY FAILURE

Disruption or impairment of regulation of the peripheral vasculature may result in circulatory failure. This includes acute sympathetic denervation, such as high quadriplegia, epidural or total spinal anaesthesia ('spinal' shock); distributive failure, such as anaphylaxis; or pathological 'vasoplegia' that occurs in severe sepsis.

These syndromes are characterized by reduced responsiveness of the peripheral circulation to endogenous or exogenous sympathetic stimulation. This results in pooling in the venous circulation due to the inability to provide a 'stressed' volume.[4]

Management of these conditions has traditionally focused on the arterial circulation with attempts to increase systemic vascular resistance, often regarded inaccurately as treatment of 'afterload failure.' This is a misnomer as the problem is predominantly impaired venous return, compounded to a lesser extent by pathological arteriolar vasodilatation.[7] Clearly, the effects of vasoregulatory failure will be exacerbated by concomitant hypovolaemia. Fluid loading to restore effective intravascular volume is essential.

Vasoactive agents have a role in restoring vasoregulatory tone once adequate volume has been established.

CLASSIFICATION

The common ultimate cellular mechanism of action of these agents involves an influence on the release, utilization or sequestration of intracellular calcium (Figure 80.2). These agents are divided into two main groups based on whether or not their actions depend upon increases in intracellular cyclic adenosine 3,5-monophosphate (cAMP) and are outlined in Table 80.2.

CATECHOLAMINES

Sympathomimetic amines are the most frequently used vasoactive agents in the intensive care unit and include the naturally occurring catecholamines dopamine, norepinephrine and epinephrine; and synthetic substances dobutamine, isoprenaline and dopexamine.

RECEPTOR BIOLOGY

PHYSIOLOGICAL

Agonists bind to populations of adrenergic receptors, largely divided into α and β subgroups. Further subgroups of α (α_{1A}, α_{1B}, α_{2A}, α_{2B}, α_{2C}) and β-receptors (β_1, β_2 and β_3) have been identified.[8]

Table 80.2 Classification of inotropes

cAMP dependent	cAMP independent
Catecholamines (β adrenergic agonists)	Catecholamines (α adrenergic agonists)
Epinephrine	Epinephrine
Norepinephrine	Norepinephrine
Dopamine	Dopamine
Dobutamine	Digoxin
Dopexamine	Calcium salts
Isoprenaline	Thyroid hormone
Phosphodiesterase inhibitors	
Amrinone	
Milrinone	
Enoximone	
Glucagon	

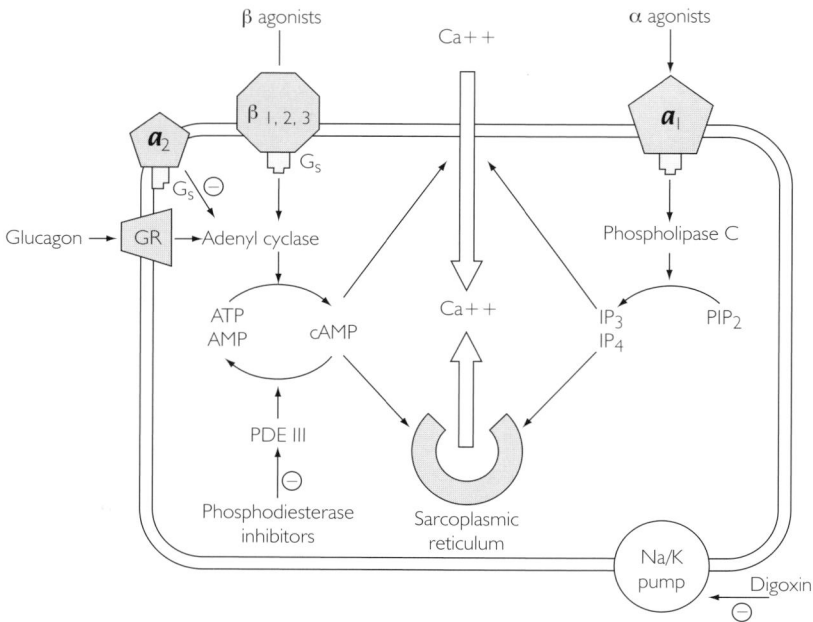

Fig. 80.2 Schematic representation of the action of inotropic drugs on intracellular calcium in myocytes. GR, glucagon receptor; Gs, G protein complex; ATP, adenosine triphosphate; AMP, adenosine monophosphate; cAMP, cyclic AMP; PDE III, phosphodiesterase III; IP$_3$, inositol phosphate 3; PIP$_2$, phosphoinositol diphosphate.

Signal transduction from agonist-receptor occupation to the effector cell is modulated by conformational changes in G proteins associated with these receptors. Under the additional influence of second messengers, such as nitric oxide, endothelin, eicosanoids, these conformational changes promote the release of calcium from intracellular stores and increase membrane calcium permeability. Subsequent phosphorylation of substrate proteins via protein kinases act as third messengers to trigger a cascade of events, which lead to specific cardiovascular effects.[8]

β-receptor occupancy predominantly activates adenyl cyclase to increase the conversion of adenosine triphosphate to cAMP. α-receptor occupancy acts independently of cAMP by activation of phospholipase C which increases inositol phosphates (IP$_3$ and IP$_4$) and diacyl glycerol.

This complex agonist-receptor-effector relationship is responsible for homeostatic mechanisms, such as physiological responses to stress and autoregulation.

PATHOPHYSIOLOGICAL

The activity and function of this system is dynamic and may be markedly influenced by pathological states. This may result in qualitative changes in the agonist-receptor-effector organ relationship (desensitization) where receptors no longer respond to physiological or pharmacological sympathetic stimulation to the same extent. Quantitative changes such as reduced receptor density, receptor sequestration and enzymatic uncoupling (downregulation) may also result in impaired responses.[9]

BIOSYNTHESIS

The biosynthesis and chemical structures of the naturally occurring catecholamines are shown in Figure 80.3a.

Catecholamines consist of an aromatic ring attached to a terminal amine by a carbon chain. The configuration of each drug is important for determining affinity to respective receptors.

Dopamine is hydroxylated to form norepinephrine, which is the predominant peripheral sympathetic chemotransmitter in man, acting at all adrenergic receptors. The release of norepinephrine from sympathetic terminals is controlled by re-uptake mechanisms mediated via α$_2$ receptors and augmented by epinephrine released from the adrenal gland at times of stress. Norepinephrine is converted to form epinephrine that is subsequently metabolized in liver and lung.[10]

All catecholamines have very short biological half-lives (1–2 min) and a steady state plasma concentration is achieved within 5–10 min after the start of a constant infusion. This allows rapid titration of drug to a clinical endpoint, such as mean arterial pressure.

Epinephrine and norepinephrine infusions produce blood concentrations similar to those produced endoge-

(a)

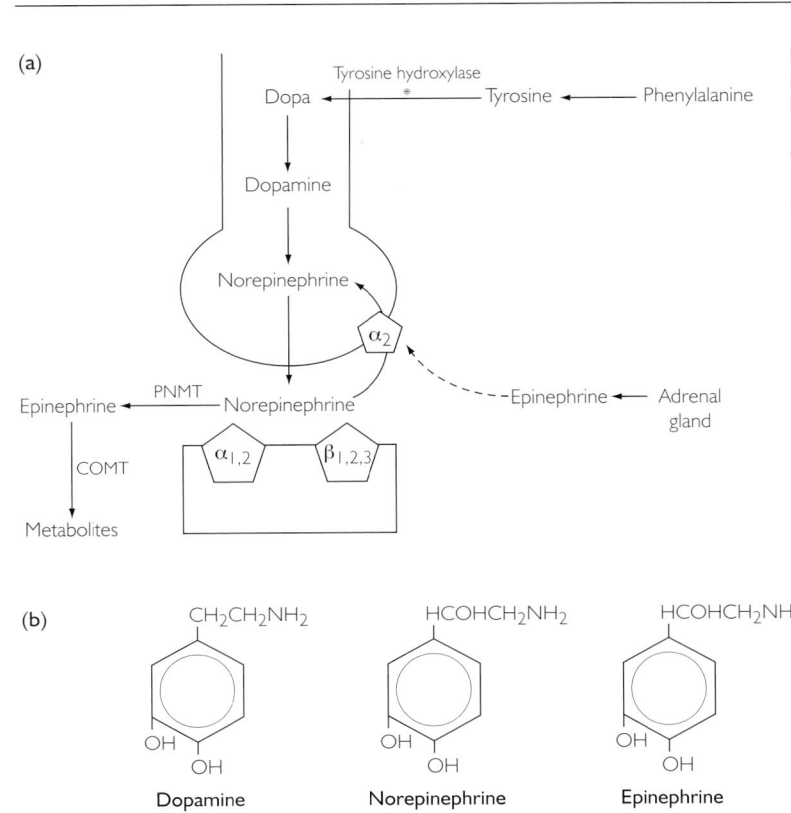

Fig. 80.3 (a) Biosynthesis of catecholamines in sympathetic terminals. *Rate limiting step by tyrosine hydroxylase. PNMT, phenethanolamine-N-methyltransferase; COMT, catechol-o-methyl-transferase. (b) Chemical structure of endogenous and synthetic catecholamines.

(b)

Dopamine

Norepinephrine

Epinephrine

Isoprenaline

Dobutamine

Dopexamine

nously in shock states, whereas dopamine infusions produce much higher concentrations than those naturally encountered. Dopamine may exert much of its effect by being converted to norepinephrine, thus bypassing the rate-limiting (tyrosine hydroxylase) step in catecholamine synthesis.

The synthetic catecholamines are derivatives of dopamine (Figure 80.3b). These agents are characterized by increased length of the carbon chain, which confers affinity for β-receptors. Dopexamine with a long carbon chain has predominantly β-effects, with no detectable α-effects. Dobutamine is a synthetic derivative of isoprenaline. These agents have relatively little affinity for α-receptors due to the configuration of the terminal amine, which differ from the endogenous catecholamines.

Epinephrine, norepinephrine and isoprenaline all have hydroxyl groups on the β-carbon atom of the side chain, and this is associated with 100-fold greater potency than dopamine or dobutamine.[10]

SYSTEMIC EFFECTS

The systemic effects of any of these agents will vary greatly between patients and within individuals at different times. Adequacy of response is often unpredictable and depends on the aetiology of circulatory failure and systemic comorbidities. In some patients, dramatic responses to small doses may occur, while in others, large doses of inotropes may be required to support the failing circulation.

The classification of sympathomimetic agents into α- and β-agonists, based on the above structure/function relationships, is only a crude predictor of systemic effects.

Epinephrine, norepinephrine and dopamine are all predominantly β-agonists at low doses, with increasing α-effects becoming evident as the dose is increased.

The synthetic catecholamines are all predominantly β-agonists.

CARDIOVASCULAR

The cardiovascular effects of the catecholamines under physiological conditions are shown in Table 80.3.

Norepinephrine, epinephrine and dopamine all tend to increase stroke volume, cardiac output and mean arterial pressure, with little change in heart rate and a low incidence of dysrhythmias. The effects on the peripheral vasculature are similar with all agents increasing venous return, without significant changes in systemic vascular resistance.

Isoprenaline increases cardiac output predominantly by increasing heart rate and by moderate inotropy. This occurs without a significant change in blood pressure due to predominant β_2-receptor induced veno- and vasodilatation.

The profile of dobutamine is similar to isoprenaline, although increases in heart rate are not as pronounced. Both of these agents may decrease mean arterial pressure, particularly in hypovolaemic patients, due to reduced venous return caused by venodilation. Dopexamine is similar in that it has mild inotropy combined with a vasodilatory effect and can cause tachycardia. The adverse effects of dobutamine, dopexamine and isoprenaline on heart rate and mean arterial pressure may compromise patients with ischaemic heart disease. However, the vasodilatory effects of dobutamine or dopexamine may be useful in selected patients with predominant systolic heart failure as means of reducing afterload.

In the failing myocardium, particularly in patients with cardiac failure, following cardiopulmonary bypass or septic shock,[11] endogenous stores of norepinephrine are markedly reduced. Furthermore, there may be significant desensitization and downregulation of cardiac β-receptors.[12] In these situations, α_1- and α_2-receptors have an important role in maintaining inotropy and peripheral vasoresponsiveness.[13] This may be expressed clinically as 'tolerance' or tachyphylaxis to catecholamines, particularly with predominantly β-agonists such as dobutamine. This phenomenon may explain the requirement for high doses of catecholamines in refractory shock states. Consequently, the role of β-agonists in patients with severe myocardial failure has been questioned.

Catecholamines have a significant effect on the venous circulation. These drugs primarily restore or maintain 'stressed volumes' of the capacitance vessels

Table 80.3 Cardiovascular effect of catecholamines

Agent	β_1-effects	β_2-effects	α_1-effects	α_2-effects
Norepinephrine Epinephrine Dopamine	+ chronotropy + dromotropy + inotropy	+ inotropy vasodilatation bronchodilatation	+ inotropy vasoconstriction	+ inotropy vasoconstriction
	β-effects predominate at low dose; α-effects predominate at high dose			
Dobutamine	+	+	(+)	–
Isoprenaline	+	(+)	–	–
Dopexamine	+	+	–	–

+, stimulation; (+), mild effect; –, no effect.

under pathological conditions, thereby maintaining or increasing cardiac output and mean arterial pressure. This is important in 'vasoplegic' states such as septic shock.

In clinically used doses, intravenously administered catecholamines have minimal direct vasoconstrictive effects on conducting arterial vessels. Consequently, derived indices such as systemic vascular resistance do not reliably reflect the effect of catecholamines on the peripheral vasculature.

The development of peripheral gangrene in refractory septic shock has been attributed to catecholamine induced vasoconstriction. There is little evidence to support this as the development of tissue gangrene in these situations primarily occurs as a consequence of intravascular thrombosis caused by sepsis mediated coagulopathy.

CEREBRAL

Under physiological conditions, catecholamines do not normally cross the blood–brain barrier.[14] Cerebral blood flow is maintained at a constant rate over a range of perfusion pressure by cerebral autoregulation. Under conditions where the integrity of the blood–brain barrier is altered, such as following traumatic brain injury and aneurysmal subarachnoid haemorrhage, or where upper and lower autoregulatory thresholds are exceeded, exogenous catecholamines may directly enter the cerebral circulation.

The degree by which these agents directly effect the cerebral circulation following head injury is unknown, although there is some evidence suggesting that dopamine has a direct effect causing increased cerebral blood flow and intracranial pressure.[15,16]

RENAL

The kidney is an efficient autoregulator, maintaining constant glomerular filtration and renal blood flow by neurohumoral mechanisms, such as the renin-angiotensin-aldosterone system. All catecholamines will increase renal blood flow to a similar extent as a consequence of increased cardiac output and mean arterial pressure with a resultant natriuresis. Catecholamine mediated increases in renal blood flow do not affect glomerular filtration rate

A direct natriuresis may also result from inhibition of cAMP in the renal tubules. This effect has been attributed primarily to low doses of dopamine (2 μg/kg per min), although this occurs to a similar extent with epinephrine, norepinephrine and dobutamine.[17–19] Despite widespread use, 'renal dose' dopamine does not prevent or ameliorate renal dysfunction in susceptible patients.[20]

SPLANCHNIC

Splanchnic autoregulation is not as robust as the brain and kidney. Perfusion is more dependent on mean arterial pressure and the duality of the mesenteric and portal systems. Concerns about catecholamine induced splanchnic vasoconstriction with mesenteric and hepatic ischaemia have been raised for many years, but remain unfounded.[21]

Dopamine and dopexamine have been promoted as selective splanchnic vasodilators, but there are no conclusive studies indicating a significant benefit over norepinephrine or epinephrine. Many studies have used gastric intramucosal pH (pHi), a surrogate measurement of splanchnic blood flow, as the primary endpoint.[22,23] However, as pHi remains an unvalidated measurement, the results of many of the comparative trials of the different sympathomimetics are inconclusive.[24,25] It would appear that all catecholamines are equally effective in increasing splanchnic perfusion by improving cardiac output and mean arterial pressure.

METABOLIC

Catecholamine mediated β-stimulation may result in hyperglycaemia, hypokalaemia and hypophosphataemia, which may need monitoring and correcting.

Epinephrine is associated with the development of lactic acidosis, due to inhibition of pyruvate dehydrogenase.[26] While pH may fall to levels around 7.2, the acidosis is not associated with impaired tissue perfusion or hypoxia. In most patients who are haemodynamically stable, this is a self-limiting phenomenon and is not associated with adverse outcomes.[27] This may become an issue in severe sepsis with the development of a severe acidosis.[28]

NON-CATECHOLAMINES

PHOSPHODIESTERASE INHIBITORS

Phosphodiesterase inhibitors are compounds that cause non-receptor mediated competitive inhibition of phosphodiesterase isoenzymes (PDE), resulting in increased levels of cAMP (Figure 80.2). Importantly, cAMP also affects diastolic heart function through the regulation of phospholamban, the regulatory subunit of the calcium pump of the sarcoplasmic reticulum. This enhances the rate of calcium re-sequestration and thereby diastolic relaxation.

For cardiovascular tissue, inhibition of isoenzyme PDE-III is responsible for the therapeutic effects. Cardiac effects are characterized by positive inotropy and improved diastolic relaxation. The latter is termed lusitropy and may be beneficial in patients with reduced ventricular compliance or predominant diastolic failure.[29,30]

These agents also cause potent vasodilatation with reductions in preload, venous return and afterload as well as a reduction in pulmonary vascular resistance. The term 'inodilation' has been used to describe this dual haemodynamic effect.

Tolerance is not a feature. These agents may have a place in the management of patients with β-receptor down-regulation by causing intrinsic inotropic stimulation and by sensitizing the myocardium to β-agonists. Other speculative actions include inhibition of platelet aggregation and reduction of post-ischaemic reperfusion injury.

Titration pharmacokinetics of phosphodiesterase inhibitors are markedly different to catecholamines. Drug half-lives may be prolonged and excretion is predominantly renal. Hypotension may result from vasodilatation and combined use with catecholamines (e.g. norepinephrine or epinephrine) may be necessary and complementary to maintain mean arterial pressure.

Phosphodiesterase inhibitors that have been used in clinical practice include the bipyridine derivatives amrinone and milrinone and the imidazolones enoximone and piroximone. The cardiovascular effects are similar.

The oral form of amrinone is no longer used clinically, due to a high incidence of thrombocytopenia, gastrointestinal and neurological side-effects.

Milrinone and enoximone are more potent agents and are currently used in clinical practice with the latter exhibiting more inotropic effects than vasodilatation.

Enoximone is more rapidly metabolized, but the metabolite is active and its cardiovascular effects persist for some hours.

There is evidence that prolonged use of these agents is associated with an increased mortality in patients with severe heart failure.

DIGOXIN

Digitalis glycosides have been used for the treatment of heart failure for 200 years and the vagotonic effects used to control the ventricular response in selected supraventricular tachyarrhythmias.

The effects of digoxin are largely mediated by an increase in intracellular calcium concentrations produced indirectly by inhibition of the Na^+/K^+ membrane pump resulting in increased myocardial contractility (Figure 80.2). The effects on impulse conduction are mediated through change in both vagal and sympathetic tone, which may also increase venous return.

Digoxin has a narrow therapeutic index, is highly protein bound and is largely excreted unchanged in the urine. Alteration in renal function may prolong the normal half-life of about 35 h to 5 d.

The role of digoxin in acute cardiac failure is questionable. It has minimal effects as an inotrope and evaluation of its efficacy is difficult. In the presence of high levels of sympathetic activity, the positive inotropic effect is negligible and there is usually a poor response in acute myocardial failure, myocarditis, advanced cardiomyopathy, shock states, and cardiac tamponade.

The potential for toxicity in the critically ill patient is increased by hypokalaemia, hypomagnesaemia, hypercalcaemia, hypoxia and acidosis. Toxicity is manifested by dysrhythmias that may assume any form including supraventricular tachyarrhythmias, bradycardia, ventricular ectopy and conduction block at any level.

Monitoring digoxin levels in critically ill patients is recommended, although interpretation of these levels is difficult. A concentration of 1–2 ng/ml represents a reasonable risk/benefit ratio, but concentrations of greater than 2 ng/ml may be associated with toxicity in some patients. However, correlation between blood concentrations, efficacy and toxic manifestations is poor. Clinical criteria remain the most reliable assessment of toxicity, but with the exception of dysrhythmias, may be difficult to elicit in ICU patients.

Commonly used drugs in the intensive care unit, such as amiodarone, calcium channel blockers and erythromycin demonstrate adverse drug interactions with digoxin. These may interfere with the radioimmune assay to reflect apparently increased digoxin blood concentrations.

The place of digoxin in the critically ill patient is therefore limited, due to unpredictable efficacy and toxicity. Careful titration of short acting inotropes and drugs such as amiodarone for control of ventricular rate in supraventricular tachycardia in critically ill patients have largely superseded its use.

The role of digoxin in chronic heart failure is well established, particularly in association with angiotensin converting enzyme inhibitors.[31] These drugs may have a role in long term intensive care patients with associated chronic cardiac failure.

In critically ill patients, digoxin should only be administered by slow intravenous injection, as oral bioavailability varies considerably due to altered gastric motility or perfusion. A loading dose (1–1.5 mg in 3 or 4 divided doses, 4–6 h apart), followed by a maintenance dose (0.125–0.5 mg/d) is a satisfactory regimen. Smaller doses should be used in the elderly, small patients, patients with renal, electrolyte and acid base disturbances, and myxoedema.

Blood for assay should be taken at least 6 h after an oral dose and 1 h after an intravenous dose.

GLUCAGON

Glucagon is a naturally occurring polypeptide that directly stimulates adenyl cyclase via specific receptors to increase cAMP concentration in myocardial cells resulting in positive inotropy without producing myocardial excitability (Figure 80.2).

Large doses are required to achieve this effect, which is associated with a high incidence of metabolic side-effects.

No definitive cardiovascular role for this agent has been established apart from anecdotal reports of its use in severe β-blocker and tricyclic poisoning.[32]

THYROID HORMONE

Thyroid hormone is required for synthesis of contractile proteins and normal myocardial contraction. It is also a regulator of the synthesis of adrenergic receptors.

Low levels of thyroid hormone have been demonstrated in brain dead organ donors, in patients with refractory cardiogenic shock particularly following cardiopulmonary bypass, and secondary to myxoedema. Preliminary studies suggest that treatment with thyroid hormone in these patients may reduce the need for inotropic agents and vasopressors to achieve satisfactory haemodynamics.[33]

VASOPRESSORS

Vascular responsiveness is mediated via adrenergic receptors: α-mechanisms predominantly cause vasoconstriction, β-mechanisms, specifically β_2-receptors, mediate vasodilatation (Table 80.3).

α-adrenergic mechanisms have an increasingly important role in the failing circulation, particularly during cardiopulmonary resuscitation. This applies at both myocardial and peripheral vascular levels.

CATECHOLAMINES

Norepinephrine, epinephrine and dopamine have variable effects on the peripheral vasculature and should not be regarded principally as vasopressors.

At high doses, depending on the individual, α-mechanisms predominate. The peripheral vascular effects are discussed below.

PHENYLEPHRINE AND METARAMINOL

These agents are direct acting α_1-agonists that are selective vasoconstrictors, both venous and arterial, with minimal β-activity. They have similar pharmacokinetics to catecholamines and may be given by infusion. In patients with normal sympathetic tone, these drugs may cause reflex bradycardia, particularly following bolus administration.

They are useful in correcting hypotension from 'pure' vasodilatory states such as epidural or spinal anaesthesia and acute spinal cord injury. They have an unproven role in patients with catecholamine resistant septic shock,[34,35] and cardiopulmonary resuscitation.

EPHEDRINE

Ephedrine is a synthetic, direct and indirect acting, non-catecholamine sympathomimetic that acts on both α- and β-receptors. Duration of action is longer than

equivalent doses of epinephrine and it is generally unsuitable as an infusion.

Modest chronotropy and inotropy make this drug popular in patients undergoing general or regional anaesthesia, but it has a limited role in intensive care patients.

VASOREGULATORY AGENTS

PATHOPHYSIOLOGY

In addition to adrenergic regulation, neurohumoral influences have a 'permissive' or regulatory role in maintaining vasomotor tone. These are mediated through renin-aldosterone-angiotensin axis and local mediators such as vasopressin, corticosteroids, nitric oxide and endothelin.

The response of the whole neurohumoral system may become blunted in conditions, such as severe sepsis, where qualitative and quantitative changes may occur. In this context, failure of vasomotor responsiveness may be considered as part of the multiple organ failure.

VASOPRESSIN

Specific vasopressinergic receptors (V_1, V_2) have been identified in association with sympathetic terminals. Vasopressin is a naturally occurring peptide secreted by the posterior pituitary gland. Reduced serum levels of vasopressin have been demonstrated in septic shock[36] and following cardiopulmonary bypass,[37] suggesting an inflammatory mediated mechanism. Levels are maintained during cardiogenic shock.[36]

A proportion of patients with severe septic shock requiring high levels of catecholamines to support the circulation will respond to low doses of infused vasopressin (0.04 U/h), by significantly reducing doses of infused catecholamine.[38] This phenomenon appears to be independent of any directly attributable vasopressor effect; rather as a supplemental 'catecholamine sparing' strategy.[39] However, the impact on mortality has not been determined in conclusive clinical trials.

STEROIDS

The role of steroid supplementation in circulatory failure has been studied for many years. Whilst immunosuppressive or anti-inflammatory doses have been shown to be ineffective, particularly in septic shock, replacement of 'stress response' doses (approximately 100–200 mg hydrocortisone per day) have been shown to improve vasoresponsiveness to catecholamine infusions in patients with refractory shock.[40]

Patients who respond to low doses of steroids may have biochemical evidence of hypoadrenalism, defined by a low serum cortisol level and/or a blunted response to intravenous adrenocorticotrophin, or functional hypoadrenalism as part of the multiple organ failure syndrome.[41,42]

NITRIC OXIDE SYNTHETASE INHIBITORS

Nitric oxide is a ubiquitous molecule that has an important role in regulation of vasomotor tone, particularly vasodilatation. 'Vasoplegic' states, such as those occurring in septic shock, may be associated with pathologically high levels of nitric oxide activity.

Inhibition of nitric oxide synthetase, the predominant enzyme in nitric oxide synthesis, with compounds, such as methylene blue, L-NMMA or L-NAME, is associated with a transient pressor response. However, clinical trials, particularly in septic shock, have not shown improvement in organ failure resolution and may be associated with increased mortality.[43,44]

Consequently, these compounds are currently not indicated in patients with circulatory failure.

CLINICAL USES

There are no definitive studies comparing the efficacy of one inotrope (or combination of inotropes) over another in terms of improving survival: there is no ideal inotrope (Table 80.1).

DRUG SELECTION

In most instances, individual experience and preference determine selection of inotrope(s).

On a pathobiological basis, exogenous catecholamines are essentially used to augment endogenous mechanisms that may be failing at a number of levels.

To this aim, norepinephrine may be considered as the first line drug in most causes of circulatory failure. epinephrine and dopamine predominantly act as a precursor of norepinephrine and may be used as alternatives to norepinephrine, although all of the endogenous catecholamines have similar pharmacodynamic profiles.

Prediction of the response of an individual to a catecholamine is problematic, as marked inter- and intra-individual variability to the response of inotropic agents may occur.

The haemodynamic and metabolic response of an agent must be carefully monitored and evaluated. If there is not a satisfactory response, or if undesirable effects are obtained, the dose or agent should be changed.

MONITORING

Accurate monitoring of the circulation is essential in patients with circulatory failure to assess baseline parameters and the response of vasoactive drugs.

Clinical assessment of the circulation remains the cornerstone of monitoring these patients and includes frequent assessment and recording of pulse rate and rhythm, blood pressure, adequacy of peripheral perfusion, skin turgor, level of consciousness and urine output.

The majority of patients with circulatory failure managed in the intensive care unit require haemodynamic monitoring as clinical signs may be masked or influenced by sedation, ventilation or organ failure. This should provide accurate information about the state of the circulation and interpreted within the context of the underlying pathophysiology.

The following principles are important in patients requiring vasoactive drugs.

BLOOD PRESSURE

All patients receiving vasoactive drugs in all but trivial doses should have accurate monitoring of mean arterial pressure, ideally with an intra-arterial catheter referenced to the aortic root.

Adequacy of tissue perfusion correlates with mean arterial pressure. Accordingly, vasoactive drugs are titrated to achieve a mean arterial pressure that is commensurate with the patient's pre-morbid blood pressure.

Circulatory dysfunction is commonly defined as a mean arterial pressure ≤ 70 mmHg for 1 hour, despite adequate fluid resuscitation, although this may vary between patients and will depend on the aetiology.

A large artery, such as the femoral artery, should be considered in haemodynamically unstable patients as radial or dorsalis pedis arterial catheters underestimate true systemic pressure in shocked patients.[45]

The measurement of systolic and diastolic blood pressures may be inaccurate in haemodynamically unstable patients, particularly if non-invasive devices are used. These devices tend to over-read in hypotensive patients and under-read in hypertensive patients.

VOLUME STATUS

Right atrial pressure monitoring via a central venous catheter provides the best assessment of volume status.[46] Accuracy may be affected by tricuspid regurgitation or pulmonary hypertension.

Left atrial pressure may be measured via direct placement of a left atrial catheter, usually during cardiac surgery. Pulmonary artery occlusion pressure may be used as an indirect measurement of left atrial pressure. However, this measurement may be affected by respiratory artefact, positive airway pressure, tachycardia, hypovolaemia and poor ventricular compliance.

The response and trend to fluid loading and/or vasoactive drug provides more useful information than absolute values.

CARDIAC OUTPUT

As cardiac output is the major determinant of mean arterial pressure, adequate pressure will usually indicate adequate flow (cardiac output). This relationship depends on the adequacy of venous return and level of afterload.

In selected patients with primary myocardial failure, an assessment of cardiac output is useful to quantify baseline function and to assess the response of the heart to drug therapy. Measurement of cardiac output may be done non-invasively using transthoracic or transoesophageal echocardiography or invasively using a pulmonary catheter, ideally using a continuous cardiac output display system.

Systemic vascular resistance is frequently calculated and used as a surrogate index of afterload. However, the clinical utility of systemic vascular resistance is limited to providing a crude estimate of global vascular tone, as it does not reflect afterload, arteriolar tone or venous return. Consequently, systemic vascular resistance should not be used as a criterion for selection of vasoactive drug or as a titratable end point.

TISSUE PERFUSION

Restoration of reduced tissue perfusion is a primary aim of inotropic therapy. This may be assessed clinically by improvements in urine output, serum urea and creatinine, reversal of metabolic acidosis and reduction in serum lactate.

Global indices of oxygenation include systemic oxygen delivery (DO_2), oxygen consumption (VO_2) and oxygen extraction ratio (VO_2/DO_2). These may be derived from pulmonary artery catheters or measured using indirect calorimetry. The utility of these indices as endpoints for intropic therapy is questionable due to the non-specificity of these measurements. Goal directed therapy directed at attaining specific values of oxygen delivery may provide an index of individual patient haemodynamic reserve, but is not associated with reduction in mortality.[47]

Measurement of regional tissue perfusion such as pHi (splanchnic) and jugular venous saturation (cerebral) are limited by poor specificity and are not used routinely.

DOSAGES AND DRUG ADMINISTRATION

Vasoactive drugs, such as catecholamines or vasopressors, are administered by continuous infusion through a dedicated central venous catheter using drug delivery systems, such as infusion pumps or syringe drivers.

Infusion lines should be free of injection portals and clearly marked with identifying labels.

Concentrations of infusions should be standardized in accordance with individual unit protocols. Suggested infusion concentrations are shown in Table 80.4.

These infusions in ml/h approximate μg/min. Absolute doses with regard to body weight are not relevant; rather the titrated clinical effect. Vasoactive drugs are usually prescribed as a titration against a desired mean arterial pressure.

SPECIFIC SITUATIONS

The following is a summary of the clinical uses of inotropes and vasopressors in common conditions of circulatory failure. Specific pharmacology and physiological effects are discussed above.

CARDIOPULMONARY RESUSCITATION

Epinephrine has been used for circulatory collapse, at least since 1907. The International Liaison Committee on Resuscitation guidelines recommend epinephrine as first line inotrope/vasopressor in cardiopulmonary resuscitation.[48] Doses are 1 mg intravenously every 3 min.

The use of 'high dose' epinephrine (5 mg), norepinephrine or phenylephrine in cardiopulmonary resuscita-

Table 80.4 Infusion concentrations of commonly used vasoactive drugs

Agent	Infusion concentration	Dose
Epinephrine	6 mg/100 ml 5% dextrose	Titrate ml/h (= μg/min)
Norepinephrine	6 mg/100 ml 5% dextrose	Titrate m/h (= μg/min)
Dopamine	400 mg/100 ml 5% dextrose	Titrate m/h ($\sim \mu$g/kg per min)
Dobutamine	500 mg/100 ml 5% dextrose	Titrate ml/h ($\sim \mu$g/kg per min)
Dopexamine	200 mg/100 ml 5% dextrose	Initially 0.5 μg/kg per h
		Dose range 1–6 μg/kg per h
Isoprenaline	6 mg/100 ml 5% dextrose	Titrate ml/h (= μg/min)
Milrinone	10 mg/100 ml 5% dextrose	Loading dose: 50 μg/kg over 20 min
		Infusion: 0.5 μg/kg per min
Phenylephrine	10 mg/100 ml 5% dextrose	Titrate ml/h (= 100 μg/h)
Metaraminol	100 mg/100 ml 5% dextrose	Titrate ml/h (= mg/h)
Ephedrine	300 mg/100 ml 5% dextrose	Titrate ml/h (= 3 mg/h)
Vasopressin	20 U/20 ml 5% dextrose	2.4 ml/h (0.04 U/min)
Hydrocortisone	100 mg/100 ml 5% dextrose	Loading dose: 100 mg
		Infusion: 0.18 mg/kg per h

tion has not been demonstrated to improve return of spontaneous circulation or survival.

Epinephrine is recommended as first line therapy for 'medical pacing' for severe bradyarrhythmias that do not respond to atropine. Isoprenaline has traditionally been used for this purpose; however its use has been superseded by epinephrine due to concerns about efficacy and lack of α-adrenergic activity.

CARDIOGENIC SHOCK

Theoretically, catecholamine infusions may confer some advantages in cardiogenic shock, particularly in association with acute myocardial infarction.[49] In patients with systolic heart failure, epinephrine, norepinephrine, dopamine and dobutamine have been shown to cause satisfactory short-term effects. This may allow the myocardium time to recover from post ischaemic 'stunning,' particularly after revascularization. However, no increased long-term survival due to their use has been demonstrated.

The role of phosphodiesterase inhibitors in acute heart failure has yet to be determined, but they may have a potential role in patients with diastolic heart failure. Due to their non-adrenergic mechanism of action, these agents may be useful in patients who are 'resistant' to catecholamines.

Norepinephrine is increasingly being used as a first line drug in patients with cardiogenic shock, although dobutamine has traditionally been used in this situation.

SEPARATION FROM CARDIOPULMONARY BYPASS

Numerous combinations of catecholamines have been used successfully to wean patients from cardiopulmonary bypass. However, there are no definitive studies demonstrating significant benefits of one catecholamine over another.[50] Similarly, the question whether mechanical support devices, such as intra-aortic counterpulsation, offer a significant advantage over inotropes following cardiac surgery remains unanswered.[51]

Epinephrine, norepinephrine and/or dopamine have been found to increase cardiac output with little increase in heart rate or afterload and are often regarded as first line drugs. At higher doses (>40 μg/kg per min), dopamine has been shown to cause more tachycardia than epinephrine and norepinephrine. Dobutamine may be associated with vasodilatation and hypotension.

There is no conclusive evidence that the catecholamines, including norepinephrine, cause vasospasm of arterial conduits in clinically used doses.

Phosphodiesterase inhibitors, such as milrinone, either as sole agents or in conjunction with epinephrine or norepinephrine have been used with success. These may have a role following mitral valve replacement in patients with pulmonary hypertension or preoperative diastolic failure.

Cardiopulmonary bypass may be associated with a systemic inflammatory response syndrome characterized by a hyperdynamic, vasodilated 'low systemic vascular resistance' state.[52,53] Norepinephrine is frequently advocated as a 'pressor' agent in this context, to restore mean arterial pressure that may be reduced as a consequence. This condition is usually self-limiting with a nadir 8 h post bypass. Although catecholamines may be required to achieve appropriate target mean arterial pressure and cardiac output, caution should be applied if high doses (e.g. >30 μg/min norepinephrine) are required. This may be associated with tachyphylaxis and potentiation of catecholamine dependency.

RIGHT VENTRICULAR FAILURE

Right ventricular infarction and major pulmonary embolism may be associated with acute right ventricular failure. Right ventricular depression may also occur in severe sepsis.[54] Restoration of preload is critical in these conditions, as the failing right ventricle is particularly susceptible to reductions in preload.[55]

Inotropes such as norepinephrine and epinephrine are regarded as first line drugs in these situations in order to maintain adequate mean arterial pressure so that right coronary artery perfusion, that occurs throughout the cardiac cycle, is maintained.

Concerns about pulmonary artery vasoconstriction and increased right ventricular afterload by norepinephrine and epinephrine appear to be unfounded. Consequently, the use of traditional vasodilators, such as isoprenaline in acute right ventricular failure has been superseded by these drugs.

SEPTIC SHOCK

The cardiovascular effects of the sepsis syndrome and septic shock are complex and range from a hyperdynamic, vasodilated state to one of increasing myocardial failure and paralysis of the peripheral vasculature (vasoplegia).[7,56,57] The latter represents inability of the venous circulation to respond to endogenous or exogenous catecholamines with resultant venous pooling.

Consequently, it is important to establish that the patient is not hypovolaemic before using a catecholamine infusion in septic shock, as 20% of patients will respond, at least initially, to intravascular volume expansion.

An increasing body of literature now supports the use of norepinephrine, epinephrine as first line agents in the septic syndrome and septic shock by effectively defending cardiac output, mean arterial pressure and thereby tissue perfusion.[58–62] Systemic vascular resistance is not significantly altered by catecholamine infusions in septic shock.[63]

Despite widespread recent use, the efficacy of dobutamine and isoprenaline in septic shock is questionable and appear to add little to the efficacy of norepinephrine or epinephrine when used in combination.[64] However, the attributable benefit of a particular catecholamine on mortality on septic shock has not been established.

Doses required to achieve this adequate mean arterial pressure may vary: norepinephrine or epinephrine infusions (up to 70 μg/min) may be necessary.

Infusions of vasopressors such as phenylephrine,[65] metaraminol or hormones, such as angiotensin[66] have been used to augment mean arterial pressure in patients with refractory septic shock with variable degrees of success.

Patients who develop marked catecholamine dependency, in the absence of other acute remediable causes such as active infection, may respond to low doses of vasopressin or 'stress response' doses of hydrocortisone[65] (see below).

ANAPHYLAXIS

Epinephrine is the drug of choice for anaphylactic reactions and for life-threatening bronchospasm, as it blocks mediator release and specifically reverses end-organ effects. A dose of 0.1 mg, as 1 ml of 1:10 000 solution, may be injected subcutaneously, intramuscularly or intravenously. Repeated doses or infusions of up to 100 μg/min may be required. A strong slowing pulse indicates a pressor effect and provides a useful clinical end-point for the rate of infusion. This α agonist effect is probably also of considerable importance in anaphylaxis, as deaths are frequently due to prolonged refractory hypotension caused by acute biventricular failure. Early intravenous fluid therapy is also important.

RENAL PROTECTION

Augmentation of mean arterial pressure in order to prevent or ameliorate acute renal failure in critically ill patients is an important use of inotropes. In addition to ensuring adequate preload, catecholamines may be used to defend renal perfusion by maintaining mean arterial pressure at appropriate levels. This is important in hypertensive patients, where higher mean arterial pressure may be required to maintain renal perfusion, particularly when these patients develop intercurrent causes of circulatory failure.

'Renal' dose dopamine (2 μg/kg per min) has been advocated for many years as a renal protective agent by causing renal vasodilatation. However, this has not been substantiated in controlled clinical trials in susceptible patients,[20] or as an adjunctive agent with other inotropes in septic shock.[17] In addition, the prolonged use of low dose dopamine is associated with suppression of anterior and posterior pituitary hormonal secretion and impairment in T-cell function.[67,68] Consequently, low dose dopamine is no longer recommended.

Equivalent renal protection has been demonstrated with dopamine, norepinephrine[18] and dobutamine[19] and it is likely that this effect relates primarily to defence of renal perfusion, rather than a specific renal effect.[69]

CEREBRAL PERFUSION PRESSURE

Augmentation of cerebral perfusion pressure is an important strategy in patients with pathological reductions in cerebral blood flow. This is well described, following traumatic brain injury and aneurysmal subarachnoid haemorrhage and is discussed elsewhere in this volume. Catecholamine interactions on the cerebral vasculature are discussed above.

Norepinephrine, epinephrine, dopamine and phenylephrine have been used to augment cerebral perfusion pressure, although there is no conclusive evidence to recommend one drug over another.[16]

REFERENCES

1 Jacobsohn E, Chorn R, O'Connor M. The role of the vasculature in regulating venous return and cardiac output: historical and graphical approach. *Can J Anaesth* 1997; **44**: 849–67.

2 Guyton AC, Lindsay AW, Kaufmann BN. Effect of mean circulatory filling pressure and other peripheral circulatory factors on cardiac output. *Am J Physiol* 1955; **180**: 463–8.

3 Bressack MA, Raffin TA. Importance of venous return, venous resistance, and mean circulatory pressure in the physiology and management of shock. *Chest* 1987; **92**: 906–12.

4 Magder S, Rastepagarnah M. Role of neurosympathetic pathways in the vascular response to sepsis. *J Crit Care* 1998; **13**: 169–76.

5 Cotter G, Kaluski E, Moshkovitz Y *et al*. Pulmonary edema: new insight on pathogenesis and treatment. *Curr Opin Cardiol* 2001; **16**: 159–63.

6 Aronow WS. Left ventricular diastolic heart failure with normal left ventricular systolic function in older persons. *J Lab Clin Med* 2001; **137**: 316–23.

7 Magder S, Vanelli G. Circuit factors in the high cardiac output of sepsis. *J Crit Care* 1996; **11**: 155–66.

8 Insel PA. Seminars in medicine of the Beth Israel Hospital, Boston. Adrenergic receptors – evolving concepts and clinical implications. *N Engl J Med* 1996; **334**: 580–5.

9 Silverman HJ, Penaranda R, Orens JB, Lee NH. Impaired beta-adrenergic receptor stimulation of cyclic adenosine monophosphate in human septic shock: association with myocardial hyporesponsiveness to catecholamines. *Crit Care Med* 1993; **21**: 31–9.

10 Runciman WB, Morris JL. Adrenoceptor agonists. In: Feldman AC, Paton W, Scurr C (eds) *Mechanisms of Drugs in Anaesthesia*. London: Edward Arnold; 1993: 262–91.

11 Jones SB, Romano FD. Myocardial beta adrenergic receptor coupling to adenylate cyclase during developing septic shock. *Circ Shock* 1990; **30**: 51–61.

12 Witkowska M, Halawa B. Beta-adrenergic receptors and catecholamines in acute myocardial infarction. *Mater Med Pol* 1989; **21**: 195–8.

13 Heusch G. Alpha-adrenergic mechanisms in myocardial ischemia. *Circulation* 1990; **81**: 1–13.

14 Hardebo JE, Owman C. Barrier mechanisms for neurotransmitter monoamines and their precursors at the blood-brain interface. *Ann Neurol* 1980; **8**: 1–31.

15 Myburgh JA, Upton RN, Grant C, Martinez A. A comparison of the effects of norepinephrine, epinephrine, and dopamine on cerebral blood flow and oxygen utilization. *Acta Neurochir Suppl (Wien)* 1998; **71**: 19–21.

16 Kroppenstedt SN, Stover JF, Unterberg AW. Effects of dopamine on posttraumatic cerebral blood flow, brain edema, and cerebrospinal fluid glutamate and hypoxanthine concentrations. *Crit Care Med* 2000; **28**: 3792–8.

17 Bersten AD, Rutten AJ. Renovascular interaction of epinephrine, dopamine, and intraperitoneal sepsis. *Crit Care Med* 1995; **23**: 537–44.

18 Desjars P, Pinaud M, Bugnon D *et al.* Norepinephrine therapy has no deleterious renal effects in human septic shock. *Crit Care Med* 1989; **17**: 426–9.

19 Duke GJ, Briedis JH, Weaver RA. Renal support in critically ill patients: low-dose dopamine or low-dose dobutamine? *Crit Care Med* 1994; **22**: 1919–25.

20 Bellomo R, Chapman M, Finfer S *et al.* Low-dose dopamine in patients with early renal dysfunction: a placebo-controlled randomised trial. Australian and New Zealand Intensive Care Society (ANZICS) Clinical Trials Group. *Lancet* 2000; **356**: 2139–43.

21 Sakka SG, Meier-Hellmann A, Reinhart K. Do fluid administration and reduction in norepinephrine dose improve global and splanchnic haemodynamics? *Br J Anaesth* 2000; **84**: 758–62.

22 Levy B, Nace L, Bollaert PE *et al.* Comparison of systemic and regional effects of dobutamine and dopexamine in norepinephrine-treated septic shock. *Intensive Care Med* 1999; **25**: 942–8.

23 Duranteau J, Sitbon P, Teboul JL *et al.* Effects of epinephrine, norepinephrine, or the combination of norepinephrine and dobutamine on gastric mucosa in septic shock. *Crit Care Med* 1999; **27**: 893–900.

24 Uusaro A, Takala J. Vasoactive drugs and splanchnic perfusion in septic shock. *Crit Care Med* 1998; **26**: 1458–60.

25 Levy B, Bollaert PE, Charpentier C *et al.* Comparison of norepinephrine and dobutamine to epinephrine for hemodynamics, lactate metabolism, and gastric tonometric variables in septic shock: a prospective, randomized study. *Intensive Care Med* 1997; **23**: 282–7.

26 Day NP, Phu NH, Bethell DP *et al.* The effects of dopamine and epinephrine infusions on acid-base balance and systemic haemodynamics in severe infection. *Lancet* 1996; **348**: 219–23.

27 Totaro RJ, Raper RF. Epinephrine-induced lactic acidosis following cardiopulmonary bypass. *Crit Care Med* 1997; **25**: 1693–9.

28 Day NP, Phu NH, Mai NT *et al.* Effects of dopamine and epinephrine infusions on renal hemodynamics in severe malaria and severe sepsis. *Crit Care Med* 2000; **28**: 1353–62.

29 Seino Y, Takano T, Hayakawa H *et al.* Hemodynamic effects and pharmacokinetics of oral milrinone for short-term support in acute heart failure. *Cardiology* 1995; **86**: 34–40.

30 Seino Y, Momomura S, Takano T *et al.* Multicenter, double-blind study of intravenous milrinone for patients with acute heart failure in Japan. Japan Intravenous Milrinone Investigators. *Crit Care Med* 1996; **24**: 1490–7.

31 The effect of digoxin on mortality and morbidity in patients with heart failure. The Digitalis Investigation Group. *N Engl J Med* 1997; **336**: 525–33.

32 Sensky PR, Olczak SA. High-dose intravenous glucagon in severe tricyclic poisoning. *Postgrad Med J* 1999; **75**: 611–2.

33 Malik FS, Mehra MR, Uber PA *et al.* Intravenous thyroid hormone supplementation in heart failure with cardiogenic shock. *J Card Fail* 1999; **5**: 31–7.

34 Gregory JS, Bonfiglio MF, Dasta JF *et al.* Experience with phenylephrine as a component of the pharmacologic support of septic shock. *Crit Care Med* 1991; **19**: 1395–400.

35 Bonfiglio MF, Dasta JF, Gregory JS *et al.* High-dose phenylephrine infusion in the hemodynamic support of septic shock. *DICP* 1990; **24**: 936–9.

36 Landry DW, Levin HR, Gallant EM *et al.* Vasopressin deficiency contributes to the vasodilation of septic shock. *Circulation* 1997; **95**: 1122–5.

37 Argenziano M, Choudhri AF, Oz MC *et al.* A prospective randomized trial of arginine vasopressin in the treatment of vasodilatory shock after left ventricular assist device placement. *Circulation* 1997; **96**: II-90.

38 Malay MB, Ashton RC, Jr., Landry DW *et al.* Low-dose vasopressin in the treatment of vasodilatory septic shock. *J Trauma* 1999; **47**: 699–703.

39 Rozenfeld V, Cheng JW. The role of vasopressin in the treatment of vasodilation in shock states. *Ann Pharmacother* 2000; **34**: 250–4.

40 Briegel J, Forst H, Haller M *et al.* Stress doses of hydrocortisone reverse hyperdynamic septic shock: a prospective, randomized, double-blind, single-center study. *Crit Care Med* 1999; **27**: 723–32.

41 Oppert M, Reinicke A, Graf KJ *et al.* Plasma cortisol levels before and during 'low-dose' hydrocortisone therapy and their relationship to hemodynamic improvement in patients with septic shock. *Intensive Care Med* 2000; **26**: 1747–55.

42 Hatherill M, Tibby SM, Hilliard T *et al.* Adrenal insufficiency in septic shock. *Arch Dis Child* 1999; **80**: 51–5.

43 Booke M, Hinder F, McGuire R *et al.* Noradrenaline and nomega-monomethyl-L-arginine (L-NMMA): effects on haemodynamics and regional blood flow in healthy and septic sheep. *Clin Sci (Colch)* 2000; **98**: 193–200.

44 Booke M, Hinder F, McGuire R *et al.* Nitric oxide synthase inhibition versus norepinephrine for the treat-

ment of hyperdynamic sepsis in sheep. *Crit Care Med* 1996; **24**: 835–44.

45 Dorman T, Breslow MJ, Lipsett PA *et al*. Radial artery pressure monitoring underestimates central arterial pressure during vasopressor therapy in critically ill surgical patients. *Crit Care Med* 1998; **26**: 1646–9.

46 Magder S. More respect for the CVP. *Intensive Care Med* 1998; **24**: 651–3.

47 Heyland DK, Cook DJ, King D *et al*. Maximizing oxygen delivery in critically ill patients: a methodologic appraisal of the evidence. *Crit Care Med* 1996; **24**: 517–24.

48 Chamberlain DA, Cummins RO. Advisory statements of the International Liaison Committee on Resuscitation ('ILCOR'). *Resuscitation* 1997; **34**: 99–100.

49 Alpert JS, Becker RC. Mechanisms and management of cardiogenic shock. *Crit Care Clin* 1993; **9**: 205–18.

50 Richard C, Ricome JL, Rimailho A *et al*. Combined hemodynamic effects of dopamine and dobutamine in cardiogenic shock. *Circulation* 1983; **67**: 620–6.

51 Moulopoulos SD, Stamateolopoulos SF, Nanas JN *et al*. Effect of protracted dobutamine infusion on survival of patients in cardiogenic shock treated with intraaortic balloon pumping. *Chest* 1993; **103**: 248–52.

52 Kristof AS, Magder S. Low systemic vascular resistance state in patients undergoing cardiopulmonary bypass. *Crit Care Med* 1999; **27**: 1121–7.

53 Gomes WJ, Carvalho AC, Palma JH *et al*. Vasoplegic syndrome after open heart surgery. *J Cardiovasc Surg (Torino)* 1998; **39**: 619–23.

54 Le Tulzo Y, Seguin P, Gacouin A *et al*. Effects of epinephrine on right ventricular function in patients with severe septic shock and right ventricular failure: a preliminary descriptive study. *Intensive Care Med* 1997; **23**: 664–70.

55 Haji SA, Movahed A. Right ventricular infarction – diagnosis and treatment. *Clin Cardiol* 2000; **23**: 473–82.

56 MacKenzie IM. The haemodynamics of human septic shock. *Anaesthesia* 2001; **56**: 130–44.

57 Carpati CM, Astiz ME, Rackow EC. Mechanisms and management of myocardial dysfunction in septic shock. *Crit Care Med* 1999; **27**: 231–2.

58 LeDoux D, Astiz ME, Carpati CM, Rackow EC. Effects of perfusion pressure on tissue perfusion in septic shock. *Crit Care Med* 2000; **28**: 2729–32.

59 Nasraway SA. Norepinephrine: no more 'leave 'em dead'? *Crit Care Med* 2000; **28**: 3096–8.

60 Tordoff SG, Thompson JL, Williams AW. Noradrenaline as a vasoactive agent in septic shock. *Intensive Care Med* 2000; **26**: 648.

61 Martin C, Papazian L, Perrin G *et al*. Norepinephrine or dopamine for the treatment of hyperdynamic septic shock? *Chest* 1993; **103**: 1826–31.

62 Martin C, Viviand X, Leone M, Thirion X. Effect of norepinephrine on the outcome of septic shock. *Crit Care Med* 2000; **28**: 2758–65.

63 Moran JL, O'Fathartaigh MS, Peisach AR *et al*. Epinephrine as an inotropic agent in septic shock: a dose-profile analysis. *Crit Care Med* 1993; **21**: 70–7.

64 Martin C, Viviand X, Arnaud S *et al*. Effects of norepinephrine plus dobutamine or norepinephrine alone on left ventricular performance of septic shock patients. *Crit Care Med* 1999; **27**: 1708–13.

65 Bellissant E, Annane D. Effect of hydrocortisone on phenylephrine – mean arterial pressure dose-response relationship in septic shock. *Clin Pharmacol Ther* 2000; **68**: 293–303.

66 Yunge M, Petros A. Angiotensin for septic shock unresponsive to noradrenaline. *Arch Dis Child* 2000; **82**: 388–9.

67 Van den Berghe G, de Zegher F. Anterior pituitary function during critical illness and dopamine treatment. *Crit Care Med* 1996; **24**: 1580–90.

68 Van den Berghe G, de Zegher F, Lauwers P, Veldhuis JD. Growth hormone secretion in critical illness: effect of dopamine. *J Clin Endocrinol Metab* 1994; **79**: 1141–6.

69 Bersten AD, Holt AW. Vasoactive drugs and the importance of renal perfusion pressure. *New Horiz* 1995; **3**: 650–61.

81

Vasodilators and antihypertensives

J A Myburgh

Vasodilators are a generic group of drugs that are primarily used in the intensive care unit for the management of acute hypertensive states and emergencies. In addition, they have an important role in the management of hypertension and cardiac failure.[1]

PHYSIOLOGY

Blood pressure is controlled by a complex physiological neurohormonal system involving all components of the cardiovascular system.[2] Traditionally, clinical practice has focused on the arterial circulation as the major regulator of systemic pressure. The importance of venous circulation in determining mean arterial pressure and cardiac output is discussed in Chapter 80.[3]

The role of the peripheral vasculature, including both arteriolar and venous systems, in the regulation of blood pressure may be conceptually regarded as a balance between vasodilation and vasoconstriction (Figure 81.1).[4]

CALCIUM FLUX

The concentration of intracellular ionized calcium is the primary determinant of vascular smooth muscle tone: increases lead to smooth muscle contraction, decreases cause relaxation. Control of calcium influx and efflux is determined by adrenergic receptor occupation and changes in membrane potential, mediated through voltage gated channels (see Ch. 80, Figure 80.2).

ENDOTHELIAL SYSTEM

The endothelium has a central role in blood pressure homeostasis by secreting substances such as nitric oxide, prostacyclin and endothelin.[5]

Nitric oxide is synthesized from L-arginine by nitric oxide synthases. It is released under the influence of endothelial agonists, such as norepinephrine, acetylcholine and substance P and in response to mechanical factors, such as endothelial shear forces and pulsatile flow. Nitric oxide diffuses into underlying smooth muscle where it activates guanylate cyclase to increase cyclic guanosine monophosphate (cGMP). Subsequent phosphorylation results in relaxation of underlying smooth muscle and vasodilation.[6]

Prostacyclin is synthesized via the arachidonic pathway and has a minor role in the control of vascular tone.

Endothelin is an endothelium derived, vasoconstrictor peptide that is associated with increases in vascular smooth muscle intracellular calcium. It acts as endogenous ligand to regulate voltage gated calcium channels, thereby producing vasoconstriction, usually in response to shear stresses, tissue hypoxia, angiotensin II and inflammatory mediators (e.g. interleukin-6 and nuclear factor $\kappa\beta$).[7]

These substances are continuously released by the endothelium and are integral in regional autoregulation.

RENIN-ANGIOTENSIN-ALDOSTERONE SYSTEM

Angiotensinogen is converted by renin to form angiotensin I, which is subsequently converted to angiotensin II by angiotensin converting enzyme (ACE). Angiotensin II has a number of effects that are responsible for blood pressure homeostasis. These include release of aldosterone, direct activation of α adrenergic receptors on vascular smooth muscle and a direct effect in the endothelium. These effects are directed at defending blood pressure and are integral in the stress response.

Angiotensin converting enzyme is also responsible for the inactivation of bradykinins that have predominantly vasodilatory effects, coupled to arachidonic acid synthesis and generation of prostacyclin.

ADRENERGIC SYSTEM

The sympathetic nervous system is integrally involved with all of the above systems, regulating vascular tone at central, ganglionic and local neural levels. Adrenergic

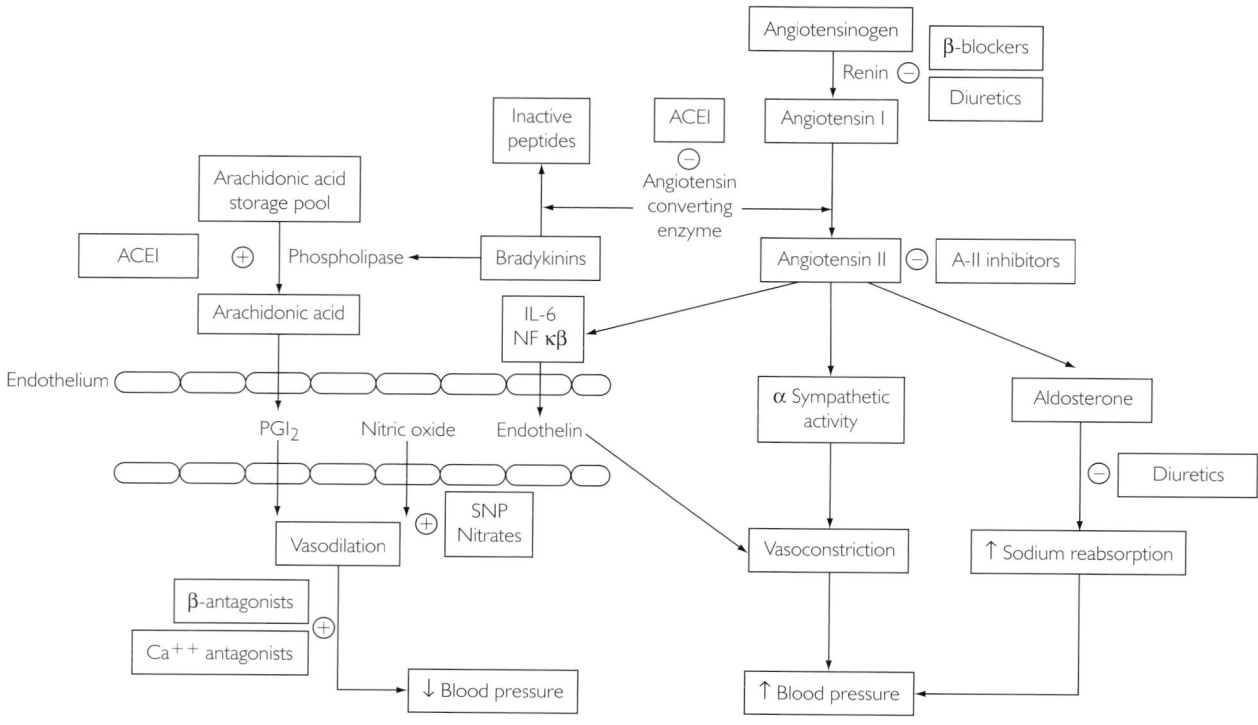

Fig. 81.1 Schematic diagram of the neurohormonal factors determining vasomotor tone. Mechanism of action of vasodilators is shown by (−) for inhibition, (+) for stimulation. ACEI, angiotensin converting enzyme inhibitors; A-II, angiotensin II; SNP, sodium nitroprusside; PGI₂, prostacyclin; IL, interleukin; NF, nuclear factor.

stimulation of β-receptors is associated with vasodilation; α receptor stimulation results in vasoconstriction. The vascular effects of the catecholamines and vasopressors are discussed in Chapter 80.

Adrenergic stimulation is the predominant system in regulating venous tone. This is due to endothelial differences in veins resulting in less production of nitric oxide and reduced responsiveness to angiotensin II.

PATHOPHYSIOLOGY

Hypertensive states develop as a result of impaired or abnormal homeostatic processes, causing an imbalance between vasoconstrictive and vasodilatory effects.

Essential hypertension is the most common cause of hypertension and is due to abnormal neurohormonal regulation, particularly exaggerated effects of renin-angiotensin activity.

Secondary causes of hypertension include structural abnormalities, such as aortic stenosis or renal artery stenosis; endocrine conditions such as phaeochromocytoma, Cushing's syndrome and pregnancy induced hypertension; or central causes such as hypertensive encephalopathy or raised intracranial pressure.

CALCIUM ANTAGONISTS

Calcium antagonists have numerous effects on the cardiovascular system, influencing heart rate conduction, myocardial contractility and vasomotor tone. Entry of calcium through voltage-gated calcium channels is a major determinant of arteriolar, but not venous tone.[8]

There are three major groups of arterioselective calcium antagonists: dihydropyridines (e.g. nifedipine, nimodipine, nicardipine and amlodipine), phenylalkylamines (e.g. verapamil) and benzothiazepines (e.g. diltiazem).

Magnesium is a physiological calcium antagonist, and is used therapeutically as magnesium sulphate.

NIFEDIPINE

Nifedipine is a predominant arteriolar vasodilator, with minimal effect on venous capacitance vessels and no direct depressant effect on heart rate conduction.

It may be administered intravenously, orally or sublingually: has a rapid onset of action (2–5 min) and duration of action of 20–30 min.

Nifedipine is frequently used to treat angina pectoris, especially that due to coronary artery vasospasm. Peripheral vasodilation results in decreased systemic blood pressure, often with associated increased peripheral sympathetic stimulation causing increased cardiac output and heart rate. The sympathetic stimulation often counters the negative inotropic, chronotropic and dromotropic effects of nifedipine. Nevertheless, nifedipine may be associated with profound hypotension in patients with ventricular dysfunction, aortic stenosis and/or concomitant β-blockade. For this reason, the use of sublingual nifedipine as a method of treating hypertensive emergencies has been questioned.[9]

Nifedipine and related drugs may cause diuretic resistant peripheral oedema that is due to redistribution of extracellular fluid rather than sodium and water retention.

NIMODIPINE

Nimodipine is a highly lipid soluble analogue of nifedipine. High lipid solubility facilitates entrance into the central nervous system where it causes selective cerebral arterial vasodilation.

It is used to attenuate cerebral vasospasm following aneurysmal subarachnoid haemorrhage. Improved outcomes have been demonstrated in patients with Grade 1 and 2 aneurysmal subarachnoid haemorrhage.[10] Systemic hypotension may result from peripheral vasodilation that may compromise cerebral blood flow in susceptible patients. Similarly, cerebral vasodilation may increase intracranial pressure in patients with reduced intracranial elastance.

It may be given by intravenous infusion or enterally with equal effect.

VERAPAMIL

The primary effect of verapamil is on the atrioventricular node and this drug is principally used as an anti-arrhythmic for the treatment of supraventricular tachyarrhythmias. For this reason, concomitant therapy with β-blockers or digoxin is not recommended.

Verapamil is not as active as nifedipine in its effects on smooth muscle and therefore causes less pronounced decrease in systemic blood pressure and reflex sympathetic activity. It has a limited role as a vasodilator.[11]

DILTIAZEM

Diltiazem has a similar cardiovascular profile to verapamil, although its vasodilatory properties are intermediate between nifedipine and verapamil. Diltiazem exerts minimal cardiodepressant effects and is unlikely to potentiate β-blockers.

MAGNESIUM SULPHATE

Magnesium regulates intracellular calcium and potassium levels by activation of membrane pumps and competition with calcium for transmembrane channels. Physiological effects are widespread affecting cardiovascular, central and peripheral nervous systems and the musculoskeletal junction.[12]

It acts as a direct arteriolar and venous vasodilator causing reductions in blood pressure. Modulation of central mediated and peripheral sympathetic tone results in variable effects on cardiac output and heart rate.

Consequently, it has an established role in the treatment of pre-eclampsia and eclampsia, perioperative management of phaeochromocytoma and treatment of autonomic dysfunction in tetanus.[13]

DIRECT ACTING VASODILATORS

These drugs act directly on vascular smooth muscle and exert their effects predominantly by increasing the concentration of endothelial nitric oxide. These drugs are also known as nitrovasodilators.[14,15]

SODIUM NITROPRUSSIDE

Sodium nitroprusside is a non-selective vasodilator that causes relaxation of arterial and venous smooth muscle. It is compromised of a ferrous ion centre associated with five cyanide moieties and a nitrosyl group. The molecule is 44% cyanide by weight.

It is reconstituted from a powdered form. The solution is light sensitive requiring protection from exposure to light by wrapping administration sets in aluminium foil. Prolonged exposure to light may be associated with an increase in release of hydrogen cyanide, although this is seldom clinically significant.

When infused intravenously, sodium nitroprusside interacts with oxyhaemoglobin, dissociating immediately to form methaemoglobin, while releasing free cyanide and nitric oxide. The latter is responsible for the vasodilatory effect of sodium nitroprusside.

Onset of action is almost immediate with a transient duration, requiring continuous intravenous infusion to maintain a therapeutic effect.

Tachyphylaxis is common, particularly in younger patients. Large doses should not be used if the desired therapeutic effect is not attained, as this may be associated with toxicity.

Sodium nitroprusside produces direct venous and arterial vasodilation resulting in a prompt decrease in systemic blood pressure. The effect on cardiac output is variable. Decreases in right atrial pressure reflect pooling of blood in the venous system, which may decrease in cardiac output. This may result in reflex tachycardia that may oppose the overall reduction in blood pressure. In patients with left ventricular failure, the effect on cardiac output will depend on initial left ventricular end-diastolic pressure. Sodium nitroprusside has unpredictable effects on calculated systemic vascular resistance. Homeostatic mechanisms in preserving cardiac output may explain tachyphylaxis to prolonged infusions.[16]

Sodium nitroprusside may increase myocardial ischaemia in patients with coronary artery disease by causing an intra-coronary steal of blood flow away from ischaemic areas by arteriolar vasodilation. Secondary tachycardia may also exacerbate myocardial ischaemia.

Due to its non-selectivity, sodium nitroprusside has direct effects on most vascular beds. In the cerebral circulation, sodium nitroprusside is a cerebral vasodilator, leading to increases in cerebral blood flow and blood volume. This may be critical in patients with increased intracranial pressure. Rapid and profound reductions in mean arterial pressure produced by sodium nitroprusside may exceed the autoregulatory capacity of the brain to maintain adequate cerebral blood flow.

Sodium nitroprusside is a pulmonary vasodilator and may attenuate hypoxic pulmonary vasoconstriction resulting in increased intrapulmonary shunting and decreased arterial oxygen tension. This phenomenon may be exacerbated by associated hypotension.[17]

The prolonged use of large doses of sodium nitroprusside may be associated with toxicity related to the production of cyanide and to a lesser extent, methaemoglobin.

Free cyanide produced by the dissociation of sodium nitroprusside reacts with methaemoglobin to form cyanmethaemoglobin; or metabolized by rhodenase in the liver and kidneys to form thiocyanate. A healthy adult can eliminate cyanide at a rate equivalent to a sodium nitroprusside infusion of 2 μg/kg per min or up to 10 μg/kg per min for 10 min, although there is marked inter-individual variability.

Toxicity should be considered in patients who become resistant to sodium nitroprusside despite maximum infusion rates and who develop an unexplained lactic acidosis. In high doses, cyanide may cause seizures.

Treatment of suspected cyanide toxicity is cessation of the infusion and administration of 100% oxygen. Sodium thiosulphate (150 mg/kg) coverts cyanide to thiocyanate, which is excreted renally. For severe cyanide toxicity, sodium nitrate may be infused (5 mg/kg) to produce methaemoglobin and subsequently cyanmethaemoglobin. Hydroxocobalamin, which binds cyanide to produce cyanocobalamin, may also be administered (25 mg/h to maximum of 100 mg).[18]

GLYCERYL TRINITRATE

Glyceryl trinitrate is organic nitrate that generates nitric oxide through a different mechanism to sodium nitroprusside.

The pharmacokinetics allow glyceryl trinitrate to be given by infusion, with a longer onset and duration of action than sodium nitroprusside. Glyceryl trinitrate may also be administered sublingually, orally or transdermally.

Tachyphylaxis is common with glyceryl trinitrate; doses should not be increased if patients no longer respond to standard doses. Glass bottles or polyethylene administration sets are required as glyceryl trinitrate is absorbed into standard polyvinylchloride sets.

The effects on the peripheral vasculature are dose dependent, acting principally on venous capacitance vessels to produce venous pooling and decreased ventricular afterload. These are important mechanisms in patients with cardiac failure.

Glyceryl trinitrate primarily dilates larger conductance vessels of the coronary circulation, resulting in increased coronary blood flow to ischaemic subendocardial areas, thereby relieving angina pectoris. This is in contrast to sodium nitroprusside that may cause a coronary steal phenomenon.[19,20]

Reductions in blood pressure are more dependent on blood volume than sodium nitroprusside. Precipitous falls in blood pressure may occur in hypovolaemic patients with small doses of glyceryl trinitrate. In euvolaemic patients, reflex tachycardia is not as pronounced as with sodium nitroprusside. At higher doses, arteriolar vasodilation occurs without significant changes in calculated systemic vascular resistance.

Glyceryl trinitrate is a cerebral vasodilator and should be used with caution in patients with reduced intracranial elastance. Headache due to this mechanism is a common side effect in conscious patients.

ISOSORBIDE DINITRATE

Isosorbide dinitrate is the most commonly administered oral nitrate for the prophylaxis of angina pectoris. It has a physiological effect that lasts up to 6 h in doses of 60–120 mg.

Mechanism of action is the same as glyceryl trinitrate. Hypotension may follow acute administration, but tolerance to this develops with chronic therapy.

HYDRALAZINE

Hydralazine is a potent, arterioselective direct acting vasodilator that acts via stimulation of cGMP and inhibition of smooth muscle myosin light chain kinase.

Following intravenous administration, hydralazine has a rapid onset of action, usually within 5–10 min. It may also be administered intramuscularly or orally. The drug is partially metabolized by acetylation, for which there is marked inter-individual variability (35% of the population are slow acetylators). While this does not have much clinical significance regarding the antihypertensive effects, it is important with respect to toxicity.

Hydralazine causes predominantly arteriolar vasodilation that is widespread, but not uniform. It is associated with direct and reflex sympathetic activity, so that cardiac output and heart rate are increased. Prolonged use of hydralazine stimulates renin release and is associated with sodium and water retention. Consequently, hydralazine is frequently administered with β-blockers and/or diuretics.

Chronic use of hydralazine may be associated with immunological side-effects, including a lupus syndrome, vasculitis, haemolytic anaemia and rapidly progressive glomerulonephritis.

DIAZOXIDE

Diazoxide is chemically related to the thiazide diuretics and is a potent, non-selective, direct acting vasodilator. The mechanism of action is unclear, but it is a predominantly arteriolar vasodilator.[21]

Diazoxide is administered intravenously or intramuscularly. It has a rapid onset (3–5 min) and prolonged duration of action (1–2 h), often with precipitous reductions in blood pressure.

Diazoxide has similar cardiovascular effects to hydralazine and is associated with significant reflex sympathetic stimulation resulting in increased cardiac output and heart rate.

It is a useful drug in accelerated hypertension associated with acute renal failure, such as glomerulonephritis and has been used in severe pregnancy induced hypertension and eclampsia. Stimulation of catecholamine release prohibits the use of diazoxide in patients with phaeochromocytoma.

It is associated with metabolic side-effects such as hyperglycaemia and sodium and water retention.

α-ADRENERGIC ANTAGONISTS

Several groups of compounds act as α adrenergic blockers with variable affinity for populations of α-receptors. Physiological and pathophysiological may influence the responsiveness of the drug-receptor-effector relationship. Receptor pathobiology is discussed in Chapter 81. Consequently, there may be marked inter- and intra-individual variability in the patient's response to these drugs.[22]

There are six main groups of α-receptor antagonists: imidazolines (e.g. phentolamine), haloalkylamines (e.g. phenoxybenzamine), prazosin, β-adrenergic antagonists with α-receptor antagonism (labetalol, carvedilol), phenothiazines (chlorpromazine) and butyrophenones (haloperidol).

PHENTOLAMINE

Phentolamine is a non-selective, competitive antagonist at α_1 and α_2 receptors. At low doses, phentolamine causes prejunctional inhibition of noradrenaline release (via α_2 receptor inhibition). At higher doses, more complete α receptor blockade is achieved, with enhancement of effects of β-agonists due to increased local concentration of norepinephrine produced by α_2 blockade (see Ch. 80, Figure 80.3a).

Phentolamine is administered intravenously and may be given intermittently or by infusion. Onset in rapid (within 2 min), with a duration of action of 10–15 min.

Arteriolar and venous vasodilators reduce systemic blood pressure, without significant changes in calculated systemic vascular resistance. Effects on cardiac output are variable, and there is modest reflex sympathetic stimulation without significant increases in heart rate.

PHENOXYBENZAMINE

Phenoxybenzamine is a non-selective, irreversible (non-competitive) α_1 and α_2-receptor antagonist. Blockade is also produced on histamine, serotonin and acetylcholine muscarinic receptors. Reuptake of norepinephrine is blocked, thereby potentiating the effects of β-agonists.

Phenoxybenzamine is usually administered orally, but may also be given intravenously. It has a long onset of action and prolonged duration of action (3–4 d).

It causes a gradual reduction in systemic blood pressure, without rapid reflex sympathetic activity. Prolonged use is associated with increased β-adrenergic effects, predominantly increased heart rate, for which combination therapy with β-blockade is used. Phenoxybenzamine is primarily used in the management of phaeochromocytoma: either preoperatively, or long term in inoperable patients. It may also used to control autonomic hyperreflexia in patients with spinal cord transection.

PRAZOSIN

Prazosin is a relatively arterioselective, competitive, α_1 receptor antagonist. It acts post-junctionally and therefore does not inhibit reuptake of norepinephrine. Consequently, it produces less tachycardia for a given reduction in systemic blood pressure.

It is administered orally and usually used for essential or renovascular (hyperreninaemic) hypertension. It is frequently used in combination β-blockers and diuretics, particularly in patients with renal dysfunction.

LABETALOL

Labetalol is a specific competitive antagonist at α_1, β_1 and β_2 adrenergic receptors. β-blockade effects predominate, with α blockade potency approximately 10% of prazosin. Labetalol has partial agonist effects on β_2-receptors. The ratio of α_1-β receptor blockade is 1:4.

It is administered intravenously, has a rapid onset of action (5–10 min) with a duration of 2–6 h. It may be given by infusion.

Systemic blood pressure and cardiac output are reduced by a combination of negative inotropy, arterial and venous vasodilation. Reflex tachycardia is attenuated by β-blockade.

Side-effects are relate predominantly to β blockade such as bronchospasm and hyperkalaemia.

CARVEDILOL

Carvedilol is a non-selective β-blocker with α_1 antagonist activity. Most of the vasodilator activity relates to α_1 antagonism, although at high concentrations it also blocks calcium entry. The ratio of α_1-β-receptor blockade is 1:10.

It is administered orally, no intravenous preparation is available.

Recent studies have demonstrated slowing of progression of congestive cardiac failure and improved mortality, particularly when used in conjunction with ACE inhibitors in patients with mild to moderate cardiac failure.[23,24] It may also be used in patients who cannot be treated with ACE inhibitors.

HALOPERIDOL AND CHLORPROMAZINE

These drugs act as competitive α receptor antagonists causing non-selective vasodilation and blockade of norepinephrine reuptake.

These drugs are primarily used as major tranquillizers or anti-psychotics; their effect on the peripheral vasculature should be regarded as a side effect, rather than a specific therapeutic action.

Reduction of systemic blood pressure is variable and may be precipitous, particularly in hypovolaemic patients with high sympathetic drive. These drugs may be useful in neurogenic hypertension, and are not regarded as first line vasodilators.

SYMPATHOMIMETICS

The peripheral vascular effects of β-adrenergic agonists such as epinephrine, norepinephrine, dopamine and synthetic catecholamines dobutamine and isoprenaline are discussed in Chapter 80.

At low doses, epinephrine, norepinephrine and dopamine are predominantly β-agonists and cause both arterial and venous vasodilation which may cause reductions in mean arterial pressure.

Dobutamine and isoprenaline are predominantly β-agonists and may cause decreases in mean arterial pressure, particularly in hypovolaemic patients or those with increased sympathetic drive. These agents may have a role in reducing left ventricular afterload in patients with systolic heart failure.

Fenoldopam mesylate is a synthetic selective dopamine agonist, binding selectively at DA_1 dopamine receptors. Its antihypertensive actions are due to a combination of

direct non-specific vasodilation and natriuresis, similar to other β adrenergic agonists. It has a short onset of action in 5–10 min, with duration of action of 10–15 min. It may be given by infusion and has been shown to be as effective as sodium nitroprusside in severe hypertension.[25]

ANGIOTENSIN CONVERTING ENZYME INHIBITORS

Angiotensin converting enzyme inhibition has become a cornerstone in the management of patients with hypertension, cardiac failure and ischaemic heart disease.[26–28] These drugs act by non-selective, competitive, irreversible, inhibition to the angiotensin I binding site.

These drugs are administered orally; there are no routinely used parenteral preparations. Doses are gradually increased over time with close monitoring of renal function.

PREPARATIONS

There are a large number of ACE inhibitors on the market.

Captopril is the prototype and is still widely used. It is administered orally in increasing doses and intervals to a maximum dose of 50 mg 8-hourly. It may be administered sublingually in acute hypertension (5–25 mg), with an onset of action in 20–30 min, duration of 4 h. There are no significant differences in the cardiovascular effects between captopril and other preparations. It is contraindicated in patients with bilateral renal artery stenosis and should be avoided in pregnancy.

Enalapril is a pro-drug, effective by hepatic metabolism to enalaprilat, producing a slower and more controlled action. It is administered orally in 5 mg increments, to a total of 20 mg b.i.d.

Enalaprilat is available as an intravenous preparation and has an undefined role in acute hypertensive states, particularly hyperreninaemic hypertension with associated left ventricular failure.[29] It has an onset of action in 15 min with a duration of 4–6 h. It must be used with caution in patients with renal dysfunction.[30]

Lisinopril is a newer preparation that has the advantage of single daily dosing.

CARDIOVASCULAR EFFECTS

The cardiovascular effects of ACE inhibition are widespread with effects that influence the peripheral vasculature, cardiac performance, and salt and water homeostasis. Consequently, ACE inhibitors are not principally regarded as vasodilators, although they have both direct and indirect effects on the peripheral vasculature.

Increased production of endothelial vasodilators such as prostacyclin and decreased production of endothelin by angiotensin result in generalized venous and arteriolar vasodilation. This occurs in the absence of reflex sympathetic activity or changes in heart rate, due to the modulation of adrenergic stimulation. Systemic blood pressure is reduced without changes in cardiac output, heart rate, or calculated systemic vascular resistance.

ACE inhibition is associated with improved myocardial performance following acute myocardial infarction due to left ventricular remodelling and improvement in neurohumoral activation. These drugs have been shown to improve survival following myocardial infarction in patients with left ventricular dysfunction.

'First dose hypotension' is described in patients receiving ACE inhibitors for the first time. This may occur particularly in patients who are salt and water depleted, or those who develop sensitivity to the drug. Sensitivity to drugs may also present as a sudden decrease in renal function following commencement of the drug (see below).

RENOVASCULAR EFFECTS

ACE inhibitors may cause renal failure, particularly in patients with renovascular disease, hyperreninaemic hypertension and acute renal dysfunction. The renal effects of ACE inhibitors may be potentiated by diuretics, non-steroidal anti-inflammatory agents and β blockers.

As a rule in intensive care patients, ACE inhibitors are started in suitable patients once renal function has stabilized and the patient is no longer requiring inotropic support.

SIDE-EFFECTS AND TOXICITY

In addition to renal dysfunction, ACE inhibitors may be associated with a number of side-effects. The most common of these is cough, which is due to the increased production of kinins.[31]

Severe angioneurotic oedema causing upper airway obstruction may occur with all ACE inhibitors, although this is less common with enalapril and lisinopril. This is due to increased activation of bradykinins. ACE inhibitors are contraindicated in patients with a history of hereditary or idiopathic angioneurotic oedema.

Neutropenia and agranulocytosis are uncommon, but potentially lethal side-effects in susceptible patients.

ANGIOTENSIN RECEPTOR BLOCKERS

These are a newer class of antihypertensive drugs that cause irreversible, selective blockade of angiotensin II at AT_1 receptors.[32]

Losartan is the prototype, which has been followed by newer compounds such as irbesartan and eprosartan.[33] These drugs are oral preparations; there is no parenteral form.

The cardiovascular profile of angiotensin receptor blockers is similar to the ACE inhibitors, although definitive studies on long term survival following acute myocardial infarction or in patients will cardiac failure have yet to be done.[34]

The selective blockade of angiotensin II offers several possible advantages over ACE inhibitors. These drugs are long acting and may be given once daily; onset of action is slow, thereby avoiding first dose hypotension; side-effects such as cough and angioneurotic oedema are less common.[35]

CENTRALLY ACTING AGENTS

These agents modulate adrenergic stimulation at central nervous system and spinal cord level.

The vasomotor centre of the medulla mainly controls sympathetic pressor influences, although other brain stem, midbrain and spinal centres have a role.

Most central responses are mediated through α_2 adrenergic receptors, which modulate the release and reuptake of norepinephrine, with subsequent effects on the peripheral vasculature and cardiac function.

CLONIDINE

Clonidine is a centrally acting α_2 agonist which stimulates inhibitory neurones in the vasomotor centre. This results in a reduction in sympathetic outflow from the central nervous system and is associated with negative inotropy and reduction in heart rate. Systemic blood pressure is reduced by this mechanism, with associated arteriolar and venous vasodilation. Clonidine has centrally acting analgesic properties, which make it a suitable drug in patients with post-operative hypertension.[36]

Peripherally, it stimulates prejunctional α_2-receptors, thereby decreasing norepinephrine release, but may also have an effect at postjunctional α_1-receptors causing vasoconstriction. This may present as rebound hypertension following initial reduction of blood pressure, as there is variable duration of the central and peripheral effects.

Clonidine is administered by intravenous administration, has a rapid onset of action (5–10 min) and duration of action of 20–30 min. It cannot be given by infusion. It has both central and peripheral effects.

METHYLDOPA

Methyldopa has been used in the treatment of hypertension for 30 years. It acts as a centrally acting 'false' transmitter following metabolism to methylnorepinephrine and subsequent stimulation of α_2-receptors, although precise mechanism is not clear.

It has no direct effect on cardiac or renal function. Cardiac output is maintained without changes in heart rate. Consequently, it may arrest or improve hypertensive nephropathy. It has a limited role in hypertensive emergencies, but is useful in accelerated essential, renovascular and pregnancy induced hypertension.

It is administered orally in doses of 250 mg–2 g/d. An intravenous preparation is available.

TRIMETAPHAN

Trimet(h)aphan is an uncommonly used ganglion blocker that blocks sympathetic and parasympathetic ganglia.

It is given intravenously, has a rapid onset of action (1–3 min) and short duration of action. It may be given by infusion and titrated to a target mean arterial pressure. It is metabolized by plasma cholinesterase. Tachyphylaxis is common.[21]

Ganglionic blockade results in reduction in vascular tone, both arterial and venous with associated decreased blood pressure and cardiac output. Heart rate is usually unchanged but may be increased by parasympathetic blockade. It causes less precipitous reductions in blood pressure compared to sodium nitroprusside.

Trimetaphan does not cross the blood–brain barrier and therefore does not affect the cerebral circulation.

Other effects of ganglionic blockade include mydriasis, ileus and urinary retention.

Its use as a vasodilator has largely been superseded by sodium nitroprusside and glyceryl trinitrate.

OTHER ANTIHYPERTENSIVE AGENTS

β-ADRENERGIC ANTAGONISTS

β-blockers have been used for the treatment of hypertension for over 30 years and have an increasingly important role in the management of cardiac failure.[37–39]

In addition to decreasing heart rate and contractility, β-blockers have other neurohumoral effects that effect vascular tone. These relate to inhibition of renin release from juxtaglomerular cells (Figure 81.1) and pre-junctional inhibition of norepinephrine that result in reduction in vascular tone and blood pressure. A central effect of β-blockers has also been proposed.

Mode of action has been described in terms of selectivity to blockade of β-adrenergic receptors – β_1 and/or β_2. While this is an appropriate pharmacological distinction, the clinical activity of these drugs is not as predictable due to mixed populations of β_1 and β_2-receptors in most organs and variable receptor responsiveness in physiological and pathophysiological conditions. Consequently, there is marked interindividual variability in the response to these drugs. In high enough doses, whether intentionally or due to toxicity, all β-blockers will cause generalized antagonism with resultant therapeutic and toxic effects.[22]

Lipid soluble β-blockers include propanolol and metoprolol that are predominantly excreted by the liver; atenolol and sotalol are predominantly renally excreted, warranting caution with these drugs in patients with renal dysfunction.

β-blockers may be given orally or intravenously – there is significant first pass metabolism so that doses for oral and intravenous administration are markedly different.

Esmolol is an intravenous β-blocker that is rapidly metabolized by red cell esterases. Its rapid onset of action and short duration allows infusion of drug, making it a useful drug in patients with acute hypertensive states associated with tachycardia. Labetalol and carvedilol are discussed above.

β-blockers are frequently used as adjuncts to vasodilators in the treatment of hypertensive emergencies and states, particularly where reflex tachycardia and sympathetic occurs, for example, hydralazine, nifedipine and prazosin.

Side-effects and toxicity of β-blockers include bradycardia, which may be profound, hypotension, bronchoconstriction, aggravation of peripheral vascular ischaemia, hyperkalaemia and masking of the sympathetic response to hypoglycaemia.

DIURETICS

As with β-blockers, diuretics have an established place in the management of hypertension. In addition to their effects on salt and water excretion and inhibition of aldosterone, direct vasodilatory effects are associated with diuretics such as frusemide and the thiazides.

These drugs have a rapid venodilatory action, which may be due to inhibition of a norepinephrine-activated chloride channel on veins. Reductions of blood pressure and right atrial pressure may occur following low doses that may occur before an associated diuresis.

All diuretics should be used with caution in patients with renal dysfunction and avoided until a euvolaemic state is achieved.

DRUG SELECTION

The clinical use of vasodilators in intensive care is different to their use in ambulatory patients. In the critically ill patient, these drugs are primarily used to control acute rises in mean arterial pressure associated with sympathetic stimulation, or as specific treatment of hypertensive emergencies.

The ideal vasodilator is therefore one that has a rapid and predictable onset of action, allows titration to achieve a desired systemic blood pressure, does not compromise cardiac output, does not cause significant reflex tachycardia and is non toxic.

The selection of drug to treat hypertensive states will depend on the predominant cause of hypertension and the mechanism of action in the homeostatic pathway outlined in Figure 81.1.

There are no large studies investigating optimum therapy in patients presenting with hypertensive emergencies. These conditions occur in a heterogenous group of patients and drug selection is essentially determined by the underlying pathophysiology, personal preference and experience.[40]

MONITORING

The principles of haemodynamic monitoring in patients receiving vasoactive drugs are outlined in Chapter 81.

Patients with severe hypertension or those receiving infusions or doses of potent vasodilators such as sodium nitroprusside, glyceryl trinitrate, diazoxide, nifedipine or trimetaphan should be monitored via an intra-arterial catheter.

The use of non-invasive measurement devices are not recommended in patients with hypertensive emergencies.

As peripheral vasodilators have significant effects on both the arterial and venous systems, measurement of volume status is important. In the majority of patients, establishing an euvolaemic state is essential before commencing a vasodilator.

DOSAGES AND DRUG ADMINISTRATION

Vasodilators administered via infusion are delivered through a dedicated central venous catheter using infusion pumps or syringe drivers and titrated to achieve a target mean arterial pressure.

Infusion lines should be free of injection portals and clearly marked with identifying labels.

Concentrations of infusions should be standardized in accordance with individual unit protocols. Suggested infusion concentrations and common drug doses are shown in Table 81.1.

SPECIFIC SITUATIONS

The following is a summary of the clinical uses of the above drugs in hypertensive states commonly encountered in the intensive care unit. Specific pharmacology and physiological effects are discussed above.

ACUTE HYPERTENSION

The most common cause of hypertension in intensive care patients is pain or agitation, particularly in postoperative patients. It is important that patients have adequate analgesia and sedation before antihypertensives or vasodilators are used.

Other common causes of hypertension include hypothermia, urinary retention, positional discomfort and omission of pre-admission antihypertensives, particularly β blockers.

The majority of instances of acute hypertension in the intensive care unit will respond to simple measures addressing the above.

Sustained hypertension may be treated acutely with incremental doses or infusions of short acting drugs such as glyceryl trinitrate, sodium nitroprusside, phentolamine, hydralazine, nifedipine or clonidine. Infusions of vasodilators may be required if hypertension persists, or if the patient in unable to take longer acting oral agents such as prazosin or amlodipine. Hypertension associated with tachycardia may be treated with β-blockers.

HYPERTENSIVE ENCEPHALOPATHY

Hypertensive encephalopathy is defined as an acute organic brain syndrome occurring as a result of failure of cerebrovascular autoregulation. There may be differences in the degree of hypertension that cause encephalopathy. It may present as confusion, visual disturbances, blindness, seizures or stroke. If not adequately treated, hypertensive encephalopathy may result in intracerebral haemorrhage, coma or death.[41]

Hypertensive encephalopathy may occur in patients with untreated or undertreated hypertension or in association with other diseases, such as renal disease (e.g. glomerulonephritis, renovascular disease), thrombotic thrombocytopenic purpura, immunosuppressive therapy, collagen vascular diseases or eclampsia. Consequently, drug treatment will depend on the context in which it occurs.

The aim of drug therapy in these patients is to reduce blood pressure in a controlled, predictable and safe way. Acutely, short acting, titratable parenteral drugs are suitable in emergency situations. Sodium nitroprusside can be used safely in most circumstances. Although sodium nitroprusside may increase intracranial pressure, associated reductions in mean arterial pressure offset this effect. Phentolamine is equally effective. Esmolol may be useful as an adjunctive agent.[42]

Other agents that are useful in controlling severe hypertension include hydralazine, diazoxide, nifedipine, clonidine and ACE inhibitors (although these must be used cautiously in patients with associated renal dysfunction). Combination therapy is usually required, although this should be done with caution to minimize additive effects with resultant hypotension.

Patients with hypertensive emergencies are frequently hypovolaemic due to excessive sympathetic stimulation. In the absence of left ventricular failure, judicious fluid replacement may reduce blood pressure and improve renal function, thereby minimizing precipitous hypotension that may result following administration of some drugs. Diuretics are generally avoided in these conditions unless there is evidence of left ventricular failure.[42]

Table 81.1 Dose and infusion concentrations of commonly used vasodilators and antihypertensives in intensive care

Agent	Infusion/Dose	Caution
Sodium nitroprusside	50 mg/250 ml 5% Dextrose; Range 3–40 ml/h	Cyanide toxicity (> total dose 0.5 mg/kg per 24 h) Photodegradation Raised intracranial pressure Rebound hypotension Shunt and oxygen desaturation
Glyceryl trinitrate	30 mg/100 ml 5% Dextrose; Range 2–25 ml/h	Drug binding to polyvinylchloride Tachyphylaxis Raised intracranial pressure
Hydralazine	10–20 mg i.v. bolus 20–40 mg 6–8-hourly	Tachycardia Myocardial ischaemia
Diazoxide	50–100 mg i.v. boluses 15–30 mg/min infusion	Precipitous hypotension Hyperglycaemia
Trimetaphan	1–4 mg/min infusion	Mydriasis, ileus Bradycardia
Phentolamine	1–10 mg i.v. boluses 5–30 mg/h infusion	Tachycardia
Phenoxybenzamine	Oral: 10 mg/d, until postural hypotension i.v.: 1 mg/kg per day	Idiosyncratic hypotension
Prazosin	2–10 mg/day, 8-hourly	
Nifedipine	5–10 mg oral/sublingual	Precipitous hypotension
Amlodipine	5–10 mg oral b.d.	Caution in renal impairment
Captopril	6.25–50 mg orally, 8-hourly Acute hypertension: 12.5–25 mg sublingually p.r.n.	Caution in renovascular hypertension and renal failure Pregnancy Angioneurotic oedema
Enalapril	5 mg–20 mg 8-hourly	
Enalaprilat	0.625–5 mg bolus	Caution in renal failure and hypovolaemia
Losartan	25–100 mg daily	Caution in renal failure
Clonidine	25 μg to 150 mg i.v. bolus	Acute, perioperative centrally mediated hypertension May cause rebound hypertension with chronic use
Atenolol	1–10 mg i.v. boluses 25–100 mg oral b.d.	Caution in poor left ventricular function, asthma Hyperkalaemia Potentiated in renal failure
Metoprolol		As for atenolol, safe in renal failure
Esmolol	Loading dose 0.5 mg/kg 10–40 mg/h infusion	
Labetalol	20–80 mg i.v. boluses 0.5–4 mg/min infusion	
Magnesium sulphate	40–60 mg/kg loading (or 6 g) 2–4 g/h infusion	Maintain serum magnesium >1.5–2 mmol/l

ACUTE STROKE

Acute stroke syndromes frequently occur in the setting of severe hypertension. The reduction of mean arterial pressure must be balanced by the maintenance of adequate cerebral perfusion pressure and cerebral blood flow. Ischaemic or infarcted brain is vulnerable to critical reductions in cerebral blood flow, while excessive mean arterial pressure may increase the risk of cerebral haemorrhage.[43]

Acutely, blood pressure should be maintained in a normal range until intracranial pathology has been identified by CT scan. Aggressive reduction in blood pressure is not recommended in patients with ischaemic stroke, while hypertension in patients with aneurysmal subarachnoid haemorrhage or intracranial haemorrhage may be managed by drugs outlined above.

AORTIC DISSECTION

Aortic dissection is the most dramatic and most rapidly fatal complication of severe hypertension. Blood pressure should be decreased as rapidly as possible to normal or slightly hypotensive levels. Titrations are usually made to achieve systolic blood pressures of 100–110 mmHg or mean arterial pressure of 65–70 mmHg. This will depend on the patient's pre-morbid blood pressure and the accuracy of blood pressure measurement. It is important to maintain blood pressure at levels compatible with adequate cerebral and renal perfusion.

This is best achieved initially combination of β-blockers (e.g. esmolol, labetalol or atenolol), then in combination with vasodilators such as sodium nitroprusside, glyceryl trinitrate or trimetaphan. Tachycardia must be avoided as this is a significant determinant of aortic shear force, $(dp/dt)_{max}$, that may exacerbate the dissection.[44]

Aortic dissection distal to the left subclavian artery is managed conservatively with antihypertensive therapy. Proximal dissections are managed surgically after acute control of blood pressure.

ACUTE MYOCARDIAL ISCHAEMIA

Myocardial ischaemia in the absence of obstructive coronary atherosclerosis may be precipitated by severe hypertension. This occurs by increased left ventricular wall stress, reduced preload, tachycardia and increased myocardial metabolic demand. Severe ischaemia may result in acute left ventricular failure.

Intravenous glyceryl trinitrate is useful in this situation and may be used in combination with β-blockers such as esmolol, labetalol or carvedilol.[45]

ACE inhibitors may be used in the acute situation and may be required for longer-term treatment.

PHAEOCHROMOCYTOMA

Tumours of the adrenal medulla secrete catecholamines that result in initial paroxysmal, then sustained, severe hypertension. They may present to the intensive care unit as a hypertensive emergency or peri-operatively for surgical ablation.[46]

Acute hypertensive crises associated with phaeochromocytoma are managed with incremental doses or infusions of phentolamine. Untreated patients may be significantly hypovolaemic and may require judicious volume replacement. β-blockers should not be used in the acute stage as these will potentiate unopposed α adrenergic stimulation.

Phenoxybenzamine forms the mainstay of treatment and preparation for surgery. This is commenced in 20–30 mg increments and continued until blood pressure is controlled. Excessive β-adrenergic effects are treated with β-blockers after sufficient α-blockade with phenoxybenzamine.[47]

Magnesium sulphate is useful in the perioperative management of phaeochromocytoma. It is given by infusion at 2–4 g/h.[13]

RENAL FAILURE

Renal insufficiency may be a cause or consequence of a hypertensive emergency. Patients on haemodialysis, particularly those receiving erythropoieitin therapy and renal transplant patients, especially those receiving

cyclosporin or corticosteroids commonly present with severe hypertension.

In patients with new onset renal failure accompanying severe hypertension, blood pressure must be controlled without potentiating renal dysfunction. Drugs such as calcium antagonists, phentolamine or prazosin may preserve renal blood flow and are appropriate in these patients.

ACE inhibitors and diuretics should be used with caution until renal function has stabilized or improved.

Patients in the recovery phase of acute renal failure are usually hypertensive. This is a normal physiological response and should not be treated unless there is associated myocardial or cerebral ischaemia.[48,49]

PRE-ECLAMPSIA AND ECLAMPSIA

In addition to delivery of the baby and placenta, parenteral magnesium sulphate is the treatment of choice to prevent the evolution of pre-eclampsia to eclampsia (seizures and deteriorating encephalopathy). Other parenteral drugs that have been used for many years for pregnancy induced hypertensive states include hydralazine, phentolamine, diazoxide and labetalol.[50,51]

ACE inhibitors and angiotensin receptor blockers are contraindicated in pregnancy.

DRUG INTERACTIONS

Severe rebound hypertension may result following abrupt cessation of antihypertensive treatment. Drugs associated with this discontinuation syndrome include clonidine, methyldopa, β-blockers, guanethidine and diuretics. The degree of rebound depends on the rapidity of withdrawal of drug, dosage, renovascular and cardiac function. Antihypertensives should be reintroduced according to the status of the patient and degree of hypertension managed accordingly.

Interaction with monoamine oxidase inhibitors and drugs such as indirect sympathomimetics, narcotics and tyramine containing foods may result in a hypertensive emergency. This is best managed acutely with α and or β-blockers.

REFERENCES

1 Erdmann E. The management of heart failure – an overview. *Basic Res Cardiol* 2000; **95**(**suppl 1**): 13–7.

2 Cohn JN. Left ventricle and arteries: structure, function, hormones, and disease. *Hypertension* 2001; **37**: 346–9.

3 Jacobsohn E, Chorn R, O'Connor M. The role of the vasculature in regulating venous return and cardiac output: historical and graphical approach. *Can J Anaesth* 1997; **44**: 849–67.

4 Gurney AM. Mechanisms of drug-induced vasodilation. *J Pharm Pharmacol* 1994; **46**: 242–51.

5 Drexler H, Hornig B. Importance of endothelial function in chronic heart failure. *J Cardiovasc Pharmacol* 1996; **27**(**suppl 2**): S9–12.

6 Sanders DB, Kelley T, Larson D. The role of nitric oxide synthase/nitric oxide in vascular smooth muscle control. *Perfusion* 2000; **15**: 97–104.

7 Gustafsson F, Holstein-Rathlou N. Conducted vasomotor responses in arterioles: characteristics, mechanisms and physiological significance. *Acta Physiol Scand* 1999; **167**: 11–21.

8 Prisant LM. Calcium antagonists – clinical considerations. *Ethn Dis* 1998; **8**: 124–7.

9 Grossman E, Messerli FH, Grodzicki T, Kowey P. Should a moratorium be placed on sublingual nifedipine capsules given for hypertensive emergencies and pseudoemergencies? *JAMA* 1996; **276**: 1328–31.

10 Nievas MN. Poor-grade subarachnoid hemorrhage patients: the use of nimodipine and other optional treatments. *Neurol Res* 1999; **21**: 649–52.

11 De Cicco M, Macor F, Robieux I *et al.* Pharmacokinetic and pharmacodynamic effects of high-dose continuous intravenous verapamil infusion: clinical experience in the intensive care unit. *Crit Care Med* 1999; **27**: 332–9.

12 Saris NE, Mervaala E, Karppanen H *et al.* Magnesium. An update on physiological, clinical and analytical aspects. *Clin Chim Acta* 2000; **294**: 1–26.

13 James MF. Use of magnesium sulphate in the anaesthetic management of phaeochromocytoma: a review of 17 anaesthetics. *Br J Anaesth* 1989; **62**: 616–23.

14 Young JD. Nitric oxide and related vasodilators. *Can J Anaesth* 1997; **44**: R23–33.

15 Harrison DG, Bates JN. The nitrovasodilators. New ideas about old drugs. *Circulation* 1993; **87**: 1461–7.

16 Friederich JA, Butterworth JF. Sodium nitroprusside: twenty years and counting. *Anesth Analg* 1995; **81**: 152–62.

17 Wood G. Effect of antihypertensive agents on the arterial partial pressure of oxygen and venous admixture after cardiac surgery. *Crit Care Med* 1997; **25**: 1807–12.

18 Johanning RJ, Zaske DE, Tschida SJ *et al.* A retrospective study of sodium nitroprusside use and assessment of the potential risk of cyanide poisoning. *Pharmacotherapy* 1995; **15**: 773–7.

19 Shapira OM, Alkon JD, Macron DS *et al.* Nitroglycerin is preferable to diltiazem for prevention of coronary bypass conduit spasm. *Ann Thorac Surg* 2000; **70**: 883–8.

20 Cotter G, Faibel H, Barash P *et al.* High-dose nitrates in the immediate management of unstable angina: optimal dosage, route of administration, and therapeutic goals. *Am J Emerg Med* 1998; **16**: 219–24.

21 Frank G. Diazoxide and trimethaphan used? *Chest* 2001; **119**: 316.

22 Runciman W B, Morris JL. Adrenoceptor antagonists. In: Feldman AC, Paton W, Scurr C (eds) *Mechanisms of Drugs in Anaesthesia*. London: Edward Arnold; 1993: 293–306.

23 Packer M, Coats AJ, Fowler MB *et al.* Effect of carvedilol on survival in severe chronic heart failure. *N Engl J Med* 2001; **344**: 1651–8.

24 Dargie HJ. Effect of carvedilol on outcome after myocardial infarction in patients with left-ventricular dysfunction: the CAPRICORN randomised trial. *Lancet* 2001; **357**: 1385–90.

25 Oparil S, Aronson S, Deeb GM *et al.* Fenoldopam: a new parenteral antihypertensive: consensus roundtable on the management of perioperative hypertension and hypertensive crises. *Am J Hypertens* 1999; **12**: 653–64.

26 Pfeffer MA, Braunwald E, Moye LA *et al.* Effect of captopril on mortality and morbidity in patients with left ventricular dysfunction after myocardial infarction. Results of the survival and ventricular enlargement trial. The SAVE Investigators. *N Engl J Med* 1992; **327**: 669–77.

27 Rodgers JE, Patterson JH. The role of the renin-angiotensin-aldosterone system in the management of heart failure. *Pharmacotherapy* 2000; **20**: 368S–78S.

28 Unger T, Azizi M, Belz GG. Blocking the tissue renin-angiotensin system: the future cornerstone of therapy. *J Hum Hypertens* 2000; **14(suppl 2)**: S23–31.

29 Schuetz WH, Lindner KH, Georgieff M *et al.* The effect of i.v. enalaprilat in chronically treated hypertensive patients during cardiac surgery. *Acta Anaesthesiol Scand* 1998; **42**: 929–35.

30 Hirschl MM, Binder M, Bur A *et al.* Clinical evaluation of different doses of intravenous enalaprilat in patients with hypertensive crises. *Arch Intern Med* 1995; **155**: 2217–23.

31 Kokkonen JO, Lindstedt KA, Kuoppala A, Kovanen PT. Kinin-degrading pathways in the human heart. *Trends Cardiovasc Med* 2000; **10**: 42–5.

32 Goodfriend TL, Elliott ME, Catt KJ. Angiotensin receptors and their antagonists. *N Engl J Med* 1996; **334**: 1649–54.

33 Beevers DG. Losartan: the first angiotensin receptor antagonist in clinical use. *J Hum Hypertens* 1995; **9(suppl 5)**: S1.

34 Grossman E, Messerli FH, Neutel JM. Angiotensin II receptor blockers: equal or preferred substitutes for ACE inhibitors? *Arch Intern Med* 2000; **160**: 1905–11.

35 Cooper ME, Webb RL, de Gasparo M. Angiotensin receptor blockers and the kidney: possible advantages over ACE inhibition? *Cardiovasc Drug Rev* 2001; **19**: 75–86.

36 Cline JC, Connelly J. Intravenous clonidine for hypertensive emergencies. *Am J Health Syst Pharm* 1999; **56**: 572–4.

37 Krum H. Guidelines for management of patients with chronic heart failure in Australia. *Med J Aust* 2001; **174**: 459–66.

38 Packer M. Current role of beta-adrenergic blockers in the management of chronic heart failure. *Am J Med* 2001; **110(suppl 7A)**: 81S–94S.

39 Gheorghiade M, Eichhorn EJ. Practical aspects of using beta-adrenergic blockade in systolic heart failure. *Am J Med* 2001; **110(suppl 7A)**: 68S–73S.

40 Hirschl MM. Guidelines for the drug treatment of hypertensive crises. *Drugs* 1995; **50**: 991–1000.

41 Mabie WC. Management of acute severe hypertension and encephalopathy. *Clin Obstet Gynecol* 1999; **42**: 519–31.

42 Vaughan CJ, Delanty N. Hypertensive emergencies. *Lancet* 2000; **356**: 411–7.

43 Goldstein LB. Should antihypertensive therapies be given to patients with acute ischemic stroke? *Drug Saf* 2000; **22**: 13–8.

44 Flachskampf FA, Daniel WG. Aortic dissection. *Cardiol Clin* 2000; **18**: 807–17, ix.

45 Ramsay JG. Cardiac management in the ICU. *Chest* 1999; **115**: 138S–144S.

46 Graham GW, Unger BP, Coursin DB. Perioperative management of selected endocrine disorders. *Int Anesthesiol Clin* 2000; **38**: 31–67.

47 Prys-Roberts C. Phaeochromocytoma – recent progress in its management. *Br J Anaesth* 2000; **85**: 44–57.

48 Klassen PS, Svetkey LP. Diagnosis and management of renovascular hypertension. *Cardiol Rev* 2000; **8**: 17–29.

49 Palmer BF. Impaired renal autoregulation: implications for the genesis of hypertension and hypertension-induced renal injury. *Am J Med Sci* 2001; **321**: 388–400.

50 Watson D. The detection, investigation and management of hypertension in pregnancy. *Aust N Z J Obstet Gynaecol* 2000; **40**: 361.

51 Dianrong S, Lirong Y, Yinglin L. A comparison of phentolamine and magnesium sulfate therapy in pre-eclampsia. *Int J Gynaecol Obstet* 2000; **68**: 259–60.

Part Fourteen

Metabolic Homeostasis

82

Acid–base balance and disorders

L I G Worthley

By affecting the charge on reactive groups of enzymes, the alteration in concentration of hydrogen ions can profoundly influence the rate of metabolic reactions.[1] Despite the abundance of hydrogen in body fluids, the concentration or chemical activity of the hydrogen ion (or hydronium ion H_3O^+) is remarkably small and constant. This is largely due to the presence of buffer systems which allow for a rapid turnover of protons with minimal alteration in hydrogen ion activity. In man, the acid–base balance is maintained and regulated by the renal and respiratory systems, which modify the extracellular fluid (ECF) pH by changing the bicarbonate pair ($[HCO_3^-]$ and PCO_2); all other body buffer systems adjust to the alterations in this pair. This relationship is best considered using the Henderson (or Henderson–Hasselbalch) equation (see below).

DEFINITIONS[2]

pH: The negative logarithm of the hydrogen ion activity (Ha^+). It is measured using a glass membrane electrode, porous only to H^+ ions, which develops a transmembrane potential proportional to the log of the H^+ ion activity (Ha^+). This potential is compared with the potential recorded using a standard solution of selected pH value. As the hydrogen ion activity coefficient is unity, and as the measurement of H^+ provides a practical scale of acidity and alkalinity, the linear consideration of the H^+ concentration has merit when compared with its logarithmic counterpart pH.[3] For example, it allows use of the Henderson equation to assess clearly the acid-base consequences of alteration in the PCO_2 and bicarbonate values[4]:

$$(H^+) = K \times CO_2/[HCO_3^-]$$

The plasma concentration of the H^+ ion at a pH of 7.4 is 40 nmol/l. Doubling or halving the H^+ concentration reduces or increases the pH by $\log_{10}$ respectively (i.e. by approximately 0.3) (Table 82.1).

- *Acid*: a proton donor or hydrogen ion donor
- *Base*: a proton acceptor or hydrogen ion acceptor

Table 82.1   Doubling or halving the H^+ concentration reduces or increases the pH by $\log_{10}$

pH	H^+ nmol/l
6.8	160
7.1	80
7.4	40
7.7	20

- *Acidaemia*: arterial blood pH less than 7.36 (H^+ greater than 44 nmol/l)
- *Alkalaemia*: arterial blood pH greater than 7.44 (H^+ less than 36 nmol/l)
- *Acidosis*: an abnormal condition which tends to decrease the arterial pH if there is no secondary changes in response to the primary disease process
- *Alkalosis*: an abnormal condition which tends to increase the arterial pH if there is no secondary changes in response to the primary disease process
- *A mixed disorder*: the presence of two or more primary acid–base abnormalities
- *Compensation*: refers to a normal body process tending to return the arterial pH to normal (respiratory or renal)
- *Acid–base balance*: refers to the difference in quantity between input and output of acids and bases (Table 82.2)
- *Buffer*: a solution containing substances which have the ability to minimize changes in pH when an acid or base is added to it
- *pKa*: the negative logarithm of the dissociation constant. If it describes a buffer system, then it is numerically equal to the pH of the system when the acid and its anion are present in equal concentrations

An analysis of acid–base chemistry has also been proposed based on the law of electroneutrality in aqueous solutions, where the total number of cations must equal the total number of anions.[5,6] The central tenet to the analysis is that only the independent variables, which are strong ions (e.g. sodium, potassium, calcium, magnesium, chloride and organic anions), PCO_2 and the non-volatile weak acids ($A_{TOT} = HA + A^-$; in plasma predominantly albuminate

Table 82.2 Daily H^+ balance

	Input (mmol/day)			Output (mmol/day)
Volatile				
CO_2	13 000	Lungs		13 000
Lactate	1500	Liver, kidney		1500
Non-volatile				
Protein SO_4	45	Titratable acid		30
Phospholipid PO_4	13			
Other	12	NH_4^+		40

ions), can change acid–base status. They then change the dependent variables of H^+ and HCO_3^- to maintain electrical neutrality. The metabolic acid-base abnormality is characterized by calculating the strong-ion difference (or SID = $[Na^+ + K^+ + Ca^{2+} + Mg^{2+}] - [Cl^- + lactate]$), a value which is essentially equal to the sum of the bicarbonate and albuminate ions[7] (i.e. $HCO_3^- = SID - A^-$) and similar to the buffer base described by Singer and Hastings 50 years ago.[7–9] This approach has not been helpful in clinical practice (e.g. it leads to the misconception that a saline induced dilution acidaemia is due to an increase in Cl^- rather than a decrease in HCO_3^-, or an elevated or reduced plasma albumin level may lead to metabolic acidosis and metabolic alkalosis, respectively).[10–12]

REGULATION OF pH [H^+] IN BODY FLUIDS

In man, despite wide variations in dietary acid and base, there seems to be no specific centre for H^+ ion regulation. The body's respiratory and renal systems co-ordinate to regulate H^+ homeostasis by regulating HCO_3^- and PCO_2. The initial body defence against a change in pH is carried out by the body's buffer systems.[13]

BODY BUFFERING

DILUTION

If the effect of adding the daily non-volatile H^+ load (70 mmol H^+) to a 70 kg man is compared to the same load added to an equal volume of non-buffered water, at the same temperature and pH (Table 82.3), it is clear that dilution is a poor defence against pH changes.

BUFFER SYSTEMS

These are present in the ECF and intracellular fluid (ICF). Their effectiveness, or capacity, is proportional to the amount of buffer, the pKa of the buffer, the pH of the carrying solutions, and whether the buffer operates as an open or closed system.

BUFFER MECHANISMS

Any chemical reaction reaching an equilibrium can be expressed by the law of mass action. In the case of a weak acid:

$$HA = (H^+) + (A^-) \tag{1}$$

At equilibrium, the product of the concentrations of H^+ and A^- is a constant fraction of the concentration of HA, or:

$$K = [H^+][A^-]/[H^+] \tag{2}$$

The value of K at equilibrium is always the same and independent of the concentrations of the reactants present initially. With the addition of another acid (H^+ donor) to the system, the ionization of the weak acid HA is reduced (maintaining K constant). If a base is added, the reduction in the H^+ ion concentration produces further ionization of the acid, HA. Both reduce the change in H^+ ion concentration (pH). However, the ionization of a weak acid is small. Thus, only a small addition of H^+ can be tolerated before the pH falls. Supplementing the ion A^- by adding a salt of a strong base (e.g. NaA) provides a reservoir for combining with the added H^+. A buffer system, therefore, can be produced by mixing a weak acid with the salt of that acid and a strong base.

Equation (2) can be rearranged as

Table 82.3 Acid–base balance refers to the difference in quantity between input and output of acids and bases

	pH (H^+ nmol/l)		
	Water volume	Before	After
70 kg man	42 l	7.4 (40)	7.39 (41)
Non-buffered water	42 l	7.4 (40)	2.78 (1 666 666)

$$[H^+] = K \times (HA)/[A^-] \qquad (3)$$
$$\text{Henderson equation}$$

The negative log of equation (3) is:

$$pH = pKa + \log[A^-]/[HA] \qquad (4)$$
$$\text{Henderson–Hasselbalch equation}$$

Most (i.e. 80%) of the buffering occurs within ±1 pH unit of the pKa value of the buffer system (Fig. 82.1). Considering equation (4), this occurs when:

$$\log(HA)/[A^-] \text{ is } ±1, \text{ i.e. BASE } 10/\text{ACID } 1 \text{ or } 1/10$$

THE BODY BUFFER SYSTEMS

The major body buffer systems involve bicarbonate, protein, haemoglobin and phosphate.

BICARBONATE-CARBONIC ACID BUFFER PAIR

The arterial H$^+$ ion activity can be represented by the Henderson equation

$$[H^+] = 24 \times PaCO_2/[HCO_3^-]$$

or the Henderson–Hasselbalch equation:

$$pH = 6.1 + \log[HCO_3^-]/PaCO_2 \times 0.03$$

Where:

24 = the numerical value of the solubility coefficient of CO$_2$ and the dissociation constant of carbonic acid
PaCO$_2$ = arterial blood partial pressure (mmHg)
[HCO$_3^-$] = arterial blood bicarbonate concentration (mmol/l)
[H$^+$] = arterial blood hydrogen ion concentration (nmol/l)
0.03 = solubility coefficient of carbon dioxide

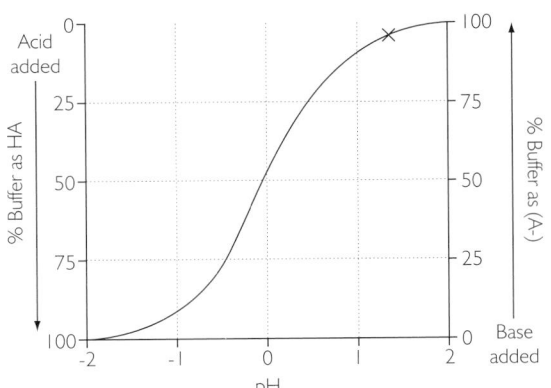

Fig. 82.1 Reaction curve for the buffer HA : (A$^-$) where pH = pKa ± 2. 'X' represents a pH of 7.4 in the bicarbonate buffer system

6.1 = negative logarithm of the dissociation constant of carbonic acid

This system is quantitatively the most important ECF buffer, and functions better as a physiological (or open system) buffer than chemical (or closed system) buffer. Its pKa is 6.1, therefore its chemical buffering capacity at a pH of 7.4 (see position 'x' in Fig. 82.1) is poor. The benefit of an open, compared to a closed, buffer system can be demonstrated if one considers both systems subjected to a pH change of 0.3 units by the addition of acid. If one considers the Henderson–Hasselbalch equation under normal conditions, when pH 7.4, PaCO$_2$ 40 mmHg, HCO$_3^-$ 24 mmol/l, then the equation is:

$$7.4 = 6.1 + \log 20/1$$

However, addition of an acid to decrease the pH by 0.3 units, will produce different effects in the closed system when compared to the open system. For example:

$$\text{Closed system: } 7.1 = 6.1 + \log 22.9/2.29$$
$$\text{Open system: } 7.1 = 6.1 + \log 12/1.2$$

In both systems, the ratio of H$_2$CO$_3^-$ to HCO$_3^-$ remains constant. In the closed system, the total amount of H$_2$CO$_3^-$ and HCO$_3^-$ remains constant (i.e. 25.2 mmol/l). In the open system, the denominator only is kept constant at 1.2 mmol/l, by increasing the ventilation and keeping the PaCO$_2$ at 40 mmHg (40 × 0.03 = 1.2). The buffer anion in the closed system falls from 24 to 22.9 whereas in the open system it falls from 24 to 12, thereby buffering more H$^+$.

The bicarbonate, carbonic acid system also has the added advantage of further CO$_2$ change with respiratory compensation, reducing even further the pH defect. These responses are shown, in stages, in Fig. 82.2.

The utility of this buffer system can be fully appreciated when it is realized that it is 'open ended' for both the numerator and the denominator. The PaCO$_2$ can be modified by change in ventilation, and the HCO$_3^-$ concentration can be regulated by renal mechanisms. All other body buffer systems adjust accordingly to alterations in this pair, an interrelationship which is known as the isohydric principle.

HAEMOGLOBIN, PROTEIN AND PHOSPHATE BUFFERS

Proteins have a series of titratable groups within their molecular structure, with the ability to buffer pH changes. The buffering characteristic of haemoglobin is almost entirely dependent upon the imidazole group of histidine, which dissociates less when haemoglobin is in the oxygenated compared to the deoxygenated form. Thus, deoxygenated blood is a better buffer than oxygenated blood; the haemoglobin molecule accommodating 0.7 mmol of H$^+$ for each mmol of O$_2$ released, without change in pH. As the respiratory quotient is normally 0.8, a slight reduction in pH usually

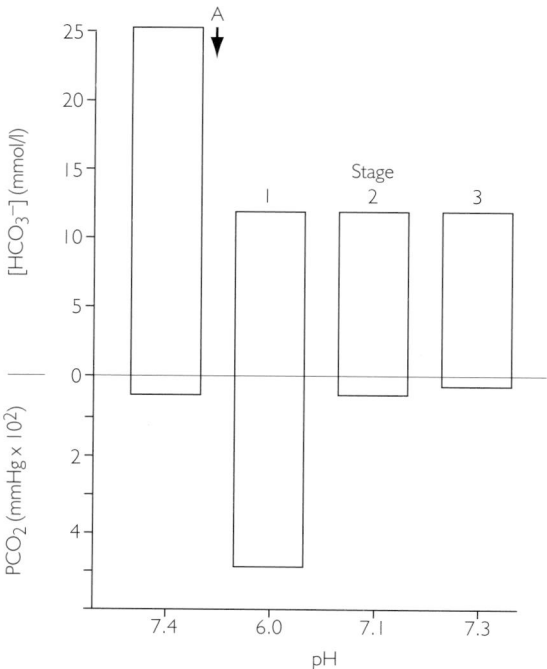

Fig. 82.2 Bicarbonate buffer system in blood if acid were added at A to reduce plasma HCO_3^- to 50%

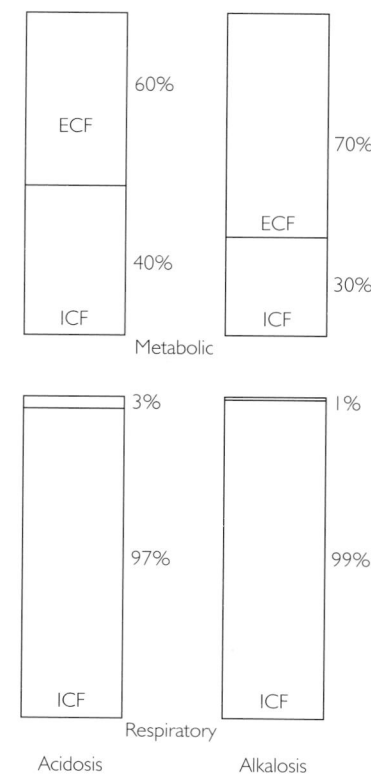

Fig. 82.3 Buffering contributions of the intracellular fluid (ICF) and extracellular fluid (ECF) with primary respiratory or metabolic acid-base changes[24]

occurs when blood travels from the arterial to the venous system.

The haemoglobin buffer is an important one, since it is involved in handling the largest daily acid load of the body (i.e. carbonic acid). Gram for gram, plasma proteins have one-third the buffering capacity of haemoglobin. However, as haemoglobin has twice the concentration of plasma protein, it has 6 times the capacity to buffer H^+.

The phosphate buffer system has a pKa of 6.8; it is a better chemical (or closed) buffer system than the bicarbonate buffer system. However, in plasma, it has 1:20 the concentration, and operates only as a closed system, so its capacity is far less than that of the bicarbonate-carbonic acid buffer. In the ICF and in urine, the phosphate buffer system assumes greater importance.

TOTAL BODY BUFFERING
The contributions of ICF and ECF buffers vary depending upon the nature of the acid or base disturbance. In dogs in which respiratory or metabolic acid base defects were produced, the respiratory pH changes were buffered mainly by ICF buffers, whereas metabolic pH changes had a greater ECF buffering component[14–16] (Fig. 82.3). Preferential utilization of extracellular buffers occurs in the initial phase of a metabolic acidosis with the contribution of ICF buffers becoming greater as the acidosis increases in severity.[17]

Experiments using rat diaphragm and human leucocytes reveal that conditions simulating respiratory acidosis or alkalosis produce a greater ICF pH change than do conditions simulating metabolic acidosis or alkalosis.[18–20] Furthermore, when metabolic acidosis or alkalosis are simulated and appropriate respiratory compensatory (carbon dioxide) changes are also included, the ICF pH remains remarkably constant, suggesting that there is a greater tolerance *in vivo* to metabolic pH change than there is to respiratory pH change.[18,21,22]

RESPIRATORY RESPONSE

It is clear, when considering the Henderson equation (Equation 1), that variations in $PaCO_2$ alter the pH. The effect is rapid and influences both the ICF and ECF. Arterial $PaCO_2$ varies inversely with alveolar ventilation and directly with CO_2 production. Normal CO_2 production is 13 000 mmol/day, and if pulmonary ventilation ceased for 20 min, $PaCO_2$ would rise to 110 mmHg (13.3 kPa) and pH would fall to 7.03. If renal function ceased for a similar period, no change in arterial pH would occur.

Regulation of ventilation involves a complex interplay between mechanical and chemical stimuli. Any change in arterial HCO_3^-, PCO_2, pH, PO_2, or stimuli from pulmonary mechanoreceptors, alters ventilation and thus $PaCO_2$ and pH. The respiratory response to a metabolic pH change follows peripheral chemoreceptor stimulation, and provides the compensatory response to metabolic pH change.

RENAL RESPONSE

This determines the final outcome to the acid or base load, by altering the denominator of the Henderson equation (i.e. $[HCO_3^-]$). The response is slow and the maximum excretory capacity of 300 mmol H$^+$ can only be reached after 7–10 days.[23]

Unlike all other ions, HCO_3^- has no permanence. It may be generated from carbon dioxide or lost with carbon dioxide excretion. The accompanying H$^+$ generated or lost is dealt with by the body's buffers. The kidney uses the bicarbonate ion for alkali reserve, and as an anion for sodium reabsorption or excretion when maintaining the ECF volume. The lungs use the bicarbonate ion for CO_2 transport and excretion.

Renal regulation of H$^+$ balance is due to reabsorption or excretion of filtered HCO_3^-, excretion of titratable acidity (TA), and excretion of ammonia. Tubular H$^+$ secretion usually involves Na$^+$ reabsorption, maintaining electrical neutrality.

REABSORPTION OF FILTERED HCO$_3^-$

About 85–90% of the filtered HCO_3^- is reclaimed by the proximal tubule. Further reabsorption occurs in the distal nephron with the luminal fluid being free of HCO_3^- at a luminal pH of 6.2.[24] The amount of HCO_3^- reaching the distal nephron is influenced by the filtered load of HCO_3^- (thus with a metabolic acidosis, the total proximal H$^+$ secretion is less than normal) and the functional ECF volume.[25] The mechanism of proximal tubular HCO_3^- reabsorption relies upon H$^+$ secretion. Cellular carbonic anhydrase (CA) supplies H$^+$ for the hydrogen pump and the brush border CA facilitates the combination of HCO_3^- with H$^+$. In the absence of the brush border carbonic anhydrase, a disequilibrium pH of 0.85–1.0 occurs, and proximal H$^+$ secretion is inhibited.

FORMATION OF TITRATABLE ACIDITY

The majority of the urinary TA is formed with the conversion of monohydrogen phosphate to dihydrogen phosphate, which occurs throughout the nephron.[24] The pKa of this system is 6.8, and at maximum urinary acidity (i.e. pH 4.5) almost all of the filtered phosphate is in the dihydrogen form. At this urinary pH, two-thirds of the filtered creatinine (pKa 4.97) and 95% of the uric acid (pKa 5.8) are in the acidic mode, and may account for 25% of the urinary TA at maximum urinary acidity. Normally, 20–30 mmol of H$^+$/day are excreted as TA,

and this is proportional to the amount of buffer excreted, the pKa of the buffer and the pH of the urine. In diabetic ketoacidosis the rate of excretion of betahydroxybutyrate (pKa 4.8) is large, and this compound forms the major component (up to 250 mmol H$^+$/day) of urinary TA. Normally, urinary excretion of phosphate is determined by the need to maintain phosphate balance rather than acid–base homeostasis. Thus, TA appears to play a supportive, rather than an active, role in H$^+$ balance.

FORMATION OF AMMONIA

Ammonia (NH_3) is formed in tubular epithelia throughout the nephron.[26] Deamidation and deamination of glutamine account for 60% of the urinary NH_3; 30–35% comes from free arterial NH_3. The NH_3 diffuses into the renal tubular lumen, where it binds a hydrogen ion to form a non-diffusable ammonium ion (NH_4^+) which is then excreted[27]. This process permits Na$^+$/H$^+$ exchange to occur without further change in urinary pH, although an acidic urine allows a greater sink into which free NH_3 can diffuse, and is therefore one of the determinants of urinary NH_4^+ excretion. Renal tubular synthesis of NH_3 is coupled to renal gluconeogenesis, which in turn is attuned to the body's acid–base requirements. Systemic acidosis, hypokalaemia, and mineralocorticoids increase ammonia production.[26] Normally, 30–50 mmol of H$^+$/day are excreted as NH_4^+, which may increase to 300 mmol/day in severe acidosis.

MECHANISMS OF PROXIMAL AND DISTAL H$^+$ SECRETIONS

Proximal H$^+$ Secretions

This is a low gradient (minimal luminal pH achievable is 7.0), high capacity system (its H$^+$ secretion is responsible for reabsorbing most of the filtered HCO_3^-, i.e. 4–5000 mmol/day). The proximal H$^+$ secretion is increased with hypokalaemia, hypercarbia, increased luminal HCO_3^-, increased tubular Na$^+$ reabsorption, the presence of non-reabsorbable anions, and increase in carbonic anhydrase activity.

Distal H$^+$ Secretion

This is a high gradient (minimal luminal pH achievable is 4.5) low capacity system (H$^+$ secretion ranges from 0–300 mmol/day). Unlike the proximal tubule, the distal nephron is influenced by mineralocorticoid activity. In hyperaldosteronism, distal Na$^+$ reabsorption and excretion of H$^+$ and K$^+$ is enhanced. In the presence of hypokalaemia, H$^+$ loss is augmented due to electroneutrality requirements for some of the distal Na$^+$ reabsorbed. In secondary hyperaldosteronism, the K$^+$ and H$^+$ loss may be less than in primary hyperaldosterone states, due to a reduction in distal luminal flow induced by avid proximal Na$^+$ reabsorption. Thus an increase in distal H$^+$ or K$^+$ urinary secretion may only become evident when distal Na^+ delivery is increased (e.g. with the use of diuretics).

CLINICAL APPROACH TO ACID–BASE DISORDERS

CLASSIFICATION OF AN ACID–BASE DEFECT

The primary defect is usually defined by its initiating process (e.g. lactic, keto, or renal tubular, acidosis). A broader classification, however, divides them into metabolic and respiratory, the latter relating to changes in carbonic acid (CO_2) only. Compensatory responses may be qualified as partial.[2] Thus, one speaks of:

1 Chronic respiratory acidosis with partial renal compensation
2 Lactic acidosis with respiratory compensation
3 Metabolic alkalosis without respiratory compensation

BIOCHEMICAL DESCRIPTION OF AN ACID–BASE DEFECT

Three values are necessary to describe an acid–base defect.

1 pH or H^+ nmol/l (a measure of acidity or alkalinity)
2 $PaCO_2$ mmHg or kPa (a measure of the respiratory component)
3 HCO_3^- mmol/l (a measure of the metabolic component)

While pH and $PaCO_2$ may be measured directly, there is no direct method to measure HCO_3^- concentration. Also, HCO_3^- concentrations may vary with changes of PCO_2. To separate the respiratory from the non-respiratory HCO_3^- components, derived indices of standard bicarbonate (i.e. the plasma bicarbonate concentration in fully oxygenated blood which has been equilibrated to a PCO_2 of 40 mmHg at 37°C), buffer base (i.e. the sum of the concentrations of all the buffer anions in the blood, which includes haemoglobin, bicarbonate, protein, and phosphate), 'strong ion difference' (similar to plasma buffer base which is the sum of the concentrations of all the buffer anions in the blood, excluding haemoglobin), base excess or deficit (i.e. the titratable base or acid, in mmol/l, needed to titrate blood to a pH of 7.4, at a PCO_2 of 40 mmHg and temperature of 37°C), and standard base excess (or *in vivo* base excess where correction factors (e.g. $0.3 \times$ the Hb value) are used to approximate the buffering effect of the ECF), have been proposed. However, these *in vitro* values have the disadvantage of not accurately reflecting the situation *in vivo*[28] and the *in vivo* corrections do not differentiate a metabolic alkalosis or acidosis from a compensatory renal

response.[29] For clinical purposes, however, in addition to the history and physical examination, the HCO_3^- concentration calculated from the Henderson equation, with the $PaCO_2$ and pH, are all that are required to fully interpret the acid–base disorder.[28, 30]

DIAGNOSIS OF AN ACID–BASE DEFECT

Here, a definition is sought of the primary attack upon the H^+ homeostasis, and an assessment of the body's compensatory response. Clinical features (e.g. Kussmaul breathing, tachypnoea, cyanosis, tracheal 'tug', hypotension, shock, ketotic breath) and biochemical data (e.g. arterial blood gas analysis, anion gap, renal and hepatic plasma 'profiles' and urinary electrolytes) should all be taken into account. The acid–base defects are usually identified as described below:

THE ARTERIAL pH, PCO_2 AND HCO_3

These values are used to detect the major acid-base defect, the likely compensatory response and the presence of mixed disorders.

THE ANION GAP

This is used to detect an anion gap acidosis (e.g. keto- or lactic acidosis) and a mixed metabolic acidosis; for example, if the decrease in HCO_3^- is greater than the increase in anion gap then both an anion and non anion gap (HCO_3^- losing) metabolic acidosis may coexist, whereas if the decrease in HCO_3^- is less than the increase in the anion gap, the patient may have both an anion gap acidosis and a metabolic alkalosis.

AN ACID–BASE DIAGRAM

This may be used as an aid to the diagnostic process. The appropriate compensatory $PaCO_2$ for the primary metabolic acid–base disorder, and the (H^+) or pH change associated with variation in primary acid-base disorders, are represented by 'confidence bands' for each disorder.[31]

In the absence of a diagram, various 'rules of thumb' have been proposed to facilitate the bedside diagnosis.[13] For example:

- *A primary metabolic acidosis* is associated with a *respiratory compensatory decrease in $PaCO_2$*, the numerical value (in mmHg) of which is usually within ±5 mmHg (0.67 kPa) of the number denoted by the two digits after the decimal point of the pH value, down to a pH of 7.15–7.10 (i.e. the $PaCO_2$ usually goes no lower than 10 mmHg, even with a profound metabolic acidosis).[32] Also as the calculated HCO_3^- halves, the pH decreases by approximately 0.1.
- *A primary metabolic alkalosis* is associated with a similar $PaCO_2$ change, increasing until the pH value reaches 7.55–7.60 (i.e. the $PaCO_2$ usually goes no higher than 60 mmHg, even with a profound metabolic alkalosis).
- In a *primary acute respiratory acidosis* the *calculated* HCO_3^- value rises 1 mmol/l for each 10 mmHg

(1.3 kPa) rise in $PaCO_2$ up to a HCO_3^- value of 30 mmol/l. The pH also decreases by approximately 0.1 for each 20 mmHg increase in $PaCO_2$.

- In a *primary respiratory alkalosis* (both acute and chronic) the *calculated* HCO_3^- decreases 2.5 mmol/l for each 10 mmHg (1.3 kPa) reduction in $PaCO_2$ down to a HCO_3^- value of 18 mmol/l. The pH also increases by approximately 0.1 for each 10 mmHg decrease in $PaCO_2$.

- In *chronic respiratory acidosis*, renal compensation elevates the *calculated* HCO_3^- 4 mmol/l for each 10 mmHg (1.3 kPa) rise in $PaCO_2$ up to a HCO_3^- value of 36 mmol/l. The pH also decreases by approximately 0.05 for each 20 mmHg increase in $PaCO_2$.

CLINICAL ACID–BASE DISORDERS

METABOLIC (NON-RESPIRATORY) ACIDOSIS

This arises from an abnormal process generating excess non-carbonic acid or abnormal loss of HCO_3^-

(Table 82.4). Characteristically, arterial gas analysis reveals pH <7.36 (H^+ >44 nmol/l), $PaCO_2$ <35 mmHg (4.7 kPa) and calculated HCO_3^- <18 mmol/l. An increased anion gap may also exist, reflecting the accumulation of unmeasured acid anions, the anion in question approximating the 'gap'.[33]

TREATMENT OF METABOLIC ACIDOSIS

Therapy in all acid–base disorders should initially focus upon treatment of the underlying disorder (e.g. insulin for diabetic ketoacidosis or measures to improve the cellular redox state in lactic acidosis). These measures terminate the production of (H^+) and allows metabolism of the organic acid present to return the pH towards normal. To maintain homeostasis of the intracellular pH while treatment takes effect, appropriate compensatory $PaCO_2$ for the metabolic acidosis should be maintained. While bicarbonate replacement is commonly used for renal tubular acidosis and gastrointestinal bicarbonate loss, sodium bicarbonate administration is now no longer recommended as a routine for the metabolic acidosis associated with diabetes[34] or cardiac arrest,[35] as there is no evidence that it reduces mortality. Furthermore, excess generation of CO_2, hyperosmolality,

Table 82.4 Aetiology of metabolic acidosis

Accumulation of acid (anion gap >16 mEq/l)	
Disorder	*Acid*
Keto-acidosis	β-hydroxybutyrate, acetoacetate
Lactic-acidosis	Lactate
Methanol	Formate, lactate
Renal failure	Sulphate, phosphate
Salycilic acid	Salycilate, lactate, keto-acids
Paraldehyde	Lactate, acetate, formate, pyruvate
Formaldehyde	Formate
Ethylene glycol	Oxalate
Toluene	Hippuric acid
Paracetamol	Lactate, pyroglutamate
Intravenous	
Fructose	Lactate
Sorbitol	Lactate
Ethanol	Lactate
Xylitol	Lactate
Accumulation of HCl (anion gap <16 mEq/l)	
Releasing HCl with metabolism	
Arginine hydrochloride, lysine hydrochloride	
NH₄Cl	
Direct administration of HCl	
Intravenous HCl	
Loss of HCO₃⁻ (anion gap <16 mEq/l)	
Gastrointestinal loss	
Small bowel, biliary or pancreatic fistula	
Diarrhoea	
Urethro enterostomy	
Renal loss	
Renal tubular acidosis	
Carbonic anhydrase inhibition	

hypocalcaemia, and rebound alkalosis, are possible hazards with its use. Small doses of 50–100 mmol $NaHCO_3$ i.v. are only used if hyperkalaemia is present. Other agents such as THAM or carbicarb (an equimolar mixture of Na_2CO_3 and $NaHCO_3$, which, during buffering, generates two-thirds of the amount of CO_2 in comparison to $NaHCO_3$) have not improved mortality in metabolic acidosis.[36, 37]

DIABETIC KETOACIDOSIS

With fluid and electrolyte therapy to correct the fluid and electrolyte losses, and insulin therapy to correct the metabolic defect, specific therapy for the metabolic acidosis is not required. If diabetic ketoacidosis has been prolonged, then the continued renal loss of ketoacids produces an effective loss of HCO_3^-. Therefore, while insulin will inhibit ketone production and allow the ketones already present to be metabolized; when the ketoacidosis is finally corrected, a normal anion gap acidosis may remain.[38,39]

LACTIC ACIDOSIS

This is defined as a metabolic acidosis associated with a high plasma concentration of lactate (>5.0 mmol/l). Plasma lactate is measured in a heparinized arterial blood sample stored on ice and assayed within 1 hour,[40] or measured on blood collected in a fluoride oxalate tube normally used for glucose assay (oxalate inhibits the glycolytic enzyme enolase). Lactic acidosis may be caused by an excess production or reduced metabolism of lactic acid. It may be classified as either type A, where an inadequate delivery of oxygen for tissue requirements generates lactate faster than it can be removed, or type B, where overt tissue hypoxia does not appear to play a major role (Table 82.5). Nevertheless, both types share mechanisms of over-production and under-utilization. While arterial blood lactate levels are often used to assess the presence or absence of lactic acidosis, assessment of the cellular redox state by measuring blood lactate : pyruvate (L : P) ratios is of questionable value since it assumes that the cytoplasmic redox state (measured by the L : P ratio) reflects the mitochondrial redox potential, which may not be so.[41] Moreover, the cytosolic and mitochondrial redox states may be reversed.[42]

Many forms of therapy for lactic acidosis have been tried, indicating a general dissatisfaction with any one form of treatment. $NaHCO_3$,[43] sodium acetate,[44] THAM,[43] insulin and glucose,[45] dichloroacetate,[46] haemo- and peritoneal dialysis, methylene blue, thiamine, pantothenic acid, biotin, and nitroprusside[47] have all been tried. Treatment should be aimed at correcting tissue perfusion. Oxygen delivery must be optimized, which often requires the use of a pulmonary artery catheter to monitor cardiac output, left and right heart pressures, and mixed venous oxygen tension. Anaemia and metabolic deficiencies of thiamine, pantothenic acid,

Table 82.5 Classification of lactic acidosis

Type A
Severe exercise
Seizures
Cardiac arrest
Shock
Hypoxia <35 mmHg (4.7 kPa)
Anaemia <30 g/l
Type B
Thiamine deficiency
Diabetes
Hepatic failure
Renal failure
Infection
Leukaemia, lymphoma
Pancreatitis
Short bowel syndrome (D-lactate)
Drug-induced
Phenformin, metformin, ethanol, methanol, salicylates
Intravenous fructose, xylitol or sorbitol
Hereditary
Glucose 6-phosphatase deficiency
Fructose 1,6-diphosphatase deficiency

biotin or magnesium should be corrected, and optimal hepatic and renal perfusion ensured, since the latter are the major sites of lactate metabolism. The traditional therapy of massive alkalinization is now no longer recommended.[48, 49]

RENAL TUBULAR ACIDOSIS (RTA)

RTA is a disorder characterized by excess urinary loss of HCO_3^-, normal anion gap, and an elevated serum level of Cl^-. It is classified into proximal or distal types[26] depending on the renal tubular site of the defect.

Distal RTA (Classic RTA or Type 1)

This arises from an inability of the distal nephron to generate and maintain a steep lumen-to-peritubular H^+ gradient. With a standard acid load of 0.1 g NH_4Cl/kg body weight, the urine pH does not fall below 5.4. There is usually evidence of nephrocalcinosis, nephrolithiasis, hypokalaemia and osteomalacia, and therapy with alkaline solutions of potassium and sodium citrate are often required.

Proximal RTA (Type 2)

This arises from a reduced proximal tubular capacity to secrete H^+ (required to reabsorb filtered HCO_3^-). Therefore, a reduced serum level of HCO_3^- is reached at which normal urinary acidification occurs, reflecting normal distal acidification mechanisms. Usually, other proximal tubular defects also exist, i.e. amino aciduria, glycosuria, and phosphaturia. Therapy with alkaline solutions is often not undertaken unless the acidosis is severe (i.e. $HCO_3^- <16$ mmol/l).

Hyperkalaemic RTA (Type 4)

Failure of the kidney to liberate renin, failure of the adrenal to synthesize or excrete aldosterone, or failure of the distal nephron to respond to aldosterone can cause hyperkalaemic hyperchloraemic metabolic acidosis, due to failure of the distal Na^+/H^+ or K^+ exchange mechanism. If there is a reduced distal delivery of sodium, distal H^+ excretion is likewise reduced. Therefore, to diagnose a distal Na^+/K^+ or H^+ exchange defect, urinary sodium should be greater than 40 mmol/l.[50] Type 4 RTA may be caused by Addison's disease, urinary tract obstruction, diabetes, interstitial nephritis, spironolactone, triamterene, amiloride, non-steroidal anti-inflammatory drugs and cyclosporin.

METABOLIC (NON-RESPIRATORY) ALKALOSIS

This condition arises from an abnormal process generating excess HCO_3^-, or an abnormal loss of non-carbonic acid. Characteristically, arterial blood gas measurements reveal pH >7.44 (H^+ <36 mmol/l), $PaCO_2$ >45 mmHg (6.0 kPa) and HCO_3^- >32 mmol/l. Normally, the kidney has a large capacity to excrete HCO_3^-; thus, once metabolic alkalosis is generated, maintenance of this state requires an abnormal retention of HCO_3^- (Table 82.6). The process of generating a metabolic alkalosis can be terminated if therapy is directed at the underlying disease.

However, correction of the pH defect only occurs with renal excretion of the excess HCO_3^-, which often requires therapy to be directed at the abnormal renal HCO_3^- retention mechanisms. Renal maintenance of the metabolic alkalosis is usually effected by a proximal or a distal mechanism.[25]

PROXIMAL MECHANISM

In the proximal tubule, there is an obligatory uptake of Na^+ controlled by the ECF volume. Normally, some of the Na^+ uptake occurs with H^+ secretion. With diminished ECF volume, this Na^+/H^+ exchange mechanism is exaggerated, and hence, if a metabolic alkalosis exists, it will be maintained. Reversal of the pH defect, even in the presence of a mild hypokalaemia, can be achieved with saline infusions, but not with Na^+ solutions of a non-reabsorbable anion. Correction of the alkalosis can also occur with the administration of saline-free albumin solutions, suggesting that nephron recognition of a diminished ECF volume is the major determinant in the maintenance of the alkalosis (and not just a chloride deficiency). Although correction of a metabolic alkalosis may be achieved without the use of saline or potassium chloride solutions, it should not be interpreted as being desirable if saline or potassium chloride deficiencies exist. Moreover, correction of an existing hypokalaemia enhances the ability of saline solutions to correct metabolic alkalosis.[13]

Table 82.6 Generation of metabolic alkalosis

Generation
(A) Loss of H^+
  (1) Renal
    Secondary hyperaldosteronism with K^+ depletion
    Conn's syndrome
    Cushing's syndrome
    Bartter's syndrome
    ACTH secreting tumours
    Drugs: corticosteroids, carbenoxolone, diuretics, liquorice
    Post-hypercarbic alkalosis
  (2) Gastrointestinal
    Nasogastric suction, vomiting
    Villous adenoma
    Congenital alkalosis with diarrhoea
(B) Gain of HCO_3^-
    $NaHCO_3$ administration
    Metabolic conversion of organic acid anions citrate, acetate, lactate
Maintenance
  Diminished functional ECF volume
  Mineralocorticoid excess with K^+ depletion
  Severe K^+ depletion >450 mmol/l
  Chronic renal failure

DISTAL MECHANISM

Under the influence of mineralocorticoids, distal Na^+ reabsorption promotes K^+ and H^+ excretion. In the presence of hypokalaemia, H^+ excretion is augmented. In primary hyperaldosteronism, mechanisms to generate and maintain the metabolic alkalosis exist, although, to generate the alkalosis, hypokalaemia is also required. In secondary hyperaldosteronism, the excess proximal Na^+ reabsorption reduces distal nephron flow, and thus reduces K^+ and H^+ loss. Hence, while the metabolic alkalosis may be maintained, it is not generated unless there is concomitant use of diuretics, which increases the distal delivery of Na^+.

TREATMENT OF METABOLIC ALKALOSIS

Therapy should be directed at correcting both proximal and distal mechanisms (Table 82.7). In the presence of renal insufficiency, these manoeuvres may be insufficient, and treatment with NH_4Cl, arginine hydrochloride or lysine hydrochloride is often recommended. However, in the presence of hepatic failure, these agents are unable to be metabolized to HCl, and may produce hyperammonaemia. In such situations, administration of i.v. HCl (200 mmol in 1 l of 5% dextrose) through a central venous line at a maximum rate of 300–350 mmol/day may be used.[51]

RESPIRATORY ACIDOSIS

This arises from an acute or chronic excess CO_2 and depends on the rate of production as well as excretion

Table 82.7 Treatment of metabolic alkalosis

Indirect
- (A) Inhibition of renal mechanisms maintaining alkalosis
  Proximal: increased functional ECF
  Saline infusions
  Blood, plasma or albumin infusions
  Inotropic agents
  Carbonic anhydrase inhibition
  Acetazolamide
  Distal: KCl
  Aldosterone inhibition (spironolactone)
  Triamterene, amiloride
- (B) Following metabolism to urea and HCl
  Arginine or lysine hydrochloride
  NH_4Cl

Direct
Intravenous HCl

of CO_2. Therapy is aimed at improving ventilation. In chronic respiratory acidosis, there often co-exists an iatrogenic metabolic alkalosis caused by corticosteroid or diuretic administration.

RESPIRATORY ALKALOSIS

This is caused by a reduction in CO_2 which often accompanies the increased ventilation associated with hypoxia, hysteria, hepatic failure, shock or sepsis. Therapy is directed at correcting the underlying abnormality causing the hyperventilation.

REFERENCES

1 Relman AS. Metabolic consequences of acid-base disorders. *Kidney Int* 1972; **1**: 347–59.
2 Anderson OS, Astrup P, Bates RG, *et al*. Report of ad hoc committee on acid-base terminology. *Ann NY Acad Sci* 1966; **133**: 251–3.
3 Campbell EJM. RIpH. *Lancet* 1962; **1**: 681–3.
4 Henderson LJ. The theory of neutrality regulation in the animal organism. *Am J Physiol* 1908; **21**: 427–48
5 Stewart PA. Modern quantitative acid-base chemistry. *Can J Physiol Pharmacol* 1983; **61**: 1444–61.
6 Fencl V, Leith DE. Stewart's quantitative acid-base chemistry: applications in biology and medicine. *Respir Physiol* 1993; **91**: 1–16.
7 Siggaard-Andersen O, Fogh-Andersen N. Base excess or buffer base (strong ion difference) as measure of a non-respiratory acid-base disturbance. *Acta Anaesthesiol Scand Suppl* 1995; **107**: 123–8.
8 Singer RB, Hastings AB. An improved clinical method for the estimation of disturbances of the acid-base balance of human blood. *Medicine (Baltimore)* 1948; **27**: 223–42.
9 Wooten EW. Analytic calculation of physiological acid-base parameters in plasma. *J Appl Physiol* 1999; **86**: 326–34.
10 Worthley LIG. Strong ion difference: a new paradigm or new clothes for the acid base emperor. *Crit Care Resuscitat* 1999; **1**: 211–4.
11 Siggaard-Andersen O, Fogh-Andersen N. Base excess or buffer base (strong ion difference) as measure of a non-respiratory acid-base disturbance. *Acta Anaesthesiol Scand Suppl* 1995; **107**: 123–8.
12 Asano S, Kato E, Yamauchi M, *et al*. The mechanism of acidosis caused by infusion of saline solution. *Lancet* 1966; **1**: 1245–6.
13 Worthley LIG. Hydrogen ion metabolism. *Anaesth Intens Care* 1977; **5**: 347–60.
14 Giebisch G, Berger L, Pitts RF. The extrarenal response to acute acid base disturbances of respiratory origin. *J Clin Invest* 1955; **34**: 231–45.
15 Swan RC, Pitts RF. Neutralization of infused acid by nephrectomized dogs. *J Clin Invest* 1955; **34**: 205–12.
16 Swan RC, Axelrod DR, Seip M, Pitts RF. Distribution of sodium bicarbonate infused into nephrectomized dogs. *J Clin Invest* 1955; **34**: 1795–801.
17 Schwartz WB, Orning KJ, Porter R. The internal distribution of hydrogen ions with varying degrees of metabolic acidosis. *J Clin Invest* 1957; **36**: 373–82.
18 Adler S, Roy A, Relman AS. Intracellular acid-base regulation. II: The interaction between CO_2 tension and the extracellular bicarbonate in the determination of muscle cell pH. *J Clin Invest* 1965; **44**: 21–9.
19 Relman AS. The participation of cells in disturbances of acid-base balance. *Ann NY Acad Sci* 1966; **133**: 160–71.
20 Levin GE, Collinson P, Baron DN. The intracellular pH of human leucocytes in response to acid-base changes in vitro. *Clin Sci* 1976; **50**: 293–9.
21 Schwartz WB, Brackett NC Jr, Cohen JJ. The response of extracellular hydrogen ion concentration to graded degrees of chronic hypercapnia: the physiological limits of the defense of pH. *J Clin Invest* 1965; **44**: 291–302.
22 Adler S, Roy A, Relman AS. Intracellular acid-base regulation. I The response of muscle cells to changes in CO_2 tension or extracellular bicarbonate concentration. *J Clin Invest* 1965; **44**: 8–20.
23 Sartorius OW, Roemmelt JC, Pitts RF. The renal regulation of acid-base balance in man. The nature of renal compensations in ammonium chloride acidosis. *J Clin Invest* 1949; **28**: 423–39.
24 Pitts RF. *Physiology of the Kidney and Body Fluids*, 2nd edn. Chicago, IL: Year Book Medical Publishers; 1968.
25 Seldin DW, Rector FC. The generation and maintenance of metabolic alkalosis. *Kidney Int* 1972; **1**: 306–21.
26 Toto RD. Metabolic acid-base disorders. In: Kokko JP, Tannen RL (eds). *Fluids and Electrolytes*. Philadelphia: WB Saunders Co; 1986: pp. 229–304.
27 Pitts RF. The role of ammonia production and excretion in regulation of acid base balance. *N Engl J Med* 1971; **284**: 32–8.
28 Schwartz WB, Relman AS. A critique of parameters used in the evaluation of acid-base disorders. *N Engl J Med* 1963; **268**: 1382–8.

29 Mizock BA. Utility of standard base excess in acid-base analysis. *Crit Care Med* 1998; **26**: 1146–7.

30 Editorial. Acids, bases and nomograms. *Lancet* 1974; **2**: 814–6.

31 Worthley LIG. A diagram to facilitate the understanding and therapy of mixed acid base disorders. *Anaesth Intens Care* 1976; **4**: 245–53.

32 Fulop M. Arterial CO_2 tension in metabolic acidosis. *Nephrology* 1998; **18**: 351–2.

33 Editorial. The anion gap. *Lancet* 1977; **1**: 785–6.

34 Morris LR, Murphy MB, Kitabchi AE. Bicarbonate therapy in severe diabetic ketoacidosis. *Ann Intern Med* 1986; **105**: 836–40.

35 Standards and Guidelines for Cardiopulmonary Resuscitation (CPR) and Emergency Medical Care (EMC). *JAMA* 1992; **268**: 2172–288.

36 Blecic S, deBacker D, Deleuze M, Vachiery J-L, Vincent J-L. Correction of metabolic acidosis in CPR: bicarbonate vs carbicarb. *Intensive Care Med* 1988; **14** (suppl. 1): 269.

37 Bleich HL, Schwartz WB. Tris buffer (THAM). *N Engl J Med* 1966; **274**: 782–7.

38 Gamblin GT, Ashburn RW, Kemp DG, Beuttel SC. Diabetic ketoacidosis presenting with a normal anion gap. *Am J Med* 1986; **80**: 758–60.

39 Adrogue HJ, Wilson H, Boyd AE III, *et al.* Plasma acid-base patterns in diabetic ketoacidosis. *N Engl J Med* 1982; **307**: 1603–10.

40 Redetzki HM, Hughes JR, Redetzki JE. Differences between serum and plasma osmolalities and their relationship to lactic acid values. *Proc Soc Exp Biol Med* 1972; **139**: 315–18.

41 Cohen RD, Simpson R. Lactate metabolism. *Anesthesiology* 1975; **43**: 661–73.

42 Williamson DH, Lund P, Krebs HA. The redox state of free nicotinamide-adenine-dinucleotide in the cytoplasm and mitochondria of the liver. *Biochem J* 1967; **103**: 514–27.

43 Woods HF. Some aspects of lactic acidosis. *Br J Hosp Med* 1971; **6**: 668–76.

44 Wain RA, Wiernik PH, Thompson WL. Metabolic and therapeutic studies of a patient with acute leukemia and severe lactic acidosis of prolonged duration. *Am J Med* 1973; **55**: 255–60.

45 Hems RA, Ross BP, Berry MN, Krebs HA. Gluconeogenesis in the perfused rat liver. *Biochem J* 1966; **101**: 284–92.

46 Alberti KG, Natrass M. Lactic acidosis. *Lancet* 1977; **2**: 25–9.

47 Taradash MR, Jacobson LB. Vasodilator therapy of idiopathic lactic acidosis. *N Engl J Med* 1975; **293**: 468–71.

48 Graf H, Arieff AI. The use of sodium bicarbonate in the therapy of organic acidosis. *Intens Care Med* 1986; **12**: 285–8.

49 Cooper DJ, Worthley LIG. Adverse haemodynamic effects of sodium bicarbonate in metabolic acidosis. *Intensive Care Med* 1987; **13**: 425–7.

50 Battle DC, von Riotte A, Schlueter W. Urinary sodium in the evaluation of hyperchloremic metabolic acidosis. *N Engl J Med* 1987; **316**: 140–4.

51 Worthley LIG. The rational use of intravenous hydrochloric acid in the therapy of metabolic alkalosis. *Br J Anaesth* 1977; **49**: 811–17.

83

Fluid and electrolyte therapy

L I G Worthley

The management of patients with fluid and electrolyte disorders requires an understanding of body fluid compartments as well as an understanding of water and electrolyte metabolism. These principles will be considered along with the commonly encountered fluid and electrolyte disturbances.

FLUID COMPARTMENTS
(Table 83.1, Fig. 83.1)

TOTAL BODY WATER

In man, water contributes approximately 60% of body weight, with organs varying in water content (Table 83.2). The variation of the percentage of total body weight as water, between individuals, is largely governed by the amount of adipose tissue. Men normally have less body fat than women, and thus have a higher percentage of body weight as water. The average water content as a percentage of total body weight is 60% for males and 50% for females. Total body water (TBW) as a percentage of total body weight decreases with age, due to a progressive loss of muscle mass, causing bone and connective tissue to assume a greater percentage of total body weight[1–3] (Table 83.3).

TBW can be measured by techniques involving dilution of substances which are distributed throughout the TBW space. Antipyrine is one such substance which is easily measured and slowly metabolized and excreted. Alternatively, isotopes of water may be used. Deuterium oxide (D_2O) is non-radioactive and thus difficult to

measure, whereas tritium (THO) is a weak β-emitter and can be easily measured. Equilibrium of a small dose takes 4–6 h and the results are predictable to within ±2%.[3,4]

TBW is commonly divided into two volumes, the extracellular fluid (ECF) volume and the intracellular fluid (ICF) volume.[2] Sodium balance regulates ECF volume, whereas water balance regulates the ICF volume. Sodium excretion is normally regulated by various hormonal and physical ECF volume sensors, whereas water balance is normally regulated by hypothalamic osmolar sensors.[5]

EXTRACELLULAR FLUID

ECF is defined as all body water external to the cell, and is commonly subdivided into plasma and interstitial fluid volumes. The ECF is normally 40% of TBW and 25% of total body weight. With acute or chronic illness, ICF volume is reduced, and ECF volume is increased and may even exceed the ICF volume. Measurement of ECF is performed by using substances which diffuse throughout the ECF space without penetrating the cell.

PLASMA VOLUME
This may be measured using Evans blue, indocyanine green, hydroxyethylstarch, or radioiodine-labelled albumin.[5,6] However, as 7–10% of ^{131}I albumin escapes from the vascular compartment per hour, plasma volume may be overestimated using this method. To counter this effect, multiple readings may be taken and extrapolation to zero time can be performed.[7]

Table 83.1 Body fluid compartments

Fluid compartment	Volume (ml/kg)	% Total body weight
Plasma volume	45	4.5
Blood volume	75	7.5
Interstitial volume	200	20
Extracellular fluid volume	250	25
Intracellular fluid volume	350	35
Total body fluid volume	600	60

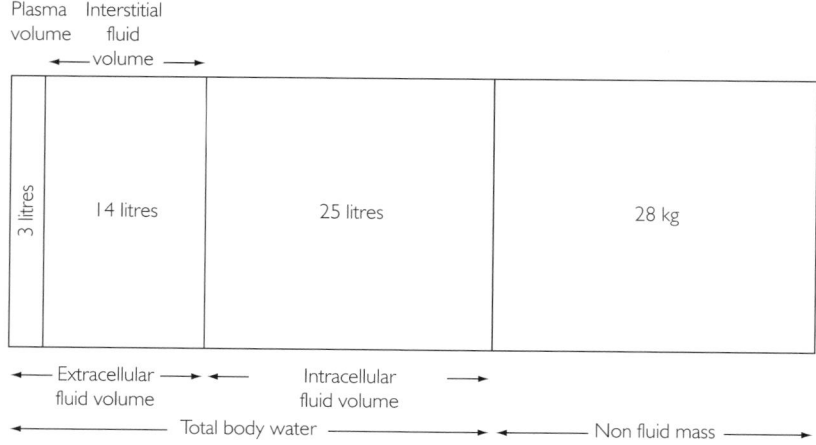

Fig. 83.1 Body fluid compartments

Table 83.2 Water content of various tissues

Tissue	% Water content
Brain	84
Kidney	83
Skeletal muscle	76
Skin	72
Liver	68
Bone	22
Adipose tissue	10

Table 83.3 Water content as a percentage of total body weight

Age (years)	Males (%)	Females (%)
10–15	60	57
15–40	60	50
40–60	55	47
>60	50	45

RED BLOOD CELL VOLUME

This is part of the ICF volume, and can be calculated from plasma volume and haematocrit values. However, total blood haematocrit is about 85–92% of venous haematocrit; therefore, estimations of red blood cell mass may be overestimated by about 5–7% using this method. Red blood cells tagged with chromium (^{51}Cr) will give a more accurate recording.[8]

EXTRACELLULAR FLUID VOLUME

Depending upon the tracer used, values ranging from 15–27% of total body weight are described. The tracers used are either ionic (e.g. isotopes of bromide, chloride, sulphate) or non-ionic (e.g. insulin, mannitol, sucrose) substances. Non-ionic substances are large molecules, and often fail to distribute throughout the ECF in a reason-able time, whereas ionic substances distribute throughout the ECF compartment and also partly through the ICF compartment. Thus, ionic substances give larger measurements of ECF volume than non-ionic substances.

Bromide equilibrates in about 20–24 h, during which time 3–5% is lost in the urine. The latter can be measured and allowed for in the calculations to give results with a variability of 2%. When reporting ECF volumes, the tracer used should be stated as well as the time taken to equilibrate (e.g. a '20-h bromide space'). Most ECF tracers show two decay curves. The first is a rapidly equilibrating pool of 20 min, delineating an ECF space which is in dynamic equilibrium with the plasma. This is about 20% of TBW or about 8–10 l in volume. The second is a slowly equilibrating ECF space (24 h), and includes the ECF of dense connective tissue and bone.

Electrical conductivity methods can be applied simply at the bedside, and have been used to measure the ratio of TBW and ECF volumes. If the TBW is also measured, then the ECF volume can be derived. However, the accuracy of these methods compared to conventional methods, particularly in patients with liver disease, has not been confirmed.[9]

Overall ECF volume, as a percentage of total body weight, shows little change with age. Therefore, most of the change in TBW due to age is from a decrease in ICF volume.

Interstitial Space

This cannot be measured directly and is often calculated as the difference between ECF volume and plasma volume.

INTRACELLULAR FLUID

ICF is defined as all the body water within cells and, unlike the ECF compartment, is an inhomogeneous, multicompartmental entity, with different pH and ionic composition depending upon the organ or tissue being considered. The ICF volume is often determined by inference, from the difference in measurements of the TBW and ECF spaces. This estimation suffers from the inaccuracies inherent in both ECF and TBW measurements. In general, the ICF is considered to be 60% of TBW and 35% of total body weight.

TRANSCELLULAR FLUID

Fluids in this compartment have a common characteristic of being formed by transport activity of cells. The fluid is extracellular in nature and will be considered as part of the interstitial volume. It may vary from 1–10 l, with larger volumes occurring in diseased states (e.g. bowel obstruction or cirrhosis with ascites), and is formed at the expense of the remaining interstitial and plasma volumes.

WATER METABOLISM

Water balance is maintained by altering the intake and excretion of water. Intake is controlled by thirst, whereas excretion is controlled by the renal action of antidiuretic hormone (ADH). In health, plasma osmolalities of about 280 mOsm/kg suppress plasma ADH to levels low enough to permit maximum urinary dilution.[10] Above this value, an increase in ECF tonicity of about 1–2% or a decrease in TBW of 1–2 l, causes the posterior pituitary to release ADH, which acts upon the distal nephron to increase water reabsorption. Maximum plasma ADH levels are reached at an osmolality of 295 mOsm/kg.[10] The osmotic stimulation also changes thirst sensation and, in the conscious ambulant man, initiates water repletion (drinking), which is more important in preventing dehydration than ADH secretion and action. Thus, in health, the upper limit of the body osmolality (and therefore serum sodium) is determined by the osmotic threshold for thirst, whereas the lower limit is determined by the osmotic threshold for ADH release.[11]

Increase in osmolality caused by permeant solutes (e.g. urea) does not stimulate ADH release. ADH may also be released in response to hypovolaemia and

Table 83.4 Drugs affecting ADH secretion

Stimulate	Inhibit
Nicotine	Ethanol
Narcotics	Narcotic antagonists
Vincristine	Dilantin
Barbiturates	
Cyclophosphamide	
Chlorpropamide	
Clofibrate	
Carbamazepine	
Amitryptylline	

hypotension, via stimulation of low and high pressure baroreceptors. The ADH release is extremely marked when more than 30% of the intravascular volume is lost. ADH may also be stimulated by pain and nausea, which are thought to act through the baroreceptor pathways.[5] ADH release may also be stimulated by a variety of pharmacological agents (Table 83.4). Renal response to ADH depends upon an intact, distal nephron, and collecting duct and a hypertonic medullary interstitium. The capacity to conserve or excrete water also depends upon the osmolar load presented to the distal nephron.[5]

WATER REQUIREMENTS

Water is needed to eliminate the daily solute load, and to replace daily insensible fluid loss (Table 83.5). With a normal daily excretion of 600 mOsm solute, maximal and minimal secretions of ADH will cause urine osmolality to vary from 1200 to 30 mOsm/kg respectively, and the urine output to vary from 500 ml to 20 l/day, respectively. Skin and lung water losses vary, and may range from 500 ml to 8 l/day depending on physical activity, ambient temperature and humidity.

DISORDERS OF OSMOLALITY

TONICITY

Osmolality is a measure of the number of osmol/kg water. The osmolality of the ECF is due largely to sodium salts. Clinical effects of hyperosmolality, due to excess solute, depends upon whether the solute distributes

Table 83.5 Daily fluid balance (for a 70 kg man at rest in a temperate climate)

	Input (ml)			Output (ml)	
	Seen	Unseen		Seen	Unseen
Drink	1000	–	Urine	1000	–
Food	–	650	Skin	–	500
Water of oxidation	–	350	Lungs	–	400
			Faeces	–	100
Total	1000	1000	Total	1000	1000

evenly throughout the TBW (e.g. permeant solutes of alcohol or urea) or distributes in the ECF only (e.g. impermeant solutes of mannitol or glucose). With impermeant solutes, hyperosmolality is associated with a shift of fluid from the ICF to the ECF compartment.[12] Hyperosmolality due to increased impermeant solutes is known as hypertonicity. This condition may also be associated with a reduction in the serum sodium concentration (see below).

WATER EXCESS

In a 70 kg man, for every 1 l excess water, ECF increases by 400 ml and ICF increases by 600 ml, on average. The osmolality also decreases by 6–7 mOsm/kg and the serum sodium falls by 3.0–3.5 mmol/l.

WATER DEFICIENCY

In a 70 kg man, for every 1 l water loss, 600 ml is lost from the ICF and 400 from the ECF. The osmolality also increases by 7–8 mOsm/kg and the serum sodium rises by 3.5–4.0 mmol/l.

ELECTROLYTES

Chemical compounds in solution may either:

- Remain intact (i.e. undissociated), in which case they are called non-electrolytes (e.g. glucose, urea)

- Dissociate to form ions, in which case they are called electrolytes. Ions carry an electrical charge (e.g. Na^+, Cl^-). Ions with a positive charge are attracted to a negative electrode or cathode, and hence are called 'cations'. Conversely, ions with a negative charge travel towards a positive electrode or anode and are called 'anions'. Each body water compartment contains electrolytes with different composition and concentration (Table 83.6)

SODIUM

Sodium is the principal cation of the ECF and accounts for 86% of the ECF osmolality. In a 70 kg man, total body sodium content is 4000 mmol (58 mmol/kg), 70% of which is exchangeable (i.e. exchanges with isotopic tracer sodium within 24 h). The majority of the exchangeable sodium (85%) resides in the ECF compartment; the remainder resides in the ICF compartment and the exchangeable bone compartment.[13] Non-exchangeable sodium resides in bone[14] (Table 83.7). ECF concentration of sodium varies between 134–146 mmol/l. The intracellular sodium concentration varies between different tissues, and ranges from 3–20 mmol/l.

The standard Western society dietary sodium intake is about 150 mmol/day, but the daily intake of sodium varies widely, with urinary losses ranging from <1 to >240 mmol/day.[15] Sodium balance is influenced by renal hormonal and ECF physical characteristics. The com-

Table 83.6 Electrolyte composition of body fluid compartments

Electrolyte	ICF (mmol/l)	ECF (mmol/l)	
		Plasma	Interstitial
Sodium	10	140	145
Potassium	155	3.7	3.8
Chloride	3	102	115
Bicarbonate	10	28	30
Calcium (ionized)	<0.01	1.2	1.2
Magnesium	10	0.8	0.8
Phosphate	105	1.1	1.0

Table 83.7 The sodium compartments in a 70 kg man

	Total (mmol)	(mmol/kg)
Total body sodium	4000	58
Non-exchangeable bone sodium	1200	17
Exchangeable sodium	2800	40
Intracellular sodium	250	3
Extracellular sodium	2400	35
Exchangeable bone sodium	150	2

plete renal adjustment to an altered sodium load usually requires 3–4 days before balance is restored.

HYPONATRAEMIA

Hyponatraemia is defined as a serum sodium less than 135 mmol/l and may be classified as isotonic, hypertonic, or hypotonic, depending upon the measured serum osmolality (Table 83.8).

ISOTONIC HYPONATRAEMIA

Plasma normally contains 93% water and 7% solids (5.5% proteins, 1% salts and 0.5% lipids). If the solid phase is elevated significantly (e.g. in hyperlipidaemia or hyperproteinaemia), any device which dilutes a specific amount of plasma for analysis will give falsely lower values for all measured compounds. This effect produces 'factitious hyponatraemia' and is associated with a normal measured serum osmolality.[16] Measurement of plasma sodium by an ion-selective electrode is not affected by the volume of plasma 'solids' and therefore 'pseudohyponatraemia' will not occur with this method.[16]

HYPERTONIC HYPONATRAEMIA

In patients who have hypertonicity due to increased amounts of impermeant solutes (e.g. glucose, mannitol, glycerol or sorbitol), a shift of water from the ICF to the ECF occurs to provide osmotic equilibration, thus diluting the ECF sodium. Such resultant hyponatraemia is often associated with an increased measured osmolality. For example, in the presence of hyperglycaemia, for every 3 mmol/l rise in glucose, the serum sodium decreases by 1 mmol/l.[17]

Table 83.8 Common causes of hyponatraemia

(1) **Misleading result**
   Isotonic
      Hyperlipidaemia
      Hyperproteinaemia
   Hypertonic
      Hyperglycaemia
      Mannitol, glycerol, glycine or sorbitol excess
(2) **Water retention**
   Renal failure
   Hepatic failure
   Cardiac failure
   Syndrome of inappropriate ADH secretion
   Drugs
   Psychogenic polydipsia
(3) **Water retention and salt depletion**
   Postoperative, post trauma or patients with excess fluid
      losses given inappropriate fluid replacement
   Adrenocortical failure
   Diuretic excess

HYPOTONIC HYPONATRAEMIA

Hyponatraemia is almost always caused by an excess of TBW, due to excessive hypotonic, or water generating i.v. fluids (eg. 1.5% glycine, 0.45% saline or 5% dextrose) or excessive ingestion of water, particularly in the presence of high circulating ADH levels. It may rarely be caused by loss of exchangeable sodium or potassium.[18] In the latter circumstances, a loss of approximately 40 mmol of sodium or potassium, without a change in TBW content, is required to lower the serum sodium by 1 mmol/l. As hyponatraemia may be associated with an alteration in both total body water and total body sodium, the ECF may be increased (hypervolaemia), decreased (hypovolaemia) or exhibit no change (isovolaemia).[10]

In health, a fluid intake up to 15–20 l may be tolerated before water is retained and hyponatraemia occurs. In psychogenic polydipsia, if the water intake exceeds the renal capacity to form dilute urine, water retention and hyponatraemia will occur. With this disorder, the plasma osmolality exceeds urine osmolality. In circumstances where ADH is increased (e.g. hypovolaemia, hypotension, pain or nausea), or where renal response to ADH is altered (i.e. in renal, hepatic, pituitary, adrenal or thyroid failure), water retention occurs with lower intakes of fluid.

TRANSURETHRAL RESECTION OF PROSTATE (TURP) SYNDROME

The TURP syndrome consists of hyponatraemia, cardiovascular disturbances (hypertension, hypotension, bradycardia), an altered state of consciousness (agitation, confusion, nausea, vomiting, myoclonic and generalized seizures) and (when using glycine solutions) transient visual disturbances of blurred vision, blindness and fixed dilated pupils, associated with TURP (although it has also been described following endometrial ablation).[19,20] It may occur within 15 min or be delayed for up to 24 h postoperatively,[21] and is usually caused by an excess absorption of the irrigating fluid which contains 1.5% glycine with an osmolality of 200 mOsmol/kg (although hyponatraemic syndromes have also been described when irrigating solutions containing 3% mannitol or 3% sorbitol have been used, both of which have an osmolality of 165 mOsm/kg). Symptomatology usually occurs when >1 l of 1.5% glycine or >2–3 l of 3% mannitol or sorbitol are absorbed.[22]

The excess absorption of irrigating fluid causes an increase in total body water (which is often associated with only a small decrease in plasma osmolality), hyponatraemia (as glycine, sorbitol or mannitol reduces the sodium component of ECF osmolality) and an increase in the osmolar gap.[23–25] When glycine is used, other features include hyperglycinaemia (up to 20 mmol/l, normal plasma glycine levels range from 0.15–0.3 mmol/l), hyperserinemia (as serine is a major metabolite of glycine), hyperammonaemia (following deamination of glycine and serine), metabolic acidosis and hypocalcaemia (due to the glycine metabolites glyoxylic acid and oxalate). Because glycine is an inhibitory neurotransmitter (by blocking chloride channels[26]), and as it passes freely into the intracellular compartment, when glycine solutions are used, hyperglycinaemia may be more important in the pathophysiology of this disorder than a reduction in body fluid osmolality and cerebral oedema,[27] as cerebral oedema is often minimal in this condition.[28]

Treatment is largely supportive with the management of any reduction in plasma osmolality being based on the measured plasma osmolality and not the plasma sodium. If the measured osmolality is >260 mOsm/kg and mild neurological abnormalities exist, if the patient is haemodynamically stable with normal renal function, close observation and reassurance (e.g. the visual disturbances are reversible and will last for less than 24 h), is usually all that is needed. If the patient is hypotensive and bradycardic with severe and unresolving neurological abnormalities, haemodialysis may be warranted.[29] Hypertonic saline is only used if the measured osmolality is <260 mOsm/kg and severe non-visual neurological abnormalities exist.

SYNDROME OF INAPPROPRIATE ADH SECRETION (SIADH)

This syndrome is a form of hyponatraemia in which there is an increased level of ADH inappropriate to any osmotic or volume stimuli that normally affects ADH secretion.[30-31] Diagnostic criteria and possible causes are listed in Tables 83.9 and 83.10, respectively.

CLINICAL FEATURES

While cerebral manifestations are usually absent when the sodium concentration exceeds 125 mmol/l, progressive symptomatology of headache, nausea, confusion, disorientation, coma and seizures are often observed when plasma sodium falls below 120 mmol/l.[32]

TREATMENT

This depends on clinical manifestations, which may also relate to the speed of onset of hyponatraemia. If the patient is asymptomatic and hyponatraemia has been present for many weeks, simple fluid restriction and

Table 83.9   Criteria for the diagnosis of syndrome of inappropriate antidiuretic hormone (SIADH)

Hypotonic hyponatraemia
Urine osmolality greater than plasma osmolality
Urine sodium excretion greater than 20 mmol/l
Normal renal, hepatic, cardiac, pituitary, adrenal and thyroid function
Absence of hypotension, hypovolaemia, oedema and drugs affecting ADH secretion
Correction by water restriction

Table 83.10   Aetiologies of syndrome of inappropriate antidiuretic hormone (SIADH)

Ectopic ADH production by tumours
    Small cell bronchogenic carcinoma
    Adenocarcinoma of the pancreas or duodenum
    Leukaemia
    Lymphoma
    Thymoma
Central nervous system disorders
    Cerebral trauma
    Brain tumour (primary or secondary)
    Meningitis or encephalitis
    Brain abscess
    Subarachnoid haemorrhage
    Acute intermittent porphyria
    Guillain–Barré syndrome
    Systemic lupus erythematosus
Pulmonary diseases
    Viral, fungal and bacterial pneumonias
    Tuberculosis
    Lung abscess

reversal of any precipitating factor may be all that is required. In hyponatraemia of rapid onset, particularly if associated with cerebral symptoms, treatment consists of i.v. hypertonic saline (50–70 mmol/h) to increase the serum sodium by 2 mmol/l per h, until a concentration of 130 mmol/l is attained.[33] If seizures are present, rapid treatment of cerebral oedema is required. While 500 ml of 20% of mannitol may be used, 250 mmol of sodium chloride i.v. over 10 min provides the same osmotic effect, and has the advantage of simultaneously increasing the serum sodium (usually by about 7 mmol/l).[34] Normally, with symptomatic hyponatraemia (serum sodium less than 120 mmol/l), the patient has both water excess (approximately 6–8 l) and sodium deficiency (200–400 mmol).

Complications reported with hypertonic saline therapy include congestive cardiac failure and central pontine- and extrapontine mylinolysis (osmotic demylination syndrome).[35] Monitoring of central venous pressure or pulmonary capillary wedge pressure throughout saline administration is required. If a spontaneous diuresis has not occurred with the administration of saline, a diuretic may be required. There is still no uniform agreement that osmotic demylination is produced by a rapid correction of hyponatraemia.[36,37] Nevertheless, serum sodium should be increased up to only 130 mmol/l, and maintained at this level for the next 24–48 h.

HYPERNATRAEMIA

Hypernatraemia is defined as a serum sodium greater than 145 mmol/l (Table 83.11). It is always associated with hyperosmolality and may be caused by:

Table 83.11 Causes of hypernatraemia

Water depletion
  Extrarenal loss
    Exposure
    GIT losses (often with excess saline replacement)
  Renal loss
    Osmotic diuresis – urea, mannitol, glycosuria
    Diabetes insipidus
      Neurogenic
        Post traumatic, fat embolism
        Metastatic tumours, craniopharyngioma, pinealoma,
          cysts
        Meningitis, encephalitis
        Granulomas (TB, sarcoid)
        Guillain–Barré syndrome
        Idiopathic
      Nephrogenic
        Congenital
        Hypercalcaemia, hypokalaemia
        Lithium
        Pyelonephritis
        Medullary sponge kidney
        Polycystic kidney
        Post obstructive uropathy
        Multiple myeloma, amyloid, sarcoid
Salt gain
  Hypertonic, saline or sodium bicarbonate

- Excessive administration of sodium salts (bicarbonate or chloride)
- Water depletion
- Excess sodium and loss of water

Excessive administration of sodium salts is rare and usually results from a therapeutic misadventure. Pure water depletion is uncommon, unless water restriction is applied to a patient who is unconscious or unable to obtain or ingest water, as the thirst response normally corrects water depletion. The serum sodium level rises, and is associated with a loss of volume in both ECF and ICF.

CLINICAL FEATURES
Hypernatraemia usually produces symptoms if the serum sodium exceeds 155–160 mmol/l (i.e. osmolality >330 mOsm/kg). The clinical features include pyrexia, restlessness, irritability, drowsiness, lethargy, confusion, and coma.[38] Convulsions are uncommon. The diminished ECF volume may reduce cardiac output, thereby reducing renal perfusion, leading to pre-renal failure.

TREATMENT
For pure water depletion, this consists of water administration. If i.v. fluid is required, 5% dextrose or hypotonic saline solutions (0.45% saline) are often used, as sterile water infusion causes haemolysis. In rare cases, i.v. sterile water may be used, by administering through a central venous catheter.[39] Since rapid rehydration may give rise to cerebral oedema, the change in serum sodium should be no greater than 2 mmol/l per h.[33]

POTASSIUM

Potassium is the principal intracellular cation and accordingly (along with its anion) fulfils the role of the ICF osmotic provider. It also plays a major role in the functioning of excitable tissues (e.g. muscle and nerve). As the cell membrane is 20-fold more permeable to potassium than sodium ions, potassium is largely responsible for the resting membrane potential. Potassium also influences carbohydrate metabolism and glycogen and protein synthesis.

Total body potassium is 45–50 mmol/kg in the male (3500 mmol/70 kg) and 35–40 mmol/kg (2500 mmol/65 kg) in the female; 95% of the total body potassium is exchangeable. The ECF potassium ranges from 3.1–4.2 mmol/l, thus the total ECF potassium ranges from 55–70 mmol. About 90% of the total body potassium is intracellular; 8% resides in bone, 2% in ECF water and 70% in skeletal muscle.[40,41] With increasing age (and decreasing muscle mass), total body potassium decreases.

The daily intake of potassium in a standard Western society diet varies from 40–150 mmol, and the urinary loss varies from 30–150 mmol/l.[15,41,42] In certain cultures, potassium ingestion may be as low as 25 mmol, or as high as 500 mmol/day.

FACTORS AFFECTING POTASSIUM METABOLISM

The potassium content of cells is regulated by a cell wall pump-leak mechanism. Cellular uptake is by the Na^+/K^+ pump which is driven by Na^+/K^+ ATPase. Movement of potassium out of the cell is governed by passive forces (i.e. cell membrane permeability and chemical and electrical gradients to the potassium ion).

Acidosis promotes a shift of potassium from the ICF to the ECF, whereas alkalosis promotes the reverse shift. Hyperkalaemia stimulates insulin release, which promotes a shift of potassium from the ECF to the ICF, an effect independent of the movement of glucose.[41] β_2-adrenergic agonists promote cellular uptake of potassium by a cyclic AMP-dependent activation of the Na^+/K^+ pump, whereas α-adrenergic agonists cause a shift of potassium from the ICF to the ECF.[43] Aldosterone increases the renal excretion of potassium, but whether it also causes a general transcellular shift of potassium is not clear. Glucocorticoids are also kaliuretic, an effect which may be independent of the mineralocorticoid receptor.

Normally, mechanisms to reduce the ECF potassium concentration (by increasing renal excretion and shifting potassium from the ECF to the ICF) are very effective. However, mechanisms to retain potassium in the presence of potassium depletion are less efficient, particularly when compared to those of sodium conservation. Even with severe potassium depletion, urinary loss of potassium continues at a rate of 10–20 mmol/day. Metabolic alkalosis also enhances renal potassium loss, by encouraging distal nephron Na^+/K^+, rather than Na^+/K^+ exchange.

HYPOKALAEMIA

Hypokalaemia is defined as a serum potassium of less than 3.5 mmol/l (or plasma potassium less than 3.0 mmol/l). It may be due to decreased oral intake, increased renal or gastrointestinal loss, or movement of potassium from the ECF to the ICF (Table 83.12).

CLINICAL FEATURES

These include weakness, hypotonicity, depression, constipation, ileus, ventilatory failure, ventricular tachycardias (characteristically *torsades de pointes*), atrial tachycardias, and even coma.[44] With prolonged and severe potassium deficiency, rhabdomyolysis and thirst and polyuria, due to

Table 83.12 Causes of hypokalaemia

Inadequate dietary intake (urine K^+ <20 mmol/l)
Abnormal body losses
  Gastrointestinal (urine K^+ <20 mmol/l)
    Vomiting, nasogastric aspiration
    Diarrhoea, fistula loss
    Villous adenoma of the colon
    Laxative abuse
  Renal (urine K^+ >20 mmol/l)
    Conn's syndrome
    Cushing's syndrome
    Bartter's syndrome
    Ectopic ACTH syndrome
      Small cell carcinoma of the lung
      Pancreatic carcinoma
      Carcinoma of the thymus
    Drugs
      Diuretics
      Corticosteroids
      Carbenicillin, amphotericin B, gentamicin
      Cisplatin
  Renal tubular acidosis
  Magnesium deficiency
Compartmental shift
  Alkalosis
  Insulin
  Na^+/K^+ ATPase stimulation
    Sympathomimetic agents with β_2 effect
    Methylxanthines
  Barium poisoning
  Hypothermia
  Toluene intoxication
  Hypokalaemic periodic paralysis

the development of renal diabetes insipidus, may occur. The ECG changes are relatively non-specific, and include prolongation of the PR interval, T-wave inversion, and prominent U-waves.

TREATMENT

Intravenous or oral potassium chloride will correct hypokalaemia, particularly if it is associated with metabolic alkalosis. If the patient has renal tubular acidosis and hypokalaemia, potassium acetate or citrate is required. Intravenous administration of potassium should normally not exceed 40 mmol/h, and plasma potassium should be monitored at 1–4-hourly intervals.[40,41] In patients with acute myocardial infarction and hypokalaemia, i.v. potassium is recommended at a rate of 10 mmol/30 min (in 50–100 ml 5% dextrose), and repeated as necessary until serum potassium is 4.0–4.5 mmol/l (or plasma potassium is 3.5–4.0 mmol/l).[45] The plasma concentration should be measured hourly during potassium replacement.

HYPERKALAEMIA

Hyperkalaemia is defined as a serum potassium greater than 5.0 mmol/l or plasma potassium greater than 4.5 mmol/l. It may be artifactual (from sampling errors), or may be due to excessive intake, severe tissue damage, decreased excretion, or body fluid compartment shift (Table 83.13).

Table 83.13 Causes of hyperkalaemia

Collection abnormalities
  Delay in separating RBC
  Specimen haemolysis
  Thrombocythemia
Excessive intake
  Exogenous (i.e. i.v. or oral KCl, massive blood transfusion)
  Endogenous (i.e. tissue damage)
    Burns, trauma
    Rhabdomyolysis
    Tumour lysis
Decrease in renal excretion
  Drugs
    Spironolactone, triamterine, ameloride
    Indomethacin
    Captopril, enalapril
  Renal failure
  Addison's disease
  Hyporeninaemic hypoaldosteronism
Compartmental shift
  Acidosis
  Insulin deficiency
  Digoxin overdosage
  Succinylcholine
  Arginine hydrochloride
  Hyperkalaemic periodic paralysis
  Fluoride poisoning

CLINICAL FEATURES

These include tingling, paraesthesia, weakness, flaccid paralysis, hypotension and bradycardia. The characteristic ECG effects include peaking of the T-waves, flattening of the P-wave, prolongation of the PR interval (until sinus arrest with nodal rhythm occurs), widening of the QRS complex, and the development of a deep S-wave. Finally, a sine wave ECG pattern develops which deteriorates to asystole, which may occur at serum potassium levels of 7 mmol/l or greater.

TREATMENT

This is directed at the underlying cause, and may include dialysis. Rapid management of life-threatening hyperkalaemia may be achieved by:

- Dextrose, 50 g i.v. with 20 U of soluble insulin
- Sodium bicarbonate, 50–100 mmol i.v.
- Calcium chloride 5–10 ml i.v. of 10% (3.4–6.8 mmol, which is used to reduce the cardiac effects of hyperkalaemia)
- Oral and rectal resonium A, 50 g

CALCIUM

Almost all (99%) of the body calcium (30 mmol or 1000 g or 1.5% body weight) is present in the bone. A small but significant quantity of ionized calcium exists in the ECF, and is important for many cellular activities, including secretion, neuromuscular impulse formation, contractile functions, and clotting. Normal daily intake of calcium is 15–20 mmol, although only 40% is absorbed. The average daily urinary loss is 2.5–7.5 mmol. The total ECF calcium of 40 mmol (2.20–2.55 mmol/l), exists in three forms. Forty percent (1.0 mmol/l) is bound to protein (largely albumin), 47% is ionized (1.15 mmol/l), and 13% is complexed (0.3 mmol/l) with citrate, sulphate and phosphate. The ionized form is the physiologically important form, and may be acutely reduced in alkalosis by causing a greater amount of the serum calcium to be bound to protein.[46,47] While the serum ionized calcium can be measured, total serum calcium is usually measured, which can vary with the serum albumin levels. A correction factor can be used to offset the effect of serum albumin on serum calcium. This is 0.02 mmol/l for every 1 g/l increase in serum albumin (up to a value of 40 g/l), added to the measured calcium level. For example, if measured serum calcium is 1.82 mmol/l, and serum albumin is 25 g/l, corrected serum calcium = 1.82 + [(40−25) × 0.02] mmol/l = 2.12 mmol/l.

Clinical features of a reduced serum ionized calcium include tetany, cramps, mental changes and decrease in cardiac output. The clinical features of hypercalcaemia, on the other hand, include nausea, vomiting, pancreatitis, polyuria, polydipsia, muscular weakness, mental disturbance, and ectopic calcification (see Ch. 53).

MAGNESIUM

Magnesium is primarily an intracellular ion which acts as a metallo-coenzyme in numerous phosphate transfer reactions. It has a critical role in the transfer, storage and utilization of energy.

In man, the total body magnesium content is 1000 mmol, and the plasma concentrations range from 0.70–0.95 mmol/l. The daily oral intake is 8–20 mmol (40% of which is absorbed) and the urinary loss, which is the major source of excretion of magnesium, varies from 2.5–8 mmol/day.[46,48]

HYPOMAGNESAEMIA

Hypomagnesaemia is caused by decreased intake or increased loss (Table 83.14). Clinical features include neurological signs of confusion, irritability, delirium tremors, convulsions, and tachyarrhythmias. Hypomagnesaemia is often associated with resistant hypokalaemia and hypocalcaemia. Treatment consists of i.v. magnesium sulphate as a bolus of 10 mmol, administered over 5 min, followed by 20–60 mmol/day.

HYPERMAGNESAEMIA

Hypermagnesaemia is often caused by excessive administration of magnesium salts or conventional doses of

Table 83.14 Causes of magnesium deficiency

Gastrointestinal disorders
    Malabsorption syndromes
    GIT fistulas
    Short-bowel syndrome
    Prolonged nasogastric suction
    Diarrhoea
    Pancreatitis
    Parenteral nutrition
Alcoholism
Endocrine disorders
    Hyperparathyroidism
    Hyperthyroidism
    Conn's syndrome
    Diabetes mellitus
    Hyperaldosteronism
Renal diseases
    Renal tubular acidosis
    Diuretic phase of acute tubular necrosis
Drugs
    Aminoglycosides
    Carbenicillin, ticarcillin
    Amphotericin B
    Diuretic therapy
    Cis-platinum
    Cyclosporin

Table 83.15   Causes of hypophosphataemia

Hyperparathyroidism
Vitamin D deficiency
Vitamin D resistant rickets
Renal tubular acidosis
Alkalosis
Parenteral nutrition
Alcoholism

Table 83.16   Causes of hyperphosphataemia

Rhabdomyolysis
Renal failure (acute or chronic)
Vitamin D toxicity
Acidosis
Tumour lysis
Hypoparathyroidism
Pseudohypoparathyroidism
Diphosphonate therapy
Excess i.v. administration

magnesium in the presence of renal failure. Clinical features include drowsiness, hyporeflexia and coma, vasodilation and hypotension, and conduction defects of sinoatrial and atrioventricular nodal block and asystole may occur. Treatment is directed towards increasing excretion of the ion, which may require dialysis. Intravenous calcium chloride may be used for rapidly treating the cardiac conduction defects.[48]

PHOSPHATE

While most of the body phosphate exists in bone, 15% is found in the soft tissues as ATP, red blood cell 2,3-DPG, and other cellular structural proteins, including phospholipids, nucleic acids and phosphoproteins. Phosphate also acts as a cellular and urinary buffer.[46,49]

HYPOPHOSPHATAEMIA

Hypophosphataemia may be caused by a decreased intake, increased excretion or intracellular redistribution (Table 83.15). While hypophosphataemia may be symptom-free, clinical features have been described which include paraesthesia, muscle weakness, seizures, coma, rhabdomyolysis and cardiac failure. Treatment consists of oral or i.v. sodium or potassium phosphate, 50–100 mmol/24 h.

HYPERPHOSPHATAEMIA

Hyperphosphataemia is usually caused by an increased intake or decreased excretion (Table 83.16). Clinical features include ectopic calcification of nephrocalcinosis, nephrolithiasis and band keratopathy. Treatment may

require haemodialysis; otherwise oral aluminium hydroxide and even hypertonic dextrose solutions to shift ECF phosphate into the ICF can be used.

REPLACEMENT THERAPY

GASTROINTESTINAL LOSSES

The daily volumes and composition of gastrointestinal (GIT) secretions in mmol/l are shown in Table 83.17. Clinical effects of fluid loss from the GIT are largely determined by the volume and composition of the fluid, and therapy is usually directed at replacing the losses. Gastric fluid loss (e.g. from vomiting and nasogastric suction) results in water, sodium, hydrogen ion, potassium, and chloride depletion. Hence, metabolic alkalosis, hypokalaemia, hypotension and dehydration develop if the saline and potassium chloride losses are not correctly replaced.

PANCREATIC AND BILIARY FLUID LOSSES
(e.g. Pancreatic or Biliary Fistula)

These may result in hyperchloraemic acidosis with hypokalaemia, hypotension and dehydration if the losses of bicarbonate, potassium and saline are not correctly replaced.

INTESTINAL LOSSES (e.g. Fistula or Ileostomy
Losses, Diarrhoea and Ileus)

These result in hypokalaemia, hypotension and dehydration if the saline and potassium losses are not replaced.

Table 83.17   Daily volume and electrolyte composition of GIT secretions

Electrolytes (mmol/l)	Vol (l)	H^+	Na^+	K^+	Cl^-	HCO_3^-
Saliva	0.5–1.0	0	30	20	10–35	0–15
Stomach	1.0–2.5	0–120	60	10	100–120	0
Bile	0.5	0	140	5–10	100	40–70
Pancreatic	0.75	0	140	5–10	100	40–70
Small and large gut	2.0–4.0	0	110	5–10	100	25

REFERENCES

1 Edelman I, Leibman J. Anatomy of body water and electrolytes. *Am J Med* 1959; **27**: 256–77.

2 Gamble J. *Chemical Anatomy, Physiology and Pathology of Extracellular Fluid*. Cambridge, Massachusetts: Harvard University Press; 1954.

3 Moore FD, Olesen KH, McMurrey JD, *et al*. *Body Composition in Health and Disease*. Philadelphia: WB Saunders Co; 1963.

4 Streat SJ, Beddoe AH, Hill GL. Measurement of total body water in intensive care patients with fluid overload. *Metabolism* 1985; **34**: 688–94.

5 Bie P. Osmoreceptors, vasopressin and control of renal water excretion. *Physiol Rev* 1980; **60**: 961–1048.

6 Thomsen J, Fogh-Andersen M, Bülow K, *et al*. Blood and plasma volumes determined by carbon monoxide gas, ^{99m}Tc-labelled erythrocytes, ^{125}I-albumin and the T 1824 technique. *Scand J Clin Lab Invest* 1991; **51**: 185–90.

7 Tschaikowsky K, Meisner M, Durst R, Rügheimer E. Blood volume determination using hydroxyethyl starch: a rapid and simple intravenous injection method. *Crit Care Med* 1997; **25**: 599–606.

8 Pain RW. Body fluid compartments. *Intensive Care Med* 1977; **5**: 284–94.

9 Holt TL, Cui C, Thomas BJ, *et al*. Clinical applicability of bioelectric impedance to measure body composition in health and disease. *Nutrition* 1994; **10**: 221–4.

10 Humes HD. Disorders of water metabolism. In: Kokko JP, Tannen RL (eds). *Fluid and Electrolytes*. Philadelphia: WB Saunders Co; 1986: pp. 118–49.

11 Phillips PJ. Water metabolism. *Anaesth Intens Care* 1977; **5**: 295–304.

12 Gennari FJ. Serum osmolality. Uses and limitations. *N Engl J Med* 1984; **310**: 102–5.

13 McKeown JW. Disorders of total body sodium. In: Kokko JP, Tannen RL (eds). *Fluid and Electrolytes*. Philadelphia: WB Saunders Co; 1986: pp. 63–117.

14 Cohn SH, Abesamis C, Zanzi J, *et al*. Body elemental composition: comparison between black and white adults. *Am J Physiol* 1977; **232**: 419–22.

15 Intersalt Cooperative Research Group. Intersalt: an international study of electrolyte excretion and blood pressure. Results for 24 hour urinary sodium and potassium excretion. *BMJ* 1988; **297**: 319–28.

16 Weisberg LS. Pseudohyponatremia: a reappraisal. *Am J Med* 1989; **86**: 315–8.

17 Katz MA. Hyperglycemia-induced hyponatremia – calculation of expected serum sodium depression. *N Engl J Med* 1973; **289**: 843–4.

18 Fuisz RE. Hyponatremia. *Medicine* 1963; **42**: 149–68.

19 Arieff AI, Ayus JC. Endometrial ablation complicated by fatal hyponatremic encephalopathy. *JAMA* 1993; **270**: 1230–2.

20 Istre O, Bjoennes J, Naess R, *et al*. Postoperative cerebral oedema after transcervical endometrial resection and uterine irrigation with 1.5% glycine. *Lancet* 1994; **344**: 1187–9.

21 Gravenstein D. Transurethral resection of the prostate (TURP) syndrome: a review of the pathophysiology and management. *Anesth Analg* 1997; **84**: 438–46.

22 Hahn RG. Irrigating fluids in endoscopic surgery. *Br J Urol* 1997; **79**: 669–80.

23 Wang JM, Creel DJ, Wong KC. Transurethral resection of the prostate, serum glycine levels, and ocular evoked potentials. *Anesthesiology* 1989; **70**: 36–41.

24 Hahn RG. Fluid and electrolyte dynamics during development of the TURP syndrome. *Br J Urol* 1990; **66**: 79–84.

25 Ghanem AN, Ward JP. Osmotic and metabolic sequelae of volumetric overload in relation to the TURP syndrome. *Br J Urol* 1990; **66**: 71–6.

26 Schneider SP, Fytte RE. Involvement of GABA and glycine in recurrent inhibition of spinal motor neurons. *J Neurophysiol* 1992; **66**: 397–406.

27 Jensen V. The TURP syndrome. *Can J Anaesth* 1991; **38**: 90–7.

28 Silver SM, Kozlowski SA, Baer JE, *et al*. Glycine-induced hyponatremia in the rat: a model of post-prostatectomy syndrome. *Kidney Int* 1995; **47**: 262–8.

29 Agarwal R, Emmett M. The post-transurethral resection of prostate syndrome: therapeutic proposals. *Am J Kid Dis* 1994; **24**: 108–11.

30 Robinson AG. Disorders of antidiuretic hormone secretion. *Clin Endocrinol Metab* 1985; **14**: 55–88.

31 Bartter FC, Schwartz WB. The syndrome of inappropriate secretion of antidiuretic hormone. *Am J Med* 1967; **42**: 790–806.

32 Arieff AI. Central nervous system manifestations of disordered sodium metabolism. *Clin Endocrinol Metab* 1984; **13**: 269–94.

33 Arieff AI, Guisado R. Effects of the central nervous system of hypernatremic and hyponatremic states. *Kidney Int* 1976; **10**: 104–16.

34 Worthley LIG, Thomas PD. Treatment of hyponatraemic seizures with intravenous 29.2% saline. *BMJ* 1986; **292**: 168–70.

35 Sterns RH, Riggs JE, Schochet SS Jr. Osmotic demyelination syndrome following correction of hyponatraemia. *N Engl J Med* 1986; **314**: 1535–42.

36 Ayus JC, Krothapalli RK, Arieff AI. Changing concepts in treatment of severe symptomatic hyponatremia. Rapid correction and possible relation to central pontine myelinolysis. *Am J Med* 1985; **78**: 897–902.

37 Tien R, Arieff AI, Kucharczyk W, *et al*. Hyponatremic encephalopathy: is central pontine myelinolysis a component? *Am J Med* 1992; **92**: 513–22.

38 Ross EJ, Christie SBM. Hypernatremia. *Medicine* 1969; **48**: 441–72.

39 Worthley LIG. Hyperosmolar coma treated with intravenous sterile water. A study of three cases. *Arch Intern Med* 1986; **146**: 945–7.

40 Stockigt JR. Potassium metabolism. *Anaesth Intens Care* 1977; **5**: 317–25.

41 Tannen RL. Potassium disorders. In: Kokko JP, Tannen RL (eds). *Fluid and Electrolytes*. Philadelphia: WB Saunders Co; 1986: pp. 150–228.

42 Kliger AS, Hayslett JP. Disorders of potassium balance. In: Brenner BM, Stein JH (eds). *Acid-base and Potassium Homeostasis in Contemporary Issues in Nephrology*, vol 2. New York: Churchill-Livingstone; 1978: pp. 168–204.

43 Sterns RH, Cox M, Felig PU, *et al*. Internal potassium balance and the control of the plasma potassium concentration. *Medicine* 1981; **60**: 339–54.

44 Phelan DM, Worthley LIG. Hypokalaemic coma. *Intensive Care Med* 1985; **11**: 257–8.

45 Standards and guidelines for cardiopulmonary resuscitation (CPR) and emergency cardiac care (ECC). *JAMA* 1992; **268**: 2172–88.

46 Thomas DW. Calcium, phosphorus and magnesium turnover. *Anaesth Intens* Care 1977; **5**: 361–71.

47 Pak CYC. Calcium disorders: hypercalcemia and hypocalcemia. In: Kokko JP, Tannen RL (eds). *Fluid and Electrolytes*. Philadelphia: WB Saunders Co; 1986: pp. 472–501.

48 Cronin RE. Magnesium disorders. In: Kokko JP, Tannen RL (eds). *Fluid and Electrolytes*. Philadelphia: WB Saunders Co; 1986: pp. 502–12.

49 Lau K. Phosphate disorders. In: Kokko JP, Tannen RL (eds). *Fluid and Electrolytes*. Philadelphia: WB Saunders Co; 1986: pp. 398–471.

84

Metabolic response to illness, injury and infection

I K S Tan

Illness, injury and infection evoke a constellation of metabolic changes in the host. The magnitude of the response is proportional to the extent of injury. Additional components of illness, such as ischaemia and reperfusion, nutrition status, surgical procedures, drugs and anaesthetic techniques, genetic polymorphisms and concurrent diseases, impact on the response. Some components of the metabolic response, or the failure to regulate the response, are destructive, and its modulation may improve patient survival.

MEDIATORS OF THE METABOLIC RESPONSE

CYTOKINES (see Ch. 13)

Cytokines are soluble, non-antibody, regulatory proteins responsible primarily for the inflammatory response. Injury and infection result in the release of cytokines from activated leukocytes, endothelial cells and fibroblasts. Interactions occur between various cytokines, and between the cytokine network and the immune, endocrine, and nervous systems. Cytokines generally exert their effects in a paracrine fashion, but in severe injury and infection, they enter the circulation and act as hormones. The following are major cytokines involved in the response to stress:

- *Tumor necrosis factor-α* (TNF-α, cachectin) is a proximal mediator. After endotoxin challenge, TNF-α concentrations peak before other mediators. The administration of monoclonal antibodies against TNF-α attenuates the increase in other mediators. TNF-α administration reproduces all features of septic shock, including hypermetabolism, fever, anorexia, hyperglycemia, decreased lipogenesis, marked protein catabolism and lactic acidosis. TNF-α activates the hypothalamic–pituitary–adrenal (HPA) axis. Soluble TNF-α receptors, a natural antagonist to TNF-α, also increase;[1] this may be a regulatory response which contributes to later immunosuppression.

- *Interleukins* (IL): IL-1 (endogenous pyrogen) produces much the same metabolic effects as TNF, and the combined effect of the two cytokines is greater than the effect of either alone. IL-1 is a potent inducer of the HPA axis as well as central and peripheral noradrenergic neurons. IL-6 is the main mediator of the acute phase response. Similar to TNF and IL-1, IL-6 levels correlate with severity of illness and outcome. IL-8 induces neutrophil adhesion, chemotaxis and enzyme release. IL-2 generation is decreased. Anti-inflammatory cytokines (IL-4, IL-10) and antagonists (IL-1 receptor antagonist) levels increase.

- *Colony-stimulating factors* stimulate the proliferation of haemopoietic cells, superoxide and cytokine production by neutrophils and macrophages.

- *Interferon-γ* (IFN-γ): IFN-γ participates in acquired cell-mediated immunity and stimulates fibroproliferation, up-regulates TNF receptors and induces TNF synthesis. IFN-γ production is synergistically induced by IL-12 and IL-18.[2]

NEUROENDOCRINE MEDIATORS

Afferent neuronal impulses and cytokine release from the site of injury or infection activate the sympathetic nervous system and hypothalamic-pituitary hormone secretion (Fig. 84.1). Administration of epinephrine, cortisol and glucagon combinations reproduce partially the metabolic response to stress. Protein catabolism is not of the magnitude observed after injury, and there is no fever or induction of the acute phase response.[3] The following hormones are involved in the response to stress:

- *Catecholamine* levels are increased, causing tachycardia and calorigenesis with increased oxygen consumption. Blood flow redistribution occurs depending on tissue receptor balance. Glycogenolysis, gluconeogenesis and lipolysis are stimulated.

- *HPA axis* activation results in gluconeogenesis, proteolysis, and lipolysis. The anti-inflammatory and cell-protective effects of cortisol attenuate damage from

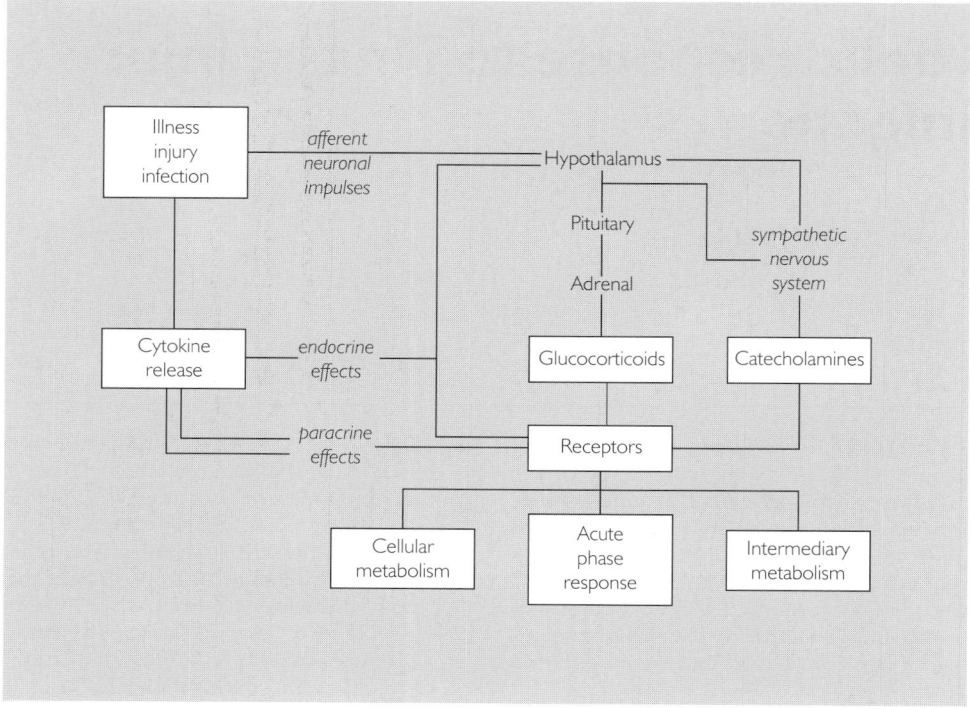

Fig. 84.1   Schema of the metabolic response to stress

excessive activation of the metabolic response.[4] A high cortisol and a poor response to a short corticotropin test is an independent predictor of death in septic shock.[5]

- *Insulin and glucagon* levels are increased but the insulin levels are inappropriately low for the level of hyperglycaemia. The increased glucagon:insulin ratio augments gluconeogenesis.
- *Growth hormone* (GH) levels increase transiently but somatomedin (insulin-like growth factor, IGF-1) activity is depressed.
- *Thyroid hormone* (T4) levels are usually low-normal. Low T3, high reverse T3 and normal TSH levels are typical of the 'sick euthyroid syndrome'.
- *Antidiuretic hormone, renin, angiotensin, aldosterone and prolactin* levels increase.

THE METABOLIC RESPONSE

The metabolic response to injury and infection begins with the activation of receptors throughout the body by the mediators discussed above. In general, a hypermetabolic-inflammatory response is produced, which is followed in time by a hypometabolic-immunosuppressive phase.[6] Many metabolic responses involve gene induction and regulation. In addition, catecholamines can initiate

rapid functional changes via protein phosphorylation, which does not require gene induction. Behavioural effects such as anorexia also affect the metabolic response. The metabolic effects may be described at three levels.

CELLULAR METABOLIC EVENTS

Heat Shock Proteins (HSPs) are synthesized in response to a variety of stress. Many HSPs are also expressed constitutively. HSPs act as 'chaperones', assisting in the assembly, disassembly, stabilization, and internal transport of other intracellular proteins. HSPs facilitate translocation of the glucocorticoid-receptor complex from the cytosol to the nucleus. HSPs have cellular protective roles in sepsis[7] and ischaemia-reperfusion.[8]

Mitochondrial abnormalities may limit cell metabolism.[9] The ketone body ratio (acetoacetate : beta-hydroxybutyrate ratio) reflects liver mitochondrial redox potential, and correlates inversely with the magnitude of stress and catabolic response.[10]

Leukocyte activation occurs systemically. Following directed adhesion to endothelium and migration into tissue, leukocytes undergo an oxidative burst, producing oxygen-derived free radicals, proteases, and arachidonic acid metabolites (leukotrienes, thromboxanes and prostaglandins).

Apoptosis, or programmed cell death,[11] may finally be induced when death receptors are engaged by their ligands. Death receptors are members of the TNF-α receptor gene superfamily.[12] TNF-α, IL-10, cortisol and nitric oxide have all been reported to induce apoptosis. Subsequent activation of caspases (cysteine containing proteases) commit the cell to death.

INTERMEDIARY METABOLISM

Protein metabolism: IL-1, TNF, related cytokines and hormonal changes trigger an extreme protein catabolism, which has been termed 'autocannibalism'.[13] Glutamine, alanine and other amino acids are mobilized from skeletal muscle and taken up by hepatocytes and gut mucosa. Glutamine depletion may occur. Increased ureagenesis and nitrogen loss occurs. Levels of branch-chained amino-acids (leucine, isoleucine, valine) fall with peripheral oxidation. The fraction of energy expenditure derived from glucose is reduced, while that derived from amino acid oxidation in the Krebs cycle is increased.[14]

Carbohydrate metabolism: hyperglycaemia results from glycogenolysis, accelerated gluconeogenesis and peripheral insulin resistance. Lactate production increases from peripheral tissue, areas of injury and the white cell mass, and serves as substrate for gluconeogenesis in hepatocytes. In the terminal phase of severe illness, hypoglycaemia may occur.

Fat metabolism: lipolysis is increased with increased turnover of triglycerides and fatty acids. TNF, IL-1 and IL-6 decrease lipoprotein lipase activity, contributing to hypertriglyceridaemia. Ketosis is suppressed, indicating that fat is not a major calorie source. Glycerol generated from lipolysis further contributes to gluconeogenesis. The action of cyclooxygenase and lipoxygenase on arachidonic acid (a tissue phopholipid) produces inflammatory leukotrienes, thromboxanes and prostaglandin E_2.

Electrolyte and micronutrient metabolism: salt and water retention occurs, with hyponatremia. Protein loss is accompanied by potassium, magnesium, and phosphate loss. Zn redistributes to liver and bone marrow. Zn deficiency is associated with impaired IL-2 production and wound healing.[15] Fe levels decrease.

SYSTEMIC PROTEIN SYSTEM RESPONSES

The acute phase response is a systemic response to injury characterized by redirection of hepatic protein synthesis and haematological alterations. Production of proteins involved in defence is increased (protease inhibitors, fibrinogen, C-reactive protein, haptoglobulin, complement C3), while synthesis of serum transport and binding molecules is reduced (albumin, transferrin). Serum levels of acute phase reactants such as C-reactive protein can be used for diagnostic, monitoring and prognostic purposes.

Complement cascade triggering produces chemo-attractants (C3a, C5a), vasoactive anaphylatoxins (C3a, C4a, C5a), opsonins (C3b), stimulation of neutrophil and monocyte oxidative burst (C3b) and neutrophil adherence to endothelium (C5a).

FACTORS AFFECTING THE METABOLIC RESPONSE

ENERGY BALANCE AND OXYGEN DELIVERY

Hypermetabolism increases oxygen demand and consumption. Inadequate oxygen delivery can lead to anaerobic metabolism and inadequate production of high energy phosphates. However, direct monitoring of intracellular pH and high energy phosphate concentration during sepsis in a number of organs do not show a fall indicative of hypoxia.[16] Inadequate oxygen delivery may be present in gut mucosa.[17] Multiple factors contribute to raised lactate levels. Aerobic glycolysis rather than anaerobic glycolysis is characteristic of the metabolic response to stress.[16]

SURGICAL PROCEDURES AND ANAESTHETIC TECHNIQUES

Total afferent neuronal blockade (somatic and autonomic block) (e.g. by epidural anaesthesia) attenuates the metabolic changes of surgical injury. Thoracic epidural blockade in addition to general anaesthesia in cardiac surgery was associated with reduced myocardial damage.[18] Minimally invasive procedures are associated with reduced cytokine release. This has translated to reduced morbidity and hospital stays.[19]

STARVATION AND NUTRITION

Starvation alone produces adaptive hypometabolism with the use of fat as the primary fuel, sparing protein. In contrast, injury and infection result in hypermetabolism with prominent protein catabolism. Starvation in combination with the metabolic changes of stress produces a hypoalbuminaemic malnourished state, not unlike 'kwashiorkor'. Malnutrition clearly contributes to morbidity and mortality. However, current forms of nutrition do not adequately reduce protein catabolism or promote protein synthesis, but result in fat and fluid gain instead.[20]

DRUGS AND DISEASE

Adverse effects of steroids include increased infection rates and myopathy (particularly in conjunction with the use of neuromuscular blocking drugs).[21] Commonly used intensive care unit (ICU) drugs such as the catecholamines, theophylline, calcium-channel blockers and antibiotics all have immunomodulatory effects. Diseases, such as diabetes, will clearly impact on the metabolic response to stress. Apart from concurrent disease, the inciting organism may itself modulate its host response by affecting cytokine mediators, their production, secretion, and elimination, or by interacting with their receptors.[22]

GENETIC POLYMORPHISMS

The mediators of the metabolic response, and their effector pathways, are under genetic control. Genetic polymorphisms in IL-1,[23] TNF-α[24] and HSPs,[25] for example, may contribute to the response to and outcome from sepsis.

SECONDARY INSULTS

Secondary insults, such as catheter-related sepsis, the use of bio-incompatible membranes for renal support, mechanical ventilator-induced lung injury, pain and hypothermia, will increase the severity and duration of the metabolic response.

VALUE OF THE METABOLIC RESPONSE

The cytokines and neuroendocrine mediators reprioritize metabolic processes, increasing the supply of substrates to active tissues involved in defense against injury. Inflammation localizes the area of injury. Cardiovascular changes divert blood flow to inflamed areas and vital organs, while salt and water retention maintains overall perfusion. Sympathectomized and adrenalectomized animals fare poorly when stressed. Etomidate, which blocks cortisol synthesis, was associated with increased mortality when used for ICU sedation.[26]

Disadvantages of the metabolic response include increased oxygen consumption and myocardial work, which is detrimental to patients with marginal cardiovascular reserves.[25] The redistribution of blood flow away from the 'non-vital' gut organ may result in translocation of bacteria and endotoxin into the circulation.[17] High catecholamine levels are arrythmogenic to the compromised heart. Systemic inflammation can result in systemic tissue destruction. Hyperglycaemia is associated with an increased incidence of infection.[30]

MODULATING THE METABOLIC RESPONSE

Modulation of the metabolic response in order to accelerate recovery, and improve morbidity and mortality is

an expanding area of research. Large multicentre trials have failed to show consistent benefits with therapies targeted at specific cytokine components of the metabolic response to infection (see Ch. 60). This has led to the development of therapies providing non-specific suppression or elimination of circulating mediators, or monitoring the state of 'immunologic dissonance',[29] in order to provide individualized therapy.

Protein catabolism leading to loss of muscle has functional consequences such as respiratory muscle weakness. A 25% body weight loss in the presence of injury may be fatal.[28] Wound healing and multiple facets of host defense are impaired, increasing the risk of nosocomial infection. Substrate nutrients may favorably influence the metabolic response to stress. A meta-analysis[31] provides some evidence that specialized nutrition including immunonutrition can reduce the hospital length of stay. Even with optimal nutrition, hypercatabolism continues. Of the anabolic agents (GH, IGF-1 and testosterone derivatives), GH has received the most attention in the setting of critical illness. Despite initial promise with GH use in severely burned children,[32] GH increased mortality in a heterogenous group of critically ill patients.[33] It is probable that patient selection, concurrent nutritional status, and dosing patterns are important in determining outcome.

In keeping with the suggestion that hyperglycaemia increases infection, a study[34] utilizing 'Intensive Insulin Therapy' to attain a glucose of 4.4–6.1 mmol resulted in a significant reduction in mortality of 4.6% compared to 8%. There was a reduction in bloodstream infections, days of mechanical ventilation, hyperbilirubinaemia, and critical illness polyneuropathy, in the population of primarily post-cardiac surgical patients.

A meta-analysis of steroid usage in septic shock which included the large trials that used high-dose steroids given over a short time concluded that steroids were not efficacious.[35] Conversely, lower doses of hydrocortisone for at least 5 days in patients with late septic shock resulted in a significant improvement in haemodynamics and survival.[36] This is supported by another study finding that hydrocortisone infusion reduced the time to cessation of vasopressor therapy, with a non-significant trend to earlier resolution of sepsis-induced organ dysfunction.[37]

Given that the extracellular fluid is the aqueous medium within which the mediators of the metabolic response function, blood purification may modulate the intensity of the metabolic response and hence influence outcome. A randomized trial of 425 ICU patients with acute renal failure to ultrafiltration doses of 20 ml/h per kg, 35 ml/h per kg and 45 ml/h per kg by continuous veno-venous haemofiltration resulted in survival at 15 days after treatment discontinuation of 41%, 57% and 58% respectively.[38] Extension of the above approach leads to the inference that high volume haemofiltration (i.e. intensive plasma water exchange) may further improve survival.[39] Other approaches to improving the clearance of larger solutes are the use of a large pore filter,[40] and the use of modes such as coupled plasma-filtration absorption[41] and albumin dialysis.[42]

In contrast to non-specific modulation of the metabolic response, the other approach is to monitor the host response so as to provide individualized therapy. Although IFN-γ did not reduce infection or mortality in burns patients,[43] it is hypothesized that monitoring HLA-DR expression may be used to identify immunosupressed patients who may benefit most from IFN-γ.[44]

REFERENCES

1 Goldie AS, Fearon KCH, Ross JA, et al., for the Sepsis Intervention Group. Natural cytokine antagonists and endogenous antiendotoxin core antibodies in sepsis syndrome. *JAMA* 1995; **274**: 172–77.

2 Lauw FN, Simpson AJH, Prins JM, et al. Elevated plasma concentrations of interferon-γ (IFN-γ) and the IFN-γ inducing cytokines interleukin-18 (IL-18), IL-12, and IL-15 in severe melioidosis. *J Infect Dis* 1999; **180**: 1878–85.

3 Gelfand RA, Matthews DE, Bier DM, Sherwin RS. Role of counterregulatory hormones in the catabolic response to stress. *J Clin Invest* 1984; **74**: 2238–48.

4 Munck A, Naray-Fejes-Toth A. The ups and downs of glucocorticoid physiology. Permissive and suppressive effects revisited. *Mol Cell Endocrinol* 1992; **90**: C1–4.

5 Annane D, Sebille V, Troche G, et al. A 3-level prognostic classification in septic shock based on cortisol levels and cortisol response to corticotropin. *JAMA* 2000; **283**: 1038–45.

6 Bone RC. Sir Isaac Newton, SIRS, and CARS. *Crit Care Med* 1996; **24**: 1125–8.

7 Villar J, Ribeiro SP, Mullen JBM, et al. Induction of the heat shock response reduces mortality rate and organ damage in a sepsis-induced acute lung injury model. *Crit Care Med* 1994; **22**: 914–21.

8 Mestril R, Chi SH, Sayen MR, et al. Expression of inducible stress protein 70 in rat heart myogenic cells confers protection against simulated ischemia-induced injury. *J Clin Invest* 1994; **93**: 759–67.

9 Dong Y, Sheng C, Herndon D, Waymack JP. Metabolic abnormalities of mitochondrial redox potential in post burn multiple system organ failure. *Burns* 1992; **18**: 283–6.

10 Kiuchi T, Shimahara Y, Wakashiro S, et al. Reduced arterial ketone body ratio during laparotomy: an evaluation of operative stress through the changes in hepatic mitochondrial redox potential. *J Lab Clin Med* 1990; **115**: 433–40.

11 Hotchkiss RS, Swanson PE, Freeman BD, et al. Apoptotic cell death in patients with sepsis, shock and multiple organ dysfunction. *Crit Care Med* 1999; **27**: 1230–51.

12 Ashkenazi A, Dixit VM. Death receptors: signalling and modulation. *Science* 1998; **281**: 1305–8.

13 Beal AL, Cerra FB. Multiple organ failure syndrome in the 1990s; systemic inflammatory response and organ dysfunction. *JAMA* 1994; **271**: 226–33.

14 Cerra FB. Metabolic manifestations of multiple systems organ failure. *Crit Care Clin* 1989; **5**: 119–31.

15 Okada A, Takagi Y, Nezu R, Lee S. Zinc in clinical surgery – a research review. *Jpn J Surg* 1990; **20**: 635–44.

16 Hotchkiss RS, Karl IE. Reevaluation of the role of cellular hypoxia and bioenergetic failure in sepsis. *JAMA* 1992; **267**: 1503–10.

17 Mythen MG, Webb AR. The role of gut mucosal hypoperfusion in the pathogenesis of post-operative organ dysfunction. *Intensive Care Med* 1994; **20**: 203–9.

18 Loick HM, Schmidt C, van Aken H, et al. High thoracic epidural anaesthesia, but not clonidine, attenuates the perioperative stress response via sympatholysis and reduces the release of troponin T in patients undergoing coronary artery bypass grafting. *Anesth Analg* 1999; **88**: 701–9.

19 Joris J, Cigarini I, Legrand M, et al. Metabolic and respiratory changes after cholecystectomy performed via laparotomy or laparoscopy. *Br J Anaesth* 1992; **69**: 341–5.

20 Streat SJ, Beddoe AH, Hill GL. Aggressive nutritional support dose not prevent protein loss despite fat gain in septic intensive care patients. *J Trauma* 1987; **27**: 262–66.

21 Zochodne DW, Ramsay DA, Saly V, et al. Acute necrotizing myopathy of intensive care: electrophysiological studies. *Muscle-Nerve* 1994; **17**: 285–92.

22 Wilson M, Seymour R, Henderson B. Bacterial perturbation of cytokine networks. *Infect Immunol* 1998; **66**: 2401–9.

23 Fang XM, Schroder S, Hoeft A, Stuber F. Comparison of two polymorphisms of the Interleukin-1 family: interleukin-1 receptor antagonist polymorphism contributes to susceptibility to severe sepsis. *Crit Care Med* 1999; **27**: 1330–34.

24 Mira JP, Cariou A, Grall F, et al. Association of TNF2, a TNF-α promoter polymorphism, with septic shock susceptibility and mortality. A multicenter study. *JAMA* 1999; **282**: 561–68.

25 Schroder S, Reck M, Hoeft A, Stuber F. Analysis of two human leucocyte antigen-linked polymorphic heat shock protein 70 genes in patients with severe sepsis. *Crit Care Med* 1999; **27**: 1265–70.

26 Ledingham IMA, Watt I. Influence of sedation on mortality in critically ill patients. *Lancet* 1983; **1**: 1270.

27 Breslow MJ. The role of stress hormones in perioperative myocardial ischemia. *Int Anesthesiol Clin* 1992; **30**: 81–100.

28 Apovian CM, McMahon MM, Bistrian BR. Guidelines for refeeding the marasmic patient. *Crit Care Med* 1990; **18**: 1030–33.

29 Bone RC. Immunologic dissonance: a continuing evolution in our understanding of the systemic inflammatory response syndrome (SIRS) and the multiple organ dysfunction syndrome (MODS). *Ann Intern Med* 1996; **125**: 680–87.

30 Rady MY, Ryan T, Starr NJ. Perioperative determinants of morbidity and mortality in elderly patients undergoing cardiac surgery. *Crit Care Med* 1998; **26**: 225–35.

31 Heys SD, Walker LG, Smith I, Eremin O. Enteral nutritional supplementation with key nutrients in patients with critical illness and cancer. A meta-analysis of randomized controlled clinical trials. *Ann Surg* 1999; **229**: 467–77.

32 Herndon DN, Barrow RE, Kunkel KR. Effects of recombinant human growth hormone on donor-site healing in severely burned children. *Ann Surg* 1990; **210**: 513–24.

33 Takala J, Ruokonen E, Webster N, *et al.* Increased mortality associated with growth hormone treatment in critically ill adults. *N Engl J Med* 1999; **341**: 785–92.

34 Van den Berghe G, Wouters P, Weekers F, *et al.* Intensive insulin therapy in the surgical intensive care unit. *N Engl J Med* 2001; **345**: 1359–67.

35 Cronin L, Cook DJ, Carlet J, *et al.* Corticosteroids for sepsis: a critical appraisal and meta-analysis of the literature. *Crit Care Med* 1995; **23**: 1430–9.

36 Bollaert P, Charpentier C, Levy B, *et al.* Reversal of late septic shock with supraphysiologic doses of hydrocortisone. *Crit Care Med* 1998; **26**: 645–50.

37 Briegel J, Forst H, Haller M, *et al.* Stress doses of hydrocortisone reverse hyperdynamic septic shock: a prospective, randomized, double-blind, single-center study. *Crit Care Med* 1999; **27**: 723–32.

38 Ronco C, Bellomo R, Homel P, *et al.* Effects of different doses in continuous veno-venous haemo-filtration on outcomes of acute renal failure: a prospective randomised trial. *Lancet* 2000; **355**: 26–30.

39 Honore PM, Jamez J, Wauthier M, *et al.* Prospective evaluation of short-term high-volume isovolemic hemofiltration on the hemodynamic course and outcome in patients with intractable circulatory failure resulting from septic shock. *Crit Care Med* 2000; **28**: 3581–7.

40 Lee PA, Weger GW, Pryor RW, *et al.* Effects of filter pore size on efficacy of continuous arteriovenous hemofiltration therapy for *Staphylococcus aureus*-induced septicemia in immature swine. *Crit Care Med* 1998; **26**: 730–7.

41 Tetta C, Cavaillon JM, Schulze M, *et al.* Removal of cytokines and activated complement components in an experimental model of continuous plasma filtration coupled with sorbent adsorption. *Nephrol Dial Transplant* 1998; **13**: 1458–64.

42 Stange J, Mitzner SR, Risler T, *et al.* Molecular Adsorption Recycling System (MARS): clinical results of a new membrane-based blood purification system for bioartificial liver support. *Artif Organs* 1999; **23**: 319–30.

43 Wasserman D, Ioannovich JD, Hinzmann RD, *et al.* Interferon-gamma in the prevention of severe burns-related infections: a European phase III clinical trial. *Crit Care Med* 1998; **26**: 434–9.

44 Kox WJ, Bone RC, Krausch D, *et al.* Interferon gamma-1β in the treatment of compensatory anti-inflammatory response syndrome. *Arch Intern Med* 1997; **157**: 389–93.

85

Enteral and parenteral nutrition

R Leonard

It is standard practice to provide nutritional support to critically ill patients in order to:

- treat existing malnutrition
- minimize wasting of lean body mass.

However, while a good case can be made that early feeding is better than late,[1-3] there is no direct evidence that any nutritional support is better than none. The rationale for nutritional support rests on the close association between malnutrition, negative nitrogen and calorie balance and poor outcome, and the inevitability of death if starvation continues for long enough. In otherwise healthy humans, this takes several weeks to occur.

It is uncertain how long hypercatabolic, critically ill patients can safely be left without nutrition. After abdominal trauma, 5 days without feeding does not increase mortality.[1] Recommendations from a conference sponsored by the US National Institutes of Health, the American Society for Parenteral and Enteral Nutrition and the American Society for Clinical Nutrition suggest that nutritional support be started in any critically ill patient unlikely to regain oral intake within 7 to 10 days.[4] The basis for this is that at a typical nitrogen loss of 20–40 g/d, dangerous depletion of lean tissue may occur after 14 days of starvation. Other clinicians use a maximum acceptable delay of 7 days.[5] This view is supported by the excess mortality observed in head-injured patients during 2 weeks of severe under-feeding.[6] Earlier support is necessary if the patient is malnourished or has already suffered a period of inadequate intake before admission to the ICU.

NUTRITIONAL ASSESSMENT

Objective assessment of nutritional status is difficult in ICU, because disease processes confound methods used in the general population. Anthropometric measures, such as triceps skin-fold thickness and mid-arm circumference may be obscured by oedema. Voluntary handgrip strength, a test of functional capacity, is impractical in unconscious patients. Laboratory measures, including transferrin, pre-albumin and albumin levels, lymphocyte counts and skin-prick test reactivity, are abnormal in critical illness. Clinical evaluation is better than objective measurement at predicting morbidity.[7] Historical features of malnutrition include weight loss, poor diet, gastrointestinal symptoms, reduced functional capacity and a diagnosis associated with poor intake. Physical signs include loss of subcutaneous fat, muscle wasting, peripheral oedema and ascites.

NUTRITIONAL REQUIREMENTS OF THE CRITICALLY ILL

Some muscle wasting and nitrogen loss are unavoidable in critical illness, despite adequate energy and protein provision.[8] Coupled with the realization that caloric requirements had previously been over-estimated, this fact has led to downward revision of intake. The aim is now to provide sufficient energy and nitrogen but to avoid the problems caused by over-feeding, which include[9]:

- uraemia (due to excess nitrogen intake)
- hypertonic dehydration (in patients fed excess nitrogen who have impaired urine concentrating ability)
- hepatic steatosis
- hypercarbic respiratory failure (due to excess CO_2 production)
- hyperglycaemia (with attendant infection risk)
- hyperosmolar non-ketotic coma
- hyperlipidaemia

ENERGY

Energy expenditure can be assessed in ICU by three methods:

- indirect calorimetry
- the Fick principle (in patients with a pulmonary artery catheter *in situ*)
- predictive equations.

Indirect calorimetry is the gold standard, and its use is increasing with the availability of devices designed for

ICU patients. It permits measurement of the resting energy expenditure (REE). This value excludes the energy cost of physical activity, which increases later in the course of an ICU admission.[10] The Fick method has shown variable correlation with indirect calorimetry, and one recent report suggested that some predictive equations may be superior.[11] Calorimetry also reveals deviations from values predicted by equations, such that two-thirds of patients in one study were being either under- or over-fed.[12] On the other hand, it could not be shown that outcomes are improved by the use of calorimetry.[13] Moreover, there are no clear data to relate measured REE to total energy expenditure in the individual patient. As a result, many units do not use calorimetry; in those that do, a target energy provision of 1.3 × measured REE is usual.[14]

There are a large number of equations claiming to predict basal metabolic rate (BMR) on the basis of weight, sex and age. The best known is the Harris-Benedict equation, which dates back more than 80 years. Schofield's equations were derived anew in the 1980s.[15] Correction factors exist to convert predictions of BMR into estimated energy expenditure by adjusting for such variables as diagnosis, pyrexia and activity. In the past, these correction factors have been excessive and may have contributed to over-feeding; a more conservative approach is now advocated. The recommendations of the British Association for Parenteral and Enteral Nutrition are[16]:

1 Determine BMR from Schofield equations (Table 85.1)
2 Adjust BMR for stress (Table 85.2)
3 Add a combined factor for activity and diet-induced thermogenesis

Table 85.1   Basal metabolic rate in kcal/day by age and gender.[15]

Age (years)	Female	Male
15–18	13.3 W + 690	17.6 W + 656
18–30	14.8 W + 485	15.0 W + 690
30–60	8.1 W + 842	11.4 W + 870
>60	9.0 W + 656	11.7 W + 585

W, weight in kg.

Table 85.2   Stress adjustment in the calculation of basal metabolic rate.[16]

Partial starvation (>10% weight loss)	subtract 0–15%
Mild infection, inflammatory bowel disease, post-operative	add 0–13%
Moderate infection, multiple long bone fractures	add 10–30%
Severe sepsis, multiple trauma (ventilated)	add 25–50%
Burns 10–90%	add 10–70%

bed-bound, immobile	+10%
bed-bound, mobile/sitting	+20%
mobile around ward	+25%

Despite the popularity of measurements or estimations of energy expenditure, it is not clear that their routine use improves outcome. Many clinicians dispense with both and simply aim to deliver 25–35 kcal/kg per day.

PROTEIN

Assessment of nitrogen balance by measuring urinary urea nitrogen has been shown to be too variable to be useful in estimating protein requirements in ICU.[17] As there is an upper limit to the amount of dietary protein that can be used for synthesis,[18] there is no benefit from replacing nitrogen lost in excess of this. A daily nitrogen provision of 0.15–0.2 g/kg/per day is therefore recommended for the ICU population; this is equivalent to 1–1.25 g protein/kg per day. Severely hypercatabolic individuals, such as those with major burns, are given up to 0.3 g nitrogen/kg per day, or nearly 2 g protein/kg per day.[16]

MICRONUTRIENTS

Critical illness increases the requirements for vitamins A, E, K, thiamine (B$_1$), B$_3$, B$_6$, vitamin C, and pantothenic and folic acids see (Tables 85.3 and 85.4).[19] Thiamine, folic acid and vitamin K are particularly vulnerable to deficiency during total parenteral nutrition (TPN). Renal

Table 85.3   Daily vitamin requirements in critical illness.[19]

Vitamin	Function	Dose
Vitamin A	Cell growth, night vision	10 000–25 000 IU
Vitamin D	Calcium metabolism	400–1000 IU
Vitamin E	Membrane antioxidant	400–1000 IU
β-carotene*	Antioxidant	50 mg
Vitamin K	Activation of clotting factors	1.5 mcg/kg per d
Thiamine (vitamin B$_1$)	Oxidative decarboxylation	10 mg
Riboflavin (vitamin B$_2$)	Oxidative phosphorylation	10 mg
Niacin (vitamin B$_3$)	Part of NAD, redox reactions	200 mg
Pantothenic acid	Part of coenzyme A	100 mg
Biotin	Carboxylase activity	5 mg
Pyridoxine (vitamin B$_6$)	Decarboxylase activity	20 mg
Folic acid	Haematopoiesis	2 mg
Vitamin B$_{12}$	Haematopoiesis	20 mcg
Vitamin C	Antioxidant, collagen synthesis	2000 mg

*Not strictly a vitamin.

Table 85.4   Daily trace element requirements in critical illness.[19]

Element	Function	Dose
Selenium	Anti-oxidant, fat metabolism	100 mg
Zinc	Energy metabolism, protein synthesis, epithelial growth	50 mg
Copper	Collagen cross-linking, ceruloplasmin	2–3 mg
Manganese	Neural function, fatty acid synthesis	25–50 mg
Chromium	Insulin activity	200 mg
Cobalt	B_{12} synthesis	
Iodine	Thyroid hormones	
Iron	Haematopoiesis, oxidative phosphorylation	10 mg
Molybdenum	Purine and pyridine metabolism	0.2–0.5 mg

Table 85.5   Basal water and electrolyte requirements/ kg per day.

Water	30 ml
Sodium	1–2 mmol
Potassium	0.7–1 mmol
Magnesium	0.1 mmol
Calcium	0.1 mmol
Phosphorus	0.4 mmol

replacement therapy can cause loss of water-soluble vitamins. Deficiencies of selenium, zinc, manganese and copper have been described in critical illness, in addition to the more familiar iron deficient state.

WATER AND ELECTROLYTES

Water and electrolyte requirements vary widely depending on the patient's condition; typical basal intakes are shown in Table 85.5.

ROUTE OF NUTRITION

Whenever possible, patients should be fed enterally. The advantages over the parenteral route are:

- lower cost
- possibly fewer infective complications.

However, the data supporting this strong recommendation for enteral feeding are less robust than many believe. Reduction in septic morbidity has only been found in certain groups, primarily abdominal trauma victims,[20,21] in whom parenteral nutrition was associated with a higher incidence of abdominal abscess and pneumonia. A third study found no difference.[22] In head-injured patients, there is one trial showing no effect and

one supporting each of the two routes. However, in the study favouring TPN the enteral nutrition group were grossly under-fed.[2,6,23] Reductions in septic complications and mortality have also been found using transpyloric feeding in pancreatitis.[24,25] In contrast, no benefit was found in sepsis, though enteral feeding was instituted late.[26] A recent review of 31 clinical trials comparing enteral with parenteral feeding found no consistent difference.[27]

Two hypotheses are advanced to support the superiority of enteral feeding. First, it is possible that TPN is immunosuppressive. In the US Veterans' Affairs Co-operative Study of peri-operative TPN, there was an excess of infective complications in those patients receiving TPN who were not severely malnourished.[28] Intravenous lipid is known to impair neutrophil and reticulo-endothelial system function. Consistent with this, a recent study comparing TPN with and without lipid in critically ill trauma patients showed a lower complication rate in those not receiving lipid.[29] More simply, hyperglycaemia due to the past tendency to over-feed parenterally may have predisposed to infection.

Second, enteral feeding may protect against infective complications. In health, the gut mucosa forms a barrier against bacteria and their toxic products. This barrier is both functional and structural, maintained by mucin, secretory IgA and intact intercellular junctions in the villi. Absence of complex nutrients from the intestinal lumen is followed in rats by villus atrophy and reduced cell mass of the gut-associated lymphoid tissue (GALT). Starved humans show these changes to a much lesser extent. Lymphocytes produced in the GALT are redistributed to the respiratory tract, and contribute heavily to mucosal immunity. In mice, this contribution is lost during TPN.

The possibility that multiple organ failure may be driven by translocation of bacteria or endotoxin across an impaired mucosal barrier has been extensively investigated in animals. While it is known that TPN is associated with increased gut permeability to macromolecules in humans,[30] this does not seem to result in translocation.[31] Although translocation does occur following surgery, and seems to be associated with sepsis,[32] a causal relation with multiple organ failure is unproven.

Enteral feeding is often associated with serious under-provision of nutrients, which may worsen outcome.[3,6] Use of protocols improves delivery.[33] Even so, some patients will plainly be unable to feed enterally, and TPN is indicated without delay. In others, there is significant clinical doubt about the practicability of feeding via the gut. This latter group is at risk of being seriously under-fed while enteral nutrition fails to be established. They are therefore exposed to the often under-estimated risks of enteral nutrition without receiving its benefits, and pose a difficult problem in clinical decision making.

A recent study randomized patients whose ability to tolerate enteral feeding within 7 days was in serious doubt to either TPN or a trial of enteral nutrition.[5] There was no reduction in septic morbidity with enteral nutrition and a higher incidence of inadequate intake and feed-related complications. The authors suggested that patients such as their study group should receive TPN early until enteral nutrition can be established. They are supported by an increasing view that the apparent excess in complications with TPN has related in the past to over-feeding TPN and under-reporting the complications of enteral access and feeding.[27] Supplementing inadequate enteral intake with TPN also seems not to increase complications, though equally no improvement in outcome has been shown.[34] The point at which one resorts to parenteral nutrition in the individual patient is a matter of clinical judgement.

ENTERAL NUTRITION

ACCESS

Nasal tubes are preferred to oral, except in patients with a basal skull fracture, in whom there is a risk of cranial penetration. A large-bore (12–14 Fr) nasogastric tube is usually used at first. Once feeding is established and gastric residual volumes no longer need to be checked, this can be replaced with a more comfortable fine-bore tube. A stylet is needed to assist in the passage of fine-bore tubes; the position must be checked on X-ray before feeding is started, as misplacement is not uncommon. Nasojejunal tubes are useful if impaired gastric emptying is refractory to prokinetic agents (see below) or in pancreatitis; they do not reduce the risk of aspiration.[35] Spontaneous passage through the pylorus is rare, but may be increased by the administration of erythromycin. However, endoscopic or fluoroscopic assistance is needed for truly reliable transpyloric tube placement.

An alternative method of access in those needing long-term enteral feeding is percutaneous gastrostomy, which is usually performed endoscopically. Percutaneous jejunal access can be obtained either via a gastrostomy or by direct placement during incidental laparotomy.

REGIMEN

Slowly increasing the rate of feeding is not proven to avoid diarrhoea or high gastric residual volumes. Head-injured patients fed from the outset with their full nutritional needs have fewer infective complications.[3] Nonetheless, standard practice is currently to start by delivering 30 ml/h and to build up to the target intake depending on tolerance, as judged by gastric residual volumes. These are assessed by aspiration of the tube every 4 h; volumes of more than 400 ml are feared to increase the risk of pulmonary aspiration, though there is no firm evidence of this. If the residual volume is consistently greater than 200–300 ml, treatment with proki-

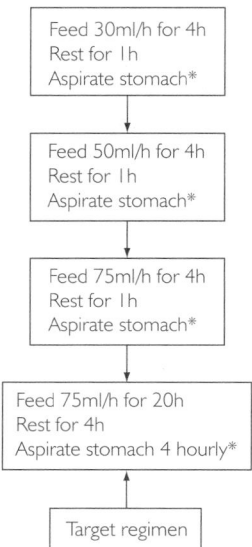

Fig. 85.1 Nasogastric feeding starter regimen (provided with the kind permission of Kumud Patel, Senior Dietitian, St Mary's Hospital, London.

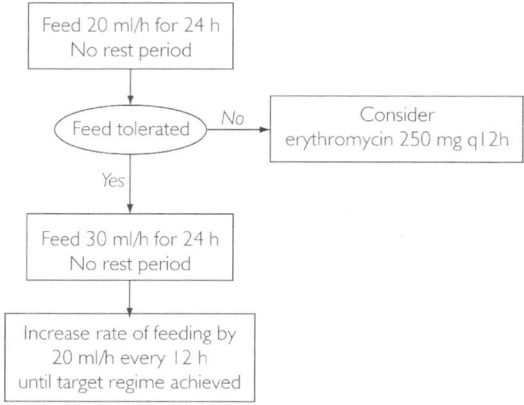

Fig. 85.2 Nasojejunal feeding (provided with the kind permission of Kumud Patel, Senior Dietitian, St Mary's Hospital, London.)

netic agents (intravenous metoclopramide 10 mg q.8 h or erythromycin 250 mg q.12 h) may be helpful. In refractory cases a nasojejunal tube often permits successful enteral nutrition, because small bowel function is resumed more quickly than gastric emptying. A nasogastric tube is still needed to drain the stomach. Diarrhoea, abdominal distension, nausea and vomiting may suggest intolerance despite low gastric volumes. Absence of bowel sounds is common in ventilated patients, and should not be taken to indicate ileus.

Fine-bore tubes should not be aspirated, as this causes them to block. Various folk remedies have been tried for unblocking tubes, including instillation of Coca-Cola™, fruit juice and pancreatic enzyme supplements. The instillates should be left *in situ* for an hour or more.

The importance of the pattern of feeding is unclear. Continuous feeding is more convenient and popular, though regimens which divide the daily intake into 4-hourly boluses, have been tried without obvious benefit. This approach may increase the risk of aspiration. Provision of a 4 or 6 h 'rest period' each day permits re-acidification of the stomach and minimizes bacterial overgrowth, possibly reducing nosocomial pneumonia.[36]

COMPOSITION

Commercially available enteral feeding solutions vary widely in composition. Polymeric feeds contain intact proteins (derived from whey, meat, soy isolates and caseinates), and carbohydrates in the form of oligo- and polysaccharides. Such formulae require pancreatic enzymes for absorption.

Elemental feeds with defined nitrogen sources (amino acids or peptides) are not of benefit when used routinely, but may enable feeding when small bowel absorption is impaired, for instance in pancreatic insufficiency or after prolonged starvation. Lipids are usually provided by vegetable oils consisting mostly of long-chain triglycerides, but some also contain more easily absorbed medium-chain triglycerides. The proportion of non-protein calories provided as carbohydrate is usually two-thirds.

Fibre reduces the incidence of diarrhoea. It is metabolized by bacteria to short chain fatty acids, which are used by colonocytes to drive water and electrolyte uptake.[37]

Vitamins and trace elements are added so that daily requirements are present in a volume containing roughly 2000 kcal. Electrolyte composition varies widely, with sodium- and potassium-restricted formulations available.

COMPLICATIONS

Enteral feeding is an independent risk factor for ventilator-associated pneumonia.[38] Contrary to popular belief, transpyloric feeding does not alter this.[35] Sinusitis due to nasogastric intubation may necessitate changing to an oro-gastric tube. Fine-bore tubes are vulnerable to misplacement in the trachea (see Chapter 32, Figure 6a) and may cause perforation of the pharynx, oesophagus, stomach or bowel. Percutaneous endoscopic gastrostomy is associated with a high 30-day all-cause mortality in acutely ill patients,[39] in whom it may be best avoided. Other complications include insertion-site infection, serious abdominal wall infection and peritonitis. Surgically-placed jejunostomies can cause similar problems, and may also obstruct the bowel.

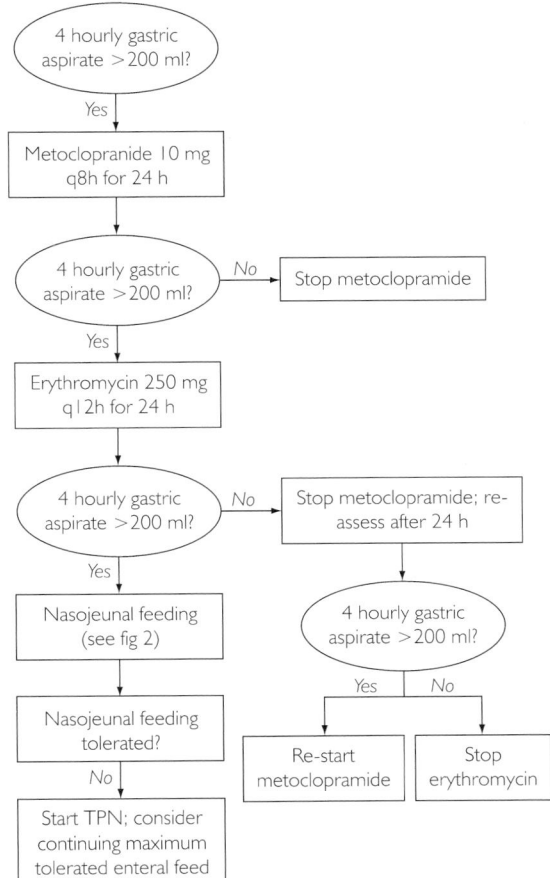

Fig. 85.3 Difficult enteral feeding algorithm (provided with the kind permission of Kumud Patel, Senior Dietitian, St Mary's Hospital, London.)

Diarrhoea is common in ICU patients, particularly those being fed enterally. It is often multi-factorial and causes considerable distress and morbidity, particularly when the patient is repeatedly soiled with watery stool. Common causes include antibiotic therapy, *Clostridium difficile* infection, faecal impaction and a non-specific effect of critical illness. Malabsorption, lactose intolerance, prokinetic agents, magnesium and medications containing large amounts of sorbitol (primarily paracetamol syrup) are occasional culprits. The composition and rate of administration of enteral feed also play a role. Fibre-containing feeds reduce the incidence of diarrhoea,[37] while malabsorption may respond to an elemental diet. Slowing the rate of feeding sometimes helps; diluting the formula does not.

Metabolic complications include electrolyte abnormalities and hyperglycaemia. Severely malnourished patients are at risk of refeeding syndrome (see below) if nutritional support is begun too rapidly.

PARENTERAL NUTRITION

Parenteral nutritional support is indicated when adequate enteral intake cannot be established. In some cases, absolute gastro-intestinal failure is obvious, while in others it only becomes apparent after considerable efforts to feed enterally have failed. There is a trend for partially tolerated, but inadequate enteral intake to be supplemented rather than replaced with parenteral nutrition. Nevertheless, the aim in all patients fed intravenously is to revert to enteral feeding as soon as possible.

Parenteral feeding solutions may be prepared from their component parts under sterile conditions. Ready-made solutions also exist, but any necessary additions must be made in the same way.

In ICU patients, the daily requirements are infused continuously over 24 hours. Careful biochemical and clinical monitoring is important, especially at the outset (Table 85.6).

ACCESS

The major concern with central venous access for TPN is prevention of infection. The following considerations apply[40]:

- *insertion site*: subclavian lines have lower infection rates than internal jugular or femoral lines
- *tunnelling* may reduce infection rates particularly in internal jugular lines. It is not recommended for routine use
- *expertise* of operator and adequacy of ICU *nurse staffing levels* affect infection rate

Table 85.6 Minimum monitoring during total parenteral nutrition. Less stable patients may require more intensive surveillance.

Nursing	Temperature
	Pulse
	Blood pressure
	Respiratory rate
	Fluid balance
	Blood sugar (4-hourly, when commencing feed)
Daily (at least)	Review of fluid balance
	Review of nutrient intake
	Blood sugar
	Urea, electrolytes and creatinine
Weekly (at least)	Full blood picture
	Coagulation screen
	Liver function tests
	Magnesium, calcium and phosphate
	Weight
As indicated	Zinc
	Uric acid

- *skin preparation*: 2% chlorhexidine in alcohol is the most effective
- *sterile technique*: maximal sterile barrier procedures (mask, cap, gown, gloves, large drape) are known to reduce catheter-related bacteraemia rates six-fold. There is a bewildering resistance to the use of these precautions outside ICUs
- *dressings*: permeable polyurethane transparent dressings are superior to impermeable
- *antimicrobial catheters*: catheters coated with either chlorhexidine and silver sulfadiazine or rifampicin and minocycline are several times less likely to cause bacteraemia than standard polyurethane catheters. The duration of the anti-infective effect appears to be longer with the antibiotic-coated catheters (2 weeks versus one)
- *scheduled exchange* has not been proven to reduce catheter-related sepsis
- *guide-wire exchange* is associated with increased bacteraemia rates, which in routine use outweigh the reduced mechanical complications

In practice, pre-existing central access is used in the first instance. Recent work has not confirmed earlier data, suggesting an increase in infections in triple lumen catheters.[41] If a multi-lumen catheter is used, one lumen should be dedicated to administration of TPN and not used for any other purpose. Three-way taps should be avoided and infusion set changes carried out daily under sterile conditions. For long-term TPN (more than two months) specialized catheters with a tunnelled cuff or a subcutaneous port are recommended.[42]

COMPOSITION

ENERGY

Energy is provided by a combination of carbohydrate and lipid. The optimal balance between the two is unknown; often 30–40% of non-protein energy is given as lipid. Alternatively, carbohydrate may be relied upon for almost all the energy, with lipid being infused once or twice a week to provide essential fatty acids.

Glucose is the preferred carbohydrate and is infused as a concentrated solution. Exceeding the body's capacity to metabolize glucose (4 mg/kg per min in the septic patient) can lead to hyperglycaemia, lipogenesis, and excess CO_2 production. Endogenous insulin secretion increases to control blood sugar levels. However, many patients require additional insulin, particularly diabetics. This may be infused separately, but when requirements are stable it is safer to add it to the TPN solution. Persistent hyperglycaemia is better addressed by reducing the glucose infusion rate than by large doses of insulin.

Lipid provides essential fatty acids (linoleic and linolenic acids) and a more concentrated energy source than glucose. It may thus avoid the complications of excess glucose administration. However, there are concerns about immunosuppression from lipid infusion, as discussed above. Current lipid preparations consist of soya-bean oil emulsified with glycerol and egg phosphatides.

NITROGEN

Nitrogen is supplied as a crystalline solution of L-amino acids. Commercially available preparations vary in their provision of conditionally essential amino acids. Glutamine, tyrosine and cysteine are absent from many because of instability.

MICRONUTRIENTS

Vitamin and trace element preparations are added to TPN solutions in appropriate amounts. Thiamine, folic acid and vitamin K are particularly vulnerable to depletion and additional doses may be necessary.

ELECTROLYTES

Amino acid preparations contain varying quantities of electrolytes; additional amounts may need to be added to the solution.

COMPLICATIONS

Parenteral nutrition has the potential for severe complications.

- *catheter-related sepsis* has been addressed above. Other complications of central venous cannulation are discussed elsewhere
- *electrolyte abnormalities* include hypophosphataemia, hypokalaemia and hypomagnesaemia, especially in the first 24–48 h
- *hyperchloraemic metabolic acidosis* may result from the use of amino acid solutions with a high chloride content. Replacing some chloride with acetate in the TPN solution will resolve this where necessary
- *rebound hypoglycaemia* may occur when TPN is discontinued suddenly. TPN should be weaned over a minimum of 12 hours. If it cannot be continued, an infusion of 10% dextrose should be started and blood sugars closely monitored
- *refeeding syndrome* may occur when normal intake is resumed after a period of starvation. It is associated with profound hypophosphataemia, and possibly hypokalaemia and hypomagnesaemia. With the restoration of glucose as a substrate, insulin levels rise and cause cellular uptake of these ions. Depletion of ATP and 2,3-DPG results in tissue hypoxia and failure of cellular energy metabolism. This may manifest as cardiac and respiratory failure, with paraesthesiae and seizures also reported. Thiamine deficiency may also play a part
- *liver dysfunction* is common during TPN. Causes include hepatic steatosis, intrahepatic cholestasis and biliary sludging from gall-bladder inactivity

- *deficiencies* of trace elements and vitamins, especially thiamine, folic acid and vitamin K, may occur.

NUTRITION AND SPECIFIC DISEASES

ACUTE RENAL FAILURE

The advent of continuous renal replacement therapy has meant that dietary fluid and protein restriction is no longer warranted in ICU. Use of specialized lipid or amino acid formulations in TPN is not supported by evidence, and in general normal nutritional support is appropriate in acute renal failure.

LIVER DISEASE

Chronic liver disease[4,43] does not alter the energy requirements of ICU patients. Lipolysis is increased, so lipid must be used with caution to avoid hypertriglyceridaemia – not more than 1 g/kg per day. Protein restriction may be required in chronic hepatic encephalopathy; starting with 0.5 g/kg per day, the dose may be cautiously increased towards a normal intake. Hepatic encephalopathy may in part be due to depletion of branched-chain amino acids (BCAAs), permitting increased cerebral uptake of aromatic amino acids, which produce inhibitory neurotransmitters. In protein-intolerant patients, the use of feeds enriched with BCAAs may permit greater protein intake without worsening encephalopathy. Thiamine and fat-soluble vitamin deficiencies are common in patients with chronic liver disease.

Fulminant hepatic failure reduces gluconeogenesis; hypoglycaemia is a common problem necessitating glucose infusion. Lipid is well tolerated. Energy and protein requirements are similar to those above. BCAAs have not been shown to be superior to standard amino-acid solutions.

RESPIRATORY FAILURE

Oxidation of fat produces less CO_2 than glucose. There have been attempts to use this to assist in weaning from mechanical ventilation by providing 50% of energy intake as lipid. The evidence is inconclusive, but such feeds may be tried if the ability to wean is marginal. Avoidance of over-feeding is much more important.

ACUTE PANCREATITIS

Until recently, TPN was a cornerstone of the management of severe acute pancreatitis in order to minimize pancreatic stimulation. This approach has begun to change with the publication of studies suggesting that jejunal feeding is safe, effective and associated with reductions in infective complications and mortality.[24,25]

Elemental feeds and pancreatic enzyme supplements are logical if malabsorption is a problem.

ADJUNCTIVE NUTRITION

Certain compounds have been used as adjuncts to feeding solutions in attempts to modulate the metabolic and immune responses to critical illness. While this is an area of much promise, no conclusive benefit has yet been shown.

GROWTH HORMONE

Small studies in patients with septic shock and burns suggested that growth hormone reduced length of stay and improved nitrogen balance. In a salutary illustration of the dangers of surrogate end-points, two large trials subsequently demonstrated increased mortality in ICU patients receiving growth hormone.[44]

GLUTAMINE

Glutamine serves as an oxidative fuel and nucleotide precursor for enterocytes and immune cells, mainly lymphocytes, neutrophils and macrophages. During catabolic illness, it is released in large quantities from skeletal muscle in order to supply this need. In these circumstances it may become 'conditionally essential' and is vulnerable to depletion, with potentially adverse effects on gut barrier and immune function. Dietary supplementation with glutamine has reduced gut mucosal atrophy in animals and humans. A small study in multiple trauma patients showed a reduction in pneumonia and bacteraemia with glutamine-enriched enteral feeding.[45]

Until recently, TPN solutions have contained no glutamine, because of problems with stability and solubility. These are now being overcome by the use of dipeptides, but results from clinical studies of intravenous glutamine supplementation during TPN have been conflicting. One study in ICU patients requiring TPN showed a reduction in late mortality that only became apparent after 20 days.[46] Another trial in a general hospital TPN population showed no benefit in either the whole sample or the ICU sub-group.[47]

BRANCHED-CHAIN AMINO ACIDS

BCAA-enriched feeds have been assessed as a means of reducing protein loss in critical illness. Despite promising animal work, no clinical benefit has been shown.

NOVEL LIPIDS

Medium chain triglycerides are less dependent than other lipids upon pancreatic enzymes for their absorption from the gut, and are metabolized more rapidly when infused intravenously. Their optimum contribution to total lipid is not known. Currently, there is interest in emulsions derived from olive oil, or enriched with either omega-3 fatty acids, structured lipids (medium and long chain triglycerides on a glycerol backbone), or vitamin E.

OMEGA-3 FATTY ACIDS

The polyunsaturated fatty acids in artificial feeding solutions are mostly omega-6 fatty acids. Replacing these with omega-3 fatty acids has anti-inflammatory effects:

- production of less inflammatory eicosanoid derivatives (leukotriene B_5 instead of B_4 and thromboxane A_3 instead of A_2)
- reduced cytokine production.

Early clinical work in patients with ARDS using enteral feed enriched in omega-3 fatty acids found a reduction in length of ventilation and ICU stay.[48]

ARGININE

Arginine is a non-essential amino acid that acts as a precursor of both nitric oxide, polyamines (important in lymphocyte maturation) and nucleotides. Animal studies suggest enhanced cell-mediated immunity and survival when arginine is supplemented.

NUCLEOTIDES

Purines and pyrimidines are precursor molecules in DNA and RNA synthesis. While they have not been considered essential to the diet, animal work suggests that a nucleotide-free diet suppresses cell-mediated immunity.

IMMUNONUTRITION

Two commercially available enteral feeding solutions combine omega-3 fatty acids, arginine, nucleotides and in one case glutamine to produce so-called immune-enhancing diets. They have been assessed in a number of trials, few of them in patient groups likely to be admitted to ICU outside North America. Only one unblinded study has shown a reduction in mortality;[49] re-analysis of another revealed increased mortality in the treatment group.[50,51] Some have found a reduction in infective complications with immunonutrition, but this usually did not reach statistical significance.

Not surprisingly, meta-analysis has failed to clarify this situation. In one study, immunonutrition had no effect on the incidence of pneumonia, but there was a reduction in other infections and in length of hospital stay. However, there was also an increase in mortality that just failed to reach statistical significance.[51] The authors did not censor for deaths, which raised the possibility that infections and length of stay were reduced by increased mortality in the treatment group. A second meta-analysis, which did censor for deaths, again found a reduction in infections and length of ventilation and hospital stay in those receiving immunonutrition. There was no discernible effect on mortality.[52]

Like all attempts to modulate the immune response in critical illness, immune-enhancing diets are a double-edged tool. There is no reason why the arbitrary mixtures of potentially antagonistic substances in currently available formulae should be optimal. The feeds are substantially more expensive than standard regimes, and the case for their use is unproven.

REFERENCES

1 Moore EE, Jones TN. Benefits of immediate jejunostomy feeding after major abdominal trauma – a prospective, randomized study. *J Trauma* 1986; **26**:874–880.
2 Grahm TW, Zadrozny DB, Harrington T. The benefits of early jejunal hyperalimentation in the head-injured patient. *Neurosurgery* 1989; **25**:729–735.
3 Taylor SJ, Fettes SB, Jewkes C, Nelson RJ. Prospective, randomized, controlled trial to determine the effect of early enhanced enteral nutrition on clinical outcome in mechanically ventilated patients suffering head injury. *Crit Care Med* 1999; **27**:2525–2531.
4 Klein S, Kinney J, Jeejeebhoy K, *et al.* Nutrition support in clinical practice: review of published data and recommendations for future research directions. *Am J Clin Nutr* 1997; **66**:683–706.
5 Woodcock NP, Zeigler D, Palmer MD, *et al.* Enteral versus parenteral nutrition: a pragmatic study. *Nutrition* 2001; **17**:1–12.
6 Rapp RP, Young B, Twyman D, *et al.* The favorable effect of early parenteral feeding on survival in head-injured patients. *J Neurosurg* 1983; **58**:906–912.
7 Baker JP, Detsky AS, Wesson DE, *et al.* Nutritional assessment. A comparison of clinical judgment and objective measurements. *New Engl J Med* 1982; **306**:969–972.
8 Streat SJ, Beddoe AH, Hill GL. Aggressive nutritional support does not prevent protein loss despite fat gain in septic intensive care patients. *J Trauma* 1987; **27**:262–266.
9 Klein CJ, Stanek GS, Wiles CE. Overfeeding macronutrients to critically ill adults: metabolic complications. *J Am Diet Assoc* 1998; **98**:795–806.
10 Plank LD, Hill GL. Sequential metabolic changes following induction of systemic inflammatory response in patients with severe sepsis or major blunt trauma. *World J Surg* 2000; **24**:630–638.
11 Flancbaum L, Choban PS, Sambucco S, *et al.* Comparison of indirect calorimetry, the Fick method, and prediction equations in estimating the energy requirements of critically ill patients. *Am J Clin Nutr* 1999; **69**:461–466.
12 Makk LJK, McClave SA, Creech PW, *et al.* Clinical application of the metabolic cart to the delivery of total parenteral nutrition. *Crit Care Med* 1990; **18**:1320–1327.
13 Saffle JR, Larson CM, Sullivan J. A randomized trial of indirect calorimetry-based feedings in thermal injury. *J Trauma* 1990; **30**:776–782.
14 Streat SJ, Plank LD, Hill GL. Overview of modern management of patients with critical injury and severe sepsis. *World J Surg* 2000; **24**:655–663.
15 Schofield WN. Predicting basal metabolic rate, new standards and review of previous work. *Hum Nutrition: Clin Nutrition* 1985; **39C(Suppl)**(1):5–41.
16 Working Party of the British Association for Parenteral and Enteral Nutrition. *Current Perspectives on Enteral Nutrition in Adults.* Maidenhead: BAPEN; 1999.
17 Konstantinides FN, Konstantinides NN, Li JC, *et al.* Urinary urea nitrogen: too insensitive for calculating nitrogen balance in surgical clinical nutrition. *JPEN* 1991; **15**:189–193.
18 Larsson J, Lennmarken C, Martensson J, *et al.* Nitrogen requirements in severely injured patients. *Br J Surg* 1990; **77**:413–416.
19 Demling RH, Debiasse MA. Micronutrients in critical illness. *Crit Care Clin* 1995; **11**:651–673.
20 Moore FA, Moore EE, Jones TN, *et al.* TEN versus TPN following major abdominal trauma – reduced septic morbidity. *J Trauma* 1989; **29**:916–922.
21 Kudsk KA, Croce MA, Fabian TC, *et al.* Enteral versus parenteral feeding: effects on septic morbidity after blunt and penetrating abdominal trauma. *Ann Surg* 1992; **215**:503–511.
22 Adams S, Dellinger EP, Wertz MJ, *et al.* Enteral versus parenteral nutritional support following laparotomy for trauma: a randomized prospective trial. *J Trauma* 1986; **26**:882–890.
23 Young B, Ott L, Twyman D, *et al.* The effect of nutritional support on outcome from severe head injury. *J Neurosurg* 1987; **67**:668–676.
24 Pupelis G, Selga G, Austrums E, Kaminski A. Jejunal feeding, even when instituted late, improves outcome in patients with severe pancreatitis and peritonitis. *Nutrition* 2001; **17**:91–94.
25 Kalfarentzos F, Kehagias J, Mead N, *et al.* Enteral nutrition is superior to parenteral nutrition in severe acute pancreatitis: results of a randomized prospective trial. *Br J Surg* 1997; **84**:1665–1669.
26 Cerra FB, McPherson JP, Konstantinides FN, *et al.* Enteral nutrition does not prevent multiple organ failure syndrome (MOFS) after sepsis. *Surgery* 1988; **104**:727–733.
27 Lipman TO. Grains or veins: is enteral nutrition really better than parenteral nutrition? *JPEN* 1998; **22**:167–182.
28 Veterans' Affairs Total Parenteral Nutrition Cooperative Study Group. Perioperative total parenteral nutrition in surgical patients. *N Engl J Med* 1991; **325**:525–532.
29 Battistella ED, Widergren JT, Anderson JT, *et al.* A prospective, randomized trial of intravenous fat emulsion administration in trauma victims requiring total parenteral nutrition. *J Trauma* 1997; **43**:52–58.

30 Hadfield RJ, Sinclair DG, Houldsworth PE, Evans TW. Effects of enteral and parenteral nutrition on gut mucosal permeability in the critically ill. *Am J Respir Crit Care Med* 1995; **152**:1545–1548.

31 Sedman PC, MacFie J, Palmer MD, *et al*. Preoperative total parenteral nutrition is not associated with mucosal atrophy or bacterial translocation in humans. *Br J Surg* 1995; **82**:1663–1667.

32 MacFie J, O'Boyle C, Mitchell CJ, *et al*. Gut origin of sepsis: a prospective study investigating associations between bacterial translocation, gastric microflora, and septic morbidity. *Gut* 1999; **45**:223–228.

33 Spain DA, McClave SA, Sexton LK, *et al*. Infusion protocol improves delivery of enteral tube feeding in the critical care unit JPEN. *JPEN* 1999; **23**:288–292.

34 Bauer P, Charpentier C, Bouchet C, *et al*. Parenteral with enteral nutrition in the critically ill. *Intensive Care Med* 2000; **26**:893–900.

35 Kearns PJ, Chin D, Mueller L, *et al*. The incidence of ventilator-associated pneumonia and success in nutrient delivery with gastric versus small intestinal feeding: a randomized clinical trial. *Crit Care Med* 2000; **28**:1742–1746.

36 Heyland DK, Cook DJ, Guyatt GH. Enteral nutrition in the critically ill patient: a critical review of the evidence. *Intensive Care Med* 1993; **19**:435–442.

37 Homann H-H, Kemen M, Fuessenich C, *et al*. Reduction in diarrhea incidence by soluble fiber in patients receiving total or supplemental enteral nutrition. *JPEN* 1994; **18**:486–490.

38 Drakulovic MB, Torres A, Bauer TT, *et al*. Supine body position as a risk factor for nosocomial pneumonia in mechanically ventilated patients: a randomised trial. *Lancet* 1999; **354**:1851–1858.

39 Abuksis G, Mor M, Segal N, *et al*. Percutaneous endoscopic gastrostomy: high mortality rates in hospitalized patients. *Am J Gastroenterol* 2000; **95**:128–132.

40 Fraenkel DJ, Rickard C, Lipman J. Can we achieve consensus on central venous catheter-related infections? *Anaesth Intensive Care* 2000; **28**:475–490.

41 Goetz AM, Wagener MM, Miller JM, Muder RR. Risk of infection due to central venous catheters: effect of site of placement and catheter type. *Infect Control Hosp Epidemiol* 1998; **19**:842–845.

42 Working Party of the British Association for Parenteral and Enteral Nutrition. *Current Perspectives on Parenteral Nutrition in Adults.* Maidenhead: BAPEN; 1996.

43 Mizock BA. Nutritional support in hepatic encephalopathy. *Nutrition* 1999; **15**:220–228.

44 Takkala J, Ruokonen E, Webster NR, *et al*. Increased mortality associated with growth hormone treatment in critically ill adults. *N Engl J Med* 1999; **341**:785–792.

45 Houdijk APJ, Rijnsburger ER, Jansen J, *et al*. Randomised trial of glutamine-enriched enteral nutrition on infectious morbidity in patients with multiple trauma. *Lancet* 1998; **352**:772–776.

46 Griffiths RD, Jones C, Palmer TEA. Six-month outcome of critically ill patients given glutamine-supplemented parenteral nutrition. *Nutrition* 1997; **13**:295–302.

47 Powell-Tuck J, Jamieson CP, Bettany GEA, *et al*. A double blind, randomised, controlled trial of glutamine supplementation in parenteral nutrition. *Gut* 1999; **45**:82–88.

48 Gadek JE, DeMichele SJ, Karlstad MD, *et al*. Effect of enteral feeding with eicosapentaenoic acid, γ-linolenic acid, and antioxidants in patients with acute respiratory distress syndrome. *Crit Care Med* 1999; **27**:1409–1420.

49 Galban C, Montejo JC, Mesejo A, *et al*. An immune-enhancing enteral diet reduces mortality rate and episodes of bacteremia in septic intensive care unit patients. *Crit Care Med* 2000; **28**:643–648.

50 Bower RH, Cerra FB, Bershadsky B, *et al*. Early enteral administration of a formula (Impact®) supplemented with arginine, nucleotides and fish oil in intensive care unit patients: results of a multicenter, prospective, randomized, clinical trial. *Crit Care Med* 1995; **23**:436–449.

51 Heys SD, Walker LG, Smith I, Eremin O. Enteral nutritional supplementation with key nutrients in patients with critical illness and cancer. A meta-analysis of randomized controlled clinical trials. *Ann Surg* 1999; **229**:467–477.

52 Beale RJ, Bryg DJ, Bihari DJ. Immunonutrition in the critically ill: a systematic review of clinical outcome. *Crit Care Med* 1999; **27**:2799–2805.

Part Fifteen

Haematological Management

86

Blood transfusion

J P Isbister

When using blood transfusion therapy, the clinical problem and patient's needs must be correctly identified and clearly understood. Blood component therapy should only be regarded as supportive therapy and rarely definitive therapy. In most circumstances, therapy is required for haematological deficiencies until the basic disease process can be corrected (e.g. surgical control for acute haemorrhage, or support for bone marrow suppression until the marrow recovers. Therapy may be given to control the effects of a deficiency or to prevent problems. In some circumstances the therapeutic indication is passive immunotherapy (e.g. Rh prophylaxis) or high dosage intravenous immunoglobulin as immunomodulatory therapy.

Homologous transfusion should not be perceived as the first line of therapy for patients with haematopoietic defects. For many patients it is possible to correct or manage the effects of deficiencies in the haematopoietic system without transfusing homologous blood components. Clearly, if homologous blood can be avoided the potential hazards need not be considered. No greater disaster can befall a patient than to be the victim of major morbidity or mortality from a transfusion or other therapy that was not clearly indicated. The decision making process for blood component therapy can be difficult and much debate continues in relation to the indications for the use of various homologous blood components.[1–3]

In considering the use of homologous blood transfusion these questions need to be addressed:

- What is the timeframe of the decision making process?
- Is it an elective decision?
- What is the haematological defect?
- What is the most appropriate therapy for the patient?
- Are there alternatives to homologous transfusion?
- What component is indicated and where should it be obtained?
- What are the potential hazards of the blood component therapy?
- Can the risk of adverse effects be avoided or minimized?
- How should the component be administered and monitored?

- What is the cost of the haemotherapy?
- Is the patient fully informed of the medical decisions?

Safe and effective transfusion requires attention to the following details (Figure 86.1).

- clearly defined indication and benefits of blood components
- accurate patient identification for compatibility
- provision of adequate amounts and quality of component/s
- communication of benefits and risk to the patient/relatives
- identification and careful management of high-risk patients
- the infusion should not be associated with any preventable ill effects
- appropriate handling, administration and monitoring
- awareness of possible transfusion-related complications
- early diagnosis and prompt action in relation to adverse events of transfusion
- accurate documentation
- input into quality assurance programmes

BLOOD STORAGE[4–6]

Whole blood is collected into closed plastic packs mixed with an anticoagulant and stabilizer, to a final volume of approximately 500 ml (70 ml preservative and 430 ml whole blood). Acid citrate dextrose (ACD) has been used since the 1940s, but in recent years, solutions with added phosphate and adenine (CPD-A) are used to increase post-transfusion viability and red cell function (e.g. 2,3 diphosphoglycerate (DPG) levels). Blood is stored at 4°C in carefully designed and monitored refrigerators. Storage shelf-life is up to 35 days with CPD-A, but it is generally advisable to use fresher blood (<2 weeks old) in critically ill patients, especially when rapid transfusion of large volumes is required or if coagulopathy is already evident. It is better to collect and store blood under appropriate conditions for each specific component. Red cells stored as whole blood are subjected to greater damage due to the presence of

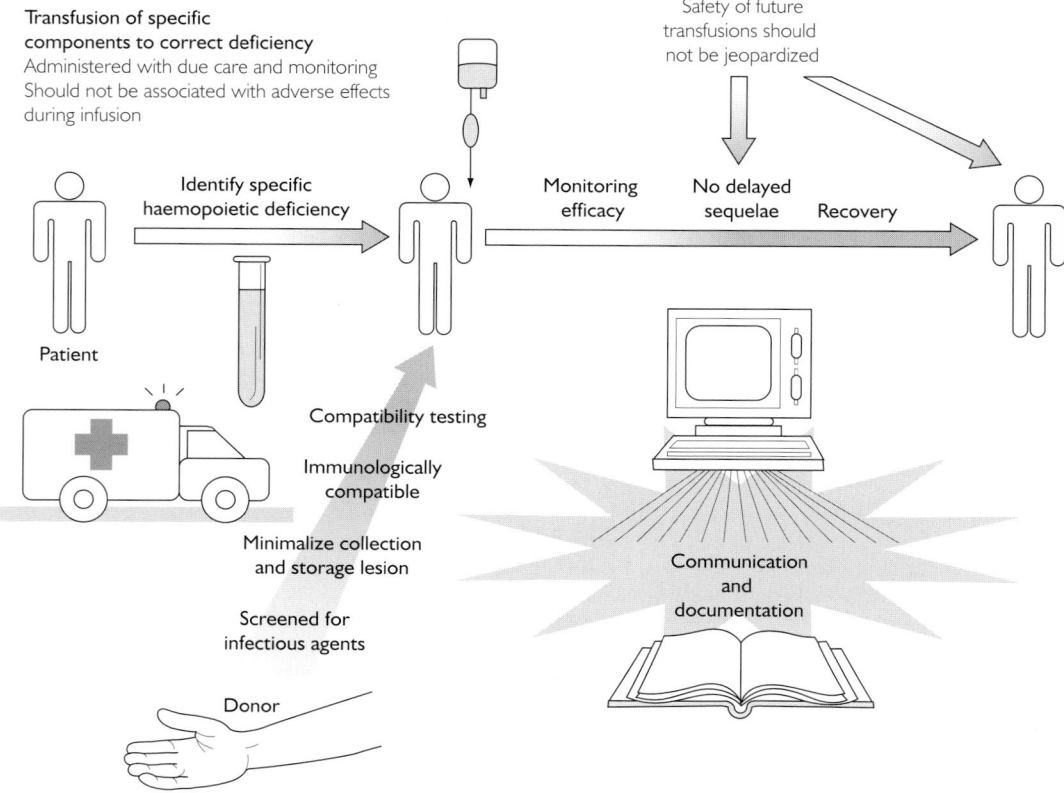

Fig. 86.1 Safe and effective blood transfusion.

neutrophils and plasma proteolytic systems. It is increasingly recognized that the presence of leukocytes (especially neutrophils) creates an adverse storage environment for most blood components and are responsible for a number of the adverse effects of blood component therapy. In some countries all blood is now leukoreduced.

POTENTIAL EFFECTS OF STORAGE ON BLOOD[7-9]

As with any biological fluid, blood degenerates with time during storage. The changes occur in both the cellular and the plasma components (Figure 86.2) .

METABOLIC EFFECTS

ATP is progressively depleted with storage and the pH rises; oxidant damage to the membrane occurs with rigid spherocyte formation, swelling and finally potassium leak. Parallel to these changes, haemoglobin (Hb) function may be altered due to falling levels of both ATP and, more significantly, 2,3 DPG resulting in increasing oxygen affinity. These changes occur earlier, and to a greater extent in whole blood than in red cell concentrates. It is now recognized that storage of blood as whole blood is associated with the greatest storage lesions and in general the only time for the use of whole blood is when it is fresh. The implications for this and the storage of autologous whole blood are still being evaluated.

Evidence would support the concept that the removal of the leukocytes prior to storage, although costly is increasingly becoming standard practice. The platelets and granulocytes in the buffy coat are the foundations for the formation of microaggregates, with various cell-damaging enzymes being released into the storage medium. Thus transfusion of large volumes of stored blood, although increasing intravascular volume, will not necessarily provide immediately available oxygen to the tissues to the degree anticipate from the post-transfusion haemoglobin rise.

MICROAGGREGATES

The plastic mesh filter used in conventional blood giving sets only removes particulate material larger than $170 \ \mu m$ in size. Microaggregates of platelet/leukocyte/fibrin thrombi, progressively form in blood during storage, ranging in size from 20 μm to >170μm. If this particulate matter is to be removed from blood, a microfilter is needed during transfusion. The adverse effects of microaggregates are still debated (Table 86.1). Nevertheless, it is generally agreed that an additional microfilter should be used when large volumes of stored blood (e.g. over 1 litre) are transfused over short periods of time. Hence the quality of stored whole blood or blood components cannot be guaranteed and the use of fresh blood products or the development of better blood preservative solutions is of paramount importance.

TRANSFUSION MANAGEMENT OF ACUTE HAEMORRHAGE

Homologous blood may be required for the restitution of blood volume and oxygen carrying capacity in the haemorrhaging patient. If blood loss has been massive or there are defects in the haemostatic system, specific component therapy may be indicated.

In previously healthy patients who have suffered an acute blood loss of less than 25% of their blood volume, restoring volume is more important than replacing oxygen carrying capacity. Plasma volume expanders may preclude the necessity for homologous transfusion, especially if bleeding can be controlled. Clear fluids also allow time for transfusion compatibility testing. In the context

Table 86.1   Potential problems from infusion of microaggregates

Impaired pulmonary gas exchange (ARDS)
Microcirculatory dysfunction
Depression of RES function
Depression of fibronectin levels
Febrile reactions
Activation of the haemostatic system
Activation of the complement system
Unnecessary antigenic stimulation
Release of vasoactive substances

of acute bleeding and hypovolaemic shock the haemoglobin level is not the primary indicator for determining the need for homologous red cell transfusion. A normal human may survive a 30% deficit in blood volume without fluid replacement, in contrast to an 80% loss of red cell mass if normovolaemia is maintained. Minimization of homologous blood transfusion is important and haemodilution to low haematocrits is now accepted practice.

Homologous red blood cell transfusion will be required if there is evidence of impaired oxygen transport, particularly when the loss of blood volume exceeds 25% and blood loss has not been adequately controlled. Loss of over 40% of blood volume is life

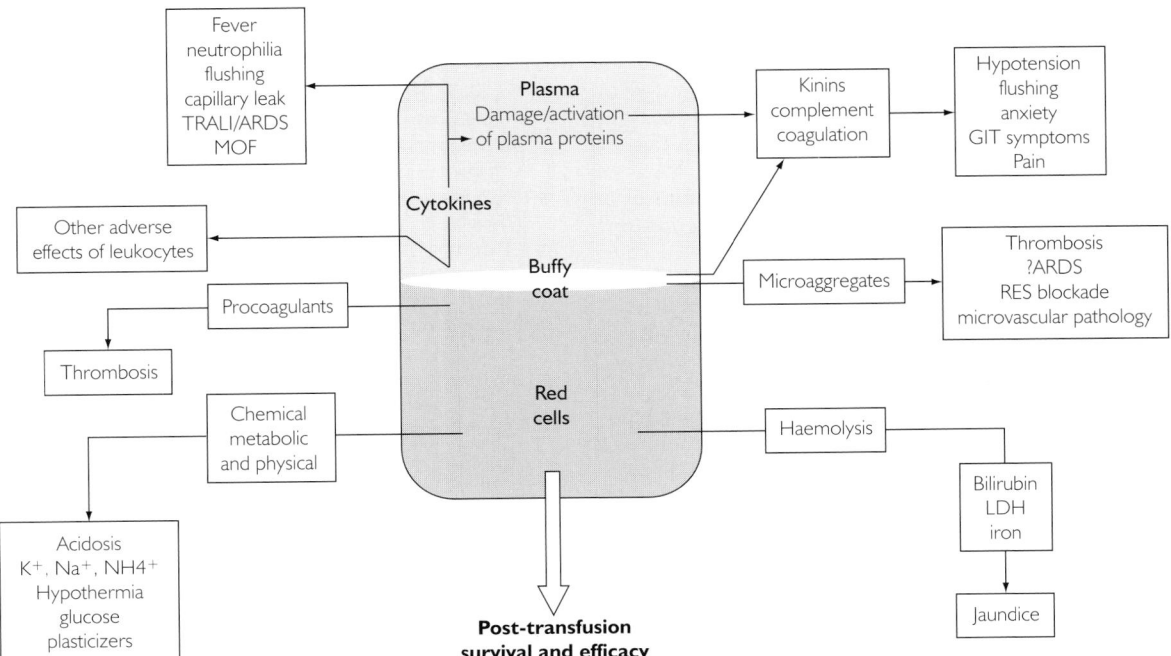

Fig. 86.2   Clinical consequences of the storage lesion.

threatening and haemotherapy is a mainstay of successful management. This requires a co-ordinated priority-orientated clinical and laboratory approach. The rapid infusion of large volumes of aged blood has potential problems, which are largely related to the storage lesion. It is not possible or necessary for fresh blood to be immediately available for all acutely haemorrhaging patients. Whenever possible, blood less than a week from the collection date is desirable in the patient continuing to bleed in order to minimize the problems of the massive transfusion syndrome and provide immediately functioning red cells. If massive blood transfusion is anticipated, the hospital transfusion service and the central blood supply agency must be alerted.

A protocol approach to blood component therapy is generally not recommended, as each patient should be treated individually. However, in an elective situation when defects can be identified in advance and appropriate blood components prescribed, a protocol approach may be justified. This should be done in close consultation with the haematologist and hospital transfusion service.

SPECIFIC HAZARDS OF MASSIVE BLOOD TRANSFUSION

Adverse effects of massive blood transfusion (usually defined as replacement of the circulating volume in 24 h) may manifest in various ways and these effects may be misinterpreted as being due to other mechanisms. Any patient receiving massive blood component therapy is likely to be seriously ill and have multiple problems. Many adverse effects must be considered in conjunction with the injuries and multiorgan dysfunction. It is not always possible to define the complications caused or aggravated by massive blood transfusion (Table 86.2).

CITRATE TOXICITY[10]

A patient responds to citrate infusion by the removal of citrate and mobilization of ionized calcium. Citrate is metabolized by the Krebs cycle in all nucleated cells, especially the liver. A marked elevation in the citrate concentration is seen with transfusion exceeding 500 ml in 5 min, the level rapidly falls when the infusion is slowed. Citrate metabolism is impaired by hypotension, hypovolaemia, hypothermia and liver disease. Toxicity may also be potentiated by alkalosis, hyperkalaemia, hypothermia and cardiac disease. The clinical significance of a minor depression of ionized calcium remains ill-defined, and it is accepted that a warm well perfused adult patient with normal liver function can tolerate a unit of blood each 5 min without requiring calcium. The rate of transfusion is more significant than the total volume transfused. Common practice is to administer 10% calcium gluconate 1.0 g i.v., following each 5 units of blood or fresh frozen plasma. Such a practice remains controversial as there is increasing concern regarding calcium homeostasis and cell function in acutely ill patients.

ACID BASE AND ELECTROLYTE DISTURBANCES
Acid-base

Stored bank blood contains an appreciable acid load and is often used in a situation of pre-existing or continuing metabolic acidosis. The acidity of stored blood is mainly due to the citric acid of the anticoagulant and the lactic acid generated during storage. Their intermediary metabolites are rapidly metabolized with adequate tissue perfusion, resulting in a metabolic alkalosis. Hence, the routine use of sodium bicarbonate is usually unnecessary and is generally contraindicated. Alkali further shifts the oxygen dissociation curve to the left, provides a large additional sodium load, and depresses the return of ionized calcium to normal following citrate infusion. Acid-base estimations should be performed and corrected in the context of the clinical situation. With continuing hypoperfusion, however, metabolism of citrate and lactate will be depressed, lactic acid production will continue, and there may be an indication for i.v. bicarbonate and calcium to correct acidosis and low ionized calcium.

Table 86.2 Potential hazards of massive and rapid blood transfusion

Impaired oxygen transport
 Microaggregates*
 Fluid overload
 Defective red cell function*
 Impaired haemoglobin function*
 Disseminated intravascular coagulation (DIC)*
 Acute respiratory distress syndrome (ARDS)*
 Multiorgan dysfunction syndrome (MODS)*
Haemostatic failure
 Dilution
 Depletion
 Decreased production
 Disseminated intravascular coagulation (DIC)*
Metabolic disturbances
 Electrolyte and metabolic disturbances*
 Hyperkalaemia or delayed hypokalaemia*
 Sodium overload*
 Acid-base disturbances*
 Citrate toxicity*
 Hypothermia*
Vasoactive reactions
 Kinin activation*
 Damaged platelets and granulocytes*
Serological incompatibility
Impaired reticuloendothelial function*

*Complications related to the method and time of storage

Serum Potassium

Although controversial, it is unlikely that the high serum potassium levels in stored blood have pathological effects in adults, except in the presence of acute renal failure. However, hypokalaemia may be a problem 24 h after transfusion as the transfused cells correct their electrolyte composition and potassium returns into the cells. Thus, although initial acidosis and hyperkalaemia may be an immediate problem with massive blood transfusion, the net result of successful resuscitation is likely to be delayed hypokalaemia and alkalosis. With CPD blood, the acid load and red cell storage lesion is less. Constant monitoring of the acid-base and electrolyte status is essential in such fluctuating clinical situations.

Serum Sodium

The sodium content of whole blood and fresh frozen plasma is higher than the normal blood level, due to the sodium citrate. This should be remembered when large volumes of plasma are being infused into patients who have disordered salt and water handling (e.g. renal, liver or cardiac disease).

HYPOTHERMIA

Blood warmed from 4°C to 37°C requires 1255 kJ (300 kcal), the equivalent heat produced by one hour of muscular work, with an oxygen requirement of 62 l. Hypothermia impairs the metabolism of citrate and lactate, shifts the oxygen dissociation curve to the left, increases intracellular potassium release, impairs red cell deformability, delays drug metabolism, masks clinical signs, increases the incidence of arrhythmias, reduces cardiac output and impairs haemostatic function. Thus a thermostatically controlled blood-warming device should be routinely used when any transfusion episode requires the rapid infusion of more than two units of blood.

JAUNDICE

Jaundice is common following massive blood transfusion. A significant amount of transfused stored blood (up to 30% if aged blood is used) may not survive, and the resulting bilirubin load will result in varying degrees of hyperbilirubinaemia. During hypovolaemia and shock, liver function may be impaired, particularly in the presence of sepsis or multiorgan failure. An important rate-limiting step in bilirubin transport is the energy-requiring process of transporting conjugated bilirubin from the hepatocyte to the biliary cannaliculus. Thus, although an increased load of bilirubin from destroyed transfused red cells may be conjugated, there may be delayed excretion, leading to a conjugated hyperbilirubinaemia. The 'paradoxical' conjugated hyperbilirubinaemia may be misinterpreted as being due to haemolysis, biliary obstruction or cholangitis, leading to unnecessary investigations. The effect of resorbing haematoma and the possibility of an occult haemolytic transfusion reaction should also be considered.

POTENTIAL ADVERSE EFFECTS OF HOMOLOGOUS TRANSFUSION[11]

The potential mechanisms of transfusion reactions include (Figures 86.3 and 86.4):

- *Immunological differences* between the donor and recipient that result in varying degrees of blood component incompatibility. In order for a reaction to occur in these circumstances, the recipient generally needs to have been previously immunized to a cellular or plasma antigen.
- *Alterations in blood products due to preservation and storage.* Storage may result in quantitative and/or qualitative deficiencies in the blood components, which will reduce transfusion efficacy.
- *Transmission of infectious disease.*

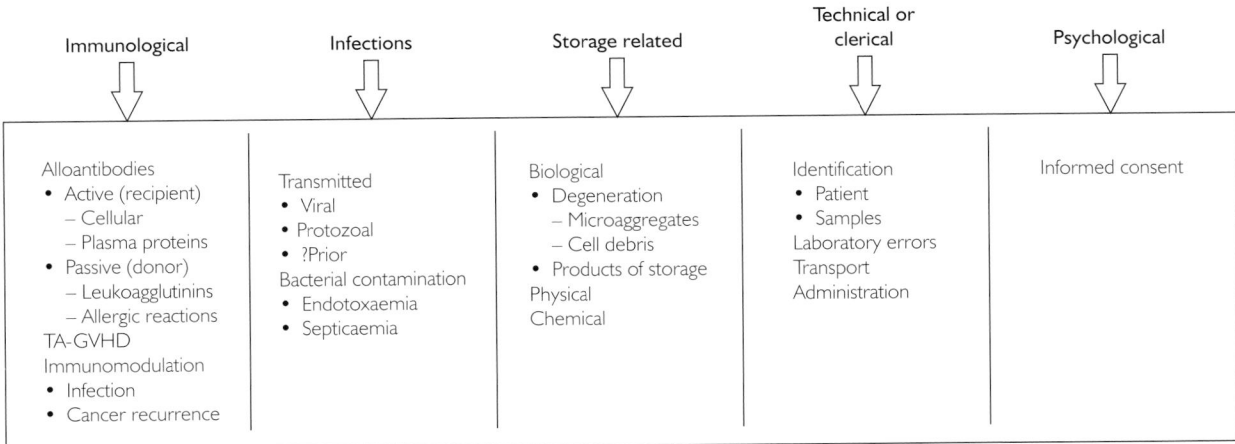

Fig. 86.3 Potential hazards of homologous blood transfusion.

PYREXIA[12]

Mild febrile reactions are not usually a matter of concern, but rigours and temperatures above 38°C should not be ignored. The majority of febrile reactions are now considered to be an immunological reaction against one or more of the transfused cellular or plasma components, usually leucocytes.

TRANSFUSION RELATED INFECTIONS[13]

For donor selection for minimizing transfusion transmitted infections, see Table 86.3.

Hepatitis

Post-transfusion hepatitis is a potential complication of homologous transfusion; serological and nucleic acid tests ensure exclusion of infective donors. Hepatitis B and C are now almost totally preventable transfusion transmitted diseases. Hepatitis C virus (HCV) is a major cause of acute and chronic hepatitis. It is claimed that up to 50% of persons with acute HCV infection seem to become chronically infected.

Human Immunodeficiency Virus

Antibody screening and more recently introduced nucleic acid testing of blood donors has almost eliminated transfusion-associated HIV infection.

Mononucleosis Syndromes

The development of swinging pyrexia with varying degrees of peripheral blood atypical mononucleosis, 7–10 d following transfusion can cause diagnostic confusion. The temperature may fluctuate markedly with associated rigours and drenching sweats, but the patient may feel reasonably well between febrile attacks. Abnormalities in liver function are common. CMV infection is the commonest cause of this syndrome.

Endotoxaemia

Bacterial contamination of stored blood has always been recognized as a potential cause of fulminant endotoxic shock. Although a rare complication, continuing reports of its occurrence, especially in relation to platelet concentrate transfusion have increased awareness. The clinical features of transfusion related endotoxic shock in the non-anaesthetized patient include rigours, fever, tachycardia, and vascular collapse, with prominent nausea, vomiting, and diarrhoea. Anaesthetized patients may have a delayed onset of symptoms (fever, tachycardia, hypotension, and cyanosis), followed by DIC, renal failure and sometimes ARDS.

HAEMOLYTIC TRANSFUSION REACTIONS

Most severe acute haemolytic transfusion reactions have a clearly identifiable and avoidable cause. Such an event may occur under several circumstances. (Table 86.4), but most delayed haemolytic reactions are immune in nature and usually cannot be prevented, unless an error has occurred.

Initial Symptoms and Signs

The classical symptoms and signs of an acute haemolytic transfusion reaction, typical of ABO incompatibility, include apprehension, flushing, pain (e.g. at infusion site, headache, chest, lumbosacral and abdominal), nausea, vomiting, rigours, hypotension and circulatory collapse.

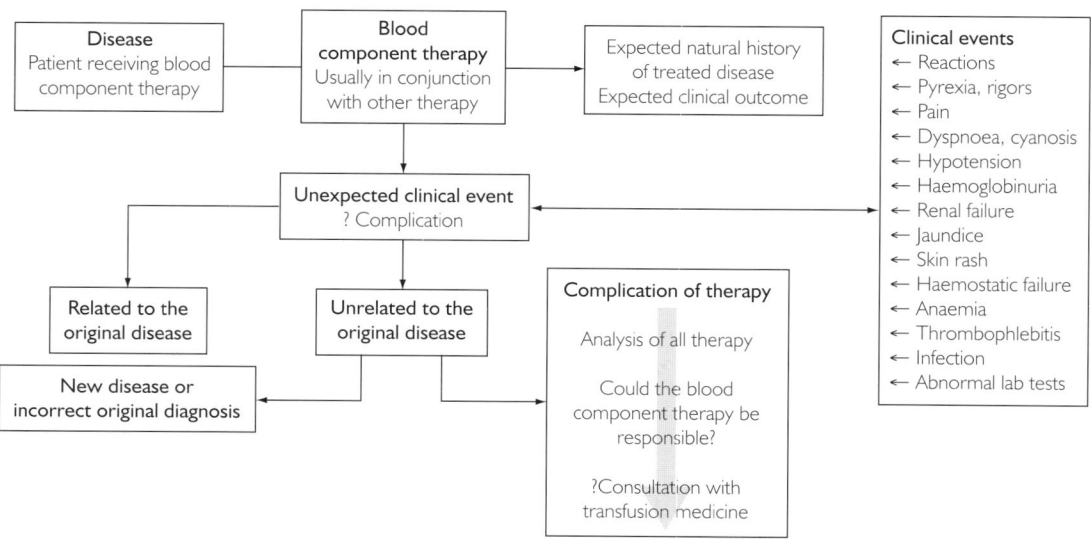

Fig. 86.4 Algorithm for analysis for the possibility of a transfusion reaction.

Table 86.3 Donor selection for minimizing transfusion transmitted infections

Infection	Donor selection by questionnaire	Donor selection by laboratory screening test
Hepatitis A	+	–
Hepatitis B	+	+
Hepatitis C	+/–	+
Cytomegalovirus infection	–	Antibody +ve blood be avoided in neonates and immunosuppressed patients
HIV	+	+
HTLV I	–	+
Epstein–Barr infection	–	–
vCJD*	+	–
Other unidentified viral agents	–	–
Toxoplasmosis	–	–
Syphilis	+	+
Parasitic disease	+	+/–
Bacterial contamination	+/–	–

*vCJD has not been proven to be transmitted by blood transfusion

Haemostatic Failure

Haemorrhagic diathesis due to disseminated intravascular coagulation (DIC) may be a feature, resulting in severe generalized haemostatic failure, with haemorrhage and oozing from multiple sites. As the responsible transfusion is likely to have been administered for haemorrhage, increasing severity of local bleeding may be the first clue to an incompatible transfusion, especially if the patient is unconscious or anaesthetized in the operating room.

Oliguria and Renal Impairment

Renal impairment may complicate a haemolytic transfusion reaction and its prevention or the appropriate management of established renal failure are important. If circulating volume and urinary output are rapidly restored, established renal failure is unlikely to occur. Death from acute renal failure directly caused by an incompatible blood transfusion is preventable, and there are usually other poor prognostic factors.

Anaemia and Jaundice

A severe haemolytic transfusion reaction may be suspected from the development of jaundice or anaemia.

ALLERGIC AND ANAPHYLACTOID REACTIONS[14,15]

Non-cellular blood (plasma and plasma derivatives) components are rarely considered to be a major cause for adverse reactions to transfusion therapy. However, the complexity of plasma and its various components and the effects from component processing results in a broader spectrum of potential adverse effects than frequently recognized. The antigenic heterogeneity of plasma proteins and the presence of antibodies does make the non-cellular components of blood responsible for a plethora of adverse effects, many of which remain poorly understood and commonly unrecognized or undiagnosed in clinical practice.

There has been debate over the years as to the classification of allergic reactions to blood components and blood substitutes. Clinical severity may range from minor urticarial reactions or flushing through to fulminant cardiorespiratory collapse and death. Many of these reactions are probably true anaphylaxis, but in others, mechanisms have been less clear and the term anaphylactoid has been used. To avoid implying the mechanism of the reaction the term immediate generalized reaction (IGR) is preferred.

The clinical syndromes of immediate reactions have been classified as follows:

- Grade I
  – skin manifestations
- Grade II
  – mild to moderate hypotension
  – gastrointestinal disturbances (nausea)
  – respiratory distress
- Grade III
  – severe hypotension, shock,
  – bronchospasm
- Grade IV
  – cardiac and/or respiratory arrest

Plasma and Plasma Components May Cause Adverse Effects by Several Pathophysiological Mechanisms

Immunological reactions to normal components of plasma may occur in two ways.

(a) Plasma proteins being antigenic to the recipient; they may contain epitopes on their molecules different from those on the recipient's functionally identical plasma proteins (e.g. anti-IgA antibodies).

(b) Antibodies in the donor plasma reacting with cellular components of the recipient's blood cells or plasma proteins.

Physicochemical characteristics and contaminants of donor plasma, such as temperature, chemical additives, medications and micro-organisms may be responsible for recipient reactions.

The preparation techniques and storage conditions of blood and blood products may potentially cause adverse reaction through:

(a) Accumulation of metabolites or cellular release products

(b) Plasma activation, ie activation of some of the proteolytic systems, importantly, the complement and kinin/kininogen systems may generate vasoactive substances and anaphylotoxins which may be responsible for reactions. Some apparently allergic reactions to blood products may be due to vasoactive substances in the infusion. Subjective sensations may be missed in an unconscious patient. Hypotension occurring during rapid infusion of a hypovolaemic patient is likely to be interpreted as further volume loss, particularly with some plasma protein fractions that have been reported as consistently producing a transient fall in blood pressure, a situation fraught with risk of overload can be produced.

(c) Histamine generation, histamine levels increase in some stored blood components and levels may be correlated with non-febrile, non-haemolytic transfusion reactions. Histamine release may be stimulated in the patient by plasma components, synthetic colloids and various medications.

(d) Generation of cytokines during storage may be responsible for non-haemolytic transfusion reactions.

(e) Chemical additives: There are various chemical additives (ethylene oxide, formaldehyde, drugs, latex) which may be responsible for immunological or non-immunological recipient reactions.

IMMUNOMODULATION[16–19]

There is evidence that homologous blood transfusion is immunosuppressive in the recipient, which has implications in relation to resistance to infection and the likelihood of cancer recurrence. Donor leukocytes probably play the most important role in this immunomodulation. Homologous transfusion has been shown to be an independent risk factor for post-operative infection. Most infections are distant from the wound site itself, suggesting a systemic reduction in host resistance to infection. The impact of the introduction of leukodepleted blood in some countries has yet to be evaluated.

TRANSFUSION ASSOCIATED GRAFT VERSUS HOST DISEASE

Transfusion associated graft-versus-host disease (TAGVHD), classically observed in relationship to allogeneic bone marrow transplantation, may occur follow-

Table 86.4   Mechanisms by which red cells may be haemolysed before or following transfusion

Immune destruction
   Donor red cell serological incompatibility
      Acute incompatible blood transfusion
      Delayed haemolytic transfusion reaction
   High-titre haemolysins in the donor plasma
   Interdonor incompatibility
   Destruction of donor red cells without detectable antibodies
Non-immune destruction
   Transfusion of incorrectly stored or outdated blood
   Inadvertently frozen blood
   Overheated blood
   Infected blood
   Mechanical destruction, e.g. infused under pressure

ing a blood transfusion due to the infusion of immuno-competent lymphocytes precipitating an immunologic reaction against the host tissues of the recipient. It is most commonly observed in immunocompromised patients, but may also be seen in recipients of directed blood donation from first degree relatives and occasionally when the donor and recipient are not related, due to homozygosity for HLA haplotypes for which the recipient is heterozygous. The syndrome usually occurs 3–30 days post homologous transfusion with fever, liver function test abnormalities profuse watery diarrhoea, erythematous skin rash and progressive pancytopenia.

TRANSFUSION RELATED ACUTE LUNG INJURY

Transfusion related acute lung injury[20] (TRALI) is a potentially fulminant complication of blood transfusion, characterized by acute respiratory distress. Symptoms usually arise within hours of a blood transfusion. In contrast to most patients with ARDS, recovery usually occurs within 48 h and patients usually make a full recovery. The pathophysiology of TRALI is classically due to the presence of leuko-agglutinins in the donor plasma. When complement is activated, C5a promotes neutrophil aggregation and sequestration in the lung microvasculature causing endothelial damage leading to an interstitial oedema. It is now recognized there is a broader spectrum of TRALI than the cases related to leukoagglutinins. The term TRALI is now being expanded to include cases of post-transfusion ARDS in which other mechanisms may be responsible (e.g. anaphylactic reactions, platelet reactions, granulocyte transfusions, DIC, poorly stored blood). Transfusion may be one factor among others predisposing a patient to ARDS.

CLINICAL GUIDELINES FOR BLOOD COMPONENT THERAPY

The following is a brief summary of the clinical guidelines for the use of commonly used blood components.[21,22] The use of specific concentrates or recombinant products is beyond the scope of this book.

RED CELL TRANSFUSIONS

The appropriate and inappropriate use of red cell transfusions[23,24] in acute medicine can be summarized. The management of chronic anaemia is a specialized subject also outside the scope of this book. The following are general broad statements about red cell concentrate transfusions:

- Use of red blood cells is likely to be inappropriate with haemoglobin levels >100 g/l unless there are specific indications.
- Use of red blood cells may be appropriate when haemoglobin is in the range 70–100 g/l. In these cases, the decision to transfuse should be supported by the need to relieve clinical signs and symptoms and prevent significant morbidity and mortality.
- Use of red blood cells is likely to be appropriate when haemoglobin is less than 70 g/l, but lower threshold levels may be acceptable in patients who are asymptomatic and/or when specific therapy is available.

PLATELET TRANSFUSIONS

Platelet transfusion[25,26] therapy may benefit patients with platelet deficiency or dysfunction. The following are the indications for platelet transfusions.

PROPHYLAXIS

- Bone marrow failure when the platelet count is $<10 \times 10^9/l$ without associated risk factors for bleeding or $<20 \times 10^9/l$ in the presence of additional risk factors
- To maintain the platelet count at $>50 \times 10^9/l$ in patients undergoing surgery or invasive procedures
- In qualitative platelet function disorders, depending on clinical features and setting (platelet count is not a reliable indicator for transfusion).

BLEEDING PATIENT

- In any haemorrhaging patient in whom thrombocytopenia secondary to marrow failure is considered a contributory factor
- When the platelet count is $<50 \times 10^9/l$ in the context of massive haemorrhage/transfusion and $<100 \times 10^9/l$ in the presence of diffuse microvascular bleeding.

The transfusion of platelet concentrates is not generally considered appropriate when:

- thrombocytopenia is due to immune-mediated destruction
- in thrombotic thrombocytopenic purpura and haemolytic uraemic syndrome
- in uncomplicated cardiac bypass surgery.

FRESH FROZEN PLASMA

There are few specific indications for fresh frozen plasma, but its use may be appropriate:

- for replacement of single factor deficiencies where a specific or combined factor concentrate is not available
- for immediate reversal of warfarin induced anticoagulation in the presence of potentially life-threatening bleeding and used in addition to vitamin K and possibly factor IX concentrate
- for treatment of the multiple coagulation deficiencies associated with acute disseminated intravascular coagulation
- for treatment of inherited deficiencies of coagulation inhibitors in patients undergoing high-risk procedures where a specific factor concentrate is unavailable
- in the presence of bleeding and abnormal coagulation parameters following massive transfusion or cardiac bypass surgery or in patients with liver disease.

The use of fresh frozen plasma is generally not considered appropriate in cases of:

- hypovolaemia
- plasma exchange procedures unless post exchange invasive procedures are planned
- treatment of immunodeficiency states.

IMMUNOGLOBULIN

Normal human immunoglobulin is available in intramuscular and intravenous forms for the treatment or prevention of infection in patients with proven hypogammaglobulinaemia. Intravenous immunoglobulin therapy also has a role in therapy of some autoimmune disorders, such as idiopathic thrombocytopenic purpura, autoimmune polyneuropathy and others (see Ch. 89).

FACTOR CONCENTRATES

There is an increasing number of plasma protein concentrates available for clinical use. Some are prepared from donor plasma and some by recombinant technology. factor VIII, and factor IX concentrates have an established role in the management of haemophilia, but others are in the process of establishing their clinical efficacy and indications. Antithrombin III concentrates are available for thrombophilia due to AT III deficiency, but their use is controversial in other disorders where ATIII may be depleted (e.g. DIC, MODS).

Of recent interest is the use of the recombinant activated haemostatic proteins and inhibitors. Recombinant activated factor VII (rFVIIa) was originally developed for the management of haemophiliac patients with coagulation factor inhibitors. Because factor VIIa is dependent on tissue factor (TF), which is usually available in limited quantities within the circulation, its clinical use is safe from a thrombosis-inducing point of view and its use is now being recommended as a panhaemostatic agent. FVIIa initiates the extrinsic coagulation pathway only when complexed to TF at sites of injury, thus bypassing the intrinsic pathway. It thus may have a role in a wide range of haemostatic disorders (e.g. massive blood transfusion, liver disease, uraemia, severe thrombocytopenia and platelet disorders). Recombinant human activated protein C has antithrombotic, antiinflammatory, and profibrinolytic properties and is likely to have a role in the treatment of patients with severe sepsis.

BASIC IMMUNOHAEMATOLOGY

Red cell serology is a highly specialized area of knowledge and it is not possible to expect clinicians to have more than a basic working knowledge essential for patient safety. The following is a summary of core knowledge for the clinician.

SALINE AGGLUTINATION

Safe red cell transfusion has revolved around this traditional serological technique. A saline suspension of red cells is mixed with serum and observed for agglutination. Saline agglutination is used for ABO blood grouping and is one of the techniques for compatibility testing of donor blood.

THE DIRECT AND INDIRECT ANTIGLOBULIN TEST

In red cell serology, the antiglobulin test (Coombs test) is used to detect IgG immunoglobulins or complement components. The direct antiglobulin test (DAT) detects immunoglobulin or complement components present on the surface of the red cells circulating in the patient. The result is positive in autoimmune haemolytic anaemia and haemolytic disease of the newborn and during a haemolytic transfusion reaction. The indirect antiglobulin test (IAT) detects the presence of non-agglutinating antibodies in the patient's plasma, usually IgG type. Antibody screening for atypical antibodies and pre-transfusion compatibility testing are the main applications of the IAT.

REGULAR AND IRREGULAR (ATYPICAL) ANTIBODIES

The regular alloantibodies (isoagglutinins) of the ABO system are naturally occurring agglutinins present in all ABO types (except AB), depending on the ABO group. Group O people have anti-A and anti-B isoagglutinins, group A have anti-B and group B have anti-A. Group A cells are the cause of the commonest and most dangerous ABO incompatible haemolytic reactions. Atypical antibodies are not normally present in the plasma, but may be found in some people as naturally occurring antibodies or as immune antibodies. Immune antibodies result from previous exposure due to blood transfusion or pregnancy. Naturally occurring antibodies more frequently react by saline agglutination and, although they may be stimulated by transfusion, are usually of minimal clinical significance. In contrast, many of the immune atypical antibodies are of major clinical significance and their recognition is the *raison d'étre* for pretransfusion compatibility testing and antenatal antibody screening. Most of the clinically significant immune atypical antibodies are detected by the IAT. Blood group antigens vary widely in their frequency and immunogenicity. The D antigen of the Rhesus blood group system is common and highly immunogenic. Thus, when an Rh negative (i.e. D negative) patient is exposed to D positive blood there is a high likelihood of forming an anti-D antibody. It is for this reason that the D antigen is taken into account when providing blood for transfusion, in contrast to the numerous other red cell antigens that are less common or less immunogenic. Beyond the Rh (D), and sometimes the Kell (K) blood group antigens, it is not practical, nor necessary, to take notice of other blood group antigens unless an atypical antibody is detected during antibody screening procedures.

THE ANTIBODY SCREEN

On receipt of a blood sample by the transfusion service the red cells are ABO and Rh D typed and the serum is screened for atypical antibodies. This screen consists of testing the patient's serum with group O screening cells. The screening panel consists of red cells obtained usually from two group O donors containing all common red cell antigens occurring with a frequency of greater than approximately 2% in the community. If an atypical antibody is detected on the antibody screen, further serological investigations are carried out to identify the specificity of the antibody. These investigations are time consuming and when possible should be carried out electively.

THE CROSSMATCH (COMPATIBILITY TEST)

The crossmatch is the final compatibility test between the donor cells and the patient's serum (Figure 86.5). The crossmatch test tends to be over-emphasized to the detriment of the antibody screen. With sophisticated knowledge of serology the emphasis in the supply of compatible blood is now concentrated on the steps prior to the final compatibility crossmatch.

THE TYPE AND SCREEN SYSTEM

As pre-compatibility testing has assumed the major role in the selection of blood for transfusion, there has been a rethinking of policies relating to the supply of blood for elective transfusions. Whenever elective surgery is

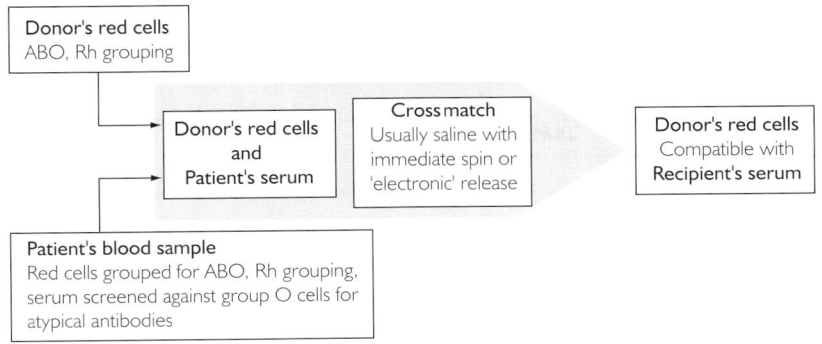

Fig. 86.5   Compatibility testing (crossmatch).

planned for a patient who is likely to require blood transfusion, the transfusion service must receive a clotted blood sample well before the anticipated time of surgery. The pre-compatibility testing should be carried out during the routine working hours when facilities are geared for large workloads and enough staff are available to handle all contingencies.

THE PROVISION OF BLOOD IN EMERGENCIES

When quick clinical and laboratory decisions are made under conditions of stress it is frequently difficult for all involved personnel to appreciate the difficulties of others. The decision to give uncrossmatched, partially crossmatched or wait for crossmatch compatible blood is not easy, and certain basic serological considerations may clarify for the clinician some of the problems faced by the serologist. Depending upon the degree of urgency and the extent of previous knowledge about the patient's red cell serology, blood can be provided with varying degrees of safety. However, it should be emphasized that when a patient is exsanguinating and likely to die, the giving of ABO compatible uncrossmatched blood, especially if the antibody screen is negative, is safe and appropriate therapy.

UNIVERSAL DONOR GROUP O BLOOD

Group O blood under normal circumstances will be ABO compatible with all recipients. The transfusions should be given as red cell concentrates screened for high titre A or B haemolysins and only used in extreme emergencies. If the recipient is in the childbearing age, every attempt should be made to give Rh D negative blood until the patient's blood group is known.

ABO GROUP SPECIFIC BLOOD

Transfusion of blood of the correct ABO type circumvents the isoagglutinin problems alluded to above. Simple as this approach may seem, its safety is dependent on meticulous attention to grouping. Previous blood group information, such as a 'bracelet' group or 'unofficial' group written in the patient's records may be incorrect, and there may be considerable risk if blood is administered on the basis of this information.

SALINE COMPATIBLE BLOOD

The administration of saline compatible blood is, for practical purposes, the administration of ABO group specific blood.

REFERENCES

1 Isbister JP. The clinicians approach to risk management. *Transfusion Science* 1994; **3**: 37–48.
2 Goodnough LT, Brecher ME, Kanter MH, *et al.* Transfusion medicine: 1. Blood transfusion. *New England Journal of Medicine* 1999a; **340**: 438–47.
3 Goodnough LT, Brecher ME, Kanter MH, *et al.* Transfusion medicine: 2. Blood conservation. *New England Journal of Medicine* 1999b; **340**: 525–33.
4 Roddie PH, Turner ML, Williamson LM. Leucocyte depletion of blood components. *Blood Rev* 2000; **14**: 145–56.
5 Brand A, van de Watering LM, Claas FH. Clinical significance of leukoreduction of blood components. *Vox Sang* 2000; **78**(suppl 2): 227–9.
6 Hamasaki N, Yamamoto M. Red cell storage function and blood storage. *Vox Sang* 2000; **79**: 191–7.
7 Timmouth A, Chin-Yee I. The clinical consequences of the red cell storage lesion. *Trans Med Rev* 2001; **15**: 91–105.
8 Moore FA, Moore EE, Sauaia A. Blood transfusion. An independent risk factor for postinjury multiple organ failure. *Archives of Surgery* 1997; **132**: 620–4.
9 Allen G, Offner PJ, Moore EE, *et al.* Age of transfused blood is an independent risk factor for postinjury multiple organ failure. *Am J Surg* 1999; **178**: 570–2.
10 Aguilera IM, Vaughan RS Calcium and the anaesthetist. *Anaesthesia* 2000; **55**: 779–90.
11 Williamson LM, Lowe S, Love EM, *et al.* Serious hazards of transfusion (SHOT) initiative: analysis of

the first two annual reports. *Brit Med J* 1999; **319**: 16–9.

12 Heddle NM. Pathophysiology of febrile nonhemolytic transfusion reactions. *Curr Opin Hematol* 1999; **6**: 420–6.

13 Dodd RY. Current viral risks of blood and blood products. *Ann Med* 2000; **32**: 469–74.

14 Isbister JP. Adverse reactions to plasma and plasma components. *Anaes Intens Care* (1993) **21**: 31–8.

15 Cyr M, Eastlund T, Blais C Jr *et al.* Bradykinin metabolism and hypotensive transfusion reactions. *Transfusion* 2001; **41**: 136–50.

16 Vamvakas EC, Blajchman MA. Deleterious clinical effects of transfusion-associated immunomodulation: fact or fiction? *Blood* 2001; **97**: 1180–95.

17 Williamson LM. Leucocyte depletion of the blood supply – how will patients benefit? *Br J Haematol* 2000; **10**: 256–72.

18 Blajchman MA, Dzik S, Vamvakas EC *et al.* Clinical and molecular basis of transfusion-induced immuno-modulation: Summary of the proceedings of a State-of-the-Art conference. *Trans Med Rev* 2001; **15**: 108–35.

19 Mynster T, Christensen IJ, Moesgaard F. Effects of the combination of blood transfusion and postoperative infectious complications on prognosis after surgery for colorectal cancer. *Brit J of Surg* 2000; **87**: 1553–62.

20 Popovsky MA. Transfusion-related acute lung injury. *Curr Opin Hematol* 2000; **7**: 402–7.

21 Goodnough LT, Despotis GJ. Establishing practice guidelines for surgical blood management. *Am J Surg* 1995; **170(suppl)**: 16S–20S.

22 Wall MH, Prielipp RC. Transfusion in the operating room and the intensive care unit: current practice and future directions. *Int Anesthesiol Clin* 2000; **38**: 149–69.

23 Spahn DR. Perioperative transfusion triggers for red blood cells. *Vox Sang* 2000; **78(suppl 2)**: 163–6 .

24 Hebert PC, Wells G, Blajchman MA, *et al.* A multicenter, randomized, controlled clinical trial of transfusion requirements in critical care. Transfusion requirements in critical care investigators, Canadian Critical Care Trials Group. *N Eng J Med* 1999; **340**: 409–17.

25 Navarro JT, Hernandez JA, Ribera JM, *et al.* Prophylactic platelet transfusion threshold during therapy for adult acute myeloid leukemia: 10 000/microL versus 20 000/microL. *Haematologica* (1998) **83**: 998–1000.

26 Rinder H, Arbini AA, Synder EL. Optimal dosing and triggers for prophylactic use of platelet transfusion. *Curr Opin Hematol* (1999) **6**: 437–41.

87

Colloids and blood products

M Mythen

Colloids are plasma expanders used to expand the blood volume. Hydrostatic and osmotic forces dictate movement of fluid between the different compartments of the body across semi-permeable membranes (Starling's forces).

The osmotic pressure generated by a solute is proportional to the number of molecules or ions of solute and independent of solute molecular size.

Colloid osmotic pressure (COP) is the osmotic pressure exerted by the macromolecules (the colloid molecules).[1,2] This can be measured using a membrane transducer system in which the membrane is freely permeable to small ions and water but largely impermeable to the colloid molecules.[3] The membrane pore size and the molecular size distribution of the colloid being studied will dictate the measured value (see Figures 87.2 and 87.3).[2,3] Capillary walls are made up of endothelial cells, which are freely permeable to small ions such as Na^+ and Cl^-, but are relatively impermeable to larger molecules such as colloids (Figure 87.3). A colloid is a homogeneous non-crystalline substance consisting of large molecules or ultramicroscopic particles of one substance dispersed through a second substance – the particles do not settle and cannot be separated out by ordinary filtering or centrifuging like those of a suspension such as blood.[2]

In practical terms, it is a fluid that when infused into the intravascular space should expand the blood volume by the volume infused.[3,4] Crystalloids have larger volumes of distribution dependent on their composition (see Figure 87.1 and Table 87.1). Colloids or plasma substitutes have molecular weights (MW) >35 kDa, and infusion results in an initial increase in blood osmotic pressure. The ideal properties of a colloid are:

- stable with a long shelf life
- pyrogen, antigen and toxin free
- free from risk of disease transmission
- plasma volume expanding effect lasts for several hours
- metabolism and excretion do not adversely effect the recipient
- no direct adverse effects, e.g. causing a coagulopathy.

COLLOID SOLUTIONS

There are two major groups of colloids – plasma derivatives or semi-synthetics.[5] Plasma derivatives include human albumin solutions, plasma protein fraction, fresh frozen plasma, and immunoglobulin solutions three principal types of semisynthetic colloid molecule commonly

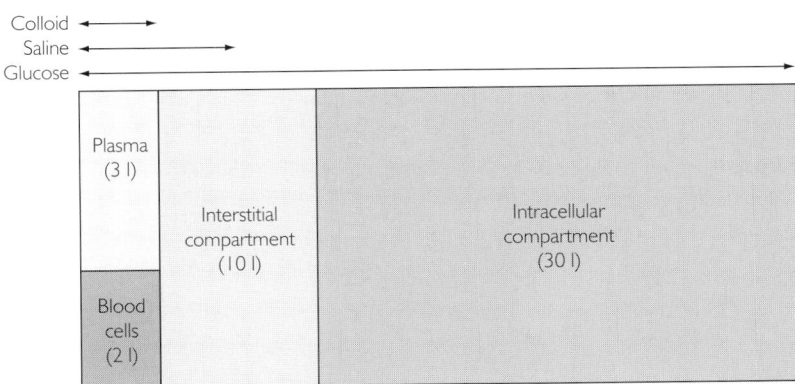

Fig. 87.1 Simplified theoretical volumes of distribution of infused isotonic solutions of an ideal colloid, saline and glucose. Reproduced with permission from ref 1.

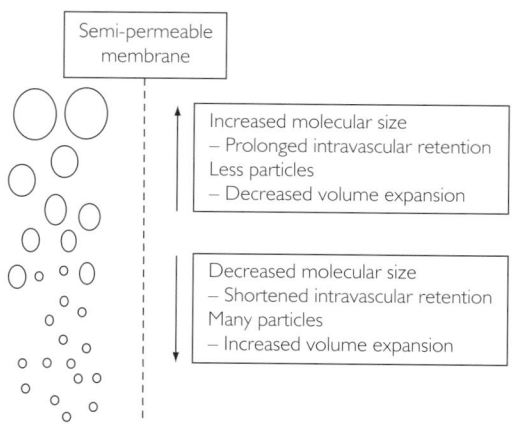

Fig. 87.2 Polydispersity of colloid molecular size. Reproduced with permission from ref 1.

Fig. 87.3 Schematic of technique for measurement of the COP50:COP10 ratio. Reproduced with permission from ref 1.

$$Cop50:Cop10 = \Delta P\ 1 : \Delta P\ 2$$

used in intravenous solutions – gelatins, dextrans and hydroxyethyl starches. All colloids are presented dissolved in a crystalloid solution. Isotonic saline is the most commonly used carrier solution but isotonic glucose, hypertonic saline and isotonic balanced electrolyte solutions are also used.

Colloids often do not consist of uniform sized molecules. Human albumin solution contains more than 95% albumin with a uniform molecular size. This is described as monodisperse. Conversely all the semisynthetic colloids have a distribution of molecular sizes and are described as polydisperse.[1,2] The size weight relationship is relatively constant although some colloids can have equivalent MW with different molecular size – succinylated and urea linked gelatins have almost identical molecular weights but the succinylated product undergoes conformational change due to an increase in negative charge and is physically larger.[2,3]

HUMAN ALBUMIN SOLUTION

Human albumin is thought of as an ideal colloid and is commonly the reference solution against which colloids are judged. Human albumin is a naturally occurring monodisperse colloid. Solutions (5% and 20%) are prepared from human plasma and heat-treated to ensure that neither hepatitis nor HIV can be transmitted. It has a relatively short (~1 year) shelf life at room temperature, but a 5-year shelf life at 2–8°C. Human albumin 5% is used for the treatment of hypovolaemia in a wide variety of clinical conditions. Concentrated salt poor 20% human albumin is used for the treatment of hypo-albuminaemia in the presence of salt and water overload (e.g. hepatic failure with ascites). Albumin has putative advantages that include limiting free radical mediated damage[6,7] but the importance of a normal serum albumin level remains uncertain.

Table 87.1 Comparison of contents, osmolarity and pH of crystalloid solutions for intravenous administration[1]

Solution	Osmolar (mosmol/l)	Ph	Na+ (mmol/l)	Cl⁻ (mmol/l)	K+ (mmol/l)	Ca²⁺ (mmol/l)	Glucose (mg/l)	HCO₃⁻ (mol/l)	Lactate (mmol/l)
Glucose 5%	252	3.5–6.5	–	–	–	–	50	–	–
Glucose 25%	1260	3.5–6.5	–	–	–	–	250	–	–
Glucose 50%	2520	3.5–6.5	–	–	–	–	500	–	–
Saline 0.9%	300	5.0	154.0	154.0	–	–	–	–	–
Glucose-saline	282	3.5–6.5	30.0	30 .0	–	–	40	–	–
Ringer's	309	5.0–7.5	147.0	156.0	4.0	2.2	–	–	–
C. Na lactate*	278	5.0–7.0	131.0	111.0	5.0	2.0	–	–	29.0
Plasmalyte B	298.5	5.5	140	98	5	–	–	50	–

*Compound sodium lactate: Hartmanns' solution or Ringer's lactate solution. Reproduced with permission from ref 1.

Human derived colloid has a number of significant disadvantages. These are expensive products and concerns have been raised about transmission of infectious agents, such as new variant Creutsfeld Jakob disease associated with BSE, that are not removed by currently available techniques. Concerns have also been raised by the conclusions of a highly controversial meta-analysis suggesting that the use of human albumin solution may be associated with increased mortality in the critically ill. These conclusions were probably unjustified,[8,9] but there is certainly no evidence that the use of human albumin has any advantages over less expensive semi-synthetic alternatives[10,11] or indeed crystalloids. However, the latter applies to all colloids[12–14].

GELATINS

Gelatins are prepared by hydrolysis of bovine collagen.[15] The commonly available preparations are succinylated gelatin (Gelofusin) and urea linked gelatin–polygeline (Haemaccel).[1,2] Because of the significant calcium content of Haemaccel, citrated blood should not be infused through a giving set that has been previously used for this product (this does not apply to SAGM blood). Gelatins are relatively inexpensive and stable, with long shelf lives. The gelatins' plasma volume expanding effect only lasts about 90–120 min.[3,4] They are mainly eliminated by renal excretion.

Incidence of reactions to gelatins are acceptable (<0.5%) and range from mild skin rash and pyrexia to life threatening anaphylaxis. The reactions appear to be related to histamine release, which is probably the result of a direct effect of gelatin on mast cells. The gelatins appear to have the least impact on haemostasis and it is not clear whether they have any impact over and above simple haemodilution of clotting factors. A specific safety issue has arisen with bovine derived gelatin products since the advent of sporadic cases of new variant Creutzfeldt-Jakob disease (CJD) associated with exposure to tissue infected with bovine spongiform encephalitis (BSE). The gelatin used in the commercially available products in the UK, for example, is sourced from the US (which is regarded as BSE free) or from certified BSE free herds in France. The UK Spongiform Encephalopathy Advisory Committee concluded that gelatin was safe to use in this context.

DEXTRANS

Dextrans are polysaccharides biosynthesized commercially from sucrose by bacterium *Leuconostoc mesenteroides* using the enzyme dextran sucrase.[1,2] This produces a high molecular weight dextran that is then cleaved by acid hydrolysis and separated by repeated ethanol fractionation to produce a final product with a relatively narrow molecular weight range. The products in current clinical use are described by their MW: Dextran 40 and Dextran 70 having MWs of 40 000 and 70 000 Da, respectively.

Dextran preparations are stable at room temperature and have long shelf lives. Dextran 70 is used as a plasma substitute for the treatment of hypovolaemia and has an intravascular volume expanding effect that lasts at least 6 h. Dextran 40 is used for its effects on microcirculatory flow and blood coagulation in some types of surgery, for example, vascular, neuro and plastic surgery. The beneficial effects on outcome when Dextran 40 is used as an 'anti-sludging agent' remain controversial. Dextran 40 should not be used as a plasma substitute for the treatment of hypovolaemia as although it produces an immediate plasma volume expansion as a result of its small molecular weight it may obstruct renal tubules and produce renal failure.[5]

Dextrans can precipitate true anaphylactic reactions, as anti-dextran antibodies may be present due to synthesis of dextrans by *Lactobacilli* that occur naturally as gut commensals. Dextran infusion, particularly of the high molecular weight products can also precipitate anaphylactoid reactions. The risk of true anaphylactic reactions can be decreased about ten-fold by pre-treatment with monovalent hapten-dextran. The Dextrans are also associated with significant haemostatic derangements. These include:

● simple haemodilution of clotting factors
● factor VIII activity is reduced
● plasminogen activation is increased
● fibrinolysis is increased
● clot strength is reduced
● impairment of platelet function.

Red cell aggregation is also reduced with the lower molecular weight Dextrans. In patients whose haemostatic function is normal prior to infusion, a maximum dose of 1.5 g/kg is often recommended to avoid risk of bleeding complications. The anti-coagulant effects of Dextrans can be utilized peri-operatively as a prophylaxis against thromboembolism.[1,2,5]

HYDROXYETHYL STARCHES

Hydroxyethyl starches (HES) are produced by hydroxyethyl substitution of amylopectin, a D-glucose polymer, obtained from sorghum or maize.[1,2] The pattern of hydroxyethyl substitution on glucose moieties influences the susceptibility to hydrolysis by non-specific amylases in the blood. A high C2 to C6 substitution ratio and a high overall degree of substitution (the proportion of glucose moieties that have been substituted) both protect against enzymatic breakdown and so prolong the effective activity of HES as a plasma volume expander.

The different HES products are commonly described by their weight-averaged molecular weight (MWw, number of molecules at each weight times the particle weight divided by the total weight of all the molecules). They are also described by their degree of substitution.[1,2–5] Hetastarches (C2/C6 ratio 0.6–0.7), pentastarches (C2/C6 ratio ≈0.5) and tetrastarches (C2/C6 ratio ≈0.4). Starch usage varies between countries. In the USA, the only starches available for clinical use are high molecular weight (>450 kDa) hetastarches presented in either normal saline or a lactate buffered, glucose containing balanced electrolyte solution (Hextend®).[16,17] There is a move in the USA towards the use of the non-saline based starch as the administration of high volumes of normal saline to humans has been associated with clinically significant acid-base disturbances.[18–21] In particular, normal saline infusion has been shown to cause a hyperchloraemic metabolic acidosis, however, the pathogenesis and significance of this phenomenon remains controversial.[18–22] Colloids presented in balanced electrolyte solutions are not currently widely available outside the USA. In the UK, medium molecular weight (220 kDa) pentastarches presented in 0.9% saline are more common, while in Continental Europe, the trend is towards the use of lower molecular weight (130 kDa) tetrastarches presented in saline.[23] Starch preparations are stable at room temperature and have long shelf lives. The duration of intravascular retention is proportional to molecular weight[3,4,24] but >6 h even for the 130 kDa tetrastarches.

HES products are associated with an acceptable incidence of adverse events including anapylactoid reactions. Tissue deposition may result in intractable itching if large volumes of HES are infused over several days.[25,26] HES products also cause a coagulopathy.[27,28] In particular HES products cause a reduction in factor VIII levels and impair platelet function causing a von Willebrand-like syndrome. These effects are greater with high molecular weight HES molecules infused at larger volumes. The effects of the high molecular weight starches on coagulation seemed to be lessened in the reformulated balanced electrolyte alternative cited above.[16]

THE ROLE OF HYPERTONIC SOLUTIONS

In recent years hypertonic (600–1800 mosmol^{-1}) crystalloid and colloid solutions have been introduced for certain clinical indications.[29–33] The theoretical advantage of these solutions is that a small volume of administered fluid will provide a significant plasma volume expansion. The high osmolarity of these solutions draws tissue fluid into the intravascular space and thus should minimize tissue oedema for a given plasma volume increment. Hypertonic crystalloids and colloids presented in a hypertonic saline carrier have been shown to achieve adequate resuscitation in a number of clinical settings.

A smaller volume of hypertonic solution is normally required to achieve similar plasma volume expansion. In particular these solutions are thought to result in reduced cerebral oedema in those patients at risk of this complication and indeed these solutions may have a place in treating refractory cerebral oedema.[31–33] Outside the peri-operative arena they are finding use in the management of burns patients and in pre-hospital resuscitation of trauma victims. They are limited at present to single dose administrations.

BLOOD SUBSTITUTES – PERFLUOROCARBON AND HAEMOGLOBIN THERAPEUTICS

In future, the use of artificial or semisynthetic oxygen carrying solutions will become increasingly common.[34] A number of products are currently under evaluation: Perflurocarbon, modified human haemoglobin (Hb), modified bovine Hb and recombinant Hb solutions. These products not only function as oxygen carriers but are also capable of sustained plasma volume expansion. Unlike Hb present in intact red cells these products often have a linear O_2Hb dissociation profile and the effects of this on O_2 uptake in the lungs and release in the tissues are not yet clearly defined. Additionally they may have specific pharmacological effects – for example, with stroma free haemaglobin nitric oxide scavenging resulting in vasoconstriction is well-recognized.

PLASMA DERIVATIVES

FRESH FROZEN PLASMA

Fresh frozen plasma (FFP) contains normal plasma levels of all the clotting factors, albumin and immunoglobulin. A unit is typically 200–250 ml and has a factor VIII level of at least 0.7 IU/ml (i.e. 70% of normal levels) and about 0.5 g of fibrinogen. It is kept at a temperature of −50°C in order to preserve coagulant levels. FFP is indicated for the replacement of multiple clotting factor deficiencies (e.g. liver disease, coumarin anticoagulant overdose and coagulopathy associated with massive blood transfusion).[35–37] An initial dose of 12–15 ml/kg (4 packs for a 70 kg adult) is appropriate. Although it is effective, FFP should not be used as a plasma volume expander solely for the treatment of hypovolaemia.

CRYOPRECIPITATE

Cryoprecipitate is usually supplied as a pool of six or so single donor units in one pack. It is prepared from FFP by using a freeze thaw method, collection of the precipitate and then re-suspending it in about 20 ml of plasma.

It contains about 50% of the coagulant factor activity of the original unit, for example, fibrinogen 250 mg, FVIII 100 IU. Cryoprecipitate is stored at −30°C and remains stable for up to a year.[35] It is indicated in the treatment of coagulation defects, including massive haemorrhage and DIC if there is microvascular bleeding associated with a fibrinogen level <0.5 g/l and as an alternative to FVIII concentrate in the treatment of inherited deficiencies of von Willebrand factor, FVIII and factor XIII.[36,37] For an adult, transfusion of 3–4 g of fibrinogen (about 16 packs) should raise the fibrinogen level by 1 g/l.

FACTOR VIII

Factor VIII concentrate is prepared from large pools of donor plasma. One freeze-dried vial contains about 300 factor VIII units.[35] The concentrates are heat or chemically treated to inactivate HIV-1. It is stable for 2 years when stored at 4°C. Further purification of the concentrate by chromatography results in high-purity factor VIII and the relative merits of high- and intermediate-purity products are being investigated. Recombinant FVIII is being increasingly commonly used in many parts of the world. Indications are the treatment of haemophilia A and von Willebrand's disease.[38] A dose of about 10–15 U/kg may be given, depending on the severity of bleeding and repeated 12-hourly, as required.

FACTOR IX

Factor IX concentrate (prothrombin concentrate) contains factors II, VII, IX and X in varying amounts, and is prepared from pools of plasma.[35] It is available as a freeze-dried preparation, and is reconstituted with water immediately before use. Factor IX concentrate of intermediate purity is used to treat haemophilia B and to correct bleeding disorders due to an overdose of coumarin anticoagulants in patients who cannot tolerate large volumes of FFP.[35] Purified factor IX concentrates are now available and are 100 times purer than the traditional concentrate, with 75% of total protein being factor IX.

OTHER PLASMA CONCENTRATES

Activated factor VII concentrate can be used in patients with inhibitors to factor VIII or IX, as it by-passes the requirement for factors VIII and IX.[35] Activated factor VII has also been used in the treatment of severe life threatening haemorrhage but this remains controversial.[39] Other concentrates, such as antithrombin III, C1 esterase inhibitor, proteins C and S are available for treating deficient patients at times of risk, such as surgery. Most of these concentrates have been used experimentally with varying success for the treatment of DIC and septic shock. Recombinant versions of most plasma factors are either clinically available or in development and will prob-ably become the standard of care. Recombinant activated protein C has been shown to be beneficial in a large human study for the treatment of septic shock[40] (see Ch. 9).

IMMUNOGLOBULINS (GAMMA-GLOBULINS)

Normal human immunoglobulin preparation is made from plasma pools obtained from normal blood donors. It contains antibodies to hepatitis A, measles, mumps, varicella, polio and prevalent bacteria.[35] Immuno-globulins are indicated in the prevention or treatment of patients with hypogamma-globulinaemia, and may have a role in the treatment of autoimmune diseases, such as thrombocytopenic purpura and myasthenia gravis. Specific immunoglobulins are available for a range of infectious agents including: tetanus, hepatitis B, rubella, measles, rabies and varicella zoster. They are made from donor plasma known to contain high levels of the specific IgG antibodies and are used for prophylaxis and treatment in patients who have not been actively immunized. Rhesus-D immunoglo-bulin is prepared from plasma containing high levels of anti Rh-D anti-bodies and it prevents sensitization of Rh-negative mothers to Rh-D positive cells that may enter their circu-lation. The principal use of Rh-D immunoglobulin is in the prevention of haemolytic disease of the newborn.[41]

REFERENCES

1 Grocott MPW, Mythen MG. Fluid therapy. In: Goldhill DR, Strunin L (eds) *Clinical Anaesthesiology*. London: Baillière Tindall; 1999: pp. 363–81.

2 Salmon JB, Mythen MG. Pharmacology and physiology of colloids. *Blood Reviews* 1993; 7: 114–20.

3 Webb AR, Barclay SA, Bennett ED. In vitro colloid osmotic pressure of commonly used plasma expanders and substitutes: a study of the diffusibility of colloid molecules. *Intensive Care Medicine* 1989; 15: 116–20.

4 Lamke LO, Liljedahl SO. Plasma volume changes after infusion of various plasma expanders. *Resuscitation* 1976; 5: 93–102.

5 Haljamae H, Dahlqvist M, Walentin F. Artificial colloids in clinical practise: pros and cons. *Clin Anaesthes* 1997; 11: 49–79.

6 Halliwell B. Albumin – an important extracellular antioxidant? *Biochem Pharmacol* 1988; 37: 569–71.

7 Strubelt O, Younes M, Li Y. Protection by albumin against ischaemia- and hypoxia-induced hepatic injury. *Pharmacol Toxicol* 1994; 75: 280–4.

8 Cochrane Injuries Group Albumin Reviewers. Human albumin administration in critically ill patients: systematic review of randomised controlled trials. *BMJ* 1998; 317: 235–40.

9 Bunn F, Alderson P, Hawkins V. Colloid solutions for fluid resuscitation (Cochrane Review). *The Cochrane Library* 4: 2000.

10 Stockwell M, Soni N, Riley B. Colloid solutions in the critically ill. A randomized comparison of albumin and

polygeline. 1. Outcome and duration of stay in the intensive care unit. *Anaesthesia* 1992; **47**: 3–6.

11 Stockwell M, Scott A, Riley B, *et al.* Colloid solutions in the critically ill. A randomised comparison of albumin and polygeline. 2. Serum albumin concentration and incidences of pulmonary oedema and acute renal failure. *Anaesthesia* 1992; **47**: 7–9.

12 Velanovich V. Crystalloid versus colloid fluid resuscitation: a meta-analysis of mortality. *Surgery* 1989; **105**: 65–71.

13 Schierhout G, Roberts I. Fluid resuscitation with colloid or crystalloid solutions in critically ill patients: a systematic review of randomised trials. *BMJ* 1998; **316**: 961–4.

14 Choi P, Yip G, Quinonez L, Cook D. Crystalloids vs colloids in fluid resuscitation; a systematic review. *Crit Care Med* 1999; **27**: 200–10.

15 Davies MJ. Polygeline. *Dev Biol Stand* 1987; **67**: 129–31.

16 Gan TJ, Bennett-Guerrero E, Phillips-Bute B, *et al.* Hextend, a physiological balanced plasma expander for large volume use in major surgery: a randomized phase III clinical trial. *Anesth Analg* 1999; **88**: 992–8.

17 Waters JH, Gottlieb A, Schoenwald P *et al.* Normal saline versus lactated Ringer's solution for intraoperative fluid management in patients undergoing abdominal aortic aneurysm repair: an outcome study. *Anesth Analg* 2001; **93**: 817–22.

18 Prough DS, Bidani A. Hyperchloremic metabolic acidosis is a predictable consequence of intraoperative infusion of 0.9% saline. *Anesthesiology* 1999; **90**: 1247–9.

19 Brill SA, Stewart TR, Brundage SI *et al.* Base deficit does not predict mortality when secondary to hyperchloremic acidosis. *Shock* 1999; **17**: 459–62.

20 Williams EL, Hildebrand KL, McCormick SA, Bedel MJ. The effect of intravenous lactated Ringer's solution versus 0.9% sodium chloride solution on serum osmolality in human volunteers. *Anesth Analg* 1999; **88**: 999–1003.

21 Wilkes NJ, Woolf R, Stephens R *et al.* The effects of balanced versus saline based intravenous solutions on acid base status and gastric mucosal perfusion in elderly surgical patients. *Anesth Analg* 2001; **93**: 811–6.

22 Healey MA, Davis RE, Liu FC *et al.* Lactated Ringer's is superior to normal saline in a model of massive hemorrhage and resuscitation. *J Trauma* 1998; **45**: 894–9.

23 Treib J, Baron JF, Grauer MT, *et al.* An international view of hydroxyethyl starches. *Intens Care Med* 1999; **25**: 258–68.

24 Degremont AC, Ismail M, Arthaud M, *et al.* Mechanisms of postoperative prolonged plasma volume expansion with low molecular weight hydroxyethyl starch (HES 200/0.62, 6%). *Intens Care Med* 1995; **21**: 577–83.

25 Morgan PW, Berridge JC. Giving long persistent starch as volume replacement can cause pruritus after cardiac surgery. *Br J Anaesth* 2000; **85**: 696–9.

26 Murphy M, Carmichael AJ, Lawler PG, *et al.* The incidence of hydroxyethyl starch-associated pruritus. *Br J Dermatol* 2001; **144**: 973–6.

27 Treib J, Baron JF. Hydroxethyl starch: effects on hemostasis. *Ann Fr Anesth Reanim* 1998; **17**: 72–81.

28 Jamnicki M, Bombeli T, Seifert B, *et al.* Low and medium molecular weight hydroxyethyl starches; comparison of their effect on blood coagulation. *Anesthesiology* 2000; **95**: 1231–7.

29 Rabinovici R, Gross D, Krausz MM. Infusion of small volume of 7.5 per cent sodium chloride in 6.0 per cent dextran 70 for the treatment of uncontrolled hemorrhagic shock. *Surg Gynecol Obstet* 1989; **169**: 137–42.

30 Oi Y, Aneman A, Svensson M *et al.* Hypertonic saline-dextran improves intestinal perfusion and survival in porcine endotoxin shock. *Crit Care Med* 2000; **28**: 2843–50.

31 Simma B, Burger R, Falk M, *et al.* A prospective, randomized, and controlled study of fluid management in children with severe head injury: lactated Ringer's solution versus hypertonic saline. *Crit Care Med* 1998; **26**: 1265–70.

32 Qureshi AI, Suarez JI. Use of hypertonic saline solutions in treatment of cerebral edema and intracranial hypertension. *Crit Care Med* 2000; **28**: 3301–13.

33 Shackford SR, Bourguignon PR, Wald SL, *et al.* Hypertonic saline resuscitation of patients with head injury: a prospective, randomized clinical trial. *J Trauma* 1998; **44**: 50–8.

34 Hill SE Oxygen therapeutics – current concepts. *Can J Anaesth* 2001; **48**: S32–40.

35 McClelland DBL (ed.) *Handbook of Transfusion Medicine.* London: HMSO; 1989.

36 Mammen EF (2000) Disseminated intravascular coagulation (DIC). *Clin Lab Sci* 2000; **13**: 239–45.

37 Mythen MG, Machin SJ. Derangements of blood coagulation. In Hanson GC (ed.) *Critical Care of the Surgical Patient.* London: Chapman and Hall; 1997: 185–94.

38 Hambleton J. Advances in the treatment of von Willebrand disease. *Semin Hematol* 2001; **38**: 7–10.

39 Moscardo F, Perez F, de la Rubia J, *et al.* Successful treatment of severe intra-abdominal bleeding associated with disseminated intravascular coagulation using recombinant activated VII. *Br J Haematol* 2001; **114**: 174–6.

40 Bernard GR, Vincent JL, Laterre PF, *et al.* Efficacy and safety of recombinant human activated protein C for severe sepsis *N Engl J Med* 2001; **344**: 699–709.

41 Greenough A. The role of immunoglobulins in neonatal rhesus haemolytic disease *BioDrugs* 2001; **15**: 533–41.

88.

Therapeutic plasma exchange

J P Isbister

Bloodletting to remove 'evil humours' has a long history of over 2000 years. Although not based on logic in the past, the removal of noxious agents from the blood remains the rationale, and now there is scientific understanding of the pathophysiology of the diseases treated by plasma exchange. Exchange transfusions revolutionized the management of haemolytic disease in the newborn, and paved the way for therapeutic plasmapheresis and plasma exchange – the removal of plasma, with replacement by albumin-electrolyte solutions or fresh frozen plasma.[1]

Plasma exchange was initially used in the management of hyperviscosity associated with malignant paraproteinaemia, but is now also used in the treatment of a wide range of autoimmune disorders (now >100). Nevertheless, it is expensive and not risk-free and debate continues on its therapeutic role in some diseases.

RATIONALE FOR PLASMA EXCHANGE

Theoretically, plasma exchange should be effective to treat any disorder in which there is a pathogenic circulating factor responsible for the disease. However, this premise is probably too simplistic, and other mechanisms may contribute to its beneficial effects (Table 88.1). It is a non-specific procedure, which brings about numerous, potentially undesirable, alterations in the plasma's *milieu interieur*.

Table 88.1 Rationale for plasma exchange

Removal of circulating toxic factor antibodies
    Monoclonal antibodies
    Autoantibodies
    Alloantibodies, immune complexes, chemicals, drugs
Depletion of the mediators of inflammation
Replacement of deficient plasma factor(s)
Potentiation of drug action
Enhanced reticuloendothelial function
Altered immunoregulation
Potentiating effects of plasma exchange on other modes of
    therapy

PATHOPHYSIOLOGY OF AUTOIMMUNE DISEASE

Autoimmune disease originates from the breakdown of immunoregulation (i.e. immune tolerance), allowing the immune system to become autoaggressive. Autoimmune diseases having underlying humoral mechanisms result from either a circulating autoantibody against a self-antigen (alone or in combination with an environmental antigen), or circulating immune complexes (which may be deposited in the microcirculation of various organs, resulting in end-organ damage). Cellular and tissue damage is effected by the autoantibody or immune complexes activating the cellular and humoral components of the inflammatory response. The circulating proteolytic systems involved include the complement, coagulation, fibrinolytic and kinin systems. On the cellular side, neutrophils and macrophages are involved, with eosinophils and basophils also playing a part.

The varied clinical manifestations of autoimmune disorders relate more to the cell, tissue or organ involved, rather than the pathophysiological process. However, basic pathophysiological mechanisms by which autoimmune disease occurs, need to be understood in order to standardize treatment. Although some cells of the host defence system, in particular the macrophages and lymphocytes, may have special differentiation appropriate to individual organs, their basic functional processes are not all that dissimilar between different organs.

In general, autoimmune disease can be an acute, self-limiting ('one hit'), intermittent or a chronic perpetuating disorder. Acute autoimmune disease may have an identifiable trigger, such as an infection, followed by a 10-day to 3-week gap until the pathogenic humoral or cellular factors appear in the circulating blood. At this point, end-organ damage commences, and clinical features of the disease appear.

The course of the disease will be determined by several factors:

- biological function and importance of the system involved
- extent of damage

- replaceability or otherwise of the cells under attack
- time course of the damaging insult

The extent of damage is a product of the:

- characteristics of the antibodies or lymphocytes involved (egg antibody affinity, complement fixing capabilities and titre)
- function of other components of the host defence system (e.g. neutrophils, platelets, proteolytic systems and reticuloendothelial system) and
- presence of other aggravating factors (e.g. infection, hormonal responses, and circulatory responses).

The kinetics of the end-cell involved in the immunological damage is relevant in determining the final outcome of the disease. Ultimate recovery of organ function after 'burn out' of a self-limiting autoimmune disease or control of a chronic autoimmune disease, is determined by the ability of the cell to replace and restore function to normal.

Cells are broadly divided into three kinetic characteristics:

- *Continuous replicators* – These cells are continuously replaced in the normal state. They are readily replaced when damaged, and if the immunological insult is removed or controlled, full replacement of the end-cells occurs. This is typically seen with the haemopoietic system, the cells lining the gut and skin cells.
- *Discontinuous replicators* – These are cells that are not being constantly replaced in the normal state, but when damaged, cell division is initiated and replacement occurs. This is seen with hepatocytes, renal tubular cells and the neuronal Schwann cell.
- *Non replicating cells* – These cells when damaged are irreplaceably destroyed with permanent loss of function. This is seen with neuronal cells, muscle cells and glomeruli.

Thus, the clinical features and final outcome of any autoimmune disease is determined by many different factors, including the ability of the end-organ to repair itself following removal/control of the immunological insult. In many self-limiting autoimmune diseases, if the end-cell is a continuous or intermittent replicator, full recovery can be expected, as long as appropriate support to end-organ function is given during the acute phase. Examples are acute tubular necrosis, acute demyelination, acute hepatic failure and some forms of marrow aplasia.

However, in disorders with non-replicating cells such as acute glomerulonephritis, therapy must be aimed to remove the immunological insult or dampen its damaging affects, so as to minimize irreparable damage to the end-cells. Immunological mediators may also produce disease without direct destruction of end-cells. This occurs when autoantibodies develop against cell receptors, with blocking or destruction of the receptor as is typically seen in myasthenia gravis and thyrotoxicosis.

Therapy in acute and chronic autoimmune disease aims to minimize irreparable end-organ damage and support patients during the acute illness. This can include:

- non-specific therapy to suppress the effector mechanisms, e.g. corticosteroids, antiplatelet therapy, non-steroidal anti-inflammatory drugs, anticoagulation and depletion of humoral effector mechanisms by plasma exchange or defibrination.
- therapy to reduce the circulating levels of a humoral factor is achieved with plasma exchange or immuno-absorption techniques.
- Specific or broad-spectrum immunosuppressive agents to suppress or block the immune response, e.g. corticosteroids, cytotoxic agents, anti-lymphocyte globulin, high-dose intravenous γ-globulin therapy.
- therapy directed at altering reticuloendothelial function, which may then have effects on autoantibody and immune complex clearance, or clearance of circulating damaged cells.

As most disorders are multifactorial, it is unlikely that a single form of therapy will be successful. A multipronged approach to therapy needs to be planned following an analysis of the basic underlying pathophysiology. The stage of the disease is also important (Figure 88.1). Clearly, plasma exchange will have a different response when autoantibody production is rising rapidly, compared with a stage when autoantibody has ceased production. Also, immunoregulation is a complex process, and therapies may interfere at different points in the immune mechanisms.

In some circumstances, specific and directed therapy may attack the most relevant link in the pathophysiological chain, but overall multiple approaches to therapy may be required. In general, plasma exchange is a temporizing procedure and concomitant immunosuppressive therapy is required to maintain control. Plasma exchange for autoimmune disease should generally be regarded as a first step in immunosuppression, and restricted to acute or fulminant situations in which autoantibodies or immune complexes are responsible for life-threatening or end-organ damaging complications. There are some situations in which the humoral factor may be only transient ('one antigen hit' disorders), and no follow up immunosuppression is required (e.g. acute post infectious polyneuritis).

TECHNICAL CONSIDERATIONS

Cell separators available for plasma exchange therapy are broadly divided into two groups:

1 Machines that use centrifugation for the separation and are also suitable for specific separation and removal of blood components (e.g. thrombopheresis and leucapheresis).

2 Machines that separate by membrane filtration and can only be used for plasma separation.

Either of these techniques for plasma exchange can be combined with immunoabsorption techniques, in which immunoglobulins are specifically or non-specifically removed.

As plasma is removed, it is replaced volume for volume with a solution of adequate colloid activity (e.g. 5% albumin) and appropriate electrolyte composition. Although the levels of other plasma proteins are reduced by plasma exchange, there are rarely clinically significant effects. However, if extremely large volumes are exchanged, or exchanges are done frequently, it may be necessary to replace some plasma proteins. In patients with coagulation factor deficiencies or immunodeficiency, fresh frozen plasma is usually required.

INDICATIONS

Acute diseases in which plasma exchange may be beneficial are shown in Table 88.2. Plasma exchange is most beneficial for immunoproliferative and auto-immune diseases. In some conditions with unclear pathophysiology, beneficial effects of plasma exchange

may be due to infusion of a deficient component in the replacement plasma, rather than removal of a circulating factor.

MONOCLONAL ANTIBODIES ASSOCIATED WITH IMMUNOPROLIFERATIVE DISEASES

Monoclonal immunoglobulins[2,3] are a classical feature of multiple myeloma and Waldenström's macroglobulinaemia, but may also be associated with other lymphoproliferative disorders. These monoclonal proteins may be associated with numerous clinical effects, many of which may be reversed by plasma exchange.

HYPERVISCOSITY SYNDROME
Characteristic clinical features of hyperviscosity in association with monoclonal proteins include visual disturbance, neurological dysfunction and hypervolaemia, all of which can be rapidly relieved by plasma exchange.

HAEMOSTATIC DISTURBANCES
Monoclonal proteins may impair haemostasis by adversely effecting platelet function or by inhibitory effects on coagulation factors. Plasma exchange is usually effective in controlling haemorrhage and may also be helpful in preparing patients for surgery.

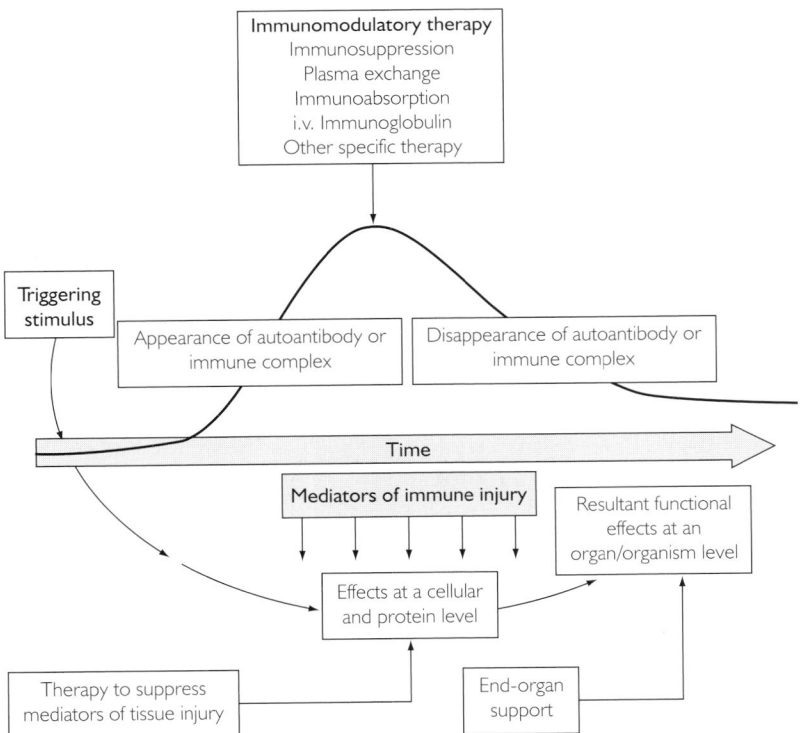

Fig. 88.1 The therapy of 'one hit' autoimmune disease.

Table 88.2 Acute diseases in which plasma exchange may be beneficial*

Immunoproliferative diseases with monoclonal immunoglobulins
> Hyperviscosity syndrome
> Cryoglobulinaemia
> Renal failure in multiple myeloma

Autoimmune diseases due to autoantibodies or immune complexes
> Goodpasture's syndrome
> Myasthenia gravis
> Guillain–Barré syndrome
> Chronic inflammatory demyelinating polyneuropathy (CIDP)
> Stiff-man syndrome
> Systemic lupus erythematosus
> Fulminant antiphospholipid syndrome
> Thrombotic thrombocytopenic purpura
> Haemolytic uraemic syndrome
> Rapidly progressive glomerulonephritis
> Coagulation inhibitors
> Autoimmune haemolytic anaemia
> Pemphigus
> Paraneoplastic syndromes

Conditions in which replacement of plasma may be beneficial ± removal of toxins[16]
> Disseminated intravascular coagulation
> Multi-organ dysfunction syndrome
> Overwhelming sepsis syndromes (e.g. meningococcaemia)

Conditions in which the mechanisms are unknown
> Reye's syndrome

Removal of protein bound or large molecular weight toxins
> Paraquat poisoning
> Envenomation?

---

*This is an incomplete list and only includes disorders which are relatively common or in which plasma exchange has a definitive role to play.

RENAL FAILURE

The development of renal failure in the course of multiple myeloma is generally regarded as a sign of poor prognosis. In most cases, the renal failure is multifactorial in origin, but some of these factors may be reversible by plasma exchange. Patients presenting acutely with hyperviscosity, dehydration and hypercalcaemia may show recovery of renal function following adequate hydration, alkaline diuresis and plasma exchange.

IMMUNOLOGICAL DISEASES

DISEASES MEDIATED BY SPECIFIC AUTOANTIBODIES

Goodpasture's Syndrome

Most cases of Goodpasture's[4,5] circulating antiglomerular basement membrane antibodies can be demonstrated.

The disease classically has a fulminant presentation with rapidly progressive renal failure and life-threatening pulmonary haemorrhage. Early diagnosis and intensive plasma exchange may be necessary to preserve renal function and control pulmonary haemorrhage. Patients who are already in anuric renal failure rarely show improvement in renal function.

Myasthenia Gravis[6,7]

Removal of the acetylcholine receptor autoantibody is associated with clinical improvement in the majority of patients with this disorder. The beneficial effects of plasma exchange are usually transient, and the procedure should usually be used in conjunction with other forms of therapy. The major role for plasma exchange is usually in myasthenic crisis, in patients whose condition is resistant to other forms of therapy, and prior to surgery. Therapy can be monitored by acetylcholine receptor autoantibody assays and respiratory function tests. Patients undergoing plasma exchange may transiently deteriorate during the procedure, due to a combination of the physical exertion and removal of medication from the circulation, and adequate ventilatory support should be available.

Stiff-man Syndrome

Stiff-man syndrome[8] is a rare neurological disorder characterized by involuntary axial and proximal limb rigidity and continuous motor unit activity on electromyography. Autoantibodies to glutamic acid decarboxylase are usually demonstrable. Plasma exchange is successful, especially in those in whom autoantibody can be demonstrated negative are less likely to respond.

Autoimmune Haematological Disorders

Haemostatic failure due to autoantibodies directed against coagulation factors may present a major management problem. Antibodies directed against factor VIII are the commonest, occurring spontaneously or in association with replacement therapy in haemophiliacs.

IMMUNE COMPLEX DISEASE
Rapidly Progressive Glomerulonephritis

Immune complex[4,9] induced rapidly progressive glomerulonephritis may occur by itself or be associated with several systemic disorders (e.g. systemic lupus erythematosus, polyarteritis nodosa, and Wegener's granulomatosis). Plasma exchange may result in improvement in renal function even in patients who present with anuria. The decomplementing and defibrinating effects of plasma exchange may be partly responsible for clinical improvement. The therapeutic role of plasma exchange in rapidly progressive glomerulonephritis is difficult to assess, but most experienced physicians feel that the procedure leads to a more rapid and complete recovery of renal function in fulminant, rapidly deteriorating cases.

However, the ultimate prognosis of the disease depends on adequate immunosuppression to inhibit immune complex formation, or spontaneous disappearance of the inciting antigen.

Systemic Lupus Erythematosus

Plasma exchange has a role in acute life-threatening or organ-damaging relapses of systemic lupus erythematosus (SLE). Rapid deterioration in renal function, cerebritis, and acute fulminant lupus pneumonitis are clinical situations in which plasma exchange should be considered.

Cryoglobulinaemia

The various forms of cryoglobulinaemia may be associated with vasculitis or hyperviscosity. In some cases, there may be an acute fulminant presentation with cutaneous vasculitis, renal failure, and neurological impairment. In this situation, plasma exchange should be considered an urgent definitive form of therapy.

OTHER IMMUNE MEDIATED DISEASES
Renal Transplant Rejection

Humoral mechanisms appear to play a part in hyperacute renal allograft rejection. Plasma exchange may be useful in tiding patients over episodes of acute graft rejection, but results of clinical trials have been conflicting. General opinion is that plasma exchange helps in a limited number of patients who cannot be currently pre-selected by any clinical or laboratory criteria.

Thrombotic Thrombocytopenic Purpura

Thrombotic thrombocytopenic purpura[10] (TTP) is a potentially fulminant and life-threatening disorder characterized by platelet microthrombi in small vessels, resulting in microangiopathy. The clinical syndrome is manifest by the pentad of thrombocytopenia, microangiopathic haemolytic anaemia, fever, renal dysfunction and neurologic abnormalities. Abdominal symptoms, hepatic dysfunction and pulmonary abnormalities may also occur. With the appropriate clinical features, thrombocytopenia and a microangiopathic blood film, diagnosis is established.

The presence of an inhibitor to vWF reducing metalloproteinase has been documented in patients with both acute TTP and those with chronic relapsing forms. In normal plasma vWF undergoes proteolysis by a specific protease and deficiency of this cleaving protease reduces or abolishes the plasma clearance of ultralarge vWF multimers resulting in intravascular aggregation of platelets, particularly at sites of intravascular shear stress. The inhibitor to the metalloproteinase has been demonstrated to be an IgG autoantibody.

There is a primary idiopathic form of the disease that usually has an acute presentation and probably has an underlying autoimmune mechanism. This form may be associated with a variety of prodromal infections (viral or bacteria). Bacterial cytotoxins, produced by *Shigella dysenteriae 1* and certain *E. coli* serotypes, have been related to TTP and HUS, probably by initiating damage to vascular endothelial cells, possibly via cytokine mechanisms. TTP may be associated with various drugs (cytotoxic agents), toxins and bites. CMV, HIV and herpes viruses have also been implicated. Chemotherapy-associated thrombotic thrombocytopenic purpura/haemolytic uraemic syndrome is being increasingly recognized and may be associated with a range of cytotoxic medications. Severe microangiopathy resembling TTP has also been reported as a complication of acute graft-versus-host disease in patients receiving cyclosporin prophylaxis following allogeneic BMT.

TTP used to be a fatal disease in 90% of patients, but dramatic improvement in its outcome has occurred over the past two decades with the development of effective therapy. Plasma exchange has become the cornerstone of the treatment with FFP replacement. Cryoprecipitate-poor plasma (depleted in vWF) may offer advantages over whole fresh frozen plasma. It is now possible to achieve remissions in the majority of patients and cures are now common, although unfortunately relapse may occur. The clinical course at relapse is usually milder than the disease at presentation and less aggressive therapy may be needed.

Haemolytic Uraemic Syndrome

Haemolytic uraemic syndrome (HUS) has many similarities to TTP, but renal involvement is the hallmark in association with microangiopathy and thrombocytopenia. The prognosis and approach to management of HUS is similar to TTP. It usually occurs in children (related to bacterial or viral infections), but may rarely be seen in adults, in whom the disease may take a more chronic and sinister course. In adult cases, medications are commonly implicated.

Inflammatory Demyelinating Neuropathies[11-14]

The acute self-limiting form of the disease (Guillain–Barré syndrome) in which an acute demyelinating neuropathy occurs (usually following a viral infection) commonly results in admission to the ICU. There is demyelination due to postinfectious autoimmunity, with both cellular and humoral arms of the immune system attacking myelin. There is now wide experience in the use of plasma exchange in Guillain–Barré syndrome, with controlled trials substantiating its benefits of shortening of the illness, and complications. Plasma exchange should be instituted early and frequently. Guillain–Barré syndrome also responds to high-dose i.v. immunoglobulin and in cases failing plasma exchange it should be the next line of therapy. In some cases the onset of recovery after plasma exchange may be delayed, probably due to time for remyelination to occur. Some patients show rapid improvement after plasma exchange, suggesting the presence of neuronal blocking factors. Chronic inflammatory demyelinating peripheral neuropathy (CIPD) is related to the GBS and plasma exchange has an important role in treatment requires long-term immunomodulatory therapy.

COMPLICATIONS

Plasma exchange is a relatively safe procedure, but close supervision by experienced physicians and nurses is essential. A sound understanding of the haemodynamic, biochemical, haematological and immunological effects of plasma exchange is of paramount importance.

Potential complications[15] of plasma exchange include: fluid imbalance, reactions to replacement fluids, vasovagal reactions, pyrogenic reactions, hypothermia, embolism (air or microaggregates), hypocalcaemia, anaemia, thrombocytopenia, haemostatic disturbances, hepatitis, hypogammaglobulinaemia, and altered pharmacokinetics of drugs. Prevention and treatment of most of these complications is usually obvious, but specific mention should be made of the following effects.

CIRCULATORY EFFECTS

Any extracorporeal procedure is likely to lead to problems of circulatory instability. Intravascular volume changes, vasovagal reactions, medications and infusion fluids may all alone, or in combination, be responsible for circulatory problems. If there are no associated oxygen transport defects, the patient will usually be able to compensate. However, if there are pre-existing defects (e.g. altered blood volume, vascular disease, or renal failure), close monitoring is essential. A strict fluid and electrolyte balance should be kept at all times, both during the plasma exchange and also as a daily tally.

PLASMA ONCOTIC PRESSURE

Most patients compensate for minor fluctuations in plasma oncotic pressure (COP). Patients who have oedema or local factors predisposing to interstitial fluid accumulation (e.g. raised intracranial pressure, interstitial pulmonary oedema, deep venous thrombosis, and renal impairment), need close attention.

INFECTION

Many patients who are undergoing plasma exchange are already immunosuppressed, either due to their disease, or secondary to drug therapy. In patients requiring recurrent and frequent plasma exchange, attempts should be made to maintain serum immunoglobulin levels. When fresh frozen plasma is not used as replacement fluid, the bacteriocidal and opsonic activities of blood are probably impaired, and it is probably advantageous to infuse at least two units of fresh frozen plasma at the conclusion of the procedure. At the completion of a course of plasma exchange consideration may need to be given to a dose of intravenous gammaglobulin.

HAEMOSTASIS

Plasma exchange causes perturbations in the haemostatic system which may result in either bleeding or thrombosis. The significance of these alterations will depend largely on the volume and frequency of exchange, pre-existing defects in the system, anticoagulation, other risk factors for thrombosis, replacement fluids and invasive procedures.

REACTIONS TO REPLACEMENT FLUIDS

The rapid infusion of any blood component may be associated with allergic or vasomotor reactions. Plasma exchange is a rather unique situation in which blood or blood products and plasma substitutes are being infused at resuscitation rates into normovolaemic, normotensive patients.

EFFECTS ON INTRAVASCULAR PROTEINS

If plasma protein fractions or albumin are being used for replacement fluids, not only will coagulation and complement components be depleted, but various transport and binding proteins in the circulation are significantly reduced. These may have significant effects on drug activity and elimination, e.g. antithrombin III levels may have effects on heparin activity. The effects of corticosteroids may be potentiated after plasma exchange owing to a reduction in binding proteins.

REFERENCES

1 Isbister JP. Plasma exchange: A selective form of blood-letting. *Aust Med J* 1979; **2**: 167–9.
2 Reinhart WH, Lutolf O, Nydegger U *et al.* Plasmapheresis for hyperviscosity syndrome in macroglobulinemia Waldenström and multiple myeloma: Influence on blood rheology and the microcirculation. *J Lab Clin Med* 1992; **119**: 69–76.
3 Isbister JP, Harris DCH, Ibels LS. The management of renal failure in multiple myeloma. *Clin Exper Haemorheology* 1984; **5**: 373–84.
4 Kaplan AA. Apheresis for renal disease. *Ther Apher* 2001; **5**: 134–41.
5 Levy JB, Turner AN, Rees AJ, Pusey CD. Long-term outcome of anti-glomerular basement membrane antibody disease treated with plasma exchange and immunosuppression. *Ann Intern Med* 2001; **134**: 1033–42.
6 Lisak RP. Myasthenia gravis. *Curr Treat Options Neurol* 1999; **1**: 239–50.

7 Qureshi AI, Suri MF. Plasma exchange for treatment of myasthenia gravis: pathophysiologic basis and clinical experience. *Ther Apher* 2000; **4**: 280–6.

8 Shariatmadar S, Noto TA. Plasma exchange in stiff-man syndrome. *Ther Apher* 2001; **5**: 64–7.

9 Pusey CD, Rees AJ, Evans DJ *et al.* Plasma exchange in focal necrotizing glomerulonephritis without anti-GBM antibodies. *Kidney Int* 1991; **40**: 757–63.

10 Knobl P, Rintelen C, Kornek G, *et al.* Plasma exchange for treatment of thrombotic thrombocytopenic purpura in critically ill patients. *Frass M Intensive Care Med* 1997; **23**: 44–50.

11 Haupt WF. Recent advances of therapeutic apheresis in Guillain–Barré syndrome. *Ther Apher* 2000; **4**: 271–4.

12 Weinshenker BG. Plasma exchange for severe attacks of inflammatory demyelinating diseases of the central nervous system. *J Clin Apheresis* 2001; **16**: 39–42.

13 van Der Meche FG, van Doorn PA. Guillain–Barré syndrome. *Curr Treat Options Neurol* 2000; **6**: 507–16.

14 Gorson KC, Chaudhry VV. Chronic inflammatory demyelinating polyneuropathy. *Curr Treat Options Neurol* 1999; **3**: 251–62.

15 Mokrzycki MH, Kaplan AA. Therapeutic plasma exchange: Complications and management. *Am J Kidney Dis* 1994; **23**: 817–27.

16 Stegmayr BG. Apheresis as therapy for patients with severe sepsis and multiorgan dysfunction syndrome. *Ther Apher* 2001; **5**: 123–7.

89.

Haemostatic failure

J P Isbister

Failure of haemostasis is common in critically ill patients and may be complex and multifactorial in pathogenesis. As haemostatic failure may complicate a wide range of medical, surgical and obstetric disorders, definitive diagnosis and specific therapy can significantly impact on outcome. Frequently, complex tests are required for definitive diagnosis, but the urgency of the situation cannot always wait for the results, and therapy may be initiated on clinical evidence with minimal laboratory information. Consultation with a clinical haematologist is strongly recommended.

NORMAL HAEMOSTASIS[1,2]

The haemostatic system is a delicately controlled component of the host defence system. Its role is to initiate haemostasis, where and when required, in adequate, but not excessive, amounts. The system closely interacts with other components of the host defence system, including the acute stress responses, inflammation, healing and immune functions. The conversion of blood from its fluid to solid state is a reasonably well-understood physiological process. The triad of vascular constriction, platelet plugging and fibrin clot formation forms haemostatic plugs and provides the framework on which haemostasis operates (Fig. 89.1) and healing occurs. Following injury, vascular constriction occurs initially reducing bleeding, and allowing time to initiate haemostasis. This constriction is further accentuated by vasoconstrictors released in association with platelet plug formation. Vascular endothelial cells play an active part by synthesizing substances which act at the membrane surface and/or interact with platelets and the coagulation system (e.g. prostacyclin, antithrombin III, plasminogen activator, Von Willebrand's factor (vWF), thrombomodulin, heparin cofactor II and nitric oxide). Following the initial vascular reactions, successful haemostasis depends on adequate numbers of functioning platelets, coagulation cascade function, and poorly understood contributions from red cells and leukocytes. Von Willebrand's factor is a multimeric glycoprotein. It plays a central role in haemostasis by mediating adhesion of platelets to the exposed subendothelium and by linking the primary vascular/platelet phase with coagulation. This occurs because it is the carrier protein for coagulant factor VIII. Factor VIII then dissociates from vWF to form a complex on the activated platelet surface with IXa (tenase complex) to activate factor X to Xa.

The coagulation system is triggered via the extrinsic pathway, by which damaged tissues expose tissue factor. Tissue factor is a membrane glyco protein present on cells surrounding the vascular bed. Factor VII and VIIa (a small amount circulates normally in the blood) are bound to tissue factor, initiating haemostasis. The concept of the intrinsic and extrinsic systems is more of historical and laboratory significance as it is now clear that such a division is artificial. However, the concept still has value in performing and assessing haemostatic laboratory tests.

The prothombinase complex (phospholipid bound Xa and Va) converts prothrombin to thrombin. Small amounts of thrombin generated activate platelets in the vicinity. The platelet surface now becomes the site for amplification of haemostasis and subsequent propagation. Thrombin is the potent proteolytic enzyme of the coagulation sequence converting fibrinogen to fibrin soluble monomers, which subsequently polymerize to form the fibrin clot. Fibrinogen is the bulk protein of the coagulation system and fibrin is the end-product of this cascade of proteolytic activity, in which precursor coagulation proteins are activated to potent proteolytic enzymes, with the aid of cofactors, to produce further activate precursors down the coagulation 'amplifier'. The polymerized fibrin is further acted on by factor XIII to form a stable fibrin clot.

The intrinsic coagulation system is initiated by activation of the contact phase (i.e. factors XII and XI). The other plasma proteolytic systems, the fibrinolytic, kinin, and complement systems, may be activated in concert with coagulation, depending on the stimulus. After contact, initial activation factors IX, VIII, calcium and platelet phospholipid, interact to form the tenase complex which activates factor X. Parallel to and within the coagulation system are

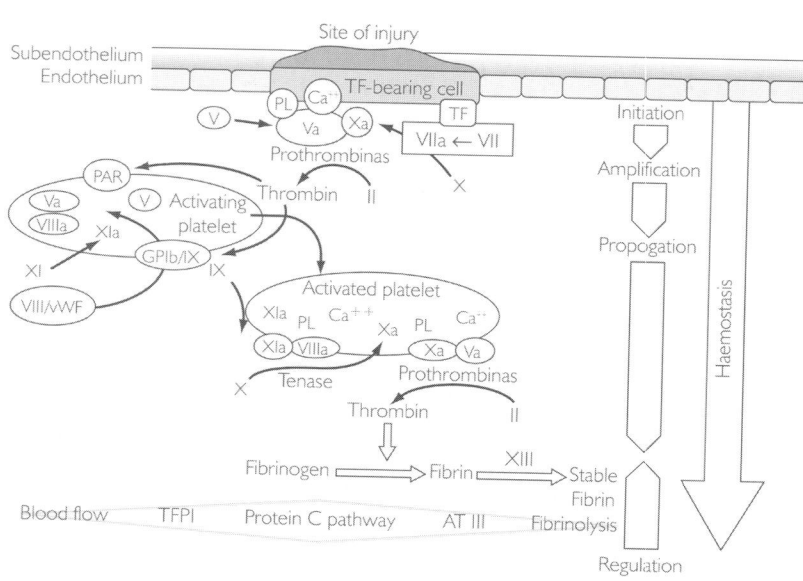

Fig. 89.1 A simplified illustration of current understanding of haemostasis. PL = Phospholipid, PAR = Protease activated receptor, TFPI = Tissue factor pathway inhibitor, ATIII = Antithrombin III

complex feedback mechanisms to ensure fine-tuning and protection against inappropriate and excessive activation (e.g. disseminated intravascular coagulation, DIC, or venous thromboembolism). There are several inhibitory proteins, including antithrombin III, thrombomodulin, protein C and S, tissue factor pathway inhibitor as well as the fibrinolytic system, which are all important in controlling the degree and site of fibrin formation. Indeed, thrombin itself acts as either a procoagulant or anticoagulant depending on context. Massive activation, as may be seen in trauma and severe infections, can precipitate systemic activation, but generally the system is well controlled and activity is localized to the area of the stimulus. Perturbations in this complex defence system can produce a wide range of clinical disorders from excessive arterial or venous thrombosis, microvascular obstruction and atheroma to haemostatic failure.

SYSTEMIC HAEMOSTATIC ASSESSMENT

There may be clinical features suggesting local or generalized failure of the haemostatic system (Fig. 89.2). Clinical history is important, especially with respect to previous bleeding problems, family history, co-morbid medical conditions and medications. The nature of surgery or an invasive intervention may have haemostatic issues that need specific consideration.

TESTS OF THE HAEMOSTATIC SYSTEM

Tests of whole blood clotting time and clot observation do not generally have a role in assessing haemosta-

sis. However, in emergency settings, while waiting for laboratory results, observation of blood collected into a glass tube and maintained at 37°C for clot formation, size, retraction and possible lysis may provide crude information of a possible coagulopathy. The thromboelastogram is a more accurate and controlled procedure for holistic assessment of the haemostatic system at the bedside, but requires close attention to technique and quality control. In most clinical settings, laboratory haemostatic screening tests are readily available, with near-patient testing techniques continuing to improve. A full blood count, prothrombin time (PT), activated partial thromboplastin time (APTT), fibrinogen level and D-Dimer ± thrombin clotting time (TCT) provide a broad screen for most clinically significant haemostatic disorders (Fig. 89.3). Based on these results, and following consultation with a haematologist, further specific tests of haemostasis may be performed (e.g. mixing studies, factor assays, platelet function tests and tests of fibrinolytic function).

In broad terms:

- PT tests integrity of the extrinsic system
- APTT the intrinsic system
- TCT fibrinogen conversion
- D-Dimer assay measures the breakdown products from lysis of fibrin

The haemostatic system optimally functions at 37°C and laboratory coagulation tests are performed at 37°C. Hypothermia may severely impair a patient's systemic and local haemostasis despite the system being structurally intact and laboratory tests normal.

The laboratory investigation of a patient with a potential haemostatic defect depends on the degree of urgency. It may be necessary to administer blood component

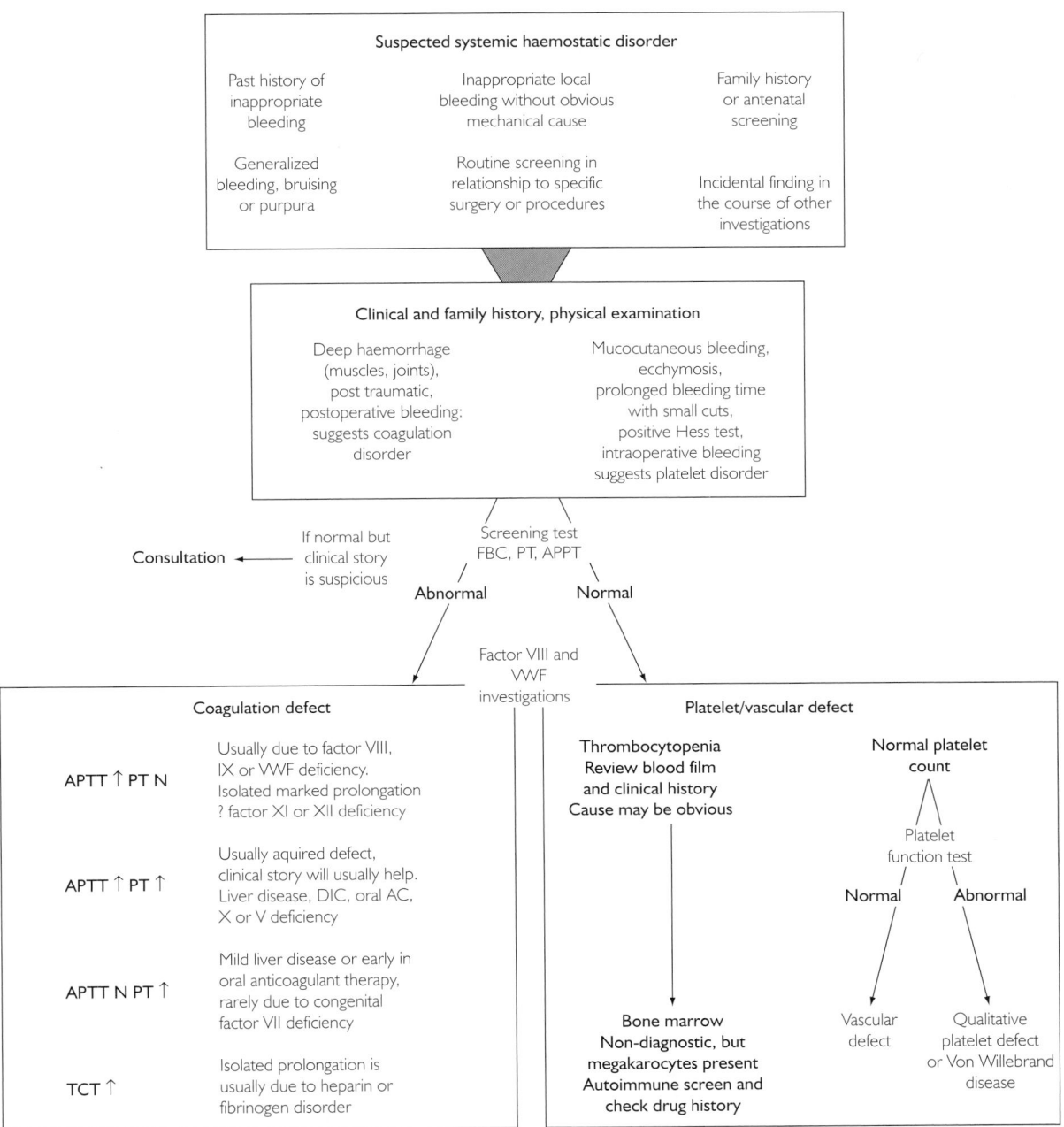

Fig. 89.2 Coagulation tests.

therapy without a definitive haemostatic defect being established. In elective settings, the defect can be accurately identified, problems pre-empted and specific blood component therapy administered prophylactically or therapeutically. A detailed clinical history and screening laboratory investigations prior to elective procedures will often avert undiagnosed emergency haemostatic crises.

There are several important principles in the collection of blood samples for haemostatic investigations. Most samples are collected into citrated tubes and the amount of anticoagulant in the tube is related to the intended amount of blood to be collected into the tube. It is important that the correct amount of blood is added to the tube and gently mixed. Attention to venepuncture technique is

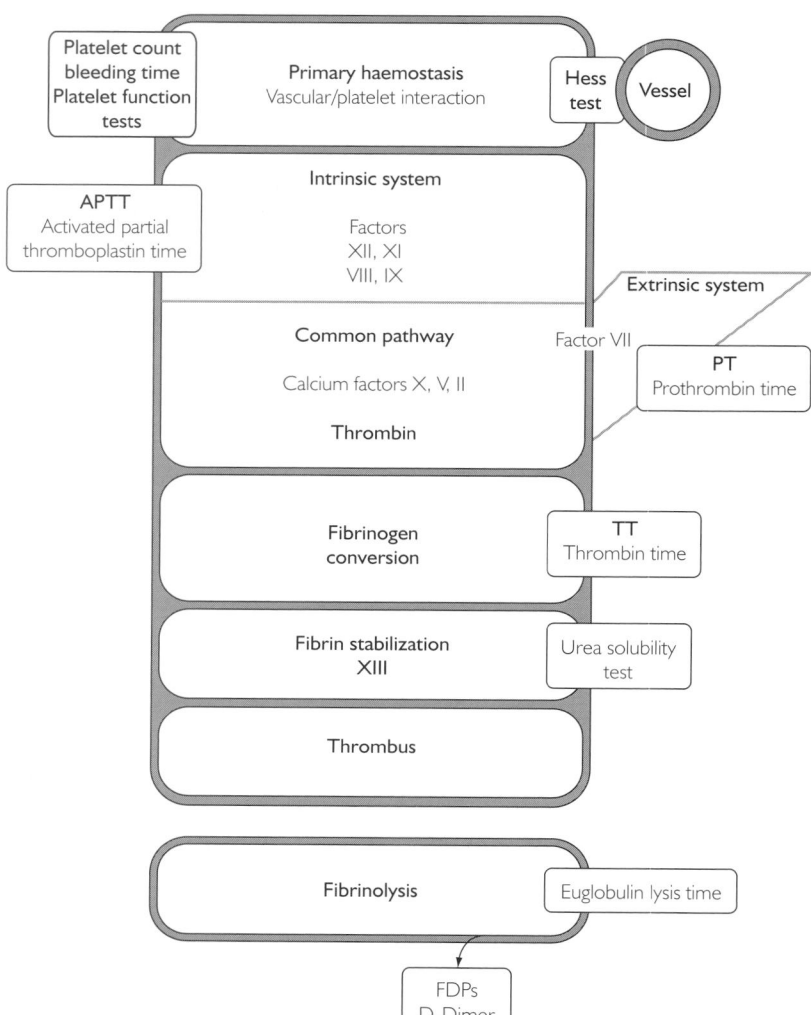

Fig. 89.3 Investigations for a suspected haemostatic defect.

crucial and rapid transfer of the sample to the laboratory is important. Contamination of the sample with tissue factor due to traumatic venepuncture will activate the sample and invalidate results. Collection from vascular access lines may result in diluted or heparin-contaminated samples. Incorrect laboratory results may be more dangerous to a patient than no results at all.

PLATELET COUNT (NORMAL 150–400 10⁹/L)

The counting of platelets is performed as part of the full blood count by automated cell counters. It is not possible to perform accurate platelet counts on 'fingerprick' blood.

BLEEDING TIME (NORMAL 3–9 MIN)

The bleeding time is progressively prolonged when the platelet count falls below 75–$100 \times 10^9/l$ assuming platelet function is normal. The bleeding time is also prolonged when platelet function is defective, in capillary/vascular disease and in some coagulation defects. The bleeding time is an invasive and operator dependent test and is not good for screening unselected patients. Its role is generally in elective settings for investigation selected patients who have good clinical evidence for a systemic haemostatic disorder. Increasingly a new test of 'closure time' platelet function screening is performed; this has better accuracy and reliability.

PROTHROMBIN TIME
(NORMAL RANGE <3 S ABOVE CONTROL)

The PT is a test of the extrinsic coagulation and prolongation may be caused by factor VII deficiency, liver disease, vitamin K deficiency or oral anticoagulant therapy. The PT is also expressed as the international normalized ratio (INR) especially when used for anticoagulant control.

ACTIVATED PARTIAL THROMBOPLASTIN TIME (APTT) (<6 S ABOVE CONTROL)

The APTT is a test of the intrinsic coagulation system but the result must be interpreted with caution. There may be significant variation in sensitivity and specificity of the test between laboratories and in unselected patients there is poor correlation between the APTT prolongation and either the presence of haemostatic failure or the likelihood of a patient bleeding. In this context, a patient suspected of having a systemic haemostatic defect and isolated prolongation of the APTT may represent deficiency or an inhibitor of factor VIII or IX. If there is a marked isolated prolongation there may be a deficiency in the contact phase of the coagulation cascade and there will also be a poor correlation with a bleeding tendency. Prolongation of APTT and PT may be due to deficiencies of factors X, V or II. A lupus anticoagulant may prolong the APTT and represent a prothrombotic state.

THROMBIN CLOTTING TIME (NORMAL < 2 S LONGER THAN CONTROL)

This is a test of the final conversion of fibrinogen to fibrin. Prolongation of TCT is due to hypofibrinogenaemia, dysfibrinogenaemia, heparin and fibrin degradation products.

D-DIMER (NORMAL <0.25 NG/L)

The D-Dimer assay measures cleavage fragments resulting from the proteolytic action of plasmin or fibrin. Elevation of D-Dimer may be seen in the postoperative state, trauma, renal impairment, sepsis and venous thrombosis. High levels of D-Dimer suggest excessive fibrinolysis, as seen in disseminated intravascular coagulation. The test is specific for fibrinolysis and not primary fibrinogenolysis.

SPECIFIC COAGULATION FACTOR ASSAYS (NORMAL 2–4 G/L)

Fibrinogen is the commonest routinely measured coagulation factor in patients suspected of systemic haemostatic failure. Other assays are usually performed in the investigation for specific defects, usually after consultation with a haematologist.

EUGLOBULIN LYSIS TIME (normal range >90 min) This test mainly reflects the presence of plasminogen activators. A shortened time is indicative of system fibrinolytic activation.

CONGENITAL HAEMOSTATIC DEFECTS[3]

Congenital bleeding disorders are relatively uncommon and are usually confined to a single defect. It is important to identify the defect so that specific replacement therapy can be given preoperatively or to arrest a particular episode of bleeding.

HAEMOPHILIA A (CLASSICAL HAEMOPHILIA)

Haemophilia A is a sex-linked disorder due to a deficiency of factor VIII. The mainstay of haemophilia treatment is coagulation factor replacement. Coagulation factor concentrates or recombinant factor VIII are given to prevent bleeding and to control existing haemorrhage. The dose of clotting factor is calculated on the basis that one unit of coagulation factor is that amount present in 1 ml of pooled normal plasma. An individual with a plasma volume of 3000 ml would have 3000 U of the clotting factor in the circulation. If such person was a haemophiliac with <1% factor VIII level in the plasma, a dose of 3000 U of factor VIII would be required to raise the plasma level to 100% of normal.

Experience has demonstrated that doses of 15–20 U/kg body weight will control most haemarthroses, but doses of up to 30 U/kg are required for muscle haematomas or for the prevention of dental bleeding. Raising clotting factor levels to 100% of normal is indicated for severe bleeding (e.g. intracranial or intraabdominal haemorrhage), but there is considerable patient variation in response to specific doses, and empirical dose-finding may be necessary. Measurement of factor VIII levels following replacement therapy is helpful. A factor VIII concentration of 25%, usually achieved with a dose of 15 U/kg, controls joint bleeding, whereas a level of 50%, generally obtained with a dose of 30 U/kg, prevents bleeding following tooth extraction. Clotting factor is given when a haemophiliac undergoes invasive procedures, including minor invasions such as arterial blood gas sampling.

The half-life of factor VIII in the circulation is approximately 12 h; on this basis, doses are repeated on a 12-hourly basis if it is necessary to maintain a specific plasma concentration of the factor. Clotting factor assays are performed near the end of this 12-h period in order to confirm that adequate levels for haemostasis are being achieved. Concentrate may also be given by continuous infusion.

HAEMOPHILIA B (CHRISTMAS DISEASE)

Haemophilia B due to factor IX deficiency is less common than classical haemophilia. The general principles of management are similar with factor IX concentrates or recombinant products being used.

VON WILLEBRAND'S DISEASE[4,5]

Von Willebrand's disease, the commonest of the hereditary haemostatic disorders, is due to a quantitative or qualitative defect in vWF. Classification of vWD is complex and controversial and therapy may be determined by the specific subtype and expert haematological consultation is important. In most cases desmopressin (DDAVP) is effective therapy, but replacement therapy may be needed for the rarer severe subtypes. DDAVP induces a haemostatic state via release of factor VIII and vWF. 0.3 μg/kg is infused slowly over 30 min immediately prior to surgery or to establish haemostasis in the bleeding patient. Antifibrinolytic agents may also be useful when not contraindicated as a thrombotic risk.

CONGENITAL PLATELET DISORDERS

Congenital platelet disorders are rare, the commonest severe disorder being Glanzmann's thrombasthenia. Platelet transfusions may be required for acute bleeds or in relation to elective surgery, DDAVP ± antifibrinolytic therapy and recombinant VIIa may all have a role.

ACQUIRED HAEMOSTATIC DISORDERS

The acquired disorders of coagulation are usually more complex and multifactorial than the hereditary disorders. A unified approach is essential for the successful management of these potentially life-threatening situations, and transfusion therapy cannot be isolated from other treatment.

MASSIVE BLOOD TRANSFUSION[6–10]

The nature and management of haemostatic defects secondary to massive blood loss and transfusion remains poorly understood. Further aggravation of the complications of massive blood transfusion can be avoided or minimized if correctable defects in the haemostatic system are identified (Table 89.1). Some degree of haemostatic failure is inevitable if stored blood, especially if more than 10 days old, is used for resuscitation. The labile factors V and VIII are not well preserved beyond 3–4 days; platelets are aggregated and non-functional, some coagulation factors may be activated during cooling and storage; and microaggregates and degenerate cells may be responsible for aggravating or initiating DIC and or multiorgan dysfunction syndrome. The relative importance of the different potential mechanisms responsible for haemostatic failure is difficult to determine, but the identification of correctable defects will avoid or minimize complications.

Haemostatic failure correlates poorly with the volume of transfusion or components administered, but better with the nature of the insult, degree of hypovolaemia and time to resuscitation. Trauma patients with major coagulopathy and microvascular haemorrhage usually have abnormal laboratory parameters prior to massive

Table 89.1 Possible factors contributing to haemostatic failure following:

Massive blood transfusion
Pre-existing haemostatic defect
Loss of coagulation factors, platelets and inhibitors
Dilution of coagulation factors, platelets and inhibitors
Impaired synthesis due to effects of shock on liver and bone marrow function
Effects of trauma: disseminated intravascular coagulation and fibrinolysis
Effects of storage lesion: depletion of coagulation factors and platelets, aggravation or precipitation of DIC
Depletion of modulators of haemostasis (e.g. antithrombin III, fibronectin and protein C)
Incompatible transfusion reaction: DIC
Hypothermia
Citrate toxicity?

Table 89.2 Potential problems with stored blood components

Failure to correct deficiency
Inadequate correction of deficiency
Blockade of RES (microaggregates, coagulation)
Microvascular pathophysiology (ARDS, MSOF)
Accentuation of free radical pathology (leukocytes, iron)
Activation and consumption of the haemostatic system
Hyperkalaemia, hypocalcaemia, hypothermia
Vasoactive effects (hypotension)
Hyperbilirubinaemia

blood transfusion. Except for severe abnormalities, haemostatic laboratory parameters correlate poorly with clinical evidence of haemostatic failure. Thrombocytopenia and impaired platelelet function are the most consistent significant haematological abnormalities; correction of which may be associated with control of microvascular bleeding. Coagulation deficiency from massive blood loss is initially confined to factors V and VIII. APTT, PT and fibrinogen assay should be performed, but the urgency of the situation does not usually allow for other specific factor assays, and fresh frozen plasma (FFP) should be infused if the test results are abnormal. A case can be made for prophylactic FFP in infusions in patients with massive blood loss which has been replaced with red cell concentrates and plasma substitutes. Hypothermia must be avoided, recognized and treated rapidly. Potential problems associated with large volume stored blood replacement are summarized in Table 89.2.

With ongoing bleeding with associated microvascular oozing, various approaches may be taken. Having ensured that all identifiable haemostatic defects have been corrected, questions arise as to the role of fresh blood and and, more recently, recombinant activated factor VII (rVIIa). There are an increasing number of anecdotal reports suggesting recombinant factor VII may be of benefit in patients requiring massive transfusion but as yet there are no definitive studies in this area.

The use of freshly collected whole blood remains controversial and is an emotive subject needing some comment. The provision of fresh whole blood can present logistic, ethical and safety problems that require consideration. Many transfusion medicine specialists categorically state there is never an indication for fresh whole blood. Such dogma can be difficult to defend in the clinical setting of the massive haemorrhage and transfusion syndrome where pathophysiology remains poorly understood and specific blood component therapy may be ineffective. The current author, from his own experience, and on the basis of current evidence, feels that the following statements reasonably summarize the current status of fresh blood transfusion:

- Fresh blood provides immediately functioning oxygen carrying capacity, volume and haemostatic factors, in the one product
- The number of homologous donors to whom a patient is exposed can be reduced
- Problems associated with infusion of massive volumes of stored blood can be minimized
- The risk of transfusion related viral infections is possibly higher than fully tested and stored blood
- The benefit in controlling haemorrhage probably relates to the presence of immediately functioning platelets

HAEMOSTATIC FAILURE ASSOCIATED WITH LIVER DISEASE

The liver is the production site of nearly all the factors involved in the formation and control of coagulation (Table 89.3). Bleeding in association with liver disease can be difficult to manage. There may be a combination of excessive consumption of coagulation factors, impaired synthesis of both clotting factors and coagulation inhibitor proteins. Excessive activation of fibrinolysis may occur and defective clearing of activated clotting factors compound the problem. Moreover, the effects of massive blood loss, shock and transfusion must also complicate the problem. Haemostatic defects due to deficient vitamin K dependent

Table 89.3 Haemostatic disturbances in liver disease

Deficiency of vitamin K dependent clotting factors II, VII, IX, X
Deficiency of fibrinogen and factor V
Dysfibrinogenaemia
Disseminated intravascular coagulation
Excessive fibrinolytic activity
Circulating anticoagulants
Platelet abnormalities

coagulation factors (in patients with predominantly cholestatic liver disease) may be rapidly reversed with vitamin K therapy, and blood transfusion may not be required. If the abnormality is not reversed by vitamin K, hepatocellular damage is likely to be present and FFP is an appropriate replacement therapy. When an elective procedure is planned, prophylactic FFP is appropriate. Low fibrinogen levels in liver disease usually indicate advanced disease and are associated with a poor prognosis, or the presence of DIC. Cryoprecipitate is the safest and most readily available form of fibrinogen.

DISSEMINATED INTRAVASCULAR COAGULATION[11-16]

Disseminated intravascular coagulation is a pathophysiological process and not a disease in itself. The disorder is an inappropriate, excessive and uncontrolled activation of the haemostatic process. Clinical manifestations of disseminated intravascular coagulation relate to occlusion of the microvessels during the obstructive phase of the syndrome and haemorrhage secondary to consumption of plasma and cellular components of the haemostatic system. The perpetuation of the process may be due to continuation of the stimulus and/or consumption of the natural inhibitors of haemostasis. DIC thus results due to inappropriate, excessive and uncontrolled activation of the haemostatic process. This may initially occur with adequate compensation when defects may only be demonstrable in the laboratory tests. If the initiating disorder is severe enough, the clinical syndrome of uncontrolled acute DIC will result with a systemic bleeding state, usually with associated end organ failure. A compensatory secondary fibrinolysis occurs, which in some cases may accentuate the bleeding.

PATHOPHYSIOLOGY

DIC is characterized by the consumption of clotting factors and platelets within the circulation, resulting in varying degrees of microvascular obstruction due to fibrin deposition (Fig. 89.4). When significant platelet and coagulation factor consumption occurs, bleeding may become a major feature.

Mechanisms which may inappropriately activate the haemostatic system include:

- Activation of the coagulation sequence by release of tissue thromboplastins into the systemic circulation (e.g. following extensive tissue trauma, during surgery, malignancy and during an acute intravascular haemolysis).
- Vessel wall endothelial injury causing platelet activation followed by activation of the haemostatic system, predominantly via the intrinsic pathway (e.g. Gram-negative sepsis from endotoxin release, viral infections, extensive burns, prolonged hypotension, hypoxia or acidosis).

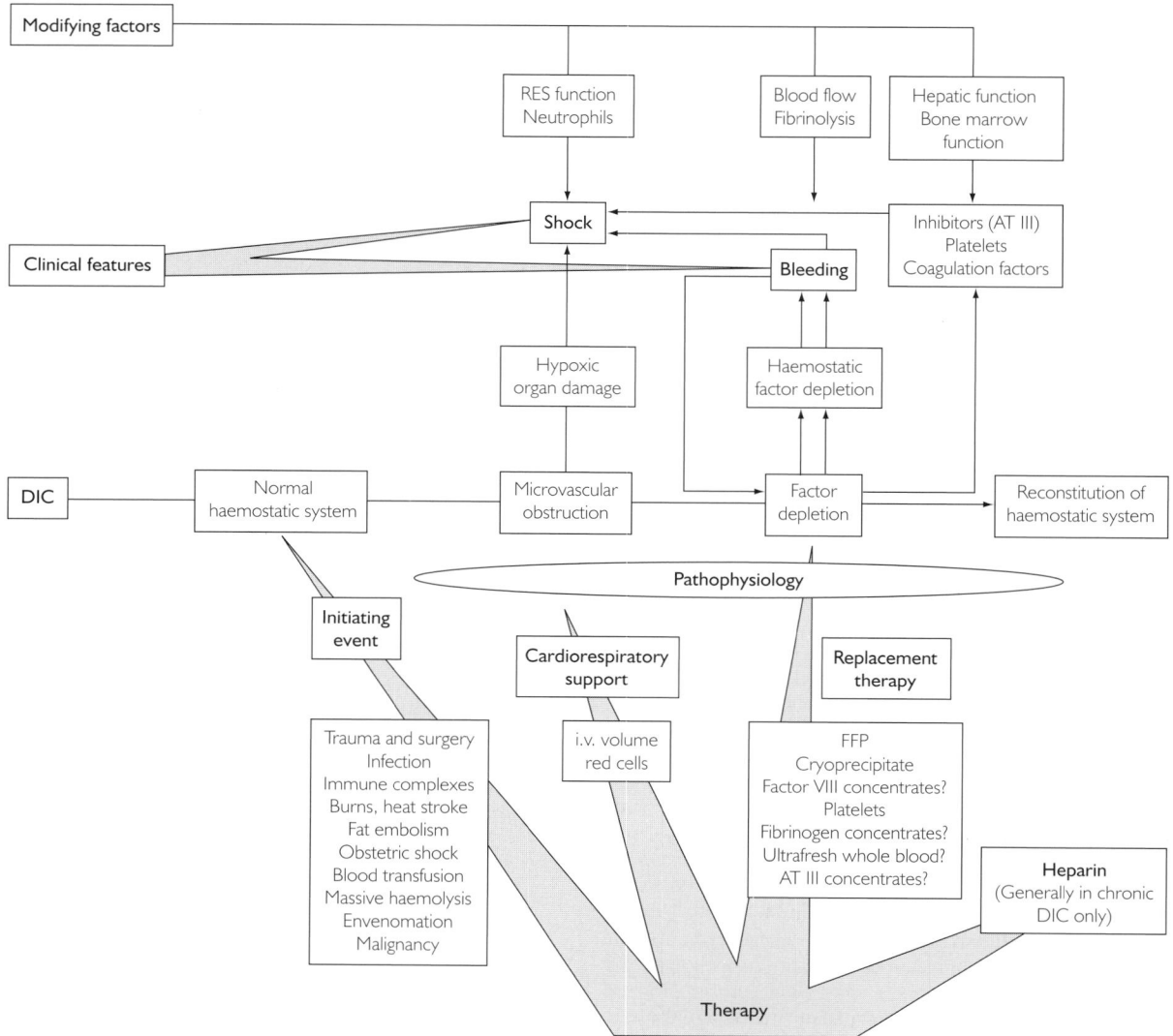

Fig. 89.4 The pathophysiology and management of disseminated intravascular coagulation (DIC).

- Induction of platelet activation (e.g. septicaemia, viraemia, antigen–antibody complexes and platelet activation).

CLINICAL FEATURES

The clinical presentation of DIC varies, with patients showing thrombotic, haemorrhagic, or mixed manifestations in various organ systems. The major clinical problem and presenting feature of acute DIC is bleeding. This may manifest as generalized bruising, bleeding at sites of therapeutic or traumatic invasion (venepuncture sites and surgical wounds). DIC may occur is association with a wide range of clinical disorders (Table 89.5). When DIC occurs in acutely ill patients with multi-

system organ failure, the prognosis is poor. In some patients, DIC may be an agonal event and should not be treated.

LABORATORY FINDINGS

Results of tests may be variable and difficult to interpret. Significant DIC can be present despite normal standard coagulation tests (i.e. PT, APTT and TCT). The key tests in diagnosis are those that provide evidence for excessive conversion of fibrinogen to fibrin within the circulation and its subsequent lysis. Platelet-fibrin clots create a mesh in the microcirculation in which passing red cells may be traumatized, resulting in red cell fragmentation and haemolysis. The blood film may

Table 89.4   Laboratory test for the diagnosis of DIC

Analysis	Early	Late
Platelet count	↑	↓↓
Activated partial thromboplastin time (APTT)	↑	↑↑
Prothrombin time (PT)	↑	↑
Thrombin clotting time (TCT)	↑	↑
Fibrin degradation products (D-Dimer assay)	↑	↑↑
Hypofibrinogen	↓	↓↓
Other coagulation factors II, VII, X, VIII,	↓	↓↓
Coagulation inhibitors – antithrombin III, protein C	↓	↓↓↓
Blood film	Usually normal in early stages	Fragmented red cells + in subacute or chronic cases
Supplementary and research tests – prothrombin fragment 1+2, thrombin–antithrombin complex (TAT–complex), procalcitonin (PCT), Plasmin-antiplasmin complexes (PAP–complex)	↑	↑

demonstrate fragmentation of the red cells (microangio-pathic haemolytic anaemia), but this is more commonly seen in chronic DIC especially in association with malignancy.

The diagnosis is usually based on a combination of the appropriate clinical picture with a supportive pattern of laboratory tests of the haemostatic system (Table 89.4). Thrombocytopenia, hypofibrinogenaemia with prolongation of the APTT, PT and TCT in conjunction with an elevation of fibrin degradation products (D-Dimer test) are supportive evidence for the diagnosis. The D-Dimer test is specific for fibrin breakdown versus primary fibrinogenolysis. More specialized tests such as elevation of fibrinopeptide A and reduced levels of antithrombin III add further weight to the diagnosis.

In chronic DIC, the laboratory findings are different from acute DIC. Many of the usual tests of haemostasis are normal or near normal. The platelet count may be normal as may be many of the haemostatic factors. However, this is a compensated state in which there is increased turnover of each of the haemostatic components. D-Dimer is elevated in this setting and a microangiopathic red cell picture is seen on the peripheral blood film.

DISORDERS ASSOCIATED WITH DIC

DIC may occur in association with a wide range of clinical disorders (Table 89.5).

THERAPY

The management of DIC remains controversial, but removal or treatment of the initiating cause is important in conjunction with general resuscitation. The early recognition of DIC and initiation of management may allow the patient to survive hours or days, granting sufficient time for definitive diagnosis and treatment of the inciting disorder. Blood component therapy should

Table 89.5   Conditions associated with disseminated intravascular coagulation

Infection
  Bacterial sepsis
  Viral haemorrhagic fevers
  Protozoal (malaria)
Trauma
  Extensive tissue injury
  Head injury
  Fat embolism
Malignancy
  Carcinoma
  Leukaemia (especially promyelocytic)
Immunological disorders
  Transplantation rejection
  Incompatible haemolytic blood transfusion reactions
  Severe allergic reaction
  Drug reactions
Extracorporeal circulations
Snake bite invenomation
Vascular disorders
  Giant haemangioma
  Aortic aneurysm
Pregnancy associated:
  Septic abortion
  Abruptio placentae
  Eclampsia
  Amniotic fluid embolism
  Placenta praevia
Burns
Hyperthermia
Liver disease and acute hepatic necrosis

be given to the haemorrhaging patient, but the use of heparin should only be considered in selected cases.

● FFP contains all the coagulation factors and the main inhibitors, antithrombin III and protein C, in near normal quantities and should be used if haemorrhage is occurring.

- Cryoprecipitate, contains all components of the factor VIII complex as well as fibrinogen, factor XIII and fibronectin in concentrated form. Five to ten units should be infused in conjunction with the fresh frozen plasma.
- Platelet transfusion may be indicated in the presence of life-threatening haemorrhage; however, this is a controversial subject and the patients tend to be resistant if the initiating cause of the DIC has not been controlled.
- It is likely that replacement therapy with antithrombin III concentrates and possibly other inhibitors of haematostasis will find a greater role in therapy. Successful treatment of the bleeding phase of DIC probably depends to a variable degree on the patient being able to 'switch off' the coagulation system. Correction of depleted coagulation inhibitor levels, reticuloendothelial blockade and impaired or excessive fibrinolysis may be important.
- In general, heparin should only be used after initial adequate replacement therapy has failed to control bleeding. The decision to use heparin should not be undertaken lightly nor without due consultation. Small doses should be used initially (e.g. 50–100 U/kg body weight followed by 10–15 U/kg per h), adjusted according to the clinical and laboratory response.

Management of sudden massive obstetric haemorrhage is similar to other cases of DIC except that the onset is more likely to be fulminant and unexpected, and associated with greater depletion of coagulation factors, especially fibrinogen, due to marked fibrinolysis. Fresh blood is possibly warranted in some of these cases where bleeding does not stop quickly. Once the uterus has been emptied and contracted, the haemostatic failure quickly resolves.

OUTCOME

Factors which may affect the outcome of DIC include:

- Nature of the initiating event.
- Host factors (e.g. state of reticuloendothelial system, levels of inhibitors of coagulation and fibrinolytic activity, hepatic synthetic function).
- The extent of end organ damage sustained during the thrombotic phase and from the shock caused during the haemorrhagic phase.

ANTITHROMBOTIC THERAPY[17]

The wider clinical use of antithrombotic therapy inevitably has resulted in an increase in iatrogenic bleeding in patients presenting with other medical conditions (e.g. trauma, surgery and invasive procedures) and inten-

sivists must be aware of the methods for rapid reversal of therapy. Bleeding problems in patients on well-controlled anticoagulation are usually due to surgery, trauma or a local lesion (e.g. peptic ulceration). Otherwise, bleeding is due to over anticoagulation, sometimes as a result of drug interactions. Elective surgery in this group of patients needs careful planning if haemorrhagic and thrombotic complications are to be avoided.

ORAL ANTICOAGULANT AGENTS

Oral anticoagulant agents induce a controlled deficiency of the vitamin K dependent clotting factors (II, VII, IX and X), the anticoagulant action being measured by prolongation of PT (INR). The indications for reversing vitamin K antagonists depends on the clinical situation and the indication for therapy. Reversal of over anticoagulation depends on the degree of overactivity and on the presence, or not, of haemorrhage. In most cases, vigorous intervention is unnecessary and the oral anticoagulation can be temporarily ceased. Short-term reversal or temporary reversal is achieved by administration of FFP. Prothrombin complex concentrate will effectively and rapidly reverse the anticoagulant effects of warfarin, including protein C correction, and has a role in anticoagulant overdose. Previous concerns about coagulation activation do not appear to be a problem with current products.

Long-term reversal requires vitamin K, but care must be taken not to give an excessive dose if it is planned that the patient needs to return to oral anticoagulation in the long-term. For most surgical interventions or invasive procedures, an INR of 1.5 or less is accepted as safe. This can usually be achieved by temporarily ceasing medication.

HEPARINS

With the wide clinical use of fractionated low molecular weight (LMW) heparins, this subject has become more complex. Heparins act by potentiating the action of antithrombin III, a natural coagulation inhibitor. Unfractionated heparin acts in neutralizing both thrombin and Xa in contrast to the LMW heparins which predominantly neutralize Xa. The anticoagulant effect of unfractionated heparin is usually measured by prolongation of the APTT. Immediate reversal of heparin activity can be achieved with protamine sulphate. Although formulas have been quoted for the reversal of heparin (e.g. 1 mg protamine sulphate will neutralize 100 U of heparin), it is better to titrate the dose using APTT after an initial empirical dose of 50 mg. Protamine sulphate should be injected slowly by the i.v. route. Protamine is not without risk, as it may itself impair coagulation and be associated with anaphylactoid reactions. LMW heparins do not prolong the APTT, are generally administered on weight basis and are not routinely monitored by a laboratory test. When monitoring is required, the anti-Xa assay is used. It is not possible to reverse effects of LMW heparins.

ANTIPLATELET AGENTS

Antiplatelet agents are being used increasingly for prophylaxis and therapy of arterial disease, and many of the non-steroidal anti-inflammatory agents are also platelet inhibitory drugs. Aspirin has an irreversible effect on platelet function and platelet function tests may show abnormalities for up to 10 days after medication. Most of the other non-steroidal anti-inflammatory drugs have a reversible effect lasting a matter of hours or occasionally days. Perioperative bleeding is usually mild, but occasionally may be serious, depending on the surgery and, in some situations, a platelet transfusion may be necessary. In other cases, the patient may already have a mild haemostatic defect (e.g. von Willebrand's disease) and aspirin may have a synergistic effect leading to major haemostatic failure.

Newer agents such as Clopidogrel act as an inhibitor of platelet aggregation by selectively inhibiting the binding of ADP to its platelet receptor by irreversibly modifying the platelet ADP receptor and, as a result, ADP mediated activation of the GPIIb/IIIa complex. As with aspirin, platelets exposed to Clopidogrel are affected for their lifespan, and recovery of normal platelet function occurs as new platelets are produced.

ACQUIRED INHIBITORS OF COAGULATION

Major haemostatic failure may be seen with rare inhibitors of coagulation factors. Autoantibodies against factors VIII (commonest), IX, X, V and vWF have been reported. A co-ordinated approach to haemotherapy is essential if bleeding is to be arrested. The patients are relatively resistant to factor replacement therapy and removal of the offending autoantibody by plasma exchange and replacement with FFP ± factor concentrates is indicated. Recombinant activated factor VII may have a role yet to be defined.

PRIMARY FIBRINOLYSIS

This rare acquired disorder of haemostasis is in reality primary fibrinogenolysis because circulating plasmin is responsible for an uncontrolled proteolytic attack on the coagulation system (particularly factor VIII and fibrinogen). The disorder may complicate specific types of surgery (e.g. neurosurgery, pulmonary and prostate) or malignancy. Rapid recognition of this potentially devastating failure of haemostasis is essential if appropriate antifibrinolytic and blood component therapy (FFP and cryoprecipitate) is to be effective. Both streptokinase and tissue plasminogen activator therapy of arterial and venous disease may cause problems and excess lysis may occur.

EXTRACORPOREAL CIRCULATION[18,19]

A range of haemostatic disturbances may be associated with extracorporeal circulation, most commonly cardiopulmonary bypass. The abnormalities are generally directly related to the time on bypass and are more likely to be seen in multiple valve replacements or re-operations. Fresh blood components have generally been advocated in cardiac bypass surgery to ensure optimal oxygen delivery and function of the haemostatic components of blood. Haemostatic failure usually becomes apparent in the operating room, or soon after, and appropriate laboratory investigations should be performed to allow logical therapy. It is pointless to infuse large volumes of plasma products or platelets if heparin has not been adequately reversed. In some cases, increased fibrinolytic activity may also contribute to bleeding.

A predictable thrombocytopenia occurs after extracorporeal blood circulation. The postoperative platelet count in the majority of cardiac bypass patients is seldom below 100 000 per μl, but platelet functional defects may contribute to bleeding and, occasionally, platelet concentrates are indicated.

THROMBOCYTOPENIA AND QUALITATIVE PLATELET DEFECTS[2–25]

IDIOPATHIC THROMBOCYTOPENIC PURPURA (ITP)

ITP is an autoimmune disorder where autoantibodies (IgG) are directed against the platelets, which are subsequently destroyed by the monocyte–macrophage system, predominantly in the spleen. ITP is typically a disease of children and young adults. The acute form is more commonly identifiable as post-infectious, and recovery over weeks to months is the usual natural history. The course of the chronic form is variable and may spontaneously recover but, more commonly, needs specific intervention.

Therapy of ITP remains controversial. Corticosteroids should generally be regarded as short-term therapy. In adults, the majority of patients respond with a rise in the platelet count. After an initial high dose of prednisolone (50–75 mg a day until response occurs), the dose is gradually reduced. There is little evidence that corticosteroids will raise the platelet count in the acute disease. However, their short-term role in reducing the incidence of bleeding, which is highest in the first weeks, may be important. High dose i.v. immunoglobulin is effective in most patients and is specifically indicated in fulminant acute disease, preoperatively and in pregnancy.

DRUG INDUCED THROMBOCYTOPENIA

The clinical presentation of drug-induced thrombocytopenia may be as variable as ITP. Some may have a dramatic and fulminant presentation with marked haemostatic failure. Drugs with a particular reputation for inducing thrombocytopenia include quinine (also in bitter drinks), quinidine, antituberculous drugs, heparin, sedormid, thiazide diuretics, penicillins, sulphonamides, rifampicin and anticonvulsants.

Heparin-induced thrombosis thrombocytopenia syndrome is an important and potentially life threatening complication of heparin therapy. An immune reaction occurs to heparin after 7–10 days of therapy, at which time the patient's platelets aggregate and thrombocytopenia develops; this reactivity can be demonstrated by a variety of laboratory tests. In contrast to other causes of drug-induced thrombocytopenia, there may be arterial, microvascular or venous thrombosis associated with the platelet aggregation. The overall incidence of this complication of heparin is unknown, but may be on the increase with the wider use of subcutaneous prophylactic heparin. The best way to avoid this potentially devastating complication is to keep heparin therapy as brief as possible, and to always be alert to the diagnostic possibility. The incidence is considerably less with the use of LMW heparins and, if cross-reactivity is not demonstrated in the heparin antibody test, the LMW heparins or heparinoids may have a part to play in therapy.

Quinine-induced immune thrombocytopenia with hemolytic uremic syndrome can be a severe drug reaction, characterized by the onset of chills, sweating, nausea and vomiting, abdominal pain, oliguria and petechiae rash following quinine or quinidine exposure. Quinine-dependent platelet-reactive antibodies can usually be identified. Plasma exchange in conjunction with renal dialysis has been found to be a beneficial adjunct to therapy.

SEPSIS

Platelets play an important role in the inflammatory response and a reactive thrombocytosis is usually seen in infection. However, if there is overwhelming sepsis, associated DIC or marrow suppressive influences, thrombocytopenia may be seen. The combination of sepsis, shock, DIC, alcoholism and nutritional deficiency are common factors contributing to thrombocytopenia in critically ill patients.

QUALITATIVE PLATELET DEFECTS

The effects of aspirin and other antiplatelet agents are discussed above. Haemostatic failure is a common manifestation of renal failure. Its mechanism is not fully elucidated, but the defect can be substantially corrected by dialysis. Prolongation of the bleeding time, defects in aggregation responses, diminished adhesion and reduced platelet factor 3 availability have all been demonstrated. A relationship between the degree of anaemia and prolongation of bleeding is usually demonstrable – increasing the haemoglobin level reduces the bleeding time. Patients with the myelodysplastic syndrome may not only have thrombocytopenia, but also a qualitative platelet function defect. Thus, they are at high risk of bleeding

in relation to any surgery or invasive procedure. β-lactam antibiotics may also be responsible for a platelet function defect.

REFERENCES

1 Dahlback B. Blood coagulation. *Lancet* 2000; **355**: 1627–32.
2 George JN. Platelets. *Lancet* 2000; **355**: 1531–9.
3 Mannucci PM, Tuddenham EGD. Medical progress: the hemophilias – from royal genes to gene therapy. *N Engl J Med* 2001; **344**: 1773–9.
4 Mannucci PM. Drug therapy: hemostatic drugs. *N Engl J Med* 1998; **339**: 245–53.
5 Mannucci PM. How I treat patients with von Willebrand disease. *Blood* 2001; **97**: 1915–9.
6 Eddy VA, Morris JA Jr, Cullinane DC. Hypothermia, coagulopathy, and acidosis. *Surg Clin North Am* 2000; **80**: 845–54.
7 Reiss RF. Hemostatic defects in massive transfusion: rapid diagnosis and management. *Am J Crit Care* 2000; **9**: 158–65.
8 Bonnar J. Massive obstetric haemorrhage. *Baillières Best Pract Res Clin Obstet Gynaecol* 2000; **14**: 1–18.
9 Stainsby D, MacLennan S, Hamilton PJ. Management of massive blood loss: a template guideline. *Br J Anaesth* 2000; **85**: 487–91.
10 Murray DJ, Pennell BJ, Weinstein SL, *et al.* Packed red cells in acute blood loss: Dilutional coagulopathy as a cause of surgical bleeding. *Anesth Analg* 1995; **80**: 336–42.
11 Levi M, ten Cate H. Disseminated intravascular coagulation. *N Engl J Med* 1999; **341**: 586–92.
12 ten Cate H. Pathophysiology of disseminated intravascular coagulation in sepsis. *Crit Care Med* 2000; **28** (suppl. 9): S9–11.
13 Bick RL. Syndromes of disseminated intravascular coagulation in obstetrics, pregnancy, and gynecology. Objective criteria for diagnosis and management. *Hematol Oncol Clin North Am* 2000; **14**: 999–1044.
14 Nizzi FA Jr, Mues G. Hemorrhagic problems in obstetrics, exclusive of disseminated intravascular coagulation. *Hematol Oncol Clin North Am* 2000; **14**: 1171–82.
15 Lee WL, Downey GP. Coagulation inhibitors in sepsis and disseminated intravascular coagulation. *Intensive Care Med* 2000; **26**: 1701–6.
16 Levi M, de Jonge E, van der Poll T, ten Cate H. Novel approaches to the management of disseminated intravascular coagulation. *Crit Care Med* 2000; **28** (suppl. 9): S20–24.
17 Hirsh J, Dalen JE, Guyatt G. The Sixth ACCP Guidelines for Antithrombotic Therapy for Prevention and Treatment of Thrombosis. *Chest* 2000; **119**: 1S–2S.
18 Woodman RC, Harker LA. Bleeding complications associated with cardiopulmonary bypass. *Blood* 1990; **76**: 1680–97.
19 Milas BL, Jobes DR, Gorman RC. Management of bleeding and coagulopathy after heart surgery. *Semin Thorac Cardiovasc Surg* 2000; **12**: 326–36.

20 Porcefijn L, von dem Borne AE. Immune mediated thrombocytopenias: basic and immunological aspects. *Baillières Clin Haematol* 1998; **11**: 331–41.

21 Drews RE, Weinberger SE. Thrombocytopenic disorders in critically ill patients. *Am J Respir Crit Care Med* 2000; **162**: 347–51.

22 Sutor AH, Gaedicke G. Acute autoimmune thrombocytopenia. *Baillières Clin Haematol* 1998; **11**: 381–9.

23 Tarantino MD, Goldsmith G. Treatment of acute immune thrombocytopenic purpura. *Semin Hematol* 1998; **35** (suppl. l): 28–35.

24 Aster R. Drug-induced immune thrombocytopenia: an overview of pathogenesis. *Semin Hematol* 1999; **36**: 2–6.

25 Kaplan KL, Francis CW. Heparin induced thrombocytopenia. *Blood Rev* 1999; **13**: 1–7.

90

Haematological malignancies

J P Isbister

The treatment of haematological malignancy has been an evolving success story. In recent years, the prognosis for patients with acute leukaemia has changed from death within 1–3 months without effective therapy to long-term survival and cure in some cases. In some diseases the potential for regular cure of patients has been realized, including Hodgkin's disease, childhood acute lymphoblastic leukaemia, some high-grade lymphomas and some adult leukaemias. These advances have predominantly resulted from the introduction of a wide range of cytotoxic chemotherapeutic regimens which permit obliteration of the disease in conjunction with comprehensive supportive therapy. In some cases, 'supralethal' therapy is necessary with the use of bone marrow transplantation (autologous or allogeneic) being used as marrow 'rescue' therapy. The development of 'engineered' highly specific and targeted drugs is offering further promise (e.g. monoclonal antibodies, tyrosine kinase inhibitors for chronic myeloid leukaemia).[1]

It is important that clinicians not regularly involved in the care of these patients do not take a nihilistic approach to management of patients with haematological malignancy. If patients can be adequately supported and complications treated during the severe neutropenic stage of chemotherapy, clinical improvement may rapidly occur following marrow recovery. However, in patients requiring prolonged ventilatory support and/or dialysis, the prognosis is poor and intensive supportive therapy can usually only be justified if marrow recovery is imminent and there is a reasonable anticipated life expectancy if the crisis can be survived.

CLASSIFICATION AND PATHOPHYSIOLOGY

The heterogeneous nature of the haemopoietic and lymphoid cells, their individual kinetic characteristics and the disseminated nature of haemopoietic and lymphoid tissue explains the complexity of haematological malignancy. The numerous confusing classification systems advocated to 'clarify' understanding have in many cases increased the confusion for the non-expert. In broad terms the haematological malignancies with origins in the marrow are classified as leukaemia or multiple myeloma and those arising in the peripheral lymphoid tissues as Hodgkin's and non-Hodgkin's lymphomas (nodal and extranodal).

The leukaemias are divided into acute and chronic, generally according to the time span of their clinical course. In general, a leukaemia that is blastic in appearance behaves in an acute and malignant manner with a rapidly fatal outcome without therapy. This is in contrast to the chronic leukaemias in which the cells are more differentiated ('benign'), with the disease following a more indolent course. Leukaemias are classified on the basis of their cell of origin with broad division into those of myeloid origin (i.e. of haemopoietic marrow origin) and those of lymphoid origin, arising from the cells of the immune system.

Most patients with acute myeloid leukaemia present with features of bone marrow failure. Acute promyelocytic leukaemia is a unique subtype of acute myeloid leukaemia which may typically present with disseminated intravascular coagulation (DIC) requiring expert haematological management. Acute lymphoblastic leukaemia is the commonest encountered in children. The lymphomas are a complex and heterogeneous group of malignancies ranging from highly malignant disorders through to low-grade indolent disease not requiring therapy.

COMPLICATIONS OF HAEMATOLOGICAL MALIGNANCY AND ITS THERAPY

METABOLIC DISTURBANCES

At presentation haematological malignancy may be associated with a range of metabolic derangements. Hyperuricaemia and hypercalcaemia are well-recognized complications, which may be associated with renal failure. The tumour lysis syndrome is a rarer complication which may occur spontaneously or shortly after the initiation of therapy. There is sudden liberation of intracellular contents in quantities, which overwhelm the excretory capacity of the kidneys resulting in hyperkalaemia, hyperphosphataemia, hypocalcaemia and occasionally lactic acidosis. Pre-empting the development of this syndrome usually allows control of the metabolic effects, especially with the maintenance of high intravenous fluid intake, alkalinizing the urine and administration of allopurinol. Multiple myeloma may be complicated by renal insufficiency, hypercalcaemia, hyperviscosity and hyperuricaemia. Most of these can be managed conventionally, however with large amounts of monoclonal protein, fluid management can be difficult due to the hypervolaemia with or without hyperviscosity and plasma exchange may be indicated.

COAGULOPATHIES

A range of haemostatic disturbances may occur in association with haematological malignancy and its therapy.

ACUTE RESPIRATORY DISTRESS SYNDROME

Acute (or adult) respiratory distress syndrome (ARDS) remains a potentially lethal complication of autoaggressive inflammation. As most of the mediators (cytokines, neutrophils, and endothelial adherence molecules) initiating the disease process are haemopoietic in origin it is not surprising ARDS may occur in haemopoietic malignancies. However, ARDS is relatively uncommon in the neutropenic septic patient, probably due to the fact that the neutrophil under normal circumstances is one of the central mediators of this syndrome. ARDS and interstitial pneumonitis may be a problem due to hyperleukocytosis, transfusion associated lung injury (TRALI), CMV infection, DIC, post marrow transplantation, and sometimes in relation to chemotherapy and radiotherapy. The use of all-trans retinoic acid (ATRA) may be associated with the development of a potentially lethal ARDS/pulmonary leukostasis syndrome (retinoic acid syndrome) usually in association with a rising leukocyte count. In all the settings mentioned early recognition of the symptom complex of fever and dyspnoea with or without a pulmonary infiltrate is important and therapy with high dose corticosteroids decreases morbidity and mortality.

SIDE-EFFECTS OF CHEMOTHERAPY

The wide range of cytotoxic chemotherapeutic agents used in the management of haematological malignancy may be responsible for a plethora of toxicities other than bone marrow suppression. The haematologists will be aware of these and should communicate necessary information to the ICU staff.

BONE MARROW FAILURE

Most of the acute leukaemias present with clinical and laboratory features of marrow failure with anaemia, bleeding or infection. If not a problem at presentation marrow failure is almost universal during remission induction and subsequent chemotherapy.

Neutropenia

Neutropenia should be considered in the following terms:

- absolute neutrophil count, the rate of fall, the nadir and duration
- duration of the neutropenia is a critical factor determining the management and outcome. Patients with profound prolonged neutropenia of $<0.1 \times 10^9/l$ granulocytes for >10 days require special attention and they may require different initial therapy.

For practical purposes neutropenia has been divided into the following groups:

- Neutropenia $<0.5 \times 10^9/l$
- Neutropenia between 0.5 and $1.0 \times 10^9/l$ and potentially falling
- Neutropenia $0.5–1.0 \times 10^9/l$ and stable or rising
- Profound prolonged neutropenia

Figure 90.1 illustrates the numerous interacting factors to be considered when managing patients with neutropenia in association with haematological malignancy and its therapy. Table 90.1 lists the organisms, which may be associated with various defects in the host defence system.

PRINCIPLES OF MANAGEMENT OF HAEMATOLOGICAL MALIGNANCIES

ICU ADMISSION

Patients with haematological malignancy may be critically ill from their disease or therapy, for brief or long periods. At times during therapy, they may require intensive supportive therapy and can develop a range of life-threatening complications. Rarely, it is necessary to admit critically ill patients with haematological disorders to the intensive care unit. Under normal circumstances, admission of such patients is to be avoided as they have severely impaired host defences and poor tolerance for invasive procedures. However, mechanical ventilation may be required for severe respiratory infections or pneumonitis. Such patients may present specific problems for the ICU staff. Most patients have severe marrow failure requiring intensive transfusion support. Severe neutropenia is the main, and most life-threatening, defect in the host defence system. Nutrition can be a challenge in these patients due to a multitude of factors. The anorexia, nausea and vomiting with chemotherapy, oral mucositis, hypermetabolism, malabsorption and diarrhoea are only some of the factors mitigating against maintaining an adequate nutritional state, and parenteral nutrition may be needed if the period of therapy is prolonged.

There must be good communication between the ICU staff and clear policies on admission and treatment. If the patient's ultimate prognosis is poor, extraordinary invasive measures cannot be justified. A palliative approach will be instituted if the patient does not respond to treatment within a specific period of time. However, if the haematological malignancy has a high likelihood of cure or long-term good-quality survival more strenuous and extended intensive care support can be justified.

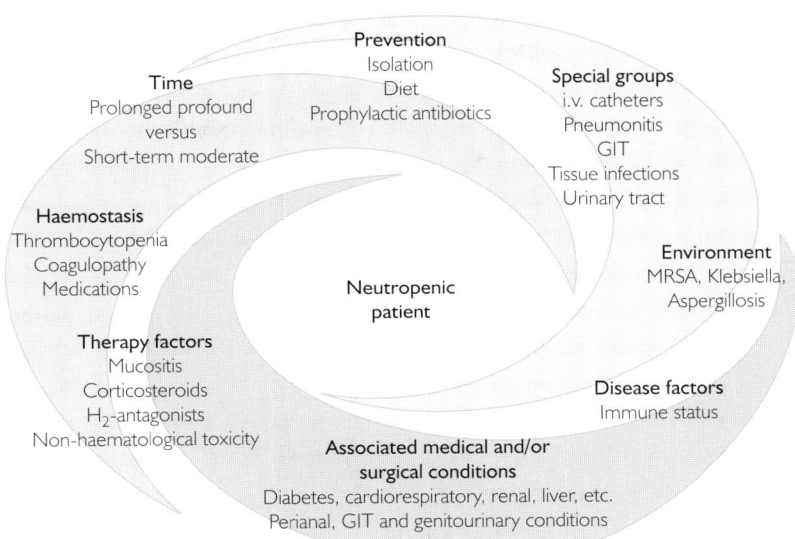

Fig. 90.1 The neutropenic patient.

INFECTION PREVENTION

Prevention of infection is extremely important and meticulous attention to sterility with invasive procedures (e.g. i.v. line insertions) is essential. Infection may be endogenously or exogenously acquired. Most patients when they are admitted to hospital become colonized with the hospital flora. The major sources of infecting organisms, however, are the patients themselves, for example, from the oropharynx, the gastrointestinal tract, i.v. line sites, lung and local lesions.

All ICUs must demand strict adherence to infection control guidelines. The most effective procedure is handwashing by all health care workers involved in the care of the immunocompromised patient.

Other preventive measures include: sterile techniques for invasive procedures by experienced staff, maintaining a clean environment, patient cooked meals, and limited use of prophylactic antibiotics. Needless to say excessive use of antibiotics is a major factor in the emergence of resistant strains and the susceptibility to colonization with hospital-acquired organisms. Many would argue that the efficacy of empirical therapy in the neutropenic patient is such that prophylaxis may be unnecessary. Reverse barrier nursing is instituted in order to minimize exposure to exogenous infection. This can be difficult in a critical care setting and will not prevent infections of endogenous origin.

INVASIVE PROCEDURES

Invasive procedures should be kept to a minimum and when performed, appropriate steps should be taken to minimize bleeding and the risk of infection. Endotracheal intubation should be avoided or minimized if at all possible. Biopsy procedures, arterial access, and other invasive procedures should be well planned and discussed with the haematologists.

BLOOD COMPONENT THERAPY[2-5]

During the period of marrow suppression, red cell concentrates need to be administered regularly to maintain the haemoglobin level around 100 g/l. If a higher oxygen delivery is desired (i.e. acute respiratory failure) the haemoglobin level should be higher (>120 g/l).

Regular platelet concentrates are required. In the presence of sepsis platelets are consumed rapidly and transfusions may be necessary on a daily basis otherwise second daily is usually adequate. The patient should be examined daily for evidence of haemostatic failure (e.g. purpura, ecchymoses, mouth, fundoscopy). Granulocyte transfusion may have a role in patients with proven unresponsive bacterial sepsis.

ANTIMICROBIAL THERAPY
The Febrile Neutropenic Patient[6-8]

After resistance of the malignant cell to therapy, infection is the commonest cause of death in patients with haematological malignancy. Patients usually tolerate neutropenia without developing infection until the count is <1.0 × 10⁹/l and it is not until the neutrophil count falls to <0.2 × 10⁹/l that spontaneous overwhelming sepsis becomes a major potentially life threatening problem. These patients must be watched closely for infection and

Table 90.1 Organisms associated with immune deficiency states

Neutropenia
  Bacteria
    Escherichia coli
    Pseudomonas aeruginosa
    Klebsiella pneumoniae
    Acinetobacter
    Staphylococcus epidermidis
    Staphylococcus aureus
    Streptococci viridans group
  Fungal
    Candida
    Aspergillus
    Mucormycosis
Cellular immune dysfunction
  Bacteria
    Listeria monocytogenes
    Salmonella
    Mycobacterium
    Nocardia asteroides
    Legionella
  Fungi
    Cryptococcus neoformans
    Histoplasma capsulatum
    Coccidioides immitis
  Viruses
    Varicella zoster
    Cytomegalovirus
    Herpes simplex
  Protozoa
    Pneumocystis carinii
    Toxoplasma gondii
    Crytosporidium
Humoral immune dysfunction
  Bacteria
    Streptococcus pneumoniae
    Haemophilus influenzae

treated early if necessary. When the neutrophil count is less than $0.5 \times 10^9/l$ any temperature above $38°C$ should be regarded as representing serious sepsis till proved otherwise. High-risk patients include those with pneumonitis, severe mucositis, an infected i.v. catheter and evidence of local sepsis. In patients with haematological malignancy and in allogeneic marrow transplant patients there may be pre-existing immunodeficiency.

Early empirical antibiotic therapy, without microbiological proof of cause, may be life-saving. With most patients fever resolves, especially if marrow function returns in the short-term. Ultimate proof of infection is frequently not established. Patients with agranulocytosis will not show the typical features of inflammation. For example, lung consolidation may not occur, cellulitis or

sputum may not be clinically obvious, and urinary tract symptoms may be minimal. The role of steroids in suppressing temperature and clinical features of inflammation must also be considered. Non-infectious fever should be borne in mind (e.g. malignancy or drugs).

The presence of rigours, hypotension and shock may point more towards Gram-negative sepsis. The value of combination therapy with a β-lactam antibiotic in combination with an aminoglycoside has been demonstrated in patients with prolonged and severe neutropenia with Gram-negative septicaemia. Gram-negative sepsis is potentially rapidly fatal in the neutropenic patient, but is less common than in the past as the less virulent Gram-positive organisms now predominate. This may be related to the increased use of permanent indwelling intravenous devices, mucositis, H_2 antagonists and the use of quinolones as antibiotic prophylaxis. However, streptococcal sepsis and staphylococcal sepsis can be severe and empiric use of vancomycin in high-risk patients is justified. *Staphylococcus epidermidis* is an indolent form of sepsis and time is usually available for adjustment of therapy, with most patients recovering.

The Choice of Empirical Antibiotic Therapy
Antibiotic therapy should be empirical, and aggressive with cover against Gram-negative sepsis as this is potentially lethal for the neutropenic patient. Anaerobic cover may need to be included when there is any problem with the gastrointestinal tract (e.g. intra-abdominal or perianal problems). This is not usually necessary when problems are confined to the mouth.

The nature and site of infection is determined by a range of factors including:

- the host defence defect
- time course of neutropenia
- local microbiological ecology
- antibiotic usage (e.g. prophylaxis)
- haemostasis
- presence of indwelling lines (i.v. endotracheal, urinary)
- type of chemotherapy
- nature of disease
- patient factors (e.g. hepatic, renal, respiratory or other factors)

Antibiotic Regimens
Initial empirical antibiotic therapy should cover: *Pseudomonas aeruginosa*, *Escherichia coli*, *Klebsiella* species, *Streptococcus viridans*, *Staphylococci* (coagulase negative and coagulase positive) depending on clinical circumstances. Other organisms should be covered after the results of cultures have been assessed or it is known that a specific organism is present in the ward (e.g. *Streptococcus viridans*) or on surveillance cultures. Coverage against *Staphylococcus epidermidis* is not necessary until bacteraemia is demonstrated.

Single-drug Therapy

Single agent therapy with a third generation cephalosporin (e.g. cefotaxime, ceftriaxone, ceftazidime) may be adequate therapy in low risk patients, i.e. neutrophil count $>0.5 \times 10^9/l$ and expected to stay above $0.5 \times 10^9/l$ or neutropenia expected to last less than 7 days.

Two-drug Therapy

Two-drug therapy with an added aminoglycoside (gentamicin, tobramycin, amikacin, netilmicin) is recommended as standard initial empirical regimen in patients with prolonged and profound neutropenia and no additional risk factors.

Three-drug Therapy

Three-drug therapy with a glycopeptide (vancomycin, teicoplanin) added to the aminoglycoside and cephalosporin is indicated for patients who are particularly likely to be infected with coagulase-negative Staphylococci, methicillin-resistant *Staphylococcus aureus*, *Corynebacterium* species and penicillin resistant *Streptococci viridans* (e.g. infected indwelling central venous catheter, pneumonitis, rash and severe mucositis).

Daily clinical assessment and review of microbiological results is essential. Antibiotic therapy is modified according to microbiological results. If no helpful microbiological information is forthcoming in the case of single or two-drug therapy, the antibiotic regimen should be re-evaluated at 48 h and if there has been no response, a glycopeptide added. If the fever has resolved and the cultures are negative the aminoglycoside may be ceased.

With patients on three-drug therapy, antibiotic reassessment at 72 hours is appropriate. If there is no response, further investigation such as a CT chest scan and broncho-alveolar lavage may be indicated. Depending on the clinical state of the patient the introduction of antifungal therapy should be considered.

Haemopoietic Growth Factors, Immunotherapy and Granulocyte Transfusions[9]

Genetically engineered haemopoietic growth factors are now widely used to minimize the degree and time of neutropenia. Granulocyte and granulocyte-macrophage colony-stimulating factors are glycoproteins which stimulate the proliferation and maturation of bone marrow progenitor cells, and increase the number and function of these committed cell populations. Treatment reduces the duration and severity of neutropenia in patients receiving chemotherapy and after haemopoietic stem cell transplantation. Growth factors do not prevent neutropenia, but shorten its duration and their use has been associated with fewer infectious febrile episodes. Intravenous immunoglobulin should be infused in patients with hypogammaglobulinaemia. Granulocyte transfusion may have a role if bacterial proven sepsis is not resolving or there is evidence of spreading local bacterial infection.

Patient Subgroups

Indwelling intravenous catheters

Indwelling intravenous silastic catheters provide a nidus for both infectious and non-infectious complications. The incidence of catheter-associated infections varies. Indwelling i.v. catheters present an increased risk of infection for both neutropenic and non-neutropenic patients. Coagulase-negative *Staphylococci* are the most common cause of catheter-associated bacteremia, but *Staphylococcus aureus*, *bacillus* species, *corynebacteria*, and gram-negative organisms (especially species of *acinetobacter* and *pseudomonas*) can also cause catheter infections and *Candida* infection can be catheter-related. Exit-site infections and infections along the subcutaneous tunnel of the catheter can be caused by aerobic bacteria, *Mycobacteria* and fungi.

If bacteraemia is thought to be catheter-related it may be possible to avoid removal of the catheter, particularly if the infection is caused by coagulase-negative *Staphylococci*. Even patients with gram-negative infections can often be successfully treated with antibiotics infused through the catheter. In patients with multiple-lumen catheters, the administration of antibiotics should be rotated through all the lumens, as infection may be restricted to only one. However, removal of the catheter is usually necessary for bacteria (e.g. species of bacillus) that may not be eradicated even though sensitive to antibiotics and with candidaemia in which there is a high incidence of dissemination. Patients with tunnel infections usually require catheter removal.

Lung infiltrates

Lung infiltrates[10] in febrile patients with neutropenia represent a high risk of treatment failure. Prolonged neutropenia has a significantly adverse effect on the outcome of infection. Incorporation of systemic antifungal agents into first-line therapy, particularly in selected high-risk subgroups, may improve the outcome. Involvement of a respiratory physician with experience in managing immunocompromised patients is important. Pulmonary investigations such as fine cut chest CT, bronchoscopy, bronchoalveolar lavage ± transbronchial biopsy may be required. Pulmonary haemorrhage can be a sudden and life-threatening cause of pulmonary infiltration and respiratory insufficiency. This usually occurs in severe thrombocytopenia associated with infection, and in patients who have become resistant to platelet transfusions.

HAEMOPOIETIC STEM CELL TRANSPLANTATION

Haemopoietic stem cell transplantation therapy is increasingly establishing a role in the treatment of a wide range of malignant and non-malignant disorders. Allogeneic bone marrow transplantation has been used as an adjunct to the treatment of acute leukaemia with an impressive success rate, which is translating into long-term survival and cure. This success is now being extended to the management of a wider range of haematological malignancies and more recently some solid tumours. Haemopoietic stem cells can be obtained from either marrow aspiration or from the peripheral blood by apheresis using a blood cell separator following stimulation of the marrow with haemopoietic growth factors ± cytotoxic chemotherapy. Allogeneic transplantation brings with it a range of potentially serious and potentially fatal complications related to graft versus host disease (GVHD). It does, however, have the advantage of using normal stem cells, which need not be stored and a limited degree of GVHD may have a beneficial anti-tumour effect. Autologous stem cell transplantation is of particular advantage when relatively normal bone marrow can be obtained in which case GVHD is not a problem.

The principles for the use of bone marrow transplantation in the management of malignancy include the following:

- The tumour must be responsive to chemotherapy and/or radiotherapy.
- The dose limitation of the chemotherapeutic agents used relate to marrow toxicity and not other end-organs.
- There should be a source of uncontaminated, or minimally contaminated haemopoietic stem cells.
- Appropriate haemopoietic supportive therapy must be available during the marrow aplastic period.
- High quality clinical and laboratory facilities must be available for the collection and preservation of haemopoietic stem cells.
- An integrated team of medical and nursing and scientific staff is essential.
- The preparation of a well-documented clinical protocol and effective implementation, with appropriate monitoring, is essential for success. The general management of the patient during the procedure is similar to the management of other patients receiving high dose chemotherapy who will have prolonged neutropenic periods.

COMPLICATIONS OF HAEMOPOIETIC CELL TRANSPLANTATION
Respiratory Failure in Haemopoietic Cell Transplant Patients

Respiratory failure[11] is the commonest cause of death in patients undergoing bone marrow transplantation. Both cytomegalovirus-induced interstitial pneumonia and the idiopathic pneumonia syndrome rarely occur in the early cytopenic phase post-transplantation. Haematological reconstitution with donor type cells seems to be a prerequisite to the development of these pulmonary complications, suggesting a key role of immunological reactions. While CMV pneumonia can be effectively treated or prevented by ganciclovir, the idiopathic syndrome is usually fatal. Due to improved prophylaxis and therapy, lethal interstitial pneumonia due to *Pneumocystis carinii, Herpes simplex, Varizella zoster* or *Toxoplasma gondii* as well as lethal pneumonia caused by bacteria or *Candida* species are generally

less common. However, *Aspergillus* species have emerged as frequent causative pathogens. Prolonged granulocytopenia and prolonged medication with corticosteroids are major risk factors for pulmonary aspergillosis, which is commonly fatal, but prophylaxis may be achieved by sterile air supply during the hospital stay and by prophylactic inhalation of amphotericin B. Pulmonary haemorrhage, as diagnosed by bronchoalveolar lavage, may develop due to the toxicity of the conditioning regimen, or may be secondary to infectious pneumonia of various kinds. Congestive heart failure or the application of cytokines might give rise to the development of pulmonary oedema. Patients with hepatic veno-occlusive disease have a high risk of subsequent pulmonary complications.

Graft-versus-host Disease

Graft-versus-host disease[12,13] (GVHD) is a major complication of allogeneic haemopoietic stem cell transplantation, especially with the increasing use of unrelated and mismatched donors. The target of the immune response in GVHD has long been regarded to be histocompatibility antigens possessed by the host, but not the donor. However it is now recognized that self-antigens have been documented in GVHD, confirming it is more complex than simple allo-reactivity. Cytokines play a central role in mediating many of the manifestations of GVHD.

Nearly all patients with GVHD have a rash. Other features include liver and gastrointestinal dysfunction. Initial therapy for low-grade disease is systemic corticosteroids. Treatment for more severe disease may include a range of therapy including; cyclosporine, antithymocyte globulin, tacrolimus, methotrexate, PUVA and thalidomide.

Veno-occlusive Disease of the Liver

Veno-occlusive disease[14] can be a major complication of haemopoietic stem cell transplantation, predominantly seen in allogeneic transplants and is a major contributor to mortality. The disorder is due to thrombotic occlusion in the small hepatic vessels, probably as a result of endothelial damage associated with high dose chemotherapy. The problem manifests as weight gain, oedema, ascites, tender hepatomegaly, jaundice and may proceed to liver failure. Prophylaxis with low dose heparin or prostaglandins may be useful. Treatment is predominantly supportive with fluid management a critical aspect. Treatment with tissue plasminogen activator and antithrombin III concentrates has been successful.

REFERENCES
1 Beutler E. The treatment of acute leukemia: past, present, and future. *Leukemia* 2001; **15**: 658–61.
2 Freireich EJ. Supportive care for patients with blood disorders. *Br J Haematol* 2000; **111**: 68–77.
3 McCullough J. Current issues with platelet transfusion in patients with cancer. *Semin Hematol* 2000; **37** (suppl 4): 3–10.

4 Murphy MF, Waters AH. Platelet transfusions: the problem of refractoriness. *Blood Review* 1990; **4**: 16–24.

5 Navarro JT, Hernandez JA, Ribera JM, *et al.* Prophylactic platelet transfusion threshold during therapy for adult acute myeloid leukemia: 10 000/microL versus 20 000/microL. *Haematologica* 1998; **83**: 998–1000.

6 Klastersky J. Empirical treatment of sepsis in neutropenic patients. *Hosp Med* 2001; **62**: 101–3.

7 Pappas PG, Rex JH. Therapeutic approach to Candida sepsis. *Curr Infect Dis Rep* 1999; **3**: 245–52.

8 Gaytan-Martinez J, Mateos-Garcia E, Sanchez-Cortes E *et al.* Microbiological findings in febrile neutropenia. *Arch Med Res* 2000; **31**: 388–92.

9 Vose JM, Armitage JO, Clinical applications of hematopoietic growth factors. *J Clin Oncol* 1995; **13**: 1023–35.

10 Maschmeyer G., Link H., Hiddemann W. Pulmonary infiltrations in febrile patients with neutropenia: Risk factors and outcome under empirical antimicrobial therapy in a randomized multicenter study. *Cancer* 1994; **73**: 2296–304.

11 Quabeck K. The lung as a critical organ in marrow transplantation. *Bone Marrow Transplant* 1994; **14**(suppl 4): S19–28.

12 Goker H, Haznedaroglu IC, Chao NJ. Acute graft-vs-host disease: pathobiology and management. *Exp Hematol* 2001; **29**: 259–77.

13 Basara N, Blau IW, Willenbacher W *et al.* New strategies in the treatment of graft-versus-host disease. *Bone Marrow Transplant* 2000; **26**(suppl 2): S12–5.

14 Carreras E. Veno-occlusive disease of the liver after hemopoietic cell transplantation. *Eur J Haematol* 2000; **64**: 281–91.

Part Sixteen

Transplants

91

Organ donation

S Streat

Many intensivists at times have responsibility for the care of organ transplant recipients and have seen the benefits of organ transplantation – one of the great medical successes of the late twentieth century.[1] Clinical results continue to improve, despite the increase in co-morbidity and case complexity that has accompanied the increase in indications for transplant and decrease in contraindications to it. This success has led to an enormous increase in demand for organ transplantation while the number of available organs has increased much more slowly, resulting in rapid growth of transplant waiting lists.[2] Many transplant centres have reported an increase in waiting times and an unacceptable number of patients dying on the waiting list.

In the absence of clinical xenotransplantation, tissue engineering or effective artificial organs, transplant programs continue to critically depend upon donated organs. This has led transplant professionals to accept organs from donors previously considered marginal, to increase transplantation from living kidney,[3] liver[4] and lung[5] donors and to vigorously champion endeavours to increase cadaveric organ donation, including non-heart-beating organ donation.[6] There has been comparatively less consideration to restricting access to waiting lists.[7]

RESPONSIBILITIES OF THE INTENSIVIST

Intensivists are in general supportive of cadaveric organ donation,[8] are responsible for the care of dying patients and their families, and should therefore be obliged to provide leadership in organ donation. This personal view is growing in intensive care medicine[8–10] but is not yet widely accepted. Intensivists must ensure that the processes involved in determination of death and facilitation of cadaveric organ donation remain of the highest standard and are publicly seen to be so. These processes include the care of the dying patient and their family, determination of brain death, identification of the potential for organ donation to occur, offering the opportunity for organ donation to the family, maintenance of physiological stability throughout the time until organ retrieval,

and aftercare for the family of the deceased, irrespective of whether organ donation took place.

CARE OF THE DYING PATIENT AND THE FAMILY

Intensivists are, in general, familiar with the care of the dying patient, including the need to avoid suffering and maintain patient dignity. The respect of the ICU staff for the humanity of the dying person is perhaps most obviously expressed in the 'patient comfort care' provided by the nursing staff and the evident compassion of the staff for the family.[11]

The intensivist has a crucial role to play in the care of the family of the dying patient. It is important to establish rapport with the family very early in the critical illness by way of a family meeting. There may need to be several 'bad news' meetings in the days to come. Such meetings should be attended by whomever the family defines themselves to include, and by the intensivist and a member of the nursing staff acting as a support role for the family (and perhaps by a chaplain or social worker if the family wish). The role of 'support person' should be kept separate from the role of the 'bearer of bad news'. These meetings should be held in a separate private room large enough to accommodate all the participants, away from the bedside and with 'protected time' against interruptions. The intensivist should convey, with evident compassion,[11] an accurate account of the sequence of events together with a realistic assessment of prognosis and the immediate care plan. Presenting CT or other visual information may assist the family to understand. There should be time to answer any questions that the family may have, and at the end of the meeting, the intensivist should ascertain that the family understand what has been said,[11] and that they are in agreement with the care plan. Ensuring that anyone who speaks with the family gives a consistent message is an essential part of maintaining trust between the family and the ICU team – ideally only one intensivist should speak with the family. This strength of the trust in the relationship will determine the ability of the ICU team and the family to deal together with the difficult and painful issues of withdrawal of intensive therapies (should that occur), the death of the patient and subsequently the consideration of organ donation.

Perhaps the most problematic issue for intensivists caring for the patient dying with severe brain injury concerns the timing of the decision to withdraw brain-oriented intensive therapies, while continuing that physiological support which preserves the possibility of organ donation in the future. It is often appropriate to withhold or withdraw brain-oriented intensive therapies (e.g. CSF drainage) when it is clear that death is inevitable. This must involve assembling definitive prognostic information, obtaining consensus of those involved in treating the patient and acceptance by the family that death is inevitable. A sedative-free clinical assessment of CNS function is an essential part of prognostication. The possibility of future organ donation has no part in the decision to withhold or withdraw specific brain-oriented therapies. This decision is guided by the ethical principles of non-malfeasance and respect for autonomy.[12] Most patients have devastating brain damage with some brain stem function, and many of them may never become brain dead. It is often appropriate to progressively withdraw, in a dignified manner, all intensive therapies from such patients, while continuing to provide 'comfort care' to the patient and support to the family.[12]

During the period of sedative-free CNS assessment, some patients will suffer apparent loss of brain stem function. However, a greater percentage of patients will have apparent loss of brain stem function, despite continuance of all available surgical and medical therapy. Brain-oriented intensive therapies should be withheld pending formal assessment of brain death. In order to meet the pre-conditions for brain death assessment,[13] extracranial homeostasis must be maintained, and these conditions also preserve the possibility of organ donation in the future.

IDENTIFICATION OF THE POTENTIAL FOR ORGAN DONATION TO OCCUR

Most ICUs admit patients with very severe brain damage where it is clear that the probability of survival is low. The primary indication for such admission is to identify that subgroup of patients who may survive and provide them with the necessary care to enable that survival. There are situations where it might be thought that the chance of that recovery is so remote that admission of the patient to ICU would not ordinarily occur. Some have advocated admitting such patients to ICU solely to allow for the future possibility that organ donation may occur, with accompanying explicit discussion with the family of this possibility.[14] Although it seems likely[14] that such a utilitarian approach might increase the number of organs available for transplant, ethical,[15] legal[16] and clinical[15] objections to the practice have all been raised.

Organ donation is possible in most situations where brain death has been confirmed. The absolute general contra-indications to organ donation are few and are absent in the majority of brain-dead patients. They include situations where there is an unacceptably high risk of the transmission to the recipient of malignancy or infection or where the function of the possible donor organs is likely to be unacceptably poor. Extracerebral malignancies and certain infections (e.g. with HIV) are likely to remain absolute contraindications but other donor factors (e.g. advanced age, recent bacterial sepsis,[17] positive HCV[18] or HBV[18] serology) are no longer thought absolute contraindications. Before deciding that organ donation is contraindicated on medical grounds, intensivists should discuss the specific issue with the appropriate agency (donor co-ordinator or organ procurement organization).

Similarly, the organ-specific contraindications to organ donation have reduced in recent years as the outcomes of recipients transplanted with donor organs formerly considered marginal have been found to be acceptable.[19] Finally, these contraindications vary somewhat between transplant centres and continue to change in a more permissive direction. In general the presence of more than mild chronic organ dysfunction or the development of severe acute organ dysfunction will likely contraindicate donation of that organ. However, intensivists should discuss these organ-specific issues with the donor co-ordinator or appropriate agency before deciding that a particular organ is unsuitable for possible donation and subsequent transplantation.

In most jurisdictions an appropriate authority (e.g. a coroner or medical examiner) may legally interdict organ donation under certain circumstances (e.g. homicide) and this issue should also be clarified with the donor co-ordinator.

The donor co-ordinator will clarify with the transplant teams whether any organ donation is possible and whether particular organs may not be suitable and the intensivist should provide the co-ordinator with the necessary information (see Table 91.1) for these decisions.

DETERMINATION OF BRAIN DEATH

This is a clinical responsibility of the intensivist and must be carried out according to appropriate codes of practice or clinical guidelines (see Ch. 45). The determination of brain death[20,21] involves several stages – first establishing the presence of a condition known to produce severe and irreversible structural brain damage, second the exclusion of possible confounding factors and finally the determination by two independent clinical examinations that there is profound unresponsive coma and persistent absence of brain stem function. The examination and determination of brain death should be documented in the medical record, which is facilitated by a pro forma. In

Table 91.1 Information likely to be required by transplant teams

Age, sex, weight, approximate height
Previous medical history (including co-morbidity, surgery, medication, alcohol, smoking, illicit drug use and allergies)
Detailed clinical history of fatal illness (including history of cardiac arrest, periods of hypotension or hypoxia)
Current clinical status (including ventilatory and inotropic support and physiological parameters)
Current investigations (including blood group, arterial blood gases, chest X-ray, ECG, urea, creatinine, electrolytes, glucose, bilirubin, transaminases, alkaline phosphatase and gamma glutamyl transpeptidase, prothrombin ratio, activated partial thromboplastin time, haemoglobin, white cell count, platelets and all microbiology results).

the circumstance where clinical examination is confounded (e.g. by barbiturate coma) then absence of cerebral blood flow must be documented by angiography or other reliable imaging.[13]

The fact of brain death and its medical and legal implications must then be conveyed to the family. It is often difficult for families to accept brain death as death, given the life-like appearance of the skin, the rise and fall of the chest and the warmth of the hands that are preserved by ventilatory and circulatory support. For some family members, the opportunity to view the second clinical examination for brain death, or the cerebral arteriogram when clinical examination is confounded, may help them to understand and accept the final awful implication of this diagnosis. Intensivists should be open to offering these options.

In the absence of organ donation, it is appropriate to remove ventilatory support at a time that allows for family needs.

OFFERING THE OPPORTUNITY FOR ORGAN DONATION TO THE FAMILY

The differentiation[9] of organ donation (an intensive care unit activity) from transplantation allows for the consideration of many perspectives that are often not considered in transplant-oriented publications. Organ donation is an activity that fundamentally modifies the human rituals surrounding death, even death in ICU. Organ retrieval is a surgical procedure carried out in the operating room and although this is done in a respectful manner with identical surgical processes to those used on living people, it is nevertheless viewed by some[22] as 'mutilating'. Discussion of organ donation is an emotionally intense activity involving a newly bereaved family and a health professional, and requires very clear and sensitive communication. It takes place at a time when the family members have only recently been told that their loved one has died and yet they must consider the

issue at this time of intense grief – there is no other time. Knowledge of organ donation varies widely in the community and some families may not previously have known that organ donation and transplantation take place. Similarly, both discussion of organ donation and acceptance and willingness to be part of it vary widely in the community. There is greater in-principle agreement with organ donation than either individual agreement or decision-making on behalf of a loved one. Discussion of organ donation among families is often promoted as a way of increasing organ donation rates with some evidence that it may do so. Some family members will have strongly held views against organ donation based on personal religious or cultural beliefs.[22]

There are several 'transplant-oriented cultural attitudes' concerning organ donation including the notion that organ donation is the only possible positive outcome that can occur in the setting of brain death,[23] that it is appropriate to refer to brain dead persons in a utilitarian way as sources of organs for transplant,[24] that for many families organ donation can assist with easing the pain of loss, and that fulfilling the previously expressed wishes of the donor should be the primary or indeed the only[25] consideration. In some jurisdictions these wishes have indeed been defined to be legally sufficient for organs to be retrieved, and are often argued to be a means of increasing the organ donation rate[26] by excluding the family from the opportunity to prohibit organ donation and 'returning control to the individual'. Implicit in this 'transplant-oriented culture' is the judgement that for a family to agree to organ donation is desirable and perhaps of greater moral value than the contrary decision, particularly if organ donation was the previously expressed wish of the dead person. This judgement implicitly denies the legitimacy of the close human relationship between the family and the deceased to determine what should happen to their loved one after death.[27] It is noteworthy that even in countries that legally allow the previously expressed wishes of the deceased to determine whether organ donation may take place, usual practice continues to involve the family and not to proceed against family objection. Furthermore, the impact on the deceased's family was rated as the most important factor determining consent practice in one such study,[28] implying an incongruity between the law and clinically acceptable decision-making under these conditions.

Intensivists should be aware of their own views on these matters, and indeed the views of others that might discuss organ donation with family members. While intensivists most often initiate discussion of organ donation with families in Australasia,[8] this is often not so elsewhere. Whoever undertakes this discussion should be skilled in communication with grieving people. An existing relationship with the family, which has been established over the previous family meetings, can make this discussion easier to initiate by the intensivist. Defining this discussion as 'offering the option of organ donation' rather than 'obtaining consent' (or even 'persuasion'[29]) is not coercive in language and frees the intensivist to providing complete and unbiased information, support the family in their decision-making and thank them for their decision, whatever that may be. The intensivist must ensure that the fact of death is understood. Then there must be sufficient time for the intensivist to inform the family of the option of organ donation and what it entails, to answer any questions and if necessary to facilitate decision-making by the family. They may take into account previously expressed wishes, previous family discussions, personal and family values and cultural and religious beliefs.

This discussion must not be coercive. Language that is potentially coercive (e.g. 'fulfilling the deceased's wishes', 'doing what he would have wanted', 'something good may come of this') can re-define the situation in terms of the family coming to fulfil the intensivist's wishes and should be avoided. Finally, some language is particularly insensitive (e.g. the use of the term 'harvest' rather than 'organ retrieval' to describe the process of organ retrieval, or 'the body' rather than the person's name to describe the brain-dead person) when viewed from the perspective of grieving families and should also be avoided.[30] The intensivist should facilitate the family spending time at the bedside prior to organ retrieval. Some tests (e.g. echocardiography or coronary arteriography) may be performed during this time and the family should be informed about the reason and implication of these. The intensivist should ensure that the family is offered an opportunity to spend time with the deceased after organ retrieval if this is desired.

MAINTENANCE OF EXTRA-CEREBRAL PHYSIOLOGICAL STABILITY IN BRAIN DEATH

Immediately prior to brain death, there is usually a period of hypertension, tachycardia and occasionally dysrhythmia, mediated by both autonomic activity and catecholamine secretion. Pulmonary oedema, biventricular dysfunction and myocardial injury may develop, but there is debate about the implications of these for subsequent cardiac graft function.[31] If treatment of this adrenergic phenomenon is thought essential then a short acting β-blocker (esmolol) should be used. Cardiac arrest can rarely occur during this phase, usually due to tachydysrhythmia, but is often reversible. This hypertension is soon followed by hypotension, associated with marked reduction in sympathetic activity and catecholamine secretion. The hypotension may be profound in the presence of simultaneous hypovolaemia or cardiac dysfunction and can lead to cardiac arrest or loss of donor organ viability, and should be promptly treated by volume expansion and inotropic support.

Diabetes insipidus due to loss of ADH production soon follows and is manifest by brisk hypo-osmolar polyuria, which will lead to hypovolaemia and hyperosmolality if untreated. Other hormone abnormalities occur but do not have serious implications in the short term. Associated with the loss of cerebral blood flow there is loss of cerebral metabolism and a fall of around 25% in oxygen consumption and carbon dioxide production.[32] This leads to a fall in the necessary ventilatory minute volume necessary for normocarbia. The fall in resting energy expenditure (heat production) together with loss of vasomotor tone and the possibility of shivering-induced thermogenesis exacerbate the risk of hypothermia developing.

Spontaneous movements and spinal motor reflexes may commonly persist in brain death.[33] These rarely include bizarre movements,[20,34] which are often reproducible. Family members may be invited to view the second brain death test in order that there can be explanation of these responses should they occur. Sympathetic responses may also occur to surgical stimulation and may justify the use of anaesthetic agents in the operating room.[35]

SUGGESTED STRATEGIES FOR MAINTAINING PHYSIOLOGICAL STABILITY

The onset of brain death is usually heralded by rises in intracranial pressure (if measured) or signs of progressive loss of brain stem function (coma, pupillary dilatation) and the need for specific support should be anticipated and planned for. This should include ensuring that central venous access is available for inotropic support and perhaps measurement of central venous pressure, that additional intravenous access is in place for rapid volume infusion and that a source of external heat (e.g. a warming blanket) is available.

VENTILATORY MANAGEMENT

The aims of ventilatory management are to maintain good oxygenation and normocarbia, minimize circulatory depression and maintain, if possible, sufficiently good lung function to allow for future lung donation to occur. The use of moderate tidal volumes (10–12 ml/kg) and addition of a low level of PEEP (5 cmH$_2$O) may prevent atelectasis. Originally a PaO$_2$ of more than 350 mmHg on 100% oxygen and 5 cmH$_2$O PEEP was thought a necessary prerequisite criterion for lung donation but recently PaO$_2$/FiO$_2$ ratios of 300 or 250 have been found to be acceptable.[36] Peak airway pressures above 30 cmH$_2$O should be avoided if possible. Usual pulmonary care including changes of position and sterile endotracheal suctioning must continue. When pulmonary dysfunction is severe higher levels of PEEP may be required to prevent airway frothing or provide adequate oxygenation. The determination of apnoea during brain death testing in such patients may require a period of mechanical hypoventilation prior to apnoea and continuation of CPAP during apnoea in such patients if serious hypoxaemia and circulatory depression are to be avoided.

CIRCULATORY MANAGEMENT

The aims of circulatory management are to maintain adequate organ perfusion and arterial pressure without producing fluid overload or excessive vasoconstriction, and without prejudicing future cardiac donation. Reasonable initial haemodynamic goals include normotension (a mean arterial pressure over 70 mmHg), heart rate of 100 or less and central venous pressure of 8 mmHg. Some inotropic support is almost always required (e.g. 224 of the 237 donors in 2000 in Australia and New Zealand[37]). Having established normotension with an inotrope infusion (norepinephrine, dopamine or epinephrine), the haemodynamic response to a controlled volume challenge should be assessed.

The choice of inotrope has been the subject of much controversy but little evidence. Dobutamine is largely ineffective and not recommended. The need for some pressor activity is common. Norepinephrine (usually less than 500 μg/h) is most commonly used in Australasia (67% of 224 donors in 2000 who received inotrope infusions[37]) without apparent detriment. Dopamine is less commonly used and may exacerbate polyuria by its tubular effect. Epinephrine may have specific benefit on renal blood flow in brain death[38] but may also increase glycaemia and thereby osmotic diuresis. Catcholamine infusion may reduce the up-regulation of organ immunogenicity that occurs in brain death and lower the incidence of acute rejection in subsequent recipients of kidney grafts.[39] Corticosteroids are sometimes used to improve haemodynamic stability, but their efficacy in this setting is unknown.

Control of excessive polyuria will minimize the risks of developing hyperosmolality,[40] hypovolaemia or hyperglycaemia secondary to infusion of large amounts of dextrose-containing fluids. Synthetic desmopressin (1-D amino-8 D arginine vasopressin) is commonly given to control diabetes insipidus and appears safe and effective.[37,41] In addition, low dose vasopressin infusion has been shown to be safe and effective in reducing the amount of catecholamine required to support arterial pressure[42] without apparent detriment to subsequently transplanted organs. It should perhaps be used in brain death if catecholamine requirements seem excessive despite adequate volume loading.[42]

Fluid therapy is similarly contentious. Control of diabetes insipidus is an essential aspect of rational fluid therapy. Hypovolaemia should be corrected with resuscitation fluids. Haemoconcentration occurs early after experimental brain death. Crystalloid infusion has been reported to worsen pulmonary function in brain death and larger volumes will be required than if colloid is used.[43] Although there is some evidence that hydroxyethylstarch may impair subsequent graft function in the kidney recipient, this is debated[44] and moderate volumes of starch are commonly given. There is a suggestion of better preservation of renal function in sepsis with polygelin rather than starch but the relevance of this situation to brain death is uncertain. At least moderate anaemia is well tolerated in brain death but red cells may be given if needed to maintain packed cell volume around 0.25 pending organ retrieval. Free water should be given as necessary (1–2 ml/kg per h as 5% dextrose) to maintain serum osmolality in the range of 280–310 mosm/kg – corresponding to serum sodium below 155 mmol/l. Severe hyperosmolality (probably a marker of inadequate donor care) is associated with poor graft function in subsequent liver recipients.[40] Failure to control diabetes insipidus will lead to increased requirements of free water to control serum osmolality. If 5% dextrose is used for this then hyperglycaemia and osmotic diuresis may result.

METABOLIC MANAGEMENT

Oxygen consumption, carbon dioxide production, heat production and glucose oxidation all fall in brain death due to the loss of cerebral metabolic activity.[32] Hypothermia may easily develop in association with vasoparesis, loss of shivering, exposure to room temperature, warm polyuria and infusion of room temperature intravenous fluids. Core temperature should be kept above the 35–36.5°C required to confirm brain death.[13,20] Keeping the ambient temperature high (24°C) and using infusion fluid warmers, heated humidifiers and external warming systems may be required. Low dose insulin infusion is occasionally required to prevent hyperglycaemia. Serum potassium should be kept above 3.5 mmol/l but potassium replacement should be given with caution as hyperkalaemia is not uncommon and may be more easily produced after brain death. Unlike the situation in sepsis, correction of hypophosphataemia does not improve haemodynamics in brain death.[45] Although levels of thyroid hormones fall after brain death this is probably the 'sick euthyroid syndrome' and replacement of thyroid hormone does not improve the circulation after brain death.[46]

NON-HEART-BEATING ORGAN DONATION

Although some transplant centres, notably Maastricht,[47] have transplanted organs from such donors for many years, non-heart-beating organ donation is being increasingly promoted. Immediate graft function in recipients of such organs is often not as good as those of organs from brain dead donors[48] but long-term recipient outcomes may be equivalent. A number of centres have developed conservative protocols for non-heart-beating organ donation and reported modest increases (commonly 10–20%) in the total number of organs, particularly kidneys, available for transplant. However, a cautious approach to non-heart-beating organ donation is still recommended as legal, ethical and medical concerns remain.[49] Non-heart-beating organ donation should only take place in the context of an institutional protocol wherein wide consultation has satisfactorily addressed these issues.

AFTERCARE OF THE DONOR FAMILY

The literature has focused on the specific needs of the donor family and there may be specific issues that need to be addressed, sometimes by way of a family meeting with an intensivist at some later stage. Most organ donation agencies and transplant programmes accept and facilitate limited anonymous information being communicated between recipients and donor families but direct contact is not recommended. However, routine aftercare for the families of all patients dying in ICUs is increasingly recommended.[50] Such aftercare programmes are well received[11] and have the potential to improve the care of subsequent families by revealing areas of inadequate or inappropriate communication.

REFERENCES

1 Groth CG, Brent LB, Calne RY, *et al.* Historic landmarks in clinical transplantation: conclusions from the consensus conference at the University of California, Los Angeles. *World J Surg* 2000; **24**: 834–43.

2 Harper AM, McBride MA, Ellison MD. The UNOS OPTN waiting list, 1988–1998. *Clin Transpl* 1999; 71–82.

3 D'Alessandro AM, Pirsch JD, Knechtle SJ, *et al.* Living unrelated renal donation: the University of Wisconsin experience. *Surgery* 1998; **124**: 604–10.

4 Trotter JF, Wachs M, Trouillot T, *et al.* Evaluation of 100 patients for living donor liver transplantation. *Liver Transpl* 2000; **6**: 290–5.

5 Cohen RG, Starnes VA. Living donor lung transplantation. *World J Surg* 2001; **25**: 244–50.

6 Daemen JW, Oomen AP, Kelders WP, Kootstra G. The potential pool of non-heart-beating kidney donors. *Clin Transplant* 1997; **11**: 149–54.

7 Frigerio M, Gronda EG, Mangiavacchi M, *et al.* Restrictive criteria for heart transplantation candidacy maximize survival of patients with advanced heart failure. *J Heart Lung Transplant* 1997; **16**: 160–8.

8 Pearson IY, Zurynski Y. A survey of personal and professional attitudes of intensivists to organ donation and transplantation. *Anaesth Intensive Care* 1995; **23**: 68–74.

9 Streat S, Silvester W. Organ donation in Australia and New Zealand – ICU perspectives. *Crit Care Resuscitation* 2001; **3**: 48–51.

10 Buckley TA. The shortage of solid organs for transplantation in Hong Kong: part of a worldwide problem. *Hong Kong Med J* 2000; **6**: 399–408.

11 Cuthbertson SJ, Margetts MA, Streat SJ. Bereavement follow-up after critical illness. *Crit Care Med* 2000, **28**: 1196–201.

12 Henig NR, Faul JL, Raffin TA. Biomedical ethics and the withdrawal of advanced life support. *Annu Rev Med* 2001; **52**: 79–92.

13 Australian and New Zealand Intensive Care Society. Recommendations on brain death and organ donation, 2nd edn. Melbourne: ANZICS; 1998.

14 Riad H, Nicholls A, Neuberger J, *et al.* Elective ventilation of potential organ donors. *BMJ* 1995; **310**: 714–8.

15 Manara A, Jewkes C. Intensive care units have good reasons not to do it. *BMJ* 1995; **311**: 121–2.

16 *F versus West Berkshire Health Authority.* 1989: 2 All ER 545–51, HL.

17 Freeman RB, Giatras I, Falagas ME, *et al.* Outcome of transplantation of organs procured from bacteremic donors. *Transplantation* 1999; **68**: 1107–11.

18 The Transplantation Society of Australia and New Zealand. Organ allocation protocols. Available at http://www.racp.edu.au/tsanz/oapmain.htm (Accessed 11 March 2002).

19 Ojo AO, Hanson JA, Meier-Kriesche H, *et al.* Survival in recipients of marginal cadaveric donor kidneys compared with other recipients and wait-listed transplant candidates. *J Am Soc Nephrol* 2001; **12**: 589–97.

20 Wijdicks EF. The diagnosis of brain death. *N Engl J Med* 2001; **344**: 1215–21.

21 Capron AM. Brain death – well settled yet still unresolved. *N Engl J Med* 2001; **344**: 1244–6.

22 Chapman JR, Hibberd AD, McCosker C, *et al.* Obtaining consent for organ donation in nine NSW metropolitan hospitals. *Anaesth Intensive Care* 1995; **23**: 81–7.

23 Murphy L. Donation – a difficult but most important discussion. *Mich Health Hosp* 1999; **35**: 20–1.

24 Fisher J. An expedient and ethical alternative to xenotransplantation. *Med Health Care Philos* 1999; **2**: 31–9.

25 May T, Aulisio MP, DeVita MA. Patients, families, and organ donation: who should decide? *Milbank Q* 2000; **78**: 323–36, 152.

26 Spital A. Mandated choice for organ donation: time to give it a try. *Ann Intern Med* 1996; **125**: 66–9.

27 Klassen AC, Klassen DK. Who are the donors in organ donation? The family's perspective in mandated choice. *Ann Intern Med* 1996; **125**: 70–3.

28 Wendler D, Dickert N. The consent process for cadaveric organ procurement: how does it work? How can it be improved? *JAMA* 2001; **285**: 329–33.

29 Siminoff LA, Gordon N, Hewlett J, Arnold RM. Factors influencing families' consent for donation of solid organs for transplantation. *JAMA* 2001; **286**: 71–7.

30 Farsides T. Winning hearts and minds: using psychology to promote voluntary organ donation. *Health Care Anal* 2000; **8**: 101–21.

31 Deibert E, Aiyagari V, Diringer MN. Reversible left ventricular dysfunction associated with raised troponin I after subarachnoid haemorrhage does not preclude successful heart transplantation. *Heart* 2000; **84**: 205–7.

32 Bitzani M, Matamis D, Nalbandi V, *et al.* Resting energy expenditure in brain death. *Intensive Care Med* 1999; **25**: 970–6.

33 Saposnik G, Bueri JA, Mauriño J, *et al*. Spontaneous and reflex movements in brain death. *Neurology* 2000; **54**: 221.

34 Ropper AH. Unusual spontaneous movements in brain-dead patients. *Neurology* 1984; **34**: 1089–92.

35 Young PJ, Matta BF. Anaesthesia for organ donation in the brainstem dead – why bother? *Anaesthesia* 2000; **54**: 105–6.

36 Gabbay E, Williams TJ, Griffiths AP, *et al*. Maximizing the utilization of donor organs offered for lung transplantation. *Am J Respir Crit Care Med* 1999; **160**: 265–71.

37 Herbertt K, Russ GR (eds) *ANZOD Registry Report 2001*. Australia and New Zealand Organ Donation Registry, Adelaide, South Australia. Available at http://www.anzdata.org.au/ (Accessed 11 March 2002).

38 Ueno T, Zhi-Li C, Itoh T. Unique circulatory responses to exogenous catecholamines after brain death. *Transplantation* 2000; **70**: 436–40.

39 Schnuelle P, Lorenz D, Mueller A *et al*. Donor catecholamine use reduces acute allograft rejection and improves graft survival after cadaveric renal transplantation. *Kidney Int* 1999; **56**: 738–46.

40 Totsuka E, Dodson F, Urakami A, *et al*. Influence of high donor serum sodium levels on early postoperative graft function in human liver transplantation: effect of correction of donor hypernatremia. *Liver Transpl Surg* 1999; **5**: 421–8.

41 Guesde R, Barrou B, Leblanc I, *et al*. Administration of desmopressin in brain-dead donors and renal function in kidney recipients. *Lancet* 1998; **352**: 1178–81.

42 Chen JM, Cullinane S, Spanier TB, *et al*. Vasopressin deficiency and pressor hypersensitivity in hemodynamically unstable organ donors. *Circulation* 1999; **100**(suppl 19): II244–6.

43 Randell T, Orko R, Hockerstedt K. Peroperative fluid management of the brain-dead multiorgan donor. *Acta Anaesthesiol Scand* 1990; **34**: 592–5.

44 Deman A, Peeters P, Sennesael J. Hydroxyethyl starch does not impair immediate renal function in kidney transplant recipients: a retrospective, multicentre analysis. *Nephrol Dial Transplant* 1999; **14**: 1517–20.

45 Riou B, Kalfon P, Arock M *et al*. Cardiovascular consequences of severe hypophosphataemia in brain-dead patients. *Br J Anaesth* 1995; **74**: 424–9.

46 Goarin JP, Cohen S, Riou B, *et al*. The effects of triiodothyronine on hemodynamic status and cardiac function in potential heart donors. *Anesth Analg* 1996; **83**: 41–7.

47 Vromen MA, Leunissen KM, Persijn GG, Kootstra G. Short- and long-term results with adult non-heart-beating donor kidneys. *Transplant Proc* 1988; **20**: 743–5.

48 Nicholson ML, Metcalfe MS, White SA, *et al*. A comparison of the results of renal transplantation from non-heart-beating, conventional cadaveric, and living donors. *Kidney Int* 2000; **58**: 2585–91.

49 Vanrenterghem Y. Cautious approach to use of non-heart-beating donors. *Lancet* 2000 12; **356**: 528.

50 Campbell ML, Thill M. Bereavement follow-up to families after death in the intensive care unit. *Crit Care Med* 2000; **28**: 1252–3.

92

Liver transplantation

E Sizer, J Wendon and S Cottam

Liver transplantation has revolutionized the care of patients, with both acute and chronic end-stage liver disease becoming the treatment of choice in the absence of contraindications. It has become an almost routine procedure, with the majority of patients having a short postoperative ICU stay and 1 year survival >90%.[1] Indications have widened, and contraindications decreased. As a consequence, the number of patients awaiting transplantation continues to outstrip cadaveric donor rates; waiting times lengthen, hence patients become critically ill before receiving a transplant, increasing risk, perioperative complications and impairing long-term outcome. Innovative strategies have evolved as possible solutions to the lack of cadaveric donor organs, including: widening the donor pool to include previously unsuitable donors (so-called marginal donors), paediatric and adult living-related donation, reduced size and splitting techniques and the use of 'non-heart beating donation'.

PATIENT SELECTION

There are currently relatively few absolute contraindications to liver transplantation and no specific age limitation. Patients must have the required cardiorespiratory reserve to tolerate the procedure. Much work has gone into the development of prognostic tools to allow accurate prediction of the need and timing for transplantation. Once multi-organ failure has developed in a debilitated patient awaiting transplantation, survival rates decrease to 20–30% and these patients often require weeks to months of postoperative hospitalization.[2]

PERIOPERATIVE ASPECTS

OPERATIVE TECHNIQUE

Orthotopic liver transplantation (OLT) involves recipient hepatectomy, revascularization of the donor graft and biliary reconstruction.

Two main techniques are used in adult liver transplantation, those with vena cava preservation ('piggy back technique') and those using portal bypass (either internal, temporary portocaval shunt or external, veno-venous bypass).[3] The advantages of the piggyback technique include haemodynamic stability during the anhepatic phase, without large volume fluid administration, and the negation of the need for venovenous bypass with its associated risks and complications. Decreased transfusion requirements, shorter anhepatic time and shorter total operating time are also observed.[4] There is no observed difference in renal function between the two techniques. The donor hepatic artery is directly anastomosed, utilizing an 'end-to end' technique or a conduit is constructed. Portal venous anastomosis must also be undertaken, in most patients this is an end-to-end anastomosis, however, portal venous thrombosis is no longer a contraindication to transplantation. These patients may undergo a re-cannulation procedure or require a jump graft technique. Such conduits and grafts are normally fashioned from donor vessels. It is imperative that all those caring for the patients are aware of the surgical technique undertaken, as complications may vary. The radiologist must be aware of the technique used to allow appropriate interpretation of subsequent investigations. This applies not just to the vascular anastomosis but also to the presence of a full graft, reduced size graft, right or left split graft or indeed an auxiliary graft. The biliary anastomosis is normally also undertaken as an end to end procedure, the donor bile duct being directly joined to the recipient duct. It is no longer standard for this to be undertaken over a T-tube, but this may be required where there is marked discrepancy between donor and recipient duct size. Some conditions (e.g. extrahepatic biliary atresia, primary sclerosing cholangitis) may preclude end-to-end anastomosis and formation of choledochojejunostomy may be required.

Auxiliary liver transplantation is a technique that involves sub-total recipient hepatectomy and implantation of a reduced size graft. It is a technically difficult procedure, as both portal and arterial supplies have to be constructed *de novo*. In addition a duplicate biliary drainage system needs to be constructed. Hepatic venous outflow is anastomosed as usual. This technique is subject to renewed interest. In acute liver failure, it has significant potential, since regeneration of the native liver may obviate the need for donor function; it also has application in the treatment of some hereditary metabolic disorders where adequate metabolic function may be achieved with an auxillary graft. The major advantage is withdrawal of immunosuppressive therapy if the patent develops severe complications, or when applicable gene therapy becomes available. The disadvantage of auxiliary transplantation in the face of acute liver failure is that the postoperative course is frequently more complicated; reasons are multifactorial, and can be due to the continued presence of a regenerating native liver or due to a smaller donor graft attempting to cope with a critical illness.

BLOOD LOSS AND COAGULOPATHY

Orthotopic liver transplantation may be associated with massive blood loss. The causes of this are multifactorial and include preoperative coagulation disorders secondary to end-stage liver disease, portal hypertension, surgical technique, adhesions related to previous surgery and intraoperative changes in haemostasis. Activation of the fibrinolytic system, especially during the anhepatic and postreperfusion phases, occurs in some recipients. Platelet dysfunction, both quantitative and qualitative, is also common. The consequences of massive bleeding and replacement are significant, both in terms of post-operative morbidity and mortality but also intraoperatively, when issues such as acute hypovolaemia, reduced ionized calcium due to citrate intoxication, hyperkalaemia, acidosis and hypothermia become important. Transfusion related acute lung injury (TRALI) is a potentially devastating complication. It is believed to result from neutrophil antibodies preformed in donor serum.[5] The immunosuppressive effects of large volume blood transfusions are well recognized and pertinent in a group of patients who are already functionally immunosuppressed. In addition to these immediate problems is the risk of transmission of, as yet, unidentified viral infections.

Much effort has gone into reducing the amount of exogenous blood products required intraoperatively. This includes the use of cell salvage techniques with autologous transfusion, near patient testing of haemostasis and the appropriate use of antifibrinolytic drugs such as aprotonin and tranexamic acid. These therapies appear to reduce intraoperative blood loss and transfusion requirements and possibly reduce the reperfusion injury sustained without increasing the incidence of thromboembolic complications or renal impairment.[6,7]

Although it is assumed that all patients with liver disease are subject to an increased risk of bleeding there are some sub-groups that are prothrombotic. Patients with preoperative portal or hepatic venous thrombosis appear to carry a higher incidence of prothrombotic mutations than the general population and patients with primary biliary cirrhosis and primary sclerosing cholangi-

tis are frequently prothrombotic. Such patients may require anticoagulation in the post-operative period.

POST-REPERFUSION SYNDROME

The post-reperfusion syndrome is a poorly understood phenomenon that occurs after reperfusion of the portal vein through the donor graft. It is characterized by hypotension, bradycardia, vasodilatation, pulmonary hypertension, hyperkalaemia and in some cases cardiac arrest.[8] The aetiology is unclear, but a sudden increase in venous return, release of vasoactive substances, and cold potassium rich preservation fluids are potentially implicated. The syndrome usually resolves within the first five minutes of reperfusion with appropriate fluid loading and electrolyte management. However, in approximately 30% of patients it lasts for significantly longer necessitating the use of inotropes and/or vasopressors. The post reperfusion syndrome seems more common in organs with longer preservation times and may well be associated with initial poor graft function

POSTOPERATIVE CARE

The postoperative care of the recipient depends to some extent on preoperative co-morbidity, the presence of any of the immediate complications listed above, recipient stability during the procedure and lastly the pre-transplant cause of liver failure.

Straightforward recipients who return to the intensive care unit in a stable condition with good graft function may be woken up and weaned immediately. The tracheal tube and some of the invasive monitoring lines should be removed as soon as no longer required to reduce risk of infection, and to encourage mobility. Close monitoring of all the physiological systems is important in the early post-op period (see Tables 92.1 and 92.2).

EARLY COMPLICATIONS

As with all post-operative surgical intensive care admissions some complications are applicable to all patients. These include haemorrhagic and pulmonary complications of any prolonged procedure in addition to specific complications pertinent to liver transplantation. These can be subdivided into technical complications, conditions and complications associated with pre-existing liver disease, complications associated with immunosuppressive agents, graft function and those associated with massive transfusion.

CARDIOVASCULAR

End stage liver disease is characterized by a hyperdynamic circulation, with a low systemic vascular resistance, high cardiac index, and a relatively reduced circulating volume. The majority of patients will return from theatre in this state and can be managed with adequate volume loading with or without vasopressor inotropes to maintain adequate perfusion pressures, however in some patients this state may compensate for degrees of cardiomyopathy (which may be difficult to detect with non-invasive preoperative investigation). The massive increase in the volume of liver transplants performed in the last decade has revealed cardiac failure as an important cause of morbidity and mortality in the transplant recipient. So-called cirrhotic cardiomyopathy, quite independent of the effects of alcohol may be multifactorial in nature, possibly due to over-production of nitric oxide, abnormal β-adrenoceptor structure and/or function, or the presence of some as yet unidentified myocardial depressant factor. Whatever the cause, OLT can impose severe stresses on the cardiovascular system: haemorrhage, third-space loss, impaired venous return due to caval clamping, hypocalcaemia and acidosis all impair myocardial contractility. Reperfusion can also be a time of profound circulatory instability, as discussed above. Haemodynamic changes after OLT are also common; hypertension with an increased systemic vascular resistance is common and may be due to the restoration of normal liver function and portal pressures, as well as the

hypertensive effect of the calcineurin immunosuppressants. The increased afterload in the early post transplant period may unmask cardiac dysfunction. Management of myocardial dysfunction post OLT is largely empirical; diuretics, afterload reduction and positive pressure ventilation may all be required.

PULMONARY

Pulmonary complications are common and occur in 40–80% of recipients. The presence of preoperative impairment (e.g. pleural effusions, hypoxaemia, pulmonary hypertension or the hepatopulmonary syndrome) is strongly associated with post-operative complications. Specific conditions related to liver transplantation include right hemidiaphragm palsy as a result of phrenic nerve damage,[9] which can occur if suprahepatic caval clamping is used intraoperatively The commonest postoperative problems are: pleural effusions, ongoing shunting secondary to the hepatopulmonary syndrome, atelectasis, and over subsequent days, infection. *De novo* acute lung injury and the acute respiratory distress syndrome are relatively uncommon at this stage. Other complications such as TRALI and pulmonary oedema are almost certainly under-recognized and under-reported.[10]

Table 92.1 Routine investigation of post transplant patient in the ICU

	FBC	LFTs	Coagulation	Drug levels	Cultures	Ultrasound
Day 1	✓	✓	✓		As indicated	Routine ultrasound including
Day 2	✓	✓	✓	✓		hepatic artery and portal vein
Day 3	✓	✓	✓	✓		flow between D1 and D3 unless
						clinically indicated at other time

Table 92.2 Monitoring of graft function in ICU

	Parameter	Comment
General	Liver perfusion	Characteristics at surgery
	Bile production	Quality ± volume if T-tube *in situ*
	Haemodynamics	Stabilization, with cessation of vasopressor requirements
Coagulation	INR/Prothrombin time (h)	8-hourly for the first 24 h, thereafter daily unless indicated. The fall in PT is more important than the actual value. FFP should be withheld to assess graft function although platelet support should be provided as usual
Biochemistry	Glucose	Hypoglycaemia is an ominous sign. 4-hourly measurement in the first 24 h. Euglycaemia or hyperglycaemia requiring insulin infusion is the norm
	Arterial blood gases and lactate	4–6-hourly depending on ventilatory requirement. Hyperlactataemia and acid base disturbance should rapidly resolve. Other causes of base deficit such as renal tubular acidosis and hyperchloraemia should be excluded
	AST	Should fall steadily (50% fall each day). The first measurement may reflect washout and thus the next may be higher. Daily measurements. The initial measurement reflects the degree of preservation injury.
	Bilirubin	Early increases reflect absorption of haematoma, does not reflect graft function. Haemolysis should be considered if the graft is not blood group matched.
	ALP/GGT	Usually normal, increases may reflect biliary complications or cholestasis of sepsis.

Respiratory complications are also seen in patients with poor muscle bulk and subsequent weakness. Similarly, the presence of osteoporosis in the pretransplant patients is frequently associated with post-operative pain and poor cough. The role of adequate analgesia is important, as in all patients, in promoting mobilization and adequate respiratory function. Regional analgesia may be efficacious in selected patients. In general the management of a protracted respiratory wean follows conventional lines.

NEUROLOGICAL

The quoted incidence of central nervous system (CNS) complications varies widely from 10–40% in the published series.[11] Most neurological complications occur within the first month of transplant. The commonest causes relate to persistent encephalopathy post transplant in a patient with pre-existing encephalopathy. The causes are multiple, including hepatic, metabolic, infectious, vascular and pharmacological. A patient with acute liver failure will remain encephalopathic in the immediate post transplant period, and is at risk for intra-cranial hypertension for 48 hours following transplantation, or longer in the face of graft dysfunction. *De novo* hepatic encephalopathy may develop in patients with severe graft dysfunction and or primary graft non-function; again the patient is at risk of cerebral oedema. The effects of sepsis, rejection (and its treatment with the high dose steroids), drug therapy (especially the sedatives and analgesics used in the ICU setting) and the presence of renal failure may all contribute to the presence of altered conscious level. The calcineurin inhibitors are particularly associated with seizures and altered conscious level. All such patients will require brain imaging to further define the aetiology of their impaired neurology. Other possible neurological complications are those of intracerebral haemorrhage. Such bleeds may relate to arterio-venous malformations, may be spontaneous or may be a complication of intracranial pressure monitoring, particularly in patients with acute liver failure. CNS infection normally presents later than the immediate post-operative period but should always be considered, especially in those patients with a prolonged and complicated postoperative course. All possible infecting agents including bacterial, viral, fungal and opportunistic should be considered. Central pontine myelinolysis is a rare, but potentially devastating complication associated with rapid sodium shifts. Modern technology and the use of haemofiltration techniques allow tight control of sodium shifts in the majority of patients, and this has become a rare neurological complication.

RENAL DYSFUNCTION

Despite intraoperative efforts, renal dysfunction can be exacerbated and acute renal function is a relatively common complication, with an incidence of between 12–50%.[12] The aetiology is multifactorial. Risk factors include: the presence of pretransplant co-morbidity (e.g. hypertension, diabetes mellitus, hepatorenal syndrome), severity of underlying liver disease, intraoperative instability, blood product requirement, drug toxicity and graft dysfunction.

Mortality in those who require renal replacement is high, and graft survival is lower. To avoid exacerbation of existing renal impairment, agents with inherent nephrotoxicity, such as the calcineurin inhibitors, may be omitted or their dose significantly reduced in the early pre-transplant period. There must be a balance between the risk of rejection and that of side-effects of drug therapies. Other agents without inherent nephrotoxicity are being assessed and may soon become standard therapy. Mycophenolate mofetil, a cytotoxic immunosuppressant, may be substituted in the post transplant course to limit or mitigate against renal dysfunction.[13]

Hepatorenal syndrome is a reversible entity following establishment of normal liver function post transplantation. There is considerable data in the literature to suggest that such patients do well with no prolongation of care or increase in mortality. Some data suggests that combined renal and liver transplant is associated with improved outcome. Patients with significant intrinsic renal dysfunction, as compared to those with functional hepatorenal dysfunction, may be offered combined liver-kidney transplantation.[14]

PRIMARY NON-FUNCTION (PNF)/INITIAL POOR FUNCTION

This is a spectrum occurring in 2–23% of cases,[15] which at worst requires urgent retransplantation. It is characterized by poor graft function from the time of reperfusion with hyperlactataemia, coagulopathy, metabolic acidosis, hypoglycaemia, hyperkalaemia and a rapid elevation in aminotransferase concentrations, accompanied by a systemic inflammatory response.

A major reason for the initial graft dysfunction is ischaemic injury to the graft, which depends on the type of preservation fluid used, and the duration of cold and warm ischaemia time. The aetiology of primary non-function remains unclear.

Vasodilator prostaglandins and antioxidants may have a role in 'rescue therapy'.[16]

SURGICAL PROBLEMS

Anastomotic thromboses are uncommon complications of liver transplantation, but can cause significant morbidity, which may require further invasive procedures and even urgent retransplantation.

Hepatic artery thrombosis occurring in the early postoperative period is associated with a similar picture to PNF. Small vessel calibre is a risk factor, and is more prevalent in the paediatric recipient where it has also been associated with prothrombotic states such as protein-C deficiency.[17] Ultrasound is the first line screening test and is undertaken both routinely in the immediate post-operative period, and if there is a sudden rise in transaminase measurements. If the vessel is not visualized the patient should proceed to angiography. If diagnosed quickly, emergency intervention can be undertaken to re-establish arterial flow; however emergency retransplantation may be required.

Venous complications such as portal thrombosis are even more uncommon, and are usually associated with intraoperative technical difficulty, recurrence of pre-operative disease or undiagnosed thrombophilia. Portal thrombosis is associated with portal hypertension and massive ascites, but may also be associated with graft dysfunction especially in the paediatric population. Treatment is dependent on the severity of the injury but ranges from diuretics to angioplasty, surgical reconstruction or ultimately retransplantation.[18]

Biliary complications post liver transplant are relatively common. The bile duct normally receives two-thirds of its arterial supply from the gastroduodenal artery and one-third from the hepatic artery. Post transplant, the only supply is from the hepatic artery, making it vulnerable to ischaemic injury whether that be at the time of retrieval, reperfusion or postoperatively. The resulting complication depends on the type of biliary anastomosis and the timing of the insult. Strictures are more commonly observed than leaks. Management of biliary complications is in the first instance endoscopic, with stent placement and/or balloon dilation. In patients with a T-tube *in situ*, cholangiography may be undertaken by that route. Open reconstruction in the early postoperative period is uncommon[19] (see Tables 92.3, 92.4 and 92.5).

ACUTE REJECTION

Acute cellular rejection becomes a risk from one-week post transplant; the clinical signs of rejection are non-specific and include fever, deterioration in graft function, and a rapid rise in serum aminotransferase concentration. Liver biopsy is the only reliable diagnostic tool; however, biopsy may be relatively contraindicated due to coagulopathy. In some circumstances transjugular biopsy offers a solution to this problem. The normal management regime for an episode of acute rejection is that of pulsed methylprednisolone, 1 g for 3 days. The differential diagnosis may be that of sepsis; there is some data to suggest that procalcitonin may be of use in the differentiation[20] (see Table 92.6).

SEPSIS AND FEVER

Transplant recipients are uniquely vulnerable to bacterial infection: preoperative colonization, prolonged and technically difficult surgery, large wounds, urinary catheterization and the frequent need for central venous access post-operatively all combine to make them at vastly increased risk.[21] However, compared with a decade ago, the overall incidence is reduced; probably due to improved immunosuppressive regimens. Sepsis remains an important and life-long complication of liver transplantation, which may require readmission to intensive care. The epidemiology of pathogens is evolving; the incidence of Gram-positive bacterial infection (enterococci and staphylococci) is now more common than Gram-negative sepsis.[22] More concerning is the emergence of multiple-antibiotic resistant bacteria in particular methicillin-resistant-*S-aureus* (MRSA), vancomycin-resistant-enterococci (VRE) and extended-spectrum-beta-lactamase (ESBL) producing

Table 92.3 Technical complications of OLT

Complication	Comment
Abdominal bleeding	
Anastomosis	Immediate
Graft surface (if cut down)	Immediate
General ooze secondary to coagulopathy	Immediate
Pseudo-aneurysm formation	Can present early or late and is usually associated with intra-abdominal sepsis and biliary leaks
Vascular complications	
Hepatic artery thrombosis	Early and late
Portal vein thrombosis	Early and late, there may also be stenosis of the portal vein rather than thrombosis
Inferior vena caval obstruction	May be infra, supra or retrohepatic in site
Biliary complications	
Biliary leak	Usually early
Biliary stricture	Usually late
Papillary dysfunction	Late
Roux-en-Y dysfunction	Usually late

Table 92.4 Biochemical and clinical features of technical problems

Complication	Features	Investigation	Management
Hepatic artery thrombosis	Early: rapid rise in transaminase, coagulopathy, graft failure	Ultrasound, angiogram	
	Differential diagnosis: Hyperacute rejection, Primary graft non/dysfunction		Thrombectomy, retransplantation
	Late: Biliary complications, strictures, sepsis, liver abscess	Ultrasound, angiogram	Angioplasty
Portal vein thrombosis	Early: rapid deterioration in graft function, acute liver failure, ascites, variceal bleeding	Ultrasound, CT, aortoportography, MRA	Thrombectomy, retransplantation
	Late: mildly abnormal LFTs, portal hypertension, varices	Investigation as for acute portal vein thrombosis	Shunt surgery, lytic therapy, endoscopic therapy

Table 92.5 Differential diagnosis of graft dysfunction In ICU

Primary non-function
Preservation injury
Rejection – hyperacute/acute
Vascular complications
Biliary complications
Drug induced liver dysfunction
Infection
Recurrent disease (normally late)

Gram-negative organisms. Mortality associated with infection caused by these multiply resistant organisms is significantly greater compared with other organisms.[23]

A decline in the incidence of both *Pneumocystis carinii* and cytomegalovirus infection is probably a result of both modulating immunosuppressive regimes and more effective prophylaxis. Opportunistic fungal infection still remain problematic (see Table 92.7).

FEVER

In transplant recipients, 76% of febrile episodes have a documented infectious aetiology, but acute rejection needs to be considered in the differential diagnosis. In the ICU transplant recipient the aetiology is even more likely to be infectious; often nosocomial and bacterial. In one study, pneumonia, catheter related bacteraemia and the biliary tree were the three most common sources in the ICU population (41%).[24] Viral infections accounted for 9% of febrile episodes, fungal infections 3% and endocarditis 3%. As mentioned above, the epidemiology of pathogens is changing and it is important to have

Table 92.6 Management of rejection in intensive care

	Comment	Characteristics	Liver biopsy	Differential diagnosis	Treatment options
Hyperacute rejection	Rare in OLT 1–10 days post transplant	Rapid deterioration in graft function. AST >1000, Coagulopathy, acidosis	Haemorrhagic necrosis	Primary non-function/ delayed function Hepatic artery thrombosis	Retransplantation Rarely: OKT3, Cyclophosphamide, plasmapheresis (unproven)
Acute rejection	30–70% Occurs at mean of 7–9 days	Often clinically silent apart from fever and RUQ pain. High AST and Bili Coagulation and acid base undisturbed	Portal inflammation Endolethitis Bile duct damage	Sepsis Viral	Methylprednisolone 1 g daily for 3 days

In those who do not respond: Consider diagnosis; if correct: Consider Tacrolimus if induction agent is Cyclosporin A, OKT3 or MMF/ Sirolimus or other new agents

thorough knowledge of local problem pathogens on which to base meaningful antibiotic policy.

This data has implications for the threshold to investigate febrile episodes, suspect bacterial infection and commence appropriate empirical antibiotic therapy. However, it should also be appreciated that immunosuppressed recipients do not always produce a febrile response to infection.

MANAGEMENT OF CYTOMEGALOVIRUS INFECTION AFTER LIVER TRANSPLANTATION

Cytomegalovirus (CMV) infection is rarely associated with symptomatic illness in healthy hosts, but is a major cause of morbidity and mortality in transplant recipients; it is the single most common opportunistic infection after solid organ transplantation. In the absence of antiviral prophylaxis the overall incidence of CMV infection after OLT ranges from 23–85%, with approximately 50% of those developing clinical disease.

CMV infection most commonly occurs in the first 3 months after OLT, with a peak incidence in the third and fourth week. Infection may be asymptomatic or it may cause a spectrum of illness including fever, thrombocytopenia, neutropenia, pneumonia and hepatitis. The indirect effects of infection probably contribute more to the adverse effects on graft function than direct effects. CMV infection further immunosuppresses the recipient leading to increased opportunistic fungal infection and also increased risk of Epstein–Barr virus (EBV) infection which can go on to be associated with post-transplant lymphoproliferative disease (PTLD). CMV infection is also implicated in increased rejection, although this is controversial.[25] In those patients who proceed to transplant who are already receiving immunosuppressive agents, or in those with acute liver failure, CMV disease may present earlier in the clinical course.

The risk of CMV infection post transplant is dependent on the serological status of both the donor and recipient, the highest risk is associated with Donor positive/Recipient negative. Because of the deleterious effects mentioned above, various prophylactic and treatment regimes including antiviral agents, pooled immune globulin, CMV immune globulin (CMVIG) and combinations of the above have been designed to prevent CMV infection in the post transplant setting. Proven prophylactic strategies in the high-risk groups include long-term intravenous (i.v.) or oral (PO) ganciclovir. Oral ganciclovir avoids the potential bone marrow suppression associated with i.v. use, however the cost-effectiveness of such a strategy is not universally accepted, and it is argued that patients should be allowed to develop CMV infection and then be treated. Currently 3 months of ganciclovir remains the gold standard in the treatment of CMV disease. In many patients, therapy will commence i.v. and then convert to oral to facilitate discharge from hospital and rehabilitation. There is no evidence to support specific immunoglobulin in addition,[26] but it is frequently added in the management of CMV pneumonitis.

MANAGEMENT OF VIRAL HEPATITIS

Hepatitis C (HCV) related cirrhosis is the commonest indication for transplantation both in Europe and the USA. Post transplant, HCV viraemia is universal. Recurrent liver disease, with a more accelerated and aggressive course, is seen in the majority; indeed 20% are cirrhotic at 5 years post transplant.[27] Those with histological evidence of recurrence also have a greater incidence of acute rejection.[28] Immunosuppression especially with steroids, directly increases the HCV RNA serum load. Most transplant programmes therefore convert to single or double agent immunosuppression regimes as soon as possible post transplant. Yet to be

Table 92.7 Infection in the intensive care unit

Aetiology:	Bacterial	Viral	Fungal	Protozoal
	Wound	HSV	Candida	Toxoplasmosis
	Nosocomial pneumonia	CMV	Aspergilla	Strongyloides
	Line sepsis	EBV	PCP	
	UTI	Varicella	Cryptococcus	
	Liver			
	Biliary			
Timing	Any time	HSV in first few weeks	Usually after 4 weeks	After 3 weeks
		CMV 3–10 weeks		
		EBV from 4 weeks		
		Varicella later		
		All may be earlier in ALF or retransplantation		

fully elucidated is the role of antiviral therapy (either interferon ± ribavirin) in the post transplant patient. Theoretically, early antiviral therapy is attractive as viral load is low, immunosuppressive therapy has just started and acute rejection necessitating pulsed steroids is relatively common. However, risk of infection and thrombocytopenia often contraindicates antiviral therapy in the early postoperative period.

Initial results of transplantation for hepatitis B infection (HBV) were discouraging, largely due to recurrent disease with rapid and fatal progression. Passive immunoprophylaxis with hepatitis B immune globulin (HBIG) peri-transplant dramatically reduces both the severity and reinfection rate, however, such therapy must be continued indefinitely following transplant to prevent disease recurrence. Nucleoside analogues such as lamivudine have been co-administered to improve the efficacy of this approach, with apparent good results.[29] In respect of modulation of immunosuppression regimes, the comments made with respect to HCV are similarly applicable.[30]

IMMUNOSUPPRESSION

As the field of transplantation evolves, new immunosuppressive regimes and drugs become available. For all combinations however there is a balance to be struck between the optimal prevention of rejection and the toxicity and unwanted effects of the drugs.

The incidence of acute rejection rises at about one week after OLT; it resembles a delayed-type hypersensitivity reaction, and immunosuppressive agents are highly effective at treating it. Chronic rejection occurs over months to years and is characterized by the 'vanishing bile-duct' syndrome, pathologic mechanisms are poorly understood and immunosuppressant agents are ineffective.

Currently, calcineurin inhibitors such as cyclosporin and tacrolimus form the mainstay drugs after liver transplantation. They have revolutionized the outcome of solid-organ transplantation, but both drugs are limited by their side-effects, predominantly nephro- and neurotoxicity, necessitating drug level monitoring. These manifestations of toxicity can be difficult in the management of post transplant immunosuppression in patients who exhibited encephalopathy or renal dysfunction pretransplant; indeed they may even be withheld, which may result in increased risk of graft rejection.

It is usual to have an induction regimen beginning in the perioperative period; this usually involves a calcineurin inhibitor and steroids, which are administered in a high dose taper regime. With time after transplantation, the level of immunosuppression required decreases and drug doses may be reduced further. Cytotoxic drugs such as azathioprine or mycophenolate mofetil (MMF) may also allow further reduction of steroids and the more toxic calcineurin inhibitors.

Another variation in the regimen is the introduction of antilymphocyte antibodies (ALA) for 10–14 days in order to delay the introduction of calcineurin inhibitors; this may be desirable in patients with impaired renal function. ALA interferes with lymphocyte function in several ways: enhanced removal of activated lymphocytes by the reticuloendothelial system, down-regulation of lymphocyte binding cell surface receptors, with decreased lymphocyte activation and proliferation.

Recently, several monoclonal antibodies have been introduced, they bind to IL-2 receptors, which are only present on activated T cells, and hence they have a more specific mode of action.

Sirolimus is a novel immunosuppressant that has been used extensively in renal transplantation and more recently in liver transplant recipients in whom the calcineurin inhibitors are contraindicated.[31] It resembles tacrolimus structurally, and binds to the same protein, but whereas cyclosporin and tacrolimus act by inhibiting Interleukin 2 gene transcription, sirolimus acts by blocking postreceptor signal transduction and IL-2 dependent proliferation. In addition to its immunosuppressive actions sirolimus is also an antifungal and antiproliferative agent. Sirolimus lacks neuro- and nephrotoxicity. However, it can raise the intracellular concentrations of cyclosporin-A and tacrolimus, indirectly potentiating their toxicity. Hyperlipidaemia has also been noted although this may be a reflection of the often higher dose steroid regimens used in combination with sirolimus. Because of its antiproliferative effects sirolimus can also cause thrombocytopenia, neutropenia and anaemia; there have also been concerns about its effects on wound healing. Sirolimus also requires therapeutic drug level monitoring, not only because serum concentrations have a high level of intraindividual and interindividual variability, but also because there are significant interactions with drugs that use the cytochrome P450 3A system.

READMISSION TO ICU/LATE COMPLICATIONS

The cause of readmission to ICU after liver transplantation varies in relation to time after transplantation. Approximately 20% of recipients require readmission, and it is correlated with actuarial reduced patient and graft survival.[32] In the period immediately after transplantation, cardiorespiratory failure is the commonest reason for readmission, both due to fluid overload and infection, indeed an abnormal pre-discharge CXR is predictive of readmission as is high CVP and tachypnoea. Other predictors of readmission are age, pretransplant synthetic function, bilirubin, amount of intraoperative blood products and renal dysfunction. Graft dysfunction, severe sepsis and postoperative care of surgical complications are other important causes of readmission. Bleeding and biliary anastomotic leaks represent the commonest surgical causes.

LIVER TRANSPLANTATION FOR ACUTE LIVER FAILURE

Acute liver failure is a syndrome associated with an acute onset coagulopathy, jaundice and encephalopathy, the causes are many and the syndrome is notable for its high morbidity and mortality. The acceptance of emergency liver transplantation in selected cases has revolutionized the clinical course, but outcome is sometimes disappointingly poor, often due to the rapid development of uncontrollable cerebral oedema, sepsis and multiorgan failure. There is also a short window of opportunity in listing these patients; despite highest priority listing they may receive 'marginal' organs or even ABO blood group incompatible organs. Early determination of prognosis and appropriate listing for transplant is clearly important. The King's College Hospital prognostic criteria for non-survival among patients with acute liver failure[33] is a tool used to identify those at high risk while sparing those in whom spontaneous recovery will otherwise occur. It has been validated both in Europe and the USA[34] (see Table 92.8).

Several advances in the supportive management of these patients have occurred since the original criteria were developed but their prognostic value holds true.

EXTRACORPOREAL HEPATIC SUPPORT

The liver has metabolic, excretory and synthetic functions all of which need to be maintained in a patient who has liver failure until either an organ becomes available or regeneration takes place. The major components of a bioartificial liver include: hepatocytes able to perform some of the functions of normal liver, a delivery system to bring blood to and from the patient and a membrane designed to allow adequate exchange between blood and hepatocytes.

Clinical trials are in progress to evaluate the place for these devices[35] and there has been some success with using them as a bridge to transplantation, and in acute liver failure in particular an improvement in neurological status and reduced cerebral oedema. Still to be elucidated is the timescale on which these devices can be used and whether they can bridge the gap to regeneration thus sparing the patient from transplantation.

PAEDIATRIC LIVER TRANSPLANTATION

OLT is the treatment of choice for children with end stage liver disease. Cholestatic disorders make up the largest indication for transplantation with extra hepatic biliary atresia plus or minus previous Kasai portoenterostomy accounting for over 50% of paediatric transplants. Metabolic diseases and primary hepatic tumours are also common indications. As in adult recipients multi-system effects of end stage liver disease are common, the occurrence of liver disease as part of a congenital syndrome (e.g. Alagille's) may warrant invasive preoperative evaluation of extrahepatic manifestation. Patient and graft survival have improved over the last decade such that 5-year patient survival is over 80%.[36] Scarce availability of paediatric donors have driven innovations such as reduced size grafts, split-liver techniques and living donor programmes which have all contributed to expand the pool of available donors and reduce the mortality for those children waiting for suitable organs. One of the biggest problems associated with paediatric transplantation is the relatively high incidence of vascular complications,[37] such as hepatic artery thrombosis, portal vein thrombosis and venous outflow obstruction.

Risk factors for these conditions include fulminant hepatic failure, long operation time, donor/recipient age and weight discrepancies, young recipient age, low recipient weight and arterial reconstruction techniques. In order to minimize these often devastating complications strategies to minimize the risk include delayed primary closure of the abdominal wall, maintaining the haematocrit at 22–25% to ensure laminar flow, avoidance of platelets and blood components combined with considered use of anticoagulants.[38]

Table 92.8 King's College Hospital prognostic criteria for non-survival among patients with acute liver failure

Paracetamol induced	Non-paracetamol induced
pH < 7.3 (irrespective of grade of encephalopathy) – following volume resuscitation and >24 h post-ingestion OR PT >100 s (INR >6.5) AND creatinine >300 μmol/l in patients with grade III–IV encephalopathy – occurring within a 24 hour time frame	PT >100 s (INR >6.5) irrespective of grade of encephalopathy OR pH < 7.3 – following volume resuscitation OR Any 3 of the following variables (in association with encephalopathy) Age <10 years or >40 years Aetiology: non-A, non-B or drug induced Jaundice to encephalopathy > 7 days PT >50 s (INR >3.5) Serum bilirubin >300 μmol/l

HEPATOPULMONARY SYNDROMES

Changes in the cardiovascular system associated with chronic liver disease may contribute to the spectrum of cardiopulmonary disease associated with chronic liver disease and portal hypertension. A hyperdynamic state with high cardiac output, longstanding portal hypertension with the development of collateral flow, together with an imbalance of vasoactive mediators either synthesized or metabolized by the liver may lead to characteristic changes in both flow and pressure through the pulmonary vasculature. This may be associated with hypoxia and orthodeoxia. Two ends of the spectrum are hepatopulmonary syndrome (HPS) and portopulmonary hypertension (PPH) the two conditions are rare but important, as they have vastly different impacts on risk associated with liver transplantation and long-term outcome[39] (see Table 92.9).

Diagnostic criteria for both conditions are summarized in the table.

HEPATOPULMONARY SYNDROME

It can be seen from the table that hypoxia is a characteristic finding in this condition, it results from intrapulmonary vascular dilatation at the pre and post capillary level leading to decreased ventilation/perfusion ratios, more uncommonly anatomical shunt is present with a-v communication. One of the postulated mechanisms of this vasodilatation is over activity of pulmonary vasculature nitric oxide synthetase; pretransplant patients have raised levels of exhaled nitric oxide that decrease post transplant with resolution of the syndrome. Medical treatment of the syndrome has been disappointing; indeed most transplant centres agree that the syndrome is an indication for transplantation in itself, as resolution is reported in up to 80% after transplantation. Risk stratification based on severity is important, as vastly increased peritransplant mortality is associated with severe hypoxia and high levels of vascular shunt. Mortality overall is 16% at 90 days and 38% at one year. Refractory hypoxia is the indirect cause of death, which may be due to multi organ failure, intracerebral haemorrhage, and sepsis due to bile leaks. Resolution of the syndrome can take months lending support to

the theory that it is vascular remodelling rather than just acute reversal of vasodilatation that reverses hypoxia.

PORTOPULMONARY HYPERTENSION

Up to 20% of pretransplant patients have pulmonary hypertension; this probably constitutes increased flow through the pulmonary vasculature and is not associated with increased resistance. These patients do well after transplantation. A much more ominous syndrome is the presence of pulmonary hypertension with high pulmonary vascular resistance (seen in <4%). The aetiology of this syndrome is complex but it is characterized by a hyperdynamic high flow state with excess central volume and non-embolic pulmonary vasoconstriction. The pathological changes associated with this syndrome match those associated with primary pulmonary hypertension except that cardiac output is high in this group. In comparison to HPS, there are several differences in terms of response to medical treatment and outcome after transplantation. The response to epoprostenol, a PGI_2 analogue, is encouraging. Decreases in pulmonary artery pressure but more importantly transpulmonary gradient (TPG) have been noted, although at least 3 months treatment seem necessary, suggesting remodelling rather than vasodilatation is the important mechanism. A limiting factor in the treatment may also be progressive thrombocytopenia and splenomegaly. Another difference is the perioperative risk and post transplant prognosis. Resolution is not associated with transplantation and progression can be a feature. Perioperatively, the higher the MPAP, PVR and TPG the greater the risk of death, usually due to acute right ventricular decompensation. If the MPAP >35 mmHG or PVR >250 dyne/s per cm^{-5} mortality reaches 40%. If MPAP >50 mmHg some have even suggested delisting or even intraoperative cancellation as the mortality is 100%.

REFERENCES

1 Transplant Patient Data Source. Richmond: United Network for Organ Sharing (28 June, 2000). http://www.patients.vnos.org/data.htm
2 Marino IR, Morelli F, Doria C, *et al*. Preoperative assessment of risk in liver transplantation: a multi-

Table 92.9 Diagnostic criteria for hepatopulmonary syndrome and portopulmonary hypertension

Hepatopulmonary syndrome	Portopulmonary hypertension
Chronic liver disease (± cirrhosis)	Portal hypertension
Arterial hypoxaemia	Mean pulmonary artery pressure (MPAP) >25 mmHg
PaO_2 <75 mmHg (10 kPa) or A-aO_2 gradient >20 mmHg	Pulmonary artery occlusion pressure (PAoP) <15 mmHg
Intrapulmonary vascular dilatation	Pulmonary vascular resistance (PVR) >120 dynes/s per cm^{-5}

variate analysis in 2376 cases of the UW Era. *Transplant Proc* 1997; **29**: 454–5.

3 Sudhakar Reddy K, Johnston TD, Putnam LA, *et al.* Piggyback technique and selective use of veno-venous bypass in adult orthotopic liver transplantation. *Clin Transplant* 2000; **14**: 370–4.

4 Parrilla P, Sanchez-Buenoa F, Figuerasb J, *et al.* Analysis of the complications of the piggyback technique in 1112 liver transplants. *Transplant Proc* 1999; **31**: 2388–9.

5 Silliman CC. Plasma and lipids from stored packed red blood cells cause acute lung injury in an animal model. *J Clin Invest* 1998; **101**: 1458–67.

6 Dalmau A, Sabate A, Acosta F, *et al.* Tranexamic acid reduces red cell transfusion better than epsilon-aminocaproic acid or placebo in liver transplantation. *Anesth Analg* 2000; **91**: 29–34.

7 Porte R, Quintus Molenaar I, Begliomini B, *et al.* Aprotonin and transfusion requirements in orthotopic liver transplantation: a multicentre randomised double-blind study. *Lancet* 2000; **355**: 1303–9.

8 Aggarwal S, Kans Y, Freeman JA, *et al.* Post-reperfusion syndrome: cardiovascular collapse following hepatic reperfusion during liver transplantation. *Transplant Proc* 1987; **19**: 54.

9 Smyrniotis V, Andreani P, Muiesan P, *et al.* Diaphragmatic nerve palsy in young children following liver transplantation. Successful treatment by plication of the diaphragm. *Transplant Int* 1998; **11**: 281–3.

10 Yost CS, Matthay MA, Gropper MA. Etiology of acute pulmonary edema during liver transplantation. *Chest* 2001; **119**: 219–23.

11 Bronster DJ, Emre S, Boccagni P, *et al.* Central nervous system complications in liver transplant recipients – incidence, timing, and long-term follow-up. *Clin Transplant* 2000; **14**: 1–7.

12 Bilbao I, Charco R, Balsells J, *et al.* Risk factors for acute renal failure requiring dialysis after liver transplantation. *Clin Transplant* 1998; **12**: 123–9.

13 Barkmann A, Nashan B, Schmidt HH, *et al.* Improvement of acute and chronic renal dysfunction in liver transplant patients after substitution of calcineurin inhibitors by mycophenolate mofetil. *Transplantation* 2000; **69**: 1886–90.

14 Morrisey PE, Gordon F, Shaffer D, *et al.* Combined liver-kidney transplantation in patients with cirrhosis and renal failure: effect of a positive cross-match and benefits of combined transplantation. *Liver Transplant Surg* 1998; **4**: 363–9.

15 Brokelman W, Stel AI, Ploeg RJ. Risk factors for primary dysfunction after liver transplantation in the University of Wisconsin Era. *Transplant Proc* 1999; **31**: 2087–90.

16 Neumann UP, Kaisers U, Langrehr JM, *et al.* Administration of prostacyclin after liver transplantation: a placebo controlled randomised trial. *Clin Transplant* 2000; **14**: 70–4.

17 Stahl RL, Duncan A, Hooks MA, *et al.* A hypercoaguable state follows orthotopic liver transplantation. *Hepatology* 1990; **12**: 553–8.

18 Settmacher U, Nussler N, Glanemann M, *et al.* Venous complications after liver transplantation. *Clin Transplant* 2000; **3**: 235–41.

19 Mosca S, Militerno G, Guardascione MA, *et al.* Late biliary tract complications after orthotopic liver transplantation: Diagnostic and therapeutic role of endoscopic retrograde cholangiopancreatography. *J Gastroenterol Hepatol* 2000; **15**: 654–60.

20 Kuse ER, Langfield I, Jaeger K, *et al.* Procalcitonin in fever of unknown origin after liver transplantation: a variable to differentiate acute rejection from infection. *Crit Care Med* 2000; **28**: 555–9.

21 Cueto G, Trigo P, Arata A, *et al.* Evaluation of prognostic factors for early infection in liver transplantation. *Transplant Proc* 1999; **31**: 3061–2.

22 Singh N. Infectious diseases in the liver transplant recipient. *Semin Gastrointest Dis* 1998; **9**: 136–46.

23 Singh N, Gayowski T, Rihs JD, *et al.* Evolving trends in multiple-antibiotic-resistant bacteria in liver transplant recipients: a longitudinal study of antimicrobial susceptibility patterns. *Liver Transplant* 2001; **7**: 22–6.

24 Singh N, Chang FY, Gayowski T, *et al.* Fever in liver transplant recipients in the intensive care unit. *Clin Transplant* 1999; **13**: 504–11.

25 Cakaloglu Y, Devlin J, O'Grady J, *et al.* Importance of concomitant viral infection during late acute allograft rejection. *Transplantation* 1995; **59**: 40–5.

26 Sampathkumar P, Paya CV. Management of cytomegalovirus infection after liver transplantation. *Liver Transplant* 2000; **6**: 144–56.

27 Burroughs AK. Posttransplantation prevention and treatment of recurrent hepatitis C. *Liver Transplant* 2000; **6**: S35–40.

28 Testa G, Crippin JS, Netto GJ, *et al.* Liver transplantation for Hepatitis C: recurrence and disease progression in 300 patients. *Liver Transplant* 2000; **6**: 553–61.

29 Angus PW, McCaughan GW, Gane EJ, *et al.* Combination low-dose hepatitis B immune globulin and Lamivudine therapy provides effective prophylaxis against post-transplantation hepatitis B. *Liver Transplant* 2000; **6**: 429–33.

30 Rizzetto M, Marzano A. Post-transplantation prevention and treatment of recurrent Hepatitis B. *Liver Transplant* 2000; **6**: S47–51.

31 Chang GJ, Mahanty HD, Quan D, *et al.* Experience with the use of sirolimus in liver transplantation – use in patients for whom calcineurin inhibitors are contraindicated. *Liver Transplant* 2000; **6**: 734–40.

32 Levy ML, Greene L, Ramsey MAE, *et al.* Readmission to the intensive care unit after liver transplantation. *Crit Care Med* 2001; **29**: 18–24.

33 O'Grady JG, Alexander GJM, Hayllar KM, *et al.* Early indicators of prognosis in fulminant hepatic failure. *Gastroenterology* 1989; **97**: 439–55.

34 Shakil AO, Kramer D, Mazariegos GV, *et al.* Acute liver failure: clinical features, outcome analysis, and applicability of prognostic criteria. *Liver Transplant* 2000; **6**: 163–9.

35 Watanabe FD, Mullon Claudy J-P, Hewitt WR. Clinical experience with a bioartificial liver in the treatment of severe liver failure. *Ann Surg* 1997; **225**: 484–94.

36 Goss JA, Shackleton CR, McDiarmid SV, *et al.* Long-term results of pediatric liver transplantation: An analysis of 569 transplants. *Ann Surg* 1998; **228**: 411–20.

37 Sieders E, Peeters PMJG, TenVergert EM, *et al.* Early vascular complications after pediatric liver transplantation. *Liver Transplant* 2000; **6**: 326–32.

38 Hammer GB, Krane EJ. Anaesthesia for liver transplantation in children. *Paediatric Anaesthesia* 2001; **11**: 3–18.

39 Krowka MJ. Hepatopulmonary syndromes. *Gut* 2000; **46**: 1–4.

93

Heart and lung transplantation

C Morgan

The first successful cardiac transplantation was performed at Groote Schuur, South Africa in 1967 and was followed by operations in other pioneer cardiac centres worldwide. However, it was not until the introduction of cyclosporine in 1979 that consistently improved long-term survival was achieved. To date, some 55 000 cardiac transplantations have been performed in over 200 centres. Further improvements in immunosuppression therapy, surgical technique, detection and treatment of rejection, and general improvements in anaesthesia and postoperative care contributed to the sustained improvements, especially in centres concentrating experience and expertise above a critical mass. Typical survival figures following cardiac transplantation are in the order of 80% survival at 1 year and 70% after 5 years. The first successful heart and lung transplantation was performed in Stanford, USA in 1981 and was followed by successful heart-lung, single-lung and double-lung transplantations, mostly at the same centres that had led the way in cardiac transplantation. With cardiac and lung transplantation accepted as standard treatment for a range of end stage cardiopulmonary diseases, a large number of recipients may potentially develop critical illness; unrelated or directly related to their original condition. Around 40% of cardiac transplant recipients are re-admitted to hospital within one year, with at least one-third requiring admission to intensive care units (ICUs).[1] Many of these patients present to the ICUs of non-transplant centres; therefore, all critical care practitioners need to be aware of the principles of management of the transplant recipient.

CARDIAC TRANSPLANTATION

The main issue with cardiac transplantation revolves around donor availability. The numbers of potential recipients who fulfil internationally accepted criteria[2] (Table 93.1) vastly outnumber the available donors, so the great majority of patients with severe end stage heart failure inevitably die before a suitable donor heart becomes available.

Table 93.1 Criteria to select cardiac transplant recipients

Clinical
  Heart Failure Survival Score (HFSS),[3] high risk
  NYHA class III/IV heart failure refractory to maximal medical treatment
  Severely limiting angina not suitable for revascularization: surgical or medical
  Recurrent symptomatic ventricular arrhythmias refractory to medical, surgical or electrophysiological treatments
Physiological
  Peak oxygen consumption less than 10 ml/kg per min after reaching anaerobic threshold
Exclusion criteria
  Age greater than 65 years
  Transpulmonary gradient (mean PAP – mean PAoP) >15 mmHg (2.0 kPa) or PVR > 5.0 Wood Units despite standardized reversibility testing with nitrates or inhaled nitric oxide
  Insulin-dependent diabetes mellitus with end organ dysfunction
  Severe psychiatric disturbance or intellectual retardation
  Current alcohol or drug abuse
  Morbid obesity
  Concurrent malignancy
  Severe hepatic or renal disease, unrelated to cardiac disease (unless being considered for combined organ transplant)
  Immunodeficiency disease
  Active systemic infection

NYHA, New York Heart Association; PAP, pulmonary artery pressure; PaoP, pulmonary artery occlusion pressure (or 'wedge' pressure); PVR, pulmonary vascular resistance.

The cardiac equivalent of dialysis, for the maintenance of the potential renal transplant recipient until an organ is available, is simply not feasible. However, there has been progress in the medical and surgical management of severe heart failure some of which are highly specialized treatments with limited availability and some more routine and commonplace (Table 93.2). The use of inotropic drugs, such as β-agonists (e.g. dobutamine), catecholamines (e.g. adrenaline) and phosphodiesterase inhibitors (e.g. milrinone), to support the failing heart

Table 93.2 Non transplant or bridge to transplant treatment of severe cardiac failure

Treatment modality	Notes	Applicability
Angiotensin-converting enzyme (ACE) inhibitors	Reduce cardiac work and improve output – beware exacerbation of renal failure	Ward setting to establish – then as outpatient
β-blockers[5, 6]	Improve β-receptor numbers and function	Ward setting to establish – then as outpatient
Inotropic support	Rescue therapy – rescue and re-stabilization sometimes possible – requires central vascular access	Coronary care unit or ICU
Intra-aortic balloon pump counterpulsation	Rescue therapy combined with inotropes – may re-stabilize and thus temporary but invasive	Coronary care unit or ICU
Anti-arrhymic treatments – implantable defibrillators and advanced pacing devices	Where recurrent or severe arrhythmias threaten life or cause general destabilizations	Cardiac centre with facilities for electrophysiology
Surgical interventions	Routine such as coronary artery bypass or complex – such as anterior ventricular remodelling, mitral reconstruction where severe mitral regurgitation complicates cardiomyopathy	Specialized cardiac centre
Ventricular assist devices (VAD)[7]	Short term and medium term mechanical support for the failed heart – extremely invasive – usually holding stage or bridge to transplant	Specialized cardiac centre
Totally implanted artificial heart[8]	Longer term version of VAD – ultimately may be instead of transplant	Specialized cardiac centre then possibly home

and circulation is widely practised, as is the use of Intra-Aortic Balloon Pump Counterpulsation. These treatment options are highly invasive but may be used as rescue therapy in a patient with severe or end-stage cardiac failure who may be waiting for a transplant but in whom some event such as infection or worsening myocardial ischaemia has resulted in a catastrophic deterioration. The response of the failing heart to β-agonists may be disappointing because of the tendency to β-receptor down-regulation from chronic over stimulation. In these cases, the phosphodiesterase inhibitor drugs such as milrinone and enoximone may have greater and more sustained potency because of their intracellular site of action. Some patients who have been deemed inoperable in conventional terms may still benefit from cardiac surgical interventions although, in the setting of severe chronic cardiac failure, the risk of death, serious morbidity and prolonged postoperative critical illness may be considered prohibitive. Sometimes, a degree of reversible myocardial ischaemia may be demonstrated by thallium scanning and guide subsequent coronary artery bypass grafting. In some cases, the degree of secondary mitral valve regurgitation caused by dilatation of the left ventricle may become a haemo-

dynamically significant lesion of itself, and reconstruction of the mitral valve or remodelling of the left ventricle may prove beneficial. In extreme cases of cardiac decompensation, and where other organ functions are maintained (an unusual combination), the use of mechanical assistance[4] to support the heart and buy time for a donor heart to become available (bridge to transplant) or to provide support while a severe but temporary process (such as some viral myocarditis episodes) subsides (bridge to recovery) may be undertaken in highly specialized centres. The logical conclusion is to develop permanent mechanical support devices obviating the need for transplantation, but this goal appears to be a long way in the future. The cost of such therapy, both in financial and human terms, has to be considered in the context of general health economics. These episodes are still at best pioneering, extremely invasive, draining on the resources of critical care, blood transfusion and pharmacy and of limited outcome benefits. On the other hand, it can be argued that the earlier use of potent mechanical assistance at a stage when other organs have yet to be irretrievably damaged should be more widely attempted outside of major cardiac specialist centres.

Table 93.3 *General criteria to select cardiac transplant donors*

Age under 60 years
Brain death criteria fulfilled
Family consent obtained
Absence of infection
Absence of chest trauma
Absence of prolonged cardiac arrest
Minimal inotropic support
Viral markers (hepatitis B, C and HIV) negative
No malignancy (except primary cerebral tumour)

DONORS AND RECIPIENTS

Most countries have seen a progressive gradual decline in the number of cardiac transplantations performed as a result of decreasing donor availability. Measures to optimize the donor pool for all solid organ transplants and care of potential donors are discussed elsewhere. Donor selection criteria are summarized in Table 93.3.

Matching of a potential cardiac donor with a recipient is determined by weight within 80% to 120% of each other, ABO blood group compatibility and negative lymphocyte cross-match. human leukocyte antigen tissue type comparisons are only available after the event and are of prognostic and theoretical interest only.

THE TRANSPLANT PROCEDURE

The care of the cardiac transplant recipient is multifaceted and should take into account the following principles:

- general preparation of a patient (and relatives) who has suffered severe chronic illness and has been under the shadow of impending death
- perioperative care for major cardiac surgery

- management of specific early postoperative complications, such as control of rejection, containment of side-effects of immunosuppression and prompt treatment of infection
- re-integration of the patient into society

The anaesthetic and perioperative care of these patients is not materially different to any other major cardiac surgery and the important principles are well described in the literature.[9-11] However, the co-ordination of the timing of surgery with the arrival of donor heart, management of the excised donor graft and the immunosuppression protocol are all crucial factors. Organ preservation after harvesting from the donor is especially important and the main factor appears to be limiting the total ischaemic time to less than 4 h (6 h at the extreme). The recipient may have to be called in from home and may have a full stomach. The recipient may be elated or extremely anxious, or both. Details of perioperative care will vary from centre to centre (e.g. the timing of components of the immunosuppression regime, exact choice of antibiotics for prophylaxis and whether or not the right internal jugular vein has to be left virgin by the anaesthetic and postoperative team so that endomyocardial biopsies may be more conveniently performed). The striking difference of the cardiac transplant recipient compared to other postoperative cardiac surgical patients is the consequences of the grafted donor heart having no nervous control. It is denervated at excision from the donor and re-innervation in the recipient does not occur.

PHYSIOLOGY AND PHARMACOLOGY OF THE DENERVATED HEART (Table 93.4)

At surgery, the sinoatrial (SA) node of the recipient is retained but does not activate the grafted heart across

Table 93.4 The pharmacology of the denervated heart

Drug	Effect on recipient	Mechanism
Digoxin	Normal increase in contractility; minimal effect on atrioventricular node	Direct myocardial effect, denervation
Adenosine	Four-fold increase in sinus and atrioventricular node blocking effect	Denervation super-sensitivity
Atropine	None	Denervation
Epinephrine	Increased contractility and chronotropy	Denervation super-sensitivity
Norepinephrine	Increased contractility and chronotropy	Denervation super-sensitivity
Isoprenaline	Normal chronotropic effect	
Glyceryl trinitrate	No reflex tachycardia	Baroreflex disruption
Quinidine	No vagolytic effect	Denervation
Verapamil	Atrioventricular block	Direct effect
Nifedipine	No reflex tachycardia	Denervation
β-blockers	Increased antagonistic effect	Denervation
Pancuronium, neostigmine, succinylcholine	No bradycardia	Denervation

the suture line. The donor heart has its own SA node but this is not innervated. It may be possible to discern two discrete P-waves on the electrocardiogram (ECG). The donor SA node controls the graft heart rate. In the absence of autonomic innervation, only drugs or manoeuvres that act directly on the heart will have an effect. For example, the Valsalva manoeuvre or carotid sinus massage will not affect heart rate, but drugs such as epinephrine, norepinephrine and isoprenaline exert a positive inotropic and chronotropic effect and β-adrenergic blockers will depress myocardial function. Quinidine and digoxin will influence conductivity through their direct effect only.

The denervated heart retains its intrinsic control mechanisms[12] (e.g. a normal Frank Starling response to volume loading, normal conductivity and intact α- and β-adrenergic receptors), possibly with enhanced responsiveness.

The coronary arteries retain their vasodilatory responsiveness to nitrates and metabolic demands. They can develop atherosclerosis in the long term, but the patient experiences no anginal pain with ischaemia or infarction because of the denervation.

Denervation results most importantly in an atypical response to exercise, hypovolaemia and hypotension. Any increase in cardiac output from increased heart rate or contractility depends on an increasing venous return and circulating catecholamines, and the response may be delayed. During exercise, muscle contraction increases venous return and the increased circulating catecholamines increase the heart rate. This is a gradual response and, as exercise ceases, the heart rate and cardiac output slowly fall as the catecholamine and the response levels decrease.[13] In pathological states, the transplanted heart is especially dependent on adequate filling volumes, and attention to preload is critical.

The denervated heart is also sensitive to extremes of heart rate; arrhythmias are unusual but may cause serious haemodynamic problems. Cardiac arrhythmias can be atrial, junctional or ventricular, and may be a sign of rejection. These may resolve if the rejection is adequately treated. Occasionally, anti-arrhythmic drugs that act directly on the conduction system (e.g. quinidine, disopyramide and procainamide) or electrical cardioversion are required. Verapamil and nifedipine have enhanced effects in the transplanted heart. Hypotension and bradycardia may be profound because of the absence of the normal cardiac sympathetic-mediated response to vasodilatation. Adenosine used for supraventricular tachycardias may induce asystole and cause profound hypotension in the transplanted heart. Amiodarone has been used successfully for ventricular and atrial arrhythmias, but its mild negative inotropy and vasodilatation can cause hypotension. Lignocaine is normally effective in the treatment of ventricular arrhythmias.

POSTOPERATIVE CARE

In the majority of cases, the immediate postoperative course is uneventful and very similar to 'routine' cardiopulmonary bypass surgery requiring sternotomy with similar duration of postoperative ventilation, and ICU length of stay, but with hospital discharge being at around 10 to 14 days if all goes well. All the usual principles of care apply with the additional concerns regarding denervation, immunosuppression, infection, and detection and treatment of rejection.

The transplanted heart may have suffered from ischaemic damage before successful reperfusion in the recipient and may require inotropic, chronotropic or even temporary mechanical support. The severity of recipient pulmonary vascular disease may have been underestimated and even modest elevations of pulmonary vascular resistance, combined with a degree of graft right ventricular myocardial dysfunction, may prove troublesome and result in haemodynamic instability or catastrophic low cardiac output states. It may be necessary therefore to tide the patient over this temporary setback with a combination of various therapeutic options selected on the basis of careful clinical examination and investigation (Table 93.5). Most complex situations are assisted by or absolutely require the use of echocardiography.

IMMUNOSUPPRESSION

The details of the immunosuppression regimen will differ between transplant centres but the principles are the same. Immunosuppression is induced just prior to transplantation and then maintained permanently with a combination of drugs aimed at maximal effect and minimal toxicity. Episodes of suspected or proven rejection prompt additional temporary treatment.

Since the early 1980s, the regime used by most centres has been triple therapy with cyclosporine, azathioprine and corticosteroids. The initial introduction of cyclosporine in 1979 was a major step, but the drug has significant problems; in addition to renal and hepatic toxicity, there is uncertain gut absorption and bioavailability (at best only 30%) which can be exacerbated by many commonly prescribed drugs.[14] Alterations in gut function may seriously reduce plasma levels to the point at which rejection may occur. Drug interactions may result in toxic levels. Plasma levels of the drug should be monitored frequently especially in the early perioperative phase and during any complicating illness. When the gut cannot be relied upon, the intravenous formulation may be used with one-third of the oral dose given by intravenous injection over 2–6 h. Recently, modified formulations of the drug have allegedly improved bioavailability and stability of plasma levels.[15]

Cyclosporine works through interleukin-2 inhibition in T-lymphocytes so its action is fairly specific. Tacrolimus is an alternative to cyclosporine, has similar

Table 93.5 Possible support options for postoperative care of the complicated cardiac transplant recipient

Treatment	Directed at	Based on
Inotropic support (e.g. milrinone or epinephrine)	Poor contractility of LV, RV or both LV and RV	Elevated filling pressures, low cardiac output, echocardiography (TTE or TOE)
Pressor support (e.g. norepinephrine)	Low systemic arterial blood pressure despite adequate filling pressures and supported contractility	Arterial pressure monitoring, cardiac output and TTE or TOE
Heart rate support with chronotropic drugs (e.g. isoprenaline or milrinone) or pacing	Low intrinsic grafted heart rate	Heart rate less than 90 in the first 48 h usually symptomatic and indication for support
Mechanical support (e.g. IABP)	Poor LV function not responsive to other measures	Elevated LAP, low cardiac output, poor response to drugs, TTE or TOE
Temporary ventricular assistance – RVAD, LVAD or BiVAD	Very poor RV, LV or biventricular function	As above, no response to less invasive measures and where recovery or retransplantation may be an option
Inhaled nitric oxide	RV failure combined with reversible elevation of PVR	Filling pressures, PAP, TTE or TOE
Resternotomy	Catastrophic states where excessive bleeding or tamponade is suspected	Combination of observations but particularly TOE

LV, left ventricle; RV, right ventricle; TTE, trans thoracic echocardiography; TOE, trans oesophageal echocardiography; IABP, intra-aortic balloon pump counterpulsation; LAP, left atrial pressure (direct or indirect); RVAD, LVAD, BiVAD, right, left or biventricular assist device support; PAP, pulmonary arterial pressure; PVR, pulmonary vascular resistance.

potency, toxicity and monitoring requirements.[16] Azathioprine is the other commonly used drug. It has a much broader T and B lymphocyte depression effect so marrow suppression is not surprisingly a major potential side effect. The intravenous alternative to the commonly used oral preparation is highly irritant and, when the oral route is not available, it is usually best omitted or an alternative used. Mycophenolate is often substituted for azathioprine. It has a much more specific effect through suppression of purine synthesis in lymphocytes, and achieves lower incidence of rejection, but at the expense of greater risk of infections.[17] Corticosteroids are very important at induction and for treatment of rejection episodes but, otherwise, the dose is tapered to minimize all the usual steroid side-effects. Immunological treatment with antithymocyte globulin (ATG) derived from various species has been traditionally reserved for the treatment of rejection episodes but newer monoclonal ATG type drugs may prove more effective and less allergenic. It is likely that newer approaches with greater specificity and lower toxicity[18] will become established, making it vital that all relevant treatment decisions are made by or discussed with the relevant transplant centre.

REJECTION

One or more episodes of rejection is experienced by the majority of recipients within the first 3 months after transplantation. The risk is subsequently negligible in successful grafts. The diagnosis may be suggested on clinical grounds but the gold standard remains histological examination of an endomyocardial biopsy. In some centres, biopsies are performed on a routine basis,

as well as when rejection is suspected. The right internal jugular vein is the preferred vascular access site for performing the biopsy and this should be considered when selecting line sites for general critical care purposes. The clinical indications or suggestions of rejection are very non-specific and include dyspnoea, weight gain, malaise, atrial arrhythmias, low voltage ECG and echocardiographic evidence of declining cardiac function. The biopsy is graded according to an internationally accepted system,[19] but some centres have moved to a more algorithm-based approach to the patient where clinical features and monitoring of the immune response helps determine the frequency of biopsies.[20]

OTHER COMPLICATIONS

The other main complications include infection, malignancy and graft atherosclerosis or cardiac allograft vasculopathy (CAV).

Infection

Opportunistic infections (commonly lung) account for many of the complications, and for a significant proportion of re-admissions. A recent study reported that 45% of infections were bacterial and less than 10% fungal; however, the associated mortalities were 40% for fungal and less than 10% for bacterial infections.[21] Opinions vary as to the current significance of cytomegalovirus (CMV) infection. Some centres believe that CMV is a problem of the past because of better matching of CMV status, and more effective and potent prophylaxis and treatment with ganciclovir when indicated.[22] However, there is still significant risk of severe acute viral illness,[23] and a possible link between acute viraemic episodes and subsequent damage to the graft and CAV.[24]

Malignancy

The transplant recipient has a hundredfold increased risk of new malignancy (around 1–2% per year) compared to age-matched controls. The majority are skin tumours and lymphomas but any neoplasm may occur. Malignancy is one of the leading causes of death or late readmission to hospital.

Cardiac allograft vasculopathy (CAV)

This is the main cause of death in the long term after heart transplantation and is a multifactorial process, resulting in diffuse obliterative coronary atherosclerosis. The diffuse nature of the lesions makes revascularization by angioplasty and stent, or by surgical bypasses difficult. Perhaps improvements in the control of rejection and management of CMV will improve the situation. In the meantime, there has been some evidence that calcium channel blockers and statins delay the process.[25]

HEART-LUNG TRANSPLANTATION

The first heart-lung transplant (HLT) was performed in Stanford in 1981. HLT was then performed for both parenchymal lung disease and pulmonary hypertension. With the advent of single- or double-lung transplantations, there is overlap between indications for these procedures. The present indications for HLT are primary pulmonary hypertension, Eisenmenger's syndrome, end-stage suppurative pulmonary disease or end-stage bilateral lung disease associated with significant cardiac failure, generally right ventricular failure.

SELECTION CRITERIA (Table 93.6)

These are similar to those for heart transplantation, except that an elevated pulmonary vascular resistance tips clinical judgement towards HLT. Exclusion criteria for recipients are also similar but probably should include a stricter age limit (i.e. 45 years), high-dose corticosteroid therapy (relative contraindication), active bronchopulmonary fungal disease, and prior sternotomy, thoracotomy or mediastinal irradiation.

Table 93.6 Heart-lung transplantation: donor selection criteria

Age and ABO blood group compatibility as per heart donors
Close size match of donor to recipient to avoid lung restriction (donor lung too big) or persistent residual space between lung and chest wall (donor lung too small)
Donor PaO_2 >100 mmHg (13.3 kPa) on FiO_2 = 0.3 or >300 mmHg (39.9 kPa) on FiO_2 = 1.0
Normal chest X-ray

THE TRANSPLANT PROCEDURE

Heart-lung transplantation is, by any definition, a massive procedure. The combination of cardiopulmonary bypass with full anticoagulation and significant likelihood of pleural adhesions tethering the explanted lungs to the chest wall make for a substantial risk of major intra-operative haemorrhage and this may continue into the postoperative phase. Preservation of nerves, such as the vagus, phrenic and recurrent laryngeal, may be difficult and result in significant morbidity when unsuccessful.

POSTOPERATIVE CARE

This is similar to that for cardiac transplant patients, with some differences. The patient is without a bronchial arterial supply or pulmonary innervation. Lymphatic drainage of the lungs is lost. Thus, patients are kept in a negative fluid balance in the early postoperative period. Active physiotherapy is required, sometimes with bronchoscopic toilet to clear secretions, as denervation prevents reflex coughing of secretions below the anastomosis (usually at around five tracheal rings above the carina). Once secretions reach the native trachea coughing may result. Immunosuppression is given as for cardiac transplantation. Antibiotic prophylaxis will depend on local policies and results of cultures of recipient and donor sputum or secretions. Rejection is more likely to manifest first in the lungs rather than the heart graft, so rejection surveillance includes frequent reassessment of pulmonary status, possibly with trans-bronchial biopsies.

COMPLICATIONS

Bleeding may occur due to extensive dissection and systemic pulmonary collaterals in congenital heart disease. Other early complications include tracheal anastomotic dehiscence and acute reperfusion lung injury (i.e. pulmonary oedema) due to long ischaemic times and infection. Heart-lung recipients have three times as many infections as heart recipients, and this contributes significantly to their higher mortality rate. Infection is the major cause of mortality in the first 6 months, and rejection thereafter.

IMMUNOSUPPRESSION

This is very similar to that used in heart transplantation, and also similar in single- and double-lung transplantation.

SINGLE- OR DOUBLE-LUNG TRANSPLANTATION

Early attempts at single-lung transplantation (SLT) yielded only short-term survival.[26] However, subsequent successes by the Toronto Group encouraged the development of double-lung transplantation,[27] initially by the *en bloc* method with tracheal anastomosis. The extensive dissection required in the recipient and the high incidence of anastomotic problems encouraged development of bilateral sequential lung transplantation (BSLT), which has found wide favour.[28] SLT is indicated for non-suppurative lung disease in a patient who does not have cardiac disease (e.g. emphysema from smoking, α_1-antitrypsin deficiency or fibrosing alveolitis). Whilst these conditions can also be managed by BLST, SLT provides satisfactory results and makes more efficient use of a limited donor pool. BSLT is indicated for suppurative and/or bilateral lung disease (e.g. cystic fibrosis and bilateral bronchiectasis). The merits of BSLT or HLT for these conditions are controversial. With HLT, the recipient's heart may be used in a 'domino' procedure as a donor heart for a second recipient.[29] Either BLST or a domino HLT allow the most efficient use of donor organs. Lung transplantation can be combined with kidney or liver transplantation.

Recipients are accepted for lung transplantation up to the age of 55 years. It is usually possible to perform SLT without cardiopulmonary bypass (CPB). The requirement for CPB is higher in BSLT (approximately 5–10%) because the first lung transplanted (usually the right) must immediately provide ventilation and gas exchange whilst the other side is transplanted. CPB increases the amount of operative blood loss and the volume of colloid required in the postoperative period. The incidence of non-cardiogenic pulmonary oedema is also increased.

PHYSIOLOGY OF THE DENERVATED LUNGS

The lungs appear to remain permanently denervated. There is evidence that the bronchial artery circulation and lymphatic system regenerate after several weeks. Control of respiration is not affected by the loss of pulmonary afferent nerves. Regulation of breathing is through chest wall afferents. Patients regain spontaneous breathing early, and are usually able to be weaned off ventilation and extubated within 48 h.

Patients who were dependent on their hypoxic drive may take time to achieve normocarbia. Arterial blood gases otherwise tend to remain normal. On exercise, minute volume, tidal volume and respiratory rate are able to increase appropriately. Bronchomotor tone is retained. The cough response is lost below the anastomosis.

POSTOPERATIVE CARE

Patients require a period of postoperative ventilation for reasons similar to all major pulmonary surgery. However, there are additional concerns regarding the temporary lung injury, which almost inevitably result from the procedure, and the worry that this injury may be compounded by infection, over generous fluid therapy, pulmonary oxygen toxicity and barotrauma or 'volutrauma' from injudicious ventilator settings. Some degree of impaired gas transfer or widened alveolar to arterial

oxygen tension gradient $(A - a)\Delta O_2$ is very common and may further widen as a result of the following complications.

IMPLANTATION RESPONSE
This manifests within a few hours. Infiltrates in the transplanted lung or lungs appear on chest X-ray, and the lungs may appear to be oedematous with increased peribronchial cuffing. In severe cases, a picture suggestive of severe acute respiratory distress syndrome is seen with widespread loss of translucency. There is an association between ischaemic time and the severity of the response. Management is supportive with fluid restriction if tolerated.

HYPERACUTE REJECTION
Fortunately, this is rare. It usually results in acute graft failure with a very poor prognosis for recovery of function. Management requires continued respiratory support and consideration of re-transplantation.

EARLY REJECTION
Episodes of rejection of the transplanted lung occur in almost all recipients in the first 3 months, but may occur very early in some recipients. Deterioration in PaO_2 and pulmonary infiltrates after 48–72 h should favour a suspicion of rejection rather than implantation response. It may be difficult to distinguish between early rejection and bacterial infection. Bronchoscopic washings may be helpful and transbronchial biopsy is essential in doubtful cases. In suspicious cases, a course of pulsed steroids is appropriate with concurrent antibiotics.

SPUTUM RETENTION
Effective analgesia, aggressive physiotherapy and early mobilization are essential to minimize this problem. Secretions below the anastomoses do not elicit a cough reflex and voluntary coughing is important.

PULMONARY INFECTION
Early pulmonary bacterial infection is common, and infection with other micro-organisms can occur later. Initially, bronchitis is more common than pneumonia. Patients with resident micro-organisms are given prophylactic antibiotics. Samples of the donor's pulmonary secretions are taken at the time of lung harvesting and may be useful in guiding the selection of antibiotics.

ANASTOMOTIC PROBLEMS
Ischaemic anastomotic ulceration is usually superficial, but occasionally deeper tissue loss eventually produces bronchial or tracheal stenosis requiring dilatation and or stent insertion in the early months. Anastomotic dehiscence is rare but often fatal. It may be preceded by fungal invasion of the anastomosis. Fibreoptic bronchoscopy to inspect the anastomoses and remove residual secretions is performed at the conclusion of surgery or after return to the ICU. This is repeated as indicated.

LONG-TERM COMPLICATIONS

Obliterative bronchiolitis,[30] which may be a manifestation of chronic rejection, may eventually lead to graft failure. Recurrent infections with *Pseudomonas* or methicillin-resistant *Staphylococcus* can be serious. After the first 6 weeks, infection with CMV, any fungus, protozoan or virus presents potential hazards. Chronic renal failure due to cyclosporine therapy may persist, but is not usually a major problem unless other complications occur. Most patients have a good quality of life with few complications. The improvement in quality of life after lung transplantation may be more important as a marker of success than bald survival figures.[31]

RESULTS OF CARDIOPULMONARY TRANSPLANTATION

A very good source of information on the results of intra-thoracic transplantation can be found both at www.ishlt.org and in more traditional publications, such as the recent summary of the results of transplantation in the UK.[32] These figures indicate that survival is considerably better after heart transplantation than heart-lung or lung transplantation. Almost 90% of heart recipients are alive at 3 months compared to around 75% of heart-lung and lung recipients. Around 70% of heart recipients are still alive after 5 years; 50% or less of heart-lung and lung recipients survive this long. While these figures are quite impressive, and may improve with current trends in immunosuppression and general care, the main issue remains the gross disparity between the numbers of patients with end-stage cardiopulmonary disease and the ever shrinking supply of donor organs. This is all the more reason to ensure that those patients who are able to benefit from such a rare and precious opportunity receive high standards of medical care throughout their remaining life.

REFERENCES

1 Brann WM, Bennett LE, Kekck BM, Hosenpud JD. Morbidity, functional status, and immunosuppressive therapy after heart transplantation: an analysis of the Joint International Society for Heart and Lung Transplantation/United Network for Organ Sharing Thoracic Registry. *J Heart Lung Transplant* 1998; **17**: 374–82.

2 Hunt SA. Twenty-Fourth Bethesda Conference: cardiac transplantation. *J Am Coll Cardiol* 1993; **22** (suppl. 1): 1–64.

3 Aaronson KD, Schwartz JS, Chen TMC, *et al*. Development and prospective validation of a clinical index to predict survival in ambulatory patients referred for cardiac transplant evaluation. *Circulation* 1997; **95**: 2660–7.

4 Glenn E, Hill DJ. Advances in mechanical bridge to heart transplantation. *Curr Opin Organ Transplant* 2000; **5**: 126–39.

5 Barnett DB. Beta blockers in heart failure: a therapeutic paradox. *Lancet* 1994; **343**: 557–8.

6 Packer M, Coats AJ, Fowler MB, *et al*. Carvedilol prospective randomized cumulative survival study group. Effect of carvedilol on survival in severe chronic heart failure. *N Engl J Med* 2001; **344**: 1651–8.

7 Rose EA, Gelinjns AC, Moskowitz AJ, *et al.*, for the REMATCH Study Group. Long-term use of a left ventricular assist device for end-stage heart failure. *N Engl J Med* 2001; **345**: 1435–43.

8 Pennington DG, Oaks TE, Lohmann DP. Permanent ventricular assist device support versus cardiac transplantation. *Ann Thorac Surg* 1999; **68**: 729–33.

9 Clark NJ, Martin RD. Anesthetic considerations for patients undergoing cardiac transplantation. *J Cardiothorac Anaesth* 1988; **2**: 519–42.

10 Stein KL, Darby JM, Grenvic A. Intensive care of the cardiac transplant recipient. *J Cardiothorac Anesth* 1988; **2**: 543–53

11 Cooper DKC, Lidsky NM. Immediate postoperative care and potential complication. In: Cooper DKC, Miller LW, Patterson GA (eds). *The Transplantation and Replacment of Thoracic Organs*. Dordrecht: Kluwer Academic Publishers; 1996; pp. 221–8.

12 Borow KM, Neumann A, Arensman FW, Yacoub MH. Cardiac and peripheral vascular responses to adreno-receptor stimulation and blockade after cardiac transplantation. *J Am Coll Cardiol* 1989; **14**: 1229–38.

13 Pope SE, Stinson EB, Daughters CT, *et al*. Exercise response of the denervated heart in long term cardiac transplant recipients. *Am J Cardial* 1980; **46**: 213–8.

14 Aziz T, El-Gamel A, Keevil B, *et al*. Clinical impact of Neoral in thoracic organ transplantation. *Transplant Proc* 1998; **30**: 1900–3.

15 Cooney GF, Jeevanandam V, Choudhury S, *et al*. Comparative bioavailability of Neoral and Sandimmune in cardiac transplant recipients over 1 year. *Transplant Proc* 1998; **30**: 1892–4.

16 Meiser BM, Uberfuhr P, Fuchs A, *et al*. Single-centre randomized trial comparing tacrolimus (FK506) and cyclosporine in the prevention of acute myocardial rejection. *J Heart Lung Transplant* 1998; **17**: 782–8.

17 Kabashigawa J, Miller L, Renlund D, *et al*. A randomized active-controlled trial of mycophenolate mofetil in heart transplant recipients. Mycophenolate mofetil investigators. *Transplantation* 1998; **66**: 507–15.

18 Beniaminovitz A Itescu S, Lietz K, *et al*. Prevention of rejection in cardiac transplantation by blockade of the interleukin-2 receptor with a monoclonal antibody. *N Engl J Med* 2000; **342**: 613–9.

19 Billingham ME, Cary NRB, Hammond ME, *et al*. A working group for the standardisation of nomenclature in the diagnosis of heart and lung rejection; heart study group. *J Heart Lung Transplant* 1990; **9**: 587–93.

20 Itescu S, Tung TC, Burke EM, *et al*. An immunological algorithm to predict risk of high-grade rejection in cardiac transplant recipients. *Lancet* 1998; **352**: 263–70.

21 Aziz T, El-Gamel A, Krysiak P, *et al*. Risk factors for early mortality, acute rejection, and factors affecting

first-year survival after heart transplantation. *Transplant Proc* 1998; **30**: 1912–4.

22 Vuylsteke A, Wallwork J. The heart-transplanted patient in the intensive care unit: last news before the millennium. *Curr Opin Crit Care* 1999; **5**: 422–6.

23 Singh N. Infections in solid organ transplant recipients. *Curr Opin Infect Dis* 1998; **11**: 411–7.

24 Valantine HA. Cytomegalovirus infection and allograft injury. *Curr Opin Organ Transplant* 2001; **6**: 305–9.

25 Kabashigawa JA, Katznelson S, Laks H, *et al.* Effect of pravastatin on outcomes after cardiac transplantation. *N Engl J Med* 1995; **333**: 621–7.

26 Derom F, Barbier F, Ringoir S, *et al.* Ten-month survival after lung homotransplantion in man. *J Thorac Cardiovasc Surg* 1971; **61**: 835–46.

27 Toronto Lung Transplant Group. Unilateral lung transplantation for pulmonary fibrosis. *N Engl J Med* 1986; **314**: 1140–5.

28 Kaiser LR, Pasque MK, Trulock EP, *et al.* Bilateral sequential lung transplantion: the procedure of choice for double lung replacement. *Ann Thorac Surg* 1991; **52**: 438–46.

29 Yacoub MH, Banner NR, Khaghani A, *et al.* Heart-lung transplantation for cystic fibrosis and subsequent domino heart transplantation. *J Heart Transplant* 1990; **9**: 459–66.

30 de Hoyos AL, Patterson GA, Maurer JR, *et al.* Pulmonary transplantation. Early and late results. *J Thorac Cardiavasc Surg* 1992; **103**: 295–306.

31 Anyanwu AC, McGuire A, Rogers CA, Murday AJ. Assessment of quality of life in lung transplantation using a simple generic tool. *Thorax* 2001; **56**: 218–22.

32 Anyanwu AC, Rogers CA, Murday AJ, The Steering Group of the UK Cardiothoracic Transplant Audit. Intrathoracic organ transplantation in the United Kingdom 1995 to 1999; results from the UK cardiothoracic transplant audit. *Heart* 2002; **87**: 449–54.

Part Seventeen

Paediatric Intensive Care

94

The critically ill child

A W Duncan

The chapters on paediatric intensive care are intended to help intensivists outside specialized paediatric centres manage common paediatric emergencies. They should be read with relevant adult chapters, as there are areas of common interest. Some common neonatal emergencies are also presented.

The differences between neonates and infants from adults render them susceptible to critical illness and alter their response to disease processes. Nevertheless, there are also similarities and many aspects of organ monitoring and support in adult ICUs have been successfully modified for use in children and are applicable to even the smallest infants.

The major differences between paediatric and adult patients are described below.

ADAPTATION

Dramatic physiological adaptation takes place as the fetus adjusts to extrauterine life. Many changes are incomplete until some time after birth and until then, reversion to fetal physiology may occur. Classically, this applies to the cardio-respiratory events at birth and the subsequent development of a transitional pattern of circulation (see below).

GROWTH AND DEVELOPMENT

There is progressive growth and development of all organ systems throughout childhood. 'Small-body technology' has evolved to cope with the technical aspects of paediatric critical care. Some aspects of growth are non-linear and contribute to the reduced cardiorespiratory reserve of the infant. Physiological differences that influence disease processes and their management are discussed in respective chapters in this section.

MATURATION

At birth, the immaturity of many systems and bio-chemical processes alters the response to pathophysio-logical stress and drugs. Thermoregulation, immune function and renal function are immature at birth, even in the full-term infant. Such immaturity is magnified in the premature infant, for example, surfactant deficiency in the lung causing hyaline membrane disease and liver glucuronyl transferase deficiency causing jaundice.

DIVERSE PATHOPHYSIOLOGICAL STATES

Developmental anomalies, inborn errors of metabolism, susceptibility to infection and various accidents and trauma provide a wide spectrum of paediatric critical illnesses. The response to these illnesses is modified by various aspects of adaption, growth and development and maturation.

PAEDIATRIC INTENSIVE CARE

The development of separate paediatric ICUs recognized the unique problems and requirements of critically ill children. The paediatric ICU (PICU) should not be seen in isolation, but as part of a tertiary paediatric centre, with well defined pre-hospital care, emergency medical services and retrieval teams. Minimum standards should be adopted. In general, a PICU should provide:

- a specialist trained in paediatric intensive care available at short notice
- a range of paediatric subspecialty support
- immediately available junior medical staff with advanced life support skills
- nursing staff with experience in paediatric intensive care
- allied health professionals and ancillary support staff
- specialized advanced life support equipment for children ranging in age from neonates to adolescents
- 24 h laboratory, radiological and pharmacy services

- purpose-built PICU, recognizing the special physical and emotional needs of critically ill children and their families
- a programme for teaching, continuing education, research and quality assurance.

Neonatal ICUs have their own particular requirements.

CARDIORESPIRATORY EVENTS AT BIRTH

During intrauterine life, 60% of blood returning to the right atrium passes directly through the foramen ovale into the left ventricle and ascending aorta. As most of this blood is from the umbilical arteries, the heart and brain are perfused with better-oxygenated blood. Pulmonary vascular resistance (PVR) is high and most of the blood reaching the right ventricle passes through the ductus arteriosus to the descending aorta. Only 10% of right ventricle output passes to the lungs which, although non-functional, require a blood supply for nutrition, growth and development of the lung vasculature.

At birth, closure of the umbilical vessels increases systemic resistance (SVR) and lung expansion leads to the dramatic fall in PVR. Pulmonary blood flow increases, leading to a rise in left atrial pressure and functional closure of the foramen ovale. The ductus arteriosus subsequently constricts and eventually thromboses.

Following the dramatic fall in PVR at birth, there is a gradual regression in muscularization of the pulmonary arterioles over the following weeks to months. This regression is prevented if high pulmonary blood flow occurs, due to congenital heart lesions (e.g. ventricular septal defect, large patent ductus arteriosus and truncus arteriosus) or lesions associated with persistent hypoxaemia (e.g. transposition of great vessels). With these lesions, progression to irreversible pulmonary vascular disease may occur at an early age.

PERSISTENT FETAL CIRCULATION

Haemodynamic adaptation at birth may be delayed or reversed by a number of factors. Persistent pulmonary hypertension and patency of the fetal channels result in right-to-left shunting through the foramen ovale and ductus arteriosus. A vicious cycle may develop, with increasing hypoxaemia and acidosis, increased PVR and further shunting. Unless the underlying disturbance is treated and the pulmonary hypertension is corrected, progression to death is likely. Pulmonary circulation pathophysiology is probably related to abnormalities of endogenous nitric oxide production and manipulation of this agent is proving useful in therapy.

CAUSES OF PERSISTENT FETAL CIRCULATION

A fetal pattern may persist due to:

- low lung volume states (e.g. hyaline membrane disease and perinatal asphyxia)
- pulmonary hypoplasia (e.g. diaphragmatic hernia and Potter's syndrome)
- meconium aspiration syndrome
- chronic placental insufficiency
- perinatal hypoxia and acidosis from any cause
- sepsis (e.g. group B streptococcal infection)
- hyperviscosity syndrome.

CLINICAL FEATURES

Hypoxaemia disproportional to the degree of respiratory distress is typical of persistent fetal circulation and suggests the possibility of congenital cyanotic heart disease. In cases without significant lung disease, echocardiography may be necessary to exclude a structural cardiac lesion. Severe respiratory distress is present in cases secondary to pulmonary disease. Differential cyanosis (i.e. increased cyanosis affecting the lower limbs when compared with the head, neck and right arm) may be seen with the right-to-left shunting at ductal level. This may be confirmed by simultaneous pre- and postductal arterial blood sampling, transcutaneous PO_2 monitoring or oximetry.

TREATMENT

It is important to treat the underlying cause (e.g. surfactant therapy for hyaline membrane disease) in addition to therapy to reduce PVR. The main steps employed are:

- maintenance of high inspired oxygen. Alveolar oxygen tension is an important determinant of pulmonary arteriolar resistance. Sudden reductions in inspired oxygen may increase shunting through fetal channels (so-called flip-flop phenomenon)
- correction of low lung volume states with continuous positive airway pressure (CPAP) or positive-pressure ventilation with positive end-expiratory pressure (PEEP)
- correction of both metabolic and respiratory acidosis
- deliberate hyperventilation using muscle relaxants to lower $PaCO_2$ and generate a respiratory alkalosis. This manoeuvre is limited by lung immaturity and risk of barotrauma. Rapid rates of ventilation (>60 breaths/min) may prove beneficial.
- maintenance of systemic arterial pressure with volume expanders and inotropic agents to reduce the pressure gradient favouring ductal shunting

- isovolaemic haemodilution with colloid, if indicated, to reduce hyperviscosity
- administration of pulmonary vasodilators, e.g. inhaled nitric oxide,[1] and i.v. tolazoline, nitroglycerin and prostaglandin E
- many centres successfully employ extracorporeal membrane oxygenation (EMCO) in this situation.

THERMOREGULATION IN THE NEWBORN

Human body temperature is maintained within narrow limits. This is achieved most easily in the thermoneutral zone – the range of ambient temperature within which the metabolic rate is at a minimum. Once ambient temperature is outside the thermoneutral zone, heat production (shivering or non-shivering thermogenesis) or evaporative heat loss processes are required to maintain body temperature within normal limits. Regulatory mechanisms are less effective in the neonate (there is no shivering or sweating), who is otherwise disadvantaged by a high surface area to body weight ratio and lack of subcutaneous tissue.

The thermoneutral zone is higher in premature infants and falls with increasing postnatal age. Oxygen consumption is minimal, with an environmental or abdominal skin temperature of $36.5°C$. Oxidation of brown fat found in the interscapular and perirenal areas (non-shivering thermogenesis) is the major source of heat production when 'cold-stressed'.

Alteration of body temperature above or below normal leads to increased or decreased metabolism respectively. Attempts by the body to maintain body temperature within normal limits are associated with increased metabolism and cardiorespiratory demands. Radiation is a major source of heat loss in the neonate and is effectively minimized by double-walled incubators or by servo-controlled radiant heaters. The latter allows better access to critically ill babies for monitoring and procedures. Cold stress *per se* increases neonatal mortality. In the presence of respiratory or cardiac disease, it may lead to decompensation.

IMMUNOLOGY OF THE INFANT

The immunological system consists of:

- non-specific mechanisms, including phagocytosis and the inflammatory response
- specific immune responses, consisting of cell mediated (T-cell) and humoral (B-cell) systems (see Ch. 59). These two components are intimately related and both may be abnormal in the newborn infant.

The inflammatory response of the newborn is attenuated. Febrile response to infection may be lacking and both cellular (chemotaxis and phagocytosis) and humoral (complement activity and opsonization) responses may be impaired. Cell-mediated immunity is completely absent in infants born without thymic function (DiGeorge syndrome). In the normal newborn, however, T-cell function appears to be quite well-developed. Rejection of skin allografts is slower in the newborn but this seems to be related mainly to the attenuated inflammatory response.

The B-cell system, responsible for antibody production, is immature at birth. The neonate has passive immunity against some infections because of transplacental transfer of maternal antibodies. Natural immunity is acquired as a result of immunoglobulin A (IgA) in breast milk and protects against some acquired gastrointestinal infections. Overall, the immaturity and inexperience of the immune system result in a markedly increased susceptibility to infection in the first 6 months of life.

RESUSCITATION OF THE NEWBORN

Some newborn infants fail to adapt from fetal to extrauterine life and require immediate cardiopulmonary and cerebral resuscitation. The Apgar scoring system (Table 94.1) scored after 1 min, remains the most widely accepted method of assessment. The best Apgar score is 10 and the worst is 0. There is an inverse relationship between the Apgar score and the degree of hypoxia and acidosis. It has been suggested that the 5 min score is a guide to ultimate prognosis but this is questioned. Collection of sequential scores must not delay the institution of resuscitation.

BIRTH ASPHYXIA

The causes of birth asphyxia may be:

- placental failure – acute or chronic (e.g. toxaemia, diabetes and antepartum haemorrhage)
- drug depression due to maternal analgesics or sedatives administered immediately prior to delivery
- obstetric complications (e.g. difficult forceps, breech, Caesarean section and prolapsed cord)
- fetal conditions (e.g. multiple births and prematurity)
- postnatal problems (e.g. respiratory distress immediately after birth from any cause).

MANAGEMENT

The principles of resuscitation are identical to those employed in other situations. Resuscitation must be started immediately after delivery. Although some cerebral insult may have occurred *in utero* or intrapartum, secondary insults from postpartum asphyxia must be avoided.

Table 94.1 Apgar scoring system

Score	0	1	2
Heart rate	Absent	< 100 beats/min	> 100 beats/min
Respiratory effort	Absent	Weak cry	Strong cry
Muscle tone	Limp	Some flexion	Active motion
Reflex irritability (in response to catheter in nose)	No response	Grimace	Grimace and cough or sneeze
Colour	Blue, pale	Body pink, extremities blue	Pink

Babies suffering mild asphyxia immediately before birth with Apgar scores between 5 and 7 usually respond to stimulation and gentle suction to the nose, mouth and pharynx although oxygen therapy is occasionally required. Babies with moderate asphyxia (Apgar 3–4) usually respond to bag-and-mask ventilation with oxygen. Acid base status should be determined and sodium bicarbonate administered to restore pH >7.25. Severely asphyxiated infants (Apgar 0–2) need urgent cardiopulmonary resuscitation (CPR). After airway suction, bag-and-mask ventilation should be followed by rapid orotracheal intubation and positive-pressure ventilation with oxygen. Fear of complications of oxygen therapy must not mitigate against the administration of 100% oxygen at this stage. If the liquor contains thick meconium, it is vital that the pharynx and trachea be suctioned prior to the onset of respiration or application of positive pressure. Meconium aspiration syndrome is a preventable condition that is often difficult to manage.

Venous access via umbilical or peripheral veins must be established immediately and followed by the administration of 1–2 mmol/kg of sodium bicarbonate. Subsequent buffer therapy should be based on arterial acid-base status if available. Rapid or excessive infusions of hypertonic solutions (e.g. sodium bicarbonate or hypertonic dextrose) or volume expanders may precipitate intracranial haemorrhage, particularly in premature infants.

Asphyxiated infants are usually volume-depleted at birth and blood pressure should be immediately restored with colloids (10 ml/kg in the first instance). External cardiac massage and additional drug therapy (see below) should be employed, if necessary, to restore cardiac rhythm. Post-resuscitative care to maintain cerebral perfusion pressure, correct abnormal serum biochemistry and control seizures is required to prevent secondary cerebral insults.[2] Myocardial dysfunction may occur secondary to asphyxia. Dopamine or dobutamine (5–10 μg/kg per min) may prove useful.

The orotracheal tube should be changed to nasotracheal to enable secure fixation once a degree of stability is attained. Radiological confirmation of tube position should be made as soon as possible. The trachea is very short in the newborn and endobronchial intubation is a particular risk.

Approximate nose to mid-trachea (T2) distances are:

1 28 weeks gestation – 7 cm
2 33 weeks gestation – 9 cm
3 term infant – 10.5 cm

CARDIORESPIRATORY ARREST IN CHILDREN

The vast majority of children lack intrinsic myocardial disease and when cardiac arrest occurs, it is usually the end-result of hypoxaemia and acidosis. The most common predisposing causes are rapidly progressive upper airway obstruction, near drowning, sudden infant death syndrome, pneumonia, sepsis, gastroenteritis and major trauma. Such children invariably arrest in asystole and this should be assumed if an electrocardiogram (ECG) is not immediately available.

Ventricular fibrillation (VF) may be anticipated in the following situations:

- congenital heart disease
- cardiomyopathies
- myocarditis
- poisoning (e.g. tricyclic antidepressant ingestion)
- hereditary prolongation of QT interval (Romano-Ward syndrome).

An international liaison committee is attempting to improve consistency of guidelines issued by international councils for paediatric resuscitation and to base the recommendations on levels of evidence.[3] The ABC of resuscitation needs modification in view of the patient's size. The management of paediatric cardiopulmonary resuscitation is discussed in detail elsewhere in this volume.

VASCULAR ACCESS

Venous access may be difficult, particularly in the collapsed, hypovolaemic or hypothermic child. The external jugular vein may be prominent when usual sites are inaccessible. Cannulation of central veins, apart from via the femoral and external jugular veins, is hazardous even in ideal situations and should not be attempted during cardiac arrest in small children and babies. Three alternatives may be considered: intraosseous infusion, intracardiac injection or endotracheal instillation.

INTRAOSSEOUS INFUSION[4]

This involves infusion into bone marrow – a non-collapsible venous system in direct communication with the circulation. In dog experiments, drugs infused in this way reach the central circulation as rapidly as those injected into a central vein. The effect of equal doses of adrenaline given by intraosseous and i.v. routes is identical in shocked dogs. The technique is simple and quick to learn.

Intraosseous infusion has been successfully used in CPR.[5]

Potential complications include:

- osteomyelitis and so conventional venous access should be established after resuscitation
- compartment syndromes requiring limb amputation have resulted from needle misplacement in muscle or influx of fluids into muscle through another bone perforation[6]
- careful placement: close observation of the limb and early removal once alternative access is achieved are recommended.

INTRACARDIAC INJECTION

Intracardiac injection reliably delivers drugs to the central circulation, but is unsuitable to correct hypovolaemia. The injection can be made using a subxiphoid approach aiming towards the left shoulder, or through the left fourth intercostal space, aiming directly posteriorly. This latter technique is easy to perform and easier to teach, but has a risk of lacerating the left anterior descending coronary artery. Stopping cardiac compression and ventilation during needle insertion and aspirating blood before injection should lessen the risk of intramyocardial injection. Other complications include pneumothorax and cardiac tamponade.

ENDOTRACHEAL INSTILLATION

Endotracheal instillation is, at best, a poor substitute for the above methods. Do not use bicarbonate and calcium as they will cause direct lung damage and cannot be administered by this route.

Adrenaline, lignocaine and atropine may be diluted in saline (newborn 1 ml, infants and pre-school children 3 ml, and older children 5 ml) and delivered into the bronchi through a catheter passed down the endotracheal tube.

PAEDIATRIC MONITORING

Technology has allowed most aspects of adult monitoring to be applied to neonatal and paediatric practice. The ideal paediatric haemodynamic and respiratory monitoring system should:

- be non-invasive, painless and readily interfaced with the child
- constitute minimal risk to the child
- provide specific data relevant to the child's status that are reproducible and readily understood
- respond rapidly to changes in status
- provide continuous visual and/or auditory display of data
- have appropriate alarms
- have facilities for recording data
- be inexpensive and require low maintenance.

ARTERIAL CANNULATION

Arterial cannulation is routine practice in paediatric intensive care, even in infants weighing <1 kg. It is indicated in all critically ill infants for continuous blood pressure monitoring and accurate blood-gas sampling. In the neonate, difficult 'stabs' may lead to significant errors in PaO_2 and $PaCO_2$. The use of umbilical arterial catheters is avoided whenever possible, because of vaso-occlusive complications (e.g. lower limb ischaemia, renal thrombosis, necrotizing enterocolitis and rarely, paraplegia).

Peripheral arteries used include radial, ulnar, brachial, femoral, posterior tibial and dorsalis pedis. Radial and ulnar or posterior tibial and dorsalis pedis vessels must never be cannulated sequentially in the same limb. The safety of brachial and femoral cannulation lies in the presence of rich collateral vessels around the elbow and hip joints. Arterial lines are kept patent by continuous flushing with 1–2 ml/h of heparinized normal saline (5 units heparin/ml flushing solution) or 5% dextrose. Complications include distal ischaemia, infection, retrograde embolization and haemorrhage. Retrograde embolization occurring with flushing is a particular risk in the small infant, depending on the length and volume of vessel and volume and speed of injection. In a 1.5 kg infant, as little as 0.5 ml of fluid injected rapidly into the right radial artery will reach the cerebral circulation. Haemorrhage from accidental disconnection can be significant because of the relatively small blood volume. Meticulous fixation is therefore required.

CENTRAL VENOUS, PULMONARY ARTERY AND LEFT ATRIAL PRESSURE MONITORING

CENTRAL VENOUS PRESSURE

All routes of central venous cannulation are applicable to infants and children and must be within the skills of paediatric intensivists. The femoral route is sometimes the safest in emergency situations. Catheters utilizing the Seldinger technique have greatly increased successful placement. Multilumen catheters are useful when infusing multiple drugs and for parental nutrition. Complications including catheter related sepsis are the same as in adults. The need for prolonged venous access may warrant regular catheter changes, or surgical implantation of a central venous device (e.g. Infusaport, Broviac or Hickman catheter). Umbilical venous cannulation and passage of the catheter through the sinus venosus to the right atrium is useful in neonatal emergencies.

PULMONARY ARTERY PRESSURE

Pulmonary artery (PA) pressure monitoring using flow-directed 4 and 5 FG catheters is feasible even in neonates. It is, however, invasive, technically more difficult and has greater risks than in the adult. It is rarely required in the neonate, as the pulmonary circulation and response to therapy can usually be gauged indirectly from the magnitude of right-to-left shunting. Systemic levels of PA pressure are usually found in neonates with severe lung disease.

The major indication for PA pressure monitoring is following surgery for congenital heart disease (e.g. repair of ventricular septal defect with pulmonary hypertension, truncus arteriosus and obstructed total anomalous pulmonary venous drainage). A catheter is inserted directly into the PA at the time of surgery. It is most useful in guiding weaning from mechanical ventilation.

LEFT ATRIAL PRESSURE

Left atrial pressure monitoring is often useful after open heart surgery for congenital heart disease, and is achieved by means of a catheter placed directly in the left atrium during surgery.

CARDIAC OUTPUT MEASUREMENT

Cardiac output determination can be performed in small children by dye dilution, thermodilution or Doppler techniques. Unfortunately, errors have been substantial, and the first two techniques are invasive, intermittent and only repeatable within finite limits. Interpretation of results is made difficult or impossible in the presence of intracardiac shunts or valvular incompetence. The dye curve may, in fact, be useful in demonstrating residual intracardiac shunts. Calculation of derived variables is only as accurate as the flow measurement.

A recently developed system (PiCCO, Pulsion Medical Systems AG, Munich, Germany) provides con-

tinuous cardiac monitoring even in small infants. Cardiac output is determined both intermittently by transpulmonary thermodilution[7] and continuously through arterial pulse contour analysis.[8] The system also derives cardiac preload volume, an index of left ventricular contractility and an estimate of intrathoracic blood volume and extravascular lung water.

TEMPERATURE MONITORING

Temperature monitoring is important in neonatal and paediatric intensive care. Prevention of cold stress requires accurate measurement of core and skin temperature. Core-to-ambient temperature gradients provide a sensitive, albeit indirect index of cardiac output and peripheral perfusion and are useful in managing fever. Toe temperature normally lies between core temperature (tympanic or oesophageal) and ambient temperature. The toe-core temperature gradient increases with low cardiac output or vasoconstriction from any cause. Toe temperature is a useful guide to the efficacy of vasodilator therapy.

PULSE OXIMETRY

Pulse oximetry provides continuous non-invasive measurement of arteriolar saturation (SaO_2) and provides a rapid indication of hypoxaemia. Accurate information is given:

- when the oxyhaemoglobin dissociation curve is shifted to the left (e.g. fetal haemoglobin and alkalosis) or to the right (e.g. sickle-cell disease and acidosis);
- in the presence of carboxyhaemoglobin (functional saturation is accurate);
- with moderately severe desaturation (e.g. cyanotic heart disease);
- with anaemia (haemoglobin concentrations above 5 g/dl);
- when skin is pigmented.

Errors occur with extreme hypoperfusion, excessive movement and rapidly changing ambient light. A range of sensors are now available to monitor children of all ages.

TRANSCUTANEOUS PO₂ AND PCO₂ MONITORING

Oxygen and carbon dioxide diffuse through well-perfused skin from the superficial capillary network and can be measured using modified polarographic and glass electrodes respectively. The electrodes are heated to 43–45°C to arterialize the capillary blood and maximize capillary blood flow. Under optimal conditions, there is good correlation between arterial and transcutaneous gas tensions. Hence continuous monitoring of blood-gas tensions is possible in a non-invasive way. The $PtcO_2$–PaO_2 gradient and the output of the heating element have been used as indices of microcirculation. The accuracy of these devices is mainly confined to the neonatal period.

DRUG INFUSIONS

All drugs used in cardiovascular and respiratory support are administered according to body weight; accurate delivery is crucial. Accurate drug infusions require accurate devices, of which syringe pumps are the most useful. Potentially lethal errors in calculating drug dilutions are minimized by the use of dose/dilution/infusion rate guidelines (Table 94.2).[9]

PAIN RELIEF AND SEDATION IN CHILDREN

Management of pain and agitation in children has received inadequate attention and has tended to be underestimated and underrated. Infants and children are often unable or unwilling to complain of pain. In the past, some believed that the neonate could not perceive pain. It is now clear that even neonates possess all the anatomical and neurochemical systems necessary for pain perception and exhibit physiological and behaviour responses to pain.[10] Stress responses associated with pain and agitation may increase morbidity and mortality in critically ill patients. Analgesia can be provided by narcotic infusions, local blocks and regional techniques in children of all ages. Painful procedures in the ICU must always be accompanied by appropriate analgesia. The addition of sedative agents such as benzodiazepines can reduce agitation, minimize harmful stress responses and result in narcotic sparing.

NEONATAL AND PAEDIATRIC EMERGENCY TRANSPORT

Care of critically ill neonates and children necessitates the use of specialized retrieval services linked to neonatal and paediatric ICUs. Retrieval services should offer facilities for specialist consultation in addition to secondary transport. Careful audit of such services is necessary to improve patient outcome.[11] The aim of retrieval services is to extend the intensive care facility to peripheral hospitals, allowing stabilization by experienced personnel prior to rapid transport to a regional centre in the most appropriate vehicle (see Ch. 3). Special considerations such as thermoregulation and

oxygen monitoring must be provided for in neonatal transport. Well-designed neonatal emergency transport services have resulted in significant reductions in morbidity and mortality.

OUTCOME OF PAEDIATRIC INTENSIVE CARE

Depending on admission criteria, mortality in paediatric ICUs ranges from 5 to 15%. If patients with pre-existing severe disabilities are excluded, the majority of survivors have a normal or near-normal life expectancy. A number of scoring systems have been developed or modified for paediatric application to predict ICU mortality. These scoring systems allow comparison between different ICUs, internal audits, stratification of patients for research purposes and analysis of cost benefit. The paediatric risk of mortality score (PRISM)[12,13] and the paediatric index of mortality score (PIM)[14] are applicable to a wide range of critically ill infants and children. Although PRISM performs marginally better, PIM is easier to collect and hence less prone to errors in data collection. PIM also has the advantage that it predicts mortality based on admission parameters whereas PRISM is based on the worst variables in the first 24 hours. As many paediatric ICU deaths occur in the first 24 hours PRISM is often recording the dying process rather than predicting it. Specialized scores have been developed for specific problems, e.g. the modified injury severity scale (MISS) and paediatric trauma score (PTS) for paediatric trauma and the modified Glasgow coma scale for neurological insults. Numerous scoring systems have been developed for meningococcaemia, the best validated being the Glasgow Meningococcal Septicaemia Prognostic Score (GMSPS).[15]

Compared with adult intensive care, children with equivalent therapeutic intervention scores (TISS) have a lower in-hospital and 1 month mortality.[16] In addition, non-survivors do not consume a disproportionate amount of resources. While multiple organ failure increases mortality, the prognosis is considerably better than for adults.[17] There is evidence that mortality is lower in specialist paediatric ICUs,[18] and that paediatric ICUs with a larger workload have better outcomes than those looking after fewer children.[19] General hospitals should therefore have facilities for urgent resuscitation of children prior to early transport to a specialized paediatric ICU. Unless unavoidable, critically ill children, particularly those requiring mechanical intervention, should not be cared for in an adult ICU for longer than 24 h. The American Academy of Pediatrics, the Society of Critical Care Medicine, the British Paediatric Association and the Australian National Health and Medical Research Council have all stated that children should receive intensive care in specialist paediatric units.

Table 95.2 Calculation of drug infusion dilutions:

1 Select desired drug dosage to be delivered in μg/kg per min.
2 Select infusion rate of syringe pump in ml/h (from centre of table)
3 Calculate number of milligrams of drug to be mixed in 50-ml syringe
    e.g.: 10-kg child, 0.1–2 μg/kg per min, infusion 1–20 ml/h: put 0.3 ml/kg (= 3 mg) in 50 ml

μg/kg per min	0.15 mg/kg in 50 ml	0.3 mg/kg in 50 ml	0.6 mg/kg in 50 ml	1.5 mg/kg in 50 ml	3 mg/kg in 50 ml	6 mg/kg in 50 ml	15 mg/kg in 50 ml	30 mg/kg in 50 ml	60 mg/kg in 50 ml
0.05	1	ml/h							
0.1	2	1	ml/h						
0.2	4	2	1						
0.3	6	3	1.5						
0.4	8	4	2	ml/h					
0.5	10	5		1					
0.6	12	6	3						
0.7	14	7							
0.8	16	8	4						
0.9	18	9			ml/h				
1	20	10	5	2	1				
1.5		15		3	1.5	ml/h			
2		20	10	4	2	1			
3				6	3	1.5			
4			20	8	4	2	ml/h		
5				10	5		1		
6				12	6	3			
7				14	7				
8				16	8	4			
9				18	9		ml/h		
10				20	10	5	2	1	
12					14	7			
14					14	7			
15					15		3	1.5	ml/h:
20					20	10	4	2	1
25							5		
30						15	6	3	1.5
40						20	8	4	2
50							10	5	
100							20	10	5
150								15	
200								20	10

Norepinephrine

Morphine

Epinephrine Isoprenaline

Dopamine Dobutamine Salbutamol

Tolazoline

Nitroglycerin-Tridilset

Nitroprusside
Max. hours of infusion

Lignocaine

Thiopentone

Ketamine

10
8
7
7
6

REFERENCES

1 Kinsella JP, Neish SR, Dunbar ID, *et al.* Clinical responses to prolonged treatment of persistent pulmonary hypertension of the newborn with low doses of inhaled nitric acid. *J Pediatr* 1993; **123**: 103–8.

2 Fletcher J, Shann F, Duncan AW. The dangers of premature extubation after severe birth asphyxia. *Aust Paediatr J* 1987; **23**: 27–9.

3 Nadkarni V, Hazinski MF, Zideman D, *et al.* ILCOR advisory statements: Pediatric resuscitation. *Circulation* 1997; **95**: 2185–95.

4 Rosetti VA, Thompson BM, Miller J, *et al.* Intraosseous infusion: an alternative route of pediatric intravascular access. *Ann Emerg Med* 1985; **14**: 885–8.

5 Saccheti AD, Linkenheimer R, Liberman M, *et al.* Intraosseous drug administration: successful resuscitation from asystole. *Pediatr Emerg Care* 1989; **5**: 97–8.

6 Moscati R, Moore GP. Compartment syndrome with resultant amputation following intraosseous infusion. *Am J Emerg Med* 1990; **8**: 470–71.

7 McLuckie A, Murdoch IA, Marsh MJ, Anderson D. A comparison of pulmonary and femoral artery thermodilution cardiac indices in paediatric intensive care patients. *Acta Paediatr* 1996; **85**: 336–8.

8 Goedje O, Hoeke K, Lichtwarek-Aschoff M, Faltchauser A, Lamm P, Reichart B. Continuous cardiac output by femoral arterial thermodilution calibrated pulse contour analysis: Comparison with pulmonary arterial thermodilution. *Crit Care Med* 1999; **27**: 2407–12.

9 Shann F. Continuous drug infusions in children: a table for simplifying calculations. *Crit Care Med* 1983; **11**: 462–3.

10 Anand KJS and Hickey PR. Pain and its effects in the human neonate and fetus. *N Engl J Med* 1987; **317**: 1321–9.

11 Henning R and McNamara V. Difficulties encountered in transport of the critically ill child. *Pediatr Emerg Care* 1991; **7**: 133–7.

12 Pollack MM, Ruttimann UE, Getson PR. Pediatric risk of mortality (PRISM) score. *Crit Care Med* 1988; **16**: 1110–6.

13 Pollack MM, Patel KM, Ruttimann UE. PRISM III: An updated pediatric risk of mortality score. *Crit Care Med* 1996; **24**: 743–52.

14 Shann F, Pearson G, Slater A, *et al.* Paediatric index of mortality (PIM): A mortality prediction model for children in intensive care. *Intensive Care Med* 1997; **23**: 201–7.

15 Thompson APJ, Sills JA, Hart A. Validation of the Glasgow meningococcal septicaemia prognostic score: a 10 year retrospective survey. *Crit Care Med* 1991; **19**: 26–30.

16 Yeh TS, Pollack MM, Holbrook PR, Fields AI and Ruttimann UE. Assessment of pediatric intensive care – application of the Therapeutic Intervention Scoring System. *Crit Care Med* 1982; **10**: 497–500.

17 Wilkinson JD, Pollack MM, Ruttimann UE, Glass NL and Yeh TS. Outcome of pediatric patients with multiple organ system failure. *Crit Care Med* 1986; **14**: 271–4.

18 Pollack MM, Alexander SR, Clarke, *et al.* Improved outcomes from tertiary center pediatric intensive care: a statewide comparison of tertiary and nontertiary care facilities. *Crit Care Med* 1991; **19**: 150–9.

19 Pearson G, Shann F, Barry P, *et al.* Should paediatric intensive care be centralized? *Trent versus Victoria. Lancet* 1997; **349**: 1213–17.

95

Upper respiratory tract obstruction in children

A W Duncan

Upper respiratory tract obstruction (URTO) is a common cause of respiratory failure in infants and children. This reflects the frequency of upper respiratory tract abnormalities and disorders, the presence of narrow airways and the structural inefficiencies of the lung and chest wall. The majority of children with critical airway obstruction are otherwise healthy, and expert management results in a normal life expectancy. Poor management can lead to cardio-pulmonary arrest and hypoxic cerebral damage.

ANATOMICAL DIFFERENCES AND CLINICAL RELEVANCE

Differences in the anatomy and function of the airway are important considerations in airway maintenance, laryngoscopy and intubation. In the newborn, the nose contributes approximately 42% of total airways resistance, which is considerably less than the adult's 63%. Thus, infants are obligatory nose-breathers. The epiglottis is longer, U-shaped and floppy, and may need to be lifted with a straight-bladed laryngoscope for visualization of the larynx and intubation. The larynx is higher in the neck (C3–4) in the neonate, and has an anterior inclination.[1] It descends over the first 3 years of life, and again at puberty, to lie opposite C6. The length of the trachea varies from 3.2 to 7.0 cm in babies weighing less than 6 kg. Accurate positioning of the tracheal tubes is required to prevent accidental extubation and endobronchial intubation. The narrowest part of the airway until puberty is the cricoid ring. This part of the airway is most vulnerable to trauma and swelling. The narrow cricoid ring also dictates tube size, and allows use of uncuffed tubes in infants and children.

PATHOPHYSIOLOGY

Although the ratio of airway diameter to body weight is relatively large in the infant, in absolute terms airway diameter is small, and a minimal reduction causes a devastating increase in airway resistance. For example, the diameter of the newborn's cricoid ring is 5 mm. A 50% reduction in radius will result in turbulent flow, and increases the pressure (and work) required to maintain breathing 32-fold.[2]

Symptoms and signs vary with the level of obstruction, the aetiology and the age of the child. Airway obstruction may be either extrathoracic or intrathoracic. Extrathoracic obstruction increases during inspiration and is characterized by inspiratory stridor and prolongation of inspiration. Intrathoracic obstruction of both large and small airways increases during expiration and is characterized by expiratory stridor, prolonged expiration, wheeze and air trapping. Biphasic stridor is characteristic of mid tracheal lesions. These features mirror the intrapleural and airway pressure changes of the respiratory cycle (Fig. 95.1). Retraction of the chest wall, an important sign of respiratory distress, reflects the negative intrapleural pressures generated combined with the compliance of the chest wall. Large negative intrapleural pressures are also transmitted to the interstitium of the lung, and may result in pulmonary oedema.[3,4] Cor pulmonale may develop secondary to chronic obstruction, hypoxia and pulmonary hypertension.[5,6]

CLINICAL PRESENTATION

Stridor is noisy breathing due to turbulent air flow. It is the cardinal feature of URTO. Parents complain that their child has noisy breathing and of 'sucking the chest in'. The pitch and timing of stridor provide information about the degree and level of obstruction.

Voice sounds may also be informative. Nasal obstruction results in hyponasality. Oropharyngeal obstruction may cause a 'hot potato' voice. Supraglottic obstruction is characterized by a muffled voice. Children with glottic lesions may be hoarse or aphonic.

Retraction of chest wall develops as obstruction progresses. Retraction is less prominent in older

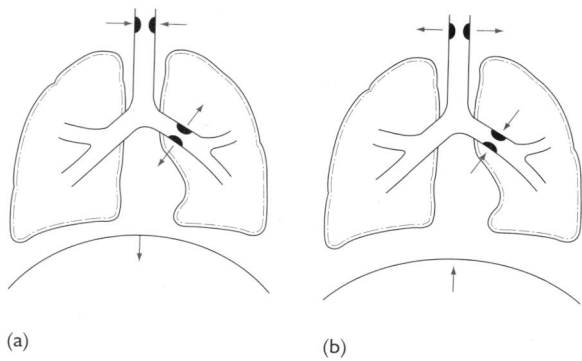

(a)   (b)

Fig. 95.1 Dynamics of (a) extrathoracic and (b) intrathoracic airways obstruction.

children, as chest-wall structure stabilizes. As obstruction worsens, the work of breathing increases and the accessory muscles become active. The alae nasi (vestigial muscles of ventilation) begin to flare. Fever increases minute volume and magnifies any degree of obstruction. Whereas infants and older children can maintain an increased work of breathing, premature infants and neonates rapidly fatigue, and may develop apnoeic episodes.[7,8]

Auscultation over the neck and larynx may identify the site of obstruction. A foreign body in the airway may produce a mechanical or slapping sound. Decreased or absent breath sounds may occur with greater degrees of obstruction. Chronic URTO is a cause of failure to thrive, chest deformity (pectus excavatum) and cor pulmonale.[5,6] Some infants present with recurrent chest infections. Abnormal posturing (head retraction) may also be a feature, particularly in infants.

Initially, the child with airway obstruction exhibits tachypnoea and tachycardia. If obstruction is severe and persistent, exhaustion eventually occurs, and the child exhibits decreased respiratory effort, decreased stridor and breath sounds, restlessness, cyanosis, pallor and eventually bradycardia.

AETIOLOGY

A classification of the causes of URTO is presented in Table 95.1. The neonatal causes are predominantly due to congenital structural lesions. Acute inflammatory lesions, foreign bodies and trauma predominate in older infants and children.

DIAGNOSIS

The cause of URTO can often be determined from the history and clinical features. Radiographic examination of the upper and lower airways with antero-posterior and lateral views may show soft-tissue swelling or the presence of foreign bodies.[9] Air shadows may indicate fixed stenotic or compressive lesions. In children with significant respiratory distress, these investigations should be undertaken in the intensive care unit (ICU) rather than the radiology department.

Table 95.1 Causes of upper airway obstruction in children

Level	Newborn	Older infant and child
Nasal	Choanal atresia	
Oropharyngeal	Facial malformations (e.g. Pierre–Robin syndrome Treacher Collins syndrome) Macroglossia Cystic hygroma Vallecular cyst	Macroglossia/post-glossectomy Angioedema Retropharyngeal abscess Tonsillar and adenoidal hypertrophy Obstructive sleep apnoea
Laryngeal	Infantile larynx Bilateral vocal cord palsy Congenital subglottic stenosis Subglottic haemangioma Laryngeal web Laryngeal cysts	Acute laryngotracheobronchitis (croup) Bacterial tracheitis Acute epiglottitis Post-intubation oedema and stenosis Laryngeal papillomata Laryngeal foreign body Inhalation burns Caustic ingestion
Tracheal	Tracheomalacia Vascular ring	External trauma Foreign body Anterior mediastinal tumours (e.g. lymphoma)

Previously, barium swallow and aortography have been used to confirm the diagnosis of vascular compression of the trachea. Computed tomography (CT) has assumed importance in the assessment of fixed lesions such as intrinsic stenosis and extrinsic compression. Magnetic resonance imaging (MRI) and CT with contrast are useful to assess vascular anomalies.[10] Tracheo-bronchography may provide excellent anatomical delineation of the proximal tracheobronchial tree and allow dynamic assessment of airway calibre.

Direct visualization of the airway may be necessary, and may also prove therapeutic (e.g. removal of a foreign body). Nasoscopy, flexible fibreoptic and rigid laryngoscopy and bronchoscopy all have a place in assessing the paediatric airway. Investigation of the child's airway should only be undertaken in specialized centres by experienced endoscopists, radiologists and anaesthetists.

Blood gas determination is rarely useful in assessment or monitoring of URTO. An exception to this is in young infants where hypercapnic respiratory failure may occur early and insidiously in URTO. It is dangerous practice to await respiratory failure before intervention. Mild hypoxaemia only may be present until fatigue, hypoventilation, cyanosis and hypercapnoea occur. Pulse oximetry may provide useful warning information. An oxygen saturation less than 90% in a patient with pure URTO is a reason for concern.

SPECIFIC AIRWAY OBSTRUCTIONS

EPIGLOTTITIS

Epiglottitis is a life-threatening supraglottic lesion which, prior to vaccination, was caused almost exclusively by *Haemophilus influenzae* type B. The prevalence of epiglottitis has fallen dramatically with the uptake of *H. influenzae* vaccination. It still occurs due to failure to vaccinate or vaccine failure. Occasional cases are caused by streptococcus, staphylococcus, pneumococcus and meningococcus, as well as by viruses. Non-infective causes include corrosive ingestion and thermal injury. The diagnosis is usually obvious from history and clinical features. There is an acute onset of high fever, toxaemia and noisy breathing. The child adopts a characteristic posture, preferring to sit with mouth open, drooling saliva. The tongue is often proptosed and immobile. Cough is usually absent. These features are the legacy of an intensely painful pharynx. Due to the accompanying septicaemia, the severity of illness often appears out of proportion to the degree of airway obstruction. Typically, a low-pitched inspiratory stridor is present, accompanied by a characteristic expiratory snore. Atypical cases with cough and without fever may obscure the diagnosis.

Sudden total obstruction is not infrequent, and may be precipitated by examination of the pharynx, the supine position or stressful procedures (e.g. cannula insertion).

When the diagnosis is in doubt, a lateral X-ray of the neck in the sitting position should be taken in the emergency department or ICU, provided that staff capable of securing the airway remain in attendance. Examination of the pharynx must not be undertaken unless personnel and facilities are available for immediate intubation.

MANAGEMENT

PARENTERAL ANTIBIOTICS

Third-generation cephalosporins are the preferred antibiotics because of emerging resistance to ampicillin and, to a lesser extent, chloramphenicol. Appropriate regimens include cefotaxime 200 mg/kg per day i.v. for 5 days, or ceftriaxone 100 mg/kg i.v. statim followed by 50 mg/kg i.v. after 24 h. Children receiving cefotaxime may be changed to oral chloramphenicol once sensitivities are available and oral intake is tolerated.

RELIEF OF AIRWAY OBSTRUCTION

All but the mildest cases require an artificial airway. Nasotracheal intubation is the optimal treatment,[11] although tracheostomy is a satisfactory alternative, depending on the available personnel. Anaesthesia for relief of airway obstruction is described below. A tube of size appropriate to age is chosen (see Ch. 102). Extubation can be undertaken when fever subsides and the child no longer appears toxic. Most cases can be extubated in less than 18 h. Only those complicated by pulmonary oedema, pneumonia or cerebral hypoxia (from delayed therapy) will require intubation for longer than 24 h. It is not necessary to re-examine the larynx prior to extubation. Nebulized epinephrine is of no benefit in this condition and may aggravate the situation.[12] Pulmonary oedema, when it occurs, is due to airway obstruction, septicaemia and increased lung capillary permeability.[3,13,14] It is managed according to conventional principles.

PROPHYLAXIS

Most invasive infections due to *H. influenzae* occur in children under 5 years of age. The risk of infection in close contacts is about 500-fold higher than in the general population. It is thus recommended that members (including adults) of any household with *H. influenzae* type B infection and with another child under 4 years should be given prophylactic antibiotics. An accepted regimen is oral rifampicin 20 mg/kg daily (maximum 600 mg) for 4 days. An alternative is a single dose of ceftriaxone 100 mg/kg i.m.

CROUP

Croup or acute laryngotracheobronchitis is due to inflammation and oedema of the glottic and subglottic regions. The narrowest part of the child's upper airway is the subglottic region, the point at which critical narrowing occurs. Retained secretions due to the bronchitic component may compound the obstruction. Three sub-groups are recognized: viral croup, spasmodic croup and bacterial tracheitis.

VIRAL CROUP

Viral croup, most commonly due to parainfluenza virus, respiratory syncytial virus and rhinovirus, is characterised by a coryzal prodrome, low-grade fever, harsh barking (croupy) cough and hoarse voice. Progression of airway obstruction in severe cases is shown in Fig. 95.2.

SPASMODIC CROUP

Spasmodic or recurrent croup occurs in children with an allergic presdisposition.[15,16] It usually develops suddenly, often at night, and without prodromal symptoms. Endoscopy reveals pale, watery oedema of the subglottic mucosa. Such children probably represent part of the asthma spectrum and wheeze, due to small airway flow limitation, may be a feature.

BACTERIAL TRACHEITIS

Bacterial tracheitis is uncommon but should be suspected in children with croup accompanied by high fever, leukocytosis and copious purulent secretions.[17] There is a significant risk of sudden complete obstruction. *Staphylococcus aureus* is usually the cause, although *H. influenzae* and group A *Streptococcus* have also been isolated.

Croup is uncommon in children under 6 months of age, and an underlying structural lesion such as subglottic stenosis or haemangioma with superimposed infection should be suspected. Endoscopy is warranted with a prior history of stridor or if symptoms persist.

MANAGEMENT

Minimal disturbance is important, as handling will increase minute ventilation, oxygen consumption and signs of obstruction.

Adequate hydration: oral fluid intake must be encouraged to avoid dehydration. Gavage feeding is contra-indicated, and i.v. fluids may occasionally be necessary. Overhydration must also be avoided. Hyponatraemia and convulsions due to inappropriate antidiuretic hormone secretion have been observed with prolonged, severe airway obstruction.

Oxygen therapy may mask signs of respiratory failure, but should be given to treat hypoxaemia. Its use can be guided by pulse oximetry (i.e. keep SaO_2 >90%). Oxygen administration may further stress the young child. The need for oxygen therapy is often an indication for intubation.

Corticosteroids have dramatically reduced the need for intubation in children with croup. They are effective in both viral and spasmodic croup.[18,19] Steroids will also shorten the duration of intubation and increase the success rate of extubation.[20,21] The dose of dexamethasone is 0.6 mg/kg statim (maximum dose 10 mg) followed, if necessary, by 0.15 mg/kg 6-hourly. In very distressed children, it is best administered i.m. or i.v. to ensure absorption. Inhaled steroids are also effective in milder cases.[22]

Humidification of inspired gases was the mainstay of supportive care for decades. Controlled studies showing efficacy are lacking. A study by Bourchier *et al.*[23] failed to demonstrate benefit and its use has been abandoned in many centres.

Nebulized epinephrine will usually provide temporary relief of acute obstruction.[24] Historically, racemic epinephrine (2.25% solution, i.e. 1 : 88 L-epinephrine), developed for use in asthma, was employed. Indications for epinephrine nebulization are:

(a) acute laryngotracheobronchitis, where relief usually lasts 1–2 h, but may be longer if secretions are expelled. It is debatable whether the natural history of the disease is altered. It is an effective temporising measure until steroids have time to work. If given prior to induction, it will facilitate inhalational anaesthesia for intubation;

(b) spasmodic croup, where one or two inhalations may produce lasting relief of airway obstruction;

(c) post-endoscopy or intubation oedema, where the benefit is often dramatic;

(d) transport, where administration will render the child safe for interhospital transfer.

The empirical dose is 0.05 ml/kg diluted to 2 ml with saline and nebulized with oxygen. A strong preparation (1%) of the L-isomer can also be used. The same mass of L-epinephrine is provided by 0.5 ml/kg of the

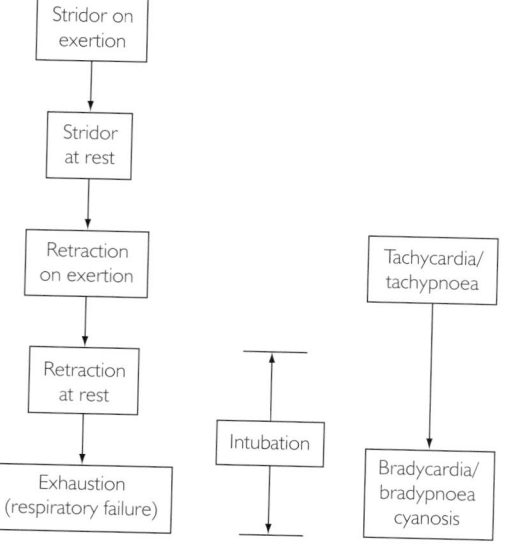

Fig. 95.2 Features of progressive upper airway obstruction

standard 1 : 1000 solution of epinephrine, and this is equally effective.

Antibiotics are indicated only for bacterial tracheitis where anti-staphylococcal cover is recommended.

Mechanical relief of airway obstruction: this requirement has been greatly reduced by early use of steroids. The need for tracheal intubation is indicated by increasing tachycardia, tachypnoea and restlessness. An SaO_2 persistently less than 90% is another reason for concern. It is important not to wait for the development of bradycardia, bradypnoea, cyanosis, exhaustion and respiratory failure. Blood gases are not a useful guide for intubation. Nasotracheal intubation is preferred. An orotracheal tube, size (inner diameter) 1 mm less than that predicted by age (Table 95.2) is first inserted under anaesthesia. A stylet through the tube is recommended to overcome the resistance of the subglottic region. The tube is changed to a nasotracheal tube immediately after aspiration of secretions.

Extubation is performed when the child is afebrile, secretions have diminished and a leak is audible around the tube with coughing or positive pressure (25 cmH$_2$O or less). The duration of intubation averages 5 days. Children under 1 year old have a higher incidence of intubation and a longer duration of intubation. Reintubation may be required in some cases. Endoscopy should be performed in cases that require repeated intubation to exclude underlying lesions and subglottic injury. Tracheostomy is a suitable alternative for some situations, although complications are more significant.

OTHER SUPRAGLOTTIC LESIONS

Retropharyngeal abscess, tonsillitis, peritonsillar abscess, infectious mononucleosis and Ludwig's angina may all mimic epiglottis. Local features will usually indicate the diagnosis. A retropharyngeal abscess can be detected by palpation and is obvious on a lateral X-ray of the neck. Airway relief, antibiotics, drainage and, rarely, neck incision form the basis of treatment for these disorders. A nasopharyngeal tube will provide relief of obstruction in most supraglottic lesions. In an emergency situation, placement of a laryngeal mask airway may be life saving. Tonsillectomy, although best performed electively, is occasionally indicated in the acute phase of tonsillar obstruction. Steroids appear to be effective in infectious mononucleosis and the response is rapid.

Table 95.2 Nasotracheal tube size in croup

Age	Size
Less than 6 months	3.0 mm
6 months to 2 years	3.5 mm
2–5 years	4.0 mm
Over 5 years	4.5 mm

TONSILLAR AND ADENOIDAL AIRWAY OBSTRUCTION

The conservative surgical view on tonsillectomy and adenoidectomy has led to an increased incidence of hypertrophy and chronic upper airway obstruction in some children.[25] Such children may present with severe, acute exacerbations due to intercurrent infection (e.g. tonsillitis). They may present in a toxic state with drooling, thereby mimicking acute epiglottitis. Obstruction is most marked during sleep. In the most severe cases, it may be necessary to relieve the obstruction with a nasotracheal tube or a nasopharyngeal tube positioned beyond the tonsillar bed. Tonsillectomy and adenoidectomy are generally contraindicated in the acute phase, because of increased risk of bleeding, but are performed when infection has settled.

OBSTRUCTIVE SLEEP APNOEA SYNDROME

Obstructive sleep apnoea (OSA) syndrome is characterized by intermittent upper airway obstruction during sleep, with heavy snoring, stertorous breathing and an abnormal, irregular respiratory pattern.[26] Frequent episodes of chest-wall motion with inadequate air flow (hypopnoea) or absent air flow (obstructive apnoea) are a feature. These episodes are most frequent during rapid eye movement sleep. They are accompanied by variable degrees of oxygen desaturation. OSA may be associated with enlarged tonsils and adenoids, a large uvula or long soft palate, macroglossia, retrognathia or various neurological disorders. Obesity is a common finding.

If OSA is severe and protracted, cardiac and pulmonary decompensation may occur. Chronic hypoxia and hypercarbia lead to pulmonary hypertension and cor pulmonale.[5,6] There may also be evidence of left ventricular failure and pulmonary oedema. Urgency of treatment is dictated by the mode of presentation. Critically ill children may require immediate relief of airway obstruction (nasopharyngeal or nasotracheal tube), oxygen therapy and diuretics. Antibiotics are indicated if there is bacterial superinfection. Surgical intervention is required after stabilization. Tonsillectomy and adenoidectomy are often dramatically beneficial. They are best removed even when not grossly enlarged. Other surgical procedures, such as uvulopalatopharyngoplasty or tracheostomy, may be required when this fails. The use of nocturnal continuous positive airway pressure (CPAP) or nasopharyngeal intubation is rarely feasible in young children.

PIERRE–ROBIN SYNDROME

This sequence consists of a posterior cleft palate, retrognathia and relative macroglossia. It is the cause of airway obstruction, feeding difficulties and failure to thrive in the newborn. Differential growth eventually reduces the significance of the deformity. Acute airway obstruction may be relieved by nursing the infant in the prone position or by passage of a nasopharyngeal tube.[27] Occasionally, nasotracheal intubation or tracheostomy is required. Tongue-lip anastomosis is sometimes beneficial.

CYSTIC HYGROMA

Although often conspicuous at birth, cystic hygroma is a relatively rare cause of upper airway obstruction in infancy. The tumours consist of masses of dilated lymphatic channels. They usually occur in the neck and may involve tissues of the tongue and larynx. Occasionally, extension into the mediastinum occurs. Airway obstruction may be due to infection or haemorrhage into the lesion. Surgical excision has been the mainstay of treatment, although complete removal is difficult and recurrence is common. Treatment using sclerosing therapy is now used. Compounds used include bleomycin emulsion or OK 432.[28,29] OK 432 is produced by lyophilization of cultures of a low virulent strain of group A *Streptococcus pyogenes* (human origin). In severe cases, long-term tracheostomy is required.

INHALATION BURNS

Respiratory complications are the major cause of mortality in children who are burnt. Direct airway burns or inhalation of products of combustion may lead to rapidly progressive oedema. The situation may be compounded by small airway and lung injury and by the need to provide adequate analgesia. Early intubation is strongly recommended prior to an emergency situation developing. Tracheal tube fixation may be problematic with extensive facial burns.

SUBGLOTTIC STENOSIS

Neonates with congenital subglottic stenosis may present with severe obstruction requiring intubation at birth. Other infants present with persistent stridor or recurrent croup due to superimposed infection. Subglottic stenosis may also occur as a complication of intubation, or as the result of pressure, mucosal ischaemia and healing by fibrosis. Prolonged intubation or tracheostomy may be required. Surgical techniques such as the cricoid split procedure or laryngotracheoplasty may be required to enlarge the airway.

SUBGLOTTIC HAEMANGIOMA

Haemangiomata are common in infancy and occur in many parts of the body. Subglottic lesions often present in the second or third month of life and owe their importance to the anatomical location. Stridor is usually both inspiratory and expiratory. A hoarse cry is indicative of vocal cord involvement. Obstruction may be severe and is aggravated by crying, struggling or superimposed infection. Cutaneous haemangiomata are present in 50%, and provide a clue to diagnosis. Definitive diagnosis rests on endoscopy. The natural history is of spontaneous resolution between the first and second years of life. Meanwhile, tracheostomy or episodes of intubation may be indicated to cover periods of obstruction. Encouraging results are being obtained with laser surgery. Intralesional steroids may be of benefit.

FOREIGN BODY OR CHOKING

A foreign body must be suspected in any acute obstruction occurring in an infant or child between 6 months and 2 years of age. Older children with neurological impairment are also at risk. A foreign body lodged in the pharynx results in gagging, respiratory distress and facial congestion. Laryngeal impaction usually produces stridor, a distressing cough and aphonia. Sudden total obstruction may occur. Symptoms usually develop while the child is playing or eating.

The technique for removal of a pharyngolaryngeal foreign body without equipment in infants and children is controversial and difficult. The American Academy of Paediatrics has made recommendations to cover various ages.[30] Gravity should be utilized by placing the child prone, straddled over your arm with the head down and a hand supporting the jaw. Four back blows between the shoulder blades should be administered. If this fails, chest thrusts or finger sweep across the pharynx should be attempted. There is some risk that the latter manoeuvre may impact the foreign body in the larynx. Abdominal thrusts (the Heimlich manoeuvre) are not recommended in infants and may be useful in children older than 1 year. Expired air resuscitation should be attempted in an emergency, although the risk of gastric distension is great. The best method of removal is extraction under direct vision using a laryngoscope, forceps, suction or a finger.

Tracheal or bronchial foreign bodies produce persistent cough and wheeze, and recurrent pneumonia. A foreign body lodged in the upper oesophagus may compress the trachea and present with either acute or, more commonly, persistent stridor. Radiopaque materials are easily shown radiologically, but both anteroposterior and lateral views may be necessary. Barium studies may prove useful for non-radiopaque material in the oesophagus. Treatment is removal at bronchoscopy or oesophagoscopy.

ANTERIOR MEDIASTINAL TUMOURS

Anterior mediastinal tumours, such as lymphoma, may compress the trachea or bronchi, causing symptoms such as dry cough, stridor or wheeze. Airway compression may become severe enough to cause hyperinflation or atelectasis. Pleural effusion is common and may add to the respiratory distress. Symptoms may be aggravated by the supine position, especially during anaesthesia for a biopsy procedure. This is likely in patients with superior vena caval syndrome. Postural symptoms or findings on flow-volume loops may allude to this risk. Sudden complete obstruction that cannot be bypassed by a standard tracheal tube has been described. The use of armoured tubes or a rigid bronchoscope may be required. Consideration should be given to leaving the tracheal tube *in situ* postoperatively until corticosteroids and chemotherapy reduce the tumour mass.

ANAESTHESIA FOR RELIEF OF AIRWAY OBSTRUCTION

Inhalational induction and anaesthesia with oxygen and halothane or sevoflurane is the preferred technique for intubation. The use of muscle relaxants is hazardous if the ability to maintain a patent airway is doubtful.

Important points are:

- A prepared induction should be undertaken with efficient suction apparatus, a range of tracheal tubes and suitable stylets. Preparations must be made to intubate without deep anaesthesia if sudden obstruction occurs.
- Inhalational anaesthesia is slow in upper airway obstruction and lower airways disease.
- Induction in the sitting position is advocated with epiglottitis. The child is laid flat after induction and prior to intubation.
- CPAP or assisted ventilation will reduce obstruction (minimize the dynamic component) and hasten induction. Care must be taken not to distend the stomach.
- Laryngoscopy is performed, and the child intubated, only when adequate depth of anaesthesia is achieved (e.g. approximately 8–10 min of 4% halothane in oxygen). Others recommend 6–8% sevoflurane.
- Orotracheal intubation is quickest and safest, and should be performed initially. After good tracheal toilet, the tube is changed to a nasotracheal one.

CARE OF NASOTRACHEAL TUBE

Successful management of URTO in children requires optimal care of nasotracheal intubation. Such children must always be nursed in an ICU. The nasotracheal tube must be positioned at the level of the clavicular heads (T2) on an antero-posterior chest X-ray. Length of the tube from 1 to 6 years of age (in cm measured at the nose) is given by age in years +13 cm. A meticulous technique of fixation must be employed to prevent accidental extubation.

Adequate humidification is difficult in the active child. Nevertheless, it is important to prevent obstruction of narrow tubes by inspissated secretions. Lightweight heat and moisture exchangers (HME) are very useful (e.g. Thermovent, Gibeck, and Humidvent, Portex).[31] The HME should be changed every 24 h to reduce contamination and increased resistance. Oxygen supplementation can be provided, if necessary. Some children will tolerate connection of a humidified T-piece.

Effective bagging and tracheal toilet is vital, and should be repeated until the airway is clear. Instillation of saline (0.5–1.0 ml) prior to suction may be necessary to remove secretions. Light sedation is used to improve tolerance of the tracheal tube and to reduce the risk of self-intubation. Midazolam, 0.1–0.2 mg/kg statim, followed by continuous infusion (0.05–0.2 mg/kg per h) is effective. Arm restraints may also be advisable, particularly in very young children. Signs of obstruction are usually relieved by intubation. Mild retraction may persist in children with high fever and increased minute ventilation in the presence of a smaller than predicted tube. Fibreoptic bronchoscopy can be performed to confirm patency. The tracheal tube must be changed or removed if there is doubt about its patency.

Nasogastric tube feeding should be commenced in children who require intubation longer than 24 h.

TRACHEOSTOMY

Tracheostomy remains a life-saving procedure and must be undertaken if tracheal intubation is impossible, or if appropriate equipment and personnel to facilitate intubation are unavailable. For chronic airway problems, it is more comfortable, allows better nasopharyngeal toilet and permits the child to leave the ICU and eventually return home. It is best performed under tracheal anaesthesia with the neck extended. When intubation is impossible, the tracheostomy can be performed under anaesthesia via a laryngeal mask airway. A longitudinal slit is made through the second and third tracheal rings without removal of cartilage. Stay sutures in the tracheal wall lateral to the incision aid recannulation if accidental dislodgement occurs prior to formation of a well-defined tract (after 4 days). A postoperative chest X-ray should be obtained to check the position of the tip of the tracheostomy tube and to exclude pneumothorax.

Care of a newly created tracheostomy is similar to that of an endotracheal tube, with the additional problem of some discomfort and blood in the airway. The first tracheostomy tube change is usually performed between 5 and 7 days.

CRICOTHYROTOMY

A wide-bore plastic i.v. cannula (14 or 16-gauge) passed into the trachea via the cricothyroid membrane may be life-saving if alternative procedures are unavailable. This should be performed with the neck extended as for tracheostomy. A system of connection to a low-pressure oxygen supply must be planned in advance. One method is to attach the hub of the cannula to the sleeve of a plastic 2–3-ml syringe (without plunger), to an adaptor from a 7.5-mm outer diameter tracheal tube, and then to a breathing circuit (e.g. Jackson Rees modification of Ayres T-piece).

REFERENCES

1 Westhorpe RN. The position of the larynx in children and its relationship to the ease of intubation. *Anaesth Intens Care* 1987; **15**: 384–8.

2 Badgwell JM, McLeod ME, Friedberg J. Airway obstruction in infants and children. *Can J Anaesth* 1987; **34**: 90–98.

3 Sofer S, Bar-Ziv J, Scharf SM. Pulmonary edema following relief of upper airway obstruction. *Chest* 1984; **86**: 401–3.

4 Stalcup SA, Mellins RB. Mechanical forces producing pulmonary edema in acute asthma. *N Engl J Med* 1977; **297**: 592–6.

5 Cox MA, Schiebler GL, Taylor WJ, *et al.* Reversible pulmonary hypertension in a child with respiratory obstruction and cor pulmonale. *J Pediatr* 1965; **67**: 192–7.

6 Luke MJ, Mehrizi A, Folger GM, Rowe RD. Chronic nasopharyngeal obstruction as a cause of cardiomegaly, cor pulmonale, and pulmonary oedema. *Paediatrics* 1966; **37**: 762–8.

7 Keens TG, Bryan AC, Levinson H, Ianuzzo CD. Development pattern of muscle fibre types in human ventilatory muscles. *J Appl Physiol Respir Environ Exercise Physiol* 1978; **44**: 909–13.

8 Muller NL, Bryan AC. Chest wall mechanics and respiratory muscles in infants. *Pediatr Clin North Am* 1979; **26**: 503–16.

9 Kushner DC, Harris GBC. Obstructing lesions of the larynx and trachea in infants and children. *Radiol Clin North Am* 1978; **16**: 181–94.

10 Siegel MJ, Nadel SN, Glazer HS, Sagel SS. Mediastinal lesions in children. Comparison of CT and MR. *Radiology* 1986; **160**: 241–4.

11 Butt W, Shann F, Walker C, *et al.* Acute epiglottitis: a different approach to management. *Crit Care Med* 1988; **16**: 43–7.

12 Kissoon N, Mitchell I. Adverse effects of racemic epinephrine in epiglottitis. *Pediatr Emerg Care* 1985; **1**: 143–4.

13 Soliman MG and Richer P. Epiglottitis and pulmonary oedema in children. *Can Anaesth Soc J* 1978; **25**: 270–5.

14 Travis KW, Todres DI, Shannon DC. Pulmonary edema associated with croup and epiglottitis. *Pediatrics* 1978; **59**: 695–8.

15 Zach M, Erben E, Olinsky A. Croup, recurrent croup, allergy and airways hyper-reactivity. *Arch Dis Child* 1981; **56**: 336–41.

16 Zach MS, Schnall RP, Landau LI. Upper and lower airway hyper-reactivity in recurrent croup. *Am Rev Respir Dis* 1980; **121**: 979–83.

17 Jones R, Santos JI, Overall JC. Bacterial tracheitis. *J Am Med Assoc* 1979; **242**: 721–6.

18 Super DM, Cartelli NA, Brooks LJ, *et al.* A prospective randomized double-blind study to evaluate the effect of dexamethasone in acute laryngotracheitis. *J Pediatr* 1989; **115**: 323–9.

19 Koren G, Frand M, Barzilay Z, Macleod SM. Corticosteroid treatment of laryngotracheitis in spasmodic croup in children. *Am J Dis Child* 1983; **137**: 941–4.

20 Tibballs J, Shann FA, Landau FI. Placebo controlled trial of prednisolone in children intubated for croup. *Lancet* 1992; **340**: 745–8.

21 Freezer N, Butt W, Phelan P. Steroids in croup: do they increase the incidence of successful extubation? *Anaesth Intens Care* 1990; **18**: 224–8.

22 Klassen TP, Feldman ME, Watters LK, *et al.* Nebulized budesonide for children with mild to moderate croup. *N Engl J Med* 1994; **331**: 285–9.

23 Bourchier D, Dawson KP, Fergusson DM. Humidification in viral croup: a controlled trial. *Aust Paediatr* 1984; **20**: 289–91.

24 Jordan WS, Graves CL, Elwyn RA. New therapy for postintubation laryngeal edema and tracheitis in children. *J Am Med Assoc* 1970; **212**: 585–8.

25 Check WA. Does drop in tonsillectomies and adenoidectomies pose new issue of adeno-tonsillar hypertrophy? *J Am Med Assoc* 1982; **247**: 1229–30.

26 Guilleminault C, Tilkian A, Dement WA. The sleep apnea syndromes. *Ann Rev Med* 1976; **27**: 465–84.

27 Heaf DP, Helms PJ, Dinwiddie MB, Mathew DJ. Nasopharyngeal airways in Pierre Robin syndrome. *J Pediatr* 1982; **100**: 698–703.

28 Tanaka K, Inomata Y, Utsunomiya H, *et al.* Sclerosing therapy with bleomycin emulsion for lymphangioma in children. *Pediatr Surg Int* 1990; **5**: 270–3.

29 Samuel M, McCarthy L, Boddy SA. Efficacy and safety of OK-432 sclerotherapy for giant cystic hygroma in a newborn. *Fetal Diagnosis Ther* 2000; **15**: 93–6.

30 American Academy of Pediatrics committee on accident and poison prevention. First aid for the choking child. *Pediatrics* 1988; **81**: 740–2.

31 Duncan A. Use of disposable condenser humidifiers in children. *Anaesth Intens Care* 1985; **13**: 330.

96

Acute respiratory failure in children

A W Duncan

Established or imminent respiratory failure is the commonest reason for admission to neonatal and paediatric ICUs. A number of structural and functional factors contribute to the high incidence of respiratory failure, particularly in the first year of life. In addition, respiratory failure is frequently a consequence of pathology primarily affecting other organ systems, e.g. congenital heart disease or central nervous system (CNS) disease.

PREDISPOSING FACTORS

Respiratory function must equate with metabolic demands. Oxygen consumption in the infant is approximately 7 ml/kg per min (3–4 ml/kg per min in the older child and adult). Fever, illness and restlessness dramatically increase demands; during periods of apnoea or respiratory depression, $PaCO_2$ rises at twice the rate of older children and adults. The lower respiratory reserve in infants and neonates is due to the following factors.

STRUCTURAL IMMATURITY OF THE THORACIC CAGE[1]

The ribs are short and horizontal and the bucket motion that increases the anteroposterior and lateral dimensions of the thorax is minimal. Thus, the infant is dependent on diaphragmatic displacement of abdominal contents to increase the length and volume of the thorax. Ribcage structure and function alter between 12 and 18 months, as the child develops the erect posture. The consequence is that any impairment of diaphragmatic function (e.g. abdominal distension) may precipitate respiratory failure.

The chest wall is soft and provides a poor fulcrum for respiratory effort. Retraction of bony structures and soft tissues, a prominent sign of respiratory distress, occurs with reduced lung compliance and increased airway resistance. Infant intrapleural pressure is –1 to –2 H_2O (–1 to –0.2 kPa) compared with –5 to –10 cm H_2O (–0.5 to –1.0 kPa) in the adult. This is due to the higher compliance of the chest wall (which tends to collapse in) and a lower elastic recoil of the lung. The result is an increased tendency to airway closure, atelectasis and intrapulmonary shunting.

In the neonate, the diaphragm and intercostal muscles have a lower percentage of type one (slow twitch and high oxidative) muscle fibres and therefore fatigue more readily. Diaphragmatic muscle mass is relatively reduced. Intercostal muscle activity is inhibited during rapid eye movement sleep further reducing ventilatory efficiency. Increased respiratory work is poorly sustained in the face of increased load and may culminate in exhaustion and apnoea.[2]

INFANT AIRWAYS

Although relatively large compared with the adult, airways of infants in absolute terms are small and more prone to obstruction. Trachea and bronchiole diameters of a 3 kg neonate are one-third and one-half respectively, those of a 60 kg adult. However, any degree of oedema or airway mucus will have a more profound effect on airway resistance in the infant.

LUNG STRUCTURE

Although the number of alveoli in the infant lung is proportionate to body size, the diffusion area is relatively small. The alveolar surface area is approximately 2.8 m^2 at birth, 32 m^2 at 8 years and 75 m^2 in the adult. Alveolar number and surface area may be reduced by *in utero* or early postnatal insults, including ventilator-induced injury. The infant lung also lacks the anatomical channels that allow 'collateral ventilation' putting the infant at greater risk of atelectasis, emphysematous changes and ventilation/perfusion abnormalities. The interalveolar pores of Kohn appear between the first and second years of life, while Lambert's channels provide communication between bronchi and adjacent alveoli beginning at 8 years.

INCREASED SUSCEPTIBILITY TO INFECTION

The immaturity and inexperience of the immune system result in a markedly increased susceptibility to infection in the first 6 months of life. Both cell-mediated (T-cell) and humoral (B-cell) systems may be impaired.

IMMATURITY OF LUNG FUNCTION

Premature infants in particular may have surfactant deficiency, resulting in alveolar instability, atelectasis, intrapulmonary shunting and reduced lung compliance.

IMMATURITY OF RESPIRATORY CONTROL

Inadequate respiratory drive from immaturity of the respiratory centre is a factor leading to apnoeic spells, particularly in premature infants. Opioid analgesics are associated with greater respiratory depression in young infants.

CONGENITAL ABNORMALITIES

Defects of the respiratory system or associated organs (e.g. heart) often present with respiratory failure shortly after birth.

PERINATAL ASPHYXIA OR INJURIES

Asphyxia or intracranial haemorrhage associated with birth may result in seizures and respiratory depression.

CLINICAL PRESENTATION

Respiratory distress is manifested by tachypnoea, distortion of the chest wall (i.e. sternal and rib retraction, recession of intercostal, subcostal and suprasternal spaces) and use of accessory muscles (e.g. flaring of alae nasi and use of neck muscles).

In young infants lethargy, pallor, apnoea, bradycardia and hypotension may be the first signs of hypoxia. The physiological anaemia of infancy may delay recognition of cyanosis, and major signs are those of CNS and cardiovascular depression. Increased work of breathing, marked by tachypnoea and chest-wall retraction, is poorly sustained; bradypnoea and apnoea are evidence of respiratory fatigue. Expiratory 'grunting' is a sign of res-

piratory distress that represents an attempt to maintain a positive expiratory airway pressure to prevent airway closure and alveolar collapse, the equivalent of pursed-lip breathing in the adult.

The older child with acute hypoxia, like the adult, demonstrates tachycardia, hypertension, mental confusion and restlessness prior to CNS and cardiovascular depression. Sweating occurs with CO_2 retention – a feature lacking in the newborn.

In the newborn, the effects of hypoxia may be compounded by the development of pulmonary hypertension and reversion to a transitional circulation, with right-to-left shunting through a patent ductus arteriosus and foramen ovale. If untreated, increasing hypoxaemia, progressive acidosis and death may occur.

Conventional clinical examination of the chest should be performed. It is, however, of limited value in the neonate, as breath sounds may be transmitted uniformly through the chest, even in the presence of tension pneumothorax, lobar collapse or endobronchial intubation. The chest X-ray is an essential part of the assessment.

AETIOLOGY

Acute respiratory failure may result from upper or lower airway obstruction, alveolar disease, pulmonary compression, neuromuscular disease or injury (Table 96.1). Upper respiratory tract obstruction is discussed in Chapter 101.

TRACHEOMALACIA, TRACHEAL STENOSIS AND VASCULAR COMPRESSION

Instability of the tracheal wall is most commonly associated with oesophageal atresia, tracheo-oesophageal fistula and various vascular anomalies. The most common causes of vascular compression are a double aortic arch and the complex of a right-sided aortic arch, left ductus arteriosus and an aberrant left subclavian artery. These produce a true vascular ring, with encirclement of the trachea and oesophagus. Anterior tracheal compression may also be due to an anomalous innominate artery. Lower tracheomalacia or tracheal stenosis may occur in association with an anomalous left pulmonary artery. The problem may extend to the major bronchi (bronchomalacia). Tracheomalacia and bronchomalacia also occur as isolated airway anomalies. In this situation, the severity of dynamic airway obstruction is aggravated by any condition that results in reduced lung compliance.

Division of the vascular ring and ligation or repositioning of the aberrant vessel, while removing the cause of the obstruction, do not immediately re-establish normal airway dimensions or stability. Although severity

Table 96.1 Causes of respiratory insufficiency in infancy and childhood

Site	Neonate	Older infant and child
Upper airway obstruction	See Chapter 101	
Lower airway obstruction		
Tracheal	Tracheomalacia	Foreign body
	Vascular anomalies	
	Tracheal stenosis	Mediastinal tumour
Bronchial	Bronchomalacia	Foreign body
Bronchiolar	Meconium aspiration	
	Congenital cystic adenomatoid malformation	Acute viral bronchiolitis
Disorders of lung function		
	Aspiration syndromes	Pneumonia
		Cystic fibrosis
	Hyaline membrane disease	
	Bronchopulmonary dysplasia	Aspiration syndromes
	Perinatal pneumonia	
	Massive pulmonary haemorrhage	Congenital heart disease
	Pulmonary oedema	Near-drowning
	Pulmonary hypoplasia	Trauma
	Diaphragmatic hernia	Burns
		Acute respiratory distress syndrome
Pulmonary compression		
	Diaphragmatic hernia	Pneumothorax
	Pneumothorax	Pleural effusion
	Repaired exomphalos or gastroschisis	Empyema
Neurological and muscular disorders		
	Diaphragmatic palsy	Poisoning
	Birth asphyxia	Meningitis
	Convulsions	Encephalitis
	Apnoea of prematurity	Status epilepticus
		Trauma
		Guillain–Barré syndrome
		Envenomation

of symptoms may be alleviated by surgery, problems may persist for some years. Tracheomalacia may sometimes be stabilized by a prolonged period of nasotracheal intubation or tracheostomy with continuous positive airway pressure (CPAP). Tracheopexy, which suspends the anterior tracheal wall from the posterior sternal surface and great vessels, is occasionally useful.

MECONIUM ASPIRATION SYNDROME

Meconium aspiration is seen in 0.3% of live births, and is most common in term or post-term infants. There is usually a history of fetal distress in labour, or prolonged and complicated delivery. Asphyxia during labour results in the expulsion of meconium into the liquor. With the first few breaths, material in the upper airway (i.e. amniotic fluid, meconium, vernix and squames) is inhaled, obstructing small airways and producing atelectasis and

obstructive emphysema. Meconium also causes a chemical pneumonitis and surfactant abnormalities. During recovery, the aspirated material is absorbed and phagocytosed.

Clinical signs include tachypnoea, retraction and cyanosis. The chest may become hyperexpanded and pneumomediastinum or pneumothorax are frequent complications. Pulmonary hypertension and persistent fetal circulation are common.

The chest X-ray confirms the diagnosis, with coarse mottling and streakiness radiating from the hila. Lungs are over-expanded, with flattened diaphragms and an increase in the chest anteroposterior diameter. The condition is largely preventable if the airway can be aspirated rapidly and completely following delivery of the head and before the first breath.

Most of these infants require oxygen therapy. Severely affected infants require controlled mechanical ventilation (CMV), which may be difficult because of the high pressures required, unevenness of ventilation, and danger of pneumothorax. Improved outcomes are now achieved using surfactant (may cause transient deterioration), inhaled nitric oxide and high frequency oscillation.[3] Extracorporeal membrane oxygenation (ECMO) is also effective in those centres that have the facility.[4] Cerebral effects of severe intrapartum asphyxia contribute to overall morbidity and mortality.

CONGENITAL CYSTIC ADENOMATOID MALFORMATION

Congenital lung cysts causing mass effects were previously termed lobar emphysema. The majority of lung cysts are now classified as congenital cystic adenomatoid malformation (CCAM). Most cases (70%) present in the first month of life, with tachypnoea, wheezing, grunting and cough. Signs include hyperresonance, decreased air entry and deviation of the trachea and heart away from the affected lobe. There may be asymmetry of the chest due to bulging of the affected hemithorax. Cyanosis may be associated with periods of increased respiratory distress.

Radiologically, the affected lobe is over-distended with compression and deviation of the surrounding structures. The pathogenesis is unknown in over 50%; 25% have localized bronchial cartilaginous dysplasia; the remainder have obstruction of a lobar bronchus from a mucous plug, redundant mucosa, aberrant vessels or localized stenosis. Lobectomy is often required. Care must be taken with positive airway pressure, because of the risk of further overdistension.

ASPIRATION PNEUMONIA

In the newborn, aspiration may result from pharyngeal incoordination or lack of protective reflexes, due to prematurity, birth asphyxia or intracranial haemorrhage. It is particularly likely to occur with abnormalities of the alimentary tract, such as oesophageal atresia, tracheo-oesophageal fistula and oesophageal reflux. Large and small airways obstruction and pneumonia may occur.

HYALINE MEMBRANE DISEASE

This is due to deficiency of lung surfactant. Predisposing factors are prematurity, maternal diabetes and intranatal asphyxia. Surfactant production is also inhibited by postnatal hypoxia and acidosis. Lack of surfactant results in alveolar instability, atelectasis, intrapulmonary shunting and increased work of breathing.

Clinical signs appear shortly after birth and consist of tachypnoea, chest-wall retraction, expiratory grunting and a progressive increase in oxygen requirements. The chest X-ray reveals a reticulogranular pattern (ground-glass appearance) with air bronchograms. In uncomplicated cases, the disease is self-limiting and resolves in 4–5 days. Respiratory failure may require increasing inspired oxygen concentrations (FiO_2), CPAP, intermittent mandatory ventilation (IMV) or CMV. CPAP is known to improve oxygenation, the pattern and regularity of respiration, retard the progression of the disease and reduce morbidity, particularly with early application in the extremely pre-term infant. In infants with persistent pulmonary hypertension, persistent fetal circulation and requiring high airway pressures, the use of inhaled nitric oxide and high frequency oscillatory ventilation are beneficial.

Instillation of surfactant into the trachea has been shown to improve oxygenation and compliance (despite some initial deterioration) and reduce the risk of pneumothorax, early mortality and morbidity.[5–8] Two types of surfactant are used, synthetic (Exosurf) and bovine (Survanta) or porcine (Curosurf).

BRONCHOPULMONARY DYSPLASIA

Bronchopulmonary dysplasia (BPD) may occur in survivors of neonatal lung disease. Its occurrence correlates with lung immaturity, high airway pressures and barotrauma. The lung architecture is abnormal with widespread fibrosis and cystic changes. There is often a reactive component to the airways disease that may be responsive to bronchodilator and anti-inflammatory therapy, such as steroids. It is a cause of chronic respiratory failure in infancy, and in severe cases progresses to cor pulmonale and death in the first 2 years of life. Prolonged low-flow home oxygen therapy may be necessary to reduce the risk of pulmonary hypertension. Superimposed bacterial and viral infection may exacerbate chronic respiratory failure and lead to further lung injury.

PNEUMONIA

Perinatal pneumonia may occur as a result of transplacental spread of a maternal infection, prolonged rupture of membranes, passage through an infected birth canal or cross-infection in the nursery. The immunoparetic state of the newborn and the need for invasive procedures increase the risk.

Clinical and radiological features may be indistinguishable from hyaline membrane disease. Antibiotics (e.g. penicillin and gentamicin) should be given until negative cultures exclude the diagnosis. The most common organisms include group B haemolytic streptococcus, *Escherichia coli*, *Pseudomonas aeruginosa*, *Klebsiella pneumoniae* and *Staphylococcus aureus*. Group B haemolytic streptococcus infection is frequently associated with septic shock and persistent fetal circulation.

Failure to suspect group B haemolytic streptococcus infections (and hence treat promptly with penicillin) will result in poor outcome. Multiresistant staphylococcal and Gram-negative bacillary infections must be suspected in longer-stay patients in neonatal ICUs.

Most pneumonia in infants and young children is of viral origin. Viruses commonly implicated are respiratory syncytial virus (RSV), influenza A1, A2 and B, and parainfluenza types 1 and 3. Adenovirus and rhinovirus are less common causes. The spectrum of illness is wide. Many infants and children have cough, fever and tachypnoea, with X-ray evidence of patchy consolidation, all of which resolve rapidly. Occasionally, infants develop life-threatening respiratory illness with extensive pneumonic changes and marked necrosis. Permanent lung damage with bronchiolitis obliterans and pulmonary fibrosis may occasionally complicate severe adenoviral pneumonia in particular.

Bacterial pneumonia also occurs. Pneumococcal pneumonia is common and usually responds dramatically to appropriate antibiotic therapy. Staphylococcal pneumonia is relatively uncommon, but may result in life-threatening respiratory failure, and is often associated with complications (e.g. empyema, pneumatocele, tension pneumothorax and suppuration in other organs). Aspiration of an effusion may be useful for diagnostic purposes. Tube thoracostomy or rib resection may be necessary to treat empyema. In severe cases with bronchopleural fistula, surgical resection of the necrotic area offers the best chance of survival.

Pneumonia due to *Haemophilus influenzae* may also occur and be associated with epiglottis, meningitis, pericarditis or middle-ear disease. The prevalence of *H. influenzae* infection has reduced dramatically since the introduction of HiB immunization.

Gram-negative pneumonia is seen mostly in infants with debilitating conditions who are hospitalized for prolonged periods. It is a particular risk for patients in ICUs with endotracheal or tracheostomy tubes. Other opportunistic infections, such as *Pneumocystis carinii*, *Candida albicans*, *Aspergillus* and cytomegalovirus, may occur in immune deficiency states.

MASSIVE PULMONARY HAEMORRHAGE

This usually presents as acute cardiorespiratory collapse, accompanied by outpouring of blood-stained fluid from the trachea, mouth and nose. It is seen in association with severe birth asphyxia, hyaline membrane disease, congenital heart disease, erythroblastosis fetalis, coagulopathy and sepsis. Hypoxia is often a precipitating factor. The condition in the newborn is believed to represent haemorrhagic pulmonary oedema due to acute left ventricular failure. Treatment is that of the underlying condition with oxygenation, CMV and correction of any coagulation disturbance.

PULMONARY OEDEMA

Pulmonary oedema in the newborn period is due mostly to congenital heart disease, especially coarctation of the aorta, patent ductus arteriosus, critical aortic stenosis and, rarely, obstructed total anomalous pulmonary venous drainage. Pulmonary oedema due to circulatory overload may also occur in erythroblastosis foetalis, the placental transfusion syndrome, or as a result of inappropriate fluid therapy. Myocarditis is a further cause seen throughout infancy and childhood.

In the newborn period, pulmonary oedema manifests as respiratory distress and feeding difficulty and specific features of congenital heart lesions may be evident. There is a spectrum of severity, from tachypnoea with a widened alveolar–arterial oxygen gradient to life-threatening respiratory failure requiring urgent support. Chest X-ray usually shows an enlarged heart (except in total anomalous pulmonary venous drainage) and a ground-glass appearance fanning out from the hilar regions.

PULMONARY HYPOPLASIA

This is seen most often in association with congenital diaphragmatic hernia, but bilateral pulmonary hypoplasia may also occur in association with renal agenesis or dysgenesis (Potter's syndrome), in babies with severe rhesus isoimmunization, and in the presence of chronic amniotic fluid leak. It may also present as an isolated malformation. Unilateral hypoplasia can occur as an isolated anomaly or in association with cardiovascular defects.

DIAPHRAGMATIC HERNIA

Congenital diaphragmatic hernia (most commonly left-sided) results in respiratory failure, partly due to lung compression but mainly related to the associated pulmonary hypoplasia (both ipsilateral and contralateral). The disturbance of pulmonary function ranges from mild to severe. In severe cases, life-threatening respiratory distress is present from birth, with cyanosis, intercostal retraction, mediastinal displacement, and poor or absent breath sounds on the affected side. The abdomen is usually scaphoid, due to much of its usual contents being in the chest. Chest X-ray shows loops of bowel in the affected hemithorax, with pulmonary compression and mediastinal displacement to the contralateral side.

Neonates presenting in the first 4 h of life have major degrees of lung hypoplasia and have a mortality of 40% despite maximal supportive therapy. Those presenting after 4 h of age should all survive. CMV may be complicated by tension pneumothorax and bronchopleural fistula on either side. Pulmonary hypertension with persistent fetal circulation and difficulties of CMV present major challenges. Many centres use ECMO[4] or high-frequency ventilation in these infants. Nitric oxide is a useful pulmonary vasodilator in this condition.[3] Prolonged ventilatory support is often required but the outlook of survivors is excellent.

PNEUMOTHORAX

Spontaneous pneumothorax may occur in normal newborns associated with the birth process, or secondary to hyaline membrane disease or meconium aspiration. Tension pneumothorax is particularly likely to occur when CMV is required in the presence of lung immaturity, lung hypoplasia, non-uniform lung disease (e.g. staphylococcal pneumonia) and diseases characterized by air trapping (e.g. meconium aspiration, bronchiolitis and asthma).

Tension pneumothorax should be suspected with any sudden deterioration of an infant on a ventilator. Classical clinical signs are evident in older children, but are of limited value in neonates. Circulatory embarrassment may be profound and rapidly progressive. Abdominal distension due to depression of the diaphragm and congestion of intra-abdominal organs and unilateral chest hyperexpansion are useful signs. Transillumination of the thorax using a bright light source is a sensitive guide in newborn infants. A chest X-ray is mandatory, but should be preceded by needle aspiration or drainage if the infant's condition is critical. Pre-existing pulmonary interstitial emphysema in one lung may also point to the side of the pneumothorax.

REPAIRED EXOMPHALOS OR GASTROSCHISIS

Complete repair of abdominal wall defects may cause marked elevation of intra-abdominal pressure when the intestines are then enclosed in a poorly developed peritoneal cavity. The diaphragm is elevated, compressing the lungs. In addition, compression of the inferior vena cava may lead to peripheral oedema, reduced cardiac output and oliguria. The associated paralytic ileus may further increase intra-abdominal pressure.

Disturbed lung function with inadequate gas exchange may require postoperative ventilation for several days. With large defects, it may be necessary to house the abdominal contents in a prosthesis, to allow gradual reduction into the abdominal cavity.

DIAPHRAGMATIC PALSY

Phrenic nerve palsy is a relatively common complication of cardiothoracic surgery. It occasionally occurs as a con-

genital abnormality, or may result from birth trauma. Paralysis and paradoxical movement of the affected diaphragm leads to reduced lung and tidal volumes, hypoxaemia and increased work of breathing. A chest X-ray taken without positive airway pressure reveals the elevated hemidiaphragm (positive pressure may mask the radiological diagnosis). Screening with ultrasound or fluoroscopy confirms the paradoxical movement.

Paralysis of the hemidiaphragm may cause respiratory failure in infants, particularly if associated with another disorder affecting lung function. Problems are greatest in children under 3 years, due to the poor stability of the chest wall. CPAP may be an effective method of increasing lung volume, stabilizing the ribcage and reducing paradoxical movement. Surgical plication of the diaphragm is usually effective in cases that fail to resolve with conservative management.

BIRTH ASPHYXIA

Birth asphyxia may result from placental failure, obstetric difficulties or maternal sedation. The resulting central respiratory depression, convulsions, intracerebral haemorrhage, meconium aspiration and persistence of fetal circulation contribute to respiratory failure. The Apgar score at 1 min is an objective means of evaluating the degree of asphyxia; the score at 5 min is a guide to prognosis. Delayed spontaneous respiration (>5 min) is also a poor prognostic sign. Further postnatal hypoxaemia, hypercapnia and brain ischaemia must be avoided. Severely asphyxiated infants need CMV after delivery, with correction of acidosis and hypovolaemia; inotropic drugs may be needed to maintain cerebral blood flow. It is important to prevent hypoglycaemia and control convulsions. Early topical hypothemia is under investigation as a protective strategy.

CONVULSIONS

Convulsions in the newborn are most frequent in the first 3 days of life. They are commonly due to birth asphyxia, trauma, intracranial haemorrhage and metabolic abnormalities such as hypoglycaemia or hypocalcaemia and meningitis. Seizures in older children commonly occur with fever, idiopathic epilepsy, CNS infection, poisoning, trauma and metabolic disturbances (e.g. hypoglycaemia, hyponatraemia and hypocalcaemia).

Generalized seizures may cause respiratory failure from airway obstruction, aspiration, apnoea or central respiratory depression. During grand mal seizures, ventilation may be inadequate, and oxygen consumption and CO_2 production may be increased by associated muscle activity. Anticonvulsant drugs may further depress respiration.

Initial management consists of ensuring a clear airway, adequate oxygenation and ventilation, and administering anticonvulsants. Oxygen should be given, because cerebral and total body oxygen consumption are increased, and it is difficult to assess adequacy of ventilation. Urgent control of seizures is important, as protracted seizures (longer than 1 h) cause cerebral oedema and may result in permanent neurological sequelae, even if hypoxaemia is avoided. The underlying cause must then be determined and treated.

APNOEA OF PREMATURITY

Recurrent apnoeic episodes (>20 s) are common in premature infants, and relate to immaturity of the brainstem, hypoxia, altered chemoreceptor responsiveness, diaphragmatic fatigue and the active (rapid eye movement) sleep state. Underlying causes such as hyaline membrane disease, hypoglycaemia, aspiration, sepsis, anaemia and intracranial haemorrhage should be sought. Mild episodes revert either spontaneously or with tactile stimulation. Severe episodes may require bag-and-mask ventilation. Apnoeic episodes may be reduced or prevented by theophylline or caffeine (central respiratory stimulants) or CPAP. IMV is necessary in some cases.

Many premature infants also suffer obstructive or mixed (central and obstructive) apnoea, both disorders of respiratory and airway musculature control. The infant airway collapses easily, and this is aggravated by neck flexion. Ex-premature infants may develop recurrent apnoea with intercurrent infection or following general anaesthesia and surgical procedures. This risk may persist until a post-conceptual age of 46 weeks, and demands close monitoring.[9] The risk may be greater in infants with a history of apnoeic episodes, bronchopulmonary dysplasia, anaemia or neurological disease. This is transient and remarkably responsive to theophylline or caffeine loading. Maintenance therapy is often unnecessary.

STATUS ASTHMATICUS

Asthma is the commonest reason for admission to most paediatric hospitals. Asthma is an inflammatory disease affecting the airways. Airway obstruction is due to mucosal oedema, mucus plugging and bronchiolar muscle spasm. Under 2 years of age, bronchiolar muscle is poorly developed, and muscle spasm is probably of less importance, with poor response to bronchodilator therapy.

Clinical and radiological features and management of asthma in small children are similar to that in adults (see Ch. 32). Blood-gas estimation is indicated for any child with acute severe asthma, if pulsus paradox greater than 20 mmHg (2.6 kPa) is present, or if the child fails to respond to optimal drug therapy. Hypoxaemia due to intrapulmonary shunt and $\dot{V}/\dot{Q}$ mismatching is the usual finding, and is the main cause of morbidity and mortality. High inspired oxygen therapy is therefore important. Hypocapnia in response to hypoxic drive is the rule; normocapnia or a rising $PaCO_2$ are signs of worsening asthma or fatigue and require increased medical therapy or mechanical ventilation.

Nebulized β_2-sympathomimetic amines, i.v. aminophylline and corticosteroids form the mainstay of drug therapy; maximal therapy should be introduced early. Salbutamol is nebulized with oxygen as 0.05 mg/kg of 0.5% solution diluted to 4 ml with sterile water, given 2–4-hourly initially, or more frequently in severe cases. A greater and more sustained response may be achieved by more frequent or continuous salbutamol nebulization.[10] Inhaled ipratropium may have additional benefit even in patients receiving maximal therapy with β_2-sympathomimetic amines.

Some centres abandoned the use of aminophylline because of its narrow therapeutic range and because of the belief that it did not add benefit to maximal therapy with salbutamol. There is evidence, however, that aminophylline does have a place in the management of severe acute asthma in children that is unresponsive to initial treatment.[11] Aminophylline is also known to possess anti-inflammatory properties. Children under 9 years have increased metabolism, and require higher doses of theophylline (0.85 mg/kg per h, equivalent to an aminophylline infusion of 1.1 mg/kg per h). Serum concentrations should be measured (therapeutic range is 60–110 μmol/l).

Continuous infusion of salbutamol has been shown to reduce the need for CMV. It should be added when $PaCO_2$ is rising or is greater than 60 mmHg (8 kPa), as an infusion of 1 μg/kg per min and increased every 20 min until $PaCO_2$ decreases by about 10%, or a maximum dose of 14 μg/kg per min is reached. An epinephrine or isoprenaline infusion (0.05–2 μg/kg per min) may be useful in refractory cases.

Metabolic acidosis may occur as a result of hypoxaemia and increased work of breathing. Epinephrine by infusion is associated with lactic acidosis. Cautious bicarbonate therapy is recommended to improve cardiovascular function and bronchomotor responsiveness to theophylline and sympathomimetic agents. Isoprenaline and theophylline may both override pulmonary hypoxic vasoconstrictor responses and thereby increase intrapulmonary shunt and worsen hypoxaemia. Salbutamol is believed to be preferable in this respect.

Particular attention should be paid to fluid balance. Dehydration may lead to inspissation of secretions, but the risks of inappropriate antidiuretic hormone (ADH) secretion and pulmonary oedema must be noted.[12,13]

With aggressive medical therapy, the need for CMV should be rare. Its use should be based predominantly on clinical features rather than solely on blood-gas analysis. It should not, however, be withheld out of fear of difficulties. CMV may worsen air trapping and lead to hypotension or pneumothorax. Controlled hypoventilation (permissive hypercapnia) with a long expiratory time is advocated to minimize airway pressures and air trapping. A trial of PEEP may be justified to reduce intrinsic (auto) PEEP and air trapping although evidence in adults suggests that PEEP may be associated with increased air trapping.[14]

ACUTE VIRAL BRONCHIOLITIS

Most cases of bronchiolitis occur in the first 6 months of life and are caused by RSV. Cough, low-grade fever, tachypnoea and wheeze are the cardinal signs. Some infants, particularly ex-premature, develop apnoeic episodes. The chest is hyperinflated with rib retraction and widespread crepitations. Clinical features are due to small airways obstruction from oedema and exudate.

Management consists of minimal handling and oxygen therapy. If respiratory distress is marked, feeds should be withheld and fluids administered i.v.. Progression of the disease leads to exhaustion and respiratory failure in 1–2% of cases. CPAP[15] and/or aminophylline therapy[16] are reported to reduce the work of breathing, lower $PaCO_2$ and eliminate recurrent apnoea. Nebulized epinephrine may also be beneficial.[17] CMV is required in some cases, particularly when the disease occurs in association with congenital heart or chronic lung disease. High airway pressures may be required, increasing the risk of pneumothorax. The antiviral agent Ribavirin is difficult to administer and has not been shown to improve outcome.[18] Bacterial coinfection is common, and justifies the use of broad-spectrum antibiotics in severe cases.[19]

RESPIRATORY FAILURE SECONDARY TO CONGENITAL HEART DISEASE

Infants with congenital heart disease may develop respiratory failure for a number of reasons.[20]

TYPE OF CARDIAC LESION

Congenital heart lesions producing acute respiratory failure fall into four main groups.

1 *Left heart obstruction* (e.g. critical aortic stenosis, interrupted aortic arch and coarctation of aorta). In this group, left ventricular failure leads to pulmonary oedema, reduced pulmonary compliance and respiratory failure.
2 *Large left-to-right shunts* (e.g. ventricular septal defect and patent ductus arteriosus). Respiratory failure in this group with excessive pulmonary blood flow results from volume overloading of the left ventricle, with pulmonary oedema, small airways obstruction,

bronchial compression or intercurrent infection. Correction of the defect is associated with improved lung mechanics.[21]
3 *Hypoxaemic lesions,* where:
(a) there is obstruction to pulmonary blood flow (e.g. tetralogy of Fallot and critical pulmonary stenosis)
(b) the pulmonary and systemic circuits are in parallel (e.g. transposition of the great vessels)
(c) there is complete mixing of systemic and pulmonary venous blood (e.g. single ventricle and truncus arteriosus).
In lesions associated with reduced pulmonary blood flow, lung compliance is high. High-pressure ventilation may further impede pulmonary blood flow, leading to increased hypoxaemia and, occasionally, CO_2 retention. Hypoxaemic lesions associated with increased pulmonary blood flow have problems of reduced lung compliance and air trapping (due to small airways disease and bronchial compression) in addition to hypoxaemia (due to mixing).
4 *Vascular lesions* associated with compression or stenosis of large airways (e.g. vascular rings and anomalous left pulmonary artery).

INTERCURRENT INFECTION

Recurrent pneumonia and bronchiolitis are common in infants with congenital heart disease, particularly those associated with high pulmonary blood flow.

POSTOPERATIVE

Respiratory failure may occur following repair of cardiac lesions due to low cardiac output state and pulmonary oedema, acute respiratory distress syndrome (ARDS), lobar collapse, pleural effusions, pneumonia, phrenic nerve palsy, respiratory depressant drugs, abdominal distension and ascites.

NEAR-DROWNING

Respiratory failure after near-drowning may result from aspiration pneumonitis or CNS depression from hypoxic-ischaemic encephalopathy. Acute gastric dilatation (associated with the immersion or resuscitation) is common and may be a contributing factor. Pulmonary oedema may be secondary to water and particulate matter inhaled, or to chemical pneumonitis from aspiration of gastric contents. Secondary infection occasionally leads to necrotizing pneumonia. Prophylactic antibiotics are not of proven benefit, but there are reports of fulminant ARDS associated with pneumococcal infection after immersion.[22] Broad spectrum antibiotic therapy should be administered early if there is significant pulmonary disease. Ongoing therapy should be guided by culture of tracheal aspirate.

Patients with both fresh- and salt-water drowning are usually hypovolaemic, hypoxic and acidotic at the time of admission. Oxygen therapy is mandatory, even in so-called dry drowning. Resuscitation usually requires volume expansion, correction of acidosis and inotropic support. Immersion hypothermia may afford some protection to the brain. Complete re-warming should not be undertaken until circulatory resuscitation is achieved. Resuscitation attempts should be sustained in the presence of severe hypothermia. CMV produces a dramatic improvement in gas exchange.

TRAUMA

Respiratory failure may follow trauma to the brain, spinal cord, chest or abdomen. High spinal cord injuries may be difficult to detect in the presence of severe brain injury. Presence of rhythmic flaring of the alae nasi without accompanying respiratory excursion is a useful sign (Duncan's sign). As the chest wall is compliant, severe pulmonary contusion can occur from blunt trauma with minimal chest-wall injury. Fractured ribs, haemothorax and pneumothorax may all precipitate respiratory failure. The diagnosis of a ruptured diaphragm is often delayed as the clinical signs are easily confused with a tension pneumothorax. CMV will effectively displace abdominal contents from the thorax and improve gas exchange prior to surgery. The chest X-ray is a mandatory investigation during resuscitation.

Acute gastric dilatation is almost invariable in the traumatized child, may mimic an acute abdomen and may exacerbate respiratory failure. Emergency decompression with a wide-bore gastric tube improves cardiorespiratory function and reduces the risk of aspiration.

ACUTE RESPIRATORY DISTRESS SYNDROME

Acute respiratory distress syndrome (ARDS) may occur in children of all ages from a variety of direct and indirect lung insults. ARDS is characterized by respiratory distress or failure, diffuse pulmonary infiltrates, reduced pulmonary compliance and hypoxaemia, in the presence of a known precipitating cause and in the absence of left ventricular failure. In children, common causes include shock from any cause, pneumonia with septicaemia, near drowning, aspiration and pulmonary contusion.

POISONING

Accidental poisoning is a common, but preventable cause of respiratory failure, particularly in the first 4 years of life. Deliberate overdose is seen in children beyond 8 years. Tricyclic antidepressants, antihistamines, anticonvulsants and benzodiazepines form the commonest CNS-depressant drugs ingested. Convulsions may aggravate the situation.

MENINGITIS AND ENCEPHALITIS

Meningitis is common in the early years of life. After the neonatal period, the usual causative organisms are *Haemophilus influenzae* (markedly reduced prevalence with immunization), *Neisseria meningitidis,* and *Streptococcus pneumoniae.* Rapid diagnosis and appropriate antibiotic therapy form the cornerstone of treatment. Respiratory failure is mainly associated with uncontrolled convulsions, altered conscious state or raised intracranial pressure (ICP). Encephalitis may also cause unconsciousness and raised ICP. Associated problems are upper airway obstruction, pulmonary aspiration and central respiratory depression. Encephalitis is usually viral in origin and may be complicated by hyperpyrexia, convulsions and cerebral oedema.

GUILLAIN–BARRÉ SYNDROME

This is the most common polyneuritis in childhood. The onset may be rapid, with respiratory failure occurring within 48 h. Intervention is based on clinical assessment of cough reflex and bulbar function, a measured vital capacity <15 ml/kg, and evidence of hypoxaemia (SaO_2 <90%). Hypoxaemia occurs relatively early due to reduced functional residual capacity, atelectasis and intra-pulmonary shunting. An elevated $PaCO_2$ is a late feature, suggesting a vital capacity in the tidal range, i.e. <5–7 ml/kg. CMV is usually necessary if intubation is required. Unless rapid recovery is anticipated, early tracheostomy is advocated for patient comfort and to allow speech. The condition is often improved by the early use of i.v. immunoglobulin therapy or plasmapheresis. Immunoglobulin is easier to deliver and probably safer. Muscle pain may require analgesic relief.

Transverse myelitis may present in a similar manner and the principles of management are the same. Nerve conduction studies and MRI may be necessary to distinguish between the two conditions.

ENVENOMATION

Some animal venoms, such as those of some snakes, ticks and blue-ringed octopus, are neurotoxic and may cause muscle weakness and respiratory insufficiency. The Sydney funnel web spider causes widespread acetylcholine release and symptoms similar to anticholinesterase poisoning. These symptoms include intense salivation, lacrimation, sweating, laryngeal and muscle spasm and pulmonary oedema. Paralysis due to tetrodotoxin may rapidly follow puffer-fish ingestion. In Australia and many other countries, specific antivenom therapy is available for most potentially lethal envenomations. Supportive therapy is required until antivenom is administered and recovery occurs.

MANAGEMENT OF ACUTE RESPIRATORY FAILURE

In some cases, definitive treatment of the underlying cause will lead to resolution of respiratory failure (e.g. relief of upper airway obstruction or reversal of drug depression). Where this is not possible, mechanical ventilatory support is required until the underlying process has resolved.

GENERAL MEASURES

GENERAL NURSING CARE

Critically ill children require a nurse:patient ratio of 1:1 and it important that the nurses are skilled in the care of a ventilated child. This is one of the important differences between a paediatric intensive care unit and a general unit that only occasionally looks after children.

THERMAL ENVIRONMENT

Maintenance of body temperature is of major importance. The immature newborn is particularly vulnerable to cold stress, which increases metabolism, rapidly depletes carbohydrate stores and causes cardiorespiratory deterioration. In a normal newborn, oxygen consumption may rise threefold on exposure to environmental temperatures of 20–25°C. Conditions are optimal when the abdominal skin temperature is 36–36.5°C.

The most satisfactory devices to maintain temperature homeostasis are servo-controlled infrared-heated open cots. These allow for observation of and access to the exposed infant. In an incubator, the environmental temperature is less stable and access is difficult. Double-glazed incubators reduce radiant heat loss. Older infants and children can be nursed in standard cots and beds.

POSTURE

Neonates are best nursed prone with the hips and knees flexed and the head turned regularly. This posture may abolish apnoeic episodes in premature infants. It also decreases gastric emptying time, making aspiration of vomitus less likely. However, if the neonate is unstable and interventions are likely, the supine position is preferred. Older infants and young children are usually

nursed in the position they find most comfortable although, as in adults, there is evidence that gas exchange is improved by prone positioning in ventilated children.

PHYSIOTHERAPY

The role of conventional chest physiotherapy with posturing, percussion and vibration in the paediatric ICU setting is unproven. Physiotherapy must be applied cautiously in children with cardiovascular instability or raised ICP. Chest compression and vibration in the newborn may result in rib fractures and possibly intracranial damage. Physiotherapy may cause a significant fall in PaO_2. FiO_2 should be increased in anticipation (caution is required in premature infants who are at risk of retrolental fibroplasia). In infants, periodic gentle pharyngeal suction removes pharyngeal secretions and may stimulate coughing. Effective bagging, tracheal suction and positioning are the most useful techniques in the intubated patient.

FLUID THERAPY

Oral feeding should be suspended with severe respiratory distress, because of the difficulty in oxygen administration and the risk of abdominal distension, vomiting and aspiration. Nasogastric feeding may be cautiously employed in infants with mild to moderate respiratory distress.

Lung and airway disease is often associated with increased secretion of ADH, leading to fluid retention. Increased airway pressure (e.g. CMV and CPAP) may also increase ADH secretion. Efficient humidification via a tracheal or tracheostomy tube prevents insensible water loss from the airway, and diminishes fluid requirements. Most patients with acute lung disease benefit from some degree of fluid restriction. Fluid balance and biochemical status must be monitored carefully. In prolonged respiratory failure, it is essential to minimize wasting of the respiratory muscles and to provide energy for increased work of breathing. High-calorie oral or nasogastric feeding may be tolerated. Parenteral nutrition is particularly useful when fluid restriction is necessary, and should be commenced early if prolonged interruption to enteral feeding is likely.

MONITORING AND ASSESSMENT

Repeated clinical observation by skilled staff is necessary to detect early signs of hypoxia, increasing respiratory distress, or onset of fatigue. Deterioration may represent a progression of disease state, development of fatigue or the presence of complications. Monitoring of cardiorespiratory parameters and respiratory therapy is imperative for optimal respiratory care.

PULSE OXIMETRY

Pulse oximetry provides essential information about the state of oxygenation (i.e SaO_2) on a continuous basis It is applicable to children of all sizes and can obviate the need for arterial cannulation in some cases. It forms part of a minimum standard for monitoring critically ill infants and children. Surprising degrees of desaturation, undetectable clinically, may be identified and treated.

BLOOD GASES

Measurement of blood gasses and acid-base status is essential in cardiorespiratory assessment. Arterial blood is obtained from an indwelling cannula or by direct puncture of peripheral arteries. The latter may be distressing to the child. Results from difficult collections may not accurately reflect the true blood-gas status. Topical anaesthesia using Emla cream should be considered for non-urgent percutaneous sampling.

Peripheral arterial cannulation is routine practice in paediatric intensive care, even in infants weighing less than 1 kg. It allows continuous blood pressure monitoring and reduces sampling errors. The radial, ulnar, brachial, femoral, posterior tibial and dorsalis pedis arteries are suitable. Radial artery cannulation by cut-down should be considered when the percutaneous method fails. Radial and ulnar or posterior tibial and dorsalis pedis vessels must not be cannulated in the same limb, even at different times, because of the danger of distal limb ischaemia. The safety of brachial and femoral cannulation lies in the collateral vessels around the elbow and hip joints. Complications of arterial cannulation include distal ischaemia, infection, haemorrhage and retrograde embolization when the cannula is flushed.

In the neonate with acute respiratory failure, a preductal vessel, such as the right radial artery, is preferred. Preductal sampling is important in premature infants, because it indicates the PaO_2 of blood perfusing the retina. Knowledge of the FiO_2 is essential to interpret information from all forms of oxygen monitoring.

CAPNOGRAPHY

Measurement of the end-tidal PCO_2 in the intubated patient provides a continuous guide to the adequacy of alveolar ventilation. In severe lung disease, the value does not reflect arterial PCO_2 (due to a wide alveolar–arterial gradient). It may still provide valuable trend information, and is also an additional means of warning of sudden reductions in cardiac output.

CHEST X-RAY

Clinical examination of the thorax may be misleading in the small infant and serial chest X-rays form a vital part of assessment. Antero-posterior supine films usually provide the necessary information. Lateral or decubitus views may be useful to localize lung pathology, or to confirm air or fluid collections. Examination should look for focal or generalized lung disease, pleural effusions, air leak phenomena, the size and shape of cardiac contour and the position of invasive devices. The tracheal tube should be level with the second thoracic vertebra or the ends of the clavicles, and take account of the neck posture. A change from extension to flexion may advance the endotracheal tube by 1 cm in the term neonate. As the trachea in the neonate is only 4 cm long, accurate placement is critical. Multiple chest X-rays may be required with rapidly changing clinical situations.

TRANSILLUMINATION

Transillumination of the thorax with a cold fibreoptic light source is a useful technique to detect pneumothorax in newborn infants. Transillumination occurs on the side of pneumothorax, but does not quantify the amount of air present. Bilateral pneumothoraces may cause confusion. In severe pulmonary interstitial emphysema, increased transillumination may be seen. A chest X-ray should be performed to confirm the pneumothorax when time permits.

VITAL CAPACITY AND MAXIMUM INSPIRATORY FORCE

In diseases such as Guillain–Barré syndrome, measurements of vital capacity and maximum inspiratory force are useful in older co-operative children. A vital capacity <15 ml/kg or a maximum inspiratory force of less than -25 cmH$_2$O (-2.5 kPa) are indications for intubation and assisted ventilation. These parameters are also useful to guide weaning.

SPECIFIC MEASURES

OXYGEN THERAPY[23]

Mode of administration is guided by patient size and required FiO_2. Neonates requiring less than 40% oxygen can be nursed in an incubator. Plastic headboxes are used to deliver higher concentrations to neonates and infants.

Older children tolerate appropriately sized facemasks but FiO_2 is rarely known. Masks incorporating a reservoir bag will deliver high concentrations in young children. Restless children do not tolerate facemasks and oxygen delivery becomes intermittent. Once positioned, nasal cannulae are usually well tolerated. A single catheter in the post nasal space (1–2 l/min) is also an effective method of delivery. With nasal cannulae, FiO_2 depends on flow rate, size of the nasopharynx, mouth-breathing and peak inspiratory flow rate. Using a single nasal cannula, a flow rate of 150 ml/kg per min provides FiO_2 about 0.5 in children under 2 years.[24] Effective humidification is difficult with nasal cannulae, and drying of mucosa and secretions may be a problem.

Therapeutic procedures, physiotherapy and handling may all increase oxygen consumption and lead to hypoxaemia and deterioration. Timing of these manoeuvres is important and a prior increase in FiO_2 may be justified.

COMPLICATIONS OF OXYGEN THERAPY IN NEONATES

RETROLENTAL FIBROPLASIA

Retinal vessels of premature infants are susceptible to vasoconstrictive effects of high arterial oxygen tension. Visual impairment is due to retinal fibroproliferative changes or to subsequent retinal detachment. While the absolute safe maximal level and duration of hyperoxia are unknown, a PaO_2 between 50 and 80 mmHg (6.6 and 10.6 kPa) is recommended.

BRONCHOPULMONARY DYSPLASIA

The development of chronic pulmonary insufficiency in mechanically ventilated neonates correlates best with lung immaturity, peak inspiratory pressures and other evidence of barotrauma. Pulmonary oxygen toxicity is probably a contributory factor. Chronic hypoxaemia, on the other hand, is a factor in the development of cor pulmonale.

INTUBATION

Tracheal intubation relieves airway obstruction, and allows accurate control of inspired oxygen, application of positive airway pressure and tracheal toilet. Nasotracheal intubation is preferred, as it allows better fixation. Implant-tested polyvinyl chloride tubes may be left in place indefinitely. For long-term use, however, tracheostomy is indicated. Disadvantages of nasotracheal intubation include bypassing nasal humidifying mechanisms, sinusitis, increased airway resistance, risk of subglottic stenosis, impaired cough reflex, loss of physiological positive end-expiratory pressure (PEEP) and impaired pulmonary defence mechanisms. In neonates, risk of laryngeal injury correlates with duration of intubation and repeated intubation trauma. The correct tracheal tube size permits a small leak when a positive pressure of less than 25 cmH$_2$O (2.5 kPa) is applied. Exceptions to the rule are:

- neonates: for unknown reasons, absence of leak rarely results in complications
- croup, where a smaller tube than predicted for age is passed, and subsequent development of a leak indicates resolution of subglottic oedema
- mechanical ventilation with low-compliance lungs, where an airtight seal may be required for effective ventilation – a risk of subglottic stenosis occurs.

MECHANICAL VENTILATORY SUPPORT

MECHANICAL VENTILATION[25]

Paediatric ventilators are discussed elsewhere in this volume. The risks of barotrauma and oxygen toxicity demand that specific ventilator settings be prescribed for rate, peak inspiratory pressure, PEEP, CPAP, flow rate, inspiratory time, minute volume and inspired oxygen. If pulmonary function progressively deteriorates, a stepwise increase of each setting should be considered. The least harmful alternative should be undertaken first (e.g. increasing FiO_2 is probably a safer alternative than increasing PEEP). Unless contraindicated, a PEEP of 3–5 cmH$_2$O (0.3–0.5 kPa) is recommended in all ventilated infants to prevent airway closure. In the presence of reduced cerebral compliance, PEEP may be associated with increased intracranial pressure. Oxygenation is a priority, however, and other means of maintaining cerebral perfusion pressure should be employed if PEEP is required. Removing or reducing PEEP must be considered if there is evidence of barotrauma. Increased PEEP demands a similar increase in peak inspiratory pressure if the same tidal volume is to be maintained. Mean airway pressure is the main determinant of oxygenation. It is dependent on rate, peak inspiratory pressure, flow rate, inspiratory time and PEEP.

In general, slow ventilatory rates (e.g. neonates 30 breaths/min, infants under 12 months 25 breaths/min, children 16–20 breaths/min) and an inspiratory time of about 1.0 s provide optimal gas exchange. Infants under 1 kg may benefit from faster ventilatory rates and shorter inspiratory times. Short inspiratory times may, however, be associated with loss of lung volume and increased intrapulmonary shunting. Strategies to recruit alveoli are important with many lung diseases particularly after suction and disconnection for bagging.

CONTINUOUS POSITIVE AIRWAY PRESSURE[26]

Continuous positive airway pressure[26] (CPAP) applies a constant pressure gradient to the spontaneously breathing patient via a special circuit. The T-piece system requires a fresh gas flow of two to three times the predicted minute ventilation to prevent rebreathing. For CPAP to be well-sustained, either flow rate must exceed peak inspiratory flow or a reservoir bag must be incorporated into the system.

Nasotracheal intubation is the safest and most efficient method of applying CPAP, although masks, nasal cannulae or a nasopharyngeal tube may be used. These latter techniques rely on neonates being obligatory nose-breathers; positive pressure is lost during crying or mouth-breathing, and abdominal distension may occur. Blood-gas sampling during mouth-breathing may lead to errors in oxygen therapy. The stomach should be decompressed continuously with a nasogastric tube.

Benefits of CPAP include the following:

- CPAP increases functional residual capacity (FRC), recruits alveoli, promotes alveolar stability and reduces intrapulmonary shunt. An increased PaO_2 results and allows a reduction in FiO_2.
- CPAP promotes the stability of large and small airways. This splinting effect is useful in airway

obstruction, bronchomalacia and tracheomalacia. CPAP has also been recommended in croup, bronchiolitis and even asthma.

- In neonates, CPAP may abolish or reduce apnoeic episodes and improve the rhythmicity of spontaneous breathing. Physiological amounts of CPAP (2–5 cmH$_2$O, 0.2–0.5 kPa) should be applied to intubated children whenever practical to prevent airway closure.

Because of the resistance of the endotracheal tube and respiratory circuit, the use of low levels of pressure support ventilation (PSV) is often more effective in minimizing work of breathing.

CPAP may reduce cardiac output or cause barotrauma. Increased ADH secretion and fluid retention are also seen, although the exact mechanism is disputed. If CPAP results in hyperinflation it may also increase pulmonary vascular resistance and right ventricular afterload. This effect is often balanced by the beneficial effect of CPAP in preventing atelectasis, optimizing lung volume and thereby reducing pulmonary vascular resistance. It is often difficult to interface CPAP and other non-invasive respiratory techniques to the non-sedated infants and children without causing excessive restlessness.

SEDATION

Sedation should be used to reduce restlessness and discomfort, and to minimize the work of breathing. In the brain-injured, sedation prevents coughing, straining, unwanted autonomic responses and increases in intracranial pressure. Heavy sedation (with or without muscle relaxants) is recommended, provided supervision and monitoring facilities are adequate.

COMPLICATIONS

Complications of mechanical ventilatory support include:

- *Reduced cardiac output:* circulatory effects of increased airway pressure may be less marked in young children.[27] Nevertheless, volume expansion (e.g. with 10–20 ml/kg of colloid) may be required at the start of CMV, particularly if muscle relaxants are employed;
- *Barotrauma* may present as:
  (a) *pulmonary interstitial emphysema* with gas in the lung interstitium, outside the alveoli. This is deleterious to gas exchange and is not amenable to drainage. It may produce intrapulmonary tension and mediastinal shift. Unfortunately, the initiating factor, positive pressure, may need to be increased further to restore gas exchange. It is a forerunner of pneumothorax. Management is to limit or remove positive pressure as early as possible. Occasionally, needle or thoracotomy decompression may be required.
  (b) *pneumothorax*
  (c) *pneumomediastinum*
  (d) *tension pneumopericardium* occasionally occurs in neonates on ventilation and may require decompres-

sion by needle aspiration or limited sternotomy and drainage
  (e) *pneumoperitoneum*, where a differential diagnosis from ruptured viscus may be difficult. Occasionally, drainage is required to reduce intra-abdominal tension and respiratory embarrassment.

Mechanical ventilation must be approached cautiously if air leak is a particular risk (e.g. in immature lungs and diseases characterized by air trapping). Permissive hypercapnia can often be tolerated, provided that oxygenation, perfusion and acid-base balance are acceptable.

WEANING

Weaning commences when the underlying process has resolved sufficiently, the cardiovascular system is stable and the child is awake or active. It is unlikely to be successful if an FiO$_2$ over 0.5 or peak airway measures greater than 25 cmH$_2$O (2.5 kPa) are required. PEEP or CPAP should be reduced to 5 cmH$_2$O (0.5 kPa) or less prior to intubation. The rate of weaning is determined by the underlying pathology and the expected response. Progression through IMV and PSV or CPAP is usually advised. Attention to the status of all organ systems must be meticulous, and some degree of fluid restriction is usually indicated. Other forms of circulatory support such as inotropic agents and vasodilators should be maintained during the weaning period. Increased work of breathing places additional demands on the cardiovascular system and may divert blood flow from other vital organs. The patient should be fasted and the abdomen decompressed prior to extubation. A period of fasting before and after long-term intubation is recommended (e.g. up to 24 h in some cases), to allow for return of laryngeal competence.

HIGH FREQUENCY OSCILLATORY VENTILATION

High frequency ventilation (HFV) refers to ventilation at respiratory rates between 4–15 Hz, with tidal volumes close to or less than anatomical dead space. Methods of HFV most commonly used are high frequency jet ventilation, high frequency flow interruption and high frequency oscillatory ventilation (HFOV). Most interest has centred on HFOV (10–15 Hz), with tidal volumes well below anatomical dead space. When combined with PEEP, all three can produce adequate oxygenation and CO$_2$ removal in infants, children and adults with restrictive lung disease, often using lower peak and mean airway pressures than in CMV. In HFOV CO$_2$ removal is very efficient and occurs by a combination of accelerated diffusion and cardiogenic mixing. Oxygenation is maintained by keeping mean airway pressure above the critical opening pressure for the alveoli. High volume cycling is avoided thereby limiting further lung injury as a result of repeated sheer stress.

Animal studies using HFOV and an 'open lung strategy' have convincingly demonstrated less of the histological changes of ARDS and less barotrauma.[28,29] Although a multi-centre trial of HFOV in preterm infants failed to show benefit, a number of single centre randomized or rescue studies have demonstrated less barotrauma in very low birth weight infants, a decreased incidence of chronic lung disease (BPD) and reduced requirement for ECMO.[30,31] The combined use of HFOV and nitric oxide therapy has led to reduced use of ECMO in many centres. HFOV has an important role in the management of severe pulmonary air leak syndromes.

REFERENCES

1 Muller NL, Bryan AC. Chest wall mechanics and respiratory muscles in infants. *Pediatr Clin North Am* 1979; **26**: 503–26.

2 Keens TG, Bryan AC, Levison H, Ianuzzo CD. Developmental pattern of muscle fibre types in human ventilatory muscles. *J Appl Physiol Respir Environ Exercise Physiol* 1978; **44**: 909–13.

3 Kinsella JP, Neish SR, Dunbar ID, *et al*. Clinical responses to prolonged treatment of persistent pulmonary hypertension of the newborn with low doses of inhaled nitric oxide. *J Pediatr* 1993; **123**: 103–8.

4 O'Rourke PP, Crone RK, Vacanti JP, *et al*. A prospective randomised study of extracorporeal membrane oxygenation (ECMO) and conventional medical therapy in neonates with persistent pulmonary hypertension of the newborn. *Pediatrics* 1989; **84**: 957–63.

5 Bose C, Corbet A, Bose G, *et al*. Improved outcome at 28 days of age for very low birth weight infants treated with a single dose of a synthetic surfactant. *J Pediatr* 1990; **117**: 947–53.

6 Long W, Corbet A, Cotton R, *et al*. A controlled trial of synthetic surfactant in infants weighing 1250 g or more with respiratory distress syndrome. *N Engl J Med* 1991; **325**: 1696–703.

7 Stevenson D, Walther F, Long W, *et al*. Controlled trial of a single dose of synthetic surfactant at birth in premature infants weighing 500–699 grams. *J Pediatr* 1992; **120**: S3–12.

8 Jobe A. Pulmonary surfactant therapy. *N Engl J Med* 1993; **328**; 861–8.

9 Sims C, Johnson CM. Postoperative apnoea in infants. *Anaesth Intens Care* 1994; **22**: 40–5.

10 Robertson CF, Smith F, Beck R, Levison H. Response to frequent low doses of nebulized salbutamol in acute asthma. *J Pediatr* 1985; **106**: 672–4.

11 Yung M, South M. Randomised controlled trial of aminophylline for severe acute asthma. *Arch Dis Child* 1998; **79**: 405–10.

12 Baker JW, Yerger SY, Segar WE. Elevated plasma antidiuretic hormone levels in status asthmaticus. *Mayo Clin Proc* 1976; **51**: 31–4.

13 Stalcup SA, Mellins RB. Mechanical forces producing pulmonary edema in acute asthma. *N Engl J Med* 1977; **297**: 592–6.

14 Tuxen DV. Detrimental effects of positive end-expiratory pressure during controlled mechanical ventilation of patients with severe airflow limitation. *Am Rev Resp Dis* 1989; **140**: 5–9.

15 Beasley JM, Jones SEF. Continuous positive airway pressure in bronchiolitis. *Br Med J* 1981; **283**: 1506–8.

16 Mezey AP. Treatment of respiratory failure associated with acute bronchiolitis. *Am J Dis Child* 1985; **139**: 650–1.

17 Sanchez I, De Koster J, Powell RE, Wolstein R, Chernick V. Effect of racemic epinephrine and salbutamol on clinical score and pulmonary mechanics in infants with bronchiolitis. *J Pediatr* 1993; **122**: 145–51.

18 Smith DW, Frankel LR, Mathers LH, *et al*. A controlled trial of aerosolized ribavirin in infants receiving mechanical ventilation for severe respiratory syncytial virus infection. *N Engl J Med* 1991; **325**: 24–9.

19 Korppi M, Leinonen M, Koskela M, *et al*. Bacterial coinfection in children hospitalized with respiratory syncytial virus infections. *Pediatr Infect Dis J* 1989; **8**: 687–92.

20 Lister G, Talner NS. Management of respiratory failure of cardiac origin. In: Gregory GA (ed.) *Respiratory Failure in the Child. Clinics in Critical Care Medicine*. New York: Churchill Livingstone; 1981: pp. 67–87.

21 Lanteri CJ, Kano S, Duncan AW, Sly PD. Changes in respiratory mechanics in children undergoing cardiopulmonary bypass. *Am J Respir Crit Care Med* 1996; **152**: 1893–900.

22 Vernon DD, Banner W, Canter P, *et al. Streptococcus pneumoniae* bacteremia associated with near drowning. *Crit Care Med* 1990; **18**: 1175–6.

23 Oh TE, Duncan AW. Oxygen therapy. *Med J Aust* 1988; **149**: 141–6.

24 Shann F, Gatchalian S, Hutchinson R. Nasopharyngeal oxygen in children. *Lancet* 1988; **1**: 1238–40.

25 Henning R. Clinical applications of mechanical ventilation. *Anaesth Intens Care* 1986; **14**: 267–80.

26 Duncan AW, Oh TE, Hillman DR. PEEP and CPAP. *Anaesth Intens Care* 1986; **14**: 236–50.

27 Clough JB, Duncan AW, Sly PD. The effect of sustained positive airway pressure on derived cardiac output in children. *Anaesth Intens Care* 1994; **22**: 30–4.

28 Hamilton PP, Onayemi A, Smyth JA, *et al*. Comparison of conventional and high-frequency ventilation: oxygenation and lung pathology. *J Appl Physiol* 1983; **55**: 131–8.

29 DeLemos RA, Coalson JJ, Gerstmann DR, *et al*. Ventilation management of infant baboons with hyaline membrane disease: the use of high-frequency ventilation. *Pediatr Res* 1987; **21**: 594–602.

30 Clark RH, Yoder BA, Sell MS. Prospective, randomised comparison of high-frequency oscillation and conventional ventilation in candidates for extracorporeal membrane oxygenation. *J Pediatr* 1994; **124**: 447–54.

31 Clark RH, Gerstmann DR, Null DM, DeLemos RA. Prospective randomised comparison of high-frequency oscillatory and conventional ventilation in respiratory distress syndrome. *Pediatrics* 1992; **89**: 5–12.

97.

Paediatric fluid and electrolyte therapy

F Shann

Children need a much higher intake of water and electrolytes per kilogram of body weight than adults. This makes children more susceptible to dehydration if they have abnormal losses of water or a reduced intake. On the other hand, an inability to excrete a water load, due to immature kidneys (in neonates) or high levels of antidiuretic hormone (ADH), means that many children in intensive care units can easily become overhydrated. Fluid and electrolyte problems in paediatric intensive care and in neonates have been well reviewed.[1-5]

WATER

The full-term neonate is 80% water. This figure falls to about 60% by 12 months of age, and then remains almost constant throughout childhood. The average intravenous (i.v.) fluid requirements for children in bed are shown in Tables 97.1 and 97.2. Substantial modification to these intakes will often be necessary (Table 97.3). For example, if a 14 kg child (maintenance fluid of 50 ml/h, Table 97.2) sustains a head injury and has evidence of high levels of ADH (maintenance fluid × 0.7),[6] is ventilated with humidified gas (maintenance × 0.75),[7] is paralysed (basal state, maintenance × 0.7) and is maintained at a rectal temperature of 36°C (maintenance − 12%), then his actual maintenance fluid requirement is (50 × 0.7 ×

$0.75 \times 0.7) - 12\% = 16$ ml/h. Even less water should be given initially if the child is overhydrated. In very small children, all fluid administered has to be taken into account – including the volume of drugs (bicarbonate, dextrose, and antibiotics) and 'flushes' used to clear i.v. lines (after blood sampling or administration of drugs).

The estimates of water requirements in Tables 97.1–3 are only approximate, and water balance must be monitored closely in any child in intensive care. Unfortunately, regular, accurate weighing of very sick children is often impractical, and hydration has to be assessed by skin turgor, urine output (minimum 0.5–1.0 ml/kg per hour), urine osmolality (maximum 600 mmol/kg), serum sodium, central venous pressure and arterial blood pressure.

Very frequent monitoring is required in very low birthweight babies. There is controversy about the degree of dehydration that is acceptable in these infants.[4,8-10] Higher fluid intakes allow a higher calorie intake, but may increase the incidence of patent ductus arteriosus (PDA), heart failure and bronchopulmonary dysplasia.[4,11] In hyaline membrane disease (HMD), improvement in lung function is preceded by diuresis.[12] Frusemide therapy may increase survival in HMD by initiating diuresis[4,13] or by some other mechanism[14]; one study has suggested that frusemide increases the incidence of PDA,[15] but a meta-analysis suggests that this is not the case.[4]

In a child with oliguria following a severe ischaemic or hypoxic insult (e.g. birth asphyxia, drowning or cardiac arrest), it may be helpful to measure urinary sodium.[16] In oliguria due to acute tubular necrosis, where restriction of fluid intake may be necessary, the urine sodium is usually more than 40 mmol/l. In

Table 97.1 Intravenous fluid requirements in infants

Day 1 of life	2 ml/kg per hour
Day 2 of life	3 ml/kg per hour
Day 3 of life	4 ml/kg per hour

Table 97.2 Intravenous fluid requirements in children

<10 kg	100 ml/kg per day
10–20 kg	1000 ml + (50 ml/kg per day for each kg over 10 kg)
>20 kg	1500 ml + (20 ml/kg per day for each kg over 20 kg)

Wt	10	12	14	16	18	20	30	35	40	50	60	70
ml/h	40	45	50	55	60	65	70	75	80	90	95	100

Table 97.3 Modifications to fluid intake

Decrease	Adjustment
Humidified inspired air	×0.75
Basal state (e.g. paralysed)	×0.7
High ADH (IPPV, brain injury)	×0.7
Hypothermia	−12% per °C
High room humidity	×0.7
Renal failure	×0.3 (+ urine output)
Increase	
Full activity + oral feeds	×1.5
Fever	+ 12% per °C
Room temperature >31°C	+ 30% per °C
Hyperventilation	×1.2
Neonate preterm (1–1.5 kg)	×1.2
radiant heater	×1.5
phototherapy	×1.5
Burns first day	+ 4% per 1% area burnt
subsequently	+ 2% per 1% area burnt

ADH, antidiuretic hormone; IPPV, intermittent positive pressure ventilation.

oliguria due to hypovolaemia, the urine sodium is usually less than 20 mmol/l.

SODIUM AND POTASSIUM

In the first one or two days of life, small preterm babies often have poor urine output and high transcutaneous fluid losses. They are therefore prone to hypernatraemia and hyperkalaemia, and such infants should usually be given 5% or 10% dextrose without sodium or potassium. From two days of age, 2–4 mmol/kg per day of sodium and potassium will usually be sufficient, but much higher intakes of sodium may be required in some preterm neonates due to their impaired renal conservation of sodium.

Sodium is a predominantly extracellular ion and so is well represented by the serum value. It must be interpreted in the context of both total hydration and the relative amount of water.

Hyponatraemia may be due to:

- poor renal conservation of sodium
- a low sodium intake (e.g. breast milk)
- diuretic therapy
- high levels of ADH (CNS disease, IPPV or lung disease)
- excessive water intake.

Hyponatraemia causes ileus, hypotension, listlessness and convulsions. Hyponatraemia due to sodium deficit should be corrected by administration of sodium (Table 97.4). Hyponatraemia due to water excess should be treated with restriction of water intake and, if symptomatic, can be corrected by administration of sodium (Table 97.4) and frusemide 0.5 mg/kg intravenously. Serum sodium should be corrected slowly; increased by no more than 0.5 mmol/l/h, and even slower in patients with long-standing hyponatraemia.[17]

Hypernatraemia may be due to:

- administration of large amounts of sodium (e.g. sodium bicarbonate)

Table 97.4 Doses and formulae in paediatric fluid and electrolyte therapy

Albumin 25%	undiluted: 2–4 ml/kg
	5% in 5% dextrose or saline: 10–20 ml/kg
Bicarbonate (number of mmol of deficit)	under 5 kg: base excess × wt(kg) × 1/2 (give 1/2 of this)
	over 5 kg: base excess × wt(kg) × 1/3 (give 1/2 of this)
Blood volume	85 ml/kg in neonate
	70 ml/kg in older children
Calcium	chloride 10% (0.7 mmol/ml Ca^{++}): maximum 0.2 ml/kg i.v. stat, requirement 1.5 ml/kg per day
	gluconate 10% (0.22 mmol/ml Ca^{++}): maximum 0.5 ml/kg i.v. stat, requirement 5 ml/kg per day.
Dextrose	for hypoglycaemia: 1 ml/kg 50% dextrose i.v.
	in neonate: 4 mg/kg per min (2.4 ml/kg per hour 10% dextrose) day 1, increasing to 8 mg/kg per min (up to 12 mg/kg per min with hypoglycaemia)
	for hyperkalaemia: 0.1 U/kg insulin and 2 ml/kg 50% dextrose i.v. stat
Magnesium	chloride 0.48 g/5 ml (1 mmol/ml Mg^{++}): 0.4 mmol (0.4 ml)/kg per dose slow i.v. 12-hourly
	sulphate 50% (2 mmol/ml Mg^{++}): 0.4 mmol (0.2 ml)/kg per dose slow i.v. 12 hourly
Mannitol	0.25–0.5 g/kg per dose i.v. (1–2 ml/kg of 25%) 2-hourly, provided serum osmolality <330 mosm/kg.
Packed cells	10 ml/kg raises Hb 3 g%, 1 ml/kg raises PVC 1%.
Potassium	maximum 0.5 mmol/kg per hour, requirement 2–4 mmol/kg per day, 1 g KCl = 13.3 mmol K$^+$.
	Hyperkalaemia: see dextrose.
Sodium	depletion: ml 20% NaCl = weight × 0.2 (140–serum Na$^+$), requirement 2–6 mmol/kg per day, 1 g NaCl = 17.1 mmol/Na$^+$.
Urine	minimum acceptable is 0.5–1.0 ml/kg per hour.

- dehydration from a large insensible fluid loss (caused by radiant heaters, or phototherapy), diarrhoea, osmotic diuresis (caused by glycosuria) or inadequate fluid intake.

With hypernatraemic dehydration, shock should be treated with rapid intravenous infusion of 10–20 ml/kg of 0.9% saline. The water deficit should then be corrected very slowly so that the serum sodium falls no faster than 0.5 mmol/l/h, to prevent cerebral oedema. Peritoneal dialysis or haemofiltration may be indicated for severe hypernatraemia without dehydration.

Potassium is a predominantly intracellular ion and is poorly represented by its serum concentration. The concentration of potassium in the serum depends on pH as well as the total body potassium (which is usually about 50 mmol/kg). A child may have hypokalaemia without a deficit of total body potassium in the presence of alkalosis and, conversely, there may be a large deficit of potassium without hypokalaemia in the presence of acidosis. Potassium should never be infused at more than 0.5 mmol/kg per hour, and it should not normally be given to a patient with severe oliguria or anuria.

CALCIUM, MAGNESIUM AND PHOSPHATE

Hypocalcaemia in children occurs in

- sick neonates in the first two days of life
- infants of diabetic mothers
- exchange transfusion with citrated blood (a temporary effect only)
- magnesium deficiency
- infants fed cows' milk (which has a high phosphate content).

Hypocalcaemia and hypomagnesaemia cause jitters, tetany, cardiac arrhythmias and convulsions. The doses of calcium and magnesium are given in Table 97.4.

Normal intravenous maintenance requirements in infants are 1 mmol/kg/day of calcium and 0.3 mmol/kg per day of magnesium.

Rickets is very common in small preterm babies, particularly those fed solely on breast milk. There is increasing evidence that this can be prevented by giving extra phosphorus (in particular) and calcium,[18] as well as the usual supplement of Vitamin D.

STANDARD PAEDIATRIC MAINTENANCE SOLUTION[1]

In the first one or two days of life, it is usual to give plain 5% or 10% dextrose if intravenous fluid therapy is required. Thereafter, a solution that is usually satisfactory is 5% or 10% dextrose with 40 mmol/l of sodium chlo-

ride (quarter normal saline) and 20 mmol/l of potassium chloride. 'Maintenance solution' is an unfortunate term, since these solutions do not provide maintenance calorie or protein requirements (see 'Parenteral nutrition', below).

DEHYDRATION AND SHOCK

Weight loss is the best guide to the degree of dehydration, if a recent weight is known. Many of the commonly used clinical signs of dehydration in children are inaccurate, and this leads to dehydration being diagnosed when it is not present, and to overestimation of the degree of dehydration.[19]

The clinical signs of mild to moderate dehydration in children are:

- decreased peripheral perfusion (as shown by pallor or reduced capillary return)
- deep breathing
- decreased skin turgor.

These signs become apparent with only 3–4% dehydration.[19]

In children with shock, intravenous access may be difficult. In these circumstances, parenteral fluid can be given rapidly into the bone marrow, which is an intravascular compartment.[20] The usual sites chosen are the junction of the upper and middle third of the tibia (0–12 months of age), the medial malleolus (1–5 years) and the iliac crest (over 5 years). A 0.9 mm (20 gauge) lumbar puncture needle or an intraosseous needle can be used; the needle is held perpendicular to the bone and pushed in *gently* with a rotary motion about its long axis – a slight decrease in resistance will be felt as the needle enters the medulla.

Shock should be treated with an initial bolus of 20 ml/kg of 0.9% albumin, followed by further boluses of 10–20 ml/kg of fluid until the intravascular volume has been restored.[21] After shock has been corrected with a rapid infusion of fluid, the remainder of the deficit is replaced over the next 24–48 hours (while giving maintenance requirements at the same time). Standard maintenance solution (see above) is usually appropriate. Thus, a 5 kg child with 10% dehydration from diarrhoea (500 ml deficit) might receive 100 ml of isotonic saline rapidly to restore the circulation, leaving a 400 ml deficit to be replaced over 24 hours. If the maintenance requirement is 500 ml/day, then the child should be given a further 900 ml of fluid in the next 24 hours (i.e. 40 ml/h) in addition to the initial 100 ml. Further fluid losses should be replaced with an appropriate fluid (see Table 97.5).

With hypernatraemic dehydration, shock should be treated as above, with rapid infusion of 10–20 ml/kg of isotonic saline. The remaining deficit should then be replaced *slowly* so that the serum sodium falls no faster

Table 97.5   Composition of some body fluids in children

Fluid	Na^{2+} mmol/l	K$^+$ mmol/l	Cl$^-$ mmol/l	HCO$_3^-$ mmol/l	Other
Gastric fluid	20–80	10–20	100–150	0	H$^+$ 30–120
Bile	140–160	3–15	80–120	15–30	
Pancreatic fluid	120–160	5–15	75–135	10–45	Basal state
Jejunal fluid	130–150	5–10	100–130	10–20	
Ileal fluid	50–150	3–15	20–120	30–50	
Diarrhoeal fluid	10–90	10–80	10–110	20–70	
Sweat					
Normal	10–30	3–10	10–35	0	
Cystic fibrosis	50–130	5–25	50–110	0	
Burn exudate	140	5	110	20	Protein 30–50 g/l
Saliva	10–25	20–35	10–30	2–10	Unstimulated

than 0.5 mmol/l/h, to prevent cerebral oedema.[2,3] It has been traditional to use 0.45% saline (with dextrose and potassium) for this slow replacement phase, but the rate of replacement is probably much more important than the type of fluid used; standard maintenance solution is satisfactory, providing it is given slowly.

In dehydration due to pyloric stenosis there is a deficit of water, hydrogen ion, chloride and potassium. Initial resuscitation should be with rapid infusion of 10–20 ml/kg of isotonic saline, then 0.45% saline in 5% dextrose with 20–40 mmol/l of potassium chloride should be given.

OEDEMA

Oedema is common in children in intensive care units. It may be due to:

- prematurity[22]
- excess water intake
- high levels of ADH (from CNS disease, IPPV or lung disease)
- capillary leak (due to the effects of hypoxia, ischaemia, acidosis or sepsis)
- heart failure
- renal failure
- hypoalbuminaemia.

Several possible causes are often present in a child, and it can be difficult to decide which is the most important.

Children with oedema and high levels of ADH will have a serum osmolality less than 270 mmol/kg (with hyponatraemia) and a urine osmolality greater than 270 mmol/kg; the appropriate treatment is fluid restriction. On the other hand, in children with oedema due to capillary leak, fluid restriction and attempts to remove water (diuretics, dialysis) are unlikely to cure the oedema, and often cause hypovolaemia; in fact, large amounts of fluid (e.g. blood and normal saline) may be needed to preserve the intravascular volume in these children – the

oedema will only disappear when the capillary damage resolves.

CRYSTALLOID OR COLLOID

There have been several reviews of the contentious issue of the relative merits of crystalloid or colloid fluids in critically ill patients. The best known review concluded that, compared with crystalloids, albumin increased mortality by 6% (95% CI 3%–9%).[23] A subsequent review had better methodology[24]: colloid was compared with isotonic crystalloid (to avoid the confounding comparison with hypertonic crystalloids). This later study found no apparent difference between isotonic crystalloid and colloid in pulmonary oedema, although there was a nonsignificant trend towards lower mortality with crystalloid in the better quality studies.[24]

There have been very few studies comparing crystalloid to colloid fluids in children, so most of the evidence comes from studies in adults. The use of albumin in paediatric and neonatal intensive care has been reviewed.[25] The meta-analyses certainly do not suggest that colloid is better than crystalloid (indeed, they suggest that it may be worse), and colloid is more expensive and carries a small risk of transmitting infection. Until more evidence is available, it seems sensible to use crystalloid as a routine, but give concentrated albumin to children with severe hypoalbuminaemia (perhaps if their serum albumin is less than 20 g/l).

PARENTERAL NUTRITION[26,27]

'Maintenance solution' is an unfortunate medical term, particularly when small children are concerned. A solution of 5% dextrose with sodium and potassium chloride provides maintenance amounts of water, sodium, potassium and chloride, but little or no calories, protein, trace elements or vitamins. For example, 100 ml/kg per day of 5% dextrose provides 20 cal/kg per day (84 kJ/kg per day), which is only 20% of the requirement of a normal infant (let alone a child with increased calorie requirements). It has been estimated that, although an adult has the energy reserve to survive for about a year on 3 l of 10% dextrose a day, a small preterm infant will survive only 11 days on 75 ml/kg per day of 10% dextrose.[28]

Many children in intensive care units are unable to absorb adequate amounts of food from the gut, and their nutritional reserves are small, so they often need parenteral nutrition. However, parenteral nutrition is difficult to administer and dangerous in small children – such patients should be referred to a specialist paediatric unit as soon as possible.

The usual requirements for amino acids, dextrose and fat in parenteral nutrition in children are shown in Table 97.6. The amino acids (Vamin in neonates, Synthamin in older children) can be mixed with dextrose in the pharmacy department to make a 'Nutrient Solution'. A standard Nutrient Solution might provide 4 mmol/kg per day of sodium, 3 mmol/kg per day of potassium, and 7.5 mmol/day of calcium and phosphate (with up to 12 mmol/l for neonates). The standard solution should also contain 4 mmol/l of magnesium, 0.2 μmol/kg per day of manganese, 3 μmol/kg per day of zinc, 0.5 μmol/kg per day of copper, 0.04 μmol/kg per day of iodide, 0.005 μmol/kg per day of chromium, 20 μg/l of hydroxycobalamin, 2 mg/l of phytomenadione, 1 mg/l of folic acid, and a multivitamin preparation. For short term nutrition, the solution need not provide fluoride, iron or Vitamins A, D and E, but MVI Paediatric should be given to children on long term parenteral nutrition. Fat can be given as a 20% emulsion (for example, Intralipid), either through a separate i.v. line or alternating with the Nutrient Solution. Nutrient Solutions for paediatric use contain high concentrations of calcium, magnesium and phosphorus, and they should not be mixed with the fat emulsion, even in a Y-connection placed just before the cannula.

In a child on parenteral nutrition, it is important that abnormal fluid losses (Table 97.5) be replaced with an appropriate solution (in addition to the Nutrient Solution), and that parenteral nutrition always be introduced and withdrawn slowly. A dislodged i.v. cannula should be replaced immediately in a child on parenteral nutrition, to prevent rebound hypoglycaemia. If Nutrient Solution is not available at any time, it should be replaced with an infusion of a similar amount of dextrose (e.g. 20% dextrose with 40 mmol/l of sodium chloride and 20 mmol/l of potassium chloride).

Children on parenteral nutrition are liable to develop:

- hyperglycaemia (with glycosuria and dehydration)
- hypoglycaemia
- sepsis
- extravasation of solutions with necrosis of tissue
- thrombocytopenia
- hypoproteinaemia
- electrolyte imbalance
- acidosis
- anaemia
- hyperlipaemia
- uraemia
- cholestatic jaundice.

Frequent, careful monitoring is essential (Table 97.7). Initially, monitoring may need to be more frequent than suggested in Table 97.7, particularly in preterm babies. Monitoring can be less frequent once a child is stabilized on parenteral nutrition.

Table 97.6 Approximate requirements in paediatric parenteral nutrition

	Total fluid ml/kg per day*	Amino acids (g/kg per day) Day			Dextrose (g/kg per day) Day			Fat (Nutralipid) (g/kg per day) Day				Total calories (kcal) needed (1 kcal = 4.2 kJ)
		1	2	3+	1	2	3+	1	2	3	4+	
Neonates	100	1.5	2	2	10	10–15	15–20	1	2	3	3	100/kg
Under 10 kg	100	1.5	2	2	10	10	15–20	1	2	3	3	100/kg
10–15 kg	90	1	1.5	2	5	10	15	1	2	3	3	1000 + (50/kg over 10 kg)
15–20 kg	80	1	1.5	1.5–2	5	10	10–15	1	2	2	3	1000 + (50/kg over 10 kg)
20–30 kg	65	1	1	1–2	5	10	10–15	1	1.5	2	2.5	1500 + (20/kg over 20 kg)
30–50 kg	50	1	1	1–2	5	5–10	10	1	1.5	1.5	2	1500 + (20/kg over 20 kg)

*One ml/kg per day of fluid is needed for each kcal/kg per day; for adjustments to requirements, see Table 97.3. [Total kcal/kg per day equals g/kg per day of (amino acids × 4) + (dextrose × 4) + (fat × 10).]

Table 97.7 Monitoring in paediatric parenteral nutrition

Daily: inspect IV site, electrolytes, acid/base, serum lipaemia (reduce Intralipid rate if lipaemia is significant).

Twice weekly: haemoglobin (transfuse if anaemia develops), platelets, proteins.

Weekly: creatinine, MG^{2+}, Ca^{2+}, phosphate, bilirubin, aspartate aminotransferase.

Dextrostix (or BM test) of blood 8 hourly until the dextrose intake is stable.

Clinitest (or BM test) of urine 8 hourly (reduce dextrose intake if more than trace).

Weigh frequently (daily if possible).

REFERENCES

1 Winters RW (ed.) *The Body Fluids in Pediatrics.* Boston: Little Brown; 1973.

2 Finberg L, Kravath RE, Hellerstein S. *Water and Electrolytes in Pediatrics: Physiology, Pathophysiology and Treatment.* 2nd edn. Philadelphia: Saunders; 1993.

3 Wood EG, Lynch RE. Fluid and electrolyte balance. In: Fuhrman BP, Zimmerman, JJ (eds) *Pediatric Critical Care,* 2nd edn. St Louis: Mosby; 1998: 703–22.

4 Bell EF. Fluid therapy. In: Sinclair JC, Bracken MB (eds) *Effective Care of the Newborn Infant.* Oxford: OUP; 1992: 59–71.

5 Seri I, Evans J. Acid-base, fluid, and electrolyte management. In: Taeusch HW, Ballards RA (eds) *Avery's Diseases of the Newborn.* 7th edn. Philadelphia: WB Saunders; 1998: 372–93.

6 Bouzarth WF, Shenkin HA. Is 'cerebral hyponatraemia' iatrogenic? *Lancet* 1982; **1**: 1061–2.

7 Sousulski R, Polin RA, Baumgart S. Respiratory water loss and heat balance in intubated infants receiving humidified air. *J Pediatr* 1983; **103**: 307–10.

8 Lorenz JM, Kleinman LI, Kotagal UR, Reller MD. Water balance in very low-birth-weight infants: relationship to water and sodium intake and effect on outcome. *J Pediatr* 1982; **101**: 423–32.

9 Baumgart S, Langman CB, Sosulski R, *et al.* Fluid, electrolyte, and glucose maintenance in the very low birth weight infant. *Clin Pediatr* 1982; **21**: 199–206.

10 Oh W. Fluid and electrolyte therapy and parenteral nutrition in low birth weight infants. *Clinics in Perinatol* 1982; **9**: 637–43.

11 Spahr RC, Klein AM, Brown DR, *et al.* Fluid administration and bronchopulmonary dysplasia. *Am J Dis Child* 1980; **134**: 958–60.

12 Engle WD, Arant BS, Wiriyathian S, Rosenfeld CR. Diuresis and respiratory distress syndrome: physiologic mechanisms and therapeutic implications. *J Pediatr* 1983; **102**: 912–7.

13 Green TP, Thompson TR, Johnson DE, Lock JE. Diuresis and pulmonary function in premature infants with respiratory distress syndrome. *J Pediatr* 1983; **103**: 618–23.

14 Najak ZD, Harris EM, Lazzara A, Pruitt AW. Pulmonary effects of furosemide in preterm infants with lung disease. *J Pediatr* 1983; **102**: 758–63.

15 Green TP, Thompson TR, Johnson DE, Lock JE. Furosemide promotes patent ductus arteriosus in premature infants with the respiratory distress syndrome. *N Engl J Med* 1983; **308**: 743–8.

16 Harrington JT, Cohen JJ. Measurement of urinary electrolytes – indications and limitations. *N Engl J Med* 1975; **293**: 1241–3.

17 Pirzada NA, Ali II. Central pontine myelinosis. *Mayo Clinic Proceedings* 2001; **76**: 559–62.

18 Specker BL, DeMarini S, Tsang R. Vitamin and mineral supplementation. In: Sinclair JC, Bracken MB (eds) *Effective Care of the Newborn Infant.* Oxford: OUP; 1992: 161–77.

19 Mackenzie A, Barnes G, Shann F. Clinical signs of dehydration in children. *Lancet* 1989; **1**: 605–7.

20 Spivey WH. Intraosseous infusions. *J Pediatr* 1987; **111**: 639–43.

21 Scheinkestel CD, Tuxen DV, Cade JF, Shann F. Fluid management of shock in critically ill patients. *Med J Aust* 1989; **150**: 508–17.

22 Wu PYK, Rockwell G, Chan L, Wang S, Udani V. Colloid osmotic pressure in newborn infants: variations with birth weight, gestational age, total serum solids, and mean arterial pressure. *Pediatrics* 1981; **68**: 814–9.

23 Roberts E. Human albumin administration in critically ill patients: systematic review of randomised controlled trials. *BMJ* 1998; **317**: 235–40.

24 Choi P, Yip G, Quinonez LG, Cook DJ. Crystalloids vs colloids in fluid resuscitation: a systematic review. *Crit Care Med* 1999; **27**: 200–10.

25 Bohn D, Carcillo JA (eds). The use of albumin in pedaitric and neonatal critical care. *Pediatr Crit Care Med* 2001; **2**(suppl 1): S1–39.

26 Baker RD, Baker SS, Davis AM. *Pediatric Parenteral Nutrition.* Aspen Publishers, 1997.

27 Heird WC. Parenteral support of the hospitalised child. In: Suskind RM, Lewinter-Suskind L. *Textbook of Pediatric Nutrition.* 2nd ed. New York: Raven Press; 1993: 225–38.

28 Heird WC, Driscoll JM, Schullinger JN, Grebin B, Winters RW. Intravenous alimentation in pediatric patients. *J Pediatr* 1972; **80**: 351–72.

98

Sedation and analgesia in children

G J Knight

All children, including preterm infants, feel and remember pain and discomfort.[1,2] Provision of adequate sedation and analgesia should therefore be a priority in the management of all critically ill children.

INDICATIONS AND BENEFITS

Pain in the paediatric intensive care unit (ICU) may be surgical in origin or due to the underlying illness or to procedures (e.g. central venous catheterization, lumbar puncture and removal of drains). Sedation is frequently necessary to allow a child to tolerate an endotracheal tube and mechanical ventilation. It may also be needed to allow sleep in a brightly lit, noisy environment. As young children are unlikely to co-operate during investigations, such as an echocardiogram or computed tomographic (CT) scan, sedation is often necessary to prevent excessive movement.

In addition to its humane benefits, sedation and analgesia can suppress non-advantageous physiological responses to noxious stimuli. Analgesic suppression of the marked post-surgery stress response has been associated with significant improvements in postoperative morbidity and mortality.[3–5] Sedation and analgesia have also been shown to blunt pulmonary hypertensive responses to stimulation in children with labile pulmonary vasculature.[6]

ASSESSMENT

Adequacy of pain relief and sedation is dependent on an accurate assessment of the degree of discomfort. This may be particularly difficult in the critically ill child for many reasons. The patient may be preverbal, developmentally delayed, intubated and/or paralysed, or simply unco-operative. Thorough assessment requires careful and frequent consideration of a number of factors. These include the nature of the noxious stimulus, variations in physiological parameters, such as heart rate and blood pressure, and interpretation of subjective clues, such as facial expressions and posture. Parental interpretations of a child's expressions are reliable and should also be considered. In older children, self-reporting measurement

scales may be useful and a number of methods have been developed to measure pain.[7,8] Although these tools are useful, particularly in research, they form only part of the overall assessment of discomfort.

APPROACH TO MANAGEMENT

The management of discomfort, anxiety and pain may take many forms. It can begin prior to the child's admission to intensive care, through orientation to the unit and clear, age appropriate explanation of a procedure or operation and its expected course. Parental presence is also important to help allay anxiety and fear. Close attention should also be paid throughout a child's admission to physiological factors, such as hunger, that may cause distress. In addition to these supportive measures, many paediatric patients require a pharmacological form of analgesia or sedation.

Patients in the paediatric intensive care unit (PICU) should have sedation and analgesic delivery tailored to their particular requirements. It is vital that there be continuous assessment and frequent adjustment of regimes so that appropriate levels of sedation and adequate analgesia are provided. This requires a clear understanding of the aims of management and of the pharmacology of the agents being administered. Relief of pain should be achieved with analgesic agents and care must be taken to avoid the over-administration of sedative agents when the patient needs pain relief (Table 98.1). Consideration should be given to optimal delivery whilst minimizing side effects. A single drug may be effective but often a combination of medications and a combination of delivery methods (e.g. i.v./oral, i.v./epidural) will be useful.

PAEDIATRIC PHARMACOLOGICAL CONSIDERATIONS

Differences in drug handling between children and adults should be considered. Drug distribution, rates of drug metabolism and relative organ blood flows differ in

Table 98.1   Single dose and infusion rates of sedative and analgesic drugs

Drug	Bolus dose	Infusion rate
Morphine	0.1–0.2 mg/kg i.v.	10–40 μg/kg per h
Pethidine	1–1.5 mg/kg i.v.	100–300 μg/kg per h
Fentanyl	1–2 μg/kg i.v.	1–10 μg/kg per h
Midazolam	0.1–0.2 mg/kg i.v.	
	0.5 mg/kg (oral)	50–200 μg/kg per h
Ketamine	1–2 mg/kg i.v.	15–20 μg/kg per h (sedation)[19]
		4 μg/kg per h (analgesia)
Propofol	1–3 mg/kg i.v.	<4 mg/kg per h (short term)
Clonidine	0.4 μg/kg (oral)	0.1–2 μg/kg per h[30]

children, particularly in young infants. These differences may result in greater concentrations of free drug and differing volumes of distribution. Neonates have relatively larger total body water, extracellular fluid volume, blood volume and cardiac output and significantly less body fat than adults.[9–11] Their blood–brain barrier is less efficient and allows more ready entry of some drugs to the brain. Mixed-function oxidases mature quickly to adult levels by 6 months of age, and acetylation and glucuronidation mechanisms mature by about 3 months.[9,10] Renal blood flow and glomerular filtration rate are low in the immediate neonatal period. However, both increase significantly in the first 2–3 days and reach adult values by 5 months.[11,12] Tubular secretory capacity reaches adult levels by 6 months of age.[10] In general, drug metabolism and clearance are relatively mature by 6 months of age but great care is required when dealing with the neonate and young infant.

NON-OPIOID AGENTS

MIDAZOLAM

Midazolam is water-soluble, has rapid onset and generally does not produce haemodynamic disturbance in children though dose-related respiratory depression does occur. Metabolism occurs in the liver and is mature by 6 months of age.[13] The standard i.v. sedative dose is 0.1–0.2 mg/kg and this is effective for uncomfortable procedures, such as echocardiography and cardioversion. The oral route (0.5 mg/kg) may also be useful though there is a 15 min delay to onset of sedation. Delivery via continuous infusion is usually effective, particularly when combined with an opioid, to facilitate mechanical ventilation. 50–200 μg/kg per h with morphine (10–40 μg/kg per h) generally provides satisfactory sedation. Midazolam may be effective as the sole sedative agent for ventilated patients.[14] Nasal administration (0.2 mg/kg) can be useful in children who do not have established i.v. access and in whom oral agents are not appropriate.[15] During continuous infusion, accumulation can occur in patients with liver dysfunction leading to delayed wakening.

KETAMINE

Ketamine is a dissociative anaesthetic agent with analgesic and amnesic properties. Biotransformation occurs by the microsomal enzyme system. Thus, there is little metabolism in the newborn and clearance is less and elimination half-life greater in infants than in older children and adults.[16,17] Usefulness in preterm infants, to a post conceptual age of 51 weeks, is limited because of an increased risk of post-anaesthetic apnoea.[18] An initial i.v. dose of 1–2 mg/kg is usually adequate to induce deep sedation. Cardiovascular disturbance is minimal and ketamine is particularly useful as the induction agent in status asthmaticus and in patients with a compromised haemodynamic state, such as tamponade. Prolonged sedation for ventilated children has been achieved with a continuous infusion of 10–15 μg/kg per min.[19] Analgesia can be provided by an infusion of 4 μg/kg per min. Concomitant use of an antisialogogue, such as glycopyrrolate, helps control the often seen increase in respiratory tract secretions. The unpleasant emergent phenomena, seen frequently in adults, occur less often in children and can be controlled by the concurrent administration of a benzodiazepine.[20]

PROPOFOL

Propofol is a rapidly acting anaesthetic agent that is used for short- and longer-term sedation in paediatric intensive care.[21] The half-life decreases with age, probably due to development of metabolizing capacity and increasing hepatic flow.[22] Rapid emergence is propofol's most attractive property. It has been safely used for short-term sedation in the spontaneously breathing patient, by using an induction dose of 1 mg/kg, followed by intermittent smaller doses.[23] Its role has been extended to that of the sedating agent for ventilated children. However, it should be used with caution because of the reported association between high dose (>4 mg/kg per h), prolonged (>29 h) infusions and a clinical syndrome consisting of metabolic acidosis, lipaemia, cardiac failure, arrhythmias and death.[24,25] The pathogenesis of the problem and the actual role of propofol remains unclear, although it has been postulated that a water-soluble metabolite is involved.[26] Thus, propofol should be limited to short-term use in the ventilated child and long-term, high-dose sedation cannot be recommended (note that the manufacturer does not recommend the use of propofol for sedation in children during intensive care).

THIOPENTONE

Thiopentone is useful as an anaesthetic induction agent in critically ill children, although its hypotensive effects limit its use in shocked patients. The standard dose is 5 mg/kg, and this should be reduced to 2–3 mg/kg when hypotension is a risk. Thiopentone is useful in the management of refractory status epilepticus and may have a role in difficult cases of raised intracranial pressure. In such cases, it is administered by continuous infusion (1–5 mg/kg per h). Accumulation can lead to prolonged sedation.

CHLORAL HYDRATE

Chloral is an effective oral hypnotic and sedative agent with no analgesic effect. The hypnotic dose is 50 mg/kg and appropriate sedation may be achieved with lower doses. Gastric irritation can be a problem in some children. Toxic doses produce depression of respiration and cardiac contractility. Despite the disadvantage of delayed onset, chloral can be useful given prior to procedures, or as a supplemental sedative agent in the ventilated child and it can effectively induce nocturnal sleep. On a cautionary note, there is some evidence that it may not be suitable in acutely wheezing infants.[27]

CLONIDINE

Clonidine is an alpha-2 adrenoreceptor agonist with significant neurological, neuroendocrine and cardiovascular effects that result in sedation, analgesia and reduced sympathetic outflow. It is rapidly absorbed after oral administration and has a half-life of 9–12 h. Metabolism is via the liver and kidney and approximately 50% is excreted unchanged in the urine.[28] A single oral dose (4 μg/kg) has been shown to provide both preoperative sedation and postoperative analgesia following moderately painful surgery.[29] An i.v. infusion (0.1–2 μg/kg per h) in combination with midazolam (50 μg/kg per h) has been shown to produce effective sedation in ventilated children without haemodynamic disturbance.[30] Clonidine may also have a role in the management of the autonomic storms seen following severe traumatic brain injury and in the management of opioid withdrawal.

OPIOID ANALGESICS

MORPHINE

Morphine is frequently used. Clearance and half-life (2 h) are at adult values by 6 months of age.[31] Marked variation in pharmacokinetics in the neonatal period has been demonstrated, but infants over 1 month of age eliminate morphine efficiently and should not be more sensitive to respiratory depression than adults.[31,32] The active metabolite is renally excreted and can therefore accumulate in renal failure. The standard i.v. dose is 0.1–0.2 mg/kg and an infusion rate of 20–40 μg/kg per h provides safe postoperative pain relief in spontaneously breathing patients. With careful titration of dose to effect, higher rates can safely be administered, particularly to the child on mechanical ventilation. Patient-controlled analgesia devices delivering fixed doses of opioid, with or without a background infusion, can be used successfully by the majority of school-aged children and may occasionally be appropriate in intensive care.[33] Morphine is commonly used in combination with a benzodiazepine in children on mechanical ventilation. Histamine related side-effects, in particular nasal itch, may warrant a change of opioid. Fentanyl is an alternative.

FENTANYL AND ALFENTANIL

Fentanyl has theoretical advantages over morphine in certain situations because of its rapid onset and its systemic and pulmonary haemodynamic stability. Termination of the effects of a single dose is by redistribution.[34] Clearance is more rapid in neonates and infants compared to adults and does not change with time during continuous infusion.[34,35] However, after prolonged infusion, unchanged fentanyl is returned to the circulation from peripheral compartments, resulting in a prolonged terminal elimination half-life of approximately 21 h.[35] The effective dose for painful procedures is 1–2 μg/kg. Fentanyl is useful as an anaesthetic agent in patients with labile pulmonary vasculature, as it can blunt changes in pulmonary vascular resistance seen with stimulation. However, it does not prevent the increase in pulmonary vascular pressure caused by hypoxia.[36] Infusions of 1–5 μg/kg per h produce effective sedation in neonates on mechanical ventilation. 1–10 μg/kg per h is required for analgesia in older children. Tolerance, noted in both neonates and older children, can develop rapidly and adjustment of the infusion rate may be necessary.[37] Fentanyl's short duration of action makes it suitable for use in epidural regimens.

Alfentanil, because of its shorter duration of action, may have advantages for analgesia or sedation for very short procedures.

'SIMPLE' ANALGESICS

The addition to an analgesic regime of either paracetamol or a non-steroidal anti-inflammatory drug (NSAID) should be considered provided there are no contraindications.

Paracetamol is useful for mild to moderate pain and, in conjunction with opioid infusions, for more severe pain. The initial dose should be 30 mg/kg and the total daily dose should be limited to 90 mg/kg. Contraindications include liver and gut dysfunction and care regarding dosages must be taken when paracetamol is given for several days.

NSAIDs should also be considered as supplemental analgesics. Care should be taken however regarding the risk of bleeding, particularly in the postoperative period and in the highly stressed patient in whom gastric bleeding is more likely. Ketorolac (0.6 mg/kg) is given i.v. and therefore has the potential to reduce the dose of opioid required in the immediate postoperative period when enteral medications are not appropriate.

INHALED AGENTS

NITROUS OXIDE

Nitrous oxide is a potent analgesic agent. It is useful in intensive care during short painful procedures such as removal of surgical drains. A mixture of 50% nitrous oxide with oxygen provides analgesia in awake and co-operative patients. It is unsuitable for repeated or continuous use because of toxicity and administration to younger children may cause distress because of the need for application of a mask.

ISOFLURANE

Isoflurane has been used for long-term sedation in intensive care in adults. As elimination is independent of hepatic and renal mechanisms, there are theoretical advantages in many critically ill patients. However, an association between isoflurane sedation in children and neurological abnormalities has been reported.[38] These abnormalities, although reversible, were a considerable clinical problem.

DRUG WITHDRAWAL SYNDROMES

Opioid withdrawal is a recognized problem and symptoms include poor feeding, tremors, agitation, poor sleeping, tachycardia, diarrhoea, sweating, increased muscle tone, dystonic posturing and seizures. It occurs particularly following prolonged high-dose infusions. Katz et al.[39] found that the risk of withdrawal following a fentanyl infusion was associated with the duration of infusion and the total dose. Infusion for >5 days duration or a total dose >1.5 mg/kg was associated with greater than 50% incidence. Benzodiazepine withdrawal (agitation, anxiety, sweating, tremor) is also seen and the risk following a midazolam infusion is associated with a total dose >60 mg/kg.[40] Although careful attention to weaning an infusion in high-risk patients can minimize symptoms, longer-term pharmacological management is occasionally required. Methadone, benzodiazepines and clonidine via i.v., oral and subcutaneous routes have been

used.[41] Although withdrawal is a significant, albeit manageable, problem adequate sedation or analgesia should never be withheld because of fears of the development of drug dependence.

LOCAL ANAESTHESIA

Local anaesthesia can produce effective analgesia without systemic effects and therefore has significant advantages in many patients, particularly the postoperative group. In the intensive care setting, it can be used as the sole method of providing analgesia or in combination with i.v. agents. The risk of toxicity is related both to the dose and rapidity of absorption, which is dependent on local blood flow. Metabolism of the amide local anaesthetics (lignocaine, bupivicaine) is via the P450 system and their half-life is longer in infants less than 6 months of age. Unbound drug does not produce analgesia but is potentially toxic as infants have lower levels of the binding protein α-glycoprotein.[42] The use of local anaesthesia in infancy therefore requires careful assessment and close monitoring.

EMLA

EMLA, an emulsion of lignocaine and prilocaine, is effective in reducing the pain associated with percutaneous procedures.[43] It needs to be applied to the skin 60 minutes beforehand and thus is unsuitable for urgent procedures. Systemic absorption of the prilocaine component and subsequent methaemoglobinaemia can occur. Neonates, because of their relative deficiency of methaemoglobin reductase, are particularly at risk and EMLA should be used with caution in this group.

LOCAL INFILTRATION

Optimal analgesia for some painful procedures is possible, particularly in older children, with careful local infiltration and minimal sedation. The total dose of local anaesthetic agent infiltrated must be monitored and maximum doses not exceeded. The total dose of lignocaine should not exceed 4 mg/kg (7 mg/kg if combined with epinephrine).

NERVE BLOCKS

Femoral nerve blockade is a simple technique that produces effective analgesia in cases of femoral shaft fracture. A single injection is effective for approximately 3 h and a technique has been developed to provide long-term analgesia.[44] Bupivacaine (0.125%) is infused continuously at 0.2–0.3 ml/kg per h through a fine catheter placed adjacent to the femoral nerve. As this technique can decrease opioid requirements, it is particularly useful in trauma patients who have suffered a coexistent head injury.

Intercostal nerve blocks are useful after thoracotomies and liver transplants in children.[45] A single dose of 0.125% bupivacaine can produce up to 8 h of analgesia. The dose must be carefully limited, because the relatively high blood flow to the area increases the risk of toxicity. The maximum single dose of bupivacaine is 2 mg/kg. Continuous infusions via an intercostal catheter can provide ongoing pain relief. These require careful monitoring in the PICU particularly regarding maximal dose. There is a risk of pneumothorax with this technique and it should therefore be avoided when there is significant coexistent lung disease.

EPIDURAL ANALGESIA

Caudal, lumbar and thoracic epidural anaesthesia can provide effective control of postoperative pain in children.[46,47] The procedures must be performed by skilled experienced staff who clearly understand the risks and benefits. A complication rate of 1.5 per 1000 has been reported with dural puncture and intravascular injection seen most commonly.[48] Other risks include cord injury, epidural infection and excessive motor blockade. Infants under 6 months are at highest risk because of their size and immature metabolism. Many epidural procedures are performed in the operating theatre and general anaesthesia is a prerequisite in most paediatric patients. PICU care may subsequently be required because of the nature of the surgery (e.g. thoracotomy, liver transplant) or because of underlying patient factors (e.g. neurological disorders, morbid obesity, age). Epidurals have been used in paediatric cardiac surgery without clear benefit over conventional postoperative analgesia.[49] Particular indications for commencing epidural analgesia in the PICU include burns in a suitable distribution (e.g. abdomen and lower limbs) and blunt chest trauma with rib fractures. Contraindications include shock, hypovolaemia, meningitis, coagulopathy and local skin infection. Bupivacaine is the most commonly used local anaesthetic. A single dose should not exceed 2.5 mg/kg and the maximum infusion rate is 0.4 mg/kg per h (0.2 mg/kg per h in infants).[42] Opioids (morphine and fentanyl) may be added and have a synergistic effect thereby allowing less local anaesthetic agent to be used. Epidural opioids can cause sedation and are associated with a decrease in the slope of the CO_2 response curve.[50] Respiratory depression is seen therefore and close observation is mandatory when epidural opioids are used.

REFERENCES

1 Anand KJS, Hickey PR. Pain in the foetus and neonate. *N Engl J Med* 1987; **317**: 1321–9.

2 McGrath PJ, Craig KD. Developmental and psychological factors in children's pain. *Paed Clin North Am* 1989; **36**: 823–36.

3 Anand KJS, Ward-Platt MP. Neonatal and paediatric responses to anaesthesia and operation. *Int Anesthesiol Clin* 1988; **26**: 218–25.

4 Anand KJS, Hickey PR. Halothane-morphine compared with high dose sufentanil for anaesthesia and postoperative analgesia in neonatal cardiac surgery. *N Engl J Med* 1992; **326**: 1–9.

5 Anand KJS, Sippell WG, Aynsley-Green A. Randomised trial of fentanyl anaesthesia in preterm neonates undergoing surgery: Effects on the stress response. *Lancet* 1987; **1**: 243–8.

6 Hickey P, Hansen DD, Wessell DL, *et al.* Blunting of stress response in the pulmonary vasculature of infants by fentanil. *Anesth Analg* 1985; **64**: 1137–42.

7 McGrath PA, deVeber L, Haarn M. Multidimensional pain assessment in children. In: Fields H, Dubner R, Cervero F (eds). *Advances in Pain Research and Therapy*, vol 9. New York: Raven Press; 1985: pp. 387–93.

8 Beyer JE, Denyes MJ, Villareul AM. The creation, validation and continuing development of the Oucher: a measure of pain intensity in children. *J Pediatr Nurs* 1992; 7: 335–46.

9 Nitowsky HM, Matz L, Berzofsky JA. Studies on oxidative drug metabolism in the full term newborn infant. *J Pediatr* 1966; **69**: 1139–49.

10 Gladtke E. The importance of pharmacokinetics for paediatrics. *Eur J Paediatr* 1979; **131**: 85–91.

11 Arant BS Jr. Developmental patterns of renal functional maturation compared in the human neonate. *J Pediatr* 1978; **92**: 705–12.

12 Leake RD, Trystad CW. Glomerular filtration rate during the period of adaptation to extrauterine life. *Pediatr Res* 1977; **11**: 959–62.

13 Lloyd-Thomas AR, Booker PD. Infusion of midazolam in paediatric patients after cardiac surgery. *Br J Anaesth* 1986; **58**: 1109–15.

14 Silvani DL, Rosen DA, Rosen KR. Continuous midazolam infusion for sedation in the paediatric intensive care unit. *Anesth Analg* 1988; **67**: 286–8.

15 Wilton N, Leigh J, Rosen D, Pandit U. Preanaesthetic sedation of preschool children using intranasal midazolam. *Anesthesiology* 1988; **69**: 927–75.

16 Chang T, Glazko T. Biotransformation and metabolism of ketamine. *Int Anesthesiol Clin* 1974; **12**: 157–77.

17 Cook DR, Davis PJ. Paediatric anaesthesia pharmacology. In: Lake CH (ed.). *Paediatric Cardiac Anaesthesia*. Norwalk, CT: Appleton and Lange; 1993: pp. 119–50.

18 Welborn LG, Rice LJ, Hannallah RS, *et al.* Postoperative apnoea in former preterm infants: Prospective comparison of spinal and general anaesthesia. *Anesthesiology* 1990; **72**: 838–42.

19 Tobias JD, Martin LD, Wetzel RC. Ketamine by continuous infusion for sedation in the paediatric intensive care unit. *Crit Care Med* 1990; **18**: 819–21.

20 Rita L, Seleny FL. Ketamine hydrochloride for paediatric premedication II. Prevention of post anaesthetic excitement. *Anesth Analg* 1974; **53**: 380–2.

21 Murdoch S, Cohen A. Intensive care sedation: a review of current British practice. *Intensive Care Med* 2000; **26**: 922–8.

22 Jones RDM, Chan K, Andrew LJ. Pharmacokinetics of propofol in children. *Br J Anaesth* 1990; **65**: 661–667.

23 Paschall A, Braner DAV, Portland OR. Sedation with propofol in the PICU. *Crit Care Med* 1993; **21**: S150.

24 Parker TJ, Stevens JE, Rice ASC *et al*. Metabolic acidosis and fatal myocardial failure after propofol infusion in children: five case reports. *Br Med J* 1992; **305**: 613–6.

25 Bray RJ. Propofol infusion syndrome in children. *Paediatr Anaesth* 1998; **8**: 491–9.

26 Cray SH, Robinson BH, Cox PN. Lactic acidaemia and bradyarrhythmia in a child sedated with propofol. *Crit Care Med* 1998; **26**: 2087–92.

27 Mallol J, Sly PD. Effect of chloral hydrate on arterial oxygen saturation in wheezy infants. *Pediatr Pulmonol* 1988; **5**: 96–9.

28 Maze M, Tranquilli W. Alpha-2 adrenoreceptor agonists: defining the role in clinical anaesthesia. *Anesthesiology* 1991; **74**: 581–605.

29 Reimer EJ, Dunn GS, Montgomery CJ, *et al*. The effectiveness of clonidine as an analgesic in paediatric adenotonsillectomy. *Can J Anaesth* 1998; **45**: 1162–7

30 Ambrose C, Sale S, Howells R, *et al*. Intravenous clonidine infusion in critically ill children: dose dependent sedative effects and cardiovascular stability. *BJA* 2000; **84**: 794–6.

31 McRori TI, Lynn AM, Nespecca MK, *et al*. The maturation of morphine clearance and metabolism. *Am J Dis Child* 1992; **146**: 972–6.

32 Bhat R, Chari G, Gulati A, Aldana O, *et al*. Pharmacokinetics of a single dose of morphine during the first week of life. *J Pediatr* 1990; **117**: 477–81.

33 Gaukroger PP. Patient controlled analgesia in children. In: Schechter NL, Berde CB, Yaster M (eds). *Pain in Infants, Children and Adolescents*. Baltimore, MD: William and Williams; 1993: pp. 203–11.

34 Johnson KL, Erickson JP, Holley FO, Scott JC. Fentanyl pharmacokinetics in the paediatric population. *Anesthesiology* 1984; **61**: A441.

35 Katz R, Kelly WH. Pharmacokinetics of continuous infusions of fentanyl in critically ill children. *Crit Care Med* 1993; **21**: 995–1000.

36 Vacanti JP, Crone PK, Murphy JP, *et al*. The pulmonary haemodynamic response to perioperative anaesthesia in the treatment of high-risk infants with congenital diaphragmatic hernia. *J Pediatr Surg* 1984; **19**: 672–9.

37 Arnold JH, Truog RD, Scavone JM, Fenton T. Changes in the pharmacodynamic response to fentanyl in neonates during continuous infusion. *J Pediatr* 1991; **119**: 639–43.

38 Kelsall AWR, Ross-Russell R, Herrick MJ. Reversible neurological dysfunction following isoflurane sedation in pediatric intensive care. *Crit Care Med* 1994; **22**: 1032–4.

39 Katz R, Kelly WH, Hsi A. Prospective study on the occurrence of withdrawal in critically ill children who receive fentanyl by continuous infusion. *Crit Care Med* 1994; **22**: 763–7.

40 Fonsmark L, Rasmussen YH, Carl P. Occurrence of withdrawal in critically ill sedated children. *Crit Care Med* 1999; **27**: 196–9.

41 Tobias JD. Tolerance, withdrawal and physical dependency after long-term sedation and analgesia of children in the paediatric intensive care unit. *Crit Care Med* 2000; **28**: 2122–32.

42 Wilder RT. Local anesthetics for the pediatric patient. *Ped Clin North Am* 2000; **47**: 545–58.

43 Sims C. Thickly and thinly applied lignocaine-prilocaine cream prior to venepuncture in children. *Anaesth Intensive Care* 1991; **19**: 343–5.

44 Johnson CM. Continuous femoral nerve blockade for analgesia in children with femoral nerve fractures. *Anaesth Intensive Care* 1994; **22**: 281–3.

45 Shelly MP, Park GR. Intercostal nerve blockade for children. *Anaesthesia* 1987; **42**: 541–5.

46 Dalens B. Lumbar epidural anasthesia. In: Dalens B (ed.). *Regional Anesthesia in Infants, Children and Adolescents*. Baltimore, MD: Williams and Wilkins; 1995: pp. 207–48.

47 Dalens B, Khandwala R. Thoracic and cervical epidural anesthesia. In: Dalens B (ed) *Regional Anesthesia in Infants, Children and Adolescents*. Baltimore: Williams and Wilkins 1995; pp. 249–260.

48 Giaufre E, Dalens B, Gombert A. Epidemiology and morbidity of regional anaesthesia in children: a one year survey of the French-language Society of Pediatric Anesthesiologists. *Anesth Analg* 1996; **83**: 897–900.

49 Biche T, Roue JC, Schlegel S, *et al*. Epidural sufentanil during paediatric cardiac surgery: effects on metabolic response and post-operative outcome. *Paed Anaesth* 2000; **10**: 609–17.

50 Attia J, Ecoffey C, Sandouk P, *et al*. Epidural morphine in children: Pharmacokinetics and CO_2 sensitivity. *Anesthesiology* 1986; **65**: 590–4.

99

Shock and cardiac disease in children

R D Henning

Most cases of shock in childhood are caused by hypovolaemia or sepsis (Table 99.1). The causes and complications of shock differ from those in adults, because the spectrum of disease is different in childhood: severe diarrhoeal disease and congenital abnormalities are common in childhood, but abdominal sepsis, pancreatitis and obstructive vascular disease occur uncommonly.

The following factors affect the epidemiology of shock in children.

SMALLER BODY FLUID COMPARTMENTS

A small volume of blood or diarrhoeal fluid loss may represent a large percentage loss of blood or extracellular fluid volume in a small child.

IMMATURE IMMUNE SYSTEM IN INFANTS AND TODDLERS[1]

In the first 6 months of life, immature and permeable gut, lung and skin barriers, low complement, immunoglobulin M (IgM) and IgA concentrations, and poor neutrophil migration and phagocyte function increase susceptibility to severe bacteraemias. Antibody response to bacterial capsular polysaccharide antigens (e.g. *Pneumococcus and Haemophilus*) remains poor until 5 years of age. Low IgG concentrations and immunological naivety predispose to frequent viral infection in the first 5 years.[2] Reduced production of cytokines in infants may alter the features and duration of the shock syndrome and causes deficiency in most T-cell functions including cytotoxicity and augmentation of B-cell differentiation.[3]

MICROBIOLOGY

In the newborn, septic shock is most often caused by *Staphylococcus aureus*, group B β-haemolytic streptococci, *Listeria monocytogenes*, Enterobacteriaceae or entero-

viruses. In childhood, *Streptococcus pneumoniae* and *Neisseria meningitidis*, Enterobacteriaceae and *S. aureus* are usually responsible. *Haemophilus influenzae* still causes septicaemia in non-immunized children under 5 years. In immunodeficient children, *S. aureus*, Enterobacteriaceae, Pseudomonas spp., *Candida albicans*, and fungi frequently cause septic shock.

SEVERE CONGENITAL ABNORMALITIES

Children with congenital heart disease, multiple congenital abnormalities, inborn errors of metabolism and the inherited immunodeficiencies are prone to develop cardiogenic, hypovolaemic or septic shock.

OTHER CHILDHOOD CONDITIONS PREDISPOSING TO SEPTIC SHOCK

Cancer and chemotherapy; burns; multiple trauma; prolonged ICU stay; indwelling vascular devices.

Most cases of septic shock in children with cancer are due to neutropenia and immune suppression after chemotherapy or bone marrow transplantation.

PATHOPHYSIOLOGY

The pathophysiology of shock is described in Chapter 9, which should be read in conjunction with this chapter. The following aspects of physiology affect the child's response to insults.

IMMATURE CARDIOVASCULAR SYSTEM[4]

The maximum force and velocity of myocardial contraction are less in infancy, because the ventricular mass per kilogram body weight is less than in adults, the immature heart has fewer myofilaments and less myofibrillar adenosine triphosphate (ATP) per unit cross-sectional area, and the myofibrils and cytoskeleton are

Table 99.1 Causes of shock in childhood

Hypovolaemia	
Bleeding	External, GI tract, body cavity, fractures
Water and electrolyte loss	
Bowel	Vomiting, diarrhoea, ileus, gastric suction
Renal	Diuretic, diabetes mellitus, diabetes insipidus
Skin	Burns, heat stroke
Plasma loss (capillary leak)	Sepsis, burns, anaphylaxis, post cardiac arrest
Water deprivation	
Distributive	
Sepsis	
Anaphylaxis	
Drugs	e.g. barbiturates, phenothiazines
Neurogenic	Injury to brainstem or high cervical spine
Cardiogenic	
Structural congenital heart disease	e.g. hypoplastic left heart syndrome
Post cardiac surgery	
Arrhythmia	Heart block, supraventricular tachycardia
Myocardial hypoxia/ischaemia	
Global hypoxia	e.g. SIDS, near-drowning
Myocardial ischaemia	Kawasaki, anomalous left coronary artery
Cardiomyopathy	
Metabolic	Storage diseases, muscular dystrophies, maternal diabetes
Endocardial fibroelastosis	
Infective	Bacteria, enteroviruses
Valvular heart disease	Congenital, infective endocarditis, rheumatic, traumatic
Sepsis	e.g. meningococcus, staphylococcal toxic shock
Drug intoxication	e.g. tricyclic antidepressants, calcium antagonists, narcotics
Tamponade	Trauma, pericarditis, right heart failure
Combined	Sepsis, drugs, pancreatitis, post cardiac arrest

GI, Gastrointestinal; SIDS, sudden infant death syndrome.

less efficiently aligned for force development. The infant therefore depends on increasing heart rate, rather than on increasing stroke volume to raise its cardiac output.

The diastolic compliance of the infant heart is poor because of immaturity of the cytoskeleton and of the dominant extracellular collagen isoform. Consequently, volume loading causes a greater increase in atrial pressures than in adults. Because most interaction between the ventricles occurs in diastole, the depression of left ventricular output by pulmonary hypertension is greater in children than in adults.

Beat-to-beat calcium release from sarcoplasmic reticulum (SR) is less than in adults, because calcium uptake, storage and release from SR are less, and trans-sarcolemmal calcium flux (which depends on the calcium concentration in extracellular fluid) has a greater effect on contractile force and velocity. This also means that systolic function is more sensitive to calcium channel blockers in infants than in adults.

Limited calcium uptake and storage in infant SR slows myocardial relaxation in diastole and reduces diastolic compliance in infancy, especially at high heart rates.

AUTONOMIC INNERVATION

The development of cardiac sympathetic innervation in infants is incomplete: there are fewer β-receptors than in the adult and myocardial noradrenaline stores are smaller, so the response to severe stress is bradycardia rather than tachycardia as in the adult, and the infant heart is relatively refractory to dopamine. Immature coupling of β-receptors to adenyl cyclase in infants means that milrinone is a less effective inotropic agent than in older children.[5]

RESPONSE TO HYPOXIA AND ISCHAEMIA

Myocardial cell survival and rate of recovery of performance after periods of hypoxia or ischaemia are greater in infants, because of lower rates of energy demand and ATP consumption or efflux, as well as higher cell glycogen reserves.[6] Glucose is the major myocardial energy source (rather than long chain fatty acids as in older children) and hypoglycaemia causes myocardial depression.

The infant with splanchnic ischaemia is more likely to develop bowel mucosal damage and sepsis syndrome due to leakage of luminal endotoxin and bacteria, because its bowel mucosa is more permeable and secretory IgA production is less than that of adults and the plasma concentration of platelet-activating factor (PAF) acetylhydrolase and levels of catalase and reduced glutathione in the colonic mucosa are low.[7,8]

CLINICAL PRESENTATION OF SHOCK IN CHILDHOOD

HYPOVOLAEMIC SHOCK

A history of blood or fluid loss and signs of dehydration, external bleeding or haematoma may be present. The presence of hypovolaemic shock implies a blood volume deficit greater than 30 ml/kg.

Signs of homeostatic compensation, such as tachycardia, narrow pulse pressure, cool mottled limbs and slow capillary refill usually precede hypotension, which tends to occur late (after loss of 15–20% of blood volume) and precipitously in young children. In severe shock of any cause, signs of multiple organ hypoperfusion (e.g. oliguria of under 0.5 ml urine/kg per hour, lethargy or coma, tachypnoea and increasing metabolic acidosis) are found. Plasma lactate is high, and bleeding due to disseminated intravascular coagulation and liver dysfunction may occur in the first 6 h. In early shock, these changes are reversible by plasma volume expansion with boluses of 20 ml/kg normal saline, colloid or blood, repeated as necessary. Failure to respond with a decrease in heart rate and capillary refill time indicates refractory shock requiring more aggressive treatment (see below).

CARDIOGENIC SHOCK

Tachycardia, hypotension, poor pulses and signs of poor organ perfusion are usually present. Cardiomegaly and a gallop rhythm may be found. Chest rales and tachypnoea indicate left heart failure, while hepatomegaly develops rapidly, and is a more reliable sign of right heart failure than a raised jugular venous pressure (JVP) (which may be hard to detect in infants).

Signs of specific heart lesions (e.g. murmurs or cyanosis, absent femoral pulses in aortic coarctation, skull, liver or renal bruits of arteriovenous fistulae, and arrhythmias) may indicate the cause of the shock although murmurs are frequently absent.

Investigation should include urgent

- chest X-ray to assess heart size and exclude pneumothorax
- electrocardiogram (ECG)
- echocardiography
- in some cases cardiac catheterization.

SEPTIC SHOCK

Septic infants younger than 6 months usually present with a hypodynamic circulation, low cardiac output and cool extremities. Early septic shock in older children is similar to that in adults: tachycardia, tachypnoea and hypotension are accompanied by warm extremities, wide pulse pressure and increased cardiac output. Lethargy, oliguria and metabolic acidosis indicate inadequate tissue oxygenation. As shock progresses, myocardial depression by endotoxin and TNF-α and IL1-β decreases cardiac output, resulting in worsening hypotension, decreased pulse pressure and cool mottled extremities.[9] Capillary leakage secondary to endothelial injury causes hypovolaemia and reduced oxygen delivery to tissues. Peripheral oedema exacerbates cellular hypoxia by increasing the diffusion distances for oxygen between capillaries and cells.

MULTIPLE ORGAN FAILURE IN CHILDHOOD SEPTIC SHOCK

Multiple organ failure in childhood septic shock consists of:

- Myocardial depression and low cardiac output. Arrhythmias are rarely clinically important.
- Acute respiratory distress syndrome can occur in a septic child of any age, including the newborn. Respiratory muscle fatigue due to poor muscle blood flow further worsens gas exchange.
- Acute renal failure occurs frequently, is usually reversible within 50 days, may require haemofiltration or peritoneal dialysis, but is not a major contributor to mortality in children with septic shock.
- Disseminated intravascular coagulation occurs very commonly, due to activation of the coagulation pathway, increased production of plasminogen activator inhibitor-1 and reduced levels of protein c, antithrombin III and thrombomodulin.[10] This contributes to multi-organ failure and combines with clotting factor dilution by fluid resuscitation to cause bleeding from puncture sites and occasionally significant upper gastrointestinal bleeding.
- Gastrointestinal failure with paralytic ileus and upper gastrointestinal bleeding.
- Plasma concentrations of liver enzymes and bilirubin are often raised but usually return to normal over a few days in survivors.
- Acalculous cholecystitis due to splanchnic ischaemia sometimes occurs in older children.
- Encephalopathy with stupor or coma occurs commonly. The appearance of seizures suggests some complication of sepsis such as glucose or electrolyte abnormality, meningitis, septic embolus or intracranial bleeding.

DISTRIBUTIVE SHOCK

The main features are vasodilatation and hypovolaemia due to plasma leakage from capillaries. The extremities

Table 99.2 Investigation of shock in children

All shocked children
  Arterial blood gases
  Plasma electrolytes, urea, creatinine, glucose, liver function
    tests
  Haemoglobin, platelet count, total and differential white cell
    count
  Coagulation screen including fibrin degradation products
  Blood group (hold serum)
If the cause of shock is unknown:
  Exclude sepsis:
    Several sets of blood cultures, percutaneous and via
      vascular catheters
    Culture and Gram stain pus
    Urine cultures from mid-stream sample or suprapubic
      aspirate of urine
    Urine, stool and nasopharyngeal aspirate for virology
    CSF bacterial and viral culture plus PCR for specific
      organisms
  Urine bacterial antigens
  To exclude cardiogenic shock: echocardiography, ECG,
    cardiac catheter
  Drug screen: urine; gastric aspirate; blood
  Metabolic screen: urinary amino acids and organic acids,
    plasma ammonia and glucose
  Short Synacthen test

CSF, cerebrospinal fluid; PCR, polymerase chain reaction; ECG,
electrocardiogram.

---

are warm and pink; blood pressure is low and pulse pressure is wide. There is tachycardia, oliguria and stupor. Other signs of anaphylaxis, spinal cord injury or drug intoxication may be present.

INVESTIGATION

See Table 99.2

MANAGEMENT

The child's airway, breathing and circulation should be secured during the initial assessment. The priorities in management are given below.

ADEQUATE PERFUSION OF BRAIN AND HEART

This requires systolic and diastolic blood pressures 80% of normal for age (Table 99.3), achieved by aggressive early blood volume expansion and by inotropic drugs. The conscious state is the best index of inadequate cerebral perfusion, while improved coronary perfusion is shown by rising blood pressure with falling atrial pressures.

Pre-load

Fluid i.v. is given in aliquots of 20 ml/kg 0.9% saline or Hartmanns solution or 10 ml/kg blood or colloid repeated every 5–10 minutes until blood pressure, heart

rate and skin vasoconstriction (i.e. skin warmth and colour, and nailbed capillary return) and indices of organ perfusion (i.e. urine output, conscious state, blood pH and lactate) improve. Heart and liver size are used to assess hypervolaemia.

If more than 40 ml/kg colloid is given,

- an inotropic drug infusion should be considered
- central venous pressure should be monitored
- arterial cannula inserted for blood pressure and bio-chemical monitoring.

The disadvantages of pulmonary artery catheterization mean that thermodilution cardiac output measurement and pulmonary artery wedge pressure measurement are rarely justified, especially in infants.

Contractility

In septic or hypovolaemic shock, infusion of dobutamine 5–10 μg/kg per minute should be started (via a peripheral i.v. or intra-osseous cannula if necessary) if volume expansion does not improve the circulation within 10–20 minutes.

If the blood pressure remains low in septic or distributive shock, infusion of norepinephrine (0.05–0.5 μg/kg per min) or vasopressin (0.0003–0.0006 U/kg per min) into a central vein may be needed to maintain adequate coronary and cerebral perfusion pressure. Vasopressin deficiency occurs commonly in septic shock.[11]

In cardiogenic shock, infusion of dopamine 5–10 μg/kg per minute is started as soon as the diagnosis is made, pending investigation and definitive treatment. If reduced cardiac output is due to systemic or pulmonary vasoconstriction, dobutamine or a phosphodiesterase inhibitor (e.g. milrinone or enoximone) may be used instead of dopamine. Dobutamine and dopamine down-regulate β-adrenergic receptors, and dopamine depletes myocardial noradrenaline stores so the dose of these drugs should be minimized as soon as possible. Catecholamines increase body oxygen consumption by increasing futile fat cycling.[12] Dopamine also suppresses prolactin, thyroid-stimulation hormone and growth hormone secretion in infants and children.[13]

In infants with severe heart failure, infusion of 10% calcium gluconate (0.2–0.5 ml/h) can increase blood

Table 99.3 Normal blood pressure and heart rate in childhood

Age	Blood pressure (mmHg (kPa))	Heart rate (beats/min)
Birth	75/40 (10.0/5.3)	125
1 year	95/60 (12.6/8.0)	120
2 years	96/60 (12.8/8.0)	110
6 years	98/60 (13.0/8.0)	110
10 years	110/70 (14.6/9.3)	90
14 years	118/75 (15.7/10.0)	80

pressure and cardiac output. Serum ionized calcium should be monitored.

ADEQUATE PERFUSION OF KIDNEYS, LIVER AND GUT

Bowel and liver ischaemia in a shocked child greatly increases the risk of bacteraemia and endotoxaemia of bowel origin,[14] and reduces detoxification of drugs and toxic metabolites. Hypovolaemia and low cardiac output must be corrected by blood volume expansion and inotropic drugs, such as dobutamine and low-dose dopamine (2 μg/kg per min). Vasoconstricting drugs (including vasopressin, norepinephrine and dopamine doses >5 μg/kg per min) should be reduced or stopped once heart and brain perfusion are secured.

Urine output >0.5 ml/kg per hour with a normal plasma creatinine concentration are the best indices of adequate renal perfusion.

Monitoring the adequacy of splanchnic perfusion is difficult. Gastric pH and gastric-arterial pCO_2 difference correlate only moderately well with outcome in septic children (but not as well as plasma lactate)[15] and are not consistently improved by measures to restore bowel perfusion.[16]

ADEQUATE PERFUSION OF MUSCLE AND OTHER TISSUES

Improvement of circulation to these tissues may require further volume expansion and infusion of vasodilators (e.g. sodium nitroprusside or milrinone) in shock states where myocardial depression is prominent, provided an adequate blood pressure can be sustained. Maintaining supranormal cardiac output and oxygen delivery has not been shown to improve survival in paediatric shock.

Afterload Reduction in Cardiogenic Shock

Vasoconstrictors and blood transfusion (to achieve a haemoglobin concentration of 120 g/l) may be required at first to ensure adequate coronary and cerebral perfusion pressure. If blood pressure is adequate (Table 99.2), cardiac output may then be improved by afterload reduction. Short-acting drugs such as sodium nitroprusside are preferred. Inhaled nitric oxide (NO) via the ventilator circuit may improve cardiogenic shock due to pulmonary hypertension after cardiac surgery, and in persistent pulmonary hypertension of the newborn.[17]

Infusion of vasodilators such as nitroglycerin, prostaglandin E_1 (PGE$_1$), prostacyclin (PGI$_2$) and sodium nitroprusside reduces systemic as well as pulmonary vascular resistance. These drugs are easier to administer than NO, but are less effective pulmonary vasodilators, and often cause systemic hypotension.

After appropriate samples are taken for investigations (Table 99.2), possible sepsis is treated aggressively with appropriate antibiotics (Table 99.4), replacement of invasive lines and drainage of collections.

Table 99.4 Suggested initial antibiotic therapy in children with septic shock

Up to 2 months of age	Older child
Benzyl penicillin 50 mg/kg i.v. 4-hourly *plus* Gentamicin 5 mg/kg i.v. daily (7.5 mg/kg after 1 week of age) *plus* Cefotaxime 50 mg/kg i.v. 6-hourly	Flucloxacillin 50 mg/kg i.v. 6-hourly *plus* Gentamicin 7.5 mg/kg i.v. daily

Supportive Measures

Early mechanical ventilation secures adequate oxygenation and pH of arterial blood. Mechanical ventilation reduces work of breathing and muscle oxygen demand, diverting the limited cardiac output away from muscles to vital organs. Airway pressures and tidal volumes should be limited to the minimum needed, as impaired venous return from positive-pressure ventilation may exacerbate hypotension.

Other measures include administration of platelets and fresh frozen plasma in consumptive coagulopathy, and early commencement of renal support with haemofiltration or peritoneal dialysis in established acute renal failure. There is convincing evidence that pooled immunoglobulin (1 g/kg i.v.) reduces mortality in adults with septic shock.[18]

In children with purpura fulminans due to *N. meningitidis* or other organisms, pressure in swollen limb compartments should be monitored with a saline-filled needle and pressure transducer. Fasciotomy is performed if the pressure approaches the diastolic blood pressure.

Controversial Measures

- *Correction of metabolic acidosis:* Administration of $NaHCO_3$ reduces myocardial intracellular pH, myocardial performance and cardiac output in adult humans and animals, but not in newborn animals.[19] $NaHCO_3/Na_2CO_3$ mixtures raise both intracellular and extracellular pH,[20] increase cardiac output and reduce pulmonary vascular resistance in some patients with systemic acidosis.[21]
- *High-dose steroids after antibiotics started:* No benefits were found in two large multicentre trials.[22]
- *Stress dose of hydrocortisone:* About 50% of children with septic shock have adrenal insufficiency on short Synacthen testing.[23] Hydrocortisone (1.5 mg/kg 8-hourly i.v. for at least 5 days) may improve the outcome of patients with septic shock, even if commenced after 12–24 hours of shock.[24,25]
- *Anti-endotoxin antibodies, anti-TNF antibody and IL-1 receptor antagonists* have not been found to be useful in clinical trials.[26]
- *Bactericidal permeability increasing protein (BPI):* a multi-centre trial in children with meningococcal

sepsis did not produce convincing evidence of reduced mortality.[27]

- *Circulatory support with extracorporeal membrane oxygenation (ECMO)* has been employed in children moribund with septic shock, with some survivors, but there is no convincing evidence of its efficacy.[28]
- *Granulocyte transfusion, exchange transfusion, plasma exchange:* There are no convincing human trials, although favourable case reports have appeared of their use in neonates and children.[28]
- *Recombinant granulocyte colony stimulating factor (rGCSF):* A randomized controlled trial in septic pre-term newborns did not show improvement in survival although the incidence of later nosocomial sepsis was less in the treatment group.[29]
- *Antithrombin III concentrate:* Controlled trials so far suggest possible reduction in all-cause mortality in septic adults. Awaiting the results of a large multi-centre trial.[30]
- *Activated protein C:* Protein C levels are low in 90% of adults with septic shock. In a randomized controlled trial in adults with severe sepsis and organ failure, 20% fewer patients died in the treatment group than the control group.[31]
- *Heparin, recombinant tissue plasminogen activator (TPA) and vasodilator drugs* have been reported in case series to improve skin perfusion and limb survival in purpura fulminans due to *N. meningitidis*, but convincing controlled trial evidence is lacking.[28]

HEART FAILURE IN CHILDREN

In cardiac failure, the cardiac output is insufficient to meet the metabolic needs of the tissues or can only become sufficient if abnormally high ventricular diastolic volumes are reached.[32]

The main causes (Table 99.5) are:

- Preload:
  (a) *excessive*, volume loading, for example, systemic arteriovenous malformation; large ventricular septal defect (VSD) or excessive fluid administration,
  or
  (b) *inadequate*, for example, mitral stenosis; pericardial tamponade or low ventricular compliance. Many conditions, which impair ventricular contractility also reduce ventricular diastolic compliance, resulting in reduced ventricular filling and high atrial pressures (e.g. ischaemia or infiltrative cardiomyopathy)
- *excessive afterload* (pressure loading, e.g. pulmonary hypertension or aortic stenosis)
- *inadequate contractility* (e.g. myocarditis or asphyxia)
- heart rate:
  (a) *too fast* (e.g. supraventricular tachycardia and atrial flutter)
  (b) *too slow* (e.g. heart block).

Table 99.5 Common causes of heart failure from infancy to adolescence

Heart failure presenting at birth
Birth asphyxia
Sepsis
Severe anaemia (hydrops fetalis)
Obstructive left-sided lesions presenting after closure of the ductus arteriosus (e.g. coarctation, aortic stenosis, interrupted aortic arch, hypoplastic left heart syndrome)
Arrhythmias: congenital SVT or heart block
Aortopulmonary window, truncus arteriosus
Systemic AV fistula (e.g. liver, brain or kidney)
Congenital cardiomyopathy
Persistent pulmonary hypertension of the newborn
Heart failure presenting in the first 8 weeks of life
Large left-to-right shunts (e.g. VSD, PDA, total anomalous pulmonary venous drainage) cause heart failure as pulmonary vascular resistance and the haematocrit decrease.
Bronchopulmonary dysplasia (causing pulmonary hypertension)
Infiltrative cardiomyopathy
Anomalous origin of the left coronary artery
Hypothyroidism
Heart failure presenting in later childhood
Congenital heart disease
  Sub-aortic stenosis
  VSD with or without aortic regurgitation
  Systemic AV valve regurgitation
  Pulmonary atresia and VSD with large aorto-pulmonary collaterals
Congenital heart disease: post-operation
  Fontan procedure
  Obstructed prosthetic valve
  Post-ventriculotomy (e.g. Fallot's tetralogy)
  Coronary artery injury
  Imperfect myocardial preservation during bypass
  Valve regurgitation after aortic or pulmonary valvotomy
  Large Blalock–Taussig shunt or aortopulmonary collaterals
Cardiomyopathy
  Infective; infiltrative; neuromuscular disease
  Asphyxia (e.g. near-drowning)
  Ischaemia (e.g. Kawasaki disease)
  Toxic: acute (e.g. tricyclic antidepressant, verapamil, flecainide)
  Toxic: chronic (e.g. anthracycline)
  Metabolic
  Heart transplant rejection
Valvular (e.g. post-rheumatic, infective endocarditis, trauma)
Arrhythmia (e.g. SVT, complete heart block)
Severe polycythaemia (haematocrit ≥70%)
Cor pulmonale (e.g. sickle cell, thalassaemia)
Acute hypertension (e.g. glomerulonephritis, haemolytic-uraemic syndrome)

SVT, supraventricular tachycardia; AV, arteriovenous; VSD, ventricular septal defect; PDA, patent ductus arteriosus.

PRESENTING SIGNS

In childhood, heart failure may present with growth failure. Feeding is slow and may cause sweating and dyspnoea. Useful signs are tachypnoea, cardiomegaly, hepatomegaly, gallop rhythm, tachycardia and cool mottled extremities. There may be clinical and X-ray signs of lung congestion, oedema and air trapping (probably due to bronchial mucosal oedema and seen in large left-to-right shunts such as VSDs). In infants, the JVP is an unreliable sign. The liver enlarges rapidly as the right atrial pressure increases, and oedema is non-pitting and located in the eyelids and the dorsum of the hands and feet.[33]

INVESTIGATIONS

After a detailed history and examination, investigations include:

- chest X-ray
- *electrocardiogram (ECG) and echocardiography* (for structural abnormality, valve stenosis or regurgitation, chamber size, wall thickness, pericardial fluid and estimates of ventricular systolic and diastolic function and left-to-right and right-to-left shunts and pulmonary artery pressure)
- *cardiac catheterization* when indicated to quantify shunts, measure pressures and demonstrate anatomy
- *others* as indicated (e.g. blood gases, chromosomes, serum digoxin, viral culture of stool, urine and throat swabs, urine screen for amino acids and ketoacids, and myocardial biopsy).

Management[34]

The development of heart failure in infancy is an emergency requiring urgent hospitalization. Management includes the following:

- *correct precipitating factors* (e.g. fever, infection, anaemia or hypertension).
- *correct the underlying cause* (e.g. repair aortic coarctation, replace a regurgitant valve, treat an arrhythmia or infection).
- *support systemic circulation* and reduce systemic and pulmonary venous congestion:
  (a) Give oxygen therapy by mask.
  (b) Reduce preload with diuretics including aldosterone inhibitors (which also reduce mortality by inhibiting ventricular remodelling),[35] fluid and salt restriction, head elevation and administration of venodilatator drugs (e.g. nitroglycerin (GTN) infusion). Preload reduction may depress the cardiac output in acute correctable lesions which obstruct ventricular inflow (e.g. cardiac tamponade).
  (c) Reduce left ventricular afterload with infusion of GTN or sodium nitroprusside or with oral phenoxybenzamine or angiotensin-converting enzyme (ACE) inhibitors. ACE inhibitors reduce mortality in early and late heart failure by improving

ventricular performance and inhibiting myocardial remodelling.[36] Vasodilators must be used cautiously in obstructive left-sided lesions to avoid myocardial ischaemia (due to reduced aortic diastolic pressure in the presence of ventricular wall hypertrophy). Vasodilators may exacerbate volume loading in VSD or aortopulmonary shunts.
  (d) Reduce right ventricular afterload with nitric oxide (NO) inhalation (0.5–10.0 parts per million) which prevents acute right ventricular failure in persistent pulmonary hypertension of the newborn and when pulmonary hypertension follows cardiac surgery.[17]
  (e) Increase contractility acutely with IV infusion of dopamine or dobutamine (2.5–20 μg/kg per min). Milrinone infusion (250–750 ng/kg per min) improves cardiac output in the short term by reducing afterload and increasing contractility.
  (f) Consider careful use of β blockers[37] when diastolic dysfunction is prominent. Start with low dose infusion of esmolol (50 μg/kg per min) and increase gradually to 200 μg/kg per minute or change to a longer-acting drug such as atenolol if esmolol is tolerated.
- *Mechanical ventilation* improves myocardial performance by improving gas exchange and reducing acidaemia, work of breathing and left ventricular afterload.[38] Sedation and muscle relaxants reduce metabolic rate and the cardiac output needed to meet metabolic demands.
- *Ventricular assist devices (VAD)*[39] can maintain life for days to weeks in very severe but reversible cardiac failure pending ventricular recovery. When severe respiratory failure complicates severe heart failure, ECMO may be needed. Aortic balloon counter pulsation is less feasible in small children than in adults.

CONGENITAL HEART DISEASE

Management of a critically ill child with congenital heart disease (CHD) before a definitive structural diagnosis is made depends on the mode of presentation. All such children should be referred immediately to a paediatric cardiac centre and a paediatric cardiologist consulted urgently before transfer. Management of acute postoperative deterioration depends on the underlying condition, nature of surgery and cause of deterioration.

Congenital heart disease in children may present in the following ways.

SHOCK IN THE FIRST FEW DAYS OF LIFE[34]

The commonest CHD causes are obstructive lesions of the left heart, including coarctation of the aorta with or without VSD, aortic stenosis, and hypoplastic left heart (HLH). Differential diagnosis includes cardiomyopathy, systemic arteriovenous malformation (AVM), septicaemia, inborn error of metabolism, anaemia, congenital heart block and supraventricular tachycardia.

In left-sided obstructive lesions, shock develops as the ductus arteriosus closes. All pulses (especially the femoral pulses in the case of coarctation) are decreased or absent. Tachycardia, tachypnoea, oliguria, cool mottled extremities, metabolic acidosis, hepatomegaly, cardiomegaly and pulmonary oedema are often present. Murmurs are often absent.

Emergency management consists of PGE_1 infusion (5–25 ng/kg per min, to provide aortic blood flow from the pulmonary artery by opening the ductus arteriosus), dopamine infusion, $NaHCO_3$ 1 mmol/kg i.v., over 1 hour, to correct metabolic acidosis and mechanical ventilation (to reduce work of breathing, maintain normocarbia and prevent apnoea due to the PGE_1). Hypocarbia and a high FiO_2 should be avoided. They reduce pulmonary vascular resistance and divert blood to the lungs, thereby reducing systemic blood flow. Normoglycaemia and normocalcaemia should be maintained.

ACYANOTIC HEART FAILURE

IN THE FIRST WEEK OF LIFE

Coarctation, aortic stenosis, cardiomyopathy (including obstructive cardiomyopathy in the infant of a diabetic mother) and endocardial fibroelastosis, anaemia, septicaemia, overtransfusion and systemic AVM can present as heart failure. Signs include poor feeding, tachycardia, tachypnoea, sweating, hepatomegaly, cardiomegaly, alar flaring, wheezing and expiratory grunt. Femoral pulses may be absent in coarctation, and bruits are audible in skull, liver or kidneys in AVM.

Emergency management includes oxygen, diuretics and fluid restriction (to 50% of maintenance requirements). In severe failure, mechanical ventilation and inotropic drug infusion are started, and the child is transferred to a paediatric cardiac unit. When femoral pulses are absent or if aortic stenosis is suspected, i.v. infusion of PGE_1 (5–25 ng/kg per min) is started.

AFTER 2–8 WEEKS OF AGE

Systolic murmurs and signs of heart failure appear in infants with lesions such as VSD, patent ductus arteriosus, aortopulmonary window and atrioventricular septal defect due to the physiological decreases of haemoglobin concentration and pulmonary vascular resistance at this time. Emergency management includes diuretics and oxygen given via a headbox. Transfusion (to haemoglobin 130–140 g/l) may reduce left-to-right shunt. If these measures fail to control heart failure, surgery is often needed, preceded if necessary by mechanical ventilation and inotropic drug infusion.

CYANOSIS

PaO_2 greater than 150 mmHg (20 kPa) breathing 100% oxygen almost completely rules out cyanotic CHD. Most cyanotic CHD have a PaO_2 less than 60 mmHg (7.98 kPa). A chest X-ray should be obtained urgently. Cyanosis occurs when:

- pulmonary blood flow is reduced (e.g. pulmonary atresia)
- pulmonary and systemic circulations are separate (e.g. transposition of the great arteries)
- saturated and unsaturated blood mix in the heart (e.g. anomalous pulmonary venous drainage).

CYANOSIS WITH PULMONARY OLIGAEMIA ON CHEST X-RAY

This is usually due to pulmonary or tricuspid valve atresia or stenosis, or tetralogy of Fallot. Deep cyanosis is present, often without murmurs or with pulmonary ejection murmur. Tachypnoea may be present. Chest X-ray shows concavity in the pulmonary artery segment of the left heart border.

Emergency Management

In the newborn: PGE_1 infusion (5–25 ng/kg per min) is used to open the ductus arteriosus and increase pulmonary blood flow. FiO_2 of 0.5 gives a small increase in oxygen delivery, and $NaHCO_3$ is used to correct a metabolic acidosis. Gentle assisted ventilation is needed if PGE_1 causes apnoea. The lungs are very compliant and airway pressures above 12–15 cmH_2O further reduce lung blood flow. The haemoglobin concentration should be kept at 120–150 g/l by transfusion if necessary. The child needs urgent echocardiographic diagnosis and most need a Blalock–Taussig shunt.

Beyond 1 month of age: If the PaO_2 is less than 30 mmHg (4.0 kPa), or if cyanotic spells occur in a child with tetralogy of Fallot despite oral propranolol, an urgent Blalock–Taussig shunt is needed. Urgent treatment in such a patient consists of a high FiO_2, knee-chest position, i.v. morphine and infusion of crystalloid or colloid 10–20 ml/kg. If these measures fail, then esmolol (0.5 mg/kg i.v., then infusion of 50–200 µg/kg per min) may be needed to reduce subpulmonary stenosis. Inotropic drugs and vasodilators should be avoided.

CYANOSIS WITH PULMONARY PLETHORA OR OEDEMA IN THE NEWBORN

The commonest cardiac causes are transposition of the great arteries (TGA), single ventricle, HLH, truncus arteriosus and total anomalous pulmonary venous drainage (TAPVD). Signs include tachypnoea, tachycardia, cardiomegaly and hepatomegaly. A murmur may be present. Differential diagnosis includes lung disease such as hyaline membrane disease and neonatal pneumonia, group B streptococcal sepsis and persistent pulmonary hypertension of the newborn.

Emergency Management[34]

Acidaemia should be corrected and FiO_2 should be high. If heart failure is present, mechanical ventilation and dopamine or dobutamine infusion are used. PGE_1 infusion (5–25 ng/kg per min) is used in all cases except when a small heart accompanies cyanosis and pulmonary oedema. These signs suggest TAPVD with obstruction of the pulmonary veins, in which PGE_1 will exacerbate the pulmonary oedema. Assessment at a paediatric cardiac centre is needed urgently. A child with TGA needs balloon atrial septostomy and the other lesions need urgent surgery.[38]

ARRHYTHMIAS IN CHILDREN[40]

SINUS BRADYCARDIA

Predisposing conditions include normal sleep, hypoxaemia, acidosis, hypotension, high intracranial pressure, cervical spinal cord injury, tracheal suction and drugs such as β blockers and digoxin (see Table 99.3, normal heart rate for age).

MANAGEMENT

No treatment is needed for asymptomatic bradycardia unless it is extreme. Correct any reversible cause. If the sinoatrial node is damaged, atropine (20 μg/kg) or isoprenaline infusion (0.1–0.5 μg/kg per min) or even temporary (oesophageal or trans-venous) pacing may be used.

BRADYCARDIA-TACHYCARDIA (SICK SINUS) SYNDROME[40]

The usual form is severe sinus bradycardia with junctional escape rhythm. It can cause syncope. Predisposing conditions include:

- congenital atrial anomalies (e.g. Ebstein's anomaly and atrio-ventricular septal defects)
- extensive atrial surgery (e.g. Fontan and Senning operations)
- viral myocarditis.

MANAGEMENT

Atrial pacing then treat tachyarrhythmias on their merits.

ATRIOVENTRICULAR BLOCK[41]

Often asymptomatic but may present with fatigue or syncope.

Predisposing conditions include congenital cardiomyopathy, myocarditis, post cardiac surgery, vasculitic conditions (e.g. rheumatic fever or maternal systemic lupus erythematosus), and carbamazepine or tricyclic overdose.

MANAGEMENT

Acquired heart block should be paced regardless of symptoms, as escape rhythms are unreliable.

Congenital in infants: temporary pacing via a transoesophageal or transvenous lead followed by implantation of a permanent pacemaker if the heart rate <55 beats/min, regardless of symptoms.

Congenital in older child: temporary, then permanent pacing if the heart rate <50 or if symptomatic or if there are ventricular ectopics or ventricular dysfunction.

Management of arrhythmias in tricyclic overdose, see below.

SUPRAVENTRICULAR TACHYCARDIA (SVT)

RE-ENTRANT SUPRAVENTRICULAR TACHYCARDIA

In younger children, an accessory atrioventricular pathway is usually present, e.g. Wolff–Parkinson–White and Lown–Ganong–Levine (no short PR interval or δ wave) syndrome. In adolescents, there may be a re-entrant pathway within the A–V node. SVT is sometimes associated with congenital defects (e.g. Ebstein's anomaly, tricuspid atresia and atrioventricular canal defects), post cardiac surgery, myocarditis, drugs, sepsis, acidosis and catecholamine administration.[42]

Management

1 Infants
   (a) Vagal stimulation (e.g. induce gag reflex and apply ice water to the whole face)
   (b) Overdrive atrial pacing via transoesophageal, transvenous or epicardial leads
   (c) Adenosine by rapid i.v. bolus 0.05 mg/kg (max 3 mg) increasing by 0.05 mg/kg (max 3 mg) every 2 min to a maximum of 0.25 mg/kg (max 12 mg)[40]
   (d) Synchronized DC cardioversion 1 J/kg
   (e) Digoxin is useful provided Wolff–Parkinson–White syndrome is absent
   (f) Amiodarone and procainamide are sometimes useful Verapamil causes profound myocardial depression and should be avoided.
2 Child – as above: verapamil (0.1 mg/kg i.v. over 30 min) or atenolol (0.05 mg/kg i.v., every 5 min until response, max 2.5 mg or 4 doses, then 0.1 mg/kg every 12–24 h), may also be used.

JUNCTIONAL ECTOPIC TACHYCARDIA (JET)[43]

Atrioventricular dissociation and ventricular rate 160–290 beats/min with narrow QRS complexes is seen on ECG.[40] JET usually follows cardiac surgery, especially when myocardial function is poor, and when surgery involves the atrioventricular node or its blood supply (e.g. Fontan operation or repair of VSD or atrioventricular septal defect). Post-operative JET can be fatal, but is usually self-limiting after 12–72 hours.

Management

1 Reduce adrenergic drug infusions
2 Induce hypothermia to 34–35°C for 2–3 days with 12-hourly normothermia, to allow assessment. Amiodarone infusion 25 μg/kg per minute is given for 4 h, then 5–15 μg/kg per minute (max 1.2 g/24 h).
JET is usually resistant to adenosine and overdrive pacing.

VENTRICULAR ECTOPIC BEATS AND TACHYCARDIA

Ventricular tachycardia (VT)[40] is uncommon in childhood, but may present as syncope, poor feeding (in infants) or heart failure. The rate is 120–300 beats/min. The QRS axis on ECG is different from that of the underlying sinus rhythm. QRS duration is usually (but not always) prolonged (>0.08 s). Supraventricular tachycardia with aberrant conduction is very rare in childhood: more than 90% of wide-complex tachycardia in children are VT. Fusion or capture beats, atrioventricular dissociation and new bundle branch block also favour the diagnosis of VT.

Predisposing conditions include congenital heart lesions and their surgery (e.g. aortic and subaortic stenosis), myocardial ischaemia, mitral valve prolapse, myocarditis, cardiomyopathy, long QT syndrome, blunt chest trauma, hypokalaemia or hypomagnesaemia and drug toxicity (including digoxin and the combination of cisapride and macrolide antibiotics).

MANAGEMENT

If symptomatic: synchronized DC cardioversion 1–4 J/kg
If asymptomatic:

- Amiodarone 5 mg/kg i.v. over 1 hour, then 5–10 μg/kg per minute
- Lignocaine 1–2 mg/kg i.v. every 5–15 minutes
- Magnesium 0.2 mmol/kg i.v. over 10 minutes (especially if torsade de pointes is present)
- Overdrive pacing if VT is associated with underlying bradycardia
- Avoid Class 1 agents if the QT interval is prolonged.

ARRHYTHMIAS IN TRICYCLIC OVERDOSES

Most arrhythmias are sinus tachycardia, multifocal ventricular ectopic beats (VEBs), VT (torsade de pointes), VF, supraventricular tachycardia or heart block.

MANAGEMENT[44]

Drug removal is accelerated by gastric lavage and charcoal. Blood is alkalinized to maintain pH at 7.45–7.50, with $NaHCO_3$ 1–3 mmol/kg. Additional sodium loading to increase the serum sodium by 2–3 mmol/kg may suppress arrhythmias.

- Class 1A and 1C anti-arrhythmic drugs exacerbate the arrhythmias by their membrane-stabilizing effects and are contraindicated.
- Magnesium chloride (0.2 mmol/kg 12-hourly i.v.), isoprenaline infusion or pacing are used to control torsade de pointes.
- β-blockers and amiodarone may be tried for supraventricular tachycardia.
- amiodarone for VEBs.
- Heart block is managed by temporary transvenous pacing.

REFERENCES

1 Tosi MF, Cates KL. Immunologic and phagocytic responses to infection. In: Feigin RD, Cherry JD (eds) *Textbook of Pediatric Infectious Diseases*, 4th edn. Philadelphia: WB Saunders; 1998: pp. 14–53.
2 Roberton DM. The child who is immunodeficient. In: Robinson MJ, Roberton DM (eds) *Practical Paediatrics*, 4th edn. Edinburgh: Churchill Livingstone; 1998: pp. 392–9.
3 Lewis DB, Wilson CB. Developmental immunology and role of host defenses in neonatal susceptibility to infection. In: Remington JS, Klein JO (eds) *Infectious Diseases of the Fetus and Newborn Infant*, 4th edn. Philadelphia: WB Saunders; 1995: pp. 20–98.
4 Mahony L. Development of myocardial structure and function. In: Allen HD, Gutgesell HP, Clark EB, Driscoll DJ (eds) *Moss and Adams' Heart Disease in Infants, Children and Adolescents*. Philadelphia: Lippincott, Williams and Wilkins; 2001: pp. 24–40.
5 Artman M, Kithas PA, Wike JS, Strada SJ. Inotropic responses change during postnatal maturation in rabbit. *Am J Physiol* 1988; **255**(Part 2): H335–42.
6 Williams CE, Mallard C, Tan W, Gluckman PD. Pathophysiology of perinatal asphyxia. *Clin Perinatol* 1993: **20**; 305–25.
7 Mannick E, Udall JN. Neonatal gastrointestinal mucosal immunity. *Clin Perinatol* 1996; **23**: 287–304.
8 Crissinger KD, Grisham MB, Granger DN. Developmental biology of oxidant-producing enzymes and antioxidants in the piglet intestine. *Pediatr Res* 1989; **25**: 612–6.
9 Kumar A, Haery C, Parillo JE. Myocardial dysfunction in septic shock. *Crit Care Clin* 2000; **16**(2): 251–87.
10 Vincent JL. New therapeutic implications of anticoagulation mediator replacement in sepsis and acute respiratory distress syndrome. *Crit Care Med* 2000; **28**(suppl 9): S83–5.
11 Landry DW, Levin HR, Gallant EM, *et al.* Vasopressin deficiency contributes to the vasodilation of septic shock. *Circulation* 1997; **95**: 1122–5.

12 Chioléro R, Flatt J-P, Revelly J-P, Jéquier E. Effects of catecholamines on oxygen consumption and oxygen delivery in critically ill patients. *Chest* 1991; **100**: 1676–84.

13 Van den Berghe G, de Zegher F, Lauwers P. Dopamine suppresses pituitary function in infants and children. *Crit Care Med* 1994; **22**: 1747–53.

14 Van Camp JM, Tomaselli V, Coran AG. Bacterial translocation in the neonate. *Curr Opin Pediatr* 1994; **6**: 327–33.

15 Duke TD, Butt W, South M. Predictors of mortality and multiple organ failure in children with sepsis. *Intens Care Med* 1997; **23**: 684–92.

16 Marshall JC. An intensivist's dilemma: support of the splanchnic circulation in critical illness *Crit Care Med* 1998; **26**: 1637–8.

17 Beghetti M, Adatia I. Inhaled nitric oxide and congenital heart disease. *Cardiol Young* 2001; **11**: 142–52.

18 Alejandria MM, Lansang MA, Dans LF, Mantaring JBV. Intravenous immunoglobulin for treating sepsis and septic shock. *Cochrane Infectious Diseases Group. Cochrane Database of Systematic Reviews*, 2000; **2**: CD001090.

19 Sessler D, Mills P, Gregory G, Litt L, James T. Effects of bicarbonate on arterial and brain intracellular pH in neonatal rabbits recovering from hypoxic lactic acidosis. *J Pediatr* 1987; **111**: 817–23.

20 Shapiro JI, Whalen M, Kucera R, Kindig N, Filley G, Chan L. Brain pH responses to sodium bicarbonate and Carbicarb during systemic acidosis. *Am J Physiol* 1989; **256**: H1316–21.

21 Leung JM, Landow L, Franks M, *et al.* for the SPI Research Group. Safety and efficacy of intravenous Carbicarb in patients undergoing surgery: comparison with sodium bicarbonate in the treatment of mild metabolic acidosis. *Crit Care Med* 1994; **22**: 1540–9.

22 Bone RC, Fisher CJ, Clemmer TP, Slotman GJ, Metz CA, Balk RA. A controlled clinical trial of high-dose methylprednisolone in the treatment of severe sepsis and septic shock. *N Engl J Med* 1987; **317**: 653–8.

23 Hatherill M, Tibby SM, Hilliard T, Turner C, Murdoch IA. Adrenal insufficiency in septic shock. *Arch Dis Child* 1999; **80**: 51–5.

24 Bollaert P-E, Charpentier C, Levy B, Debouverie M, Audibert G, Larcan A. Reversal of late septic shock with supraphysiologic doses of hydrocortisone. *Crit Care Med* 1998; **26**: 645–50.

25 Briegel J, Forst H, Haller M, *et al.* Stress doses of hydrocortisone reverse hyperdynamic septic shock: a prospective, randomized double-blind, single-center study. *Crit Care Med* 1999; **27**: 723–32.

26 Kox WJ, Volk T, Kox SN, Volk HD. Immunomodulatory therapies in sepsis. *Intens Care Med* 2000; **26**(suppl 1): S124–8.

27 Levin M, Quint PA, Goldstein B, *et al.* Recombinant bactericidal/permeability increasing protein (rBPI$_{21}$) as adjunctive treatment for children with severe meningococcal sepsis: a randomised trial. rBPI$_{21}$ Meningococcal Sepsis Study Group. *Lancet* 2000; **356**: 961–7.

28 Leclerc F, Leteurtre S, Cremer R, Fourier C, Sadik A. Do new strategies in meningococcemia produce better outcomes? *Crit Care Med* 2000; **28**(suppl 9): S60–3.

29 Miura E, Procianoy RS, Bittar C, *et al.* A randomized, double-masked, placebo-controlled trial of recombinant granulocyte colony-stimulating factor administration to preterm infants with the clinical diagnosis of early-onset sepsis. *Pediatrics* 2001; **107**: 30–5.

30 Fourrier F, Jourdain M, Tournoys A. Clinical trial results with antithrombin III in sepsis. *Critical Care Medicine* 2000; **28**(suppl 9): S38–43.

31 Bernard GR, Vincent J-L, Laterre P-F, *et al.* Efficacy and safety of recombinant human activated protein C for severe sepsis. *New Engl J Med* 2001; **344**: 699–709.

32 Braunwald E. Heart failure. In: Fauci AS, Braunwald E, Isselbacher KJ, Wilson JD, Martin JB, Kasper DL, Hauser SL, Longo DL (eds) *Harrison's Principles of Internal Medicine*, 14th edn. 1998: pp. 1287–98.

33 O'Laughlin MP. Congestive heart failure in children. *Pediatr Clin North Am* 1999; **46**(2): 263–73.

34 Penny DJ, Shekerdemian LS. Management of the neonate with symptomatic congenital heart disease. *Arch Dis Child* 2001; **84**: F141–5.

35 Francis GS. Aldosterone inhibition and heart failure: too good to be true? *Am Heart J* 2001; **141**: 1–2.

36 Armstrong PW, Moe GW. Medical advances in the treatment of congestive heart failure. *Circulation* 1993; **88**: 2941–52.

37 Braunwald E. Expanding indications for beta-blockers in heart failure. *N Engl J Med* 2001; **344**: 1711–2.

38 Bohn D. Cardiopulmonary interactions. In: Chang AC, Hanley FL, Wernovsky G, Wessel DL (eds) *Pediatric Cardiac Intensive Care*. Baltimore: Williams and Wilkins; 1998: pp. 107–25.

39 Reddy M, Hanley FL. Mechanical support of the myocardium. In: Chang AC, Hanley FL, Wernovsky G, Wessel DL (eds) *Pediatric Cardiac Intensive Care*. Baltimore: Williams and Wilkins; 1998: pp. 345–9.

40 Vetter V. Arrhythmias. In: Moller JH, Hoffman JIE (eds). *Pediatric Cardiovascular Medicine*. New York: Churchill Livingstone; 2000: pp. 833–83.

41 Lawrence JH, Kanter RJ, Wetzel RC. Pediatric arrhythmias. In: Nichols DG, Cameron DE, Greeley WJ, Lappe DG, Ungerleider RM, Wetzel RC (eds) *Critical Heart Disease in Infants and Children*. St Louis: Mosby; 1995: pp. 217–53.

42 Ludomirsky A, Garson A. Supraventricular tachycardia. In: Gillette PC, Garson A (eds) *Pediatric Arrhythmias: Electrophysiology and Pacing*. Philadelphia: WB Saunders; 1990: pp. 380–426.

43 Perry JC, Walsh EP. Diagnosis and management of cardiac arrhythmias. In: Chang AC, Hanley FL, Wernovsky G, Wessel DL (eds) *Pediatric Cardiac Intensive Care*. Baltimore: Williams and Wilkins; 1998: pp. 461–81.

44 Pimentel L, Trommer L. Cyclic antidepressant overdoses. A review. *Emerg Med Clin North Am* 1994; **12**: 533–47.

Neurological emergencies in children
G J Knight and A J Slater

Neurological emergencies are the most common life-threatening emergencies in children. In developed societies, after the first year of life, the leading cause of death in childhood is injury, particularly traumatic brain injury. There is a range of conditions affecting the brain, spinal cord and peripheral nervous system that require prompt recognition, resuscitation and definitive management. The pathophysiology, clinical features, treatment and outcome of these acute neurological emergencies are influenced by several important differences between adults and children. These differences include response to injury, developmental maturity and capacity for growth and recovery.

PATHOPHYSIOLOGY OF BRAIN INJURIES IN CHILDREN

Brain injuries are usually caused by a primary event (e.g. trauma, ischaemia, infection or metabolic disturbance) and are frequently accompanied by secondary injuries including oedema, altered cerebrovascular autoregulation, tissue hypoxia or other cytotoxic events. It is unlikely that therapy administered after the event will influence the outcome of the primary injury. However, appropriate resuscitation and treatment and the avoidance of iatrogenic complications may prevent or reduce the impact of secondary injuries.

Features of brain injury particular to the paediatric patient are described below.

DIFFUSE CEREBRAL SWELLING

Diffuse brain swelling in the absence of oedema is a frequent early finding in paediatric brain injury, and is due to generalized cerebral vasodilation. It often resolves in 1–2 days if there is no other significant brain injury. With more severe primary traumatic injury, diffuse cerebral swelling may be accompanied by areas of contusion, multifocal petechial haemorrhage and vasogenic oedema that progress over several days.

CEREBRAL BLOOD FLOW AND METABOLISM

The cerebral perfusion pressure (CPP) represents the difference between mean arterial pressure (MAP) and intracranial pressure (ICP).

$$CPP = MAP - ICP$$

If autoregulation is disturbed as part of the illness, CPP becomes the major determinant of cerebral blood flow, particularly in areas with more severe damage. The ideal CPP in childhood is not known. The normal range of mean arterial pressure varies with age from 40 mmHg in a term neonate to 90 mmHg in an adult. The target CPP is usually adjusted with age taking into consideration the normal blood pressure for age. For example, for an adolescent patient, therapy may be directed at maintaining a CPP of 70 mmHg, while for a child aged 5 years, the aim may be to maintain a CPP of 50 mmHg.

In conditions where vasogenic oedema occurs, arterial hypertension may increase vascular shift of fluid and worsen brain swelling. However, treatment aimed at lowering arterial pressure (e.g. with vasodilators) may interfere with homeostatic mechanisms and should be used cautiously.

The brain comprises up to 12% of body weight in infancy compared with 2–3% in adulthood. Cerebral oxygen and glucose consumption is therefore proportionately greater in childhood while glycogen stores are readily depleted. Hypoglycaemia occurs commonly in severe illnesses such as sepsis, therefore blood glucose should be monitored regularly.

HYPOVOLAEMIA

Children have small blood volumes and commonly develop hypovolaemia from scalp bleeding or intracranial haemorrhage. For example, hypovolaemia will develop in a 5-kg infant (blood volume 400 ml) following blood loss of only 100 ml. Hypovolaemia should be treated aggressively with fluid boluses of 20 ml/kg to ensure adequate cerebral perfusion.

RELATIVE GROWTH

The child's short stature and proportionately large head confer a number of risks. The toddler's head is at the level of the front of a motor vehicle and isolated head injury is subsequently common following pedestrian injury in this age group. The neck muscles are relatively weak in infancy and they support a large head. This renders the brain prone to deceleration injury in motor vehicle crashes and in cases of domestic violence. Injury inflicted by shaking an infant by the shoulders snaps the head to and fro leading to compression of brain tissue and rupture of delicate bridging veins.

BONE DEVELOPMENT[1]

The skull bones in the first year of life are thin with open sutures and open fontanelles. Beyond the age of 2 years, the skull sutures close and the cranial vault thickens. In young children, there tends to be less bony protection from high impact trauma, while the non-rigid skull may expand to partially decompress expanding lesions.

UNDIAGNOSED COMA

An ordered approach to diagnosis and treatment is required for a child with depressed conscious state of unknown origin. This approach must consider common life-threatening and rare treatable diseases (Table 100.1).

INITIAL MANAGEMENT

Management should always begin with rapid assessment of the adequacy of airway, ventilation and circulation. If

Table 100.1 Causes of coma in children

Structural	Metabolic
Trauma	Post-ictal state
accidental	Infection
inflicted	meningitis
Hydrocephalus	encephalitis
Haemorrhage	Drugs and toxins
AVM	Hypoxia-ischaemia
aneurysms	Circulatory shock
tumour	Biochemical
Tumour	hypoglycaemia
Cerebral abscess	electrolyte disorders
	sodium/water
	calcium
	acid-base disturbance
	Hyperthermia
	Hepatic failure
	Haemolytic-uremic syndrome
	Inborn errors of metabolism
	Reye's syndrome

inadequacies are detected, interventions aimed at correcting them should occur immediately. Once venous access is obtained, blood should be drawn for routine tests including immediate measurement of bloodglucose. If hypoglycaemia is demonstrated 2 ml/kg of 25% glucose or 5 ml/kg of 10% glucose should be given intravenously as the neurological sequelae of unrecognized hypoglycaemia can be profound.

Concurrent with the initial assessment and resuscitation, relevant details of the present and past history should be obtained. A detailed neurological and general physical examination should be performed. It is important to document accurately the conscious state so that changes over time, particularly deterioration, can be easily recognized. The Glasgow Coma Scale (GCS) is appropriate for this purpose. The responses of children change with development and therefore the GCS requires modification for paediatric use (Table 100.2). After completing the clinical assessment, the likely diagnosis is often apparent and appropriate investigation and treatment can commence. Multiple factors may compound to produce coma. For example, a child with severe gastroenteritis may have hyperthermia, hyponatraemic dehydration, metabolic acidosis and hypovolaemic shock.

CONTROLLED VENTILATION

Indications for ventilating a comatose child are:

- Upper airway obstruction or loss of airway reflexes
- Apnoea, respiratory failure
- Rapidly worsening coma
- Signs of progressive elevation of ICP (ie bradycardia, hypertension, abnormal pupillary light reflexes and localizing signs)

Once ventilation is initiated the stomach should be drained with a gastric tube and blood pressure checked every 5 min. Raised ICP should be considered in any case of rapidly progressive coma. Intracranial hypertension should be managed with moderate hyperventilation and intravenous (i.v.) mannitol (0.25 g/kg). Hypertonic saline given as 0.5 ml/kg of 20% solution (3.4 mmol/ml) can also rapidly reduce ICP.[2] Once stability is achieved, adequate sedation and analgesia is required. Muscle relaxants may be necessary to facilitate ventilation and prevent straining; however, their use precludes further neurological assessment and therefore, if long acting muscle relaxants are continued, ICP monitoring is advisable. Hyperventilation is a short-term manoeuvre and following the early resuscitation phase, gradual return to a low-normal arterial blood partial pressure should be the aim. This is best achieved with endtidal CO_2 and ICP monitoring. Particular attention should be paid to restoring intravascular volume and maintaining an adequate cerebral perfusion pressure.

Table 100.2 Glasgow Coma scale for children

Glasgow Coma Scale (4–15 years)		Child's Glasgow Coma Scale (< 4 years)	
Response	Score	Response	Score
Eye opening		Eye opening	
Spontaneously	4	Spontaneously	4
To verbal stimuli	3	To verbal stimuli	3
To pain	2	To pain	2
No response to pain	1	No response to pain	1
Best motor response		Best motor response	
Obeys verbal command	6	Spontaneous or obeys verbal command	6
Localizes to pain	5	Localizes to pain or withdraws to touch	5
Withdraws from pain	4	Withdraws from pain	4
Abnormal flexion to pain (decorticate)	3	Abnormal flexion to pain (decorticate)	3
Abnormal extension to pain (decerebrate)	2	Abnormal extension to pain (decerebrate)	2
No response to pain	1	No response to pain	1
Best verbal response		Best verbal response	
Orientated and converses	5	Alert, babbles, coos, words to usual ability	5
Disorientated and converses	4	Less than usual words, spontaneous irritable cry	4
Inappropriate words	3	Cries only to pain	3
Incomprehensible sounds	2	Moans to pain	2
No response to pain	1	No response to pain	1

CRANIAL COMPUTERIZED TOMOGRAPHY (CT)

A CT scan is required in comatose children with localizing signs and in those in whom the diagnosis is not clear. A CT should also be performed if the conscious state is abnormal and there is history of trauma. Even if the general condition does not warrant controlled ventilation, a CT is often best performed under general anaesthesia. Unwanted movement will cause poor quality images and sedation alone may place the child at risk of hypoventilation or aspiration.

LUMBAR PUNCTURE

Lumbar puncture (LP) should be performed when there is reasonable suspicion of meningitis or encephalitis. The risks and contraindications to LP are discussed under bacterial meningitis.

ADDITIONAL INVESTIGATIONS

Additional investigations include arterial blood gas analysis, electrolytes, urea and creatinine, liver function tests, serum ammonia, serum and cerbrospinal fluid (CSF) lactate and pyruvate and urine analysis. Appropriate screening of blood and urine will exclude common poisons and drug intoxications.

SPECIFIC TREATMENT

The clinical signs and results of investigations generally guide treatment. If hypoglycaemia occurs, after initial correction, care should be taken to ensure that it does not recur by the administration of appropriate glucose containing i.v. fluid and regular blood glucose monitoring. Herpes simplex encephalitis can present in many ways and is not excluded by the absence of CSF pleocytosis. Acyclovir therapy should therefore be considered in any patient in whom herpes cannot be confidently excluded.

STATUS EPILEPTICUS

Status epilepticus is usually defined as a continuous convulsion lasting 30 min or longer or repeated convulsions lasting 30 min or longer without recovery of consciousness between convulsions.[3] The common causes of status epilepticus in children are:

- prolonged febrile convulsion
- epilepsy associated with either first presentation or anticonvulsant withdrawal or intercurrent illness, often with fever
- central nervous system infection (i.e. meningitis or encephalitis)
- metabolic disturbance (e.g. hypoglycaemia, hyponatraemia, hypocalcaemia)
- trauma, including inflicted injury.

PATHOPHYSIOLOGY

Many physiological changes occur during prolonged seizures. There is an initial phase of compensation lasting less than 30 min. Following a period of transition, there is a phase of decompensation commencing between 30 and 60 min and evolving over hours. Physiological changes during the compensated phase include tachycardia, hypertension, increased catecholamine release and increased cardiac output. Changes within the brain include increased cerebral blood flow and increased cerebral utilization of glucose and oxygen. After 30–60 min, the mechanisms for homeostatic compensation fail. During the decompensated phase, there may be falling blood pressure and cardiac output, hypoglycaemia, hypoxia, acidosis, electrolyte disturbance and rhabdomyolysis. The cerebral physiology is characterized by failing autoregulation and reduced cerebral blood flow and oxygen and glucose utilization. Over hours, a deficit in brain energy develops and this is associated with the development of brain damage.[4]

EXCITATORY AMINOACIDS AND BRAIN INJURY

Mesial temporal sclerosis is the most common acquired brain lesion following status epilepticus. There is evidence that the accumulation of a number of excitatory and inhibitory amino acids have a role pathophysiology of neuronal injury. In particular, glutamate accumulation and stimulation of N-methyl-D-aspartate receptors leads to an influx of intracellular calcium, which triggers a number of cytotoxic events and, ultimately, cell death.[5]

MANAGEMENT

The initial management is as for other neurological emergencies with attention to airway and oxygenation. Most seizures in childhood cease spontaneously in a short time, but if they persist for 5 min or continue after presentation to an emergency department, they should be stopped to avoid metabolic and ischaemic neuronal damage. Hypoglycaemia should be excluded or detected early. If i.v. access cannot be obtained rapidly, drugs can be administered intramuscularly, rectally or via the intra-osseous (i.o.) route. Specific drug treatment is described below.

BENZODIAZEPINES

Diazepam, midazolam and lorazepam are the most useful agents. Diazepam is given initially as 0.2 mg/kg i.v./i.o., and repeated up to 0.5 mg/kg. If venous access cannot be secured it can be given per rectum. The recommended rectal dose is higher than the i.v. dose (0.5 mg/kg p.r.). Excessive sedation and respiratory depression occur with larger doses and must be dealt with effectively. Lorazepam (0.05–0.1 mg/kg i.v.) may have advantages over diazepam as it is as effective, has a longer half-life, and causes less respiratory depression.[6,7] Midazolam and clonazepam are also effective. When i.v. access is not available, intramuscular administration of midazolam is an alternative to rectal diazepam.[8] In children presenting to

an emergency department who are still convulsing, 0.2 mg/kg i.m. of midazolam has been reported to control 83% of seizures within 5 min of administration and 93% of seizures within 10 min[9]. Midazolam has also been used by constant i.v. infusion (1–5 µg/kg/min) to control refractory status epilepticus in children.[10,11]

PHENYTOIN

Phenytoin should be commenced if benzodiazepines are not effective. It is given as 20 mg/kg i.v. over 30 min, which is followed by a maintenance dose (4 mg/kg 8-hourly past the neonatal period). It causes minimal sedation or respiratory depression, but is not suitable in neonates and in patients who are already on maintenance doses. Because it is given slowly, phenytoin will not have rapid effects and, if generalized status epilepticus persists, consideration should be given to the use of thiopentone (see below). Fosphenytoin, a prodrug of phenytoin, can be administered intramuscularly and has less irritant effect when given i.v.[12] Its place in the management of status epilepticus in children is not yet clear.[13]

PHENOBARBITONE

When phenytoin is contraindicated, phenobarbitone (20 mg/kg i.v. over 30 min) should be given. Respiratory depression and hypotension occur, particularly after benzodiazepines. Further doses can be safely administered to the ventilated child who has ongoing seizures.

THIOPENTONE

If seizures are prolonged and are not controlled by benzodiazepines, thiopentone 2–5 mg/kg slowly i.v., then 1–5 mg/kg per hour by continuous infusion into a central vein can be given. Appropriately skilled staff and suitable equipment are necessary as thiopentone necessitates endotracheal intubation and mechanical ventilation, and possibly inotropic drugs to counter its myocardial depressant effects. Blood concentrations need to be monitored during prolonged use. Whenever muscle relaxants are used, they should be short-acting to ensure ongoing seizure activity is not masked. Seizures are only controlled by anaesthetic doses of thiopentone.

PARALDEHYDE

In many centres, rectal paraldehyde (0.4 ml/kg mixed with an equal quantity of olive oil) is frequently used in the management of status.[13] One advantage of paraldehyde is that, similar to diazepam, it can be administered rectally if i.v. access is difficult to obtain.

OTHER MANAGEMENT

The patient must be protected from self-injury during seizures. Severe respiratory and metabolic acidosis are common and are best managed by rapid control of the seizure and maintenance of adequate ventilation and oxygenation. Once seizures are controlled, the cause should be sought. A detailed history is invaluable. A CT scan should reveal structural lesions. An LP should be deferred if the child is unconscious after a seizure. However, if the conscious state improves, and there are no signs of raised ICP (see below), an LP will confirm or exclude meningitis. When the diagnosis remains unclear, viral encephalitis (herpes, enterovirus), metabolic encephalopathy, poisoning and inflicted injury should be considered.

OUTCOME

The outcome of status epilepticus is dependent on the aetiology. Neurologically normal children in whom status epilepticus is precipitated by fever are considered to have a good prognosis. The incidence of neurological deficits or cognitive impairment in this group is very low.[5] Persistent neurological deficits occur more frequently when seizures are symptomatic of other brain pathology; however, in this setting, it is very difficult to tease out the extent to which prolonged seizures contribute to neurological sequelae.

BACTERIAL MENINGITIS

PATHOPHYSIOLOGY

Bacterial meningitis (BM) usually occurs following haematogenous spread of organisms carried in the nasopharynx. In childhood, the common bacteria causing BM are *Streptococcus pneumoniae*, *Neisseria meningitidis* and *Haemophilus influenza* type b (Hib). Immunization has significantly reduced the incidence of Hib meningitis.[14,15] *Group B streptococcus*, *E. coli* and *Listeria monocytogenes* are the most common causative organisms of neonatal BM. Occasionally, meningitis occurs as a complication of other pathology such as base of skull fracture, chronic middle ear infection or infection of a congenital dermoid sinus.

In the early stages of the disease, cerebral hyperaemia occurs. This can be followed by cerebral ischaemia, which may occur by several different mechanisms. Local vasculitis of vessels transversing the subarachnoid space can progress to arterial thrombosis and focal infarction. Other vascular abnormalities, including vasospasm and sagittal sinus thrombosis, can also occur. Cerebral oedema is relatively common in meningitis and is caused by a combination of vasogenic, cytotoxic and hydrostatic factors. If cerebral oedema is severe, raised ICP and impaired cerebral perfusion can occur leading to global cerebral ischaemia.

CLINICAL FEATURES

In children, the typical features of BM are fever, headache, photophobia, neck stiffness and vomiting. The history may extend over several days; however, in fulminant cases, the time from first symptom to coma

and death may be only a few hours. Neonates and young infants do not present with the typical localized symptoms and signs. Instead, they present with generalized signs of illness including lethargy, poor feeding and pallor. Generalized or focal convulsions or apnoea may be present at presentation. Tuberculous meningitis usually presents with a more insidious onset of symptoms and may be associated with focal neurological signs.

Complications occur commonly in BM. During the early phase, meningitis may be associated with septic shock and disseminated intravascular coagulation. Fluid and electrolyte abnormalities are relatively common, particularly hyponatraemia and hypoglycaemia. Focal and generalized convulsions are relatively common and may progress to status epilepticus. During the recovery phase, subdural effusions or hydrocephalus may occur.

INVESTIGATIONS

LP for CSF microscopy, culture and bacterial antigen testing is required for definitive diagnosis of BM and to guide antibiotic therapy. While a lumbar puncture can be performed safely in the majority of children with BM, LP may precipitate brainstem herniation if raised ICP is present.[16] Identifying children at risk of this complication is difficult; however, it is generally recommended that empiric antibiotic therapy be commenced and LP deferred if any of the following clinical features are present: depressed conscious state, decorticate or decerebrate posturing, focal neurological signs or other signs of raised ICP. A normal CT scan does not exclude the possibility of elevated ICP.[16] Therefore, the decision to defer an LP should be based on clinical rather than radiological signs. In addition to signs of increased ICP, other indications for deferring the LP include cardiorespiratory instability and severe coagulopathy.

If LP is deferred, alternative methods of establishing a bacterial diagnosis include blood culture and bacterial antigen testing in urine and polymerase chain reaction (PCR) testing of blood.[17,18]

MANAGEMENT

RESUSCITATION

Severely ill patients require rapid resuscitation. Comatose patients require intubation and ventilation to prevent airway obstruction and hypoventilation. Hypovalaemia should be treated rapidly with boluses of fluid. Patients with septic shock will also require inotropic support.

CEREBRAL RESUSCITATION

General principles of supporting brain injury apply to BM. These include optimizing cerebral oxygen delivery, controlling ICP and preventing cerebral metabolic stress. The role of ICP monitoring is controversial. There is some anecdotal evidence to support the use of ICP monitoring in a small number of selected cases. Unfortunately, there are no large studies that assess the benefit or harm of ICP monitoring and ICP targeted therapy in BM.

ANTIBIOTIC THERAPY

Empiric broad-spectrum antibiotics should be selected based on likely pathogens and local resistance patterns. A common protocol for BM is to use ampicillin plus cefotaxime for the first month of life and to use a third generation cephalosporine (cefotaxime or ceftriaxone) after the first month.[19] In regions where penicillin and cephalosporin resistant pneumcoccus occurs, vancomycin should be added to the initial empiric antibiotics until the causative organism is identified and the antibiotic sensitivities are known.

ADJUVANT THERAPY

A number of adjuvant therapies have been investigated experimentally; however, the only one that is commonly used clinically is dexamethasone. If dexamethasone is used, it should ideally be given before the first dose of antibiotics and continued for 48 hours (0.4 mg/kg 12-hourly).[20] There is evidence that dexamethasone reduces the incidence of neurological sequelae and sensineural deafness; however, the benefits have only been reported in Hib meningitis.[21,22] Now that immunization has changed the epidemiology, and antibiotic resistant pneumococcal strains are more common, it is possible that the relationship between risk and benefit of dexamethasone therapy has changed. Therefore, the role of dexamethasone in BM remains controversial.[23]

FLUID THERAPY

There is consensus that hypovolaemia should be treated rapidly and aggressively; however, fluid therapy after the initial resuscitation is controversial. Restriction of maintenance fluids has been commonly practised. Hyponatraemia is common in BM and, if it is assumed that this is secondary to the syndrome of inappropriate antidiuretic hormone secretion (SIADH), then fluid restriction is logical. However, recent evidence suggests that ADH is appropriately elevated in response to hypovolaemia[24] and that hyponatraemic patients with BM tend to be more dehydrated than normo-natraemic patients.[25] Compared to fluid restriction, fluid therapy aimed at providing maintenance plus the fluid deficit has been reported to result in a more rapid correction of sodium and ADH.[24,26] Although these studies suggest fluid restriction may not benefit all children with BM, it is important that fluid is restricted in patients with BM and true SIADH, as maintenance fluid therapy in these patients will cause the serum sodium to fall further. This complication is potentially life-threatening, with the progressive fall in sodium precipitating seizures and

worsening cerebral oedema. Therefore, sodium should be monitored closely during the first 24–48 h of therapy in all patients with BM.

CHEMOPROPHHYLAXIS FOR CONTACTS

Prophylaxis is required for every household member in cases of meningococcal infection, and in cases of haemophilus infection when there is another child in the household aged under 5 years who is unimmunized. Rifampicin (10 mg/kg to a maximum of 600 mg b.d.) for 2 days in meningococcal disease or 4 days in haemophilus disease is appropriate. Neonates require 10 mg/kg per day. Pregnant women can be effectively managed with a single intramuscular dose of ceftriaxone (250 mg). Ciprafloxacillin (15 mg/kg to a maximum of 750 mg) is also effective and has the advantage of single dose therapy.[27]

OUTCOME

BM is associated with significant mortality and morbidity. Overall mortality for BM in childhood is 5–10 %; however, in children requiring mechanical ventilation, a mortality rate of 30% has been reported with major neurosequelae occurring in 33% of survivors.[28]

ENCEPHALITIS

Common causes of encephalitis include enteroviruses, mycoplasma, cytomegalovirus, herpes, Epstein–Barr and respiratory viruses (adenovirus and parainfluenzae). The most significant causes world-wide are the insect transmitted arbovirus encephalitides including Australian, Japanese B and St Louis. These can cause profound coma and are associated with significant incidence of residual neurological deficit.

Presenting symptoms of encephalitis include seizures, focal neurological deficits in the setting of an acute febrile illness, confusion and coma. Meningeal irritation may not be obvious. CSF analysis may show a pleocytosis and, in the early phase, this can consist predominantly of neutrophils. As previously mentioned, herpes is the most important diagnosis to make, because it is treatable. Electroencephalography, CT and magnetic resonance imaging (MRI) are helpful in making the diagnosis. MRI is more sensitive than CT for detecting signs of encephalitis, particularly during the early stages of the illness. PCR on CSF may also aid rapid diagnosis[29,30.] Acyclovir used early improves outcome and should be commenced when the diagnosis is suspected.

The enteroviruses are important causes of encephalitis in children. In addition, they cause other acute neurological illnesses including acute flaccid paralysis due to transverse myelitis and Guillain–Barré syndrome.[31] Pleconaril is a promising new antiviral agent that appears to have clinical benefit in enteroviral infections, including central nervous system disease.[32] Outcome of viral encephalitis is worse in infancy than in older age groups.[33]

NON-TRAUMATIC INTRACRANIAL HAEMORRHAGE

Non-traumatic intracranial haemorrhage (ICH) is uncommon in children. Arteriovenous malformations (AVM) are a more common cause of haemorrhage in children than aneurysms[34] (Table 100.3). The presenting features are similar to those seen in adults, and include sudden severe headache, altered conscious state and seizures. Diagnosis can usually be made by CT scan. Raised ICP, if present, is managed in the usual manner. A mass lesion or acute obstructive hydrocephalus requires neurosurgical assessment. Following diagnosis of ICH, further investigations may be required to clarify the underlying cause. These include coagulation profile and platelet count. Angiographic images can be obtained with CT, magnetic resonance angiography or digital subtraction. In some cases, definitive cerebral angiography may be required to define the underlying vascular malformation or tumour. Definitive surgery or endovascular treatment of an AVM can be planned once the underlying lesion has been defined. A period of close observation is required as children may be at greater risk of rebleeding from an AVM than adults.[35] The efficacy of therapies (e.g. calcium channel blockers) used to prevent vasospasm in adults has not been studied in children with aneurysmal haemorrhage. Sequelae of ICH include hemiparesis, aphasia, seizures and hydrocephalus.

Table 100.3 Aetiology of spontaneous intracranial haemorrhage in children

Vascular malformations
  AVM
  capillary telangiectasia
  cavernous malformation
  venous malformation
Aneurysm
  'berry'
  mycotic
  post-traumatic
Coagulopathy
  thrombocytopaenia
  haemophilia
  anticoagulant therapy
Tumours
  gliomas
Hypertension

HYPOXIC-ISCHAEMIC ENCEPHALOPATHY

AETIOLOGY

The most common causes of hypoxic-ischaemic encephalopathy outside the neonatal period are:

- near-miss sudden infant death syndrome
- immersion
- accidents, including drug ingestion and strangulation
- inflicted injury.

PATHOLOGY

The brain depends on an uninterrupted supply of oxygen and glucose to produce, via aerobic glycolysis, sufficient high-energy adenosine triphosphate (ATP) to maintain neuronal membrane and synthetic function. Under anoxic conditions, anaerobic glycolysis occurs which produces lactic acid but less ATP (by 18 times). Because there are virtually no stores of ATP, rapid neuronal failure ensues. If ischaemia accompanies hypoxia, there is associated failure of both substrate delivery and metabolic waste removal, which amplifies the cellular insult. Ischaemia produces coma in less than 10 s and cerebral damage in as little as 2 min.

Following restoration of cerebral blood flow, there is a period of relative hyperaemia followed by relative hypoperfusion. Animal studies suggest that the blood flow during this phase of post-ischaemic hypoperfusion is determined by the metabolic needs of the brain.[36] Cytotoxic cerebral oedema may subsequently develop, but significant elevation of ICP is unusual unless ischaemia and damage are profound.

MANAGEMENT

The principles of therapy are similar to those for other brain injuries. It is mandatory to provide rapid cardio-pulmonary resuscitation and prevent secondary insults. In cases of out of hospital cardiac arrest, full resuscitation must be attempted while the history is sought. A number of factors need to be addressed during this phase. The stomach may contain large volumes of water and air following immersion and should be drained. Pulmonary aspiration of water or gastric contents is also common although, in 10–15% of children, early laryngospasm causes 'dry drowning'. Haemodynamic disturbance may develop because of primary cardiac dysfunction or hypovolaemia secondary to bowel fluid loss (ischaemic diarrhoea). Circulating volume should be restored and inotropic agents considered. Normothermia should be achieved but care taken to avoid hyperthermia. Comatose patients with hyper or hypotonia and a GCS <8 are probably best managed by mechanical ventilation, sedation and paralysis for 1–2 days although benefits are not proven. The role of ICP measurement is limited as correlation between ICP and outcome is poor.[37] Barbiturate coma and induced hypothermia are also of no proven value and increase the risk of sepsis.[38] Hyperglycaemia has been associated with a worse prognosis and, although it may simply be a marker of injury severity, active treatment has been advocated.

PROGNOSIS

The major determinants of recovery are:

- ischaemic time
- cerebral metabolic rate
- quality of resuscitation.

In immersion injuries in young children, full recovery may be possible despite prolonged ischaemia if sufficient rapid cerebral cooling has occurred. In these cases, the onset of ischaemia may be delayed by bradycardia with preferential cerebral flow (the 'diving reflex'). In general, survival from out of hospital cardiac arrest is unlikely, even with expert cardiopulmonary resuscitation (CPR), if asystole is present on arrival at hospital.[39] The rare exception is the hypothermic child who presents following immersion; prolonged CPR may be justified in selected cases when profound hypothermia was induced rapidly. If cardiac output is present on arrival at hospital, with either flexion or extension to pain, recovery is likely. Normothermic patients, who present apnoeic, flaccid and unresponsive to pain, are likely to die or have serious neurological deficits. This group is also prone to further deterioration several days after the insult, with progression of cerebral oedema.[37] Coma persisting for more than 24 h is a predictor of poor prognosis and minimal long-term improvement is likely in this group.[40] Residual neurological deficits present at the end of the first week are less likely to improve following ischaemic injury than following traumatic brain injury.

A number of ancillary tests have been investigated as predictors of neurological outcome. Somatosensory evoked potentials (SEPs) performed at the bedside are the most useful aid to prediction. One report of 109 children with severe brain injury concluded that, with appropriate patient selection, the positive predictive value for poor outcome of bilaterally absent SEPs is 100% (95% confidence interval 0.92–1.0).[41]

GUILLAIN–BARRÉ SYNDROME

CLINICAL FEATURES

Guillain–Barré syndrome (GBS) is the most common cause of acute motor paralysis in children. Although most patients develop typical ascending, symmetrical areflexic weakness, GBS may present insidiously with apparent lethargy or loss of motor milestones in the young child. There may also be rapid progression and admission criteria to the intensive care unit include respiratory failure, bulbar palsy, severe autonomic disturbance or rapidly progressive weakness. Sensory loss is usually minimal and transient. Pain in the back and legs, possibly neurogenic in origin, is common and may be the presenting feature.[42] This pain may be severe and is often difficult to control. Papilloedema and encephalopathy occasionally occur.[43] The complications of deep venous thrombosis and thromboembolism are not common problems in children.

INVESTIGATIONS

CSF protein is generally elevated after the first week and nerve conduction studies may also be useful.

MANAGEMENT

Adequate respiratory care is the basis of minimizing morbidity and mortality in GBS. Up to one-third of patients require ventilatory support and, ideally, mechanical ventilation should be undertaken electively. Early indications are an apparent increased work of breathing, fatigue, poor cough and progressive bulbar palsy. Hypercarbia is a late sign and should be avoided. In children that are old enough to co-operate, forced vital capacity (FVC) should be monitored during the progressive phase of the illness. Mechanical ventilation should be considered if FVC falls below 15–20 ml/kg. Careful frequent clinical assessment is necessary. Once mechanically ventilated, many patients require some degree of hyperventilation to prevent 'air hunger'. Although nasotracheal intubation is satisfactory initially, a tracheostomy should be performed if recovery is delayed. This will improve comfort and allow speech via pressure-generated ventilation and an air leak around the tracheostomy tube. Successful weaning is unlikely unless vital capacity exceeds 12 ml/kg and maximum negative inspiratory force is at least 20 cmH$_2$O (2 kPa).

Autonomic dysfunction is an important cause of morbidity and mortality in children with GBS. Airway manipulation or induction of anaesthesia, particularly in the presence of hypoxia, may provoke serious cardiac arrhythmias. Fluctuating blood pressure, urinary retention and gut dysfunction also occur.

Plasmapheresis and i.v. immunoglobulin (IVIG) are effective therapies. The indications for either are rapid progression, respiratory insufficiency or weakness to the point of being unable to walk unassisted. Plasmapheresis reduces the duration of ventilation required in adults and small studies support its efficacy in children.[44,45] However IVIG is as effective as plasma exchange in adults and, in a study in children, IVIG (1 g/kg for 2 days) appeared as effective as daily plasma exchanges of 200–250 ml/kg.[46,47] Because it has significant potential advantages over plasmapheresis, IVIG is generally the first line therapy in children. Both therapies have been used concurrently or sequentially, although additional benefit of the combination has not been proven.

The problems of long-term ventilation in a conscious patient compounded by emotional immaturity, speech failure, fear of procedures and family disruption make the management of a child with GBS and their family particularly challenging. A sensitive team approach is essential.

PROGNOSIS

The prognosis in acute GBS may be better for children than adults. Full recovery is likely if the time from maximal deficit to onset of recovery is less than 18 days. However, complete recovery, despite a longer plateau phase, has been reported.[48] Good recovery can occur in patients who have required ventilation and the need for ventilation may not be a poor prognostic factor in children.[44] Those presenting with a subacute course are at risk of relapses and permanent motor deficits.

METABOLIC ENCEPHALOPATHY

Approximately 0.1% of babies have an inborn error of metabolism. Acute encephalopathy is one of the many ways neurometabolic diseases present in childhood.[49,50] In general, acute presentations occur in the neonatal period and early infancy. Symptoms are often vague and include lethargy, poor feeding and vomiting. Older infants and children more commonly present with a chronic encephalopathy, with features that may include seizures, long-tract signs, visual impairment and loss of milestones.

APPROACH TO DIAGNOSIS

A careful history and examination may elicit clues to a possible metabolic problem. Family history and history of drug exposure are extremely important. Valproate, in particular, has been associated with a Reye-like illness. The following readily available investigations are useful to allow a broad categorization and direct further detailed investigations: blood gas analysis, blood sugar,

Table 100.4 Biochemical markers of metabolic disorders

Biochemical marker	Disorder
Hypoglycaemia	Organic acidurias
	methylmalonic/propionic
	acidaemia
	Reye's syndrome
	Fat oxidation defects
	MCAD
Ketoacidosis	Diabetes mellitus
	Organic acidurias
Lactic acidosis	Mitochondrial encephalomyopathies
	respiratory chain disorders
	pyruvate carboxylase deficiency
Hyperammonaemia	Reye's syndrome
(2–3 × normal)	Urea cycle defects
	Fat oxidation defects
	MCAD
	Organic acidurias

serum ammonia, serum lactate, urine metabolic screen and urine ketones. While lactic acidosis and hypoglycaemia can occur in a number of disease states, including sepsis, persisting abnormalities require further investigation. This is best performed in collaboration with a metabolic disease specialist or a clinical biochemist.

Lactic acidosis can be further assessed with measurement of lactate : pyruvate ratio and urine biochemical analysis may provide further diagnostic information (Table 100.4).

ASSESSMENT

Metabolic coma can be staged using Lovejoy's classification for Reye's syndrome (Table 100.5).[51]

MANAGEMENT

Initial management is largely supportive. Metabolic derangements, such as acidosis and hypoglycaemia, should be corrected. Acute intracranial hypertension should be managed with mechanical ventilation while the

Table 100.5 Staging in metabolic encephalopathy

Stage	Coma	Pain response	Reflexes
1	lethargy	normal	normal
2	combative	variable	pupils sluggish
3	coma	decorticate	pupils sluggish
4	coma	decerebrate	pupils sluggish
			abnormal occulocephalic
5	coma	flaccid	no pupil response
			absent occulocephalic

Adapted from NIH, modification of Lovejoy.[51]

role of ICP monitoring is controversial. Hyperammon-aemia should be managed with limited protein intake initially. In certain circumstances, increasing ammonia metabolism using agents such as arginine and sodium benzoate is helpful. In some settings, providing calories intravenously in the form of glucose and fat may help limit the extent of catabolism and thereby help to curtail the metabolic crisis. Dialysis is used to control severe hyperammonaemia and acidosis. Continuous venovenous haemodiafiltration is considered more effective than peritoneal dialysis.[52]

REYE'S SYNDROME AND REYE-LIKE ILLNESS

Reye's syndrome is a rare disorder, occurring almost exclusively in children. It is characterized by an acute encephalopathy with brain swelling and fatty degeneration of viscera, especially the liver. Typically, the patient presents with intractable vomiting followed by progressive encephalopathy. There is an association with aspirin use and a preceding varicella infection. Diagnosis can be made when a compatible history accompanies hyperammonaemia and elevation of serum hepatocellular enzymes to at least twice normal, but with a normal bilirubin concentration. Hypoglycaemia occurs in patients aged under 2 years. Management consists of correction of hypoglycaemia, neurological monitoring and management of raised ICP.

A wide range of conditions has been described that closely mimic typical Reye's syndrome. Ten percent of cases originally described as being Reye's syndrome were subsequently found to be due to an inherited metabolic disorder.[53] A careful approach is mandatory to ensure detection of inherited disorders.

The introduction of neonatal screening programs using tandem mass spectrometry will see many inherited metabolic diseases diagnosed in the neonatal period, often before the onset of symptoms. This technology is particularly useful for detecting fatty acid oxidation defects (e.g. medium-chain acyl-coenzyme A dehydrogenase deficiency) and disorders of amino acid metabolism (e.g. methylmalonic acidaemia).[54]

SPINAL INJURY

INCIDENCE

Paediatric spinal trauma is relatively rare, comprising <5% of all spinal injuries. Approximately 5% of children with severe head trauma will have a cervical spine injury. However, a high proportion of children who die following motor vehicle trauma, particularly those who suffer immediate cardiorespiratory arrest, or who die before arrival at hospital, have disruption of the spinal cord above C3, particularly at the cervico-medullary junction.[55,56]

AETIOLOGY

The commonest causes of paediatric spinal trauma are motor vehicle accidents, either as a pedestrian or passenger, falls and especially diving accidents. Sports related injuries are uncommon.

PATHOPHYSIOLOGY

The patterns of spinal injury in children differ from those seen in adults in many ways. Spinal cord injury without radiographic abnormality (SCIWORA) occurs almost exclusively in children (20–60% of spinal cord injuries). It is associated with a high incidence of complete neurological deficit. Spinal injury in the first decade occurs most commonly in the first two cervical segments, with atlanto-axial rotatory subluxation, bony or ligamentous injuries, or SCIWORA and severe cord injury. However, lower cervical injuries below C4 do occur and have been reported to comprise up to 50% of cases.[57] Injury may occur at more than one level. Atlanto-axial rotatory subluxation is rarely associated with neurological deficit and ligamentous injury is more likely than high cervical fractures to be associated with permanent neurological deficit.[58] As the bony spine matures, the pattern of injury becomes more adult-like with lower cervical and thoracic injuries seen in the second decade.[59]

CLINICAL FEATURES

The immediate effects of spinal cord damage are similar at any age. Frequently, an associated head injury can render clinical assessment extremely difficult; and confirmation of cord injury is sometimes delayed. Clues to the diagnosis in the unconscious patient include:

- flaccidity, immobility and areflexia below the level of the lesion
- hypoventilation with paradoxical chest movement; this occurs if intercostal muscles are paralysed and the phrenic nerves are intact (in the absence of airway obstruction)
- apnoea with rhythmic flaring of the alae nasi (Duncan's sign), seen when the lesion is above C3
- hypotension with inappropriate bradycardia and cutaneous vasodilatation below the level of injury, due to absent spinal sympathetic outflow
- priapism, which occurs frequently.

There may be visible or palpable evidence of trauma to the spine and surrounding soft tissues, including retropharyngeal or retrolaryngeal haematomas. Spinal shock is common with temporary complete loss of function. As this resolves after 3–5 days, reflexes progressively return, usually starting with bulbocavernosus and anal reflexes.

Incomplete lesions, including the Brown–Sequard cord hemisection, and anterior and central cord syndromes may become apparent at this stage.

INVESTIGATIONS

Resuscitation, including emergency intubation, should not be delayed to perform X-rays. However, the entire spinal column should subsequently be X-rayed to demonstrate the presence of subluxation, fractures, or dislocations. MRI is useful in both the acute setting and in assessment at later stages and is now accepted as the standard for identifying haemorrhage, contusion or compression of the cord. CT produces better definition of bony injuries, and may also show cord involvement by haematomas, bone fragments and foreign bodies. In cases of SCIWORA, metrizamide myelography with CT examination may reveal cord injury with soft tissue or disc involvement and dural tears. Somatosensory evoked potentials may be useful to evaluate the integrity of the spinal cord, particularly in the comatose patient.

MANAGEMENT

Achieving control of airway, ventilation and circulation is always of first priority. If tracheal intubation is indicated, and if stability of the neck is unknown, skilled assistance is necessary to immobilize the head and neck and prevent flexion or extension. Because of the sympathectomized state in high cord injuries, a relatively low blood pressure can be expected even after hypovolaemia is corrected. Significant hypotension becomes more likely the higher the lesion and the younger the patient. Haemodynamic support with a vasoconstrictor such as noradrenaline is useful if hypotension is problematic following restoration of intravascular volume. Because up to 20% of patients will have multiple trauma, many will require major surgical procedures, during which the spinal cord must remain protected. If muscle relaxants are required 2–3 days following the injury, suxamethonium, which may cause fatal hyperkalemia, should be avoided.

The use of steroids is controversial and there are no studies specific to children. Results of a controlled study in adults, demonstrated that high-dose methyl prednisone administered within 8 h of the injury (30 mg/kg initially followed by 5.4 mg/kg per hour for the following 23 h) improved outcome.[60] The study has significant limitations and the results have not been universally accepted.[61]

As with brain injuries, preventing secondary injury is vital. Adequate perfusion of the cord should be ensured, as autoregulation of blood flow is lost after trauma. Immobilization can be maintained by skull tongs with axial traction or external bracing. Operative intervention is controversial with little evidence of neurological improvement from decompressive surgery. Laminectomy and decompression in children with complete cord injuries carry significant mortality. There should be early consultation with a specialized spinal injuries unit. Optimal rehabilitation requires a team of orthopaedic and neurosurgeons, rehabilitation specialists, nurses, physiotherapists, occupational therapists, psychiatrists, social workers and schoolteachers.

PROGNOSIS

The prognosis of all spinal injuries in children may be better than in adults. In one series of 113 children with spinal column injuries, 55 (48%) had no neurological deficit and 38 (34%) had an incomplete deficit. Of these, 23 (20%) made a complete recovery and 11 (10%) improved.[55] The remaining 20 (18%) children had a complete cord injury and, of these, four improved and three died. In a smaller series, 44% had neurological deficits, SCIWORA was seen in 21% and 11% of injuries were immediate, complete and permanent. Of the 18 children with SCIWORA, four had a permanent, complete deficit.[58]

REFERENCES

1 Mann KS, Chan KH, Yue CP. Skull fractures in children: their assessment in relation to developmental skull changes and acute intracranial hematomas. *Childs Nerv Sys* 1986; **2**: 258–61.

2 Suarez JI, Qureshi A, Bhardwaj A, *et al.* Treatment of refractory intracranial hypertension with 23.4% saline. *Crit Care Med* 1998; **26**: 1118–22.

3 Hanhan UA, Fiallos MR, Orlowski JP. Status epilepticus. *Pediatr Clin North Am* 2001; **48**: 683–94.

4 Lothman E. The biochemical basis and pathophysiology of status epilepticus. *Neurology* 1990; **40** (suppl. 2): 13–23.

5 Scott RC, Surtees RAH, Neville BGR. Status epilepticus: pathophysiology, epidemiology, and outcomes. *Arch Dis Child* 1998; **79**: 73–7.

6 Chiulli DA, Terndrup TE, Kanter RK. The influence of diazepam or lorazepam on the frequency of endotracheal intubation in childhood status epilepticus. *J Emerg Med* 1991; **9**: 13–7.

7 Appleton RE, Sweeney A, Choonara I, *et al.* Lorazepam versus diazepam in the treatment of epileptic seizures and status epilepticus. *Dev Med Child Neurol* 1995; **37**: 682–8.

8 Chamberlain JM, Altieri MA, Futterman C, *et al.* A prospective, randomized study comparing intramuscular midazolam with intravenous diazepam for the treatment of seizures in children. *Pediatr Emerg Care* 1997; **13**: 92–4.

9 Lahat E, Aladjem M, Eshel G, *et al.* Midazolam in treatment of epileptic seizures. *Pediatr Neurol* 1992; **8**: 215–6.

10 Rivera R, Segnini M, Baltodano A, Pérez V. Midazolam in the treatment of status epilepticus in children. *Crit Care Med* 1993; **21**: 991–4.

11 Koul RL, Raj Aithala G, Chacko A, *et al.* Continuous midazolam infusion as treatment of status epilepticus. *Arch Dis Child* 1997; **76**: 445–8.

12 Wheless JW. Paediatric use of intravenous and intramuscular phenytoin: lessons learned. *J Child Neurol* 1998; **13**: S11–4.

13 Appleton R, Choonara I, Martland T, *et al.* The Status Epilepticus Working Party. The treatment of convulsive status epilepticus in children. *Arch Dis Child* 2000; **83**: 415–9.

14 McIntyre PB, Chey T, Smith WT. The impact of vaccination against invasive haemophilus influenzae type b disease in the Sydney region. *Med J Aust* 1995; **162**: 245–8.

15 Adams WG, Deaver KA, Cochi SL *et al.* Decline of childhood Haemophilus influenzae type b (Hib) disease in the Hib vaccine era. *JAMA* 1993; **269**: 221–6.

16 Rennick G, Shann F, de Campo J. Cerebral herniation during bacterial meningitis in children. *BMJ* 1993; **306**: 953–5.

17 Seward RJ, Towner KJ. Evaluation of a PCR-immunoassay technique for detection of Neisseria meningitidis in cerebrospinal fluid and peripheral blood. *J Med Microb* 2000; **49**: 451–6.

18 Newcombe J, Cartwright K, Palmer WH, McFadden J. PCR of peripheral blood for diagnosis of meningococcal disease. *J Clin Microbiol* 1996; **34**: 1637–40.

19 Feigin RD, Pearlman E. Bacterial meningitis beyond the neonatal period. In: Feigin RD, Cherry JD (eds). *Textbook of Paediatric Infectious Diseases*. Philadelphia: WB Saunders; 1998; pp. 400–29.

20 Odio CM, Faingezicht I, Paris M *et al.* The beneficial effects of early dexamethasone administration in infants and children with bacterial meningitis. *N Engl J Med* 1991; **324**: 1525–31.

21 McCracken GH, Label MH. Dexamethasone treatment for bacterial meningitis in infants and children. *Am J Dis Child* 1989; **143**: 287–9.

22 Schaad UB, Lips U, Gnehm HE, *et al.* Dexamethasone therapy for bacterial meningitis. *Lancet* 1993; **342**: 457–61.

23 McIntyre PB, Berkey CS, King SM *et al.* Dexamethasone as adjunctive therapy in bacterial meningitis. A meta-analysis of randomised clinical trial since 1988. *JAMA* 1997; **278**: 925–31.

24 Powell KR, Sugarman LI, Eskenazi AE *et al.* Normalisation of plasma arginine vasopressin concentrations when children with meningitis are given maintenance plus replacement fluid therapy. *J Pediatr* 1990; **117**: 515–22.

25 Bianchetti MG, Thyssen HR, Laux-End R, Schaad UB. Evidence for fluid volume depletion in hyponatraemic patients with bacterial meningitis. *Acta Paediatr* 1996; **85**: 1163–6.

26 Singhi SC, Singhi PD, Srinivas B *et al.* Fluid restriction does not improve the outcome of acute meningitis. *Pediatr Infect Dis* 1995; **14**: 495–503.

27 Cuevas LE, Kazembe P, Mughogho GK, *et al.* Eradication of nasopharyngeal carriage of Neisseria meningitidis in children and adults in rural Africa: a comparison of ciprofloxacin and rifampicin. *J Infect Dis* 1995; **171**: 728–31.

28 Madagame ET, Havens PL, Bresnahan JM, *et al.* Survival and functional outcome of children requiring mechanical ventilation during therapy for acute bacterial meningitis. *Crit Care Med* 1995; **23**: 1279–83.

29 Aurelius E, Johansson B, Skoldenberg B, *et al.* Rapid diagnosis of herpes simplex virus encephalitis by nested polymerase chain reaction assay of cerebrospinal fluid. *Lancet* 1991; **337**: 189–92.

30 Troendle-Atkins J, Demmler GJ, Buffone GJ. Rapid diagnosis of herpes simplex encephalitis by using polymerase chain reaction. *J Paediatr* 1993; **123**: 376–80.

31 McMinn P, Stratov I, Nagarajan L, Davis S. Neurological manifestations of enterovirus 71 infection in children during an outbreak of hand, foot, and mouth disease in Western Australia. *Clin Inf Dis* 2001; **32**: 236–42.

32 Rotbart HA, Webster AD. Treatment of potentially life-threatening enterovirus infections with Pleconaril. *Clin Inf Dis* 2001; **32**: 228–35.

33 Koskiniemi M, Vaheri A. Effect of measles, mumps, rubella vaccination on pattern of encephalitis in children. *Lancet* 1989; **00**: 31–4.

34 Al-Jarallah A, Al-Rifai MT, Riela AR, Roach S. Nontraumatic brain hemorrhage in children: etiology and presentation. *J Child Neurol* 2000; **15**: 284–9.

35 Stein BM, Wolpert SM. Arteriovenous malformation of the brain II: Current concepts and treatment. *Arch Neurol* 1980; **37**: 69–75.

36 Michenfelder JD, Milde JH. Post-ischaemic canine cerebral blood flow appears to be determined by cerebral metabolic needs. *J Cereb Blood Flow Metab* 1990; **10**: 71–6.

37 Sarnaik AP, Preston G, Lieh-Lai M, Eisenbrey AB. Intracranial perfusion pressure in near-drowning. *Crit Care Med* 1985; **13**: 224–7.

38 Bohn DJ, Biggar W D, Smith CR, *et al.* Influence of hypothermia, barbiturate therapy and intracranial pressure monitoring on morbidity and mortality after near-drowning. *Crit Care Med* 1986; **14**: 529–34.

39 Schindler MB, Cox PN, Jarvis A, Bohn DJ. Factors influencing outcome from out of hospital paediatric cardiopulmonary arrest. *Anaesth Int Care* 1995; **23**: 381–2.

40 Kriel RL, Krach LE, Luxenberg MG, *et al.* Outcome of severe anoxic/ischaemic brain injury in children. *Paediatr Neurol* 1994; **10**: 207–12.

41 Beca J, Cox PN, Taylor MJ, *et al.* Somatosensory evoked potentials for prediction of outcome in acute severe brain injury. *J Pediatr* 1995; **126**: 44–9.

42 Manners PJ, Murray KJ. Guillain-Barré syndrome presenting with severe musculoskeletal pain. *Acta Paediatr* 1992; **81**: 1049–51.

43 Cole GF, Matthew DJ. Prognosis in severe Guillain-Barré syndrome. *Arch Dis Child* 1987; **62**: 288–91.

44 Jansen PW, Perkin RM, Ashwal S. Guillain-Barré syndrome in childhood: Natural course and efficacy of plasmapheresis. *Pediatr Neurol* 1993; **9**: 16–20.

45 Lamont PJ, Johnston HM, Berdoukas VA. Plasma-pheresis in children with Guillain-Barré syndrome. *Neurology* 1991; **41**: 1928–31.

46 Van der Meche FGA, Schmitz PIM, Dutch Guillain-Barré Study Group. A randomised trial comparing intravenous immune globulin and plasma exchange in Guillain-Barré syndrome. *N Engl J Med* 1992; **326**: 1123–9.

47 Vajsar J, Sloane A, Wood E, Murphy EG. Plasma-pheresis vs intravenous immunoglobulin treatment in childhood Guillain-Barré syndrome. *Arch Pediatr Adolesc Med* 1994; **148**: 1210–2.

48 Briscoe DM, McMeniman LB, O'Donohoe. Prognosis in Guillain-Barré syndrome. *Arch Dis Child* 1987; **62**: 733–5.

49 Neville BGR. Paediatric neurology. In: Walton J (ed.). *Brain's Diseases of the nervous System*. Oxford: Oxford Medical Publications; 1993; pp. 453–77.

50 Chaves-Carballo E. Detection of inherited neuro-metabolic disorders. A practical clinical approach. *Pediatr Clin North Am* 1992; **39**: 801–19.

51 National Institutes of Health Conference on Reye's Syndrome: diagnosis and treatment of Reye's Syndrome. *JAMA* 1981; **246**: 2441.

52 Schaffer F, Straube, Oh J, *et al*. Dialysis in neonates with inborn errors of metabolism. *Nephrol Dial Transplant* 1999; **14**: 918–9.

53 Green A, Hall S. Investigation of metabolic disorders resembling Reye's syndrome. *Arch Dis Child* 1992; **67**: 1313–7.

54 Andresen BS, Dobrowolski SF, O'Reilly L *et al*. Medium-chain acyl CoA dehydrogenase deficiency (MCAD) mutations identified by MS/MS-based screening of newborns differ from those observed in patients with clinical symptoms: Identification and characterization of a new, prevalent mutation that results in mild MCAD deficiency. *Am J Hum Genet* 2001; **68**: 1408–18.

55 Hadley MN, Zabramski MD, Browner CM, *et al*. Paediatric spinal trauma. Review of 122 cases of spinal cord and vertebral column injuries. *J Neurosurg* 1988; **68**: 18–24.

56 Swan PK, Bohn DJ, Sides CA, Armstrong P. Cervical spine damage associated with severe head injury in the paediatric patient: implications for airway management. *Anaesth Int Care* 1987; **15**: 115–6.

57 Givens TG, Policy KA, Smith GF, Hardin WD Jr. Pediatric cervical spine injury: a three year experience. *J Trauma* 1996; **41**: 310–4.

58 Ruge JR, Sinson GP, McLone DG, Cerullo LJ. Pediatric spinal injury: the very young. *J Neurosurg* 1988; **68**: 25–30.

59 Birney TJ, Hanley EN. Traumatic cervical spine injuries in childhood and adolescence. *Spine* 1989; **14**: 1277–82.

60 Bracken MB, Shepard MJ, Collins WF Jr *et al*. Methylprednisolone or naloxone treatment after acute spinal cord injury: 1 year follow-up data. Results of the second National Acute Spinal Cord Injury Study. *J Neurosurg* 1992; **76**: 23–31.

61 Short DJ, Elmasry WS, Jones PW. High-dose methyl-prednisone in the management of acute spinal cord injury – a systematic review from a clinical perspective. *Spinal Cord* 2000; **38**: 273–86.

101

Paediatric trauma

N T Matthews

Paediatric patients presenting with trauma have clinical symptoms and examination findings, which differ from adults, and vary across the range of their ages. Trauma is the leading cause of death in children over 1-year-old, and the third leading cause under 1 year after sudden infant death syndrome and congenital abnormalities.[1] Causes of trauma and patterns of injury are determined by age-related behaviour, with falls and assaults most common in younger children, and motor vehicle accidents most common in older children. In general, blunt trauma with multiorgan injury is most likely.

As with adults, there are three peak mortality periods after injury:

- *minutes* at the scene, from airway obstruction, bleeding and fatal primary brain injury
- *hours* during resuscitation and transport from airway obstruction, aspiration, haemorrhage and the head injury
- *days to weeks* later from head injury or complications.

None-the-less, there are differences from adults in injury patterns, pathophysiology and management.

PREVENTION STRATEGIES

Paediatric trauma requires resources and co-ordinated efforts to successfully reduce mortality and morbidity.[2] New emphasis has seen the development of prevention strategies (Table 101.1), including:

- injury surveillance, prevention research, legislation and public safety campaigns
- education programmes directed at care givers
- nationally co-ordinated approaches to trauma care.

HEAD INJURY

Significant head injury occurs in 75% of children admitted with blunt trauma,[4] and 70% result in death. Causes of injury are determined by behaviour patterns, which change with age and are commonly due to falls and assaults in infants, and motor vehicle accidents (including bicycle-related injuries) in older children.

ASSESSMENT

The Glasgow Coma Scale (GCS) requires different interpretation in children, where scores tend to be more subjective and prone to misinterpretation. When using the original GCS described for adults, children under 5 years are unable to score normally for verbal and motor responses. Normal aggregate scores for age are:

- 9 at 6 months
- 11 at 12 months
- 13–14 at 5 years.

This has led to attempts to modify the scale by either changing the scoring assessment signs, or by reducing the total score (i.e. eliminating some response categories).[5] The latter does not allow for comparison of outcome data.

An example of a commonly used scale modified for infants is shown in Table 101.2. However, difficulties remain as regards the accuracy and reproducibility of GCS for infants. Clinical assessment must also look for signs and symptoms of cerebral oedema or raised intracranial pressure (Table 101.3).

Table 101.1 Prevention strategies[3]

Paediatric injuries	Preventative strategies
MVA – occupant	Child car seat
	Seatbelt restraint
MVA – pedestrian	Safety programmes in schools
Bicycle	Helmet
Drowning	Surround pool fencing
Burns	Smoke detectors
	Water tap regulator
	Flammable fabric legislation
Poisoning	Preventative packaging
Violence	Handgun legislation
	Crisis resolution counselling

Table 101.2 Glasgow Coma Scale modified for infants

Glasgow Coma Scale			Glasgow Coma Scale modified for infants		
Activity	*Best response*	*Scale*	*Activity*	*Best response*	*Scale*
Eye opening	Spontaneous	4	Eye opening	Spontaneous	4
	To speech	3		To speech	3
	To pain	2		To pain	2
	None	1		None	1
Verbal	Orientated	5	Verbal	Coos, babbles	5
	Confused	4		Irritable, cries	4
	Inappropriate words	3		Cries to pain	3
	Non-specific sounds	2		Moans to pain	2
	None	1		None	1
Motor	Obeys commands	6	Motor	Spontaneous activity	6
	Localizes pain	5		Withdraws to touch	5
	Withdraws to pain	4		Withdraws to pain	4
	Abnormal flexion	3		Flexion to pain	3
	Extensor response	2		Extension to pain	2
	None	1		None	1

Table 101.3 Signs of raised intracranial pressure

Depressed level of consciousness
Changes in respiratory pattern, blood pressure and pulse rate
Increased head circumference (less than 18 months age)
Full or bulging fontanelle
Motor weakness
Cranial nerve palsies
Decorticate or decerebrate posturing
Vomiting
Headache
Papilloedema (late)

MANAGEMENT

The aims of therapy are to minimize secondary effects on the primary brain injury by maintaining adequate cerebral blood flow and oxygen supply, and preventing secondary ischaemic injury and herniation from raised ICP.

- Deterioration in level of consciousness and the appearance of signs of herniation must be rapidly recognized.
- Airway, oxygenation and respiration should be optimized and intubation performed when the airway is compromised.
- Controlled ventilation with muscle relaxation and sedation should be instituted in the presence of hypoventilation, seizures and signs of raised ICP (Table 101.3).
- Hypotension significantly increases mortality in children and the systemic circulation must be maintained.
- Management of blood pressure is difficult because the exact ranges of cerebral autoregulation are unknown in children.[6] Hypotension is most likely from blood

loss (especially from scalp lacerations) and not brain injury, and fluid management needs to balance the need for volume resuscitation with the attempt to avoid hypovolaemia.

- Hypotonic and glucose containing solutions should be avoided because of poor outcomes.[7]
- Hyperthermia should be avoided with a servo-controlled cooling blanket and adjustment of humidifier temperature because each 1°C temperature rise increases cerebral metabolic rate by 5%.[8]
- Cerebral venous return should be optimized by neutral head positioning. Cerebral perfusion pressure may be best with the bed flat.[9]
- Treatment of seizures with phenytoin (20 mg/kg i.v.) provides less central nervous system depression than barbiturates or benzodiazepines. Monitoring for seizures to guard against resulting increases in cerebral blood flow and oxygen consumption is difficult in the paralysed patient. Systems for continuous electroencephalogram monitoring are complex to interpret at the bedside and provide limited information. Posttraumatic seizures are more common under 2 years of age,[10] but their long-term incidence is not reduced by acute prophylaxis.[11]
- Continuous measurement of jugular venous oxygen saturation (Sjo_2) via fibreoptic reflection oximetry can identify global cerebral hypoperfusion and ischaemia.[12] However, its use in children is subject to technical difficulties, mainly related to catheter position. Its use is not clinically routine in paediatrics.

DIAGNOSTIC INVESTIGATIONS

Supportive investigations can be performed while emergency assessment and therapy proceed. These include pH and acid-base, serum glucose, osmolality, electrolytes, calcium, magnesium and phosphate, complete blood profile and blood cross-match.

X-rays of skull and cervical spine (both anteroposterior, lateral and C_1-C_2 views), chest and pelvis are needed. Ultrasound of the skull, where the fontanelle is open, measures ventricular size, and can detect intracranial haemorrhage. It is useful for repeated assessment in the unstable patient.

A cranial computed tomography (CT) scan in stable patients is useful to exclude surgically treatable lesions, to assess the size of cerebrospinal fluid (CSF) spaces, including the basal cisterns, to detect herniation and shift, and to show the presence of hyperaemia, oedema, intracerebral haematomas, contusions and fractures. A normal CT scan does not exclude raised ICP. Intracranial blood collections are less common than in adults.[13] The following are poor prognostic signs:

- subdural haemorrhage (as an indication of severe trauma and damage to underlying brain tissue)
- ablated basal cisterns and midline shift
- reversal of grey/white differentiation.

CEREBRAL PERFUSION PRESSURE

Maintenance of cerebral perfusion pressure (CPP) in children is important and has significant implications, but the minimal required CPP in children has not been determined. CPP depends on the difference between mean systemic blood pressure and ICP. These values vary with age. In particular, blood pressure assumes great importance in the younger age group, where physiological systolic pressures are lower:

- 85 mmHg (11.3 kPa) at 6 months
- 95 mmHg (12.6 kPa) at 2 years
- 100 mmHg (13.3 kPa) at 7 years.[14]

In addition, normal ICP is lower,[15] being up to 5 mmHg (0.67 kPa) at 2 years and up to 10 mmHg (1.3 kPa) at 5 years. Thus, in younger age groups, relative hypotension has a more profound effect on CPP and outcome,[16] and hypotension may be the main cause of cerebral ischaemia. For adolescents, therapy should aim to sustain CPP over 70 mmHg (9.3 kPa), with maintaining normal blood volume and adequate blood pressure (with pressor agents if required). A CPP less than 40 mmHg (5.3 kPa) reduces the likelihood of intact survival. Younger patients should have therapeutic targets adjusted to age related realistic end points.

INTRACRANIAL PRESSURE

Mechanisms of raised intracranial pressure (ICP) in childhood trauma are listed in Table 101.4. If ICP remains persistently raised and uncompensated, cerebral ischaemia and herniation result. This herniation can be cingulate, uncal (temporal lobe), cerebellar tonsillar, upward cerebellar (posterior fossa hypertension) or transcalvarian (through vault defects). Signs of herniation are as for raised intracranial pressure (Table 101.3).

MEASUREMENT OF INTRACRANIAL PRESSURE

As with adults, measurement of ICP is indicated when intracranial hypertension is likely or potential (e.g. GCS 8 or less), or where signs are hidden by muscle relaxation. However, measurement in children can be more difficult. Subdural catheters and intracranial transducers are widely used, but require careful placement in children. Subarachnoid bolts, such as the Richmond screw, need special threads to maintain stability in thin cranial bone, are difficult to insert under 12 months of age, and fail at high pressures. Ventricular catheters allow removal of CSF to reduce ICP, but are difficult to insert when ventricles are small, and readings are difficult to interpret when ventricles collapse. Non-invasive applanation devices over the anterior fontanelle allow trend recording of pressure in neonates,[17] but have not been widely accepted. Development of new strain-gauge technology will allow easier and more meaningful measurement of ICP (including intracerebral pressure).

Increased ICP above 40 mmHg (5.3 kPa) indicates poor outcome.[18] However, regional pressure and perfusion are not linked to total cerebral blood flow and focal oedema affects local cerebral blood flow despite normal limits of ICP and CPP.

REDUCTION OF RAISED INTRACRANIAL PRESSURE

Several mechanisms allow physiological compensation for raised ICP in children (Table 101.5). In the child under 18 months of age, a gradual increase in intracranial volume is achieved by an increase in head circumference. Measurement of this circumference is important, because this compensation can delay recognition of clinical signs and diagnosis in emerging intracranial pathology. The important factor in the rate of change in compliance and ICP is the elasticity of the dura, which is dependent on the rate of change in intracranial volume.

Table 101.4 Mechanisms of raised intracranial pressure

Increased intracranial blood volume
  Intracranial bleeding (epidural, subdural, subarachnoid, intracerebral)
  Cerebral hyperaemia (in the first 1–2 days postinjury[19])
  Increased cerebral blood flow (increased $PaCO_2$, decreased PaO_2, convulsions)
Cerebral oedema (after day 2[20])
Hydrocephalus from intraventricular blood

Table 101.5 Physiological compensatory mechanisms for raised intracranial pressure in children

Displacement of CSF to distensible spinal subarachnoid space
Compression of intracranial venous system
Increased CSF reabsorption
Reduced CSF production
Stretching of dura, unfused skull bones and skin (less than 18 months age)

Hyperventilation is effective in lowering raised ICP. However, excessive hyperventilation may cause cerebral ischaemia, and $PaCO_2$ should be maintained between 35 and 40 mmHg (4.7–5.3 kPa). Weaning from hyperventilation should be slow, to minimize rebound rises in ICP.[21] Fluid restriction is helpful, provided circulating blood volume is maintained.

Mannitol (0.25–0.50 g/kg i.v. slowly) reduces raised ICP by increasing the osmotic gradient across the intact blood–brain barrier and reducing cerebral oedema. Its effects may also be due to reduced blood viscosity and induced cerebral vasoconstriction. Serum osmolality should be monitored to avoid hyperosmolar states.

Frusemide (1 mg/kg) reduces cerebral water and CSF production, but excessive diuresis from mannitol or frusemide may compromise the circulation. The use of hypertonic saline in children requires further evaluation. CSF drainage is possible if a ventricular drain is *in situ*. Surgical decompression or removal of cerebral contusion in the face of intractably raised ICP in head trauma are advocated,[22] with improved results in unremitting focal oedema.

SPINAL CORD INJURY

Anatomical differences in children under 8 years render their spines more mobile and subject to stress. The cervical spine in this age group has less muscular support. Its ligaments and joint capsules are more flexible, and facet joints more horizontal. In addition, the relatively large head mass increases momentum, with the fulcrum of mobility at C2–C3 as opposed to C4–C5 in the adult. Thus paediatric cervical spine injuries tend to be above C4. The use of seat belts has led to an increase in lumbar spinal cord injury in children.[23]

ASSESSMENT

Assessment can be difficult in the clinical examination of neurological deficits in the young child, and in the interpretation of radiological investigations. Despite improved detection of abnormalities with combined X-ray and CT scan examinations, spinal cord injury without obvious radiological abnormality (SCIWORA) may be present.[24] Sensory evoked potentials can be a valuable adjunct to diagnosis. Spinal cord injury can only be dismissed after imaging assessments (which may include magnetic resonance imaging in the non-acute setting) and careful and repeated examination of the lucid patient. Delayed onset of spinal neurological signs has been reported in children.[25]

MANAGEMENT

From the time of injury, the spine should be assumed to be unstable until proved otherwise. Immobilization is necessary from the time of injury in the presence of:

- signs or symptoms suggesting neurological spinal deficit
- a history of loss of consciousness
- altered mental status
- history of a high-speed accident or significant fall (including diving)
- significant head or chest trauma.

It is often difficult to decide whether the spinal-injured child is initially best cared for in a paediatric ICU or a specialized spinal unit. This decision will be ultimately determined on the age of the child and the stability of the spine. Certainly, infants should not be managed in adult spinal units, whereas for older children, expertise in spinal care may be more important. However, once spinal column stability and surgical fixation have been achieved, children are best managed in paediatric facilities for ongoing management and rehabilitation.[26] Ongoing care is complex, and requires a multi-disciplinary approach. Attention to pressure areas, bladder and bowel care and training, nutrition and prevention of contractures is essential. Symptoms of hypercalcaemia (eg. vomiting, anorexia, nausea and malaise) can be distressing and difficult to control. Depression is common in adolescents.

With high spinal cord injury, chin-operated battery-powered wheelchairs, portable ventilators and computer-activated environment control devices allow for relative independence and a functional lifestyle.

THORACIC TRAUMA

Despite a low incidence in children, thoracic trauma is usually associated with multiorgan injury and high mortality.[27] The mechanism of injury is almost entirely related to motor vehicle accidents, with penetrating trauma being uncommon. The child's small size and more elastic chest wall allow transmission of more kinetic energy to intrathoracic structures, with a high incidence of pulmonary contusions without rib fractures or flail chest. Despite this, the incidence of pneumothorax with or without tension can be high.[28]

As for adults, life-threatening injuries which require immediate intervention are upper airway obstruction, tension pneumothorax, open pneumothorax, flail chest, pericardial tamponade and massive haemothorax (see

Ch. 68). Potentially life-threatening injuries are airway rupture, pulmonary contusion, ruptured aorta, diaphragmatic rupture, oesophageal perforation and myocardial contusion. Contrast CT scan and/or angiography is the method of choice in diagnosing aortic rupture in children.

ABDOMINAL TRAUMA

Abdominal trauma is usually associated with blunt injury[29] and recognition may be difficult in the presence of multisystem injury. The abdominal wall and thoracic cage of children provide less protection to intra-abdominal organs. Also, the liver and spleen are relatively large and more exposed below the rib cage. Forces need not be excessive to cause rupture of either organ. Lap seat belt injuries are an important cause of abdominal injury in restrained children.

Improvements in radiological imaging techniques have allowed blunt abdominal trauma to be managed conservatively in children.[30] This approach requires appropriate monitoring and supervision in a paediatric setting, with an awareness of the need for urgent intervention, e.g. laparotomy (Table 101.6).

- Ultrasonography is an important screening tool for detecting free fluid[31] and confirming intra-abdominal bleeding. However, it cannot detect organ injury.
- CT scan assessment with intraluminal and i.v. contrast is indicated with clinical suspicion of abdominal injury or when physical examination is unreliable. It allows for examination of solid organs and renal tract, and detection of intraperitoneal blood and free air.
- Diagnostic peritoneal lavage has become less important, and is only indicated when the source of continued bleeding is undetermined, when an urgent procedure is required for a non-abdominal injury or when a prolonged observation period is anticipated, when ultrasonography or CT scan is not available.

NON-ACCIDENTAL INJURY

Non-accidental injuries to children are seen in younger age groups, and include physical assault, sexual and emotional

Table 101.6 Indications for laparotomy in paediatric abdominal trauma

Profound hypovolaemia
Persistent haemorrhage
Haemodynamic instability after replacement 40 ml/kg[32]
Penetrating injury
Gastrointestinal perforation
Signs of peritonism
Pancreatic injury

abuse and neglect (especially inadequate supervision and deprivation of nutrition and medical care). Injuries resulting from intentional assault can be difficult to diagnose, unless a high index of awareness is maintained.

With regard to the history, suspicion should be raised when:

- the cause of the injury cannot be explained
- there is discrepancy between the volunteered history and the sustained injury, especially when the child's stage of development is taken into account
- there is a history of repeated injuries
- it is alleged that he injury is self-sustained; or
- there is a delay in seeking care.

Physical examination should be thorough, to establish a pattern of injury. Multiple bruises in differing stages of development can be separately estimated for age.[33] Patterns for burns are typical for forced immersion in hot water (with sparing of the groin area) and from cigarettes. Suspicion should be raised where cerebral trauma is associated with retinal haemorrhages, subdural haematomas or fractures. Retinal haemorrhages are typical of head-shaking, but are also caused by cardiopulmonary resuscitation.[34] The most common intra-cranial pathology is subdural and sub-arachnoid haemorrhage, and account for the higher morbidity and mortality. A whole-body X-ray series and bone scan will detect fractures in differing stages of healing from multiple assaults.

Whenever non-accidental injury is suspected or diagnosed, a multidisciplinary approach is required by a specialized child protection unit to deal with medical and legal issues, and with the counselling. Urgent intervention may be necessary where the safety of other siblings is threatened.

TRANSPORT

The outcome of trauma in remote locations is optimal, when advice, pre-hospital stabilization and transport are provided by teams based in tertiary paediatric ICUs.[35] Secondary insults occur more frequently when paediatric-trained personnel are not used for transport.[36] A referral and retrieval infrastructure which links a tertiary centre to outlying areas within the region is necessary. Local health care providers must have sufficient skills to stabilize any critically ill child adequately. The transport team must offer a leave of care during the stabilization and transport phases that is equivalent to that of the receiving paediatric ICU.

It is important for regional hospitals not used to routinely caring for paediatric trauma patients to recognize and acknowledge their individual abilities and limitations. A relationship with a tertiary PICU is essential to allow appropriate and timely communication regarding advice on clinical care, pre-hospital stabilization, and safe transport for individual patients.

BRAIN DEATH

Determination of brain death in children has different implications.[37] Isoelectric EEGs have been reported in neonates with partially preserved clinical brain function, and brain death can occur without marked increase in intracranial pressure, allowing partial cerebral blood flow in the presence of brain death criteria and electrocerebral silence. In addition, partial brain recovery has been demonstrated after prolonged periods of clinical unresponsiveness. Thus, for determination of brain death, consideration needs to be given to longer observation periods, more frequent use of confirmatory tests, and an emphasis on the history and clinical findings. The American Academy of Pediatrics has set longer observation times, which include the requirement for two separate EEGs or one EEG and a cerebral radionucleotide angiogram. These longer observation times depend on the child's age, specifically: over 1 year of age – 12 hours observation; ages 2–12 months – 24 hours observation; ages 7 days to 2 months – 48 hours observation; no recommendation for patients under 7 days age. The Australian and New Zealand Intensive Care Society recommendations on brain death and organ donation only make reference to the under 2 months age group when 'determination of brain death may be more difficult and different time periods may be required'.[38] Importantly, there is a lack of evidence for any required observation periods, and usual practice is to apply the same brain death criteria for newborns, infants, children and adults.[39] The most important factors when determining brain death are knowing the cause of coma, and being certain of its irreversibility. Time must be allowed for relatives to come to terms with the diagnosis, and there is a responsibility to discuss organ donation. Having relatives watch the physical examination for brainstem testing is helpful.

ORGAN DONATION

During the process of brain death determination and consideration of organ donation, there are significant emotional implications for both the care givers and the relatives:

- There is a critical time when the hopelessness of the child's outcome becomes apparent and consideration is about to be given for the declaration of brain death.
- The treatment plan previously focused on cerebral resuscitation, and intensive care staff reach a pivotal decision point when treatment is deemed unsuccessful.
- If organ donation is to be considered, then some therapies must be withdrawn to allow for an assessment of cerebral function.

This moment can be a very stressful time for the professional caregivers involved, because they need to shift from a cerebral resuscitation paradigm to withdrawal of support to allow for declaration of brain death, and then institute protocols aimed at organ resuscitation for possible organ donation.

Parents and relatives have to deal with:

- their child being taken from them unexpectedly
- the death being surrounded by tragic circumstances
- intensive medical therapy and critical decisions concerning interventions
- discussions on withdrawal of support
- confronting the issue that their child who outwardly looks no different is clinically dead; and
- subliminal conflicts of blame and guilt which can lead to conflict within family relationships.

Success in asking for paediatric organs from parents is associated with:

- knowing the certainty of death
- a willingness to do good for others
- previous discussion of organ donation within the family unit
- a knowledge of the patient's wishes before death.

Factors inhibiting a willingness to donate by parents include:

- an uncertainty in the parents understanding the diagnosis
- insufficient information and counselling from health professionals
- a fear of mutilation.

WITHDRAWAL OF SUPPORT

The emotion surrounding a child's impending death can be overwhelming for both relatives and intensive care staff. Children are involved in sudden and catastrophic events that at times seem unreasonable and unfair. For parents, the grieving process begins before or during the intensive care admission, and intensive care staff are intimately involved in helping parents and relatives through this process. The death of any child is a tragedy, and communication between staff is important to ensure appropriate emotional support. Intensive care staff need to understand that withdrawal of therapy can be appropriate. Ensuring the process has dignity and helping relatives through their grieving process are important facets of the intensive care commitment.[40]

REFERENCES

1 Klauber MR, Barrett-Conner E, Marshall LF, Bowers SA. The epidemiology of head injury: a prospective of an entire community – San Diego County, California, 1978. *Am J Epidemiol* 1981; **113**: 500–9.

2 National Road Trauma Advisory Council. *Report of the Working Party on Trauma Systems.* Canberra: Australian Government Publishing Service, 1993.

3 Stylianos S, Eichelberger MR. Pediatric trauma prevention strategies. *Ped Clin N Am* 1993; **40**(6): 1359–68.

4 Lam WH, Mackersie A. Paediatric head injury: Incidence, aetiology and management. *Paediatr Anaesth* 1999; **9**: 377–85.

5 Simpson D and Reilly P. Paediatric coma scale (letter). *Lancet* 1982; **2**: 450.

6 Kokoska ER, Smith GS, Pittman T. Early hypotension worsens neurological outcome in pediatric patients with moderately severe head trauma. *J Pediatr Surg* 1998; **33**(2): 333–8.

7 Michaud LJ, Rivara FP, Longstreth WT, Grady MS. Elevated initial blood glucose levels and poor outcome following severe brain injuries in children. *J Trauma* 1991; **31**(2): 1362–6.

8 Ross AK. Pediatric trauma. *Anaesth Clin N Am* 2001; **19**(2): 309–37.

9 Rosner MJ, Cotey IB. Cerebral perfusion pressure, intracranial pressure and head elevation. *J Neurosurg* 1986; **65**: 636–41.

10 Hahn YS, Chyung C, Barthel MJ, *et al.* Head injuries in children under 36 months of age. Demography and outcome. *Childs Nerv Syst* 1988; **4**: 34–40.

11 Temkin NR, Dikmen SS, Winn HR. Management of head injury. Posttraumatic seizures. *Neurosurg Clin N Am* 1991; **2**: 425–35.

12 Dearden NM, Midgley S. Technical considerations in continuous jugular venous oxygen saturation measurement. *Acta Neurochir Suppl Wien* 1993; **59**: 91–7.

13 Lam WH, Mackersie A. Paediatric head injury: Incidence, aetiology and management. *Paediatr Anaesth* 1999; **9**: 377–85.

14 Horan MJ. Report of the second task force on blood pressure in children. *Pediatrics* 1987; **79**: 1–25.

15 Welch K. The intracranial pressure in infants. *J Neurosurg* 1980; **52**: 693–9.

16 Raju TN, Vidyasagar D, Papazafiratou C. Cerebral perfusion pressure and abnormal intracranial waveforms: their relation to outcome in birth asphyxia. *Crit Care Med* 1981; **9**: 449–53.

17 Colditz PB, Williams GL, Berry AB, Symonds PJ. Fontanelle pressure and cerebral perfusion pressure: continuous measurement in neonates. *Crit Care Med* 1988; **16**: 876–9.

18 Longfitt TW, Gennarelli TA. Can the outcome from head injury be improved? *J Neurosurg* 1982; **56**: 19–25.

19 Bruce DA, Alavi A, Bilaniuk L, Dolinskas C, Obrist W, Uzzell B. Diffuse cerebral swelling following head injuries in children: the syndrome of 'malignant brain edema'. *J Neurosurg* 1981; **54**: 170–8.

20 Snoek JW, Minderhoud JM, Wilmink JT. Delayed deterioration following mild head injury in children. *Brain* 1984; **107**: 15–36.

21 Havill JH. Prolonged hyperventilation and intracranial pressure. *Crit Care Med* 1984; **12**: 72–4.

22 Lam WH, Mackersie A. Paediatric head injury: incidence, aetiology and management. *Paediatric Anaesthesia* 1999; **9**: 377–85.

23 Newman KD, Bowman LM, Eichelberger MR. The lap belt complex: intestinal lumbar spin injury in children. *J Trauma* 1990; **30**: 1140–4.

24 Dickman CA, Rekate HL, Sonntag VKH, Zabramski JM. Pediatric spinal trauma: vertebral column and spinal cord injuries in children. *Pediatr Neurosci* 1989; **15**: 237–56.

25 Pang D, Wilberer JE. Spinal cord injury without radiological abnormalities in children. *J Neurosurg* 1982; **57**: 114–29.

26 Sherwin ED, O'Shanick GJ. The trauma of paediatric and adolescent brain injury: issues and implications for rehabilitation specialists. *Brain Injury* 2000; **3**: 267–84.

27 Peclet MH, Newman KD, Eichelberer MR, *et al.* Thoracic trauma in children: an indicator of increased mortality. *J Pediatr Surg* 1990; **25**: 961–6.

28 Nakayama DK, Ramenofsky ML, Rowe MI. Chest injuries in childhood. *Ann Surg* 1989; **210**: 770–5.

29 Cooper A, Barlow B, DiScala C, String D. Mortality and truncal injury. The pediatric perspective. *J Pediatr Surg* 1994; **29**: 33–8.

30 Erin S, Shandling B, Simpson J, Stephens C. Nonoperative management of traumatised spleen in children. *J Pediatr Surg* 1978; **13**: 117–9.

31 Akgur FM, Aktug T, Olguner M, Kovanlkaya A, Hakguder G. Prospective study investigating routine use of ultrasonography as the initial diagnostic modality for the evaluation of children sustaining blunt abdominal trauma. *J Trauma* 1997; **42**(4): 626–8.

32 Rance CH, Singh SJ, Kimble R. Blunt abdominal trauma in children. *J Paediatr Child Health* 2000; **36**: 2–6.

33 Wilson EF. Estimation of the age of cutaneous contusions in child abuse. *Pediatrics* 1977; **60**: 750–2.

34 Goetting MG, Sowa B. Retinal haemorrhage after cardiopulmonary resuscitation in children: an etiological re-evaluation. *Pediatrics* 1990; **89**: 585–8.

35 Pearson G, Shann F, Barry P, *et al.* Should paediatric intensive care be centralised? Trent versus Victoria. *Lancet* 1997; **349**: 1213–7.

36 McNab JM. Optimal escort for interhospital transport of pediatric emergencies. *J Trauma* 1991; **31**: 205–9.

37 Fishman MA. Validity of brain death criteria in infants. *Pediatrics* 1995; **96**: 513–5.

38 ANZICS. Recommendations Concerning Brain Death and Organ Donation. *Working Party on Brain Death and Organ Donation Report*, March, 1998.

39 Farrell MM, Levin DL. Brain death in the pediatric patient: historical, sociological, medical, religious, cultural, legal and ethical consideration. *Crit Care Med* 1993; **21**: 1951–65.

40 Matthews NT. Issues of withdrawal of therapy and brain death in paediatric intensive care. *Critical Care and Resuscitation* 1999; **1**: 7–12.

102

Equipment for paediatric intensive care

J Tibballs

This chapter discusses equipment and its performance required in paediatric and neonatal intensive care. How to use equipment is not discussed. Examples of equipment are given, but exhaustive lists are not intended. Only essential equipment is considered.

Not discussed includes equipment for aerosol therapy, anaesthesia, bronchoscopy, cardiovascular monitoring, cardiac output measurement, echocardiography, electroencephalographic monitoring, extracorporeal membrane oxygenation, home mechanical ventilation, hyperbaric treatment, negative pressure ventilation, nitric oxide therapy, phrenic nerve pacing, prevention of shock, suction devices, tracheostomy and ventricular assistance.

All equipment should be purchased, used and maintained in accordance with recognized local standards and manufacturers' instructions. Medical and nursing staff should read the manuals accompanying all items of equipment and receive instruction on safe use.

AIRWAY MANAGEMENT

ENDOTRACHEAL TUBES

TUBE TYPES

Polyvinyl chloride or silastic tubes are suitable for long-term intubation. They should be cuffless and be of the Magill type – curved but neither preformed nor of variable diameter. Cuffs on tubes may damage subglottic tracheal mucosa, and reduce the tube diameter, which would otherwise be available for gas flow. High-volume low-pressure cuffed tubes may be used after puberty when the cricoid region of the trachea has enlarged and is no longer a narrow region at special risk. The cuff should be inflated with the minimum volume of air necessary to maintain a seal, and checked every 4–8 hours. Recording of pressure in the cuff is desirable.

Preformed tubes (e.g. Rae and Childs) make suction difficult and automatically stipulate length in relation to diameter and circumference. Tubes of non-uniform diameter (e.g. Cole and Oxford) may damage the vocal cords, and do not prevent endobronchial intubation.

- Radio-opacity is necessary for correct positioning.
- All tubes should have length markings and a Murphy eye, that is, a side aperture at the distal end, allowing gas to flow if the tip abuts against the tracheal wall.

TUBE SIZE

A selection of sizes, one larger and one smaller than the anticipated size, should be available at intubation. Tube sizes according to body weight and age are given in Table 102.1 and Table 102.2. A rough guide for internal diameter size in the child is age (in years)$/4 + 4$ mm.

Correct selection of size is necessary to avoid pressure-induced ischaemia/ulceration of tracheal mucosa and to limit aspiration around the tube. The correct size should allow a small leak on application of moderate inflation pressure (25 cmH$_2$O, 2.5 kPa) but also enable adequate pulmonary inflation and expiration. When lung compliance is poor, it is permissible to use a cuffless tube without a leak or a cuffed tube to achieve lung inflation.

PLACEMENT

Oral or nasal tubes may be used. Orally placed tubes are preferred in acute resuscitation and when only a short duration of intubation is required, e.g. for anaesthesia during insertion of a central venous cannula. Nasal placement of tubes is preferred in the setting where spontaneous or mechanical ventilation is required for prolonged periods.

Nasal tubes are more comfortable and manageable for the awake patient and are more easily secured to the face, but pose risks, which include sinus infection and necrosis of the ala nasi. Oral tubes are difficult to fix, uncomfortable and are easily occluded by biting by conscious/semi-conscious patients.

TUBE LENGTH (DEPTH)

The endotracheal tube tip should be located in the mid-trachea so that the risks of accidental extubation and endobronchial intubation are minimized. Correct positioning of the tube should always be checked by auscultation in the axillae, by chest X-ray immediately after intubation and daily thereafter.[1] At intubation, visualization

Table 102.1 Orotracheal and nasotracheal tube lengths for premature neonates

Birth weight (g)	Gestation (weeks)	Oral depth (cm)	Nasal depth (cm)
750	24–25	5–5.5	6.5
1,000	27	5.5	7
1,500	30–31	6	8
1,750	31–32	6.5	8.5
2,000	33	7	9
2,250	34–35	7–7.5	9.5
2,500	35–36	7.5	9.5–10
2,750	36–37	8	10.5
3,000	37–38	8–8.5	10.5
3,500	40	9	11–11.5

ETT sizes: BW <1 kg 2.5 mm; 1–3.5 kg 3.0 mm; >3.5 kg 3.5 mm

of the depth of the tube passed through the cords should be a guide only, since the tube advances when the head is released from extension as the laryngoscope is removed.[2]

The lengths (depths) at which orotracheal and nasotracheal tubes can be chosen initially on the basis of weight or gestation in premature neonates are given in Table 102.1, and on the basis of age for infants and children in Table 102.2. The lengths are at the lips for oral tubes and at the exit from the nose for nasal tubes. For oral tubes, a guide to correct depth for 2 years and over is given by the formula: (age in years/2 + 12 cm), while for nasal tubes the formula is: (age in years/2 + 15 cm). The depth of insertion of any tube should be documented or marked on the tube.

LARYNGOSCOPES

The adult curved Macintosh blade is suitable for all paediatric patients except neonates and infants, in whom a straight blade is needed to displace the relatively large epiglottis anteriorly from the laryngeal inlet. A straight flat blade, e.g. Miller (size 0 or 1) or Seward blade or a straight blade with a medial flange (Magill, Robertshaw, Oxford or Wisconsin) is equally suitable for this purpose. The latter blades displace the tongue medially and give a better view of the larynx, but leave less room for instrumentation with a sucker, introducer or forceps.

SUCTION CATHETERS

Sizes 5, 6, 8, 10 and 12 FG should be available. The suction catheter should be large enough to remove secretions but not too large to occlude the endotracheal/tracheostomy tube lumen (Table 102.3). Many suitable types are available – differing in number and location of suction ports (end and side ports are needed) and whether the tip is angled or straight. Angle tips facilitate entry into the left main bronchus. Satin-finish types with smooth port edges are needed. Single use suction catheters may be re-used up to 24 hours without adding to the risk of pneumonia.[3] Closed suction systems permit suction without disconnection from ventilator as may be indicated during nitric oxide therapy, severe lung disease or frequent suction.

Table 102.2 Endotracheal tube sizes (internal diameter) and orotracheal and nasotracheal depths for infants and children

Body weight/age	Size (mm)	Oral depth (cm)	Nasal depth (cm)
Newly-born 3.5 kg	3.0	9	11–11.5
1–6 months	3.5	9.5–11	12–13
6–12 months	4.0	11.5–12	13–14
2–3 years	4.5	13–13	15–16
4–5 years	5.0	14–14	17–18
6–7 years	5.5	15–15.5	19
8–9 years	6.0	16–16	20
10–11 years	6.5	17–17	21
12–13 years	7.0	18–18	22
14–16 years	7.5	19	23

OROPHARYNGEAL AIRWAYS

A range of Guedel airways (sizes 000, 00, 0, 1, 2 and 3) constructed of polyvinyl chloride with a metal insert should be available. An airway which is too small may be occluded by the surface of the tongue or displace the tongue backwards to obstruct the airway. An airway which is too large may enter the oesophagus. The correct size, when placed alongside the cheek, extends from the centre of the lips to the angle of the mandible. Nasopharyngeal airways are available for the older child, but any size can be constructed from an endotracheal tube. A guide to length is from the tip of the nose to the tragus of the ear.

LARYNGEAL MASK AIRWAYS

Sizes are available to suit body weight (kg) of newborns, infants and children:

- size 1   <5 kg
- size 1½   5–10 kg
- size 2   10–20 kg
- size 2½   20–30 kg
- size 3   30–50 kg
- size 4   50–70 kg
- size 5   70–100 kg
- size 6   >100 kg

They have complementary roles in paediatric intensive care practice which are as airways under anaesthesia, a limited role during CPR and as emergency relief of upper airway obstruction.

MECHANICAL VENTILATION

RESUSCITATOR 'BAGGING' CIRCUITS

Manual pulmonary inflation is often necessary via a mask or endotracheal/tracheostomy tube. Two types of devices are available: flow-inflated and self-inflated bags.

Table 102.3 Recommended suction catheters

Internal diameter (mm) of ETT or tracheostomy	Recommended suction catheter (FG)
2.5	5
3.0	6
3.5–5.5	8
6.0–6.5	10
7.0 and larger	12

ETT, endotracheal tube.

FLOW-INFLATED BAGS

These are exemplified by Jackson–Rees modified Ayre's T-piece. Gas flow must exceed 220 ml/kg per min for children and 3 l/min for infants, to prevent rebreathing during manual ventilation. It is possible to control precisely the concentration of inspired oxygen, which is an advantage, especially for the premature neonate at risk of oxygen-induced retrolental fibroplasia. However, considerable experience is necessary to provide adequate ventilation without barotrauma in the intubated infant. The circuit has neither a valve nor any pressure-relief device. A pressure gauge should be incorporated in the circuit to help prevent barotrauma.

SELF-INFLATED BAGS

These bags are designed to give positive pressure ventilation attached to either a mask or endotracheal/tracheostomy tube. Rebreathing is prevented by one-way duck-bill valves, spring disk/ball valves or diaphragm/leaf valves. The Laerdal bag series (infant, child, adult), typify these devices. A pressure-relief valve (infant and child size) opens at 35 cmH$_2$O (3.5 kPa). A pressure monitor can be incorporated in the circuit. Supplemental oxygen is added to the ventilation bag, with or without attachment of a reservoir bag, whose movement may serve as a visual monitor of tidal volume during spontaneous ventilation when intubated. However, the valve may offer too much resistance for spontaneous ventilation and they should not be used to provide supplemental oxygen to a spontaneously breathing patient via a mask placed loosely over the face. With Laerdal and Partner bags, negligible amounts of oxygen (0.1–0.3 l/min) issue from the patient valve when 5–15 l/min of oxygen is introduced into bags unconnected to patients.[4] The valve is unlikely to open unless the mask is sealed well on the face. The delivered oxygen concentration is dependent on the flow rate of oxygen, use of the reservoir bag, and the state of the pressure relief valve (whether open or closed).

With use of the reservoir bag and oxygen flow greater than the minute ventilation, 100% oxygen is delivered.

Without the reservoir bag the delivered gas is only 50% oxygen, despite oxygen flow rate at twice minute ventilation.

At an oxygen flow rate of 10 l/min to the infant resuscitator bag, the delivered gas is 85–100% oxygen without the use of the reservoir bag.

Other self-inflated bags include the Combibag, Ambu, AirViva and Hudson RCI.

MASKS

Masks should facilitate an airtight seal on the face with minimal dead space.

- For neonates, Rendell–Baker Soucek masks (sizes 0 and 1) or Bennett masks (sizes 1 and 2) are suitable.
- For infants and small children, the larger Rendell–Baker Soucek masks (sizes 2 and 3) or small masks with inflatable rims, such as CIG (sizes 2 and 3) or MIE (sizes 0 and 1), are suitable.
- For older children, masks with inflatable rims are preferred.

Masks with rims created by infolding of the body are more difficult to use.

MECHANICAL VENTILATORS

CONVENTIONAL VENTILATORS

Some ventilators are designed specifically for neonates and infants. A few adult ventilators are also satisfactory. In addition to general requirements of ventilators, the paediatric ventilator should have:

- low circuit volume, compliance and resistance
- minimal dead space within the ventilator and circuit
- rapid response time for gas flow during spontaneous respiratory effort
- a light-weight circuit
- inspiratory time adjustment independent of the inspiratory/expiratory ratio
- capability for a ventilation rate up to 60 breaths/min (excluding capability for high-frequency ventilation)
- variable gas flow at least up to 2–3 l/kg per min
- electronic display of inspiratory pressure wave
- accurate measurement of low tidal volume.

A generic classification of ventilators, their operational characteristics and by their modes of ventilation has been proposed.[5] It is described here briefly to enable functional description and comparison of some ventilators (Table 102.4).

Ventilators may be operationally classified as pressure, volume, flow or time controllers. These are the independent or control variables. Since only one variable can be controlled at a given time, i.e. predetermined, the remaining features of the waveform are dependent variables. If pressure, volume or flow are not predetermined the ventilator is presumed to be a time controller in which only the timing of the inspiratory and expiratory phases is controlled.

Pressure controller: the pressure waveform does not change when resistance or compliance changes, but volume waveform will.

Volume and flow controllers: the volume waveform does not change when resistance and compliance change but the pressure waveform changes.

In a volume controller the volume is measured and used in control whereas it is not in a flow controller. In a flow controller it is flow that is used.

Time controller: both pressure and volume waveforms change when resistance and compliance change.

These concepts allow understanding of any mode of ventilation and to interpret bedside pulmonary mechanics, that is, resistance, compliance, time constants etc. The manner of controlling the independent variable may be an open loop system, in which no feedback occurs during inspiration to achieve the target goal, or a closed-loop or feedback or servo control system in which the independent variable is modified according to progress during inspiration.

During inspiration, dual control may be used and may be altered from one independent variable to another. For example in the VAPS mode (volume assured pressure support mode) of the Bird VIP Gold ventilator, control is switched from pressure to flow control if a preset tidal volume has not been achieved. In another example using the Pmax feature of the Drager Evita 4, if in flow control a pressure limit has been reached, control is passed to pressure while the tidal volume is monitored and the inspiratory time increased until the preset tidal volume has been achieved.

PHASE VARIABLES

The manner of initiation of inspiration (triggering), sustaining inspiration (limit variables), initiation of expiration (cycling) and sustaining expiration are the phase variables. Initiation of inspiration, or triggering, may be dictated by machine or patient. Usual triggers are the elapse of time or generation of pressure or flow by the patient. Flow triggering during spontaneous ventilation is more energy efficient and better tolerated than other variables, particularly when the flow sensor is located at the endotracheal tube. Mandatory breaths are all those triggered by a pre-set frequency or minimum minute ventilation, or terminated by a pre-set frequency or tidal volume. Spontaneous breaths are those initiated by the patient and terminated by lung mechanics or ventilatory drive. The quantification of the inspiratory phase is by time, pressure or volume. Initiation of expiration (termination of inspiration) or cycling is achieved by elapse of time, pressure, volume or flow. Expiration is sustained usually by pressure alone.

Modes of ventilation may be described on the following generic basis. It is derived from the controller variables. It should not be assumed that a manufacturer's mode terminology accurately defines its functional attributes or is intuitively obvious. Terminology is not necessarily interchangeable between different manufacturers. Although some new modes are genuine inventions, another purpose appears to be differentiation of product from competition. The capabilities of any ventilator can be defined by the following:

- The controller variable (pressure, volume, dual)
- The pattern of mandatory breaths versus spontaneous breaths:

Table 102.4 Major characteristics of some ventilators (adapted from Branson et al., 1999[5]).

	Bear Cub BP2001	Bear Cub 750vs	Bird T Bird	Bird VIP Gold	Drager Babylog 8000	Drager Evita 4	Infant Star 950	Sechrist IV-100B	Sechrist IV-200 SAVI	Siemens Servo 900C	Siemens Servo 300
Controller (generator) variables											
Pressure	●	●	●	●	●	●	●	●	●	●	●
Volume							●				
Flow	●	●	●	●	●	●	●	●	●	●	●
Time											
Phase variables											
Trigger variables											
Pressure			●	●		●				●	●
Volume											
Flow		●	●	●	●	●	●		●	●	●
Time	●	●	●	●	●	●	●	●	●	●	●
Manual	●	●		●			●	●		●	●
Other						●					
Inspiration limit variables											
Pressure	●	●	●	●	●	●	●	●	●	●	●
Volume											
Flow		●	●	●	●	●	●	●		●	●
Cycle variable											
Pressure				●	●	●	●	●	●		
Volume		●	●	●		●				●	●
Flow											
Time	●	●	●	●	●	●	●	●	●	●	●
Other											
Modes											
Volume/flow control											
CMV			●	●		●				●	●
SIMV			●	●		●				●	●
Pressure control/limited											
CMV	●	●		●	●	●	●	●	●	●	●
SIMV		●		●	●	●			●		
CSV						●					
Unassisted	●	●			●		●	●	●		
Pressure support			●	●		●				●	●

Table 102.4 Major characteristics of some ventilators (adapted from Branson et al., 1999[5]) (continued)

	Bear Cub BP2001	Bear Cub 750vs	Bird T Bird	Bird VIP Gold	Drager Babylog 8000	Drager Evita 4	Infant Star 950	Sechrist IV-100B	Sechrist IV-200 SAVI	Siemens Servo 900C	Siemens Servo 300
Dual (volume/flow + pressure) control											
CMV											
SIMV			∞	∞		∞					∞
CSV			∞	∞		∞					
Mandatory minute ventilation						∞				∞	∞
Sigh			∞			∞					
Apnoea backup			∞								
Output displays (measured)											
Pressures											
Peak		∞	∞	∞	∞	∞	∞	∞		∞	
Mean		∞		∞	∞	∞	∞				∞
Baseline (PEEP)			∞	∞	∞	∞	∞	∞	∞		∞
AutoPEEP						∞					
Volumes											
Tidal volume		∞	∞	∞	∞	∞					
Leak		∞		∞	∞	∞				∞	∞
Deadspace											
Minute ventilation		∞	∞	∞	∞	∞	∞				
CO$_2$ production				∞		∞				∞	∞
Times											
Inspiratory (I)	∞	∞	∞	∞	∞	∞	∞	∞	∞		
Expiratory (E)	∞	∞						∞	∞		
Breath rate	∞	∞	∞	∞			∞	∞	∞	∞	∞
I:E ratio	∞	∞	∞								∞

∞, characteristic present; CMV, continuous mandatory ventilation; SIMV, synchronized intermittent mandatory ventilation; CSV, continuous spontaneous ventilation; PEEP, positive end expiratory pressure. These are examples of ventilators. Not all features are included (waveform, gas concentrations, mechanics, alarms are omitted).

– CMV is continuous mandatory ventilation (conventional IPPV)
– SIMV is synchronized intermittent mandatory ventilation
– CSV is continuous spontaneous ventilation.
- The phase variable for mandatory breaths, especially trigger and cycle variables
- Whether spontaneous breaths are assisted.

If conditional variables exist, these act to change the pattern of ventilation, for example, to give a sigh breath based on elapse of time, or switching from patient-triggered breaths to machine-triggered breaths in the SIMV mode or mandatory minute ventilation modes.

Volume/flow-control modes are suitable for conditions in which lung compliance and resistance are variable. In these circumstances, the peak inspiratory pressure attained is a valuable observation. However, when a pressure limit is imposed, such information is lost. A mode consisting of flow control, time triggering, pressure limitation and time cycling is commonly used, because of the relative ease of operation. However, relatively small leaks may severely compromise tidal volume, mean airway pressure and oxygenation. Large leaks may also delay attainment of preset pressure until late in the inspiratory cycle. Thus, it is helpful to display the volume and pressure waveforms. Some ventilators do however provide leak compensation, e.g. Bird VIP Gold. Gas flow should be set above 2 l/kg per min to achieve the preset pressure early in the inspiratory period. This flow rate is also suitable for peak inspiratory flow rate during spontaneous respiratory effort with intermittent mandatory ventilation.

Pressure in the circuit should be monitored in close proximity to the endotracheal tube. Changes in endotracheal tube resistance from encrustation or kinking have a major adverse effect on tidal volume.[6]

Neonates and infants have small tidal volumes (5–50 ml), and are therefore prone to alveolar hypoventilation when variable air leaks occur around the endotracheal tube and from the ventilator-humidifier circuit. Moreover, the internal compliance and compressible volume of the circuit may exceed the tidal volume. Small tidal volumes are difficult to set and maintain when the lung compliance and resistance are abnormal.[7]

Most neonatal ICUs use pressure control modes which in hyaline membrane disease achieves adequate oxygenation with minimal barotrauma.[8] The pressure-control mode is more appropriate than volume-control for neonates and infants 0.5–5.0 kg body weight. Ventilators, which are pressure controllers, deliver a variable flow dependent on lung and airway characteristics.

Improvements in ventilatory management of newborns are observed with a new generation of ventilators, which utilize changes in airway pressure, airway gas flow or abdominal movement to trigger inspiration, and which have ultrashort trigger delays.[9] Previously, ventilators were unable to cope with the very short inspiratory times (mean 0.31, SD 0.06 s) of newborns with respiratory distress syndrome.[10] Patient-triggered ventilation (PTV) permits synchronous ventilation with better gas exchange, prevents the patient fighting the ventilator and reduces the need for neuromuscular paralysis.[11,12]

HIGH FREQUENCY VENTILATORS

Ventilation at least 4 times normal rate high frequency and may be classified into 5 types[5]:

- high-frequency positive pressure ventilation (HF-PPV)
- high-frequency jet ventilation (HFJV)
- high-frequency flow interruption (HFFI)
- high-frequency oscillation (HFO)
- high-frequency percussive ventilation (HFPV).

High-frequency oscillatory ventilation (HFO) at 15 Hz has been shown to achieve better gas exchange with less barotrauma than conventional mechanical ventilation in infants with respiratory distress.[13,14] Examples of high-frequency oscillators are the Sensor Medics and 3100A and 3100B (adult) and the Humming series models, of which the latest is Atom Humming V. The latter also offers a synchronized intermittent mandatory ventilation mode. An example of a high frequency jet ventilator is the Bunnell Life Pulse jet ventilator which is used in conjunction with a conventional ventilator to provide PEEP and humidified gas for spontaneous ventilation. An example of a high frequency positive pressure ventilator is the Nellcor Puritan-Bennett Infant Star 950, which operates as a flow interrupter.

TRANSPORT VENTILATORS

Although 'hand-bagging' may be used during transport from the field to hospital, between hospitals and within hospitals, it is highly desirable to utilize a purpose-designed transport ventilator to ensure consistent ventilation and cardiorespiratory stability. Ventilation by machine also enables personnel to attend to other tasks. Whether pneumatic or electronically powered, it must be compact, light, rugged, easy to operate and yet provide a standard and mode of ventilation required by a wide variety of patient illnesses and equivalent to that required by any patient in the intensive care unit. Electrically powered ventilators should have both mains and battery power. The ventilator should be capable of providing SIMV, CPAP, PEEP, time or flow cycling, flow or pressure-triggered and provide 21–100% oxygen. Controls for rate, inspiratory time, flow, tidal volume and pressure should be independent. It should be unaffected by altitude and be operable in an MRI environment. It should incorporate alarms for low and high pressure, disconnection, apnoea and disconnection. All these aims are difficult if not impossible to fulfil. Examples of ventilators are Drager Oxylog 2000, Pulmonetic Systems LTV1000 and Newpot HTSO.

NON-INVASIVE VENTILATION

The application of ventilation 'BiPAP' (bilevel positive airways pressure) or CPAP by mask has become an essential part of paediatric intensive care practice. Although a proprietary name (Respironics), 'BiPAP' has become synonymous with non-invasive ventilation. It is distinct from BIPAP (biphasic positive airway pressure), a mode available in some conventional ventilators in which spontaneous ventilation is permitted during all phases of mechanical ventilation. CPAP or BiPAP is given by an interface of a nasal or oronasal (full face) mask with harnesses with or without a chin strap (headgear). Other interface devices such as mini-masks, nasal pillows, nasal cushions or a mouthpiece/lipseal are uncommon in paediatrics. CPAP is commonly used to relieve upper airway obstruction or improve oxygenation in lung disease. BiPAP is commonly used to provide ventilation in central hypoventilatory states although BiPAP machines are primarily intended for use in adult patients with obstructive sleep apnoea and are not in general intended for use as life support. Most are not licensed to provide ventilation via endotracheal tube or tracheostomy. The defining characteristics of BiPAP are the automatic breath-by-breath compensation for air leaks and the ability to trigger and cycle by flow or time in synchronization with patient effort. The devices can be set to provide a spontaneous (assisted) mode, timed (mandatory) mode or a combined mode. When the inspiratory positive airway pressure (IPAP) is set the same as the expiratory positive airway pressure (EPAP), CPAP is provided. Examples of CPAP machines are Tranquility (Healthdyne) and CPAP S6 series (Resmed). Examples of BiPAP machines are the BiPAP S/T, S/T-D, S/T-D 30, Harmony and Synchrony series (Respironics), the KnightStar 335 (Nellcor-Puritan-Bennett) but not suitable for children <30 kg, and the Sullivan VPAP II and VPAP II ST (Resmed).

OXYGEN THERAPY AND MONITORING

OXYGEN CATHETERS

Sizes 6, 8 and 10 FG should be available and placed in the same nostril as the nasogastric tube, to limit airway resistance. Size 6 FG is suitable for neonates; 8 FG for infants and small children and 10 FG for older children. It should be appreciated that oxygen catheters placed in the nasopharynx provide a small amount of PEEP, and indeed may be used for that purpose.[15] Nasal cannulae (two-pronged) are not recommended. Excessive flow may cause gastric distension. Flow rate for infants should be regulated by a low-flow metre, graduated 0–2.5 l/min.

OXYGEN MASKS

Masks may not be well-tolerated by the infant or small child; oxygen catheters are preferable.

HEAD BOXES AND INCUBATORS

A clear perspex head box is the best way of administering a high concentration of oxygen to the unintubated neonate and infant. Precise oxygen therapy is possible but rebreathing, heat loss and desiccation are potential problems. To avoid rebreathing, a large flow rate 10–12 l/min) of fresh gas with predetermined oxygen content should be introduced. The practice of introducing a low flow rate of 100% oxygen into a head box (to gain a lesser concentration) may cause rebreathing and hypercarbia. If 100% oxygen is the only compressed gas available, lesser concentrations of oxygen may be attained without rebreathing by using a flow of 100% oxygen and a Venturi device. The relatively large capacity of an incubator precludes the attainment of a high concentration of oxygen, but limited oxygen therapy, up to 60%, can be achieved.

OXYGEN ANALYSERS

These are essential to regulate oxygen therapy via incubator or head box. The devices utilize either a polarographic electrode or galvanic cell (microfuel cell) as oxygen sensor. The polarographic types require a source of power (battery or mains), are more expensive to buy but cheaper to run, and have a faster response time.[13,16] An incorporated alarm is recommended. The sensing electrode should be placed close to the patient's head.

An oxygen analyzer capable of monitoring deliberate hypoxic gas mixtures (e.g. OX60+, Parker Healthcare Pty Ltd) is required if nitrogen is to be used, for example to increase pulmonary vascular resistance in management of post-Norwood repair of hypoplastic left heart syndrome.

TRANSCUTANEOUS GAS ANALYSERS

Transcutaneous gas tensions in paediatric patients equate well with arterial gas tensions. However, PaO_2 is underestimated by $PtcO_2$ during mild hyperoxaemia in neonates.[17] Transcutaneous gas values are dependent on both arterial gas tensions and on blood flow. During normovolaemia with adequate flow, $PtcO_2$ reflects PaO_2 and $PtcCO_2$ reflects $PaCO_2$. However, during circulatory failure, a reduction in $PtcO_2$ reflects a reduction in flow, provided PaO_2 is normal.[18] Likewise, during circulatory failure, $PtcCO_2$ exceeds $PaCO_2$ and is flow-dependent.[19] Typical transcutaneous dual function single electrodes are Hewlett Packard Virida $tcpO_2/tcCO_2$, Sensormedics FasTrac SaO_2/CO_2 monitor.

Continuous-pulse oximetry (SpO_2) has evolved to be an integral part of monitoring in neonatal and paediatric intensive care. Transcutaneous pulse oximetry is more convenient than transcutaneous partial pressure measurement. Each patient should have a pulse oximeter. The value of pulse oximetry is detection of hypoxaemia, not hyperoxaemia. They cannot be used accurately to titrate oxygen therapy, which requires blood or transcutaneous partial pressure measurement. The accuracy of pulse oximetry at low SaO_2 (<75%) is poor.[20] Numerous devices are available.

BLOOD-GAS ANALYSERS

In many neonatal and paediatric conditions, frequent blood-gas analysis is essential for optimal management. A blood-gas analyser utilizing small volumes (<0.2 ml) is essential. The instrument should he located within or near the ICU, so that tests can be performed and the results known without delay. Hand-held bedside devices are available, e.g. i-Stat.

APNOEA MONITORS

Infant apnoea is often due to upper airway obstruction, seizures or gastro-oesophageal reflux[21] although it may be idiopathic and is commonly associated with prematurity. Short apnoeic spells (<15 s) are normal during sleep and feeding. Significant apnoea is associated with bradycardia, cyanosis and hypotonia. The detection and treatment of apnoea in intensive care are dependent on cardiovascular monitoring and constant nursing observation. In the home or ward, where observation is less than that available in the ICU, apnoea may be detected by the use of a pressure sensor in a pad or mattress under the infant, or by impedance pneumography, in which diaphragmatic movement causes a change in resistance between two electrodes on the skin. Apnoea of central origin is detected early by these devices but obstructive apnoea, resulting in paradoxical respiratory effort, is detected late. Some devices incorporate electrocardiogram monitoring and rely upon bradycardia as evidence of hypoxaemia, which is a useful but late sign in obstructive apnoea, when both hypoxaemia and movement of the diaphragm are present. False-positive alarms are not uncommon.

THERMOREGULATION

RADIANT HEATERS AND INCUBATORS

Adequate temperature regulation is essential in neonates and infants to avoid cold stress, and to maintain a thermoneutral environment.[22] Numerous heaters and incubators are available with special features for transport, resuscitation, intensive care and regular ward nursing. Open-type radiant heaters (e.g. Drager Babytherm 8000 OC, Air Shields Vickers IICS-90, Datex Ohmeda 4000 series) are more suitable for use in intensive care. The ideal radiant heater should incorporate:

- servo-controlled overhead heating device with alarm for overheating

- open tilt bed of adequate area
- clear perspex removable/hinged sides
- adequate illumination
- adjustable height
- facility for X-ray examinations
- facility for phototherapy.

Additional features may include facilities for bottled oxygen, positive pressure, resuscitation and suction equipment.

Incubators are less suitable for use in intensive care because of limited access, but are better for transportation. Heating is via a conductive mattress. Double-walled infant incubators (e.g. Air-Shields Isolette C2000) reduce heat loss, attain preset temperature rapidly, do not produce excessive air currents or sound levels, and do not permit carbon dioxide accumulation.[23] Oxygen therapy and mechanical ventilation are possible with both types of units, but are technically easier with all open-cot radiant heater.

HUMIDIFIERS

Adequate humidification of ventilator circuits is of utmost importance in the paediatric patient. Unless adequately humidified, the relatively narrow endotracheal and tracheostomy tubes are prone to encrustation and blockage. Insensible water and heat loss are also prevented with adequate humidification. High-flow heated humidifiers provide near 100% humidification (44 mg H_2O/l gas, 47 mmHg) at body temperature and are preferred. They are easily adapted for use into ventilator circuits, face and tracheostomy masks, T-piece circuits and oxygen head boxes. When used in ventilator circuits, it is important to realize that they contribute to internal compliance and a compressible volume, which produce errors in both volume-preset and pressure-preset ventilators. Ideally, the compliance should not exceed 1.0 ml/cmH$_2$O for infants less than 10 kg body weight.[24] Several methods exist to maintain the water level including an airlock system, parallel-fill system, float-system and a pinch-clamp system.[5] Systems that automatically maintain a constant level are preferred for the aforementioned reasons. Incorporation of servo-control is also important. A thermistor probe incorporated into the proximal inspiratory circuit and heating of the inspiratory limb ensures that gas is delivered to the patient at body temperature. However, because some heat loss may occur along the inspiratory limb and much more along the expiratory limb (which is not heated), significant condensation (rain out) occurs. A water trap must be incorporated to gather 'rain-out' and the circuit, particularly the expiratory limb, positioned in a dependent manner to prevent aspiration by the patient. Such water, although potentially contaminated by airway bacteria, does not pose nosocomial infection risk and may be allowed to drain into the humidifier where high temperature inhibits bacterial growth. Circuits may be changed infrequently. Examples of servo-controlled heated humidifiers are Puritan-Bennett Cascade II and Fisher and Paykel MR600, 700, 720, 850 series.

Condenser-type humidifiers or 'artificial noses' have a role in intensive care. They are passive humidifiers capturing exhaled water vapour and heat permitting its re-use on inhalation (heat and moisture exchangers, HME). Numerous devices exist, some incorporating filters and/or hydroscopic materials leading to subclassifications of heat and moisture exchanging filter (HMEF), hydroscopic heat and moisture exchanger (HHME) and hydroscopic heat and moisture exchanging filter (HHMEF). They are often added to tracheostomy or endotracheal tubes of spontaneously breathing patients or inserted into the inspiratory limb of a ventilator circuit for short periods, e.g. for transport. They cannot replace full humidification. HMEs provide approximately one-quarter to one-third relative humidity whereas HHME/HHMEFs provide approximately one-half to three-quarters relative humidity.[5] Problems with these devices include deterioration of performance with time, resistance and deadspace. The appropriate size for the patient (adult, paediatric, neonatal) must be used. They are not suitable for use if the patient is hypothermic, has thick or bloody secretions or requires frequent changes. They should never be used in conjunction with heated water humidifiers because of potential circuit blockage. They should not be moistened and the addition of oxygen, although sanctioned by some manufacturers, will compromise performance. Unheated humidifiers of the passover, bubble, bubble diffuser and jet types are inefficient and have limited applicability in the intensive care setting. Other types of humidifiers such as jet nebulizers and ultrasonic nebulizers have little role in intensive care.

MISCELLANEOUS EQUIPMENT

INFUSION DEVICES

Numerous electromechanical devices have been developed to overcome the deficiencies of gravity-fed i.v. infusion sets. They enable constant and accurate infusion of predetermined volumes. These devices have wide clinical application and are used to control the administration of potent drugs, hormones and parenteral nutrition. Performance and application are variable.[25,26]

FLOW REGULATORS

With these devices (e.g. Dial-A-Flow and Helix), flow is manually regulated. They are simple, cheap, easy to adjust and are more suited to infusion at high flow rates. However, they do not overcome the main deficiencies of gravity-fed i.v. giving sets, such as the effects of venous pressure and fluid viscosity. Their accuracy is poor at low flow rates, and they are not suitable for administration of concentrated potent drugs.

VOLUMETRIC PUMPS

These regulate flow rate by delivering a pre-measured bolus under pressure. In some the delivery is not smooth. They utilize disposable closed cassettes. The risk of air pumping is minimal and alarms indicate infusion failure. High (up to 999 ml/h) and low flow rates (1 ml/h) are possible. Examples are IVAC Neo-mate 565, Alaris Medical Systems Gemini PC-1, PC-2, Abbott Lifecare 5000 'Plum' Pump, B/Braun Infusomat fm.

SYRINGE PUMPS AND DRIVERS

These are suitable for infusion of potent drugs in concentrated form at very low rates (down to 0.1 ml/h). They are mains electricity and/or battery-powered. The latter are suitable for use during transport and miniaturized models are suitable for ambulant use. These devices are suitable for i.v., intra-arterial, intramuscular, subcutaneous infusion or enterogastric feeding, being particularly suitable for use in neonates and infants. They are not suited to infusion of large volumes and offer no safeguard against extravasation unless an overpressure alarm is incorporated. Generally, the pumps utilize specified syringes unless recalibrated. Some syringe brands do not run smoothly. At low flows (<1 ml/h) infusion line compliance contributes to irregular drug delivery associated with vertical displacement of the pump.[27] Examples of syringe infusion pumps are B/Braun Perfusor, Graseby 3100, IVAC Alaris P3000, P6000.

INDIRECT MEASUREMENT OF BLOOD PRESSURE

Measurement of blood pressure in the critically ill neonate and infant is important in cardiovascular monitoring. Continuous direct intra-arterial measurement is preferred in cardiovascular instability, but adequate monitoring can be achieved with Doppler ultrasonography (e.g. Roche Arteriosonde) or with microprocessor analysis of oscillometric signals (e.g. Critikon Dinamap, Nippon-Colin, Ohio NIMP, Narco Scientific and Vita-Stat, Kenz BPM). The latter devices provide time-automated analysis of systolic, diastolic and mean blood pressure, as well as heart rate at specified intervals. Some portable monitoring devices provide additional data, such as invasive pressure measurement, electrocardiogram, heart rate, pulse oximetry, capnography, respiratory rate and temperature (e.g. Nellcor Propaq, Datascope Passport, Schiller Argus TM-7, S & W Diascope, BCI 6100).

Continuous non-invasive measurement of blood pressure may be measured with the Ohmeda Finapres non-invasive blood pressure monitor. Blood pressure measured with these non-invasive devices correlates well with simultaneous measurement by direct intra-arterial measurement in neonates,[28] infants and children.[29] Generally, systolic pressure is underestimated by only 2–4 mmHg (0.3–0.5 kPa), while the diastolic pressure is overestimated by a similar amount. Venostasis and radial nerve compression are occasional complications.[30]

NASOGASTRIC TUBES

These are mandatory in all intubated and/or ventilated patients as aids to prevent aspiration, and are a useful means of providing nutrition and medication. A range of sizes should be available: 5–6 FG for neonates; 8 FG for infants; 10 FG for small children and 12 FG for larger children.

PLASMAPHARESIS/HAEMOFILTRATION

Generally, the techniques described in dialytic therapy are applicable to infants and children. Although separate veins, or an artery and a vein may be cannulated, it is common to perform these procedures via a double lumen catheter inserted into a large vein (femoral, jugular, subclavian), that is, to perform continuous venovenous haemo/diafiltration (CVVH, CVVHD), plasmafiltration or haemoperfusion. In infants (0–1 year), this requires a 6.5 FR catheter to achieve blood flow of 25–40 ml/min, small children (1–8 years) an 8.5 FR to achieve 30–60 ml/min and in large children (>8 years) an 11 FR catheter to achieve 50–100 ml/min via a blood pump, for example, Gambro MPM 10. Typically, the filtration rate is one third of the blood flow while the size of the molecules appearing in the filtrate is determined by filter size. To remove molecules up to 30 000 Daltons, Gambro FH 22, 55, 66, 77 or 88 are used. To remove molecules up to 3 million Daltons, Gambro PF1000, PF2000 are used.

REFERENCES

1 Greenbaum DM, Marshall KE. The value of routine daily chest X-rays in intubated patients in the medical intensive care unit. *Crit Care Med* 1982; **10**: 29–30.
2 Bosman YK, Foster PA. Endotracheal intubation and head posture in infants. *South Afr Med J* 1977; **52**: 71–8.
3 Scoble MK, Copnell B, Taylor A, Kinney S, Shann F. Effect of reusing suction catheters on the occurrence of pneumonia in children. *Heart and Lung* 2001; **30**: 225–33.
4 Tibballs J, Carter B, Whittington N. A disadvantage of self-inflating resuscitation bags. *Anaesth Intens Care* 2000; **28**: 587.
5 Branson RD, Hess DR, Chatburn RL. *Respiratory Care Equipment*. Philadelphia: Lippincott Williams & Wilkins, 1999.
6 Abrahams N, Fisk GC, Vonwiller JB, Grant GC. Evaluation of infant ventilators. *Anaesth Intens Care* 1975; **3**: 6–11.

7 Simbruner G, Gregory GA. Performance of neonatal ventilators: the effects of changes in resistance and compliance. *Crit Care Med* 1981; **9**: 509–14.
8 Reynolds EOR, Taghizadeh A. Improved prognosis of infants mechanically ventilated for hyaline membrane disease. *Arch Dis Child* 1974; **49**: 505.
9 Greenough A, Milner AD. Respiratory support using patient triggered ventilation in the neonatal period. *Arch Dis Child* 1992; **67**: 69–71.
10 South M, Morley CJ. Respiratory timing in intubated neonates with respiratory distress syndrome. *Arch Dis Child* 1992; **67**: 446–8.
11 Hird MF, Greenough A. Patient triggered ventilation using a flow triggered system. *Arch Dis Child* 1991; **66**: 1140–2.
12 Cleary JP, Bernstein G, Mannino FL, Heldt GP. Improved oxygenation during synchronized intermittent mandatory ventilation in neonates with respiratory distress syndrome: a randomized, crossover study. *J Pediatr* 1995; **126**: 407–11.
13 Ogawa Y, Miyasaka K, Kawano T, *et al*. A multicenter randomized trial of high frequency oscillatory ventilation as compared with conventional mechanical ventilation in preterm infants with respiratory failure. *Early Human Dev* 1993; **32**: 1–10.
14 HiFO study group. Randomized study of high-frequency oscillatory ventilation in infants with severe respiratory distress syndrome. *J Paediatr* 1993; **122**: 609–19.
15 Shann F, Gatachalian S, Hutchinson R. Nasopharyngeal oxygen in children. *Lancet* 1988; **2**: 1238–40.
16 Cole AGH. Small oxygen analysers. *Br J Hosp Med* 1983; **29**: 469–71.
17 Martin RJ, Robertson SS, Hopple MM. Relationship between transcutaneous and arterial oxygen tension in sick neonates during mild hyperoxaemia. *Crit Care, Med* 1982; **10**: 670–2.
18 Tremper KK, Shoemaker WC, Shippy CR, Nolan LS. Transcutaneous oxygen monitoring of critically ill adults with and without low flow shock. *Crit Care Med* 1981; **9**: 706–9.
19 Tremper KK, Shoemaker WC, Shippy CR, Nolan LS. Transcutaneous PCO_2 monitoring on adult patients in the ICU and operating room. *Crit Care Med* 1981; **9**: 752–5.
20 Carter BG, Carlin JB, Tibballs J, Mead H, Hochmann M, Osborne A. Accuracy of two pulse oximeters at low arterial hemoglobin-oxygen saturation. *Crit Care Med* 1998; **26**: 1128–33.
21 Brown LW. Home monitoring of the high-risk infant. *Clin Pediatr* 1984; **11**: 85–100.
22 Hull D, Chellappah G. On keeping babies warm. In: Chiswick ML (ed.) *Recent Advances in Perinatal Medicine*. Edinburgh: Churchill Livingstone; 1983: pp. 153–68.
23 Bell EF, Rios GR. Performance characteristics of two double-walled infant incubators. *Crit Care Med* 1983; **11**: 663–7.
24 Holbrook PR, Taylor G, Pollak MM, *et al*. Adult respiratory distress syndrome in children. *Pediatr Clin North Am* 1980; **27**: 677–85.

25 Shyam VSR, Tinker J. Recent developments in infusion devices. *Br J Hosp Med* 1981; **25**: 69–75.

26 Dickenson JR. Syringe pumps. *Br J Hosp Med* 1983; **29**: 187–91.

27 Weiss M, Banziger O, Neff T, Fanconi S. Influence of infusion line compliance on drug delivery rate during acute line loop formation. *Intens Care Med* 2000; **26**: 776–9.

28 Lui K, Doyle PE, Buchanan N. Oscillometric and intra-arterial blood pressure measurements in the neonates: evaluation and comparison of methods. *Aust Paediatr J* 1982; **18**: 32–4.

29 Savage JM, Dillon MJ, Taylor JFN. Clinical evaluation and comparison of the infrasonde, arteriosonde and mercury sphygmomanometer in measurements of blood pressure in children. *Arch Dis Child* 1979; **54**: 184–9.

30 Showman A, Betts EK. Hazard of automatic noninvasive blood pressure monitoring. *Anesthesiology* 1981; **55**: 717–9.

103

Paediatric poisoning

J Tibballs

EPIDEMIOLOGY

The peak incidence of poisoning in childhood is among 1–4 year olds. It usually occurs in the home when the child ingests a single prescribed or over-the-counter medication or a household product. Over 3600 children of this age are admitted to hospital each year in Australia.[1] This mode of poisoning is called 'accidental' – erroneously because it is usually the result of inadequate supervision or improper storage of poisons. The mortality is very low and if hospitalization is required, it is usually brief (1–3 days). In this circumstance, care must be taken to ensure that whatever treatment is applied, it does not impose additional risk.

Occasionally, poisoning in childhood is either truly accidental or is part of a syndrome of child abuse, or is iatrogenic as when a parent mistakes medications at home or when medical or nursing staff make errors in drug administration in hospital. Medication errors occur in approximately 5% of paediatric in-patient medication.[2] Self-poisoning in older children is usually with the intention to manipulate their psychosocial environment or to commit suicide, or is the result of substance abuse. All circumstances of poisoning require remedial action.

DIAGNOSIS

Commonly, the diagnosis of poisoning in paediatric practice is self evident and supported by a history detailed by parents or guardians. Although a single poison is usually involved, the possibility of several or multiple poisons should be considered. Occasionally the diagnosis is unknown on presentation. Any child who presents with otherwise unexplained obtundation, fitting, hypoventilation or hypotension should have the diagnosis excluded.

OPTIONS FOR TREATMENT

The treatment should be determined by the seriousness of poisoning, as judged by the observed and expected effects of the poison, by the amount ingested, by the interval between ingestion and presentation and by the existence or otherwise of an antidote.

The range of treatment options is to: discharge home, observe for a short duration in the emergency department or ward, provide intensive nursing care or to treat medically. The task is to match the intensity of treatment to the severity of the poisoning thereby avoiding under and over-treatment.

PRINCIPLES OF MANAGEMENT

The four basic principles in management of poisoning are:

- support vital functions
- confirm the diagnosis
- remove the poison from the body
- administer an antidote. Few poisons have antidotes (Table 103.1).

Individual poisons may require specific measures. Consult toxicology texts[3–5] for details.

The vast majority of poisoning in childhood is by ingestion. The correct choice of a gastrointestinal decontamination technique is crucial to uncomplicated recovery. The choices are induced emesis, gastric lavage, activated charcoal, whole bowel irrigation or a combination of these techniques. The efficacy, indi-cations, contra-indications and disadvantages and complications of these techniques are discussed below. A general plan of management is presented in Figure 103.1.

A crucial point in management is initial recognition that the patient is in a state of either 'full-consciousness' or 'less-than-full consciousness'. Traditionally, management has been dependent on a judgement of whether the gag reflex is present or absent, but in practice this is rarely tested. Since aspiration pneumonitis is a common feature of poisoning management, particularly among (but not confined to) CNS obtunded patients, it is prudent to regard all obtunded patients as having incompetent pharyngeal reflexes.

Table 103.1 Antidotes to some serious poisons

Poison	Antidotes	Comments
Amphetamines	Esmolol i.v. 500 µg/kg over 1 min, then 25–200 µg/kg/min	Treatment for tachyarrhythmia
	Labetalol i.v. 0.15–0.3 mg/kg or	Treatment for hypertension
	Phentolamine i.v. 0.05–0.1 mg/kg every 10 min	
Benzodiazepines	Flumazenil i.v. 3–10 µg/kg, repeat 1 min, then 3–10 µg/kg per h.	Specific receptor antagonist. Beware convulsions.
Beta blockers	Glucagon i.v. 7 µg/kg, then 2–7 µg/kg per min	Stimulates non-catecholamine cAMP, preferred antidote
	Isoprenaline i.v. 0.05–3 µg/kg/min	Beware β_2 hypotension
	Noradrenaline i.v. 0.05–1 µg/kg/min	
Calcium channel blocker	Calcium chloride i.v. 10%, 0.2 ml/kg	
Carbon monoxide	Oxygen 100%	Decreases carboxyhaemoglobin May need hyperbaric oxygen
Cyanide	Dicobalt edetate i.v. 300 mg over 1 min, then 300 mg at 5 min	Give 50 ml 50% glucose after each dose
	Amyl nitrite 0.2 perles by inhalation until Sodium nitrite 3% i.v. 0.33 ml/kg over 4 min, then Sodium thiosulphate 25% i.v. 1.65 ml/kg (max 50 ml) at 3–5 min	Nitrites form methaemoglobin-cyanide complex. Beware excess methaemoglobin >20%. Thiosulphate forms non-toxic thiocyanate from methaemoglobin-cyanide
Digoxin	Magnesium sulphate i.v. 25–50 mg/kg (0.1–0.2 mmol/kg)	
	Digoxin Fab i.v: acute: 10 vials per 25 tablets (0.25 mg each), 10 vials per 5 mg elixir; steady state: vials, serum digoxin (ng/ml) × BW(kg)/100	
Ergotamine	Sodium nitroprusside infusion 0.5–5.0 µg/kg per min	Treats vasoconstriction. Monitor BP continuously
	Heparin i.v. 100 U/kg then 10–30 U/kg per h	Monitor partial thromboplastin time
Lead	Dimercaprol (BAL) i.m. 75 mg/m² 4-hourly 6 doses, then i.v. CaNa₂edetate (EDTA) 1500 mg/m² over 5 days if blood level >3.38 µmol/l. If asymptomatic and blood level 2.65–3.3 µmol/l infuse CaNa₂EDTA 1000 mg/m² per day, 5 days or oral succimer 350 mg/m² 8-hourly 5 days, then 12-hourly 14 days	
Heparin	Protamine 1 mg/100 units heparin	
Iron	Desferrioxamine 15 mg/kg per h, 12–24 h if serum iron >90 µmol/l (500 µg/dl) or >63 µmol/l (350 µg/dl) and symptomatic.	Give slowly, beware anaphylaxis.
Methanol. Ethylene glycol, Glycol ethers	Ethanol i.v. loading dose 10 ml/kg 10% diluted in glucose 5%, then 0.15 ml/kg per h to maintain blood level 0.1% (100 mg/dl).	
Methaemoglobinaemia	Methylene blue i.v. 1–2 mg/kg over several min	
Opiates	Naloxone i.v. 0.01–0.1 mg/kg, then 0.01 mg/kg per h as needed.	
Organophosphates and Carbamates	Atropine i.v. 20–50 µg/kg every 15 min until secretions dry	Blocks muscarinic effects
	Pralidoxime i.v. 25 mg/kg over 15–30 min, then 10–20 mg/kg per h for 18 h or more. Not for carbamates	Reactivates cholinesterase
Paracetamol	N-acetylcysteine i.v. 150 mg/kg in dextrose 5% over 60 min then 10 mg/kg per h for 20–72 h OR oral 140 mg/kg then 17 doses of 70 mg/kg 4-hourly (total 1330 mg/kg over 68 h)	Restores glutathione inhibiting metabolites. Give if serum paracetamol exceeds 1500 µmol/l at 2 h, 1000 at 4 h, 500 at 8 h, 200 at 12 h, 80 at 16 h, 40 at 20 h. Beware anaphylaxis

Table 103.1   Antidotes to some serious poisons   (*continued*)

Poison	Antidotes	Comments
Phenothiazine dystonia	Benztropine i.v or i.m. 0.01–0.03 mg/kg	Blocks dopamine re-uptake
Potassium	Calcium chloride 10% i.v. 0.2 ml/kg	Antagonizes cardiac effects
	Sodium bicarbonate i.v. 1 mmol/kg	Decreases serum potassium, beware hypocalcaemia
	Glucose i.v. 0.5 g/kg plus insulin i.v. 0.05 U/kg	Decreases serum potassium. Monitor serum glucose
	Salbutamol aerosol 0.25 mg/kg	Decreases serum potassium
	Resonium oral or rectal 0.5–1 g/kg	Absorbs potassium
Tricyclic antidepressants	Sodium bicarbonate i.v. 1 mmol/kg to maintain blood pH > 7.45	Reduces cardiotoxicity.

The decision to attempt removal of a poison should always be made with due reference to two facts:

- The vast majority of childhood poisonings recover with merely supportive care or no treatment at all.
- Aspiration pneumonitis is more serious than most poisonings.

Occasionally, removal from the circulation by charcoal haemoperfusion, plasmafiltration or haemofiltration is indicated.

INDUCED EMESIS

Induced emesis is quickly disappearing from hospital practice and should not be performed routinely in this setting.[6] It does not improve outcome and may reduce effectiveness of the alternative treatments of activated charcoal, oral antidotes and whole bowel irrigation.

Specific contraindications include actual or impending loss of full consciousness or ingestion of corrosives or hydrocarbons.[6]

Syrup of Ipecacuanha has succeeded other more injurious substances as emetic agents. It contains alkaloids, mainly emetine and cephaeline, which induce emesis by stimulation of the chemoreceptor trigger zone of the medulla and by irritation of the gastric mucosa.

The efficacy of ipecacuanha is limited and decreases with time from ingestion. Although it causes vomiting in a high percentage (93–100%) of children within 25 minutes, the percentage of stomach contents ejected is small (28%) even when administered immediately after ingestion.[7] Moreover, solids are retained in the stomach or may even be propelled into the duodenum.[8]

In experimental drug ingestions, approximately 50–83% of ingested experimental drug is removed if ipecac is given after 5 minutes,[9] but falling to 2–44% if

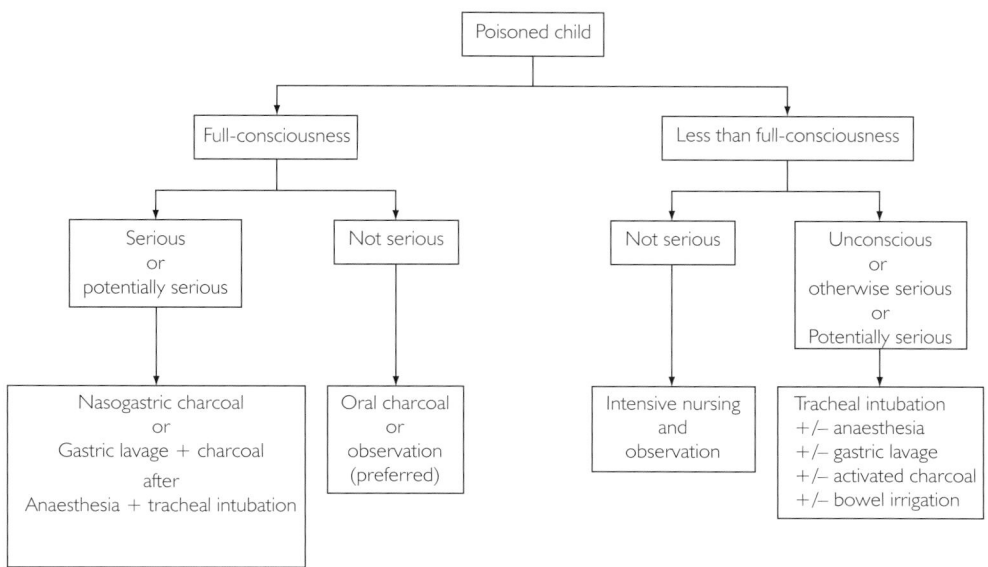

Fig. 103.1   General management of the poisoned child.

given at 30 or 60 minutes.[10–14] In paediatric paracetamol poisoning, the 4-hour post-ingestion serum level was approximately 50% of controls if ipecac-induced vomiting occurred within 60 minutes of ingestion, but no benefit was derived if emesis occurred beyond 90 minutes after ingestion.[15] Similarly, serum levels of paracetamol were reduced approximately 50% if ipecac was administered at home, inducing emesis at a mean of 26 minutes after ingestion, compared with ipecac administered at a medical facility at a mean of 83 minutes.[16]

In adults, ipecac is even less useful and has to be given immediately to have quantifiable effects.[17]

Induced emesis appears superior to gastric lavage but inferior to activated charcoal. In children poisoned with salicylate, emesis retrieved twice as much compared with gastric lavage.[18] In adult volunteers ipecac-induced vomiting, occurring at an average of 19 minutes after ingestion removed 54% of a tracer compared with 30% with gastric lavage performed at the equivalent times after ingestion.[19–21]

The use of ipecac has potential complications:

- Time-related lack of efficacy
- protracted vomiting (17%),
- diarrhoea (13%)
- lethargy (12%).[22]

More serious, but rare complications include:

- gastric, oesophageal or brain haemorrhage
- pneumomediastinum
- aspiration pneumonitis may occur, even in the fully conscious
- delayed onset of vomiting which is a threat if loss of consciousness subsequently occurs
- abuse in bulimia which may cause cardiotoxicity as well as the sequelae of associated with repetitive vomiting.

Critics claim that induced emesis merely creates work, delays discharge from the emergency department[23] and increases complications[24] and does not benefit the patient who presents more than one hour after ingestion.[25] Importantly, ipecac did not alter the clinical outcome of patients who presented awake and alert to the emergency department.[25]

Induced emesis has been largely abandoned by emergency departments but its use in the home is safe and is associated with less paediatric emergency department attendances.[26] Its use at home is still recommended by authoritative paediatric health organizations in USA[27] and by approximately half of poison centre staff.[28] Although ipecac was recommended inappropriately in 20% of cases to poisons information centres, it caused little morbidity.[29]

CONCLUSION

In hospital, it has no practical role. Even when a child presents very early after significant poisoning, oral or nasogastric charcoal is preferred. Whenever induced emesis is used the child must be fully conscious on administration and expected to be fully conscious when vomiting occurs.

GASTRIC LAVAGE

Its place in the management of the poisoned victim has also been curtailed. It is an invasive technique with questionable efficacy. Moreover, it is potentially harmful and should be reserved for the child who presents soon after life-threatening poisoning such as ingestion of iron or colchicine.

It involves passage of a large bore oro- or nasogastric tube into the stomach and the repeated instillation of fluid, usually water but some authorities advocate normal or half-normal saline. The oral route is preferred because of less potential for traumatic injury but an oropharyngeal airway may be needed to prevent tube occlusion by biting. A smaller tube may be used if the poison is a liquid. Traditionally, the child should be placed in the left lateral position to limit stomach emptying but volume of intragastric contents rather than body position determines gastric emptying.[30]

Experimental studies with therapeutic substances in volunteers or with liquid medicines or substances instilled into the stomachs of overdose victims, reported that gastric lavage retrieved 90% at 5 minutes,[31] 45% at 10 minutes[20] and 30% at 19 minutes[19] and reduced absorption or bioavailability by 20–32% at 1 hour after ingestion.[10,32] When gastric lavage was performed 5 minutes after ingestion of tablet drugs, it failed to prevent absorption presumedly because the tablets had not disintegrated.[33] In true overdose situations, gastric lavage within 4 hours of admission reduced serum paracetamol levels by 39%.[34]

Efficacy of gastric lavage, even with large bore tubes is poor because tablets are not removed and lavage encourages propulsion into the duodenum.[8] In symptomatic patients, gastric lavage alone compared with gastric lavage and activated charcoal increased pneumonic aspiration and did not alter the duration of intubation or the stay in the emergency department or in ICU,[35] and was not beneficial unless performed within one hour of ingestion.[25] A prospective randomized trial of gastric lavage in acute overdose,[36] although criticized on methodological grounds,[36,37] suggested that it made no difference to outcome of obtunded patients when preceding activated charcoal.

CONTRAINDICATIONS

- Less-than-full consciousness patient (unless already intubated) because of the risk of aspiration pneumonitis – which is not negligible even during full consciousness.[35]

- After ingestion of corrosives because of the risk of perforation
- After ingestion of hydrocarbons or petrochemicals because of the risk of pneumonitis.

COMPLICATIONS

- aspiration pneumonitis
- water intoxication
- minor trauma to oropharynx (gastro-oesophageal perforation occurs rarely)
- intra-bronchial instillation of lavage fluid.

As expected, infants and children never co-operate fully for gastric lavage, thus increasing risks of complications and the degree of psychological trauma.

If lavage is indicated, that is, for life-threatening poisoning, rapid sequence induction of anaesthesia with intubation is advised. The largest possible lubricated tube of diameter similar to an appropriate sized endotracheal tube should be used and correct placement in the stomach confirmed. Small volumes (1–2 ml/kg) of warm tap water may be used to lavage until clear. However, most water should be retrieved to avoid hyponatraemia.

ACTIVATED CHARCOAL

Charcoal is a substance which adsorbs many drugs and is regarded as a 'universal antidote'. It is advocated as the sole treatment in most poisonings although it is overused for minor poisonings. For many poisons no data exists regarding efficacy.

Treatment of charcoal with chemicals and heat increases its surface area to approximately 950 m²/g in so-called low surface area activated charcoal and to 2000 m²/g in super-activated charcoal. The latter adsorbs paracetamol better[38] and is more palatable.[38,39] Activated charcoal is not pleasant to drink and alone caused vomiting in 6–8% of subjects.[40]

It is superior to induced emesis and gastric lavage in treatment of symptomatic poisoned patients.[21,25,35] Its efficacy diminishes with time after ingestion. Activated charcoal reduces absorption of ingested experimental drugs in volunteers by 85–100% when administered 5 minutes after ingestion,[9,33,41] by 40–75% at 30 minutes[9] and by 30–50% at 60 minutes.[13,41] At a mean time of 98 minutes (SD 44) or more than 2 hours after poisoning, it was not effective at all.[42,43]

Studies have suggested that charcoal alone is as effective as when combined with either emesis or with lavage.[36,37] Furthermore, combined methods have a higher incidence of aspiration, 8.5% versus none.[33] Activated charcoal failed to show a benefit in asymptomatic poisoned patients.

Repeated doses of activated charcoal enhances elimination of some drugs by increasing adsorption and by achieving post-absorption elimination by interrupting enterohepatic circulation and by removing drug from the gastrointestinal mucosa ('gastrointestinal dialysis'). Although there are multiple reports in experimental and clinical practice (see Table 103.2), there is no hard evidence to show that this therapy reduces mortality or morbidity. Only in life-threatening poisoning by carbamazepine, dapsone, phenobarbital, quinine or theophylline should multiple dose activated charcoal be considered.[44]

A suitable single dose is 1–2 g/kg. A multiple-dose regimen for children is 1–2 g/kg stat followed by 0.25–0.5 g/kg 4–6-hourly. An alternative is 0.25 g–0.5 g/kg hourly for 12–24 hours.[45]

CONTRAINDICATIONS

- if ileus is present
- a less-than-fully conscious patient unless already intubated
- substances not adsorbed include strong corrosive acids and alkalis, cyanide, metals (iron, lithium, mercury, lead), alcohols, glycols, petroleum distillates (not all) and essential oils.[3–5]

Table 103.2 Elimination and lack of elimination of drugs by multiple dose activated charcoal[44]

Elimination increased in experimental and clinical studies	Elimination increased in volunteer studies	Elimination not increased in experimental or clinical studies
Carbamazepine	Amitryptyline	Astemizole
Dapsone	Dextropropoxyphene	Chlorpropamide
Phenobarbital	Digitoxin	Doxepin
Quinine	Digoxin	Imipramine
Theophylline	Disopyramide	Meprobamate
	Nadolol	Methotrexate
	Phenylbutazone	Phenytoin
	Phenytoin	Sodium valproate
	Piroxicam	Tobramycin
	Sotalol	Vancomycin

See text for details.

COMPLICATIONS

Aspiration of charcoal causes severe and often fatal pneumonitis, bronchiolitis obliterans and adult respiratory distress syndrome. Intratracheal instillation of activated charcoal causes a significant increase in lung microvascular permeability and arterial blood gas derangements.[46]

Constipation is common after charcoal but bowel obstruction is fortunately rare. The addition of a laxative (e.g. sorbitol or magnesium sulphate) is not recommended because although transit time through the gut is decreased, efficacy of the charcoal is reduced and life-threatening fluid and electrolyte imbalance may occur.[47]

WHOLE BOWEL IRRIGATION

Irrigation of the bowel with an iso-osmolar solution of polyethylene glycol and electrolytes is effective in reducing absorption of experimental drug by 24–67% at 1 hour after ingestion[48,49] and up to 73% at 4 hours after ingestion.[50] However, it has not been shown conclusively to improve the outcome of poisoned patients. The technique has limited applications to sustained-release or enteric-coated drugs and remains a theoretical option for ingestions of iron, lead, zinc (substances not adsorbed by activated charcoal), packets of illicit drugs[51] and for lithium.[52] Whole bowel irrigation may be useful in delayed presentations when poisons have progressed beyond the stomach.

Irrigation solutions are adsorbed by activated charcoal and cause desorption of drug – necessitating prior administration of charcoal if a combined technique is used.[53] However, whole bowel irrigation did not add to the benefits of activated charcoal in an experimental model of sustained-release theophylline poisoning.[54]

A suitable regimen is approximately 30 ml/kg per hour for 4–8 hours until rectal effluent is clear. A regimen of 25 ml/kg per hour has been used safely for 5 days (total 44.3 litres),[55] but a total of 3 litres performed as well as 8 litres in a simulated poisoning.[56]

CONTRAINDICATIONS

- in less-than-full consciousness
- during bowel obstruction or ileus because of risk of aspiration pneumonitis.

PLAN OF MANAGEMENT

A general plan of management is suggested in Figure 103.1, but each case of poisoning mandates a specific plan of management according to circumstances. The primary determinant is the state of consciousness which relates to the risk of aspiration. Apart from that, the timing of presentation in relation to the severity of poisoning and the existence or otherwise of an effective antidote dictate if removal should be attempted, and by what means.

POISONING BY SPECIFIC SUBSTANCES

Like adults, children are poisoned regularly by therapeutic prescription or over-the-counter therapeutic drugs and substances. The poisons probably reflect their availability in the home. In a recent survey, the most common agents responsible for hospital admission were benzodiazepines, anticonvulsants, anti-parkinsonism drugs, paracetamol, major tranquillizers, antidepressants and cardiovascular drugs.[57] The inquisitive nature of young children, however, may lead to poisoning by substances not normally regarded as dangerous – a few of these and others which have notably different management from similar poisoning in adults, are considered here, briefly.

BUTTON OR DISC BATTERIES

Ingestion may cause electrolytic injury and potentially corrosive, toxic or pressure injury. There are many types of batteries that contain a variety of substances: the most important are lithium, mercury, and potassium hydroxide.

Impaction in the oesophagus is the most significant situation; this can result in oesophageal perforation and tracheo-oesophageal fistula or aorto-oesophageal fistula. An impacted battery must be removed endoscopically as soon as possible. Lithium batteries are large and impact readily and they have higher voltages than other types. Electrolysis commences as soon as the battery surfaces are immersed in oesophageal fluid. The consequence is local and surrounding tissue destruction, including the trachea.[58] Strong alkali is produced at the cathode and strong acid is produced at the anode. Mercury batteries are more likely to fragment[59] but mercury poisoning is very uncommon.

Sufficient follow-up is necessary to exclude oesophageal and tracheal damage and to ensure that a battery in the stomach or distal bowel is eliminated.

PETROLEUM DISTILLATES

Numerous by-products of petroleum distillation are utilized in industrial and domestic purposes. Ingestion of these hydrocarbons may cause CNS toxicity, (comprising obtundation and convulsion), gastro-intestinal irritation, occasional hepato-renal toxicity, and pneumonitis.

Pneumonitis is the most significant and it may occur during ingestion or subsequent vomiting. Although variable, these substances have low surface tensions which enables their rapid dispersement throughout contiguous mucosal surfaces which includes the respiratory tree. Prime examples are petrol, kerosene, lighter fluid, lamp oil and mineral spirits. Any child who ingests a distillate must be assessed for pneumonitis and this should include clinical examination, a chest X-ray and at least a non-invasive measurement of oxygenation such as pulse oximetry. Although most children who ingest petroleum distillates do not develop pneumonitis the onset of this complication may be within 30 minutes[60] and progress rapidly to severe lung disease. An adequate period of observation (6 hours) is necessary to exclude this complication. There is a poor correlation between the amount ingested and the severity of pulmonary toxicity.

Deliberate inhalation of volatile hydrocarbons such as petrol or aerosolized paint have the additional toxicity on myocardial tissues such that fatal tachydysrhythmia, possibly due to sensitization to endogenous catecholamines. The deliberate inhalation of paint fumes, usually via a plastic bag, is called 'chroming'.

ESSENTIAL OILS

The oils from certain plants contain mixtures of terpenes, alcohols, aldehydes, ketones and esters, which are used domestically for various purposes. The well known oils are eucalyptus, turpentine, citronella, cloves, melaleuca, peppermint, wintergreen and lavender. In general, small amounts cause depression of conscious state, irritation of gastro-intestinal tract, liver dysfunction and pneumonitis if inhaled. Each has different toxicity. For example, as little as 5 ml of eucalyptus oil[61] or 15 ml of turpentine may cause depression of conscious state.

Emesis should not be induced and gastric lavage performed only if airway protection is required.

LEAD

Children are more susceptible to lead poisoning after ingestion than are adults, possibly because of better absorption.

Acute poisoning usually occurs after ingestion of a lead salt or metallic foreign body or a lead-containing product, such as paint or traditional remedy or cosmetic. Acute poisoning by a salt may cause life-supporting cardiovascular collapse, and encephalopathy.

Chronic poisoning can occur with ingestion of lead-contaminated water, or by inhalation of leaded petrol fumes or contaminated house dust. Chronic poisoning causes multi-organ dysfunction including neuromuscular dysfunction and encephalopathy.

Treatment consists of gastric decontamination in the case of recent ingestion of lead salts. The use of chelating agents may be indicated. In the case of ingestion of a lead foreign body, serial X-rays should be taken to ensure elimination, otherwise surgical removal is indicated. In the case of multiple embedded gun shot pellets and in all cases of chronic poisoning,

serum lead levels should be measured to guide chelation therapy (see Table 103.1).

PARACETAMOL

This is the most common drug ingested by children either in an accidental, iatrogenic or deliberate overdose situation. Overdose has the potential for hepatic failure and less commonly, renal failure. The onset of toxicity is delayed – up to several days. Consequently, the need for acute gastric decontamination is uncommon, but would be justifiable for acute large dose presentations. The toxicity in part is caused by the hepatic metabolite of the drug (N-acetyl-p-benzoquinoneimine), which accumulates when endogenous glutathione, which normally facilitates conversion of N-acetyl-p-benzoquinoneimine to non-toxic substances, becomes exhausted. Adequate supply of glutathione is ensured by administration of the antidote, N-acetylcysteine, a glutathione precursor which can be administered intravenously or orally (see Table 103.1).

The time of presentation after ingestion, as well as the dose, determines the management. If presentation is within an hour of ingestion, effective gastric removal or administration of activated charcoal may be all that is required pending a serum paracetamol level. In contrast, if presentation is several hours after ingestion, administration of the antidote, according to serum paracetamol level, takes precedence and although it may be administered orally or intravenously, the intravenous route is preferred.[62] Near-simultaneous administration of activated charcoal may be of some benefit but it may also cause vomiting or desorption thus decreasing the effectiveness of the antidote. If presentation is many hours after the poisoning, activated charcoal would not be indicated, so the antidote could be administered orally if necessary according to serum paracetamol levels. In all cases, evidence of liver dysfunction mandates administration of the antidote.

The threshold single toxic dose of paracetamol indicating N-acetylcysteine administration is generally regarded as 150 mg/kg, although it has been suggested that a single dose less than 200 mg/kg in children less than 6 years of age may be safely managed at home.[63] However, in situations of repeated sub-150 mg/kg doses hepatotoxicity has a high mortality among children[64] and in adults.[65] Unfortunately, toxic overdosing by chronic administration is not uncommon even in paediatric institutions.[66] No sufficient data exists on which to firmly base a decision to administer N-acetylcysteine to children. Time-related serum levels of paracetamol should be measured and reference made to a guideline to administer the antidote (Table 103.1) as derived from single toxic dose adult data.[67] The serum paracetamol level indicating antidote has been predicted as >225 mg/l (1500 μmol/l) at 2 hours after ingestion of a single overdose of elixir in children 1–5 years of age.[42] If serum levels of paracetamol cannot be obtained and >150 mg/kg has been ingested as a single dose or liver dysfunction is present after chronic poisoning, the antidote should be given.

Adverse reactions to N-acetylcysteine (approximately 8%) respond to an antihistamine[68] and its temporary cessation.

IRON

Small quantities of elemental iron (>20 mg/kg) are toxic to children. This dose may be reached by ingestion of few iron tablets. The initial effects are gastrointestinal, which may include gastric erosion, followed sometimes by an interval before cardiovascular failure occurs at 6–24 hours and then followed by multi-organ failure including encephalopathy and hepatic and renal failure up to some 48 hours after ingestion. In addition to general supportive measures, specific management should include abdominal X-ray to determine if unabsorbed tablets are present in which case gastric lavage or whole bowel irrigation may be useful. Activated charcoal is useless. Chelation therapy with desferrioxamine (see Table 103.1) should be guided by serum iron level and clinical status.

CAUSTIC SUBSTANCES

In a study of 743 children,[69] the incidence of oesophageal burns caused by ingestion of automatic machine dishwashing detergents was 59%, caustic soda 55% and drain cleaners 55%. All are strongly alkaline and are corrosive. Dishwasher detergents are presented as liquids, powders or tablet blocks and are commonly accessed in an open dishwasher.[70] Pharyngeal and oesophageal irritation, burns or corrosion may occur. There may be simultaneous ocular and dermal toxicity. Any child presenting with a history of ingestion of a caustic substance, irrespective of clinical signs, should be considered for oesophagoscopy and follow-up since the correlation between symptoms and signs and oesophageal burns is poor[69] and significant oesophageal damage may occur in the absence of more proximal injury.[71]

REFERENCES

1 Australian Department of Health and Aged Care. *Injury Prevention.* At: http:// www.health.gov.au/pubhlth/ strateg/injury/index.htm.
2 Kaushal R, Bates DW, Landrigan C, *et al.* Medication errors and adverse drug events in paediatric inpatients. *JAMA* 2001; **285**: 2114–20.
3 Haddad LM, Shannon MW, Winchester JF. *Clinical Management of Poisoning and Drug Overdose.* 3rd edn. Philadelphia: WB Saunders; 1998.
4 Ellenhorn MJ, Schonwald S, Ordog G, Wasserberger J, Ellenhorn SS. *Ellenhorn's Medical Toxicology.* 2nd edn. Baltimore: Williams and Wilkins; 1997.
5 Bates N, Edwards N, Roper J, Volans G. *Paediatric Toxicology.* London: Macmillan; 1997.
6 Krenzelok EP, McGuigan M, Lheur P. Position statement: ipecac syrup. American Academy of Clinical Toxicology; European Associations of Poisons Centres and Clinical Toxicologists. *J Toxicol Clin Toxicol* 1997; **35**: 699–709.
7 Corby DG, Decker WJ, Moran MJ, Payne CE. Clinical comparisons of pharmacologic emetics in children. *Pediatr* 1968; **4**: 361–4.
8 Saetta JP, March S, Gaunt ME, Quinton DN. Gastric emptying procedures in the self-poisoned patient: are we forcing gastric content beyond the pylorus? *J Roy Soc Med* 1991; **84**: 274–6.
9 Neuvonen PJ, Vartiainen M, Tokola O. Comparison of activated charcoal and ipecac syrup in prevention of drug absorption. *Eur J Clin Pharmacol* 1983; **24**: 557–62.
10 Tenenbein M, Cohen S, Sitar DS. Efficacy of ipecac-induced emesis, orogastric lavage, and activated charcoal for acute drug overdose. *Ann Emerg Med* 1987; **16**: 838–41.
11 Curtis RA, Barone J, Giacona N. Efficacy of ipecac and activated charcoal/cathartic. Prevention of salicylate absorption in a simulated overdose. *Arch Intern Med* 1984; **144**: 48–52.
12 Danel V, Henry JA, Glucksman E. Activated charcoal, emesis, and gastric lavage in aspirin overdose. *Brit Med J* 1988; **296**: 1507.
13 McNamara RM, Aaron CK, Gemborys M, Davidheiseer S. Efficacy of charcoal cathartic versus ipecac in reducing serum acetaminophen in a simulated overdose. *Ann Emerg Med* 1989; **18**: 934–8.
14 Vasquez TE, Evans DG, Ashburn WL. Efficacy of syrup of ipecac-induced emesis for emptying gastric contents. *Clin Nucl Med* 1988; **13**: 638–9.
15 Bond GR, Requa RK, Krenzelok EP, *et al.* Influence of time until emesis on the efficacy of decontamination using acetaminophen as a marker in a pediatric population. *Ann Emerg Med* 1993; **22**: 1403–7.
16 Amitai Y, Mitchell AA, McGuigan, MA, Lovejoy FH Jr. Ipecac-induced emesis and reduction of plasma concentrations of drugs following accidental overdose in children. *Pediatrics* 1987; **80**: 364–7.
17 Saincher A, Sitar DS, Tenenbein M. Efficacy of ipecac during the first hour after drug ingestion in human volunteers. *J Toxicol Clin Toxicol* 1997; **35**: 609–15.
18 Boxer L, Anderson FP, Rowe MD. Comparison of ipecac-induced emesis with gastric lavage in the treatment of acute salicylate ingestion. *Ped Pharmacol Ther* 1969; **74**: 800–3.
19 Young WF Jr, Bivins HG. Evaluation of gastric emptying using radionuclides: gastric lavage versus ipecac-induced emesis. *Ann Emerg Med* 1993; **22**: 1423–7.
20 Tandberg D, Diven BG, McLeod JW. Ipecac-induced emesis versus gastric lavage: a controlled study in normal adults. *Am J Emerg Med* 1986; **4**: 205–9.
21 Albertson TE, Derlet RW, Foulke GE, Minguillon MC, Tharratt SR. Superiority of activated charcoal alone with ipecac and activated charcoal in the treatment of acute toxic ingestions. *Ann Emerg Med* 1989; **18**: 56–9.

22 Czajka PA, Russell SL. Nonemetic effects of ipecac syrup. *Pediatics* 1985; **75**: 1101–4.

23 Kornberg AE, Dolgin J. Pediatric ingestions: charcoal alone versus ipecac and charcoal. *Ann Emerg Med* 1991; **20**: 648–51.

24 Foulke GE, Albertson TE, Derlet RW. Use of ipecac increases emergency department stays and patient complication rates. *Ann Emerg Med* 1990; **17**: 402.

25 Kulig K, Bar-Or D, Cantrill SV, Rosen P, Rumack BH. Management of acutely poisoned patients without gastric emptying. *Ann Emerg Med* 1985; **14**: 562–7.

26 Bond GR. Home use of syrup of ipecac is associated with a reduction in pediatric emergency department visits. *Ann Emerg Med* 1995; **25**: 338–43.

27 Quang LS, Woolf AD. Past, present, and future role of ipecac syrup. *Curr Opin Ped* 2000; **12**: 153–62.

28 Marchbanks B, Lockman P, Shum S, Beard D. Trends in ipecac use: a survey of poison center staff. *Vet Hum Toxicol* 1999; **41**: 47–9.

29 Wrenn K, Rodewald L, Dockstader L. Potential misuse of ipecac. *Ann Emerg Med* 1993; **22**: 1408–12.

30 Doran S, Jones KL, Andrews JM, Horowitz M. Effects of meal volume and posture on gastric emptying of solids and appetite. *Amer J Physiol* 1998; **275**: R1712–8.

31 Auerbach PS, Osterich J, Braun O, *et al.* Efficacy of gastric emptying: gastric lavage versus emesis induced with ipecac. *Ann Emerg Med* 1986; **15**: 692–8.

32 Grierson R, Green R, Sitar DS, Tenenbein M. Gastric lavage for liquid poisons. *Ann Emerg Med* 2000; **35**: 435–9.

33 Lapatto-Reiniluoto O, Kivisto KT, Neuvonen PJ. Gastric decontamination performed 5 min after ingestion of temazepam, verapamil and moclobemide: charcoal is superior to lavage. *Brit J Clin Pharmacol* 2000; **49**: 274–8.

34 Underhill TJ, Greene MK, Dove AF. A comparison of the efficacy of gastric lavage, ipecacuanha and activated charcoal in the emergency management of paracetamol overdose. *Arch Emerg Med* 1990; **7**: 148–54.

35 Merigian KS, Woodard M, Hedges JR, Roberts JR, Stuebing R, Rashkin MC. Prospective evaluation of gastric emptying in the self-poisoned patient. *Am J Emerg Med* 1990; **8**: 479–83.

36 Pond SM, Lewis-Driver DJ, Williams GM, Green A. C, Stevenson NW. Gastric emptying in acute overdose: a prospective randomised controlled trial. *Med J Aust* 1995; **163**: 345–9.

37 Whyte IM, Buckley NA. Progress in clinical toxicology: from case reports to toxicoepidemiology. *Med J Aust* 1995; **163**: 340–1.

38 Roberts JR, Gracely EJ, Schoffstall JM. Advantage of high-surface-area charcoal for gastrointestinal decontamination in a human acetaminophen ingestion model. *Acad Emerg Med* 1997; **4**: 167–74.

39 Fischer TF, Singer AJ. Comparison of the palatabilities of standard and superactivated charcoal in toxic ingestions: a randomized trial. *Acad Emerg Med* 1999; **6**: 895–9.

40 Boyd R, Hansen J. Prospective single blinded randomised controlled trial of two orally administered activated charcoal preparations. *Emerg Med J* 1999; **16**: 24–5.

41 Neuvonen PJ, Elonen E. Effect of activated charcoal on absorption and elimination of phenobarbitone, carbamazepine and phenylbutazone in man. *Eur J Clin Pharmacol* 1980; **17**: 51–7.

42 Anderson BJ, Holford NHG, Armishaw JC, Aicken R. Predicting concentrations in children presenting with acetaminophen overdose. *J Paediatr* 1999; **135**: 290–5.

43 Yeates PJ, Thomas SH. Effectiveness of delayed activated charcoal administration in simulated paracetamol (acetaminophen) overdose. *Brit J Clin Pharmacol* 2000; **49**: 11–4.

44 Anonymous. Position statement and practice guidelines on the use of multi-dose activated charcoal in the treatment of acute poisoning. American Academy of Clinical Toxicology; European Association of Poisons Centres and Clinical Toxicologists. *J Toxicol Clin Toxicol* 1999; **37**: 731–51.

45 Ohning BL, Reed MD, Blumer JL. Continuous nasogastric administration of activated charcoal for the treatment of theophylline intoxication. *Ped Pharmacol* 1986; **5**: 241–5.

46 Arnold TC, Willis BH, Xiao F, Conrad SA, Carden DL. Aspiration of activated charcoal elicits an increase in lung microvascular permeability. *J Toxicol Clin Toxicol* 1999; **37**: 9–16.

47 Palatnick W, Tenenbein M. Activated charcoal in the treatment of drug overdose. *Drug Safety* 1992; **7**: 3–7.

48 Smith SW, Ling LJ, Halstenson CE. Whole bowel irrigation as a treatment for acute lithium overdose. *Ann Emerg Med* 1991; **29**: 536–9.

49 Tenenbein M, Cohen S, Sitar DS. Whole bowel irrigation as a decontamination procedure after acute drug overdose. *Arch Intern Med* 1987; **147**: 905–7.

50 Kirshenbaum LA, Mathews SC, Sitar DS, Tenenbein M. Whole-bowel irrigation versus activated charcoal in sorbitol for the ingestion of modified-release pharmaceuticals. *Clin Pharmacol Ther* 1989; **46**: 264–71.

51 Tenenbein M. Position statement: whole bowel irrigation. American Academy of Clinical Toxicology; European Association of Poisons Centres and Clinical Toxicologists. *J Toxicol Clin Toxicol* 1997; **35**: 753–62.

52 Scharman EJ. Methods used to decrease lithium absorption or enhance elimination. *J Toxicol Clin Toxicol* 1997; **35**: 601–8.

53 Makosiej FJ, Hoffman RS, Howland MA, Goldfrank LR. An in vitro evaluation of cocaine hydrochloride adsorption by actvated charcoal and desorption upon addition of polyethylene glycol electrolyte lavage solution. *J Toxicol Clin Toxicol* 1993; **31**: 381–95.

54 Burkhart KK, Wuerz RC, Donovan JW. Whole bowel irrigation as adjunctive treatment for sustained-release theophylline overdose. *Ann Emerg Med* 1992; **21**: 1316–20.

55 Kaczorowski JM, Wax PM. Five days of whole-bowel irrigation in a case of pediatric iron ingestion. *Ann Emerg Med* 1996; **27**: 258–63.

56 Olsen KM, Gurley BJ, Davis GA, Archer SR, Ma FH, Ackerman BH. Comparison of fluid volumes

with whole bowel irrigation in a simulated overdose of ibuprofen. *Ann Pharmacotherapy* 1995; **29**: 246–50.

57 Hoy JL, Day LM, Tibballs J, Ozanne-Smith J. Unintentional poisoning hospitalizations among young children in Victoria. *Injury Prevention* 1999; **5**: 31–5.

58 Tibballs J, Wall R, Velandy Koottayi S, *et al.* Tracheo-oesophageal fistula caused by electrolysis of a button battery impacted in the oesophagus. *J Paediatr. Child Health* 2002; **38**: 201–203.

59 Litovitz T, Schmitz BF. Ingestion of cylindrical and button batteries: an analysis of 2382 cases. *Pediatrics* 1992; **89**: 747–57.

60 Anas N, Namasonthi V, Ginsburg CM Criteria for hospitalizing children who have ingested products containing hydrocarbons. *JAMA* 1981; **246**: 840–3.

61 Tibballs J. Clinical effects and management of eucalyptus oil ingestion in infants and young children. *Med J Aust* 1995; **163**: 177–80.

62 Buckley NA, Whyte IM, O'Connell DL, Dawson AH. Oral or intravenous N-acetylcysteine: which is the treatment of choice for acetaminophen (paracetamol) poisoning. *J Toxicol Clin Toxicol* 1999; **37**: 759–67.

63 Bond GR, Krenzelok EP, Normann SA, *et al.* Acetaminophen ingestion in childhood – cost and relative risk of alternative referral strategies. *J Toxicol Clin Toxicol* 1994; **32**: 513–25.

64 Heubi JE, Barbacci MB, Zimmerman HJ. Therapeutic misadventures with acetaminophen: hepatotoxicity after multiple doses in children. *J Paediatrics* 1998; **132**: 22–7.

65 Schiodt FV, Rochling FA, Casey DL, Lee WM. Acetaminophen toxicity in an urban county hospital. *NEJM* 1997; **337**: 1112–7.

66 Hynson JJ, South M. Childhood hepatotoxicity with paracetamol doses less than 150 mg/kg per day. *Med J Aust* 1999; **171**: 497.

67 Smilkstein MJ, Bronstein AC, Linden C, Augenstein WL, Kulig KW, Rumack BH. Acetaminophen overdose: a 48 hour intravenous N-acetylcysteine treatment protocol. *Ann Emerg Med* 1991; **20**: 1058–63.

68 Schmidt LE, Dalhoff K. Risk factors in the development of adverse reactions to N-acetylcysteine in patients with paracetamol poisoning. *Brit J Pharmacol* 2001; **51**: 87–91.

69 Bautista Casasnovas A, Estevez Martinez E, Varela Cives R, Villanueva Jeremias A, Tojo Sierra R, Cadranel S. A retrospective analysis of ingestion of caustic substances by children. Ten-year statistics in Galicia. *Eur J Pediatrics* 1997; **156**: 410–4.

70 Cornish LS, Parsons BJ, Dobbin MD. Automatic dishwasher detergent poisoning: opportunities for prevention. *Aust New Zealand J Pub Health* 1996; **20**: 278–83.

71 Krenzelok EP, Clinton JE. Caustic esophageal and gastric erosion without evidence of oral burns following detergent ingestion. *JACEP* 1979; **8**: 194–6.

104

Paediatric cardiopulmonary resuscitation

J Tibballs

This chapter concerns basic and advanced cardiopulmonary resuscitation (CPR) for newly-born infants, infants and children. The recommendations are based on publications of several authoritative resuscitation organizations[1-3] and are intended primarily for use by medical and nursing personnel in hospital. To add ability to knowledge, it is advisable to undertake a specialized paediatric cardiopulmonary resuscitation course, such as the Advanced Paediatric Life Support (APLS) or Paediatric Advanced Life Support (PALS) courses. This chapter should be regarded as an addendum to Chapters 15 (Cardiopulmonary resuscitation), 95 (The critically ill child) and 103 (Equipment for paediatric intensive care).

Distinctions within the term paediatric are based on combinations of physiology, physical size and age. Some aspects of CPR are different for 'the newly born', infant, small (younger) child and large (older) child. 'Newly-born' refers to the infant at birth or within several hours of birth. 'Infant' refers to an infant outside the 'newly-born' period up to the age of 12 months. Other terms, such as newborn or neonate do not enable that distinction. 'Small/young child' refers to a child of pre-school and early primary school from the age of 1–8 years. 'Large/older child' refers to a child of late primary school from the age of 9 up to 14 years. Children older than 14 years may be treated as adults but they do not have the same propensity for ventricular fibrillation as do adults. One guideline[2] regards children of 8 years and over as adults specifically for use of out-of-hospital semi-automatic external defibrillators.

EPIDEMIOLOGY

The causes of cardiopulmonary arrest in infants and children are many and include any cause of hypoxaemia or hypotension or both. Common causes are trauma (motor vehicle accidents, near drowning, falls, burns, gunshot), drug overdose and poisoning, respiratory illness (asthma, upper airway obstruction, parenchymal diseases), post-operative (especially cardiac), septicaemia and sudden infant death syndrome. As many as 10% of newly-born infants require some form of resuscitation for varied conditions of which birth asphyxia is the most common.

MANAGEMENT – BASIC LIFE SUPPORT

ASSESSMENT OF AIRWAY AND BREATHING

On determining that the patient is not responsive to tactile and auditory stimulation, airway opening manoeuvres and assessment of breathing should be performed. This is usually done in the supine position but one organization[1] recommends that the patient be turned onto the side to assess breathing. This is potentially time wasteful and in practice, the airway and breathing can be assessed effectively in either the supine or lateral position in which the patient is found.

Obvious causes of airway obstruction in the pharynx should be removed. Fluids such as vomitus or blood, should be aspirated with a Yankauer sucker. Solid or semi-solid objects, such as food particles or foreign objects, should be removed with an instrument, e.g. Magill's forceps. Since the most common cause of airway obstruction in an obtunded state is the tongue, first aid manoeuvres to elevate it should be performed. The manoeuvres are backward head tilt, chin lift and jaw thrust. Head tilt and chin lift are often combined. If neck injury is present or suspected, neither the head tilt nor chin lift manoeuvre should be used. Then the presence of absence of adequate breathing is assessed by inspection of movement of the chest and abdomen, and by listening and feeling for escape of exhaled air from the mouth and nose (look, listen and feel). If adequate breathing is occurring the patient should be placed on the side in a coma position.

EXPIRED AIR RESUSCITATION

There is no evidence to dictate the number of initial breaths. However, at least two are recommended by all authorities with some stating up to five. While maintaining the airway, slow breaths over 1–1.5 s should be given with enough air to achieve adequate chest inflation. In children of all sizes, a mouth-to-mouth technique is possible while pinching the nostrils closed. In newly-born and infants, a mouth-to-mouth-and-nose technique is recommended, but if the rescuer has a small mouth, a mouth-to-nose technique is an alternative. Lack of chest rise may signify obstruction of the airway requiring repositioning of the head and neck.

PULSE CHECK AND COMMENCEMENT OF EXTERNAL CARDIAC COMPRESSION

If a pulse cannot be detected or is less than 60 beats/min, external cardiac compression should be commenced. Although the pulse check has been discarded in guidelines for lay-person CPR, because of inability to reliably check the pulse, it has been retained in guidelines for health-care personnel. Of interest are some studies that also question the reliability of pulse detection by health-care personnel. No more than 10 s should be spent attempting to palpate a pulse. Palpation of any major pulse (carotid, brachial, femoral) is appropriate. Information derived from the pulse check should be combined with any evidence of 'signs of life' (movement, breathing, coughing) to help decide whether external cardiac compression should be commenced. If no signs of life are present or the pulse is absent or inadequate, external cardiac compression should be commenced.

EXTERNAL CARDIAC COMPRESSION (ECC)

Different techniques are used for children of different sizes. For newly-born infants and infants, two techniques are in common use. In the 'two-finger technique', the middle and forefingers are used to compress the lower sternum. This technique is taught to lay-persons and is also the preferred technique by a single health-care rescuer. With the 'two-thumb technique', the hands encircle the thorax, approaching the chest from either above or below, and the thumbs are placed either opposite, alongside or atop one another. With this technique, care must be taken to avoid restriction of chest inflation by the hands. With premature newly-borns and small infants, the rescuer's encircling fingers can reach and stabilize the vertebral column, without limiting chest inflation. With both techniques, the sternum is compressed above the xiphoid to a depth approximating one-third the depth of the chest. For young children, ECC can be performed with the heel of one hand. For older children, a bimanual technique as per adults may be used. In all ages, the lower sternum is compressed. Approximately 50% of each cycle should be compression.

For infants and children, compressions should be delivered at a rate of 100/min, i.e. one compression every 0.6 s. This does not mean that 100 actual compressions are given each minute. When ventilation is interposed between compressions, the actual compressions will be less than 100 but at least 60/min should be achieved.

More compressions and breaths each minute are possible with efficient inflations and changeovers between compression and ventilation. The time for a breath or breaths plus the changeovers should be no more than 2 s for infants and small children and no more than 3 s for older children. Essentially, five compressions are given in 3 s followed by an effective breath (for infants and small children) and 15 compressions are given in 9 s followed by two effective breaths (for older children).

RATIO OF COMPRESSION TO VENTILATION

After every 5 compressions, a pause should allow delivery of a breath whenever expired air resuscitation or any type of mask ventilation is given. ECC can be given during exhalation. Strict co-ordination of compression and ventilation is not as crucial when ventilation is given via endotracheal or tracheostomy tube when effective ventilation can be given against resistance imposed by chest compression.

The ratio of compression to breaths should be 5:1 given by one or two rescuers. However, a single rescuer may not be able to physically sustain this requirement using a bimanual technique for an older child and hence the adult ratio of 15:2 (whether one or two rescuers) is acceptable. For newly-born infants the total number of recommended 'events' per minute is 120, with the aim of achieving 90 compressions and 30 inflations each minute, that is, in a ratio of 3:1.

MANAGEMENT – ADVANCED LIFE SUPPORT

As soon as practicable, mechanical ventilation with added oxygen should be commenced with either a bag-valve-mask or via endotracheal intubation. Although intubation is preferred (see below), valuable time should not be wasted in numerous unsuccessful attempts. Initial effective bag-valve-mask ventilation is a necessary prerequisite for successful paediatric CPR. Bags of appropriate sizes should be available for infants, small children and large children. A bag of ~500 ml volume should be available for newly-born infants. Insertion of an oropharyngeal (Guedel) airway may be necessary to facilitate bag-valve-mask ventilation. Access to the circulation and display of the electrocardiograph should also be achieved as soon as possible. Thereafter treatment should be guided by the cardiac rhythm. Underlying causes of cardiopulmonary arrest (CPA) should be sought and treated.

AIRWAY MANAGEMENT

If attending personnel are skilled, the trachea should be intubated as soon as possible. This action establishes and maintains an airway, facilitates mechanical ventilation with

100% oxygen, minimizes the risk of pulmonary aspiration, enables suctioning of the trachea and provides a route for the administration of selected drugs. If difficulty is experienced at initial intubation, oxygenation should be established with bag-valve-mask ventilation before a re-attempt at intubation. Initial intubation should be via the oral route, not via the nasal route.

Intubation via the oral route

- is invariably quicker than via the nasal route
- is less likely to cause trauma and haemorrhage
- enables the endotracheal tube to be more easily exchanged if the first choice is inappropriate.

On the other hand, a tube placed nasally:

- can be better affixed to the face and so is less likely to enter a bronchus or be subject to inadvertent extubation
- is preferred for transport and long-term management.

A nasogastric tube should be inserted after intubation to relieve possible gaseous distension of the stomach sustained during bag-valve-mask ventilation.

Correct placement of the endotracheal tube in the trachea must be confirmed. In the hurried conditions of emergency intubation at cardiopulmonary arrest, it is not difficult to mistakenly intubate the oesophagus or to intubate a bronchus. There is no substitute for:

- visualizing the passage of the tip of the endotracheal tube through the vocal cords at intubation
- confirmation of bilateral pulmonary air entry by auscultation in the axillae
- continuous observation of rise and fall of the chest on ventilation.

It is recommended that correct placement of the endotracheal tube be confirmed by capnography or CO_2 detection after initial placement with the realization that CO_2 excretion can only occur with effective pulmonary blood flow. This implies that CO_2 detection cannot be expected unless spontaneous cardiac output returns or unless external cardiac compression is effective. Oxygenation should be confirmed with use of a pulse oximeter or measurement of arterial gas tension.

Tube size

- 2.5 mm tube is used for a premature newborn <1 kg
- 3.0 mm for infants 1–3.5 kg
- 3.5 mm for infants >3.5 kg and up to age of 6 months
- size 4 mm for infants 7 months to 1 year
- For children over 1 year, the size is approximately determined by the formula: size (mm) = age (years)/4 + 4.

Tubes larger and smaller should be available. The correct size should allow a small leak on application of moderate pressure but also enable adequate pulmonary inflation.

The tube is inserted a specific depth to avoid accidental extubation or endobronchial intubation. Assessment of the depth of insertion at laryngoscopy is not reliable because this is performed with the neck extended. When the laryngoscope is removed the head assumes a position of neutrality or flexion and the tube depth increases.

The appropriate depth of insertion measured from the centre of the lips for an oral tube is:

- 9.5 cm for a term newborn
- 11.5 cm for a 6 month old infant
- 12 cm for a 1 year old.

An alternative formula for oral tube depth of insertion is: depth (cm) = size (mm) × 3. After one year the depth is given by the formula: depth (cm) = age (years)/2 + 12. The appropriate depth of insertion for a nasal tube in this age group is: depth (cm) = age (years)/2 + 15. On a chest X-ray taken with the head in neutral position, the tip of the tube should be at the interclavicular line.

A laryngeal mask airway (LMA) may be used to establish an airway in the setting of CPA. However, its role in provision of mechanical ventilation remains uncertain. Like bag-valve-mask ventilation, it does not protect the airway from aspiration. Although insertion of an LMA is easier to learn than endotracheal intubation, training should not replace mastery of bag-valve-mask ventilation. It is unsuitable for long term use or during transport when endotracheal intubation is mandatory.

ELECTROCARDIOGRAPH

The electrocardiograph (ECG) should be displayed with either leads or paddles. Drug therapy or immediate direct current shock is administered according to the existing rhythm.

ACCESS TO THE CIRCULATION

According to the skills of the personnel, access to the circulation via a peripheral or central vein should be attempted immediately. Any site is acceptable. Visible or palpable peripheral veins are to be found on the dorsum of the hand, wrist, forearm, cubital fossa, chest wall, foot and ankle. In infants, scalp veins are accessible and the umbilical vein can be used up to about a week after birth. The external jugulars are usually distended at CPR but cannulation may be impeded by performance of intubation. Cannulation of femoral, subclavian, or internal jugulars are options. Surgical cutdown onto a long saphenous, saphenofemoral junction or basilic is a valuable skill sometimes required in traumatic exsanguination. Any pre-existing functioning line can be used provided it does not contain any drug or electrolyte precipitating the CPA.

INTRAOSSEOUS INJECTION

If intravenous access cannot be rapidly achieved, say within 60 s, intra-osseous access should be obtained. This route has been used for patients of all ages and provides rapid, safe and reliable access to the circulation. It serves as an adequate route for any parenteral drug and fluid administration.

A metal needle with a trocar (e.g. disposable intraosseous needle, Cook, Illinois, USA) is preferable although a short lumbar puncture type of needle with an inner trocar may suffice. Although many sites have been used for bone marrow injection, the easiest to identify is the antero-medial surface of the upper or lower tibia, especially in children less than 6 years. The site of the latter is a few centimetres below the anterior tuberosity and the former a few centimetres above the medial malleolus. The handle of the device needle is held in the palm of the hand while the fingers grip the shaft about a centimetre from the tip. It is inserted perpendicular to the bone surface and a rotary action is used to traverse the cortex. Sudden loss of resistance signifies entry to bone marrow. Correct positioning of the needle is confirmed by aspiration of bone marrow (which may be used for biochemical and haematological purposes) but that is not always possible. Bone injection guns (Wais Med Ltd.), which fire a needle a pre-set distance according to size of the patient, enable easy intraosseous injection for infants, children and adults.

Volume expanders need to be given by syringe to gain rapid access to the central circulation. This is best achieved using a 10 ml syringe with a three-way tap in the i.v. tubing.

Care should be exercised to avoid complications particularly cutaneous extravasation, compartment syndrome of the leg, and osteomyelitis. Contra-indications include local trauma and infection.

ENDOTRACHEAL ADMINISTRATION OF DRUGS

Lipid-soluble drugs (epinephrine, atropine, lignocaine and naloxone) may be administered via the endotracheal tube if neither intravenous nor intraosseous access are possible. Although the optimal doses of these drugs by this route are not known, work in animal models suggests doses should be 10 times the intravenous doses. The drugs should be diluted in normal saline up to 2 ml for infants, 5 ml for small children and 10 ml for large children. It is acceptable and simplest to squirt the drugs from the syringe (after removing the needle) directly into the endotracheal tube and disperse them throughout the respiratory tree with bagging.

Neither sodium bicarbonate nor calcium salts should be administered via the tracheal route because they injure the airways.

DC SHOCK

Unsynchronized DC shock is required as first treatment for ventricular fibrillation (VF) and pulseless ventricular tachycardia (VT). If effective for VF it is called defibrilla-

tion. Synchronized DC shock may also be required for pulsatile VT and haemodynamically unstable supraventricular tachycardia (SVT).

Defibrillators should have paediatric paddles of cross sectional area 12–20 cm² for use in children <10 kg BW. For others, adult sized paddles (50–80 cm²) are satisfactory provided the paddles do not contact each other. Selectable energy levels should enable delivery of doses 0.5–4 J/kg. The closest level to the dose should be selected. One paddle is placed over the mid-axilla opposite the xyphoid or nipple, the other to the right of the upper sternum below the clavicle. Conductive gel (confined to the area beneath the paddles) or gel pads and firm pressure are needed to deliver optimum energy to the heart without causing skin burns. Rescuers should maintain the paddles on the chest and be prepared to deliver a series of three shocks in quick succession, pausing only to verify the rhythm. Using a monophasic waveform, the initial dose and mode for VF and pulseless VT is unsynchronized 2 J/kg progressing to 4 J/kg if required. The mode and dose for pulsatile VT and SVT is synchronized 0.5 J/kg initially progressing to 2 J/kg. The paediatric doses required for biphasic waves are as yet unknown although likely to be less than for monophasic waves. In the treatment of refractory arrhythmias, equipment failure should be excluded. An antero-posterior position of the paddles (one over cardiac apex, one over left scapula) may be efficacious in refractory arrhythmia. Dextrocardia may be present with congenital heart disease and the position of the paddles should be altered accordingly.

Monophasic and biphasic semi-automatic external defibrillators (SAEDs) with energy doses of 150–200 J may be used in children older than 8 years of age or 25 kg BW. However, their use in younger children cannot be recommended since the dose would exceed the maximum 4 J/kg. Moreover, although they can detect VF in children of all ages, they cannot reliably distinguish tachycardia in infants and hence their use poses a risk of harmful DC shock.

TREATMENT OF SPECIFIC ARRHYTHMIAS

The following discussion assumes that mechanical ventilation with oxygen and external cardiac compression have been commenced and continued if an adequate pulse rate is not detectable. The treatment of pulseless arrhythmias are summarized in Figure 104.1. Causes of arrhythmias should be treated.

For example:

- calcium channel blockade toxicity is treated with calcium i.v. or i.o. (chloride 10% 0.2 ml/kg, gluconate 10% 0.7 ml/kg)
- hyperkalaemia treated with calcium salt, sodium bicarbonate, hyperventilation, insulin and dextrose.

All drugs should be flushed into the circulation with a small bolus of isotonic fluid. To prevent inactivation, drugs should not be mixed in the syringe or in infusion lines.

ASYSTOLE AND BRADYARRHYTHMIA

Asystole should be treated with epinephrine 10 μg/kg intravenous (i.v.) or intraosseous (i.o.). If these routes are not available, epinephrine 100 μg/kg should be administered via endotracheal tube (ETT).

Unresponsive asytole should be treated with similar doses (10 μg/kg i.v., i.o.; 100 μg/kg ETT) every 3–5 min. Higher doses, up to 200 μg/kg i.v. or i.o. may be used but have not altered outcome and predispose to complications (post-arrest myocardial dysfunction, hypertension, tachycardia). In newly born infants, the initial bolus dose is 100–300 μg/kg.

Recurrent bradyarrhythmia or asystole may require an infusion of epinephrine at 0.05–3 μg/kg per min. Doses of <0.3 μg/kg per min are predominantly beta-adrenergic, doses >0.3 μg/kg per min are predominantly alpha-adrenergic. Infuse into secure large vein. If sinus rhythm cannot be restored, sodium bicarbonate 1 mmol/kg i.v. or i.o. may be helpful but do not allow mixing with epinephrine since catecholamines are inactivated in alkaline solution.

In all age groups, bradycardia is defined as a heart rate <60/min or rapidly declining rate with poor perfusion. Sinus bradycardia, sinus arrest with slow junctional or idioventricular rhythm and atrioventricular block are the most common preterminal arrhythmias in paediatric practice. Untreated, bradycardia progresses to asystole.

The treatment is:

- reversal of the cause (hypoxaemia, hypotension, acidosis, hypothermia, intracranial hypertension)
- if unresponsive, epinephrine 10 μg/kg i.v. or i.o. or 100 μg/kg ETT.
- Bradycardia caused by vagal stimulation should be managed with cessation of the stimulus and/or atropine 20 μg/kg i.v. or i.o. (minimum dose 100 μg).
- Persistent vagal-mediated bradycardia should be treated with epinephrine 10 μg/kg i.v. or i.o. If facilities are available, pacing (oesophageal, transcutaneous, transvenous, epicardial) may be effective if sinus node dysfunction or heart block exist. It is not helpful in asystole.

VENTRICULAR FIBRILLATION AND PULSELESS VENTRICULAR TACHYCARDIA

As soon as recognized, VF or pulseless VT should be treated with DC shock. No other treatment takes precedence. If onset is witnessed, a precordial thump may be given but its efficacy has not been proven. The initial shock is 2 J/kg increasing up to a maximum of 4 J/kg in a series of three shocks if the arrhythmia persists.

Failure to revert to sinus rhythm should be treated with epinephrine 10 μg/kg i.v. or i.o. or 100 μg/kg ETT followed by another 1–3 shocks, if necessary, all at 4 J/kg after an interval of 30–60 s. Persistent (refractory) or recurrent VF or VT may be also treated with antiarrhythmics (amiodarone, lignocaine, magnesium) interpersed with DC shock. Irrespective of other drug therapy, epinephrine should be administered every 3–5 min. The dose of lignocaine (lidocaine) is 1 mg/kg i.v. or i.o. bolus followed by an infusion if successful at 20–50 μg/kg/min. The dose of amiodarone is 5 mg/kg i.v. or i.o. over several to 60 min. It may be repeated to maximum of 15 mg/kg. Magnesium, 25–50 mg/kg (0.1–0.2 mmol/kg) is indicated for polymorphic VT (torsades de pointes). The alternative to epinephrine as a vasopressor, vasopressin, has not been adequately investigated for use during CPR for children.

PULSATILE VENTRICULAR TACHYCARDIA

Haemodynamically stable VT may be treated with antiarrhythmic agent such as amiodarone (5 mg/kg i.v. over 20–60 min) or procainamide (15 mg/kg i.v. over 30–60 min). Both drugs prolong QT interval and should not be given together. If torsades de pointes is present, magnesium (25–50 mg/kg, 0.1–0.2 mmol/kg i.v.) may be used. If cardioversion is needed, it should be synchronized at 0.5–2 J/kg under sedation/anaesthesia.

PULSELESS ELECTRICAL ACTIVITY AND ELECTROMECHANICAL DISSOCIATION

A normal ECG complex without pulses is called electromechanical dissociation (EMD). If untreated, the ECG initially deteriorates to an abnormal but still recognizable state when it is called pulseless electrical activity (PEA). Both conditions should be treated as for asystole and their cause ascertained and treated.

SUPRAVENTRICULAR TACHYCARDIA

SVT is the most common spontaneous arrhythmia in childhood and infancy. It may cause life-threatening hypotension. It is usually re-entrant with a rate of 220–300/min in infants, less in children. The QRS complex is usually narrow (<0.08 s) making it difficult sometimes to discern from sinus tachycardia. However, whereas ST is a part of other features of illness, SVT is a singular entity and whereas the rate in ST is variable with activity or stimulation, it is uniform in SVT. In both rhythms, a P wave may be discernible. SVT with aberrant conduction (wide QRS) may resemble VT.

If haemodynamically stable (adequate perfusion and blood pressure), initial treatment of SVT should be vagal stimulation. For infants and young children, application to the face of a plastic bag filled with iced-water is usually effective. Older children may be treated with carotid sinus massage or perform a Valsalva – such as blowing through a narrow straw. If unsuccessful, give adenosine

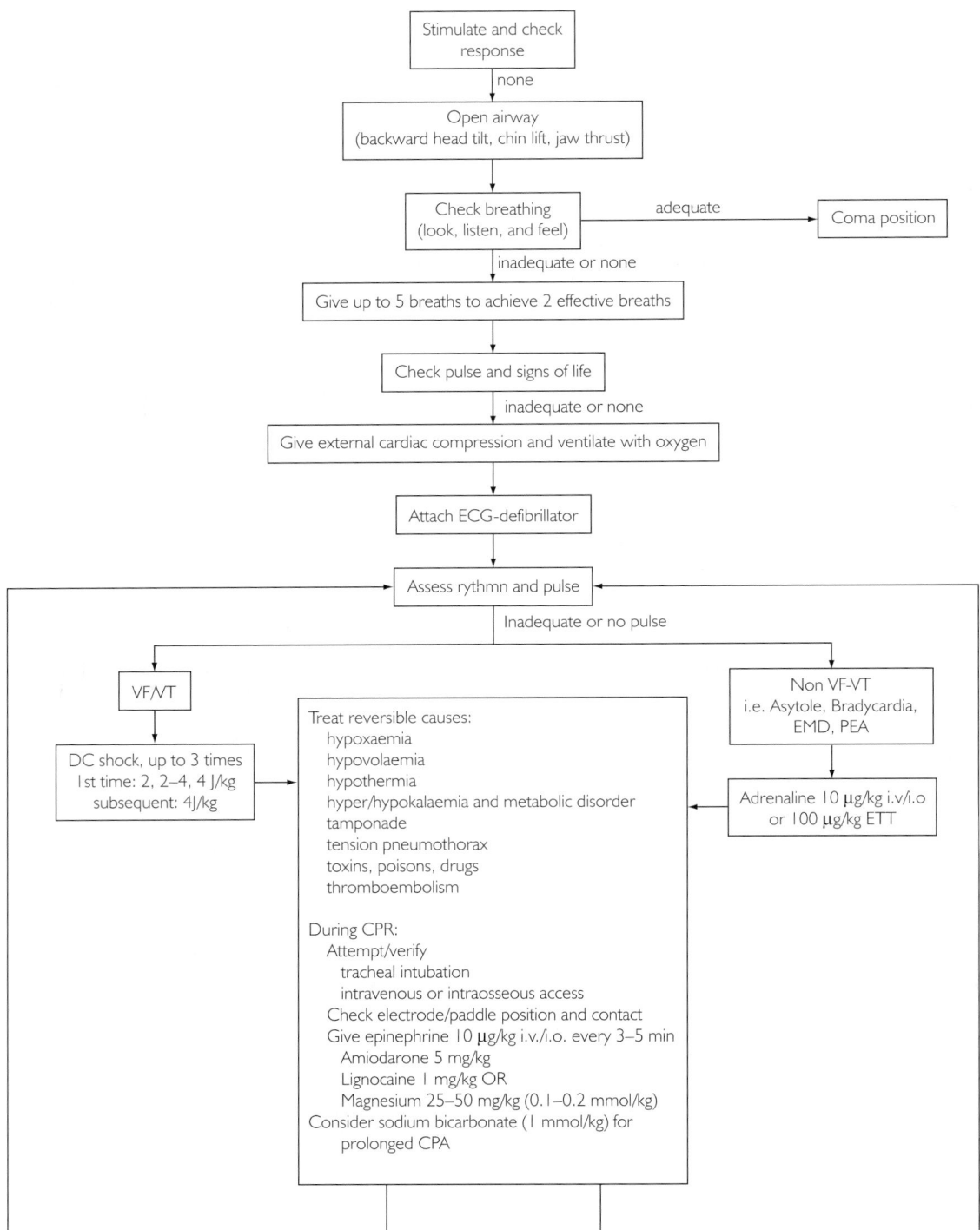

Fig. 104.1 Paediatric basic and advanced cardiopulmonary resuscitation.

100 μg/kg i.v. by rapid bolus (max dose 6 mg), doubling once to 200 μg/kg. If unsuccessful, give synchronized DC shock (cardioversion) commencing with 0.5 J/kg progressing if unsuccessful to 2 J/kg. If SVT is accompanied by haemodynamic instability, that is, hypotension, proceed to cardioversion (synchronized 0.5–2 J/kg) immediately although vagal stimulation or adenosine (i.v. or i.o.) may be used provided they do not delay cardioversion. Verapamil should not be used to treat SVT in infants and should be avoided in children because its induces hypotension and cardiac depression.

POST RESUSCITATION CARE

Supportive therapy should be provided until there is recovery of function of vital organs. This may require provision of oxygen therapy, mechanical ventilation, inotropic/vasopressor infusion, renal support, parenteral nutrition and other therapy for several days or longer. Recovery of infants and children is usually slow because cardiorespiratory arrest is often secondary to prolonged global ischaemia or hypoxaemia which implies that other organs sustain damage before cardiorespiratory arrest.

Particular care should be taken to ensure adequate cerebral perfusion with well-oxygenated blood. Hyperventilation is not useful for this purpose. Although post-ischaemia hypothermia (33–36°C) may have beneficial effects there is as yet insufficient evidence to recommend deliberate hypothermia for infants and children. Inadvertently hypothermic patients, provided temperature is above 33°C, should not be actively warmed and hyperthermia should be aggressively treated. The optimal duration of such requirement however, is unknown.

- Shivering should be prevented with sedation and/or neuromuscular blockade.
- Seizures should be actively sought and treated with anticonvulsant.
- The cause of the CPA should be investigated and treated appropriately, e.g. sepsis or drug overdose.

Complications of CPR should be sought especially if secondary deterioration occurs. A chest X-ray should be obtained to check the position of the endotracheal tube, to exclude pneumothorax, lung collapse, contusion or aspiration and to check the cardiac silhouette although an echocardiographic examination is preferable to specifically check contractility and to exclude a pericardial effusion. Measurement of haemoglobin, pH, gas tensions, electrolytes and glucose are important.

CESSATION OF CARDIOPULMONARY RESUSCITATION

Long-term outcome from paediatric CPR is poor, but better if arrest is respiratory alone or if CPA occurs in hospital. The decision to cease CPR should be based on a number of factors including the duration of resuscitation, response to treatment, pre-arrest status of the patient, remediable factors, likely outcome if ultimately successful, opinions of personnel familiar with the patient and whenever appropriate the wishes of the parents. In general, unless hypothermia or drug toxicity exists, survival to normality is most unlikely if there has been a failure to respond to full CPR after 30 min and several doses of epinephrine. In the newly-born infant, discontinuation of treatment is appropriate if CPR does not establish a spontaneous circulation within 15 min. Family members should be kept informed, allowed to be present or asked if they want to be present during resuscitation.

POST RESUSCITATION STAFF MANAGEMENT

Unfortunately, CPA occurring in hospital is often unexpected as when for example a moribund patient arrives unannounced in the emergency department, or a patient's condition deteriorates rapidly on the ward or when a mishap occurs under anaesthesia. These situations test the readiness, training, abilities and skills of individuals and the organization of the institution. It is prudent to monitor performance with a view to improvement and not ignore the psychological impact which such events have on individuals. Sensitive debriefing sessions should be encouraged.

REFERENCES

1 Australian Resuscitation Council, Melbourne. *Policy Statements* 7.1.2, 7.2, 12.1–12.9.
2 American Heart Association. Guidelines 2000 for cardiopulmonary resuscitation and emergency cardiovascular care. International consensus on science. *Circulation* 2000, **102**(**suppl**): I253–357.
3 Advanced Life Support Group. *Advanced Paediatric Life Support*. London: *BMJ* Books; 2001.

Normal biochemical values

I BLOOD CHEMISTRY

S = serum		
P = plasma		
HWB	= heparin whole blood	
α_1 Acid glycoprotein (S)		0.5–1.4 g/l
Aldosterone (S)		Supine – 140–530 pmol/l
		Erect – 220–970 pmol/l
Ammonia (P) to lab without delay		4–50 μmol/l
Amylase (S or P)		70–300 U/l
α_1 Antitrypsin (S or P)		2.1–4.0 g/l
Aspartate aminotransferase (AST) (P)		6–42 U/l
Bicarbonate (P)		22–32 mmol/l
Bilirubin (total) (S or P)		3–17 μmol/l
Bilirubin (direct) (S or P)		2–9 μmol/l
Caeruloplasmin (S or P)		0.20–0.60 g/l
Calcium (S or P)		2.25–2.65 mmol/l
Carotene (S or P)		1.0–4.8 μmol/l
Chloride (S or P)		98–108 mmol/l
Cholesterol (S or P)		3.1–6.5 mmol/l
Copper (S or P)		11–23 μmol/l
Cortisol (S or P)	8–9 am	300–800 nmol/l
	4–5 pm	100–600 nmol/l
Creatinine (P)		50–120 μmol/l
Creatinine clearance		>1.3 ml/s
Creatinine kinase (P)		20–130 U/l
Creatinine kinase isoenzymes – qualitative		
Digoxin (S)	toxic	>2 μg/l
Effective thyroxine ratio (ETR) (S)		0.90–1.09
FSH (S) Male		3–19 U/l
Female follicular		5–20 U/l
Mid-cycle		15–30 U/l
Luteal		5–15 U/l
Post-menopausal		50–100 U/l
Glucose (fasting) (fluoride) (P)		3.9–6.2 mmol/l
γ-Glutamyl-transferase (γGT) (P)	F	7–30 U/l
	M	10–50 U/l
Growth hormone (fasting, resting) (S)	M	<6 mU/l
	F	<16 mU/l
	Child	<10 mU/l
Insulin (fasting) (S)		3–28 mU/l
Iron (S or P) (1) Iron	M	14–31 μmol/l
8–10 am	F	11–29 μmol/l
(2) Iron binding capacity	M	41–70 μmol/l
	F	37–77 μmol/l

Lactate (special collection)		0.3–1.3 mmol/l
LDH (S or P)		<80 U
Lead (HWB)		<2 μmol/l
Lithium (S) not plasma		0.8–1.2 mmol/l (therapeutic range)
Magnesium (S or P)		0.7–1.1 mmol/l
Oestriol (pregnancy) (S)		Depends on gestation
Osmolality (S or P)		275–295 mosm/kg
Phosphatase		
A. Prostatic (S or P)		0–4 U/l
(stabilize plasma with 5 mg/ml of NaHSO₄ or freeze)		
B. Alkaline (S or P)		100–350 U/l
Phosphate (inorganic) (P)		0.8–1.4 mmol/l
Porphyrins (red cell) (HWB)		<1.2 μmol/l
Potassium (P)		3.4–5.0 mmol/l
Prolactin (S) (resting)		25 μg/l
Proteins		
A. (1) Total (S)		63–78 g/l
(2) Albumin (S)		35–45 g/l
B. Electrophoresis (S) not plasma:		
Albumin		35–45 g/l
α_1 Globulin		2–4 g/l
α_2 Globulin		5–9 g/l
β Globulin		6–10 g/l
γ Globulin		8–16 g/l
Pyruvate (special collection)		30–80 μmol/l
Renin (special tubes – keep blood cold)		
100–180 mmol Na intake –		
Supine (6 h)		<0.58 ng/s/l
Upright (4 h)		0.28–1.25 ng/s/l
Sodium (P)		134–146 mmol/l
Thyroxine (S)		60–150 nmol/l
Transferrin (S or P)		2.1–3.5 g/l
Triglyceride (fasting) (P)		1.80 mmol/l
Tri-iodothyronine (S)		1.3–2.9 nmol/l
TSH (S)		1–11 mU/l
Urea (P)		3.0–8.0 mmol/l
Uric acid (P)	M	0.18–0.48 mmol/l
	F	0.12–0.42 mmol/l
Zinc (P)		12–20 μmol/l

II URINE

AA = 20 ml 50% acetate
d = 24 h collection
Sp = spot urine

Aldosterone (d, AA)		14–55 nmol/d
ALA (delta amino laevulinic acid) (Sp or d, AA)	Sp:	<50 μmol/l
	d:	10–50 μmol/d
Amylase (Sp or d, NO ACID)	Sp:	<900 U/l
	d:	100–1000 U/d
Calcium (d, AA)		<7.5 mmol/d
Catecholamines and derivatives (d, 20 ml 50% HCL):		
1. HMMA (VMA) Hydroxymethoxymandelic acid		<35 μmol/d
2. Metadrenaline		<5.6 μmol/d
3. Catecholamine		<1.6 μmol/d
Copper (d, AA)		<1.6 μmol/d
Coproporphyrin (collect 24 hr urine into 8 g sodium carbonate)		<245 nmol/d
Creatinine (d, AA)		10–20 mmol/d

5 Hydroxyindole-acetic acid (5-HIAA) (d, AA)		5–37 μmol/d
Hydroxyproline (d, AA)		<0.35 mmol/d (gelatin-free diet)
Indican (d, AA)		0.04–0.36 mmol/d
Lead (d, AA)		0.4 μmol/d
Magnesium (d, AA)		2.0–6.6 mmol/d
Melanin (fresh Sp)		Qualitative
Oestriol (in pregnancy) (d, AA)		50–160 μmol/d
		at 36 weeks' gestation
Osmolality (Sp)		300–1300 mosm/kg
Oxalate (d, AA)		<300 μmol/d
Phosphorus (d, AA)		10–42 mmol/d
Porphobilinogen (fresh Sp)		Qualitative
Potassium (d or Sp, AA)		25–100 mmol/d
Protein (d or Sp, AA)		0.02–0.06 g/d
Sodium (d or Sp, AA)		40–210 mmol/d
Steroids (d, AA):		
1. 17-Oxosteroids	M	28–80 μmol/d
	F	14–60 μmol/d
2. 17-Hydroxy corticosteriods	M	14–70 μmol/d
	F	7–50 μmol/d
Urea (d or Sp, AA)		170–500 mmol/d
Uric acid (d, 8 g sodium carbonate)		<3.6 mmol/d (purine-free diet)
Urobilinogen (fresh Sp)		Qualitative
Uroporphyrin (collect as for Coproporphyrin)		<50 nmol/d
Xylose absorption:		
Xylose excretion in 5 h		>27 mmol
Plasma value at 2 h		1.7–3.4 mmol/l

III FAECES

Fat (3 d collection)	<5 g/l
Porphyrins (single stool)	
Coproporphyrins	<30 nmol/g dry wt
Protoporphyrins	<135 nmol/g dry wt

IV CSF

Protein	0.15–0.45 g/l
Glucose	2.7–4.2 mmol/l
IgG	<0.05 g/l
IgG: Total protein ratio	5–14%

Appendix 2

Système International (SI) units

BASIC SI UNITS

PREFIXES

Physical quantity	Name	Symbol	Factor	Name	Symbol	Factor	Name	Symbol
Length	Metre	m	10^{18}	Exa-	E	10^{-18}	Atto-	a
Mass	Kilogram	kg	10^{15}	Peta-	P	10^{-15}	Femto-	f
Time	Second*	s	10^{12}	Tera-	T	10^{-12}	Pico-	p
Electric current	Ampere	A	10^{9}	Giga-	G	10^{-9}	Nano-	n
Thermodynamic temperature	Kelvin	K	10^{6}	Mega-	M	10^{-6}	Micro-	μ
Luminous intensity	Candela	cd	10^{3}	Kilo-	k	10^{-3}	Milli-	m
Amount of substance	Mole	mol	10^{2}	Hecto-	h	10^{-2}	Centi-	c
			10^{1}	Deca-	da	10^{-1}	Deci-	d

* Minute (min), hour (h) and day (d) will remain in use although they are not official SI units.

DERIVED SI UNITS

Quantity	SI units	Symbol	Expression in terms of SI base units or derived units
Frequency	Hertz	Hz	$1\ Hz = 1\ cycle/s\ (1\ s^{-1})$
Force	Newton	N	$1\ N = 1\ kg.m/s^2$
Work, energy, quantity of heat	Joule	J	$1\ J = 1\ N.m\ (1\ kg.m^2.s^{-2})$
Power	Watt	W	$1\ W = 1\ J/s\ (1\ J.s^{-1})$
Quantity of electricity	Coulomb	C	$1\ C = 1\ A.s$
Electric potential, potential difference, tension, electromotive force	Volt	V	$1\ V = W/A\ (1\ W.A^{-1})$
Electric capacitance	Farad	F	$1\ F = 1\ A.s/V\ (A.sV^{-1})$
Electric resistance	Ohm	W	$1\ W = 1\ V/A\ (1\ V.A^{-1})$
Flux of magnetic induction, magnetic flux	Weber	Wb	$1\ Wb = 1\ V.s$
Magnetic flux density, magnetic induction	Tesla	T	$1\ T = 1\ Wb/m^2\ (1\ Wb.m^{-2})$
Inductance	Henry	H	$1\ H = 1\ V.s/A\ (V.s.A^{-1})$
Pressure	Pascal	Pa	$1\ Pa = 1\ N/m^2\ (1\ N.m^{-2})$ $= 1\ kg/m^2.s^2\ (1\ kg.m^{21}.s^{-2})$

The litre (1) (10^{-3} m^3 = dm^3), though not official, will remain in use as a unit of volume as also will the dyne (dyn) as a unit for force (1 dyn = 10^{-5} N).

PRESSURE MEASUREMENTS

		Conversion factors	
SI unit	Old unit	Old to SI (exact)	SI to old (approx.)
kPa	mm Hg	0.133	7.5
kPa	1 standard atmosphere (approx 1 Bar)	101.3	0.01
kPa	cm H$_2$O	0.0981	10
kPa	Ibs/sq in	6.894	0.145

HAEMATOLOGY

			Conversion factors	
Measurement	SI unit	Old unit	Old to SI	SI to old
Haemoglobin (Hb)	g/dl	g/100 ml	Numerically	equivalent
Packed cell volume	No unit*	Per cent	0.01	100
Mean cell Hb conc	g/dl	Per cent	Numerically	equivalent
Mean cell Hb	pg	uug	Numerically	equivalent
Red cell count	Cells/litre	Cells/mm^3	10^6	10^{-6}
White cell count	Cells/litre	Cells/mm^3	10^6	10^{-6}
Reticulocytes	Per cent	Per cent	Numerically	equivalent
Platelets	Cells/litre	Cells/mm^3	10^6	10^{-6}

* Expressed as decimal fraction.

pH	H1
pH	nmol/litre
6.80	158
6.90	126
7.00	100
7.10	79
7.20	63
7.25	56
7.30	50
7.35	45
7.40	40
7.45	36
7.50	32
7.55	28
7.60	25
7.70	20

Respiratory physiology symbols and normal values

SYMBOLS

Primary		*Secondary symbols for gas phase*	
C	Concentration of gas in blood	A	Alveolar
F	Fractional concentration in dry gas	B	Barometric
f	Frequency of respiration (breaths/min)	D	Dead space
P	Pressure or partial pressure	E	Expired
Q	Volume of blood	I	Inspired
Q̇	Volume of blood per unit time	L	Lung
R	Respiratory exchange ratio	T	Tidal
S	Saturation of haemoglobin with O_2		
V̇	Volume of gas per unit time		

Secondary symbols for blood phase

a	arterial
c	capillary
ć	end-capillary
i	ideal
v	venous
v̄	mixed venous
⁻	above any symbol denotes a mean value
·	above any symbol denotes a value per unit time

NORMAL VALUES

1. **Blood**
   - (a) *Arterial*

pH	:	7.36–7.44	(H^+ = 44–36 nmol/l)
PaO_2	:	85–100 mm Hg	(11.3–13.3 kPa)
$PaCO_2$	:	36–44 mm Hg	(4.8–5.9 kPa)
O_2 content	:	20–21 vols%	(8.9–9.4 nmol/l)
CO_2 content	:	48–50 vols%	(21.6–22.5 nmol/l)

   - (b) *Venous*

pH	:	7.34–7.42	(H^+ = 38–46 nmol/l)
PO_2	:	37–42 mm Hg	(5–5.6 kPa)
PCO_2	:	42–50 mm Hg	(5.6–6.7 kPa)
O_2 content	:	15–16 vols%	(6.7–7.2 mmol/l)
CO_2 content	:	52–54 vols%	(23.3–24.2 mmol/l)

2. Gases

(a) *Inspired air*

O_2	:	20.93%	
PIO_2	:	149 mm Hg	(19.9 kPa)
N_2	:	79.04%	
PIN_2	:	563 mm Hg	(75 kPa)
CO_2	:	0.03%	

(b) *Expired air*

O_2	:	16–17%	
PEO_2	:	113–121 mm Hg	(15–16 kPa)
N_2	:	80%	
PEN	:	579 mm Hg	(77 kPa)
CO_2	:	3–4%	
$PECO_2$	:	21–28 mm Hg	(2.8–3.7 kPa)

3. Ventilation:perfusion

(a) *Alveolar–arterial oxygen gradient*:

5–20 mm Hg   (0.7–2.7 kPa) breathing air
25–65 mm Hg   (3.3–8.6 kPa) breathing 100% oxygen

(b) *Venous admixture* ($\dot{Q}_S:\dot{Q}_T$): 5% of cardiac output

(c) *Right to left physiological shunt*: 3% of cardiac output

(d) *Anatomical dead space*: 2 ml/kg body weight

(e) *Dead space: tidal volume ratio* $V_D:V_T$): 0.25–0.4 or $33 + \dfrac{Age}{3}$ per cent

4. Lung volumes

Approximate values in adults are listed. Values are less in smaller subjects and in females.

Tidal volume	:	500 ml or 7 ml/kg
Inspiratory capacity	:	3.6 litres
Inspiratory reserve volume	:	3.1 litres
Expiratory reserve volume	:	1.2 litres
Functional residual capacity	:	2.4 litres
Residual volume	:	1.2 litres
Total lung capacity	:	6.0 litres
Vital capacity	:	4.8 litres

or 2.5 l/sq m body surface or 2.5 l/m height in males
    2.0 l/sq m body surface or 2.0 l/m height in females
or 65–75 ml/kg

5. Lung mechanics

(a) *Peak expiratory flow rate*   :   450–700 l/min (males)
                                       :   300–500 l/min (females)

(b) *Forced expiratory volume in 1 sec* (FEV$_1$)   :   70–83% of vital capacity

(c) *Compliance* (approximate values)   :

(i) Lung compliance (C_L)   :

		Static	Dynamic
conscious (erect)	:	200 ml/cm H_2O	180 ml/cm H_2O
paralysed anaesthetized (supine)	:	160 ml/cm H_2O	80 ml/cm H_2O

(ii) Chest wall compliance (C_{CW})   :   200 ml/cm H_2O

(iii) Total compliance (C_T):

conscious (erect)	:	150 ml/cm H_2O	100 ml/cm H_2O
*paralysed anaesthetized (supine)	:	74 ml/cm H_2O	56 ml/cm H_2O

(d) *Airways resistance*   :

conscious   :   0.6–3.2 cm H_2O/l/sec

sedated, partially paralysed and ventilated (includes resistance of endotracheal tube and catheter mount): 10–15 cm H_2O/l/sec

(e) *Work of breathing*: 0.3–0.5 kg m/min
    or oxygen consumption of 0.5–1 ml/l ventilation

* Compliance values would be lower for the sedated, partially paralysed, ventilated patient in the Intensive Care Unit, i.e. Effective dynamic compliance = 40–50 ml/cm H_2O

6. **Cardiovascular** – pressures in kPa are given within brackets

(a)	Cardiac index	:	2.5–3.6 l/min/m²
(b)	Stroke volume	:	42–52 ml/m²
(c)	Ejection fraction	:	0.55–0.75
(d)	End diastolic volume	:	75 ± 15 ml/m²
(e)	End systolic volume	:	25 ± 8 ml/m²
(f)	Left ventricular stroke work index	:	30–110 g-m/m²
(g)	Left ventricular minute work index	:	1.8–6.6 kg-m/min/m²
(h)	Oxygen consumption index	:	110–150 ml/l
(i)	Right atrial pressure	:	1–7 mm Hg (0.13–0.93)
(j)	Right ventricular systolic pressure	:	15–25 mm Hg (2.0–3.3)
(k)	Right ventricular diastolic pressure	:	0–8 (0–1)
(l)	Pulmonary artery systolic pressure	:	15–25 mm Hg (2.0–3.3)
(m)	Pulmonary artery diastolic pressure	:	8–15 mm Hg (1–2)
(n)	Pulmonary artery mean pressure	:	10–20 mm Hg (1.3–2.7)
(o)	Pulmonary capillary wedge pressure	:	6–15 mm Hg (0.8–2.0)
(p)	Systemic vascular resistance	:	770–1500 dyne-s/cm⁵
		:	77–150 kPa-s/l
(q)	Pulmonary vascular resistance	:	20–120 dyne-s/cm⁵
		:	2–12 kPa-s/l
(r)	Systolic time intervals		

Appendix 4

Physiological equations

RESPIRATORY EQUATIONS

(a) *Oxygen consumption* (250 ml/min)

Oxygen consumption = amount of oxygen in inspired gas minus amount in expired gas

i.e. $\dot{V}O_2 = (\dot{V}I \times FIO_2) - (\dot{V}E \times F\bar{E}O_2)$

(b) *Carbon dioxide production* (200 ml/min)

Volume CO_2 eliminated in expired gas = expired gas volume times CO_2 concentration in mixed expired gas

i.e. $\dot{V}CO_2 = \dot{V} \times F\bar{E}CO_2$

As expired volume is made up of alveolar and dead space gas,

$\dot{V}CO_2 = (\dot{V}A \times FACO_2) + (\dot{V}D \times FICO_2)$

As $FICO_2$ is negligible, especially if there is no rebreathing,

$\dot{V}CO_2 = \dot{V}A \times FACO_2$

or $FACO_2 = \dfrac{\dot{V}CO_2}{\dot{V}A}$

or $PACO_2 \text{ (mmHg)} = \dfrac{\dot{V}CO_2 \text{ (ml/min STPD)}}{\dot{V}A \text{ (1/min BTPS)}} \times 0.863$

or $PACO_2 \text{ (kPa)} = \dfrac{\dot{V}CO_2 \text{ (mmol/min)}}{\dot{V}A \text{ (1/min BTPS)}} \times 2.561$

STPD: Standard temperature (0°C) and pressure (760 mm Hg or 101.35 kPa) dry gas
BTPS: Body temperature and ambient pressure, saturated with water vapour

(c) *Physiological dead space*

Bohr's equation, $\dfrac{V_D}{V_T} = \dfrac{PACO_2 - P\bar{E}CO_2}{PACO_2}$

or $\dfrac{V_D}{V_T} = \dfrac{PaCO_2 - P\bar{E}CO_2}{PaCO_2}$

(d) *Alveolar oxygenation*

$PAO_2 = PIO_2 - \dfrac{PaCO_2}{R}$ where R is the Respiratory Quotient (normally 0.8)

$PAO_2 = PIO_2 - PACO_2 \dfrac{(PIO_2 - P\bar{E}O_2)}{(P\bar{E}CO_2)}$

or $\quad PAO_2 = PIO_2 - PACO_2 \left(FIO_2 + \dfrac{1 - FIO_2}{R} \right)$.

when $FIO_2 = 1.0$ (patient breathing 100% oxygen),
then $PAO_2 = (PB - \text{saturated water vapour pressure}) - PACO_2$
$\qquad\quad = (PB - 47) - PaCO_2$

(e) *Venous admixture*

$$\dfrac{\dot{Q}_S}{\dot{Q}_T} = \dfrac{C\acute{c}O_2 - CaO_2}{C\acute{c}O_2 - C\bar{v}O_2}$$

$$= \dfrac{(PAO_2 - PaO_2) \times 0.0031}{CaO_2 + (PAO_2 - PaO_2) \times 0.0031 - C\bar{v}O_2}$$

$$= \dfrac{(PAO_2 - PaO_2) \times 0.0031}{(PAO_2 - PaO_2) \times 0.0031 + 5} \quad \text{(simplified)}$$

$$= C\acute{c}O_2 - C\bar{v}O_2$$

(f) *Fractional inspired oxygen concentration*

$$FIO_2 = \dfrac{O_2 \text{ flow in l/min} + (\text{Air flow in l/min} \times 0.21)}{\text{Total } O_2 + \text{Air flow in l/min}}$$

(g) *Henderson–Hasselbalch equation*

$$pH = pK_A + \log \dfrac{(HCO_3^-)}{(CO_2)}$$

$$pH = 6.1 + \log \dfrac{(HCO_3^- \text{ in mmol/l})}{(PCO_2 \text{ in mm Hg}) \times 0.03}$$

$$[H^+] \text{ nmol/l} = 24 \times \dfrac{(PCO_2 \text{ in mm Hg})}{(HCO_3^- \text{ in mmol/l})}$$

$$[H^+] \text{ nmol/l} = 180 \times \dfrac{(PCO_2 \text{ in kPa})}{(HCO_3^- \text{ in mmol/l})}$$

CARDIOVASCULAR EQUATIONS

(a) *Mean blood pressure* $(BP = DBP + 1/3 \, (SBP - DBP)$
(b) *Rate pressure product* $(RPP) = P \times SBP$
(c) *Body surface area* (BSA) in $m^2 = (Ht)^{0.725} \times (Wt)^{0.425} \times 71.84 \times 10^{-4}$

(d) *Cardiac Index* $(CI) = \dfrac{CO}{BSA} = ml/min/m^2$

(e) *Stroke volume* $(SV) = \dfrac{CO}{P} = ml/beat$

(f) *Stroke volume index* $(SVI) = \dfrac{SV}{BSA} = ml/beat/m^2$

(g) *Left ventricular stroke work index* $(LVSWI) = (BP - PCWP)\,(SVI)\,(0.0136) = g\text{-}m/m^2/beat$

(h) *Systemic vascular resistance* $(SVR) = \dfrac{BP - RAP}{CO}$ resistance units

(Multiply $\times 79.9$ to convert to absolute resistance units, dynes sec cm^{-5})

(i)   *Pulmonary vascular resistance* (PVR) $= \dfrac{\text{PAP} - \text{PCWP}}{\text{CO}}$ resistance units

(Multiply $\times$ 79.9 to convert to absolute resistance units, dynes sec cm^{-5})

(j)   *Left ventricular pre-ejection period* (PEP) $= QS_2 - LVET$ m sec

(k)   *Other systolic time index ratios* may easily be calculated:

$$\frac{1}{PEP^2} \quad \text{and} \quad \frac{PEP}{LVET}$$

* For interpatient comparisons and reference standards, the 'index' term, output normalized to body surface, may be used when

SBP   = systolic blood pressure in mm Hg
DBP   = diastolic blood pressure in mm Hg
P   = heart rate in beats/min
Ht   = height in cm
Wt   = weight in kg
CO   = cardiac output in ml/min
PCWP = pulmonary capillary wedge pressure in mm Hg
RAP   = right atrial pressure in mm Hg
PAP   = mean pulmonary artery pressure in mm Hg
LVET = left ventricular ejection time in m sec
QS_2 = total electromechanical systole in m sec

RENAL EQUATIONS

(a)   *Standard creatinine clearance* (ml/min/1.73 m^2)

$$= \frac{\text{urine creatinine (mmol/l)}}{\text{serum creatinine (mmol/l)}} \times \text{urine volume (ml/min)} \times \frac{1.73}{\text{body surface area (m}^2)}$$

(b)   *Per cent filtered Na$^+$ excreted*

$$= \frac{\text{urine Na}^+ \text{ (mmol/l)}}{\text{serum Na}^+ \text{ (mmol/l)}} \times \frac{\text{serum creatinine (mmol/l)}}{\text{urine creatinine (mmol/l)}} \times 100$$

(c)   *Free water clearance* (ml/min)

$$= \text{urine vol (ml/min)} - \frac{\text{urine osmolality (mosm/kg)}}{\text{plasma osmolality (mosm/kg)}} \times \text{urine vol (ml/min)}$$

(d)   *Additional calculated parameters*:

(i) $\dfrac{\text{urine}}{\text{plasma}}$ osmolality ratio

(ii) $\dfrac{\text{urine}}{\text{serum}}$ creatinine ratio

(iii) $\dfrac{\text{blood urea}}{\text{serum creatinine}}$ ratio

(iv) $\dfrac{\text{urine}}{\text{Plasma}}$ urea ratio

(v)   urinary Na$^+$ and K$^+$ excretion (mmol)

(vi) $\dfrac{\text{urinary Na}^+}{\text{urinary K}^+}$ ratio

Plasma drug concentrations and American nomenclature

PLASMA DRUG LEVELS

Drug	Normal or therapeutic concentration mg/l	Toxic concentration mg/l	Lethal or potentially lethal concentration mg/l
Acetazolamide	10–15	–	–
Acetohexamide	21–56	–	–
Acetone	–	200–300	550
Aluminium	0.13	–	–
Aminophylline (Theophylline)	10–20	20	–
Amitriptyline	50–200 μg/l	400 μg/l	10–20
Ammonia	500–1700	–	–
Amphetamine	20–30 μg/l	–	2
Arsenic	0.0–20 μg/l	1.0	15
Barbiturates			
Short-acting	1	7	10
Intermediate-acting	1–5	10–30	30
Phenobarbitone	15	40–70	80–150
Benzene	–	any measurable	0.94
Beryllium	Tissue levels generally used (lung & lymph)	–	–
Boric acid	0.8	40	50
Bromide	50	0.5–1.5 g/l	2 g/l
Brompheniramine	8–15 μg/l	–	–
Cadmium	0.1–0.2 μg/l	50 μg/l	–
Caffeine	–	–	100
Carbamazepine	6–12	12	
Carbon monoxide	1% saturation of Hb	15–35% saturation of Hb	50% saturation of Hb
Carbon tetrachloride	–	20–50	
Chloral hydrate	10	100	250
Chlordiazepoxide	1.0–2.0	6	20
Chloroform	–	70–250	390
Chlorpromazine	0.3	1–2	3–12
Chlorpropamide	30–140	–	–
Codeine	25 μg/l	–	–
Copper	1–1.5	5.4	–
Cyanide	0.15	–	5
DDT	13 μg/l	–	–
Desipramine	0.59–1.4	–	10–20
Dextropropoxyphene	50–200 μg/l	5–10	57
Diazepam	0.5–2.5	5–20	50
Dieldrin	1.5 μg/l	–	–
Digitoxin	20–35 μg/l	–	320 μg/l
Digoxin	1–2 μg/l	2–9 μg/l	–

Dinitro-o-cresol	–	30–40 μg/l	75
Diphenhydramine	5	10	–
Disopyramide	3–7	–	–
Ethosuximide	40–80	–	–
Ethyl chloride	–	–	400
Ethylene glycol	–	1.5 g/l	2–4 g/l
Fluoride	0.5	–	2
Gentamicin	5–8	10–12	–
Glutethimide	1–5	10–30	30–100
Gold (sodium aurothiomalate)	3–6	–	–
Hydrogen sulphide	–	–	0.92
Hydromorphone (Dihydromorphinone)	–	–	0.1–0.3
Imipramine	0.1–0.3	0.7	2
Iron	500 (erythrocytes)	6 (serum)	–
Lead	0.05–1.3	1.3	–
Lignocaine	2–4	6	–
Lithium	0.8–1.2 mmol/l	1.5 mmol/l	4 mmol/l
LSD (lysergic acid diethylamide)	–	1–4 μg/l	–
Magnesium	0.7–1.1 mmol/l	–	–
Manganese	0.15	4.6	–
Meprobamate	10	100	200
Mercury	60–120 μg/l	–	–
Methadone	480–860 μg/l	2	4
Methanol	–	200	890
Methapyrilene	2 μg/l	30–50	50
Methaqualone	1–2	5–30	30
Methsuximide	2.5–7.5	–	–
Methylamphetamine	–	5	40
Methyprylone	10	30–60	100
Mexiletine	0.6–2.5	–	–
Morphine	0.1	–	0.5–4
Nickel	0.41	–	–
Nicotine	–	10	5–52
Nitrofurantoin	1.8	–	–
Nortriptyline	50–200 μg/l	400 μg/l	10–20
Orphenadrine	–	2	4–8
Oxalate	2	–	10
Papaverine	1	–	–
Paracetamol	5–25	30	250 at 4 h 50 at 12 h
Paraldehyde	50	200–400	500
Paramethoxy-amphetamine (PMA)	–	–	2–4
Pentazocine	0.1–1	2–5	10–20
Perphenazine	–	1	–
Pethidine	600–650 μg/l	5	30
Phenacetin	5–25	30	400
Phencyclidine	–	0.5	1
Phensuximide	10–19	–	–
Phenylbutazone	100	–	–
Phenytoin (Dilantin)	8–20	30	100
Phosphorus	Concentration in tissues usually used	–	–
Primidone	10	50–80	100
Probenecid	100–200	–	–
Procainamide	3–8	10	–
Prochlorperazine	–	1	–
Promazine	–	1	–
Propoxyphene	0.1–1	5–20	57
Propranolol	0.025–0.1	–	8–12

Propylhexedrine	–	–	2–3
Quinidine	3–6	10	30–50
Quinine	–	–	12
Salicylate (acetylsalicylic acid)	100–350	350–400	500
Strychnine	–	2	9–12
Sulphadiazine	80–150	–	–
Sulphafurazole	90–100	–	–
Sulphaguanidine	30–50	–	–
Sulthiame	4–10	–	–
Theophylline	10–20	20	–
Thioridazine	1–1.5	10	20–80
Tin	0.12	–	–
Tobramycin	5–8	10–12	–
Tolbutamide	53–96	–	–
Toluene	–	–	10
Tribromoethanol	–	–	90
Tricyclics	50–200 $\mu g/l$	400 $\mu g/l$	10–20
Trimethobenzamide	1.0–2.0	–	–
Valproate	50–100	–	–
Warfarin	1.0–10	–	–
Zinc	0.68–1.36	–	–
Zoxazolamine	3–13	–	–

AMERICAN NOMENCLATURE

Drug	American equivalent
Adrenaline	Epinephrine
Amethocaine	Tetracaine
Cinchocaine	Dibucaine
Corticotrophin	Corticotropin
Desferrioxamine	Deferoxamine
Dextropropoxyphene	Propoxyphene
Dihydromorphinone	Hydromorphone
Ergometrine	Ergonovine
Frusemide	Furosemide
Hydrallazine	Hydralazine
Hyoscine	Scopolamine
Isoprenaline	Isoproterenol
Lignocaine	Lidocaine
Meclozine	Meclizine
Mepivacaine	Carbocaine
Methohexitone	Methohexital
Methylamphetamine	Methamphetamine
Methyprylone	Methyprylon
Noradrenaline	Norepinephrine, Levarterenol
Orciprenaline	Metaproterenol
Oxybuprocaine	Benoxinate
Paracetamol	Acetaminophen
Pethidine	Meperidine
Phenobarbitone	Phenobarbital
Salbutamol	Albuterol
Thiopentone	Thiopental
Thyroxine	Levothyroxine

REFERENCES

1. Koch-Weser J. Serum drug concentrations as therapeutic guides. N Engl J Med 1972, 287:227–31.
2. Winek CL. Tabulation of therapeutic, toxic and lethal concentrations of drugs and chemicals in blood. Clin Chem 1976, 22:832–6.
3. Richens A, Warrington S. When should plasma drug levels be monitored? Curr Therapeutics 1979, 20:167–85.
4. Koch-Weser J. The serum level approach to individualization of drug dosage. Eur J Clin Pharm 1975, 9:1–8.
5. Davies DS, Prichard BNC. Biological Effects of Drugs in Relation to their Plasma Concentrations. London, Macmillan, 1973.

Appendix 6

Confirmation of intubation

This is a frequently performed procedure in anaesthesia, in the ICU and in a wide range of emergency situations with very variable availability of sophisticated equipment. It is also the cause of significant morbidity and mortality.
This is a simple check list which can be modifed depending on the equipment available.

Always:

- Visualise the passage of the tip of the endotracheal tube through the vocal cords at intubation; where possible.

- Observe. Continuous observation of rise and fall of the chest on ventilation.

- Auscultate. Confirm air entry by auscultation in the axillae and also listen over the stomach. The axillae will confirm bilateral air entry (and indicate endo-bronchial intubation if air entry is unilateral). Auscultation over the stomach will allow differential breath sounds between axillae and stomach and may indicate oesophageal tube placement if the stomach sounds are louder.

- Observe the patients colour. They should remain pink.

  Equipment may be available that will also assist.

- Capnography. There should be CO_2 in the exhaled air

- Oximetry helps confirm oxygenation.

'If in doubt, take it out.' Sometimes some of the 4 basic signs are unconvincing but if there is any doubt the tube should be replaced or mouth to mouth/mask ventilation should be used.

Paramters monitored and measured by the PiCCO monitor

New non-invasive monitors have introduced some new 'measurements' into clinical practice.

Parameter normal value	Symbol
Pulse Contour Cardiac Output/index CI 3.0-5.0l/min/m^2 Pulse contour cardiac output is calibrated by means of a simple trans-cardiopulmonary Thermodilution measurement	PCCO/PCCI
Global End Diastolic Volume/index 680 – 800 ml/m^2(indexed) the total end diastolic volume of all four chambers of the heart	GEDV/I
Intrathoracic Blood Volume/index 850 – 1000 ml/m^2 (indexed) The global end diastolic volume plus the pulmonary blood volume	ITBV/I
Extravascular Lung Water/index 3.0 – 7.0 ml/kg (indexed) Quantifies lung status in terms of pulmonary permeability	EVLW/I
Cardiac Function Index 4.5 – 6.5 l/min (indexed) CO/GEDV = preload independent variable of heart function	CFI
Stroke Volume/index 40 –60ml/m^2	SV/I
Stroke Volume Variation <10% Percentage difference of biggest to smallest stroke volumes over the last 30 seconds	SVV
Left Ventricular contractility 1200 – 2000mmHg/sec Maximum velocity of blood pressure curve corresponds to maximum power or Contractility of the left heart	dP/dtmax
Systemic vascular resistance/index 1200 – 2000dyn/s/cm-5/m^2 (indexed)	SVR/SVRI

EVLW
The two mechanisms by which the EVLW may be raised are either increased intravascular filtration pressure (left heart failure, volume overload) or increased pulmonary vascular permeability as in endotoxic shock and sepsis.
There is a direct relationship between the mortality of intensive care patients with ARDS and high extravascular lung water.

SVV
Large variations in stroke volume are an indication of reduced intravascular volume (also AF, heart valve disease)

Appendix 8

Pediatric Risk of Mortality (PRISM) score. Mortality risk assessment.

Parameter	Age limit	Ranges	Points
Systolic blood pressure (mmHg)	Infants	130–160	2
		55–65	2
		> 160	6
		40–54	6
		< 40	7
	Children	150–200	2
		65–75	2
		> 200	6
		50–64	6
		< 50	7
Diastolic blood pressure (mmHg)	All ages	> 110	6
Heart rate (beats/min)	Infants	> 160	4
		< 90	4
	Children	> 150	4
		< 80	4
Respiratory rate (breaths/min)	Infants	61–90	1
		> 90	5
		apnea	5
	Children	51–70	1
		> 70	5
		apnea	5
PaO_2/FIO_2	All ages	200–300	2
		< 200	3
$PaCO_2$ in torr (mmHg)	All ages	51–65	1
		> 65	5
Glasgow coma score	All ages	< 8	6
Pupillary reactions	All ages	unequal or dilated	4
		fixed and dilated	10
PT/PTT	All ages	1.5 times control	2
Total bilirubin mg/dL	> 1 month	> 3.5	6
Potassium in mEq/L	All ages	3.0–3.5	1
		6.5–7.5	1
		< 3.0	5
		> 7.5	5
Calcium in mg/dL	All ages	7.0–8.0	2
		12.0–15.0	2
		< 7.0	6
		> 15.0	6
Glucose in mg/dL	All ages	40–60	4
		250–400	4
		< 40	8
		> 400	8
Bicarbonate in mEq/L	All ages	< 16	3
		> 32	3

Infants: 0–1 years of age. PRISM score = (systolic blood pressure points) + (diastolic blood pressure points) + (heart rate points) + (respiratory rate points) + (oxygenation points) + (Glasgow coma score points) + (pupillary reaction points) + (coagulation points) + (bilirubin points) + (potassium points) + (calcium points) + (glucose points) + (bicarbonate points).

The Sepsis-related Organ Failure Assessment (SOFA) score. Easy to calculate, describes the sequence of complications in a critically ill patient rather than predicting outcome.

Organ system	Measure
Respiration	PaO$_2$ to FIO$_2$ ratio
Coagulation	Platelet count
Liver	Serum bilirubin
Cardiovascular	Hypotension
Central nervous system	Glasgow coma score
Renal	Serum creatinine or urine output

Measure	Finding	Points
PaO$_2$ to FIO$_2$ ratio	≥ 400 (mmHg)	0
	300–399 (mmHg)	1
	200–299 (mmHg)	2
	100–199 (mmHg)	3
	< 100 (mmHg)	4
Platelet count	≥ 1500/µL	0
	1000–149 999/µL	1
	500–99 999/µL	2
	200–49 999/µL	3
	< 200 per µL	4
Serum bilirubin	< 1.2 mg/dL	0
	1.2–1.9 mg/dL	1
	2.0–5.9 mg/dL	2
	6.0–11.9 mg/dL	3
	≥ 12.0 mg/dL	4
Hypotension	Mean arterial pressure ≥ 70 (mmHg)	0
	Mean arterial pressure < 70 then (no pressor agents used) (mmHg)	1
	Dobumatine any dose	2
	Dopamine <= 5 µg/kg per min	2
	Dopamine > 5–15 µg/kg per min	3
	Dopamine > 15 µg/kg per min	4
	Epinephrine <= 0.1 µg/kg per min	3
	Epinephrine > 0.1 µg/kg per min	4
	Norepinephrine <= 0.1 µg/kg per min	3
	Norepinephrine > 0.1 µg/kg per min	4
Glasgow coma score	15	0
	13–14	1
	10–12	2
	6–9	3
	3–5	4
Serum creatinine or urine output	Serum creatinine < 1.2 mg/dL	0
	Serum creatinine 1.2–1.9 mg/dL	1
	Serum creatinine 2.0–3.4 mg/dL	2
	Serum creatinine 3.5–4.9 mg/dL	3
	Urine output 200–499 mL/day	3
	Serum creatinine > 5.0 mg/dL	4
	Urine output < 200 mL/day	4

PaO$_2$ is in mmHg and FIO$_2$ in percent, from 0.21 to 1.00.
Adrenergic agents as administered for at least 1 h with doses in µg/kg per min.
A score of 0 indicates normal and a score of 4 indicates most abnormal.
Data can be collected and the score calculated daily during the course of the admission.
Interpretation: minimum total score: 0; maximum total score: 24.
The higher the organ score the greater the organ dysfunction.
The higher the total score the greater the multiorgan dysfunction.

Mortality rate by SOFA score.[1]

Organ system	0	1	2	3	4
Respiratory	20%	27%	32%	46%	64%
Cardiovascular	22%	32%	55%	55%	55%
Coagulation	35%	35%	35%	64%	64%
CNS	32%	34%	50%	53%	56%
Renal	25%	40%	46%	56%	64%

LOGISTIC ORGAN DYSFUNCTION SYSTEM (LODS)

Assess patients for severity of critical organ dysfunction. To predict the probability of death for the patient.

Data collection	During the first 24 h in the ICU.
Data point	If not measured then it is assumed to be normal for scoring purposes.
	If several measurements, use the most severe value.

LOD score = (neurologic score) + (cardiovascular score) + (renal score) + (pulmonary score) + (hematologic score) + (hepatic score).

Neurologic score.

Glasgow coma score	Points
14–15	0
9–13	1
6–8	3
< 6	5

Use lowest value. If sedated estimate the score prior to sedation.

Cardiovascular score.

Heart rate (beats/min)		Systolic BP in (mmHg)	Points
30–139	*and*	90–239	0
≥ 140	*or*	240–269	1
		70–89	1
		≥ 270	3
		40–69	3
<30	*or*	< 40	5

The most abnormal value for heart rate or systolic blood pressure either minimum or maximum.

Renal score.

Serum urea nitrogen mg/dL		Creatinine mg/dL		Urine output (L/d)	Points
< 17	*and*	< 1.20	AND	0.75–9.99	0
17–27.99	*or*	1.2–1.59			1
28–55.99	*or*	≥ 1.60	OR	≥ 10	3
				0.5–0.74	3
≥ 56					5
				< 0.5	5

Highest value for urea nitrogen and for creatinine.
If the urine output data is for less than a 24-h period, adjust that value to 24 h, assuming the same rate of excretion.
On hemodialysis, use the value of urine output prior to initiating hemodialysis

Pulmonary score.

On ventilation or CPAP?		Ratio (PaO$_2$ in mmHg)/(FIO$_2$)	Points
No			0
Yes	*and*	≥ 150	1
Yes	*and*	< 150	3

Respiratory support; use the lowest ratio of PaO$_2$ to FIO$_2$.

Hematologic score.

White blood cell count 10^9/l		Platelet count 10^9/l	Points
2.5 to 4.9/µL	*and*	≥ 50/µL	0
≥ 50/µL			1
1 to 2.4/µL	*or*	< 50/µL	1
< 1/µL			3

Note: Most abnormal value for the white cell count either minimum or maximum.
minimum platelet count if several values are available.

Hepatic score.[2]

Bilirubin		Prothrombin time	Points
< 2.0 mg/dL (< 34.2 µmol/L)	*and*	<= 3 seconds above standard (≥ 25% of standard)	0
≥ 2.0 mg/dL (≥ 34.2 µmol/L)	*or*	> 3 seconds above standard (< 25% of standard)	1

Highest value for bilirubin available. Highest value for prothrombin time in seconds.

MPM II , MORTALITY PROBABILITY MODELS.[3,4]

Excluded
  Age < 18 years
  Burn patients
  Coronary care patients
  Cardiac surgery patients
(The scoring is either present or not present)
Definitions
  Coma or deep stupor at time of ICU admission
  ● Not due to drug overdosage
  ● If patient is on paralyzing muscle relaxant awakening from anesthesia or heavily sedated, use best judgment of the level of consciousness prior to sedation
  ● *Coma*: no response to any stimulation; no twitching, no movements in extremities, no response to pain, or command Glasgow coma: scale 3
  ● *Deep stupor*: decorticate or decerebrate posturing; posturing is spontaneous or in response to stimulation or deep pain; posturing is not in response to commands; Glasgow coma: scale 4 or 5
Heart rate at ICU admission
  Heart rate ≥ 150 beats/min within 1 h before or after ICU admission
Systolic blood pressure at ICU admission
  Systolic blood pressure <= 90 mmHg within 1 h before or after ICU admission
Chronic renal compromise or insufficiency
  Elevation of serum creatinine > 2 mg/dL and documented as chronic in the medical record
  If there is the acute diagnosis on chronic renal failure then only record yes for acute renal failure
Cirrhosis
  History of heavy alcohol use with portal hypertension and varices
  Other causes of liver disease with evidence of portal hypertension and varices
  Biopsy confirmation of cirrhosis
Metastatic malignant neoplasm
  Stage IV carcinomas with distant metastases
  Do not include involvement only of regional lymph nodes

Include if metastases are obvious by clinical assessment or confirmed by a pathology report

Do not include if metastases not obvious, or if pathology report is not available at the time of ICU admission

Acute hematologic malignancies are included

Chronic leukemias are not included unless there are findings attributable to the disease or the patient is under active treatment for the leukemia. Findings include sepsis anemia stroke, caused by clumping of white blood cells tumor lysis syndrome with elevated uric acid following chemotherapy pulmonary edema or lymphangiectatic form of ARDS

Acute renal failure

Acute tubular necrosis or acute diagnosis on chronic renal failure

Prerenal azotemia is not included

Cardiac dysrhythmia

Cardiac arrhythmia paroxysmal tachycardia fibrillation with rapid ventricular response second or third degree heart block

Do not include chronic and stable arrhythmias

Cerebrovascular incident

Cerebral embolism occlusion CVA stroke brain-stem infarction cerebrovascular arteriovenous malformation (acute stroke or cerebrovascular hemorrhage not chronic arteriovenous malformation)

Gastrointestinal bleeding

Hematemesis melena

A perforated ulcer does not necessarily indicate GI bleeding; may be identified by obvious 'coffee grounds' in nasogastric tube

A drop of hemoglobin by itself is not sufficient evidence of acute GI bleeding

Intracranial mass effect

Intracranial mass (abscess tumor hemorrhage subdural) as identified by CT scan associated with any of the following: (1) midline shift (2) obliteration or distortion of cerebral ventricles (3) gross hemorrhage in cerebral ventricles or subarachnoid space (4) visible mass > 4 cm or (5) any mass that enhances with contrast media

If the mass effect is known within 1 h of ICU admission, it can be indicated as yes

CT scanning is not mandated and is only indicated for patients with major neurological insult

Age in years

Patient's age at last birthday

CPR within 24 h prior to ICU admission

CPR includes chest compression defibrillation or cardiac massage

Not affected by the location where the CPR was administered

Mechanical ventilation

Patient is using a ventilator at the time of ICU admission or immediately thereafter

Medical or unscheduled surgery admission

Do not include elective surgical patients (surgery scheduled at least 24 h in advance) or pre-operative Swan-Ganz catheter insertion in elective surgery patients

REFERENCES

1. Vincent JL, Moreno R, *et al*. The SOFA (Sepsis-related Organ Failure Assessment) score to describe organ dysfunction/failure. *Int Care Med* 1996; **22**:707–710.
2. Le Gall J, Klar J, *et al*. The Logistic Organ Dysfunction System. *JAMA* 1996; **276**:802–810.
3. Lemeshow S, Teres D, *et al*. Mortality Probability Models (MPM II) based on an international cohort of intensive care patients. *JAMA* 1993; **270**:2478–2486.
4. Lemeshow S, Le Gall J-R. Modeling the severity of illness of ICU patients. *JAMA* 1994; **272**:1049–1055.

Index

Notes: This index is presented in a letter-by-letter order, whereby hyphens and spaces between words are ignored. Cross-references in *italics* refer to general references (e.g. *see also specific drugs*).

Abbreviations used in sub-entries: ALI, acute lung injury; ARDS, acute respiratory distress syndrome; COPD, chronic obstructive pulmonary disease; CPR, cardiopulmonary resuscitation; DIC, disseminated intravascular coagulation; ECG, electrocardiography; EEG, electroencephalography; HIV, human immunodeficiency virus; MI, myocardial infarction; MODS, multiple organ dysfunction syndrome; PEEP, positive end-expiratory pressure; TBI, traumatic brain injury.